CLINICAL PHARMACOLOGY AND NURSING

CLINICAL PHARMACOLOGY AND NURSING

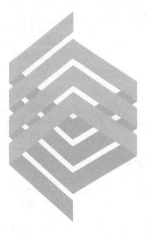

Charold L. Baer, RN, PhD
Professor, Department of Adult Health
and Illness, Oregon Health Sciences
University, School of Nursing, Portland,
Oregon

Bradley R. Williams, PharmD
Assistant Professor of Clinical Pharmacy
and Clinical Gerontology, University of
Southern California, Schools of
Pharmacy and Gerontology, Los Angeles,
California

SPRINGHOUSE PUBLISHING COMPANY
Springhouse Corporation
Springhouse, Pennsylvania

STAFF

CLINICAL STAFF

Director, Nursing Textbooks
Minnie B. Rose, RN, BSN, MEd

Consultant
Helene Nawrocki, RN, MSN Candidate

Clinical Editors
Joanne DaCunha, RN, BS
Barbara McVan, RN
Diane Schweisguth, RN, BSN, CEN, CCRN

Advisory Board
Kathleen G. Andreoli, DSN, FAAN, Vice-President, Nursing Affairs and The John L. and Helen Kellogg Dean of the College of Nursing, Rush-Presbyterian–St. Luke's Medical Center/Rush University, Chicago

Elnora D. Daniel, RN, EdD, FAAN, Dean, School of Nursing, Hampton (Va.) University

Kathleen Dracup, RN, DNSc, CCRN, FAAN, Associate Professor, School of Nursing, University of California, Los Angeles

Rhetaugh G. Dumas, RN, PhD, FAAN, Dean, School of Nursing, University of Michigan, Ann Arbor

Elizabeth Grossman, RN, EdD, FAAN, Dean, Indiana University School of Nursing, Indianapolis

Evelyn R. Hayes, RN, PhD, Associate Professor, University of Delaware, College of Nursing, Newark

Mary D. Naylor, PhD, FAAN, Associate Dean and Director of Undergraduate Studies, University of Pennsylvania School of Nursing, Philadelphia

PUBLICATION STAFF

Executive Director, Editorial
Stanley Loeb

Executive Director, Creative Services
Jean Robinson

Design
John Hubbard (art director), Stephanie Peters (associate art director), Lynn Foulk, Julie Carleton Barlow, Mary Stangl

Editing
Diana Potter, Richard Stull, Nancy Priff, Leslie Brennan

Copy Editing
David Moreau (manager), Edith McMahon (supervisor), Nick Anastasio, Keith de Pinho, Mary Durkin, Diane Labus, Doris Weinstock, Debra Young

Art Production
Robert Perry (manager), Mark Marcin, Loretta Caruso, Anna Brindisi, Donald Knauss, Robert Wieder, Christina McKinley, Christopher Buckley

Typography
David Kosten (manager), Diane Paluba (assistant manager), Nancy Wirs, Brenda Mayer, Joyce Rossi-Biletz, Alicia Dempsey, Mary T. Madden

Manufacturing
Deborah Meiris (manager), T.A. Landis, Lisa Weiss

Production Coordination
Susan Hopkins Rodzewich, Vikky Person

Library of Congress Cataloging-in-Publication Data
Clinical pharmacology and nursing.
　　Includes bibliographies and index.
　　1. Pharmacology.　2. Nursing.　I. Baer, Charold Lee Morris, 1946-　. II. Williams, Bradley R.
[DNLM: 1. Drug Therapy—nurses' instruction.
2. Pharmacology, Clinical—nurses' instruction. QV 38 C6413]
RM301.C53　1988　615'.1　87-26744
ISBN 0-87434-137-X

CONTENTS

UNIT ONE: GENERAL PHARMACOLOGY

UNIT TWO: PHARMACOTHERAPEUTICS AND THE NURSING PROCESS

CONTRIBUTORS

Steven R. Abel, PharmD, RPh, Assistant Director of Pharmacy, Clinical and Educational Services, Indiana University Hospitals, Indianapolis

Kathleen G. Andreoli, DSN, FAAN, Vice President, Nursing Affairs and The John L. and Helen Kellogg Dean of the College of Nursing, Rush-Presbyterian–St. Luke's Medical Center/Rush University, Chicago

Charold L. Baer, RN, PhD, Professor, Department of Adult Health and Illness, Oregon Health Sciences University, School of Nursing, Portland

Naomi R. Ballard, RN, MA, MS, Associate Professor, Department of Adult Health and Illness, Oregon Health Sciences University, School of Nursing, Portland

Carol L. Beck, PharmD, RPh, Assistant Professor of Pharmacy Practice, North Dakota State University, College of Pharmacy, Fargo

Rebecca E. Boehne, RN, MSN, Assistant Professor, Adult Health and Illness, Oregon Health Sciences University, School of Nursing, Portland

Karna Bramble, RN, MS, CGNP, Assistant Professor of Nursing, California State University, Department of Nursing, Long Beach

Barbara Gross Braverman, RN, MSN, CS, Instructor of Psychiatry and Clinical Nurse Specialist, Medical College of Pennsylvania, Philadelphia

Linda P. Brown, RN, PhD, Assistant Professor, University of Pennsylvania, School of Nursing, Philadelphia

Kathleen C. Byington, RN, MSN, Pediatric Clinical Specialist, Vanderbilt Children's Hospital, Vanderbilt University, Nashville, Tenn.

James D. Carlson, PharmD, RPh, Associate Director, Pharmacology Research and Clinical Studies Institute, Fargo, N.D.

Bruce C. Carlstedt, BSPh, PhD, RPh, Associate Professor of Clinical Pharmacy, Purdue University, School of Pharmacy and Pharmacal Sciences, West Lafayette, Ind.

Vivian Hayes Churness, RN, DNSc, Assistant Professor, University of Southern California, Department of Nursing, Los Angeles

Teresa Lyon Coluccio, RN, MN, Clinical Nurse Specialist, Oncology, Providence Medical Center, Seattle

Carol Solomon Dalglish, RN, MSN, Clinical Specialist, Center for Fertility and Reproductive Research; and Adjunct Faculty, School of Nursing, Vanderbilt University, Nashville, Tenn.

N. Michael Davis, MS, RPh, Coordinator, Drug Information Center, University of Miami; Jackson Memorial Medical Center, Miami

Robin Donohoe Dennison, RN, MSN, CS, Cardiopulmonary Nursing Consultant and President, Continuing Education for Health Professionals, Inc., Huntington, W.Va.

Patricia A. Diehl, RN, BSN, MA, Associate Professor, West Virginia University, School of Nursing, Morgantown

Laura D'Oria, PharmD, Assistant Professor of Pharmacy Practice, University of Arkansas for Medical Sciences, College of Pharmacy; and Clinical Coordinator, Arkansas Children's Hospital, Department of Pharmacy, Little Rock

Belle Erickson, RN, MS, Assistant Professor, Villanova (Pa.) University, College of Nursing

Carmel A. Esposito, RN, MSN, Medical-Surgical Chairperson, Ohio Valley Hospital, School of Nursing, Steubenville

Janet M. Farahmand, RN, MSN, EdD, Assistant Professor, Widener University, School of Nursing, Chester, Pa.

C. Cecil Fuselier, MSc, RPh, Associate Professor of Pharmacy Practice, University of Arkansas for Medical Sciences, College of Pharmacy, Little Rock

Corre J. Garrett, RN, EdD, CCRN, Assistant Professor, East Carolina University, School of Nursing, Greenville, N.C.

Anna Gawlinski, RN, MSN, CCRN, Cardiovascular Clinical Nurse Specialist, University of California Medical Center, Los Angeles

Martin R. Giannamore, PharmD, RPh, Clinical Pharmacist, Grant Medical Center, Columbus

Richard K. Gibson, RN, MN, JD, CCRN, Clinical Nurse Specialist, Veterans Administration Medical Center, San Diego

Barbara Given, RN, PhD, FAAN, Director of Nursing Graduate Program, College of Nursing, Michigan State University, East Lansing

Dean E. Goldberg, PharmD, Assistant Professor of Pharmacy Practice, University of Minnesota, College of Pharmacy, Minneapolis

Mary Elizabeth Greipp, RN, MSN, EdD, Assistant Professor of Nursing, Rutgers University, Camden (N.J.) College of Arts and Sciences

Kathleen Whittaker Groves, RN, MS, Instructor II, Johns Hopkins Hospital, Baltimore

Bridget A. Haupt, PharmD, Assistant Director of Pharmacy, Temple University Hospital; and Assistant Professor of Clinical Pharmacy, Temple University, College of Pharmacy, Philadelphia

David W. Hawkins, PharmD, Associate Professor and Assistant Dean, University of Georgia, College of Pharmacy, Athens

Marcia J. Hill, RN, MSN, Manager, Dermatologic Therapeutics, Methodist Hospital, Houston

Phyllis G. Hummel, RN, MSN, Chairman, Department of Nursing, North Dakota State University, Fargo

Sande Jones, RNC, MS, Inservice Education Coordinator, Mount Sinai Medical Center, Miami Beach

Lynne Kreutzer-Baraglia, RN, MS, Assistant Professor, West Suburban College of Nursing, Oak Park, Ill.

Eileen Hayes Lantier, RN, MSN, Assistant Professor, Syracuse (N.Y.) University, College of Nursing

Jan L. Lee, RN, MN, CS, Adjunct Assistant Professor of Nursing, University of Southern California, Department of Nursing, Los Angeles

Colleen Lucas, RN, MN, CNS, Medical-Surgical Clinical Nurse Specialist, Good Samaritan Hospital and Medical Center, Portland

Brenda L. Lyon, RN, DNS, Associate Professor of Nursing, School of Nursing; and Chairperson, Graduate Department of Nursing Adults with Biodissonance, Indiana University, Indianapolis

Mary Y. Ma, PharmD, Antimicrobial Clinical Pharmacist, Veteran Administration West Los Angeles Medical Center; and Associate Clinical Professor of Pharmacy, University of Southern California, Los Angeles

Meredith Ann McCord, RN, MS, Assistant Professor, Oregon Health Sciences University, School of Nursing, Portland

Barbara L. MacDermott, RN, MS, Associate Professor and Assistant Dean, Syracuse (N.Y.) University, College of Nursing

Sara Lynn Machowsky, RN, MS, Clinical Administrator, Ophthalmic Pavilion, Easton, Pa.

Gary Milavetz, PharmD, RPh, Assistant Professor of Pharmacy, University of Iowa, College of Pharmacy, Iowa City

Rita Short Monahan, RN, MSN, EdD, Assistant Professor, Oregon Health Sciences University, School of Nursing, at Easton Oregon State College, LaGrande

John Nagelhout, RN, PhD, CRNA, Assistant Professor of Anesthesia and Pharmacology, Wayne State University, Detroit; and Clinical Nurse Anesthetist, Detroit Receiving Hospital

Brenda Marion Nevidjon, RN, MSN, Manager, Cancer Program, Providence Medical Center, Seattle

Patricia O'Leary, RN, MSN, Assistant Professor, East Carolina University, School of Nursing, Greenville, N.C.

Nina Hubej Olesinski, RN, MSN, Clinical Nurse Consultant, Ophthalmology and Otolaryngology, University of Illinois Hospital, Chicago; and Faculty, University of Illinois, Chicago

Keith M. Olsen, PharmD, Assistant Professor of Pharmacy Practice, University of Arkansas for Medical Sciences, College of Pharmacy, Little Rock

C. Lynne Ostrow, RN, MS, EdD, Associate Professor, West Virginia University, School of Nursing, Morgantown

Karen P. Padrick, RN, MN, Doctoral Student, Oregon Health Sciences University, School of Nursing, Portland

Patricia Peschman, RN, MS, Clinical Nurse Specialist, Renal and Gastrointestinal, Abbott Northwestern Hospital, Minneapolis

Larry A. Pfeifer, BSPh, RPh, LT. COMMANDER U.S. PUBLIC HEALTH SERVICE, Chief, Pharmacy Services, Gillis W. Long Hansen's Disease Center, Carville, La.

Colleen S. Pfeiffer, RN, MS, CCRN, Doctoral Candidate, University of Illinois at Chicago Medical Center, School of Nursing

David Pipher, PharmD, Assistant Director of Pharmacy, Western Psychiatric Institute and Clinic, Pittsburgh

Beverly A. Post, RN, MS, CIC, Infection Control Coordinator, Louis A. Weiss Memorial Hospital, Chicago

Carol B. Pugh, PharmD, Assistant Professor of Clinical Pharmacy, Philadelphia College of Pharmacy and Science

Mark C. Pugh, PharmD, Clinical Pharmacist, Thomas Jefferson University Hospital, Philadelphia

Frances W. Quinless, RN, PhD, CCRN, Chairperson, Department of Nursing Education, University of Medicine & Dentistry of New Jersey, School of Health Related Professions, Newark

Ann Ziegler Sedore, RN, MA, Associate Professor, Syracuse (N.Y.) University, College of Nursing

Thomas R. Simpson, PharmD, RPh, Director of Pharmacy, Humana Hospital, Huntington Beach, Calif.

Lilliam Sklaver, PharmD, Clinical Coordinator of Pharmacy Services, St. Francis Hospital, Miami Beach

Gary D. Smith, PharmD, RPh, Clinical Pharmacist, Minneapolis Children's Health Center

Brenda M. Splitz, RN, MSN, GNP, Clinical Coordinator, Nurse Practitioner Program, George Washington University Medical Center, Washington, D.C.

Joseph F. Steiner, PharmD, RPh, Professor of Clinical Pharmacy, University of Wyoming College of Health Sciences, Wyoming Family Practice Residency Program, Casper

Susan B. Stillwell, RN, MSN, CCRN, Instructor, Arizona State University, College of Nursing, Tempe

Margot T. Stock, RN, MSN, Instructor, East Carolina University, School of Nursing, Greenville, N.C.

David M. Stuart, BSPh, PhD, Professor of Clinical Pharmacy, Ohio Northern University, College of Pharmacy, Ada

Catherine M. Todd, RN, MS, Assistant Professor, Villanova (Pa.) University, College of Nursing

Paul J. Vitale, PharmD, Assistant Director of Pharmacy and Clinical Services, The Anne Arundel General Hospital, Annapolis, Md.

Bradford G. Wallenberg, PharmD, RPh, Assistant Professor of Clinical Pharmacy, South Dakota State University, College of Pharmacy, Brookings

Margaret Wallhagen, RN, MSN, Doctoral Candidate, University of Washington, School of Nursing, Seattle

Lisa J. Woodard, BSPh, MPH, RPh, Clinical Staff Pharmacist, Providence Medical Center, Seattle

REVIEWERS

Steven R. Abel, PharmD, RPh, Assistant Director of Pharmacy, Clinical and Educational Services, Indiana University Hospitals, Indianapolis

Stephen C. Adams, BS, PharmD, RPh, Coordinator of Drug Information Services, St. Luke's Episcopal Hospital and Texas Heart Institute, Houston

Robert J. Anders, PharmD, Cardiovascular Research Fellow, University of Illinois at Chicago, Department of Pharmacy Practice, College of Pharmacy

Wendy L. Baker, RN, MS, CCRN, Trauma Clinical Nurse Specialist, Vanderbilt University Hospital, Nashville, Tenn.

Alan D. Barreuther, PharmD, RPh, Clinical Associate Professor, University of Arizona, College of Pharmacy, Tucson; and Supervisor, Drug Information, Tucson Medical Center

Shirley K. Bell, RN, MSN, EdD, Assistant Professor, Ohio State University, College of Nursing, Columbus

Joy Boarini, RN, MSN, ET, Clinical Nurse Specialist and Program Director, ET Nursing Education Program, Abbott Northwestern Hospital, Minneapolis

Ruth Ann Lindsey Bowen, RN, MS, Lecturer, Texas Woman's University, College of Nursing, Denton

Alan J. Braverman, PharmD, Scientific Project Administrator, Smith Kline & French Laboratories, Philadelphia

Gerald G. Briggs, BPharm, Clinical Pharmacist, Women's Hospital, Memorial Medical Center; and Assistant Clinical Professor of Pharmacy, University of California, Long Beach

Karen E. Burgess, RN, MSN, Neuroscience Clinical Nurse Specialist, Huntington Memorial Hospital, Pasadena, Calif.

Bruce C. Carlstedt, BSPh, PhD, RPh, Associate Professor of Clinical Pharmacy, Purdue University, West Lafayette, Ind.

Barry L. Carter, PharmD, Assistant Professor, University of Iowa, College of Pharmacy, Iowa City

Vivian Hayes Churness, RN, DNSc, Assistant Professor, Department of Nursing, University of Southern California, Los Angeles

Bruce D. Clayton, PharmD, RPh, Professor and Chairman, Department of Pharmacy Practice, University of Arkansas for Medical Sciences, Little Rock

Michael R. Cohen, MS, RPh, Director of Pharmacy, Quakertown (Pa.) Community Hospital

Susan E. Costello, RN, MSEd, DNSc, Nursing Education and Research Director, Georgetown University Hospital, Washington, D.C.

Linda Crosby, RN, MSN, Program Director, Nurse Recovery Program, Tampa Area Hospital Council, Tampa, Fla.

Judith Hopfer Deglin, PharmD, RPh, Assistant Clinical Professor, University of Connecticut, School of Pharmacy, Storrs

Jeffrey C. Delafuente, MS, RPh, Associate Professor of Pharmacy and Medicine, University of Florida, Colleges of Pharmacy and Medicine, Gainesville

Janet K. Dickerson, RN, Research Assistant III, University of Arizona, College of Medicine, Tucson

Grace Ann Ehlke, RN, DNSc, Assistant Professor, George Mason University, Department of Nursing, Fairfax, Va.

Alexander M. Gilderman, PharmD, Assistant Professor of Clinical Pharmacy, University of Southern California, School of Pharmacy, Los Angeles

Edward J. Haas, PharmD, Director of Drug Information Services, University of Maryland Medical System, Department of Pharmacy Services, Baltimore

Joe E. Haberle, BSPh, PhD, RPh, Professor and Director, Division of Pharmacy, St. Louis College of Pharmacy

Clare Hastings, RN, MS, Director of Marketing and Communications, National Institutes of Health, Nursing Department, Clinical Center, Bethesda, Md.

David W. Hawkins, PharmD, Associate Professor and Assistant Dean, University of Georgia College of Pharmacy, Athens

Cynthia S. Heister, RN, MN, OCN, Instructor of Clinical Nursing, University of Southern California, Department of Nursing, Los Angeles

Anne Cowley Herzog, RN, BSN, CCRN, Education Coordinator, Quakertown (Pa.) Community Hospital

Kathleen Hill-Besinque, PharmD, Clinical Pharmacist, Kenneth Norris Cancer Hospital; and Course Coordinator, University of Southern California, School of Pharmacy, Los Angeles

Alan W. Hopefl, PharmD, Assistant Professor of Clinical Pharmacy, St. Louis College of Pharmacy; and Assistant Professor of Pharmacy in Internal Medicine, St. Louis University School of Medicine

Priscilla Deming Houck, RN, MSN, Oncology Clinical Nurse Specialist, Philadelphia Hematology and Oncology Associates, Inc.

Ruth Susan Kitson, RN, BAA, MBA, Director of Nursing, Critical Care Services, Toronto Western Hospital

Barbara N. Klaus, RN, MN, Patient Education Coordinator, Ambulatory Services, York (Pa.) Hospital

Karen Landis, RN, MS, CCRN, Pulmonary Clinical Nurse Specialist, Lehigh Valley Hospital Center, Allentown, Pa.

Bruce H. Livengood, PharmD, RPh, Clinical Pharmacy Specialist, Mercy Hospital of Pittsburgh; and Associate Professor of Clinical Pharmacy, Duquesne University, Pittsburgh

Sharon Lock, RN, MSN, Clinical Instructor, Pitt County Memorial Hospital and East Carolina University School of Nursing, Greenville, N.C.

Janet McCombs, PharmD, RPh, Clinical Pharmacology Associate, University of Georgia, College of Pharmacy, Athens

Marlene McNemar-Ciranowicz, RN, MSN, Diabetes Clinical Nurse Specialist, Hahnemann Medical College and Hospital, Philadelphia

Terry T. Martinez, BSPh, PhD, Associate Professor of Pharmacy and Toxicology, St. Louis College of Pharmacy

Margaret E. Miller, RN, MSN, Head and Neck Nurse Coordinator, Illinois Masonic Medical Center, Chicago

Patricia Gonce Morton, RN, MS, Doctoral Candidate and Assistant Professor, University of Maryland, School of Nursing, Baltimore

Madeline A. Naegle, RN, PhD, Associate Professor, Division of Nursing, New York University, School of Health, Education, Nursing and the Arts Professions, New York

Sandra Ludwig Nettina, RN, MSN, CRNP, Nurse Practitioner, Department of Emergency Medicine, Temple University Hospital, Philadelphia

Donald S. North, PharmD, Assistant Professor of Clinical Pharmacy, University of Wyoming, School of Pharmacy, Laramie

John D. Ostrosky, PharmD, Drug Information Specialist and Drug Utilization Review Coordinator, Medical College of Virginia Hospitals, Department of Pharmacy Services and Drug Information Service, Richmond, Va.

Theresa S. Richmond, RN, MSN, CCRN, Trauma Nurse Coordinator, Thomas Jefferson University Hospital, Philadelphia

Dorothy A. Ruzicki, RN, PhD, Patient Education and Research Coordinator, Sacred Heart Medical Center, Spokane, Wash.

Jeanne L. Sawyer, BSN, MA, Instructor, Midland Lutheran College, Division of Nursing, Fremont, Neb.

William Simonson, PharmD, Associate Professor of Pharmacy, Oregon State University, College of Pharmacy, Corvallis

Irving Steinberg, PharmD, Assistant Professor of Clinical Pharmacy and Clinical Pediatrics, University of Southern California, Schools of Pharmacy and Medicine, Los Angeles

Joseph F. Steiner, PharmD, RPh, Professor of Clinical Pharmacy, University of Wyoming, College of Health Sciences, Wyoming Family Practice Residency Program, Casper

Thomas F. Turco, PharmD, Drug Information Specialist, University of Maryland Medical System, Department of Pharmacy Services, Baltimore

Susan A. Turner-Savage, RN, MSN, Pediatric Nursing Instructor, Northeastern Hospital School of Nursing, Philadelphia

Paul J. Vitale, PharmD, Assistant Director of Pharmacy and Clinical Services, The Anne Arundel General Hospital, Annapolis, Md.

Frederick P. Zeller, PharmD, Assistant Professor, Department of Pharmacy Practice, University of Illinois at Chicago, College of Pharmacy; and Instructor in Medicine, Section of Cardiology, University of Illinois at Chicago, Department of Medicine

PREFACE

Medication therapy is an essential component of health care today. Indeed, most patients receive a number of different types of medications several times a day. Thus, dealing with medication therapy constitutes a major portion of the nurse's activities. Specifically, the nurse is directly responsible for:
• knowing the pharmacokinetic, pharmacodynamic, and pharmacotherapeutic information about each drug that the patient receives
• using appropriate procedures and techniques to administer various medications
• using appropriate safeguards to prevent errors during medication administration
• assessing the patient's clinical responses to medication therapy, including observing for adverse reactions
• documenting the patient's clinical responses to medication therapy.

These activities require an extensive pharmacologic knowledge base and familiarity with a growing number of references and other resources. *Clinical Pharmacology and Nursing* was designed to meet both of those requirements: it can be used by the student nurse in a basic pharmacology course and in subsequent clinical courses; it is also a general reference book for the practicing clinician.

One of the major needs for students of basic clinical pharmacology is an appropriate conceptual framework that organizes the information for clinical application. This text provides such a framework. Unit I gives an overview of pharmacology. Unit II relates medication therapy to the nursing process and provides the context for the clinical application of the content. Units III through XVII present specific drug classes used in providing patient care. Consistently structured, these units present essential pharmacokinetic, pharmacodynamic, pharmacotherapeutic, and adverse drug reaction information. Additionally, each drug class includes:
• contraindications and precautions
• techniques for preventing and treating adverse reactions
• essential specific interventions
• proper drug preparation and administration techniques
• patient education information.
Numerous graphs, illustrations, and summary charts facilitate learning.

This text exists to provide students and clinicians with essential pharmacologic principles and data for patient care. Therefore, all contributors are at least master's degree–prepared, practicing clinicians, academicians, or pharmacologists. These experts represent the various specialty areas of nursing and pharmacology, providing the most current, accurate, and clinically applicable information. Their collective efforts have produced a resource that is greater than the sum of its parts.

Charold L. Baer
Bradley R. Williams

FOREWORD

At last, a publisher has produced an unusually comprehensive and readable textbook on pharmacology for student nurses, nursing educators, and clinical nurses. *Clinical Pharmacology and Nursing* is a welcome choice among today's pharmacologic nursing textbooks. It stands out as a text and reference that organizes relevant scientific content into conceptual frameworks with related information for clinical application. Organizing vast amounts of information in a clear format streamlines learning and makes it enjoyable. An impressive group of specialists in nursing and pharmacology is represented in the book's 76 contributing authors and 53 clinical reviewers; these experts ensure accurate, current, complete, and clinically applicable content. Moreover, the authors have related details on specific drugs to a broad base of pharmacologic concepts and perspectives, thereby enhancing student understanding and application of information and providing faculty with organized approaches for teaching. The book is an indispensable text for a basic pharmacology course and for more advanced clinical courses and practice.

Clinical Pharmacology and Nursing successfully combines pharmacology theory and clinical application. Pharmacologic theory is presented through general pharmacologic principles, including pharmacokinetics, pharmacodynamics, pharmacotherapeutics, toxicity and poisoning, and drug abuse, dependence, and addiction. A conceptual framework controls the presentation. Clinical application details pharmacologic products that treat, control, and prevent disorders in individuals across the life span including pediatric, young and mid-life, pregnant, lactating, and geriatric patients. Medication therapy in emergency situations also is covered.

Overview chapters are organized by the nursing process, and that process is reflected, when applicable, in the drug classification chapters. These describe assessment data, intervention strategies, drugs' interactions and effects, and nursing implications. Nursing responsibilities are outlined clearly for the drug selected; its mechanism of action; predictable patient reactions; method of administration; signs of dependence, overdose, or toxicity; steps in the event of an untoward reaction; and patient and family education. "Reader-friendly" information in this classic textbook makes difficult decisions easier.

The student's study and learning needs also have been given full consideration. Theory, interwoven throughout, helps establish and reinforce a strong conceptual foundation. Each chapter offers learning objectives and summaries and includes graphics, charts, and tables that summarize drug information, illustrate procedures, and succinctly explain complicated pharmacodynamics and physiology. The two-color design enhances the presentation. The 17 unit introductions provide overviews for the drugs covered, including necessary anatomy and physiology and a glossary of terms. The comprehensive index aids the student in easily locating general information and generic and brand-name drugs.

Although each chapter is a valuable reference and may be read as an independent selection, the book's organization sequences and reinforces learning. For example, an overview of the fundamental principles of pharmacology is presented in the first 6 chapters (Unit One). Unit Two, containing 10 chapters, presents the principles and applications of pharmacology in the context of the nursing process. The 15 other units, including chapters 17 to 82, use a format that includes drug class, pharmacokinetics, pharmacodynamics, pharmacotherapeutics, adverse drug reactions, nursing implications, and a chapter summary. So much important information gives the reader a sense of security in its ownership.

Drug therapy is a major part of health care practice today, and the nurse is the major provider in the administration of this therapy. Given the dynamic nature of biomedical knowledge and technology and the extensive and growing knowledge base in clinical pharmacology, the nurse is challenged to remain up to date in medication therapy. Yet, how can the student and the practicing nurse exercise informed nursing judgments and provide safe, high-quality care? One way is to draw on resources like *Clinical Pharmacology and Nursing*. It is the newest and finest authoritative reference in its field for nursing students, faculty, and clinical nurses. No nurse should practice without it.

Kathleen G. Andreoli, DSN, FAAN
Vice-President, Nursing Affairs
and the John L. and Helen Kellogg Dean
of the College of Nursing
Rush-Presbyterian—St. Luke's Medical Center/Rush
University, Chicago

GENERAL PHARMACOLOGY

Today, many people use pharmacotherapeutic agents (drugs) rather liberally. For many people, using drugs encompasses a wide range of products, from over-the-counter (OTC) substances such as aspirin to controlled substances such as morphine.

Nurses must consider routine drug use a major health problem for patients. The problem usually involves interactions and toxic effects from drug combinations. As a result, nurses must know the physiologic and psychological alterations produced by specific drugs and their interactions. Furthermore, nurses must know how certain patient traits influence pharmacokinetics, pharmacodynamics, and pharmacotherapeutics. Such information is as necessary for providing optimum patient care as knowing the name, classification, onset and duration of action, dosage range, administration route, contraindications, potential adverse interactive effects, and predicted outcomes of a specific drug. The information in Unit One provides a framework for understanding pharmacology; toxicity and poisoning; and drug abuse, dependence, and addiction.

Chapter 1
Introduction to Pharmacology
Chapter 1 defines the scope of the science of pharmacology and graphically depicts its five branches: pharmacokinetics, pharmacodynamics, pharmacotherapeutics, toxicology, and pharmacognosy. It introduces terminology and drug nomenclature that the nurse needs to make drug therapy decisions. It also describes chronologic events significant to the evolution of pharmacology. The chapter concludes with an overview of the development process for a new drug and the legal regulations and standards governing drug use.

Chapter 2
Pharmacokinetics
Chapter 2 presents the pharmacokinetic properties of a drug, including the time course of drug absorption, distribution, metabolism, and excretion. It investigates the relationship between these properties, which determine the plasma concentration level of a drug at any given time, and the intensity and onset of action of the drug's therapeutic and adverse effects. It also includes the pharmacokinetic-related concepts of a drug's time course of action, its half-life, and its accumulation plateau. This chapter applies pharmacokinetic principles to daily patient care.

Chapter 3
Pharmacodynamics
Chapter 3 describes drug pharmacodynamics, or the mechanisms by which drugs produce a biochemical or physiologic change in the body. It differentiates between drug action in cells and drug effects in the body (systemic). It also explains the interaction between a drug and a receptor, and the role of agonistic and antagonistic drugs. It graphically depicts various dose-response curves and relates drug potency and efficacy to those curves. Therapeutic index and adverse effects are also discussed, and the chapter concludes by detailing the implications of pharmacodynamics in implementing the nursing process.

Chapter 4
Pharmacotherapeutics
Chapter 4 explores the pharmacotherapeutics of drugs, or their usefulness in preventing or treating disease. It describes further the concept of therapeutic index and its relevance in patient care. It also includes the various effects of interactions between drugs and the factors that affect a patient's clinical response to a drug. It concludes with a discussion of the implications of pharmacotherapeutics in the nursing process and in patient care.

Chapter 5
Toxicity and Poisoning
Chapter 5 discusses adverse drug reactions and poisoning. It presents information about predisposing factors related to the patient, such as age, weight, genetic variations, and disease state; to the drug, such as bioavailability, administration routes, and multiple drug therapy; and to exogenous factors, such as diet and environment.

Glossary

Absorption: process by which a drug leaves an administration site, passes through or across tissue into the general circulation and becomes biologically available.

Active transport: use of cellular energy to move a drug from an area of low concentration to one of higher concentration.

Addiction: drug-seeking behavior in which the abuser is unable to control the desire or craving for the drug.

Adverse reaction: undesirable patient response ranging from mild effects to severe, life-threatening hypersensitivity reactions. These reactions can be predictable (dose-related) or unpredictable (non-dose-related).

Agonist: drug that has an affinity for a receptor and enhances or stimulates the receptor's functional properties.

Alcoholism: pattern of alcohol use, leading to impaired social or occupational functioning.

Antagonist: drug that occupies a receptor and inhibits the receptor's functional properties.

Autocoid: general term for various physiologically active endogenous substances that are otherwise unclassified pharmacologically, such as serotonin, angiotensin, histamine, and prostaglandins.

Bioavailability or **Biological availability:** degree to which a drug is absorbed and reaches the general circulation.

Controlled substance: drug designated by the Controlled Substance Act as having the potential for abuse or user dependence.

Distribution: degree to which an absorbed or intravenous drug is delivered to various body fluids and tissues.

Drug: pharmacologic agent or medication capable of interacting with living organisms to produce biological effects.

Drug abuse: self-directed detrimental use of drugs for nontherapeutic purposes.

Drug action: interaction between a drug and cellular constituents.

Drug dependence: loss of physiologic or psychological control over drug intake.

Drug effect: response from a drug's action.

Drug excretion: process of drug elimination from the body.

Drug interactions: relationships between concurrently administered drugs that result in alterations in the therapeutic effects of any or all of the drugs.

Drug misuse: improper drug use that leads to acute and chronic toxicity.

First-pass effect: process by which orally administered drugs progress from the intestinal lumen to the hepatic system before entering the general circulation.

Habituation: state that results from drug-induced psychological dependence.

Half-life: time required to reduce the total amount of a drug in a person's body by 50%.

Ligands: endogenous substances, such as hormones, neurotransmitters, or autocoids, that interact with a receptor to produce a response.

Metabolism or **Biotransformation:** biological process of altering or converting a drug from its present form to an inactive substance.

Nonprescription drug or **Over-the-counter drug:** drug considered safe and effective when used according to proper direction by consumers without the supervision of a physician.

Orphan drug: useful for treating disease but a drug that no company has developed, usually because of a limited market (such as a drug for a rare disease) or high-risk adverse effects.

Passive transport: movement of a drug from an area of high concentration to one of lower concentration without expending cellular energy.

Peak concentration level: point at which drug absorption and elimination are equal.

Pharmacodynamics: study of the biochemical and physical effects and mechanisms of action of drugs in living organisms.

Pharmacognosy: study of the natural sources of drugs, such as plants, animals, and minerals, and their products.

Pharmacokinetics: study of a drug's alterations as it is absorbed into, distributed through, metabolized in, and excreted from a living organism.

Pharmacology: scientific study of the origin, nature, chemistry, effects, and uses of drugs.

Pharmacotherapeutics: use or clinical indications of drugs to prevent, diagnose, and treat disease in living organisms.

Pinocytosis: movement of a drug by cellular engulfment.

Predictable adverse reactions: undesirable drug effects that are dose-related.

Prescription drug: drug safely used only under the supervision of a person licensed to prescribe and dispense in accordance with a state's laws.

Receptor: specialized reactive substance or large group of molecules that interlocks with a drug molecule. The interaction of a drug and its receptor should result in a drug effect, or pharmacologic response.

Safety or **Toxicity:** drug standard that measures incidence and severity of reported adverse effects following drug use.

Therapeutic index or **Margin of safety:** relationship between a drug's therapeutic effects and adverse effects.

Tolerance: decreased response or sensitivity of a receptor to a drug ligand at the same dose over a period of time.

continued

> ### Glossary continued
>
> **Toxicity:** condition caused by a poison or by a substance that does not cause adverse effects in smaller amounts.
> **Unpredictable adverse reactions:** allergic or idiosyncratic drug effects that are non-dose-related.
> **Volume of distribution:** concept that relates the
>
> amount of a drug in the body to the concentration of the drug in the blood.
> **Withdrawal syndrome:** unpleasant, sometimes life-threatening signs and symptoms that occur when certain drugs are stopped after prolonged, regular use.

It describes the classification system for adverse drug reactions and the nurse's role in relation to those patient reactions. The chapter also investigates mechanisms of action of poisons, clinical assessment of systemic manifestations of poisoning, poison prevention techniques, and treatment principles.

Chapter 6
Drug Abuse, Dependence, and Addiction

Chapter 6 examines substance abuse. It begins with essential terminology and then explores the effects of frequently abused substances. The clinical assessment of substance abuse is detailed as well as the signs and symptoms of withdrawal and the various types of treatment programs. The chapter concludes with a discussion of the impaired nurse.

Nursing diagnoses for acute poisoning or drug abuse

The nurse must formulate nursing diagnosis based on a patient's drug therapy. The chart below lists selected nursing diagnosis for patients who experience poisoning or abuse drugs. These nursing diagnoses are based on the classifications from Seventh National Conference of the North American Nursing Diagnosis Association (NANDA).

• Alteration in bowel elimination; diarrhea related to withdrawal from opiates
• Alteration in cardiac output: decreased, related to acute cocaine toxicity; withdrawal from benzodiazepines
• Alteration in cardiac output: decreased, related to cardiovascular manifestations—disruption of electrical conduction
• Alteration in comfort; pain related to acute amphetamine toxicity
• Alteration in nutrition: less than body requirement related to withdrawal from opiates or cannabis; abuse of alcohol
• Alteration in thought processes related to abuse of opiates, benzodiazepines, alcohol, cannabis, or psychotomimetics

• Alteration in thought processes related to central nervous system (CNS) manifestations—cognitive and behavioral changes
• Alteration in tissue perfusion related to cardiovascular manifestations—vasodilation
• Alteration in urinary elimination patterns related to renal manifestations—oliguria due to tubular necrosis
• Disturbance in self-concept related to abuse of cocaine, amphetamines, or alcohol
• Fear related to psychological manifestations—the unknown effects of poisoning
• Fluid volume deficit related to withdrawal from opiates, alcohol, or cannabis
• Fluid volume excess related to renal manifestations—oliguria due to tubular necrosis
• Impaired physical mobility related to abuse of alcohol
• Impaired physical mobility related to CNS manifestations—disruption of motor activity
• Impaired verbal communication related to abuse of opiates
• Impairment of skin integrity related to abuse of opiates or cocaine
• Ineffective breathing patterns related to respiratory manifestations—ineffective respiratory center
• Ineffective coping related to withdrawal from cocaine, alcohol, or nicotine
• Knowledge deficit related to techniques for prevention of poisoning
• Potential for injury related to abuse of benzodiazepines, alcohol, or cannabis; withdrawal from alcohol
• Potential for injury related to CNS manifestations—increased seizure activity
• Potential for violence related to acute cocaine toxicity; abuse of benzodiazepines or psychotomimetics
• Sensory-perceptual alteration related to abuse of opiates, benzodiazepines, alcohol, cannabis, or psychotomimetics
• Sensory-perceptual alteration related to CNS manifestations—altered level of consciousness
• Sleep pattern disturbance related to withdrawal from opiates or cannabis

INTRODUCTION TO PHARMACOLOGY

OBJECTIVES

After reading and studying this chapter, you should be able to:

1. Differentiate among the five branches of pharmacology: pharmacokinetics, pharmacodynamics, pharmacotherapeutics, toxicology, and pharmacognosy.

2. Briefly define prescription, nonprescription, controlled, and recreational drugs.

3. Explain the difference between a drug's chemical, generic, and trade names.

4. Trace the history of drug research from traditional natural materials—plants, animals, minerals—to chemicals, enzymes, and hormones.

5. Explain why orphan drugs can be unprofitable, even though they may be needed.

6. Describe the four phases required by the FDA for approval and marketing of a new drug.

7. Describe at least three consequences of the Federal Food, Drug and Cosmetic Act of 1906.

8. Define the five schedules of controlled drugs.

9. Explain these five drug properties: purity, bioavailability, potency, efficacy, safety, and toxicity.

10. List several sources of relevant drug information, including pharmacopeias and compendia, available to nurses.

INTRODUCTION

Chapter 1 defines pharmacology and describes its scope. Beginning with the historical evolution of pharmacology as a science, the chapter presents important terminology, drug nomenclature (names), drug sources, drug types, drug development, drug regulations, and drug standards. All are vital information nurses must have to fulfill their major responsibilities.

The increasing numbers, kinds, and complexities of new drugs require that one's knowledge of pharmacology be continually updated. Practicing nurses frequently need to consult sources included in the chapter that offer the latest drug information.

DEFINITION AND SCOPE

You have just begun the study of one of the most dynamic aspects of nursing—pharmacology. Pharmacology represents the scientific study of the origin, nature, chemistry, effects, and uses of drugs. (See *Five branches of pharmacology* for an illustration of the different categories that constitute this complex science.)

Pharmacokinetics refers to the absorption, distribution, metabolism, and excretion of a drug in a living organism. *Pharmacodynamics* is the study of the biochemical and physical effects of drugs and the mechanisms of drug actions in living organisms. *Pharmacotherapeutics* (clinical pharmacology) is a general term covering the use of drugs (clinical indications) in the prevention and treatment of disease. The majority of a nurse's drug-related functions fall under the heading of pharmacotherapeutics. *Toxicology* represents the study of poisons, including the adverse effects of drugs on living organisms. Detailed discussions of pharmacokinetics, pharmacodynamics, pharmacotherapeutics, and toxicology appear in Chapters 2, 3, 4, and 5 respectively. *Pharmacognosy,* the fifth branch of pharmacology, deals with natural drugs—that is, plants, animals, or minerals and their products. A discussion of pharmacognosy follows later in this chapter.

Pharmacology is an interdisciplinary science. Although most students traditionally associate chemistry

Five branches of pharmacology

An extensive science, pharmacology includes absorption, distribution, metabolism, and excretion (pharmacokinetics); biochemical and physical effects, and mechanism of action (pharmacodynamics); clinical indications or uses (pharmacotherapeutics); toxicity and adverse reactions (toxicology); and natural sources of drugs (pharmacognosy).

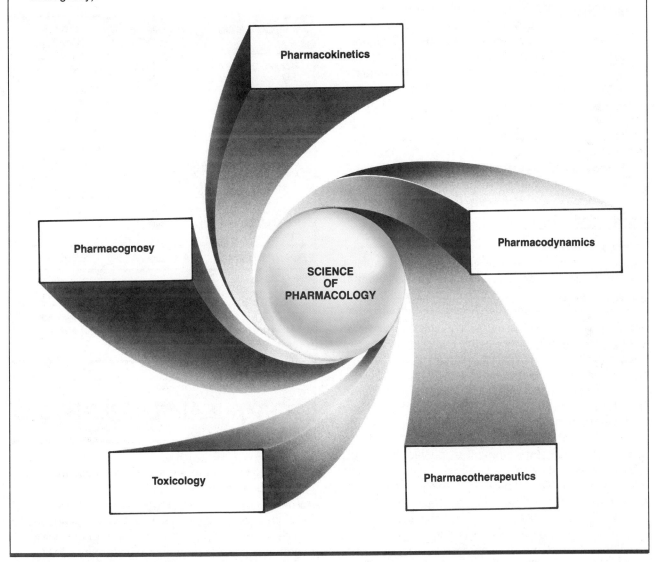

Pharmacokinetics

Pharmacognosy

Pharmacodynamics

SCIENCE OF PHARMACOLOGY

Toxicology

Pharmacotherapeutics

with pharmacology, the physical, biological, and social sciences also contribute information on using drugs to achieve and maintain optimum health without causing toxicity or patient dependence.

TERMINOLOGY

Nurses must know the following terminology both to aid their own understanding and to enable them to interpret information for patients.

A *drug* (medication) is a pharmacologic agent that is capable of interacting with living organisms to produce biological effects.

A *prescription drug* can only be used safely under the supervision of a health care practitioner who is licensed to prescribe or dispense drugs according to state laws.

A *nonprescription drug* (over-the-counter, or OTC, drug) can be used by consumers safely without the supervision of a licensed health care practitioner, provided consumers follow the directions.

A *controlled drug* is so called because it can lead to drug abuse or drug dependence and because its use is actually controlled by various federal, state, and local laws.

Drug abuse describes the self-directed use of drugs for nontherapeutic purposes, a practice that does not comply with sociocultural norms within a given culture.

Drug dependence results when a person loses the ability to keep drug intake under control. Drug dependence may be physiologic, psychological, or both.

Drug misuse refers to the improper use of common drugs, leading to acute and chronic toxicity with such problems as gastrointestinal bleeding, kidney damage, or liver damage.

A *recreational drug* is one used for its pleasant psychological or physical effects with no therapeutic intent.

DRUG NOMENCLATURE

The *chemical name* of a drug precisely describes the drug's atomic and molecular structure. The manufacturer who first developed the drug usually assigns it a *generic name.* The generic name, in most cases derived from the chemical name, is shorter—abbreviated for simplicity. The drug company selling the product selects its *trade name* (also known as the brand name or proprietary name). Trade names are protected by copyrights. The symbol ® following the trade name indicates that the name is registered by and restricted to the drug manufacturer. Because pharmacies stock various trade-name drugs, nurses can avoid confusion by always using the generic name when speaking or writing about a drug. In 1962, the federal government mandated the use of *official names* so that only one official name would represent each drug. The official names (the generic names) are listed in the United States Pharmacopeia (USP) and National Formulary (NF). (See *Drug nomenclature* for examples of various names assigned to drugs.)

Drugs that share similar characteristics are also grouped together as classes (families), such as penicillins, beta blockers, and benzodiazepines. A second grouping is the therapeutic classification, illustrated by antihypertensives. Thiazides and vasodilators are both antihypertensives, but they share very few characteristics. Discussions of the different drug classes appear in Chapters 17 through 82 in this book.

Drug nomenclature

A drug has at least three names. The surest way to avoid confusion is to use the drug's generic name. Note that a drug may have many trade names. The ones listed here are examples only, not inclusive.

CHEMICAL NAME	GENERIC NAME	TRADE NAME
6-chloro-2*H*-1,2,4-benzo-thiadiazine-7-sulfona-mide 1,1-dioxide	chlorothia-zide	Diuril®
7-chloro-1,3-dihydro-1-methyl-5-phenyl-2H-1,4-benzodiazepin-2-one	diazepam	Valium®
ethyl 1-methyl-4-phenyli-sonipecotate hydrochloride	meperidine	Demerol®
[2,3-dichloro-4-(2-methy-lene-butyryl)-phenoxy] acetic acid	ethacrynic acid	Edecrin®
acetylsalicylic acid	aspirin	Ecotrin®
17,21-dihydroxypregna-1,4-diene-3,11,20-trione	prednisone	Deltasone® Meticorten®
magnesium hydroxide Mg(OH)$_2$	magnesium salts	Phillips Milk of Magnesia®

HISTORICAL PERSPECTIVE

History helps nurses to see the development and uses of drugs in religious, social, and political contexts. (See *Historical development of pharmacotherapeutics,* pages 8 and 9, for a chronologic list of important contributions in this branch of pharmacology and the names of the individuals or groups of people responsible for the contributions.)

Before 3000 B.C.

Early in the development of pharmacotherapeutics, people relied primarily upon empirical methods (trial and error) when dealing with illness. Observations of animals and their eating habits helped primitive humans conclude that what was eaten provided either nutritional or medicinal benefits, or both. Hunters learned to smear vegetable substances, such as ouabain, on arrowheads to stun or kill animals. Others learned how to ferment carbohydrate substances, such as grapes, potatoes, or rice, to yield alcohol, which they then used for its anesthetic effects.

At times, illness became so severe that tribes or settlements needed an expert to provide therapy. Thus emerged the physician figure, called in various societies a shaman, medicine man, or witch doctor. Since illness was equated with possession by evil spirits, the physician figure commonly gave his patients a vile-tasting concoction (often purgatives or laxatives) to drive out the evil spirits. Such "magical remedies" were orally passed on from generation to generation.

From 2700 B.C. through the beginning of the Christian era

The earliest known written accounts of mixtures used for medicinal purposes appeared in Sumeria in 2100 B.C. The Sumerians, who lived in the Valley of the Euphrates River (now Iraq), preserved their prescriptions in cuneiform script on clay tablets. Although the Sumerians are credited with the first written prescriptions, the Chinese compiled a textbook dated about 2700 B.C. that documented the medicinal uses of plants and other natural substances. Some of the textbook's suggestions, such as the effectiveness of rhubarb and senna as laxatives, are still used today. Less effective remedies, such as the use of rhinoceros horn as an aphrodisiac, also appear in the text.

During his reign, the Babylonian ruler Hammurabi developed a code of laws used in the courts. Some of the laws in Hammurabi's code protected citizens from unskilled physicians and unnecessary medical procedures. The laws specified penalties and rewards for unsuccessful or successful treatments of disease.

Around the same time, Indian civilizations in both North and South America were using herbs for ceremonial and medicinal purposes. For example, in North America, the Iroquois tribe chewed herbs to stimulate the sense of taste. In South America, the Incas used herbs as diuretics and for relief of respiratory distress.

In 1874, Georg Ebers, a German Egyptologist, edited a medical papyrus that he had discovered on an expedition to Egypt. Ebers' Medical Papyrus, a scroll about 22 feet long, indicates that some drug preparations had been standardized as early as 1500 B.C. While Ebers' papyrus primarily contains information about substances that prevent decay of a body after death, it also gives many prescriptions for substances used to treat the living. Ebers' Medical Papyrus also indicates that remedies were prepared in various forms, including tablets, powders, gargles, salves, and poultices.

By 1500 B.C., the Hebrew civilization in Palestine had developed remarkable hygienic and sanitary practices. The Mosaic Health Code addressed many aspects of life in the society, from personal hygiene to environmental protection.

The Persians, a group of Iranian tribes welded into a nation by Cyrus the Great in 600 B.C., practiced a religion known as Zoroastrianism. The Zoroastrians' sacred book, the Avesta, contains ceremonial rites relating to the events of birth and death that were performed by Zoroastrian priests. Besides the priests, three types of physicians practiced medicine in Persia, those who healed with the knife, with herbs, and those who healed with holy words.

The Greeks were leaders in many creative areas including art, architecture, philosophy, and medicine. Hippocrates, commonly known as the Father of Medicine, practiced an early form of patient-centered (holistic) medicine. Hippocrates mentioned many drugs in his writings, but his clinical studies indicate that he used only a few of what we consider important drugs. For example, Hippocrates prescribed opium for pain relief.

Around 200 B.C. in India, Hindu priests wrote about pharmacology, citing such preparations as colchicum, gentian, castor beans, and digitalis.

From the 1st century through the 19th century

Greeks who emigrated to Rome from the 1st to the 3rd centuries A.D. took the practice of medicine with them. Galen, a Greek physician living in Rome, pioneered the preparation of vegetables as medicinal aids (galenicals). Dioscorides, another Greek physician who journeyed to Rome, specialized in the study of botany and wrote a text on drugs and their uses, *De Materia Medica*.

For several hundred years after the fall of the Roman Empire, Arabs settled throughout the Holy Land, Egypt, North Africa, and Spain. The Arabs were especially interested in medicine, chemistry, and pharmacy. They blended the scientific knowledge of the Greeks, Romans, and Jews with the ancient astrology of Egypt and India. The Arabs concocted many new drugs, using musk, myrrh, tamarind, and cloves and originated syrups, juleps, and aromatic water. In the Arab culture, pharmacy was practiced separately from medicine, and Arab pharmacists set up the prototype for the London Pharmacy.

The Middle Ages, a term commonly applied to the period between the 5th century and the middle of the 15th century, saw little advancement in the science of pharmacology, which returned to a primitive empiricism. Priests in the monasteries throughout Europe were almost solely responsible for the preservation of ancient texts and prescriptions. In the monastery gardens (particularly those of the Benedictine order), the monks per-

(Text continues on page 10.)

Historical development of pharmacotherapeutics

Interest in and experiments with plants, animals, and minerals as drugs began early in our history. Much later, in the 19th century, drug research shifted from traditional natural materials to chemical synthesis and manipulation of enzymes and hormones.

PERIOD OF HISTORY	DEVELOPERS	CONTRIBUTIONS
Before 3000 B.C.	Early physician figures known in various cultures as shamans, witch doctors, medicine men	Toxins to kill animals for food Cathartics and emetics Alcohol for anesthesia Bark of willow tree to relieve joint stiffness Salt as an essential ingredient for health
From 2700 B.C. through the beginning of the Christian era		
2700 B.C.	Chinese	Textbook of medicine recommending plants, such as rhubarb and senna, as laxatives
2100 B.C.	Inhabitants of the Euphrates River Valley (now Iraq)	Clay tablets written in cuneiform script containing medical prescriptions
2000 B.C.	Inhabitants of Babylonia, also located along the Euphrates River	Hammurabi's code of law protecting patients from medical malpractice
2000 B.C.	North American Indians (Iroquois)	Herbs used to stimulate a sense of taste
2000 B.C.	South American Indians (Incas of Peru)	Herbs used for diuretics, to relieve respiratory distress
1500 B.C.	Egyptian medical papyrus, known today as Ebers' Medical Papyrus	Scroll containing prescriptions for over 700 drugs, including aloe, castor oil, vinegar, opium, and peppermint; remedies were prepared as pills, powders, gargles, salves, and poultices
1500 B.C.	Hebrew priest-physicians and health inspectors living in what was then known as Palestine, now divided between Israel and Jordan	Wine and vinegar used for medicine Fig poultices Mosaic Health Code
600 B.C	Zoroastrian priest-physicians of Persia (now Iran)	Drugs used to stimulate uterine contractions; specialized medical practice divided among three groups—one specialty group used herbs for treatment
400 B.C.	The Greek physician, Hippocrates (Father of Medicine)	Mentions 400 drugs in his writings; however, used drugs very selectively
200 B.C.	Hindu priests in India	Recognized colchicum, castor beans, and digitalis

PERIOD OF HISTORY	DEVELOPERS	CONTRIBUTIONS
From the 1st century through the 19th century		
100 A.D.	Dioscorides, a Greek living in Rome	Authored *De Materia Medica,* a definitive textbook on medical materials
200 A.D.	A Greek living in Rome named Galen (disciple of Hippocrates)	Originated many preparations from vegetables (galenicals), such as cold cream
500 A.D.	Arabs living in Palestine, Egypt, North Africa, and Spain	Spread their knowledge of many drugs such as musk, myrrh, tamarind, and cloves Originated syrups, juleps, and aromatic water Pharmacy practiced separately from medicine
610 A.D.	The Arab physician Avicenna	Wrote *Canon of Medicine*
1000 to 1500 A.D.	Monastery gardeners of Europe	Cultivated herbs, such as clover, primrose, and belladonna, for medicinal purposes
1500 through 1700 A.D.	Scientists working during the Renaissance in Europe	Beginnings of empirical chemistry—plants were classified; relationship of drug dose to toxicity was recognized
1526	German physician and alchemist Paracelsus	Investigated use of metals for medicinal purposes
1618	English scientists	First London pharmacopeia was published
1785	English, William Withering	Described medical uses of foxglove
1815	German, Frederick Sertürner	Isolated the alkaloid of morphine from opium
1842	American, Crawford Long	Used ether as a general anesthetic
In the 20th century		
1907	German, Paul Ehrlich	Discovered Salvarsan as a treatment for syphilis
1908	German, Gelmo	Discovered sulfanilamide
1922	Canadians, Banting, Best, and Macleod	Discovered insulin for treatment of diabetes mellitus
1929	English, Sir Alexander Fleming	Discovered penicillin
1955	American, Jonas Salk	Discovered poliomyelitis inactivated vaccine
1970s and 1980s	Scientists worldwide	Purified drugs are prepared from the traditional natural materials; the drugs include oral contraceptives, synthetic analogues of human sex hormones Chemical synthesis of drugs and manipulation of biological products, such as enzymes and hormones

petuated the ancient practice of growing herbs for medicinal purposes.

With the Renaissance in the 15th century came a renewed interest in the accomplishments of the past. The revival applied to the visual arts, architecture, and literature, as well as to science, including pharmacology. Paracelsus, the son of a German physician and chemist, traveled widely throughout Europe, studying folk medicine and investigating the use of metals for medicinal purposes.

In the years following the Renaissance, pharmacologic advancements occurred more frequently. In London, the first pharmacopeia was published in 1618. The London College of Physicians sponsored the pharmacopeia, with King James I mandating its use throughout the British realm. In the late 18th century, William Withering described the medicinal uses of foxglove.

In the 19th century, pharmacology started to become a highly specialized science. The first great pharmaceutical discovery occurred in 1815 when Frederick Sertürner isolated the alkaloid morphine from opium. This led to considerable research into the isolation of active components of drugs. Researchers conducted enthusiastic studies on vegetable drugs. Research in the 19th century also focused on the effects of chemicals on organs and tissues. In 1842, in the United States, Crawford Long first used ether as a general anesthetic.

In the 20th century

During the 20th century, drugs have become more chemical than botanical. In 1907, the German Paul Ehrlich introduced Salvarsan to treat syphilis; in 1922, Banting, Best, and Macleod discovered insulin. Both developments represent landmarks in the history of the 20th century. Gelmo's discovery of sulfanilamide in 1908 provided a breakthrough for other research workers who had hoped that chemotherapeutic agents would effectively combat infectious diseases. Still, the therapeutic effect of sulfanilamide was not fully recognized until 1932. Likewise, Sir Alexander Fleming's discovery of penicillin in 1929 did not immediately lead to use of the drug in therapy. Penicillin was finally used for treating patients in 1942, when Dr. Howard Florey of Oxford University came to the United States and asked for the assistance of the National Research Council in studying penicillin. In 1955, the new poliomyelitis vaccines were hailed as providing relief from that dreaded disease.

In 1962, the Kefauver-Harris drug amendment was passed. The amendment requires proof of a drug's efficacy as well as its safety. Since passage of the amendment, the introduction of new drugs has slowed down. Despite the slower pace, new drugs valuable to the prevention and treatment of diseases continually become available. Although scientists still use the traditional natural materials as ingredients for drugs, researchers increasingly develop drugs through chemical synthesis or the manipulation of biological products, such as enzymes and hormones. Twentieth-century pharmacology has grown into a complex science involving a vast drug-manufacturing industry.

At the same time, many people have remained or become interested in natural products, including the commonly referred to "natural" foods and herbal remedies. The administration of and experimentation with herbal medicines may lead to the discovery of new and valuable drugs, although not without risk. For example, impurities in a newly discovered natural drug may cause adverse physical reactions. Therefore, care must be taken to ensure that the manufacturers of new natural drugs comform to all drug control laws and labeling regulations.

The future of pharmacology necessitates a balance between technology and the natural order. While promoting technology to improve the quality of life, scientists and manufacturers must take care to avoid toxic effects on patients and the environment. The readily available drug supply also creates a tremendous potential for drug abuse and misuse, which drains human productivity, increases crime, and overburdens law enforcement agencies.

PHARMACOGNOSY

Traditionally, *pharmacognosy* refers to the study of natural drug sources, such as plants, animals, or minerals and their products. Today, however, chemicals developed and used in the laboratory allow researchers to increase the number of drug sources. For example, oral contraceptives, which are synthetic analogues of human sex hormones, are manufactured chemically. Chemically developed drugs are free of the impurities found in natural substances.

Researchers and drug developers also can now manipulate the molecular structure of substances, such as antibiotics, so that a slight change in the chemical structure makes the drug effective against different organisms. The first-generation cephalosporins, produced by an organism cultured in seawater, were effective against the organisms of *Streptococcus*, *Staphylococcus*, *Escherichia coli*, *Proteus mirabilis*, and *Shigella*. Subsequent chemically altered structures of cephalosporin (second and third generation) effectively treat infections caused by *Bacteroides fragilis* and *Hemophilus influenzae* (second generation) and *Pseudomonas* (third generation).

The hormone insulin, used to treat diabetes mellitus, was customarily obtained from the pancreata of slaughtered animals, mainly cattle and pigs. While animal insulin is not chemically identical to human insulin, it is physiologically active in humans. Porcine insulin (derived from pigs) most nearly resembles human insulin. The chemical alteration of three amino acids in porcine insulin makes it identical to human endogenous insulin. The chemically altered porcine insulin is marketed and usually referred to as "human insulin." Drug developers can also manufacture human insulin from bacteria.

Plant sources of drugs

In most cases, the earliest concoctions using plants as drug sources consisted of the entire plant, including leaves, roots, bulb, stem, seeds, buds, and blossoms. Much extraneous material, some of it often harmful to human tissues, found its way into the mixture. The active components in the crude mixture caused the drug's effect. As the understanding of plants as drug sources became more sophisticated, researchers sought to isolate the active components and avoid the extraneous material.

The active components consist of several types and vary in character and effect. The most important are alkaloids (one of the largest groups of active components), which act as alkali. The organic alkaloids react with acids to form a salt. This salt, a neutralized or partially neutralized form, is thus more readily soluble in body fluids. The names of alkaloids and their salts usually end in *-ine*, for example, atropine, caffeine, and nicotine.

Other active principles include glycosides, gums, resins, and oils. As glycosides decompose, they yield sugars and an aglycon, or the noncarbohydrate group of a glycoside molecule. Names of glycosides usually end in *-in*, for example, digitoxin and digoxin. Gums, usually polysaccharides producing viscous solutions, constitute another group of active components. Gums give products the ability to attract and hold water. Examples include seaweed extractions and seeds with starch. Resins, of which the chief source is pine tree sap, often act as local irritants or as laxatives and caustic agents. Oils, thick and sometimes greasy liquids, are classified as either volatile or fixed. Examples of volatile oils include peppermint, spearmint, and juniper. Fixed oils, not easily evaporated, include castor oil and olive oil.

Animal sources of drugs

The body fluids or glands of animals can act as sources of drugs. The drugs obtained from animal sources include hormones, such as insulin; oils and fats (usually fixed), such as cod-liver oil; and enzymes, produced by living cells, which act as catalysts. Enzymes include pancreatin and pepsin. Vaccines (suspensions of killed, modified, or attenuated microorganisms) are also obtained from animal sources.

Mineral sources of drugs

Metallic and nonmetallic minerals provide various inorganic materials not available from plants or animals. The mineral sources are used as they occur in nature or are combined with other ingredients to provide drugs to form acids, bases, or salts. For example, coal tar, an acid, yields salicylic acid, aluminum hydroxide (a base), and sodium chloride (a salt).

Laboratory-produced (chemical) sources of drugs

Today's researchers produce an ever-increasing number of drugs in the laboratory. The new drugs may be organic (from living organisms) or inorganic substances or a combination of the two. Examples of drugs produced in the laboratory include penicillin (organic), sulfonamides and oral contraceptives (inorganic), and propylthiouracil (combination organic and inorganic). Recombinant DNA research has led to another chemical source of organic compounds: the reordering of genetic information enables scientists to develop bacteria that produce insulin for humans.

NEW DRUG DEVELOPMENT

Although drugs were once found by trial and error, they are now primarily developed by systematic scientific research. Scientists still search for new organic and inorganic sources, however they now focus the greater part of their attention on the laboratory to discover drugs needed for the future.

The Food and Drug Administration (FDA) carefully monitors the process of new drug development, which can take many years to complete. New drug development begins with animal tests to determine the drug's pharmacologic use, dosage ranges, and possible toxic effects. Only after reviewing extensive animal studies and data on the safety and effectiveness of the proposed drug will the FDA approve the application for an Investigational New Drug (IND).

Four phases of clinical evaluation involving human subjects follow approval of the IND. The clinical studies are intended to provide information on purity, bioavailability, potency, efficacy, safety, and toxicity. Depending upon the results of testing, the studies can be stopped at any phase.

Phase I

In phase I, a clinical pharmacologist supervises studies involving a small number of healthy volunteers. All effects of the drug on the volunteers are recorded. The recorded clinical data determine the need for further testing.

Phase II

A small number of individuals who have the disease for which the drug is purported to be diagnostic or therapeutic are then given the drug. Supervisors carefully document both toxic effects and side effects to determine the drug's proper dosage. Researchers then review and compare data from the animal studies and human studies, closely monitoring drug effects on both animal and human fertility and reproduction.

Phase III

In phase III, large numbers of patients in medical research centers receive the drug. This larger sampling provides information about infrequent or rare adverse effects. Information collected during this phase helps determine any risks associated with the new drug. Researchers must also perform various tests that take into account those patients who are so emotionally involved that they experience relief of symptoms based on suggestion. The administration of a placebo, a medically inert substance, to some patients provides control for such psychological responses. In one frequently used procedure, one half of the patients receive the drug and one half receive the placebo. To remove all bias, neither the patients nor the physician knows who has received the drug and who has received the placebo until completion of the study, known as a double-blind study. In another type of study (crossover study), patients receive the drug for part of the time and a placebo for the rest of the time.

After the first three phases, the FDA evaluates the results. If the FDA announces a favorable evaluation, the company developing the drug then completes a New Drug Application (NDA). Approval of the company's NDA by the Food and Drug Administration means that the new drug has been accepted.

Phase IV

After approval by the NDA, the drug company begins surveillance or post-market surveillance. The drug company receives from physicians reports concerning the therapeutic results of the drug. The company must communicate adequately with the FDA and with the public during the drug's use. Some medications, such as benoxaprofen (Oraflex), have been found to be toxic and have been removed from the market after their initial release. At times, manufacturers have contended that a drug's benefits for a certain segment of the population outweigh its risks. Such was the manufacturer's response when the antidepressant tranylcypromine was withdrawn from the market. Eventually but with certain restrictions, the FDA reinstated tranylcypromine in the market for use by severely depressed patients.

ORPHAN DRUGS

Some drugs useful to treat various diseases never reach the market. Drug companies do not adopt and develop the drugs, appropriately referred to as "orphans." The reasons for this vary. Some orphan drugs useful for rare diseases have a limited market; others produce high-risk side effects that make insurance costs prohibitive. Many useful drugs remain orphans because the manufacturers cannot hope to make back the huge amounts of money spent in developing a new drug.

In 1983, Congress signed the Orphan Drug Act, which offers substantial tax credits to companies that develop orphan drugs. Small companies may receive federal financial grants to assist them in researching and developing orphan drugs. As a result, thousands of patients may now use drugs that until recently were unavailable. Despite the legislation, many orphan drugs remain without developers.

LEGAL REGULATIONS AND STANDARDS

As a society develops and uses drugs, it needs to establish controls regulating the manufacture, distribution, and use of those drugs. Religious and social mores provide informal controls on drug use. In most cases, a society's attitudes and values more strictly determine the acceptable limits of drug use than formal controls. Formal drug controls range from the policies of individual institutions to governmental legislation.

International controls

The United Nations, through its World Health Organization, attempts to influence international health by providing technical assistance and encouraging research for drug use. One committee has been established to cope with the problems associated with habit-forming drugs. Drug enforcement agencies in various nations do cooperate, but no administrative or judicial structures enforce controls. As a result, control of international drug trade depends largely upon the voluntary cooperation of nations.

Controls in the United States

Legislative drug control in the United States began in 1906 with the passage of the Federal Food, Drug and Cosmetic Act (FFDCA). While the FFDCA primarily addressed the issue of food purity, it also designated the United States Pharmacopeia (USP) and the National Formulary (NF) as the official standards for drugs. (See *Federal drug legislation* for a list of laws and amendments adopted since 1906 and a summary of each.)

In 1912, the Sherley Amendment to the FFDCA increased federal involvement in drug control by prohibiting the use of fraudulent claims by drug companies.

Because of a less than rigorous enforcement of the Sherley Amendment, drug companies continued to advertise the wide-ranging efficacies of their products.

In 1914, Congress passed the Harrison Narcotic Act. The legislation classified certain drugs, such as marijuana, opium, cocaine, and their derivatives, as habit-forming narcotics. The act also placed regulations on the importation, manufacture, sale, and use of habit-forming narcotics. The Harrison Narcotic Act was the first narcotic control legislation passed by any nation.

In the 1930s, the need for more stringent drug regulations became apparent when more than 100 people died from ingesting sulfanilamide (an antibacterial drug). Researchers discovered that a sulfanilamide had been prepared with a previously uninvestigated toxic substance called diethylene glycol. After the sulfanila-

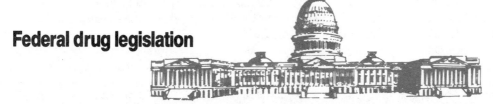

Federal drug legislation

Since 1906 when Congress passed the Federal Food, Drug and Cosmetic Act, the federal government has legislated drug manufacture, sales, and use. The following list gives the major legislative acts and their significance.

YEAR	LEGISLATION	SIGNIFICANCE TO THE PUBLIC
1906	Federal Food, Drug and Cosmetic Act (FFDCA)	Designated official standards for drugs (United States Pharmacopeia and National Formulary)
1912	Federal Food, Drug and Cosmetic Act—Sherley Amendment	Prohibited drug companies from making fraudulent claims about their products
1914	Harrison Narcotic Act	Classified certain habit-forming drugs as narcotics and regulated their importation, manufacture, sale, and use
1938	Federal Food, Drug and Cosmetic Act—Amendment	Provided for governmental approval of new drugs before they enter interstate commerce; defined labeling requirements
1945	Federal Food, Drug and Cosmetic Act—Amendment	Provided for certification of certain drugs through testing by the Food and Drug Administration
1952	Federal Food, Drug and Cosmetic Act—Durham-Humphrey Amendment	Distinguished between prescription and over-the-counter drugs; specified procedures for the distribution of prescription drugs
1962	Federal Food, Drug and Cosmetic Act—Kefauver-Harris Amendment	Provided assurance of the safety and effectiveness of drugs and improved communication about drugs
1970	Comprehensive Drug Abuse Prevention and Control Act (the Controlled Substance Act)	Outlined controls on habit-forming drugs; established governmental programs to prevent and treat drug abuse; assisted with the campaign against drug abuse by developing a classification that categorized drugs according to their abuse liability; placed drugs into schedules

mide incident, Congress passed the 1938 amendment to the Federal Food, Drug and Cosmetic Act. The amendment established regulations for approval by the federal government of all new drugs and specified requirements for drug labeling. According to the 1938 amendment to the FFDCA, drug labels were to consist of the following elements before the products could enter interstate commerce:

• A statement accurately describing the package's contents

• The usual names of the drugs, both official (preparations listed in the pharmacopeia and adopted by the government as meeting pharmaceutical standards) and nonofficial drugs (those drugs not listed in the pharmacopeia)

• Indication of the presence, quantity, and proportion of certain drugs (such as alcohol, atropine, digitalis, and bromides)

• A warning of habit-forming drugs in the product and of their effects

• The names of the manufacturer, packager, and distributor

• Directions for use and warnings against unsafe use, including recommendations for dosage levels and frequency

• A statement on all new drugs not yet approved for interstate commerce, for example: "Caution: New Drug—Limited by Federal Law to Investigational Use."

Finally, no false or misleading statements were to appear on the label.

In 1945, the Federal Food, Drug and Cosmetic Act was further amended to provide for direct governmental supervision and inspection of pharmaceuticals during production. According to the 1945 amendment, governmental certification of certain drugs, such as antibiotics, could not be granted until each batch of the drug produced was tested. The Durham-Humphrey Amendment to the FFDCA in 1952 distinguished between prescription and over-the-counter drugs. The Durham-Humphrey Amendment also specified procedures for the distribution of prescription drugs.

In the 1960s, the public became aware of the potential dangers of drugs when 200 cases of poliomyelitis developed from hastily prepared batches of poliomyelitis vaccine. Birth defects in some European countries that were linked to the ingestion by pregnant women of the drug thalidomide also caused great public concern. Media exposure of the poliomyelitis and thalidomide incidents and of the huge profits earned by many drug companies triggered the 1962 passage of the Kefauver-Harris Amendment. The amendment attempted to control the safety and effectiveness of drugs and to assure the public of necessary and timely drug information.

Schedules of controlled drugs

The Controlled Substances Act of 1970 classified drugs into categories (schedules) according to their abuse liability. Health care practitioners must be aware of these schedules to ensure the proper handling of controlled substances.

Schedule I Research use only.	**Narcotics** • Heroin **Hallucinogens** • LSD • Mescaline **Depressants** • Methaqualone
Schedule II Written prescriptions required. No telephone renewals. In an emergency, a physician may prescribe over the telephone.	**Narcotics** • Opium poppy • Codeine **Stimulants** • Amphetamine • Phenmetrazine **Depressants** • Secobarbital
Schedule III Prescriptions required to be rewritten after 6 months or 5 refills. Physician may prescribe over the telephone.	**Narcotics** • Opium 25 mg/5 ml • Codeine of less than 1.8 g/100 ml **Stimulants** • Benzphetamine • Mazindol **Depressants** • Butabarbital • Glutethimide • Methyprylon • Talbutal
Schedule IV Prescription required to be rewritten after 6 months or 5 refills.	**Narcotics** • Pentazocine • Propoxyphene **Stimulants** • Phentermine • Fenfluramine **Depressants** • Benzodiazepines • Chloral hydrate
Schedule V Dispensed as any other (nonnarcotic) prescription drug. Some Schedule V drugs may also be dispensed without prescription unless additional state regulations apply.	Primarily small amounts of narcotics, such as codeine, dihydrocodeine, and diphenoxylate, when used as antitussives or antidiarrheals in combination products.

In 1970, Congress passed the Comprehensive Drug Abuse Prevention and Control Act (CSA or Controlled Substance Act) designed to contain the rapidly increasing problem of drug abuse. The Controlled Substance Act promoted drug education programs and research into the prevention and treatment of drug dependence. The act also provided for the establishment of treatment and rehabilitation centers and strengthened drug enforcement authority. Further, it designated categories, or schedules, that classified controlled drugs according to their abuse liability. (See *Schedules of controlled drugs,* which lists examples of drugs in each of the five schedules.)

Schedule I contains drugs that have a high abuse potential, have no currently accepted medical use in the United States, or pose unacceptable dangers. Clearance from the FDA is necessary to obtain Schedule I drugs.

Schedule II represents drugs with high abuse potential, but with currently acceptable therapeutic use.

Sources of drug information

Many types of publications help fulfill the need of physicians, nurses, and pharmacists for up-to-date and detailed drug information. The nurse in a clinical situation may need to consult various references to obtain all of the necessary information. The following are reliable sources:

Pharmocopeia—Official
- The United States Pharmacopeia (USP) and National Formulary (NF)
- The British Pharmacopeia (BP)
- The British National Formulary (BF)

Compendia—Nonofficial
- Martindale: The Extra Pharmacopeia
- Drug Information—American Hospital Formulary Service, published by authority of American Society of Hospital Pharmacists
- Facts and Comparisons
- USP Dispensing Information

Pharmaceutical Firms
- Physicians' Desk Reference (PDR)
- Package inserts—brochures required by law. Content is approved by the FDA.

Journal
- The Medical Letter on Drugs and Therapeutics

The use of Schedule II drugs may lead to physical or psychological dependence, or both.

Schedule III drugs have a lower abuse potential than those in Schedules I or II. Schedule III drugs also have currently acceptable therapeutic use in the United States. Abuse of Schedule III drugs may lead to moderate or low physical or psychological dependence, or both. Some drugs in Schedule III are compounds containing limited amounts of certain narcotic and nonnarcotic drugs. Schedule III also includes certain depressants and barbiturates not listed in another schedule.

Schedule IV drugs have a low abuse potential compared to the drugs in Schedule III. Schedule IV drugs also have an acceptable therapeutic use in the United States.

Schedule V includes drugs with a lower abuse potential and with currently acceptable therapeutic use in the United States. Abuse of the drugs in Schedule V leads to a more limited physical or psychological dependence compared to the drugs in Schedule IV.

State, local, and institutional controls
Although state drug controls must conform to federal laws, states usually impose additional regulations, such as those determining the legal age for drinking alcohol. Local drug regulations imposed by counties or municipalities usually involve restrictions on the sale or use of alcohol or tobacco.

Institutional drug controls must conform to federal, state, and local regulations. Both public and private institutions adopt and impose drug controls primarily to prevent health problems and legal violations by people within the institution.

Legislation in Canada
The control of drugs in Canada falls under the direct supervision of the Department of National Health and Welfare. The 1953 Canadian Food and Drugs Act (amended yearly) provides regulations for drug manufacture and sale. In 1965, the Canadian Narcotic Control Act restricted the sale, possession, and use of narcotics. It further restricts narcotic possession to authorized personnel. Under the law, legal possession of narcotics by a nurse is limited to occasions when the nurse administers the drug to a patient under a physician's order, when the nurse serves as a custodian of narcotics in a health care agency, or when the nurse personally uses the narcotic as part of a prescribed treatment.

DRUG STANDARDS

The federal government establishes and enforces drug standards to ensure the uniform quality of drugs. The standards pertain to the following drug properties:

• *Purity* refers to the uncontaminated state of a drug containing only one active component. In reality, a drug consisting of only one active component rarely exists because manufacturers usually must add other ingredients both to facilitate drug formation and to determine absorption rate. Extraneous substances from the manufacturing plant may also contaminate the pure drug. As a result, standards of purity do not demand 100% pure active ingredients but specify the type and acceptable amount of extraneous material.

• *Bioavailability* describes the degree to which a drug becomes absorbed and transported to its target site in the body. Factors affecting bioavailability include the particle size, crystalline structure, solubility, and polarity of the compound. The blood or tissue concentration of a drug at a specified time after administration usually determines bioavailability.

• *Potency* of a drug refers to its strength or its power to produce the desired effect. Potency standards are set by testing laboratory animals to determine the definite measurable effect of an administered drug.

• *Efficacy* refers to the effectiveness of a drug used in treatment. Objective clinical trials attempt to determine efficacy, but absolute measurement remains difficult.

• *Safety and toxicity* are determined by the incidence and severity of reported adverse effects after the use of a drug. Some harmful effects may not appear for a considerable time. Safety and toxicity standards are constantly being refined as past experiences illuminate deficiencies in the standards.

The modern laboratory testing procedures of bioassay significantly help to determine drug standards and assure adherence to the standards. Still, much remains to be improved in testing procedures, some of which remain expensive and unreliable.

Research constantly adds to the body of drug information already known. (See *Sources of drug information* on page 15 for a list of the major sources available to health care practitioners.)

CHAPTER SUMMARY

Chapter 1 defined the science of pharmacology and identified and explained its five branches: pharmacokinetics, pharmacodynamics, pharmacotherapeutics, toxicology, and pharmacognosy. Here are the highlights of the chapter:

• Drug terminology assists nurses and their patients in making decisions about drug therapies.

• The drug nomenclature system classifies drugs into four categories according to: (1) the drug's chemical structure, (2) the name assigned by the manufacturer that developed the drug (generic name), (3) the official name (listed in the United States Pharmacopeia) as mandated by federal legislation, and (4) the trade name or proprietary name registered and copyrighted by the company that developed the drug.

• Drugs can also be categorized by families or classes that share similar characteristics. Examples of classes of drugs are penicillins, beta-blockers, and benzodiazepines. An example of a therapeutic classification of drugs is antihypertensives.

• A historical perspective of pharmacotherapeutics shows its development from early societies to modern times and helps the nurse understand the evolutionary development of drugs in religious, social, and political contexts. Historical perspective also explains how some natural sources of early medicinal products have evolved into today's modern drugs prepared by chemical synthesis and biological manipulation.

• A discussion of pharmacognosy, the study of the sources of drugs, reveals that active component in drugs traditionally were found in plants, animals, and minerals. Today, chemical sources produced in laboratories provide active component in drugs. Laboratory methods also provide means to purify, alter, or synthesize active component found in nature.

• The process whereby a newly developed drug reaches the market is discussed. The Food and Drug Administration approves an application for an investigational new drug (IND). After the manufacturer has conducted extensive animal studies, phase I of the new drug development involves testing the drug on healthy volunteers. Phase II involves trials with human subjects who have the disease for which the drug is thought to be effective. The tests determine the proper dosage as well as effects of the drug on fertility and reproduction. Phase III involves large numbers of patients in medical research centers, using unbiased research methods to detect infrequent or rare adverse effects. The FDA will approve a New Drug Application (NDA) if phase III studies are satisfactory. Phase IV involves post-market surveillance of the drug's therapeutic effects at the completion of phase III.

• The chapter also explores the difficulties in researching and developing orphan drugs that offer little financial gain. The Orphan Drug Act of 1983 has tentatively helped, providing tax incentives and monies for research to drug companies.

• Drug regulations and standards have been developed to control drug use and promote public safety. The passage of the Federal Food, Drug and Cosmetic Act (FFDCA) in 1906 designated the United States Pharmacopeia (USP) and the National Formulary (NF) as the official standards for drugs. In 1912, the Sherley Amendment to the FFDCA attempted to prohibit the use of fraudulent claims. The Harrison Narcotic Act of 1914 regulated the importation, manufacture, sale, and use of habit-forming narcotics. The 1938 amendment to the Federal Food, Drug and Cosmetic Act established regulations whereby the federal government approved the development and marketing of all new drugs.

• The 1938 amendment also established the elements of drug labeling. Labels had to give the package contents and the usual names of the drugs, as well as the presence, quantity, and proportion of certain drugs (alcohol, atropine, digitalis, bromides). Labels also had to include the names of habit-forming drugs; a warning that the drugs were habit forming; names of manufacturer, packager, and distributor; directions for use, including recommended amounts and frequency of dosage; and a warning statement on all new drugs not approved for interstate commerce. No false or misleading statements could appear on the label. The 1945 amendment to the FFDCA mandated the federal government to supervise and inspect the production of certain drugs by testing each batch. The Durham-Humphrey Amendment in 1952 distinguished between prescription and over-the-counter drugs. In 1962, the Kefauver-Harris Amendment gave assurance to the public concerning drug safety and effectiveness. The Kefauver-Harris Amendment also ensured that the public would receive pertinent information about drug safety. In 1970, the Comprehensive Drug Abuse Prevention and Control Act (CSA, the Controlled Substance Act) attempted to control the drug abuse problem. The CSA aided drug education, research, treatment, and enforcement.

• The classification of controlled drugs (Schedules I through V) describes their abuse liability.

• Drug control in Canada falls under the direct supervision of the Department of National Health and Welfare. Canadian laws mandate that nurses may legally possess narcotics only when nurses administer a narcotic to a patient under a physician's order, when nurses act as custodians of narcotics in a health care agency, or when nurses receive the narcotic as prescribed treatment for themselves.

• Drug standards help achieve uniform quality with respect to purity, bioavailability, potency, efficacy, safety, and toxicity.

• Sources of drug information for physicians, nurses, and pharmacists who need current data include pharmacopeias (official), compendia (nonofficial), pharmaceutical firms, and journals.

BIBLIOGRAPHY

Aikman, L. "Nature's Healing Arts: From Folk Medicine to Modern Drugs." In *Folk Medicine: An Enduring Art.* Washington, D.C.: National Geographic Society, 1977.

Austin, A. *History of Nursing Source Book.* New York: G.P. Putnam Sons, 1957.

DeMarco, C. *Pharmacy and the Law,* 2nd ed. Rockville, Md.: Aspen Systems Corp., 1984.

Dolan, J., et al. *Nursing in Society: A Historical Perspective,* 15th ed. Philadelphia: W.B. Saunders Co., 1983.

Federal, Food, Drug, Cosmetic Law Reporter. New York: Commerce Clearing House, 1985.

Fink, J.L., III, ed. *Pharmacology Law Digest.* Media, Pa.: Harwal Publishing, 1985.

Gilman, A.G., et al. *The Pharmacological Basis of Therapeutics,* 7th ed. New York: Macmillan Co., 1985.

Goth, A. *Medical Pharmacology,* 11th ed. St. Louis: C.V. Mosby Co., 1984.

Leake, C.D. *An Historical Account of Pharmacology to the Twentieth Century.* Springfield, Ill: Charles C. Thomas, 1975.

Levine, R. *Pharmacology: Drug Actions—Reactions,* 3rd ed. Boston: Little, Brown & Co., 1983.

Remington's Pharmaceutical Sciences, 17th ed. Easton, Pa.: Mack Publishing Co., 1985.

Thorwald, J. *Science and Secrets of Early Medicine.* New York: Harcourt, Brace and World, 1963.

Tyler, V. *Pharmacognosy,* 8th ed. Philadelphia: Lea & Febiger, 1981.

CHAPTER 2

PHARMACOKINETICS

OBJECTIVES

After reading and studying this chapter, you should be able to:

1. Describe how the different oral formulations, including compressed tablets, sustained-release formulations, and the osmotic pump, release active drug for absorption.

2. Describe how drug dosage forms—including orally administered drugs (tablets, capsules, sublingual, and buccal formulations) and parenteral drugs, such as intravenous injections—affect drug absorption.

3. Describe what happens during passive drug absorption, active transport, and pinocytosis.

4. Describe the effect of the following variables on drug absorption: surface area, blood flow, pain, first-pass effect, enterohepatic recycling, solubility, body pH, gastrointestinal motility, dosage form, interactions between drugs (drug-drug), and interactions between drugs and food (drug-food).

5. Compare the absorption rates for the oral, buccal, sublingual, rectal, transdermal, intradermal, subcutaneous, intramuscular, intrathecal, intraarticular, and intravenous routes.

6. Discuss how decreased binding between plasma proteins and active drug causes an excess of free active drug in the body.

7. Explain how a large volume of drug distribution causes a lower plasma concentration level of the drug and how a small volume of distribution causes a higher plasma concentration level.

8. Describe the general purpose of drug metabolism and the various kinds of metabolites that can result.

9. Explain the significance of a drug's half-life in terms of the frequency of a dosing schedule and the patient's clinical responses.

10. Identify how a drug's minimum effective concentration level, toxic concentration level, and therapeutic range relate to each other.

11. Explain the significance of applying pharmacokinetic data to guide therapeutic drug regimens in patient care.

INTRODUCTION

Chapter 2 focuses on pharmacokinetics, defining terminology and describing related concepts. Pharmacokinetics deals with a drug's actions as it is absorbed into, distributed to, metabolized within, and excreted from a living organism. The chapter explores the many variables that affect a drug's: (1) absorption, (2) onset of action, (3) time of peak action, (4) duration of action, (5) ability to maintain an effective blood concentration level, and (6) the dosage schedule. All of the factors have an impact on the patient's response to drug therapy.

The discussion of pharmacokinetics in Chapter 2 encompasses two additional disciplines: pharmaceutics and biopharmaceutics. Pharmaceutics describes different dosage formulations, such as tablets and syrups, and their components. Biopharmaceutics describes the interactions between the biological system and the dosage formulation that result in a biologically available drug for therapeutic use. Pharmacokinetics as well as pharmaceutics and biopharmaceutics uses mathematical formulas to describe drug movement into and throughout the system. Chapter 2, however, explains the concepts rather than the mathematics, while developing in the nursing student an appreciation for the application of pharmacokinetics and related disciplines involved in drug administration.

APPLYING PHARMACOKINETICS

The use of pharmacokinetics as a tool to assess a patient's response to drug therapy stems from observations that a strong relationship exists among a patient's positive responses to a drug (positive effects), the patient's blood concentration level of the drug, and the patient's toxic responses at specific blood concentration levels.

The primary pharmacokinetic factors affecting the patient's responses and the blood concentration levels of a drug include: (1) the rate of drug absorption, (2) the amount of drug absorbed by the body, (3) the distribution of the drug throughout the body, (4) the process and timing of drug metabolism, and (5) the rate and route of drug excretion from the body.

For some of the pharmacokinetic factors, physicians, pharmacists, and nurses need additional information. To determine drug absorption rates, they need to know how much of a drug both ill and healthy patients will absorb. The amount of drug absorbed by the body is determined partly by which body tissues accept the drug and which exclude it. The process and timing of drug metabolism depend on how and where a drug is metabolized and whether the metabolites are active or inactive compounds.

Drugs can be measured in body fluids such as blood (serum, plasma, or red blood cells), urine, cerebrospinal fluid, sputum, and other miscellaneous and accessible specimens. Recent technologic improvements in the tests used for analyzing body fluid specimens provide rapid and precise results, both quantitative and qualitative, for an increasing number of frequently administered drugs. Not all drugs require blood level monitoring, nor do assays (measurement of the drug concentration levels in blood or serum) currently exist for every drug. Nonetheless, when possible and appropriate, the inclusion of drug concentration data enhances patient assessment and helps physicians, pharmacists, and nurses to refine a patient's drug therapy.

Monitoring end-organ response can also provide information concerning pharmacokinetic factors. End-organ tests involve comparing body functions before drug therapy with the same functions when appropriate drug concentration levels are achieved. Physicians often monitor pulmonary or renal function to evaluate end-organ response.

DRUG ABSORPTION

Drug absorption encompasses a drug's progress from its pharmaceutical dosage form to a biologically available substance that can then pass through or across tissues. The transformation from dosage form to a biologically available substance must occur before the active drug ingredient reaches the systemic circulation. After a tablet or capsule disintegrates in the stomach or small intestine, enough liquid must be available for the active drug ingredients to dissolve before systemic absorption. The body requires a solution of the drug's active ingredients because tissues cannot absorb dry powders or dry crystals. (Pinocytosis, the exception to the rule, is discussed on page 22.) Because syrups and suspensions occur in dosage form as solutions, their progress from drug administration to drug absorption is more rapid, leading to a quicker onset of drug action.

ORAL DRUG ABSORPTION

A brief account of the most common types of drug formulations and their components provides a useful base for the study of drug absorption. A discussion of commonly used formulations will also help the student understand why certain tablets and capsules may not provide the anticipated response in selected situations.

Formulations

A *compressed tablet*, the most frequently dispensed form of a drug, provides a readily administered, standard dosage form. Compressed tablets, which may be engraved with a company symbol and code number for identification, usually have a thin, shiny coating that reduces dust during manufacturing and helps the patient swallow by decreasing the tablet's tendency to stick to the mouth or throat. The tablet may or may not be scored for dividing the dose. An unscored tablet should not be broken. Leaving an unscored tablet intact can protect the patient's stomach from a potentially irritating drug and protect the drug from the damaging stomach acid. Leaving the tablet intact also prevents too-rapid release of the drug from an otherwise sustained-release tablet.

Sustained-release formulations release drugs in a controlled, predictable manner, providing safe and effective drug absorption throughout the entire alimentary tract. Unless physicians and nurses completely understand the type of sustained-release tablet or capsule formulation being administered, they should never break or divide a drug formulation to provide a lower dose for a patient.

Manufacturers employ several processes to produce the many sustained-release formulations on the market. The oldest method involves applying an enteric coating to a tablet. By not dissolving in the stomach or upper intestinal tract, the enteric coating creates a barrier between the drug and the acids in the stomach or intestinal mucosa. The coating allows the tablet to pass undisturbed through the stomach to the lower small intestine, where a more basic pH safely dissolves it.

Another process uses beads or granules with varying thicknesses of protective coating over the different particles. The various coatings dissolve at different times, thereby releasing the drug at different rates over an extended period of time. Spansules by SmithKline and French Laboratories and sequels by Lederle Laboratories represent such formulations. Capsules containing coated granules should never be opened, nor should the product be chewed, because doing so immediately releases active drug into the body. The instant total dose may cause adverse reactions.

Manufacturers also produce sustained-release formulations by embedding the drug in a slowly eroding matrix. Both drug and matrix are formulated together in tableting machines. The matrix slowly breaks down during intestinal transit, releasing the drug. (Slow-K tablets by CIBA Pharmaceutical Company represent a drug in an eroding matrix.) Manufacturers sometimes embed the drug in an insoluble plastic matrix. The drug is then slowly leached from (absorbed through) the insoluble plastic matrix, and the intact plastic matrix passes through the alimentary tract. (Fero-Gradumet Filmtabs by Abbott Laboratories use the plastic matrix process.)

"Repeat action" tablets carry an initial dose in an outer "shell" and a second dose within an inner "shell." The inner shell of a "repeat action" tablet disintegrates later in the intestinal tract. (Chlor-Trimeton Repetabs by Schering Corporation are "repeat action" formulations.)

The newest process for manufacturing sustained-release formulations produces the *osmotic pump*. Osmotic pumps usually are tablets with special semipermeable membrane coverings. The tablet's covering allows water to enter. The drug in solution can then leave the tablet, but only through a single small hole made by a laser beam during the formulation process. The osmotic pump formulation provides controlled release of a drug for several hours. (Acutrim by CIBA Consumer Pharmaceuticals uses the osmotic pump formulation.)

Other novel kinds of formulations improve patient compliance with oral tablets. Chewable tablets were developed for a few products, such as children's aspirin and acetaminophen, to simplify administering the products to children. Cardiac patients can now take sublingual or buccal tablets. The soft tablet compression of sublingual and buccal tablets combined with a sufficient lactose content causes rapid, almost instantaneous disintegration of the drug when the patient places the tablet sublingually or buccally. Nitroglycerin sublingual tablets produced by various manufacturers provide good examples of the method. Sublingual and buccal formulations are especially useful for drugs requiring a rapid patient response. By dissolving in the mouth, the drug quickly passes through the mucosa into the patient's bloodstream, avoiding the destructive effects of stomach acid and various other barriers, such as food in the stomach.

Inert ingredients

Tablets and capsules contain multiple inert ingredients, including diluents, lubricants, disintegrating agents, binders, and coloring agents. The inert ingredients assist the pharmaceutical manufacturer by: (1) forming a powder that readily flows through the manufacturer's tableting equipment, (2) increasing the dimensions of a finished tablet to a manageable size for the patient, (3) binding the tablet to avoid crumbling in shipment, (4) enhancing in vivo disintegration in the stomach or small intestine, and (5) providing an aesthetically pleasing product. Furthermore, combinations of inert ingredients in a tablet or capsule stimulate disintegration, dissolution, and drug availability in the body.

Although inert ingredients do not normally produce a biological effect, some patients experience allergic reactions to such inert ingredients. For example, tartrazine yellow, a common coloring agent used in prescription and over-the-counter drugs, may precipitate an acute asthma attack in sensitive, asthmatic individuals. For this reason, manufacturers have removed tartrazine yellow from antiasthma medications.

PARENTERAL DRUG ABSORPTION

Fewer formulation variables affect the release of a parenteral drug into the system. Clear liquid solutions for direct entry into the venous or arterial circulatory system usually pose no absorption problems because they become instantaneously available to the appropriate target tissue. Differences in absorption occur, however, depending on the parenteral route selected. For example, intravenous (I.V.) administration requires no absorption time, although intramuscular (I.M.) and subcutaneous (S.C.) injections do.

Parenteral drugs indicated for any route other than intravenous or intrathecal, however, can pose absorption problems, although such problems occur rarely. For example, I.M. injections that provide a "long-acting" effect may be formulated in an oil or as microfine crystals. The nurse should never administer either formulation into a vein or an artery because the crystals or oil diluent may create emboli. The general principle regarding formulations is *If the formulation looks cloudy or "thick," do not inject it into a vein or an artery.* The oral route of drug administration remains the preferred route for drug therapy, especially because it promotes patient comfort, safety, and ease of use.

THE PHYSIOCHEMICAL BASIS OF DRUG ABSORPTION

Drug absorption varies, depending on the absorptive surface. Damaged, impaired, or surgically removed ab-

Cellular drug absorption

In most cases, drug absorption follows the same pathways as nutrient absorption. Passive mechanisms of absorption, including diffusion, convective absorption, and carrier-mediated absorption, require no energy and involve drug movement from an area of higher concentration to an area of lower concentration. Active transport for drug absorption requires energy to move drugs against a concentration gradient. Pinocytosis facilitates absorption by engulfing the drug particles and moving them across the cell membrane.

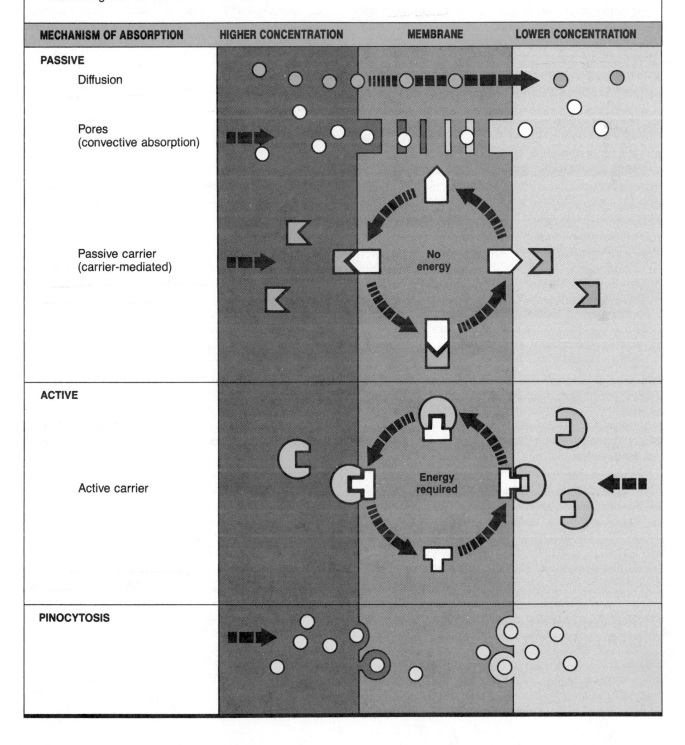

MECHANISM OF ABSORPTION	HIGHER CONCENTRATION	MEMBRANE	LOWER CONCENTRATION
PASSIVE Diffusion			
Pores (convective absorption)			
Passive carrier (carrier-mediated)		No energy	
ACTIVE Active carrier		Energy required	
PINOCYTOSIS			

sorptive surfaces can increase or decrease the amount of drug absorbed into the body and alter a patient's response. To predict the result of drug activity accurately, physicians consider the drug absorption site, whether it is the intestinal lumen or a target cell wall. Drug absorption occurs either passively or actively or by pinocytosis. (See *Cellular drug absorption* on page 21 for the three general types of drug absorption.)

Passive drug absorption, a simple diffusion action, requires no cellular energy because the drug moves from an area of high concentration, such as a disintegrated tablet's or capsule's location in the alimentary tract, to an area of lower concentration, such as the bloodstream. Administering additional amounts of a drug causes more of the drug to be absorbed.

In passive drug absorption, small water-soluble molecules diffuse across membranes or, to a lesser degree, through pores. Drugs with larger molecular sizes will pass across membranes more slowly.

Carrier-mediated diffusion, or facilitated transport, represents a second form of passive drug absorption without using cellular energy. The classic example is dietary vitamin B_{12}, which binds with intrinsic factor produced by the stomach wall. The vitamin B_{12}–intrinsic factor complex is selectively but passively carried from an area of high concentration to an area of lower concentration (gut lumen). A third and also minor passive absorption method occurs with convective absorption. During convective absorption, small drug molecules, like those of some electrolytes, move along with fluid through the pores in cell walls.

Active transport for drug absorption requires cellular energy to move the drug from an area of low concentration to one of higher concentration. Active transport is the cellular mechanism used during the absorption of the electrolytes sodium and potassium as well as some drugs, such as levodopa.

Pinocytosis, the third method of drug absorption, is a uniquely different form of active transport that occurs when a cell engulfs a drug particle in a manner comparable to phagocytosis. During pinocytosis, the drug need not be dissolved because the cell forms a vacuole or vesicle for the drug transport across the cell membrane and into the inner cell. Cells commonly employ pinocytosis to transport fat-soluble vitamins (vitamins A, D, E, and K).

OTHER VARIABLES AFFECTING DRUG ABSORPTION

Besides the type of drug formulation, the condition of the absorptive surface, and the mechanism of absorption, other variables affect the rate of absorption as well as the amount of drug absorbed.

Surface area. Most absorption of orally administered drugs occurs in the small intestine, where the mucosal villi provide extensive surface area. If large sections of the small intestine have been surgically resected, drug absorption decreases because of the reduced surface area. In some cases, the shortened intestine reduces intestinal transit time, which in turn diminishes the time that a drug is exposed to the intestinal lumen for absorption. Not all areas of the intestine absorb drugs well. For example, the decreased number of villi in the distal small intestine and the absence of villi throughout the large intestine reduce the amount of absorption possible in these locations.

Blood flow. Drug absorption also depends on blood flow to the absorption site. During normal oral drug absorption, the drug moves rapidly from the blood capillary side of the intestinal lumen. A slow rate of oral drug absorption probably indicates a low availability of the drug at the intestinal lumen wall. Food stimulates blood flow (splanchnic blood flow) to the gastrointestinal (GI) viscera and may enhance drug absorption. Strenuous physical exercise diminishes splanchnic blood flow by diverting blood to the muscles and, therefore, slows drug absorption.

With intramuscular drug absorption, drugs administered in the deltoid muscle are absorbed faster than drugs administered in the larger gluteal muscle because of the increased blood flow in the deltoid muscle. The more rapid absorption leads to a quicker onset of drug action.

Pain and stress. Pain, such as that with a migraine headache, can decrease the total amount of drug absorbed. Although the exact cause of the decreased absorption remains unknown, it is probably from a change in blood flow, reduced GI motility, or gastric retention triggered by autonomic nervous system activity that causes pyloric sphincter contraction. Decreased drug absorption can also occur during periods of stress, possibly from similar causes.

First-pass effect. Orally administered drugs do not go directly into the systemic circulation after absorption. They move from the intestinal lumen to the mesenteric vascular system to the portal vein and into the liver with its elaborate enzyme system before passing into the general circulation. During this passage, part of a drug dose may be metabolized. (See *Oral drug absorption* for the progress of an orally administered drug.) Enzymes in the liver and in the terminal portal vein may metabolize a significant portion of the drug to an inactive form before it passes into the circulatory system and to the site of action.

Oral drug absorption

Oral drugs absorbed in the GI tract are exposed to the first-pass effect of metabolism. If the enzyme system in the terminal portal vein does not metabolize the drug, it may pass into the systemic circulation and the biliary system. Drugs in the bile may be reabsorbed from the intestine and eventually sent into the systemic circulation.

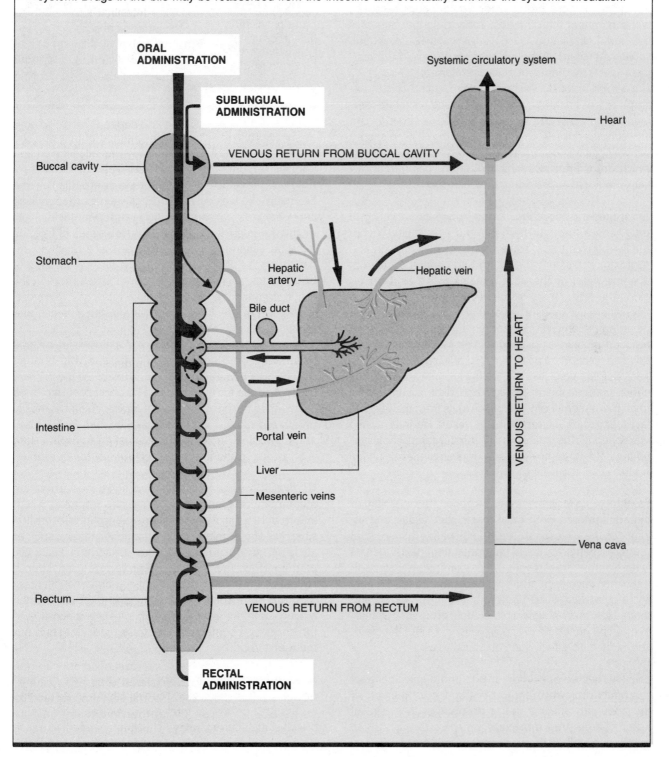

The metabolic change of a drug before it reaches the systemic circulation is referred to as the first-pass effect. (See *First-pass effect drugs* for a list of some drugs susceptible to the process.) Although many drugs may undergo some metabolism during the first pass through the liver, this process is significant only for a few. For drugs undergoing a significant first-pass effect, the orally administered dose required for a therapeutic response is much greater than the dose for a route that bypasses the portal circulation (such as the vaginal, parenteral, sublingual route). Although such routes avoid the first-pass effect, they are not always preferred.

Propranolol hydrochoride represents a classic example of a first-pass effect drug. The usual recommended *oral* anti-arrhythmic dose is 40 to 120 mg. The *intravenous* dose is usually 1 to 3 mg. The disparity between the two dosage ranges points out how knowing which drugs are susceptible to the first-pass effect can help the nurse avoid drug administration errors.

Enterohepatic recycling. In enterohepatic recycling, a drug moves through the body and eventually reaches the liver. From there, some drugs, such as digoxin and digitoxin, enter both the biliary and general circulatory systems. Most of the drug remains active as it travels along the biliary tract, eventually returning to the intestine, where it is reabsorbed and recycled. Enterohepatic recycling becomes important when the patient requires reduced digoxin or digitoxin levels to alleviate serious adverse reactions. The system typically removes digoxin and digitoxin very slowly. However, orally administered cholestyramine binds digoxin and digitoxin in the GI tract, permanently removing the drugs from the bile and facilitating their excretion in the feces. By interrupting enterohepatic recycling, orally administered cholestyramine helps to reduce digoxin or digitoxin levels within hours rather than days.

Solubility. To facilitate drug absorption, the solubility of the administered drug must match the cellular constituents of the absorption site. Lipid-soluble (fat-soluble) drugs can penetrate lipoid (fat-containing) cells, whereas water-soluble drugs cannot. For example, a water-soluble drug, such as penicillin, cannot penetrate the highly lipoid cells that act as barriers between the blood and brain. However, a highly lipid-soluble drug, such as thiopental, can penetrate the lipoid cells, cross into the brain, and induce an effect, such as anesthesia.

pH. The degree of acidity, or pH, in the intestinal tract can affect drug absorption; pH throughout the rest of the body can affect a drug's distribution to its site of action. Large drug molecules can pass through a cell membrane only if they are un-ionized; that is, if they

---

First-pass effect drugs

The following drugs are susceptible to the first-pass effect, which reduces the amount of orally administered drug to reach the circulatory system:

- coumadin
- dopamine
- imipramine
- isoproterenol
- lidocaine
- morphine
- nitroglycerin
- propranolol
- reserpine

---

are not positively or negatively charged at that site. Because most drugs exist in the body partially ionized and partially un-ionized, local pH can partly determine if a drug will move across a membrane at a particular site. For example, weakly acidic drugs such as theophylline and phenytoin, are ionized less in the low (acidic) pH of the stomach than in the high (alkaline) pH of the intestine. Therefore, absorption of these drugs is enhanced in the stomach. Conversely, weakly alkaline, or basic, drugs, such as quinidine, are ionized more in the acidic stomach than in the alkaline intestine. Therefore, absorption of quinidine is inhibited in the stomach and enhanced in the intestine.

A major factor in drug absorption is the surface area to which the drug is exposed. The intestine, with its larger surface area compared with the stomach, is the primary absorption site for most drugs. The effect of surface area is illustrated by the absorption of aspirin. Aspirin is mostly un-ionized in the stomach and is more than 99% ionized in the intestine. In spite of this, most of an aspirin dose is absorbed in the larger surface area of the intestine.

GI motility. High-fat meals and solid food affect alimentary transit time by delaying gastric emptying, which in turn delays initial drug delivery to intestinal absorption surfaces. The administration of anticholinergics, such as atropine, scopolamine, and the belladonna alkaloids, may slow intestinal motility and prolong intestinal transit time. The prolonged intestinal transit time may increase total drug absorption. Cathartics and diarrhea shorten a drug's contact time with small intestine mucosa, and this shortened contact time may decrease drug and nutrient absorption.

Dosage form. The drug absorption rate and the time needed to reach peak blood concentration levels depend on the type of dosage form used. Tablets and capsules dissolve at different rates. The time needed to reach peak effect for sublingual tablets is less than the time needed for compressed tablets and sustained-release tablets. Using sublingual and I.V. bolus administration routes results in the most rapid onset of drug action.

Drug interactions. Combining the drug with another drug or with food can cause interactions that affect drug absorption. For instance, administering tetracycline with an antacid reduces the amount of tetracycline available for absorption. Similarly, tetracycline administered with milk also reduces tetracycline's availability. To avoid undesirable interactions between drugs (drug-drug interactions) or between drugs and food (drug-food interactions), nurses should consult the appropriate current compendia or the pharmacist before administering a new drug or educating patients about that drug.

ROUTES FOR DRUG ABSORPTION

The three routes of drug administration discussed here are the enteral, parenteral, and topical. The enteral route is used when drugs are administered by mouth or rectum or directly into the intestinal system (such as by a gastrostomy tube). The parenteral route is used for drugs administered as injections into a vein, an artery, a muscle, a joint, or a skin layer or into the spinal column. The topical route is any administration to the skin or mucous membranes. Each drug administration route presents advantages and disadvantages that affect the drug's pharmacokinetics. (See Chapter 10, Intervention: Routes and Techniques of Administration, for a detailed discussion of these administration routes.)

Enteral route. Drug absorption after enteral drug administration can occur in the oral mucosa, gastric mucosa, small and large intestine, or rectum. Drug administration for absorption through the oral mucosa is usually restricted to small quantities of sublingual and buccal preparations. The preparations themselves are also restricted to water-soluble drugs, drugs with little flavor, and drugs requiring a rapid onset of action. For example, the sublingual absorption of nitroglycerin results in a rapid onset of action for a drug that would not survive exposure to gastric acid or the hepatic metabolic system.

The gastric mucosa is usually not employed for drug absorption because of the small gastric surface area (1 m²) and the unremarkable capillary blood flow (150 ml/minute). The gastric region is, however, an important site for disintegrating and dissolving tablets or capsules in preparation for absorption in the small intestine. Physical activity and body position may either slow or hasten

gastric emptying time, which will lengthen or shorten the time the drug is in contact with the gastric mucosa. A patient lying on the left side has a slower gastric emptying time because the body position causes the pyloric sphincter to lie above the stomach contents. In contrast, lying on the right side hastens gastric emptying time. Stomach fluid volume, viscosity, and contents can also affect gastric emptying time. For example, fat slows gastric emptying time, whereas liquids and carbohydrates hasten it. Strongly hypertonic solutions slow gastric emptying time because the body is attempting either to remove the hypertonic substance through emesis or to dilute the stomach contents with body fluids. Gastric pH, which ranges from about 1 to 2, may enhance or impair drug absorption, depending on the effect of pH on ionization, as was previously discussed.

The major site of drug absorption for drugs administered by enteral routes is the small intestine. From the small intestine, the active drug passes into the systemic circulation. The relatively large surface area (about 200 m²) and rapid intestinal capillary blood flow (estimated at 1 liter/minute) facilitate the efficient, rapid absorption of most drugs. Furthermore, the pH of the acidic gastric secretions increases in the intestines to about 4 or 5 because of the alkalinizing secretions of the pancreas and the neutralizing capacity of the bile. The large intestine primarily reabsorbs water and electrolytes rather than drugs.

Rectal drug absorption advantageously circumvents the first-pass effect, but only if the drug is administered in the lower rectum. Administration in the lower rectum is an alternative enteral route if oral administration poses a problem because of potential emesis or mechanical obstacles. Rectal absorption may be erratic because retention of the dosage form by the patient varies. Furthermore, the lack of fluid in the rectum inhibits a drug's disintegration and dissolution and retards its transfer across the intestinal mucosa, further delaying absorption. Another problem with administering drugs in the lower rectum is local drug-induced irritation.

Parenteral route. The administration routes for parenteral drugs include intradermal, S.C., I.M., intrathecal, intraarticular, and I.V. Nurses do not usually administer drugs by the intrathecal and intraarticular routes. Compared with orally administered drugs, parenteral drugs—usually liquid formulations—must overcome fewer barriers between the sites of drug administration and drug action. Parenteral drugs, however, still must be absorbed into the tissues or cells to exert an effect on the system.

Employing the intradermal route usually involves administering parenteral drugs between the skin layers just below the surface stratum corneum. The drugs diffuse slowly from the injection site into the local microcapillary system. In most cases, the intradermal route is limited to allergens of various strengths used in diagnostic allergy testing. A faster introduction of an allergen into a sensitive person could cause a life-threatening allergic reaction.

Using the S.C. route involves administering drugs in the region below the epidermis. S.C. administration facilitates drug diffusion to the capillary vascular system at a rate much faster than that achieved by the intradermal route. Adding vasoconstrictors slows the uptake of the drug by the circulation. The administration of mixtures, such as a combination of epinephrine (a vasoconstrictor) and lidocaine hydrochloride (a local anesthetic), prolongs the local anesthetic effect of lidocaine by slowing the removal of the drug from the blood. In contrast, gently massaging the area or applying warm compresses increases drug uptake. Gentle massage and warm compresses improve the blood flow and facilitate drug absorption from the injection site. In rare cases, physicians increase drug dispersion and absorption by administering S.C. hyaluronidase, an enzyme that breaks down tissue barriers.

Parenteral drug absorption from I.M. sites depends on whether an I.M. solution, suspension, or emulsion is used. Solutions, which are clear preparations containing one or more substances dissolved in a fluid, provide an immediate therapeutic effect. Suspensions, which contain crystalline particles causing a cloudy appearance, and emulsions, which have an oil-like base, prolong drug activity by slowing active drug absorption from the I.M. injection site. The muscle area selected for I.M. administration may also make a difference in the drug absorption rate. For example, blood flows faster through the deltoid muscle than through the gluteal muscle; however, the gluteal muscle can accommodate a larger volume of drug (up to 5 ml) than can the deltoid muscle (up to 2 ml).

Intrathecal administration places the parenteral drug directly into the cerebrospinal fluid, thereby avoiding the absorption barrier between the blood and the brain. The drug is absorbed directly into the target brain tissue. Bypassing the blood-brain barrier necessitates omitting stabilizers and buffers routinely used in injectables. Such stabilizers and buffers may produce serious adverse reactions, such as seizures, when placed directly in the patient's central nervous system. Physicians using intrathecal administration use only those drugs compatible with the intrathecal route and clearly specified on the product label "For Intrathecal Use Only."

Intraarticular drug administration involves placing the solution directly into the synovial joint fluid to provide a local effect. Systemic drug absorption after intraarticular drug administration is usually negligible. In most cases, corticosteroids prescribed for arthritis are admin-istered intraarticularly in a crystalline form to slow absorption and prolong the drug's effect.

Administering drugs by the I.V. route bypasses the absorption barriers and provides an immediate systemic response. Physicians mostly prescribe I.V. drug administration for an immediate response or for drugs not tolerated or absorbed by other administration routes. Nurses should always read the product brochure before administering an I.V. drug to determine the method and diluent for reconstitution, the rate of administration, and any restrictions. I.V. drugs should not be administered too rapidly because sensitive target tissues can absorb an excessive amount, possibly resulting in such effects as fatal heart block.

Topical route. Using topical routes of drug administration involves applying drugs to various body surfaces. In recent years, the transdermal drug delivery system (TDDS) has gained popularity. With this system, the nurse usually applies a multilayered laminate to the skin, covering an area about the diameter of a U.S. quarter. A protective film from the contact adhesive is removed and applied to an unshaven, preferably hairless, skin area. Shaving alters the skin's integrity and allows the drug to penetrate faster. Some TDDS formulations rely on intact skin to help slow drug entry to the body.

The TDDS provides continual drug delivery to achieve a constant, steady blood concentration level of the drug. The continual but regulated drug delivery should help avoid high blood concentration levels of the drug and the associated potential adverse reactions sometimes experienced by the patient during systemic therapy with oral or parenteral drugs. A disadvantage of TDDS application, however, is the slow onset of drug action from initiation until a steady blood concentration level of the drug is attained (up to several hours). The drug used for TDDS is available as a gel solution in a drug reservoir and migrates from the reservoir across the skin. The nurse should rotate application sites to avoid tissue irritation, which could change the drug absorption rate as well as damage the skin. The nurse should also review the manufacturer's recommendations for placing the transdermal patch before application, because different areas of the skin have different permeabilities. (See *Transdermal drug absorption.*)

Topical ointments, creams, and gels typically provide local rather than systemic effects. Ointments, usually occlusive-type topical preparations, are used to treat chronic dry skin conditions. The ointments resist removal by water and readily attain and maintain hydrated skin; however, systemic absorption from ointments usually is poor. Creams, also called "vanishing creams," are easier

Transdermal drug absorption

Transdermal absorption of drugs through different skin sites varies. Product literature usually itemizes appropriate application sites.

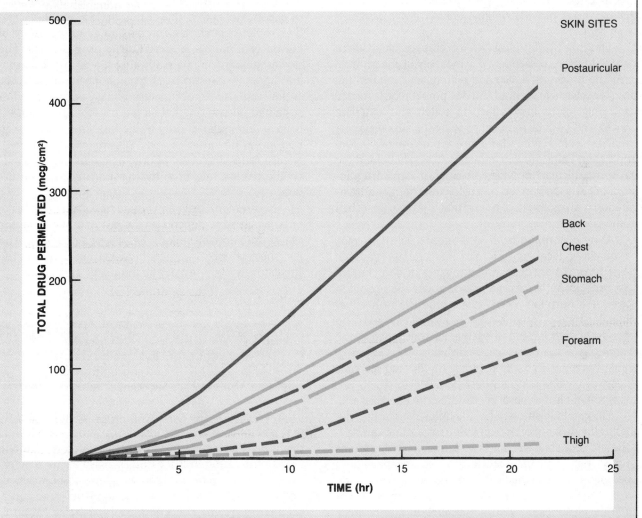

Reprinted with permission from "Transdermal Therapeutic Systems" by Jane E. Shaw in: *Dermal and Transdermal Absorption*. Brandau, R., and Lippold, B.H. (eds.), Stuttgart, Germany, 1982, Wissenschaftliche Verlagsgesellschaft mbH Stuttgart.

to apply and easier to remove with water than ointments. Gels contain large amounts of water for easy spreading of a water-soluble drug. Topical preparations can cause some systemic adverse reactions, and adequate skin hydration for optimal drug absorption may be difficult to maintain without a protective covering over the applied ointment, cream, or gel. Because drug absorption of topical ointments, creams, and gels to treat systemic disorders is unreliable, physicians seldom use or encourage the use of the topical route.

Rapid local drug absorption usually accompanies ophthalmic preparations because the drug is typically administered in solution. However, ophthalmic drugs can be administered to the eyes as solutions, ointments, or ophthalmic inserts. Because of the eye's ability to remove foreign substances rapidly, ophthalmic solutions and ointments usually require reapplication every 2 to 4 hours. Application frequency depends on the disease or disorder, the drug, and the type of formulation. Systemic drug absorption of ophthalmic solutions can occur, causing adverse reactions. For example, timolol maleate ophthalmic drops can exert a beta-blocker effect on a patient's cardiac system. Ophthalmic inserts (small elliptic disks placed directly on the eyeball behind the lower eyelid) provide a sustained-release preparation for drug absorption. Some ophthalmic inserts (Pilocarpine Ocuserts by Alcon Laboratories) can remain on the eye for several days. The local release and absorption of ophthalmic drugs provide optimal control if the patient is compliant.

Drugs applied topically to the ears usually result in negligible drug absorption. Permeation of the stratum corneum proceeds slowly and with difficulty unless the drug is occlusively secured. An otic preparation is mostly used only for its local effect, to soften and solubilize earwax and ease its removal or to treat a superficial ear canal rash or infection. Warming otic preparations before application helps prevent earaches. The skin behind the ear (postauricular) provides an area for rapid drug absorption. A scopolamine patch for transdermal administration is an example of a drug that is rapidly absorbed in the postauricular area.

Drug absorption from local nasal instillations may cause either local or systemic drug effects. Although nasal decongestant drops and sprays act locally to induce vasoconstriction, excessive use or abuse may result in systemic absorption. Using nasal products with either phenylephrine or pseudoephedrine can increase blood pressure. Other intranasal agents, like beclomethasone dipropionate, can ease seasonal rhinitis with only negligible systemic effects. In contrast, the desired systemic effects of vasopressin can best be achieved by its administration via the nasal route for some conditions.

Drug administration by the inhalation route demands the delivery of micron-size particles that can navigate the bronchial tree and reach the affected portions of the lung. The small particle size also enhances drug absorption because only a thin membrane separates the air and the drug in each pulmonary alveolus from the capillary blood flow. Drug administration by the inhalation route provides either local effect in the bronchial tree (isoproterenol administered to asthmatics) or systemic effect (inhalation of vasopressin to treat diabetes insipidus).

RATE OF DRUG ABSORPTION

The drug absorption rate determines when peak concentration levels of a drug will be reached. Although a dosage form (such as a solution) may make a drug immediately available, the onset of drug activity may be rapid, intermediate, or slow, depending on the administration route and the number of barriers between the drug and the site of action. If only one or a few cells separate the active drug from the systemic circulation,

rapid absorption will occur. Hence, a predicted rapid onset of action usually means that drug absorption occurs within seconds or minutes of administration via the sublingual, I.V., or inhalation route. Drugs with an intermediate absorption rate usually demonstrate an onset of activity within 1 to 2 hours. In most cases, they are administered by the oral, I.M., or S.C. route. The onset of action occurs at a slower rate by the oral, I.M., and S.C. routes because the complex membrane systems of GI mucosa, muscle, and skin delay drug passage. The slowest absorption rate may cause the drug to take several hours or days to reach peak concentration levels. A slow rate usually occurs with rectally administered or sustained-release drugs. Using a solution to disperse a rectally administered drug to the intestinal mucosa can accelerate the onset of drug activity. With sustained-release drugs, the onset of drug action usually depends on the release rate from the system used, not on the drug.

In summary, drug absorption and drug availability, or bioavailability, depend on the drug dosage form, the site of drug administration, the patient's condition, and the physiochemical barriers between the drug and the circulatory system, especially the portal circulation.

DRUG BIOAVAILABILITY

Bioavailability is the fraction of an administered drug that reaches the systemic circulation. Important factors related to drug bioavailability include peak concentration levels of the drug in the blood or plasma, the time required for that peak concentration level to be reached, and the area under the concentration level–time curve. (See *Drug plasma concentration–time curve* for an illustration of the factors that determine a drug's bioavailability.) The following discussion is limited to pharmacokinetic principles because these will help the nurse identify and interpret therapeutic benefits and problems with drugs.

PEAK CONCENTRATION

After a drug is administered and absorbed, its concentration level rises and then begins to fall. The time when this level is greatest is called *peak concentration*. While the concentration level is increasing, the absorption rate exceeds the elimination rate; at the peak concentration level, the rates are equal; when the level is decreasing, the elimination rate exceeds the absorption rate.

Drug plasma concentration–time curve

Plotting the drug plasma concentration levels against time provides useful information about a drug's bioavailability (peak concentration, time of peak concentration, and the area under the concentration-time curve). The illustrations at the bottom demonstrate the differences in two drugs' bioavailability.

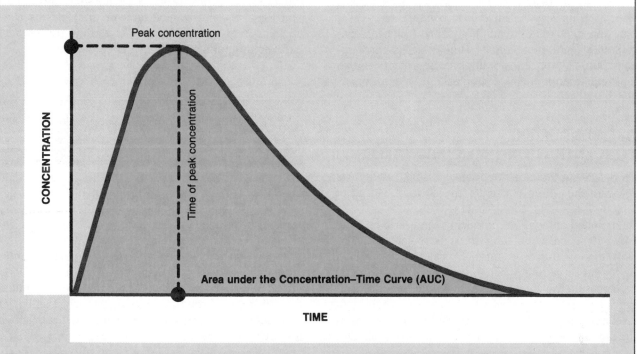

Interpreting drug plasma concentration–time curves

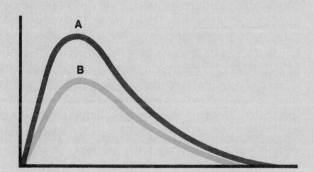

The bioavailability of A is greater than that of B, as shown by the larger AUC.

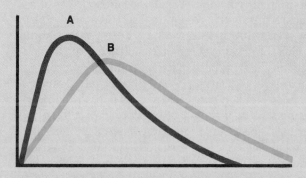

The bioavailability of products A and B are equal. However, product A peaks higher and earlier than B. This may be an advantage in acute situations that need rapid achievement of concentration levels, but it will probably offer no significant advantage with long-term dosing of the drug.

TIME OF PEAK CONCENTRATION

The time of peak concentration is determined by the absorption rate. The absorption rate primarily relates to the route of administration; it is not affected by the dose. For example, because I.V. administration bypasses the absorption phase, the time of peak concentration occurs as soon as the dose is administered. Sublingual doses also reach peak levels rapidly. In contrast, I.M., S.C., oral, and rectal routes of administration reach peak concentration levels more slowly. Time of peak concentration is usually not of major importance except in cases that require an immediate drug action, as in an emergency.

AREA UNDER THE CONCENTRATION-TIME CURVE (A.U.C.)

To determine the bioavailability of a drug, researchers measure the serum concentration levels of a drug at various times after administration. This information is then plotted on a graph, producing a curve. (See *Drug plasma concentration–time curve* on page 29 for an illustration of this procedure.) By calculating the area under this curve (the AUC), the physician or pharmacist can measure the bioavailability of a drug and can compare it to other formulations of the same drug. This calculation sometimes shows significant differences in the amount of drug delivered to the system by different products.

Another important reason for examining the concentration-time curve is that some drugs show a relationship between the blood concentration level and a patient's therapeutic response. The curve may explain why a patient responds to one preparation but not to another. For example, the bronchodilator drug theophylline produces its best effects when the serum concentration level is between 8 and 20 mcg/ml. Examining the concentration-time curves of two preparations of theophylline may show that one formulation has a significantly smaller area under the curve than the other, meaning that it is less bioavailable. The curve could also show that, even though the two AUCs are roughly equivalent, the absorption rate for one drug is too slow to reach a sufficient peak concentration level for bronchodilation.

Although different drug preparations may differ in bioavailability, the difference is usually not great enough to cause therapeutic problems. Sometimes though, the drug's bioavailability is significant clinically, as with drugs that have a narrow range among ineffectiveness, therapeutic activity, and toxicity. Theophylline is an exam-

ple: a preparation with a poor bioavailability probably will not produce therapeutic benefit. Conversely, a preparation absorbed too rapidly might deliver too much drug at one time and produce toxic effects shortly after administration. Other drug examples are digoxin, levothyroxine sodium, and phenytoin. The best way to avoid patient problems with these drugs is to keep a stabilized patient on one brand and not substitue another one. Also, the nurse must monitor drug plasma concentrations and check for proper storage procedures, because drug deterioration can affect bioavailability.

DRUG DISTRIBUTION

Distribution of an absorbed drug within the body depends on several factors: blood flow, the drug's affinity for lipid or aqueous tissue, and protein binding. How efficiently a drug is distributed throughout the body affects the concentration level of the drug remaining in the circulatory system and at the site of action. Evaluating the blood concentration level of a drug helps determine the efficiency of drug absorption, the achievement of therapeutic blood concentration levels, and the time that the drug will remain in the body.

BODY DRUG STORAGE

During drug distribution through the vascular or lymphatic system, the drug comes in contact with various proteins and either remains free or binds to plasma carrier protein, storage tissue, or receptor protein. As soon as a drug binds to plasma carrier protein or storage tissue protein, it becomes inactive, rendering it unavailable for binding to a receptor protein and incapable of exerting therapeutic activity. However, a bound drug can rapidly free itself to maintain a balance between the amounts of free and bound drug. Only the free, or unbound, percentage of the drug remains active.

The percentage of drug that remains free and available for activity depends on the amount of plasma protein available for binding. The major intravascular source for carrier protein binding is plasma albumin.

The percentage of free drug is usually constant for a single drug but differs between drugs. For example, about 50% to 60% of the total gentamicin sulfate in the plasma usually remains free, whereas only about 0.5% to 1% of the total warfarin sodium in the plasma remains free. Administering a single dose of aspirin to a patient on long-term warfarin therapy causes competition for storage protein binding between the two drugs. As a result, the amount of free warfarin in the plasma increases from about 1% to 2%. Although the 1% increase appears minuscule, the amount of free warfarin available to exert a therapeutic effect increases by approximately 100%, with possible life-threatening consequences.

The amount of free drug in the plasma also differs among patients, depending on their medical conditions. For example, malnutrition, which directly affects the liver, deprives the body of protein building blocks and decreases plasma albumin production. This decrease in plasma albumin and the consequent decrease in protein-binding sites boosts the amount of free drug in the plasma, which may be undesirable. The nurse must note any changes in the patient's status that could alter the percentage of free drug in the patient's plasma. Unfortunately, the procedure for distinguishing between free and bound drug is too detailed and expensive to use routinely in the clinic or hospital, so it is performed in only selected cases. Someday it may be a routine test for some drugs.

DRUG VOLUME OF DISTRIBUTION

This concept represents body areas or compartments (such as blood, total body water, or fat) in which drugs distribute and localize. Although it is mathematically determined, volume of distribution does not refer to real volume. Rather, it is a convenient way to measure the size of a compartment that would be filled by the amount of a drug in the same concentration as that found in the blood or plasma.

A highly water-soluble drug possesses a small volume of distribution and has a high blood concentration level. A highly fat-soluble drug possesses a large volume of distribution and has a low blood concentration level. Factors that tend to keep a drug in the circulatory system, such as high water solubility and high serum protein binding, result in a lower volume of distribution and a higher blood concentration level. Conversely, factors that promote the movement of a drug from the blood to other compartments, such as high lipid solubility (promoting storage of the drug in fat) or high degrees of binding to body tissues, result in a higher volume of distribution and lower blood concentration levels.

Other factors also can influence a drug's volume of distribution, such as blood flow through different types of tissues that absorb a drug or a drug's ability to cross different barriers (such as the blood-brain or blood-milk barrier). If a drug's ability to cross certain barriers temporarily changes (as in a lactating patient), both the volume of distribution and the blood concentration level will change.

Drug volume of distribution is unrelated to a drug's effectiveness or duration of action. A large volume of distribution lets the physician and clincial pharmacist know that: (1) the drug may take a long time to move to and from the patient's body compartments, (2) a partly stored drug may be unavailable to exert an effect, and (3) the patient's system may require hours or days to accumulate or excrete the drug.

Volume of distribution in a patient is used primarily by clinical pharmacists, who incorporate the values into logarithmic calculators or computer equations to determine adjustments in drug dosages. The adjustments depend on the relationship among the patient's drug concentration level and dosing regimen, the patient's physical characteristics and state of health, and the goals of therapy.

PROBLEMS WITH DISTRIBUTION

The physician should never assume that a drug distributes well throughout the body system. Abscesses, exudates, glands, and tumors can all affect drug distribution adversely. For example, antibiotics typically do not distribute to abscesses and exudates. Glands, such as the prostate, tend to be impermeable to most antibiotics, rendering a prostatic infection difficult to treat effectively.

Variable drug concentrations among different organs and sometimes different tissues within a single organ can also complicate drug distribution. The differences in tissue drug concentration levels result from such variables as tissue affinity for the drug, blood flow, and protein-binding sites.

Another drug distribution problem can occur because some drugs become trapped in tissues and accumulate. Drug accumulation may pose a potential hazard if the amount exceeds the usual doses or exposure levels. For example, fluoride is absorbed well and distributed adequately to bone, but the system eliminates only about half of the drug. Long-term exposure to significant amounts of fluoride could lead to fluoride toxicity and brittle bones.

DRUG METABOLISM

Drug metabolism, or biotransformation, refers to the body's ability to change a drug biologically from its dosage or parent form to a more water-soluble form. The resulting metabolite is usually an inactive form of the

Drug metabolism

Drug metabolism usually changes active parent drugs into inactive metabolites. Many drugs, however, are biologically transformed from an inactive parent drug to an active metabolite. Metabolism changes still other drugs from active parent drugs into more active metabolites. Some examples of parent drugs that are biologically transformed into active metabolites include the following.

PARENT DRUG	ACTIVE METABOLITE
acetohexamide	hydroxyhexamide
allopurinol	alloxanthine
amitriptyline	nortriptyline
chloral hydrate	trichloroethanol
cortisone acetate	hydrocortisone
diazepam	desmethyldiazepam
flurazepam hydrochloride	N-desalkyl-flurazepam
imipramine	desipramine
mephobarbital	phenobarbital
prednisone	prednisolone
procainamide hydrochloride	N-acetylprocainamide
propranolol hydrochloride	4-hydroxypropranolol
spironolactone	canrenone

parent drug; however, the metabolism of some drugs results in the ability of one or all of the metabolites to demonstrate some degree of drug activity.

Through metabolism, the body detoxifies and disposes of foreign substances. Because drugs are unnatural to the body, they are disposed of as are other body toxins. In most cases, the enzyme system increases the water solubility of a drug so that the renal system can excrete it. The lipid solubility of some drugs may be enzymatically altered so that the end products enter into and are excreted through the biliary system. Using either the renal or the biliary pathway for disposal, the body usually transforms the drug into a readily eliminated, pharmacologically inactive product.

The metabolism of some parent drugs may, however, result in metabolites capable of drug activity. For example, the liver metabolizes imipramine to both inactive metabolites and the active metabolite desipramine. (Discovery of the active desipramine led to the commercial marketing of desipramine as an active parent drug.) In a few cases, the body metabolizes an inactive parent drug to an active metabolite. For example, dopamine hydrochloride is the drug of choice for treating parkinsonism; however, it cannot cross the blood-brain barrier. Levodopa, an inactive precursor to dopamine, readily crosses the blood-brain barrier into the central nervous system, where it is metabolized to dopamine with therapeutic results. (See *Drug metabolism* for a list of some other parent drugs and their active metabolites.)

Not all drugs are metabolized to the same extent or by the same mechanisms. Some drugs, such as the aminoglycosides, are unmetabolizable; they pass through the body and are excreted in unchanged form. Other drugs, such as barbiturates, stimulate or induce enzyme metabolic activity, thus reducing the amount of active drug in the body. For example, repeated administration of phenobarbital induces enzyme metabolism, which increases drug metabolism. In such cases, the drug stimulates its own metabolism, a process referred to as autoinduction. In a related process, called foreign induction, one drug stimulates the metabolism of another. For example, if hexobarbital or theophylline therapy were added to an existing phenobarbital regimen, the phenobarbital-induced enzyme activity would stimulate the metabolism of the hexobarbital or theophylline.

In contrast, some drugs inhibit or compete for enzyme metabolism, which may cause the accumulation of concurrently administered drugs. The accumulation increases the potential for an adverse reaction or drug toxicity. Cimetidine, for example, inhibits the enzyme system that metabolizes theophylline in the liver, causing an elevated theophylline level within the vascular system. The increased theophylline may cause such adverse reactions as tachycardia or seizures. (See *Factors and drugs affecting metabolism* for some drugs that produce autoinduction and foreign induction and some drugs that inhibit enzyme metabolism.) Before interpreting a drug response or altering therapy because of an inappropriate blood concentration level of an active drug, the physician usually investigates the possibility of drug-induced changes in drug metabolism.

Disease-induced physiologic changes can negatively affect drug metabolism. When end-stage cirrhosis damages the liver enough to reduce or alter liver blood flow, the supply of a drug to liver enzyme metabolic sites decreases. When congestive heart failure causes the patient to retain excessive fluid, drug metabolism decreases because the drug delivery to liver metabolic sites becomes inefficient. Genetics may also alter the efficiency of drug metabolism, as evidenced by the ability of some individuals to metabolize drugs rapidly while others metabolize them more slowly. Slowed metabolism of a drug may cause it to accumulate to toxic levels.

Factors and drugs affecting metabolism

Drug metabolism may be affected by autoinduction (a drug induces its own metabolism), foreign induction (one drug stimulates the metabolism of another), and enzyme inhibition (a drug inhibits enzyme metabolism, possibly leading to drug accumulation).

Drugs producing auto induction

glutethimide	nitroglycerin	probenecid
hexobarbital	phenobarbital	tolbutamide
meprobamate	phenylbutazone	

Drugs producing foreign induction

INDUCER	DRUGS WITH INDUCED METABOLISM
alcohol	pentobarbital sodium tolbutamide
antihistamines	hydrocortisone phenobarbital
DDT and chlordane	barbiturates warfarin
ethchlorvynol	warfarin sodium
glutethimide	barbiturates dipyrone warfarin
griseofulvin	warfarin
haloperidol	warfarin
meprobamate	warfarin
phenobarbital and other barbiturates	androstenedione bilirubin chloramphenicol digitoxin doxorubicin hydrochloride estradiol griseofulvin hexobarbital and other barbiturates phenytoin progesterone testosterone thyroxine tolbutamide
phenytoin	hydrocortisone
tolbutamide	barbiturates

Drugs causing enzyme inhibition

ENZYME INHIBITORS	DRUGS WITH INHIBITED METABOLISM
allopurinol	mercaptopurine
aspirin	chlorpromazine
chloramphenicol	hexobarbital
chlorpromazine	hexobarbital
cimetidine	benzodiazepines theophylline warfarin
codeine	hexobarbital
cyclophosphamide	chloramphenicol
desipramine hydrochloride	amphetamines
disulfiram	alcohol
meperidine hydrochloride	oral contraceptives
6-mercaptopurine	allopurinol
MAO inhibitors	barbiturates tyramine sympathomimetic amines
morphine	hexobarbital
nortriptyline	hydrocortisone

Environment, too, may affect drug metabolism. For example, cigarette smokers metabolize theophylline much more rapidly than nonsmokers do. Developmental changes, particularly during infancy and old age, can also affect drug metabolism. (Chapters 12 and 13 examine the changes in detail.)

In summary, drug metabolism varies for different types of drugs. Physicians pay careful attention to the way in which the body removes a drug, to drugs that may affect hepatic metabolic function, and to drugs that may affect the metabolism of concurrently administered drugs. Finally, physiologic, genetic, environmental, and developmental factors also may alter drug metabolism.

DRUG EXCRETION

The body eliminates drugs by metabolism (usually hepatic) and excretion (usually renal). Physiologically, drugs can be eliminated via the lungs, exocrine glands (sweat, salivary, or mammary glands), kidneys, liver, skin, and intestinal tract. Drugs may also be artificially removed by direct interventions, such as peritoneal dialysis or hemodialysis. Artificial interventions are typically reserved for drug overdose patients or those with

Determining drug half-life

Drug half-life can be determined from a drug blood level curve by measuring the time required for a drug blood concentration level to decrease by one half. For example, this illustration shows a drug's concentration of l00 mcg/ml at 2 hours; a half-life of 4 hours (a concentration of 50 mcg/ml).

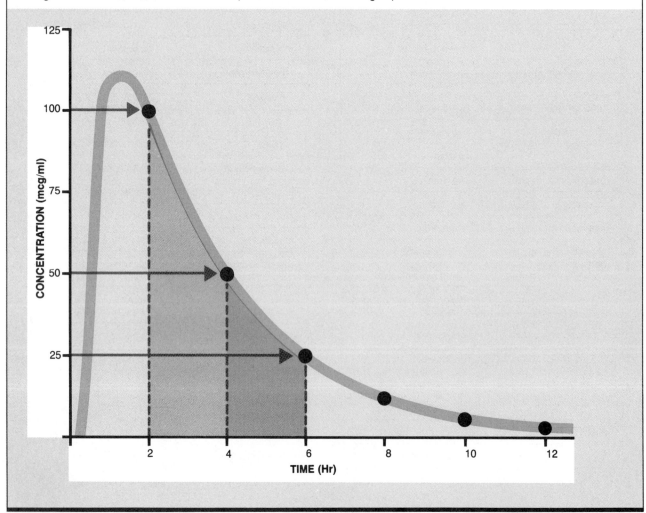

renal dysfunction. Both short- and long-term peritoneal dialysis and hemodialysis, however, may inadvertently complicate patient care because routine dialysis removes wastes nonspecifically and, in the process, may remove active drugs.

DRUG HALF-LIFE

To predict the frequency of the drug dosage schedule, the physician must determine how long a drug will remain in the body. Usually, the rate of drug loss from the body can be estimated by determining the half-life of the drug. Drug half-life represents the time required for the total amount of a drug in the body to diminish by one half. The half-life of a drug can be determined from a blood drug curve. (See *Determining drug half-life.*)

If a single 100-mg dose of theophylline is administered to a patient and the half-life of the theophylline in the patient is 5 hours, the total amount in the body would diminish by one half after 5 hours. The drug amount would continue to decrease accordingly with each subsequent half-life. Most drugs are essentially eliminated after five half-lives because the amount remaining is probably too low to exert any beneficial or adverse effect. This concept is useful in many situations. For example, if a drug overdose occurs and the excretion rate of the drug is not compromised, about 97% of the original dose will be eliminated after five half-lives.

DRUG ACCUMULATION

Drug half-life also proves to be a useful tool when assessing drug accumulation. A drug that is not readministered is almost completely eliminated after five half-lives, but a regularly administered drug reaches a "constant" total body amount, or steady state, after five half-lives. (See *Steady-state curves* on page 36 for an illustration of the blood concentration levels of drugs using two different dosing regimens.)

Having once reached a steady state, the serum concentration levels of the drug will fluctuate below the "average" concentration level. This means that, although the drug was once at steady state, drug concentration levels do not remain uniform; rather, they increase, peak, and decline, although within a constant range. (See *Steady-state dosing* on page 37 for a discussion of the range of blood concentration levels that can occur after successive doses of a drug.)

For some drugs, the time required to reach therapeutic blood concentration levels may be too long. For example, when using digoxin with a half-life of about 1½ (1.6) days, the physician could not wait 8 days (1.6 days times 5 half-lives) to achieve steady-state blood concentration levels to control a life-threatening dysrhythmia, such as atrial fibrillation. Therefore, an initial large dose, called a loading dose, would be rapidly administered to reach the desired therapeutic blood concentration level. Subsequently, smaller "maintenance doses" would be given daily to replace the amount of drug eliminated since the last dose. These doses maintain a therapeutic blood concentration level in the body at all times.

Amount of drug remaining

Drug half-life can be used to estimate the amount of drug remaining in the body after the last dose. With the discontinuation of drug therapy, all drug activity usually ceases after a period of five half-lives.

NUMBER OF HALF-LIVES	TOTAL AMOUNT OF DRUG REMAINING	PERCENT OF ORIGINAL DOSE
Dose	100 mg	100%
1	50 mg	50%
2	25 mg	25%
3	12.5 mg	12.5%
4	6.3 mg	6.3%
5	3.1 mg	3.1%
6	1.6 mg	1.6%
7	0.8 mg	0.8%

DRUG CLEARANCE

Drug clearance refers to the removal of a drug from the body. A drug is said to have a low clearance rate if it is removed from the body slowly. A drug is said to have a high clearance rate if it is removed from the body rapidly. A drug with a high clearance may require more frequent administration and higher doses than a comparable drug with a low clearance. Drugs with a low

Steady-state curves

A steady-state drug blood concentration level can be reached by initiating a constant dosing regimen and waiting five half-lives (see solid line). This level can be achieved much more rapidly by giving a calculated loading dose (dotted line) followed by a routine maintenance dose. The maintenance dose is the same as the dose in a constant regimen. The dashed line shows the elimination pattern of a drug when only a single dose is given.

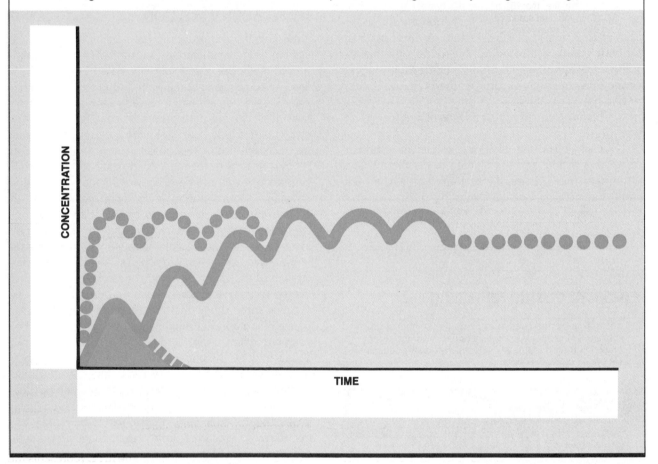

clearance can accumulate to toxic concentration levels in the body unless they are administered less frequently or at lower doses.

Physicians, pharmacists, and nurses must consider drug clearance when assessing dosing regimens. If a particular drug is normally removed by a metabolic process, determining the efficiency of the metabolic system before administering the first dose is difficult. As a result, physicians may base the maintenance dose and dosing frequency calculations on a "best estimate," which cor-

relates with information gained from similar cases involving patients with comparable diseases or disorders.

If the kidneys eliminate the drug, an estimate of the drug's renal clearance can be determined with simple bedside formulas that account for the patient's body size and creatinine clearance, or renal function. For example, if the kidneys normally eliminate 100% of a drug and the patient's renal function decreases by 50%, the physician can appropriately decrease the drug dose by 50% or double the dosing interval to maintain safe and effective blood concentration levels.

Steady-state dosing

Drugs accumulate in the body during multiple dosing until they reach a plateau, or a steady state. Drug input then equals drug output during the dosing interval. The following example illustrates a drug that is dosed every half-life. If the drug is given in 100 mg doses and is completely absorbed, the total amount in the body is 100 mg. At the next dose, one half-life later, the amount has decreased to 50 mg. The next dose of 100 mg increases the amount in the body to 150 mg. At the next dose, one more half-life, the 150 mg has decreased by 50% to 75 mg. A third dose increases the amount in the body to 175 mg. This continues until steady state is reached, as shown in the table. The maximum and minimum amounts listed illustrate the fluctuations of drug levels after a dose.

DOSE NUMBER	DOSE AMOUNT	MAXIMUM AMOUNT IN BODY (IMMEDIATELY AFTER DOSE)	MINIMUM AMOUNT IN BODY (IMMEDIATELY BEFORE NEXT DOSE)
1	100 mg	100 mg	50 mg
2	100 mg	150 mg (50 mg + 100 mg dose)	75 mg (½ of 150 mg)
3	100 mg	175 mg (75 mg + 100 mg dose)	88 mg (½ of 175 mg)
4	100 mg	188 mg	94 mg (½ of 188 mg)
5	100 mg	194 mg	97 mg (steady state)
6	100 mg	197 mg	99 mg (½ of 197 mg)
7	100 mg	199 mg	100 mg (½ of 199 mg)
8	100 mg	200 mg	100 mg (½ of 200 mg)
9	100 mg	200 mg	100 mg (½ of 200 mg)

DRUG BLOOD CONCENTRATION LEVELS

The concentration level of a drug in the blood helps determine whether the therapeutic goals have been reached with the drug regimen. (See Chapter 4, Pharmacotherapeutics, for a more detailed discussion of drug blood levels.) Drug concentration levels are most often measured in plasma or serum; however, the same principles apply whether levels are taken from blood or any other fluid, such as cerebrospinal fluid or saliva.

By correlating the plasma concentration level–time curve with a patient's response, the physician and clinical pharmacist can gain valuable information about the minimum effective concentration (MEC), minimum toxic concentration (MTC), and therapeutic range for a drug. (See *Therapeutic range* on page 38 for a typical plasma concentration level–time curve.) The MEC represents the necessary plasma concentration level for the drug to be effective in most patients. The MTC represents the lowest blood concentration level at which significant adverse reactions to the drug generally occur. The therapeutic range is bordered at the low end by the MEC and at the high end by the MTC. The time during which the drug concentration remains between these values represents the drug's duration of action.

One goal of therapy is to maximize the duration of action while avoiding the MTC. Obtaining serum drug levels is often useful in monitoring this goal. Shortly after a drug is administered, the highest, or "peak," level of the drug in the system can be measured. Just before

Therapeutic range

The minimum effective concentration (MEC) and the minimum toxic concentration (MTC) represent the lower and upper borders of the plasma concentration level–time curve. Drug blood level concentration determinations help the physician and clinical pharmacist make drug therapy decisions. The peak drug level is represented by the square on the graph; the trough level is represented by the triangle. The time during which the plasma drug concentration curve remains between the MEC and the MTC represents the duration of drug activity.

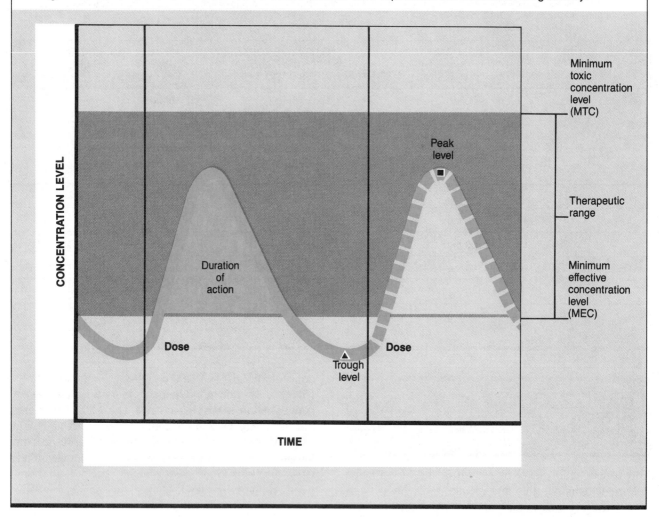

administration of the next dose, the lowest, or "trough," level of the drug can be measured. For a drug like theophylline, the therapeutic range is between 8 and 20 mcg/ml. This means that the drug's peak level needs to be less than 20 mcg/ml and the trough level to be greater than 8 mcg/ml.

For many drugs, the blood concentration levels correlate with the anticipated therapeutic response. Unfortunately, commercial assay methods have not been developed for most drugs. Those with a narrow thera-

peutic range—that is, where the concentration level differences between the MEC and MTC are small—are most likely to have easily available assay methods because even a small dosage error may cause drug toxicity.

Obtaining drug blood concentration levels does not guarantee trouble-free therapy. Some patients will develop toxicity even at concentration levels below the MTC, and not every patient will benefit when a drug's concentraion in the blood is above the MEC. Drug blood levels serve as a valuable tool in monitoring, but they do not substitute for good medical and nursing practice.

USING PHARMACOKINETICS

Pharmacokinetics allows the physician and clinical pharmacist to incorporate known information about the patient when estimating how to achieve a positive response to a drug therapy regimen. Known information about a patient may include drug concentration levels in the blood, the dosing regimen, or the patient's clearance rate of the drug.

Understanding pharmacokinetics helps physicians and nurses avoid arbitrary changes in drug therapy and dosing regimens prompted by the lack of patient response. Using pharmacokinetics, the nurse may find that the problem involves: (1) a blood level curve below the therapeutic range, (2) an as-yet unachieved steady-state concentration level, or (3) lack of drug absorption from pathophysiologic abnormalities. Knowing the patient's condition and the drug's pharmacokinetics also assists the physician in estimating when toxic drug concentration levels have diminished safely, making the reinstitution of drug therapy possible while avoiding unnecessary drug exposure.

CHAPTER SUMMARY

Chapter 2 explored the concepts of pharmacokinetics, explaining the ways in which drug absorption, distribution, metabolism, and excretion affect a patient's response to drug therapy. The chapter also described how understanding pharmacokinetics enhances the nurse's ability to participate in a therapeutic drug regimen. Here are the highlights of Chapter 2:

• Drug absorption depends on several variables, including the drug dosage form, the site and route of drug administration, physiochemical factors affecting drug transport into the circulatory system, and the physiologic status of the patient.

• Orally administered drugs include capsules, compressed tablets, osmotic pumps, and sublingual, buccal and sustained-release formulations. Orally administered drugs disintegrate at different rates. Although parenteral drugs administered by I.V. or intrathecal routes present few drug absorption problems, oral drugs remain the preferred dosage form.

• Physiochemical factors that influence drug absorption refer to the ways in which absorption occurs. Drugs are absorbed by passive drug absorption, active transport, or pinocytosis.

• Other factors affecting drug absorption include the surface area at the absorption site, blood flow to the absorption site, pain and stress, first-pass effect, enterohepatic recycling, drug solubility, body pH, GI motility, dosage form, and interactions between drugs and between drugs and food.

• The major routes for drug absorption include the enteral, parenteral, and topical routes. Drugs administered by enteral routes are absorbed by the oral mucosa, gastric mucosa, small intestine, and rectum. Parenteral routes include the intradermal, S.C., I.M., intrathecal, intraarticular, and I.V. routes. Topical routes are used for transdermal drugs, ophthalmic preparations, and otic preparations and for drugs used for local nasal instillation.

• Drug bioavailability, an important factor in drug therapy, describes how well a drug is absorbed and reaches the systemic circulation. The pharmacokinetic variables in drug bioavailability are peak concentration levels, the time of peak concentration, and the area under the concentration level–time curve.

• Drug distribution within the body depends on several factors, such as blood flow, the drug's affinity for lipid or aqueous tissue, and protein binding.

• When absorbed, many drugs bind to plasma proteins (albumin) for distribution. If the patient has had a protein-poor diet for a prolonged period or if the patient cannot metabolize food appropriately, the patient's system will possess fewer protein "building blocks," making the body's protein levels low. When adequate protein binding cannot occur, the excess free drug in the body may cause a magnified drug response.

• Drug volume of distribution represents the extent of drug distribution throughout the body. When a drug is being distributed throughout the body, the volume of distribution is large, but the drug concentration level is small. Inversely, a drug restricted to a smaller area has a small volume of distribution but a high concentration level of drug in the blood.

• Drug metabolism occurs as the body changes a drug from the dosage or parent form to a more water-soluble form. Drug metabolism creates metabolites, which may or may not be able to demonstrate drug activity. Drug metabolism transforms a drug so that the renal and biliary systems can more readily excrete it.

• Various illnesses can alter drug metabolism. Cirrhosis can result in adverse drug reactions because the liver cannot remove the drug, leaving the active drug in the blood for prolonged periods.

• Usually, the renal system excretes metabolized drugs from the body. Drugs can also be eliminated via the lungs, exocrine glands, liver, skin, and GI tract. Direct intervention, such as peritoneal dialysis, removes drugs artificially.

• Drug half-life represents the time required for the total amount of a drug in the body to diminish by one half. Knowing the half-life of a drug can help the nurse predict the frequency of drug dosing and assess drug accumulation in the system.

• The physician and clinical pharmacist can measure the concentration level of a drug in the blood by using the plasma concentration level–time curve. The plasma curve indicates the minimum effective concentration (MEC), the minimum toxic concentration (MTC), and the therapeutic range. The therapeutic range falls between the MEC and the MTC.

BIBLIOGRAPHY

Alvan, G. "Individual Differences in the Disposition of Drugs Metabolized in the Body," in *Handbook of Clinical Pharmacokinetics, Section I.* Edited by Gibaldi, M., and Prescott, L. New York: ADIS Health Science Press, 1983.

Ansel, H.C. *Introduction to Pharmaceutical Dosage Forms,* 4th ed. Philadelphia: Lea & Febiger, 1985.

Banker, G.S., and Chalmers, R.K. *Pharmaceutics and Pharmacy Practice.* Philadelphia: J.B. Lippincott Co., 1982.

Gennaro, A.R., ed. *Remington's Pharmaceutical Sciences,* 17th ed. Easton, Pa.: Mack Publishing Co., 1985.

Nies, A.S., et al. "Altered Hepatic Blood Flow and Drug Disposition," in *Handbook of Clinical Pharmacokinetics, Section I.* Edited by Gibaldi, M., and Prescott, L. New York: ADIS Health Science Press, 1983.

Ritschel, W.A. *Handbook of Basic Pharmacokinetics.* Hamilton, Ill.: Drug Intelligence Publications, 1982.

Rowland, M., and Tozer, T.N. *Clinical Pharmacokinetics: Concepts and Applications.* Philadelphia: Lea & Febiger, 1980.

Shargel, L., and Yu, A.B.C. *Applied Biopharmaceutics and Pharmacokinetics,* 2nd ed. East Norwalk, Conn.: Appleton-Century-Crofts, 1985.

Shaw, J.E. "Transdermal Therapeutic Systems," in *Dermal and Transdermal Absorption.* Edited by Brandau, R., and Lippold, B.H. Stuttgart, Germany: Wissenschaftliche Verlagsgesellschaft mbH Stuttgart, 1982.

Volans, G.N. "Migraine and Drug Absorption," in *Handbook of Clinical Pharmacokinetics, Section III.* Edited by Gibaldi, M., and Prescott, L. New York: ADIS Health Science Press, 1983.

Winter, M.E., et al. *Basic Clinical Pharmacokinetics.* Spokane, Wash.: Applied Therapeutics, 1980.

PHARMACODYNAMICS

OBJECTIVES

After reading and studying this chapter, you should be able to:

1. Describe the relationship between a drug's pharmacodynamic properties and the patient's response.
2. Differentiate between drug action and drug effect.
3. Explain the mechanisms of action involved in the physical, chemical, and nutrient modifications of the cell function and environment.
4. Describe how drugs modify cell function either by drug-receptor interactions or drug-enzyme interactions.
5. Differentiate between the actions of agonistic and antagonistic drugs.
6. Identify the principles used to classify drug receptors.
7. Differentiate between up-regulation and down-regulation as these terms apply to receptors.
8. Identify the characteristics represented by an ideal dose-response curve.
9. Differentiate between drug potency and drug efficacy.
10. Identify the causes of the five different types of adverse drug effects, including predictable, unpredictable, allergic, idiosyncratic, and iatrogenic.
11. Identify the activities in each step of the nursing process that result from an understanding of pharmacodynamics.

INTRODUCTION

Pharmacodynamics is the study of the mechanisms by which specific drug dosages produce biochemical or physiologic changes in the body. The pharmacodynamic phase is one of the four phases involved in the disposition of a drug. (See *Drug disposition* on page 42 for a depiction of the four phases of drug activity.) The pharmacodynamic phase of drug action progresses concurrently with the pharmacokinetic processes of: (1) drug absorption from the administration site, (2) drug distribution throughout the body via the body fluids, (3) metabolism of the parent drug to inactive, active, or more active metabolites, and (4) drug excretion.

After a drug penetrates the cellular barriers and reaches its site of action within the target cell, tissue, or body organ system, the resulting drug action is effected by one or more mechanisms. The drug action, or physiologic change, in turn leads to an overall response, or pharmacologic effect. The response observed represents the outcome of what may be a complex sequence of physical and chemical interactions between the drug and specific cellular components at the site of action. The cellular components affected at the site of action are usually referred to as the *drug receptors*. As the final result, the function of the target cell changes to produce the desired pharmacologic response.

Attaining the objectives of drug therapy depend upon an understanding of the pharmacodynamics of the administered drug, including both the mechanisms of action and the expected pharmacologic responses. To assess a patient's responses and to maximize the role of drug therapy in a treatment plan, nurses must know the pharmacodynamics of the drugs administered.

MECHANISMS OF ACTION

To understand pharmacodynamics, the nurse must differentiate between drug action and drug effect. The interaction at the cellular level between a drug and cellular components, such as the complex proteins that make up the cell membrane, enzymes, or target receptors, represents *drug action*. The response resulting from drug action represents the *drug effect,* which may affect total body function. For example, when insulin is administered, the expected drug action is the transport of glucose across the cell membrane. The lowering of the blood glucose level represents the expected drug effect.

By modifying cell function, a drug causes a response that may lead to either a positive therapeutic outcome

Drug disposition

The phases between drug administration and drug effect include the pharmaceutical, pharmacokinetic, pharmacodynamic, and pharmacotherapeutic. The following illustration depicts the activities involved in each of the phases, as well as the various factors that have an impact on those activities.

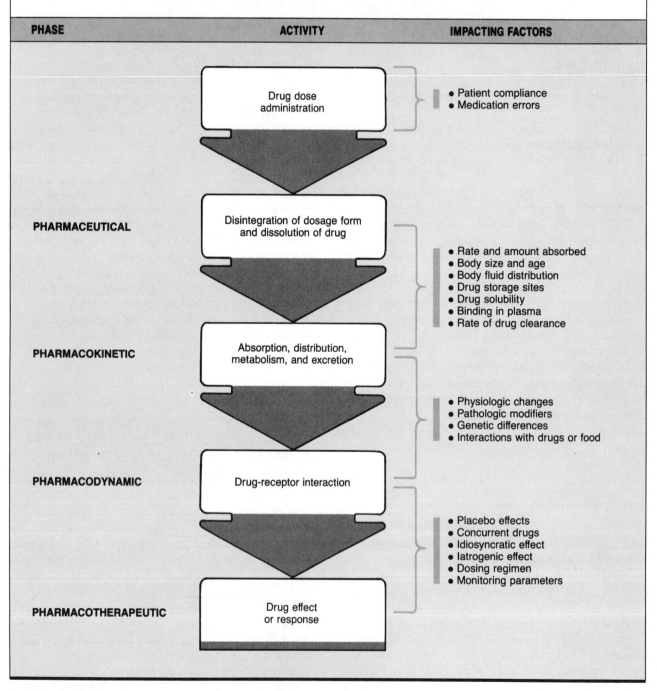

PHASE	ACTIVITY	IMPACTING FACTORS
	Drug dose administration	• Patient compliance • Medication errors
PHARMACEUTICAL	Disintegration of dosage form and dissolution of drug	
		• Rate and amount absorbed • Body size and age • Body fluid distribution • Drug storage sites • Drug solubility • Binding in plasma • Rate of drug clearance
PHARMACOKINETIC	Absorption, distribution, metabolism, and excretion	
		• Physiologic changes • Pathologic modifiers • Genetic differences • Interactions with drugs or food
PHARMACODYNAMIC	Drug-receptor interaction	
		• Placebo effects • Concurrent drugs • Idiosyncratic effect • Iatrogenic effect • Dosing regimen • Monitoring parameters
PHARMACOTHERAPEUTIC	Drug effect or response	

or an adverse drug effect. Remember that a drug may modify cell function or the rate of function, but *a drug cannot impart a new function to a cell or target tissue.* Therefore, the drug effect or response depends upon what the cell should be capable of accomplishing.

An alteration in cell function to cause a response in the target tissue may be initiated by one of two mechanisms of action. A drug may alter the cell function of its target cell by either modifying the cell environment or modifying cell function.

A modification of the cell environment results from drugs that produce their therapeutic responses by affecting the cells externally. The mechanism of drug action occurs through either a physical or chemical change in the cell environment. Drugs that produce responses by affecting the cell externally are considered to be structurally nonspecific. Some of these drugs act by biophysical means that do not change cell or enzyme functions.

By contrast, modification in cell function occurs when a drug molecule interacts with macromolecules within the target tissue. These macromolecules consist of either a receptive substance or a configuration of molecules that acts as a receptor. Regardless of the target area, the process, referred to as a drug-receptor interaction, may either accelerate or slow cell function in the target tissue.

NONSPECIFIC MODIFIERS OF CELL ENVIRONMENT

Drugs that modify the cell environment do not specifically attach to the cell. Such drugs, however, accumulate on or pass through cell membranes, where they physically or chemically interfere with some of the metabolic processes of the cell. Because nonspecific modifiers do not demonstrate any structural attachment to the cell or drug receptors, they seem to act nonspecifically on cell membranes and the cellular processes. Thus, the drug effects are induced externally by changing the physical or chemical environment of the cells.

Physical modification of cell environment

Various drugs with structurally nonspecific mechanisms of action act by biophysical means that do not change cell or enzyme functions. Rather, the drugs physically modify the cell environment. The modification of cell environment may create a barrier, reduce surface tension, or lubricate. For example, applying petrolatum (Vaseline) reduces diaper rash by providing a barrier

between the skin and ammoniacal urine. Sunscreen lotion acts by providing a barrier between the skin and damaging ultraviolet sun rays. Surfactant stool softeners, such as docusate calcium or docusate sodium, reduce the surface tension of fecal matter. Such stool softeners allow water to penetrate the feces to promote stool softening and regularity. The administration of mineral oil facilitates the passage of feces by lubricating the contents of the bowel.

Chemical modification of cell environment

Although structurally nonspecific drugs do not usually alter cell function, chemical modification of the cell environment by nonspecific modifiers may alter cell function if the drug reacts with other chemicals or invokes changes in the components of the body fluids. For example, the intravenous administration of sodium bicarbonate in a patient with severe diabetic ketoacidosis results in improved cellular function when the body pH approaches normal. A less dramatic chemical change in the cell environment may be induced when antacids, administered orally to neutralize increased gastric acid levels, promote ulcer healing.

Cell environment can also be changed by altering vascular osmolality. For example, intravenous mannitol administration increases the intravascular osmotic load, which in turn draws water into the vascular system to dilute the mannitol. The dilution of mannitol leads to an osmotic diuresis that removes excess water from the body and changes the cell environment.

Another example of chemical modification at the cell level involves lipid-soluble (fat-soluble) drugs, including some general anesthetics, hypnotics, and sedatives. The fat-soluble drugs enter the lipoid nerve cell membrane and inhibit nerve conduction. The drugs are not, however, structurally specific to any receptor; their presence merely overwhelms the cell and alters cell function.

A deleterious change in the cell environment may also be induced by alcohol, detergents, certain disinfectants, and hydrogen peroxide. These agents act by irreversibly destroying the functional integrity of the living cell.

SPECIFIC MODIFIERS OF CELL FUNCTION

The drug-receptor interaction is the second major mechanism of drug action. A receptor consists of either a specialized reactive substance or a macromolecule (a large group of molecules, such as a cell membrane, protein, or enzyme) that will interlock with a drug molecule. The interaction of the drug and its receptor should result in a drug effect, or pharmacologic response. The binding of a drug to a receptor can involve many different types of binding forces and may or may not be reversible. The drug-receptor interaction can be visualized as a key fitting a lock. (See *Drug-receptor interaction* for an illustration of this mechanism of action.)

Drug-receptor interactions occur within the target cell, tissue, or organ. The receptor primarily consists of protein. The molecular structure of protein allows each specific receptor to assume a different shape. The differing shapes among receptors support the theory of a structure-specificity relationship between the receptor and the drug. The structure-specificity relationship demonstrates the tendency of receptors to interact only with those drugs that are exactly compatible structurally.

The structure-activity relationship between a drug and a receptor is more complex. According to this relationship, if the structure of the drug is changed even slightly, the receptor may still interact with the drug, but the response elicited from the altered drug will differ from the response of the unaltered drug. The modified response could be either a positive therapeutic outcome or an adverse reaction. (See *Structure-activity relationship* for a depiction of this kind of binding.)

Drug-enzyme interactions may also result in a drug response. An enzyme is a protein-based substance whose catalytic action can promote or accelerate a biochemical reaction with a substrate (substance acted on by an enzyme) molecule. Sometimes, the enzyme mistakenly identifies the drug as the usual substrate, and a drug-enzyme interaction occurs. This interaction could be the source of a drug response that increases or decreases the rate of a cellular biochemical reaction. For example, neostigmine, an anticholinesterase, interacts with the enzyme acetylcholinesterase and inhibits the destruction of acetylcholine released from the parasympathetic nerves. Thus, acetylcholine accumulates and increases the activity in the target tissue. The response may lead to increased gastric contractions or gastric acid secretion.

Nutrient effect on cell function

Nutritional substances, such as vitamins and trace elements, can modify cell function. As a result, they must be considered pharmacologically active. Vitamins and trace elements in small quantities promote daily cell function, though excessive amounts may cause deleterious effects. For example, proper amounts of vitamin A pro-

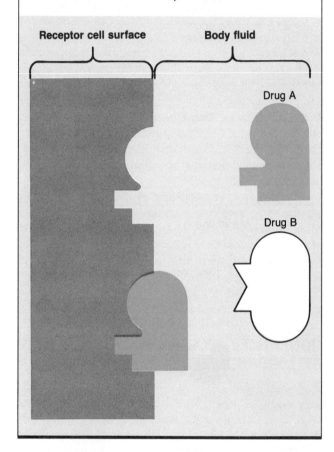

Drug-receptor interaction

The two receptors shown in the following illustration are structurally compatible with drug A. Drug B will not interact with these receptors.

Receptor cell surface   **Body fluid**

Drug A

Drug B

mote the homeostasis of multiple organ systems, including the eyes, skin, liver, pancreas, and lungs; however, excessive doses may induce papilledema, dry skin, headache, fatigue, vomiting, irritability, and other adverse reactions.

DRUG RECEPTORS

Several basic concepts help explain the action of drugs at receptor sites. A drug attracted to a receptor displays

Structure-activity relationship

Some receptors are less selective of the drugs with which they will interact. Therefore, a receptor may interact with a drug that has been structurally altered. The response to the altered drug, however, will usually differ from the original drug response. Also, all of the receptors need not be occupied for a response to occur.

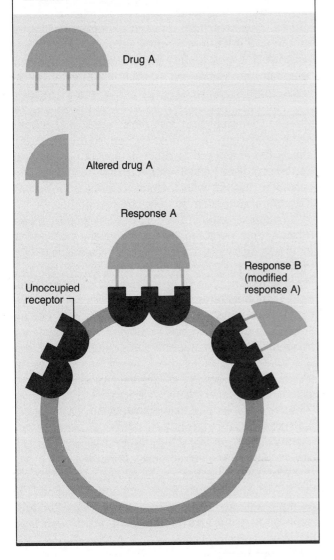

Drug A

Altered drug A

Response A

Response B (modified response A)

Unoccupied receptor

an affinity for that receptor. The drug's ability to initiate a response after binding with the receptor is referred to as intrinsic activity. When a drug displays an affinity for a receptor and then enhances or stimulates the functional properties of the receptor, the drug acts as an *agonist.* A drug that is not an agonist can compete with an agonist for a receptor by occupying the receptor, thereby preventing the action of the agonist. Such a drug, called an *antagonist,* does not initiate an effect. Instead, the antagonist prevents a response from occurring.

Antagonists consist of two types. The first, a competitive antagonist, competes with the agonist for receptor sites. If the concentration of the competitive antagonist increases without a change in the amount of agonist available, the affinity of the competitive antagonist for the receptor will displace the agonist. Eventually, the competitive antagonist will completely inhibit receptor activity. For example, naloxone is a competitive antagonist with an affinity for the opioid receptor. The parenteral administration of naloxone reverses opioid respiratory depression within 1 to 2 minutes, thereby reversing the effects of opioid overdose. The opposite result may occur when the concentration of a competitive antagonist remains constant. In such circumstances, receptor activity slowly resumes, and increasing amounts of agonist displace the antagonist.

The second type of antagonist, the noncompetitive antagonist, inhibits agonist response regardless of agonist concentration. The affinity of the noncompetitive antagonist for the receptor is so high that the receptor becomes essentially unavailable for the agonist or normal substrate. For example, the noncompetitive antagonist phenoxybenzamine protects the patient from the intermittent release of large amounts of catecholamines from adrenal tumors.

FUNCTION OF RECEPTORS

Receptors can either change the rate of body functions or initiate an activity. Ligands (endogenous substances, such as hormones, neurotransmitters, or autacoids) interact with a receptor, binding with it to cause a response. A drug will mimic a ligand when the drug's structure resembles the ligand's or when the receptor is not appropriately selective. When ligand binding occurs, the activity rate of bodily functions is either enhanced or inhibited.

CLASSIFICATION OF RECEPTORS

Drug receptors are usually classified by the effects produced. However, a nonselective drug may interact with more than one receptor type, thereby causing multiple effects. Also, some receptors are classified further by their specific effects. For example, the *beta receptors* usually produce increased heart rate and bronchial relaxation, besides other systemic effects.

Beta receptors, however, can be subdivided into beta$_1$ receptors (act primarily on cardiac tissue) and beta$_2$ receptors (act primarily on smooth muscles and gland cells). A dominance of beta$_1$ receptors occurs in the heart, whereas beta$_2$ receptors primarily appear in the lungs. Administering a nonselective beta antagonist, or beta blocker, such as propranolol, to a patient with tachycardia will decrease the heart rate. Unfortunately, the nonselectivity of propranolol will also block beta$_2$ receptors, which could precipitate an asthmatic attack in susceptible patients. Administering a selective beta$_1$ antagonist, such as metoprolol or atenolol, will reduce the risk of receptor nonselectivity and specifically decrease heart rate, but should not affect pulmonary function.

Epinephrine is a nonselective beta agonist used to treat acute asthmatic disorders. Unfortunately, when administered subcutaneously, epinephrine will interact with both beta$_1$ and beta$_2$ receptors and further increase the asthmatic patient's accelerated heart rate. Therefore, terbutaline, administered parenterally, is a preferred drug: it is more selective for beta$_2$ receptors. The physician assesses the patient's responses to selective versus nonselective drugs before determining the best drug for each patient.

RECEPTOR NUMBERS AND RESPONSE

The number of receptors and their affinity for binding with a ligand may actually increase or decrease in some situations. An increased number of receptors, termed up-regulation, is associated with receptors that are triggered by hormones and neurotransmitters. For example, thyroid hormone is thought to increase the number of selective cardiac receptors, which would explain why in thyrotoxicosis the number of beta$_1$ receptors in the heart increases, and why propranolol, a beta$_1$ antagonist, is effective treating tachycardia. In contrast, a decreased number of receptors, or their decreased affinity for the

ligand, is termed down-regulation. The concepts of up-regulation and down-regulation help explain the sometimes mysterious changes in response that occur during routine drug therapy.

Besides a patient's receptors varying in their affinity for ligand binding, a patient's overall responsiveness to a drug can vary considerably. (See Chapter 4, Pharmacotherapeutics, for a more detailed explanation of overall patient responsiveness.) A patient may also exhibit different responses to the same drug at different times during the treatment program. This variable can range from a heightened response to relatively no response. Hyperreactivity refers to a more magnified response to a drug dose than the response seen in most patients. (Do not confuse hyperreactivity with hypersensitivity, an immediate, possibly life-threatening, allergic drug response.)

Hyporeactivity refers to the less-than-usual response to a normal drug dose, which usually necessitates an unusually large drug dose to produce the usual drug effect. The resistance to drug therapy of patients with hypothyroidism typically reflects hyporeactivity. The condition resolves with thyroid hormone supplements that return the patient to normoreactivity.

Tolerance refers to a decreased response or sensitivity of the receptor to a drug. Though the mechanisms for this modification in response are not completely clear, tolerance seems to occur when a patient has had previous exposure to a drug. Tolerance may also result from increased rates of drug metabolism or from the receptor's adaptation to the local drug action. For example, using hypnotics and sedatives over a long period frequently becomes ineffective in producing sleep; that is, a tolerance to sedative induction at initial doses develops. Other examples of tolerance-producing agents include barbiturates, alcohol, nitrates, tobacco, and opiates. A cross-tolerance between drugs can also develop, as demonstrated by alcohol and general anesthetics. The tolerance that develops from chronic alcohol use increases the usual required dose of anesthetic.

Immunity describes a reduced response only when the modification results from antibody formation. For example, tetanus toxoid initiates a low-grade immune response that will later protect the human body from the life-threatening response that follows exposure to the tetanus bacterium.

Occasionally, patients demonstrate an idiosyncratic, or unusual, response to a drug. Idiosyncratic responses, which occur infrequently, are usually associated with genetic differences in enzyme activity or immunologic mechanisms.

OUTCOME OF DRUG ACTION

The major factors determining the outcome of drug action include the location and function of the receptors with which the drug interacts and the drug concentration at the receptor site. If the drug interacts with common receptors located throughout the body, the drug effects will be widespread. The use of drugs exhibiting such widespread response can be particularly dangerous because potential toxicity may affect many organ systems. The margin of safety for such drugs can be narrow, as in chemotherapeutic drugs. (See Chapter 4, Pharmacotherapeutics, for further discussion of the concept of margin of safety under the topic of therapeutic index.)

If the drug interacts with specific receptors that are unique for highly differentiated cells, the response should be quite predictable. For example, the careful use of controlled doses of radioactive iodine, which has a strong affinity for receptor sites within the thyroid gland, affectively treats hyperthyroidism.

The drug treatment outcome may also depend upon whether the drug affects the target organs and tissues directly or indirectly. For example, in the treatment of asthma, theophylline directly modifies the bronchodilator receptors within the lung to improve ventilation. This direct effect provides a rapid onset of action and allows the physician to use theophylline blood concentration levels to correlate the therapeutic outcomes and drug dosages. In contrast, levodopa indirectly affects the target tissue within the central nervous system. Dopamine, the active metabolite of levodopa, cannot cross the blood-brain barrier and bind with the target tissue to elicit a response. Therefore, levodopa, which freely crosses the blood-brain barrier, must be used to produce dopamine within the central nervous system.

Outcome also depends upon the drug concentration at the receptor site. The amount of drug at the site usually affects the intensity of the drug-induced response. The effect of drug concentration at the receptor site on outcome is best reflected in the dose-response curve.

DOSE-RESPONSE CURVE

Understanding the previously discussed fundamentals concerning drug response and its dependence upon the receptor affinity of the active drug is necessary to understand the dose-response curve. As its name implies, a dose-response curve represents graphically the relationship between the dose of a drug and the response elicited. (See *The dose-response curve* on page 48 for an illustration of the following discussion.)

On a dose-response curve, an initial low dose usually corresponds with a low response. As the dose increases incrementally, the corresponding response usually increases. A high correlation between the dose and the response indicates that the dose regimen can be increased to reach a point where receptor sites are saturated without causing adverse reactions. At this point, further increase in dose will not increase response. In short, the maximal response to the drug has been attained.

The administration of theophylline reflects a high correlation between dose and response. The incremental increase in dose corresponds to an incremental increase in the blood concentration of the drug. Furthermore, the theophylline regimen can be increased without adverse reactions until the pulmonary function of the asthmatic patient improves. Eventually, however, the maximal response is attained; the pulmonary bronchi can dilate no further. At this point, any further increase in theophylline dose will not improve ventilation.

All drugs elicit more than one response. Morphine at low doses may calm an irritable bowel; higher doses of the drug can serve as a narcotic analgesic. Unfortunately, some adverse reactions usually occur at normal therapeutic doses. On a dose-response curve, the curve representing the doses of morphine used as a narcotic analgesic would overlap the curve representing the drug's adverse effects. In the case of morphine, respiratory depression may preclude the continual increase in dose to achieve pain relief.

Ideally, a drug will possess a low-dose-response curve, a high-dose-response curve, and an adverse effect–dose-response curve, none of which overlaps the other. The three curves would be adequately separated, thus reducing exposure of the patient to any risk of an adverse drug reaction. (See *Ideal dose-response curves* for an illustration of this concept.) Unfortunately, this treatment goal has yet to be achieved for the majority of drugs.

The dose-response curve

Most drugs demonstrate a high correlation between the dose and the response (effect A). All drugs, however, usually exert more than one effect. Unfortunately, with some drugs, the occurrence of adverse effects does not permit the use of a wide dosage range to achieve the desired effect (effect B). In fact, with some drugs, the onset of adverse effects may preclude using the drug even to obtain effect B.

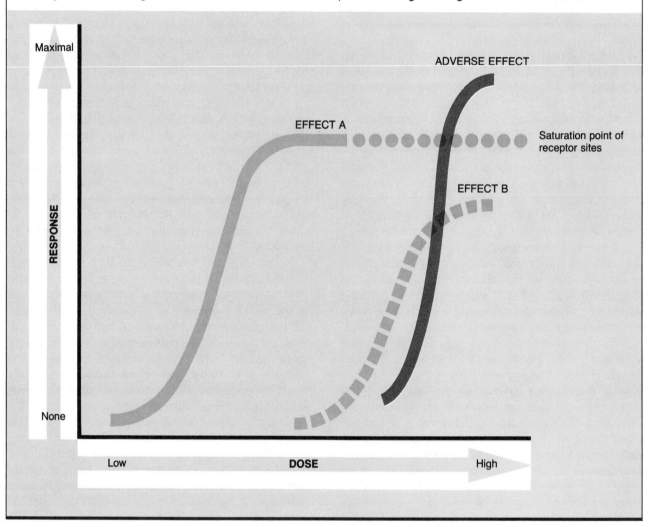

DRUG POTENCY

Drug potency, a frequently used and misunderstood term, refers to the relative amount of a drug required to produce the desired response. Comparing the drug potency of one drug with that of another drug can reveal the more potent drug. For example, comparing the usual doses of two diuretics shows that chlorothiazide requires 500 to 1,000 mg daily to achieve a therapeutic effect whereas hydrochlorothiazide requires only 50 to 100 mg daily. Because hydrochlorothiazide achieves comparable effects at a lower dose, it is the more potent of the two diuretics. (See *Drug potency and efficacy* on pages 50 and 51 for an illustration of the differences in dosages needed between drug A and drug B to attain the desired effect.) The drug potency is relatively unimportant in clinical practice unless the quantity required for administration is unpalatable.

Ideal dose-response curves

Ideally, the doses needed to achieve effect A and effect B will differ sufficiently to avoid overlap in the response. The adverse effect curve also would not overlap the therapeutic response curves.

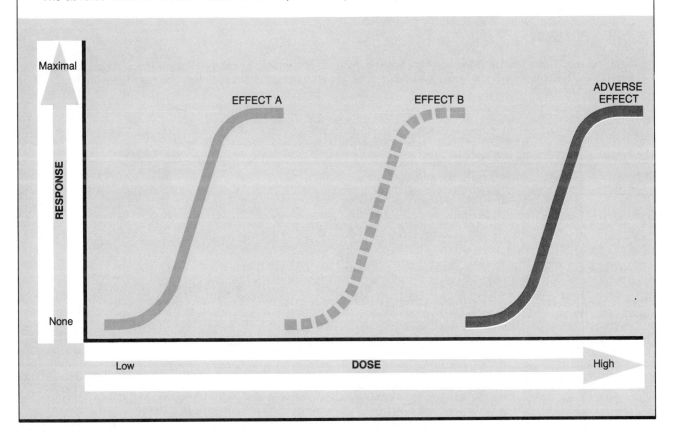

DRUG EFFICACY

Drug efficacy differs from drug potency in that it relates to the maximal response or effect achieved when the dose-response curve reaches its plateau. For example, compare the use of morphine and aspirin to treat pain. Aspirin is effective only for mild to moderate pain, while morphine is effective for all pain levels. (See *Drug potency and efficacy* on pages 50 and 51 for the dose-response curves of morphine and aspirin.) Unfortunately, other factors may affect this dose-response–plateau relationship. For instance, the incidence and severity of adverse reactions before the plateau is attained can reduce a drug's efficacy. Furthermore, a drug's pla-

teau may fall short of the maximal amount needed for effective therapeutic treatment.

THERAPEUTIC INDEX

Most drugs produce multiple effects. For example, morphine acts as an analgesic, cough suppressant, and sedative, and also causes respiratory depression, constipation, and other adverse reactions. The relation-

(Text continues on page 52.)

Drug potency and efficacy

Potency and efficacy are often confused. A more potent drug achieves comparable effects of another drug but at smaller doses. Ideally, a drug should exhibit potency, a high efficacy, and a low incidence of adverse effects.

DRUG POTENCY

Drug potency is the relative difference between the doses of two drugs necessary to achieve a comparable drug response. The potency comparison of two drugs is of little importance clinically unless the needed quantity of drug B is unpalatable.

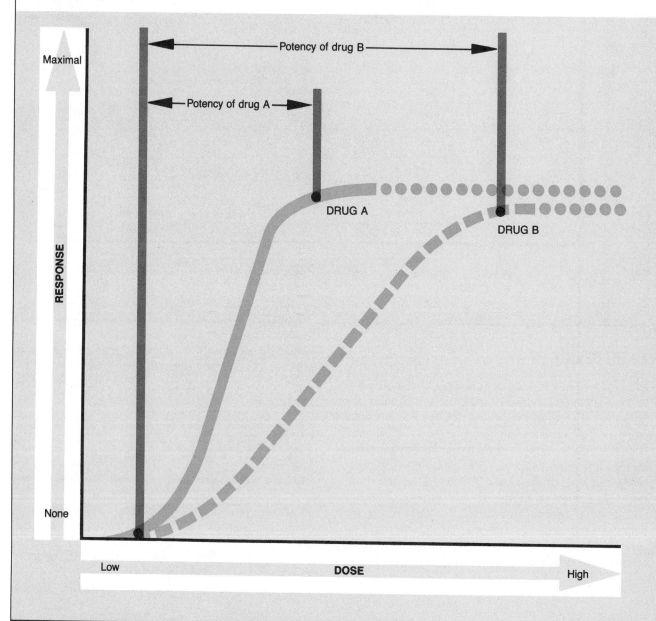

DRUG EFFICACY

Drug efficacy reflects the comparative differences in the maximal responses of two drugs. The physician must evaluate the incidence and severity of the patient's adverse reactions in determining the efficacy of a drug.

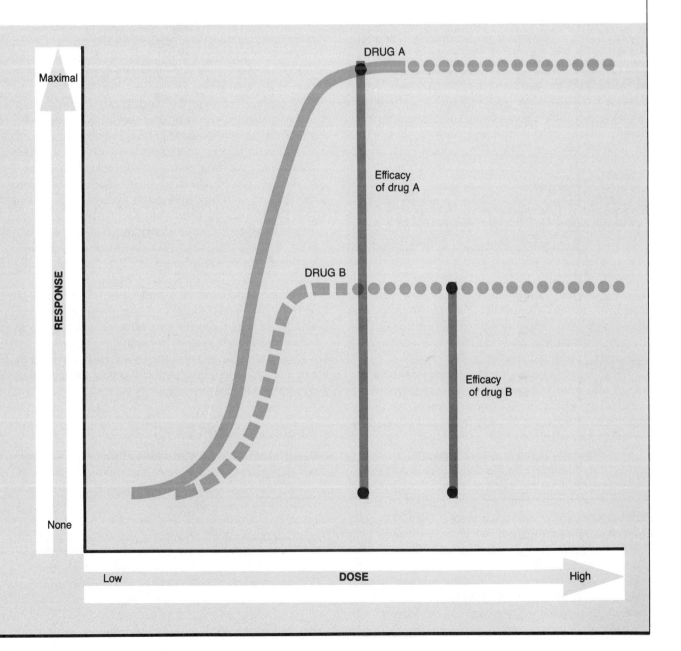

ship between a drug's desired therapeutic effects and its adverse effects is interchangeably termed the drug's therapeutic index, its selectivity, or its margin of safety.

A review of how the therapeutic index is determined in animals illustrates the concept. In animal experiments, researchers compare the effective treatment dose for 50% of the animals to the dose that resulted in 50% of the animals succumbing to the drug's adverse effects. If the difference between the two doses is significant, the therapeutic index is wide. If the difference between the two doses is narrow, the therapeutic index is narrow. A narrow therapeutic index probably precludes the drug's use in humans.

Obviously, using this method to determine the therapeutic index in humans is not acceptable. Therefore, the human therapeutic index usually represents a measure of the difference between an effective dose for 50% of the patients treated and the minimal dose at which adverse reactions occur. All drugs with a narrow therapeutic index should be routinely and thoroughly monitored.

ADVERSE DRUG EFFECTS

Most drugs produce a spectrum of effects that ranges from the desired, predictable, and routinely anticipated response to the unpredictable, potentially life-threatening, and unexplainable response. In all drug therapy, physicians must weigh the benefits of the drug against its possible adverse effects.

The desired effects of a drug represent those expected responses that benefit the patient's therapy. Adverse drug effects encompass a broad range of undesirable responses, ranging from mild adverse reactions in the patient, such as stomach upset, to severe or life-threatening hypersensitivity reactions.

Distinguishing an effect as desired or adverse sometimes depends upon the medical disorder being treated. For instance, for the common cold, diphenhydramine reduces nasal stuffiness and rhinorrhea. Unfortunately, the drug causes drowsiness, which may interfere with the patient's safe driving of a vehicle. In this case, the reduced nasal stuffiness represents the desired effect, and drowsiness represents the adverse reaction. In contrast, when diphenhydramine is indicated for insomnia, the drug's ability to induce drowsiness becomes the de-

sired effect. The adverse reaction in using diphenhydramine for insomnia is dry mucous membranes. Predictable adverse reactions may be anticipated by knowing the effect of patient variables (genetic differences, health status, age, weight, renal or hepatic disease, psychological status, and immune system status) on drug activity and effect.

Toxic drug effect describes an adverse reaction that occurs when the drug concentration in susceptible tissue reaches levels that may cause either a reversible or irreversible damaging effect. Toxic drug effects, which may be dangerous to the patient, can be anticipated when the drug's threshold level is exceeded. Excess drug concentration in susceptible tissues usually elicits an additional or exaggerated response to the primary effect of the drug within the target tissue. For example, if an elderly patient with a dysrhythmia ingested more than the prescribed dosage of digoxin, the drug would not only continue to slow the cardiac rate but might also slow the cardiac electrical conduction pathways to the point of inducing a potentially fatal complete heart block.

Several factors other than an excess of the drug can initiate toxic drug effects; for example, drug receptor sensitivity, inadequate drug distribution, altered drug metabolism, and inadequate drug excretion. A patient with liver or kidney disease may experience toxic drug effects because the disease can alter the drug's metabolism and excretion. In such circumstances, the unmetabolized or unexcreted drug would accumulate in the body and reach potentially toxic levels.

Unpredictable adverse effects or idiosyncratic effects are not related to the expected pharmacodynamic effects. Instead, unpredictable adverse effects seem to be unique to each patient. Because these unpredictable effects cannot be prevented or anticipated, physicians continually and effectively must evaluate the responses of a patient to drug therapy.

ALLERGIC RESPONSES

Allergic responses, or hypersensitivity reactions to a drug, are exaggerated responses to an antigen-antibody reaction and occur in the body as defensive reactions to foreign substances, particularly protein. In most cases, an allergic response to a drug can follow only a previous sensitizing exposure. In an antigen-antibody reaction, the body recognizes an antigen, or a foreign molecule, and the immune system reacts exaggeratedly by producing an antibody. Antibodies are specific immuno-

Drug allergies

Drug allergies are divided into four basic groups: Types I, II, III, and IV.

TYPE	RESPONSES	EXAMPLES
I	Immediate reactions to stings and drugs	Anaphylaxis, urticaria, angioedema
II	Drug-induced autoimmune disorders	Sulfonamide-induced granulocytopenia, quinidine-induced thrombocytopenic purpura, hydralazine-induced systemic lupus erythematosus
III	Reactions to penicillins, sulfonamides, iodides; antibody targeted against tissue antigens	Urticarial skin eruptions, arthralgia, lymphadenopathy, fever
IV	Reexposure to an antigen	Poison ivy and its resulting contact dermatitis

globulins that help protect the body from foreign molecules, such as bacteria, viruses, and other foreign substances. (See *Drug allergies* for the classification and characteristics of allergic responses.)

An idiosyncratic allergic reaction to a drug is rare and occurs during the first known exposure to the drug. Patients can unknowingly expose themselves to the offending drug again by ingesting trace amounts in food and dairy sources. For example, meat derived from livestock treated with a drug may carry trace amounts of the drug into humans. A drug's pharmaceutical ingredient may also initiate allergic reactions. One pharmaceutical ingredient that can initiate allergic responses is the dye tartrazine yellow, used to color tablets and capsules. Susceptible asthmatic patients suffer asthma exacerbation upon ingestion of products containing tartrazine yellow.

IATROGENIC DRUG EFFECTS

Some adverse drug effects induced by the prescribed drug, known as iatrogenic effects, may mimic pathologic disorders. As a result, the physician may inadvertently treat an iatrogenic effect as a concurrent pathology. For example, some drugs, such as antineoplastics, aspirin, corticosteroids, and indomethacin, frequently cause gastrointestinal irritation and bleeding. Other examples of iatrogenic effects include propranolol-induced asthma,

methicillin-induced nephritis, gentamicin-induced deafness, and thiazide-induced dizziness. Obtaining complete medical and drug histories from the patient helps reduce the risk of iatrogenic effects.

NURSING IMPLICATIONS

Whereas pharmacokinetics describes the movement of a drug through the body system and identifies the variables affecting drug movement, pharmacodynamics evaluates the mechanisms by which a drug initiates its action. The nurse who understands a drug's mechanism of action knows how the drug acts to bring about its effect and can apply this knowledge to the patient's total treatment program. The nurse can make pertinent assessments of the expected therapeutic drug effects and initiate nursing interventions that will enhance the patient's response to the drug. Also, the nurse who understands a drug's pharmacodynamics can anticipate potential adverse effects and institute appropriate monitoring and intervention procedures.

The nurse can integrate pharmacodynamic principles into patient treatment by including the following nursing actions in each corresponding step of the nursing process.

Assessment

● Evaluate the subjective and objective patient assessment data in terms of the expected therapeutic drug response.

● Assess the variables that can modify a patient's response to the usual dose of a drug, including genetic differences, health status, age, weight, evidence of renal or hepatic pathology, psychological status, and immune system status.

● Document any known drug allergies of the patient.

● Assess the margin of safety of each drug for each patient.

● Formulate a nursing diagnosis based on actual or potential patient problems related to drug responses.

Planning

● Determine the appropriate interventions to deal with the identified patient problems related to drug therapy.

● Determine if the patient runs a high risk of developing adverse drug reactions, and develop an appropriate monitoring schedule for detecting such reactions.

● Anticipate possible adverse drug reactions and their effects on the patient's psychological and physiologic status, activities of daily living, occupation, and social activities.

Implementation

● Consult with the physician about any potential problems before drug administration.

● Implement for the patient a teaching plan that includes the following information:

—the expected drug action and therapeutic effects

—the probability of adverse drug reactions

—the importance of reporting immediately any unexpected reactions (low-grade fever, sore throat, cough, itching), even if they seem minor, because such minor responses could indicate a severe adverse drug effect

—the importance of seeking a physician's assistance in treating adverse reactions rather than using home remedies (such as iron preparations for a "lack of pep," baking soda for an upset stomach, or aspirin for fever) that can mask the symptoms and delay the recognition of serious adverse drug effects.

● Administer all drugs cautiously because they may elicit multiple responses. Furthermore, any drug can cause toxic effects, and a patient's response to the same drug may vary during treatment.

● Be prepared to treat adverse reactions, assuring that all emergency equipment is readily accessible and in working order.

Evaluation

● Correlate the patient's drug response with the expected drug response.

● If the drug is not initiating the expected response, consult the physician about possibly altering the therapeutic regimen.

CHAPTER SUMMARY

Chapter 3 presented pharmacodynamics, that is, the mechanisms of action by which drugs produce biochemical or physiologic changes in the patient's body. Here are the highlights of the chapter:

● Drug action represents the interaction between a drug and cellular components; drug effect describes the responses from the interaction. Drug action occurs at the cellular level; drug effect may affect total body function.

● Drugs do not change the functions of target cells in the body. Instead they regulate the rates of those cell functions either by altering the cell environment or by interacting with receptors.

● Receptors are specialized reactive substances or large groups of molecules, such as a cell membrane, a protein, or an enzyme. The specificity of drug-receptor interaction may be represented by the analogy of a lock and key.

● Drugs that display affinity for receptors and enhance or stimulate the receptors' functional properties are called agonists. Drugs that occupy receptor sites and prevent the action of agonists are called antagonists. Agonists stimulate a drug response whereas antagonists inhibit such a response. Two types of antagonists exist (competitive and noncompetitive). When an agonist and a competitive antagonist are both present, the one in the highest concentration causes the response. The noncompetitive antagonist inhibits agonist response regardless of agonist concentration.

● Drug receptors are classified by the effects they produce.

● A dose-response curve represents graphically the relationship between the dose of a drug and the response it elicits.

● Drug potency refers to the amount of a drug required to produce a response, whereas drug efficacy relates to the maximal response achieved when the dose-response curve reaches its plateau. Ideally, a drug should provide potency, a high efficacy, and a low incidence of adverse effects.

● The therapeutic index, selectivity, and margin of safety all refer to the relationship between a drug's desired therapeutic effects and its adverse effects.

● Adverse effects may be predictable (dose-related), unpredictable (not dose-related), allergic, idiosyncratic, or iatrogenic.

● The nurse must consider the pharmacodynamics of a patient's therapeutic drug regimen in each step of the nursing process.

BIBLIOGRAPHY

Avery, G. *Drug Treatment: Principles and Practice of Clinical Pharmacology and Therapeutics,* 2nd edition. New York: ADIS Press, 1980.

Gilman, A.G., et al. *Goodman and Gilman's The Pharmacological Basis of Therapeutics,* 7th edition. New York: Macmillan Publishing Co., 1985.

Goth, A. *Medical Pharmacology,* 11th edition. St. Louis: C.V. Mosby Co., 1984.

Katzung, B.G. *Basic and Clinical Pharmacology,* 2nd edition. Los Altos, Calif.: Lange Medical Publications, 1984.

Knoben, J.E., and Anderson, P.O. *Handbook of Clinical Drug Data,* 5th edition. Hamilton, Ill.: Drug Intelligence Publications, Inc., 1983.

Shinn, A.S., and Shrewsbury, R.P. *Evaluations of Drug Interactions,* 3rd edition. St. Louis: C.V. Mosby Co., 1985.

PHARMACOTHERAPEUTICS

OBJECTIVES

After reading and studying this chapter, you should be able to:

1. Describe the types of drug therapy and explain the factors that determine which types a patient receives.

2. Give examples of drugs used to prevent, diagnose, and treat diseases.

3. Explain the concept of the therapeutic index and its importance in drug therapy.

4. Discuss the effects of gastrointestinal (GI), renal, hepatic, thyroid, and cardiovascular diseases on drug action.

5. Describe how age, genetics, weight, gender, body build, and circadian variations affect a patient's response to drugs.

6. Differentiate between drug tolerance and dependence.

7. Discuss the effects of three kinds of drug interactions and their effects on the patient.

8. Explain how incompatibilities among parenteral drugs can alter a drug's pharmacologic activity.

9. Explain how the nurse uses the nursing process to meet a patient's drug needs.

INTRODUCTION

This chapter presents an overview of pharmacotherapeutics, or the use of drugs to treat disease, and an examination of factors that may alter a patient's response to drug therapy.

Therapeutics describes the science and art of treating disease. A patient's treatment may include one or a combination of therapies. Therapeutics begins with the assessment of the nature and extent of the patient's health problem. This assessment is based on a patient history obtained by the nurse, as well as on diagnostic procedures, laboratory tests, and careful clinical observation. Assessing the options and selecting the therapy or therapies are based on a knowledge of the patient,

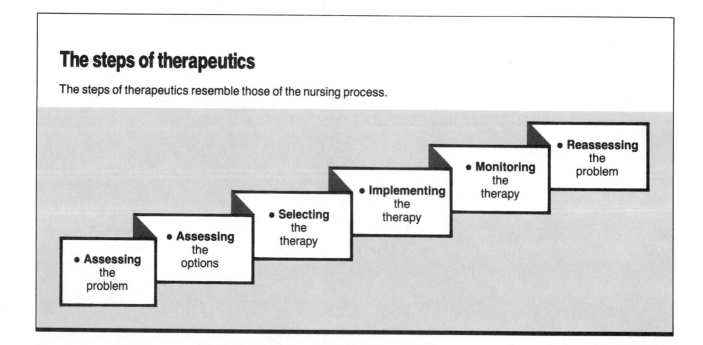

The steps of therapeutics

The steps of therapeutics resemble those of the nursing process.

• **Assessing** the problem

• **Assessing** the options

• **Selecting** the therapy

• **Implementing** the therapy

• **Monitoring** the therapy

• **Reassessing** the problem

related socioeconomic factors, and the risks and benefits of the various medical therapies.

During treatment, the nurse monitors the patient for adverse and therapeutic effects, recording both expected and unexpected reactions. The frequency of assessment depends on the severity and urgency of the patient's condition. Therapy is adjusted if the patient's problem resolves or progresses, if adverse effects occur, or if the therapy proves unsuccessful. (See *The steps of therapeutics* for a summary of the activities involved.)

TYPES OF THERAPY

The required therapy depends upon the severity, urgency, and prognosis of the patient's condition. The patient's therapy may be acute, empiric, supportive, palliative, maintenance, supplemental, or replacement.

Critically ill patients require acute intensive therapy. For example, a trauma patient may require antibiotics to prevent or treat infection, pressor agents to treat hypotension, volume expanders to treat blood loss, and analgesics to relieve pain.

Empiric therapy is based on practical experience rather than on pure scientific data. Physicians frequently treat fever spikes in hospitalized patients initially with empiric antibiotic therapy, selecting the antibiotic from a deduction about the microorganisms the patient is most susceptible to—basing their deduction on the patient's general health, hospital stay, or chronic diseases instead of waiting for the results of culture and sensitivity tests.

Some diseases require supportive therapy, which does not treat the cause of the disease but maintains other threatened body systems until the patient's condition resolves. For example, no antiviral agents are available to treat acute viral gastroenteritis, which causes nausea, vomiting, and diarrhea. Instead, patients with this virus receive fluid and electrolyte replacements to prevent dehydration until the condition resolves.

Palliative therapy is often used for patients with end-stage or terminal diseases, to make the patient as comfortable as possible. For example, high-dose continuous infusions of narcotic analgesics may be used to manage pain in a terminal cancer patient, or home oxygen may be supplied for a patient with end-stage pulmonary disease.

Maintenance therapy is used for patients with chronic conditions that do not resolve. This therapy seeks to maintain the patient's level of well-being while preventing further progression of the disease, if possible. An example is hypertension, in which the long-term effects can include decreased renal function, impaired vision, cerebrovascular accident, myocardial infarction, cardiac enlargement, and cardiac failure if maintenance therapy is not instituted.

Supplemental or replacement therapy may be short- or long-term. A patient with iron deficiency anemia, for example, may receive iron supplements until hemoglobin and hematocrit levels are corrected and the body stores of iron are repleted, which may take approximately 6 months. However, a patient with diabetes mellitus who cannot produce adequate amounts of insulin may require lifelong injections that substitute the missing hormone.

Other medical conditions may require continual supplemental or replacement therapies. A patient taking a potassium-depleting diuretic, such as furosemide, often requires daily potassium replacement, and a patient with hypoactive thyroid glands needs daily replacement of thyroid hormones.

PHARMACOTHERAPEUTICS/ USES OF DRUGS

Therapeutics includes all forms of medical therapy; pharmacotherapeutics is the study of drug use to prevent, diagnose, and treat diseases. Some drugs are used to prevent, diagnose, and treat, whereas others are used for only one or two of these purposes. (See *Pharmacotherapeutic uses of drugs* on page 58 for examples of specific drug uses.)

Drugs for prevention
Vaccinations are administered to prevent infectious diseases, either before or after patient exposure to the disease. School systems in the United States require that children be immunized against commonly occurring infectious diseases. Some vaccines consist of weakened infectious agents or antigens that stimulate the body to produce its own antibodies (active immunity). Other vaccines provide the body with actual antibodies against the infectious agent (passive immunity).

Hepatitis B immune globulin (HBIG) is given to health care professionals to prevent hepatitis B after accidental needle sticks or close contact with patients with hepatitis B viral infections. The injections of HBIG contain antibodies isolated from the blood plasma of hepatitis B patients. Thus, a vaccination of HBIG provides passive immunity to and nearly instant protection from hepatitis B. Heptavax-B, a vaccine for hepatitis B, consists of inactivated viral antigens that stimulate the immune system to manufacture antibodies, thus providing active immunity.

Physicians often prescribe antibiotics to prevent infections. Patients may receive antibiotic injections before surgery to decrease the risk of postoperative infections. The antibiotic rifampin, which prevents meningitis, may be given prophylactically to patients with a high susceptibility to meningitis who have been exposed to *Hemophilus influenzae*.

Drugs for diagnosis

Radiologic studies using iodine-based dyes are used to diagnose abnormalities in organ function. For example, intravenous pyelography using iodine-based dyes allows visualization of the kidneys, ureters, and bladder, enabling the physician to check for structural abnormalities and obstruction.

Substances, like barium, that are clearly visible on X-rays are used in radiographic diagnostic studies. In one such test, the patient swallows a barium-containing suspension that outlines the inner lining of the upper GI tract on X-rays. This test can reveal ulcerations and structural abnormalities in the upper GI tract and the esophagus.

Radiopharmaceuticals, drugs labeled with radioactivity, are used in diagnostic studies of the liver, heart, spleen, bones, and other organs to determine alterations in function that occur secondary to organ damage or disease.

Cosyntropin (Cortrosyn), a synthetic hormone that stimulates the adrenal glands to produce cortisol, is used to diagnose adrenal abnormalities. Cortisol levels are measured immediately before and 30 or 60 minutes after the injection of cosyntropin. In patients with normal adrenocortical function, the adrenal cortex responds by secreting cortisol. Patients with adrenal insufficiency do not respond with increased cortisol levels and will require exogenous corticosteroids in periods of stress or illness.

Drugs for treatment

Physicians prescribe drugs to treat the causes of diseases or to alleviate symptoms if the causes are unknown, undetermined, or untreatable. Antineoplastic agents are used, often in combination, to treat malignant neoplasms. Cisplatin (Platinol), chlorambucil (Leukeran), and doxorubicin (Adriamycin) are antineoplastic agents used to treat many kinds of malignant neoplasms.

Laxatives, such as milk of magnesia and bisacodyl, are used to treat constipation, a frequent symptom of unknown origin or of a specific disease or drug therapy. Antibiotics used prophylactically to prevent disease are also used to treat microbial infections.

Pharmacotherapeutic uses of drugs

Drugs are used to prevent, diagnose, and treat diseases. Here are specific examples of these different uses.

DRUG	CONDITION
Prevention	
hepatitis B vaccine	• Hepatitis B
amantadine	• Influenza
antibiotics	• Postoperative infection • Urinary tract infections • Otitis media
estrogens	• Contraception • Osteoporosis
Diagnosis	
iodine dye	• Organ system abnormalities
purified protein derivative (PPD)	• Tuberculosis
technetium 99	• Bone alterations
Treatment	
methyldopa	• Hypertension
digoxin	• Dysrhythmias • Heart failure
iron	• Anemia
thiamine	• Deficiency • Wernicke-Korsakoff syndrome
folate	• Megaloblastic anemia
quinidine	• Dysrhythmias
insulin	• Diabetes mellitus
estrogens	• Menopause

FACTORS INFLUENCING THE CHOICE OF THERAPY

Several factors help a physician choose a patient's therapy, including an analysis of a drug's potential risks and benefits, the likelihood of patient compliance, and the cost of the therapy.

Analyzing risks and benefits

Both the physician and the patient must analyze the therapeutic value of a drug against its inherent risks. The physician considers the seriousness of the disease and the availability of less toxic and more reliable drugs. The physician or nurse should inform the patient that every beneficial therapy involves risks.

For example, a physician may consider using cyclosporine, which helps prevent patient rejection of transplanted organs, with a patient about to receive a transplant. Its benefits, which could lead to a longer, more productive life after transplant surgery, may outweigh the risks of its nephrotoxicity.

Patient compliance

Compliance describes the degree to which a patient follows the prescribed treatment regimen. Patient compliance is extremely important to a therapy's success or failure. Compliance can be improved by using drugs that simplify the regimen, such as those that require only one or two daily doses, come in palatable liquid dosage forms, dissolve easily, or are available as transdermal patches.

Cost

The physician needs to consider the cost to the patient when selecting a drug since the cost of drugs may interfere with patient compliance.

CLINICAL RESPONSE TO DRUGS

Several drug-related factors, including adverse and cumulative effects, influence the patient's response to drugs during therapy. The nurse must consider these factors when planning and implementing the patient's care.

The therapeutic index of a drug represents the ratio between its effective and toxic plasma concentrations. The therapeutic index is a quantitative measure of a drug's safety. A low therapeutic index indicates a narrow range between a therapeutically active dose and a toxic dose. Examples of drugs with low therapeutic indices include phenytoin, theophylline, and lidocaine. When administering any medication with a low therapeutic index, the nurse must check the dosage and monitor the patient closely. Monitoring activities include assessing the patient's response and laboratory tests (including drug levels) to evaluate the drug's effects. Although the nurse usually includes monitoring and teaching activities in every nursing care plan, these elements are especially important for the patient taking a drug with a low therapeutic index.

A physician prescribes a drug to benefit the patient; however, adverse reactions do occur. Recognizing them and knowing their effects on the patient are integral components of monitoring drug therapy. (See Chapter 3, Pharmacodynamics, for information about patient hypersensitivity and idiosyncratic adverse reactions to drugs.) A drug may also produce undesirable responses because of cumulative effects, sometimes resulting in toxicity. Cumulative effects may occur when the drug is excreted more slowly than it is absorbed or when another dose of the drug is administered before the previous dose is metabolized, or cleared from the body.

Toxic drug concentration levels may result when standard drug doses normally eliminated by the kidneys are administered to patients with decreased renal function. Because diseased or damaged kidneys cannot effectively remove the drug from the body, the drug accumulates and leads to toxicity. For example, normal doses of aminoglycoside antibiotics administered at normal intervals to patients with decreased renal function may result in nephrotoxicity and ototoxicity. The physician will need to decrease the drug dosage to prevent toxicity.

Drugs that undergo extensive hepatic metabolism may become toxic in patients with impaired or immature hepatic function. Neonates, for example, must receive reduced doses of the antibiotic chloramphenicol. If given normal doses of chloramphenicol, they might develop concentration-related toxic effects, such as bone marrow suppression, because the neonate's immature hepatic enzyme system cannot metabolize the drug sufficiently to avoid the toxic effects.

Although a new drug undergoes extensive testing before receiving Food and Drug Administration (FDA) approval, its adverse effects cannot be reliably predicted until it has received widespread exposure in the general population. In recent years, some newly FDA-approved drugs have been withdrawn from the market after some unpredicted, serious adverse effects became evident.

Factors affecting a patient's response

Because no two people possess identical physiologic or psychological compositions, drug response varies greatly, depending upon the following factors:

- Disease
- Infection
- Immunization
- Occupational exposures
- Drug interactions
- Circadian variations
- Diet
- Cardiovascular function
- GI function
- Immunologic function
- Hepatic function
- Renal function
- Albumin concentration
- Genetic constitution
- Enzyme induction
- Stress
- Fever
- Starvation
- Alcohol intake
- Age
- Pregnancy
- Lactation
- Exercise
- Sunlight
- Barometric pressure
- Smoking
- Hypersensitivity
- Trauma

Other factors, many related to the patient's overall health, can alter the patient's response to a drug. As a result, a physician must consider a patient's concurrent diseases and other medical conditions when selecting an appropriate drug therapy. (See *Factors affecting a patient's response* for more details.)

DISEASES AND DISORDERS

Diseases and disorders of the major body systems or glands will alter a patient's response to drugs. Altered pharmacokinetic properties (absorption, distribution, metabolism, and excretion) can influence drug effect and necessitate alterations in drug dosages.

Gastrointestinal system

Drugs are primarily absorbed not from the stomach, but from the small intestine. Consequently, alterations in gastric emptying or in the environment of the small intestine may affect the absorption of many orally administered drugs.

Hypomotility, or decreased GI movement, can slow or delay drug absorption. Several diseases are associated with hypomotility. In the long-term diabetic patient, for example, hypomotility is secondary to autonomic neuropathy of the GI tract. Patients with the eating disorder anorexia nervosa may exhibit delayed gastric emptying of a standard meal.

Achlorhydria, a condition characterized by the absence of hydrochloric acid in the gastric juices, may lead to the decreased absorption of drugs like ketoconazole that require an acidic pH.

GI surgery, particularly gastrectomy and vagotomy, can result in decreased absorption of nutrients and deficiencies of iron, folic acid, and vitamin B_{12}. Gastrectomy (partial removal of the stomach) and vagotomy (severing the nerves that stimulate acid production in the stomach) lead to decreased acid production and increased pH. Iron absorption decreases because dietary iron is converted to a more absorbable form in the stomach's acidic environment. The inability to absorb dietary iron eventually leads to iron deficiency.

Drug absorption is also altered in patients with inflammatory bowel disease (Crohn's disease and ulcerative colitis).

Renal system

Because most drugs are excreted at least partially by the kidneys, decreases in renal function can significantly influence the therapeutic and toxic effects of a drug. Renal insufficiency can result from disorders, such as acute tubular necrosis, drug-induced renal failure, and diabetes mellitus. It may also result from aging. On the average, the glomerular filtration rate decreases 35% to 45% between ages 20 and 90. Creatinine clearance, estimated either from 24-hour urine collections or formulas, is used to gauge the glomerular filtration rate. The physician determines dosages for patients with decreased renal function based on the creatinine clearance.

Hepatic system

Because the liver is extensively involved in drug metabolism, impaired hepatic function can alter drug metabolism and excretion. Impaired hepatic function may result from acute or chronic inflammatory or degenerative or neoplastic processes. Because the liver synthesizes protein, its function can affect drug distribution, particularly highly protein-bound drugs. Patients with cirrhosis or ascites may experience alterations in the volume of distribution.

Unlike renal insufficiency, hepatic dysfunction does not lend itself to reliable guidelines for adjusting drug dosage, partly because no noninvasive methods for estimating hepatic function exist (as compared to using creatinine clearance to estimate renal function) and partly because the liver has an enormous reserve capacity. Large amounts of liver tissue can be destroyed before physiologic changes appear.

As a basic principle, the half-life of a drug that is extensively metabolized in the liver will increase in patients with hepatic disease, depending on the extent of damage to the hepatic cells and blood flow in the liver. A patient with liver disease will require closer monitoring during the first few days of drug therapy.

Thyroid gland

Abnormal functioning of the thyroid gland can affect the metabolism of drugs. Patients with hypothyroidism or hyperthyroidism metabolize drugs at slower and faster rates, respectively. As drugs, surgery, or radiation brings patients to the euthyroid (normal thyroid function) state, metabolic rates adjust. For example, a hyperthyroid patient may require large doses of digoxin to maintain a therapeutic level. As the hyperthyroid state is treated, the patient's metabolism slows, as does clearance of the digoxin. When the patient becomes euthyroid, the digoxin dose must be decreased. Throughout the process, the nurse must closely monitor the patient.

Circulatory system

Alterations in the integrity of the circulatory system can affect the availability of drugs within the body. For a drug to act therapeutically, it must reach the site of action. Drug transport is hampered in patients with peripheral vascular disease, which can develop secondarily to diabetes mellitus, and atherosclerosis.

Shock, characterized by hypoperfusion throughout the body, can compromise circulation and significantly affect the administration and pharmacokinetics of emergency drugs. Emergency drugs should not be given intramuscularly to hypotensive patients because of the unpredictable muscle perfusion and consequent erratic absorption of the drug.

OTHER FACTORS

Physiologic factors that most determine and modify drug activity in a patient include age, genetics, gender, body build, and circadian variations.

Age

The level of organ function changes throughout life. Premature infants (less than 36 weeks gestational age), neonates (1st month of postnatal life), and infants (age 1 to 12 months) are extremely susceptible to the effects of drugs because of immature organ systems (especially the liver and kidneys), which significantly affect the metabolism and excretion of drugs. Elderly patients, with decreased organ function secondary to aging, are also susceptible to drug effects. The decline in renal function is one example of the effect of aging on normal physiologic functioning.

The percentage of total body water varies from 85% in a premature infant to 75% in a full-term infant, decreases to the adult value of 55% by age 12, and progressively decreases thereafter. Changes in total body water affect drug distribution and necessitate dosage adjustments. For example, neonates and infants require larger mg/kg doses of water-soluble aminoglycoside antibiotics than adults do.

Although total body water decreases with age, the percentage of body fat increases. A younger patient with less body fat obtains a higher plasma concentration of fat-soluble drug and a more rapid response than an older patient does. In patients with increased body fat, fat-soluble drugs are distributed more to tissues and less to plasma, resulting in delayed responses because of redistribution from tissue to plasma. Fat-soluble drugs include benzodiazepines, phenothiazines, and barbiturates.

The physician and the pregnant patient must give special consideration to the effects of drugs on the fetus. Highly fat-soluble drugs may cross the placenta to the fetus in significant amounts, sometimes producing undesirable effects or even birth defects (teratogenicity). A pregnant patient should avoid all unnecessary drugs, especially during the first 3 months.

Children. Because of immaturity and incomplete development of certain functions, children under age 12 metabolize some drugs in ways that cause unusual effects. For example, the adult stimulant methylphenidate (Ritalin) calms hyperactive children. Also, children metabolize phenobarbital at a faster rate than adults do, thus requiring larger doses to achieve the same effects. Theophylline is metabolized to caffeine in newborns, but very little is so metabolized in adults. (See Chapter 12, Intervention: The Pediatric Patient, for further discussions of the effects of drugs on children.)

Elderly. Disease or aging can decrease organ function in the elderly, altering a drug's pharmacokinetic properties (absorption, distribution, metabolism, and excretion). For example, because of altered pharmacokinetics, the elderly may demonstrate increased sensitivity to the effects of depressants on the central nervous system (CNS). Such sensitivity leads to a high incidence of oversedation and paradoxical psychotic reactions when elderly patients receive a usual adult dose of a sedative-hypnotic instead of a reduced dose. Similar effects occur with other sedatives and CNS depressants.

Genetics

Genetically determined variability in rates of acetylation (one of several drug metabolic pathways) can affect the therapeutic effects and adverse reactions produced by a drug. Procainamide (Procan SR, Pronestyl), an antiarrhythmic drug, is reduced to a metabolite that contributes to the drug's effects. Thus, the physician must consider both procainamide and its metabolite to calculate drug concentrations accurately, because a patient with a rapid acetylation rate may have low procainamide levels but adequate combined levels of procainamide and its metabolite.

Patients with a slow acetylation rate are at risk of developing toxic reactions to some drugs. For example, when receiving the antihypertensive hydralazine, they may develop antinuclear antibodies and a drug-induced form of systemic lupus erythematosus.

Lack of enzymes or coenzymes can also cause toxicity and alter therapeutic effects. For example, drugs that require glucose-6-phosphate dehydrogenase (G6PD) for metabolism can cause hemolytic anemia if given to patients lacking the enzyme. (G6PD deficiency is a hereditary defect commonly affecting the Mediterranean peoples and about 10% of American blacks.) Drugs requiring G6PD for metabolism include quinidine, an antiarrhythmic agent; sulfa antibiotics; and antimalarial agents such as primaquine and quinacrine.

Gender

Females generally possess a greater percentage of adipose tissue and a smaller percentage of total body water than males. As a result, they may require drug dosage alterations.

Body build

A patient's body build directly influences the drug dosage required. Muscle mass and fat content significantly affect drug activity.

Muscle. A decreased muscle mass leads to decreased production of creatinine from muscle breakdown. An overestimation of creatinine clearance in debilitated and elderly patients could lead to overdosing.

Fat. Lean body weight is important in determining doses of highly fat-soluble drugs; some drugs may require adjustments for obesity greater than 20% above ideal body weight. For example, doses of highly fat-soluble anesthetics may require adjustment in obese patients. The need for adjusted dosing of theophylline and aminoglycoside antibiotics in obese patients is a controversial issue; at the least, the nurse should carefully monitor the serum levels of such patients to ensure adequate therapy.

Circadian variations

Variations caused by circadian or daily rhythms may affect a patient's metabolic processes and responses to drug therapy. Researchers have noted recently that the pharmacokinetics of the hypnotic triazolam differed significantly in the daytime as compared to the evening, when the drug is normally administered: administered at night, it had a slower absorption rate and a longer half-life.

Concentration levels of cortisol vary according to the time of day. The highest concentration levels occur in early to mid-morning. This fact is clinically significant for hormone drugs, such as corticosteroids and thyroid drugs. For example, one daily corticosteroid dose given in early to mid-morning will minimize adrenal suppression and most closely mimic normal physiologic activity.

DRUG ADMINISTRATION

The route and timing of drug administration affect drug activity. (See Chapter 2, Pharmacokinetics, for a discussion of how the routes influence drug activity.)

The timing of drug administration is an important nursing responsibility, whether the nurse administers the drug or teaches the patient to self-administer it.

The dosing schedule of a drug can significantly influence the patient's response to therapy. Therapeutic serum levels of antibiotics, antiarrhythmics, and anticonvulsants must be maintained to achieve therapeutic effects. When these drugs are prescribed four times a day, the nurse should administer doses every 6 hours (q6h) to maintain therapeutic levels. If more time separates the last dose of the day from the first dose of the next day, the patient may experience breakthrough effects during the night. Evenly spaced dosing intervals are not as essential for drugs with extremely long half-lives, such as digoxin or levothyroxine; however, the nurse should encourage the patient on long-term therapy with such a drug to take the dose at the same time each day. Observing a regular dosing schedule also improves patient compliance.

Onset and duration of action

A drug's onset of action and duration of action depend largely upon the drug's pharmacologic characteristics, such as lipid solubility. The formulation of the drug and the route of administration can, however, alter the onset of action. (See Chapter 2, Pharmacokinetics, for further discussions of onset of action and duration of action.)

STABILITY OF PHARMACEUTICAL PREPARATIONS

To ensure that a drug is as potent and therapeutically effective as intended, the nurse must carefully observe expiration dates and follow storage recommendations provided by the manufacturer or pharmacy.

Expiration dates are required by federal regulations to appear on all drug containers. The regulations stipulate that at least 90% of the active ingredient must be available up to the expiration date, ensuring that patients do not receive drugs that are no longer therapeutically active or that have degraded to toxic compounds. Hospital pharmacists relabel expiration dates on oral drugs that are repackaged for hospital administration. Parenteral drugs are given new expiration dates after being reconstituted or mixed with intravenous fluids.

Drug storage can affect stability and, ultimately, therapeutic effectiveness. Drugs degrade more rapidly in warm, humid conditions. Tablets and capsules can usually be stored safely at room temperature, unless otherwise specified. Liquid dosage forms and injectable drugs sometimes require refrigeration. Some drugs must also be protected from light. For example, nitroglycerin should be stored in light-resistant bottles. The nurse should always check the label for storage requirements.

PSYCHOLOGICAL AND EMOTIONAL FACTORS

Besides the physiologic factors that affect drug activity, psychological and emotional factors are also at work. These include the placebo effect, patient compliance, and health beliefs. The nurse must consider these factors during drug therapy.

Placebo effect. Placebos are inert or inactive substances sometimes administered in place of drugs. Because they satisfy the patient's psychological need for a drug, placebos may actually elicit therapeutic responses. In one study, 35% of patients taking placebos experienced satisfactory pain relief. (See Chapter 8, Intervention: Administration Processes, for more information about placebos.)

Patient compliance. The nurse must carefully monitor compliance, particularly in the ambulatory adult patient with little supervision. Many factors influence a patient's conscious or unconscious decision to take drugs as prescribed. Patient education about drug therapy (preferably by the nurse, pharmacist, *and* physician) can significantly promote patient compliance. (See Chapter 16, Evaluation, for further discussion of compliance.)

Health beliefs. A patient's health beliefs reflect what the patient considers a normal healthy state and what the patient believes can be accomplished by medical care. A patient who does not perceive abdominal upset and cramping after every meal as abnormal probably will not seek medical atttention. Health beliefs vary among cultures, age-groups, and regions of the country and affect compliance, especially in patients with long-term diseases like hypertension who may never feel sick. The nurse should consider health beliefs when assessing a patient's condition and counseling patients and family members.

TOLERANCE AND DEPENDENCE

Tolerance, a patient's decreased response to a repeated drug dose, differs from dependence. A drug-dependent patient displays a physical or psychological need for the drug. For example, an alcohol-dependent patient not only needs increasing quantities of alcohol to achieve the same effects, but also risks physical and psychological withdrawal symptoms if the alcohol use is discontinued.

A cancer patient using a narcotic analgesic for severe pain can display both tolerance and dependence. However, the psychological aspects differ from those of the substance abuser. The cancer patient usually is concerned with maintaining a reasonable level of pain relief, whereas the substance abuser desires the euphoric effects of the drug. (See Chapter 6, Drug Abuse, Dependence, and Addiction, for more information about this concept.)

DRUG INTERACTIONS

Drug interactions may occur between drugs or between drugs and foods. They may involve prescribed drugs or over-the-counter (OTC) products. The nurse should always ask the patient specifically about the use of OTC products when obtaining the patient history because the patient may not realize that many OTC products contain drugs.

Drug interactions may interfere with the results of a laboratory test or produce physical or chemical incompatibilities. The more drugs a patient receives, the greater the probability of a drug interaction. The nurse should particularly monitor elderly patients, who are more sensitive to drug effects and often receive several medications. The average ambulatory patient over age 65 takes 2 to 3.4 medications each day, and approximately 25% of patients over age 65 are discharged from the hospital with 6 or more prescription drugs. (See Chapter 13, Intervention: The Geriatric Patient, for more information about drug effects on the elderly.)

INTERACTIONS BETWEEN DRUGS

Interactions involving two drugs usually produce a combined effect equal to the single most active component of the mixture. Such an interaction, called indifference, does not alter the therapeutic effects of either drug, nor does it produce any unpredictable adverse reactions.

Two or more drugs administered to a patient can also produce additive effects that are usually equivalent to the sum of the effects of either drug administered alone in higher doses. The concept of additive pharmacologic response is illustrated by the two analgesics acetaminophen and codeine. Acetaminophen 325 mg and codeine 30 mg are equal in analgesic effect. When combined, as in Codeine #3, their analgesic effect is the same as either acetaminophen 650 mg or codeine 60 mg. The advantages of giving the combination drug are lower doses of each drug can be given, decreasing the likelihood of adverse effects, and patients report a greater decrease in pain intensity than when one of these drugs is given alone. This is probably because they have different mechanisms of action.

A synergistic effect occurs when two drugs producing the same qualitative effect are combined to produce a greater response than either drug given alone. For example, ethanol depresses the CNS, leading to sedation and drowsiness. When ethanol and other drugs that have a CNS-depressant effect are combined, the sedative effect is enhanced and psychomotor skills are impaired. For that reason, patients taking barbiturates, benzodiazepines, or other drugs that cause drowsiness or sedation are cautioned against ingesting moderate to heavy amounts of ethanol.

An antagonistic drug interaction occurs when the combined response of two drugs is less than the response produced by either drug administered singly. Physicians prescribe levodopa to decrease the stiffness, rigidity, and other symptoms of Parkinson's disease. When pyridoxine (vitamin B_6) is combined with levodopa, levodopa's effects are reversed, or antagonized. This effect may occur because pyridoxine may enhance the metabolism of levodopa, making less drug available to the sites of action within the brain.

Pharmacokinetic interactions

Many drug interactions alter the pharmacokinetic characteristics of the drugs involved, including absorption, distribution, metabolism, and excretion.

Alterations in absorption. Two drugs given concurrently may change the rate or extent of absorption of one or both of the drugs. For example, the combination of antacids and the nonsteroidal anti-inflammatory drug naproxen slows the absorption rate of naproxen, but produces no effect on the total amount absorbed. This interaction does not require any dosage adjustments.

In contrast, antacids administered with the antibiotic tetracycline decrease the extent, or total amount, of tetracycline absorbed. To prevent this interaction, the nurse should space doses and avoid giving tetracycline within 1 to 2 hours of antacids.

Alterations in distribution. Concurrent administration of two drugs can alter the volume of distribution by changes in protein binding. For example, the oral anticoagulant warfarin (Coumadin) is highly protein-bound (>97%), and the nonsteroidal anti-inflammatory drug phenylbutazone (Butazolidin) successfully competes with warfarin for protein-binding sites. Combining these two drugs increases the amount of active warfarin available, which significantly increases the risk of bleeding in patients receiving both drugs.

Alterations in metabolism and excretion. Drug interactions can alter both the metabolism and excretion of the drugs. For example, in the antagonistic interaction between pyridoxine and levodopa, pyridoxine increases the metabolism of levodopa.

Barbiturates stimulate the hepatic microsomal enzymes, increasing the metabolism and excretion and decreasing the therapeutic effects of other drugs that are significantly metabolized in the liver. Tobacco smoke also stimulates the hepatic enzymes, causing faster theophylline metabolism and excretion in smokers than in nonsmokers. Propoxyphene (Darvon), a weak narcotic analgesic, is also metabolized faster in smokers than in nonsmokers. Rifampin is another drug noted for inducing hepatic metabolism.

Drug interactions affecting metabolism and excretion commonly lead to toxic levels of the inhibited drug. For example, the antiulcer drug cimetidine inhibits the hepatic metabolism of the bronchodilator theophylline, thereby decreasing theophylline metabolism and excretion and increasing theophylline's half-life and serum concentration levels. This interaction can result in toxic theophylline serum concentration levels if the theophylline doses are not adjusted.

Alterations in hepatic blood flow resulting from drug interactions and disease also affect drug metabolism and excretion. The antiulcer drug cimetidine reduces hepatic blood flow, as do chronic liver disease and cirrhosis. Decreased hepatic blood flow affects drugs, such as propranolol (Inderal), whose metabolism and excretion depend more on blood flow than on enzyme activity. Conversely, drugs whose metabolism and excretion depend on intrinsic enzyme activity are generally not affected by changes in hepatic blood flow.

Some drug interactions affect excretion only. For example, the interaction between the uricosuric drug probenecid (Benemid) and penicillin can produce therapeutic effects. Combining probenecid and penicillin decreases the renal excretion of penicillin and increases the drug's half-life and plasma concentration levels.

When therapy with the antiarrhythmic drug quinidine is initiated in patients already on digoxin, quinidine reduces the excretion of digoxin (primarily renal clearance) and may also displace digoxin from tissue binding sites. The interaction results in increased serum digoxin levels and must therefore be closely monitored to determine if dosage adjustments are necessary.

Pharmacodynamic interactions

Drug interactions also produce pharmacodynamic alterations. The synergistic interaction and the enhanced sedation produced by combining ethanol and barbiturates is an example of such a pharmacodynamic alteration.

Administered concurrently, the bronchodilator theophylline may sensitize pulmonary beta-adrenergic receptors, increasing response to beta-adrenergic agonists, such as terbutaline or albuterol.

When combined with opiates, the narcotic antagonist naloxone (Narcan) competes with opiates for opiate receptor sites. As a result, naloxone can reverse opiate-induced respiratory depression.

DRUG INTERACTIONS AND LABORATORY TESTS

Drug interactions can alter laboratory tests. Health care professionals assess renal function by using a laboratory test that measures serum creatinine levels. The test uses a colorimetric method. Many cephalosporins, such as cefazolin (Kefzol) and cefoxitin (Mefoxin), contain non-creatinine chromogens that are not differentiated by the colorimetric method. As a result, the laboratory test may overestimate the creatinine levels, possibly leading to inadequate drug dosages.

Physicians use guaiac testing of feces to check for the presence of occult, or unseen, blood. A positive guaiac stool indicates blood in the feces. Patients taking large amounts of iron supplements may produce false-positive results for this test.

Blood glucose testing is the preferred method of monitoring diabetes. However, some stable diabetic patients monitor their diabetes using urine testing for glucose. Drugs that interfere with urine glucose testing include cephalothin (Keflin), isoniazid, levodopa (Larodopa), probenecid (Benemid), and large amounts (1 to 2 grams/day) of ascorbic acid. False-positive results indicating high glucose levels could cause a patient to decrease sugar intake or to increase insulin doses when the blood glucose level is stable.

Drug effects on the EKG

Some drugs, particularly cardiac drugs, produce visible effects on the electrocardiogram (EKG) that can lead to misinterpreted results. For example, the antiarrhythmic quinidine can widen the QRS complex and prolong the Q-T interval. The prolongation of the Q-T interval can be up to 35% greater than the baseline value without representing toxicity. EKG changes of this significance require medical attention in patients not taking quinidine. The EKG also provides information about electrolyte imbalances that may be related to drug therapy.

DRUG AND FOOD INTERACTIONS

Interactions between drugs and food can produce alterations in the therapeutic effects of the drug or in the utilization of nutrients.

Alterations in bioavailability. Food can alter the rate and amount of drug absorbed from the GI tract. These alterations affect the bioavailability, the amount of a drug dose that is available to the systemic circulation. (See Chapter 2, Pharmacokinetics, for further discussion of bioavailability.) For example, the bioavailability of the antifungal drug griseofulvin increases when the drug is administered with a high-fat meal, and the bioavailability of theophylline increases with a low-protein, high-carbohydrate diet.

Drugs can also bind with foods and impair vitamin and mineral absorption. For example, cholestyramine (Questran), used to treat hyperlipidemia, forms a complex with folate, thereby decreasing the amount of folate available to the body. Absorption of vitamins A, D, and K is also lowered, and some patients may require vitamin supplements. Mineral oil, an emollient laxative, forms an insoluble complex with the fat-soluble vitamins A, E, D, and K. The insoluble complex passes through the gut before absorption can occur. Because fat-soluble vitamins help maintain skin integrity, the long-term excessive use of mineral oil can eventually interfere with wound healing.

Induction of enzymes. Some drugs induce or stimulate enzyme systems, and this induction increases both metabolic rates and the demand for vitamins that are enzyme cofactors. For example, in alcoholics, the increased demand for thiamine, a cofactor in the metabolism of alcohol, decreases serum levels and places alcoholics at high risk for thiamine deficiency and associated neurologic complications.

Alterations in sites of action. Broad-spectrum antibiotics interfere with vitamin K synthesis by altering the GI flora. Microorganisms in the colon are the normal sites for the GI production of vitamin K, important for coagulation. Prolonged use of broad-spectrum antibiotics kills the synthesizing microorganisms and can result in bleeding problems, especially in debilitated or elderly patients, if not accompanied by vitamin K supplements.

Increased toxicity. The antiacne drug isotretinoin (Accutane) is a structural isomer of vitamin A. Therefore, patients taking isotretinoin must avoid taking vitamin A supplements or increasing dietary vitamin A since vitamin A overdose is a risk.

Many foods also produce pharmacologic activities. For example, aged cheddar cheese and wine contain tyramine. A patient taking a monoamine oxidase inhibitor (an antidepressant) should avoid foods containing tyramine because intake of these foods could cause a release of catecholamines that are present in large amounts in nerve endings and the adrenal medulla, precipitating a hypertensive crisis.

INCOMPATIBILITIES OF PARENTERAL DRUGS

The nurse must carefully consider drug incompatibilities when administering drugs via parenteral (intravenous, intramuscular, or subcutaneous) routes. Drug incompatibility can produce either a physical reaction or a chemical inactivation.

Physically incompatible drugs interact before the drugs reach the site of action, usually interfering with the pharmacologic activity of one or both drugs. Mixing incompatible drugs can form precipitates or change a drug's color. Precipitate formation is especially dangerous for the patient if the solution is to be infused intravenously.

The anticonvulsant phenytoin is administered intravenously to control seizures in status epilepticus as well as those of unknown origin. The drug remains stable in an intravenous solution of normal saline (0.9% sodium chloride). However, when phenytoin is mixed with I.V. solutions of dextrose 5% in water, a cloudy, white precipitate forms. The precipitate also forms if the line from the dextrose-containing I.V. fluid is not flushed with saline solution before the nurse starts the phenytoin infusion.

Some light-sensitive drugs may change color if they are not protected. Whether the changed color indicates a decreased drug activity is not known. Usually, the nurse should not administer drugs that have changed color.

Exposing an aminoglycoside antibiotic (amikacin, gentamicin, tobramycin) to penicillins for a prolonged time inactivates the aminoglycoside. This chemical inactivation can occur: (1) if the two drugs are combined in the same I.V. administration bag, (2) if both drugs are being given to a patient with severe renal failure, and (3) if aminoglycoside blood levels drawn from a patient with renal failure are not assayed promptly. In the third instance, the inactivation by the penicillin results in lower reported serum levels of aminoglycoside and dosage adjustments that could be toxic.

MONITORING RESPONSE

The nurse can maintain an effective therapeutic drug regimen by understanding the prescribed drug and closely monitoring the patient. Knowing the biological half-life of a drug and the physiologic factors that may alter the half-life enables the nurse to understand the appropriate dosing interval for a patient.

When developing a drug therapy that will not interfere with the patient's life-style, the nurse must also consider the adverse reactions of the drug, which can lead to noncompliance. For example, hypertensive patients who operate vehicles or heavy machinery on the job may choose not to take antihypertensives that cause drowsiness and CNS disturbances. Knowledge of adverse reactions is also necessary for accurate patient monitoring and effective patient education.

Therapeutic drug monitoring. For drugs with low therapeutic indices, toxic and therapeutic levels are close. When the therapeutic response and toxicity of a drug can be related to serum concentrations, the nurse uses serum drug concentration levels to monitor drug therapy.

Obtaining samples for plasma drug concentration levels

The nurse may be responsible for drawing blood samples from the patient for drug level analysis. The following represents therapeutic and toxic levels or some commonly administered drugs. Values may differ from institution to institution.

DRUG	HALF-LIFE	TIME REQUIRED TO ACHIEVE STEADY STATE	TIME TO DRAW SAMPLE	ADULT THERAPEUTIC RANGE	POTENTIALLY TOXIC LEVELS
Antibiotics					
amikacin kanamycin gentamicin netilmicin tobramycin	0.5 to 3 hours (<30 years) 1.5 to 15 hours (>30 years)	2.5 to 15 hours (<30 years) 7.5 to 15 hours (>30 years)	Trough: before dose Peak concentration level: 15 to 30 min after I.V. dose; 1 hour after I.M. dose	Amikacin, kanamycin: 7.5 to 10 mcg/ml 20 to 30 mcg/ml Gentamicin, netilmicin, tobramycin: 0.5 to 2 mcg/ml 4 to 10 mcg/ml	Trough: Amikacin, kanamycin: >10 mcg/ml Gentamicin, netilmicin, tobramycin: >2 mcg/ml Peak concentration level: Amikacin, kanamycin: >30 mcg/ml Gentamicin, netilmicin, tobramycin: >10 mcg/ml
Anticonvulsants					
carbamazepine	5 to 27 hours	>2 weeks	Trough: before dose Peak concentration level: 3 hours after dose	4 to 12 mcg/ml	Single drug regimen: >12 mcg/ml Multiple drug regimen: >8 mcg/ml
phenobarbital	50 to 120 hours	10 to 25 days	4 hours after dose	15 to 40 mcg/ml	>40 mcg/ml
phenytoin (Dilantin only)	20 to 40 hours	1 to 2 weeks	Trough: before dose Peak concentration level: oral, 3 to 9 hours; I.V., 2 to 4 hours	10 to 20 mcg/ml	>20 mcg/ml
Cardiovascular Drugs					
digoxin	1.6 days	1 to 2 weeks	5 to 8 hours after dose	0.8 to 2 ng/ml	>2 ng/ml
lidocaine	75 to 140 min	6 to 12 hours	12 hours after starting I.V. drip or toxicity suspected	1.5 to 5 mcg/ml	>5 mcg/ml
quinidine	6 to 8 hours	30 to 35 hours	Trough: before next dose	2.3 to 5 mcg/ml	>5 mcg/ml
Respiratory Drugs					
theophylline	4.4 hours (smoker) 8.7 to 16 hours (nonsmoker)	1 to 2 days	Peak concentraton level: 2 hours (solution/solid dosage); 4 to 6 hours (slow-release dosage); 12 hours after start of I.V. infusion, then every 24 hours	10 to 20 mcg/ml	>20 mcg/ml

Drug level analysis. When serum or plasma concentration levels need to be drawn for drug monitoring, the nurse should refer to a current laboratory manual for appropriate procedures and therapeutic levels. Such specifics as when to draw blood or infuse drugs and how to draw blood for monitoring after intravenous infusion are covered there. (See *Obtaining samples for plasma drug concentration levels* on page 67 for a summary of this information as it relates to some commonly administered drugs.)

To interpret drug levels accurately, the nurse must understand peak concentration (time when drug absorption and drug elimination are equal), blood level of a drug, and steady-state duration of action. (See Chapter 2, Pharmacokinetics, for more details about these concepts.)

NURSING IMPLICATIONS

The effective, safe use of drugs in treating diseases requires the cooperation of all those involved, including the patient, physician, pharmacist, and nurse. The nurse must be able to apply knowledge about which drugs are used to prevent, diagnose, and treat a disease in specific patient situations. The nurse must also know the goals of the prescribed therapy, its benefits and adverse effects, and its pharmacotherapeutic measurement.

The nurse should base assessments, planning, interventions, and evaluations relating to pharmacotherapeutics on scientific data about a drug and on a comprehensive patient drug history. The nurse needs to know how each drug is absorbed, distributed, metabolized, and excreted by the body, as well as the various factors that can alter these processes. With knowledge of these processes, the nurse can anticipate and possibly halt any adverse reactions and can accurately assess each drug's effectiveness. Because no one can know everything about every drug, the nurse must be conscientious in consulting current reference books and research findings as well as asking questions of peers when unsure about anything related to the patient's therapy.

The drug therapy of a patient needs to be integrated into the nursing process and become a part of the total plan of care. The nurse must exercise objectivity and sensitivity when administering drugs and relating to patients.

Questions to ask

Asking the patient or family to repeat information can help you assess their understanding of drug information. Important points to emphasize are:
● Why is the drug being given?
● How does the drug work? What are the drug's expected effects?
● What are the symptoms of possible adverse drug reactions or ineffective drug therapy?
● Which route of drug administration are you going to use?
● When should you take your drug?
● Should you avoid over-the-counter medications during your drug therapy? If yes, why?
● Should you avoid any foods that could result in decreased therapeutic effect(s) or increased toxicity? If yes, which ones?
● Should you check the labels on foods and drugs? If yes, why?

ASSESSMENT

Carefully assessing the patient's problem and the options for therapy helps establish the most effective, appropriate care. To do so, the nurse follows these steps:
1. Obtain a drug history before administering any drug. The patient should include any drugs currently being used (prescription drugs, OTC drugs, vitamins, tobacco, marijuana, alcohol, coffee, tea, cola, and home remedies). The patient should also mention any exposure to chemicals and pollutants.
2. Assess the patient's expectations of drug therapy.
3. Assess the patient's level of compliance with previous drug regimens.
4. Assess the appropriateness of the prescribed drug and dosage for the patient's condition. Consider:
● What should the drug prevent, diagnose, or treat?
● Is the prescribed dose within recommended, safe limits?
● Is the prescribed route compatible with the patient's condition?
● Is the drug compatible with other drugs the patient is taking? If a probable drug interaction exists, notify the physician before administering the prescribed drug.
● Does the patient have any diseases that affect drug absorption, distribution, metabolism, or excretion?
5. Assess the risks and benefits of the drug therapy as well as its cost and probable patient compliance.
6. Formulate a nursing diagnosis that relates to the drug therapy and reflects the strengths and weaknesses of the patient and family.

PLANNING

Having completed the assessment, the nurse then develops a plan of care for the patient. The nurse includes the following:

1. Assist the patient and family in formulating realistic goals related to the prescribed drug therapy.

2. Collaborate with the physician, pharmacist, and patient when selecting the regimen best suited to the socioeconomic factors, life-style, likes and dislikes, physiologic condition, and psychological state of the patient and family.

3. Consider possible interactions between the prescribed drug and food or other drugs, the effects of the prescribed therapy on any necessary laboratory tests, and any drug's incompatibilities with parenteral drugs.

4. Institute precautions to ensure patient safety during drug therapy, such as checking the patient's pulse or blood pressure or raising the side rails on the patient's bed.

5. Incorporate specific assessment and surveillance times into the care plan, especially for a drug with a narrow therapeutic range.

INTERVENTIONS

The following general guidelines can be applied to the specific interventions devised for a patient's drug therapy:

1. Administer drugs accurately and safely, correlating the route of administration and the therapeutic effects with the patient's condition and ability to take drugs.

2. Implement a patient-teaching plan that includes the cognitive (acquiring new knowledge), the psychomotor (acquiring skill in drug administration), and the affective (interests, likes, dislikes, values, attitudes, and beliefs). (See Chapter 11, Intervention: Patient Education, for more information.)

• Present cognitive drug information at a level the patient and family can understand. Encourage questions about the prescribed drug regimen, potential adverse reactions, and the influence of the drug therapy on life-style. Check to see that the patient understands these matters. (See *Questions to ask.*)

• Teach the patient or family the skills of safe drug administration. Using teaching aids, such as charts, films, and models, can help. Then have the patient demonstrate the drug administration skills.

• Help design a drug regimen that the patient understands and appreciates—one that incorporates the patient's likes, dislikes, beliefs, and attitudes as it presents the route of administration, dosing schedule, and dosage formulations. As part of the teaching plan, verify with the patient that appropriate follow-up evaluations (lab-

oratory tests, blood levels, and examinations) are scheduled and that the patient understands the importance of these evaluations.

EVALUATION

Evaluation is a major component of the nurse's role and includes the following activities:

1. Evaluate the subjective and objective data related to the effectiveness of the drug therapy. Include in the evaluation predictable, unpredictable, adverse, and beneficial effects.

2. Evaluate the patient's progress in meeting the identified goals (outcome criteria) related to the drug therapy.

3. Correlate the patient's response to therapy with drug plasma levels when appropriate.

4. Evaluate the patient's compliance with the drug regimen. If the patient is noncompliant, help the patient to identify the causes.

5. Maintain an ongoing evaluation, and modify the care plan as necessary to meet the changing needs of the patient.

CHAPTER SUMMARY

Chapter 4 explored pharmacotherapeutics, using drugs to treat diseases. The chapter began by defining therapeutics and its relationship to the nursing process. Here are highlights:

• Patients may receive acute, empiric, supportive, palliative, maintenance, supplemental, or replacement therapy—depending on the severity, urgency, and prognosis of the patient's condition.

• Drugs are used to prevent, diagnose, or treat diseases; some, for more than one purpose.

• A physician considers many factors when selecting a drug for a patient, including an analysis of the drug's risks and benefits, the likelihood of patient compliance, and the cost of drugs and therapy.

• The therapeutic index of a drug represents the ratio between its effective and toxic plasma concentration levels.

• Certain diseases of the GI, renal, hepatic, and circulatory systems and of the thyroid gland affect the absorption, distribution, metabolism, and excretion of drugs. These diseases may necessitate dosage adjustments. Age, genetics, weight, gender, body build, and circadian variations also affect a patient's response to a drug. The very young and the elderly are most susceptible to these alterations.

• The nurse should always check the expiration date before administering any drug. The nurse and patient should follow the manufacturer's suggestions for storage of the drug.

• Patient compliance and a patient's health beliefs significantly affect the results of drug therapy.

• A patient who develops drug tolerance requires more of the drug to produce the same effect. A drug-dependent patient displays a physical or psychological need for the drug.

• Drug interactions involve other drugs or food and can affect laboratory test results. The nurse should carefully monitor the patient for all these interactions. Interactions between drugs alter the absorption, distribution, metabolism, and excretion of the drug. Interactions between a drug and food alter the bioavailability of the drug.

• Incompatibilities between parenteral drugs can interfere with the pharmacologic activity of one or both drugs or chemically inactivate the drugs.

• The nurse must consider all the factors that affect the pharmacotherapeutic action of a drug and patient responses to drug therapy when developing and implementing a care plan.

BIBLIOGRAPHY

American Hospital Formulary Service. *Drug Information 87.* Edited by McEvoy, G.K. Bethesda, Md.: American Society of Hospital Pharmacists, 1987.

American Medical Association. *Drug Evaluations,* 6th ed. Philadelphia: W.B. Saunders Co., 1986.

Braunwald, E., et al., eds. *Harrison's Principles of Internal Medicine,* 11th ed. New York: McGraw-Hill Book Co., 1986.

Clark, D.W.J. "Genetically Determined Variability in Acetylation and Oxidation: Therapeutic Implications," *Drugs* 29:342, April 1985.

Gilman, A.G., et al. *Goodman and Gilman's The Pharmacological Basis of Therapeutics,* 7th ed. New York: Macmillan Publishing Co., 1985.

Green, L.W., et al. "Programs to Reduce Drug Errors in the Elderly: Direct and Indirect Evidence from Patient Education," *Journal of Geriatric Drug Therapy* 1:3, Fall 1986.

Hansten, P.D. *Drug Interactions,* 5th ed. Philadelphia: Lea & Febiger, 1985.

Katcher, B.S., et al. *Applied Therapeutics: The Clinical Use of Drugs,* 3rd ed. San Francisco: Applied Therapeutics, Inc., 1983.

Knoben, J.E., and Anderson, P.O. *Handbook of Clinical Drug Data,* 5th ed. Hamilton, Ill.: Drug Intelligence Publications, Inc., 1983.

Nimmo, W.S. "Drugs, Diseases and Altered Gastric Emptying," in *Handbook of Clinical Pharmacokinetics.* Edited by Gibaldi, M., and Prescott, L. New York: ADIS Health Science Press, 1983.

Oversen, L. "Drugs and Vitamin Deficiency," *Drugs* 18:278, October 1979.

Pucino, F., et al. "Pharmacogeriatrics," *Pharmacotherapy* 5:314, November/December, 1985.

Ravel, R. *Clinical Laboratory Medicine: Clinical Application of Laboratory Data,* 4th ed. Chicago: Year Book Medical Publishers, 1984.

Roe, D.A. *Drug-Induced Nutritional Deficiencies,* 2nd ed. Westport, Conn.: Avi Publishing Co. Inc., 1985.

Smith, R.B., et al. "Temporal Variation in Triazolam Pharmacokinetics and Pharmacodynamics after Oral Administration," *Journal of Clinical Pharmacology* 26:120, February 1986.

Vessell, E.S. "On the Significance of Host Factors that Affect Drug Disposition," *Clinical Pharmacology and Therapeutics* 31:1, January 1982.

Wilkinson, G.R. "Influence of Hepatic Disease on Pharmacokinetics," in *Applied Pharmacokinetics: Principles of Therapeutic Drug Monitoring,* 2nd ed. Edited by Evans, W.E., et al. San Francisco: Applied Therapeutics, Inc., 1986.

CHAPTER 5

TOXICITY AND POISONING

OBJECTIVES

After reading and studying this chapter, you should be able to:

1. Discuss how genetic variations, drug characteristics, and exogenous factors can predispose a patient to adverse drug reactions.

2. Provide examples of each of the predisposing factors.

3. Differentiate between predictable and unpredictable adverse drug reactions.

4. Describe the nurse's role in treating the patient for adverse drug reactions.

5. Describe frequent causes of acute poisoning among infants, children, preteens, adolescents, adults, and the elderly.

6. Describe the nurse's role in assessing, managing, and preventing acute poisoning.

7. Discuss methods used to treat complications of acute poisoning.

INTRODUCTION

Along with the growing use of drugs that improve life and health has come an increasing incidence of adverse drug reactions and poisonings. This development has occurred primarily because every drug can be toxic. This chapter covers specific types of drug toxicity, including adverse drug reactions and acute poisoning. Drug-specific adverse reactions are covered in other chapters. (See Chapter 4, Pharmacotherapeutics, for a discussion of drug interactions, and Chapter 6, Drug Abuse, Dependence, and Addiction, for information on the toxic effects of abused substances.)

ADVERSE DRUG REACTIONS

An adverse drug reaction is a harmful, undesirable patient response to a specific drug therapy; it may result from any clinically useful drug. Adverse drug reactions can range from mild ones that disappear when the drug is discontinued to debilitating diseases that become chronic. Some adverse reactions are predictable and may be preventable with careful prescription and administration practices or may be inseparable from a particular drug's primary therapeutic effects. Others are unpredictable. In this era of sophisticated, complex pharmacotherapy, physicians and nurses must be alert to and know how to respond to adverse drug reactions. (See *Common adverse drug reactions* on page 72, which lists adverse reactions to some widely used drugs and drug classes.)

Although physicians, nurses, and pharmacists cannot always predict who will experience an adverse drug reaction, they can identify factors that increase the patient's risk and may prevent or minimize the patient's adverse response.

FACTORS THAT LEAD TO ADVERSE DRUG REACTIONS

A patient's therapeutic responses to a drug result from the interplay among patient characteristics, drug characteristics, and exogenous (external) factors. Patient, drug, and exogenous factors can alter that interplay to produce adverse drug reactions, as this section illustrates.

Predisposing patient factors

These include extremes of age, extremes of body weight, genetic variations, temperament and attitudes, circadian

Common adverse drug reactions

This chart correlates certain adverse reactions and the drug or drug groups that cause that reaction.

ADVERSE REACTIONS	DRUGS INVOLVED
Rashes, hives, lesions	penicillin, sulfonamides, thiazide diuretics
Hemolytic anemia, thrombocytopenia, agranulocytosis	quinidine, meprobamate, chlorpromazine, phenylbutazone
Hepatitis, biliary obstruction, hepatic necrosis	tetracycline, halothane, acetaminophen
Glomerulonephritis, acute and chronic renal failure	aminoglycoside antibiotics, aspirin
Blurred vision, blindness, cataract development, corneal and retinal changes	chloroquine, phenothiazines, corticosteroids
Deafness, dizziness, loss of balance, tinnitus	salicylates, quinine, aminoglycoside antibiotics
Delirium, disorientation, lethargy	hypnotics, sedatives, antidepressants
Psychomotor retardation, subjective feelings of loss and sadness	reserpine, corticosteroids, methyldopa, indomethacin
Birth defects, fetal and neonatal functional abnormalities	antineoplastic drugs, narcotics, isotretinoin

rhythms, changes associated with disease status, and changes associated with pregnancy.

Extremes of age. The absorption, distribution, metabolism, and excretion of drugs are different in infants and elderly patients than in young adults. Infants lack certain drug-metabolizing enzymes and have decreased renal blood flow. These physiologic factors increase drug and metabolite blood levels. The breast-feeding infant also may develop adverse reactions to drugs that pass into the mother's breast milk (see Chapter 14, Intervention: The Pregnant or Lactating Patient, for specific drugs that pass into breast milk). Elderly patients have decreased blood flow to all organs, especially hepatic and renal blood flow. These conditions result in increased drug concentration levels as well as changes in drug distribution and greater risk of toxicity.

Extremes of body weight. Recommended dosages are typically based on the average-sized adult. Therefore, the extremely thin or obese patient requires an individualized dosage calculation to prevent overdosing or underdosing. Abnormal thinness or obesity may alter drug distribution, resulting in either higher- or lower-than-expected drug concentration levels in tissues and at receptor sites.

Genetic variations. Genetic variations that alter enzyme activity or cause enzyme deficiency affect drug metabolism or drug action. For example, isoniazid, hydralazine, and procainamide are metabolized in the liver by a pathway known as acetylation, a process that proceeds at a partially genetically-determined rate. Most patients are either fast or slow acetylators. A slow acetylator will display a higher blood level of a given drug dose than a fast acetylator and may experience an adverse drug reaction as a result. Glucose-6-phosphate dehydrogenase (G6PD) plays a vital role in red blood cell stability; its deficiency is an inherited enzyme defect that alters the action of drugs. In a patient with a deficiency of this stabilizing enzyme, aspirin and other drugs can precipitate hemolysis. (See *Genetic variations* for a list of such variations, their frequency, the drugs involved, and the usual adverse reactions to them.)

An inherited predisposition to allergies increases the patient's risk of an allergic response to a drug. Especially at risk is the patient with a history of eczema, angioedema, asthma, hay fever or hives. (See the discussion of drug allergy on page 75 for more information on allergic responses to drugs.)

Temperament and attitudes. Psychological factors and personal values and beliefs can predispose a patient to adverse drug reactions. For example, patients who exhibit emotional, excitable, and hypochondriacal behavior may report adverse drug reactions more frequently than patients without these psychological factors. Attitudes can shape a patient's patterns of drug taking and can lead to erratic and unsafe self-medication. The patient also may feel community and cultural pressures when interpreting drug effects and reporting undesirable reactions. Patient expectations of a drug's action also can affect response. These patient characteristics can affect both the incidence of self-diagnosed adverse reactions and the frequency and thoroughness of reporting patterns.

Circadian rhythms. Normal physiologic rhythms can influence drug action and lead to adverse drug reactions. Research suggests that normal human biological rhythms can alter the absorption, metabolism, and excretion of certain drugs. Researchers are studying the contribution of sleep rhythms, hormone secretion, urinary excretion, and other regulatory processes to drug effectiveness and adverse drug reactions.

Changes associated with disease. Pathophysiologic changes associated with various diseases may cause adverse drug reactions. Diseases of organs responsible for drug absorption, metabolism, and excretion can alter drug actions and effects. For instance, cirrhosis of the liver may alter a drug's pharmacokinetic properties, especially its metabolism, thereby leading to abnormal drug concentration levels in the system.

Diseases also can alter physiologic states unfavorably. For example, hypoalbuminemia can alter the availability of protein-binding drugs by decreasing the number of available plasma protein-binding sites. As a result, the drug's distribution, binding, and excretion are altered.

Genetic variations

This chart lists genetic variations, their frequency, the drugs that the variations affect, and the patient's probable adverse reactions. The nurse must realize the importance that genetic variations play in the patient's response to certain drugs.

GENETIC VARIATION	FREQUENCY	AFFECTED DRUGS	ADVERSE REACTION
Slow acetylation	50% of U.S. population	isoniazid, phenelzine, dapsone, hydralazine	Polyneuritis
Decreased cholinesterase	Approximately 1 in 2,500 patients	succinylcholine	Apnea
Warfarin insensitivity	Rare	warfarin	Insufficient anticoagulation response to usual drug dose
Glaucoma	Common	corticosteroids	Increased intraocular pressure
Malignant hyperthermia	Approximately 1 in 20,000 anesthetized patients	such anesthetics as halothane, succinylcholine, methoxyflurane, ether, cyclopropane	Severe hyperpyrexia, muscle rigidity, death
Unstable hemoglobin Zurich	Rare	sulfonamides	Hemolysis
Unstable hemoglobin H	Rare	sulfisoxazole	Hemolysis
Glucose-6-phosphate dehydrogenase (G6PD) deficiency	Common in persons of African, Mediterranean, or Asiatic origin	analgesics, sulfonamides, antimalarials, nitrofurantoin, other drugs	Hemolysis

Adapted from Harrisons Principles of Internal Medicine, 11th ed., (New York: McGraw-Hill Book Company, 1987) with permission of the publisher.

Changes associated with pregnancy. Although numerous physiologic changes occur in pregnancy, the pregnant patient is not necessarily at higher risk for adverse drug reactions. However, pregnant patients can experience decreased serum concentration levels of drugs such as anticonvulsants, necessitating dosage adjustments. Changes in drug distribution and excretion rates probably produce the decrease in serum concentration levels.

During a patient's pregnancy, physicians and nurses are concerned with the potential adverse effects of drugs on the fetus. While many drugs cross the placenta, the type of drug, its concentration level, and fetal age determine the potential for adverse reactions in the fetus. (See Chapter 14, Intervention: The Pregnant or Lactating Patient, for further information on this subject.)

Predisposing drug factors
Several drug factors influence adverse reactions, including bioavailability, additives, degradation, dosage, administation, and the number of drugs administered.

Bioavailability, additives, and drug degradation. Among different brands of the same drug, bioavailability may vary because of manufacturing processes. Differences in onset of action, peak serum concentration levels, and duration of action among different products may lead to adverse drug reactions. The physician and pharmacist must exercise caution when substituting different forms of antiepileptic drugs, anticoagulants, digitalis, and endocrine agents.

Dyes, buffering preparations, stabilizing agents, and other additives can produce adverse drug reactions in certain patients. When an additive produces widespread problems, the manufacturers may reformulate the product by removing the offending substance or substituting a less toxic compound.

Although uncommon, adverse drug reactions can occur when a patient uses a drug after its expiration date or uses one that has been stored in an unfavorable environment.

Drug dosage factors. Patients receiving higher dosages for longer periods of time usually have an increased probability for an adverse reaction. For example, patients who take the antihypertensive hydralazine are more likely to develop drug-induced lupus erythematosus when the dosage is greater than 200 mg P.O./daily and the therapy lasts longer than 6 months.

Administration routes and techniques. Parenteral drug administration, especially intravenous, causes more frequent adverse reactions than other administration routes. A parenterally administered drug does not have to be absorbed through the gastrointestinal (GI) tract before distribution into the blood, which makes it more quickly available at receptor sites. Toxicity and hypersensitivity occur more frequently in these circumstances.

Drugs are made for safe administration via designated routes. Administration via unrecommended routes may cause adverse drug reactions. For example, instilling an otic solution into the eye may cause pain and irritation because the otic solution is not formulated to the pH of the eye. Suspensions intended for intramuscular or subcutaneous use may be lethal if administered intravenously.

Even when the appropriate route is used, improper administration can cause adverse drug reactions. For example, administering some intravenous drugs too rapidly can alter distribution and produce a toxic response. Administering an excessive amount intramuscularly may cause tissue necrosis.

Number of drugs administered. The risk of adverse drug reactions increases in direct relationship to the number of drugs administered to the patient. Complex interactions between drugs also may minimize some therapeutic effects and enhance others. (See Chapter 4, Pharmacotherapeutics, for the specific dynamics of drug interactions.)

Predisposing exogenous factors
Dietary and environmental factors also influence a patient's predisposition to adverse drug reactions.

Dietary factors. Substances in foods may interfere with the activity of certain drugs. For example, tyramine in some cheeses, beer, and red wine can precipitate a hypertensive crisis when ingested while a patient is taking monoamine oxidase inhibitors. Green leafy vegetables may interfere with oral anticoagulants because of their high vitamin K content.

Dietary factors can also influence the pharmacokinetics of a drug. Certain foods, such as charcoal-broiled meats, vegetables from the *Brassica* family (cabbage and broccoli), and those containing caffeine can stimulate the activity of liver enzymes, thereby increasing drug metabolism rate.

A poor diet resulting in malnutrition also can alter drug action by impairing microsomal enzyme activity. For example, the effects of some barbiturates are prolonged in patients with protein malnutrition. The presence of food in the patient's stomach can alter drug absorption. Tetracycline absorption is decreased by food; carbamazepine absorption is increased. Foods can bind drugs and delay gastric emptying times.

Environmental factors. A patient's environment may influence the relationship between physiologic function and drug effects and contribute to adverse reactions. Pesticides, tobacco, and alcohol may alter the pharmacokinetics of certain drugs and increase the patient's risk of adverse drug reactions.

CLASSIFICATION OF ADVERSE DRUG REACTIONS

The various adverse drug reactions can be grouped as predictable, which are usually dose-related, or unpredictable, which are usually related to patient sensitivity.

Predictable adverse drug reactions

Most adverse drug reactions result from the known pharmacologic effects of a drug and are typically dose-related. Therefore, the physician and nurse can predict them in most cases.

Excessive therapeutic effect. Such effects occur most frequently from miscalculations and overdose of a drug that requires precise, individualized dose calculation. For example, a diabetic patient being treated with insulin may easily experience hypoglycemia from even a slight miscalculation of the insulin dose.

Secondary reactions. A drug typically produces not only a major therapeutic effect, but also additional and inseparable secondary pharmacologic actions that can be adverse. For example, morphine for pain control may lead to two undesirable secondary effects: constipation and respiratory depression. Physicians occasionally employ drugs for their secondary pharmacologic effects. For example, the physician may prescribe an antihistamine, typically used for allergies, to induce sleep because the secondary reaction of an antihistamine is drowsiness from CNS depression.

Hypersusceptibility to pharmacologic actions. Some patients are extremely susceptible to either the primary or secondary pharmacologic actions of a drug. Even when given a usual therapeutic dose, a hypersusceptible patient can experience an excessive therapeutic response or augmented secondary effects. Hypersuscep-

tibility frequently results from altered pharmacokinetics, which leads to higher-than-expected drug serum concentration levels. Increased receptor sensitivity also may increase the patient's response to therapeutic or adverse effects.

Overdose toxicity. Most drugs produce toxicity if given in large enough doses, or when drug concentration levels exceed the threshold needed for therapeutic effect. Predictable toxic effects may result from the local accumulation of a drug, as when chemotherapeutic agents accumulate in and damage hair follicle cells, which leads to alopecia (hair loss). Systemic drug effects also can produce predictable toxicity. For example, rapid I.V. administration of aminophylline can precipitate severe hypotension and circulatory collapse.

Toxic effects may seriously damage tissues and organs and precipitate drug-induced diseases. Such conditions result from treatment with a variety of drugs and can lead to serious, long-lasting health problems. Toxic effects may cause only transient changes in affected organs or more serious, irreversible changes, such as the tardive dyskinesias associated with antipsychotic therapy. Such effects can be more serious than the original illness.

Unpredictable adverse drug reactions

A less common type of adverse reaction, neither dose-related nor predictable, results from a patient's unusual and extreme sensitivity to a drug or its components. These unpredictable adverse reactions arise from unique tissue response rather than from an extension or alteration of the expected pharmacologic action. Extreme patient sensitivity may be manifested as a drug allergy or as an idiosyncratic response.

Drug allergy. Occasionally, a patient's immunologic system identifies a drug, a drug metabolite, or a drug contaminant as a dangerous foreign substance that must be neutralized or destroyed. Previous exposure to the drug or to one with similar chemical characteristics sensitizes the patient's immune system, and subsequent exposure mobilizes the system and causes an allergic reaction (hypersensitivity). An allergic reaction not only directly injures cells and tissues, but also produces broader systemic damage by initiating cellular release of vasoactive and inflammatory substances.

A drug allergy can be categorized according to the underlying immunologic mechanism it provokes. The adverse reaction may vary in intensity from an immediate, life-threatening anaphylactic reaction to penicillin, to a contact dermatitis secondary to the topical application of a neomycin cream.

Idiosyncratic response. Unpredictable adverse drug reactions that do not result from known pharmacologic properties of a drug or from patient allergy but are peculiar to the patient are called idiosyncratic responses. For example, a patient may experience nervousness and excitability after ingesting phenobarbital, normally a tranquilizing agent. A patient's idiosyncratic response sometimes has a genetic cause.

ADVERSE DRUG REACTIONS: THE NURSE'S ROLE

Drug treatment is a significant part of therapies used to cure disease, manage symptoms, and alleviate discomfort. Because the potential for adverse reactions accompanies virtually all drug administration, the nurse must act to minimize their likelihood and manage any that develop.

The nurse must learn about the patient, drug, and situational factors that increase the patient's risk. The nurse can routinely identify a variety of predisposing factors during the assessment phase of the nursing process. Information obtained from the patient's physical assessment and history enables the nurse to collaborate with the physician during the prescriptive phase and later should modifications in the patient's drug regimen be necessary. The nurse's, physician's, and pharmacist's knowledgeable analysis of patient, drug, and situational factors helps determine a therapeutic regimen with the least potential for triggering adverse drug reactions.

The nurse also helps by educating the patient and family about a drug. The nurse should teach the patient and family the effects of a prescribed drug, the details of its administration, and any necessary precautions. The patient who understands correct dose, route, timing, and required precautions can minimize the risk of adverse drug reactions.

Despite meticulous assessment and precautions, the nurse cannot prevent all adverse drug reactions. Should a patient experience an adverse reaction, the nurse assumes responsibility for its early detection and management of symptoms. Because of frequent, close contact with the patient, the nurse is usually the first to detect signs and symptoms. By quickly and accurately reporting the evolving problem to the physician, the nurse ensures prompt attention to necessary changes in the drug regimen and efforts to control or treat the adverse reactions.

At times, the patient must tolerate adverse reactions as part of drug therapy, as when a drug that can cure a disease or maintain life causes unavoidable reactions. In such circumstances, the nurse can develop interventions to offset or minimize patient discomfort. Common adverse reactions that the nurse will encounter in patients include anorexia, nausea and vomiting, itching, constipation, and diarrhea.

The nurse has an essential role in preventing, detecting, and treating adverse drug reactions. By working closely with the physician, the patient, and the patient's family, the nurse can ensure more precise, individualized prescription; more knowledgeable and accurate administration practices; and the most comfortable and safest course of drug treatment possible.

ACUTE POISONING

Despite an extensive campaign against it, poisoning remains a serious problem in the United States. The National Clearinghouse for Poison Control Centers estimates that 2 to 3 million poisonings occur annually, resulting in approximately 5,000 deaths.

Although some poisonings result from the intentional ingestion of toxic substances and others from homicidal actions, most incidents are accidental. Drug ingestion, often in conjunction with alcohol, frequently causes accidental poisoning as does the ingestion of household substances used for cleaning and maintenance. Industrial poisonings from environmental pollutants, pesticides, and radioactive substances pose a growing threat.

Patterns of poisoning vary according to age. Poisoning in children under age 1 typically results from an accidental drug overdose administered by parents. Exploration and experimentation by toddlers and preschoolers lead to poisonings not only from prescription and over-the-counter drugs, but from almost any other substance that can be ingested. The most common agents involved in poisonings in children are aspirin, insecticides, plants, soaps, detergents, bleaches, and solvent cleaners. Older children, vulnerable to peer pressure, may ingest poisonous substances on a dare or as part of an evolving pattern of drug and alcohol abuse.

Antidotes for selected poisons

This chart outlines potential poisons, their antidotes, and how each antidote works to remove or neutralize the poison.

POISON	ANTIDOTE	TYPE AND EFFECT OF ANTIDOTE
strychnine	diazepam, barbiturates	Physiologic antagonists: offset central nervous system stimulation
methanol	ethanol	Dispositional antidote: slows formation of toxic products
	sodium bicarbonate	Physiologic antagonist: offsets acidosis
narcotics and derivatives	naloxone	Receptor antidote: displaces narcotic from receptor
anticholinesterases (organophosphates)	atropine	Receptor antidote: blocks muscarinic receptors
	pralidoxime	Dispositional antagonist: reactivates cholinesterase
anticholinergics	physostigmine	Receptor antidote: blocks receptors
acetaminophen	acetylcysteine	Dispositional antagonist: hastens detoxification
carbon monoxide	oxygen	Dispositional antagonist: hastens carboxyhemoglobin breakdown
iron	sodium bicarbonate (before absorption)	Chemical antidote: forms insoluble iron carbonate
fluoride	calcium	Chemical antidote: precipitates fluoride

From the preteen years on, intentional poisoning may result from depression and despair. The most common poisoning agents in adults include benzodiazepines, alcohol, barbiturates, opiates, and aspirin. Carelessness, inattention, and inadvertent contact with noxious substances in the workplace, as well as intoxication and sedation, may lead to adult poisoning. The elderly are particularly vulnerable to poisoning because frequently they take several drugs for various medical conditions; in such circumstances, confusion or disorientation can cause excessive ingestion.

ASSESSMENT OF ACUTE POISONING

Successful management of the patient experiencing acute poisoning requires rapid assessment of the condition's severity. The physician or nurse should observe vital signs and perform a brief physical examination fo-

cusing on CNS and pulmonary functions and on cardiovascular status. If necessary, basic life support measures should be started. The treatment of many poisonings is symptomatic, and most patients will detoxify themselves if their vital functions are adequately supported.

The physician or nurse should obtain information about the drug or substance ingested, the amount and time of ingestion, and any significant medical problem that the patient had before the poisoning. If this information is not available, the physician or nurse must assume that multiple substances might have been ingested. The stabilized patient should have a complete physical examination, with careful observation for needle marks and trauma.

Laboratory tests are important in evaluating the poisoned patient. Routine tests including electrolyte, blood glucose, and serum creatinine levels; complete blood count; and arterial blood gas analysis should be monitored. A chest X-ray will detect the presence of aspiration pneumonia or pulmonary edema, and an EKG will detect drug-induced dysrhythmias. Routine toxicologic screening is controversial because the results rarely modify patient treatment and specific antidotes are available for only a few drugs. (See *Antidotes for selected poisons* on page 77 for a list of poisons and their antidotes.)

Knowledge of the blood concentration level of certain drugs can help the physician or nurse determine the severity of the poisoning and choose the most effective treatment. For example, hemoperfusion is suggested when the serum theophylline concentration level exceeds 20 mcg/ml. If the theophylline concentration level is below this value, care is limited to supportive and symptomatic therapy.

MANAGEMENT OF THE POISONED PATIENT

Because most poisonings result from oral ingestion, preventing absorption minimizes toxic effects. Based on the average rate of absorption of most substances, the patient's GI tract will contain removable quantities even as long as 6 hours after ingestion. Drugs such as phenothiazines, tricyclic antidepressants, antihistamines, belladonna alkaloids, some antiparkinsonian agents, and over-the-counter sleep preparations produce significant anticholinergic action, thereby slowing GI motility and prolonging gastric-emptying time. As a result, these sometimes can be removed from the GI tract up to 12 hours after ingestion.

Several methods are used to remove a toxic substance from a patient's GI tract. Emetics, agents that induce vomiting, are the most widely used because they can be administered at home by nonprofessionals. Syrup of ipecac, a local and centrally acting emetic, is available without a prescription and is effective in producing emesis when used appropriately. The usual dose of syrup of ipecac is 10 ml P.O. in children under age 1, 15 ml P.O. in older children, and 15 to 30 ml P.O. in adolescents and adults. Concomitant administration of water or fruit juice is necessary because syrup of ipecac is less effective when the stomach is empty. Apomorphine is an alternative agent but requires parenteral administration and may produce CNS and respiratory depression.

Emetics are contraindicated in patients who have lost their gag reflex secondary to CNS depression, because of the risk of aspiration; patients experiencing seizures or at risk of having them, also because of the risk of aspiration; and patients who have ingested caustics, such as strong acids or bases, because of the risk of further damaging the mouth and esophagus. The use of emetics for petroleum distillate poisoning is controversial because of the risk of aspiration. Their use is also questionable in antiemetic overdoses, such as might occur with the phenothiazines, because of the antagonism between the effect of the emetic and that of the toxic substance. If syrup of ipecac is not expelled by emesis, it may be absorbed, leading to systemic toxicity, specifically GI or cardiovascular effects.

When the use of emetics is inappropriate, the physician or nurse may remove the toxic substance by gastric lavage. An adsorbant such as activated charcoal is administered after successful emesis or lavage to prevent further absorption of any toxic substance remaining in the GI tract. Because activated charcoal binds with and inactivates syrup of ipecac, the two should not be administered together.

Cathartics are frequently given to speed the passage of toxic substance through the GI tract, but no evidence indicates that they decrease the absorption of toxic substances. Moreover, the diarrhea after cathartics may cause significant fluid and electrolyte losses.

Once a toxic substance has been absorbed, the patient must excrete it. The success of methods to aid excretion depends largely on the underlying pharmacokinetics of the toxic compound. Drugs with a large volume of distribution, such as digoxin, tricyclic antidepressants, phenothiazines, and benzodiazepines, are extensively distributed in tissues; the blood will contain very little of these drugs in the body.

Transfer of these drugs from the tissue to the blood is necessary before excretion. Therefore, the physician or nurse can use procedures such as altering the pH of the urine, forced diuresis, hemodialysis, or hemoperfusion to remove substances such as ethanol, salicylates, theophylline, barbiturates, ethylene glycol, and paraquat; however, these procedures are not without complications. Attempts to alter urine pH may result in metabolic acidosis or alkalosis. Forced diuresis with large volumes of saline solution may produce pulmonary edema and electrolyte disturbances. Hemoperfusion may be associated with thrombocytopenia, hypocalcemia, and hypothermia.

Complications and their management

Appropriately treating the poisoned patient includes recognizing and managing complications. CNS depression and coma are the most common complications in the poisoned patient. The physician or nurse should evaluate the patient for other possible causes for CNS depression, such as head trauma, cerebrovascular disease, and infection. Comatose patients are usually treated with naloxone, which will reverse narcotic effects, and I.V. glucose, which will reverse excess insulin effects. If the patient responds to naloxone or glucose, the nurse will have some idea of what the poisoning agent was. Patients in a coma should receive supportive treatment, but not CNS stimulants because of the risk of inducing dysrhythmias and seizures.

Overdoses of amphetamines, cocaine, phencyclidine, LSD, or anticholinergics may produce a toxic delirium. Patients with this condition are at risk of harming themselves and others; prompt treatment is necessary.

A seizure may occur with an overdose of stimulants, theophylline, antidepressants, antipsychotics, or anticholinergics. It may be caused by the drug's effect on the brain or by other effects of the drug. For example, hypoglycemia or acidosis, which may follow an overdose, contribute to the development of seizures. Treating the underlying condition usually terminates the seizure; otherwise, anticonvulsant therapy may be indicated.

Cardiac manifestations of acute poisoning include hypotension, hypertension, and dysrhythmias. Hypotension is usually corrected when other problems are treated, but severe hypotension may require pressor drug therapy. Similarly, hypertension may cause cerebrovascular accident, and antihypertensive therapy may be necessary, depending on blood pressure elevation and the substance ingested.

Dysrhythmias frequently occur with overdoses of antidepressants, digoxin, or stimulants. Since the dysrhythmias may be life-threatening, they require prompt treatment with appropriate antiarrhythmic drugs. The nurse should monitor the patient for recurring dysrhythmias. Other complications of acute poisoning that may require drug therapy include pulmonary edema, bronchoconstriction, renal failure, and pulmonary infections secondary to aspiration.

Treating acute poisoning is often complex because specific systemic antidotes are available for only a small number of drugs and toxic substances, and even available antidotes should be used as only one part of a comprehensive treatment plan. Supportive and symptomatic measures remain the cornerstone of treatment.

PREVENTION OF ACUTE POISONING

The incidence of acute poisoning among children under age 5 has actually decreased over the last few years because of the concerted efforts of health care professionals, and nurses play a key role in this prevention. Family education remains a significant element in efforts to prevent acute poisoning among children. The nurse should emphasize the careful use and storage of drugs, alcohol, and household chemicals. The community health nurse can greatly benefit families by identifying and correcting dangerous practices. Decreasing the incidence of intentional poisoning should receive equal priority. The nurse can instruct families about how to recognize and respond immediately to signs of depression and suicidal intent.

Preventing poisoning in the workplace remains a high priority. Businesses and industries frequently hire nurses to promote employee health. In this capacity, the nurse can monitor the work environment for poison risks and implement corrective or preventive action. The nurse also can educate employees about poison risks and protective actions.

CHAPTER SUMMARY

Chapter 5 covered adverse drug reactions and acute poisonings. Chapter highlights include:
• An adverse drug reaction is a harmful, undesirable patient response to a specific drug therapy.
• Adverse drug reactions may result from any clinically useful drug. Some are dose-related, predictable, and preventable with careful prescription and administration practices, or unavoidable if primary therapeutic effects are to be achieved. Others are unpredictable.
• Most predictable adverse drug reactions are caused by pharmacologic toxicity, excessive therapeutic effect, or hypersusceptibility; unpredictable ones are caused by an allergic or idiosyncratic response.
• A patient's therapeutic responses to drugs result from the interplay among patient characteristics, drug characteristics, and external factors. The interplay can alter a drug's action or the patient's response, producing adverse drug reactions.

• Patient factors that predispose to adverse drug reactions include extremes of age, extremes of body weight, genetic variations, temperament and attitudes, circadian rhythms, disease, and pregnancy. Drug-related factors include bioavailability, additives, degradation, dosage, administration, and the number of drugs administered. Diet and environment also may predispose the patient to adverse reactions.

• Successful management of an acutely poisoned patient begins with the nurse's assessment.

• Treatment goals for the poisoned patient should include supporting vital functions, decreasing further absorption of the toxic substance, promoting excretion of the toxin, and managing complications.

• Specific antidotes are available for a few poisonings only. They should be used in conjunction with, not as a substitute for, supportive and symptomatic treatment.

BIBLIOGRAPHY

Bayer, M., and Rumack, B. *Poisoning and Overdose.* Rockville, Md.: Aspen Systems Corp., 1983.

Fox, D. "Nonsteroidal Anti-inflammatory Drugs and Renal Disease," *Journal of the American Medical Association* 251:1299, 1984.

Gossel, T., and Bricker, J. *Principles of Clinical Toxicology.* New York: Raven Press Pubs., 1984.

Jick, H. "Adverse Drug Reactions," in *Topics in Clinical Pharmacology and Therapeutics.* Edited by Maronde, R. New York: Springer-Verlag, 1986.

Jick, H., et al. "Tricyclic Antidepressants and Convulsions," *Journal of Clinical Psychopharmacology* 3:182, 1983.

Jonsson, S., et al. "Acute Cocaine Poisoning," *American Journal of Medicine* 75:1061, 1983.

Levine, R. *Pharmacology: Drug Actions and Reactions,* 3rd ed. Boston: Little, Brown & Co., 1983.

Matsumura, F. *Toxicology of Insecticides,* 2nd ed. New York: Plenum, 1985.

McCarron, M. "Diagnosis and Treatment of Drug Overdose," in *Topics in Clinical Pharmacology and Therapeutics.* Edited by Maronde R. New York: Springer-Verlag, 1986.

Nriagu, J., ed. *Changing Metal Cycles and Human Health.* New York: Springer-Verlag, 1984.

Pentel, P. "Toxicity of Over-The-Counter Stimulants," *Journal of the American Medical Association* 75:1061, 1984.

Randall, B. "Reacting to Anaphylaxis," *Nursing86* 16:86, 1986.

CHAPTER 6

DRUG ABUSE, DEPENDENCE, AND ADDICTION

OBJECTIVES

After reading and studying this chapter, you should be able to:

1. Identify the physical and psychological effects caused by abuse of opiates, stimulants, central nervous system (CNS) depressants, alcohol, tobacco, cannabis, and psychotomimetics.

2. Identify the drugs used to treat opiate abuse.

3. Explain why withdrawal from CNS depressants should be done under medical supervision.

4. Describe how metabolic rate contributes to the effects of alcohol on the user.

5. Describe what the nurse should look for in assessing a patient for alcohol abuse.

6. Describe the positive and negative outcomes associated with the treatment of psychotomimetic abusers.

INTRODUCTION

A pharmacology textbook would be incomplete without mentioning the problems that can occur with the misuse of drugs and alcohol. Drug abuse, dependence, and addiction have become a national problem: alcoholism involves at least 10% of the adult population, the United States Department of Health and Human Services estimates that 18 million people use marijuana, more than 22 million Americans have tried cocaine once, and approximately 4 to 5 million currently use cocaine regularly. Drug abuse has a major economic impact on society. Workers who abuse drugs and alcohol waste or miss work time; accidents result from the use of these substances; and the financial burden of treating related health problems and rehabilitating abusers grows each year.

Drug abuse can also produce detrimental effects on a family. Money normally used to support the family may be diverted to support the abuser's habit. Children may lose the attentive care of one or both of their parents because of problems associated with drug abuse.

This chapter discusses terminology necessary for the study of drug abuse; the physiologic and psychological effects of drugs on individuals; and the effects of drug abuse on society and the nursing profession. Also discussed are seven general categories of commonly abused drugs, including opiates, stimulants, CNS depressants, alcohol, tobacco (nicotine), cannabis, and psychotomimetics.

Terminology

Drug abuse describes the nonmedical use of drugs, including alcohol and nicotine. Such use can become detrimental to the user, family, and society. Commonly abused drugs are usually self-administered to: (1) alter the user's mood or perception of the world, (2) produce unusual sensations, (3) enhance the user's perceived ability to function in certain social situations, or (4) alleviate pain.

A person who abuses drugs can develop *physical dependence* or *psychological dependence* or both. With physical dependence, withdrawal from the drug produces physical effects ranging from nausea and vomiting to convulsions and even death. A psychologically dependent drug abuser desires the drug during withdrawal but does not experience physical effects. This psychological drug dependence may be referred to as *habituation*.

Addiction refers to drug-seeking behavior in which the abuser is unable to control the desire or craving for the chemical substance. It is possible to be physically dependent on drugs without being addicted.

Body tissues display *tolerance* when they adjust to the presence of a drug in a way that the person requires increasing amounts to produce the same effect. Tolerance increases the risk of reaching toxic drug levels in the effort to produce the desired effects.

Alcoholism is characterized by a pattern of alcohol use leading to impaired social and occupational functioning. This pattern may include the daily need for alcohol, an inability to reduce or stop drinking, binges, and/or an inability to recall what occurred during intoxication.

OPIATES

Opiates are used therapeutically as pain relievers and sedatives; in larger doses, they induce sleep. Opiates can be classified according to their origin as naturally occurring opiates, semisynthetic agents, and synthetic agents. The two naturally occurring opiates, morphine and codeine, are obtained from the opium poppy, *Papaver somniferum*. Semisynthetic agents, chemical derivatives of morphine and codeine, include heroin, hydromorphone (Dilaudid), and oxymorphone (Numorphan). Synthetic agents include meperidine (Demerol) and methadone (Dolophine).

GENERAL EFFECTS OF OPIATES

The intensity of an opiate's effect depends upon the amount taken, the route of administration, the interval between doses, and the degree of drug tolerance the user has developed. Opiates may be ingested, inhaled through the nose, smoked, or administered subcutaneously or intravenously. Subcutaneous and intravenous administration produce the most immediate effects.

After an opiate is taken intravenously, a release of histamine produces itching, reddening of the eyes, and a drop in blood pressure. CNS depression follows, causing extreme sedation until the opiate user develops tolerance to the drug. Sedative effects include lethargy, decreased vision, decreased physical activity, light sleep, and feelings of euphoria. Once tolerance develops, sedative effects are no longer obtained.

Assessment of abuse
The nurse should use sensitivity and discretion when asking a patient about drug-taking habits as part of the drug history. The nurse first asks less intrusive questions about caffeine and cigarette use, proceeding to the use of prescription and nonprescription medications and finally asking about the patient's use of illicit drugs. The nurse should explain to the patient that this information may affect diagnosis and treatment.

A physical examination may reveal needle marks on the arms, legs, hands, and neck; between the toes and under the tongue; behind the knees; or at the site of a tattoo. These marks are generally hyperpigmented, linear, and raised, with a dry, rough texture. Recent injection sites may appear red, warm, and swollen—the effects of local inflammation.

With an opiate overdose, the patient may be unconscious. Other signs of overdose include constricted pupils, respiratory depression, cold and clammy skin, confusion, convulsions, dizziness, drowsiness, nervousness or restlessness, hypotension, bradycardia, and severe weakness.

Withdrawal syndrome
Abrupt withdrawal from opiates produces varying physiologic symptoms and degrees of psychological distress. Withdrawal consists of four phases, each with a different set of symptoms.

Symptoms first appear approximately 4 to 8 hours after the last dose of the opiate and usually include rhinorrhea, lacrimation, yawning, diaphoresis, insomnia, and generalized anxiety. The drug user may describe these symptoms as "flulike." In the second phase, which occurs about 15 hours after the last dose, the opiate user may fall into a restless sleep. The user generally awakens unrefreshed and experiences loss of appetite, nausea, vomiting, and diarrhea. In the third phase, the patient experiences rebound CNS excitability manifested by pupillary dilation, increased heart rate, elevated blood pressure, and involuntary twitching and kicking. The final phase is characterized by dehydration, hypoglycemia, and possible acid-base imbalances. At this point, cardiovascular collapse may occur, but this is very rare. Symptoms usually decrease in intensity after 48 to 72 hours. All withdrawal symptoms should disappear in approximately 7 to 10 days. The withdrawal syndrome can be reversed at any time with an injection of the opiate.

Treatment
Treatment of opiate addiction usually includes detoxification and rehabilitation. During detoxification, the addict is withdrawn from the drug, either with or without pharmacologic support. (See "Drugs to treat opiate abuse.") After detoxification, the patient should not experience any physical need for the drug; however, the psychological need may persist. Rehabilitation may include vocational counseling, psychotherapy, drug education, pharmacologic support, and/or emotional support. The aim of rehabilitation is to eliminate the patient's psychological need for the drug. A patient may

undergo detoxification and rehabilitation on an inpatient or an outpatient basis.

Drugs to treat opiate abuse

Physicians may prescribe methadone, clonidine, and narcotic antagonists to treat opiate abuse. Methadone and clonidine are used to decrease withdrawal symptoms. Methadone blocks withdrawal symptoms via a maintenance mechanism; clonidine does so via an adrenergic mechanism. The narcotic antagonists inhibit the euphoria experienced with opiates, and in emergency situations they reverse opiates' effects.

methadone (Dolophine). A Schedule II drug used to treat opiate addiction since the 1960s, methadone prevents withdrawal symptoms. The patient can be detoxified with methadone over a 21-day period, with the dosage being gradually decreased. The patient then may be placed on methadone maintenance and given a small amount of the drug daily. Success rates for methadone treatment vary from program to program and depend on the patient's ability to learn to live without using chemical agents.

clonidine (Catapres). In the late 1970s, clonidine, a drug used to treat hypertension, was found to suppress the signs and symptoms of opiate withdrawal. Clonidine has since been used to increase the rate of detoxification from opiates. Patients taking clonidine may be detoxified in 7 to 14 days as compared to the usual 21 days needed for methadone treatment. Because clonidine can produce hypotension, the nurse should monitor the patient's blood pressure just before administration and again at the drug's peak concentration level, which occurs approximately 2 hours after administration. Clonidine does not eliminate every withdrawal symptom of opiate addiction; lethargy and insomnia may persist. Clonidine has also been used to treat alcohol or benzodiazepine withdrawal.

narcotic antagonists. Noted for its use in emergencies, the narcotic antagonist naloxone (Narcan) is used to reverse narcotic-induced respiratory depression from overdose. More long-acting than naloxone, naltrexone (Trexan) is used to block the euphoria opiates produce. (Some physicians believe that blocking drug-induced euphoria decreases the user's desire for the drug.) Naltrexone should not be used to treat drug overdose but can be used as adjunct therapy during rehabilitation.

Inpatient and outpatient treatment

The components of inpatient treatment programs vary. In one method, called the *therapeutic community,* for-mer drug addicts and abusers work with other drug abusers and try to rehabilitate them. The program lasts 12 to 18 months, and the patient dropout rate is high. Inpatient treatment programs should include vocational counseling, problem-solving strategies, psychotherapy, and drug education—an important component of all treatment.

Methadone maintenance clinics and drug-free aftercare clinics are common outpatient treatment centers. Patients receive methadone daily at one of these treatment centers. The programs at drug-free aftercare clinics usually emphasize counseling and referral services for various problems.

CENTRAL NERVOUS SYSTEM STIMULANTS

Amphetamines and cocaine are commonly abused stimulants. Amphetamines have been used therapeutically to suppress appetite and manage mild depression. Some physicians question the usefulness of amphetamines for these purposes, however, and usage has decreased. Cocaine is a white, odorless alkaloid powder manufactured from the leaves of the coca plant. Therapeutically, it is used as a local anesthetic for ear, nose, and throat surgery. The drug produces feelings of omnipotence and self-confidence, along with a high energy level.

GENERAL EFFECTS OF STIMULANTS

Amphetamines can be taken orally or intravenously, or they may be inhaled. The drugs produce feelings of euphoria, enhanced self-confidence, increased alertness, greater energy, an increased ability to concentrate, and reduced hunger and fatigue. Users are continually active and talkative and see themselves as rapid and effective thinkers. With continued use, however, the user becomes restless and irritable. Amphetamines also increase heart rate and blood pressure, and widen pulse pressure. The user may experience palpitations, a dry mouth, and dilated pupils. As the drug's effects begin to wear off, fatigue and drowsiness set in, and the user may fall asleep. A chronic user may experience a hangover upon awakening.

With long-term amphetamine use, manic paranoia may develop. Eventually, the drug user develops delusions of persecution; auditory, visual, and tactile hallucinations; and compulsive behavior. Tolerance to amphetamines appears to develop rapidly.

Cocaine's effects resemble those of amphetamines but do not last as long. Cocaine increases the heart rate and blood pressure by vasoconstriction; it may affect the cardiovascular system, even to the point of cardiac arrest; it can be taken via nasal inhalation (sniffing or snorting), intravenous administration, and smoking. Nasal inhalation constricts the blood vessels in the nose. When the drug wears off, the user experiences nasal stuffiness and tender nasal membranes. Extended use results in scarred nasal membranes and damaged nasal passages.

Assessment of abuse

The nurse should obtain a general health history as well as a specific drug history documenting the frequency and amount of each drug used. Physical examination of an intravenous user of amphetamines will probably reveal needle marks. A user with acute amphetamine toxicity may exhibit violent behavior, psychotic reactions, muscular tremors and tics, restlessness, anxiety, apprehension, dizziness, confusion, irritability, chest pain, hallucinations, hypertension, and diaphoresis. Convulsions, hyperpyrexia, and shock may result in death.

Acute cocaine toxicity is commonly characterized by convulsions and cardiac dysrhythmias; death from cardiac arrest may occur.

Withdrawal syndrome

Controversy exists about whether amphetamines and cocaine cause physical dependence. Physical symptoms associated with stimulant withdrawal include anorexia, irritability, fatigue, and depression. Much of the discomfort from stimulant withdrawal, however, is caused by the psychological craving for the drug's effects.

The depression from cocaine withdrawal varies in severity, probably in proportion to the quantity used and the duration of habitual use. Because of the depression, withdrawal treatment should include suicide assessment and prevention measures.

Treatment

No known pharmacologic agent blocks the euphoric effects of stimulants, but the depression sometimes experienced during withdrawal can be treated with tricyclic antidepressants. The psychotic reaction that can occur during amphetamine withdrawal may be treated with phenothiazines or antipsychotic agents, such as haloperidol (Haldol). Acute toxicity to amphetamines and cocaine can be treated with chlorpromazine (Thorazine).

Diazepam (Valium) can be administered to control convulsions. Local support groups, such as Cocaine Anonymous, and professional psychological therapy can also help users.

CENTRAL NERVOUS SYSTEM DEPRESSANTS

CNS depressants include barbiturates, nonbarbiturate nonbenzodiazepine sedative-hypnotics, benzodiazepines, and alcohol. The shorter-acting barbiturates, such as pentobarbital (Nembutal), secobarbital (Seconal), and amobarbital (Amytal), are frequently abused. Because longer-acting barbiturates, such as phenobarbital, have a longer onset of action, they are not abused so frequently.

Nonbarbiturate nonbenzodiazepine sedative-hypnotics that are frequently abused include methaqualone, ethchlorvynol (Placidyl), and glutethimide (Doriden). Although methaqualone is no longer commercially available in the United States, it is produced illegally.

Benzodiazepines are frequently prescribed antianxiety agents. Diazepam (Valium) is the most often prescribed *and* abused benzodiazepine. (See Chapter 32, Antianxiety Agents, for details about these drugs.)

Alcohol is also a CNS depressant. However, because of its social acceptance and the prevalence of its abuse, it warrants discussion as a separate entity. The discussion of alcohol follows this section.

GENERAL EFFECTS OF CNS DEPRESSANTS

Generally, the CNS depressants produce sedation and decrease inhibitions; they may also produce some feelings of euphoria. In large doses, CNS depressants decrease mental acuity and physical coordination and produce slurred speech, impaired thinking, poor memory and judgment, and a limited attention span. The user may also experience mood swings and become aggressive or violent.

Assessment of abuse

Chronic abusers of CNS depressants experience neurologic changes, including diplopia, nystagmus, slurred speech, positive Romberg's sign (inability to maintain balance while standing with eyes closed and feet together), ataxic gait, decreased reflexes, and hypotonia. They also exhibit somnolence and lethargy and may be severely disoriented and apprehensive.

Tolerance to CNS depressants develops rapidly, so users must increase the dose needed to achieve the desired effect. As a result, the range between an intoxicating and a fatal dose narrows significantly. At toxic levels, arousal may be difficult, response to noxious stimuli may be absent, respiratory depression may occur, and death may ensue. Combining CNS depressants with alcohol is particularly hazardous and a common cause of accidental deaths and suicides.

Withdrawal syndrome

Both physical and psychological dependence develop with the use of CNS depressants. Medical supervision is recommended during withdrawal, which is usually more severe for users of other CNS depressants than for benzodiazepine users. Symptoms, which appear approximately 24 hours after discontinuation of the drug, initially include trembling, anxiety, restlessness, abdominal cramping, nausea, vomiting, and orthostatic hypotension. Life-threatening tonic-clonic seizures or respiratory arrest may occur with all of the CNS depressants except the benzodiazepines. A psychotic delirium may also develop during which the user hallucinates and is extremely agitated. Hyperthermia, cardiovascular collapse, and death may result.

Treatment

Initial detoxification should be performed in a supervised setting. To facilitate withdrawal by decreasing the physiologic reflex response, a similar depressant is administered to replace the abused one and the dosage is gradually decreased. When this method is used for a barbiturate abuser, the replacement drug of choice is usually a benzodiazepine or phenobarbital. The nurse administers the prescribed substitute drug based on the observed signs and symptoms indicating the severity of withdrawal. The nurse should keep the patient alert while administering sufficient medications to control the tremulousness and anxiety.

Once the patient has been successfully withdrawn from the barbiturate, the benzodiazepine or phenobarbital dose is gradually reduced until the patient is drug-free. A subsequent rehabilitation program can help the patient become psychologically drug-free as well.

ALCOHOL

Alcohol, also a CNS depressant, is the most widely abused drug in the United States, and its use is increasing. According to the United States Department of Health and Human Services, the average consumption of alcohol for all people over age 14 increased 10% from 1973 to 1983. This figure is significant, especially since other studies estimate that individuals report ingesting only 50% of the alcohol that they actually consume.

Alcoholism ranks third among all health care problems. Conservative estimates are that 90 million people use alcohol, that 9 to 10 million are alcoholics, and that at least 30 million are affected by a friend's or relative's alcohol use. These figures indicate that alcoholism is also a major social problem, an indication further supported by the estimated $43 billion annual economic loss experienced by industries because of alcoholism.

GENERAL EFFECTS OF ALCOHOL

Affecting almost every tissue in the body, alcohol is readily absorbed from the stomach and small intestine. The rate of absorption is modified by the stomach contents and the amount and kinds of fluid mixed with the alcohol. Alcohol is metabolized in the liver at a constant rate, which remains stable even if the amount of intake varies. Therefore, if alcohol intake exceeds the amount metabolized, the alcohol level in the blood increases, and drunkenness results. Because only 5% of alcohol intake is excreted unchanged in the urine, frequent urination does not rid the body of alcohol.

The initial psychological effects of alcohol are euphoria, a feeling of well-being, decreased inhibitions, and increased self-confidence. As more alcohol is consumed, motor coordination, equilibrium, judgment, and decision-making abilities become impaired. Eventually, stupor, coma, and death from respiratory depression may occur.

Chronic alcohol abuse can result in many vitamin and mineral deficiencies because of decreased food intake, malabsorption, and enhanced urinary excretion of vitamins and minerals. Zinc, vitamin A, magnesium, phosphorus, and calcium deficiencies commonly occur in chronic alcoholics.

Numerous gastrointestinal (GI) effects may also occur, including GI bleeding, reflux esophagitis and pancreatitis. Alcohol interferes with liver function and can lead to cirrhosis and fatty infiltration of the liver, resulting in cell necrosis. Regeneration, associated with scarring, distorts liver structure and function and may result in portocaval hypertension and esophageal varices.

Regular consumption of alcohol during pregnancy increases the risk of fetal alcohol syndrome. Affected infants exhibit slow growth; brain abnormalities; intellectual deficits; heart defects; and atypical facial features, such as a short nose, an underdeveloped upper lip, and short eyelid folds. This syndrome reflects the ability of alcohol to depress the normal growth of fetal tissue.

Assessment of abuse

The nurse can assess the individual for potential alcohol abuse by recognizing certain psychological, physiologic, social, and personal indicators. Psychological indicators include low self-esteem, depression, a sense of inadequacy, high anxiety levels, feelings of loneliness and inferiority, and a dependent personality. Physiologic indicators include insomnia, unexplained bruises and broken bones (possibly sustained during alcoholic binges), and gastritis. Social indicators may include a lack of social support and solitary drinking. The nurse can assess for personal indicators by obtaining a thorough patient history. With a nonjudgmental attitude, the nurse should ask the patient specific questions about alcohol. For example, "Do you drink alcoholic beverages?" "How much do you drink?" "How often?" "Do you drink beer?" "Do you drink wine?" "When do you drink?" "Do you drink by yourself or with others?"

Withdrawal syndrome

Alcohol withdrawal progresses through several stages, which vary among patients. Symptoms of the first stage begin to appear approximately 24 to 48 hours after discontinuation of alcohol use and include tremulousness, diaphoresis, weakness, anxiety, nausea, vomiting, and abdominal cramps. The alcoholic becomes restless and agitated but remains alert. During the next stage, the alcoholic may experience tonic-clonic seizures. These seizures can occur within 24 hours of alcohol discontinuation but may also occur 2 to 3 days later.

The final stage of withdrawal is characterized by delirium tremens (DTs). In DTs, auditory, visual, and tactile hallucinations occur; the alcoholic becomes extremely agitated and sleeps little; and tachycardia, profuse diaphoresis, disorientation, restlessness, and fever develop. Once it begins, this state is difficult to reverse. Current treatment includes I.V. glucose, thiamine, and other B complex vitamins. DTs can be fatal as a result of hyperthermia or peripheral vascular collapse. The alcohol withdrawal syndrome usually lasts 5 to 7 days.

Treatment

For treatment to be successful, the physiologically dependent alcoholic must first undergo withdrawal in a medically supervised setting. Withdrawal from alcohol is managed in the same manner as withdrawl from CNS depressants. Once again, care must be taken to balance the need for medication with the risk of oversedation.

Although the physician prescribes the appropriate sedatives, the nurse administers them based on the patient's changing signs and symptoms. The nurse also monitors the patient's mental status and vital signs to avoid oversedation and to determine the patient's progress. Diazepam (Valium) is the usual drug of choice for sedation, but oxazepam (Serax) may be given to patients with severe liver disease.

The nurse must also carefully monitor the patient's hydration and electrolyte balance, because diaphoresis and diuresis can cause extreme fluid loss leading to hypokalemia. Because the nutritional status of the alcoholic is usually very poor, thiamine should be administered to prevent Korsakoff's psychosis (a dementia syndrome caused by CNS depression and destruction of nerve cells from chronic alcohol ingestion).

The safety of the patient must be considered at all times. If restraining the patient is necessary to prevent injury, care should be taken to ensure that the restraints are properly applied, the bed rails are up, and the patient is closely monitored.

After successful withdrawal, the goal of an alcoholic's treatment program is abstinence. Treatment options for attaining this goal include Alcoholics Anonymous (AA), disulfiram (Antabuse) therapy, behavioral therapy, and therapeutic support groups. AA, an organization of alcoholics who offer each other support and understanding in an effort to lead lives of abstinence, is a voluntary, lifelong self-help program. Members are encouraged to follow 12 steps which, when implemented, provide guidance for personal change.

Aversion or deterrent therapy employs a daily oral dose of disulfiram. Disulfiram inhibits the enzyme responsible for the oxidation of acetaldehyde, a metabolite of alcohol. The resulting accumulation of acetaldehyde produces symptoms if the disulfiram-treated patient ingests alcohol. The symptoms include increased heart rate, cold sweat, facial flushing, pulsating headache, nausea, and vomiting. Severe symptoms, such as respiratory depression, cardiac dysrhythmias, acute congestive heart failure, myocardial infarction, and cardiovascular collapse, may also occur.

Disulfiram should be given only with the patient's knowledge. Patients taking disulfiram should be instructed to avoid all substances containing alcohol, such as elixirs, tonics, wine vinegars, mouthwashes, gargles, cough syrups, and certain sauces. They also should not apply alcohol-containing substances, such as after-shave lotion, rubbing alcohol, liniments, cologne, toilet water, or after-bath preparations, because the skin may absorb the alcohol.

Behavioral modification, associating negative images or sensations with the consumption of alcohol, has also been used in the treatment of alcoholism. Other behavioral treatment includes assertiveness training to provide alcoholics with alternative methods for solving their problems.

Therapeutic communities that treat opiate abusers also treat alcoholics, using treatment regimens very similar to those used for drug abusers.

TOBACCO AND NICOTINE

An estimated 54 million Americans smoke cigarettes even though cigarette smoking is associated with an increase in coronary artery disease; arteriosclerotic peripheral vascular disease; chronic obstructive pulmonary disease; and cancer of the larynx, esophagus, and oral cavity. Cigarette smoking is also the major identifiable factor contributing to residential deaths and injuries by fire.

GENERAL EFFECTS OF NICOTINE

Nicotine is the primary habit-forming substance in tobacco smoke. The physiologic effects of nicotine include stimulation of the sympathetic nervous system, increased heart rate and blood pressure, and constriction of blood vessels in the heart, extremities, and placenta. Nicotine also increases platelet aggregation, accelerates the atherosclerotic process, and increases cardiac work load. Also, nicotine has serious deleterious effects on the fetus. As a result, nicotine use should be discouraged during pregnancy.

The psychological effects of smoking vary. Some smokers feel that cigarettes relax them; others find smoking to have a stimulating effect.

Assessment of abuse

The nurse can use numerous assessment tools for detecting nicotine abuse. One instrument, the Fagerstrom inventory, was developed in 1918 by Fagerstrom, a Swedish psychologist who worked in a smoking ces-

sation clinic. The Fagerstrom inventory can help the nurse determine the degree of nicotine dependence in a patient. Questions from the inventory include: (1) How many cigarettes do you smoke per day? (2) Do you smoke more in the morning than at other times during the day? (3) Do you find it difficult to refrain from smoking in places where it is forbidden, such as in church?

The more cigarettes a patient smokes, the greater the dependence on nicotine. A patient who smokes more in the morning, when nicotine levels are low, displays a greater physiologic need for nicotine. The patient who has difficulty controlling the urge to smoke in places where smoking is socially unacceptable displays extreme psychological dependence on nicotine.

Withdrawal syndrome

Smokers develop physiologic dependence on nicotine. Withdrawal symptoms include irritability, mental depression, difficulty concentrating, headache, weight gain, restlessness, and muscle aches and pains. The weight gain some former smokers experience may be from increased food intake, decreased metabolic rate, or increased food transit time through the body.

Treatment

The nurse can help patients who want to quit smoking by informing them about the dangers of smoking and providing support during their efforts to stop. The nurse can help ex-smokers by informing them of the benefits of continued abstinence. An estimated 95% of ex-smokers stop on their own. Many simply quit abruptly; others gradually decrease the number of cigarettes, follow published regimens, or use other aids such as nicotine gum (see below).

A number of treatment programs are also available to help people stop smoking. Some behavioral treatments use aversion therapy, which associates smoking with a negative thought or sensation, such as an electric shock. A number of support groups and formal programs are available through community organizations, such as the American Cancer Society, the American Lung Association, and the American Heart Association. Some private organizations also provide programs for people who want to stop smoking.

Nicotine gum can help some people stop smoking, but the nurse needs to inform the patient that nicotine gum is an aid, not a panacea, and is a prescription medication. The patient must first decrease the number of cigarettes smoked each day to 12 to 15 before beginning to use the gum. The patient then stops smoking entirely and chews the gum whenever the urge to smoke occurs. The gum replaces the nicotine that cigarettes normally provide, taking effect in 15 to 20 minutes.

Most smokers require 10 pieces of gum each day during the 1st month of treatment, then decrease the number of pieces required until gum is no longer needed. The patient should not use more than 30 pieces of nicotine gum a day or use the gum longer than 6 months.

CANNABIS

Marijuana and hashish are produced from the *Cannabis sativa,* or hemp plant. These drugs have been used for their intoxicating effects for more than 2,500 years. They have also been used to treat numerous physical ailments, including gout. Until the early 1900s, these agents were included in the list of prescription organic compounds. Although only available illegally, both drugs are frequently abused. (See Chapter 49, Emetic and Antiemetic Agents, for the therapeutic use of a synthetic derivative of delta-9-tetrahydrocannabinol [Δ^9-THC], the principal hallucinogen in marijuana.)

GENERAL EFFECTS OF CANNABIS

In low doses (20 mg of Δ^9-THC or a cigarette containing 2% Δ^9-THC), cannabis produces feelings of euphoria and well-being, relaxation, and altered perceptions. Short-term memory becomes impaired, and the user experiences difficulty performing complicated tasks such as driving. Balance, stability, information processing, and decision making are also impaired for 4 to 8 hours.

Users of cannabis report that the drug produces increased hunger, dry mouth and throat, vivid visual imagery, and a keener sense of hearing. Increased heart rate and peripheral blood flow, reddening of the conjunctiva, and decreased intraocular pressure also occur.

Higher doses of cannabis may produce paranoia, delusions, and psychosis. Performance of complex motor tasks is impaired, and reaction time is slowed. The slowed reaction time makes driving under the influence of cannabis as dangerous as driving under the influence of alcohol. The user's thinking may become confused and disorganized. Toxic psychosis with hallucinations and loss of insight may occur with very high doses.

Chronic smoking of cannabis has been associated with bronchitis and asthma. Pulmonary function decreases, and the bronchial epithelium is physiologically altered.

Assessment of abuse

Chronic marijuana use may result in amotivational syndromes characterized by apathy; dullness; and impairment of judgment, concentration, and memory. Severe abuse may result in loss of interest in personal appearance and in the pursuit of personal goals. Other adverse effects may range from frequently occurring panic reactions to less frequently occurring episodes of toxic psychosis. During toxic psychosis, the patient is disoriented and confused and experiences visual and auditory hallucinations. The psychosis is self-limiting; when most of the marijuana is metabolized from the body, the symptoms disappear. Metabolites of marijuana are retained in lipid tissues for several days or weeks. This retention does not provide a cumulative drug effect.

Withdrawal syndrome

Physical dependence on cannabis does not develop in occasional users; the effect on long-term users is currently being studied. Abrupt discontinuation after long-term use produces withdrawal symptoms, which may include loss of sleep, irritability, restlessness, decreased appetite, weight loss, hyperactivity, and diaphoresis.

Treatment

Talking and listening to the patient experiencing an adverse reaction to cannabis are preferred to administering antipsychotic medication. Treatment of long-term users involves psychotherapy, counseling, and self-help programs.

PSYCHOTOMIMETICS

The psychotomimetics, often referred to as *hallucinogens* or *psychedelics,* include three general drug classes: indolealkylamines, phenylethylamines, and arylcyclohexylamines. The term psychotomimetics is somewhat misleading for these drugs because all of them except phencyclidine (an arylcyclohexylamine) produce a state that only superficially resembles psychosis. Individuals using phencyclidine, however, have been misdiagnosed as having schizophrenia.

Effects of psychotomimetics

The increased use of psychotomimetics necessitates that the nurse know about their effects.

DRUG	DRUG SOURCE	ADMINISTRATION	EFFECTS
mescaline	Peyote cactus	Dried cactus disks are chewed or ground into powder for oral or intravenous use	Fight or flight response, hyperactivity, hallucinations, altered color and space perceptions
psilocin, psilocybin	Mushroom (*Psilocybe mexicana*)	Taken orally	Hallucinations, time and space distortions, perceptual alterations
lysergic acid diethylamide (LSD)	Synthetic	Taken orally	Increased blood pressure, tachycardia, trembling, pupillary dilation, feelings of derealization, perceptual alterations, impaired judgment
phencyclidine (PCP)	Synthetic	Taken orally, smoked, snorted, or injected intravenously	Hostile and bizarre behavior, blank stare, staggering gait, nystagmus, agitation, increased blood pressure and heart rate, catatonic muscular rigidity, slurred speech, diaphoresis; severe hypertension may lead to cerebral hemorrhage

The most frequently abused indolealkylamines are lysergic acid diethylamide (LSD), psilocin, and psilocybin. The major phenylethylamine is mescaline; DOM, STP, MMDA, and DMT are synthetic forms of mescaline. The major arylcyclohexylamine is phencyclidine (PCP). This drug was used therapeutically as an anesthetic and analgesic until its deleterious effects were discovered.

GENERAL EFFECTS OF PSYCHOTOMIMETICS

The effects of psychotomimetics vary. Generally, these drugs induce a state of altered perceptions, ideas, and feelings. Indolealkylamines decrease the turnover rate of serotonin in the brain. (Serotonin is a neurotransmitter involved in the regulation of body temperature, sensory perception, and sleep.) After oral administration, indolealkylamines have an onset of action of approximately 30 to 40 minutes and a duration of action of 8 hours or longer.

The site of action of the phenylethylamines is probably the norepinephrine synapse. Mescaline is rapidly and completely absorbed after ingestion; effects begin in 30 to 90 minutes and last up to 12 hours. High doses of mescaline usually are not toxic. However, high doses of the synthetic mescalines (DOM, MMDA, and TMA) can produce gross hyperactivity and hyperexcitability.

Tremors may progress to convulsions and death. PCP is well absorbed after all routes of administration. Its onset of action varies; its duration of action is 6 to 8 hours.

Because of the analgesia produced by PCP, self-inflicted injuries and injuries from physical restraint may go unnoticed. The patient is also unaware of the surroundings and unresponsive to noxious stimuli. (See *Effects of psychotomimetics* for more details.)

Assessment of abuse

Obtaining a thorough drug use history and performing a complete physical examination are major components of the assessment process for detecting psychotomimetic abuse. The most helpful tool to determine the psychotomimetic a patient has used is a toxicologic urine screening; a blood screening is used to assess the amount of drug in the blood.

Withdrawal syndrome

Psychotomimetics do not produce physical dependence. Consequently, no withdrawal syndrome occurs with discontinuation of the drugs.

Treatment

A calm environment and reassurance are advocated for the initial treatment of psilocybin and psilocin overdose. If these measures fail, diazepam or chlorpromazine may be used. Diazepam is usually administered for sedation in LSD and mescaline overdose; these patients require clinical monitoring to prevent self-injury.

Treatment of PCP overdose can be problematic for health care providers, who must avoid becoming victims of the patient's violent behavior. Usually, gastric lavage is performed to remove any unabsorbed drug, and the urine is acidified to a pH of 5.5 to help accelerate the excretion of the drug. Increased fluids and diuretics may be administered to force diuresis, and diazepam is used for sedation.

IMPAIRED NURSES

Nurses are statistically a high-risk group for engaging in substance abuse. They work in stressful situations and have access to potentially abused prescription drugs. Some nurses may believe that their professional knowledge renders them invulnerable to drug abuse. When nurses abuse drugs, their clinical performance becomes ineffective or impaired. Many professional groups, including nurses, have adopted the term "impaired" to describe those group members who are ineffective in their performance because of substance abuse.

Assessment

The impaired nurse may be able to conceal substance abuse for a while, but because substance abuse is progressive, a change in job performance eventually will become apparent. Changes in job performance include decreased productivity, mistakes in carrying out procedures, poor judgment in clinical decision making, frequent absenteeism, and discrepancies in the documentation of administered medications. The impaired nurse often requests work situations that involve little supervision or contact with co-workers. Patients may report episodes of inadequate pain relief, and co-workers may complain of problems created by the nurse's tardiness or frequent absences from work. The nurse who is addicted to prescription medications is often identified through omitted or fraudulent documentation of administered drugs.

Treatment

First, the impaired nurse must realize that substance abuse has become a problem. Denial is a primary char-

acteristic of the disease of addiction that must be recognized before treatment can begin. The denial may be weakened by a realistic presentation of documented observations of the impaired nurse taking the drug or being negligent on the job. Once the nurse acknowledges the problem, referral to a treatment program for the nurse with substance abuse problems can occur. Any comprehensive drug treatment program is acceptable for an impaired nurse; however, factors related to recovery and reentry into practice and professional membership must also be addressed. Some communities have impaired-nurse peer support groups to aid the recovering nurse.

In 1982, the American Nurses Association House of Delegates adopted a resolution directing the association to support: (1) the development of guidelines for assistance programs for impaired nurses, (2) the education of nurse administrators and employers of nurses about the needs of impaired nurses, and (3) the ongoing collection and dissemination of information about substance abuse by nurses. Many state nurses' associations have developed nurse-assistance referral and treatment programs. Also, many specialty nursing organizations have programs to provide assistance.

CHAPTER SUMMARY

Chapter 6 presented discussions about drug abuse, dependence, and addiction. Drugs that are commonly abused, the effects of those drugs, withdrawal symptoms, and treatments were presented. Here are the major highlights of the chapter:
• *Drug abuse* describes the nonmedical use of drugs and other substances that can become detrimental to the user, family, and society.
• A person who is physically dependent on a drug experiences physical effects, such as nausea and vomiting, when the drug is withdrawn.
• A person who is psychologically dependent desires the drug upon withdrawal but may not experience any physical effects.
• *Addiction* refers to drug-seeking behavior in which the drug abuser is unable to control the desire or craving for the chemical substance.
• When body tissues adjust to a drug, tolerance develops, so the person requires increasing amounts of the drug to produce the same effect.

• Upon discontinuing a drug, the drug abuser experiences characteristic signs and symptoms known as *withdrawal syndrome*.

• Opiates include morphine, codeine, heroin, hydromorphone, oxymorphone, meperidine, and methadone. Opiate use results in itching, reddening of the eyes, a drop in blood pressure, lethargy, decreased vision, and sedation.

• Methadone, clonidine, and narcotic antagonists are the major pharmacologic agents used for treating opiate abuse on either an inpatient or outpatient basis.

• Amphetamines and cocaine are frequently abused stimulants. Physiologic effects of stimulant abuse include increased heart rate and blood pressure, widened pulse pressure, dry mouth, palpitations, and dilated pupils.

• Barbiturates, nonbarbiturate sedative-hypnotics, and benzodiazepines are the frequently abused CNS depressants. These drugs, which usually produce sedation, include pentobarbital, secobarbital, amobarbital, ethchlorvynol, glutethimide, and diazepam.

• Alcohol acts as a CNS depressant.

• The general classes of psychotomimetics are indolealkylamines, phenylethylamines, and arylcyclohexylamines.

• Caution must be exercised when caring for patients using psychotomimetics because behavior may be violent and unpredictable.

• Nicotine in cigarettes remains a major health concern in the United States.

• Nurses are at high risk for substance abuse because: (1) they work in stressful situations, (2) they have access to potentially abused prescription drugs, and (3) they may believe that their professional knowledge renders them invulnerable to drug abuse.

Chychula, N.M. "Screening for Substance Abuse in a Primary Care Setting," *Nurse Practitioner* 9:15, July 1984.

Cross, L. "Chemical Dependency in Our Ranks: Managing a Nurse in Crisis," *Nursing Management* 16:15, November 1985.

Efinger, J.M. "Women and Alcoholism," *Topics in Clinical Nursing* 4:10, January 1983.

Farquhar, J.W. "What Role for the New Nicotine Gum?" *Patient Care* 18:196, June 1984.

Halikas, J.A., et al. "A Longitudinal Study of Marijuana Effects," *The International Journal of the Addictions* 20:701, May 1985.

Mennies, J.H. "Smoking: The Physiologic Effects," *American Journal of Nursing* 83:1143, August 1983.

Preston, K.L., and Bigelow, G.E. "Pharmacological Advances in Addiction Treatment," *The International Journal of the Addictions* 20:845, June/July 1985.

Seixas, F.A. "Alcoholism in the 1980s," *Family and Community Health* 7:28, August 1984.

Strasen, L. "Acute Alcohol Withdrawal Syndrome in the Critical Care Unit," *Critical Care Nurse* 2:24, November/December 1982.

U.S. Department of Health and Human Services. *Drug Abuse and Drug Abuse Research*. Washington, D.C.: U.S. Government Printing Office, 1984.

U.S. Department of Health and Human Services. *Health—United States and Prevention Profile*. Washington, D.C.: U.S. Government Printing Office, 1983.

Vellman, W.P., and Jorden, R.C. "History, Metabolism, and Pathophysiology of Alcohol," *Topics in Emergency Medicine* 6:1, July 1984.

Washton, A.M., et al. "Opiate and Cocaine Dependencies," *Postgraduate Medicine* 77:293, April 1985.

BIBLIOGRAPHY

Allison, M., and Hubbard, R.L. "Drug Abuse Treatment Process: A Review of the Literature," *The International Journal of the Addictions* 20:1321, 1345, September 1985.

Bragg, C., and Hughes, G.H. "Understanding and Managing Patients who Smoke," *Family and Community Health* 7:12, May 1984.

Cami, J., et al. "Efficacy of Clonidine and of Methadone in the Rapid Detoxification of Patients Dependent on Heroin," *Clinical Pharmacology and Therapeutics* 38:336, September 1985.

PHARMACOTHERAPEUTICS AND THE NURSING PROCESS

Most nurses will agree that medication administration is the most challenging, and sometimes most frightening, new experience for a nursing student. It is challenging because safe therapeutic medication administration requires technical competence, sound judgment, and meticulous attention to detail. (See *Nursing responsibilities associated with medication administration* for more information.) It can be frightening because it is a complex activity that can directly harm the patient if not implemented properly.

Nurses are legally responsible for maintaining patient safety, ethically responsible for making moral nursing decisions, and professionally responsible for facilitating the therapeutic effects of medications. To meet these responsibilities, the nurse must apply a broad knowledge base to all aspects of care and must be aware of the related legal and ethical implications of nursing care.

Nursing responsibilities associated with medication administration

When giving medication to any patient, the nurse must:
1. Assess the patient's physiologic and psychosocial status.
2. Form nursing diagnoses that identify actual or potential responses that require nursing intervention.
3. Administer the right drug in the right dose to the right patient at the right time by the right route.
4. Assess the patient's responses to drug therapy and determine if the drug is producing therapeutic or adverse effects.
5. Question medication orders that are not clear or that appear to be inappropriate for the patient.
6. Inform the physician of any necessary deviations in medication administration and of any adverse patient reactions to drug therapy.
7. Ensure that the patient is properly educated in the safe, therapeutic self-administration of drugs.
8. Evaluate the effectiveness of nursing interventions.

Unit Two provides the basic information necessary for the nurse to become knowledgeable and competent in safe, therapeutic drug administration. Although learning to administer medications is a complex task, the information contained in Unit Two should help the nurse successfully meet the challenge.

Chapter 7
Assessment, Diagnosis, and Planning
Chapter 7 describes the nursing process as a framework for delivering nursing care. It focuses primarily on the first three steps of the nursing process—assessment, diagnosis, and planning—in relation to drug administration. It also details the use of drug history information in the nursing process and the formulation of nursing diagnoses. The chapter concludes with a discussion of outcome criteria and nursing care plans for specific drug therapy problems.

Chapter 8
Intervention: Administration Processes
Chapter 8 describes the essential components of a medication order and presents the common standardized abbreviations in medication administration. It also presents the seven types of medication orders typically used in hospitals as well as the five rights of medication administration and the procedural safeguards that prevent medication errors. Later, the chapter explores four types of drug delivery systems. It concludes with a discussion of malpractice, moral principles, and the use of placebos.

Chapter 9
Intervention: Dosage Measurements and Calculations
Chapter 9 first surveys the common measurement systems used in clinical situations (metric, apothecaries', and household systems). It then discusses the formulas for converting measurements from one system to another and for calculating drug dosages. The chapter con-

Glossary

Ampule: small, sterile, sealed glass or plastic container that holds a single drug dose.

Anaphylaxis: exaggerated and possibly life-threatening response to an exogenous protein or substance.

Arrest: cessation of cardiac, respiratory, or other physiologic function.

Bradycardia: heart rate of less than 60 beats per minute.

Buccal route: oral medication administration in tablet form on the inside of the cheek.

Capsule: gelatin shell that dissolves in the stomach and contains drug in a powder, sustained-release bead, or liquid form.

Cardiogenic shock: heart failure and peripheral tissue necrosis caused by the heart's inability to contract with sufficient force.

Colloid: state in which high-molecular-weight particles are dispersed in a solution, such as albumin.

Compliance: degree to which a patient follows the advice of a health care professional.

Cream: thick emollient (substance that softens tissue) that contains a paste-drug mixture of oil and water; designed for topical use.

Crystalloid: state in which low-molecular-weight particles are dispersed in a clear solution, such as normal saline solution.

Dermal route: topical medication administration by application to the skin.

Drops: medicated liquid administration in minute spheres.

Drug delivery system: institutional mechanism for obtaining medications from a general stock pharmacy for administration to patients in a clinical unit; also refers to dosage forms.

Elixir: flavored, sweetened hydroalcoholic (water and alcohol) liquid that contains a medicinal agent.

Endotracheal route: medication administration into an endotracheal tube.

Enteric-coated tablet: tablet with a thin coating that prevents release and absorption of its contents until it reaches the small intestine.

Epidural route: medication administration through a catheter inserted into the space around the dura mater of the spinal column.

Ethical responsibility: duty that a nurse has to use fundamental moral values when making nursing decisions.

Evaluation: part of the nursing process in which the nurse judges the effectiveness of care based on preestablished criteria.

Formulary: listing of drugs and information about them.

Gestalt or **cognitive learning theory:** theory that learning is related to an individual's ability to think, process information, form concepts, make decisions, and solve problems.

Goal: statement of the objective or aim of directed nursing care efforts.

Humanistic learning theory: theory that learning is related to the self, to emotional status, and to self-actualization.

Hypodermic route: medication administration by injection into subcutaneous tissue.

Hypovolemia: deficit of extracellular fluid volume.

Inhalant: medicinal vapor administered through the nose, trachea, or respiratory system.

Injection: act of introducing a liquid into the body using a syringe; a solution of a medicine suitable for injection.

Intraarticular route: medication administration by instillation or injection into a joint.

Intradermal route: medication administration by injection of small amounts of solution, usually antigens, between the epidermal and dermal (skin) layers.

Intramuscular route: medication administration by injection of a solution into a muscle.

Intrathecal route: medication administration by direct injection through the theca of the spinal cord into the subarachnoid space.

Intravenous route: medication administration by injection or infusion into a vein.

Learning: acquiring knowledge or skills through study, practice, or experience, which may be demonstrated by behavior change.

Legal responsibility: duty that a nurse has to abide by nursing practice acts and court decisions.

Lotion: medicated liquid applied topically to protect the skin or treat a dermatologic disorder.

Lozenge or **troche:** tablet containing a drug, flavoring, sweetener, and mucilage that is made to dissolve in the mouth.

Malpractice: professional acts of commission or omission, such as negligence and other types of misconduct, that give rise to liability.

Milliequivalent: number of grams of a solute in one milliliter of a normal solution.

Nebulization: treatment by an aerosol spray consisting of particles inhaled into the nose or trachea.

Nurse practice act: state (or Canadian provincial) legislation that describes educational requirements for professional licensure and professional scope of nursing practice.

Nursing care plan: written plan that includes prioritized goals, nursing interventions, and outcome criteria for a specific patient.

Nursing diagnosis: part of the nursing process in which the nurse uses a standard nomenclature to describe actual and potential patient care problems, their etiologies, and their signs and symptoms.

continued

Glossary continued

Nursing process: framework for nursing care that includes assessment, diagnosis, planning, implementation, and evaluation.

Ointment: semisolid preparation that contains a medication for topical application.

Operant conditioning or **reinforcement theory:** theory that learning is behavioral change produced by a system of rewards.

Outcome criteria: statement of desired results that contains a content description, an action verb, a time line, and criterion modifiers.

Over-the-counter drug: drug available without a prescription.

Parenteral route: medication administration by a route other than the alimentary canal and by injection, such as intradermal, intramuscular, and intravenous injection.

Paste: soft, semisolid substance that contains medication in a fatty base, a viscous (sticky) base, or a mixture of petroleum and starch; usually applied topically.

Patch: thin membrane or gel base applied to the skin that releases a measured dose of medication over an extended period.

Percentage solution: solution in which the solute (solid) represents a percentage of the solution's total weight. For example, *0.9% saline solution* means that every 100 milliliters of solution contains 0.9 grams of sodium chloride (or every liter of solution contains 9 grams of sodium chloride).

Placebo: inactive substance, such as normal saline solution, or a less-than-effective dose of a substance, such as a vitamin, prescribed as if it were an effective medication dose.

Powder: small particles of medication obtained by grinding a solid drug.

Prescription: order for medication, therapy, or a therapeutic device given by a properly authorized person to a person properly authorized to dispense or perform the order.

Professional responsibility: duty that a nurse has to the standards of practice established by the profession as its code of ethics.

Rectal route: medication administration by insertion, injection, or infusion into the rectum.

Social learning theory: theory that learning occurs through imitation, role modeling, and role assumption.

Subcutaneous route: medication administration by injection of a substance under the skin into the layer of loose connective tissue.

Sublingual route: medication administration by placement of a tablet under the tongue.

Suppository: medicated mass, usually cone-shaped, that melts or dissolves after insertion into a body cavity.

Suspension: preparation in which small particles of a solid drug are dispersed—but not dissolved—in a liquid for administration. Stirring or shaking the mixture maintains dispersal.

Syrup: concentrated solution that contains a medication, flavoring, sugar, and water.

Tablet: solid preparation in which medication is combined with inert ingredients and compressed into a shape.

Tachycardia: heart rate of more than 100 beats per minute.

Teaching: system of actions intended to produce learning.

Teratogenesis: development of physical defects in an embryo or fetus.

Tincture: liquid preparation that contains a medication and alcohol or water and alcohol.

Vaginal route: medication administration by insertion or injection into the vagina.

Vial: small, glass, multidose medication container sealed with a rubber diaphragm.

Wax matrix tablet: wax, honeycomb structure that contains medication slowly released as the comb dissolves.

cludes with pediatric dosage calculations and with special considerations for geriatric patients and those receiving chemotherapy.

Chapter 10
Intervention: Routes and Techniques of Administration

Chapter 10 defines the oral and parenteral forms of liquid drugs and explains the mechanisms of absorption for suppository and inhalant drugs. Then it details the procedures and techniques for administering drugs by the oral, buccal, sublingual, rectal, vaginal, parenteral, dermal, nasal, ophthalmic, and respiratory routes, and

by nasogastric and gastrostomy tubes. This chapter emphasizes the rationales underlying nursing decisions about medication administration routes and techniques.

Chapter 11
Intervention: Patient Education

Chapter 11 focuses on patient education that fosters patient compliance with drug therapy. It explores four major learning theories (operant conditioning, Gestalt, humanistic, and social learning) as well as three teaching and three learning principles: establishing nurse-patient rapport aids patient teaching; effective communication is essential; environmental control can influence teaching; objectives guide the teaching session; cultural, ethnic, and religious beliefs must be considered in planning teaching sessions; and evaluation is an essential part of the teaching process. Then it describes how to use the three learning domains in teaching about medication therapy. It also details the components of a teaching plan and explains how to use them to meet a specific patient's education needs. Finally, the chapter differentiates between formative and summative evaluation of patient teaching.

Chapter 12
Intervention: The Pediatric Patient
Chapter 12 examines the special considerations for medication administration to pediatric patients. First, the chapter describes age-related changes that affect a drug's pharmacokinetics, pharmacodynamics, and pharmacotherapeutics in pediatric patients. It illustrates these variations with specific examples and discusses the effects of drugs on normal growth and development. The chapter also explores variations in pediatric medication administration techniques and procedures. Lastly, it discusses family education and drug therapy.

Chapter 13
Intervention: The Geriatric Patient
Chapter 13 presents special considerations for geriatric patients. It begins by discussing age-related changes that affect a drug's pharmacokinetics, pharmacodynamics, and pharmacotherapeutics in geriatric patients. Next, it explores the factors that predispose the elderly to adverse drug reactions and the common signs and symptoms of these reactions. Then it discusses the nurse's role in reviewing medication regimens for geriatric patients and reviews ways to help cognitively impaired patients self-administer medication.

Chapter 14
Intervention: The Pregnant or Lactating Patient
Chapter 14 explores the pharmacokinetic changes that occur when a drug is given to a pregnant or lactating woman. It explains placental transport and the relationship between teratogenicity and drug administration at different gestational ages of the fetus. This chapter also discusses medications used to treat pregnancy-related symptoms, such as heartburn, nausea, constipation, and headache. It describes breast-milk formation and drug transport to this milk. It concludes with guidelines to help the nurse counsel the pregnant or lactating patient who needs drug therapy.

Chapter 15
Intervention: Emergencies
Chapter 15 discusses drug administration during emergency situations, such as cardiac arrest, cardiogenic shock, hypovolemia, hypertensive crisis, anaphylactic shock, and narcotic overdose. It emphasizes decision-making rationales in these situations. It discusses the rationale for use, administration procedures and dosages, and nursing precautions of code drugs. It describes alpha- and beta-adrenergic receptors and differentiates between adrenergic receptor stimulation and blockade. It includes information on endotracheal drug administration and discusses various volume expanders used to manage hypovolemic states.

Chapter 16
Evaluation
Chapter 16 defines and illustrates evaluation and evaluation criteria related to medication administration—part of the nursing process. Then it elaborates on evaluating the outcomes of, and the patient's compliance with, drug therapy. It includes questions the nurse can use to evaluate the effectiveness of a patients's drug therapy, and it includes factors that help the nurse evaluate patient compliance. The chapter concludes by discussing the importance of documenting the evaluation of drug therapy.

Nursing diagnoses
Unit Two deals with several components of the nursing process and their relationship to drug therapy and suggests a number of related nursing diagnoses that would be used to plan patient care, including:
- Alteration in comfort: pain related to medication administration routes
- Alteration in comfort: pain related to medication administration techniques
- Alteration in health maintenance related to long-term medication therapy
- Alterations in oral mucous membranes related to buccal medication administration
- Anxiety related to medication therapy
- Anxiety related to self-medication administration
- Disturbance in self-concept: self-esteem related to long-term medication therapy
- Fear related to medication therapy
- Fear related to self-medication administration
- Impaired tissue integrity related to poor medication administration techniques
- Knowledge deficit related to medication administration techniques and routes
- Knowledge deficit related to medication therapy

- Knowledge deficit related to self-medication administration techniques
- Noncompliance related to medication therapy
- Potential for infection related to poor medication administration techniques
- Potential for injury related to medication administration techniques
- Potential for injury related to medication therapy
- Self-care deficit related to medication administration
- Sensory-perceptual alterations related to medication therapy
- Skin integrity, impaired: potential related to medication administration
- Sleep pattern disturbances related to medication therapy

ASSESSMENT, DIAGNOSIS, AND PLANNING

OBJECTIVES

After reading and studying this chapter, you should be able to:

1. Explain the nursing process as a logical sequence involving assessment, diagnosis, planning, implementation, and evaluation.

2. Collect appropriate data during the assessment step to serve as the basis for subsequent decisions about the patient's drug regimen.

3. List the three major categories—general information, prescription drugs, and over-the-counter drugs—that must be included when obtaining a drug history.

4. Explain why the following areas should be investigated when gathering general information for a drug history: allergies, medical history, habits, socioeconomic status, life-style and beliefs, and sensory deficits.

5. Explain why a patient's use of prescription drugs and over-the-counter drugs can alter the patient's responses to a prescribed drug regimen.

6. Explain the effect of a patient's cognitive abilities on the patient's ability to participate successfully in drug therapy.

7. Formulate a nursing diagnosis using the PES method and its components: the problem statement, the etiology, and the signs and symptoms.

8. Identify the six types of errors that most frequently occur when formulating a nursing diagnosis.

9. Apply three diagnostic labels in developing a nursing care plan for a patient's drug therapy.

10. Write outcome criteria, which contain the content area, an action verb, a time frame, and criterion modifiers.

INTRODUCTION

This chapter investigates the nursing process in relation to drug therapy. The nursing process, a framework that aids in the development, implementation, and evalua-

tion of patient care, consists of five essential steps: assessment, identification of a nursing diagnosis (identifying a patient's health need), planning, implementation of the nursing plan of care, and evaluation. (See *The nursing process* on page 98 for an illustration of the five steps and their relation to one another.)

During assessment, the nurse focuses on direct data collection by obtaining: (1) a history from the patient, spouse, parent, or significant other, (2) physical examination of the patient, (3) previous medical records, and (4) laboratory or diagnostic test results. The nurse continually updates the assessment step as information is collected during each patient interaction. Because the subsequent steps depend upon the information collected during assessment, this first step is crucial in the nursing process.

In the second step, the nurse identifies the actual or potential nursing diagnosis or health need. An analysis of the essential assessment data, the specific signs or symptoms (defining characteristics), and the probable cause (etiology) helps the nurse identify a particular nursing diagnosis.

Having formulated a nursing diagnosis, the nurse then begins the planning step. The nursing plan of care consists of two major components: the outcome criteria, or patient goals, and nursing interventions. Outcome criteria describe the desired patient behaviors or responses resulting from the nursing care. The nurse focuses the outcome criteria on patient education and management of the specific drug regimen. The nurse might want the patient to verbalize knowledge of a particular drug. The patient might also be expected to demonstrate how to give subcutaneous injections or how to administer antibiotics intravenously. The nurse should state each outcome criterion as a measurable, objective statement. For example, ''The patient will state the major action of furosemide (Lasix)'' or ''The patient's lungs

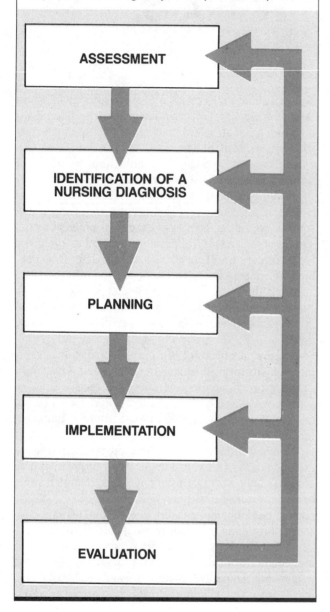

The nursing process

The nurse proceeds through the five steps of the nursing process, moving from assessment to evaluation. Depending on the evaluation findings, the nurse may update or change any of the previous steps.

ASSESSMENT

IDENTIFICATION OF A NURSING DIAGNOSIS

PLANNING

IMPLEMENTATION

EVALUATION

dependent. For example, altering the drug schedule to coincide with the patient's daily routine represents an independent intervention, whereas consulting with the physician and pharmacist to change a patient's medication because of adverse effects represents an interdependent intervention. Administering an already prescribed drug on time is a dependent intervention. The choice of which of the three types of nursing actions to use depends on the proposed outcome criteria for each stated nursing diagnosis.

In the fourth step of the nursing process, the nurse implements the developed plan of care. During the implementation step, the nurse administers the prescribed drug regimen and monitors its effectiveness. The nursing staff implements the established plan of care, whether it involves patient knowledge of drugs and skills in administering drugs, assessment of the patient for the regimen's effectiveness, or discussions focusing on the reasons for noncompliance. In implementing the nursing plan of care, the nurse may need to use various resources, including other health care professionals.

During evaluation, the fifth step, the nurse notes progress toward and possible resolution of the desired outcome criteria. The nurse's evaluation assures that the best possible plan is being implemented. Chapter 16, Evaluation, presents a detailed discussion of the evaluation step.

Evaluation is a critically important, ongoing component of the nursing process and of the care delivered to the patient. Continual reassessment, updating, and change occur in each of the five steps of the nursing process. Depending upon the findings of the evaluation step, the nurse may return to any step in the process. The nurse may find that more assessment information is needed or that outcome criteria are not established at an appropriate level. The nursing interventions may need revision to meet the outcome criteria or the nurse may find that the outcome criteria have been accomplished.

The nursing process is a dynamic process that allows the nurse to develop and modify a total plan of care in a logical sequence for a particular patient.

THE NURSE'S ROLE IN ASSESSMENT

During the assessment step of the nursing process, the nurse gathers information for a patient's drug therapy. One important information source is the patient's drug

will clear to auscultation by the time of discharge from the hospital.''

Nursing interventions, determined by the nurse, depend upon the established outcome criteria; that is, the nurse devises interventions to help the patient achieve the outcome criteria. Nursing interventions are classified according to type as independent, interdependent, or history, which the nurse obtains from data given by the patient, spouse, parent, or significant other. The nurse also obtains information by performing a physical examination to detect any potential adverse reactions to the patient's drug regimen and by consulting the patient's previous medical records. Furthermore, the nurse examines the laboratory or diagnostic test results, noting any unusual findings that may: (1) indicate a possible adverse reaction, such as a toxic level of digoxin, or (2) document drug efficacy, such as a therapeutic increase in clotting time secondary to the use of anticoagulants.

The nurse continuously updates the assessment data by collecting information during each patient interaction. Assessment represents a crucial step in the nursing process because all subsequent steps depend upon the information collected.

COMPONENTS OF A DRUG HISTORY

The nurse must obtain a thorough patient drug history upon the patient's admission to either the hospital or the outpatient setting. Currently, instead of depending on one family physician for overall medical care, a patient may have numerous specialists, such as an internist, cardiologist, or pulmonologist. Seeking the care of specialists in different fields can be beneficial for the patient, but can also present some difficulties. Usually with various physicians participating in the care of one patient, no one physician may be designated to oversee and coordinate the care and, with several physicians prescribing drugs, conflicting or incompatible drug regimens may occur. The potential for conflicting or incompatible drug regimens makes obtaining a thorough drug history essential for those patients new to the hospital or outpatient setting, including those admitted for the monitoring and regulating of particular drug regimens and those with drug complications.

The nurse compiling a comprehensive drug history should ask specific questions that cover the patient's background, for example, allergies and socioeconomic status, prescription drugs, and over-the-counter drugs. (See *Critical components of a drug history* on page 100.)

General information

General information covers background data related to the patient. The major components are allergies, medical history, habits, socioeconomic status, life-style and beliefs, and sensory deficits.

Allergies. To obtain a comprehensive profile of a patient's allergies, the nurse should investigate the patient's reactions to both drugs and foods. While discussing allergic reactions to drugs, the nurse must inquire about

the type of drug, when the allergic reaction occurred, the situation and setting at the time of the reaction, the type of reaction that occurred, and any other contributing factors. Examples of contributing factors might include the use of alcohol or recreational drugs, a change in eating or nutritional habits, environmental agents (such as pollens or poison oak), and newly prescribed drug regimens. The patient's responses may provide the nurse with some insight into the factors and circumstances that contributed to the allergic reaction.

The patient's description of an allergic reaction can help the nurse determine whether the patient actually reacts adversely to a particular drug or simply dislikes the drug. For example, one patient may "identify" an allergic reaction to all major pain medications because they cause an "out of control" feeling. Another patient may develop a body rash and experience difficulty breathing after receiving certain pain medications. The first patient does not have a true drug allergy and may need education concerning the effects of the different drugs. The second person has experienced an allergic reaction. When a patient has a drug allergy, the nurse needs to document the specific drug and reaction in the patient's chart and other pertinent patient records.

The nurse also needs to assess for allergies to foods because such allergies can also affect a patient's drug regimen and care. Many of the dyes used for various medical procedures contain iodine or are by-products of shellfish. As a consequence, a patient's information regarding shellfish allergies becomes an important part of the assessment. Some vaccines are also derived from animal proteins. For example, chick embryo tissue cultures are sometimes used to prepare mumps vaccines. A patient's information regarding allergic reactions to eggs will help ensure proper treatment.

Finally, the nurse should discuss with the patient any possible environmental causes of allergies, such as pollens, feathers, or cat or dog hair.

Medical history. Examining a patient's medical history particularly helps the nurse understand any particular drug regimen the patient may be following. In gathering data, the nurse should note any chronic or long-term diseases or disorders the patient may have. Such diseases may include hypertension, cancer, emphysema, or renal failure. For each chronic illness experienced by the patient, the nurse should note the following: (1) the diagnosis date, (2) the initial prescribed treatment, (3) the current treatment, and (4) the physician in charge of the patient's care. Finally, the nurse should find out how often the patient seeks consultation with a physician on each particular drug regimen.

Critical components of a drug history

When formulating the patient's drug history, the nurse must investigate certain components essential to proper nursing practice. The major components include general information, prescription drugs, and over-the-counter drugs. The following list serves as a guide for obtaining a drug history.

GENERAL INFORMATION

Allergies
- Medications
- Food

Medical history
- Associated illness and diseases

Habits
- Dietary
- Recreational drug use
—alcohol
—smoking
—stimulants (e.g., caffeine)
—illicit drugs

Socioeconomic status
- Age
- Educational level
- Occupation
- Insurance coverage

Life-style and beliefs
- Marital status
- Childbearing status
- Personal support systems
- Attitudes toward health and health care
- Locus of control
- Utilization of the health care system
- Typical pattern of daily activities

Sensory deficits

PRESCRIPTION DRUGS

Reason for use

Knowledge of drugs

Frequency or dosage

Effectiveness or reactions

Pattern and route of administration

OVER-THE-COUNTER DRUGS

Reason for use

Knowledge of drugs

Frequency or dosage

Effectiveness or reactions

Pattern and route of administration

The nurse should also record any acute episodes of illnesses or disorders experienced by the patient. Examples include colds, gastric upsets, and headaches. The nurse should note the frequency and patterning of the acute episodes, as well as the treatment used for each. Treatments include any home remedies that have been used, as well as prescription or over-the-counter drugs. The nurse should also record those remedies the patient found successful.

Habits. Documenting certain habits directly related to drug therapy represents another important step in compiling a patient's drug history. Two major areas that the nurse should consider are the patient's dietary habits and use of recreational drugs, including alcohol, tobacco, caffeine, and illicit drugs, such as marijuana, cocaine, and heroin.

Dietary intake can directly affect the effectiveness of many drugs. For example, a person taking calcium supplements must maintain a diet that meets the daily requirements of vitamin D, which aids in the absorption and utilization of calcium. For a patient on warfarin (Coumadin) therapy, the intake of green leafy vegetables should not fluctuate significantly, because these vegetables contain certain levels of vitamin K that antagonize the action of Coumadin.

The use of recreational drugs can profoundly affect a patient's health and inhibit the effectiveness of a particular drug regimen. For alcohol intake, the nurse needs to note the frequency of use, as well as the type and amount of alcohol consumed. Many people consider themselves to be "social drinkers," a phrase that can differ in meaning. For example, a social drinker may take one drink with each meal, two or three drinks in the evening, or one drink a month. Each of the circumstances involves different amounts of alcohol consumption. The nurse must therefore quantify the amount of alcohol consumed when the patient uses such descriptive phrases as "social drinker," "weekend drinker," "occasional drinker," or "heavy drinker." The nurse should also note whether the patient primarily drinks beer, wine, cocktails, or hard liquor, because equal amounts of the various types of alcoholic beverages contain differing amounts of alcohol and affect each person differently.

For smoking, the nurse should document the following: (1) the length of time the patient has been smoking, (2) what the patient smokes (cigarettes, cigars, a pipe), (3) the amount smoked per day (packs of cigarettes, number of cigars), and (4) the brand of cigarettes or cigars the patient smokes. Different brands may or may not have filters, which supposedly block some of the nicotine intake. The nurse must also note whether or not the patient chews tobacco, and if so, how much per day and the type of tobacco.

A patient's smoking history can be easily expressed in terms of pack years. To calculate pack years, the nurse multiplies the number of packs the patient smokes per day by the number of years the patient has smoked. A patient who has smoked 2 packs of cigarettes per day for 25 years would have a 50 pack-year history of smoking. Another patient who smoked 1 pack per day for 5 years, then 1½ packs per day for 20 years, would have a 35 pack-year history of smoking (1 pack per day × 5 years + 1½ packs per day × 20 years).

Next the nurse must document the intake of stimulants, such as caffeine, because stimulants can significantly affect a patient's cardiovascular status and nervous system. The nurse should record the form in which the stimulant appears (coffee, tea, soda, or chocolate), the frequency of intake, and the amount consumed. The nurse should note if the individual experiences any unusual sensations, such as palpitations or shakiness, after ingesting the stimulant.

When assessing the use of illicit drugs, the nurse must document the type of drug used, the frequency with which it is used, the amount used, and the route of administration. Each type of illicit drug can produce a different and profound effect on a person, depending on the drug, the route of administration, and the individual. Chapter 6, Drug Abuse, Dependence, and Addiction, discusses specific reactions to different types of illicit drugs.

Socioeconomic status. The factors related to a patient's socioeconomic status include age, educational level, occupation, and insurance coverage. Although socioeconomic factors may not be directly related to compliance, they can be quite significant when developing a successful nursing care plan for a particular patient. Knowing the patient's age can assist the nurse in determining whom to include in the plan, such as parents or other family members, and what level of information to provide. When initiating a care plan for a pediatric or geriatric patient, the nurse will need to consider special nursing actions or interventions. (See Chapters 12 and 13 for detailed discussions of these considerations.)

Knowing the patient's educational background helps the nurse focus selected interventions at an appropriate level and determine specific strategies to use in the nursing plan of care. Besides understanding a patient's educational level, the nurse should know the patient's occupation. Knowing about a patient's job can help the nurse determine appropriate examples to use when explaining various facts about the drug regimen. Knowing the patient's occupation can also help the nurse plan a drug regimen that fits the patient's schedule, thus minimizing the chances of disrupting the patient's daily routine. Individualized scheduling will positively affect the patient's adherence to the prescribed regimen.

Knowing a patient's type of insurance coverage can help the nurse calculate the potential length of hospital stay, especially if the patient has Medicare, a program that sets standards for its participants through DRGs (Diagnosis-Related Groups). Knowing the patient's type of insurance coverage can also help the nurse determine the potential need for extra funds or financial counseling.

Life-style and beliefs. In assessing a patient's life-style, the nurse should obtain information about the following subjects: support systems, marital status, childbearing status, attitudes toward health and health care, use of the health care system, and daily activities patterns. Positive, strong support systems at home and in other areas of life can help a patient adhere to a specific drug regimen. Noting the type of support systems available to the patient is critical.

The patient's support system may consist of a spouse, other family members, or significant others. Compliance literature has documented that people who isolate themselves from society and from potential support systems are less likely to comply with prescribed drug regimens. Marital status is also important because married patients exhibit a positive correlation with increased patient compliance. The nurse also can use information on the female patient's childbearing status and use of contraceptives because of the potential for some medications to cause fetal damage.

Numerous research studies also have shown that a patient's attitudes toward health and health care have a significant effect on compliance. Therefore, the nurse needs to assess the patient's beliefs and knowledge in this area. Research indicates that if the patient believes that the physiologic, psychological, or economic benefits of the prescribed health care regimen outweigh the disadvantages, the patient will be more likely to comply with the drug regimen.

Another issue that the nurse needs to consider is the patient's locus of control, or the degree to which an individual perceives events that occur as being a consequence of the individual's own actions. Research indicates that those people who possess an internal locus of control believe that they exercise direction over events in their lives. Both mental and emotional reinforcements for persons with an internal locus of control come from within. On the other hand, research indicates that people who have an external locus of control believe that outside factors control their lives. People with an external locus of control tend to derive reinforcement from abstractions, such as fate or chance, which they perceive as lying outside themselves. Studies further indicate that patients with an internal locus of control are more likely to be compliant because they seek information and help to make the best decision for their particular circumstances.

The nurse must also consider how each patient uses the health care system. One patient may see a physician regularly, while another patient may depend on the emergency department for primary care. Still other patients may be seeing a specialist for each body system, consulting regularly with the different specialists. If a patient has numerous specialists, the nurse must find out if one physician is responsible for coordinating the patient's total care. Contacting the physican in charge can help the nurse avoid implementing conflicting drug regimens. The nurse must also consult with the physician in charge to determine the type of follow-up care that the patient will need.

The last factor related to life-style is the patient's daily activities pattern. The nurse can address this issue by asking the patient to describe what occurs during a typical day and using that information to educate the patient and establish the least disruptive health care regimen for home use. Considering all of the factors related to the patient's life-style and beliefs can help the nurse decrease a drug regimen's complexity and increase patient compliance.

Sensory deficits. The presence or absence of any sensory deficits can significantly shape the development of an appropriate health care plan for the patient. The nurse should first note the obvious sensory deficits, such as impaired vision or hearing, the paralysis of one or more extremities, or the loss of a particular limb. Besides noting the more obvious deficits, the nurse should explore such things as diseases or decreased sensations in the extremities, any of which can interfere with the patient's ability to give self-administered injections, break scored tablets, and open medication containers. Another sensory deficit that can significantly affect patient compliance is color blindness. In many cases, color helps identify a drug, particularly when the size and shape of different drugs are similar. The nurse must consider all types of sensory deficits when planning to implement a prescribed drug regimen.

Prescription drugs

The nurse must also determine the patient's knowledge about previously prescribed drug regimens. In assessing a patient's history of prescription drug use, the nurse should explore the following: the reason for using the drug; the patient's knowledge of when the drug should be taken, dosage, and efficacy; and the route of administration.

The nurse needs to know if the patient understands why a particular drug has been prescribed, what type of adverse effects the drug might cause, and when to contact a physician. The nurse should also note any special monitoring that the patient must perform in relation to the drug regimen, such as comparing the radial pulse rate with specified parameters before digoxin administration or implementation of glucose self-monitoring tests for insulin therapy.

The nurse should also find out if the patient knows the prescribed dosage and the particular schedule of each drug. The nurse should discuss the effectiveness of the drug regimen with the patient, noting any symptoms or unpredicted adverse effects that have occurred since the regimen began.

The nurse should also note the pattern of administration that the patient follows at home, because it may provide insight into reasons why a particular drug regimen succeeds or fails. Information about the pattern of administration can also aid the physician and nurse in developing a realistic plan for the patient. Consider the following example:

A truck driver named Tom Dunlop was admitted to the hospital for regulation of his insulin regimen. Mr. Dunlop usually adheres to the following daily pattern: he arises at 3:00 a.m., eats breakfast at 3:30 and is on the road from 4:00 a.m. to 8:00 a.m., at which time he stops for lunch. Then he drives till noon, eats supper at about 2:00 p.m., and goes to bed around 7:00 p.m.

During his stay in the hospital, Mr. Dunlop's insulin administration and meals should not be timed according to the hospital routine, because as soon as he leaves the hospital, he will return to his previous schedule. Deviating from the previous schedule of insulin administration may make it difficult for Mr. Dunlop to adjust to and maintain appropriate control of his diabetes. In Mr. Dunlop's case, the nurse should follow the patient's normal pattern of administration during his stay in the hospital to ensure proper regulation and compliance.

Over-the-counter drugs

To obtain a comprehensive assessment of the patient's drug regimen, the nurse must explore what type of over-the-counter drugs the patient is taking. Many over-the-counter drugs can inhibit or potentiate the effects of a prescribed drug. For instance, patients taking anticoagulants, such as warfarin, should not take aspirin or any drugs containing aspirin because aspirin potentiates the anticoagulant effects. Patients taking tetracycline or its derivatives should know that antacids may decrease the drug's effectiveness.

Over-the-counter drugs include a wide range of products, from common aspirin to nutritional supplements to cleansing agents, such as douches and enemas. Over-the-counter products may come in solid, liquid, cream, and powdered forms. The patient may not even think of all these products as drugs.

The nurse, in acquiring information concerning over-the-counter drug use, should explore why the patient is taking the drugs and if the patient knows the drug actions and effects. The nurse should also note the frequency and dosage of the over-the-counter drug use. The nurse also should discuss the administration pattern because it can provide insights into how the patient uses the drug and may help determine the success or failure of the prescribed regimen.

Finally, the nurse should note whether or not the patient considers the drug effective and if the patient experiences any unusual effects while taking it. If the patient reports any unusual effects, the nurse should record their frequency and severity, noting whether the effects worsened with each exposure to the drug.

CLINICAL BEHAVIORS

Besides obtaining a drug history during assessment, the nurse needs to consider two other important matters that affect drug administration: the patient's cognitive abilities and the body systems that may be affected by the prescribed drugs.

A patient's cognitive abilities need to be intact to ensure that the patient can understand and implement the actions necessary for compliance. The nurse initially notes whether the patient appears alert and oriented. Both qualities can readily be assessed while obtaining the patient's drug history. The nurse must also note the patient's ability to interact and the appropriateness of the conversation. The nurse must ascertain whether the patient can think clearly, integrate those thoughts into a logical process, and then express those thoughts in a coherent and efficient manner.

The nurse must check both short-term and long-term memories because the patient uses both when following a specified drug regimen. The nurse can assess the patient's long-term memory while obtaining the drug history by noting the patient's ability to describe past experiences, such as illnesses or drug regimens. Short-term memory can be assessed by various methods. For example, while obtaining the drug history, the nurse can give the patient new information, such as the visiting hours or the patient's room number, and then ask the patient to recall this information later in the interview.

If a patient's cognitive abilities are not intact, the nurse must determine the probable cause, which can range from a drug-related effect to a pathophysiologic condition. Whatever the cause, the nurse must determine whether or not the patient possesses the ability to carry out the prescribed drug regimen. If the patient's cognitive abilities are impaired, the nurse must determine another way to ensure that the patient will comply. The nurse may need to educate a family member or significant other, obtain a visiting nurse referral, use a day-care setting, or consider admitting the patient to an extended-care facility.

Having completed the drug history, the nurse needs to assess those body systems that may be affected by the patient's prescribed drug regimen. Every drug produces a particular effect on a specific body system or systems. Some of the effects may represent the desired action of the drug. At the same time, however, every drug can potentially affect other body systems in adverse ways. For instance, chemotherapeutic drugs destroy cancerous cells, yet they also destroy normal cells and lead to nausea, loss of appetite, hair loss, and diarrhea. The nurse must closely monitor the potentially harmful adverse effects of a drug to ensure that the patient does not become seriously compromised.

The nurse must have a thorough understanding of the pharmacology of each prescribed drug. No nurse can possess a complete knowledge of all available drugs, but the nurse can assume responsibility for locating references or resources that provide necessary information for understanding new or unfamiliar drugs. Examples of some of these references are discussed in Chapter 1, Introduction to Pharmacology.

FORMULATING A NURSING DIAGNOSIS

Formulating a nursing diagnosis occurs after the assessment or data collection step in the nursing process. Very little mention of nursing diagnosis appeared in the literature until the 1970s. In 1973, the First National Conference-Group on Nursing Diagnosis convened in St. Louis. Since that time, the group, now called the North American Nursing Diagnosis Association (NANDA), has met every 2 years to discuss the ongoing classification system for nursing diagnosis. The classification system aids in defining the scope of nursing practice as it relates to patient care and enables nurses to communicate in a universal language. One of the most widely published definitions of nursing diagnosis, proposed by Gordon in 1976, states that a nursing diagnosis represents an "actual or potential health problem, which nurses, by virtue of their education and experience, are capable and licensed to treat."

Nursing diagnoses help the nurse to identify patient problems or health needs and to establish priorities of care for each patient. Currently, NANDA has approved 84 diagnostic labels that nurses should use in developing nursing diagnoses. (See *NANDA taxonomy of nursing diagnoses* on pages 106 and 107 for a list of the diagnostic labels.) The list of diagnostic labels does not represent an end but a beginning; it is continually being updated and strengthened as it is tested and used in clinical practice.

THE COMPONENTS OF A NURSING DIAGNOSIS

Several methods of writing a nursing diagnosis exist. Gordon developed one of the most straightforward methods, which includes the problem, its etiology, and its signs and symptoms, known as the PES method. (See *The PES method for developing a nursing diagnosis* on page 108 for an illustration of this method and its components.)

According to Gordon, the first component, the problem statement, identifies the actual or potential health problem or patient need. In writing the problem statement, the nurse can use the taxonomy of nursing diagnoses developed and accepted by NANDA. Remember, the information collected during the assessment phase of the nursing process forms the basis for identifying the nursing diagnosis. Therefore, the problem component of the PES method represents the stated diagnostic label, such as "Knowledge deficit," "Impaired home maintenance management," or "Noncompliance." The identified problem needs to fall within nursing's realm; that is, the problem should be something that nurses are licensed to treat. The nurse should write the problem statement as clearly and concisely as possible to avoid confusion. One purpose of a nursing diagnosis is to communicate to other nurses, as well as to other health care professionals, what is occurring with a particular patient.

The etiology statement, the second component, consists of the factors related to the development of the problem or the possible cause of the patient's identified health needs. The etiology statement determines the specific outcomes and interventions for each nursing diagnosis. To illustrate, "Knowledge deficit" and "Impaired home maintenance management" both give the nurse an idea of what major area to focus on, but neither statement gives direction concerning what care plan to develop for a specific patient. By connecting the etiology statement to the problem statement, the nurse can determine what the specific care plan should be. For example, the etiology statements "Knowledge deficit, related to a new diagnosis of lung cancer and chemotherapy" and "Knowledge deficit, related to the actions and schedule of the patient's anticoagulant therapy" require very different types of interventions and outcome criteria, even though both of the statements address knowledge deficits.

The etiology component determines the plan of action. The nurse must write the etiology statement as concisely as possible to ensure that other nurses and health care professionals will understand the cause of the patient problem and the reason for the nursing diagnosis. The etiology statement also dictates the type of outcome criteria and interventions that should be developed for each particular nursing diagnosis.

The third component of the PES method, the signs and symptoms or the defining characteristics, represents the specific factors that led to identifying the particular diagnostic label or problem statement. In other words, the defining characteristics comprise the supporting data for the stated problem or health need. The nurse identifies the defining characteristics during the assessment phase of the nursing process. For example, with a diagnosis of "Potential for injury, related to chlorpromazine administration," such defining characteristics as "dizziness" and "feeling light-headed when sitting up and ambulating" may be patient statements obtained while documenting the drug history. The nurse may also note orthostatic changes in the blood pressure and an unsteady gait. Thus, the defining characteristics can be subjective or objective.

In writing a nursing diagnosis, the nurse uses only the first two components, the problem statement and the etiology statement, connecting the two statements with the phrase "related to." An example of a correctly worded diagnosis would be "Knowledge deficit, related to the management of nausea." The defining characteristics or signs and symptoms supporting such a diagnosis would include the patient's inability due to nausea to eat more than 10% of the scheduled meals, a weight loss of 5 pounds (2 kg) in 1 week, and the patient's ingestion of metoclopramide (Reglan) and prochlorperazine (Compazine), antiemetics, every 2 to 4 hours. The nurse should document the defining characteristics in the patient's data base in the history and physical examination report or in the nurses' notes. Remember, the defining characteristics help to determine the appropriate nursing diagnosis.

Common pitfalls of nursing diagnoses

Errors frequently occur as nursing students and nurses learn to formulate nursing diagnoses. Those errors include using a medical diagnosis instead of a nursing diagnosis, stating a diagnostic test or procedure rather than a nursing diagnosis, stating a nursing need rather than a nursing diagnosis, using a diagnostic label and a synonymous etiology, using two diagnostic labels in the same problem statement, and stating the nursing diagnosis in terminology that could cause legal problems.

The most frequent error occurs when the nursing diagnosis is stated as a medical diagnosis. For example, "Congestive heart failure, related to cardiomyopathy" is not a nursing diagnosis because it refers to a patient response or problem for which a nurse cannot independently develop a care plan or nursing interventions. However, a patient with congestive heart failure may experience significant difficulty in breathing or gas exchange. As a consequence, the nurse would identify the nursing diagnosis as "Alteration in gas exchange." Another patient with congestive heart failure may have problems with excess fluid or peripheral edema, so the nurse would work with a "Fluid volume excess" or an "Alteration in skin integrity" problem. In essence, nurses deal with the varied responses a patient may have to an alteration in health status.

The nurse needs to ensure that the nursing diagnosis is not stated as a diagnostic test or treatment, such as "Hyperalimentation." In a situation involving hyperalimentation, the nurse may be concerned about the patient's nutritional status, although the nutritional status encompasses much more than just hyperalimentation. The nurse also needs to monitor overall caloric intake, which may include oral or nasogastric supplements. The nurse would also monitor the patient's daily weight and instruct either the patient or some significant other about the importance of increasing the nutritional intake, if necessary. The nurse would work with the patient to determine the patient's likes and dislikes and, if possible, have the family bring in favorite foods. Depending upon the assessment data, the nurse also may be concerned about the potential complications that might occur while the patient is receiving hyperalimentation.

The nursing diagnosis relates to the assessment of the patient and directs the care for the patient's particular health need or problem. Nursing diagnoses, however, are sometimes mistakenly stated as nursing needs or actions. For example, "Need for frequent interaction to decrease patient isolation" relates to a nursing intervention or need rather than a patient health problem. The actual nursing diagnosis for the patient might be better stated as "Alterations in sensory-perceptual areas, related to isolation."

Writing an etiology statement synonymous with the problem statement represents another frequent mistake. For example, "Activity intolerance, related to the patient's inability to tolerate activity" is a redundant etiology statement; it does not inform the nurse about the causes of the problem, which is "Activity intolerance." As a result, the nurse cannot develop a care plan for the patient based on the nursing diagnosis. The activity

NANDA taxonomy of nursing diagnoses

A taxonomy for discussing nursing diagnoses has evolved over a number of years. The following list contains the approved diagnostic labels of the North American Nursing Diagnosis Association, as of summer 1986.

Acivity intolerance

Activity intolerance: Potential

Adjustment, impaired

Airway clearance, ineffective

Anxiety

Body temperature, altered: Potential

Bowel elimination, altered: Constipation

Bowel elimination, altered: Diarrhea

Bowel elimination, altered: Incontinence

Breathing pattern, ineffective

Cardiac output, altered: Decreased

Comfort, altered: Pain

Comfort, altered: Chronic pain

Communication, impaired: Verbal

Coping, family: Potential for growth

Coping, ineffective family: Compromised

Coping, ineffective family: Disabled

Coping, ineffective individual

Diversional activity, deficit

Family processes altered

Fear

Fluid volume excess

Fluid volume deficit: Actual (1)

Fluid volume deficit: Actual (2)

Fluid volume deficit: Potential

Gas exchange, impaired

Grieving, anticipatory

Grieving, dysfunctional

Growth and development, altered

Health maintenance, altered

Home maintenance management, impaired

Hopelessness

Hyperthermia

Hypothermia

Incontinence, functional

Incontinence, reflex

Incontinence, stress

Incontinence, total

Incontinence, urge

Infection: Potential for

Injury, potential for

Injury, potential for: Poisoning

Injury, potential for: Suffocating

Injury, potential for: Trauma

Knowledge deficit (specify)

Mobility, impaired physical

Noncompliance (specify)

Nutrition, altered: Less than body requirements

Nutrition, altered: More than body requirements

Nutrition, altered: Potential for more than body requirements

Parenting, altered: Actual

Parenting, alterated: Potential

Post-trauma response

Powerlessness

Rape-trauma syndrome

Rape-trauma syndrome: Compound reaction

Rape-trauma syndrome: Silent reaction

Role performance, altered

Self-care deficit: Bathing/hygiene

Self-care deficit: Dressing/grooming

Self-care deficit: Feeding

Self-care deficit: Toileting

Self-concept, disturbance in: Body image

Self-concept, disturbance in: Personal identity

Self-concept, disturbance in: Self-esteem

Sensory-perceptual alteration: Visual, auditory, kinesthetic, gustatory, tactile, olfactory

Sexual dysfunction

Sexuality, altered patterns

Skin integrity, impaired: Actual

Skin integrity, impaired: Potential

Sleep pattern disturbance

Social interaction, impaired

Social isolation

Spiritual distress (distress of the human spirit)

Swallowing, impaired

Thermoregulation, ineffective

Thought processes, altered

Tissue integrity, impaired

Tissue integrity, impaired: Oral mucous membrane

Tissue perfusion, altered: Renal, cerebral, cardiopulmonary, gastrointestinal, peripheral

Unilateral neglect

Urinary elimination, altered patterns

Urinary retention

Violence, potential for: Self-directed or directed at others

intolerance identified in the problem statement could be from shortness of breath from a recent bout with pneumonia, from paralysis of the left leg, or from recovery from coronary artery bypass surgery. For each of the potential etiologies, the nursing care plan would be different. Remember, the etiology component determines the care plan for each identified nursing diagnosis.

Nurses must also take care not to put two diagnostic labels into one nursing diagnosis, such as "Alteration in gas exchange and alteration in mobility, related to copious secretions and left hemiplegia." The plan for each of the two health concerns would be completely different. If both problems are important, the nurse should address each one in a separate nursing diagnosis.

In phrasing a nursing diagnosis, the nurse must avoid statements that may cause legal problems. The diagnoses "Knowledge deficit of chemotherapy, related to inadequate health teaching" and "Alteration in skin integrity, related to continually lying on the back" both raise definite legal questions about the care given or not given to the patient. For the "Knowledge deficit" diagnosis, the nurse might be assessing that the patient had never received chemotherapy before or that the patient was either too ill or anxious to remember the information taught at previous sessions. Therefore, a more correct statement of the nursing diagnosis would be "Knowledge deficit of chemotherapy, related to a new drug regimen" or "Knowledge deficit of chemotherapy, related to anxiety due to newly diagnosed cancer." In the case of the "Alteration in skin integrity" diagnosis, the nurse may be trying to indicate that an alert patient did not understand the importance of changing positions. The correct statement of this nursing diagnosis would be "Knowledge deficit, related to the importance of position changes for maintaining skin integrity." For all nursing diagnoses, the nurse must document the defining characteristics or signs and symptoms that led to the stated diagnosis.

By being aware of the frequent errors that occur while formulating nursing diagnoses, the nurse can avoid such problems. Knowing the list of diagnostic labels, understanding how to use the available reference handbooks for nursing diagnoses, and practicing formulating diagnoses will prove most beneficial to nursing students and nurses learning how to develop nursing diagnoses.

NURSING DIAGNOSES RELATED TO DRUG THERAPY

"Knowledge deficit," "Noncompliance," and "Alteration in health maintenance" are the most common diagnostic labels used by the nurse to develop care plans

The PES method for developing a nursing diagnosis

The following summary presents the key elements of the PES method, the most frequently used method for developing a nursing diagnosis.

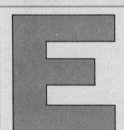

Problem statement

Problem statement—identifies the actual or potential health problem of a patient. When choosing a problem statement, the nurse can use the NANDA list of diagnostic labels. The problem statement should fall within nursing's realm, with the nurse writing the problem statement in clear, concise terms.

Etiology

Etiology—consists of factors related to the problem's development or possible cause. The etiology helps the nurse determine the type of care plan to develop for each nursing diagnosis.

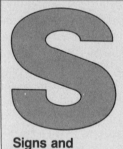

Signs and symptoms

Signs and symptoms or the defining characteristics—identify the cluster of cues that define a diagnostic label or problem statement applicable for a particular patient. The defining characteristics are a part of the subjective and objective assessment data, which the nurse collects for each patient.

Adapted from *Nursing Diagnosis: Process and Application*, 2nd ed., Marjory Gordon, McGraw-Hill Book Co., 1987. Reprinted with permission from McGraw-Hill Book Co.

for the management of a patient's drug regimen. The nurse may also identify other nursing diagnoses depending upon the potential risks or adverse effects occurring secondary to drug therapy. A "Knowledge deficit" can occur for a variety of reasons. Remember, the specific nursing diagnosis depends on the etiologies and defining characteristics that the nurse identifies. (See *Parameters for knowledge deficit* for NANDA-approved etiologies and defining characteristics applicable to the "Knowledge deficit" diagnostic label.)

The nursing diagnosis depends upon the assessment data and drug regimen of each patient. The following case illustrates how a knowledge deficit can result from several causes:

Mrs. Kaminsky, age 71, entered the hospital with shortness of breath and difficulty walking due to edema and pain in her legs. She was diagnosed as having congestive heart failure and was started on the following medications: digoxin 0.25 mg P.O. daily, furosemide (Lasix) 40 mg P.O. daily, and potassium chloride (K-Tab) 2 P.O. twice a day. Mrs. Kaminsky's only significant past medical history is a 2-year history of hypertension, which is being monitored by her family internist. Mrs. Kaminsky takes no other drugs except for a calcium supplement and daily vitamins.

At the present time, she can perform her routine daily activities without shortness of breath. Her legs remain slightly swollen, though greatly decreased in size from the time of admission, and her weight remains 3 pounds (1.5 kg) above her expected dry weight. She is to be discharged in about 3 days if no complications arise.

Mrs. Kaminsky lives alone, although her son and his family live nearby. She wants to return to her home and asks questions regarding her drugs, diet, disease, and activity levels.

In Mrs. Kaminsky's case, the nurse may be dealing with a "Knowledge deficit, related to the new drug regimen," a "Knowledge deficit, related to the prescribed diet," or a "Knowledge deficit, related to the self-management of congestive heart failure" diagnosis.

"Noncompliance" is another diagnostic label that can occur when the nurse deals with a patient and a specified drug regimen. Some defining characteristics of "Noncompliance" include:
● behavior indicating failure to follow a regimen, supported by direct observation or statement by the patient or significant other
● failure on objective tests
● evidence of the development of complications
● exacerbations of the symptoms
● failure to keep appointments
● failure to progress
● inability to set or maintain mutual goals.

The following example illustrates some of the various identifying characteristics of noncompliance:

Mr. Miller, age 65, is admitted to the hospital with an exacerbation of his emphysema. Within the past 12 months, Mr. Miller has entered the hospital three times with the same medical diagnosis. Each time, he received I.V. antibiotics, steroids, and oxygen.

During Mr. Miller's present admission, the nurse noted the following characteristics as part of the assessment. "The patient is alert, exhibits circumoral cyanosis, has a respiratory rate of 32 with the use of accessory muscles, has breath sounds with scattered inspiratory and expiratory wheezes throughout and crackles in the posterior bases, has a cough productive of thick yellow-green secretions, and states his shortness of breath has increased over the past 2 weeks, until he now needs assistance to perform his ADLs (activities of daily living). The patient has a 50 pack-year history of smoking; he smokes 1 pack per day and has refused to decrease this. He states that he quit taking his drugs 2 weeks before admission because they did not seem to make any difference in how he felt and were expensive. Upon further discussion, Mr. Miller could not state the effects of his drugs and treatments."

Mr. Miller lives with his wife, who also has several medical problems that require treatment. He is on a fixed income; he has insurance, the benefits of which are almost exhausted; Medicare; and Social Security. During the present admission, the patient's respiratory status has improved. He performs his ADLs with a minimal shortness of breath, although he needs oxygen at night. Upon discharge, he is to take prednisone 40 mg P.O., which should be tapered over the next 2 weeks according to a set schedule, theophylline (Theo-Dur), metaproterenol (Alupent Inhaler), beclomethasone (Vancenase Inhaler), furosemide (Lasix), potassium chloride (K-Lor), and cephalexin (Keflex) for 10 days, and use oxygen at night.

The defining characteristics for Mr. Miller include his repeated admissions for the exacerbation of emphysema, discontinuance of treatment, questionable understanding of the prescribed treatment, minimal resources to pay for treatment, and the nurse's assessment findings, including shortness of breath, wheezes and crackles, the use of accessory muscles for breathing, and an increased respiratory rate. The nurse needs to collect more information about Mr. Miller's disease knowledge and his beliefs about the effects of the treatment. The nurse may be dealing with "Noncompliance, related to a misunderstanding of the importance of the prescribed drug regimen" or "Noncompliance, related to a lack of financial resources."

For "Alteration in health maintenance," a third commonly used diagnostic label, the identified defining characteristics include:
• a demonstrated lack of knowledge about basic health practices
• a demonstrated lack of adaptive behaviors to internal or external environmental changes
• a reported or observed inability to take responsibility for meeting basic health practices in any or all functional pattern areas
• a history of lacking health-seeking behavior
• an expressed interest in improving health behaviors
• a reported or observed lack of equipment or financial resources or other resources
• a reported or observed impairment of personal support systems.

In other cases, possible nursing diagnoses related to "Alteration in health maintenance" may resemble the following: "Alteration in health maintenance, related to the patient's inability to comprehend the established drug

---

Parameters for knowledge deficit

A nurse must be able to differentiate among the various diagnostic labels. The differentiating parameters usually consist of the etiologies and defining characteristics. The following shows a diagnostic label, its associated etiologies, and its defining characteristics.

DIAGNOSTIC LABEL
• Knowledge deficit

ETIOLOGIES
• Lack of exposure
• Information misinterpretation
• Unfamiliarity with information resources
• Lack of recall
• Cognitive limitation
• Lack of interest in learning or request for information

DEFINING CHARACTERISTICS
• Statement of misconception
• Verbalization of the problem
• Request for information
• Inaccurate follow-through of instruction
• Inadequate test performance
• Inappropriate or exaggerated behaviors

regimen," "Alteration in health maintenance, related to paralysis of the patient's right side," and "Alteration in health maintenance, related to a cognitive inability to manage the prescribed drug regimen."

The nurse may formulate and use many other nursing diagnoses, depending upon the potential or actual adverse effects of drug regimens. Some further nursing diagnoses the nurse might use include: "Potential for injury, related to anticoagulant therapy," "Alteration in skin integrity, related to a reaction to the prescribed medication," and "Alteration in oral mucous membranes, related to a superimposed infection," which could be from steroids, chemotherapy, or antibiotic use. "Alteration in nutrition: less than body requirements, related to nausea, anorexia, and chemotherapy" and "Sexual dysfunction, related to prescribed medications," such as propranolol (Inderal), represent still other diagnoses that the nurse might use.

With such nursing diagnoses, the defining characteristics will depend upon the patient's specific reaction to the particular drug regimen. For example, with the diagnosis "Potential for injury, related to anticoagulant therapy," the defining characteristics may include the presence of petechiae, increased bruising, an elevated prothrombin time above therapeutic levels, or the use of aspirin. For the diagnosis concerning "Alteration in nutrition," the defining characteristics may include decreased weight, eating less than 50% of meals, weakness, or a change in the way foods taste.

THE PLANNING STEP

Once the nursing diagnosis is formulated, the nurse can proceed to the planning step of the nursing process, determining the nursing plan of care for the patient. This consists of two major components: the outcome criteria, or patient goals, and nursing interventions.

DEVELOPING OUTCOME CRITERIA OR PATIENT GOALS

The outcome criteria, the first critical component of the nursing plan of care, represent patient goals and state the desired patient behaviors or responses that should result from the nursing care.

The nurse should ensure that outcome criteria exhibit certain characteristics. Each outcome criterion should be measurable and objective, concise, realistic for the patient, and attainable by nursing management. Furthermore, for each criterion, the nurse should include only one behavior, express that behavior in terms of patient expectations, and indicate a time frame.

More important, the nurse must express each outcome criterion as a measurable, objective statement. Each outcome criterion statement should be able to be answered with "yes" or "no." Typical outcome criteria are: "The patient verbalizes the major adverse effects related to his chemotherapy drugs prior to discharge" or "The patient demonstrates the proper administration of her antibiotic regimen prior to discharge." Outcome criteria should also be realistic for each patient. The nurse could not realistically or appropriately expect a patient with a PO_2 chronic respiratory disorder to have a PO_2 in the 80s, although a PO_2 in the 50s would be acceptable.

The nurse should use only one behavior for each outcome criterion, thereby reducing the chance of ambiguity and clarifying the patient goal for other nurses as well as for the patient. For example, the outcome criterion "The patient lists and demonstrates the steps necessary to use the Alupent Inhaler" contains two behaviors. The patient may be able to list but not demonstrate the necessary steps for using the inhaler, thus producing ambiguity about whether the patient has met the goal. The statement should be written as two criteria: "The patient lists the steps necessary for using the Alupent Inhaler" and "The patient demonstrates the steps necessary for using the Alupent Inhaler."

The nurse can attain further clarity by being as concise as possible. When developing a care plan for the patient, the nurse needs to express the outcome criteria in terms of patient expectations. For example, "Cephalothin (Keflin) 2 g will be given q 6 hours" or "The patient will be turned q 2 hours" represent nursing interventions, not patient goals or outcome criteria. Remember, an outcome criterion states what the nurse wants the patient to achieve after the nursing care. In the first intervention about the Keflin administration, a possible outcome criterion may be: "Patient will be free of infection in left leg ulcer" or "Patient verbalizes the proper sequence for Keflin administration." In the intervention about turning the patient, a possible outcome criterion may be written as "Patient is free of any redness over bony prominences."

Finally, each outcome criterion should be attainable by nursing management, with a time frame designated by the nurse. Designation of time frames, such as "by the time of discharge" or "after the initial teaching session," helps the nurse decide how to implement the interventions necessary for a desired outcome. Stated time frames also help the nurse evaluate patient performance for a specific outcome criterion.

Components of an outcome criterion

The nurse must consider four major components in writing outcome criteria: the content area, an action verb, a time frame, and criterion modifiers.

The content area describes the subject that the patient will focus on or the physiologic or psychological response to be elicited. The focus of the content area may be "the steps of I.V. administration of penicillin," "the adverse effects of prednisone," or "the condition of the lungs upon auscultation."

The action verb, the second component of the outcome criterion, describes how the patient will achieve the goal of the content area. Using action verbs with the three previously mentioned content areas would result in "Demonstrate the steps of the I.V. administration of penicillin," "State the adverse effects of prednisone," and "The lungs sound clear upon auscultation." Notice that the action verbs call for patient behaviors or responses that the nurse can measure against standards of success. The following lists contain verbs commonly used in outcome criteria:

Difficult to measure	Easy to measure
• adequately understand	• contrast
• know	• demonstrate
• believe	• differentiate
• fully appreciate	• identify
• internalize	• state

The first list consists of verbs that are difficult to measure; the second list contains verbs that are easy to measure. The nurse should avoid using weak action verbs, such as understand, appreciate, and think, which do not call for the patient to act in a way that the nurse can accurately measure.

A time frame gives the nurse a target date for the completion of the expected outcome criteria and assists the nurse in evaluating the patient's progress. For example, the statements "Demonstrate the steps of the I.V. administration of penicillin by the time of discharge," "State the adverse effects of prednisone by the end of the second review session," and "Lungs remain clear upon auscultation for 3 consecutive days prior to discharge" include specific time frames that tell the nurse when the patient should achieve the stated goals.

The time frames also help the nurse determine when to initiate the different parts of the nursing plan. For instance, in a cardiac rehabilitation program, the nurse may establish outcome criteria in progressive steps, such as "The patient sits on the side of the bed on the second day post-myocardial infarction," "On the fifth day, the patient ambulates in her room with assistance," and "On the seventh day, the patient ambulates in the hall 25 yards (22 meters) with assistance."

Finally, the nurse must consider the criterion modifiers, which specify each outcome criterion. In some cases, the criterion modifiers clarify what the patient should achieve by delineating specified limits for a specific action. For example, "The patient accurately demonstrates the steps of the I.V. administration of penicillin by the time of discharge" specifies that the patient must demonstrate the behaviors accurately. The following outcome criteria also contain criterion modifiers: "The patient selects from a menu a meal plan consistent with a 2-g sodium diet by discharge" and "The patient's respiratory pattern returns to baseline within 10 minutes after ambulating 200 yards (180 meters)."

Remember, when writing an outcome criterion, the nurse must include the content area, the action verb, and the time frame. Criterion modifiers are not essential, but are helpful. (See *Writing outcome criteria* on page 114 for a summary of the components.)

Common pitfalls in writing outcome criteria

Four errors frequently occur when writing outcome criteria. The errors include writing criteria that: (1) are not measurable or objective, (2) contain more than one behavior, (3) include nursing interventions rather than patient behaviors or responses, and (4) are meaningless statements. The first three of these common errors have been discussed previously; the fourth requires elaboration. A nurse or nursing student may use all of the correct components when forming an outcome criterion, yet fail to write a meaningful statement. Sometimes, the nurse may write what Robert Mager has called "jibberish" statements. An example of such a statement that, nonetheless, contains all of the correct components of an outcome criterion follows:

> "The patient will develop critical thinking in relation to the emergency procedures to follow when adverse effects of the chemotherapy occur at home."

The statement looks and sounds impressive, yet no nurse could accurately measure "Develop critical thinking." Remember, each outcome criterion should represent a concise statement that calls for one objective, measurable patient behavior or response.

DEVELOPING INTERVENTIONS

After developing the outcome criteria, the nurse determines the interventions needed to help the patient reach the desired behavior or response goals. Interventions are the actions that the nurse implements to meet the identified outcome criteria. The types of interventions and strategies depend upon the identified nursing diagnosis and outcome criteria. If the nursing diagnosis states "Knowledge deficit, related to newly prescribed Lasix," the nurse may focus interventions on patient education for the actions, adverse effects, and scheduling of Lasix, as well as the monitoring of daily weights. If the diagnosis states "Knowledge deficit, related to the administration of daily insulin," the nurse might develop interventions that focus on education for the action and adverse effects of insulin, steps to take in case of an insulin reaction, demonstration of self-injection techniques, and observation and guidance for the patient when administering self-injections.

Remember, the type of strategies or interventions depend upon the established nursing diagnosis, outcome criteria, and the individual patient. (See *Three nursing care plans* for examples that illustrate the progression from diagnosis to outcome criteria to intervention.)

CHAPTER SUMMARY

Chapter 7 presented the relationship between drug administration and the nursing process. The chapter focused on the assessment, diagnosis, and planning steps of the nursing process, detailing how each step relates to drug therapy. The text also delineated the nurse's role in drug therapy. The nurse's responsibilities include obtaining a drug history, assessing pertinent body systems, identifying an appropriate nursing diagnosis, and developing a plan that focuses on patient education and the management of the established drug regimen. The nurse also monitors the regimen's effectiveness and the drug's potential adverse effects. Here are the highlights of Chapter 7:
• The nursing process involves assessment, diagnosis, planning, implementation, and evaluation.

Three nursing care plans

The first example gives the nursing care plan for Mrs. Kaminsky, for whom the nurse diagnosed "Knowledge deficit, related to the new drug regimen." The second example gives Mr. Miller's nursing care plan for his diagnosis "Noncompliance, related to a misunderstanding of the importance of the prescribed drug regimen." The third nursing care plan is for a diagnosis of "Potential for injury, related to anticoagulant therapy."

Knowledge deficit, related to the new drug regimen

NURSING DIAGNOSIS
Knowledge deficit, related to the new drug regimen (includes digoxin, furosemide [Lasix], and potassium chloride [K-Tab])

OUTCOME CRITERIA
Mrs. Kaminsky will:
• State the major action of each drug before discharge.
• Identify before discharge at least three adverse reactions that should be brought to the immediate attention of a health care practitioner.
• Describe the importance of monitoring daily weight.
• Demonstrate the ability to take her pulse accurately before discharge.

NURSING INTERVENTIONS
• Instruct Mrs. Kaminsky in the major actions of and possible adverse reactions to each drug.
• Instruct Mrs. Kaminsky about adverse reactions that need immediate medical attention, such as a sudden change in weight, nausea, loss of appetite, change in affect, palpitations, or lethargy.
• Provide Mrs. Kaminsky with a list of this information for home use.
• Discuss the importance of monitoring daily weight and noting more than a 2- to 3-pound (1- to 1.5-kg) increase.
• Provide Mrs. Kaminsky with written instructions concerning the major actions and adverse reactions of each drug as a guide for home use.
• Include Mrs. Kaminsky's son and/or significant other in the teaching, if possible.
• Instruct Mrs. Kaminsky on methods for taking her pulse, using demonstration and practice.

Noncompliance, related to a misunderstanding of the importance of the prescribed drug regimen

NURSING DIAGNOSIS
Noncompliance, related to a misunderstanding of the importance of the prescribed drug regimen (includes theophylline [Theo-Dur], metaproterenol [Alupent Inhaler], beclomethasone [Vancenase Inhaler], furosemide [Lasix], potassium chloride [K-Tab], and cephalexin [Keflex])

OUTCOME CRITERIA
By discharge, Mr. Miller will:
• State two reasons why he has exacerbations of his emphysema.
• Identify at least three signs that may indicate exacerbations of his emphysema.
• Verbalize the major actions of the prescribed drugs.
• Describe the difference between adverse reactions to the drugs and the signs of exacerbations of his emphysema.
• Describe the relationship between his drug regimen and his emphysema.
• Verbalize the importance of taking his prescribed drugs as ordered.

NURSING INTERVENTIONS
• Discuss emphysema with Mr. Miller, noting the disease process and why exacerbations occur—discontinuation of his drugs, progression of his disease, or exposure to cold viruses.
• Instruct Mr. Miller about the signs and symptoms that indicated a need for medical attention prior to hospitalization and how to monitor the signs, including increased shortness of breath, increased use of oxygen, inability to perform ADLs, and changes in the color of secretions.
• Discuss and provide written information on the drug actions.
• Discuss the relationship of the prescribed drugs to his disease.
• Discuss the difference between the adverse reactions to the drugs and signs and symptoms that indicate an exacerbation of his emphysema or progression of the disease state. Provide Mr. Miller with a list of the information.
• Contact the home health agency for follow-up care.
• Involve Mr. Miller's wife in the teaching sessions.
• Contact social services to assess the family finances, and refer Mr. Miller to hospital and community resources.

Potential for injury, related to anticoagulant therapy

NURSING DIAGNOSIS
Potential for injury, related to anticoagulant therapy

OUTCOME CRITERIA
The patient will:
• Describe the action of warfarin (Coumadin).
• State the importance of self-monitoring for signs of bleeding.
• List the signs of bleeding to report to the physician.
• Identify the reasons for carrying a medication alert identification card and/or bracelet.
• Verbalize the importance of the blood tests (prothrombin time) in monitoring the warfarin dose.
• State the importance of not using products that contain aspirin.
• List at list three safety precautions to follow while on anticoagulant therapy.

NURSING INTERVENTIONS
• Instruct the patient concerning the actions of warfarin.
• Discuss the signs and symptoms of bleeding that the patient should be aware of, such as bleeding of the gums and increased bruising, and when to report these signs to the physician.
• Provide the patient with the medication alert information and discuss it.
• Discuss the need for follow-up blood tests (prothrombin time) to adjust the warfarin dose.
• Provide the patient with a booklet on anticoagulant therapy.
• Discuss the reasons for not using products that contain aspirin.
• Discuss the safety factors related to anticoagulant therapy, such as the use of a soft toothbrush and the careful use of razors.

Writing outcome criteria

The essential components of outcome criteria and examples of those components are:

CONTENT AREA

describes the subject that the patient will focus on or the response to be elicited, such as
- Action of digoxin
- Pulse taking

ACTION VERB

describes how the patient will achieve the content area aim, such as
- *Verbalize* the action of digoxin
- *Demonstrate* pulse taking

TIME FRAME

gives a target date for completion of the outcome criteria, such as
- Verbalize the action of digoxin *after the initial teaching session*
- Demonstrate pulse taking *by discharge*

CRITERION MODIFIERS

add specificity to the subject, action, or time, such as
- Verbalize *correctly the major* action of digoxin after the initial teaching session
- Demonstrate pulse taking before discharge *with a degree of accuracy within 4 beats of the pulse the nurse takes*

• In assessing the clinical behaviors of a patient before drug administration, the nurse determines the patient's cognitive abilities and body systems that may be affected by prescribed drugs. The nurse must know if the patient possesses the appropriate cognitive abilities to manage the prescribed drug regimen. The nurse's assessment of body systems, such as the cardiovascular or the integumentary system, helps determine the potential effectiveness of a particular drug regimen.

• When developing a nursing diagnosis, the nurse can use the PES method identified by Gordon. The PES method includes the following major components of a nursing diagnosis: the problem statement, etiology, and signs and symptoms. The problem statement identifies the patient's health problem or need. The nurse may use the NANDA taxonomy of nursing diagnoses to form the problem statement. The etiology component states the probable cause of the identified health problem and determines the type of plan to be used. The third component, the signs and symptoms, represents defining characteristics that help the nurse determine which diagnostic label to use.

• An outcome criterion states a patient goal, or the desired patient behavior or response to be reached with nursing care. An outcome criterion should specify a content area and include an action verb and a time frame. The content area determines what the patient should achieve or which response should be elicited. The action verb determines how the patient will achieve the designated goals. The time frame determines when the patient should achieve the desired outcome criterion. The nurse should write measurable, objective outcome criteria.

• The development of nursing interventions helps the patient achieve the goals of the outcome criteria.

• The three major information categories used to compile a drug history include general information, prescribed drugs, and over-the-counter drugs. General information covers allergies, medical history, habits, socioeconomic status, life-style and beliefs, and sensory deficits. With prescribed drugs and over-the-counter drugs, the nurse must assess the reason for use, the patient's knowledge of the drugs, frequency of use, dosage, drug efficacy, pattern of administration, and drug reactions. The patient's use of prescription drugs and over-the-counter drugs can affect the patient's response to a prescribed drug regimen.

BIBLIOGRAPHY

Adams, Carolyn. "Nursing Diagnosis in Patient Care Planning," *Military Medicine* 149:202, April 1984.

Carpenito, Lynda Juall. *Nursing Diagnosis: Application to Clinical Practice.* Philadelphia: J.B. Lippincott Co., 1983.

DiNicola, Dante, and DiMatteo, M. Robin. "Practitioners, Patients, and Compliance with the Medical Regimens: A Social Psychological Perspective," in *Hand Tools of Psychology and Health,* 4th ed. Edited by Taylor, S., and Jirger, J. Hillside, N.J.: Erlbaum, 1984.

Doenges, Marilyn, and Moorhouse, Mary. *Nurse's Pocket Guide: Nursing Diagnoses with Interventions.* Philadelphia: F.A. Davis Co., 1986.

Emanuelsen, Kathy Lynn, and Rosenlicht, Jacqueline McQuay. *Handbook of Critical Care Nursing.* New York: John Wiley & Sons, 1986.

Gordon, Marjory. "Nursing Diagnosis and the Diagnostic Process," *American Journal of Nursing* 76(8):1298, August 1976.

Gordon, Marjory. *Nursing Diagnosis: Process and Application.* New York: McGraw-Hill Book Co., 1987.

Guzzetta, Cathie, and Dossey, Barbara. "Nursing Diagnosis: Framework, Process and Problems," *Heart & Lung* 12:281, May 1983.

Haynes, Robert Brian, et al. *Compliance in Health Care.* Baltimore: Johns Hopkins University Press, 1979.

Kim, Mija, et al. *Pocket Guide to Nursing Diagnoses.* St. Louis: C.V. Mosby Co., 1984.

Luckenbaugh, Phyllis. "An Overview of Nursing Diagnosis and Suggestions for Use with Chronic Hemodialysis Patients," *Nephrology Nurse* 5:58, November/December 1983.

Mager, Robert. *Preparing Instructional Objectives,* 2nd ed. Belmont, Calif.: Fear-Pitman Publishers, 1975.

McCord, Meridith. "Compliance: Self-Care or Compromise?" *Topics in Clinical Nursing* 7(4):1, January 1986.

North American Nursing Diagnosis Association (NANDA). *Classification of Nursing Diagnoses: Proceedings of the Seventh Conference.* St. Louis: C.V. Mosby Co., 1987.

Redman, Barbara. *The Process of Patient Education,* 5th ed. St. Louis: C.V. Mosby Co., 1984.

Tartaglia, Michael. "Nursing Diagnosis: Keystone of Your Care Plan," *Nursing84* 15:34, March 1984.

Warren, Judith. "Accountability and Nursing Diagnosis," *Journal of Nursing Administration* 13(10):34, October 1983.

CHAPTER 8

INTERVENTION: ADMINISTRATION PROCESSES

OBJECTIVES

After reading and studying this chapter, you should be able to:

1. Identify the eight essential components of a properly written medication order.

2. State the meanings of the standardized abbreviations most frequently used in medication orders.

3. Describe the purposes of the seven types of medication orders routinely used in the hospital.

4. Describe standard nursing practices that help the nurse achieve the five "rights" of drug administration.

5. Identify at least six other procedural safeguards against medication errors listed in the text.

6. Describe the nurse's responsibilities when using each of the four types of drug delivery systems.

7. Define malpractice and discuss its relation to the administration of medications.

8. Explain how the nurse applies autonomy, paternalism, truthfulness, beneficence, fidelity, and respect for property to professional practice.

9. Identify the advantages and disadvantages of using placebos.

INTRODUCTION

Chapter 8 investigates how nursing intervention applies to drug administration. The chapter presents essential background information about requirements for medication orders, the nurse's responsibilities in receiving and transcribing medication orders, and the proper procedures for preventing errors during drug administration. Various systems for delivering medications from the pharmacy to the nursing unit for administration are examined for their advantages and disadvantages. The chapter also explores various legal expectations, such as what the nurse should know and do to administer medications safely. The nursing student will also learn the components that constitute malpractice and the special nursing responsibilities related to controlled drugs. Chapter 8 concludes with a discussion of some of the fundamental values and moral principles that guide nursing practice in medication administration.

MEDICATION ORDERS

Under the law, as outlined in the medical practice act of each state, licensed physicians as well as dentists, podiatrists, and in some states optometrists may prescribe, dispense, and administer drugs. In selected circumstances and within certain protocols, other health care professionals, such as nurses or physicians' assistants, may legally prescribe and dispense drugs. Nevertheless, physicians write the vast majority of medication orders. Pharmacists dispense the drugs, and nurses usually administer the drugs to patients.

REQUIREMENTS FOR MEDICATION ORDERS

A medication order may take one of two forms, depending on whether the physician is treating a hospitalized patient or an outpatient. For the hospitalized patient, the physician can order medications, along with all other orders such as those for diet, X-rays, and laboratory work, on the physician's order sheet in the patient's chart. The physician can also use a separate medication order sheet. For outpatients, the physician usually writes medication orders on prescription pad sheets, which the physician then gives directly to the patient. The patient takes the medication order to a hospital or community pharmacy to be filled. (*See Components of a medication order* for a complete, properly written medication order for a hospitalized patient.)

The physician's order sheet lists the patient's full name for identification purposes. The order sheet may be stamped with complete identifying information including the patient's birth date, the hospital number, room number, and date of admission. Physicians and nurses must take extreme care in identifying patients, particularly if two or more patients with the same or similar names appear on the unit.

The physician should give either the generic or trade name of the drug and its dosage form, if more than one form of the drug is available. The physician should ex-

press the dose to be given at each administration in metric, apothecaries', or household measures. The most common administration routes are oral, intra-muscular, subcutaneous, and intravenous, although additional routes involving other body structures and cavities exist. Oral medications, representing the majority, tend to be the safest, the least expensive, and the most convenient for the patient to take.

Physicians usually state the time schedule for administration as the number of times per day that the medication is to be administered. Upon noting the time schedule, the nurse then schedules the specific hours according to how quickly a supply of the medication can be procured, the medication's characteristics, and institutional policies. The medication's characteristics, in-

Components of a medication order

The physician writes medication orders for hospitalized patients on the physician's order sheet in the patient's chart. The medication order should give the patient's full name, the name of the drug, the dosage form, the dose amount, the administration route, the time schedule, the prescriber's signature, as well as the date and time of the order.

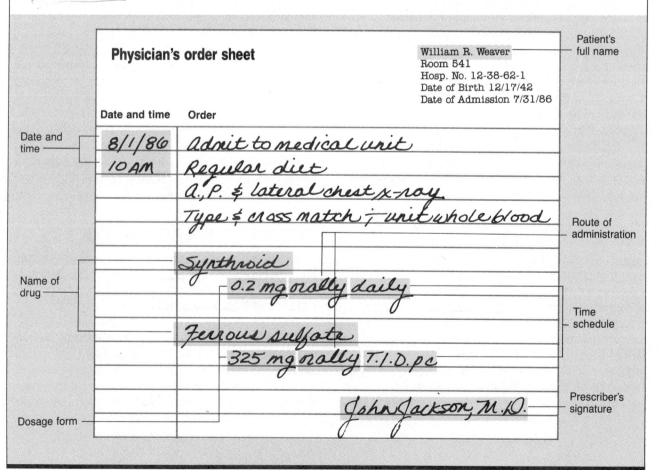

cluding its nature, onset of action, and duration of action, primarily determine the schedule. For instance, if regular, intermittent peak blood concentration levels of antibiotics must be maintained to combat infections, the physician will schedule the drug administration at regular intervals around the clock.

To a lesser extent, institutional policy determines the schedule. For example, policy may dictate a 10 a.m. administration for all drugs given only once a day. Sometimes, the specific responses of the patient to the illness and treatment determine the administration schedule. For example, the nurse may receive an order to administer 5 units of regular insulin to a diabetic patient whenever routine urine glucose tests indicate that 2% glycosuria (glucose in the urine) is present.

The prescriber's signature, along with the date and time of day the order was written, should also appear. The date and time are often referred to when the order has an expiration date. For example, a narcotic order valid for 72 hours, written at noon on August 21, will expire at noon on August 24.

To implement a medication order properly, the nurse must understand dosage forms, measurement systems, administration routes, and accepted abbreviations. Prescribers should adhere strictly to the abbreviations approved by their specific institution. Adherence to approved abbreviations becomes particularly important in large institutions where practitioners come from many different areas. Nonstandardized abbreviations lead to guesswork, which significantly increases the possibility of error. (See *Frequently used abbreviations* on pages 120 and 121 for a list of many of the standardized, widely accepted abbreviations used today.)

Physicians usually write outpatient medication orders as prescriptions. Before the patient leaves the outpatient setting, the nurse should clarify for the patient any abbreviations used in the prescription. By clarifying any doubtful abbreviations, the nurse can help avoid subsequent misinterpretation of the prescription by the patient. (See *Frequently misinterpreted abbreviations* on pages 124 and 125 for a list of abbreviations that patients often misunderstand.)

Like orders for hospitalized patients, prescriptions for outpatients identify the patient's name and address, and the date the prescription was written. Physicians and nurses sometimes refer to the identifying information as the superscription. (See *Outpatient medication order* on page 122 for an illustration of how the prescriber writes a medication order for an outpatient.)

After Rx, which means "take thou," the prescriber writes the name, form, and dosage of the drug, along with instructions on amount to be dispensed. The prescriber often calculates the amount to provide the patient with an adequate supply, which should last until the patient's next visit to the physician. Prescribing an adequate supply also enables the physician to evaluate the patient's clinical response to the drug. In evaluating the patient's response, the physician may decide to change the medication. In such a case, by prescribing no more than an adequate supply, the physician saves the patient from incurring the unnecessary expense of the unused medication.

After the abbreviation *Sig.,* which means "let it be labeled," the physician writes directions to the patient for taking the medication. The directions are followed by the physician's signature, address, and telephone number. Finally, the prescriber indicates the number of times the prescription can be refilled. On some prescriptions, the physician's state medical license number may also appear. A prescription for any federally controlled drug must also include the physician's registration number with the Drug Enforcement Agency (DEA).

Outpatients must fill prescriptions for controlled substances within 6 months of the date written and cannot refill the prescription more than five times. Many prescriptions will also indicate whether the pharmacist should fill the prescription with generic or trade name products. If unspecified, most states allow the pharmacist to dispense the generic form of the drug, thereby sometimes decreasing the patient's expense. Patients should be aware that they have the right to ask the physician to write the prescription for the generic drug.

Besides the previously mentioned prescription requirements, all states now require the pharmacist to label each prescription container with the name, strength, and drug amount dispensed. These requirements contribute significantly to the patient's knowledge and understanding of the treatment regimen.

TYPES OF MEDICATION ORDERS

The following seven types of medication orders are routine in the hospital: standard written orders, single orders, stat orders, p.r.n. orders, standing orders, verbal (or oral) orders, and telephone orders.

Standard written orders apply indefinitely until the prescriber writes another order to alter or discontinue the first one. In some cases, the prescriber may specify on the standard written order a particular termination date. A standard written order with a termination date might read as "Ergotrate (ergonovine) 0.2 mg P.O. q 4 hours × 3 days." In many cases, hospitals establish policies that indicate how long orders for certain classes of drugs remain valid. Examples of drugs with controlled termination dates include narcotic orders for 3 days and antibiotic orders for 7 days. If the patient still needs the drug after the expiration date, the physician must rewrite the order. The physician must also rewrite standard written orders postoperatively, if the medications are to be continued.

Single orders for medications are given only once. For example, a physician may order one tetanus toxoid injection for a patient with a laceration or puncture wound who received a primary tetanus toxoid series more than 10 years earlier.

Stat orders call for medications that are to be administered immediately for an urgent patient problem. For instance, a physician may order a single dose of an antianxiety drug to calm an acutely agitated patient.

P.R.N. orders derive their name from a Latin phrase that means "as the occasion arises." Prescribers write p.r.n. orders for medications that are to be given when needed. The administration time results from the collaborative judgments of the nurse and the patient. Sometimes, a p.r.n. order delineates the reason for giving the drug. For example, the prescriber may write "Tylenol 500 mg P.O. p.r.n. for a temperature above 101.3° F. (38.5° C.)." If an ordered drug, such as acetaminophen (Tylenol), serves multiple purposes, some hospital policies state that the nurse administer the drug only for the specific condition mentioned in the order. Under such a policy, the nurse would not give Tylenol ordered only for fever if the patient complained of a headache but had no fever. Other institutions allow the nurse to determine when to administer p.r.n. ordered drugs. When administering p.r.n. medications, the nurse should describe in the patient's record the reason for their use and their degree of subsequent effectiveness.

Standing orders, or protocols, establish guidelines for the treatment of a particular disease or set of symptoms. Standing orders require considerable judgment and expertise in assessing both the patient's need for the medication and any predictable reactions that might occur. In clinics, standing orders frequently serve as guides for nurse practitioners when they prescribe treatment for many patients with the same needs. For example, nurse practitioners in family-planning clinics commonly prescribe vaginal creams for minor infections and contraceptives for birth control. The nurses usually follow standing orders for such prescriptions, using predetermined guidelines and working under a physician's general supervision.

Although not strict protocols, certain developed routines may exist to guide the care rendered to patients in acute emergencies. Physicians and nurses formulate routines in advance for predictable emergencies. For example, in an emergency, the nurse should always assess the patient for any *contraindications* to a routine order. To illustrate, patients in diabetic ketoacidotic coma usually require large amounts of I.V. fluids with added drugs such as potassium chloride. To prevent life-threatening cardiac dysrhythmias resulting from potassium intoxication, the nurse must be certain that the patient has an adequate urinary output to eliminate excess potassium before the I.V. fluid potassium is given.

Special care areas of the hospital, such as the coronary care unit (CCU), routinely establish standing orders that apply to such drug therapies as morphine sulfate for chest pain and anxiety, lidocaine (Xylocaine) for ventricular tachycardia, and furosemide (Lasix) for pulmonary congestion. Hospitals may also institute medication protocols that specifically designate drugs that a nurse may *not* give. Medication protocols may also state that only specially prepared nurses working in special care units be allowed to give certain drugs, such as intravenous phenytoin (Dilantin), which can cause cardiac arrest if administered too rapidly. Historically, as technology has advanced and health care professionals have gained more experience with new drugs, nurses have assumed greater responsibility for drug administration.

Verbal orders are medication orders given orally rather than in writing. Physicians and nurses try to avoid using verbal orders because such orders can lead to miscommunication. In urgent situations, the nurse should write and sign the order dictated by the physician. Then, the nurse should repeat the order aloud for the physician's verification and request the physician to spell the drug name if necessary. The physician should sign the verbal order that the nurse has written as soon as possible. The institution should have a policy that dictates the time in which the physician must sign a verbal order. If a patient experiences hypoglycemic or insulin shock and the physician instructs the nurse to prepare immediately 50 ml of 50% glucose for I.V. administration, the nurse should show the physician the label on the empty glucose vial while simultaneously stating the drug's name and handing the syringe to the physician. Such actions allow the physician to confirm the accuracy of the drug and its dose.

(Text continues on page 122.)

Frequently used abbreviations

These abbreviations may be used, in institutions that approve them, in transcribing medication orders and documenting drug administration.

a̅a̅	of each		g, gm or GM	gram (quantity usually expressed in Arabic numerals)
a.c.	before meals			
A.D.	right ear		gr	grain (quantity usually expressed in Roman numerals)
ad lib	as desired		gtt	drop
A.M./a.m.	morning		h or hr	hour
aq	aqueous (water)		h.s.	at bedtime
A.S.	left ear		HT	hypodermic tablet
A.U.	each ear		I.M.	intramuscular
b.i.d.	twice a day		in or ″	inch
c̅	with		I.V.	intravenous
caps	capsules		IVPB	intravenous "piggyback"
cc	cubic centimeter		kg	kilogram
cm	centimeter		Ⓛ	left
comp	compound		L	liter
d	day		LA	long acting
/d	per day		lb or #	pound
D/C or dc	discontinue		m or M_x	minim
disp	dispensary		mcg	microgram
DS	double strength		mEq	milliequivalent
D_5W	5% dextrose in water		mg	milligram
EC	enteric coated		ml	milliliter
elix	elixir		mm	millimeter
et	and		MR × 1	may repeat once
ext	extract		Noct.	night
fl or fld	fluid		N.P.O.	nothing by mouth

NR	no refills		**Rx**	treatment, prescription
NS or **N/S**	normal saline (0.9%)		**s̄**	without
¼NS	¼ normal saline (0.225%)		**s̄s̄**	one-half
½NS	½ normal saline (0.45%)		**sat**	saturated
O.D.	right eye		**S.C., SQ**	subcutaneous
os	mouth		**sec**	second
O.S.	left eye		**Sig.**	write on label
OTC	over the counter		**SL** or **sl**	sublingual
O.U.	each eye		**sp.**	spirits
p̄	after		**SR**	sustained release
p.c.	after meals		**stat**	immediately
per	by or through		**supp**	suppository
P.O. or **p.o.**	by mouth		**syr.**	syrup
pt	pint		**T, Tbs., tbsp.**	tablespoon
q	every		**t, tsp.**	teaspoon
q a.m. or **Q.M.**	every morning		**tab**	tablet
q.d.	every day		**t.i.d.**	three times a day
q.h.	every hour		**tinct** or **tr**	tincture
q.i.d.	four times a day		**U**	unit
q3h, q4h, etc.	every 3 hours/every 4 hours, etc.		**ung.**	ointment
q.o.d.	every other day		**vag**	vaginal
QS	quantity sufficient		**VO**	verbal order
QNS	quantity not sufficient		**×**	times, multiply
qt	quart		**ʒ**	dram
Ⓡ	right		**oz** or **ℨ**	ounce
R or **PR**	by rectum			

Outpatient medication order

Community pharmacies usually fill outpatient medication orders. The following represents a typical prescription, showing its basic components:

HILLCREST MEDICAL ASSOCIATES

John Jackson, M.D. AJ 6051281
Richard Turner, M.D. AT 4051552

2813 Hillcrest Drive
Mayfield, PA 19682
Telephone: 814/613-5409

NAME: *Marie Fletcher*   AGE: *38*

ADDRESS: *206 Elmwood Drive*   DATE: *8/16/86*

Rx: *Penicillin VK 500 mg tablets orally*
Dispense #6

Sig.: *Take 4 tablets 1 hour before dental*
extractions;
then 2 tablets 6 hours later

_____*John Jackson*_____ M.D.   _____ M.D.
Generic equivalent permitted   Dispense as written

Refill: ___*2*___ times

Telephone orders, verbal orders given to a nurse by a staff physician over the telephone, may result in dangerous errors from mechanical problems involving the telephone and from the lack of nonverbal communication clues between the physician and nurse. Nurses should avoid telephone orders whenever possible. When a nurse must take a telephone order, the nurse should ask another nurse to monitor the call on an extension telephone. By monitoring the call, the second nurse can confirm the order. Unfortunately, nurses cannot always include such monitoring on the clinical unit. Besides verifying the drug name given during a telephone order,

the nurse should orally repeat the individual digits of the dose. For instance, having understood the order to be 15 milligrams of meperidine (Demerol), the nurse might inquire, "You did say one-five milligrams of meperidine, Doctor? Is that correct?" Repeating the order gives the physician the opportunity to confirm or correct the order, as in "No, that should be *fifty,* five-0, milligrams of meperidine." The nurse then writes the order, indicating that it was a telephone order. The physician must later co-sign the order within the time period established by institutional policy.

Unusual circumstances

The nurse will encounter situations related to the standard written order that require considerable nursing judgment in deciding whether and how to give the drug. On some occasions, the nurse may omit or at least delay a medication dose. This frequently occurs for patients prohibited from ingesting anything in preparation for certain diagnostic tests. In such cases, the nurse should confer with the physician. The nurse and physician may decide to omit the drug, give the drug orally with a very small amount of water, administer the drug by another route, or give the drug orally after completion of the test. Other circumstances may arise in which the nurse intentionally omits a dose of medication because the patient no longer needs it. For example, the nurse may omit a laxative dose if the patient has had a bowel movement since the medication order. The nurse sometimes omits medications because the patient refuses to take them.

Since the consumer movement of the 1960s, both health care professionals and the public have placed considerable emphasis on the inclusion of the patient and family in making decisions about health care. Most physicians and nurses recognize a patient's right to know about specific drugs and to participate in making the decision to use the drugs. Before participating in decisions about a drug, however, the patient should be accurately informed about the drug and its effects. The patient can then make an informed decision. Health care professionals must assume the responsibility of supplying the necessary information and fully discussing the information with the patient.

Despite having the right to collaborate in the decision-making process, the patient may still refuse a drug, for many and varied reasons. Patients may complain that the drug tastes bad and produces nausea, that injections hurt, that they do not understand the drug's purpose, and that they remain unconvinced that the drug will help. Patients may also believe that they are receiving the wrong medication. Some patients base their refusals on religious or cultural beliefs. In any case, the nurse should try to determine the patient's reason for refusing a medication.

The nurse may resolve problems by exploring the patient's feelings, listening to the patient's fears, and talking honestly to the patient about the need for the medication. Though the patient may still refuse the medication, the nurse should *never* give the medication by deceptive means, such as disguising it with food. In all instances in which patients do not receive an ordered medication, the nurse should indicate the omission on the medication administration record, describe the reason for the omission, and notify the patient's physician immediately if appropriate to do so.

PREVENTING MEDICATION ERRORS

The safe, accurate administration of medications demands that nurses possess current, pertinent drug knowledge and follow safe procedures. From the beginning of a nursing student's professional training, educators make every effort to ensure the progressive accumulation of adequate knowledge about drug therapy.

Nursing educators encourage students to read pharmacology textbooks, examine brochures in medication packages, and consult clinical pharmacists. Some nursing educators require students to purchase or develop a file of drug cards containing essential information about different drugs. The information usually entered on a drug card includes the drug category, generic and trade names, clinical actions and uses, mechanisms of action, pharmacokinetics, adverse effects, contraindications, usual dosage ranges, nursing implications, and patient education information. (See *A nursing drug card* on page 126 for an example of how this information is organized.) Because new medications constantly come into use, nurses *must* continue throughout their professional careers to seek drug information and develop the habit of pursuing continuing education offerings to maintain current drug knowledge.

Knowing about drugs, as well as the factors to observe when preparing and administering each drug, helps the nurse avoid medication errors. The nurse should prepare all medications in a quiet area, conducive to concentration. Noise, interruptions, and confusion increase the chance of error. The nurse should limit the traffic through a medication room while preparing medications. Frequently used equipment, such as stethoscopes and sphygmomanometers, should not be stored in the medication room since their retrieval for use distracts and diverts the nurse's attention from the task at hand. Co-workers should avoid interrupting a nurse who is preparing medications.

After receiving a written order, the nurse transcribes it onto the appropriate working document approved by the hospital. The working document may be a medication administration record (the MAR), a medication Kardex, medication cards or tickets, or a computer printout. Because the chance for error increases with the repeated copying of orders, the nurse must read each order carefully and prepare the medications directly from the approved document. The nurse *never* relies on memory or personal worksheet notations. As a precaution

(Text continues on page 126.)

Frequently misinterpreted abbreviations

Physicians and nurses should use only approved abbreviations, writing each clearly and avoiding those that a patient or pharmacist might misinterpret, even if they are approved. Here are some frequently misinterpreted abbreviations.

ABBREVIATION	INTENDED MEANING	MISINTERPRETATION
A.U.	*auris uterque* (each ear)	Has been mistaken for "OU" (*oculus uterque*—each eye).
Chemical Symbol Na	Sodium	Not understood or misread.
D/C	discharge discontinue	Patients' medications have been prematurely discontinued when D/C, intended to mean "discharge," was misinterpreted as "discontinue" when followed by list of drugs.
M_x	minim	Not understood or misread.
Drug names MTX CPZ HCl DIG MVI HCTZ ARA-A	methotrexate Compazine (prochlorperazine) hydrochloric acid digoxin multivitamins *without* fat-soluble vitamins hydrochlorothiazide vidarabine	Mustargen (mechlorethamine HCl) chlorpromazine potassium chloride (The "H" is misinterpreted as "K.") digitoxin multivitamins *with* fat-soluble vitamins hydrocortisone (HCT) cytarabine (ARA-C)
μg	microgram	When handwritten, this can easily be mistaken for "mg."
o.d.	once daily	Frequently misinterpreted as "right eye" (OD—*oculus dexter*), so that oral medication is administered in a patient's right eye.
OJ	orange juice	Has been mistaken for "OD" (*oculus dexter*—right eye) or "OS" (*oculus sinister*—left eye). Medications that were meant to be diluted in orange juice and given orally have been given in a patient's right or left eye.
i/d	once daily	Mistaken as "t.i.d."
per os	orally	The "os" can be mistaken for left eye.
q.d.	every day	The period after the "q" has sometimes been mistaken for an "i," and the drug has been given q.i.d. rather than daily.
qn	nightly or at bedtime	Misinterpreted as "every hour" when poorly written.
q.o.d.	every other day	Misinterpreted as "q.d." or "q.i.d." if the "o" is poorly written.
sub q	subcutaneous	The "q" has been mistaken for "every." In the example, a prophylactic heparin dose meant to be given 2 hours before surgery was given every 2 hours before surgery.
U or u	unit	Seen as a zero or a four, causing a tenfold or greater overdose.

EXAMPLE	CORRECTION
Colymycin gtts iii ou tid	Write clearly.
Na comincden 5 mg today	Write it out.
D/c meds Digoxin 0.25mg Lasix 40 mg KCl 20mEq	Write out "discharge" and "discontinue."
Elexophyline 3T tid Tr opium 10 mx	Use the metric system or write out minim.
	Use the complete spelling for drug names.
Vit B12 1 mg IM Now	Use mcg.
KCl 15 mEq OD	Don't abbreviate "daily." Write it out.
Lugol's sol'n gtts x̄ in OJ	Write out "orange juice."
Diabinese 250mg q̄ 1d	Write it out.
Lugol's sol'n gtts x̄ per os	Use "P.O." or "by mouth" or "orally."
Digoxin 0.25mg q.d.	Write it out.
Librium 10mg qh	Use "h.s." or "nightly."
digoxin 0.25 mg q. 1. d.	Use "q other day" or "every other day."
Heparin 5000 units subc q2hrs before surgery	Use SC, SQ, or write out "subcutaneous."
NPH 6 u Now SC NPH 44 now SC	Write it out for clarification.

A nursing drug card

Nursing students and nurses use drug cards repeatedly; however, the nurse should always consider the information in relation to the individual patient. The following illustrates a typical drug card for hydrochlorothiazide:

Generic name: hydrochlorothiazide   **Category:** thiazide diuretic

Trade names: HydroDiuril, Esidrix, Oretic, Diaqua, Zide

Clinical actions and uses: diuretic used mainly for control of edema in congestive heart failure, and in hypertension.

Mechanism of action: promotes diuresis by inhibiting reabsorption of sodium, chloride, and water in the distal tubule of the nephron. Inhibits carbonic anhydrase. Increases potassium excretion, retains calcium, and decreases uric acid excretion. Antihypertensive action thought to be from diuresis and vasodilation.

Pharmacokinetics: onset of action 2 hours, peak concentration levels 4 hours, duration of action 6 to 12 hours. Food believed to increase absorption. Eliminated unchanged by kidneys.

Adverse reactions: fluid and electrolyte imbalances.
• Fluid: thirst, weakness, weight loss, hypotension, tachycardia
• Hyponatremia: nausea, headache, malaise, lethargy, seizures, coma
• Hypokalemia: nausea, weakness, fatigue, leg cramps, palpitations, abdominal distention, constipation
• Other: orthostatic hypotension, hyperuricemia, precipitation of acute gout, latent diabetes mellitus

Drug interactions: may increase lithium toxicity, and potentiates some antihypertensives. Increases risk of digitalis toxicity, decreases action of antidiabetic drugs.

Usual dose: edema—adults 25 to 200 mg initially, then 25 to 100 daily or b.i.d.; children 1 to 2 mg/kg/day, infants may require 3 mg/kg/day.

Patient education: Tell the patient to take a diuretic early in the day to avoid sleep loss from frequent urination; to take with food to increase absorption and decrease gastric irritation; and that bananas and orange juice will relieve mild symptoms of potassium loss (if renal function is normal). If electrolyte imbalances become severe, replacement therapy may be required. Have the patient weigh daily; instruct the patient to rise slowly from sitting and lying positions to avoid orthostatic hypotension. Tell the patient to seek ongoing professional supervision for blood pressure and electrolyte monitoring.

against omitted orders, the established practices of many hospitals require the nurse to check periodically all medication administration records against the original order sheet. Also, the nurse preparing the change-of-shift report usually alerts the oncoming staff to any new medication orders.

THE FIVE "RIGHTS" OF MEDICATION ADMINISTRATION

Classic safeguards, known as the five "rights," exist to ensure accurate medication administration. Even though the five "rights"—the right drug, dose, patient, time, and route—address a variety of issues, health care professionals generally regard the safeguards as the minimum requirements for safety. Much additional forethought is required before any medication is administered.

The right drug. While working with the vast number of today's available drugs, the nurse must carefully discriminate among similar-sounding names. For example, digoxin (Lanoxin), digitoxin (Crystodigin), and Desoxyn (methamphetamine) all have similar-sounding names but are very different drugs. Digoxin and digitoxin represent different forms of the cardiac drug digitalis, while Desoxyn is a drug used for weight reduction. The nurse should always compare the name of the drug on the container label to the medication order. As part of standard practice, the nurse should mentally pronounce the drug name and check the label three times, first when removing the container from the shelf, then when pouring the medication, and again when returning the container to the shelf. For medications that are individually wrapped in single doses, the nurse should check the name when removing the drug from the drawer and again when unwrapping and giving the drug to the patient.

Anytime a patient comments that the medication seems unusual, the nurse should recheck the drug name and strength. For example, a patient may say, "Nurse, this can't be my medication. I always take one pink pill, but you've given me two yellow pills." As a result, the nurse may discover a medication error or need to explain to the patient that the pink pill contains 10 mg of the drug whereas one yellow pill contains 5 mg of the same drug. Any patient comment mandates that the nurse explore the situation before administering the drug.

The right dose. The widespread use of unit-dose medications, individually wrapped and labeled single doses, has alleviated many problems related to drug dosage. Also, the many commercially prepared medications, available in various size tablets, decreases the number of calculations that the nurse must make to determine the dosage. The nurse should develop the standard practice of first mentally calculating the approximate dose, then calculating the actual dose in writing, using the correct formulas. For example, when giving 75 mg of a drug labeled 50 mg per ml, the nurse can mentally estimate the dosage to be 1½ ml. The nurse can then calculate the definitive dose by using the following formula:

$$50 : 1 :: 75 : X$$
$$50X = 75$$
$$X = 1.5 \text{ ml}$$

The nurse should recheck all calculations with another nurse or the pharmacist when possible. Many hospitals require double checks of dosage calculations for children's medications and for all drugs with narrow safety margins, such as heparin and insulin. Because a nurse rarely needs more than one or two dosage units to prepare a prescribed dose, the nurse should always recheck the dosage if the calculations call for more than one tablet for a single dose or for a very small fraction of a dosage. The nurse must also be especially careful using decimal points since a misplaced or obscured decimal point can increase the dose many times or decrease it to a tiny fraction of the intended dose. The nurse should always write a zero in front of a decimal point so that no one misreads a figure such as 0.25 mg as 25 mg.

Likewise, a zero should never follow a decimal point because it could be easily misread and could increase the dosage tenfold.

Occasionally, the nurse encounters unusual situations that cause difficulty in measuring the precise dose because of the supplied drug's form. The nurse should not break unscored tablets, since the resulting dosages will not be exact. The nurse should confer with the pharmacist to have an inconvenient form of a drug changed into a form that the nurse can accurately measure. The nurse must be able to handle competently the basic arithmetic involved when working with the decimal system, common fractions, ratios and proportions, and percentages. Most medication orders and labels appear in the metric system; however, a nurse may sometimes need to convert an order from one system of measurement to another. Consequently, the nurse must be familiar with all of the systems of measurement discussed in Chapter 9, Intervention: Dosage Measurements and Calculations.

To measure doses of oral liquid drugs accurately, the nurse uses a medicine glass or cup. The nurse first sets the glass or cup at eye level when pouring, then reads the meniscus against the appropriate scale, i.e., milliliters, drams, or ounces. (See *Measuring oral liquid medications* on page 128 for the proper technique of measuring liquids.) By holding the bottle with the label toward the palm of the hand and pouring from the opposite side, the nurse avoids obliterating the label with dripping medication. The nurse should send bottles with illegible labels to the pharmacy and procure a new supply.

When measuring injectable medications, the nurse must carefully read the correct scale on the syringe. Most syringes are marked in milliliters or cubic centimeters. Insulin syringes, marked according to the strength of insulin, may measure 40 or 100 units per cubic centimeter. The nurse must be sure to use the scale that correlates to the concentration of the insulin being used.

The nurse must never alter the dosage specified in the physician's order. For example, at the time of surgery, a physician orders 75 mg of meperidine (Demerol) for pain for the postoperative patient. The nurse later observes that the patient remains in excruciating pain and that the 75 mg of Demerol does not seem to be sufficient. The nurse may believe that 100 mg of Demerol would alleviate the patient's pain, but the nurse does *not* have the prerogative to change the dose. The nurse should consult with the physician and obtain a new written order. In many instances, physicians now write medication orders with dosage ranges so that the nurse can decide the appropriate dosage within the specified range.

Measuring oral liquid medications

Oral liquid medications are accurately measured by reading the fluid level at the lower line of the convex curve. Note that some medication adheres to the side of the glass, forming a *meniscus,* a crescent shape on the liquid's surface.

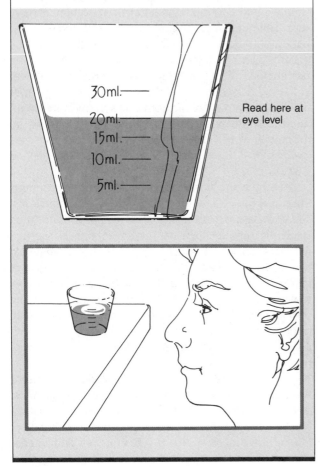

30ml.

20ml.

15ml.

10ml.

5ml.

Read here at eye level

The right patient. The nurse should always carefully check the patient's identification bracelet against the medication administration record before giving any medication. As a further check, the nurse should ask the patient to state his or her name. Nursing students sometimes feel awkward about asking the patient's name, especially when they have been working closely with a patient. However, both patient and nursing student can appreciate the reason for the precaution, and the feelings of awkwardness soon disappear when the patient sees that the procedure is standard practice. The nurse should not suggest the patient's name, since some patients may misunderstand the name or become confused and an-

swer to the wrong name. Furthermore, the nurse should never assume that the patient in a correctly labeled bed is the right patient. Confused patients sometimes get into the wrong bed.

The right time. Most hospitals establish routine times for drug administration. When administering drugs for which a consistent blood concentration level must be maintained to achieve therapeutic effects, nurses observe equal time intervals around the clock. For example, nurses may give the antiarrhythmic drug procainamide (Pronestyl) q 4 hours at 8 a.m., 12 noon, 4 p.m., 8 p.m., 12 midnight, and 4 a.m. A nurse may also have to measure certain patient responses to a therapy before administering another dose. For instance, the nurse should take the patient's apical pulse rate before giving digitalis preparations and measure the patient's respiratory rate before administering drugs such as morphine.

For drugs with no dictating features, the nurse may simply space the divided doses over the patient's waking hours. The nurse may give such drugs four times a day (q.i.d.) at 8 a.m., 12 noon, 4 p.m., and 8 p.m. Spacing the daily dose serves to prevent adverse effects, which might be caused by a too-high concentration of the drug in the bloodstream at any given time. Bradycardia from propranolol (Inderal) use is an example of an adverse effect that the nurse can prevent by spacing daily doses. Sometimes, nurses must consider other events, such as mealtime, when administering drugs. For example, a nurse giving a patient aspirin for a headache may administer the drug *before* meals to enhance absorption and the quick pain relief. On the other hand, the nurse may deliberately give other medications after meals to reduce gastric irritation caused by the drug. For example, a nurse would give large doses of aspirin, such as those commonly taken by arthritic patients, *after* meals. The large doses given after meals relieve pain more slowly but safely over a long period of time.

By administering all drugs at evenly spaced intervals and at consistent times each day, the nurse can prevent errors and accommodate the patient's daily schedule. For example, quinidine gluconate (Quinaglute Dura-Tabs), used to treat certain cardiac dysrhythmias, acts for 12 hours. Scheduling the drug for 8 a.m. and 8 p.m. administration maintains the necessary blood level without interfering with the patient's sleep. Routine administration schedules also help the patient develop the habit of taking the drug at a regular time. As a result, the patient is less likely to forget the drug after returning home.

To decrease further the risk of error in drug administration time, some institutions have policies that require the nurse to use different ink colors when recording information about drugs. The ink color depends upon whether the drug is to be given in the morning or evening. The nurse must pay attention to both the hour of administration and the color of the ink. Errors can result even with the color coding system. Other hospitals use the 24-hour system to decrease the number of medication errors related to timing. For example, the nurse would note a 10 p.m. medication time as 2200. By using the 24-hour system, the nurse cannot confuse 10 a.m. with 10 p.m.

The nurse should avoid scheduling medication administration at busy hours on the nursing unit, such as during the change of shift. Instead of scheduling a b.i.d. medication for 8 a.m. and 6 p.m., the nurse might better schedule the administration for 9 a.m. and 7 p.m. to avoid the busy 8 a.m. hour after the shift change. Regardless of the exact schedule, the nurse should follow standard practice and allow one half hour before and after the designated time for medication administration. In many institutions, medications given beyond these time limits are considered errors.

The right route. The nurse must pay careful attention to the administration route specified in the medication order and on the product label. Some drugs must be given in certain manufactured forms to be appropriate for particular entry routes into the body. For example, the eye, with its delicate nature, requires special preparations. Also, the nurse should never inject a solution anywhere into the body unless the label clearly indicates that the solution is *for injection.*

The administration route may also affect the amount of the medication given. If given intramuscularly, 10 mg of morphine sulfate, a frequently used adult dose, relieves pain. If the drug is ordered to be given I.V., the equivalent dose would decrease to 2 to 4 mg. If ordered orally, the dose of morphine sulfate would need to be greater than 10 mg.

The procedure used to administer a drug may also affect the rate of the drug's absorption into the bloodstream. Some topical ointments, such as nitroglycerin paste, enter the bloodstream more rapidly and completely if spread over a large surface area and covered with plastic wrap or special paper supplied with the medication. On the other hand, crushing enteric-coated tablets or opening sustained-action capsules and dissolving the drug in liquid will result in improper absorption of the drug into the bloodstream and, possibly, unintended effects. (See *Sustained-action drugs* for more information about administering these types of drugs.) Chapter 10, Intervention: Routes and Techniques of Administration, discusses proper techniques of medication administration.

Sustained-action drugs

Nurses increasingly encounter drugs designed to achieve an extended action over many hours. Prepared to dissolve at different rates, the drugs are gradually but continuously released into the bloodstream. Convenient for the patient, sustained-action drugs require fewer doses per day and provide more even control of symptoms.

Sustained-action drugs are supplied as plain tablets, coated tablets, and capsules filled with tiny granules. These drugs may be identified by "SA" after the drug name or by many prefixes used in the drug name to indicate prolonged effect. Common examples include Quinaglute *Dura-Tabs,* Dimetapp *Extentabs,* Chlor-Trimeton *Repetabs,* and Desoxyn *Gradumets.* Other names sometimes used include spansules, gyrocaps, and plateau caps.

The nurse must know that sustained-action tablets should *never* be *split, crushed,* or *chewed,* and that capsules should *never* be *emptied* into foods or beverages because doing so may alter the absorption rates, causing adverse effects or a subtherapeutic level of activity. The nurse must be certain that the patient understands the importance of taking the sustained-action drug in its supplied form.

Errors regarding the administration route can occur if a nurse uses improper equipment or technique while giving injections. Injections intended to be intramuscular may become subcutaneous if the nurse does not inject the needle deeply enough. If the nurse injects the needle too deeply, the needle may strike underlying bone. Although specific needle lengths exist for I.M. injections, the lengths are based upon average body masses. If the patient's body mass is greater or less than average, the nurse must make appropriate adjustments when choosing the needle. For example, a nurse would need a longer I.M. needle for a robust, 250-pound (113-kg) man than for a frail, 90-pound (51-kg) man. Similarly, injections intended to be intradermal can become subcutaneous if the nurse injects the needle at an improper angle.

PROCEDURAL SAFEGUARDS

Besides acknowledging the minimum requirements of the five "rights," nurses practice other procedural safeguards to prevent errors. The following section discusses several special precautions, but the list is not all-inclusive. Nurses should always think of safety and analyze situations that could lead to medication errors.

care professionals should handle and store
refully to maintain the drugs' stability and
strength. Because temperature, air, moisture, and light
may all affect a drug's stability, the nurse should follow
these precautions. Always keep drugs in the containers
in which the pharmacy dispensed them. Bottles should
be tightly capped and stored away from sources of heat,
light, and moisture. Some drugs are kept in brown bottles, and some I.V. medication bags are wrapped in
aluminum foil to protect them from light during infusion.
Some bottles of tablets contain small cylinders that absorb moisture and keep the product fresh. Ordinarily,
drugs are stored at room temperature. Only those drugs
that require cool temperatures are refrigerated, since
refrigeration causes moisture formation through con-
densation. Usually allow refrigerated drugs to reach room
temperature before administration.

• The law requires that narcotics and controlled substances be kept under double lock and key.

• The nurse should always note a drug's expiration date,
the date after which the original potency of the drug is
believed to change. The nurse should never give an
outdated drug, nor should the nurse give a drug that
looks or smells unusual. If the manufacturer's drug package appears to have been tampered with, the nurse
should not give the drug but should return the package
to the pharmacy for investigation. Drugs to be dispensed
as powders may be reconstituted by the nurse at administration time. The nurse should label any unused
medication with the date, time, strength, and the nurse's
initials or signature. The nurse should discard any drug
that will remain stable for only a short time and will reach
its expiration date before another dose is due. The nurse
should never give a drug that has not been properly
labeled following reconstitution. If a nurse finds an un-
labeled syringe containing a medication, the nurse should
discard it since nothing about the syringe (drug, dose,
sterility, etc.) can be assured.

• When delivering drugs to a patient's room, the nurse
stays with the medication cart or tray. If the nurse must
leave, the nurse should lock the cart and take it or the
tray back to the medication room or to the usual storage
place. The nurse remains with the patient until the patient
takes the medication. By remaining with the patient, the
nurse can verify that the patient took the medication as
directed. The nurse never leaves doses of medication
at the patient's bedside unless a specific order to do so
exists.

• The nurse should administer only medications prepared personally or by the pharmacist, unwrapping individual doses (unit doses) at the patient's bedside just
before ingestion. The nurse then discards the wrappers
at the medication cart, later using the discarded wrappers
to double-check what was administered. The nurse

should administer to a patient only the unit doses prepared for that patient.

• Before administering medications based on new orders, the nurse should review the patient's medication
history to detect any known allergies or other idiosyn-
cracies. The chart of any patient who has allergies should
be clearly labeled.

• When administering oral drugs, the nurse should encourage the patient to drink a full glass of water, if appropriate. The water helps to move the tablets through
the esophagus and into the stomach and dilutes the drug,
reducing the chance of gastric irritation.

• The physician must order those drugs that are to be
left at the patient's bedside for self-administration. Drugs
left at the patient's bedside should be marked with the
patient's name, the drug name, dose, and instructions.
Drugs frequently left at the patient's bedside include
antacids, which the patient may take repeatedly, and
nitroglycerin tablets, which the patient may need immediately for chest pain. The nurse remains responsible
for supervising a patient whose drugs are left at the
bedside. For example, the nurse must know how many
nitroglycerin tablets the patient took, the exact times of
self-administration, whether the patient obtained relief,
and any unusual reactions to the drug. The nurse must
record the information in the chart and report it to the
physician.

• The nurse should chart drugs immediately after giving
them. Delayed charting, especially of p.r.n. medications,
can result in an error of repeated doses, while early
charting (charting before giving the medication) may
result in omitted doses.

• The nurse should record observations of the patient's
responses, both positive and negative, to the medication.
For instance, for a patient receiving an antibiotic for
pneumonia, charted comments describing positive responses, such as a decreased amount of sputum, the
absence of fever, and easier breathing, would confirm
the drug's effectiveness. Negative reactions might include skin eruptions or gastric disturbances. Severe adverse reactions may prompt the physician to substitute
another drug.

If an error occurs, the nurse must: (1) report the
error immediately upon discovery to the physician and
the nursing supervisor, (2) render whatever care is necessary to safeguard the patient from further harm, and
(3) initiate a medication error incident report.

DRUG DELIVERY SYSTEMS

Several systems currently exist for procuring ordered drugs from the pharmacy. In each system, the nurse serves a vital coordinating function between the physician and the pharmacist.

The floor stock system

The floor stock system, the oldest system in use, features the maintenance of a stock supply of medications on the nursing unit. Stock supplies are usually kept in a medication room and may be arranged alphabetically or in groups according to drug action. Upon receiving a medication order, the nurse immediately transcribes it onto the medication cards and a special medication Kardex. The medication cards or tickets give the patient's name, room, and bed number; the name, dose, and administration schedule of the medication; the name or initials of the nurse who noted the order; and the date of the order. The medication cards may also be color coded to call attention to the administration time schedule.

After transcribing the medication order, the nurse prepares the appropriate medication dose from the available stock supply, places the dose into individual medication cups, and transports the medication to the patient on a tray or medication cart. If the nurse must dispense a large number of regularly scheduled medications, the nurse performs the charting in the nurses' station after administering all the medications for that hour. The chief advantage of the floor stock system is that nurses can implement medication orders quickly because the drug is immediately available on the unit. The floor stock system, however, presents at least three distinct disadvantages: (1) the nurse must interpret the order and requisition of the medication alone, with no input from the pharmacist, (2) transcription errors can easily occur, particularly if many different nurses have transcribed the drug orders, with no safeguard or check by the pharmacist, and (3) errors of omission can also occur if nurses misplace medication cards.

Individual prescriptions

When using the individual prescription system, the nurse transcribes the medication order and sends it to the pharmacy. The pharmacist fills the prescription using a container labeled for the particular patient. The nurse then administers the drug directly from the container. The nurse is less likely to commit the error of giving the drug to the wrong patient because the drug supply is designated for only one patient. Implementation, however, is slow in the individual prescription system because the medication order must travel from the nurse to the pharmacy and back to the nurse.

Unit-dose system

When using the unit-dose system, the nurse transcribes the order on the patient's medication administration record (MAR) and sends a carbon copy of the physician's order sheet directly to the pharmacy. The pharmacy may consist of a single centralized department serving the entire hospital, or it may consist of several substations, or satellites, with a substation staffed by a pharmacist available on each nursing unit. The pharmacist transcribes the order and dispenses a supply of single doses, wrapped and labeled, of all forms of drugs, oral as well as injectable preparations, and I.V. solutions with additives. The pharmacist usually dispenses drugs and I.V. solutions sufficient to last 24 hours and may also prepare trays of medications for administration by the nurse at specified hours. The pharmacist may either prepare unit doses or purchase them commercially. The pharmacist usually places drugs for each patient in individual drawers of a portable medication cart. The nurse keeps the drugs in their labeled wrappers until the actual administration time. (See *The medication cart* on page 132 for features of the cart and how drugs may be stored.)

The nurse keeps the MAR in a Kardex or notebook on the medication cart and records all drugs immediately as they are given to each patient. As a safeguard against errors from illegible longhand, the nurse prints the medication information on the MAR. The nurse should check the physician's order sheet and recopy the MAR anytime it becomes soiled or otherwise unreadable.

Using the unit-dose system reduces the chances for drug errors because: (1) the physician and nurse collaborate with the pharmacist on the total drug regimen and teaching plan for an individual patient, (2) the physician, nurse, and pharmacist can more readily foresee and prevent therapeutic incompatibilities, possible adverse reactions, and incorrect dosages because the clinical pharmacist keeps a detailed Kardex or record on each patient, (3) the system provides a double check for all medications, (4) practitioners using the method waste fewer medications, and (5) nurses chart medications immediately. Furthermore, using the unit-dose system reduces the risk of medication contamination because the pharmacist wraps medications as single doses and prepares I.V. medications under laminar airflow conditions in the pharmacy to assure sterility. The unit-dose system conveniently relieves the nurse of some

The medication cart

A medication cart provides important advantages when the nurse distributes drugs:
• The nurse can complete the entire medication procedure, from checking the order to documenting administration, at each patient's bedside, thus reducing probability of medication errors.

• The medications for other patients are covered and protected from contamination.
• The cart itself can be left at the patient's doorway, reducing the risk of transferring bacteria from one room to another.

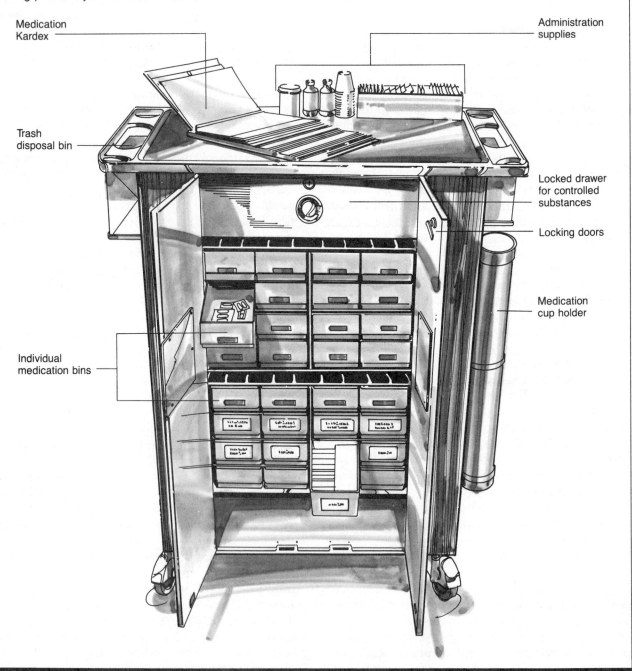

Medication Kardex

Trash disposal bin

Individual medication bins

Administration supplies

Locked drawer for controlled substances

Locking doors

Medication cup holder

of the preparation activities, thus enabling the nurse to devote more time to other aspects of patient care. The system proves particularly useful in hospitals that do not have 24-hour pharmacy service since pharmacists may prepare drugs for later administration by the nurse.

For the unit-dose system to work properly, some hospitals may have to increase their numbers of pharmacy personnel. Some institutions may view the increased staffing as a disadvantage of the unit-dose system.

Automated systems

Automated systems essentially represent computerized versions of the unit-dose system. A mechanical medication-dispensing unit delivers individually wrapped and labeled medications upon command by the nurse. The pharmacist fills the unit and keeps it locked. A computer records all drug transactions on electronic tape and furnishes requested printouts. The automated system greatly simplifies the maintenance of accurate drug records because the system's computer can monitor and track drugs in every respect, from the original inventory to the billing of patients. The efficiency of the system saves time and allows pharmacy personnel to expand their role to include more consultation and teaching. The system also relieves the nurse of the responsibilities of transcribing the medication order and procuring and storing the drug. The time saved frees the nurse to attend to other aspects of patient care.

Unfortunately, implementing an automated system can be extremely expensive, and all mechanical systems are subject to failure. Because of possible computer downtime, hospitals using automated systems devise backup plans for administering and recording medications.

Although hospitals usually select and use one drug delivery system, some institutions follow two systems. For example, an institution primarily using the unit-dose system may maintain small supplies of stock drugs in special care units for patients whose conditions may change rapidly, thus requiring that drugs be immediately available.

Regardless of the drug delivery system used in a hospital, the hospital's nurses, physicians, and pharmacists must work collaboratively. Although many hospitals are instituting automated systems, nurses in most hospitals continue to note medication orders and to administer medications. The drug delivery system does not relieve the nurse of traditional responsibilities in giving medications, nor can the delivery system substitute for the nurse's judgment required in unusual patient circumstances where routine procedures do not apply.

LEGAL RESPONSIBILITIES

Chapter 1 discussed the sources and types of laws governing drug administration. The following section deals only with specific nursing responsibilities imposed by the law. Practice acts passed by the legislature of each state govern the practice of each of the major health professions. Therefore, the nurse practice act, medical practice act, and pharmacy practice act of each state represent statutory laws and determine the scope of practice for those professionals. Essentially, practice acts allow physicians to prescribe, dispense, and administer drugs; pharmacists to prepare, dispense, and furnish drugs on the retail market; and nurses to administer medications. Also, the Controlled Substances Act, a federal legislation, regulates the manner in which narcotics and other controlled substances are dispensed and administered, thus directly affecting nursing practice.

EXPECTATIONS OF THE LAW

The law expects nurses who administer drugs to patients to know about those drugs. The nurse should know the goals of the drug therapy, the drug's mechanism of action, expected and unusual effects, dosage, proper administration methods, and any contraindications. The nurse also should assess the patient's medication responses and teach the patient about self-administration. The nurse practice acts in some states now specifically include patient teaching as a legal expectation.

On receiving a medication order, the nurse should consider it carefully. If any part of the order seems unusual, the nurse should not implement it until clarifying the problem with the prescriber. Under no circumstances should the nurse *ignore* the medication order and fail to carry it out. The nurse has an obligation to seek clarification of any questions concerning the order. Sometimes nurses are reluctant to approach a physician and question an order for fear of being rebuked. Questioning a medication order requires a combination of assertiveness and tact on the nurse's part. Frequently, nurses consult pharmacists or approved published drug references to confirm their knowledge of the drug before approaching a physician. When questioning an order, the nurse should discuss the matter with the physician privately, professionally, and with an attitude of objective scientific inquiry. If the physician's explanation is unacceptable, the nurse must notify the supervisor and withhold the medication until further clarification of the order is received.

MALPRACTICE

Malpractice refers to the negligence or dereliction of a professional person in the rendering of services. Under the law, nurses are judged to be responsible for their own actions. Thus, upon the implementation of an incorrect order, the nurse, as well as the physician and the hospital, may be held legally liable. Medication errors resulting in malpractice may take two forms: errors of omission and errors of commission. An error of omission occurs when the nurse entirely omits an important part of care. For example, a nurse who overlooks a patient's 2 p.m. dose of cimetidine (Tagamet) commits an error of omission. An error of commission occurs when the nurse performs a procedure improperly. For example, a nurse administers 3 ml (0.15 mg) of digoxin (Lanoxin) to an infant I.M., rather than orally, and the infant suffers cardiac arrest. The nurse has committed an error of commission.

While malpractice may sound harsh, especially to the beginning nursing student, the student may feel reassured by learning that the law does not expect the nurse to be infallible. The law does expect sound knowledge, good judgment, and due care. Because medication errors, along with falls, rank at the top of the list of causes of malpractice suits, the nurse must safeguard against medication errors by carefully considering and following the five "rights" of medication administration.

Further legal expectations of the nurse arise when an error occurs. Upon discovery of the error, the nurse should: (1) immediately notify the physician, the nursing supervisor, and the pharmacist, that is, *only* those personnel who can do something to rectify the error, (2) carefully assess the patient's condition and render care as necessary, and (3) complete a medication error incident report.

Medication error incident reports

Most hospitals include medication error incident reports among their unusual incident forms. The medication error incident report typically requires a clear description of the event, including the time and date of the error, and what the nurse did about it. The physician completes a section describing the patient's condition and any medical action taken. Nurses should not neglect to fill out medication error incident reports for fear that the reports will be used in disciplinary action against them. Administrative personnel can use the medication error incident reports to help improve patient care through the implementation of policies or procedures to prevent similar errors from occurring in the future.

Circulation of a medication error incident report should be limited to administrative personnel who need to know the facts about a specific incident. The medication error incident report is usually not placed in the patient's chart, but the nurse's charting on the patient's record should explain what happened and which actions subsequently were taken.

CONFLICTS BETWEEN PRACTICE ACTS

A few special circumstances necessitate that the nurse must operate exactly within the provisions of the practice act and not infringe on the practice of one of the other professions. Nurse practice acts typically state that the nurse implements orders written by *licensed* physicians, podiatrists, and dentists. Medication orders written by physician's assistants do not meet the criterion. Therefore, a licensed physician must countersign any order written by a physician's assistant before the nurse implements the order.

Possible conflicts with pharmacy practice acts occasionally restrict nursing actions. For example, transferring medications from one bottle to another or relabeling bottles falls within the realm of pharmacy, not the realm of nursing. Also, nursing supervisors who need drugs from the pharmacy when it is closed may only procure enough medication for one dose. Pharmacy practice acts regard the taking of larger quantities as dispensing, a clear function of the pharmacist.

The emerging role of the nurse practitioner sometimes conflicts with medical practice acts. In 1981, the *Sermchief versus Gonzales* case in Missouri set a precedent. Under prescribed protocols and under the general guidance of staff physicians, two nurses employed as nurse practitioners in a family-planning clinic frequently diagnosed reproductive tract conditions and prescribed medications, such as antibiotic creams and contraceptive drugs and devices. A charge of practicing medicine without a license was brought against the two nurse practitioners. The state supreme court upheld the nurse practitioners' actions by ruling that they were operating within the provisions of the nurse practice act, which had been recently revised to allow for expanded nursing roles. All of the examples emphasize the need for the nurse to understand clearly the provisions of the nurse practice act established by the state in which the nurse is practicing.

CONTROLLED SUBSTANCES

The Controlled Substances Act of the federal government imposes a few special responsibilities on the nurse. Under its provisions, the nurse must account for the proper use of controlled drugs with specific patients. Thus, when administering a narcotic, a barbiturate, or another controlled drug, the nurse must sign for the drug on a special narcotics record. Every dose that the pharmacy dispenses must be accounted for, whether the dose was used for a particular patient or was discarded accidentally.

Most hospitals require change-of-shift controlled substance or narcotics counts to assure that the supply on hand correlates exactly with the records. A nurse going off duty and a nurse coming on duty cooperatively make the controlled substance or narcotics count, and both sign the form verifying the accuracy of the count. If the count indicates a discrepancy between the supply and the record, the reason for the discrepancy must be traced immediately. Someone simply may have forgotten to sign for a dose that was given to a patient, a dose may have been somehow contaminated and wasted without an explanation on the narcotics record, or someone may have removed a dose from the supply without authorization.

The law also requires that controlled drugs be stored in locked cabinets. The nurse maintains the narcotics supply under double lock and key. The nurse should always carry the narcotics keys, never leaving them in a drawer or hung on a hook where unauthorized persons could have access to them.

ETHICAL OBLIGATIONS

Nursing ethics represent the application of moral principles and values to professional practice. Whereas legal affairs concern rights and correlated responsibilities, ethics deal with the duties and obligations that the nurse has to self, patients, and professional colleagues. Conflicts of value can occur when the nurse, patient, and physician express differences of opinion about what actions to take in a particular situation. Consider the following:

A nurse is caring for a patient with advanced cancer, and the patient's physician orders chemotherapy. The patient is reluctant to begin the chemotherapy and asks the nurse many questions regarding its efficacy and adverse effects. The nurse knows that the patient's disease is terminal and that the therapy may cause hair loss as well as severe nausea and vomiting. The nurse wants to be truthful and believes in the patient's right to refuse the therapy and live as desired. Yet the nurse also knows that the physician recommends the chemotherapy. Under the circumstances, the nurse's strong belief in the patient's right to self-determination, the role of the nurse as a patient advocate, and the nurse's sincere desire to be honest can produce ethical conflicts for the nurse.

Ethical conflicts have always existed in nursing but have become prominent today because of the quality of life issue. Rapidly advancing technology often prolongs life, resulting in conditions that some people may want to avoid.

Moral principles

The nurse applies six moral principles when considering all types of patient care, including medication administration. Those principles include autonomy, paternalism, truthfulness, beneficence, fidelity, and respect for property. In analyzing ethical issues involving these principles, the nurse emphasizes:

- What is morally right and therefore ought to be done?
- What benefits and harms would result from this action?
- Who would be benefited or harmed?

Autonomy refers to the right of every person to make rational decisions about one's life. The nurse's belief in autonomy leads to a respect for the patient's decisions. The nurse actively helps the patient to overcome fear, pain, and knowledge deficits that might interfere with the patient's rational thinking. The nurse must assess each patient and consider the patient's decision regarding the medication administration.

Paternalism results when someone decides what is best for another person and acts without consulting the person. Anyone acting paternalistically toward a patient must consider whether the action is justifiable. Unjustified paternalism in no way supports the patient.

The nurse may practice justified paternalism when administering pain medication to a terminally ill patient who may refuse medication because the drug causes drowsiness. The nurse knows the positive and negative consequences of the medication and convinces the patient to take the medication by deemphasizing the drug's sedative effects. In such a situation, the nurse's justified paternalism benefits the patient.

Truthfulness refers to being honest. The nurse displays truthfulness by not withholding information. For example, if a patient's drug produced adverse effects, such as severe nausea and vomiting, the nurse would disclose the full information about the adverse effects while focusing on the positive benefits of the therapy and reassuring the patient that the nausea can be treated. The nurse must answer all questions honestly and seek further information if necessary.

Beneficence refers to the concept that nursing actions should always cause beneficial effects, never harmful ones. All nursing procedures are based on the principle of beneficence. The nurse should always plan and implement actions that assure safe outcomes for the patient and avoid negative consequences, which might cause harm. Hence, the nurse reads drug labels repeatedly, double-checks dosage calculations, and compares the patient's identification band to the medication order.

Fidelity requires the nurse to be faithful and truthful and to keep promises made to self, patients and families, co-workers, and employers. A nurse should not make a promise to a patient without absolute certainty that the promise can be kept.

Respect for property refers to the safekeeping of the patient's personal possessions. If a patient brings medications to the hospital, most hospitals require that the nurse take the medications from the patient upon admission and store them to prevent double dosing or undesirable drug interactions. The patient, however, must consent to the storage, and the nurse must return the medications to the patient upon discharge. Medications ordered from the pharmacy become the patient's personal property even though the nurse keeps the drugs in the medication cart and administers them. Therefore, the nurse would violate the patient's property rights by administering the drugs to another patient or by destroying the patient's drugs brought from home.

Placebos

Placebos, substances used for nonspecific, psychological effects without the patient's immediate knowledge that a placebo is being given, create certain ethical quandaries. In some respects, placebo use is deceptive. Traditionally, physicians and nurses have not told patients about placebos because doing so usually diminishes the chance of the placebo producing the desired effect. The success of placebo use seems to depend upon a patient's susceptibility. Physicians and nurses sometimes use glucose pills and saline solution injections as placebos.

Advocates contend that placebos present less danger to the patient than active drugs. They might argue that relieving pain with 1 ml of normal saline solution is safer than injecting an opiate, which might cause dependence. Opponents argue that physicians and nurses giving placebos practice unethical deception, which is unjustifiably paternalistic. Other people occupy a moderate position and believe that the use of placebos can serve a legitimate function in therapy and need not be deceptive.

Other practitioners believe that some patients can learn to mobilize natural pain-relief responses using placebos to stimulate endorphins, which are endogenous opiate-like substances stored in the brain and spinal cord. The physician and nurse devise a treatment plan and tell the patient that they are administering either an active or an inert drug. They also explain that they will give the patient an active pain reliever if the placebo does not stimulate the endorphins. The patient participates with full knowledge and consent.

Practitioners who use placebos should acknowledge the extenuating circumstances and comply with the following guidelines:

- Use placebos only after careful diagnosis.
- Use only inert substances.
- Answer questions as truthfully as possible.
- Honor the patient's request if the patient specifically asks not to receive placebos.
- Never give placebos when other treatment is indicated or before exploring all treatment options.

Researchers use placebos extensively, both in blind studies, in which the patient doesn't know whether a substance is active or inert, and in double-blind studies, in which neither the patient nor the researcher knows if the patient is receiving an active or inert substance. Researchers thoroughly explain the study to the patient, and the patient agrees to participate.

CHAPTER SUMMARY

Medication orders usually originate with the physician and vary in form, depending on whether they apply to a hospitalized patient or to an outpatient. Physicians write medication orders for hospitalized patients along with or in addition to all other medical orders. Requirements of the medication order include the patient's name, the name and dose of the drug, the administration route, the schedule, the prescriber's signature, and the date and time. Physicians write medication orders for outpatients as prescriptions. Prescriptions must include the patient's name and address, the drug name, form and dose, directions for taking the drug, as well as the physician's signature, address, phone number, and registration numbers. The chapter discussed nursing considerations as they apply to each of the following types of medication orders: standard written, single, stat, p.r.n., standing, verbal, and telephone. Other highlights of Chapter 8 include:

• Safeguards exist to help the nurse avoid medication errors. Using the five "rights" of medication administration, nurses ensure that they are giving the right drug and the right dose of the drug. Nurses should also check the patient's identification to ensure that they are giving the drug to the right patient. They must also establish and verify the right time for drug administration. Finally, nurses must be sure that they use the right administration route when giving a drug to a patient. The medication order and the drug product label specify the administration route. Other procedural safeguards, such as checking expiration dates, staying with the patient until the patient has taken the medication, and recording any observations of patient responses to the drugs, can help the nurse prevent medication errors.

• Different systems are used for delivering medications from the pharmacy to the patient. With the floor stock system, each nursing unit maintains a stock supply of medications. By having the medications on hand, the nurse can quickly implement medication orders. Using the individual prescription system, the pharmacist fills a single order, using a container labeled for the particular patient. The nurse then administers the drug directly from the container. When using the unit-dose system, the pharmacist dispenses medication supplies, storing the medications either on trays or in a medication cart. The nurse then takes the medication cart or tray from room to room, administering the drugs. Hospitals using automated systems must also establish a backup system for times during which the computers are nonfunctional.

• The law expects the nurse administering medications to possess sound knowledge and good judgment and to exercise due care in executing procedures. The nurse is obligated to clarify any unusual or unclear medication orders with the prescriber before implementing them. The nurse cannot ignore a medication order, but the nurse can refuse to give a medication if the prescriber cannot satisfactorily explain the order.

• Causes of malpractice include errors of omission, in which the nurse fails to give necessary care, and errors of commission, in which the nurse renders necessary care in an improper way. The nurse can be held liable for a patient's injury if the injury directly results from the nurse's action.

• Nurses must apply fundamental values and moral principles to their professional nursing practice. Six moral principles that the nurse applies when considering patient care relate to autonomy, paternalism, truthfulness, beneficence, fidelity, and respect for property. Placebos pose potential ethical dilemmas because of the deceptive nature required for their administration. Placebos, however, can be legitimately used in some situations.

BIBLIOGRAPHY

Bok, S. "The Ethics of Giving Placebos," *Scientific American* 231(5):17, November 1974.

Creighton, H. *Law Every Nurse Should Know.* Philadelphia: W.B. Saunders Co., 1986.

Cushing, M. "Drug Errors Can Be Bitter Pills," *American Journal of Nursing* 86:895, August 1986.

Cushing, M. "Incident Reports: For Your Eyes Only?" *American Journal of Nursing* 85:873, August 1985.

Davis, A.J., and Aroskar, M.A. *Ethical Dilemmas and Nursing Practice.* Norwalk, Conn.: Appleton-Century-Crofts, 1983.

Dugas, B.W. *Introduction to Patient Care.* Philadelphia: W.B. Saunders Co., 1983.

Marchewka, A.E. "When is Paternalism Justifiable?" *American Journal of Nursing* 83:1072, July 1983.

McGovern, K. "10 Steps for Preventing Medication Errors," *Nursing86* 16:36, December 1986.

Rabinow, J. "Six Legal Safeguards vs. Drug Errors," *NursingLife* 4:56, January/February 1984.

Scherer, J.C. *Nurses' Drug Manual.* Philadelphia: J.B. Lippincott Co., 1985.

Templin, M.S., et al. "Placebos: How Much Do You Know About Them?" *NursingLife* 4:52, November/December 1984.

CHAPTER 9

INTERVENTION: DOSAGE MEASUREMENTS AND CALCULATIONS

OBJECTIVES

After reading and studying this chapter, you should be able to:

1. Discuss age, size, integrity of the body systems, and the type and virulence of the patient's disease as important factors when determining a drug dosage.

2. Give the advantages of the metric system, including its international use and exact equivalents, over the apothecaries' and household systems of measurement.

3. Give at least two clinical examples of how each of the three systems of measurement is used in medication administration.

4. Identify two drugs that use special systems of measurement developed by the manufacturers.

5. Perform the proper calculations for a drug ordered in one system of measurement but available only in another system of measurement.

6. Use the fraction and ratio methods to convert measurements from one system to another and to calculate drug dosages.

7. Use the fraction and ratio methods to calculate the necessary amounts for reconstitution of powdered drugs for injection, for percentage solutions, and for intravenous infusion rates.

8. Identify the two most effective methods for computing a pediatric drug dose.

INTRODUCTION

This chapter contains information related to administering safe, accurate dosages of drugs—a major responsibility for nurses. The chapter begins by discussing factors that determine variations in drug dosages, followed by information regarding the major systems of drug weights and measures. The chapter includes the characteristics of each system of drug weights and measures, the units for both liquid and solid measures within each system, and examples of physicians' orders for drugs measured in each system. Conversions between

the systems of measurement are explained, and methods for calculating drug dosages within each system of drug weights and measures are presented. Sample problems and their solutions appear throughout the chapter to assist in the step-by-step approach needed to calculate correct dosages. Practice computations and their answers are also presented. The chapter also explores special problems, such as the calculation of drug doses for children, for adults with special needs, and for individuals receiving chemotherapeutic drugs.

FACTORS INFLUENCING DRUG DOSAGES

Several major factors influence the amount of a drug that would prove most effective and safe for each patient.

Age

The first factor, the patient's age, predetermines to some extent body size and affects the functioning of the various body systems.

Health care professionals must give special consideration to both infants and elderly patients. In an infant, immature body systems impede pharmacokinetics—the absorption, distribution, metabolism, and excretion of drugs. Elderly patients may experience age-related changes involving the degeneration of one or more of the major body systems. The degeneration of body systems increases the likelihood of chronic illnesses involving these systems. The resulting chronic illnesses may subsequently alter the absorption, distribution, metabolism, and excretion of drugs. The alterations in pharmacokinetics can adversely affect the effectiveness and safety of an administered drug.

Size

A patient's size is determined by body weight and body-surface area. Both factors affect drug dosages. In most cases, a larger patient requires a larger dose of medication. For example, adult patients usually receive larger drug doses than pediatric patients. In some instances, the patient's weight determines the drug amount prescribed. In other cases, the patient's body-surface area affects drug dosage.

Integrity of body systems

The proper functioning of body systems is another important consideration when determining the drug dosage needed by a patient. Alterations in gastrointestinal functioning affect the time and amount of absorption of orally administered drugs. Alterations in cardiovascular functioning affect the absorption of injected medications. The integrity of the cardiovascular system also affects the transport of drugs from the absorption site to the action site. Because the liver metabolizes the majority of drugs, any alteration in hepatic function disturbs the normal rate of such metabolism. Alterations in hepatic function and the resulting effects on drug metabolism lead to increasing blood concentration levels of a drug and the likelihood of a toxic effect, despite the administration of the drug within a safe dosage range.

Excretion of drugs occurs via the gastrointestinal and renal systems and to a lesser extent, the respiratory system. Alterations in renal function most significantly and adversely affect drug excretion. Patients with kidney pathology retain drugs and the end products of drug degradation. The retention causes increased blood concentration levels of the drug and end products and consequently increases the risk of toxicity.

Type and virulence of disease

The type and virulence of a patient's disease also affects the drug dosage. The same medication may be given for several purposes; however, the dose varies according to the desired effect. For example, the antianxiety drug diazepam (Valium) may be given in a small dose to control a patient's anxiety, but it may also be given in a larger dose to produce an anesthetic effect. Similarly, the dose of an antibiotic can vary, depending upon the extent of infection evident.

Safe drug dosages

Drug companies and researchers extensively test each new drug before its approval for distribution to the general public. The research provides information about the drug's activities, effectiveness, side effects, and toxicity, as well as about the drug's dosage ranges that yield desired outcomes. Drug manufacturers provide their research results to physicians for use in determining drug dosages. The nurse's responsibilities include ensuring that all administered drugs fall within the safe ranges determined by manufacturers. To fulfill their responsibilities, nurses must be able to: (1) determine equivalent measurements from among the metric, apothecaries', and household systems of measurements and (2) use appropriate mathematical formulas to calculate drug dosages, percentage solutions, and intravenous infusion rates. Mastery of the information presented in this chapter will provide an essential knowledge base for implementing these important nursing skills. (Additional information regarding the effects of patient characteristics on drug dosages and pharmacokinetics appears in Chapter 2, Pharmacokinetics.)

SYSTEMS OF DRUG WEIGHTS AND MEASURES

Physicians use several systems of measurement when ordering drugs. The three systems of measurement most often used in clinical situations are the metric system, the apothecaries' system, and the household system. The avoirdupois system is used for ordering and purchasing pharmaceutical products. Nurses also use the avoirdupois system in the clinical setting when weighing patients.

THE METRIC SYSTEM

The metric system, the most widely used and international system of measure, is also the system of measure used by the United States Pharmacopoeia. Among its many advantages, the metric system affords a way to achieve accuracy in calculating small drug dosages. Furthermore, the metric system uses Arabic numerals, which are commonly used by health care professionals throughout the world. Finally, most manufacturers calibrate newly developed drugs in the metric system.

Unfortunately, the general population in the United States has shown little eagerness to adopt the metric system. As a consequence, nurses and student nurses often view the metric system as a new and complicated concept. However, when they understand the general principles of this system, nurses can easily make drug calculations and conversions within it.

Metric measures

This table shows the relationships among some commonly used measures. Several less commonly used measures, such as the hectogram, also appear.

LIQUIDS	SOLIDS
1 ml = 1 cc	1,000 mg = 1 g
1,000 ml = 1 liter	1,000 g = 1 kilogram
100 centiliters = 1 liter	100 centigrams = 1 g
10 deciliters = 1 liter	10 decigrams = 1 g
10 liters = 1 dekaliter	10 g = 1 dekagram
100 liters = 1 hectoliter	100 g = 1 hectogram
1,000 liters = 1 kiloliter	

Liquid measures

The liter of the metric system approximates 1 quart in volume. A milliliter equals one one-thousandth of a liter. Liters are often used when ordering and administering intravenous solutions. Milliliters are used in the administration of parenteral and some oral drugs. (See *Metric measures* for a breakdown of liquid measurements in liters and subdivisions of liters called milliliters [ml].)

Solid measures

In the metric system, the gram (g) serves as the basis for solid measures or units of weights. A milligram (mg) equals one one-thousandth of a gram. Physicians order many drugs in milligrams. Body weight is recorded in kilograms (kg). A kilogram equals 1,000 grams.

The following examples represent possible physicians' orders using the metric system:
- 1 liter of 5% dextrose solution I.V. per 8 hours
- 30 ml (milliliters) Milk of Magnesia P.O. h.s.
- Ancef 1 g (gram) I.V.P.B. q6h
- Lanoxin 0.125 mg P.O. daily
- Maintain 10 kg (kilogram) continuous traction

THE APOTHECARIES' SYSTEM

Though older than the metric system and still used to measure several medications, the apothecaries' system is slowly being phased out of use. The apothecaries' system possesses two unique features: the use of Roman numerals and the placement of the unit of measurement before the Roman numeral. For example, *5 grains* would be written as *grains v.* Within the apothecaries' system, the equivalents among the various units of measure are close approximations. When using equivalents for calculations and conversions, keep in mind that the calculations, though not precise, will fall within acceptable standards. The apothecaries' system is the only system of measurement that uses symbols besides abbreviations to represent several of the units of measure.

Liquid measures

Visualize the minim, the smallest of the units, as the approximate size of a drop of water. Fifteen to 16 minims comprise about 1 milliliter. (Note the approximation of the measure.) Sixty minims equals 1 fluidram. Eight fluidrams equals 1 ounce. The symbol f$\mathfrak{z}$ represents the fluidram, and the symbol f$\mathfrak{z}$ represents the fluidounce. Remember that the larger unit, the fluidounce, also has an extra line in its symbol. (See *Apothecaries' measures* for liquids measured in minims [M_x], fluidrams [f$\mathfrak{z}$], fluidounces [f$\mathfrak{z}$], pints [pt], quarts [qt], and gallons [gal].)

Solid measures

The grain (gr) represents the solid measure or unit of weight in the apothecaries' system. Historians claim that the weight of an average grain of wheat originally determined the grain of the apothecaries' system.

Apothecaries' measures

This table displays the relationships between measures, both liquid and solid, within the apothecaries' system.

LIQUIDS	
60 minims (M_x)	= 1 fluidram (f$\mathfrak{z}$)
8 fluidrams (f$\mathfrak{z}$)	= 1 fluidounce (f$\mathfrak{z}$)
16 fluidounces (f$\mathfrak{z}$)	= 1 pint (pt)
2 pints	= 1 quart (qt)
4 quarts	= 1 gallon (gal)

SOLIDS	
20 grains (gr)	= 1 scruple ($\mathfrak{z}$)
3 scruples ($\mathfrak{z}$)	= 1 dram ($\mathfrak{z}$)
8 drams ($\mathfrak{z}$)	= 1 ounce ($\mathfrak{z}$)
12 ounces ($\mathfrak{z}$)	= 1 pound (lb)

The following examples represent possible physicians' orders using the apothecaries' system:
- multivitamin elixir M_x (minims) xii P.O.
- Robitussin f3 (fluidrams) iv P.O. q6h
- Mylanta f3 (fluidounce) i P.O. 1 hour p.c.
- Tylenol gr (grains) x P.O. q4h p.r.n. headache

THE HOUSEHOLD SYSTEM

Most people in the United States are familiar with the household system of weights and measures. In most cases, food products, recipes, over-the-counter drugs, and home remedies use the household system. Although the units of measure in the household system may be the most familiar, great discrepancies exist about quantities attributed to each measure and conversions between the measures. In the clinical setting, health care professionals seldom use the household system for drug administration; however, some household measures may prove useful.

Liquid measures

Liquid measurements in the household system most often used in the clinical setting are teaspoons (tsp) and tablespoons (tbs). (See *Devices of the household system* for an illustration of that system's spoon, which represents a more exact measure than the spoon used in the home for food preparation.) The clinically used teaspoon and tablespoon have been standardized to equal 5 ml and 15 ml, respectively. Thus, 3 teaspoons equals 1 tablespoon, and 6 teaspoons equals 1 ounce.

Liquids
- 1 teaspoon (tsp) = 5 ml
- 3 teaspoons (tsp) = 15 ml or 1 tablespoon (tbs)
- 6 teaspoons (tsp) = 1 ounce

Patients with prescribed medications to be taken in dosages of teaspoons or tablespoons should obtain clinical equipment calibrated in these measures to receive the exact prescribed dosage.

The following examples represent possible physicians' orders using the household system:
- 2 tsp (teaspoons) elixir of terpin hydrate P.O. b.i.d.
- Riopan 2 tbs (tablespoons) P.O. 1 hr. a.c. and h.s.

THE AVOIRDUPOIS SYSTEM

The solid measures or units of weight in the avoirdupois system include the ounce (437.5 grains) and the pound (16 ounces or 7,000 grains). Note that the apothecaries' pound equals 12 ounces in contrast to the 16-ounce pound of the avoirdupois system.

Devices of the household system

To ensure the accuracy of dosages measured in teaspoons and tablespoons, the patient should receive information about obtaining proper measuring devices and the proper method of administration.

1. Obtain a spoon with hollow handle calibrated in teaspoons and tablespoons.

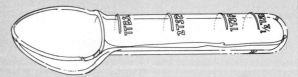

2. Check dose after filling. Hold spoon upright. Shaded area indicates dose of 2 tsp.

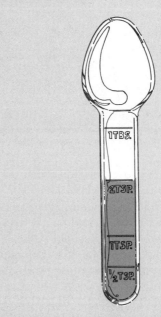

3. Administer by tilting the spoon so the medication (shaded area) fills the bowl of spoon. Then place the spoon in mouth.

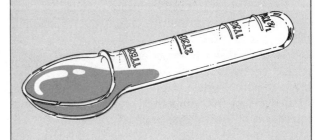

Measuring drops

When held vertically, a standard medication dropper is usually calibrated to deliver 20 drops of water or other solution per milliliter. Standard intravenous solution administration sets usually deliver 10 to 20 drops per milliliter, while microdrip units deliver 60 drops per milliliter.

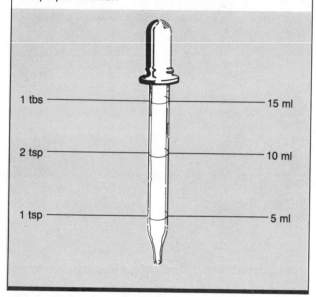

1 tbs — 15 ml

2 tsp — 10 ml

1 tsp — 5 ml

MIXED SYSTEMS

Several units of measure may arbitrarily appear in the apothecaries', household, or avoirdupois systems. Two such units of measure, the drop and ounce, appear in both the apothecaries' and household systems. The *drop*, traditionally considered equal to a drop of water, is an inexact measure that varies in size depending on the physical characteristics of the liquid being measured and the equipment used to form the drop. The drop is the unit of measure used when instilling liquid medication into areas such as the ear, nose, or conjunctival sac of the eye. (See *Measuring drops* for an illustration of a standard dropper used for instilling liquids.) Nurses also use the drop as the unit of measure when monitoring intravenous solutions.

The pound and the ounce appear in both the apothecaries' and avoirdupois systems. While the determination of which system to place the pound and ounce within may vary from authority to authority, the size and equivalents of the measures remain consistent.

OTHER MEASURES

Some drugs require special systems developed by the manufacturers for measuring their quantities. The following discussion addresses special systems of measurement.

Units

Insulin, a drug used by many diabetic patients to assist in controlling blood sugar, is measured in units (U). Many types of insulin exist; however, all are measured in units. The international standard of U-100 insulin means that 1 milliliter of insulin solution contains 100 units of insulin regardless of type. (See *U-100 insulin syringes* for an illustration of syringes typically used for insulin administration.)

Heparin, an anticoagulation drug, is also measured in units. Heparin exists in liquid form containing 100, 1000, 5000, or 10,000 units per milliliter for parenteral (subcutaneous or intravenous) use.

Several antibiotics, available in liquid, solid, and powder forms for either oral or parenteral uses, also have units as their basis of measure. The drug manufacturer provides information about the number of metric units required to provide the number of special units. For example, nystatin, an oral liquid preparation, contains 100,000 U per milliliter. The antibiotic penicillin, also measured in units, is manufactured in powdered form, to be reconstituted later for parenteral or oral ad-

U-100 insulin syringes

Several different syringes labeled in units are available for the administration of insulin. Here are two examples.

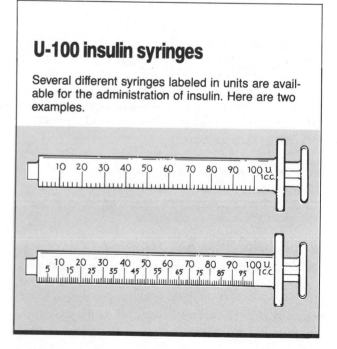

ministration. Penicillin also exists in tablet form for oral use and in liquid form prepackaged in syringes for intramuscular injection.

The following examples represent possible physicians' orders using units:
- 14 U NPH insulin S.C. this a.m.
- heparin 5,000 Units S.C. b.i.d.
- nystatin 200,000 Units P.O. q6h
- 300,000 U procaine penicillin I.M. q4h

International Units

International Units (IU) represent the unit of measurement of biologicals, such as vitamins, enzymes, and hormones. For instance, the activity of calcitonin (Calcimar), a synthetic hormone used in calcium regulation, is stated in International Units.

Milliequivalents

Electrolytes may be measured in milliequivalents (mEq). The drug manufacturers provide information about the number of metric units required to provide the prescribed number of milliequivalents, for example, 1 ml equals 4 mEq. Physicians usually order the electrolyte potassium chloride in milliequivalents. Potassium preparations for intravenous, oral, or other use come in liquid (elixir and parenteral) and solid (powder and tablet) forms.

The following examples represent possible physicians' orders using milliequivalents:
- 30 mEq (milliequivalents) KCl P.O. b.i.d.
- 1 liter of 5% dextrose in 0.9% saline solution with 40 mEq KCl to run at 125 ml per hour

EQUIVALENTS AMONG THE SYSTEMS OF MEASUREMENT

In the clinical setting, nurses must sometimes make conversions from one system of drug measurement to another. The necessity for conversions occurs when a drug is ordered in one system of measurement but is available only in another system. To perform the calculations involved in making conversions, the nurse must know the equivalents among the different systems of measurement. When first learning to make conversions, nursing students should use a small number of the most common equivalents to calculate other equivalents. (See *Units of exchange among systems of drug measurement* on page 144 for key equivalents useful when calculating conversions.)

Key conversion equivalents

For rough estimates, 1 liter (1,000 milliliters) approximately equals 1 quart. For more exacting measurement,

1 quart equals 0.946 liters or 946 milliliters (ml). (See *One-liter containers* on page 145, which shows a glass bottle and a plastic bag calibrated in milliliters of the metric system.)

One milliliter represents 15 to 16 minims. Thirty milliliters equals 1 fluidounce (f3), which equals 8 fluidrams (f3), which equals 2 tablespoons (tbs). (See *Medication cup* on page 145, which shows a container resembling the one used in many clinical settings to dispense liquids.) The calibration on the medication cup is useful as a source of information about measurement system equivalents.

One kilogram (kg) in the metric system equals 2.2 pounds (lb) in the avoirdupois system, which nurses need to know when converting patients' weights from one system to another.

When calculating solid medication equivalents between the metric and the apothecaries' systems, use the following standard equivalents: 1 gram (g) equals approximately 15 grains (gr), and 60 or 65 milligrams (mg) equals approximately 1 grain.

CONVERSIONS BETWEEN SYSTEMS OF MEASUREMENT

Several methods can be used to convert a drug measurement from one unit to another. Use the method you feel most comfortable with. Remember, you may be converting measurements from one measure to another within the same system, or you may be converting a unit of measure from one system to the equivalent measurement in another system. Making conversions associated with drug administration is a skill nurses frequently use.

The fraction method for conversions

The fraction method for conversions requires an equation consisting of two fractions. Set up the first fraction by placing the ordered dosage you need to convert over X units of the available dosage. For example, a physician orders 300 mg of aspirin. The bottle you have is labeled aspirin gr v per tablet. The milligram dosage represents the ordered dosage, and the grain dosage represents the available dosage. Because the amount of the available dosage is still unknown, it is represented by an X. The first fraction of the equation appears as:

$$\frac{300 \text{ mg}}{X \text{ gr}}$$

Then set up the second fraction of the equation. The second fraction consists of the standard equivalents between the ordered and available measures. Since you

Units of exchange among systems of drug measurement

The following shows some approximate liquid equivalents among the household, apothecaries', and metric systems.

HOUSEHOLD	APOTHECARIES'	METRIC
1 teaspoonful (tsp)	1 fluidram (f₃)	5 ml
1 tablespoonful (tbs)	½ fluidounce (f₃)	15 ml
2 tablespoonfuls	1 fluidounce	30 ml
1 measuring cupful	8 fluidounces	240 ml
1 pint (pt)	16 fluidounces	473 ml
1 quart (qt)	32 fluidounces	946 ml (1 liter)
1 gallon (gal)	128 fluidounces	3,785 ml

The following shows some approximate solid equivalents between the metric system and the apothecaries' system.

APOTHECARIES'	METRIC
15 grains	1 gram (g) (1,000 mg)
10 grains	0.6 g (600 mg)
7½ grains	0.5 g (500 mg)
5 grains	0.3 g (300 mg)
3 grains	0.2 g (200 mg)
1½ grains	0.1 g (100 mg)
1 grain	0.06 g (60 mg) or 0.065 g (65 mg)
¾ grain	0.05 g (50 mg)
½ grain	0.03 g (30 mg)
¼ grain	0.015 g (15 mg)
1/60 grain	0.001 g (1 mg)
1/100 grain	0.06 mg
1/120 grain	0.5 mg
1/150 grain	0.4 mg

The following lists some approximate solid equivalents among the avoirdupois, apothecaries', and metric systems.

AVOIRDUPOIS	APOTHECARIES'	METRIC
1 gr	1 gr	0.065 g
15.4 gr	15.4 gr	1 g
1 ounce	480 gr	28.35 g
437.5 gr	1 ounce	31 g
1 lb	1.33 lb	454 g
0.75 lb	1 lb	373 g
2.2 lb	2.7 lb	1 kg

want to convert milligrams to grains, the second fraction appears as:

$$\frac{60 \text{ mg}}{1 \text{ gr}}$$

since 60 mg equals 1 gr. Remember, the same unit of measure appears in the numerator of both fractions. Likewise, the same unit of measure appears in both denominators. The entire equation should appear as follows:

$$\frac{300 \text{ mg}}{X \text{ gr}} = \frac{60 \text{ mg}}{1 \text{ gr}}$$

To solve for X, cross multiply:

$$300 \text{ mg} \times 1 \text{ gr} = 60 \text{ mg} \times X \text{ gr}$$
$$300 = 60 X$$
$$\frac{300}{60} = \frac{60 X}{60}$$
$$5 \text{ gr} = X$$

The patient should receive 5 gr (gr v) of aspirin, which in this case equals 1 tablet.

The ratio method for conversions

When using the ratio method to make conversions, first express the ordered dosage and available dosage as a ratio. For example, a physician's order calls for ASA (aspirin) gr x, but the aspirin is available in tablets measured in milligrams. As a result, the first ratio appears as 10 gr : X mg. The X represents the unknown dosage of milligrams. The second ratio represents the standard equivalents between the ordered and available measures. Since 60 mg equals 1 gr, the second ratio appears as 1 gr : 60 mg. Note that the same unit of measure (gr) appears in the first half of each ratio, and the same unit (mg) appears in the second half. The equation should appear as:

$$10 \text{ gr} : X \text{ mg} :: 1 \text{ gr} : 60 \text{ mg}$$

To solve for X, multiply the means of the ratio and the extremes (the outer portions of the ratio and the inner portions):

$$X \text{ mg} \times 1 \text{ gr} = 10 \text{ gr} \times 60 \text{ mg}$$
$$X = 600 \text{ mg}$$

Ten grains equals 600 milligrams.

One-liter containers

The calibrated glass bottle and plastic bag shown here are typically used to hold intravenous solutions.

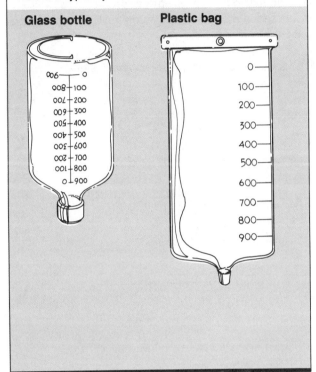

Glass bottle   **Plastic bag**

Medication cup

Notice that the medication cup is calibrated in measures from the metric, apothecaries', and household systems.

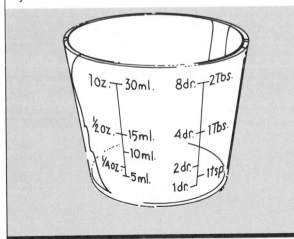

Practice conversions with answers

1. The physician orders 15 grains of a drug. The drug label states that the tablets are measured in milligrams. Fifteen grains equals how many milligrams?

2. The physician orders 2 ml of a drug. The drug is available in minims. Two ml equals how many minims?

3. One-half ounce of a drug is ordered. The drug is dispensed in milliliters. How many milliliters should the patient receive?

The answers to the practice conversions are:

1.

$$\frac{15 \text{ gr}}{X \text{ mg}} = \frac{1 \text{ gr}}{60 \text{ mg}}$$

$$15 \text{ gr} \times 60 \text{ mg} = X \text{ mg} \times 1 \text{ gr}$$

$$900 \text{ mg} = X$$

Fifteen grains equals 900 milligrams.

2.

$$2 \text{ ml} : X \text{ M}_x :: 1 \text{ ml} : 15 \text{ M}_x$$

$$X \text{ M}_x \times 1 \text{ ml} = 2 \text{ ml} \times 15 \text{ M}_x$$

$$X = 30 \text{ M}_x$$

Two milliliters equals 30 minims.

3.

$$\frac{0.5 \text{ oz}}{X \text{ ml}} = \frac{1 \text{ oz}}{30 \text{ ml}}$$

$$0.5 \text{ oz} \times 30 \text{ ml} = X \text{ ml} \times 1 \text{ oz}$$

$$15 \text{ ml} = X$$

Fifteen milliliters equals ½ oz. Therefore, the patient should receive 15 milliliters.

COMPUTATION OF DRUG DOSAGES

Determining the drug dosage to be administered occurs after verification of the physician's order. Computing drug dosages is a two-step process. During the first step, ascertain if the drug ordered is available in units within the same system of measurement. If the ordered drug is available only in another system of measurement, perform the conversion between the two systems. Use the fraction method or the ratio method explained in the previous section. If the physician orders the drug in units that are available, proceed directly to the next step.

If the ordered units of measurement are available, calculate the quantity of a particular dosage form to be administered. For example, if the dose to be given calls for 250 mg, determine the quantity of tablets, powder, or liquid equal to 250 mg. To determine the quantity, use either the fraction or ratio method, similar to the methods used for converting units of measure. Explanations of the fraction and ratio methods follow.

The fraction method

When using the fraction method to compute drug dosage, write an equation consisting of two fractions. First, set up a fraction showing the number of units to be given over X, which represents the quantity of the dosage form, or the number of tablets or milliliters. On the other side of the equation, form a fraction showing the number of units of drug in its dosage form over the quantity of dosage forms that contain the measure stated in the numerator. (Information provided on the drug label should supply the details needed to form the second fraction. The number of units and the quantity of dosage form are specific for each drug. In most cases the stated quantity equals 1 ml or 1 tablet.) An example of the fraction method for computation follows: If the number of units to be administered equals 250 mg, then the first fraction in the equation is:

$$\frac{250 \text{ mg}}{X \text{ tab}}$$

The drug label states that each tablet contains 125 mg. The second fraction is:

$$\frac{125 \text{ mg}}{1 \text{ tab}}$$

The same units of measure must appear in the numerator of each fraction. Likewise, each denominator should show the same units of measure. The units of measure in the denominators will differ from the units in the numerators. The entire equation should appear as:

$$\frac{250 \text{ mg}}{X \text{ tab}} = \frac{125 \text{ mg}}{1 \text{ tab}}$$

Solving for X determines the quantity of the dosage form (number of tablets, in this example) to give to the patient.

The ratio method

First, write the amount of the drug to be given and the quantity of the dosage (X) as a ratio. Using the example shown for the fraction method, in which the drug ordered equaled 250 mg, write the ratio as 250 mg : X tab. Next, complete the equation by forming a second ratio consisting of the number of units of the drug in the dosage form and the stated quantity of the dosage form. (Remember, the manufacturer's label provides information for the second ratio.) If, for example, each tablet contained 125 mg, write the second ratio as 125 mg : 1 tab. The entire equation is:

$$250 \text{ mg} : X \text{ tab} :: 125 \text{ mg} : 1 \text{ tab}$$

Solving for X determines the quantity of the dosage form.

The following example uses the ratio method for conversion between systems of measurement, then uses the fraction method to compute drug dosage. A physician orders 15 mg of phenobarbital for a patient. The drug is available in scored tablets containing gr ss (½ grain). How many tablets should the patient be given?

First, convert the milligrams of the metric system into grains of the apothecaries' system. The standard conversion is: 60 mg = 1 gr. Using the ratio method, the equation is:

$$15 \text{ mg} : X \text{ gr} :: 60 \text{ mg} : 1 \text{ gr}$$

To solve for X, multiply the means and the extremes:

$$X \text{ gr} \times 60 \text{ mg} = 15 \text{ mg} \times 1 \text{ gr}$$
$$60 X = 15$$
$$X = \frac{15}{60}$$
$$X = \frac{1}{4} = 0.25 \text{ gr}$$

Next, determine the drug dosage, in this case the number of tablets to administer. The drug label states that each tablet contains ss or ½ (0.5) grain of phenobarbital. The patient is to receive ¼ (0.25) grain. Using the fraction method, the equation is:

$$\frac{0.25 \text{ gr}}{X \text{ tab}} = \frac{0.5 \text{ gr}}{1 \text{ tab}}$$

To solve for X, cross multiply:

$$0.25 \text{ gr} \times 1 \text{ tab} = 0.5 \text{ gr} \times X \text{ tab}$$
$$0.25 = 0.5 X$$
$$\frac{0.25}{0.5} = X$$
$$0.5 \ (½) = X$$

The patient should receive ½ tablet of phenobarbital.

The "desired-available" method

The "desired (ordered)-available" method, also known as the dose over on-hand method (D/H), represents a third way to compute drug dosages. The desired-available method combines the conversion of ordered units into available units and the computation of drug dosage into one step. The equation for doing this is:

$$\begin{array}{c} \text{ordered} \\ \text{units} \end{array} \times \begin{array}{c} \text{conversion} \\ \text{fraction} \end{array} \times \frac{\begin{array}{c} \text{quantity of} \\ \text{dosage form} \end{array}}{\begin{array}{c} \text{stated quantity} \\ \text{of drug within} \\ \text{each dosage} \\ \text{form} \end{array}} = \begin{array}{c} \text{X quantity} \\ \text{to give} \end{array}$$

The following situation shows how the equation works. A physician orders 10 grains of a drug. The drug, however, is available only in 300-mg tablets. To determine the drug dosage, or the number of tablets to give to the patient, substitute 10 gr (the ordered number of units) for the first element of the equation. Then use the conversion fraction

$$\frac{60 \text{ mg}}{1 \text{ gr}}$$

as the second portion of the formula. The measure in the denominator of the conversion fraction must be the same as the measure in the ordered units. In this instance, the physician ordered 10 grains. As a result, grains appear in the denominator of the conversion fraction.

The third element of the equation shows the dosage form over the stated drug quantity within each dosage form. Since the drug is available in 300-mg tablets, the equation is:

$$\frac{1 \text{ tab}}{300 \text{ mg}}$$

The dosage form, in this case tablets, should always appear in the numerator, while the quantity of drug in each dosage form should always appear in the denominator. The completed equation is:

$$10 \text{ gr} \times \frac{60 \text{ mg}}{1 \text{ gr}} \times \frac{1 \text{ tab}}{300 \text{ mg}} = X \text{ tab}$$

Solving for X shows that the patient should receive 2 tablets.

The desired-available method has the advantage of requiring only one equation. The method, however, requires memorizing an equation more elaborate than the one used in the fraction or ratio methods. Having to memorize a more complicated equation may increase the chance of error. (See *Using the desired-available method* for another example of calculating a dosage.)

Using the desired-available method

A physician orders 15 mg of phenobarbital. The drug is available only in tablets containing gr ss. Determine the drug dosage by solving for *X* as follows:

The ordered units would be 15 mg.

The conversion fraction is: $\dfrac{1\text{ gr}}{60\text{ mg}}$

$\dfrac{\text{The dosage form}}{\text{stated quantity}}$ is $\dfrac{1\text{ tab}}{0.5\text{ gr}}$

Use the information in the equation:

$$15\text{ mg} \times \frac{1\text{ gr}}{60\text{ mg}} \times \frac{1\text{ tab}}{0.5\text{ gr}} = X\text{ tab}$$

Solve for *X*:

$$15 \times \frac{1}{60} \times \frac{1}{0.5} = X$$

$$\frac{15}{60 \times 0.5} = X$$

$$\frac{15}{30} = X$$

$$0.5\text{ tab} = X$$

The patient should receive ½ tablet of phenobarbital.

---

from the units in which the dosage form will be administered. For example, if a patient is to receive 1,000 milligrams of a drug available in liquid form and measured in milligrams, with 100 milligrams contained in 6 milliliters, how many milliliters would the patient receive? Since both the ordered and the available doses occur in milligrams, no initial conversion calculations need be made. Simply use the ratio or fraction method to determine the number of milliliters of drug the patient should receive. The ratio method would be: 1,000 mg : X ml :: 100 mg : 6 ml. Solving for *X* determines that 60 milliliters of the drug should be given.

Next, because the drug is to be administered in ounce form, determine the number of ounces needed, using a method of conversion. For the fraction method for conversion, the equation is:

$$\frac{60\text{ ml}}{X\text{ oz}} = \frac{30\text{ ml}}{1\text{ oz}}$$

Solving for *X* indicates that the patient should receive 2 ounces of the drug.

To use the desired-available method, simply change the order of the elements in the equation to correspond with the situation. The revised equation is:

$$\text{ordered units} \times \frac{\text{quantity of dosage form}}{\text{stated quantity of drug within each dosage form}} \times \text{conversion fraction} = X\text{ quantity to give}$$

Placing the given information into the equation results in:

$$1,000\text{ mg} \times \frac{6\text{ ml}}{100\text{ mg}} \times \frac{1\text{ oz}}{30\text{ ml}} = X$$

Solving for *X* indicates that the patient should receive 2 ounces of the drug.

SPECIAL COMPUTATIONS

The fraction, ratio, and desired-available methods can each be used to compute drug dosage when the ordered drug and available form of the drug occur in the same units of measure. The three methods can also be used when the quantity of the particular dosage form differs

Computing drug dosages in special systems

Any of the three methods for drug dosage calculation may be used to calculate dosages of drugs measured in special systems. For example, a physician orders 3,000,000 U of penicillin for a patient. The penicillin is available in liquid form for intramuscular use, with 5,000,000 U per milliliter; however, the dosage is to be administered in minims. When determining the number of minims to administer, first write the dosages as 5 m.U and 3 m.U instead of 5,000,000 and 3,000,000 units. The shorter notation eliminates the need for all the zeros in each dosage and makes the computation appear more manageable. The shorter notation also reduces the chance of error in miscopying the number of zeros during the calculation.

Using the fraction method, set up the initial equation as:

$$\frac{3 \text{ m.U}}{X \text{ ml}} = \frac{5 \text{ m.U}}{1 \text{ ml}}$$

Solving for X indicates that the patient should receive 0.6 milliliters of penicillin.

Using the ratio method to determine the number of minims to administer, set up the equation as:

$$0.6 \text{ ml} : X \text{ M}_x :: 1 \text{ ml} : 15 \text{ M}_x$$

Solving for X determines that the patient should receive 9 minims of the penicillin.

Using the desired-available method, the equation is:

$$3 \text{ m.U} \times \frac{1 \text{ ml}}{5 \text{ m.U}} \times \frac{15 \text{ M}_x}{1 \text{ ml}} = 2 \text{ M}_x$$

Solving the equation results in the same number of minims (9).

(See *Computing dosages of heparin* for a problem using the fraction method to calculate the dosage of a drug measured in a special system.)

Inexact nature of conversions and computations

Converting drug measures from one system to another and then determining the amount of a dosage form to give can easily produce inexact dosages. A rounding error during computation or discrepancies in the dosage to give may occur, depending upon the conversion standard used in calculation. The nurse may determine a precise drug amount to be given, only to find that administering the amount is impossible. The nurse may determine, for example, that a patient should receive 0.97 tablet. Administering such an amount is impossible. The following general rule helps avoid calculation errors and discrepancies between theoretical and real dosages: *No more than 10% variation should exist between the dosage ordered and the dose to be given.* Following the rule, a nurse who determined that 0.97 tablet should be given could permissibly give 1 tablet.

The nurse often encounters such discrepancies when administering aspirin and acetaminophen (Tylenol). Physicians usually order aspirin and acetamino-

---

Computing dosages of heparin

A physician orders 5,000 U of heparin S.C. for a patient. On hand is heparin 10,000 U/ml. How many milliliters should the patient receive?

Using the fraction method, the equation is:

$$\frac{10,000 \text{ U}}{1 \text{ ml}} = \frac{5,000 \text{ U}}{X \text{ ml}}$$

After cross multiplying, the equation becomes:

$$10,000 \text{ X} = 5,000$$

Solving for X provides the answer:

$$X = \frac{5,000}{10,000} = 0.5 \text{ ml}$$

The patient should receive 0.5 or ½ ml of heparin.

---

phen in grains (gr x being the usual adult dose); however, both drugs are usually available in 325-mg tablets. Converting gr x to milligrams indicates that 600 mg should be given, but two tablets would equal 650 mg, not 600 mg. To apply the rule concerning such discrepancies, first calculate 10% of 600 mg, which equals 60 mg. Adding 60 mg to 600 mg indicates that giving up to 660 mg is permissible. Since two tablets equals only 650 mg, the dosage would be safe to administer.

Practice computations with answers

1. The physician orders 30 mg of a drug available in tablets, each of which contains 1 grain. How many tablets should the patient receive?
2. The physician orders 200 mg of a drug available in an elixir that contains 100 mg/30 ml. How many ounces of the drug should be given?
3. The physician orders 5,000 units of a drug for a patient. The drug is available in a solution that contains 10,000 units per ml. How many minims should the patient receive?
The answers to the practice computations are:

1. Using the ratio method
$$30 \text{ mg} : X \text{ gr} :: 60 \text{ mg} : 1 \text{ gr}$$
$$X \text{ gr} \times 60 \text{ mg} = 30 \text{ mg} \times 1 \text{ gr}$$
$$X = \frac{30}{60}$$
$$X = 0.5 \text{ gr}$$

Thirty milligrams equals 0.5 grains.

$$0.5 \text{ gr} : X \text{ tab} :: 1 \text{ gr} : 1 \text{ tab}$$
$$X \text{ tab} \times 1 \text{ gr} = 0.5 \text{ gr} \times 1 \text{ tab}$$
$$X = 0.5 \text{ tab}$$

The patient should receive ½ tablet.

2. Using the desired-available method

$$200 \text{ mg} \times \frac{30 \text{ ml}}{100 \text{ mg}} \times \frac{1 \text{ oz}}{30 \text{ ml}} = X \text{ oz}$$

$$200 \times \frac{30}{100} \times \frac{1}{30} = X$$

$$\frac{2}{1} = X$$

$$2 \text{ oz} = X$$

Two ounces of the drug should be given.

3. Using the fraction method

$$\frac{5,000 \text{ U}}{X \text{ ml}} = \frac{10,000 \text{ U}}{1 \text{ ml}}$$

$$5,000 \text{ U} \times 1 \text{ ml} = X \text{ ml} \times 10,000 \text{ U}$$

$$\frac{5,000}{10,000} = X$$

$$0.5 \text{ ml} = X$$

One-half of 1 milliliter contains 5,000 U.

$$\frac{0.5 \text{ ml}}{X \text{ M}_X} = \frac{1 \text{ ml}}{15 \text{ (or 16)} \text{ M}_X}$$

$$0.5 \text{ ml} \times 15 \text{ (or 16)} \text{ M}_X = X \text{ M}_X \times 1 \text{ ml}$$

$$7.5 \text{ or } 8 \text{ M}_X = X$$

The patient should receive 7.5 or 8 minims.

COMPUTATION OF DRUGS FOR PARENTERAL ADMINISTRATION

The methods for computing drug dosages can be used for oral or parenteral routes. The following example shows how to determine drug dosages to be given via the parenteral route.

The physician orders 75 mg of Demerol. The package label reads: meperidine (Demerol), 100 mg/ml. Using the fraction method to determine the number of milliliters the patient should receive, the equation is:

$$\frac{75 \text{ mg}}{X \text{ ml}} = \frac{100 \text{ mg}}{1 \text{ ml}}$$

To solve for X, cross multiply:

$$75 \text{ mg} \times 1 \text{ ml} = X \text{ ml} \times 100 \text{ mg}$$

$$75 = 100 \text{ X}$$

$$\frac{75}{100} = X$$

$$0.75 \text{ or } \frac{3}{4} \text{ ml} = X$$

The patient should receive 0.75 or ¾ ml.

A nurse might need to know the number of minims that would deliver the same dosage. The equation for the ratio method is:

$$0.75 \text{ ml} : X \text{ M}_X :: 1 \text{ ml} : 15 \text{ M}_X$$

To solve for X, multiply the means and the extremes:

$$X \text{ M}_X \times 1 \text{ ml} = 0.75 \text{ ml} \times 15 \text{ M}_X$$

$$X = 12 \text{ M}_X$$

Twelve minims equals 0.75 ml, which would contain the 75 mg of Demerol ordered by the physician.

RECONSTITUTION OF POWDERS FOR INJECTION

Although the pharmacist usually reconstitutes powders for parenteral use, nurses sometimes perform the function. The nurse also often computes intravenous fluid rates. The following discussion addresses both the reconstitution of powders for injection and the computation of intravenous drip rates.

When reconstituting powders for injection, consult the drug label for the needed information. The label gives the total quantity of drug in the vial or ampule, the amount and type of diluent to add to the powder, and the strength and shelf life (expiration date) of the resulting solution. When diluent is added to a powder, the powder increases the fluid volume. For this reason, the label calls for less diluent than the total volume of the prepared solution. For example, a nurse may have to add 1.7 ml of diluent to a vial of powdered drug to obtain a 2-ml total volume of prepared solution. Reconstituting a powdered drug simply requires following the directions on the drug label.

To determine the amount of solution to administer, use the manufacturer's information about the concentration of the solution. For example, if the nurse wants to administer 500 mg of a drug, and the concentration of the prepared solution is 1 g (1,000 mg) per 10 ml, the nurse can set up a fraction or ratio equation as follows:

Fraction method

$$\frac{500 \text{ mg}}{X \text{ ml}} = \frac{100 \text{ mg}}{10 \text{ ml}}$$

Ratio Method

500 mg : X ml :: 100 mg : 10 ml

(*See Reconstitution of a powder* for another example of how a nurse might perform the required computations.)

Reconstitution of a powder

The physician orders 500 mg of ampicillin for a patient. A 1-g vial of powdered ampicillin is available. The label states, "Add 4.5 ml sterile water to yield 1 g/5 ml." How many milliliters of reconstituted ampicillin should the patient be given?

The nurse first dilutes the powder according to the instructions on the label. The concentration listed on the label provides the first portion of the equation:

$$\frac{1 \text{ g}}{5 \text{ ml}}$$

The nurse then needs to assure that the same units of measure appear in both numerators of the equation. In this case, the units must both be grams or milligrams; either choice is acceptable. If the nurse chooses to use milligrams and chooses the fraction method, the equation would be:

$$\frac{1{,}000 \text{ mg}}{5 \text{ ml}} = \frac{500 \text{ mg}}{X \text{ ml}}$$

The nurse then cross multiplies:

$$1{,}000 \text{ X} = 2{,}500$$

Then, to solve for *X*, the nurse divides:

$$X = \frac{2{,}500}{1{,}000}$$

$$X = 2.5 \text{ ml}$$

After computation, the nurse finds that 2.5 ml of reconsitituted ampicillin provides 500 mg.

Intravenous drip rates and flow rates

For these special computations, first set up a fraction showing the volume of solution to be delivered over the number of minutes in which that volume is to be infused.

For example, if a patient is to receive 100 milliliters of solution within 1 hour, the fraction would be written as

$$\frac{100 \text{ ml}}{60 \text{ min}}$$

Next, multiply the fraction by the drip factor (the number of drops contained in 1 ml) to determine the number of drops per minute to be infused. The drip factor varies among different intravenous sets and appears on the package containing the intravenous tubing administration set. Following the manufacturer's directions for drip factor is an extremely important step. (*See Intravenous flow rates* on page 152 for a discussion of the drip factors of several well-known intravenous administration sets.) Standard administration sets have drip factors of either 10 or 20 drops per milliliter. A microdrip (minidrip) set has a drip factor of 60 drops per milliliter.

Use the following equation to determine the drip rate of an intravenous solution:

$$\frac{\text{total no. of ml}}{\text{total no. of min}} \times \text{drip factor} = \frac{\text{drops per}}{\text{minute}}$$

Calculating intravenous drip rate

The physician's order states: 1,000 ml 5% dextrose in 0.45% sodium chloride to infuse over 12 hours. The administration set delivers 15 drops per milliliter. What should the drip rate be?

Use the equation:

$$\frac{\text{Total no. of ml}}{\text{Total no. of min}} \times \text{drip factor} = \text{drip rate}$$

Set up the equation using the given data:

$$\frac{1{,}000 \text{ ml}}{12 \text{ hrs} \times 60 \text{ min}} \times 15 \text{ gtt/ml} = \text{X gtt/min}$$

After multiplying the number of hours by 60 minutes in the denominator of the fraction, the equation is:

$$\frac{1{,}000 \text{ ml}}{720 \text{ min}} \times 15 \text{ gtt/ml} = \text{X gtt/min}$$

After dividing the fraction, the equation is:

$$1.39 \text{ ml/min} \times 15 \text{ gtt/ml} = \text{X gtt/min}$$

The final answer is 20.85 gtt/min, which can be rounded to 21 gtt/min. The drip rate is 21 drops per minute.

Intravenous flow rates

When calculating the flow rate of I.V. solutions, remember that the number of drops required to deliver 1 ml varies with the type of administration set used and the manufacturer. The illustration at left shows a standard (macrodrip) set, which delivers from 10 to 20 drops/ml. The illustration at right shows a pediatric (microdrip) set, which delivers about 60 drops/ml.

To calculate the flow rate, you must know the calibration of the drip rate for each manufacturer's product. As a quick guide, refer to the chart below.

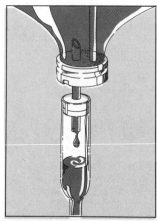
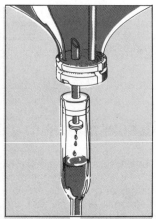

CO. NAME	DROPS/ML	DROPS/MINUTE TO INFUSE					
		500 ml/ 24 hr	1,000 ml/ 24 hr	1,000 ml/ 20 hr	1,000 ml/ 10 hr	1,000 ml/ 8 hr	1,000 ml/ 6 hr
		21 ml/hr	42 ml/hr	50 ml/hr	100 ml/hr	125 ml/hr	166 ml/hr
Abbott	15	5 gtt	10 gtt	12 gtt	25 gtt	31 gtt	42 gtt
Baxter-Travenol	10	3 gtt	7 gtt	8 gtt	17 gtt	21 gtt	28 gtt
Cutter	20	7 gtt	14 gtt	17 gtt	34 gtt	42 gtt·	56 gtt
IVAC	20	7 gtt	14 gtt	17 gtt	34 gtt	42 gtt	56 gtt
McGaw	15	5 gtt	10 gtt	12 gtt	25 gtt	31 gtt	42 gtt

The equation applies to intravenous solutions that infuse over many hours or to small-volume infusions such as those used for antibiotic administration, which are administered in less than 1 hour. (See *Calculating intravenous drip rate* on page 151 to see how the equation works in a specific situation.)

The nurse can modify the equation by first determining the number of milliliters to be infused over 1 hour (the flow rate). The nurse then divides the flow rate by 60 minutes. The resulting calculation is then multiplied by the drip factor to determine the number of drops per minute. The nurse will also use the flow rate when working with intravenous infusion pumps to set the number of milliliters to be delivered in 1 hour.

Quick methods for calculating drip rates

Besides the equation and its modified version, quicker methods exist for computing intravenous solution administration rates. To administer intravenous solutions via a microdrip set, adjust the flow rate (number of milliliters per hour) to equal the drip rate (number of drops per minute). Using the equation, divide the flow rate by 60 minutes and then multiply by the drip factor, which also equals 60. Because the flow rate and drip factor are equal, the two arithmetic operations "cancel out" each other. For example, if 125 ml of fluid per hour represented the ordered flow rate, the equation would be:

$$\frac{125 \text{ ml}}{60 \text{ min}} \times 60 = \text{drip rate (125)}$$

Rather than spend the time calculating the equation, the nurse can simply use the number assigned to the flow rate as the drip rate.

For intravenous solution administration sets that deliver 15 drops per milliliter, the flow rate divided by 4 equals the drip rate. For sets with a drip factor of 10, the flow rate divided by 6 equals the drip rate.

Practice computations with answers

1. The patient is to receive 2 g of a drug available in powdered form. The drug label states: *Contains 3 g. Add 17 ml of sterile water to yield 1 g per 6 ml.* How many milliliters of solution should the patient receive?

2. The patient is to receive 3 liters of intravenous solution over 24 hours. The drip factor for the intravenous infusion set is 15 gtt (drops) per ml. How many milliliters should be infused each hour? What is the drip rate for the solution?

3. The physician orders 50 ml of a drug to be infused over 25 minutes. The intravenous infusion set has a drip factor of 10 gtt per ml. What is the drip rate for the solution?

The answers to the practice problems follow:

1.
$$2 \text{ g} : X \text{ ml} :: 1 \text{ g} : 6 \text{ ml}$$
$$X \text{ ml} \times 1 \text{ g} = 2 \text{ g} \times 6 \text{ ml}$$
$$X = 12 \text{ ml}$$

The patient should receive 12 milliliters of solution.

2.
$$\frac{3{,}000 \text{ ml}}{24 \text{ hr.}} = \frac{X \text{ ml}}{1 \text{ hr}}$$
$$3{,}000 \text{ ml} \times 1 \text{ hr} = 24 \text{ hr} \times X \text{ ml}$$
$$\frac{3{,}000}{24} = X$$
$$125 \text{ ml} = X$$

The flow rate equals 125 ml per hour.

$$\frac{125 \text{ ml}}{60 \text{ min}} \times 15 \text{ gtt per ml} = X \text{ gtt per min}$$
$$\frac{125}{60} \times 15 = X$$
$$31.25 = 31 \text{ gtt per min} = X$$

As an alternative, divide the flow rate by 4 (the quick method for sets with a drip factor of 15):

$$\frac{125}{4} = 31.25 = 31 \text{ gtt per min (drip rate)}$$

The drip rate equals 31 drops per minute.

3.
$$\frac{50 \text{ ml}}{25 \text{ min}} \times 10 \text{ gtt per ml} = X \text{ gtt per min}$$
$$\frac{50}{25} \times 10 = X$$
$$2 \times 10 = X$$
$$20 \text{ gtt per min} = X$$

The drip rate equals 20 drops per minute.

PERCENTAGE SOLUTIONS

In most clinical settings, either the pharmacy department or pharmaceutical companies prepare solutions containing drugs for topical use (for example, wound irrigation and the soaking of infected or inflamed body parts). Nurses, however, must prepare special percentage solutions for emergencies, such as resuscitation attempts after cardiac arrest. Furthermore, community health nurses working in home settings may need to prepare large-volume solutions if prepared solutions are not accessible to the patient.

Calculation of percentage solutions

An example of a percentage solution is 0.9% saline, which indicates that every 100 milliliters of solution contains 0.9 grams of sodium chloride. Expressed as a fraction, the figures would appear as

$$\frac{0.9}{100}$$

The ratio form would appear as 0.9 : 100. A liter of 0.9% saline would contain 9 grams of sodium chloride. The figures for 1 liter would be

$$\frac{9}{1{,}000}$$

in fraction form, and 9 : 1,000 in ratio form.

The nurse may prepare percentage solutions by adding solutes (solid or liquid forms of drugs) to solvents (diluents). The solvents usually used include sterile water, normal saline solution, and 5% dextrose in water. As a general rule when preparing solutions, the nurse should consider the solid form, whether crystals, powders, or tablets, to be 100% strength. The liquid form, also known as the stock solution, may vary in strength.

The nurse may use the following formulas to calculate the strength of percentage solutions. The fraction method offers two usable formulas:

$$\frac{\text{weaker solution}}{\text{stronger solution}} = \frac{\text{solute}}{\text{solvent}}$$

$$\frac{\text{small \% strength}}{\text{large \% strength}} = \frac{\text{small volume}}{\text{large volume}}$$

The ratio method also offers two formulas:

$$\text{weaker : stronger :: solute : solvent}$$

$$\text{small \% strength : large \% strength :: small volume : large volume}$$

Although a solid combined with a diluent will increase the total volume of the prepared solution, the increase is usually insignificant and may not need to be calculated. The increase, however, will prove significant and should be considered when adding either a large amount of solid or a small amount of diluent. When adding a liquid, subtract the amount of the liquid from the total volume desired. The calculation tells the amount of diluent to add. For example, if the preparation of 1 liter of solution requires 50 ml of a liquid drug, add the 50 ml of liquid drug to 950 ml of diluent.

As an example, the nurse must prepare 500 ml of a 0.5% lidocaine (Xylocaine) solution and finds on hand a 2% Xylocaine solution and 5% dextrose in water, which is the diluent. The nurse must determine the number of milliliters of Xylocaine solution to use, and the number of milliliters of dextrose solution to use.

Using the ratio method, the nurse sets up the following equation:

$$0.5\% : 2\% :: X \text{ ml} : 500 \text{ ml}$$

Multiplying the means and the extremes gives $2X = 250$. The nurse then divides to solve for X:

$$X = \frac{250}{2}$$
$$X = 125 \text{ ml of 2\% xylocaine solution}$$

Since the nurse wants a total volume of 500 ml and must use 125 ml of Xylocaine solution, the nurse must next determine the amount of dextrose solution to use as the diluent. Subtracting 125 from 500 yields the amount of dextrose solution to use:

$$500 \text{ ml} - 125 \text{ ml} = 375 \text{ ml of dextrose solution}$$

Practice computations with answers

1. An irrigation treatment scheduled for a patient requires the use of 500 milliliters of a 5% solution. The drug is available in solid form. How many grams of the drug are needed to prepare the solution for one treatment?
2. A nurse needs to prepare a liter of 4% solution. On hand is a 20% stock solution. How much of the stock solution should the nurse use? How many milliliters of water should the nurse add to the portion of the stock solution to obtain 1 liter of 4% solution?

3. A nurse is preparing 4 liters of 2% solution. The stock solution is 100% strength. How many milliliters of the stock solution does the nurse need? How many milliliters of water will the nurse add to prepare 4 liters of the desired solution?

The answers to the practice computations follow:

1.
$$5\% : 100\% \quad :: X \text{ g} : 500 \text{ ml}$$
$$100 X = 5 \times 500$$
$$100 X = 2,500$$
$$X = 25 \text{ g}$$

The nurse needs 25 grams of the drug to prepare enough solution for one treatment.

2.
$$\frac{4\%}{20\%} = \frac{X \text{ ml}}{1,000 \text{ ml}}$$
$$4 \times 1,000 = 20 \times X$$
$$4,000 = 20X$$
$$\frac{4,000}{20} = X$$
$$200 \text{ ml} = X$$

The nurse should use 200 milliliters of stock solution.
$$1,000 - 200 = X \text{ ml}$$
$$800 \text{ ml} = X$$

The nurse should add 800 milliliters of water to the stock solution.

3.
$$2\% : 100\% :: X \text{ ml} : 4,000 \text{ ml}$$
$$100 X = 2 \times 4,000$$
$$X = \frac{8,000}{100}$$
$$X = 80 \text{ ml}$$

The nurse needs 80 milliliters of stock solution.
$$4,000 \text{ ml} - 80 \text{ ml} = X \text{ ml}$$
$$3,920 \text{ ml} = X$$

The nurse will add 3,920 milliliters of water to the 80 milliliters of stock solution.

COMPUTATION FOR PEDIATRIC DOSES

Special rules for calculating drug dosages for children have been developed. One frequently used method involves the child's weight in kilograms; a second recommended method involves the child's body-surface area. Other methods of dosage calculations are not recommended.

Physicians and nurses use pediatric rules primarily to determine the safe pediatric dosage range when the safe adult range is known. The nurse should determine the safe dosage range to verify that the physician's order is appropriate for a particular child. The nurse's professional and legal responsibility requires such dosage verification in the administration of drugs.

Dosage range per kilogram of body weight

Currently, many pharmaceutical companies provide information on the safe dosage ranges for drugs given to children. The companies usually provide the dosage ranges in milligrams per kilogram of body weight, and, in many cases, give similar information for adult dosage ranges. The following example and explanation indicates how to calculate the safe pediatric dosage range for a drug, using the company's suggested safe dosage range provided in milligrams per kilograms.

A physician orders for a pediatric patient a drug with a suggested dosage range of 10 to 12 mg per kilogram of body weight per day. The child weighs 12 kg. What is the safe daily dosage range for the child?

The nurse must calculate both the lower and upper limits of the dosage range provided by the manufacturer. The nurse first calculates the dose based on 10 mg per kilogram of body weight, then calculates the dose based on 12 mg per kilogram of body weight. The answers represent the lower and upper limits of the daily dosage range, expressed in milligrams per kilogram of the child's weight. (See *Calculating pediatric dosages* for a depiction of a similar problem and its solution.)

Body-surface area

A second method for calculating safe pediatric doses uses the child's body-surface area as a factor. This method may provide a more accurate calculation because the child's body-surface area is thought to be closely related to the child's metabolic rate. The nurse determines the body-surface area of a child by using a three-columned chart called a nomogram. (See Chapter 12, Intervention: The Pediatric Patient, for details on how to use a nomogram.) The nurse marks the child's height in the first column and the child's weight in the third column, then draws a line between the two marks. The point at which the line intersects the vertical scale in the second column indicates the estimated body-surface area of the child in square meters. To calculate the child's approximate dose, the nurse uses the body-surface area measurement in the following equation:

$$\frac{\text{body-surface area of child}}{\text{average adult body-surface area (1.73 m}^2)} \times \frac{\text{average}}{\text{adult}} \text{dose} = \text{child's dose}$$

The following example illustrates the use of the equation. Using a nomogram, a nurse finds that a 25-pound child 33 inches tall has a body-surface area of 0.52 square meters. The nurse needs to determine the

---

Calculating pediatric dosages

The physician orders 150 mg of a drug to be given q6h to an 18-kg child. (Remember that 1 kg equals 2.2 lb). The literature provided by the manufacturer indicates that the safe dosage range for the drug is 30 mg/kg to 35 mg/kg per day, to be given in divided doses. Can the nurse safely administer the ordered dose?

Using the ratio method to determine the lower limit of the safe dosage range, the nurse sets up the following:

30 mg : X mg :: 1 kg : 18 kg

After cross multiplying the means and the extremes, the nurse finds that X = 540 mg; the 540 mg represents the low dose.

Using the same method, the nurse then calculates the upper limit of the safe dosage range:

35 mg : X mg :: 1 kg : 18 kg

After cross multiplying the means and the extremes, the nurse finds that X = 630 mg, the high dose.

The safe dosage range for the child is 540 to 630 mg per day. Since the physician ordered 150 mg to be given every 6 hours, the child would receive four doses per day, or a total daily dosage of 150 mg x four doses per day = 600 mg per day. This daily dosage falls within the safe range, so the nurse can safely administer 150 mg q6h.

---

child's dose of a drug with an average adult dose of 100 mg. The equation would appear as:

$$\frac{0.52 \text{ m}^2}{1.73 \text{ m}^2} \times 100 \text{ mg} = 30.06 \text{ mg (child's dose)}$$

The child should receive 30 mg of the drug.

Other rules

Because drug companies provide dosage ranges, nurses calculate pediatric dosages primarily to check and verify them. The importance of verifying dosages necessitates the nurse's understanding of the rules. Three other rules for calculating and verifying pediatric doses follow:
• Clark's rule (for children over age 2), based on *body weight* only:

$$\frac{\text{child's weight (lb)}}{150 \text{ lb (average adult weight)}} \times \frac{\text{average}}{\text{adult}} \text{dose} = \frac{\text{child's}}{\text{dose}}$$

● Fried's rule (for infants under age 1), based on child's *age* only:

$$\frac{\text{child's age (months)}}{\text{150 months (age at which an adult dose would be appropriate)}} \times \frac{\text{average adult dose}} = \frac{\text{child's dose}}$$

● Young's rule (for children age 2 to 12), based on child's *age* only:

$$\frac{\text{child's age (yrs)}}{\text{child's age (yrs)} + 12} \times \frac{\text{average adult dose}} = \frac{\text{child's dose}}$$

Clark's rule, Fried's rule, and Young's rule use an average adult dose as the standard from which to derive pediatric doses. The results are approximate. In practice, a safe adult dose of a particular drug usually falls within a range of doses, and depends on the individual. Therefore, the average adult dose used in the rules as a standard represents a somewhat imprecise number.

Each rule also depends on an average developmental level of the child. For example, Fried's rule and Young's rule rely solely on the child's age. Fried's rule considers a child of 150 months (12.5 years) to be an adult, whereas Young's rule uses 12 years as the measure. Both rules assume that the child's body systems and functions achieve a particular level of maturity consistent with the child's chronologic age. The assumption is somewhat unreliable because children at any age display a range of normal maturational levels. Furthermore, Fried's rule and Young's rule do not consider the child's weight and body size. The following example illustrates what can occur when using Fried's rule or Young's rule to calculate pediatric drug doses for a child of 15 months who does not fall within the age range for either of these rules.

A child of 15 months is to receive a drug usually given to adults in 100-milligram doses. If using Fried's rule, the nurse would calculate the following:

$$\frac{15 \text{ months}}{150 \text{ months}} \times 100 \text{ mg} = 10 \text{ mg (child's dose)}$$

With Young's rule, the calculations would be:

$$\frac{1.25 \text{ yrs.}}{1.25 \text{ yrs.} + 12 \text{ yrs.}} \times 100 \text{ mg} = 9.43 \text{ mg (child's dose)}$$

Using Fried's rule and Young's rule to calculate for the same situation results in a discrepancy of 0.57 mg.

Clark's rule considers the child's weight but not the child's age. By not considering the child's age, Clark's rule ignores individual differences in body system maturity. If the child of 15 months in the previous example weighed 27 pounds, calculating with Clark's rule would result in the following:

$$\frac{27 \text{ lb}}{150 \text{ lb}} \times 100 \text{ mg} = 18 \text{ mg (child's dose)}$$

Using Clark's rule results in a significantly larger dose than the doses calculated using Fried's rule or Young's rule. The child's dose could vary from 9.43 mg to 18 mg, almost twice the first amount. The discrepancies underscore that pediatric doses calculated using specific equations represent, at best, approximations. Therefore, calculating with equations other than those involving dosage ranges per kilogram of body weight or body-surface area should be done only to verify dosages, *not* to determine dosages.

Many institutions have adopted guidelines that determine the acceptable calculation method. Nurses in pediatric settings must familiarize themselves with the particular institution's policies regarding pediatric dosages. Chapter 12 addresses the special considerations necessary when administering drugs in pediatric settings.

Special considerations related to chemotherapy

Chemotherapeutic drugs used for malignant neoplasms also require special dosage calculations. Most chemotherapy is given in accordance with the patient's body-surface area. The body-surface area is estimated by plotting the patient's height and weight on a nomogram. Patients usually achieve the desired blood concentration level of chemotherapeutic drugs when the drugs are given in accordance with body-surface area. Therefore, accurate recording of a patient's height and weight is essential throughout the course of chemotherapy. The manufacturer provides information about the dosage specific for each chemotherapeutic drug. The dosage information, the height and weight data, and body-surface area help determine the dosage for any particular patient. Chapters 73 through 77 provide information regarding drugs used to treat malignant neoplasms.

Special considerations for geriatric patients

Geriatric patients may require drug dosages that differ from the usual adult dosages because of chronic illnesses. As a result, the physician determines doses for individual geriatric patients. No general rules exist. Because of the individual nature of the aging process and the unique medical history of each geriatric patient, nurses in gerontologic settings must consistently assess patients' responses to drugs. Although patients may receive average adult doses, such doses do not account for individual differences. Chapter 13 addresses the special considerations needed when working with geriatric patients.

Special needs related to weight

Physicians and nurses must also make special considerations when determining drug dosages for an adult patient whose weight varies significantly from the average adult weight of 150 pounds. For example, an 80-pound patient receiving an average adult dose may very likely experience toxic effects. Similarly, a 350-pound patient receiving an average adult dose will probably not experience the desired therapeutic response from the drug.

PRACTICE COMPUTATIONS WITH ANSWERS

1. A patient weighing 65 kilograms is to receive 15 milligrams per kilogram of body weight of a drug. How many milligrams of the drug should the patient receive?

2. A child weighs 44 pounds. The physician orders a drug to be administered in a dose of 30 milligrams per kilogram of body weight. How many milligrams of the drug should be given?

3. A child has a body-surface area equal to 0.6 square meters. The adult dose of a drug is 1 gram. How many milligrams of the drug should the child receive?

The answers to the practice problems are:

1.
$$65 \text{ kg} : X \text{ mg} :: 1 \text{ kg} : 15 \text{ mg}$$
$$X \text{ mg} \times 1 \text{ kg} = 65 \text{ kg} \times 15 \text{ mg}$$
$$X = 975 \text{ mg}$$
The patient should receive 975 milligrams of the drug.

2.
$$\frac{44 \text{ lb}}{X \text{ kg}} = \frac{2.2 \text{ lb}}{1 \text{ kg}}$$
$$44 \text{ lb} \times 1 \text{ kg} = X \text{ kg} \times 2.2 \text{ lb}$$
$$\frac{44}{2.2} = X$$
$$20 \text{ kg} = X$$
The child weighs 20 kilograms.
$$\frac{20 \text{ kg}}{X \text{ mg}} = \frac{1 \text{ kg}}{30 \text{ mg}}$$
$$20 \text{ kg} \times 30 \text{ mg} = X \text{ mg} \times 1 \text{ kg}$$
$$600 \text{ mg} = X$$
The child should receive 600 milligrams of the drug.

3.
$$\frac{\text{body-surface area}}{1.73} \times \text{adult dose} = \text{child's dose}$$
$$\frac{0.6}{1.73} \times 1,000 \text{ mg} = \text{child's dose}$$
$$346.8 = \text{child's dose}$$
The child should receive 346.8 milligrams (rounded to 350 mg) of the drug.

CHAPTER SUMMARY

Chapter 9 explored the responsibilities of a professional nurse in administering safe and accurate doses of drugs. Information about the various ways to calculate drug dosages should assist the student nurse in reaching the goal of safe, accurate drug administration. Here are highlights of the chapter:

• Factors that help determine the amount of a drug dosage include the patient's age, size, integrity of the body systems, and the type and virulence of the patient's disease. The purpose, action, and pharmacokinetic properties of a drug also affect the dosage ordered. Nurses must familiarize themselves with the recommended dosage ranges provided by pharmaceutical companies.

• The metric system is used internationally for ordering drugs, and most new drugs are measured in metric units. The use of the metric system is advantageous because equivalents within the system are exact rather than approximate. The metric system uses liquid measures based on the liter. The gram forms the basis of solid measures. Drugs measured in the metric system are frequently available in liters, milliliters, grams, and milligrams.

• The apothecaries' system, older and less precise than the metric system, is used less often. Equivalents within the apothecaries' system are approximate rather than exact. Liquids are measured in minims, fluidrams, fluidounces, pints, quarts, and gallons; solids are measured in grains.

• The household system, familiar because of its use in the measurement of food substances, is the least used system of measurement in the clinical area. In many cases, over-the-counter medications are measured in the household system. Liquids are measured in teaspoons and tablespoons. The household system also includes pints, quarts, and gallons.

• Some drugs are measured in special systems developed by the manufacturer. Units, milliequivalents, and drops represent special drug measures. The labels of products manufactured in special measures give information on the size of the measures. Some drugs, such as insulin, require special equipment for measuring dosages.

• The nurse must make conversions from one system of drug measurement to another when a drug is ordered in one system but is only available in another system. The nurse must know the equivalents between the systems of measurement to make the conversion calculations.

• The fraction method for conversion uses an equation made up of two fractions. The first fraction shows the ordered dosage to be converted over X units of the available dosage. The second fraction consists of the standard equivalents between the ordered and available measures. The ratio method for conversion uses the same information; however, it is set up as ratios.

• If the physician orders the drug in available units, the nurse proceeds directly to computing the drug dosage. The nurse may use the fraction method, the ratio method, or the desired-available method to perform the calculation.

• When reconstituting powdered drugs before parenteral administration, the nurse should consult the drug label for needed information.

• Nurses often calculate intravenous fluid rates regulated manually or by an intravenous fluid pump. The nurse must know how to calculate the hourly rate, or flow rate, as well as the drip rate, or number of drops per minute. Intravenous administration sets vary in the size of the drop produced. The nurse must, therefore, be familiar with the equipment in use and aware of the drip factor, or number of drops per milliliter that the equipment delivers.

• Sometimes the nurse must prepare special percentage solutions for emergencies. To prepare such solutions, the nurse adds solutes (solid or liquid forms of drugs) to solvents, such as normal saline solution. The nurse can use the fraction method or ratio method to calculate the amount of drug, or solute, and the volume of the solvent to use when preparing a solution of desired concentration.

• Nurses use special methods for computing pediatric doses. Because of children's varying sizes, immature body systems, and maturational patterns, nurses must carefully calculate and verify such doses. Many pharmaceutical companies provide guidelines on the range of acceptable doses of particular drugs. Traditionally, nurses have used Clark's rule, Fried's rule, and Young's rule to calculate children's doses, but each of these rules is limited in the data used to calculate an acceptable dose. The most accurate method for pediatric dose calculation considers the child's body-surface area. Another accurate method involves the dose range per kilogram of body weight.

• Past medical history and individual aging process affect the type and amount of drugs to be given to a geriatric patient.

• Patients receiving chemotherapy may have their drug dosages calculated based upon their body-surface area. A nomogram is used to calculate the patient's body-surface area.

BIBLIOGRAPHY

Drugs, 2nd ed. Springhouse, Pa.: Springhouse Corporation, 1984.

Malseed, Roger T. *Pharmacology: Drug Therapy and Nursing Considerations,* 2nd ed. Philadelphia: J.B. Lippincott Co., 1985.

Nursing88 Drug Handbook. Springhouse, Pa.: Springhouse Corporation, 1988.

Stoklosa, M.J., and Ansel, H.C. *Pharmaceutical Calculations,* 7th ed. Philadelphia: Lea & Febiger, 1980.

INTERVENTION: ROUTES AND TECHNIQUES OF ADMINISTRATION

OBJECTIVES

After reading and studying this chapter, you should be able to:

1. Differentiate among the following solid drug forms in terms of their disintegration sites and absorption rates: tablets, capsules, enteric-coated tablets, and wax matrix tablets.

2. Identify the composition of each of the following oral liquid drug forms: syrups, suspensions, tinctures, and elixirs.

3. Describe how suppository and inhalant drug forms are absorbed.

4. Identify the procedure for administering the following drug forms via the oral route: tablets, capsules, liquids, and lozenges.

5. Describe the procedures for using liquid parenteral drugs packaged as vials, ampules, and self-contained or prefilled syringes.

6. Differentiate between the procedures for administering a drug via a nasogastric tube or a gastrostomy tube.

7. Describe the procedures used to administer sublingual and buccal medications.

8. Explain the rationale for administering medications via the rectal route, and describe the technique for giving a retention enema.

9. Differentiate between the procedures for reconstituting a powdered medication from a vial and from an ampule.

10. Differentiate among the techniques for administering medications via the following parenteral routes: intradermal, subcutaneous, intramuscular, and intravenous.

11. Explain the importance of rotating injection sites when administering parenteral medications.

12. Explain the rationales for using the intrathecal and epidural routes of drug administration.

13. Describe the procedures used to administer the following drug forms via the dermal route: cream, lotion, ointment, powder, and patch.

14. Explain how liquid and powdered nasal medications are administered.

15. Explain the techniques for urethral and vaginal medication administration.

16. Describe the procedures for using the updraft and metered-dose nebulizers for administering drugs via the respiratory route.

INTRODUCTION

The complexity and variety of available medications make proper administration a task requiring knowledge and care. Before administering a medication, the nurse must know the pharmacokinetics, pharmacodynamics, pharmacotherapeutics, drug interactions, adverse effects, dosage range, and nursing implications related to the specific drug. In addition, the nurse must ensure that the five rights of medication administration are observed: the right patient, right drug, right route, right dose, and right time. (See Chapter 8, Intervention: Administration Processes, for further discussion of the five rights.)

Chapter 10 presents techniques as well as rationales for administering medications in the clinical setting.

DRUG FORMS AND PACKAGING

Drugs are manufactured in many different forms and are packaged in numerous styles. The nurse must be knowledgeable about the different effects of the many drug forms to administer drugs safely. For example, nitroglycerin administered sublingually, allowing it to dissolve under the tongue, can relieve chest pain in less than 1 minute. The same drug administered as an ointment applied to the chest wall may not relieve acute pain at all; it may, however, be used prophylactically for chest pain.

The nurse must also consider packaging differences. Drugs may be packaged in unit-dose format, in which one dose of a drug comes in a labeled container or wrapper. They can also be packaged in bulk format, in which multiple doses of a drug are packaged in a container, bottle, or wrapper. The nurse should always remember to *read the label*. Valuable information appears on the label, and reading it assists the nurse in administering medications properly. Other important information may appear in the package insert. For example, the insert may include information about changes in drug actions related to the consumption of food or alcohol with the drug. It may also identify certain interactions between drugs given to the same patient via different routes.

The drug chlordiazepoxide serves as a good example of how reading package information can make a difference. When administering chlordiazepoxide intravenously, the nurse dilutes the drug with sterile water or saline solution. If, however, chlordiazepoxide is to be injected intramuscularly, the nurse must reconstitute the drug with the special diluent supplied by the manufacturer. If the nurse does not use the supplied diluent, the injection can result in severe pain.

SOLIDS

The solid drug forms include tablets, capsules, enteric-coated tablets, and wax matrix tablets. A tablet is the result of compressing a drug, usually combined with inert ingredients, into one of many different shapes. Chewable tablets offer several advantages over other types of drug formulations: palatable taste, enhanced absorption, and easier ingestion for patients who have difficulty swallowing large tablets. Disintegration and some dissolution of chewed tablets take place in the mouth, and some absorption occurs in the stomach. Most of the absorption of the drug, however, occurs in the small intestine.

When swallowed, uncoated tablets disintegrate and dissolve in the stomach. Drug absorption from uncoated tablets usually occurs in the small intestine. Sublingual tablets are directly absorbed into the bloodstream by the blood vessels under the tongue; buccal tablets are absorbed by blood vessels in the cheek.

A capsule is either a hard or soft gelatin shell that contains a drug in a powder, in sustained-released beads, or in liquid form. Capsules dissolve in the stomach and release medication into the small intestine. Usually, solid

drugs are contained in hard gelatin shells and liquid medications are contained in soft gelatin shells. Swallowed capsules disintegrate and dissolve in the stomach; absorption occurs in the small intestine. The precise degree of dissolution and absorption, as well as the site of those activities, depends upon the specific drug.

Enteric-coated tablets have a thin coating that allows the tablet to pass through the stomach and disintegrate and dissolve in the small intestine, where the drug is absorbed. Unscored tablets, enteric-coated tablets, and capsules should *never* be divided. Each of these products may contain inert or other ingredients along with the drug, and dividing the drug form could result in incorrect dosage administration or damage to the stomach mucosa. In addition, dividing an enteric-coated tablet destroys the enteric barrier, allowing stomach secretions to act on the medication and alter its absorption.

In the wax matrix form of an orally administered drug, the drug is deposited throughout a honeycomb-like structure made of a wax material. Many of these tablets are then covered with an enteric-coated shell, allowing disintegration and absorption to occur in the small intestine. The wax matrix allows for the sustained release of a drug, which in turn provides a more constant blood level of the drug. The nurse should inform the patient taking a wax matrix preparation that the indigestible casing may be expelled in the feces. The enteric-coated drug form delivers a concentrated dose of drug to the intestinal mucosa, which may result in irritation or ulceration to the intestinal mucosa.

LIQUIDS

Liquid medications are usually given via a parenteral route or orally. The nurse may also administer liquid medications as irrigations, soaks, enemas, or gargles. Orally administered liquids, which contain the drug mixed with some type of fluid, are classified as syrups, suspensions, tinctures, or elixirs.

Syrups are drugs mixed in a sugar-water solution. Cough syrup is a medication frequently given in this form.

Suspensions consist of finely divided drug particles suspended in a suitable liquid medium. The nurse or patient administering a suspension should shake the preparation thoroughly before using it. Shaking the suspension ensures that the drug particles are dispersed uniformly throughout the liquid. Antacids are commonly manufactured in suspension form.

Tinctures and elixirs are two types of alcoholic solution. Tinctures are hydroalcoholic drug solutions, while elixirs are hydroalcoholic solutions plus glycerin, sorbitol, or another sweetener. The nurse or patient should not mix alcoholic solutions with a liquid other than water without first consulting a pharmacist. The nurse should never give alcoholic solutions to patients who also take the drug disulfiram (Antabuse) or other drugs that can cause disulfiram-like effects when taken with alcohol, such as metronidazole.

Liquids given parenterally are available in three packaging styles: vials, ampules, and self-contained systems or prefilled syringes.

Vials, which are bottles sealed with a rubber diaphragm, can contain a single dose or several doses. Multidose vials contain preservatives that enable them to be used for more than one dose, whereas single-dose vials do not contain such agents. The nurse must discard single-dose vials after one use or dose. The medication in vials may come in a liquid form or in a powder that the nurse must reconstitute before use.

An ampule contains a single dose of medication. The ampule is a glass container with a thin neck, which is usually scored so it can be snapped off. Ampules usually contain liquid medications.

Self-contained systems, or prefilled parenteral medications, contain a single dose of a drug in a plastic bag or in a prefilled syringe with an attached needle. Nurses and physicians use prefilled syringes for narcotics and other analgesics as well as for drugs used during cardiopulmonary resuscitation or advanced life-support activities. Prefilled syringes are also used in unit-dose drug administration systems.

SUPPOSITORIES

Administered rectally and vaginally, suppositories carry medications in a solid base that melts at body temperature. Suppositories produce local (analgesic, laxative, and antipruritic) and systemic (antiemetic, antipyretic, and analgesic) effects. Usually bullet-shaped, most suppositories are about 1 inch (2.5 cm) long and require lubrication for insertion. Because they melt at body temperature, suppositories usually require refrigeration until administration.

INHALANTS

Inhalants are powdered or liquid forms of a drug that are given via the respiratory route and are rapidly absorbed by the rich supply of capillaries in the lungs. Powdered forms must be broken into fine particles by means of a mechanical device before inhalation. Several frequently used methods of inhalation include metered-dose nebulizers, ultrasonic nebulizers, turbo inhalers, and vaporizers. Beclomethasone is a frequently used powdered inhalant medication.

Other drug forms and packaging described in this chapter include sprays, which are used via several administration routes; creams, lotions, and patches, which are administered topically; and lozenges, which are used for local effects via the oral route. Antifungal remedies are frequently administered as lozenges.

GASTROINTESTINAL TRACT ADMINISTRATION TECHNIQUES

The gastrointestinal (GI) tract provides a fairly safe, but relatively slow-acting, site for drug absorption. Oral and rectal preparations are given via the GI tract.

ORAL

Orally routed drug forms include tablets, capsules, liquids, and lozenges. As long as the patient is alert and able to swallow, oral administration is relatively simple. For this reason and because oral medications are convenient, relatively safe, and economical, both the patient and the nurse usually feel comfortable with the oral administration route.

After checking the five rights of medication administration, the nurse must gather the necessary equipment. To administer tablets or capsules, the nurse needs a souffle cup (medicine cup), a glass of water or other suitable liquid, and the medication container. When using a bottle, the nurse should follow the instructions: (1) Shake the correct number of tablets or capsules comprising a dose into the lid, then transfer them to the souffle cup. Do not touch the medication directly, to avoid contamination of other tablets or capsules. (2) Take the souffle cup containing the appropriate number of tablets or capsules and the glass of water to the patient. If the tablets or capsules come in a unit-dose form, take the appropriate dose to the patient's bedside and remove the tablets or capsules from the individually sealed unit. (3) Identify the patient by checking the patient's armband and name tag and stating the name and action, or use, of the drug; then instruct the patient to place the tablets or capsules in the mouth and swallow them with the water. The patient may take the tablets or capsules one at a time or all at once. For the patient who has difficulty swallowing medications, suggest that the patient sit in an upright position and drink liquid both before and while swallowing the capsules or tablets. The patient should drink at least 3 ounces (90 ml) of liquid after swallowing the medication to ensure that the medication travels down the esophagus and to decrease the risk of local irritation by the medication, particularly in elderly patients. (4) Remain at the bedside until the patient swallows all of the medication, thus ensuring that the patient has not aspirated the medication and that it has entered the GI tract. In addition, never leave the medication at the patient's bedside. This precaution ensures that the medication is not hoarded, lost, discarded, or ingested by someone other than the intended patient.

Giving medications through a gastric tube, such as a nasogastric (NG) tube or a gastrostomy tube, involves special techniques. When drugs are given by mouth, saliva and esophageal juices mix with the medication, and some disintegration and dissolution occur. Drugs administered through a gastric tube enter the stomach directly, thus bypassing the mouth and esophagus and the disintegration processes that occur there. To administer a drug appropriately via the NG or gastrostomy tube, the nurse must reproduce the disintegration and dissolution processes by crushing a tablet and preparing a liquid form. When using the NG or gastrostomy tube, the nurse must know how the action of a medication changes when a tablet is crushed. A crushed tablet disintegrates immediately, and absorption from the GI tract occurs very rapidly. These changes may not produce significant differences in blood levels and absorption rate if the tablet was designed for rapid disintegration and absorption. If, however, the tablet was designed for slow release and absorption, crushing can significantly alter the effect of the drug. In some cases, the nurse may consult the physician about using a different form of the drug or a different route to achieve the intended effect.

The nurse must never place an intact tablet or capsule in a gastrostomy or NG tube. The small diameter of most NG tubes prohibits most tablets and capsules from passing through the lumen.

To determine which drugs should and should not be crushed, the nurse should read the label, consult a pharmacist, or check the package insert information. In general, uncoated tablets or those with sugar coatings designed only to camouflage a bitter taste can be crushed. The nurse should not crush enteric-coated tablets, because the coating is designed to protect the drug from stomach acids and ensure that the drug reaches and dissolves in the small intestine. When these tablets are crushed, gastric or esophageal irritation as well as altered drug action can result. Wax matrix tablets should not be crushed because the drug would dissolve faster,

thereby increasing the serum level of the drug and causing the drug to be excreted much more rapidly. The intended sustained-release action of the wax matrix tablet would become unpredictable.

The beads in sustained-release capsules should not be crushed because all of the drug would be released at once; the sustained-release action of the drug would be altered in much the same way as in crushing a wax matrix tablet. The nurse who must administer a sustained-release drug through a gastric tube should obtain and use a liquid form of the drug if possible. Otherwise, the patient may require more frequent doses, which may result in toxic effects. Capsules that contain a powder can be emptied for easy administration by gastric tube.

If crushing the tablet is necessary, the nurse should use a glass mortar and pestle or a special pill-crushing device. The hospital pharmacy may perform this service for patients who cannot take medications orally. Ideally, the tablet would be available in a unit-dose package and the nurse would crush it without opening the package. When a unit-dose package is not available, the nurse crushes the medication using a clean, dry mortar and pestle or places the tablet in a souffle cup and uses the pill-crushing device. The nurse then removes the uniformly crushed powder from the unit-dose package, mortar and pestle, or souffle cup, mixes it with a liquid, and administers the dose to the patient through the NG or gastrostomy tube. The mortar and pestle should then be cleaned with an ethyl alcohol swab.

Powders can be dissolved in lukewarm water. For capsules containing a liquid, the nurse can prick the capsule in one end with a needle and squeeze the contents into the gastric tube. The nurse can also dissolve the whole capsule in a small amount of lukewarm water and then administer the dose. Dissolving the capsule ensures administration of the entire dose, but the dissolution process can take a long time.

Many medications that require administration via a gastric tube are available in liquid form, the use of which is always preferable to crushing tablets. Some of these medications may also be given parenterally. When using a gastric tube, the nurse should administer only room-temperature liquids. Liquids going through a gastric tube bypass the mouth and esophagus, which normally help warm or cool fluid entering the stomach. A burning or cramping sensation can occur in the stomach if the patient receives a liquid that is too hot or too cold via a gastric tube. (See *Administering medication via an NG tube* for step-by-step procedures.)

Administering medication via an NG tube

Before administering medication, the nurse identifies the patient by checking the patient's armband and name tag and states the name and action of the drug. To administer medication via an NG or gastrostomy tube, the nurse will need these supplies: a 50-ml syringe with a catheter tip that fits snugly into the gastric tube, a plastic medicine cup (containing the medication), a tissue or washcloth, a stethoscope, and a glass of tap water.

1 Check for NG tube displacement by connecting the NG tube to the syringe and aspirating a small amount of stomach contents into the syringe. If stomach contents do not return upon aspiration, or if the diameter of the feeding tube is too small, insert a bolus of 10 cc of air into the tube while auscultating the abdomen midline, just below the xiphoid process. The stomach will emit a loud gurgle when the bolus of air enters. Patients with gastrostomy tubes will not require this procedure because the gastrostomy tube is placed directly into the stomach through a surgical incision.

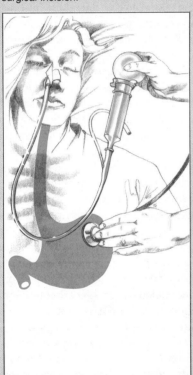

2 Remove the syringe from the tube. Then remove the plunger or bulb from the syringe and place the syringe back into the NG tube, making sure that it fits snugly.

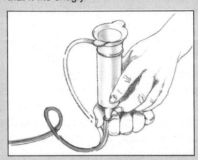

4 After the medication enters the gastric tube, measure 30 to 50 ml of room-temperature water in the medicine cup and pour it into the syringe. The amount of water needed depends upon the length and diameter of the tube. Usually a large-bore tube requires 30 to 50 ml, and a small-bore tube needs 15 to 25 ml. Flow into the gastric tube should occur by gravity. The water will help ensure that all medication is rinsed from the sides of the syringe, the gastric tube, and the medicine cup. This additional fluid also assists in maintaining tube patency. Any residue in the tube lumen may occlude the tube.

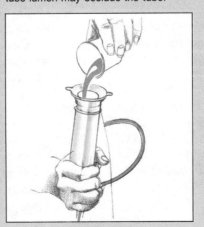

3 Slowly pour the medication into the syringe, which acts as a funnel.

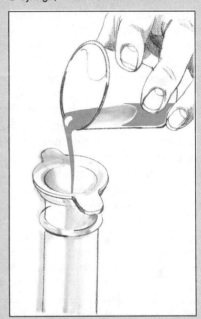

5 Remove the syringe from the tube while keeping a tissue or washcloth below the connection to catch any excess liquid. Then recap or clamp the gastric tube.

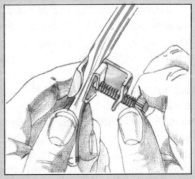

Some patients require special assistance or slightly altered techniques for oral administration. If the patient has difficulty swallowing medications, the nurse can encourage the patient to drink some liquid before and during swallowing of capsules or tablets. If the medication can be crushed, the nurse can place it in a small amount (usually a tablespoon) of applesauce, jelly, mashed potatoes, or other semisolid food. The nurse should use only small amounts of food because some medication may be lost if the patient does not ingest all of the food. This technique works well with toddlers and small children. It is also preferred for patients with dysphagia because they experience more difficulty swallowing liquids than semisolids.

A confused patient may refuse medication, but the nurse must distinguish between a patient who experiences confusion and one who makes an informed choice to refuse the medication. If the patient is confused, the nurse should return and offer the medication a few minutes later. The nurse may obtain the medication in a liquid form or may crush and mix it with a food or beverage. Under no circumstance should the nurse physically force the patient to swallow medication; doing so is illegal and unprofessional and could lead to aspiration or other injuries.

Physicians prescribe all oral medications for infants in liquid form. Small infants can take medications through a bottle after the drug has been diluted with water or other liquid. Medications may also be given using a dropper, which is the preferred method. An infant taking medication through a bottle may receive an incomplete dose if all the liquid in the bottle is not ingested. When administering medications to an infant by the dropper method, the nurse must first identify the patient by checking the armband and name tag. Then the nurse follows these steps: (1) Place a bib on the infant to protect the clothing. (2) Hold the infant in one arm with the head at a 45-degree angle, taking care to restrain the infant's extremities. With the free hand, remove the correct dose of medicine from the bottle and hold the dropper to the infant's lips. (3) Instill the medication in the pocket between the infant's cheek and gum: instilling the drops in that location helps deter the infant from spitting out the medication. (4) Replace the dropper in the medication bottle if the bottle and medication are for an individual patient and the dropper is attached to the bottle cap. If the dropper is not attached to the bottle cap, rinse the dropper in warm water, dry it with a clean paper towel, and store it in a clean airtight container for later use by the same patient.

SUBLINGUAL AND BUCCAL

Uncoated tablets are used for sublingual and buccal routes, which differ from the oral route. Because the patient does not swallow the tablets, they do not enter the GI tract. Instead, the tablets disintegrate and dissolve in the mouth, either under the tongue (sublingual) or between the cheek and gum (buccal). Furthermore, orally routed drugs are absorbed mainly in the small intestine. Sublingual and buccal drugs are absorbed directly into the bloodstream from the oral mucosa, thus bypassing the hepatic and GI systems.

When a drug bypasses the liver, first-pass metabolism cannot significantly reduce the percentage of drug that reaches the systemic circulation. (See Chapter 2, Pharmacokinetics, for a more detailed description of the first-pass effect.) The time required for a drug to begin therapeutic action also greatly diminishes when the drug bypasses the GI tract. The reduced time needed for therapeutic action can be advantageous in certain circumstances. For example, nitroglycerin given sublingually for acute chest pain dissolves under the tongue, where it enters the bloodstream directly. The onset of action can occur in seconds. The same drug orally routed via a gastrostomy tube takes up to 30 minutes to produce effective action.

The time difference produced by sublingual and buccal routing also influences peak serum levels and the duration of action. The duration of action of sublingual nitroglycerin for acute chest pain is approximately 5 minutes. A patient experiencing acute chest pain lasting longer than 5 minutes may need another dose of sublingual nitroglycerin. Therefore, sublingual nitroglycerin is not given to prevent chest pain throughout the day. In that case, a drug form with a longer duration of action would be used. Nitroglycerin applied to the skin surface as paste or patch provides a duration of action of 4 and 24 hours respectively. These forms of the drug would be appropriate for the long-term prevention of chest pain.

Drugs frequently given via the sublingual or buccal route include nitrates, such as nitroglycerin or isosorbide dinitrate, ergotamine, and the liquid contents of a capsule of the calcium channel blocker nifedipine.

Another major drug form used for sublingual administration is the spray. In administering the spray form of nitroglycerin, for example, the nurse dispenses the liquid by completely depressing the plunger on the pressurized aerosol container once. Doing so provides the patient with a metered dose of the drug. The nurse should deliver the dose while the patient maintains an open mouth with or without the tongue raised toward the roof of the mouth. The spray is deposited on the floor of the mouth, in the same location as a sublingual tablet. The patient then closes the mouth and resumes normal activity.

To administer drugs via the sublingual route, the nurse follows these steps: (1) Place the tablet in a souffle cup. (2) Identify the patient by checking the armband and name tag. (3) State the name of the drug and its action. (4) Ask the patient to open the mouth and touch the tip of the tongue to the roof of the mouth. (5) Place the tablet on the floor of the mouth and have the patient close the mouth. Instruct the patient not to swallow the tablet, but rather to hold it in place until it has been absorbed.

For administration via the buccal route, the nurse follows these steps: (1) Place the medication in a souffle cup. (2) Identify the patient using the standard procedure. (3) State the name of the drug and its action. (4) Have the patient open the mouth. (5) Place the tablet between the gum and cheek near the back of the mouth, and instruct the patient to close the mouth and keep the tablet against the cheek until it is absorbed.

Sublingual and buccal medications are frequently kept at the patient's bedside for immediate use. In those instances, the medications are self-administered. Self-administration necessitates that the nurse provide adequate patient education and supervision.

RECTAL

Nurses administer medications via the rectal route for a variety of reasons. A postoperative patient may have an NG tube connected to continuous suction to keep the stomach decompressed, thus prohibiting the use of the oral route. In such circumstances, suppositories can provide a relatively convenient, painless route for some necessary drugs. Antiemetics given rectally to the nauseated patient are frequently effective when the oral route cannot be used. Using a promethazine suppository can be as therapeutically effective as an injection for the patient.

The rectal route is also the route of choice for circumstances in which certain local and systemic effects are desired. For example, bisacodyl suppositories are given to treat constipation. These suppositories produce a local irritant effect that stimulates peristalsis within a relatively short time. The nurse can administer an enema such as sodium polystyrene sulfonate (Kayexalate) to decrease serum potassium levels. Kayexalate works locally in the large intestine to exchange sodium for potassium ions in the GI tract. This local action also affects systemic potassium levels, resulting in decreased serum levels.

The rectal route may also represent the route of choice for unconscious patients. Because unconscious patients cannot swallow, using the rectal route helps avoid potential aspiration.

Using the rectal route for administering medications poses several disadvantages. Receiving drugs rectally may embarrass the patient. Using the rectal route can also result in incomplete drug absorption if the patient cannot retain the medication or if the rectum contains feces. Also, pain can result from hemorrhoids or an irritating drug. (See *Inserting a rectal suppository* on page 166 for an explanation and illustration of this procedure.)

The technique used for administering medications by enema depends upon the time the patient must retain the fluid in the rectum. Medicated fluid that requires retention for at least 30 minutes is called a retention enema. In most cases, a retention enema contains between 100 and 200 ml of fluid for adults and 75 to 150 ml of fluid for children over age 6. Children younger than age 6 should not receive retention enemas because they will not be able to voluntarily retain the fluid.

For patients who require a retention enema but cannot retain the fluid, the nurse may need to use a catheter with an inflatable balloon for administration. The nurse inserts the catheter into the rectum, inflates the balloon with the appropriate amount of air or saline solution, and administers the medication. Following administration, the nurse clamps the catheter, thereby helping the patient retain the fluid. Following the retention period, the nurse unclamps and removes the catheter. Expulsion of the retained fluid usually occurs simultaneously with catheter removal.

Nonretention enemas, which are either medicated or unmedicated, are given to evacuate the lower bowel. Nonretention enemas contain between 750 and 1,000 ml of fluid for adults and lesser amounts for children and infants. Ideally, the adult and older child retain the fluid for 10 minutes. To administer the nonretention enema, the nurse uses an enema bag. The procedure is not discussed in this chapter because any basic medical/surgical nursing text covers the administration of nonretention enemas.

The equipment that the nurse needs to administer a retention enema includes a rectal tube (14 or 20 French for adults and 12 to 14 French for children), water-soluble lubricant, a bedsaver pad, a 4 × 4 gauze pad or tissue, a rubber-tipped hemostat, a bedpan, a 200-ml catheter tip or bulb syringe with the plunger or bulb removed, and a paper towel. To administer the retention enema, the nurse follows these steps: (1) After identifying the patient and explaining the purpose of the med-

Inserting a rectal suppository

Before administering the medication, the nurse identifies the patient by checking the patient's armband and name tag and states the name and action of the drug. To administer a suppository, the nurse will need these supplies: a finger cot or nonsterile disposable examination glove, a water-soluble lubricant, the foil-wrapped or unwrapped suppository, and a tissue or clean 4 × 4 gauze pad. The nurse should draw the curtains or close the door to ensure the patient's privacy.

1 Assist the patient into a comfortable position in which the anus is exposed. Then place the glove or finger cot on the index finger of the dominant hand, remove the foil wrapper, if present, hold the suppository in the gloved hand, and lubricate the tapered end of the suppository with approximately 1 teaspoon (5 ml) of lubricant.

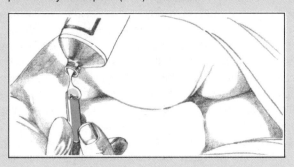

2 Spread the patient's buttocks and insert the suppository, tapered end first, into the anal opening, gently advancing the suppository past the anal sphincter. Use the index finger with the glove or the finger cot to advance the suppository. In an adult, advance the suppository approximately 3 inches (7 cm) to pass the internal anal sphincter. Clean the excess lubricant from the anal area with the 4 × 4 gauze pad or tissue, and encourage the patient to retain the suppository for at least 20 minutes. If the suppository is not a cathartic, the patient may feel very little or no urge to expel it. If, however, the suppository is intended to relieve constipation, the patient may want to expel it as soon as an urge to defecate occurs.

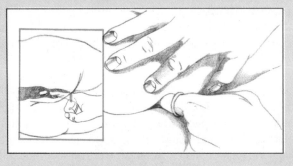

ication and the procedure, ensure the patient's privacy by closing the door or drawing the curtains. (2) With the bed flat, assist the patient onto the left side with the right knee flexed. This position allows the medication to flow from the rectum into the colon. If the patient cannot assume this position, assist the patient to lie on either the right side or the back. (3) Place the bedsaver pad well under the patient's buttocks to protect the bed linen. (4) Insert the tip of the syringe into the rectal tube. (The syringe will act as a funnel.) Purge the air from the rectal tube by first turning the tip of the tube upward and pinching it off with the fingers. (5) Pour a small amount of the medicated solution into the syringe, slowly lowering the tip of the tube until the solution flows out. Immediately turn the tip upward and attach the hemostat, or close the clamp, about 8 inches (20 cm) from the tip. *Do not* lay down the syringe and tube from this point until the medication is instilled and the tube removed from the patient. Laying these items down would allow the fluid to flow out, and the procedure would need to begin again. (6) After purging the air from the tube, lubricate the tip of the tube with the water-soluble lubricant. Place approximately 1 tablespoon (15 ml) of lubricant on the paper towel and roll the distal 2 inches (5 cm) of the tip of the tube in the lubricant. (7) Separate the patient's buttocks and insert the tube into the anus. Advance the tube about 4 inches (10 cm) (2 to 3 inches [5 to 7 cm] in children), directing it toward the umbilicus. This technique can be awkward because the tube must be inserted with the same hand that is holding the syringe. To help alleviate awkwardness, hold the tube and syringe in the dominant hand and spread the patient's buttocks with the nondominant hand. (8) Slowly pour the prescribed solution into the syringe, holding the tip of the syringe about 4 to 5 inches (10 to 13 cm) above the anus. Release the clamp and allow the fluid to flow into the patient by gravity. If the fluid level rises too far above the anus, the patient may experience cramping or a strong urge to defecate. Instruct the patient to take deep breaths during the insertion and instillation to help the patient relax and avoid the urge to defecate. After instilling all of the solution, clamp the tubing. Inform the patient that you are going to remove the tube. (9) Instruct the patient to take a deep breath. As the patient inhales, quickly remove the tube. Firmly apply pressure against the anus with the 4 × 4 gauze pad or tissues for about 10 to 20 seconds or until the urge to defecate passes. (10) Cleanse the area of any solution or lubricant, and encourage the patient to wait the prescribed length of time (usually at least 30 minutes) before evacuating the enema. Leave the bedsaver pad in place and the bedpan near the patient until the patient has defecated.

PARENTERAL ADMINISTRATION TECHNIQUES

Administration via the parenteral route can involve all routes other than the GI tract. The discussion in this chapter, however, concentrates on those medications given by injection. Nurses use the parenteral route to provide a rapid onset of action and to ensure high blood levels of the drug. The parenteral route is also used when the GI route would inactivate the drug, in unconscious patients, and in unstable or seriously ill patients who require precise administration and monitoring.

Medications can be injected into several body spaces, and the type of injection depends upon the body space that is utilized. The techniques and equipment used for each injection type vary. All injections require a liquid form of the prescribed drug and some type of syringe and needle; the nurse must know and use the correct type of needle and syringe for the different kinds of injections. For example, an intramuscular injection requires a long intramuscular needle. A short subcutaneous needle would not reach the muscle, and pain or tissue damage could result. Using an incorrect needle could also alter the drug action and decrease the efficacy of the drug. (See *Syringes and needles* on pages 168 and 169 for illustrations and descriptions of the different types.)

Dead space

After selecting the correct needle and syringe, the nurse must prepare the syringe. Part of this preparation includes consideration of the dead space in the syringe. Dead space refers to the volume of fluid in a syringe and needle that remains after the plunger has been completely depressed. (See *Syringes and needles* on pages 168 and 169 for an illustration.) One way to compensate for dead space is to withdraw 0.2 cc of air after drawing the correct dose of a medication into the syringe. The nurse then administers the injection. The air bubble remains in the syringe hub and needle while the patient receives all the medication (and perhaps a very small amount of air).

For an intramuscular (I.M.) injection, the added 0.2 cc of air provides two major benefits. The patient receives the entire dose of medication, and the medication does not track or seep into subcutaneous tissue. The method, however, can cause problems. Syringes are calibrated to deliver a specific dose of medication, and the man-

ufacturer does not include the hub of the syringe in these calibrations. Because the manufacturer assumes that the drug in the hub of the syringe is not expelled during injection, the addition of an air bubble can result in an overdose of medication, which may be hazardous to some patients, especially children and elderly patients. Furthermore, some syringes, such as insulin syringes, are designed to eliminate dead space. As this discussion suggests, adding an air bubble for the purpose of clearing the hub and needle of the entire dose is not usually recommended.

Nonetheless, adding an air bubble to keep the medication from tracking into the subcutaneous tissues is valuable for some medications. The package inserts of iron dextran and aluminum-adsorbed toxoids and vaccines recommend use of the air bubble. With iron dextran, an air bubble and the Z-track method of injection help prevent permanent staining of the patient's skin should the solution leak into the subcutaneous tissue. Tracking of aluminum toxoids can cause abscesses and tissue necrosis, and the sealing action of the air bubble technique helps prevent these problems.

The nurse should not use the air bubble method with other types of I.M. injections or with any subcutaneous (S.C.) injections. The Z-track method of injection effectively seals the needle track with I.M. injections. (See *The Z-track method for I.M. injections* on page 179 for details on giving these injections.) In addition, no scientific evidence supports the use of an air bubble to prevent bruising after S.C. heparin injections. Nor does the air bubble decrease the pain associated with I.M. injections.

Vial reconstitution and withdrawal

Both liquid and powdered medications for parenteral administration are packaged in sterile vials or ampules. Antibiotics are frequently packaged as powders in vials, but powdered drugs are rarely packaged in ampules. The nurse can simply withdraw liquid medication into the syringe, but powdered forms must first be reconstituted. The nurse must use sterile technique during all medication preparations and injection procedures because injection will interrupt the patient's skin integrity.

The nurse may have to reconstitute powdered medications and prepare them for injection. (See *Reconstituting and withdrawing medications* on page 170 for a complete explanation and illustration of the procedure.)

Small air bubbles may adhere to the interior surface of the syringe when medication is withdrawn from a vial. This small amount of air would not harm the patient if injected; however, it could change the dose of medi-

Syringes and needles

SYRINGES

Standard syringes are available in 3-, 5-, 10-, 20-, 25-, 30-, 35-, and 50-ml sizes. They are used to administer a wide variety of medications in numerous settings. Each one consists of a plunger, barrel, hub, needle, and dead space. The dead space in a syringe is the volume of fluid remaining in the syringe and needle when the plunger is completely depressed. Some syringes, such as insulin syringes, do not have dead space areas.

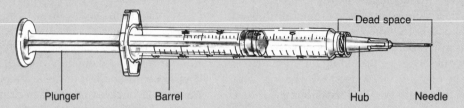

Plunger   Barrel   Dead space   Hub   Needle

The insulin syringe has an attached 25-gauge (25G) needle and no dead space. The syringe is divided into units rather than milliliters for measurement. This syringe should be used only for insulin administration.

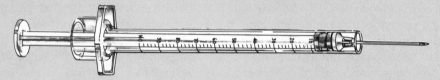

The tuberculin syringe holds up to 1 ml of medication. Used most frequently for intradermal injections, it is also used to administer small volumes of medication, such as might be required in pediatric and intensive care units.

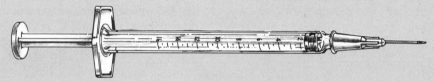

NEEDLES

When choosing a needle, the nurse must consider the needle gauge, bevel, and length. Gauge refers to the inside diameter of the needle. The smaller the gauge, the larger the diameter. Bevel refers to the angle at which the needle tip is opened, and length is the distance from the tip to the hub of the needle.

Needles usually used for **intradermal** injections are 3/8 to 5/8 inch (1 to 1.5 cm) long and are 25G in diameter. Such needles usually have short bevels.

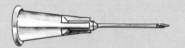

Needles for **subcutaneous** injections are 5/8 to 7/8 inch (1.5 to 2 cm) long, have medium bevels, and are 23G to 25G in diameter.

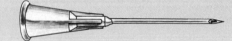

Needles for **intramuscular** use are 1 to 3 inches (2.5 to 7.5 cm) long, have medium bevels, and are 23G to 18G in diameter.

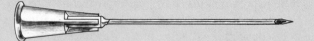

Syringes and needles continued

Needles for **intravenous** use are 1 to 3 inches long, have long bevels, and are 25G to 14G in diameter.

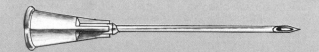

Microscopic pieces of rubber or glass may enter the solution when the nurse punctures the diaphragm of a vial with a needle or when the nurse snaps open an ampule. The nurse can use a **filter needle** with a screening device contained within the hub to remove minute particles of foreign material from a liquid solution. Filter needles should not be used for injection. Filter needles are 1½ inches (4 cm) long, have medium bevels, and are 20G in diameter.

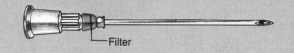
Filter

A **closed system device** comes with the needle in place. These devices come either with the plunger attached (prefilled syringe) or as a cartridge to be inserted into a barrel with a plunger attached (cartridge-needle unit). Emergency drugs, such as atropine and lidocaine, are manufactured in prefilled syringes. Narcotic analgesics, heparin, and injectable vitamins are manufactured in cartridge-needle units.

To prepare the prefilled syringe, hold the medication chamber in one hand and the syringe and needle in the other. Flip the protective caps off both ends. Insert the medication chamber into the syringe section. Remove the needle cap and expel any air in the system.

To prepare the cartridge-needle unit for use, insert a cartridge into the reusable syringe. Twist the barrel until it is engaged. Then, insert the plunger and twist until the barrel rotates in the reusable syringe. Remove the needle cap and purge the device of air and any extra medication.

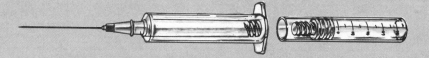

cation actually administered. Therefore, the nurse should remove the air bubbles. To do so, hold the syringe with the needle pointed upward, tap the side of the syringe until the bubbles accumulate at the hub, then slowly push the plunger until the air is expelled. If the amount of medication is not accurate after this procedure, withdraw more of the drug to complete the prescribed dose.

Ampule reconstitution and withdrawal

The procedure for reconstituting and withdrawing medication from an ampule resembles that for vials, with one major difference. The nurse does not inject air into the ampule. Capillary action holds the liquid inside an inverted ampule. Injecting air would disrupt this capillary action, and the fluid would flow out of the inverted ampule. (See *Withdrawing solution from an ampule* on page 171 for an illustrated description.)

Mixing drugs

The nurse must frequently mix drugs in one syringe. Probably the most commonly mixed drugs are insulin preparations. Because the onset of action, peak concentration level, and duration of action of insulin preparations vary, the nurse may have to combine a rapid-acting and a longer-acting type to manage a patient's diabetes. (See Chapter 55, Hypoglycemic Agents and Glucagon, for a detailed discussion of insulin.) Rather than administer two injections, the nurse mixes the two insulins together and administers a single injection. For example, the nurse might mix 10 units of regular insulin with 33 units of NPH insulin.

Reconstituting and withdrawing medications

To reconstitute and withdraw medication from a vial, the nurse will need these supplies: the medication vial, a vial or ampule of an appropriate diluent, an iodophor or ethyl alcohol swab, a syringe, two needles of appropriate size, and a filter needle, if available, to screen particulate matter that may accumulate from the reconstitution process.

1 Place the medication vial on a counter top. Wipe the rubber diaphragm with the alcohol or iodophor swab. Do not rub the diaphragm vigorously, because doing so can introduce bacteria from the nonsterile rim of the vial. Repeat the process with the vial of diluent.

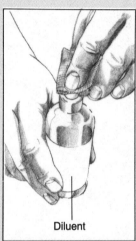

Diluent

2 Pick up the syringe, uncap the needle, and pull back on the plunger until the space inside the syringe equals the amount of diluent desired. Puncture the rubber diaphragm of the diluent vial with the needle, and inject the air. Injecting the air counters the fluid volume and creates a positive pressure. The positive pressure allows the fluid to be easily withdrawn from the vial and prevents a vacuum from forming after the contents are withdrawn. Invert the vial, and withdraw the desired amount of diluent.

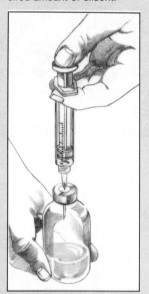

3 Inject the diluent into the medication vial, and withdraw the needle. Roll or shake the vial to thoroughly mix the medication. If a filter needle is available, remove the first needle, and attach the filter needle to the syringe and uncap it. If a filter needle is not available, leave the first needle attached to the syringe.

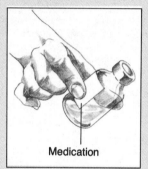

Medication

4 Pull back the plunger until the volume of air in the syringe equals the volume of medication to be given. Puncture the diaphragm of the medication vial, and inject the air. Invert the vial, and withdraw the correct amount of solution. Replace the original needle or the filter needle with a clean sterile needle because medication that may have adhered to the needle when the solution was withdrawn from the vial can irritate the patient's tissues. The syringe filled with medication is now ready to label and administer to the patient. If the medication is already in a liquid form, withdrawing it from a vial involves the same steps as previously described in handling a medication after reconstitution.

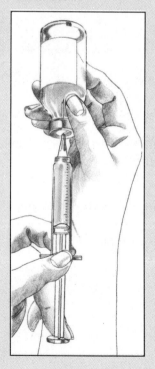

Withdrawing solution from an ampule

To reconstitute and withdraw medication from an ampule, the nurse will need these supplies: an ampule with the medication, a vial or ampule of the appropriate diluent, an ampule file if the ampule is not scored, a syringe, two needles of appropriate size, two filter needles (if available), and a dry 2×2 gauze pad.

1 Make sure that all of the fluid is located in the base of the ampule; if any remains in the stem, or top portion, gently tap the stem to cause the liquid to flow through the thin neck to the base. If tapping the stem does not work, grasp the base of the ampule, raise it to approximately eye level, and quickly lower it an arm's length.

Serrate the neck of an unscored neck of the ampule with an ampule file if necessary. Cover the ampule stem with the 2×2 gauze pad to protect your fingers from cuts as the neck is snapped. When snapping the neck of an ampule, always point it away from you and others.

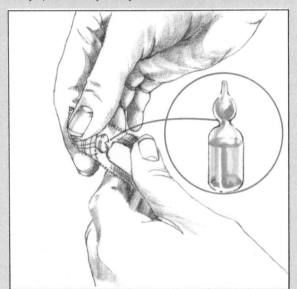

2 Place the filter needle (or a regular needle if the filter needle is not available) on the syringe. Insert the needle into the fluid, and withdraw the appropriate amount of medication. Finally, replace the filter needle with the needle for administering the medication. The medication is now ready for injection.

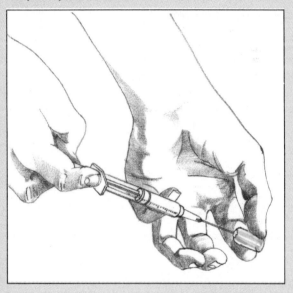

To mix 10 units of regular insulin and 33 units of NPH insulin in one syringe, the nurse will need these supplies: an insulin syringe calibrated in units equal to the insulin concentration, two alcohol swabs, a vial of NPH insulin, and a vial of regular insulin. The nurse follows these steps: (1) Gently roll the NPH insulin vial between the hands to mix the particles into suspension. This action is not necessary for regular insulin. (2) Cleanse the tops of the vials with the alcohol wipes. (3) Remove the needle cap and withdraw the plunger until 43 units of air, which equals the total insulin dose,

are in the syringe. (4) Carefully inject 33 units of air into the NPH insulin vial and then inject the remaining 10 units into the regular insulin vial. Do not inject air into the solution itself because doing so may produce air bubbles that can alter the dosage. Without removing the needle, invert the vial of regular insulin and withdraw exactly 10 units of regular insulin. (5) Insert the needle into the vial of NPH insulin. Invert the vial, and withdraw 33 units of NPH insulin. The plunger should be at the 43-unit calibration. The medications are now mixed in one syringe and ready for injection.

Skin preparation

After filling the syringe, the nurse must prepare the patient's skin for injection. Giving an injection disrupts the skin, the body's first line of defense, and provides an entry route for bacteria. In preparing the skin for injection, the nurse removes as many bacteria as possible; that is, disinfects the skin.

If the injection site is soiled, wash and dry the site thoroughly. Then use one of several antiseptic agents to disinfect the skin. Ethyl alcohol and iodophor are two of the most frequently used antiseptic agents. Use alcohol with intradermal injections because iodophor discolors the skin and can interfere with interpretation of skin test results. Also use alcohol with patients who are allergic to iodine.

Take care not to touch the patient's skin with anything except the sterile swab, cotton, or gauze impregnated with the disinfectant. When using a disinfectant, always begin at the point where the needle will be inserted and wipe in a spiral pattern from the center outward. Cleansing from the puncture site outward carries bacteria away from the site.

Before injecting the medication, allow the disinfected area to dry for about 1 minute. Do not blow on or fan the area to hasten the drying process, because these activities increase the risk of contamination. Injecting while the skin is still moist introduces alcohol or iodophor into the tissues and causes irritation. Allowing the skin to dry before injection in many cases reduces injection pain.

INTRADERMAL

Intradermal injections are used for skin tests, such as the tuberculin or histoplasmin test. The results of the test are usually interpreted about 24 to 48 hours after the injection. Specific guidelines for each antigen determine whether a patient shows a positive or negative response. In general, an induration of 5 mm or greater indicates a positive response. However, the nurse should consult the package insert or drug reference manual for details on each test.

Most nurses do not give intradermal injections frequently; however, when they do, they should administer the injection in the area of the scapula, upper chest, dorsal upper arm, or the ventral forearm. The ventral forearm is the site of choice. (See *Giving an intradermal injection* for a description of how to find the site on the ventral forearm.) Any area with scars, blemishes, or abundant hair should not be used because they could make interpretation of the test results difficult. Before

Giving an intradermal injection

Before giving an injection, the nurse must identify the patient by checking the patient's armband and name tag and must state the drug's name and action. To give the injection, the nurse will need acetone, a gauze pad, an alcohol swab, a syringe containing the medication, and a needle of appropriate size.

1 To identify the injection site on the ventral forearm, have the patient extend the forearm and rest it on a table with the palm up. Measure 2 to 3 finger-widths distal from the antecubital space. Then measure a hand-width proximal from the wrist. The space between these measures represents the area available for injection.

Prepare the injection site with an acetone-soaked gauze pad and then with an alcohol swab.

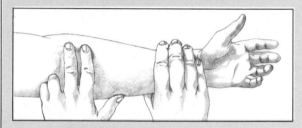

2 Hold the patient's forearm and stretch the skin taut with one hand. With the other hand, place the syringe almost flat against the patient's skin (approximately at a 15 degree angle) with the bevel up. Insert the needle by pressing it against the skin.

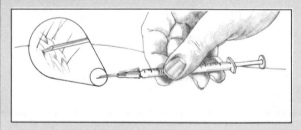

3 Inject the medication slowly and gently. During injection, the needle should be visible through the skin, and you should encounter resistance.

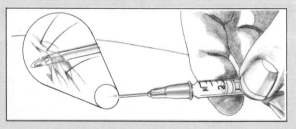

giving the injection, identify the patient by checking the identification armband and name tag; then explain the medication and the procedure.

To administer an intradermal injection, the nurse will need an alcohol wipe for skin preparation and a tuberculin syringe with the appropriate type and amount of antigen. The nurse follows these steps: (1) After properly preparing the skin, expel any air in the needle. With the nondominant hand, retract the patient's skin proximal to the injection site until the skin is taut. Be careful not to contaminate the injection site by touching it. (2) Grasp the syringe with the thumb and index finger, with the barrel extending across the other fingers. Insert the needle at approximately a 15-degree angle with the bevel up. (See *Giving an intradermal injection* for an illustration of the proper technique.) (3) Slowly insert the needle through the epidermis and slowly inject the antigen. Blanching and the formation of a wheal about 6 mm in diameter should occur. (4) Withdraw the needle and apply gentle pressure but do not massage the area. Massaging could lead to site irritation and interfere with the results.

SUBCUTANEOUS

Nurses use S.C. injections to provide a slow, sustained release of medication, a longer duration of action, or to deliver no more than 1 ml of liquid. Many medications, including insulin, heparin, and epinephrine, are given by the S.C. route.

Subcutaneous injection sites, all areas relatively distant from bones and major blood vessels, include the area over the scapulae, the lateral aspects of the upper arms and thighs, and the abdomen. At least a 1-inch (2.5-cm) pinched fold of skin and tissue is necessary for administering an S.C. injection. The nurse should not use burned, edematous, or scarred skin as an S.C. injection site. Nor should the nurse use the area 2 inches (5 cm) in diameter around the umbilicus or the belt line. However, the abdomen is the site of choice for S.C. heparin injections.

The nurse should ensure that injection sites are rotated and that a rotation pattern is established for patients who receive frequent S.C. injections. Site rotation helps promote adequate absorption of the medication and prevents the formation of hard nodules in the subcutaneous tissue. Because site rotation is especially critical for diabetic patients, the nurse must include it as part of the teaching plan for self-care. The nurse must also help each patient establish an individual rotation pattern. Patients who self-administer S.C. injections require different rotation patterns from patients who do not self-administer. For example, the scapular

areas and upper arms are impractical injection sites for the patient who self-administers these injections.

The nurse should establish with the patient the convenient injection site areas, instruct the patient to use each of the injection sites on a given area once before moving on to the next area, and encourage the patient to use the injection sites one after another in an orderly fashion. The nurse needs to stress the importance of establishing and using a systematic pattern.

One effective method of rotating sites is to utilize a diagram to represent the patient's pattern. (See *Sites for subcutaneous injections* on page 174 for a record-keeping diagram.)

When patients do not self-administer injections, the rotation pattern being used must be communicated to other nurses. Most facilities have special flow sheets available to record the rotation patterns used for a specific patient. Notations can also be made on medication sheets.

Heparin and insulin are frequently administered via the S.C. route using the abdominal sites. The administration technique for these sites resembles that used for the general S.C. injection, and the nurse or patient usually gives the injection holding the needle at a 90-degree angle. (See *Giving a subcutaneous injection* on page 175 for the step-by-step procedure.) Grasping a skin fold, however, is not always necessary at the abdominal site. If the patient is dehydrated, cachectic, or frail, the abdominal site may not provide adequate subcutaneous tissue for injections.

Aspiration is not necessary with S.C. injection because subcutaneous tissue usually contains only small blood vessels. Therefore, the danger of unintended intravenous injection is minimal. In fact, aspirating S.C. injections may cause tissue damage that could adversely affect drug absorption. Aspiration is also not recommended with heparin or insulin injections. Aspiration during an insulin injection may result in tissue trauma that may lead to nodule formation in the subcutaneous tissue.

Insulin pumps

Nurses currently use two major types of insulin pumps in providing patient care. The closed-loop system, sometimes called an artificial pancreas, consists of several parts. It includes a device that constantly measures blood glucose levels and sends information to a small computer, which calculates the needed dose of insulin and triggers the battery-powered delivery system. The insulin is then delivered through a subcutaneous needle that is usually implanted in the abdomen.

Sites for subcutaneous injections

The nurse or patient can use a number of administration sites in several areas for subcutaneous injections. Systematic rotation of injections helps maintain those sites. In documenting a patient's site rotation pattern, the nurse frequently uses a diagram similar to this one.

In a typical patient, the nurse would administer the first injection in the site represented by a dot on the upper right quadrant and administer the next injection in the area represented by the second dot in that row. This continues until the sites represented by the top row of dots have been used once, then proceeds with the site represented by the dot on the figure's right side in the center row. When the sites on the abdomen have each been used once, injections may begin in the right leg and follow a similar pattern. When all right leg sites have been used, injections can begin in another area.

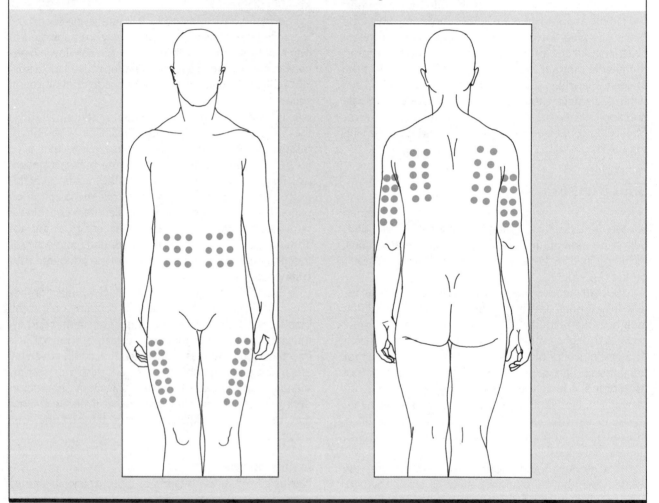

The second, more frequently used type of insulin pump is the open-loop system. With this system, the patient measures the blood glucose levels throughout the day and calculates any necessary adjustments in the baseline infusion rate.

The patient places the day's supply of insulin in a syringe and inserts the syringe into the pump. A length of special tubing is connected to the hub of the syringe, and a subcutaneous needle is attached to the distal end.

The patient inserts the needle into the abdomen in the same manner used for an S.C. injection. The needle is then taped in place and the infusion begins.

The patient should change the insertion site every 2 days and keep the site dry to prevent bacterial contamination. Using an insulin pump provides greater control of blood glucose levels and decreases the number of injections necessary to obtain normal glucose levels.

Giving a subcutaneous injection

Before administering the medication, the nurse identifies the patient by checking the patient's armband and name tag and states the name and action of the drug. To administer an S.C. injection, the nurse will need a syringe with a 23G to 25G needle and the medication and two alcohol or iodophor swabs.

1 Identify and prepare the injection site using an alcohol swab.

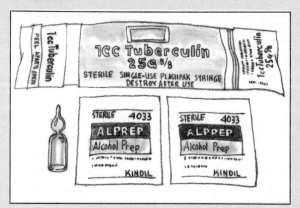

2 Open a second alcohol swab. To keep the swap accessible and maintain sterility of the portion that will contact the insertion site, remove the swab from the wrapper while touching only a corner. Place that same corner between the index and middle finger of the nondominant hand while administering the injection. Grasp at least a 1-inch (2.5-cm) skin fold of the prepared skin area between the thumb and first two fingers of the nondominant hand. Remember, the swab is also in this hand.

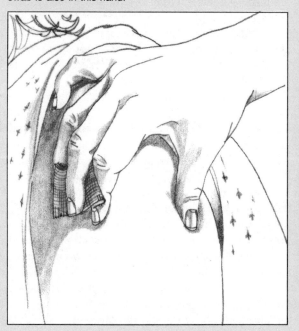

3 In the dominant hand, hold the syringe like a pencil with the bevel of the needle up. If the needle is ½ inch or shorter, hold it at a 90-degree angle to the skin fold. If the needle is ⅝ inch, as in the illustration, hold it at a 45-degree angle.

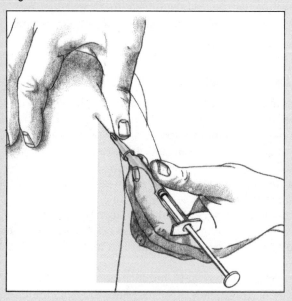

4 Insert the needle using a quick, dartlike motion. Then release the skin fold, and slowly inject the medication. When the plunger is completely depressed and all medication has been injected, place the sterile portion of the second alcohol swab over the insertion site. While gently applying downward pressure, quickly withdraw the needle and syringe. Continue to apply gentle pressure to the site for a few seconds.

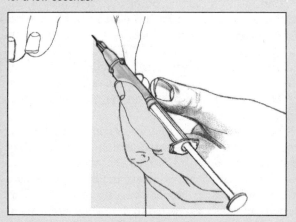

However, the battery pack can be cumbersome, and keeping the insertion site dry and sterile can limit some patient activities.

INTRA-ARTICULAR

Intra-articular injections are not given frequently because of their high risk of infection. Furthermore, intra-articular injections may reduce the chances of success of future joint replacement surgery. Occasionally, patients with severe joint inflammation receive an intra-articular injection of corticosteroids, but these injections are usually not repeated. When giving an intra-articular injection, the physician uses a long needle to deposit the medication directly into the joint and observes strict aseptic technique.

INTRAMUSCULAR

Intramuscular injections are given for various reasons, especially when the rapid absorption of medication is desired. In general, the onset of action is within 10 to 15 minutes following an I.M. injection. However, the blood flow to the injection site affects the absorption rate. Intramuscular injections of drugs that irritate subcutaneous tissues cause less pain than S.C. injections. In addition, a larger amount of fluid can be administered in an I.M. injection. The recommended volume for a single I.M. injection for an adult is a maximum of 3 to 5 ml.

Frequently used I.M. injection sites include the dorsogluteal, ventrogluteal, vastus lateralis, rectus femoris, and deltoid muscles. The nurse needs to identify I.M. injection sites accurately. Major blood vessels and nerves traverse the muscle groups used for I.M. injection; therefore, using an inappropriate injection site could result in permanent damage to the patient. (See *Intramuscular injection sites* for the correct anatomic identification of the various injection sites.)

Damage to a muscle can also occur if the muscle group is overused for injections, which can be avoided by rotating sites. For example, if a nurse gives an injection in the left ventrogluteal muscle, the next injection might be in the left dorsogluteal or right ventrogluteal site, and a third injection might be given in the right dorsogluteal site. The nurse should record on the medication sheet each I.M. site utilized.

The injection technique for administering I.M. injections to infants is the same as that for adults. (See *Giving an intramuscular injection* on page 178 for the procedure.) Positioning an infant requires special care so that the knees are flexed and arms restrained. This position provides easy access to the rectus femoris and vastus lateralis sites. Gentle restraint should be used to prevent the infant from jerking, which may cause trauma. Restraining and positioning an infant often requires a second adult. The nurse should use the rectus femoris and vastus lateralis sites for I.M. injections in infants and small children. The deltoid, ventrogluteal, and dorsogluteal sites are not used because of the immature muscle size at both sites and the increased risk of injury. (See Chapter 12, Intervention: The Pediatric Patient.)

The nurse should use the Z-track method for I.M. injection when a medication, such as iron dextran (Imferon), can irritate or discolor subcutaneous tissue. This method prevents leakage of medication from the muscle into the subcutaneous tissue by using an air bubble to help seal the medication into the muscle. (See *The Z-track method for I.M. injections* on page 179 for a depiction of the technique.)

INTRAVENOUS

Nurses administer medications intravenously to obtain an immediate onset of action, to attain the highest possible blood concentration levels of a drug, and to treat conditions that require the constant titration of medication. Life-threatening situations, such as shock, often require such constant titration. Intravenous (I.V.) administration is also used when the medication is not available in another form and when the patient cannot tolerate the medication via other routes.

Sites used for I.V. administration include the veins on the hand and wrist, the forearm veins that transverse the antecubital fossa, the veins in the scalp and the umbilical vessels (for infants), the subclavian and internal and external jugular veins (for long-term administration or for medications that require rapid blood dilution), and the superficial veins of the leg and foot when other sites cannot be used. (See *Sites for I.V. injection* on page 180 for an illustration.)

The equipment used for an I.V. injection depends on several factors. The vein chosen for the injection or infusion in part determines the type of needle used. For a one-time bolus of a medication, the nurse may use an antecubital vein because of the vein's accessibility and large size. For a bolus type of injection at an antecubital site, the nurse may use a syringe with a needle. For continuous or intermittent infusions lasting a few days, the nurse would select a vein of the hand, wrist, forearm, scalp, or umbilicus. For such an infusion, the nurse would use a cannula or scalp vein needle (also called a butterfly, because of the winglike tabs used to hold the needle during insertion). If the solution is irritating, a smaller gauge needle is recommended to create greater dilution by the blood flow.

Intramuscular injection sites

Ventrogluteal

Used for all patients, this site is desirable because it is not only relatively free of large nerves and adipose tissue, but is also remote from the rectum (which minimizes the risk of contamination).

For this site, position the patient on the back or side.

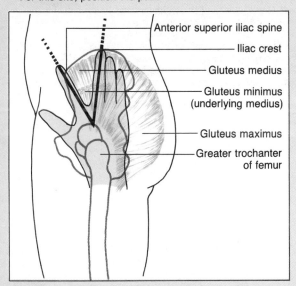

- Anterior superior iliac spine
- Iliac crest
- Gluteus medius
- Gluteus minimus (underlying medius)
- Gluteus maximus
- Greater trochanter of femur

Deltoid

Not frequently used because the muscle is small and can accommodate only small doses of medications, the deltoid is also near the radial nerve.

For this site, seat the patient upright or have the patient lie flat with the arms apart.

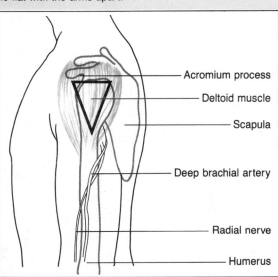

- Acromium process
- Deltoid muscle
- Scapula
- Deep brachial artery
- Radial nerve
- Humerus

Dorsogluteal

Frequently used for adults, the dorsogluteal site is not used for infants and children under age 3 because these muscles are not well developed.

Position the patient flat on the stomach with the toes pointed inward and the arms apart and flexed toward the head.

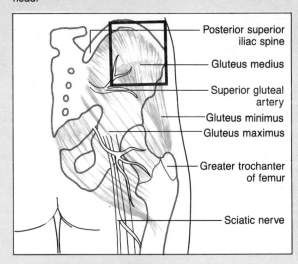

- Posterior superior iliac spine
- Gluteus medius
- Superior gluteal artery
- Gluteus minimus
- Gluteus maximus
- Greater trochanter of femur
- Sciatic nerve

Vastus lateralis and rectus femoris

The vastus lateralis is used for all patients, especially children. It is well developed and has few major blood vessels and nerves. The rectus femoris is most often used for self-injection because of its accessibility.

For this site, position the patient in bed either sitting up or lying flat.

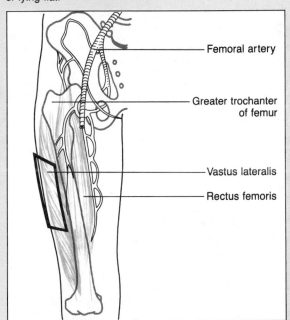

- Femoral artery
- Greater trochanter of femur
- Vastus lateralis
- Rectus femoris

Giving an intramuscular injection

Before administering the medication, the nurse identifies the patient by checking the patient's armband and name tag and states the name and action of the drug. To administer a medication via an I.M. injection, the nurse will need two alcohol swabs, a syringe containing the medication to be injected, and a needle of appropriate size.

1 Expose the area where the injection will be administered. Remember to provide privacy for the patient if any site other than the deltoid muscle is being used. Palpate the appropriate anatomic landmarks, and identify the exact site for the injection. In this illustration, the vastus lateralis muscle is being used.

Prepare a 2-inch (5-cm) diameter area of skin around the injection site using an alcohol swab. Open a second alcohol swab and place it between the index and second finger of the nondominant hand.

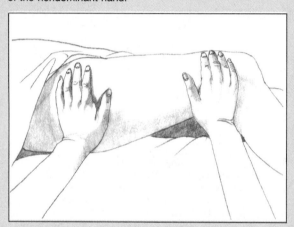

2 Grasp the syringe like a pencil in the dominant hand, and remove the needle cap. With the nondominant hand, spread the skin surrounding the injection site until it is taut. This action helps displace the subcutaneous tissue and brings the muscle closer to the surface.

With a quick, dartlike motion, insert the needle at a 90-degree angle into the muscle. Release the skin surrounding the injection site and use the nondominant hand to steady the syringe for aspiration.

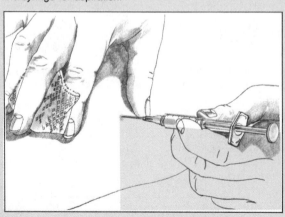

3 Gently aspirate; aspiration is used to determine if the inserted needle has entered a vessel. Pull back slightly on the plunger after inserting the needle into the injection site. If the needle has entered a vessel, blood will flow into the syringe. If blood is aspirated, remove and discard the syringe. Then start the procedure again. If no blood is aspirated, slowly inject the medication. Steady the syringe with the nondominant hand during aspiration and injection.

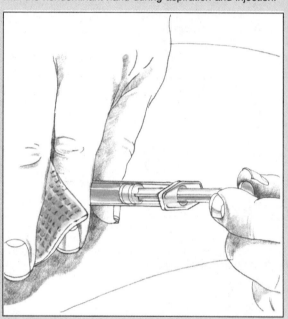

4 When the injection is completed, place the second alcohol swab over the insertion site and apply gentle downward pressure while quickly withdrawing the needle. Massage the site with the alcohol swab to help promote circulation to the area and decrease pain.

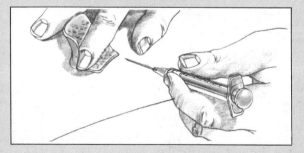

The Z-track method for I.M. injections

The Z-track method for I.M. injections involves pulling the skin in such a way that subcutaneous layers are staggered, causing the needle track to be sealed off after the injection, minimizing subcutaneous irritation and discoloration.

1 After withdrawing the appropriate amount of medication, draw 0.2 cc of air into the syringe. Then replace the needle with a sterile 3-inch (7.5-cm) needle.

Pull the skin laterally away from the intended injection site to ensure the needle's proper entry into the muscle tissue.

2 After cleansing the site, insert the needle, and inject the medication slowly.

When the injection is completed, wait 10 seconds before withdrawing the needle. Waiting prevents medication seepage from the site.

3 Withdraw the needle and syringe, and allow the retracted skin to resume its normal position, which effectively seals the needle track.

Never massage the site or allow the patient to wear tight-fitting clothing over the site immediately after an injection. Either action could force the medication into the subcutaneous tissue and cause irritation.

To increase the patient's absorption rate, encourage physical activity, such as walking. For subsequent injections, remember to rotate the sites.

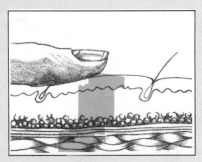
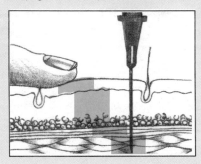
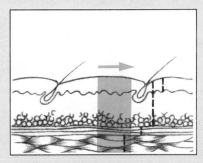

Infusions that require rapid blood dilution and infusions or injections administered frequently and long-term require that special catheters be inserted into large veins. Hyperalimentation is an example of this type of infusion. A physician usually inserts hyperalimentation catheters, frequently in the operating room, to reduce the probability of infection. The Hickman catheter is an example of this type of venous access device.

After determining the appropriate site and needle, the nurse performs a venipuncture. (See *Performing a venipuncture* on pages 181 and 182 for the procedure for inserting a butterfly needle into a dorsal hand vein.)

After completing the venipuncture, the nurse documents the date and time of the insertion, the type and gauge of needle inserted, and the initials of the person inserting the I.V. on the tape that secures the gauze pad. Once a venipuncture has been performed, the administration of medication via the I.V. route can begin.

Direct bolus

To administer medication by direct bolus, the nurse will need a syringe and a 20-gauge (20G) or smaller needle filled with 1 ml of saline solution, a syringe and needle with the prescribed medication, a syringe and needle with 1 ml of heparin flush solution, and three iodophor or alcohol swabs.

The nurse follows these steps to administer the bolus: (1) Identify the patient and explain the medication and procedure. (2) Cleanse the intermittent infusion port with a swab. Puncture the center of the port with the syringe and needle containing the medication, and gently aspirate. A small amount of blood should return to ensure correct placement of the I.V. needle. Slowly inject the medication over the recommended time interval. (3) Withdraw the medication syringe, and cleanse the port with a second swab. Inject the saline-filled syringe to rinse all medication from the port and needle. (4) Remove the syringe and needle used to inject the

Sites for I.V. injection

The primary sites for I.V. injection in the hand include the basilic, dorsal metacarpal, and cephalic veins. All of these vessels are relatively easy to locate. As the cephalic and basilic veins traverse the forearm, they branch into other vessels that are also easily accessible for I.V. injections.

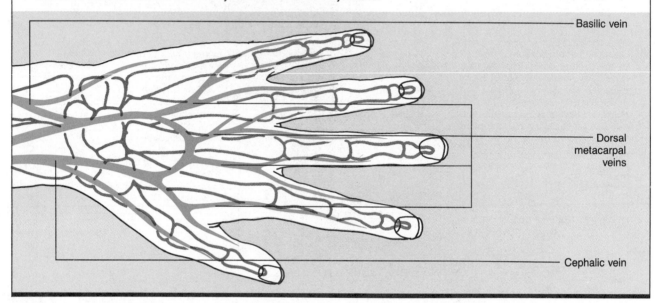

Basilic vein

Dorsal metacarpal veins

Cephalic vein

saline solution. Swab the port a third time, and inject the heparin flush solution. Remove the needle and syringe.

Intermittent infusion

To administer medication using the intermittent infusion method, the nurse will need three alcohol or iodophor swabs, a syringe and needle with 1 ml of heparin flush solution, a syringe and needle with 1 ml of saline solution, I.V. administration tubing, a 20G or smaller needle, the I.V. bottle or bag of medication, and an I.V. pole.

The nurse follows these steps to administer the infusion: (1) Identify the patient and explain the procedure. Remove the I.V. administration tubing from the container and the protective cover from the medication bottle or bag. Close the roller clamp, which regulates fluid flow through the tubing. Remove the cap from the I.V. tubing spike, and insert it into the diaphragm of the medication bag or bottle. Invert the bag or bottle and hang it from the I.V. pole. (2) Fill the drip chamber of the administration tubing. Remove the protective cap on the end of the tubing, and replace it with the 20G needle. Remove the needle cap, and slowly open the roller clamp, allowing the fluid to clear the tubing of air. Close the roller clamp when the liquid has reached the

tip of the needle, and replace the needle cap. (3) Cleanse the intermittent infusion port. Remove the needle cap, and insert the needle into the port. Secure the needle with tape for the duration of the infusion. Open the roller clamp slightly, and lower the medication bag or bottle below the I.V. site. A backflow of blood confirms correct placement of the needle. Return the bottle or bag to the I.V. pole, and infuse the medication over the recommended time interval. (4) When the infusion is completed, remove and cap the infusion needle, cleanse the port with the second swab, and inject the saline solution. Use the third swab to cleanse the port, and inject the heparin flush solution.

Continuous infusion

The procedure for administering a continuous I.V. infusion is very similar to that used for the intermittent infusion, the only difference being the longer duration of infusion. The I.V. administration tubing is usually used for a 24- to 48-hour period; however, the medication bottle or bag may need to be replaced during that period. To do so, the nurse inserts the sterile spike into the new bottle or bag of medication and continues the infusion.

Continuous I.V. medication administration is often facilitated by using an infusion pump. The nurse sets the electric or battery-powered infusion pump to deliver a constant amount of solution per minute or hour. To

Performing a venipuncture

Before beginning a venipuncture, the nurse identifies the patient by checking the patient's armband and name tag and explains the procedure. For a venipuncture into a dorsal hand vein, the nurse will need these supplies: a tourniquet, a butterfly needle (the gauge must be slightly smaller than the lumen of the vein), an iodophor swab, an alcohol swab, a sterile 2×2 gauze dressing, paper or silk tape, a package of antiseptic ointment, and a bedsaver pad.

1 Place the bedsaver pad under the patient's hand to be used for the venipuncture. Apply a tourniquet about 8 to 10 inches (20 to 25 cm) proximal to the needle insertion site.

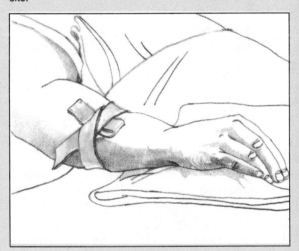

2 Prepare the injection site, using the iodophor swab first, then repeating the process with the alcohol swab. Using the alcohol swab removes some of the iodophor, allowing the vein to appear more clearly.

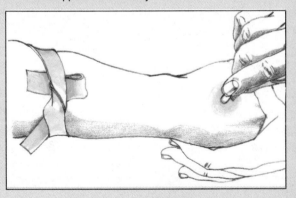

3 Remove the needle cover, and grasp the butterfly needle by its wings with the bevel up, using the thumb and forefinger of the dominant hand.

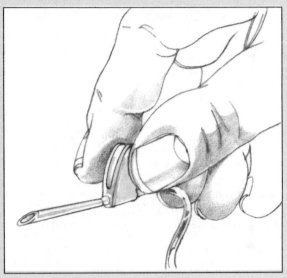

4 Stabilize the vein by gently retracting the skin just distal to the puncture site, using the thumb of the nondominant hand.

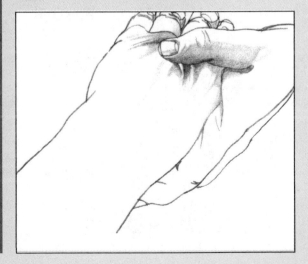

continued

Performing a venipuncture continued

5 Direct the needle at a 30- to 45-degree angle to the skin and puncture the skin just to the side of the vein, using a slow, steady motion.

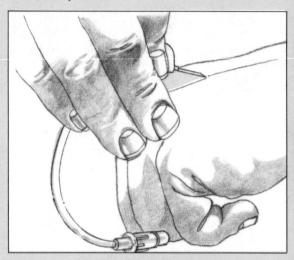

6 Once the entire bevel has penetrated the skin, reposition the needle slightly by directing it toward the vein and decreasing the angle until the needle is almost flat. Then, puncture the vein wall. A backflow of blood confirms that the vein has been entered. Continue to insert the needle its full length.

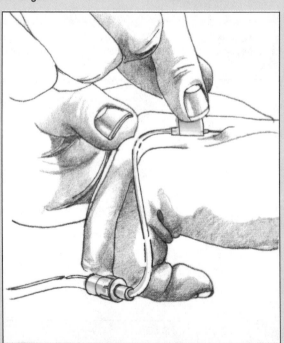

7 Secure the wings by placing a strip of tape over each side. Remove the protective cap on the end of the tubing, and attach an infusion set or intermittent infusion port.

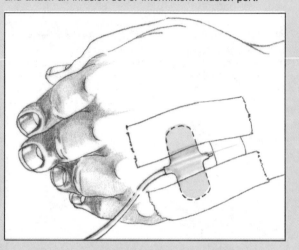

8 Do not cover the insertion site with the tape. Instead, place a small amount of iodophor or other antibiotic ointment over the site and cover it with the gauze pad or another occlusive dressing. Apply a 2-inch-wide (5-cm) strip of tape over the gauze pad to hold it in place. Then loop the tubing and secure it with tape.

Leave the hub of the needle exposed so that it is easy to see and use. Remember to document the needle gauge, date and time of insertion, and your initials on the tape covering the site.

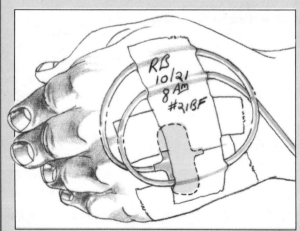

determine the pump settings, the nurse considers the total amount of fluid to be given and the interval over which it must be infused. Each of the different infusion pumps available comes with its own set of operating instructions. The nurse must follow the manufacturer's guidelines to ensure adequate functioning of the pump.

Hickman catheter administration

The Hickman catheter, one of the oldest and best-known venous access devices, is used when the patient requires frequent venous access over a sustained period. During such time, the nurse may obtain blood samples or administer medications or hyperalimentation.

The Hickman catheter and other similar venous access devices are implanted in a large vein, such as the cephalic or internal jugular vein. The tip of the catheter is introduced into the right atrium, and the end of the catheter exits the vessel through the chest wall. The end of the catheter has an intermittent infusion port attached to it.

The procedures for injecting or infusing medication resemble those used for I.V. infusion or injection. The volume of the heparin flush solution, however, is greater (3 ml). Furthermore, the catheter requires special care for maintenance.

OTHER ROUTES OF ADMINISTRATION

Eight other routes are used for medication administration: intrathecal, epidural, dermal, nasal and sinus, ophthalmic, urethral, vaginal, and respiratory.

INTRATHECAL ADMINISTRATION

During intrathecal administration, an access device implanted beneath the scalp delivers medication to the brain. The access device, which consists of a dome-shaped reservoir and a ventricular catheter, is surgically implanted below the scalp on the top portion of the head. The catheter is threaded into the lateral ventricles. (See *The intrathecal access device* for a depiction of this device.) A bolus of medication is then injected into the pliable reservoir. When the filled reservoir is compressed, medication is ejected through the catheter into the brain. Intrathecal reservoir injections are not usually administered by nurses.

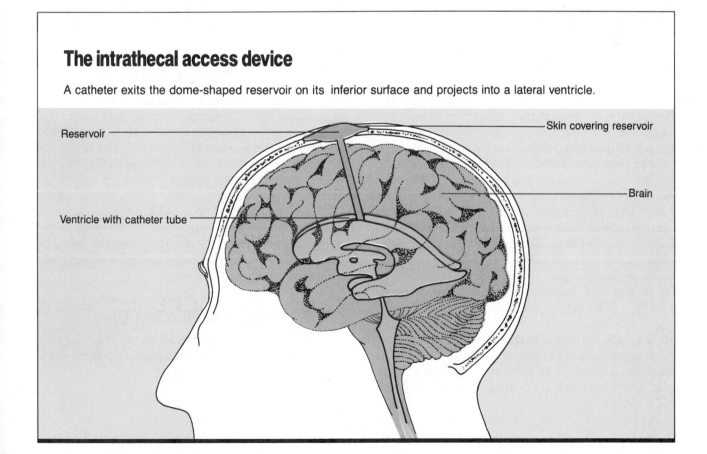

The intrathecal access device

A catheter exits the dome-shaped reservoir on its inferior surface and projects into a lateral ventricle.

Reservoir

Skin covering reservoir

Brain

Ventricle with catheter tube

Physicians use intrathecal administration for patients requiring frequent chemotherapy treatments for lymphoma, leukemia, or meningeal metastases. The intrathecal device delivers chemotherapeutic agents at regular intervals and also provides greater patient mobility and freedom from repeated lumbar punctures. It is also used to administer antibiotics to patients with CNS infections.

EPIDURAL ADMINISTRATION

Using the epidural route requires that a catheter be placed into the spinal column via a lumbar puncture. Physicians use the epidural route to administer anesthesia and narcotic analgesics, such as morphine. The route is also used postoperatively. Patients in intensive care units often require epidural catheters. The procedure for injecting or infusing medication via the epidural catheter follows that used for the I.V. route. The epidural route requires much lower doses of medication than the I.V. route; in addition, the effects of the medication last longer.

DERMAL ADMINISTRATION

The dermal route is also referred to as the dermatomucosal route and, more frequently, the topical route. Physicians and nurses usually use dermal medications for their local rather than systemic effects. One of several exceptions, nitroglycerin is given via the dermal route for its systemic rather than local effect.

Medication forms given via the dermal route include creams, lotions, ointments, powders, and patches. The medication is absorbed through the epidermal layer into the dermis. The extent of absorption depends upon the vascularity of and circulation in the region. After applying a cream, lotion, or ointment, the nurse should usually rub the medication into the patient's skin. Powders should not be rubbed into the skin. Patches contain a measured dose of medication that is delivered over an extended time. Medications in patch form include nitroglycerin, scopolamine, clonidine, and estrogen. The nurse should apply the patch over clean, dry skin. Removal of excessive hair will ensure proper absorption. The drug is released through a thin membrane or from a gel base in the patch.

For the dermal administration of a cream, the nurse will need one to three bedsaver pads, one pair of nonsterile gloves, one sterile tongue depressor, and a jar of the ordered cream. The nurse follows these steps to administer the cream: (1) Identify the patient, explain the procedure, and close the patient's door or draw the curtains for privacy. Protect the bed linens with bedsaver pads. (2) Assist the patient into a comfortable position and expose the area (or a section, if the whole body is to be covered) where the cream will be applied. Check for cream residue from previous applications, and remove any residue with clear water and a sterile gauze pad. Mineral oil may also be used to remove residue. (3) Put on the nonsterile gloves. Using a sterile tongue depressor, remove an ample amount of cream from the container. The tongue depressor helps prevent the introduction of bacteria into the container. Rub the cream between the fingers to warm it. Apply the cream beginning in the midline and work downward. Massage the cream to improve its absorption. Use a new sterile tongue depressor to remove additional cream from the container as necessary. Finally, use the sterile gauze pad to remove any excess cream from the patient's skin. (See Chapter 78, Integumentary System Agents, for an illustration of the application patterns for topical agents.)

Nitroglycerin is prepared in ointment form and supplied in a tube. The chest, upper arm, and upper back are frequently used administration sites. Other sites, such as the lower leg or abdomen, are also acceptable if cutaneous circulation is adequate. Administration sites should be rotated to decrease cutaneous irritation. Applying nitroglycerin involves several special considerations. (See Chapter 36, Antianginal Agents, for a depiction of this special process.)

NASAL AND SINUS ADMINISTRATION

The nurse administers both liquid and powdered forms of medications via the patient's nose and sinuses by instillation or by an atomizer or nasal aerosol device. Vasoconstrictors represent one kind of drug frequently administered by this route. (See Chapter 46, Decongestant Agents, for instructions on instilling medication into the nose and sinuses.)

The nasal aerosol device is not frequently used. The technique for its use resembles that for the atomizer and drop instillation methods. The package insert provides specific information regarding the administration technique for this device.

OPHTHALMIC ADMINISTRATION

Liquid and ointment medications are administered topically into the eye. The nurse usually instills liquid medications by the drop method. (See *Ophthalmic agent administration,* Chapter 79, Ophthalmic Agents, for an illustration and explanation of this procedure.)

URETHRAL ADMINISTRATION

Physicians and nurses most frequently use urethral administration for local antibiotic or antifungal therapy. Using sterile technique, the nurse instills the liquid medication into the urethra through a small-diameter urinary catheter. The nurse then removes or clamps the catheter so the medication can reach and bathe the bladder walls. How long the catheter remains clamped determines the duration of medication retention in the bladder. Occasionally, an intracath (the type used for intravenous administration), with the needle removed, is inserted into the urethra for the instillation of liquid medication. Severe cases of epididymitis may be treated in this manner.

Urethral administration may be repeated several times a day for about a week or only performed once. For repeated treatment, the nurse will probably use a special urinary catheter with an extra lumen for medication instillation. The volume of medication can range from a few milliliters to almost a liter.

VAGINAL ADMINISTRATION

Vaginal administration is used for topical antibiotic or antifungal medications, either in liquid or suppository form. When administering drugs in liquid form, the nurse performs what is frequently called a douche or vaginal irrigation. The procedure resembles that used for a rectal retention enema except for the use of a special vaginal catheter. (See the section on rectal drugs for a description of the procedure for a retention enema.) When the nurse inserts the catheter tip into the vagina, the patient should be on a bedpan or toilet, because no sphincter controls the vagina and the fluid will flow immediately out of the vaginal vault.

To administer a vaginal suppository, the nurse will need the ordered medication and its applicator, gloves, a sheet or drape, water-soluble lubricant, a paper towel, cotton balls, a bedsaver pad, and soap and water. The nurse should: (1) Identify the patient and explain the procedure and medication. Then close the door or pull the curtains to ensure privacy. Instruct the patient to lie on her back with her feet flat on the bed and knees apart. Place the bedsaver pad under her buttocks and cover her knees with the sheet or drape. (2) Expose the perineal area. Using one cotton ball per stroke, cleanse the perineum with soap and water. Cleanse the center last while spreading the labia. Place some lubricant onto the paper towel, and lubricate the suppository. (3) Spread the labia with one hand, and insert the applicator

Inserting a vaginal suppository

Before inserting a suppository, the nurse identifies the patient by checking her armband and name tag and states the drug's name and action. To administer the suppository, the nurse will need these supplies: the prescribed medication (suppository, cream, ointment, tablet, or gel), applicator, sterile gloves, water-soluble gel, a paper towel, bedpan, bedsaver pad, several cotton balls, perineal pads, drape, and soap and water. The nurse should provide for the patient's privacy and explain the procedure to her. Ask her to empty her bladder.

Help the patient lie down, with her knees flexed and legs spread apart. Place a bedsaver pad under the patient to protect the bed linen, and drape over her legs, leaving only her perineum exposed.

To administer a vaginal suppository, insert the medication into the applicator, lubricate the applicator tip (and suppository, if applicable), advance it about 2 inches (5 cm) into the vagina, and then depress the plunger of the applicator to deposit the suppository.

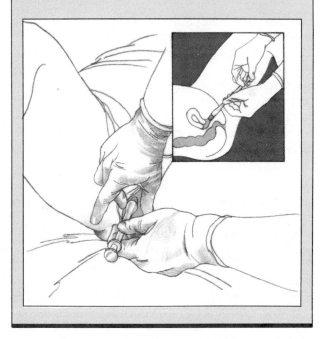

into the vagina with the other. Advance the applicator about 2 inches (5 cm) while angling it toward the sacrum. (See *Inserting a vaginal suppository* for an illustration of this procedure.) Release the labia and push the plunger, releasing the suppository from the applicator. (4) Remove the applicator and wipe any excess lubricant from the perineum. Instruct the patient to remain supine for about 30 minutes to retain the suppository. (5) Provide patient with tissues to wipe away any unabsorbed medication present upon assuming an upright position.

RESPIRATORY ADMINISTRATION

Almost all drugs given via the respiratory route produce a systemic effect because of the rich blood supply in the lungs. The drug forms administered via this route include gas, such as oxygen; liquid, such as isoproterenol; and powder, such as cromolyn sodium.

Powder is administered with a turbo inhaler. The nurse places a capsule of powdered drug inside the inhaler, and the patient inhales deeply through the mouth. As a result, the contents of the capsule are delivered in a fine powdered form to the lungs.

Nebulization is another frequently used method for administering drugs via the respiratory route. The two major kinds of nebulizers are the updraft nebulizer and the metered-dose nebulizer or inhaler. The updraft nebulizer uses a small volume of medication (usually under 1 ml) combined with about 3 ml of saline solution. Air forced through the nebulizer delivers the medication in a fine mist, which the patient inhales by breathing deeply through a mouthpiece attached to the nebulizer.

Administering drugs via a metered-dose nebulizer requires only the nebulizer, which is prefilled by the manufacturer with several doses of the drug. Each patient receives an individual nebulizer filled with the appropriate medication and dose. (See *Cromolyn sodium* in Unit Nine Introduction for instructions on using the metered-dose aerosol and turbo inhaler.)

CHAPTER SUMMARY

Chapter 10 presented the different drug forms and routes of administration, including detailed descriptions of techniques used for the different routes. Here are the highlights of the chapter:

- The major drug forms include solids, liquids, suppositories, and inhalants. The form of a drug affects the way the patient utilizes the drug.
- Drugs are packaged in the unit-dose format (one dose in a labeled container) and bulk style (multiple doses in a labeled container).

- Solids include tablets, capsules, enteric-coated tablets, and wax matrix tablets. Solid drug forms are given orally and via the sublingual and buccal routes.
- Liquids include syrups, tinctures, elixirs, and suspensions. Liquids are administered orally or parenterally via injection.
- Suppositories are administered via the rectal and vaginal routes.
- The technique for administering an enema depends on whether the drug requires retention.
- Inhalants are either powdered or liquid forms of a drug, which are administered via the respiratory route using either an updraft or metered-dose nebulizer.
- Most medications are administered via the oral route because it is the safest, most convenient, and most economical. Other administration routes include sublingual and buccal, rectal, parenteral, dermal, nasal, ophthalmic, urethral, vaginal, and respiratory.
- Enteric-coated and wax matrix tablets should not be crushed because doing so alters the drug action and may result in irritation to the esophageal and gastric mucosa.
- Buccal and sublingual medications are absorbed into the bloodstream without going through the GI tract.
- Parenteral medications are administered via intradermal, subcutaneous, intra-articular, intramuscular, and intravenous routes. Rotating injection sites improves absorption and minimizes patient discomfort.
- Parenteral liquids are packaged in vials, ampules, and self-contained or prefilled syringes. Parenteral medications often come in powdered form and must be reconstituted prior to administration.
- The nurse must match the type of syringe and appropriate needle size with the correct parenteral administration route. Alcohol is the substance most frequently used to cleanse the skin before administration of parenteral medications.
- Intravenous medications may be administered as a bolus, intermittent infusion, or continuous infusion. Infusion pumps may be used to deliver intravenous medications.
- Intrathecal administration delivers medication to the brain through an access device implanted under the scalp.
- Epidural administration delivers medication to the spinal cord through a catheter.
- Medications administered via the dermal route include creams, lotions, ointments, powders, patches, and pastes.

• Nasal drops and ophthalmic medications are administered topically into the nose and eyes.

• Urethral administration is frequently used for local antibiotic and antifungal therapy and involves instillation of liquid medication through a catheter.

BIBLIOGRAPHY

Birdsall, C., and Uretsby, S. "How Do I Administer Medication by NG?" *American Journal of Nursing* 84:1259, October 1984.

Brenner, Z., et al. "Effects of Alternative Techniques of Low-dose Heparin Administration on Hematoma Formation," *Heart and Lung* 10:657, July/August 1981.

Chaplin, G., et al. "How Safe is the Air Bubble Technique for I.M. Injections?" *Nursing85* 15:59, July 1985.

Giving Medications. Nursing Photobook series. Springhouse, Pa.: Springhouse Corporation, 1984.

Goodman, M., and Wickham, R. "Venous Access Devices: An Overview," *Oncology Nursing Forum* 2:16, September/October 1984.

Hubbard, S., and Seipp, C. "Administering Cancer Treatment: The Role of the Oncology Nurse," *Hospital Practice* 20:167, July 15, 1985.

Intramuscular Injections: A Guide to Sites and Technique. Philadelphia: Wyeth Laboratories, 1985.

Monahan, F. "When Swallowing Pills is Difficult," *Geriatric Nursing* 5:88, March/April 1984.

Vanbree, N., et al. "Clinical Evaluation of Three Techniques for Administering Low-Dose Heparin," *Nursing Research* 33:15, January/February 1984.

Winfrey, A. "Single Dose I.M. Injections: How Much is Too Much?" *Nursing85* 15:38, July 1985.

Zenk, K.E. "Medication Error Caused by Use of Technique for Intramuscular Injection," *American Journal of Hospital Pharmacy* 40:1154, July 1983.

INTERVENTION: PATIENT EDUCATION

OBJECTIVES

After reading and studying this chapter, you should be able to:

1. Explain how patient characteristics, including demographic, physiologic, and psychosocial factors, influence patient compliance.

2. Describe how the nurse-patient relationship and the therapeutic regimen affect compliance.

3. Describe how the operant conditioning theory, Gestalt-cognitive theory, humanistic theory, and social learning theory influence the nurse's development of a teaching plan.

4. Differentiate between learning and teaching principles in describing how the nurse uses them to develop and implement a teaching plan.

5. Explain why patient education is the responsibility of the entire health care team.

6. Explain why documenting patient-teaching procedures and results is important.

INTRODUCTION

Chapter 11 addresses the importance of patient education in fostering compliance. The chapter also covers learning-teaching theories and learning principles as well as the role of the nursing process in patient education. Whether providing comprehensive care in the hospital or follow-up home care, the nurse must educate the patient about procedures, hospital routines, and prescribed drug regimens.

In today's climate of tightly controlled hospital costs, patient education plays a critical role in ensuring optimal patient recovery despite limited hospital reimbursement, increased patient acuity, and decreased lengths of stay. A nurse's educational background and constant contact with a patient and significant others create an ideal environment for patient education. Thus, the nurse has

become a primary resource for teaching patients the importance of taking responsibility for their own health care, including compliance.

Working in a health care environment characterized by decreased lengths of stay, the nurse must often care for patients too debilitated to learn or so swiftly discharged that the nurse has inadequate time for patient education. This should not discourage nurses, however: Miller and Shank (1986) have found that groups of patients educated by nurses displayed an increased level of compliance compared to other groups.

COMPLIANCE

To achieve the optimal effects from drug therapy, the patient must comply with the prescribed regimen. *Compliance* describes the extent to which a patient follows medical or health advice about taking drugs, following diets, or implementing life-style changes. Many factors, categorized as either patient characteristics or clinical characteristics, can affect patient compliance. (See *Compliance characteristics* for a summary of the following discussion.)

PATIENT CHARACTERISTICS

Patient characteristics include demographic factors, physiologic factors, and psychosocial factors. How these factors influence patient compliance is discussed below.

Demographic factors

Demographic factors include the patient's age, sex, culture or race, and educational level. Although the relationship between such factors and compliance has not

Compliance characteristics

This table lists patient and clinical characteristics that affect patient compliance. Understanding these characteristics helps the nurse develop and implement effective patient education programs.

Patient characteristics

Demographic factors
- Age
- Sex
- Culture or race
- Educational level

Physiologic factors
- Disease severity
- Disease duration
- Knowledge of disease

Psychosocial factors
- Support systems
- Locus of control
- Attitudes and beliefs
- Participation in prescribed treatment

Clinical characteristics

Nurse-patient relationship
- Patient satisfaction
- Communication
- Caring
- Effective use of time

Therapeutic regimen
- Complexity
- Cost
- Adverse reactions
- Impact on patient's life-style

Adapted with permission of Aspen Publishers, Inc., from McCord, M.A. *Topics in Clinical Nursing,* "Compliance: Self-Care or Compromise," vol. 4, January 1986.

been clearly established, the nurse should consider them when developing the patient's teaching plan. This approach can also help the nurse present information at the appropriate level for each patient.

Physiologic factors

Physiologic factors include the severity and duration of the disease state as well as the patient's knowledge about it. The relationship between each of these factors and compliance varies; duration is the only physiologic factor that has been clearly shown to affect compliance. In contrast, disease severity has not been found to alter patient compliance significantly.

Duration of disease does affect compliance. For example, a patient with chronic renal failure or chronic lung disease usually takes a multitude of drugs for extended periods of time, sometimes for life. In comparison, a patient with a bladder infection may take only a 14- or 21-day course of antibiotics. The patient requiring the longer duration of treatment is less likely to maintain compliance and—lacking an adequate understanding of the prescribed therapy's desired outcome—may stop taking medications if the disease appears to progress.

Research findings relating the patient's knowledge of the disease state to compliance remain controversial: some studies find no positive correlation. Although controversy remains, the nurse can probably improve patient compliance by assessing and evaluating the patient's learning needs in relation to the patient's knowledge of the disease state and drug regimen.

Psychosocial factors

Support systems, locus of control, patient attitudes and beliefs, and patient participation in treatment are important psychosocial factors that affect compliance. A patient with a strong support system of family members and/or significant others usually maintains high self-esteem, which promotes compliance.

A patient's locus of control also affects compliance. Individuals with an *internal* locus of control, feeling they control their own lives, will seek medical information and follow treatment regimens. Patients with an *external* locus of control believe that factors such as fate, chance, and luck control their lives. These patients are less likely to seek medical information and less likely to be compliant than patients with an internal locus of control.

Positive attitudes and beliefs also strongly affect compliance. For example, a patient who believes that the benefits of a prescribed regimen outweigh its disadvantages, such as adverse effects and high cost, usually is compliant. In addition, patients who have a positive outlook for recovery and accept responsibility for their care tend to be more compliant than patients with negative attitudes.

Increased patient participation in the prescribed therapy and increased contact with the health care professional may positively affect compliance. For example, a patient who is taught self-regulation of insulin dosage should monitor blood glucose levels. After initial instruction, the patient should demonstrate the proper method of checking blood glucose levels. Then, during the 1st week at home, the patient should call in the daily blood glucose levels and obtain the required insulin dosage. During the next step, the patient should receive different blood glucose ranges with corresponding insulin dosages. The patient should also keep a log of blood glucose levels and amounts of insulin administered and share this information with the nurse weekly, then monthly, then as needed.

CLINICAL CHARACTERISTICS

Like patient characteristics, clinical characteristics can affect patient compliance. The nurse must consider them when planning and implementing patient teaching. The two major groups of clinical characteristics are the nurse-patient relationship and the therapeutic regimen.

Nurse-patient relationship

Factors that constitute the nurse-patient relationship include patient satisfaction and communication. A nurse-patient relationship characterized by a trusting, informative interaction promotes patient satisfaction—and compliance. The nurse who communicates a sense of concern for the patient's well-being instills confidence and trust in the patient—also a key to compliance.

Because of increased patient acuity and shorter hospital stays, the nurse must use time with the patient wisely and creatively to teach the patient while providing care. For example, while administering a medication, the nurse can educate the patient about it, including any adverse reactions that must be reported.

Therapeutic regimen

The therapeutic regimen affects a patient's compliance through its complexity, cost, and adverse reactions; the patient's life-style also affects compliance. Complex drug regimens often lead to patient noncompliance: the patient may become discouraged by the variety of schedules when taking multiple medications, such as theophylline twice daily, digoxin daily, beclomethasone dipropionate inhaler 2 puffs three times a day, and prednisone daily. Even taking one drug several times a day, such as penicillin four times a day, can lead to noncompliance.

The effects of a drug regimen's cost and adverse reactions on patient compliance remain controversial. Some studies have shown that decreased cost leads to increased patient compliance; however, other studies find no such relationship. The same mixed results have

occurred in studies of adverse reactions. If the patient views the adverse reactions as being unexpected or more traumatic than the disease, noncompliance may occur.

The patient whose life-style routines are interrupted by the prescribed drug regimen may become noncompliant. For example, suppose a telephone operator is scheduled to take digoxin at breakfast time, warfarin sodium at 2 p.m., isosorbide dinitrate four times a day (at 8 a.m., 1 p.m., 6 p.m., and 10 p.m.), and furosemide at 9 a.m. During work hours, 7 a.m. to 4 p.m., the patient must take four medications at different times. In addition, the patient will need to void frequently for several hours after taking furosemide. These interruptions may disturb the work schedule to such an extent that the patient may believe job performance is compromised and self-esteem is lost. Such conditions promote noncompliance. To avoid interfering with the patient's routine when establishing a drug regimen, the nurse or physician discusses the times most convenient for the patient to take medication.

TEACHING AND LEARNING THEORIES AND PRINCIPLES

When assessing, developing, and implementing patient teaching, the nurse should be aware of the prevalent major teaching-learning theories. The following section covers the operant conditioning theory, Gestalt-cognitive theory, humanistic theory, and social learning theory. Each presents a different perspective of teaching and improving learning, but all focus on the ability to acquire knowledge and change behaviors. The nurse may combine several theories to formulate a patient-teaching plan.

OPERANT CONDITIONING THEORY

The operant conditioning theory focuses on providing rewards, or reinforcements, to produce the desired behavior in the patient. Using this theory, the nurse rewards wanted behavior but not unwanted. Withholding the reward moves the patient toward correcting unwanted behavior.

To use operant conditioning, the nurse divides an expected patient behavior into several small steps building toward the goal. Success at each step is rewarded to ensure that learning occurs. This step-by-step progression structures patient learning and provides the nurse with specific criteria for evaluating the patient's success. The operant conditioning theory also provides many opportunities for compliance-promoting interactions between nurse and patient. According to this theory, learning occurs more quickly if reinforcements are given at each step, and retention is prolonged if rewards are given intermittently once the patient has learned the behavior.

For example, the nurse may use operant conditioning when instructing a patient about self-administration of an intravenous antibiotic. Such a program might involve the following steps: (1) determining the supplies needed for administration of the antibiotic, (2) gathering all the desired supplies, (3) washing the hands, (4) connecting the intravenous tubing to the antibiotic bag, (5) connecting the needle to the tubing, (6) priming the tubing with the fluid, (7) cleansing the I.V. access site with alcohol, (8) inserting the needle into the access site, (9) turning on and timing the infusion, and (10) securing the tubing in place with tape. As the patient successfully demonstrates each step, the nurse provides a reward in the form of positive reinforcement. This varies with each patient and nurse and might include oral or written praise or a more tangible reward, such as a button or sticker that publicizes the patient's success.

GESTALT-COGNITIVE THEORY

The key components of the Gestalt-cognitive theory are the patient's cognitive and problem-solving abilities. Cognitive abilities (thinking) help the patient understand concepts, so this theory focuses on the way a patient thinks—on understanding the relationships necessary to learn information and make expected behavioral changes. According to this theory, each patient's perceptions are based on physical factors, such as diseases, as well as on social and environmental interactions. For this reason, the nurse must carefully assess these factors and use this assessment data when organizing and presenting information to the patient. How the nurse presents information is a key variable, because cognitive processes are structured hierarchically (progressing from simple to complex), which allows learning to occur. The nurse should present information to be learned in a logical, sequential manner.

When using the Gestalt-cognitive theory, the nurse must accurately assess the patient's cognitive level as it relates to the material being taught. For example, the nurse developing a teaching plan for a patient taking quinidine sulfate every 6 hours needs to find out if the patient has ever taken quinidine sulfate (or any other

medication). This information provides a reference point for teaching. The nurse would also assess the patient's education level, age, and occupation to develop a teaching plan meaningful to the patient.

The teaching plan for quinidine sulfate would focus on the importance of the drug's therapeutic effects on the patient. In discussing the drug schedule, the nurse would explain that around-the-clock dosing maintains therapeutic blood levels to prevent dysrhythmias.

Once the nurse has accurately assessed the patient's cognitive level, the stage is set for presenting the patient-teaching material in a logical sequence and relating the material to the patient's age and background.

HUMANISTIC THEORY

The humanistic theory focuses on the patient as a total being, emphasizing emotional status over cognitive ability. In applying this theory, the nurse serves as a resource person who helps patients become aware of their attitudes, feelings, and values. Such awareness increases the patient's ability to deal with life and make the appropriate behavioral changes for successful health care. To use the humanistic theory, the nurse should develop a friendly, nonthreatening, and trusting relationship with the patient and offer support.

Using this approach in patient teaching, the nurse must be careful not to control the learning situation. Instead, the nurse should encourage the patient to discover learning experiences independently as they arise from increased self-awareness. For example, a nurse might incorporate the humanistic theory into teaching a patient who has recently had coronary bypass surgery and has subsequently developed cardiac dysrhythmias. The nurse would focus on developing a trusting relationship with the patient and would help explore the patient's values and feelings about the dysrhythmias and the drugs needed to control them. The nurse would also serve as an information resource, offering various teaching materials, such as written or oral information, to help the patient clarify or, if necessary, change attitudes toward the prescribed regimen.

SOCIAL LEARNING THEORY

The social learning theory, focusing on imitation and role taking or modeling, is based on the belief that much of behavior is shaped by social (role) models. The patient's response to role models may be conscious or unconscious. Using this theory, the nurse serves as a role model and may provide additional role models to help the patient alter or learn health behaviors. The nurse may also incorporate strategies from the other teaching-learning theories, such as operant conditioning (offering rewards as reinforcement for desired behavior) or the Gestalt-cognitive theory (structuring information based on the patient's cognitive ability).

The nurse can use a variety of teaching tools, including live models (other people with the same illness), a series of still pictures, a slide-audio tape program (a slide show narrated by an audiotape), written and illustrated examples, or video presentations. For example, when instructing a patient before discharge about the use of a bronchial inhaler, the nurse would first separate the procedure into several steps. The nurse would next demonstrate each step several times, allowing the patient to observe, and then have the patient demonstrate it with the nurse's guidance. Before discharge, the patient would demonstrate the procedure without guidance. (See *Major learning theories* for a comparison of the theories discussed in this chapter.)

LEARNING PRINCIPLES

Using learning principles strengthens patient teaching by providing information about factors that influence patient learning. The following discussion covers important learning principles.

The patient needs to be motivated to learn. This principle stresses the importance of the nurse's awareness of the patient's motivation level. The nurse may try different activities or approaches to encourage the patient to learn about the drug regimen, but success ultimately depends on the patient's motivation to learn: without adequate motivation, the patient is less likely to retain and use information. The nurse can increase the patient's motivation by knowing the patient and applying the Gestalt-cognitive theory.

Physical and emotional readiness are essential for learning. This principle focuses on the patient's physical, intellectual, and emotional capabilities, which the nurse must assess. For example, with a patient recovering from a recent cerebrovascular accident, the nurse would assess any residual effects that might interfere with learning ability—such as receptive aphasia, right-sided paralysis, fatigue, pain, anxiety, and adverse reactions to prescribed drugs (especially analgesics). All these factors can affect the patient's physical and emotional readiness to learn.

Active participation can be critical to learning. The most effective way for the patient to develop new skills

Major learning theories

This chart compares the major learning theories and outlines the nurse's role in those theories.

OPERANT CONDITIONING THEORY	GESTALT-COGNITIVE THEORY	HUMANISTIC THEORY	SOCIAL LEARNING THEORY
(Skinner, Watson, and Guthrie)	(Ausubel, Bruner, and Piaget)	(Rogers and Kohl)	(Bandura and Walters)
Premise	**Premise**	**Premise**	**Premise**
The expected behavioral change is produced by a system of rewards (reinforcements). This is a structured and controlled approach.	The focus is on the patient's cognitive, or thinking, abilities. The patient's cognitive processes and organization are key elements.	The focus is on the patient's whole being, with an emphasis on emotional aspects. The patient ultimately determines what information to learn and how to learn it. A strong nurse-patient relationship is essential.	Learning occurs by means of imitation (role modeling). Behavior is shaped by social models and may be a conscious or unconscious effort on the part of the learner.
Nurse's role	**Nurse's role**		**Nurse's role**
Develop the structure for the expected behavior. Break the task into successive steps. Provide rewards (reinforcement) to promote learning.	Assess the patient's cognitive abilities. Present information in an organized, logical sequence, progressing from simple to complex.	**Nurse's role** Facilitate learning by helping the patient become aware of attitudes, feelings, and values so that adjustments can occur. Develop a friendly, trusting relationship that creates a nonthreatening learning environment.	Act as a role model or provide role models to aid the patient in learning the desired behavior.

or change behavioral patterns is to take an active role in the education process. For example, a patient who is to administer intravenous antibiotics at home can learn this function more efficiently by practicing with the appropriate materials and demonstrating the proper procedure to the nurse. The patient can use this method to learn psychomotor skills (how to mix the antibiotic solution) as well as cognitive information (how much drug to mix and administer over what period of time).

Learning should be based on prior experiences and knowledge. Learning is more effective when it builds on ideas and practices familiar to the patient. That is why assessing the patient's educational level, occupation, and cultural or ethnic beliefs is so important: doing so helps the nurse determine the type and level of information to include in patient teaching. For example, if assessment data indicate that a diabetic patient's mother was also a diabetic, the nurse should question the patient to see what was learned from that experience and build on it.

Learning is more effective when knowledge can be applied immediately. For example, when instructing a patient to monitor pulse rate before digoxin administration, the nurse should demonstrate the procedure for counting a pulse rate while explaining the steps to follow. Then the nurse should have the patient demonstrate the procedure. This allows the nurse to give immediate feedback to enhance patient learning.

Information presented to the patient must be congruent with the patient's expectations and goals. Before beginning patient teaching, the nurse should assess the patient's expectations and goals for the prescribed therapy. The nurse's goals must incorporate the patient's—and the patient must feel secure in this—before the patient will readily receive and learn information. The nurse should discuss the patient's goals and expectations at each teaching session. For example, the nurse may be focusing teaching on cast care for a patient with a full leg cast and crutches who is most concerned about how to go up and down steps. Instead, the nurse should assess the patient's expectations and goals and adjust the teaching plan accordingly.

Repetition can reinforce learning. The amount of repetition needed to learn new information or behavior varies from patient to patient. Repetition not only gives the patient opportunities to practice but also allows for feedback between nurse and patient. Thus, repetition reinforces the patient's ability to learn, retain, and use the new information.

TEACHING PRINCIPLES

To develop and implement effective patient education, the nurse needs to be aware of principles that influence teaching techniques and strategies. The following section presents important teaching principles.

Establishing nurse-patient rapport aids patient teaching. The patient's relationship with the nurse can significantly affect patient compliance. If the patient and nurse establish an effective, therapeutic rapport, the nurse will be better able to assess the patient's learning needs and to identify the most effective teaching strategies.

Effective communication is essential. Earlier in this chapter, the importance of communication regarding compliance was discussed along with the need for nurses to express caring and concern for patients. When presenting new information, the nurse needs to assess the patient's educational level, occupation, and vocabulary to ensure that the information is being presented at an appropriate level. Many patients become noncompliant because they misunderstand the instructions and actions of the health care professional.

Environmental control can influence teaching effectiveness. Noise level, temperature, lighting, and patient privacy and comfort can enhance or interfere with the effectiveness of a teaching session. These factors are not always under the nurse's control, but whenever possible, the nurse should take action to minimize distracting factors that could interfere with the patient's ability to participate in the teaching session. The goal is to make both patient and nurse as comfortable as possible.

Behavioral objectives can guide the teaching session and aid in evaluation. Behavioral objectives, or outcome criteria, are a critical component of each teaching plan; they serve as guidelines for the nurse and the patient. By developing objectives, the nurse determines what needs to be covered in the teaching sessions. By allowing the patient to participate in development of the objectives, the nurse promotes patient motivation and informs the patient of the expected outcomes of the teaching session. After the session, the objectives serve as a basis for evaluating the effectiveness of the teaching and learning. Predeveloped teaching plans with objectives and content outlines that can be adapted to specific patients are available.

Nursing process and patient teaching

This flow chart demonstrates the steps of patient teaching as they relate to the nursing process.

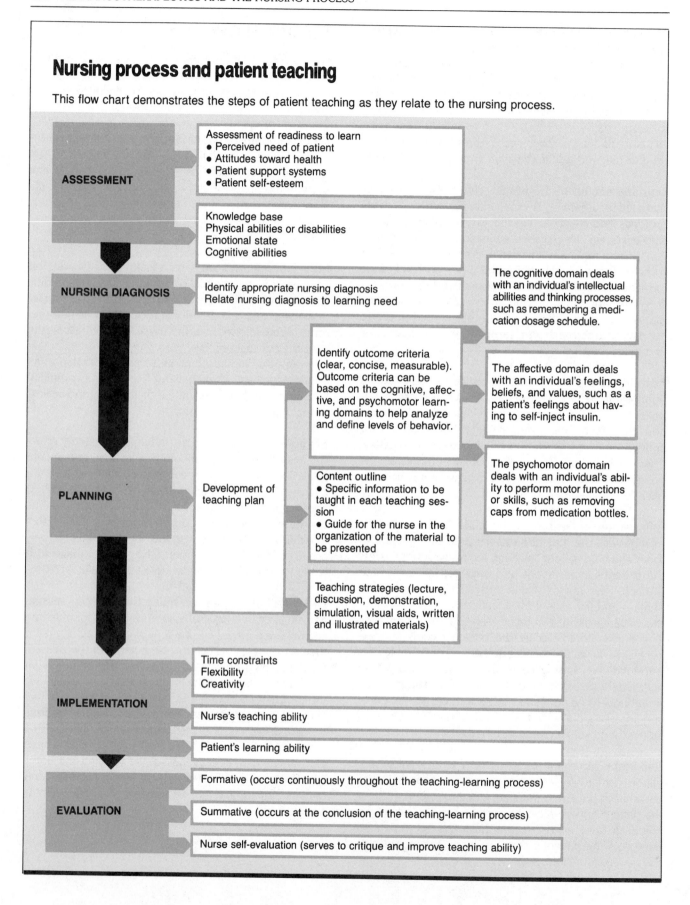

ASSESSMENT

Assessment of readiness to learn
- Perceived need of patient
- Attitudes toward health
- Patient support systems
- Patient self-esteem

Knowledge base
Physical abilities or disabilities
Emotional state
Cognitive abilities

NURSING DIAGNOSIS

Identify appropriate nursing diagnosis
Relate nursing diagnosis to learning need

The cognitive domain deals with an individual's intellectual abilities and thinking processes, such as remembering a medication dosage schedule.

PLANNING

Development of teaching plan

Identify outcome criteria (clear, concise, measurable). Outcome criteria can be based on the cognitive, affective, and psychomotor learning domains to help analyze and define levels of behavior.

The affective domain deals with an individual's feelings, beliefs, and values, such as a patient's feelings about having to self-inject insulin.

Content outline
- Specific information to be taught in each teaching session
- Guide for the nurse in the organization of the material to be presented

The psychomotor domain deals with an individual's ability to perform motor functions or skills, such as removing caps from medication bottles.

Teaching strategies (lecture, discussion, demonstration, simulation, visual aids, written and illustrated materials)

IMPLEMENTATION

Time constraints
Flexibility
Creativity

Nurse's teaching ability

Patient's learning ability

EVALUATION

Formative (occurs continuously throughout the teaching-learning process)

Summative (occurs at the conclusion of the teaching-learning process)

Nurse self-evaluation (serves to critique and improve teaching ability)

Cultural, ethnic, and religious beliefs must be considered in planning teaching sessions. Cultural, ethnic, and religious beliefs can significantly influence the success of a teaching plan; the nurse must collect the appropriate data during assessment. For example, in some cultures men are expected to maintain a rugged, strong image. They may view illness as a weakness and, therefore, deny it. Learning will not take place until the patient can resolve his self-image conflict.

Evaluation is an essential part of the teaching process. Evaluation enables the nurse to determine how effective the teaching was and what the patient gained from it. Evaluation can also help the nurse identify areas where additional teaching is needed and determine the effectiveness of teaching strategies, such as lectures, discussions, and role playing. The overall purpose of evaluation is to strengthen the teaching-learning process.

NURSING PROCESS AND PATIENT EDUCATION

The nursing process serves as the basic framework for developing, implementing, and evaluating a teaching program. The nurse uses the nursing process to assess patient learning needs; to develop a nursing diagnosis; to develop a teaching plan that includes objectives, a teaching content outline, and teaching strategies; to implement the plan; and to evaluate the teaching and learning that occurred.

The Teaching Plan

Development of a teaching plan is an essential part of the education process. Each teaching plan includes outcome criteria or behavioral objectives, teaching content, teaching strategies, and evaluation methods.

Outcome criteria. Outcome criteria are the desired patient behaviors or responses that result from the teaching. They guide and focus the teaching and serve as evaluation criteria.

Outcome criteria fall into three learning domains: cognitive, affective, and psychomotor. Within each domain, levels of behavior progress from simple to complex.

The cognitive domain addresses an individual's intellectual abilities and thinking processes. For example, the learner would be expected to know the actions and adverse effects of medications. The affective domain addresses an individual's feelings, beliefs, and values. In this domain, for example, the patient expresses feelings and beliefs about how medications affect daily routines and life-style. The psychomotor domain addresses an individual's ability to perform motor functions or skills, such as giving insulin injections. The level of the taxonomy helps determine the outcome criteria and the type of teaching strategies necessary.

Teaching content outline. The content outline identifies the specific information to teach in each session. Detail varies with the learner's needs and the teacher's knowledge of the topic. A more complete outline decreases the probability of omitting important ideas and information.

Teaching strategies. The teaching strategies selected, such as lecture, discussion, demonstration, or simulation, depend on the patient and the content. The learning domains can assist in determining the type of teaching strategies. The nurse may need to use more than one teaching method to enhance learning. For example, when instructing an individual about the importance of monitoring the pulse rate and blood pressure before administering propranolol, the nurse may use various teaching methods or strategies, because the greater the number of senses (sight, hearing, touch) that the learner uses in the session, the greater the retention of information.

Media selection is another important component to consider. When selecting different types of media, the nurse needs to remember the focus of the presentation. The selected media should support major concepts and highlight essential ideas.

When selecting learning materials for a patient, the nurse can go beyond prepackaged or published ones. The nurse's own informal materials, such as medication schedules, written lists, or drawings, also may be used. Whether the materials are prepackaged or handwritten, the nurse needs to verify that they are clear, concise, and written at the patient's level of understanding.

Evaluation. Evaluation, a critical component of the teaching plan, examines what the learner has accomplished. To evaluate the learner, the nurse uses outcome criteria or behavioral objectives. Behaviors specified in the outcome criteria determine how the evaluation should be conducted. For example, if the patient was to "state the action of digoxin at the end of the session," then the evaluation would be based on what the patient said; but if the patient was to "demonstrate how to mix NPH and regular insulin in one syringe," the evaluation would be based on what the patient did. Other forms

Sample teaching plan

The following sample presents a teaching plan for Mrs. Davis, a patient with cancer and the nursing diagnosis of knowledge deficit related to chemotherapy.

OUTCOME CRITERIA	CONTENT	TEACHING METHODS	EVALUATION
Mrs. Davis will state the major action of chemotherapy drugs after the initial teaching session. After the teaching session, Mrs. Davis will identify major adverse reactions to the chemotherapy drugs with 100% accuracy. Before discharge, Mrs. Davis will list the adverse reactions that warrant contacting the physician. By discharge time, Mrs. Davis will describe when she is at the greatest risk for infection.	Actions of chemotherapy drugs (fluorouracil, cisplatin): • attack and destroy the rapidly growing cancer cells • interfere with the ability of cancer cells to divide and grow. Adverse reactions to chemotherapy drugs: • occur mainly because chemotherapy drugs also affect other rapidly growing or dividing cells • most commonly involved areas include hair (alopecia), mucous membranes (mouth sores), GI tract (nausea, vomiting, diarrhea). Serious, unpredictable reactions: If any of the following occurs at home, the patient should contact her physician—chills, fever, sore throat, unusual bleeding or bruising, swelling of feet or legs, difficulty hearing. Other adverse reactions occur because of destruction of rapidly growing cells, including red blood cells, white blood cells, and platelets. • These adverse reactions cause fatigue and weakness and increase the risk of infection. • The patient needs to protect herself from persons who have infections and must take care to avoid injury that could cause bleeding. • The peak effect of these actions is 7 to 14 days after chemotherapy.	Use lecture and discussion format. Plan two sessions, each 15 minutes long: • first session to cover the major actions and adverse reactions of chemotherapy • second session to cover the remaining content information and review the first session's main points. Use a variety of media materials. • Give "Chemotherapy and You" slide-tape presentation • Give the patient the "Chemotherapy and You" book; underline the two drugs she is receiving.	After the initial teaching session, Mrs. Davis will be able to: • state the major actions of the chemotherapy drugs • select the major adverse reactions when provided with a list. By discharge time, Mrs. Davis will be able to: • list adverse reactions that warrant contacting the physician • describe when she is at risk for an infection.

of evaluation include paper and pencil tests, crossword puzzles, case studies, role playing, and simulations or games.

Two other types of evaluation use outcome criteria. Formative (or concurrent) evaluation occurs continuously throughout the teaching and learning process. One benefit of this type of evaluation is that the nurse can adjust teaching strategies as necessary to enhance learning. Summative (or retrospective) evaluation occurs at the conclusion of the teaching and learning session. This evaluation, where feedback is given at the end of the session, does not allow for adjustment until after teaching and learning are finished. (See *Nursing process and patient teaching*, page 194, for an illustration of how the nursing process helps structure patient education.)

Documentation

The nurse must document each teaching session in the patient's chart so that other nurses and members of the health care team know what was covered, what patient learning resulted, and what areas need refinement and/or further instruction. The nurse must remember that the patient's education is the concern of the entire health care team, each member having a different area of expertise: to provide optimal patient education, the nurse must work closely with all other members.

The chart is one method of sharing information. Other methods include informal health care team meetings, educational rounds, family conferences with the health care team, and discharge planning rounds. Above all, the patient's medical record must include complete documentation of all teaching efforts. (See *Sample teaching plan*, which incorporates the points covered in this chapter.)

CHAPTER SUMMARY

Chapter 11 covered the importance of patient education in fostering compliance. Various factors that can influence learning were also discussed. Here are the highlights of the chapter:

• The overall goal of patient education is to promote compliance.

• Factors that significantly influence patient compliance can be divided into two major categories: patient characteristics and clinical characteristics. Patient characteristics include demographic factors, physiologic factors, and psychosocial factors. Clinical characteristics include the nurse-patient relationship and the therapeutic regimen.

• Nurses can strengthen their teaching abilities by being aware of the major teaching and learning theories that describe the different ways patients learn. Important theories include the operant conditioning theory, Gestalt-cognitive theory, humanistic theory, and social learning theory. The nurse can use these theories separately or in combination during teaching sessions.

• The nurse should also be aware of the teaching principles that have been developed to strengthen the teaching plan and provide the nurse with information that can positively affect patient learning.

• To provide the most effective patient education, the nurse must develop a specific teaching plan for each patient. The nurse accomplishes this goal by first assessing the patient's learning needs. This assessment focuses on the patient's readiness to learn and knowledge base as well as on the patient's physical, intellectual, and emotional abilities. The initial assessment is critical, because subsequent steps and the potential effectiveness of the teaching plan depend on it.

• The nurse then identifies the nursing diagnosis based on the patient's established learning needs.

• Next, the nurse develops a teaching plan that consists of behavioral objectives, a content outline, specific teaching strategies, and evaluation methods. The teaching plan helps the nurse identify the content to be taught, patient goals and expectations, and the most effective teaching strategies.

• The evaluation step helps the nurse determine the effectiveness of the teaching session. The nurse can also assess which points need refinement and/or additional teaching.

• All members of the health care team participate in patient teaching, so the nurse must document all teaching sessions.

BIBLIOGRAPHY

Becker, M., and Marman, L. "Strategies for Enhancing Patient Compliance," *Journal of Community Health* 6:113, 1980.

Devine, E., and Cook, T. "Clinical and Cost-Saving Effects of Psychoeducational Interventions with Surgical Patients: A Meta-Analysis," *Research in Nursing and Health* 89, 1986.

Edwards, M., and Pathy, J. "Drug Counseling in the Elderly and Predicting Compliance," *The Practitioner* 228:291, 1984.

Eraker, S., et al. "Understanding and Improving Patient Compliance," *Annals of Internal Medicine* 100:258, 1984.

Felsenthal, G., et al. "Medication Education Program in an Inpatient Geriatric Rehabilitation Unit," *Arch. Phys. Med. Rehab.* 67:27, 1986.

Franz, R. "Selecting Media for Patient Education," *Topics in Clinical Nursing* 77, 1980.

Haynes, R.B., et al. *Compliance in Health Care.* Baltimore: Johns Hopkins University Press, 1979.

Huckabay, L. *Conditions of Learning and Instruction in Nursing.* St. Louis: C.V. Mosby Co., 1980.

McCord, M. "Compliance: Self-care or Compromise," *Topics in Clinical Nursing* 1, January 1986.

Miller, G., and Shank, J.C. "Patient Education: Comparative Effectiveness by Means of Presentation," *Family Practice* 22:178, 1986.

Moree, N. "Nurses Speak Out on Patients and Drug Regimens," *American Journal of Nursing* 51, January 1985.

Muhlenkamp, A., and Sayles, J. "Self-Esteem: Social Support and Positive Health Practices," *Nursing Research* 35:334, 1986.

Pohl, M. *Teaching Function of the Nursing Practitioner.* Wm. C. Brown Company Publishers, 1984.

Redman, B. *The Process of Patient Education.* St. Louis: C.V. Mosby Co., 1984.

Sackett, D., and Haynes, R.B. *Compliance with Therapeutic Regimens.* Baltimore: Johns Hopkins University Press, 1976.

Tarnow, K. "Working with Adult Learners," *Nurse Educator* 34, September/October 1979.

Wartman, S., et al. "Patient Understanding and Satisfaction as Predictors of Compliance," *Medical Care* 21:886, 1983.

Yoos, L. "Factors Influencing Maternal Compliance to Antibiotic Regimens," *Pediatric Nursing* 10:141, 1984.

Youssef, F. "Compliance with Therapeutic Regimens: A Follow-Up Study for Patients with Affective Disorders," *Journal of Advanced Nursing* 8:513, 1983.

CHAPTER 12

INTERVENTION: THE PEDIATRIC PATIENT

OBJECTIVES

After reading and studying this chapter, you should be able to:

1. Explain how absorption, distribution, metabolism, and excretion of a drug differ between a child and an adult.

2. Describe how a drug's pharmacodynamics and pharmacotherapeutics are influenced by a child's age and individual response to the drug and by the route of administration.

3. Calculate a correct pediatric dosage by weight and body-surface area.

4. Identify probable sources of drug toxicity for a pediatric patient.

5. Describe how to administer oral medications to children in different age-groups.

6. Select an appropriate intramuscular (I.M.) injection site and needle size for a pediatric patient.

7. Explain how to administer an intravenous (I.V.) medication safely to a pediatric patient.

8. Identify appropriate sites for subcutaneous (S.C.) drug administration in a child.

9. Describe how to apply a topical medication, and explain how its absorption may differ with the patient's age.

10. Explain why a drug may be given rectally, and tell how to administer it.

11. Explain how to administer eye, ear, and nose drops to a child.

12. Develop a plan for teaching a pediatric patient and family members about the child's medications.

INTRODUCTION

Children are not small adults. Although the medication administration routes for children and adults are the same, pediatric injection sites, administration techniques, and especially dosages can differ greatly. Medication dosages for pediatric patients cannot be derived or scaled down from adult dosages, because the pharmacokinet-ics, pharmacodynamics, and pharmacotherapeutics of drugs in children vary substantially from those in adults. Physiologic differences and immature body systems exaggerate these variances and make medication effects less predictable—sometimes even risky. So the nurse must base all drug therapy on the child's physiologic and psychosocial development.

PEDIATRIC PHARMACOLOGY

In a pediatric patient, many factors can influence the pharmacokinetic, pharmacodynamic, and pharmaco-therapeutic processes that occur in the body. (See Chapter 2, Pharmacokinetics; Chapter 3, Pharmacodynamics; and Chapter 4, Pharmacotherapeutics, for general information about these processes.)

PHARMACOKINETICS

A child's age, physiologic state, body composition, immature organ function, and other factors can affect the absorption, distribution, metabolism, and excretion of a drug.

Absorption

After a drug is administered orally, its absorption depends on the child's age, the underlying disease, the dosage form, and the presence of other drugs or foods taken concurrently.

In a young child, the gastric pH is higher, or less acidic, than in an adult. It drops to an adult level sometime between ages 3 and 7. Therefore, a child under age 3 will absorb more of those medications which react positively in a low-acid environment. For example, an infant would absorb more penicillin—a drug that is un-

Differences in body composition

Total body water and extracellular fluid volume differ by age-group. These differences can significantly affect a drug's distribution. In a neonate, for example, the area for drug distribution and fluid volumes are proportionately greater than those in an adult. Because most drugs travel through extracellular fluid to reach their receptors, a drug is likely to become less concentrated and less effective in a neonate as it becomes more widely distributed.

AGE-GROUP	TOTAL BODY WATER	EXTRACELLULAR FLUID VOLUME
Neonate	85% to 90%	35% to 40%
Infant	75%	35% to 40%
Child	64%	16% to 22%
Adult	59%	16%

stable in an acid environment—than an older child or an adult would. As the child develops, gastric pH decreases, acidity increases, and drug absorption is altered. Milk and formula can also affect gastric pH and may alter absorption. For these reasons, most pediatric medications are administered when the child's stomach is empty.

Several other factors can influence drug absorption from the gastrointestinal (GI) tract and make it less predictable and less efficient in a child under age 2. The shortness of the intestine and the presence of diarrhea can reduce the amount of time a drug is available for absorption. Decreased transit time through the GI tract can also decrease drug absorption.

Absorption of I.M. medications in infants may be unpredictable because of vasomotor instability, shock, and decreased muscle tone. Pain medications, such as morphine, are usually administered I.M. to children, producing analgesic effects in 30 to 45 minutes. When morphine is administered I.V., pain relief results within minutes. If I.V. morphine is given too rapidly, however, the child may experience a rapid decrease in respiratory rate—a risk less likely after I.M. administration because the morphine must be absorbed before it can be distributed.

A child in shock may absorb a drug poorly when it is given I.M., S.C., or topically, because shock decreases cardiac output and peripheral circulation. For this reason, most drugs are given I.V. to a child in shock.

A child will absorb a topical drug at about the same rate as an adult, but will absorb it more completely

because of a greater body-surface area relative to total body mass. An occlusive dressing will further enhance topical absorption. Because young children absorb more medication topically, they are more likely than adults to experience adverse reactions to some topical drugs. Steroid creams can cause mild to severe reactions, depending on the amount absorbed into the systemic circulation. These drugs can even suppress the pituitary-adrenal axis in a child when used to treat dermatitis. For that reason, a pediatric patient should receive the least amount of steroid cream in the lowest concentration for the shortest time possible.

Adverse reactions may also result from topical application of silver sulfadiazine if it is absorbed systemically, which is likely to happen if it is applied to burns that cover 20% or more of the body surface. Adverse reactions may include blood dyscrasias and impaired renal function. Topical application of salicylic acid can also produce systemic toxicity even when applied to intact skin. Mild toxicity produces skin reactions, edema, GI symptoms, tinnitus (ringing in the ears), and hyperventilation. Severe toxicity produces skin eruptions, acid-base and electrolyte imbalances, and central nervous system (CNS) changes that can progress to respiratory failure.

Distribution

A drug's distribution is affected by its dilution in the body. In a neonate and an infant, total body water and extracellular fluid volume are higher than those of an older child or an adult. (See *Differences in body composition* for a comparison by age-group.) The higher percentage of water in neonates and infants dilutes water-soluble drugs, making them less effective. That is why neonates and infants often require higher mg/kg dosages to achieve therapeutic drug levels.

Body composition also affects the distribution of fat-soluble drugs, although to a lesser degree than water-soluble ones. As the percentage of fat increases with age, so does the distribution of fat-soluble drugs. Therefore, distribution of these drugs is more limited in children than in adults.

In a newborn, the immature liver may also affect drug distribution by decreasing formation of plasma proteins, which results in hypoproteinemia and edema. The edema increases the volume of distribution and can dilute the drug. Infants produce fewer plasma proteins for drugs to bind to than adults do. Since only unbound, or free, drugs produce a pharmacologic effect, the infant's decreased protein binding can intensify drug effects and possibly cause toxicity. Other adverse drug effects can occur when drugs, such as salicylates and sulfonamides, compete for the same protein-binding sites as endogenous substances, such as bilirubin and free fatty acids. Any medication that competes with bilirubin for protein-binding sites or inhibits the binding of bilirubin increases the risk of kernicterus (bilirubin accumulation in the CNS).

Metabolism

In most people, the liver adequately metabolizes drugs. But an infant's immature liver may interfere with drug metabolism. As the liver matures during the first year of life, drug metabolism improves.

Dosage and choice of therapeutic agent may be altered for an infant with immature liver function or liver disease. The immature liver function increases the risk of toxicity with some drugs, such as chloramphenicol. When the liver fails to inactivate this drug, toxic levels can accumulate in the blood and produce gray baby syndrome, characterized by rapid respirations, ashen gray cyanosis, vomiting, loose green stools, progressive abdominal distention, vasomotor collapse, and possibly death. Fortunately, discontinuation of the drug can reverse the syndrome.

Children typically metabolize drugs that require oxidation, such as theophylline, caffeine, phenobarbital, and phenytoin, more rapidly than adults. The rate of metabolism for drugs such as aspirin and the sulfonamides that are catalyzed by microsomal or nonmicrosomal enzymes can vary among individuals and may be genetically determined.

In early infancy, drug metabolism and hepatic enzyme activity differ between the sexes and may be related to changes in diurnal rhythms. Before puberty, other sex-related differences in drug metabolism occur, especially in the microsomal enzymes that catalyze gonadal steroid metabolism.

Excretion

The rate of renal excretion of a drug depends on the rate of glomerular filtration, tubular reabsorption, and tubular secretion. Because most drug excretion occurs in the urine, the degree of renal development can affect drug excretion and, ultimately, dosage requirements for a pediatric patient.

At birth the kidneys are immature, renal excretion is slow, and drug dosages must be carefully adjusted. As the kidneys mature during the first few months of life, renal excretion of drugs increases, although the rate of increase is slow for a premature neonate. At about age 3 months, the kidneys can concentrate urine at the adult level. (See *Physiologic characteristics of pediatric patients* for a summary of these developments.)

Before the renal system matures completely, two drugs need particularly careful dosage adjustments: gentamicin, filtered by the glomerulus and excreted almost entirely by the kidneys; and penicillin, excreted by the renal tubules, which are functionally immature in the newborn.

Some drugs, such as nafcillin, are excreted by the biliary tree into the intestinal tract. In the first few days of life, however, biliary blood flow is low, which can prolong the effects. Administering the drug in lower doses can prevent toxicity. Interactions with other drugs may also affect drug excretion. The nurse must be cognizant of these facts and familiar with possible drug interactions.

Physiologic characteristics of pediatric patients

Body system immaturity and other physiologic characteristics of a pediatric patient can influence drug therapy.

AREA AFFECTED	CHARACTERISTIC
Renal system	• From birth until about age 3 months, the immature system has a decreased ability to concentrate urine. • Urinary excretion remains low until about age 2½, when the kidneys become functionally mature.
Gastrointestinal system	• Transit time through the GI tract increases until the toddler years, when it nears the adult rate. • Stomach acidity increases as the child becomes a toddler. • Immature liver interferes with the child's ability to metabolize drugs until about age 1. • The digestive processes mature by the preschool years.
Body-surface area	• The relationship between surface area and body weight changes as the child grows. The proportion of body-surface area to weight in an infant age 2 months may be 2½ times that of an adult, decreasing in a child age 1 to 3 to roughly 2 times that of an adult. By age 12, the child's body-surface area to weight proportion is only slightly greater than an adult's.
Metabolism	• Metabolism is increased during infancy and childhood in relation to body weight.

PHARMACODYNAMICS

Biochemically, a drug will display the same mechanism of action in all individuals. For example, if a drug normally inhibits the transfer of a substance into a cell, it will perform this action in anyone, child or adult. The response to a drug, however, can be affected by the maturity of the target organ and may require a dosage adjustment for a neonate, infant, or child. In addition, receptor sensitivity varies in infants and young children; it may be increased or decreased for certain drugs. Therefore, an infant or child may require a lower or higher dose of a drug than expected.

PHARMACOTHERAPEUTICS

The goal of medication administration is to achieve and maintain a therapeutic drug level without producing toxicity. Achievement of a therapeutic level depends on the drug's absorption, distribution, metabolism, and excretion. For example, children between ages 2 and 6 clear and excrete theophylline much faster than adults or neonates do, and boys clear and excrete the drug faster than girls do. For this reason, the child may need higher doses more frequently or may need sustained-release preparations to achieve therapeutic drug levels.

To maintain therapeutic levels, the patient must receive repeated doses at intervals that may vary according to age. For example, a neonate would probably receive gentamicin every 12 hours initially, because of an immature renal system that cannot excrete the drug as well as an older child's. An infant or child would be more likely to receive gentamicin every 8 hours initially because the more mature renal system can excrete the drug efficiently. But because the response to drugs is individual, the specific dosage for a pediatric patient is best determined by serum gentamicin levels.

The nurse must exercise extreme caution to achieve therapeutic effects without producing toxicity in a child. The nurse must calculate drug dosages and monitor the child very carefully.

Several drugs that are commonly used in pediatric patients have low therapeutic indexes (differences between therapeutic and toxic serum concentrations) and should be monitored by serum concentration levels. These drugs include aminoglycosides, digoxin, phenytoin, and chloramphenicol. Phenobarbital and other anticonvulsants can be monitored in the same way, although they have higher therapeutic indexes.

Dehydration and acid-base or electrolyte imbalances can alter the therapeutic and toxic effects of a medication. The nurse must closely monitor a child with these disorders for adverse reactions.

DRUG EFFECTS ON GROWTH AND DEVELOPMENT

Some drugs can adversely affect a child's growth and development. Long-term treatment with steroids, which may be necessary for a child with an organ transplant or asthma, may stunt growth. In these cases, the benefits of drug therapy must be evaluated against the effects on growth. A jaundiced infant who receives drugs that compete with bilirubin-binding sites may develop kernicterus, which may result in mental retardation. Tetracycline can produce tooth stains if given before the permanent teeth have formed. It can also bind calcium and phosphates and temporarily depress bone growth during the last half of gestation and during childhood from birth to age 8.

Drug excretion in breast milk

Many drugs are excreted in breast milk, and some can have an adverse effect on an infant. The nurse should advise a lactating woman to avoid taking medications, if possible. Drugs that can produce adverse effects in breast-feeding infants include diazepam, oral contraceptives, laxatives, and tetracyclines. (See Chapter 14, Intervention: The Pregnant or Lactating Patient, for more detailed information.)

PEDIATRIC NURSING CONSIDERATIONS

When caring for a pediatric patient, the nurse must pay particular attention to dosage calculations, administration techniques, and education of patients and their families.

PEDIATRIC DOSAGE CALCULATIONS

To determine the correct pediatric dosage of a medication, physicians and nurses usually use two computation methods. One is based on the child's weight in kilograms; the other uses the child's body-surface area. Other methods are less accurate and are not recom-

Calculating pediatric dosages by body-surface area

The nurse can determine a correct pediatric drug dose by estimating the child's body-surface area. If the child is average size, find the child's weight and corresponding surface area on the first, boxed scale. Otherwise, use the nomogram to the right. To do this, mark the child's height in the first column and weight in the third column; then draw a line between the two marks. Where the line intersects the scale in the second column indicates the estimated body-surface area of the child in square meters.

To calculate the child's dosage, complete this equation:

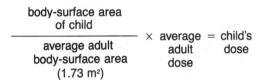

$$\frac{\text{body-surface area of child}}{\text{average adult body-surface area } (1.73 \text{ m}^2)} \times \text{average adult dose} = \text{child's dose}$$

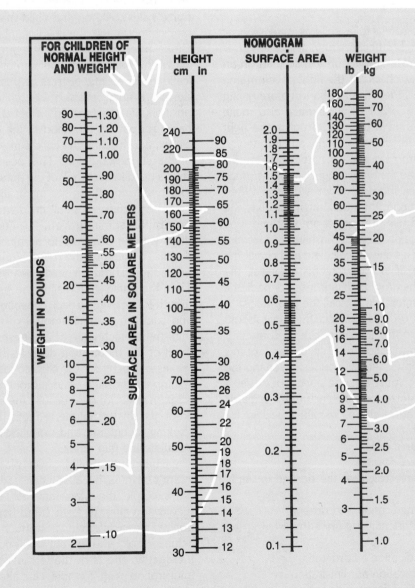

FOR CHILDREN OF NORMAL HEIGHT AND WEIGHT

WEIGHT IN POUNDS

90	1.30
80	1.20
70	1.10
60	1.00
50	.90
	.80
40	.70
30	.60
	.55
	.50
20	.45
	.40
15	.35
	.30
10	.25
9	
8	
7	
6	.20
5	
4	.15
3	
2	.10

SURFACE AREA IN SQUARE METERS

NOMOGRAM

HEIGHT cm in | **SURFACE AREA** | **WEIGHT** lb kg

HEIGHT cm	in
240	90
220	85
200	80
190	75
180	70
170	65
160	60
150	
140	55
130	50
120	45
110	
100	40
90	35
80	30
70	28
	26
60	24
	22
50	20
	19
	18
	17
40	16
	15
	14
	13
30	12

SURFACE AREA:
2.0, 1.9, 1.8, 1.7, 1.6, 1.5, 1.4, 1.3, 1.2, 1.1, 1.0, 0.9, 0.8, 0.7, 0.6, 0.5, 0.4, 0.3, 0.2, 0.1

WEIGHT lb	kg
180	80
160	70
140	60
130	
120	50
110	
100	
90	40
80	
70	30
60	25
50	
45	20
40	
35	15
30	
25	
	10
20	9.0
18	8.0
16	7.0
14	6.0
12	5.0
10	
9	4.0
8	
7	3.0
6	2.5
5	
	2.0
4	
3	1.5
	1.0

mended. (See Chapter 9, Intervention: Dosage Measurements and Calculations, for further information about pediatric dosage computations based on body weight.)

A child's body-surface area is thought to be related to the child's metabolic rate. To determine a child's dosage using this method, the nurse must estimate the child's body-surface area with a nomogram and use the resulting figure in a dosage calculation. (See *Calculating pediatric dosages by body-surface area* on page 203 for details on how to use a nomogram.)

PEDIATRIC ADMINISTRATION TECHNIQUES

Administering drugs safely to a child requires special attention to the five rights, because any medication error can have a much greater impact on a child than on an adult. The nurse must check for the right patient name by reading the child's identification band before giving each dose of medication. The nurse must also make sure that the medication is the right drug, in the right dose, for the right route, at the right time and frequency.

Checking the drug's dosage is particularly important. The nurse can use the body weight or body-surface area method to check the dosage for accuracy. When preparing the medication, the nurse must calculate the dosage carefully and use the correct amount and type of diluent. When digoxin, heparin, insulin, or narcotics are ordered, two nurses should calculate and check the dosage for accuracy. If an order seems incorrect, the nurse should check the drug's package insert or pediatric and pharmacologic references or call the pharmacist to verify the order. If the order is incorrect, the nurse should notify the physician so that the order can be corrected.

Administering medication to a child also requires careful attention to other details. Besides observing the five rights, the nurse must also be aware of adverse reactions and drug interactions. To ensure the pediatric patient's safety, the nurse should use this checklist for medication administration:
- Check the physician's order.
- Calculate the correct dosage.
- Have a second nurse calculate the dosage to verify accuracy.
- Prepare the right medication and dosage.
- Verify the patient's identity before administering the medication.
- Administer the medication as ordered.
- Document the medication administration.
- Observe the patient for therapeutic and adverse effects of the medication.

For each route of administration, the nurse must modify adult administration techniques for a pediatric patient. No matter what route is used, the nurse should try to elicit the child's cooperation to make medication administration as easy as possible. If the child is unable to cooperate, the nurse should enlist help to hold the child still during administration. (See *Administering pediatric medications* for further information.)

Oral administration

Although absorption from the GI tract is less predictable than by other routes, oral administration is often ordered because it is the least expensive and traumatic for the child. But oral administration to a child can challenge a nurse's skills. Although a child may willingly swallow a medication at first, the child may begin to spit, drool, or choke after realizing that the medication tastes bad. When this happens, the nurse must try to give the medication with as little distress as possible to the child. To do this, a nurse might hold a child in a bottle-feeding position, placing the child's inner arm behind the nurse's back, supporting the head in the crook of the nurse's elbow, and holding the child's free hand with the hand of the supporting arm. This position immobilizes the child's head in the crook of the nurse's arm and prevents the child from spilling the medication with either hand.

If an infant or small child must be restrained for medication administration, the nurse should use a syringe without a needle to administer small, controlled doses. To minimize the risk of choking or aspirating, the nurse should hold the child's head upright or to the side. Then the nurse should slide the syringe into the child's mouth about halfway back between the gums and cheeks and squirt in a small amount of medication. This administration technique offers several advantages. Placement of the medication deep in the side of the mouth makes it difficult for the child to lose the medication by spitting or drooling. And although medication administration takes longer because the drug is given in small amounts, this technique reduces the risk of the child's choking, coughing, and vomiting because it does not stimulate the gag reflex.

The nurse should never place medication in an infant's formula, because it can lead to several problems. For example, the infant may not take the feeding if the medication alters its taste. If this happens, the nurse will not be able to determine how much medication the child actually took, and the child will not receive the drug's therapeutic effects or the formula's nutrition. Also, administration with formula can alter the absorption of

Administering pediatric medications

To administer pediatric medications effectively, the nurse must understand how children of different ages think about and react to drugs and know how to intervene appropriately.

AGE-GROUP	PATIENT CHARACTERISTICS AND REACTIONS TO MEDICATION	NURSING INTERVENTIONS
Infant	• In a very young infant, lack of experience eliminates fear; the infant may take medication willingly. • Between ages 5 and 8 months, the infant begins to observe visual cues and anticipate unpleasant events. • By age 10 months, the infant will try to get away from anticipated unpleasantness and may spit, drool, or choke to avoid taking medication.	• Hold the infant still when giving an oral medication. • Make the medication palatable; if appropriate, mix it with syrup or applesauce. • Administer medication in a syringe placed in the side of the mouth or from a spoon placed far back on the tongue. • Allow the infant to suck medication from a nipple. • Give medication slowly to prevent choking and spitting. • Ask the parent or a co-worker to hold the infant still during a painful administration. • Cuddle, rock, and speak soothingly to the infant after a painful procedure.
Toddler	• A toddler has a limited ability to express anger in words, but will protest loudly. • A toddler may try to escape from the nurse or physician. • A toddler has a limited understanding of explanations and a poor concept of time. • The child may not be able to cooperate and may squirm because of a lack of self-control.	• Explain the procedure very simply just before performing it. • Mention that the child has no options about taking the medication. • Tell the child that you realize the procedure is unpleasant. Warn the child before a painful procedure. • Let the toddler exercise some control over the situation by allowing a choice of a spoon, straw, cup, or syringe to take an oral medication. • Try to improve the medication's taste by mixing it with a small amount of syrup or food, if appropriate. • Use the child's rituals to administer medication whenever possible. • Hold the child still, if necessary. Praise any attempts the child makes to hold still. • Encourage the child to express feelings, and offer reassurance that the child is not being punished. • Allow the parents to comfort the child after the procedure.
Preschooler	• A child in this age-group has a limited ability to understand a detailed explanation. • A preschooler will attempt to cooperate. • After an I.M. injection, a preschooler may think that body fluids will leak out of the injection site.	• Express faith in the child's ability to cooperate even with an unpleasant procedure. • Provide options, whenever possible, to give the child a sense of control over the situation. • Explain the procedure simply. • Warn the child before a painful procedure. • Praise the child for all attempts to cooperate. • Encourage the child to express feelings. • Offer the child an adhesive bandage after an I.M. injection. • Allow the parents or caregiver to comfort the child after the procedure. • Use therapeutic play before and after the procedure. Listen carefully to the child's play. Clear up any misconceptions, and provide further explanations, as needed.
School-age child	• The older the school-age child, the greater the ability to exercise restraint and to cooperate.	• Explain the procedure in detail. • Allow the child to make choices, whenever possible. • Warn the child in advance when a painful procedure is scheduled. • Reassure the child that no one likes the procedure. • Praise the child for cooperating. • Listen to the child's concerns and feelings.
Adolescent	• An adolescent's reaction to medication is similar to an adult's. The ability to cooperate is highly developed.	• Include the adolescent in discussions and decisions about the procedure. • Allow the adolescent to make choices and to exercise as much control as possible. • Give support and encouragement, but do not treat the adolescent like a child.

some medications. For example, Osmolite can inhibit the absorption of phenytoin suspension.

During oral administration, the nurse can use certain techniques to enhance the pediatric patient's cooperation, depending on the child's development. An infant or small child may squirm less if the nurse talks soothingly and holds the child's head securely. Obviously, an explanation will not help an infant to cooperate, but it may reassure the child's caregiver. An explanation may help a toddler react better if it is given just before the nurse administers the medication. However, it will not help the toddler to cooperate. To promote cooperation, the nurse should praise the toddler's efforts. After receiving an explanation, preschoolers will attempt to cooperate. Young school-age children should be able to exercise more restraint and a greater degree of cooperation. The nurse should not shame preschool and young school-age children if they have difficulty cooperating but should help them gain some control by allowing choices when possible. For example, the nurse may ask if the child would like to take the medicine in a cup or a spoon.

Intramuscular administration

For an I.M. injection, the nurse should use the smallest gauge needle appropriate for the medication. This is usually a needle that is 22G to 25G and 1 to 1½ inches (2.5 to 3.8 cm) long. A needle length should not exceed 1 inch (2.5 cm), except for an adult-size adolescent, who may require a 1½-inch (3.8-cm) needle.

The recommended injection sites vary with age. The vastus lateralis and rectus femoris muscles are the recommended sites for an infant or toddler. For a child who has been walking for about 1 year, the nurse can give an I.M. injection in the ventrogluteal or dorsogluteal area. Walking develops these muscles, thus reducing the risk of sciatic nerve damage during an I.M. injection. (See *Intramuscular injection sites* for illustrations of these areas.) For an older child, the nurse may use an adult I.M. injection site, such as the deltoid, gluteus maximus, ventrogluteal, vastus lateralis, or rectus femoris muscle.

After selecting an injection site appropriate to the patient's age, the nurse should cleanse it with alcohol or antiseptic in a circular motion from the center out. Then the nurse should do the following: (1) Grasp the skin firmly, pull it taut, and insert the needle quickly at a 90-degree angle. (2) To ensure that the needle is not in a blood vessel, pull back on the plunger slightly. (3) If blood appears in the syringe, remove the needle and prepare another injection. (4) If no blood appears, inject the medication slowly to allow it to disperse in the muscle. (5) Withdraw the needle only after all of the medication has been injected to avoid injecting it along the insertion track. To prevent medication from leaking into the subcutaneous tissue, the nurse should use the Z-track method. (See Chapter 10, Intervention: Routes and Techniques of Administration, for detailed information about the Z-track method.) (6) Massage the injection site and encourage the patient to use the muscle to increase drug absorption. (7) Document the medication administration, noting the injection site so that different sites can be used for subsequent injections.

The air bubble technique, which uses an air bubble to clear the needle and hub after medication is drawn into the syringe, is not recommended for pediatric I.M. injections. Because the calibration on most syringes does include the amount in the hub and needle, an overdose can occur with the air bubble technique. Only the Becton-Dickinson insulin syringe with a permanent needle and the Wyeth Tubex system can now deliver an accurate dose when the air bubble technique is used.

The nurse giving an I.M. injection can use certain techniques to help ensure a child's cooperation and safety. Before entering the child's room, the nurse should prepare the medication and syringe. The nurse should provide an explanation for all children regardless of age or ability to understand or cooperate. For the infant, the explanation will be helpful to the parent or primary caregiver. Although the toddler's understanding may be limited, the nurse should give a simple explanation immediately before the injection. The toddler will not be able to cooperate and may protest loudly. So the nurse should make the explanation brief, perform the injection quickly, and allow the caregiver to comfort the child. If the child is alone, the nurse should hold and comfort the child after the injection. Before administering an injection to a preschooler, the nurse should explain that the shot will hurt and that it is OK to cry. The nurse should emphasize that the child will need to hold still and that another nurse will help the child hold still, if necessary. (See *Positioning a child for an intramuscular injection* on page 209 for an illustration of this technique.) Then the nurse should give the injection and praise the child for any cooperative efforts. A preschooler has a poor concept of body integrity and may think that body fluids will leak out of the injection site. To relieve this fear, the nurse should give the child an adhesive bandage. The school-age child should benefit from an explanation of the procedure and probably will be able to hold still. However, a young school-age child or one who is stressed might need help to hold still. The nurse must never shame the child, but should praise every attempt at cooperation. The adolescent child generally has enough self-control to cooperate and benefits greatly from an explanation.

Subcutaneous administration

Subcutaneous administration is the same in a child as in an adult. The needle should be 23G to 27G and ⅜ to ⅝ inch (1 to 1.5 cm) long. The nurse must remember to provide an age-appropriate explanation and to po-

sition the child properly, as described under "Intramuscular administration."

Intravenous administration

Pediatric intravenous administration poses several challenges for the nurse. For example, the nurse must assist with or perform the I.V. insertion, which can be traumatic for the child and parents. The nurse must also monitor the I.V. closely to maintain its patency.

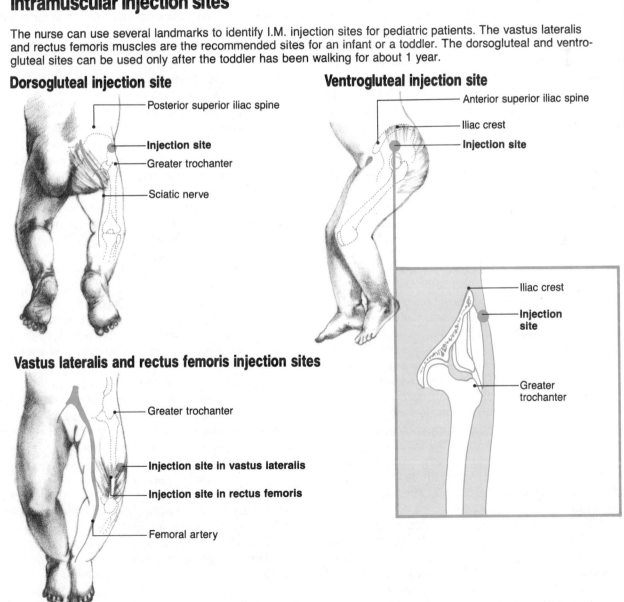

Intramuscular injection sites

The nurse can use several landmarks to identify I.M. injection sites for pediatric patients. The vastus lateralis and rectus femoris muscles are the recommended sites for an infant or a toddler. The dorsogluteal and ventrogluteal sites can be used only after the toddler has been walking for about 1 year.

Dorsogluteal injection site

- Posterior superior iliac spine
- **Injection site**
- Greater trochanter
- Sciatic nerve

Ventrogluteal injection site

- Anterior superior iliac spine
- Iliac crest
- **Injection site**

- Iliac crest
- **Injection site**
- Greater trochanter

Vastus lateralis and rectus femoris injection sites

- Greater trochanter
- **Injection site in vastus lateralis**
- **Injection site in rectus femoris**
- Femoral artery

The nurse should explain the procedure to the parents of a neonate or an infant, to prepare them for the necessity of the I.V. and the possibility that the infant's head will be shaved if the I.V. catheter is inserted in the scalp. The nurse should also tell the parents that the procedure may take some time so that they do not expect to see the infant again in a few minutes. For a toddler, the nurse should briefly explain the procedure immediately before taking the child to the treatment room, because the toddler's concept of time is not fully developed. A toddler probably will not be able to cooperate, so the nurse should plan to restrain the child carefully to ensure safe insertion of the I.V. catheter. For a preschooler, who has a better concept of time, the nurse may explain the procedure a short time before performing it. A preschooler especially needs to know that crying is permitted, but that he or she is expected to hold still. Although a young school-age child should be able to hold still without help for a painful procedure, the nurse should offer to help, by holding the child's hand, for instance. Generally, an older school-age child or an adolescent can hold still for this procedure.

For infants and small children, the nurse uses 22G to 24G I.V. catheters. For older children, the nurse may use 18G to 20G catheters. Silastic catheters are preferred because they are less irritating to the vein.

Before starting the I.V. catheter insertion, the nurse should: (1) tear off strips of tape and keep them ready to secure the inserted catheter; prime the I.V. tubing, removing all of the air bubbles, and cover the end with a sterile capped needle, a sterile capped T-connector, or the tubing's protective cover; and observe the I.V. fluids for contaminants and glass bottles for cracks or breaks. If irregularities are detected, the nurse should obtain a new container of I.V. fluid.

(2) Select a site for I.V. catheter insertion. The antecubital fossa is not the first choice for a pediatric I.V. site, because the child can bend the arm with the inserted I.V. and dislodge the needle. Instead, start with the veins of the hand and lower arm to identify a site, and work from the distal to more proximal areas. That way, if an I.V. infiltrates in the lower hand, the nurse can use the veins of the wrist and forearm for other sites. The same rule applies to selecting an I.V. site in a lower extremity. Use the veins on the dorsum of the foot first and proceed upward to the ankle, if necessary.

(3) After inserting the I.V. catheter, secure it with the pretorn tape, restrain the extremity, and assess the circulation in the digits. At the end of the procedure, ensure that any tourniquets have been removed that were used to try starting the I.V. in different extremities. A tourniquet inadvertently left in place can seriously impair sensation and circulation in the affected extremity.

If a head vein is used for I.V. access in an infant, apply a mummy restraint, which holds the infant's head firmly in place and prevents body movement during the procedure, leaving the nurse's hands free to insert the catheter. Make sure that the infant can breathe adequately with this restraint in place.

If an extremity is used for I.V. access, use a padded board to secure the hand or foot. Some nurses prefer to secure the extremity to the board before starting the I.V., but others prefer to secure it afterward.

With either method, tape the I.V. in such a way to leave the insertion site visible for frequent monitoring. If the extremity must be immobilized by pinning the arm board to the sheet or using a sandbag, be careful to secure the I.V. so that hourly observation of the site can verify no signs of complications. Listen to the child to detect complications. If the child complains of pain at the I.V. site or if an infant or young child becomes unusually irritable, check closely for signs of infiltration or phlebitis, such as redness or swelling.

Infants, small children, and children with compromised cardiopulmonary status are particularly vulnerable to fluid overload with I.V. medication administration. To prevent this problem, the nurse should use a volume control set (a volume-control device in the I.V. tubing) and an infusion pump or syringe and place no more than 2 hours' worth of I.V. fluid in the volume control set at a time. These techniques help ensure that a limited amount of fluid is infused in a controlled manner.

Other factors can influence the amount and rapidity of medication administration. In tubing with a narrow lumen, the medication will reach the child faster than in tubing with a wide lumen because of increased pressure in the narrow tubing. If a child has a delicate fluid balance, an infusion (auto) syringe can deliver small amounts of fluid. With this technique, a syringe containing medication is secured in the cradle of an autoinfusion mechanism. The nurse can set the correct rate on the syringe to infuse the medication automatically.

Careful monitoring of intake and output can help prevent fluid overload and ensure that the child gets the amount of fluid ordered. Careful observation of the infusion will detect clot formation in the catheter, which is especially likely with a slow I.V. rate. Frequent assessment of the flow rate—particularly with gravity infusion—is important because position changes, crying, and restraints can impede the flow of fluids.

With all I.V. medications, the nurse must flush the volume control set and tubing before and after administration. Some medications are not compatible, and if they are mixed, they may form a precipitate in the I.V. administration set. If a precipitate forms, the nurse must stop the infusion immediately and change all of the tubing.

Positioning a child for an intramuscular injection

Administration of an I.M. injection to a small child usually requires two people. One person flexes the child's knee and holds the child without restraining the arms. With the child in this position, the other person can easily administer the I.M. injection at the rectus femoris or vastus lateralis site.

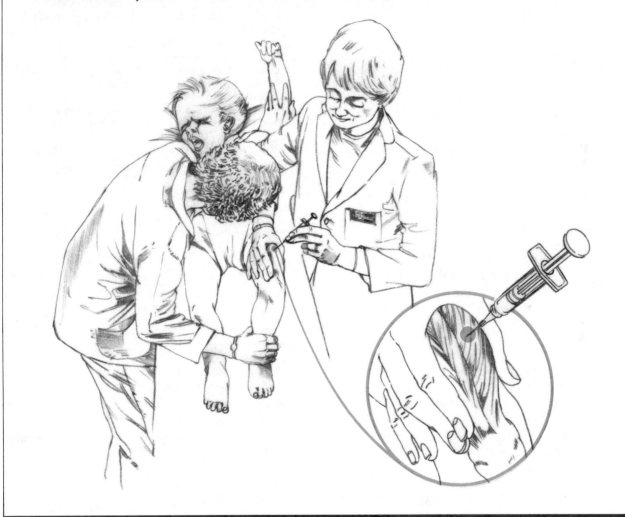

Topical administration

In a neonate, infant, or small child, thin epidermis and large body-surface area allows for increased drug absorption of topical medications and explains why a young pediatric patient is more likely to develop a toxic, systemic drug reaction than an older patient. Topical corticosteroids can produce particularly severe reactions. To decrease the risk of toxic effects, the nurse should wash a cleansing solution off an infant's skin, unless otherwise ordered, and apply a topical medication as thinly as possible and to as small a body-surface area

as possible. When removing a topical medication from a jar, the nurse should use a tongue depressor to avoid contaminating the medication with the hand that applies it.

Rectal administration

Drug absorption from the rectum is unpredictable. The presence of stool in the rectum can delay, decrease, or block drug absorption. Nevertheless, medications are often administered rectally when oral administration is contraindicated or when they are designed for rectal administration. Children who are neutropenic or thrombocytopenic, however, should not receive rectal medications because of the increased risk of infection and bleeding.

Before administering the rectal medication, the nurse should explain the procedure and the importance of retaining the suppository rather than expelling it. To administer the medication, the nurse uses a gloved hand to insert the unwrapped, lubricated suppository past the rectal sphincters. Then the nurse should hold the buttocks together so the child cannot expel the medication.

Some suppositories are scored and can be halved easily and accurately, if necessary. If an unscored suppository must be halved, the nurse should split it lengthwise to ensure even distribution of its medication.

Administration of eye, ear, and nose drops

To administer eyedrops, the nurse may need to have a co-worker restrain an infant or toddler. For any pediatric patient, the nurse places the hand that holds the dropper on the child's forehead so that it will move as the child's head moves and decrease the risk of injury. With the other hand, the nurse can pull down the lower lid to expose the conjunctival sac. If the child is old enough to cooperate, the nurse should ask the child to look up and then instill the drops in the lower conjunctival sac. If the child will not cooperate, the nurse can place the eyedrops at the inner canthus while the child's eyes are closed. As the child's eyes open, the drops will be dispersed. After instillation, the nurse should encourage the child to blink or close the eyelids and rotate the eyes to distribute the medication.

Before administration, the nurse should warm ear drops almost to body temperature to prevent pain or vertigo when the drops come in contact with the child's tympanic membrane. The nurse should assist the child into a supine position with the head turned to the side and the affected ear up. For a child under age 3, the nurse will have to pull the pinna down and back to straighten the external auditory canal. For a child over age 3, the nurse should pull the pinna up and back. Then the nurse can administer the drops and massage the area in front of the tragus to promote their entry into the ear. If only one ear is affected, the child should lie on the unaffected side for several minutes after administration. If both ears are affected, the nurse should place a cotton ball in each external canal to prevent the medication from escaping.

To prevent nose drops from entering the throat rather than the nasal passages, the nurse should administer them to a child whose head is suspended over the edge of a pillow or bed or to an infant who is being held in the football position (tucked against the nurse's side with the infant on its back, its head at the nurse's

head, and its feet against the nurse's waist). The nurse should keep the child in this position for 1 minute after medication administration to allow the drops to come in contact with the nasal passages.

PATIENT AND FAMILY EDUCATION

Whether the child is treated in an outpatient or acute care setting, the nurse will probably be responsible for patient and family education. Education can help increase medication compliance. Whenever patient or family education is required, the nurse should remember these teaching tips:
- Keep the instruction simple.
- Keep each session short.
- Repeat information.
- Allow time for questions.
- Provide written information.

(See *Steps for effective patient and family education* for further details.)

Medication information should include the drug's name; its correct dosage, administration route, and frequency of administration; its therapeutic and adverse effects; and instructions for any required administration devices.

In this written information, the nurse should spell the name of the drug correctly and explain, simply and clearly, why the drug is being given. The nurse should

---

Steps for effective patient and family education

To make patient and family education as effective as possible, the nurse should consider any psychosocial, physiologic, or cognitive deficits. Follow these steps:
- Decide who needs to be taught.
- Assess readiness to learn.
- Determine the necessary information to be taught.
- Present the information at a level that the learner can understand.
- Reinforce the teaching with printed materials.
- Assess the learner's ability to solve problems by asking "What if..." questions.
- Provide the necessary resources to meet the educational goals.
- Evaluate the learning, and review information, as necessary.

instruct the family about the correct dosage and demonstrate how to prepare the correct amount for administration.

The nurse should describe the route of administration simply. For example, the nurse would use the phrase "by mouth" rather than "P.O." when talking to the parents and the patient. The nurse should also explain why the drug must be given in the exact way it is ordered. For example, the nurse might caution the parents to give a capsule without opening it because the capsule protects the medication from destruction by stomach acids and allows it to be absorbed properly in the intestine. The frequency of administration requires careful discussion, too. If the timing of the doses presents a problem, the nurse should help the parents develop a schedule that will interfere as little as possible with their daily routine.

The parents and child must also learn what therapeutic and adverse reactions to expect from the medication. For example, if theophylline is prescribed to treat a child's asthma, the nurse should explain that this drug should decrease or eliminate the wheezing; that the medication must be given at regular intervals to achieve the maximum effect; and that adverse effects, such as irritability and nausea, may occur. Finally, the nurse should make sure that the family knows when to contact their physician about the drug therapy. (See Chapter 11, Intervention: Patient Education, for additional information.)

CHAPTER SUMMARY

This chapter provided information on drug dosage calculations, routes and techniques of administration, and nursing techniques that are specific to the pediatric patient. Here are the highlights of the chapter:

• Children require different medication administration techniques than adults do. Drug absorption, distribution, metabolism, and excretion are affected by the route of administration and the child's age, condition, and individual response to the drug.

• Children may require wide variations of drug dosages to achieve therapeutic effects. Because of this, the nurse must monitor a pediatric patient closely to detect therapeutic and adverse effects. Pediatric patients are at particularly high risk for drug toxicity.

• Immature body systems, differences in body composition, and other physiologic characteristics can significantly affect drug therapy in pediatric patients. Failure

to take these characteristics into account during drug therapy can result in adverse effects or reduced therapeutic effects.

• The nurse should base accurate drug dosages on the child's weight or body-surface area.

• The nurse must administer medications carefully, delivering the right medication to the right patient at the right time by the right route and in the right amount.

• Although pediatric and adult routes of medication administration are the same, pediatric sites and techniques of administration vary considerably with age. The nurse must be familiar with the drug to be administered as well as the appropriate administration techniques for the child's age.

• Whenever possible, the nurse should explain the administration procedure to the patient and parents and try to elicit their cooperation in administering medications safely and effectively.

• Patient and family education is essential for compliance with a medication regimen at home. The nurse should provide oral and written instructions as a part of patient and family education.

BIBLIOGRAPHY

Banner, W. "Why Read a Pharmacokinetic Article?" *American Journal of Diseases of Children* 140:104, February 1986.

Bartels, H. "Drug Therapy in Childhood: What Has Been Done and What Has to Be Done?" *Pediatric Pharmacology* 3:131, May 27-28, 1983.

Behrman, R.E., and Vaughn, V.C., eds. *Nelson Textbook of Pediatrics,* 12th ed. Philadelphia: W.B. Saunders Co., 1983.

Bennett, H.L. "Why Patients Don't Follow Instructions," *RN* 45, March 1986.

Boréus, L.O. "The Role of Therapeutic Drug Monitoring," *Pediatric Pharmacology* 3:145, May 27-28, 1983.

Cohen, S.N., and Strebel, L. "Drug Therapy," in *Nelson Textbook of Pediatrics,* 12th ed. Edited by Behrman, R.E., and Vaughn, V.C. Philadelphia: W.B. Saunders Co., 1983.

Cole, C.H., ed. *The Harriett Lane Handbook,* 10th ed. Chicago: Year Book Medical Pubs., 1984.

Dale, J.C. "A Multidimensional Study of Infant's Response to Painful Stimuli," *Pediatric Nursing* 12:27, January/February 1986.

Dayton, P.B., and Sanders, J.E. "Dose-Dependent Pharmacokinetics: Emphasis on Phase 1 Metabolism," *Drug Metabolism Reviews* 14:347, May 1983.

DiFlorio, I.A., and Duncan, P.A. "Design for Successful Patient Teaching," *MCN* 11:246, July/August 1986.

Gilman, A.G., et al. *Goodman and Gilman's The Pharmacological Basis of Therapeutics,* 7th ed. New York: Macmillan Publishing Co., 1985.

Hazinski, M.F. *Nursing Care of the Critically Ill Child.* St. Louis: C.V. Mosby Co., 1984.

Kauffman, R.E. "The Clinical Interpretation and Application of Drug Concentration Data," *Pediatric Clinics of North America* 28:35, February 1981.

Keithley, J.K., and O'Donnell, J. "Look Out for These Drug-Nutrient Interactions," *Nursing86* 16:42, February 1986.

Koren, G., et al. "Tenfold Errors in Administration of Drug Doses: A Neglected Iatrogenic Disease in Pediatrics," *Pediatrics* 77:848, June 1986.

Kramer, M.S., et al. "Antibiotic-Associated Gastrointestinal Symptoms in General Pediatric Outpatients," *Pediatrics* 76:365, September 1985.

Lutz, W.J. "Helping Hospitalized Children and Their Parents Cope with Painful Procedures," *Journal of Pediatric Nursing* 1:24, February 1986.

MacLeod, S.M., and Radde, I.C. *Textbook of Pediatric Clinical Pharmacology.* Littleton, Mass.: John Wright PSG, 1985.

McGowan, D., and Parks, B. "Pediatric Drug Information," *Pediatric Nursing* 11:298, July/August 1985.

Mott, S.R., et al. *Nursing Care of Children and Families: A Holistic Approach.* Menlo Park, Calif.: Addison-Wesley Publishing Co., 1985.

Pedersen, S., and Moller-Petersen, J. "Erratic Absorption of a Slow-Release Theophylline Sprinkle Product," *Pediatrics* 74:534, October 1984.

Roberts, R.J. "Intravenous Administration of Medications in Pediatric Patients: Problems and Solutions," *Pediatric Clinics of North America* 28:23, February 1981.

Schanzer, H., and Jacobsen, J.H. "Tissue Damage Caused by the Intra-Muscular Injection of Long-Acting Penicillin," *Pediatrics* 75:741, 1985.

Shope, J.T. "Medication Compliance," *Pediatric Clinics of North America* 28:5, February 1981.

Stewart, C.M., and Stewart, L.B. *Pediatric Medications: An Emergency and Critical Care Reference.* Rockville, Md.: Aspen Systems Corp., 1984.

Trang, J.M., et al. "Pharmacokinetics for Pediatric Nurses," *Pediatric Nursing* 10:267, July/August 1984.

Waechter, E.H., et al. *Nursing Care of Children,* 10th ed. Philadelphia: J.B. Lippincott Co., 1985.

Wester, R.C., and Maibach, H.I. "Cutaneous Pharmacokinetics: 10 Steps to Percutaneous Absorption," *Drug Metabolism Reviews* 14(2):169, 1983.

Whaley, L.F., and Wong, D.L. *Nursing Care of Infants and Children.* St Louis: C.V. Mosby Co., 1983.

CHAPTER 13

INTERVENTION: THE GERIATRIC PATIENT

OBJECTIVES

After reading and studying this chapter, you should be able to:

1. Describe the atypical signs and symptoms of disease characteristic of geriatric patients.

2. Describe the characteristics of reduced reserve capacity.

3. Explain how age can alter drug absorption, distribution, metabolism, and excretion.

4. Explain how age can alter a drug's mechanism of action.

5. Describe the risk factors that a nurse can use to help identify patients prone to adverse drug reactions.

6. Describe the common signs and symptoms of adverse drug reactions in a geriatric patient.

7. Describe the expected changes in organ function that accompany normal aging.

8. Devise safe and efficient systems to help the impaired geriatric patient self-medicate at home.

INTRODUCTION

The geriatric population in the United States, which is growing faster than that of any other age-group, is expected to nearly double—from about 11% to 21%—by the year 2030. As the geriatric population grows, so will its need for nurses with advanced knowledge and skills in geriatric health care, especially in pharmacology.

This chapter covers the geriatric population, aging effects, age-related changes in pharmacokinetics and pharmacodynamics, and nursing interventions for geriatric patients at high risk for adverse drug reactions.

THE GERIATRIC POPULATION EXPLOSION

Traditionally, the geriatric population has been defined as people aged 65 or older. This definition persists, even though longevity has increased and the concept of "old age" has changed. Some people under age 65 may also be considered part of the geriatric population because they appear and act old and have geriatric medication needs.

The geriatric population has three main subgroups: the young-old, age 65 to 75; the middle-old, age 75 to 85; and the old, age 85 and older. Because the old group is the fastest growing and neediest, it has a major impact on the rest of society. One additional group, the frail elderly, includes all people over age 65 who suffer from a debilitating condition. Members of this group are at especially high risk for adverse drug reactions.

Why is the geriatric population growing? Medical advances have contributed greatly by decreasing mortality; new treatments have decreased mortality from acute and chronic disease; improved medical care has reduced infant mortality, allowing more infants to survive and possibly live to old age; and, as survivorship has increased, the birth rate has decreased, amplifying the population shift.

Initially, the young-old group experienced the greatest growth, spurring the development of nursing care facilities and educational, training, and medical assistance programs to support and care for the young-old. As this group has aged, the growth surge has extended into the middle-old and old groups, and the higher numbers of older individuals should continue growing beyond 2030. The old may even live to age 105 to 120, which, according to some scientists, is the natural end point for human life when unencumbered by disease or other adverse conditions.

THE NEED FOR NURSES

As the old and frail elderly groups become larger, the demand—and the challenges—for geriatric health care nurses will grow. Geriatric patients can require intensive nursing intervention in hospitals and other institutions to manage their diseases and age-related changes. They sometimes need nurses to assist them in noninstitutional settings, especially in those communities designed for and populated by elderly people. In these settings, nurses may act autonomously and as members of interdisciplinary teams to provide skilled care, promote optimum functioning, and ensure the highest possible quality of life for geriatric patients.

Traditionally, the nurse has been responsible for administering and monitoring prescribed medication regimens. This responsibility assumes even greater importance with geriatric patients, especially in long-term care facilities, where several physicians may prescribe drugs for each patient. The nurse must work closely with geriatric patients every day to be aware of their health and cognitive status. The informed nurse is in the best position to detect subtle symptoms of an illness or of adverse drug reactions and to begin interventions.

THE EFFECTS OF AGING

The aging process is usually accompanied by a decline in organ function, which profoundly affects drug metabolism and detoxification, among other things. This physiologic decline is likely to be exacerbated by a pathologic one, produced by a disease or chronic disorder. As a result, the geriatric patient has a significantly higher risk of drug toxicity and adverse reactions. (See *A geriatric case study* for an example.) Aging also produces a wide range of general effects, including effects on pharmacokinetic and pharmacodynamic processes.

GENERAL EFFECTS

With age, a patient may develop atypical signs and symptoms of disease, multiple health problems, reduced reserve capacity, and confusion. The nurse must be aware of these aging effects to assess the geriatric patient properly.

Atypical signs and symptoms

A geriatric patient is likely to have complicated, yet subtle, health problems that differ from the diseases that affect a younger patient. These atypical signs and symptoms of a disease or drug toxicity often complicate assessment. For example, a geriatric patient may display decreased or absent pain perception. As a result, a "silent" myocardial infarction can occur, especially in a middle-old patient. This type of infarction does not trigger the mechanism that alerts the body. Therefore, the infarction may remain undiscovered until the nurse performs a routine physical examination or an examination for an unrelated illness.

A geriatric patient may also display an altered ability to regulate body temperature. This alteration not only causes susceptibility to hypothermia and heat stroke, but also decreases the body's ability to produce a fever in response to infection. In a geriatric patient, a low-grade fever is an ominous sign and may indicate a severe infection. If this atypical sign is not assessed properly, the patient may receive insufficient treatment and develop serious complications. Although temperature assessment is a routine matter in a younger adult, it deserves special consideration in a geriatric patient.

In some cases, the presence of atypical symptoms can increase the risk of misdiagnosis and result in unintentional mistreatment. For example, hyperthyroidism (Graves' disease) can produce signs and symptoms of hypothyroidism (apathy and inactivity) in an elderly patient. If assessment and diagnosis do not account for these effects in the patient, treatment may be administered for hypothyroidism—the exact opposite of the treatment needed for hyperthyroidism.

Multiple health problems

The geriatric patient may experience multiple pathologies and age-related changes and may take several medications. All of these characteristics complicate the assessment. Because of the complex nature of geriatric health problems, the physician and the nurse must carefully determine which etiology or combination of etiologies is causing the symptoms. To determine the etiology, the physician and the nurse must decide whether a new or previous disease is causing the symptoms. They must also determine if the symptoms are

A geriatric case study

In this case study, a geriatric patient develops adverse drug reactions when she adds over-the-counter (OTC) remedies to her prescription regimen.

Rose Greenwald, age 78, lives alone on a fixed income and has been taking the same heart medications for years. When she developed a mild upper respiratory tract infection, she worried about the expense of seeing her physician to treat this problem, which she thinks is a cold. So Rose decided to purchase OTC remedies for symptomatic relief. She bought Nyquil, a cough suppressant that contains alcohol, to relieve her nighttime cough, and Dristan, an antihistamine, for her rhinorrhea and congestion. To relieve her fatigue, Rose opted for bed rest.

After Rose took the OTC medications and her usual medicines as directed on the bottles, her appetite decreased, she felt too weak to prepare meals, and she ate and drank less. She also felt depressed, but attributed this to the illness and continued to take the medications. She did not realize that the alcohol in the cough medicine decreased the appetite and cough reflex essential to her recovery. She did not know that the antihistamine increased her feeling of lethargy and produced urinary retention. In fact, she was glad that she did not need to get up to urinate so often. After a few days, a neighbor noticed that Rose had not been outside lately. Upon investi-gation, the neighbor found her in bed, disoriented and incontinent.

Like many other elderly people, Rose Greenwald put herself at risk for adverse drug reactions in several ways. She diagnosed and treated herself, which could have been dangerous if her symptoms had been related to her history of congestive heart failure and not to a mild respiratory infection. She mixed OTC and prescription medications without consulting her physician or the pharmacist about potential drug interactions or adverse reactions. Rose decreased her nutritional and fluid intake, which increased the concentration and effect of the medications. She also misjudged her reserve capacity to recover from this illness. Also, she did not keep track of the situation as it changed or alert her physician when her condition worsened. Finally, she did not realize that her decreased activity reduced her ability to eliminate the medication.

Then Rose experienced disorientation and depression, two common symptoms of adverse drug reactions. If she had had anemia, low albumin levels, or a renal, hepatic, or cardiovascular dysfunction, the risk of a severe adverse reaction would have been high.

---

associated with normal aging or are the result of one drug or a combination of drugs. Basic knowledge of age-related changes and common pharmacotherapeutics helps the physician and the nurse to appropriately assess and treat the geriatric patient.

Reduced reserve capacity

Normal aging can also reduce normal body maintenance functions. Elderly people, especially frail ones, often cope poorly with illness or injury because they have a lowered reserve capacity when challenged by adverse conditions. Their responses to illness or injury tend to be more catastrophic, especially when they experience a rapid onset of disease or several adverse conditions simultaneously.

The reduced reserve capacity is frequently overlooked, however, because most geriatric patients maintain homeostasis fairly well when they are unchallenged. However, the nurse must be alert to this deficit because a geriatric patient who seems quite well may suddenly become a high-risk patient when threatened by a con-dition as simple as a urinary tract infection. A sign of reduced reserve capacity is the presence of orthostatic hypotension, a common geriatric condition in frail elderly people. Many factors may lead to orthostatic hypotension, including diseases, medications such as diuretics and autonomic inhibitors, immobility, and dehydration. In some patients, all of these factors are present simultaneously. The nurse's alertness to reduced reserve capacity and prompt intervention can avert a potentially fatal incident.

Confusion

Most people consider forgetfulness to be a natural part of aging, but the nurse must remember that the onset of confusion or a sudden increase in forgetfulness is the most common symptom of drug toxicity. Any changes in a patient's health status require investigation to determine if the changes are related to illness or drug toxicity. For example, a fall that caused an injury may have resulted from confusion. The nurse's astute history taking, observation, and knowledge of drug effects and adverse reactions will help determine if the confusion is a symptom of an underlying health problem or a normal part of aging.

The nurse may experience difficulty in assessing a confused or cognitively impaired patient. If so, the nurse should initiate a medication review and obtain information from the patient's family or friends, as necessary.

EFFECTS ON PHARMACOKINETICS

Many physiologic changes of aging affect drug absorption, distribution, metabolism, and excretion. The nurse must be especially aware of these changes when administering medications to a geriatric patient and when observing for adverse drug reactions.

Absorption

Age-related changes in the gastrointestinal (GI) system can alter drug absorption by decreasing gastric acid secretion and GI motility. When the pH of gastric contents is neutral or alkaline, medications formulated to dissolve in an acid medium will dissolve poorly, decreasing absorption. In a geriatric patient, the stomach empties slowly and intestinal contents move slowly. This slower action lengthens exposure of GI mucosa to an orally administered drug and may increase absorption.

Distribution

The aging process alters body composition and produces cardiac and hematologic changes that can affect drug distribution. In most geriatric patients, total body mass, lean body mass, and total body water decrease, and total body fat increases. These changes in body composition can affect a drug's concentration and solubility in the body. A water-soluble drug, such as gentamicin, is distributed primarily in the aqueous parts of the body and the lean tissue. Because the geriatric patient has relatively less water and lean tissue, more of the water-soluble drug stays in the blood, which can increase blood concentration levels and require dosage reduction.

Distribution of a fat-soluble drug is also affected by age. Because the geriatric patient has a higher proportion of body fat, more of a fat-soluble drug is distributed to the fatty tissue. This produces misleadingly low blood levels and may cause the dosage to be incorrectly increased. The fatty tissue slowly releases the stored drug into the bloodstream. This phenomenon explains why a fat-soluble sedative, such as phenobarbital, may produce a hangover effect.

After age 30, cardiac output normally declines approximately 1% per year, reducing the circulatory function and drug distribution. Other factors, such as cardiovascular insufficiency, dehydration, hypotension, inactivity, and bed rest, also reduce cardiac output and drug distribution.

The aging process may alter blood levels of hemoglobin and albumin, blood proteins that bind with and transport many drugs. In a geriatric patient, albumin and hemoglobin concentrations are slightly decreased. These decreases can significantly inhibit drug-binding capability and may cause toxicity. Low albumin and hemoglobin levels allow a greater percentage of drug to circulate unbound in the blood. When unbound, some drugs, such as warfarin, phenytoin, tolbutamide, and salicylates, are especially likely to cause adverse reactions, even in small doses, and must be used cautiously. The nurse must closely monitor the patient who is receiving such drugs and must teach the patient and the family to recognize signs of toxicity.

Metabolism

The aging process slightly reduces the liver's ability to metabolize drugs. (This reduced ability may result from decreased cardiac output, redistribution of blood flow, or decreased enzyme function.) Poor nutrition, a common problem in the geriatric population, may also influence drug metabolism. A patient on a low-protein, high-carbohydrate diet metabolizes medications slower than a patient on a balanced diet.

The liver has two major pathways for drug metabolism. Phase I, the nonsynthesis pathway, involves oxidation, reduction, and hydrolysis. Phase I is inhibited by the aging process much more than Phase II, the synthesis pathway, which involves coupling of the drug or its metabolite with glucuronic, acetic, sulfuric, or amino acid. Some medications may be detoxified by the liver, whereas others maintain high blood concentration levels even after the first pass through the liver. This can lead to uneven drug metabolism. For example, a patient who does not metabolize a medication well in Phase I may develop signs of toxicity from one medication but experience therapeutic effects of another drug that was metabolized in Phase II. The patient may develop mildly toxic effects from increased levels of both medications. Cimetidine demonstrates a profound effect on Phase I metabolism, slowing this pathway's reactions and inhibiting hepatic circulation. When combined with other medications that require hepatic metabolism, cimetidine dramatically increases their risk of toxicity.

Reduced blood flow to the liver, possibly resulting from decreased cardiac output, also decreases the rate at which the liver metabolizes medications. This decreased rate increases the risk of toxicity.

The symptoms of altered metabolism are difficult to predict. Observation skills can help the nurse detect signs of toxicity, and a knowledge of pharmacology can help relate these signs to a particular drug. An awareness of metabolic pathways will help the nurse formulate a care plan to monitor carefully for adverse drug reactions.

Excretion

In any patient, renal function is the most important factor in drug clearance and excretion. With aging, a significant decline occurs in the renal system with loss of 40% to 50% of its function by age 80. This age-related decline may reduce the drug excretion rate and elevate drug concentration levels—a problem in an older patient in whom high medication concentration levels can cause toxic symptoms even before reaching the usual toxic levels.

Other factors, such as decreased circulatory volume and the use of multiple drugs, frequently further the physiologic decrease in renal function. If decreased circulatory function delivers less blood-borne medication to the kidneys, medication may accumulate in the blood, leading to toxicity.

Numerous medications can inhibit renal function even when given in low doses. They may cause retention of a specific drug or of all drugs. Drugs frequently used in geriatric patients, such as digoxin, cimetidine, lithium, procainamide, and some penicillin-like antibiotics, commonly diminish renal function.

Alcohol consumption and cigarettes can cause unpredictable changes in drug elimination in a geriatric patient.

EFFECTS ON PHARMACODYNAMICS

A geriatric patient may experience an increase or decrease in a drug's mechanism of action—that is, how a drug acts on a target organ. In the target organ, the receptor site's ability to respond to medication may change, caused by a shift in the number, function, or sensitivity of receptor sites that control the response. Receptor-site dysfunction may drastically alter the effects of some medications, but not others.

Receptor-site sensitivity usually increases with age, causing an increase in a drug's effect, which may help explain the high incidence of toxic reactions in geriatric patients. Usual adult dosages, based on research using young, healthy adults, should be used with caution in a frail elderly patient. The normal dose for a patient age 20 could cause adverse reactions in a patient age 80. (See *Drugs that commonly cause adverse reactions in geriatric patients.*)

Decreased receptor-site sensitivity may develop, causing a geriatric patient to have a reduced therapeutic response to a medication. Two important medications, lidocaine and propranolol, are less potent in a geriatric patient, probably because of decreased receptor sensitivity in the myocardium. To obtain a therapeutic response, a larger dose must be given, but the risk of toxicity increases with the size of the dose. The nurse must be vigilant in observing for signs of toxicity.

Physiologic and pathophysiologic changes in organ function may affect response to medication, even if the receptor is functioning properly. The pathologic changes may prevent an organ from responding to the action at the receptor.

NURSING CONSIDERATIONS

Whenever a geriatric patient takes medications, the risk of medication errors and adverse reactions is high. Well planned nursing interventions can help prevent drug-related problems.

HIGH-RISK FACTORS

Although elderly people constitute only about 11% of the population, they annually use 25% to 30% of all prescription drugs sold. Also, the elderly purchase up to

---

Drugs that commonly cause adverse reactions in geriatric patients

The nurse should administer the following drugs cautiously to geriatric patients since normal adult dosages may cause adverse reactions.

• allopurinol	• codeine
• amphetamines	• digoxin
• antidepressants	• flurazepam
• antihypertensives	• gentamicin
• aspirin	• heparin
• barbiturates	• indomethacin
• chlordiazepoxide	• phenothiazines
• cimetidine	• warfarin

40% of nonprescription medications. Not only do elderly people use medications frequently, they also experience adverse drug reactions two to seven times more frequently than younger people.

Geriatric patients tend to use more than one medication concurrently. In some studies of institutionalized geriatric patients, nearly 10% were taking 12 or more medications before admission. The average nursing home patient takes three to six prescription drugs a day. At this high rate of drug use, patients are likely to have adverse drug reactions.

Medication errors may further increase the risk of drug reactions. A quarter to a half of noninstitutionalized patients make medication errors, usually because of medication knowledge deficits. Geriatric patients are no exception. About 25% of all medication errors lead to a worsening of health problems and require medical care or hospital admission.

Several risk factors help identify geriatric patients who are prone to adverse drug reactions. Identification of high-risk geriatric patients can allow the nurse to protect them by monitoring closely, preventing medication errors, identifying drug-related problems promptly, and intervening as needed. The risk factors include advanced age, small physique, multiple illnesses, multiple medications, previous adverse drug reactions, living alone, and malnutrition.

Many of the risk factors are interrelated. A geriatric patient who takes multiple medications is prone to medication errors and will probably have a history of adverse drug reactions. An elderly patient who lives alone is more likely to be malnourished and dehydrated than one who lives with family or in an institution. A patient who lives alone and has multiple illnesses may also lack support systems that assist with medication problems. Financial problems and lack of access to a pharmacy to obtain medications may compound these problems for a patient who lives alone.

NURSING INTERVENTIONS

To help a geriatric patient comply with the medication regimen and avoid adverse reactions, the nurse should simplify the medication schedule, educate the patient and family, review medications periodically, help the patient to overcome cognitive and functional impairments, assess the patient's ability to obtain medications, plan for medical follow-up care, and assess the patient's risk level.

Simplify the medication schedule

Compliance drops sharply when more than three medications are prescribed. This drop may result from confusion about multiple medication schedules, concern about taking too much medication, or concern about the cost of medications. Cost is especially important for patients who live on fixed incomes.

Devising the simplest possible medication schedule is the best way to increase compliance and reduce medication errors. The nurse should help the patient associate medications with meals, daily activities, or bedtime, if possible, to aid memory and establish a routine.

If the patient has a memory or sensory deficit, the nurse may introduce a system to administer medication safely. For example, the nurse may suggest the use of prefilled insulin syringes for a diabetic patient with decreased vision. The syringes contain the correct amount of medication, can be stored in the refrigerator, and allow the patient to take the insulin safely every day. For another, slightly impaired patient, the nurse may suggest individual prefilled envelopes or containers labeled with the medication, day of the week, and time of administration. The envelopes or containers, which can be refilled at scheduled intervals, allow the nurse to see how much medication has been taken. Medicine boxes based on this system are commercially available. They all provide compartments that hold medication doses, and the expensive models have programmable alarms that sound when medications are due. Of course, a labeled egg carton can serve the same compartmentalizing purpose at a much lower cost.

Another way to simplify the medication schedule is to give as few doses of a medication as possible. Although a simple schedule is best, high drug doses given at longer intervals may be dangerous to a geriatric patient because this schedule can produce a pattern of toxic blood levels followed by subtherapeutic ones. To avoid this toxic-subtherapeutic pattern and maintain even blood levels, the nurse may suggest using the drug in a sustained-release form. Or the nurse may recommend adjusting the dosage to twice a day, depending on the drug's half-life. A drug with a long half-life, such as digoxin, should be given once a day. A drug with a short half-life, such as acetaminophen, should be given several times a day, although perhaps not as frequently as a younger person might receive it.

Educate the patient and family

With geriatric patients, nurses frequently encounter a lack of knowledge about medications, including the reason for the prescription and the important therapeutic and adverse effects. These patients sometimes have difficulty learning about one drug, much less several. Hospitalized patients typically have little chance to learn about the medications that are administered to them or to make decisions about how to take them. All too often, insufficient patient education involves only a quick drug description during the intense activity that accompanies discharge. Because most individuals remember less than half of what they hear, and even less when under stress, many patients arrive home with little information about their medications. In a geriatric patient, who may be affected by sensory deficits, multisystem disease, and the stress of recent illness and hospitalization, retention of knowledge about medications is even less likely.

To avoid these pitfalls, the nurse must begin to teach the patient and the family about the prescribed medications well before discharge. To reinforce this teaching, the nurse can provide written information in large print and in simple terms geared to the patient's educational level and suitable for patient and family review at home. (See *Using a medication card* on page 220 and Chapter 11, Intervention: Patient Education, for additional patient-teaching ideas and information.)

Review medications periodically

The nursing care plan should include regular medication reviews even if the physician has prescribed no new medications. The nurse must determine which drugs the patient is taking, because a geriatric patient may stray from a regimen in several ways.

A geriatric patient may: (1) experiment with self-treatment by taking the medication of a friend who seems to have similar symptoms, (2) take a medication that was discontinued long ago if old symptoms reappear, or discontinue a medication as symptoms improve, (3) have drugs prescribed by a physician who may not know all the medications that the patient is taking, and (4) take one or more OTC medications that may cause serious drug interactions or toxicity. A periodic medication review allows the nurse to evaluate the total medication regimen, to report potential problems, and to coordinate the medication therapy safely. The potential for drug interactions requires special attention, and medications that follow the same metabolic pathways or that have long half-lives need careful consideration. The nurse should report any adverse reactions to the physician immediately.

The medication review is especially important for a home care nurse who may be the only health care professional to see what medications the patient is taking and to ensure that all drugs are currently and appropriately prescribed. As part of the medication review, the home care nurse should inspect the medicine cabinet and other storage areas to remove out-of-date or dangerous drugs.

Overcome cognitive and functional impairments

An impaired patient, especially one with a progressive disorder such as dementia, requires special consideration. The nurse must assure this patient's safety, while promoting dignity and independence. The nurse can help a cognitively impaired patient by prepouring medications and putting away the excess. Strategies for overcoming a functional impairment depend on its nature, which may range from an inability to open containers to decreased vision or limited mobility. The nurse must carefully question the patient to form a workable plan for overcoming the impairment. For example, a patient who has difficulty reaching the bathroom may want to omit diuretics. The nurse may suggest that the patient closely watch intake of fluids to reduce the need for the diuretic.

Assess the ability to obtain medications

A geriatric patient is usually discharged from the hospital with a variety of prescriptions. The hospital nurse can facilitate compliance by assessing the patient's ability to obtain medications. If the patient will be homebound, the nurse should develop a system that involves family, friends, or visiting nurses in obtaining medications. The nurse may also suggest the use of a pharmacy that delivers. Also, the nurse should assess the patient's financial status to ensure that the patient can pay for needed medications. Referral to a social worker may be necessary to obtain financial assistance.

Plan for medical follow-up

Anyone who receives medications needs medical follow-up. A homebound, confused, or isolated geriatric patient is more likely to take a prescribed medication improperly, have adverse reactions, or combine prescription and OTC medications. The nurse should help the patient plan for medical follow-up before discharge. If the patient has several physicians, the nurse should clarify which one will be the primary physician. The nurse should also ensure that the patient can contact this physician or arrange for special assistance, if needed.

Assess the patient's risk level

When assessing a geriatric patient, the nurse can use the high-risk factors described earlier as a guide for interventions. An isolated or malnourished patient may

Using a medication card

As follow-up to patient teaching, the nurse can compile drug information on a card, including the dose, the frequency of administration, and other information as shown on the sample card below. Taping a tablet or capsule on the card may also be helpful in identifying the drug. The medication card can help the patient and family remember and comply with the drug regimen and serve as a guide to reordering the medication, if necessary. It can also help inform the physician about the patient's medications and be invaluable if an emergency arises or if the patient cannot communicate.

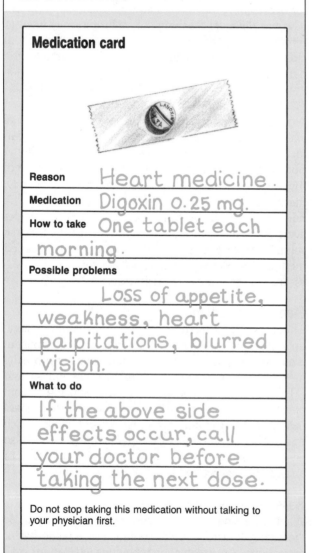

Medication card

Reason	Heart medicine.
Medication	Digoxin 0.25 mg.
How to take	One tablet each morning.
Possible problems	Loss of appetite, weakness, heart palpitations, blurred vision.
What to do	If the above side effects occur, call your doctor before taking the next dose.

Do not stop taking this medication without talking to your physician first.

benefit from Meals on Wheels, meal programs at senior centers, or, possibly, nursing home placement. A patient who has experienced several adverse drug reactions may benefit from prepoured medications, frequent nursing visits, reduced drug doses, or discontinuation of medications, as prescribed.

CHAPTER SUMMARY

This chapter has concentrated on the special medication needs of geriatric patients. Here are its highlights:
- Atypical signs and symptoms of diseases and drug toxicities make the diagnosis of health problems in geriatric patients difficult and require special knowledge.
- The metabolism of a geriatric patient differs greatly from that of a younger patient. Age-related changes, accumulated illnesses, concurrent use of many drugs, and other factors increase the incidence of health problems in the elderly. Many of these health problems result from adverse drug reactions and drug toxicity.
- An etiology may be particularly difficult to determine because it can be caused by normal aging processes, pathology, or medications and because cognitive impairment can adversely influence the patient's ability to describe symptoms or medication use.
- Geriatric patients commonly use multiple medications, which puts them at a higher risk for toxic reactions.
- Age-related changes may affect various organ systems at different rates, especially the renal, hepatic, and cardiovascular systems. In turn, age-related changes can disrupt pharmacokinetic processes. With multiple deficits, diminished function in one system can reduce the function of other systems.
- The nurse can further patient compliance with a self-medication regimen and reduce the likelihood of adverse reactions by simplifying the patient's medication schedule, educating the patient and family, reviewing medications periodically, helping the patient to overcome cognitive and functional impairments, assessing the patient's ability to obtain medications, planning for follow-up care, and assessing the patient's risk level.

BIBLIOGRAPHY

Anderson, W. F., and Judge, T.G., eds. *Geriatric Medicine.* New York: Academic Press, 1974.

Conrad, K.A., and Bressler, R., eds. *Drug Therapy for the Elderly.* St. Louis: C.V. Mosby Co., 1982.

Garnett, W.R., and Barr, W.H. *Geriatrics Pharmacokinetics.* Richmond, Va.: Department of Pharmacy and Pharmaceutics, Medical College of Virginia, 1984.

Hodkinson, H.M. *Outline of Geriatrics.* New York: Academic Press, 1981.

Jarvik, L.F., and Greenblatt, D.J. *Clinical Pharmacology and the Aged Patient,* vol. 16. New York: Raven Press Pubs., 1981.

Judge, T.G., and Caird, F. *Drug Treatment and the Elderly Patient,* 2nd ed. New York: Pitman Books Ltd., 1982.

Krupp, M.A., et al. *Current Medical Diagnosis and Treatment* 1986. Los Altos, Calif.: Lange Medical Pubns., 1986.

O'Malley, K., and Waddington, J.L., eds. "Therapeutics in the Elderly: Scientific Foundations and Clinical Practice," *Proceedings of the Symposium on Pharmacology and Therapeutics in the Elderly.* Dublin, March 20-21, 1985.

Pearson, L.J., and Kotthoff, E.M. *Geriatric Clinical Protocols.* Philadelphia: J.B. Lippincott Co., 1979.

Steinberg, F., ed. *Care of the Geriatric Patient.* St. Louis: C.V. Mosby Co., 1984.

Walshe, T.M. *Manual of Clinical Problems in Geriatric Medicine.* Boston: Little, Brown & Co., 1985.

CHAPTER
14

INTERVENTION: THE PREGNANT OR LACTATING PATIENT

OBJECTIVES

After reading and studying this chapter, you should be able to:

1. Identify factors that alter absorption, distribution, metabolism, and excretion of a drug ingested by a pregnant or lactating patient.

2. Describe the effects of drug exposure on the fetus at different times during gestation.

3. Describe the components the nurse should include in the patient education of a pregnant or lactating patient.

4. Describe the clinical indications for antacids, antiemetics, laxatives and stool softeners, and nonnarcotic analgesics during pregnancy.

5. Describe the nurse's role when drugs are administered during labor and delivery.

6. Describe the anatomy and physiology of the breast and how drugs pass through breast milk.

INTRODUCTION

Pregnant and lactating patients require special consideration during drug therapy. Throughout gestation, especially during the first trimester, the fetus is sensitive to substances ingested by the mother. After birth, the breast-feeding infant may also be sensitive because of immature metabolism and excretion systems.

Despite increasing recognition of the potential adverse effects of drugs administered during pregnancy and lactation, pregnant and lactating women are increasing their drug consumption. Almost 50% of all pregnant women have used at least one drug during their pregnancy. (Comparable statistics for lactating women are not available.) Many of these women took their drugs without medical supervision and without knowledge of the potential adverse effects on the fetus and infant.

Precise data for the effects of drugs on pregnant and lactating women remain unavailable. Consequently, most pharmaceutical compounds approved for use in the United States carry disclaimers that the safety of the

Pregnancy drug risk categories

The following summarizes the Food and Drug Administration (FDA) risk-factor categories for drugs used during pregnancy.

Category A: Controlled studies in women fail to demonstrate a risk to the fetus in the first trimester (no evidence of a risk in later trimesters); the possibility of fetal harm appears remote.

Category B: Animal-reproduction studies have not demonstrated a fetal risk (no controlled studies in pregnant women), or animal-reproduction studies have shown an adverse effect other than decreased fertility that was not confirmed in controlled studies with women in the first trimester; no evidence of a risk in later trimesters.

Category C: Studies in animals have revealed teratogenic, embryocidal, or other effects on the fetus, or no controlled studies in women or animals are available. Drugs should be administered only if the potential benefit justifies the potential risk to the fetus.

Category D: Positive evidence of human fetal risk exists, but the benefits from use in pregnant women may be acceptable despite the risk (for example, if the drug is needed in a life-threatening situation or for a serious disease for which safer drugs cannot be used or are ineffective).

Category X: Studies in animals or women have demonstrated fetal abnormalities, or evidence of fetal risk exists based on human experience, or both, and the risk in pregnant women clearly outweighs any possible benefit. The drug is contraindicated in women who are or may become pregnant.

Category NR: No rating available.

Adapted with permission from Briggs, G., Freeman, R., and Yaffe, S. *Drugs in Pregnancy and Lactation,* 2nd ed. Baltimore: Williams and Wilkins Co., 1986.

drug has not been established for use in pregnant and lactating women. Physicians and nurses are thus faced with the responsibility of counseling these patients without the benefit of well-documented, research-based information.

In 1979, the Food and Drug Administration (FDA) established five categories (A, B, C, D, X) to indicate the level of risk to a fetus posed by drugs. While these categories are helpful, they may not be entirely accurate. (See *Pregnancy drug risk categories* for the FDA risk categories.)

THE PREGNANT PATIENT

Most drugs ingested by a pregnant patient cross the placenta to the fetus. A number of pregnancy-related changes and structures can alter the absorption, distribution, metabolism, and excretion of a drug ingested by the pregnant patient. The fetus also significantly influences drug distribution and disposition.

PHARMACOKINETICS

During pregnancy, the tone and motility of the gastrointestinal (GI) tract decrease, probably from increased progesterone production and decreased motilin levels (an intestinal hormone that causes increased intestinal motility and also stimulates pepsin secretions). These effects prolong the gastric emptying and intestinal transit times. The formation of hydrochloric acid in the stomach also decreases. All these factors delay absorption of drugs that require an acidic environment or that are absorbed in the small intestine.

Absorption of drugs administered parenterally may also be altered during pregnancy. Because of peripheral vasodilation, drugs administered subcutaneously, intramuscularly, or intradermally may be absorbed more rapidly.

The physiologic changes of pregnancy also alter drug distribution. Influencing factors include increased interstitial and cellular water and increased blood volume, elevated nearly 45% by the end of gestation. These increases change the ratios of blood constituents that affect drug distribution. For example, the ratio of albumin to water decreases during pregnancy. This decrease further dilutes the free drug in tissue and plasma and affects protein-binding capacity, thereby increasing the level of free drug available from a dose.

During pregnancy, estrogen and progesterone levels also rise, as do those of free fatty acids (triglycerides, cholesterol, and phospholipids) from increased fatty tissue metabolism. These effects are accompanied by increased competition for protein-binding sites. With fewer binding sites, a larger percentage of drug remains free to move to receptor sites or across the placenta.

Numerous changes in the urinary system occur during pregnancy and can affect drug excretion. The glomerular filtration rate and renal plasma flow (RPF) increase early in pregnancy, and the former persists to birth. Because of the increased RPF, drugs that normally are easily excreted may be eliminated even more rapidly.

The term "placental barrier" can be misleading because it implies that the placenta protects the fetus from drug effects. In fact, many drugs ingested by the pregnant patient will cross the placenta and reach the fetus. Although some drugs, such as insulin, do not cross the placenta, most do when administered at therapeutic levels.

Placental transport of substances to and from the fetus begins at approximately the fifth week of gestation. Substances of low molecular weight diffuse freely across the placenta, driven primarily by the concentration gradient, although active transport, facilitated diffusion, and other transport processes also are involved.

Any condition that alters placental circulation, such as pregnancy-induced hypertension or diabetes mellitus, can affect drug transport. Differences in maternal and fetal pH will also increase the rate of transfer and reabsorption of drugs.

Because the placenta is metabolically active, it can affect drug disposition. The placenta appears to be capable of several enzymatic reactions, including reduction, hydrolysis, and conjugation, that can reduce the potency of a drug's metabolites. Conversely, these reactions may produce a more potent and toxic metabolite, thereby increasing fetal danger.

The fetus may also significantly affect drug distribution and disposition by fetal circulation, binding of plasma and tissue proteins, and excretory activity. Furthermore, enzyme systems that are normally deficient during fetal life can be stimulated by certain drugs. The fetus also has slower drug clearance than the adult, and drugs persist longer in the fetus' tissues and blood than in the mother's.

DRUG ADMINISTRATION

Drug effects on the fetus depend upon the timing of drug administration in relation to gestational age. During the first week to the end of the second week of pregnancy, fertilization, implantation, and rudimentary placental formation occur. During the embryonic period,

Known teratogens

The following known teratogens are not recommended for use during pregnancy under any circumstances (FDA classification category X).

AGENT	ADVERSE EFFECTS
methotrexate (anti-neoplastic)	Meningoencephalocele, cranial anomalies, cleft lip or palate, low-set ears, malpositioned extremities
disulfiram (used to prevent alcohol consumption in patients with a history of alcohol abuse)	Clubfoot, multiple anomalies with VACTERL syndrome (radial aplasia, vertebral fusion, tracheoesophageal fistula), phocomelia
diethylstilbesterol	*In the female:* vaginal adenosis, vaginal and cervical clear cell adenocarcinoma, cervical or vaginal fornix defects, vaginal defects, uterine or fallopian defects *In the male:* reproductive dysfunction, altered semen analysis, infertility
alcohol (sedative), category X if used in large amounts or for prolonged time	Fetal alcohol syndrome: craniofacial deformities, mild to moderate retardation, growth deficiency; cardiac, renogenital, cutaneous, skeletal, and muscular defects
oral contraceptives (estrogenic and progestogenic hormones)	Progesterone-related effects: masculinization of female infants, increased serum bilirubin

AGENT	ADVERSE EFFECTS
phencyclidine [PCP] (hallucinogen)	Depressed newborn, craniofacial abnormalities, weakened muscular function of eyes and neck
sodium iodine ^{125}I or ^{131}I (radiopharmaceutical or diagnostic agent)	Anomalies involving head, skin, and limbs have been observed, but a causal relationship has not been proven; if administered at 12 weeks or beyond, abolition of fetal thyroid gland
measles vaccine	Increased abortion, congenital malformations (theoretical risk only)
mumps vaccine	Increased first trimester abortion, fibroelastosis of the newborn (theoretical risk only)
rubella vaccine	Congenital rubella syndrome (theoretical risk only)
smallpox vaccine	Fetal death
isotretinoin (vitamin A isomer)	Central nervous system, facial, cardiovascular defects
vitamin A (category X if used in dosages greater than RDA)	Congenital xerophthalmia, anophthalmia, other eye anomalies; with high dosages, urinary tract defects

Adapted with permission from Briggs, G., Freeman, R., and Yaffe, S. *Drugs in Pregnancy and Lactation*, 2nd ed. Baltimore: Williams and Wilkins Co., 1986.

from the second through the eighth week, the major organ systems form (organogenesis). The fetal period, from the ninth week to the end of pregnancy, is one of rapid body growth. Some tissue differentiation also occurs. Functional maturation continues after birth.

The fetus is most susceptible to the adverse effects of drugs from the time of implantation to the embryonic period, with limb formation defects potentially occurring through the end of the first trimester. During conception and implantation, the ovum is bathed in fallopian tube fluid. At that time, any damage to the ovum from drug exposure is usually lethal; however, the ovum can recover completely from damage inflicted by a sublethal dose. During the embryonic period, major structural anomalies may occur after only a single exposure to a toxic drug. Teratogenic drug exposure (causing fetal anomalies) during the fetal period usually slows cell growth and retards growth of the exposed part or of the entire fetus. Such an effect is called intrauterine growth retardation.

The care with which a drug is administered to the mother and infant during the intrapartum period is critical to the infant's safety. Maternal-fetal equilibrium of drug levels is usually reached within 40 minutes after drug ingestion and more rapidly with parenteral or intravenous administration.

Drug teratogenesis

Drug exposure during pregnancy probably accounts for only about 1% of all congenital anomalies. Almost 60% of congenital anomalies have no known cause, and 20% are probably from hereditary tendencies and unknown environmental factors.

The mechanisms whereby drugs exert teratogenic effects are poorly understood. Drugs may alter maternal tissues with indirect effects upon the fetus, or they may directly affect the embryonic cells, resulting in specific abnormalities. Drugs may also interfere with nutrient transport or alter placental metabolism, both of which may interfere with fetal nutrition.

Health care professionals are increasingly concerned with the adverse effects of drugs on the intellect and the social and functional behavior of the child; however, determining just how a drug produces such anomalies is difficult, especially given the number of intervening variables not related to drug use. Identifying causal relationship for drugs that may produce delayed effects following intrauterine exposure is also difficult. For example, researchers suspect that the maternal ingestion of diethylstilbestrol leads to an increased risk of adenocarcinoma of the vagina in female offspring or abnormalities of the reproductive system in male offspring. However, an exact link has not been established. (See *Known teratogens* for some other drugs that may cause adverse effects.)

PHARMACOTHERAPEUTICS

When counseling the pregnant patient, the physician should evaluate each drug to determine whether equivalent benefits can be obtained through alternative measures. The patient should actively participate in these decisions. If a drug must be used, the physician should prescribe one that has been widely used in pregnancy for many years rather than a recently introduced drug with inadequately established effects.

The physician will substitute alternative measures, if possible, during the pregnancy time when a drug is likely to produce teratogenic effects. For example, a pregnant patient with thromboembolic disease might receive anticoagulants, such as warfarin. However, warfarin exposure during the first 6 to 9 weeks of gestation carries an 8% incidence of warfarin embryopathy, characterized by hypoplasia (underdevelopment) of the nose and stippled epiphyses (faulty growth and ossification of ends of long bones). Exposure after the first trimester may produce central nervous system (CNS) defects. The physician can reduce the risks by substituting heparin during the first trimester, followed by warfarin between weeks 13 and 36 and heparin for the last weeks of pregnancy.

The physician and nurse should educate both pregnant and nonpregnant patients of childbearing age about the use of drugs, including the array of over-the-counter medications. The nonpregnant patient should be instructed to be aware of her last menstrual period so that she can recognize a pregnancy at the earliest possible time; many women self-medicate without knowing they are pregnant. Those women attempting to conceive should discuss with their physician, nurse, midwife, or pharmacist any drug they are taking or considering. The pregnant patient should never self-medicate without consultation with her physician.

Pregnancy usually produces some discomfort. The most frequent complaints involve the GI tract, including heartburn, nausea and vomiting, and constipation. The patient may also need a nonnarcotic analgesic throughout gestation to relieve headaches and minor muscle discomforts. The drugs frequently used to alleviate these symptoms include antacids, antiemetics, laxatives and stool softeners, and nonnarcotic analgesics. The nurse should be aware of these agents and the implications associated with their use.

Antacids. Antacids are used by approximately 50% of pregnant women for relief of heartburn and other reflux symptoms. Unfortunately, little data are available on the antacid effects on the fetus. Physicians currently consider most aluminum-, magnesium-, and calcium-containing antacids safe in therapeutic doses during the second and third trimesters. Sodium bicarbonate and magnesium trisilicate, however, should be avoided. The nurse counseling a pregnant patient about reflux symptoms should encourage the patient to avoid behaviors that aggravate heartburn (overeating, consuming fatty or fried foods, and lying down too soon after meals). Milk, hot tea, chewing gum, good posture, and small meals can prevent or minimize such symptoms.

Antiemetics. The antiemetic prochlorperazine maleate (Compazine) has been linked to an increased risk of cardiovascular and other malformations. Diphenhydramine hydrochloride (Benadryl) may cause cleft palate, and trimethobenzamide hydrochloride (Tigan) may produce other congenital anomalies. Phosphorated carbohydrate solution (Emetrol), an over-the-counter liquid preparation used to treat morning sickness, has not been linked to toxicity.

The nurse counseling a pregnant patient about the nausea and vomiting associated with pregnancy can encourage nonpharmacologic practices to minimize the symptoms, including eating small, frequent meals; con-

(Text continues on page 228.)

Drugs used during labor and delivery

This chart supplies important information on drugs used during labor and delivery and their effects on the labor, the mother, the fetus, and the newborn.

DRUG OR CLASS	USE	ADVERSE LABOR OR FETAL EFFECTS
Analgesics		
narcotics	Relieve pain	May increase uterine activity (meperidine), fetal distress, labor secondary to reduced tone and contractions
Antianxiety agents		
benzodiazepines (diazepam)	Sedate just before or after delivery; usually not used during delivery	May cause loss of beat-to-beat variability in fetal heart rate, decreased fetal movements, fetal tachycardia
phenothiazines (promazine, promethazine)	Relieve pain and sedate when combined with narcotic; control nausea and vomiting	May increase or decrease uterine activity
Anesthetics		
inhalation nitrous oxide	Reduces loss of pain perception during labor and delivery	May cause maternal and fetal hypoxia if concentration exceeds 70%
ether	Reduces loss of pain perception during labor and delivery	May cause uterine relaxation, fetal depression
local, regional	Relieve pain through blockage of nerve impulse initiation and conduction	Local: may cause fetal bradycardia. Regional: may impede labor if administered too early; may cause fetal distress secondary to maternal hypotension

ADVERSE MATERNAL EFFECTS	ADVERSE NEWBORN EFFECTS	NURSING IMPLICATIONS
Respiratory depression, restlessness, decreased oxygen consumption, postural hypotension, tachycardia, nausea, vomiting, urinary retention	Respiratory depression (time and dose dependent)	• Observe the patient for progress of labor, signs of fetal distress, signs of respiratory depression, and hypotension. • Observe the newborn for signs of depression. • Have available a narcotic antagonist, such as naloxone (Narcan), recommended for infants.
Ataxia, drowsiness, lethargy	Dose-dependent response: frequency of newborn complications increases when doses exceed 30 mg or ingested long-term. Two major syndromes noted: floppy infant syndrome (hypotonia, lethargy, sucking difficulties) and withdrawal syndrome (intrauterine growth retardation, tremors, irritability, hypertonicity, diarrhea and vomiting, vigorous sucking); may alter thermogenesis	• Because transplacental passage is rapid, time the I.V. dose during contraction to reduce the amount of drug transferred to fetus. • Observe the newborn for adverse effects.
Possible stimulation or inhibition of respirations; hypotension, tachycardia	Respiratory depression, rare impairment of platelet aggregation, possible relationship between promazine use and hyperbilirubinemia	• Assess uterine activity and maternal vital signs frequently during labor. • Observe for signs of fetal distress from maternal hypotension. • Observe newborn for bleeding tendency, jaundice, and respiratory depression.
Nausea and vomiting	Possible hypoxia	• Monitor the mother for nausea and vomiting. • Monitor the newborn for signs and symptoms of hypoxia.
Respiratory tract irritation, postoperative nausea and vomiting, depresses central nervous system (CNS), increases secretions, decreases renal function	Depression	• Continuously monitor maternal and fetal status, including maternal urinary output. • Assess newborn for signs of CNS depression. • Assess mother for increased postpartum bleeding.
Local: vasodilation with sustained hypotension possible, CNS stimulation. Regional: may cause hypotension, urinary retention; some techniques may interfere with urge to bear down	Bradycardia with local; fetal distress with regional	• Assess fetal heart tones before and for 30 minutes after administration. • Continuously monitor mother and fetus for signs of hypotension and fetal distress, respectively. • Monitor the mother for urinary retention.

continued

Drugs used during labor and delivery continued

DRUG OR CLASS	USE	ADVERSE LABOR OR FETAL EFFECTS
Other agents		
oxytocin	Stimulates uterine contraction	Speeds labor; if overdosed, may cause fetal distress from impaired uteroplacental blood flow secondary to uterine hypertonus
magnesium sulfate	Prevents eclamptic seizures in patients with pregnancy-induced hypertension; inhibits contractions in preterm labor	Inhibits myometrial activity of uterus, may slow labor, decreases variability of fetal heart tones
ritodrine (FDA-approved for inhibition of preterm labor)	Inhibits uterine contractions	Increases heart rate, increases blood pressure

suming liquid and dry foods separately; avoiding fried, odorous, spicy, greasy, or gas-forming foods; and keeping crackers or other dry food at the bedside to be eaten in the morning before arising.

Laxatives and stool softeners. The pregnant patient may require a laxative or stool softener to treat the constipation and painful hemorrhoids that accompany pregnancy. Certain laxatives are not safe during pregnancy. Castor oil may initiate premature uterine contractions; hyperosmotic saline cathartics, such as magnesium hydroxide and Milk of Magnesia, may promote sodium retention in the mother. Frequent use of lubricants, such as mineral oil, can lead to a decreased absorption of fat-soluble vitamins, resulting in neonatal hypoprothrombinemia and hemorrhage.

Some stimulant laxatives, such as bisacodyl and senna, may be safe during pregnancy, as may stool softeners containing docusate sodium. Bulk-forming laxatives containing psyllium hydrophilic mucilloid may also be safe during pregnancy. As a component of patient teaching, the nurse should encourage nonpharmacologic measures to alleviate constipation or hemorrhoids, such as increasing fluid intake, walking as much as possible during the day, increasing dietary fiber, and avoiding straining while defecating.

Nonnarcotic analgesics. Headaches and minor muscle aches occur frequently during pregnancy. In therapeutic doses, acetaminophen is safe for short-term use during pregnancy for analgesic and antipyretic actions. Prolonged use at high doses, however, has been associated

ADVERSE MATERNAL EFFECTS	ADVERSE NEWBORN EFFECTS	NURSING IMPLICATIONS
Uterine hypertonicity, which if uncorrected may lead to uterine rupture, cervical tears; in large doses may have transient hypotension followed by a sustained rise in blood pressure; water intoxication	Possible hyperbilirubinemia	• Continuously observe mother and infant for signs of uterine hypertonicity, altered vital signs, fetal distress, and signs of water intoxication. • Discontinue infusion and notify physician if indicated by maternal or fetal condition. • Carefully administer medication using infusion pump for better dose titration.
CNS depression resulting from hypermagnesemia: flushing, sweating, sedation, confusion, depressed reflexes, muscle weakness	Potential for depression and hypotonia; aminoglycoside use in newborns exposed near birth may cause respiratory arrest	• Monitor mother for signs of CNS depression; check vital signs, patellar reflex, clonus, and mental status frequently (every 1 to 4 hours, depending on route). • Withhold drug and notify physician if reflexes are absent, respirations below 12, marked decrease in pulse rate, or urine output below 30 ml/hour. • Monitor labor progress. • Keep antidote (calcium gluconate) and syringe available. • Monitor for fetal distress; monitor newborn for weak cry, hyporeflexia, respiratory depression, and flaccidity.
Tachycardia; increased systolic pressure and decreased diastolic pressure; tremor; palpitations; nervousness; pulmonary edema	Hypoglycemia	• Monitor and assess maternal and fetal vital signs. • Monitor the patient's intake and output. • Monitor intensity and frequency of contractions. • Assess newborn for signs of hypoglycemia. • Carefully administer medication with an infusion pump for better dose titration.

with fatal kidney disease in infants. High doses, especially during the first trimester, may also result in severe liver damage in the fetus.

Aspirin, the drug most frequently ingested by pregnant women, has been associated with maternal anemia, antepartum and postpartum hemorrhage, and prolonged gestation and labor. The prolonged gestation and labor result from aspirin's inhibition of prostaglandin synthetase. Aspirin may also delay the induced-abortion time in nulliparous women and complicate delivery.

The adverse effects of aspirin on the fetus and newborn include increased perinatal mortality, intrauterine growth retardation, congenital salicylate intoxication, and depressed albumin-binding capacity. Aspirin given in low doses during the week prior to delivery may affect the newborn's clotting ability.

DRUGS DURING LABOR AND DELIVERY

The need to relieve pain during labor must be balanced with the delivery time and the drug dose to protect the infant from a potentially toxic dose.

When administering an analgesic during labor and delivery, the nurse carefully monitors the maternal and fetal condition by frequent assessment of vital signs, careful observation, and assessment of internal or external monitor information. The nurse also assesses the progress of labor and prepares, if necessary, for a depressed infant. (See *Drugs used during labor and delivery* on pages 226 to 229 for a summary of these drugs.)

THE LACTATING PATIENT

Because most drugs and chemicals ingested by a mother appear in breast milk, physicians must evaluate drug effects on the lactating mother and the infant. Unfortunately, several factors complicate this evaluation: systematic, complete information on individual drugs is lacking; available information is generally questionable because of unscientific studies; measurements of drug concentration are often unrelated to dose timing; conclusions are based on studies of animals whose physiochemical milk properties differ from humans'; and reports on toxic effects do not include the quantity of the drug in breast milk.

Breast anatomy and physiology

A brief review of breast anatomy and physiology and of the process of milk formation indicates how drugs pass through breast milk. The breast is composed of approximately 15 to 20 lobes embedded in fatty stroma. The lobes are drained by the lactiferous ducts near the nipple. In the nipple, the ducts dilate slightly to form the lactiferous sinuses. Each lobe is separated by connective tissue septa through which blood vessels, lymphatic vessels, and nerves pass. This connective tissue further subdivides the lobes into lobules, each with its own excretory or interlobular duct. (See *Anatomy of the breast* for an illustration.)

The basic secretory units of the lobes are the alveoli, surrounded in a basketlike fashion by myoepithelial cells. With the proper stimulus, these cells contract and eject milk from the alveoli and alveolar ducts. Prolactin is the hormone responsible for milk secretion, and oxytocin regulates the let-down (milk-ejection) reflex. Both of these hormones are under neurohormonal control.

Breast milk is a suspension of fat in a protein-mineral-carbohydrate solution; lactose is the carbohydrate. The milk's curds and whey contain many proteins, including alpha-lactalbumin, lactoferrin, albumin, lysozyme, and immunoglobulin A, that may serve as molecules for drug binding and drug transport. The fat structure may also promote drug transport. In the protein-lactose-mineral aqueous phase of milk, the lipid structure is suspended in fat globules that contain lipid surrounded by a lipoprotein membrane. Drugs may be transported by binding to the lipoprotein or be trapped within the milk-fat globule during fat formation.

Milk pH, another important variable affecting drug passage, ranges from 7.0 to 7.6, with an average of 7.2.

Drug characteristics

Before a drug can enter an alveolar cell from the maternal circulation, it must cross the capillary endothelium, extracellular water, cell basement membrane, and cell plasma membrane. Drugs are usually transported by passive diffusion and active transport.

Drug characteristics that affect the degree and rate of transport include molecular weight, solubility, maternal plasma protein-binding, and ionization. A drug with a molecular weight greater than 200 displays difficulty crossing cell membranes. Highly lipid-soluble drugs cross the lipoprotein cell membrane more readily than more water-soluble drugs. Those bound to maternal plasma proteins are not readily transported; a nonprotein-bound (free) drug passes more easily into the milk.

Because most drugs are either weak acids or bases, their crossing of a biological membrane is greatly influenced by ionization characteristics and pH differences. (See Chapter 2, Pharmacokinetics, for more specific information.) Because breast milk has a slightly lower pH than plasma, the milk's ions trap the basic drug compounds. The nonionized portion of a drug, however, can cross the lipid cell membrane.

Other factors that influence a drug's passage into breast milk include the route of administration, absorption rate, and drug half-life.

Maternal factors

Volume composition of breast milk may alter the amount of free drug available. Maternal factors, including nutrition, concurrent diseases, and infant intake, affect milk volume. Also, a high mammary blood flow during peak drug absorption could deliver a greater drug quantity to the milk. Milk fat content, which peaks between 6 a.m. and 10 a.m. and drops to its lowest level in the late evening, can affect drug availability, too. The composition of breast milk also varies depending on the infant's age. These changes in the milk may alter the amount of free (unbound) drug.

Infant characteristics

Unlike the fetus, the infant cannot depend on the placenta for the metabolism and excretion of maternally ingested drugs.

Infant sucking behavior, the amount consumed per feeding, and the frequency of breast-feeding affect the amount of drug the infant ingests. Low gastric acidity and slower absorption rates in the infant also play a role. Changes in plasma protein-binding in the infant may alter drug concentration levels at receptor sites. Further,

Anatomy of the breast

This illustration of the breast anatomy and neurohormonal control depicts the lactation process.

Clavicle

Alveoli

Intralobular duct

Single lobule

Lobes of breast

Lactiferous duct

Lactiferous sinus

Myoepithelial cells

Cavity of alveolus

Nipple — Areola

Single alveolus

Montgomery's tubercle

Fat cells

Rib

Hormonal preparation of breast postpartum for lactation

PIF (prolactin inhibiting factor)

Prolactin releasing factor(s)

Adenohypophysis
Prolactin synthesis increases and prolactin releases into the circulation.

Prolactin

Hypothalamus
Withdrawal of placental and luteal sex hormones and the infant's sucking depress PIF or stimulate prolactin releasing factor(s).

Supportive metabolic hormones
Insulin, cortisol, thyroid hormone, parathyroid hormone, and growth hormone are released.

Breast
Milk is synthesized and released into the mammary alveoli.

Let-down reflex

Neurogenic stimulation

Neurohypophysis
Suckling induces synthesis and release of oxytocin.

Oxytocin

Drugs that affect lactation

Certain drugs ingested by the mother may not adversely affect the infant but may interfere with the hormones controlling milk secretion and let-down (ejection), namely prolactin and oxytocin.

DRUG	EFFECT
anesthetics, sedatives alcohol	Decrease let-down reflex
antihypertensive, cardiovascular agents reserpine	Galactorrhea
diuretics (thiazides) bendroflumethiazide, chlorothiazide	May suppress lactation
hormones contraceptive pill with estrogen and progesterone	Decrease milk production and protein content
antipsychotics neuroleptics	Galactorrhea
stimulants nicotine	Decrease milk production

Adapted with permission from American Academy of Pediatrics, *Pediatrics* 72(3):376-377, 1983.

drugs that are insufficiently metabolized and excreted by immature neonatal systems may accumulate, increasing the risk of toxicity.

Counseling guidelines

The nurse should inform the lactating patient that all drugs should be screened by a physician, nurse, or pharmacist for safety. The nurse should inform the patient about drugs that affect milk secretion. The amount of drug that usually crosses to the milk is small, about 1% to 2% of the maternal dose. Because of the well-established advantages of breast-feeding, it should be discontinued only when substantial evidence exists that the mother's drug treatment may harm the infant. (See *Drugs that affect lactation* for a list of drugs and effects.)

To minimize the amount of a prescribed drug received by the infant, the mother should ingest the drug immediately after breast-feeding and postpone the next breast-feeding for four hours, if possible. Altering the administration schedule is another way to minimize the

infant's drug exposure. For example, if the drug is to be administered once a day, the mother may take the dose before the infant's longest sleep period.

Should an infant become sick or fail to thrive for reasons that cannot be otherwise explained, the mother should discontinue the drug and temporarily discontinue breast-feeding. The mother may use a breast pump to maintain lactation while the infant's responses are monitored. The nurse should obtain samples of maternal plasma, breast milk, and infant plasma for drug assay.

The nurse should teach the lactating patient the potential toxic effects of drugs on the infant. Easily recognizable effects include sedation, poor feeding, diar-

Drugs contraindicated during breast-feeding

Several drugs are contraindicated during breast feeding. The nurse should be aware of these drugs to provide adequate patient education.

DRUG	SIGN OR SYMPTOM IN INFANT
methotrexate*	Possible immune suppression; unknown effect on growth or association with carcinogenesis
cimetidine†	May suppress gastric acidity in infant, inhibit drug metabolism, and produce CNS stimulation
clemastine	Drowsiness, irritability, refusal to feed, high-pitched cry, neck stiffness
cyclophosphamide*	Possible immune suppression; unknown effect on growth or association with carcinogenesis
ergotamine	Vomiting, diarrhea, convulsions (doses used in migraine medications)
gold salts	Rash, inflammation of kidney and liver
methimazole	Potential for interfering with thyroid function

*Data unavailable for other cytotoxic agents.
†Drug is concentrated in breast milk.

Adapted with permission from American Academy of Pediatrics Committee on Drugs, "Transfer of Drugs and Other Chemicals into Human Breast Milk," *Pediatrics* 72(3):375, 1983.

Adverse effects from social drugs during pregnancy or lactation

The nurse should be aware that some socially used drugs can affect the fetus and breast-feeding newborn. This chart contains some drugs that may cause adverse effects during pregnancy, postpartum, and lactation.

DRUG	ADVERSE EFFECTS During pregnancy and postpartum	During lactation
alcohol	Fetal alcohol syndrome	Large doses inhibit let-down reflex and may cause alcohol intoxication in newborn
caffeine	High intake (more than 6 to 8 cups daily) may be associated with complications, including infertility	Heavy maternal use produces irritability and poor sleeping patterns in infant
cocaine*	Depressed interactive abilities; impaired organizational abilities; increased rate of spontaneous abortion; with I.V. use, onset of labor with placental abruption	Newborn exhibits tremors and exaggerated startle response
heroin*	Intrauterine death may occur from meconium aspiration syndrome; potential increase in major fetal anomalies; low birth weight, underdevelopment for gestational age; impaired behavioral, perceptual, and organizational activities	Withdrawal of drug from mother induces withdrawal symptoms in infant; sufficient quantities can cause addiction in infant
marijuana (THC—active ingredient)	Not documented	May impair DNA and RNA formation and proteins essential for proper growth and development
smoking (nicotine and carbon monoxide—active ingredients)	Reduced birth weight	May interfere with let-down reflex

*Effects of these drugs may be complicated by multiple drug use.

rhea, rash, and CNS stimulation. Some drugs may be contraindicated during breast-feeding. (See *Drugs contraindicated during breast-feeding* for a list of drugs and their effects.) Others may require a temporary cessation of breast-feeding. The nurse should also include the effects of social drugs. (See *Adverse effects from social drugs during pregnancy or lactation* for a summary of the documented adverse effects of these drugs.)

CHAPTER SUMMARY

Chapter 14 covered the use of drugs during pregnancy and lactation. The fetus throughout gestation and the breast-feeding infant are sensitive to drugs ingested by the mother. Even so, maternal drug consumption is increasing. Here are the chapter highlights:

• Maternal, placental, and fetal factors alter the absorption, distribution, metabolism, and excretion of a drug. Maternal factors include decreased tone and motility of the GI tract, increased blood volume, altered fat and carbohydrate metabolism, increased glomerular filtration rate, and increased renal plasma flow. Placental factors include the transport of drugs across the placenta and the occurrence of reduction, hydrolysis, conjugation, and oxidation. Fetal factors include fetal circulation and excretion and the stimulation of normally deficient enzyme systems.

• The timing of drug administration during gestation can help prevent teratogenic drug exposure for the fetus.

• When counseling the pregnant woman, the physician and nurse should discuss the benefits and risks of each drug. The patient should be encouraged to use alternative nonpharmacologic measures and alternative drug treatments.

• Antacids, antiemetics, laxatives and stool softeners, and nonnarcotic analgesics should be used with caution by the pregnant patient, who should consult the physician or nurse before using any over-the-counter product.

• When drugs are used in labor and delivery, the nurse must monitor vital signs and assess the progress of labor.

• Most drugs and chemicals ingested by the mother appear in breast milk. When evaluating the use of drugs in a lactating patient, the physician considers drug characteristics, maternal factors, and infant characteristics.

• The nurse should inform the lactating patient about the signs and symptoms of drug toxicity that the infant may exhibit. Drug exposure during lactation may require the temporary discontinuation of breast-feeding.

BIBLIOGRAPHY

American Academy of Pediatrics. Committee on Drugs. "The Transfer of Drugs and Other Chemicals into Human Breast Milk," *Pediatrics* 72:375, 1983.

Balkam, J. "Guidelines for Drug Therapy During Lactation," *Journal of Obstetric, Gynecologic, and Neonatal Nursing* 15:65 January/February 1986.

Briggs, C., et al. *Drugs in Pregnancy and Lactation*, 2nd ed. Baltimore: Williams & Wilkins Co., 1986.

King, C. "Genetic Counseling for Teratogen Exposure," *Obstetrics & Gynecology* 67:843, 1986.

Ledward, R., and Hawkins, D. *Drug Treatment in Obstetrics*. London: Chapman and Hall, 1983.

Lewis, J., et al. "The Use of Gastrointestinal Drugs During Pregnancy and Lactation," *American Journal of Gastroenterology* 80:912, 1985.

Neville, M., and Neifer, M. *Lactation, Physiology, in Nutrition and Breast-Feeding*. New York: Plenum Press, 1983.

Phillans, P., and Coetzee, E. "Anticoagulation During Pregnancy," *South African Medical Journal* 69:469, 1986.

Pritchard, J., et al. *Williams Obstetrics*, 17th ed. Norwalk, Conn.: Appleton-Century-Crofts, 1985.

United States Pharmacopeial Convention. *Drug Information for the Health Care Provider*, vol. 1, 6th ed. Rockville, Md.: USPC, 1986.

CHAPTER 15

INTERVENTION: EMERGENCIES

OBJECTIVES

After reading and studying this chapter, you should be able to:

1. Describe the locations and functions of the alpha-, beta$_1$-, and beta$_2$-adrenergic receptors.

2. Contrast the effects produced by adrenergic-receptor stimulation with those produced by adrenergic blockade.

3. Distinguish among drugs used to correct acidosis, restore heartbeat and increase contractility, correct bradycardia, correct ventricular dysrhythmias, and increase blood pressure and cardiac output.

4. Describe the rationale for use, administration dosages and procedures, and nursing precautions for each of the following drugs: sodium bicarbonate, epinephrine, atropine, isoproterenol, lidocaine, procainamide, bretylium, dopamine, dobutamine, norepinephrine, nitroglycerin, and calcium chloride.

5. Identify those drugs that can effectively be administered endotracheally, and describe the circumstances in which endotracheal administration is recommended.

6. Describe the procedure involved in administering medications endotracheally.

7. Explain the appropriate uses for the following volume expanders in managing hypovolemia: whole blood, plasma products, crystalloids, and colloids.

8. Describe the rationale for use, administration dosages and procedures, and nursing precautions for the following drugs used to treat a hypertensive crisis: nitroprusside, nifedipine, and labetalol.

9. Describe the physiology of anaphylaxis.

10. Describe the rationale for use, administration dosages and procedures, and nursing precautions for the following drugs used in managing anaphylactic shock: epinephrine, aminophylline, theophylline, and diphenhydramine.

11. Describe the administration procedures, dosages, and nursing precautions for naloxone, which is used in managing narcotic overdoses.

INTRODUCTION

All emergencies have in common the need for immediate intervention. Emergencies, however, vary in type and severity. Furthermore, the number of drugs available to treat emergencies continues to grow. Because no one can remember all of the emergency drugs, the nurse must take a more practical approach and know the physiologic response required during an emergency and the pharmacologic drug class that facilitates that response.

This chapter discusses specific physiologic responses involving the adrenergic nervous system and drugs that affect that system. The pharmacologic management of cardiac arrest, cardiogenic shock, hypovolemic states, hypertensive emergencies, anaphylaxis, and narcotic overdose are also discussed. To provide quality patient care, the nurse must know the drug classes, the physiologic rationale for administration, and exact dosages. The nurse who knows the drug classes can assign each newly marketed drug to an existing family, which makes learning about the new drug easier.

ADRENERGIC RECEPTORS: TYPES, LOCATION, AND FUNCTION

The three basic types of adrenergic, or sympathetic, receptors are alpha receptors, beta$_1$ receptors, and beta$_2$ receptors. Alpha receptors are located throughout the body, primarily in the smooth muscle of the peripheral arterioles. Beta$_1$ receptors are concentrated in the myocardium, primarily in the sinoatrial (SA) node and throughout the atrioventricular (AV) conduction system. Beta$_2$ receptors are concentrated in the smooth muscle of the arterioles in the lung as well as in all other smooth muscles and in some gland cells. (To distinguish between beta receptors, remember that each person has *one* heart, which is where beta₁ receptors are located, and *two* lungs, which is where beta₂ receptors are concentrated.)

Stimulation of any of the adrenergic receptors provokes the familiar fight or flight response. More specifically, stimulation of alpha receptors, located throughout the peripheral arterioles, results in peripheral vasoconstriction and increased blood pressure. Peripheral vasoconstriction leads to the shunting of blood to more vital organs such as the heart and brain.

The stimulation of beta₁ receptors produces four effects on the heart: (1) the heart rate increases from an increased conduction rate, thereby producing what is called a positive chronotropic effect; (2) the force of atrial and ventricular contractions increases, and the heart beats more forcefully, a condition referred to as a positive inotropic effect; (3) the heart's excitability, or automaticity, increases, which may result in ectopic or skipped beats; and (4) the oxygen demands of the heart increase from the increased heart rate and force of contraction. Stimulation of beta₂ receptors results in peripheral vasodilation and relaxation of the bronchial smooth muscle, which facilitates breathing.

Adrenergic blockade produces effects opposite to those produced during stimulation. If alpha receptors are blocked, smooth muscle in the peripheral arterioles relaxes, producing peripheral vasodilation and resulting in decreased blood pressure. Beta₁ blockade decreases the heart rate (a negative chronotropic effect), decreases the force of myocardial contraction (a negative inotropic effect), and decreases myocardial oxygen demands. Excessive beta₁ blockade can result in congestive heart failure from significant decreases in myocardial contractility. Beta₂ blockade produces constriction of bronchial smooth muscle, an action that may result in wheezing and increased respiratory distress.

ADRENERGIC STIMULANTS

In emergencies, such as cardiac arrest, alpha- and beta-receptor stimulation is usually the desired physiologic response; however, few drugs provide both alpha- and beta-receptor stimulation. Furthermore, the amount of alpha- and beta-receptor stimulation may vary. For example, epinephrine provides some beta₂-receptor stimulation but produces its major effect on alpha and beta₁ receptors. Isoproterenol, on the other hand, provides beta₁- and beta₂-receptor stimulation but produces no alpha-receptor effect. (See *The effects of adrenergic stimulants* for the effects of these drugs on the various receptors.)

The effects of adrenergic stimulants

The stimulation of sympathetic alpha and beta receptors is often necessary when managing an emergency. Therefore, the nurse must know which drugs stimulate which receptors to produce the desired physiologic responses.

DRUG	RECEPTOR		
	α	β₁	β₂
epinephrine 1 to 4 mcg/min	+ +	+ +	+
dopamine 0.5 to 2 mcg/kg per min*	0	0	0
2 to 10 mcg/kg per min	0	+ +	0
> 10 mcg/kg per min	+ +	+	0
dobutamine 1 to 10 mcg/kg per min	+	+ +	0
isoproterenol 1 to 5 mcg/min	0	+ +	+ +
norepinephrine 8 to 12 mcg/min (initially)	+ +	+ +	0
1 to 5 mcg/min (maintenance)	+ +	+ +	0

*Dopaminergic effect results in vasodilation of renal, mesenteric, and coronary vascular beds.

KEY:
+ + = major effect
  + = minor effect
  0 = no change

EMERGENCY DRUGS

Drugs are a major component of the therapeutic management of patients in emergencies. The drugs discussed in this chapter are used to manage the following emergencies: cardiac arrest, cardiogenic shock, hypovolemic states, hypertensive emergencies, anaphylactic shock, and narcotic overdose.

MANAGEMENT OF CARDIAC ARREST

The American Heart Association classifies all code drugs (drugs used in cardiac arrest) into five categories based on their therapeutic effects. The categories include:
- drugs to correct acidosis
- drugs to restore heartbeat and increase contractility
- drugs to correct bradycardia
- drugs to correct ventricular dysrhythmias
- drugs to increase blood pressure and cardiac output.

Because the drugs in these five categories are discussed in depth elsewhere in the text, only their actions and use in emergencies are presented in the following section. (See *Drugs used to manage a cardiac arrest* on pages 240 and 241 for the dosages and administration routes for the drugs.)

Drugs to correct acidosis

Acidosis, defined as a serum pH less than 7.35, results in a decreased fibrillatory threshold, which means that the heart is more likely to beat in an uncontrolled fashion. This makes converting a fibrillatory pattern into a functional rhythm more difficult. Acidosis also produces a decreased sensitivity to catecholamines, such as epinephrine. Hyperventilation with 100% oxygen administered through an Ambu bag is the recommended method to correct acidosis. If hyperventilation, which removes carbon dioxide, fails to correct acidosis, limited and prudent use of sodium bicarbonate may be instituted to treat acidosis caused by hypoperfusion.

Sodium bicarbonate is usually administered to correct acidosis only after other arrest interventions have been implemented without success. The use of sodium bicarbonate depends upon the arterial blood gas values. Furthermore, because sodium bicarbonate does not cross the blood-brain barrier, hyperventilation with oxygen is the only means to prevent cerebral dysfunction from acidosis.

Because sodium bicarbonate inactivates catecholamines, it should not be mixed with I.V. solutions of dopamine, dobutamine, epinephrine, or norepinephrine. Also, sodium bicarbonate should not be mixed with calcium chloride because a precipitate will form.

Drugs to restore heartbeat and increase contractility

Epinephrine is the major drug used to restore heartbeat and increase contractility during a cardiac arrest.

Epinephrine stimulates the alpha-adrenergic and beta-adrenergic receptors. The resulting alpha effects increase the blood pressure, which leads to increased blood flow to the coronary arteries and to the brain. The beta effects increase the rate, force of contraction, and automaticity of the heart.

Epinephrine is used primarily for its alpha-stimulating effects. The stimulating effects on beta receptors remain controversial, because the effects may increase the oxygen demands of the myocardium and decrease subendocardial perfusion.

Because of peripheral vasoconstriction, administer epinephrine through a central line. Epinephrine should not be mixed with alkaline solutions, such as sodium bicarbonate, which inactivate the drug. Because of the beta-stimulating effects of epinephrine, the drug should not be used in patients with ventricular tachycardia.

Drugs to correct bradycardia

The major drugs used to correct bradycardia during a cardiac arrest include atropine and isoproterenol.

Atropine is used to treat bradycardia because of the drug's anticholinergic effect, which increases the heart rate. The parasympathetic blockade provided by atropine decreases cardiac vagal tone, enhances the rate of discharge of the SA node, and facilitates AV conduction. These effects lead to an increased heart rate. Physicians use atropine to treat bradycardia accompanied by severe hypotension and frequent ventricular escape beats. Atropine may also be used to treat AV block at the nodal level as well as ventricular asystole.

Dosages less than 0.5 mg I.V. may produce paradoxical slowing of the heart, caused by parasympathomimetic effects. The physician or nurse should administer atropine cautiously when treating patients with myocardial ischemia or acute myocardial infarction because the increased heart rate could increase the ischemia or the zone of infarction.

Isoproterenol is used for its beta-adrenergic receptor stimulation, which increases heart rate and cardiac output. Isoproterenol is usually administered to maintain the heart rate while preparing for pacemaker insertion in patients with hemodynamically significant bradycardia that is refractory to atropine. Isoproterenol increases the myocardial work load and exacerbates the ischemia and dysrhythmias associated with ischemic heart disease. The drug is contraindicated when a pulse cannot be established.

Excessive beta stimulation with isoproterenol may precipitate ventricular dysrhythmias. Isoproterenol is incompatible with sodium bicarbonate.

Drugs to correct ventricular dysrhythmias

Lidocaine, procainamide, and bretylium are usually administered in emergencies to correct ventricular dysrhythmias.

Lidocaine is used to correct ventricular dysrhythmias because it depresses conduction in the reentrant pathways, decreases the automaticity of the Purkinje fibers, and decreases excitability. Lidocaine also raises the ventricular fibrillation threshold. Physicians use lidocaine primarily to treat premature ventricular contractions (PVCs) that are frequent, or greater than six per minute; close coupled; multiform; or occurring in short bursts of two or more in succession.

The drug is also used to treat ventricular tachycardia and ventricular fibrillation. Lidocaine proves particularly effective in treating ventricular fibrillation that is resistant to defibrillation; in such circumstances, lidocaine may improve the myocardial response to electrical stimulation.

Lidocaine is not used to treat PVCs secondary to bradycardia (ventricular escape beats); in such situations, atropine is the drug of choice. When the patient is unconscious during a cardiac arrest, seizures may occur as the first sign of lidocaine toxicity.

Procainamide is used to suppress PVCs and recurrent ventricular tachycardia. Procainamide decreases cardiac irritability and is the second-line drug to treat ventricular ectopy (misplaced beats) when lidocaine is contraindicated or when the patient does not respond to lidocaine.

Hypotension, the major adverse reaction to procainamide therapy, occurs especially when procainamide is administered too rapidly. The nurse should closely monitor the electrocardiogram (EKG) for widening of the QRS complex and Q-T interval secondary to a slowing of intraventricular conduction. Procainamide is not the drug of choice for treating PVCs secondary to bradycardia; in such circumstances, atropine should be used.

Bretylium initially releases catecholamines from adrenergic nerve endings. This action increases the heart rate and blood pressure. However, postganglionic adrenergic blocking action follows such increases and frequently results in profound hypotension.

Physicians use bretylium to treat ventricular fibrillation and ventricular tachycardia, although it is not the first-line drug of choice for these dysrhythmias. Bretylium is used when: (1) lidocaine and defibrillation fail to convert ventricular fibrillation, (2) ventricular fibrillation occurs despite the use of lidocaine, or (3) lidocaine and procainamide fail to control ventricular tachycardia in patients with an established pulse.

Hypotension is the major adverse reaction to bretylium. If the drug is administered too rapidly, nausea and vomiting may occur.

Drugs to increase blood pressure and cardiac output

The drugs used to increase blood pressure and cardiac output during a cardiac arrest include dopamine, dobutamine, and norepinephrine.

Dopamine, a chemical precursor of norepinephrine, stimulates alpha, beta, and dopaminergic receptors. Dopamine dilates renal and mesenteric blood vessels at low doses (1 to 2 mcg/kg per minute) and preserves renal blood flow, glomerular filtration rate, and urine output in low cardiac output states. Physicians also use dopamine in emergencies to maintain the patient's blood pressure and cardiac output when an organized rhythm is established. At moderate doses (5 to 10 mcg/kg per minute), beta effects predominate, producing increased contractility and cardiac output. At higher doses (>10 mcg/kg per minute), alpha effects predominate, resulting in peripheral vasoconstriction and increased blood pressure.

Because of vasoconstriction, the physician infuses higher doses of dopamine through a central line. Doing so also prevents extravasation, which may occur with a peripheral line. Because monoamine oxidase (MAO) inhibitors potentiate dopamine's effects, patients receiving MAO inhibitors require one-tenth the normal dose of dopamine to prevent hypertensive crisis. Dopamine should not be mixed with alkaline solutions, such as sodium bicarbonate, because these solutions will precipitate. Finally, dopamine therapy should be gradually tapered; abruptly discontinuing the drug can cause rebound effects.

Dobutamine is administered for its beta$_1$ stimulation without alpha effect, which results in increased myocardial contractility. Because dobutamine is cardiac specific, it does not produce peripheral vasoconstriction or renal hypoperfusion. Instead, dobutamine induces a reflex peripheral vasodilation. Physicians primarily use dobutamine to maintain the patient's blood pressure and cardiac output when a rhythm has been established.

Dobutamine should not be mixed with alkaline solutions because such solutions inactivate the drug. Higher doses of dobutamine may cause tachycardia and ventricular ectopy.

Norepinephrine, which acts more rapidly than dopamine or dobutamine, is used for its profound alpha and beta effects. Its profound alpha effect produces vasoconstriction of the renal and mesenteric vascular beds and peripheral vasculature. The strong beta effects increase the force of myocardial contraction but also increase myocardial oxygen consumption.

When using norepinephrine, the physician and nurse should observe the patient for reflex bradycardia, which may occur secondary to profound increases in blood pressure. The nurse should monitor the patient's fluid volume because norepinephrine is contraindicated in hypovolemic patients. Norepinephrine should be administered through a central line because peripheral infiltration causes severe tissue necrosis. Norepinephrine should not be mixed with sodium bicarbonate because alkaline solutions inactivate norepinephrine.

Other drugs to manage cardiac arrest

Calcium chloride is used to correct hyperkalemia, hypocalcemia, and calcium channel blocker toxicity. Administering it during a cardiac arrest is controversial because calcium chloride may exacerbate cellular ischemia.

Because of its possible detrimental effect, calcium chloride is no longer used for its positive inotropic effect, which made the drug useful in treating electromechanical dissociation (the presence of an electrical rhythm but no effective pumping action or pulse). Physicians currently use calcium chloride to treat the patient's electromechanical dissociation only when a calcium abnormality coexists with the asystole (lack of pulse).

Because calcium precipitates when combined with most other emergency drugs, the nurse should flush all I.V. lines well and not mix calcium chloride with other drugs.

ENDOTRACHEAL ADMINISTRATION OF CODE DRUGS

A central line is the route of choice for administering drugs during a cardiac emergency. When using a central line is not possible, the American Heart Association recommends the endotracheal tube as the second route of choice because it facilitates rapid, reliable administration of drugs. Intracardiac routing is not recommended.

The procedure for administering code drugs via the endotracheal tube is predicated on delivering them as deeply as possible into the tracheobronchial tree for absorption by the alveoli. For endotracheal administration: (1) a 3½- inch (9-cm) needle or catheter is attached to a drug-filled syringe, (2) three to five forced ventilations are delivered to the patient using an Ambu bag or ventilator, (3) the drug is rapidly and deeply instilled into the endotracheal tube, (4) 2 to 3 ml of sterile saline solution are administered into the endotracheal tube, and (5) five additional ventilations are delivered to the patient using the Ambu bag or ventilator; these additional ventilations help to distribute the drug as well as to oxygenate the patient.

Drugs currently considered to be effective by endotracheal administration are epinephrine, lidocaine, and atropine. The dosages of these drugs for endotra-

cheal administration are the same as those used for intravenous administration. (See *Drugs used to manage a cardiac arrest* on pages 240 and 241 for I.V. dosages.) Though not approved for endotracheal administration, naloxone and diazepam are being studied for use via this route. Drugs that are not effective when given through an endotracheal tube include sodium bicarbonate, because of the large volume and high pH; calcium and norepinephrine, because they produce tissue necrosis; and bretylium, because it is poorly absorbed.

MANAGEMENT OF CARDIOGENIC SHOCK

The drugs used to treat cardiogenic shock are classified according to their therapeutic effects. The two specific classes important in this therapy are the vasopressors (dopamine and dobutamine) and the vasodilators (nitroglycerin and nitroprusside).

Dopamine is used for its beta-stimulating effects. At moderate doses (5 to 10 mcg/kg per minute), the positive inotropic effect of dopamine increases the force of myocardial contractility. Lower doses (<3 mcg/kg per minute) produce renal artery dilation, which may promote diuresis and sodium loss. Dopamine is a more effective vasopressor than dobutamine and, therefore, may be used to treat patients with severe hypotension.

One major goal in treating cardiogenic shock is to minimize the heart's oxygen requirements. These requirements are increased more by the increase in heart rate (positive chronotropic action) than by the increase in force of contraction (positive inotropic action) produced by vasoactive drugs. Thus, low doses of dopamine are appropriate for treating cardiogenic shock because high doses cause both increased heart rate and increased force of contraction. Regardless of the dosage, the physician does not abruptly withdraw the drug but decreases dopamine therapy gradually.

The optimal dose of dopamine to treat cardiogenic shock is 5 to 10 mcg/kg per minute. At this dose, cardiac function and blood pressure increase without excessively increasing myocardial oxygen consumption.

Doses as high as 10 mcg/kg per minute may be required to maintain cardiac output and blood pressure. At this dose, however, increased beta effects often increase heart rate and myocardial irritability. At doses greater than 10 mcg/kg per minute, both the beta and alpha effects of dopamine result in increased myocardial oxygen consumption.

Dobutamine is used to manage cardiogenic shock because of its specific beta$_1$-stimulating properties. Because dobutamine is a more potent inotropic drug than

Drugs used to manage a cardiac arrest

The following summarizes the dosages, administration routes, and administration tips for the drugs presented in this chapter. The drugs are listed in the order of their discussion in the chapter.

DRUG	DOSAGE AND ROUTE	ADMINISTRATION TIPS
sodium bicarbonate	**I.V. bolus:** 1 mEq/kg I.V. push. Repeat no more than one half of the initial dose every 10 minutes.	● Prepare all I.V. infusions using minidrip or microdrip tubing. ● Base repeated doses on arterial blood pH or laboratory values.
epinephrine	**I.V. bolus:** 0.5 to 1 mg (5 to 10 ml of a 1:10,000 solution) I.V. push. Repeat every 5 minutes until myocardial contractility is restored. **Endotracheal:** 1 mg (10 ml of a 1:10,000 solution) followed by 2 to 3 ml of sterile saline solution. **I.V. infusion:** 1 to 4 mcg/minute, titrated according to the effect. Add 1 mg to 250 ml of D_5W. This provides 4 mcg/ml. Therefore, using minidrip tubing: 1 mcg/min = 15 drops 2 mcg/min = 30 drops	● Do not mix with alkaline solutions.
calcium chloride	**I.V. bolus:** 2 ml of 10% solution administered over 1 to 2 minutes. May repeat up to 10 ml of 10% solution. Not a first-line drug.	● Administer I.V. into a large vein; severe necrosis and sloughing of tissues follows extravasation.
calcium gluceptate	**I.V. bolus:** 5 to 7 ml of 22% solution given over 1 to 2 minutes. Not a first-line drug.	● Administer I.V. into a large vein.
calcium gluconate	**I.V. bolus:** 5 to 8 ml of 10% solution given at 1 to 2 ml/minute. Not a first-line drug.	● Administer I.V. into a large vein, though this drug is less irritating than calcium chloride.
atropine	**I.V. bolus:** for asystole, 1 mg I.V. push, repeated in 5 minutes if asystole persists; for bradycardia, 0.5 mg I.V. push. May repeat every 5 minutes until a total dose of 2 mg is achieved. **Endotracheal:** 1 mg followed by 2 to 3 ml of sterile saline solution.	● Prepare all I.V. infusions using minidrip or microdrip tubing.
procainamide	**I.V. bolus:** 50 to 100 mg I.V. push over 5 minutes. May repeat every 5 minutes to a maximum dose of 1 gram. **I.V. infusion:** 1 to 4 mg/minute. Add 1 gram to 250 ml of D_5W to provide 4 mg/ml.	● The dosage should be decreased in patients with renal dysfunction. ● Continued dosage levels are dependent upon blood concentration levels. ● Prepare all I.V. infusions using minidrip or microdrip tubing.
isoproterenol	**I.V. infusion:** 2 to 10 mcg/minute, titrated according to heart rate and rhythm response. Add 1 mg to 500 ml of D_5W. This provides 2 mcg/ml. Therefore, using minidrip tubing: 1 mcg/min = 30 drops 2 mcg/min = 60 drops	● Drug is no longer recommended for use during a cardiac arrest, but for treating bradycardia in patients resistant to atropine. ● Prepare all I.V. infusions using minidrip or microdrip tubing.

Drugs used to manage a cardiac arrest continued

DRUG	DOSAGE AND ROUTE	ADMINISTRATION TIPS
lidocaine	**I.V. bolus:** 1 mg/kg I.V. push. Additional 0.5 mg/kg boluses may be given every 8 to 10 minutes until a total of 3 mg/kg has been reached. **I.V. infusion:** after successful resuscitation, 2 to 4 mg/minute. Add 1 gram to 250 ml of D_5W. This provides 4 mg/ml. Therefore, using minidrip tubing: 1 mg/min = 15 drops 2 mg/min = 30 drops	● Prepare all I.V. infusions using minidrip or microdrip tubing.
bretylium	**I.V. bolus:** 250 to 500 mg or 5 mg/kg I.V. push. May double-dose (10 mg/kg) and repeat every 15 to 30 minutes to a maximum dose of 30 mg/kg. **I.V. infusion:** 1 to 2 mg/minute. Add 5 to 10 mg/kg to 50 ml of D_5W.	● Bretylium may take 2 minutes to reach the central circulation. ● Prepare all I.V. infusions using minidrip or microdrip tubing.
dopamine	**I.V. infusion:** 2 to 5 mcg/kg per minute. Add 400 mg to 500 ml of D_5W. This provides 800 mcg/ml. Therefore, using minidrip tubing: 400 mcg/min = 30 drops 800 mcg/min = 60 drops	● Do not mix with sodium bicarbonate because it is inactivated by alkaline solutions. ● Prepare all I.V. infusions using minidrip or microdrip tubing.
dobutamine	**I.V. infusion:** 2.5 to 10 mcg/kg per minute. Add 250 mg to 500 ml D_5W. This provides 500 mcg/ml. Therefore, using minidrip tubing: 250 mcg/ml = 30 drops 500 mcg/ml = 60 drops	● Do not mix with sodium bicarbonate because it is inactivated by alkaline solutions. ● Doses greater than 20 mcg/kg per minute increase the risk of tachycardia, dysrhythmias, and worsening myocardial ischemia. ● Prepare all I.V. infusions using minidrip or microdrip tubing.
norepinephrine	**I.V. infusion:** 2 to 4 mcg/minute, titrated to effect. Add 4 mg to 500 ml D_5W. This provides 8 mcg/ml. Therefore, using minidrip tubing: 2 mcg/min = 15 drops 4 mcg/min = 30 drops	● Do not mix with sodium bicarbonate because it is inactivated by alkaline solutions. ● Extravasation results in tissue ischemia, necrosis, and sloughing. ● Prepare all I.V. infusions using minidrip or microdrip tubing.

dopamine, it proves more useful in managing borderline hypotension when inotropic support rather than pressor support is needed. Dobutamine predominantly stimulates beta$_1$ receptors, thereby increasing cardiac contractility with less chronotropic effects and with little or no vasoconstriction.

Administration is the same as that used for dobutamine treatment of a cardiac arrest. (See *Drugs used to manage a cardiac arrest* for dosage and route.)

Nitroglycerin is used because of its major effect (decreases preload) and its minor effect (decreases afterload). Preload represents the stretch on the ventricular muscle fiber at the end of diastole. Afterload is the amount of force the left ventricle must generate to pump blood through the arterial systems.

Nitroglycerin decreases preload by dilating venous vessels, allowing them to hold larger quantities of fluid. This action decreases cardiac output and myocardial oxygen consumption. Nitroglycerin also dilates the vessels that supply collateral circulation to the coronary arteries. Afterload may be slightly reduced secondary to arterial dilation, but the venous effects usually predominate.

Headache and hypotension are the most frequent adverse reactions to nitroglycerin therapy. While administering I.V. nitroglycerin, the nurse must monitor blood pressure continuously. If the systolic pressure falls below 90 mm Hg, the nurse should decrease the dose or stop the infusion. Intravenous nitroglycerin is absorbed by PVC (polyvinyl chloride) tubing and the I.V. bag. Therefore, the nurse must mix I.V. nitroglycerin in glass bottles and administer the drug through non-PVC tubing. If PVC tubing is used, higher doses need to be administered. In most cases, the nurse uses minidrip tubing and an infusion pump when administering nitroglycerin. Note that the I.V. solution of nitroglycerin is light sensitive.

For I.V. infusion, the nurse adds 50 mg nitroglycerin to 250 ml D_5W to obtain 200 mcg/ml. Using this infusion in minidrip tubing provides the following:

$$10 \text{ mcg/min} = 3 \text{ drops}$$
$$25 \text{ mcg/min} = 7.5 \text{ drops}$$
$$50 \text{ mcg/min} = 15 \text{ drops}$$
$$75 \text{ mcg/min} = 22.5 \text{ drops}$$
$$100 \text{ mcg/min} = 30 \text{ drops}$$

The nurse usually begins the infusion at 5 mcg/minute and increases by 5 mcg every 3 to 5 minutes up to 20 mcg/minute. If no response occurs, the dosage can continue to be increased by 20 mcg/minute until desired effect is achieved. Nitroglycerin has no maximum dose; therefore, the dose may be increased until the desired clinical results are achieved.

Nitroprusside is a potent, direct peripheral vasodilator used to manage heart failure and hypertension. The drug acts by relaxing arterial smooth muscle, which reduces peripheral arterial resistance and increases cardiac output. Overall, nitroprusside administration results in the following: (1) increased cardiac output, (2) direct venous dilation, which decreases left ventricular filling, relieves pulmonary congestion, and decreases left ventricular volume and pressure, (3) increased systolic ejection or emptying, (4) decreased pulmonary pressures, and (5) decreased myocardial oxygen consumption.

The rapid, profound decrease in blood pressure produced by nitroprusside requires continuous hemodynamic monitoring via an arterial line. Nitroprusside should not be infused with another I.V. because even a small bolus can decrease blood pressure. Nitroprusside is always administered through minidrip tubing, using an infusion pump. The drug should be reconstituted every 24 hours, and the I.V. solution should be protected from light by wrapping the I.V. bag in opaque material. Because one nitroprusside metabolite is thyocyanate, a chemical precursor to cyanide, the nurse should monitor the patient for cyanide toxicity, which can occur after the rapid administration of high doses. Thyocyanate toxicity can also occur after the prolonged use of high doses of nitroprusside. For I.V. infusion, the normal dose is 0.5 to 10 mcg/kg per minute. The nurse should reconstitute nitroprusside in D_5W only. The I.V. solution often is reconstituted according to weight, using the following procedure: (1) multiply the patient's weight (in kg) by 1.5, and (2) add this amount (mg) to 250 ml D_5W. This procedure results in a solution with the concentration of 6 mcg/kg per minute. Using minidrip tubing gives the following amounts:

$$1 \text{ mcg/kg per min} = 10 \text{ drops}$$
$$2 \text{ mcg/kg per min} = 20 \text{ drops}$$
$$6 \text{ mcg/kg per min} = 60 \text{ drops.}$$

MANAGEMENT OF HYPOVOLEMIC STATES

The goal of fluid resuscitation is the rapid restoration of intravascular fluid volume and tissue perfusion with minimal deterioration of organ function. But fluid volume replacement is a controversial topic. Only in the case of acute hemorrhage do physicians agree that fluid resuscitation should be performed, in part, with whole blood or blood components. Physicians have not yet reached a consensus about the volume replacement for patients with hypovolemic sepsis, trauma, burns, or peritonitis. Many support the use of crystalloids (such as normal saline solution), while others advocate the use of colloid (such as dextran) therapy.

The major area of controversy centers around pulmonary capillary membrane permeability. Briefly, one group of physicians contends that capillary permeability changes during shock, thereby allowing proteins to leave the intravascular space and enter the interstitial space, taking fluid with them. This premise supports the use of crystalloids in shock treatment.

The proponents of colloid therapy believe that colloid solutions do not adversely affect the capillary membrane damage that has already been caused by shock. This group supports the use of colloids for volume expansion. Only continuing research and documentation will resolve these fundamental issues. In the meantime, however, physicians use four types of volume expanders to treat hypovolemic states. The four types of volume expanders include whole blood, plasma products, crystalloids, and synthetic colloids.

Volume expanders to treat hypovolemic states
Whole blood is the fluid of choice in replacing acute massive *blood* losses because of its large fluid volume and oxygen-carrying capacity. Each unit of whole blood is approximately 450 ml in volume.

Blood-typing and cross-matching are required before administering whole blood. In some emergencies, there may not be sufficient time to have this test performed in the laboratory. Under such circumstances, whole blood is an inappropriate fluid replacement choice. During the administration of whole blood, the potential danger of transmitting infectious diseases, such as hepatitis or acquired immune deficiency syndrome (AIDS), always exists. Also, whole blood contains no functioning platelets and possesses low concentrations of coagulation factors usually caused by the long storage time of blood bank blood. Therefore, when transfusing large quantities of blood, the physician must consider additional platelet and plasma transfusions.

Plasma products include albumin and fresh frozen plasma. Albumin is available in three different forms: purified albumin, human albumin, and plasma protein fraction. Physicians use purified albumin and human albumin primarily to treat chronic hypoalbuminemia. Plasma protein fraction, which is 92% albumin, has a volume-expanding capacity that is slightly greater than the volume infused. The effective half-life of plasma protein fraction is approximately 15 hours. Plasma protein fraction is beneficial in maintaining normal blood volume, but it has not been proven effective in maintaining oncotic pressure (the pressure that proteins exert within the circulatory system to hold fluid in the system).

Fresh frozen plasma (FFP) is used as a source of active coagulation factors or when dilution of clotting factors has occurred after massive blood transfusions or fluid replacement. FFP should never be used strictly for volume replacement.

Cost is a considerable disadvantage of plasma products. Of the three major volume expanders, albumin is by far the most expensive.

Crystalloids given by rapid infusion (normal saline solution or lactated Ringer's solution) is the accepted *initial* treatment when fluid losses are expected to be small or short term. Because only 25% to 30% of the infused volume will remain in the intravascular space, three to four times the amount of blood lost needs to be replaced. Movement of fluid from the intravascular space to the interstitial space results in edema.

Administering large quantities of crystalloids may lead to peripheral edema and, possibly, pulmonary edema. Although crystalloids rapidly correct interstitial and cellular fluid shifts, they do not prove effective in supporting blood volume. Ineffective blood volume support can result in prolonged tissue hypoxia and progressive cellular injury.

Synthetic colloids are macromolecular substances suspended in electrolyte solutions. The two main groups of colloids available in the United States are dextrans and hetastarch. The duration of action and oncotic potential of the synthetic colloids depend on their macromolecular sizes. Smaller macromolecular substances, such as Dextran 40, initially exert a more potent oncotic effect. However, the smaller macromolecular substances are more rapidly eliminated than larger macromolecular substances, such as Dextran 70.

Unlike crystalloids, synthetic colloids rapidly restore intravascular volume without producing edema, thereby reducing the time the tissue is hypoxic (reduced oxygen content).

Dextran 40, a 10% solution, provides an initial volume-expanding capacity nearly double the volume infused. Because of its small macromolecular size, Dextran 40 is rapidly eliminated within 2 to 3 hours.

Dextran 70 is available as a 6% solution. Its initial oncotic effects provide volume expansion nearly equal the volume infused. The drug's larger macromolecular size prevents rapid elimination, thereby retaining 20% to 30% of its volume-expansion properties for 24 to 36 hours.

Both Dextran 40 and Dextran 70 shorten thrombin time, reduce plasma levels of Factor VIII, and decrease platelet adhesiveness. These effects may benefit microcirculation in certain shock states, but they also increase the risk of hemorrhage. Dextran 40 may also obstruct the renal tubules, thereby precipitating renal failure in patients with hypovolemic shock.

Hetastarch is available as a 6% solution in normal saline solution. The solution is marketed under the trade name Hespan. The volume-expanding capacity of Hespan equals the volume infused. Hespan retains 30% to 35% of its effect for 24 to 36 hours.

The infusion of large volumes of hetastarch may prolong prothrombin, partial thromboplastin, and clotting times. Also, serum amylase levels may double, but this increase is clinically insignificant.

The infusion of large quantities of any colloid solution may precipitate pulmonary edema. Therefore, do not use colloids in patients with congestive heart failure.

THE MANAGEMENT OF HYPERTENSIVE EMERGENCIES

Life-threatening elevations of systolic and diastolic blood pressure require immediate intervention to prevent acute left ventricular failure or cerebral dysfunction. Because of their rapid onset of action, nitroprusside, nifedipine, and labetalol are used as initial therapy in hypertensive crisis.

Drugs used to manage hypertensive emergencies

The drugs most frequently used to manage hypertensive crises are discussed in the following chart. Because these drugs act rapidly and produce a significant effect on the patient's blood pressure, the nurse must know how to administer them properly to ensure patient safety.

DRUG	DOSAGE AND ROUTE	ADMINISTRATION TIPS
nitroprusside	**I.V. infusion:** 0.5 to 10 mcg/kg per minute. Reconstitute in D_5W only. To mix according to weight: 1. Multiply weight (in kg) by 1.5. 2. Add this amount (mg) to 250 ml D_5W. This provides a solution that equals 6 mcg/kg per minute. Therefore, using minidrip tubing: 1 mcg/kg per min = 10 drops 2 mcg/kg per min = 20 drops 6 mcg/kg per min = 60 drops	• Rapid, profound decrease in blood pressure requires continuous blood pressure monitoring. • Do not piggyback into another I.V. • Protect I.V. solution from light by wrapping the I.V. bag in opaque material. • Drug expires 24 hours after reconstitution. • Cyanide toxicity can occur after rapid use of high doses. • Administer using minidrip tubing and an infusion pump.
nifedipine	**Sublingual:** 10 to 20 mg every 2 hours. Cut the top off of the capsule or use a sterile needle and make a hole in one end; then squeeze the liquid center under the patient's tongue. Remind the patient not to swallow the medication, but to keep it under the tongue. **Oral:** 10 to 20 mg P.O. every 8 hours.	• Monitor blood pressure frequently after administration. • Drug decreases the excretion of digoxin and quinidine, so observe for signs of digitalis toxicity. • Give cautiously with nitrates because of the hypotensive effects of both drugs. • Drug can be given safely with beta blockers. • Observe for noncardiogenic peripheral edema. • Headache and facial flushing are common adverse reactions.
labetalol	**I.V. bolus:** 10 to 20 mg I.V. push over 2 minutes. May repeat every 10 minutes until 300 mg is accumulated.	• Monitor blood pressure frequently during and after administration. • Give cautiously to patients with sinus bradycardia or heart block. • Drug may produce wheezing or respiratory difficulty in patients with asthma or chronic obstructive pulmonary disease. • Drug may cause congestive heart failure, so observe the patient closely. • Monitor the patient's blood glucose levels because this drug may mask the normal signs of hypoglycemia. • Dizziness is the most frequent adverse reaction.

Nitroprusside sodium provides immediate vasodilating effects. The drug can only be given I.V., with the patient constantly monitored. Because of the restriction of I.V. administration and the required constant monitoring, nitroprusside is unsuitable for the long-term management of hypertension.

Nifedipine offers the distinct advantage of sublingual administration. When I.V. access is difficult or immediate action is necessary, nifedipine can be given sublingually. The drug's rapid onset of action starts lowering blood pressure within 10 minutes.

Labetalol is both an alpha blocker and a beta blocker. When given I.V., its onset of action occurs within 2 to 3 minutes. Because labetalol can be given orally, it is suitable for maintenance therapy. Because of its nonspecific beta effects, labetalol can produce respiratory difficulties in patients with asthma or chronic obstructive pulmonary disease, and congestive heart failure in patients with a history of heart failure. (See *Drugs used to manage hypertensive emergencies* for a summary of these drugs.)

MANAGEMENT OF ANAPHYLACTIC SHOCK

Anaphylaxis occurs when two or more antibodies simultaneously recognize a single antigen. This occurrence triggers a reaction that decreases intracellular adenosine 3':5'-cyclic phosphate (cyclic AMP). The decrease in cyclic AMP stimulates the release of the mediators (histamine, heparin, and other products) that produce the anaphylactic reaction.

In humans, anaphylaxis affects two major systems: the cardiovascular and pulmonary. The cardiovascular effects include myocardial depression and vascular collapse due to sudden intravascular volume loss from dilation of venous capacitance vessels. The primary pulmonary effects are upper airway obstruction caused by laryngeal edema and acute emphysema.

The goal of anaphylaxis treatment is to: (1) prevent further release of histamine and other mediators, (2) prevent the effects of already-released mediators on end organs, and (3) reverse any physiologic effects that have occurred. Drugs used to treat anaphylaxis are classified according to their therapeutic effects. The two specific drug classes involved are vasopressors and drugs used as adjunct therapy, specifically bronchodilators and antihistamines. The vasopressor used to treat anaphylactic shock is epinephrine.

Epinephrine and isoproterenol. Epinephrine and isoproterenol prevent histamine release and provide alpha- and beta-receptor stimulation. Through the beta stimulation of adenylate cyclase, epinephrine increases intracellular cyclic AMP. Increased levels of cyclic AMP inhibit histamine release. The beta effects also relax bronchial smooth muscle and increase heart rate and myocardial contractility. The alpha effects of epinephrine increase peripheral vascular resistance.

The rapid I.V. administration of epinephrine may cause dysrhythmias.

The nurse should use either subcutaneous or intramuscular administration. To prevent gas gangrene from occurring, the nurse should avoid the I.M. administration of epinephrine in oil in the buttocks. When administered in this way, epinephrine reduces oxygen tension of the tissues, thereby encouraging the growth of contaminating organisms. The dosage for both routes is 0.3 to 0.5 ml of 1:1,000 strength. This dose may be repeated every 15 minutes. If hypotension exists, 3 to 5 ml of 1:10,000 solution may be given slowly (over 5 minutes) I.V. push. This dose may be repeated every 15 minutes.

Isoproterenol by nebulizer and racemic epinephrine by inhaler are used as adjunctive therapy to treat anaphylactic shock.

Theophylline, aminophylline, and antihistamines. The bronchodilators (theophylline and aminophylline) and antihistamines are used strictly as adjunct therapy to treat anaphylactic shock. The physician uses these drugs *after* epinephrine, not in place of it.

Theophylline and aminophylline are used to relieve bronchospasm. Theophylline directly relaxes the smooth muscle of the bronchial airways by inhibiting the breakdown of cyclic AMP. Theophylline and aminophylline also block adenosine receptors and inhibit the release of histamine.

The nonspecific beta stimulation of the bronchodilators may produce tachycardia, palpitations, or dysrhythmias.

Aminophylline is administered via an I.V. infusion. The loading dose of aminophylline is 6 mg/kg, while the maintenance dose is 0.4 to 0.7 mg/kg per hour.

Antihistamines, such as diphenhydramine, are used for symptomatic relief in minor reactions. They may also help prevent a recurrence of symptoms.

Antihistamines may cause drowsiness, especially in elderly patients.

When using I.V. or I.M. routes for diphenhydramine, the dose is 10 to 50 mg with a maximum daily dose of 400 mg. The oral dose is 25 to 50 mg every 4 to 6 hours.

MANAGEMENT OF NARCOTIC OVERDOSE

Narcotic overdose, whether accidental or deliberate, is a common occurrence. For this reason, the nurse must know how it is treated.

Naloxone hydrochloride (Narcan). Naloxone provides immediate reversal of narcotic-induced respiratory depression, including the effects of pentazocine and propoxyphene. Naloxone also reverses the central nervous system depression produced by opiates. More recently, naloxone has been used in attempts to reverse alcohol-induced coma and benzodiazepine overdoses.

Naloxone may produce rapid onset of the signs and symptoms of narcotic withdrawal, including sweating, tremors, agitation, severe pain, confusion, tachycardia, and hypertension.

The usual dose of naloxone is 0.4 mg I.V., S.C., or I.M. The dose may be repeated every 2 to 3 minutes for three doses. Although naloxone has been successfully administered experimentally through an endotracheal tube, definitive recommendations depend upon further research.

CHAPTER SUMMARY

This chapter emphasized the rationale for drug administration during different emergency situations. The nurse must be familiar with the broad classifications of emergency drugs and their pharmacologic actions. Here are the highlights of the chapter:

• The three types of adrenergic receptors in the body are alpha receptors, located in the smooth muscle of the peripheral arterioles; beta₁ receptors, concentrated in the myocardium; and beta₂ receptors, located in the smooth muscle of the lungs and in other body systems and glands.

• Stimulation of the adrenergic receptors produces the fight or flight response, including increased heart rate, force of contraction, and blood pressure.

• The code drugs used in the management of a cardiac arrest are classified as: (1) drugs to correct acidosis, (2) drugs to restore heartbeat and increase contractility, (3) drugs to correct bradycardia, (4) drugs to correct ventricular dysrhythmias, and (5) drugs to increase blood pressure and cardiac output.

• The management of cardiogenic shock requires the use of vasopressors, such as dopamine and dobutamine, and vasodilators, such as nitroglycerin.

• When using a central line (the optimal route for administering drugs during a cardiac emergency) is impossible, the endotracheal route proves effective for epinephrine, lidocaine, and atropine.

• Various types of volume expanders are used to manage hypovolemia. The volume expanders include whole blood, plasma products, crystalloids, and colloids.

• Nitroprusside, nifedipine, and labetalol are used to manage a hypertensive crisis.

• The management of anaphylactic shock centers around the use of vasopressors, such as epinephrine, and adjunct therapy involving bronchodilators and antihistamines.

• Naloxone is used to manage a narcotic overdose.

BIBLIOGRAPHY

American Heart Association. "Standards and Guidelines for Cardiopulmonary Resuscitation and Emergency Cardiac Care," *Journal of the American Medical Association* 255:2891, June 6, 1986.

Anderson, J.L. "Bretylium Tosylate: Profile of the Only Available Class III Anti-Arrhythmic Agent," *Clinical Therapeutics* 7:205, 1984.

Bauman, E.C. "Code Drugs," *Nursing85* 15:50, December 1985.

Fath, J.J., and Cerra, F.B. "The Therapy of Anaphylactic Shock," *Drug Intelligence and Clinical Pharmacy* 18:14, January 1984.

Greenberg, M.I. "The Use of Endotracheal Medication in Cardiac Emergencies," *Resuscitation* 12:155, November 1984.

Groeneveld, A.B. "Controversies in Pharmacotherapy During a Cardiopulmonary Resuscitation: A Pathophysiological Approach," *Netherland Journal of Medicine* 28:208, 1985.

Haljamae, H. "Rationale for the Use of Colloids in the Treatment of Shock and Hypovolemia," *Acta Anaesthesiology Scandanavia* 29:48, 1985.

Jones, S., and Bass, A. "What to Do after CPR: The Drugs You'll Use in a Code," *RN* 48:43, July 1985.

Macintyre, E., et al. "Fluid Replacement in Hypovolemia," *Intensive Care Medicine* 11:23, 1985.

Mortberg, A. "Aspects on Crystalloid Fluid Therapy," *Acta Anaesthesiology Scandanavia* 29:45, 1985.

Mueller, H.S. "Inotropic Agents in the Treatment of Cardiogenic Shock," *World Journal of Surgery* 9:3, February 1985.

Norsen, L. "Using Emergency Drugs Correctly, Part II," *NursingLife* 5:31, November/December 1985.

Nursing87 Drug Handbook. Springhouse, Pa.: Springhouse Corp., 1987.

Powers, R.D., and Donnowitz, L.G. "Endotracheal Administration of Emergency Medication," *Southern Medical Journal* 77:340, March 1984.

Rude, R.E. "Acute Myocardial Infarction and Its Complications," *Cardiology Clinics* 2:163, May 1984.

Scherer, P. "ACLS Guidelines: What Nurses Are Saying About the Drug Changes," *American Journal of Nursing* 86:1352, December 1986.

Shock. Nursing Now Series. Springhouse, Pa.: Springhouse Corp., 1984.

Sturm, J.A., and Wisner, D.H. "Fluid Resuscitation of Hypovolemia," *Intensive Care Medicine* 11:27, 1985.

EVALUATION

OBJECTIVES

After reading and studying this chapter, you should be able to:

1. Identify the major areas assessed during a patient's drug therapy.

2. Explain the nurse's use of outcome criteria during evaluation.

3. Define therapeutic effect, adverse drug reaction, and drug interaction, and discuss the importance of each in evaluation.

4. Explain how various patient-related factors and drug therapy factors can affect patient compliance.

5. Explain the importance of documenting evaluation data.

INTRODUCTION

An integral part of the nursing process, evaluation is a formal and systematic process for determining the effectiveness of nursing care. Hagen defines evaluation as a process used to provide descriptive data that enable the nurse to understand the patient's present status and thereby make better informed decisions about what to change and what to keep the same. This chapter discusses evaluation as it relates to patients receiving drug therapy.

EVALUATION CRITERIA

Often considered the final step in the nursing process, evaluation helps the nurse determine the optimum care for the patient. Earlier in the process, the nurse has used the nursing diagnosis, or problem statement, to define the patient's current and potential problems and deter-

mine outcome criteria, or patient goals. The outcome criteria also suggest what nursing interventions may help the patient achieve these goals.

Interventions may be *independent* nursing actions, such as turning an unconscious patient every hour. They may be *interdependent* nursing actions requiring a physician's order but also requiring the nurse to exercise judgment, such as administering a pain medication p.r.n. They may be *dependent* nursing actions requiring a physician's order, such as administering a prescribed medication.

The nurse performs evaluation to determine whether the outcome criteria have been met. For example, the nurse might ask the patient if headache relief was achieved within 1 hour after administering a p.r.n. analgesic. If the headache was relieved, the outcome criterion was met. If the headache was better but not completely relieved, the outcome criterion was only partially met. If the headache was the same or worse, the outcome criterion was not met. In this stage of the evaluation, the nurse assesses only the outcome criteria.

To complete the evaluation, the nurse must reassess unmet or partially met outcome criteria, applying appropriate steps in the nursing process, to determine what changes are required. This reassessment may indicate the need for replanning or may yield new data that invalidate the nursing diagnosis or that indicate why the outcome criteria were not met. The reassessment may also suggest new nursing interventions more specific or acceptable to the patient. Finally, the nurse reapplies the nursing process to determine whether the patient is still at risk for a specified nursing diagnosis.

Evaluation enables the nurse to design and implement a revised nursing care plan, reevaluating outcome criteria continuously and replanning until each nursing diagnosis is resolved.

EVALUATING DRUG EFFECTS, REACTIONS, AND INTERACTIONS

The nurse can use evaluation to determine whether nursing interventions for drug administration are effective. To do so, the nurse reassesses for therapeutic effects, adverse drug reactions, and drug interactions. To evaluate these factors properly as they relate to the outcome criteria, the nurse must understand the physiologic actions of the drug or drugs being administered.

One recommended method for acquiring information about drugs involves first learning about specific drug classes. By studying and learning about a drug class, the nurse or nursing student acquires general information about a number of drugs. For example, learning the mechanism of action, potential adverse drug reactions, drug interactions, and indications for use for the antibiotic class aminoglycosides provides the nurse with information about seven different antibiotics. Although differences among these seven antibiotics exist, the nurse possesses general information for planning and evaluating outcome criteria for therapy with any of them.

For example, a nurse who understands the interactions between drugs, such as between aminoglycosides and penicillins (another antibiotic class), knows never to administer drugs from these two antibiotic classes through the same I.V. site: the patient would receive little or no beneficial antibiotic therapy because the two drug classes inactivate each other. Similarly, knowledge of the possible interaction between aminoglycosides and heparin (because heparin's highly acidic nature inactivates the aminoglycoside) should alert the nurse to always flush the I.V. heparin lock with saline solution before and after administration of any drug belonging to the aminoglycoside class.

Learning about the different drug classes can also help the nurse develop appropriate outcome criteria and interventions. The nurse must, however, remember to examine each specific drug for information that distinguishes it from the other drugs in its class. The following sections explain how drugs exert their therapeutic effects and what happens in adverse drug reactions and drug interactions.

THERAPEUTIC EFFECTS

The therapeutic effect is the body's response to a drug's pharmacologic action when that action produces a benefit for the patient. To understand how a drug produces its therapeutic effect, the nurse must understand the drug's mechanism of action. For example, some laxatives work by altering surface tension; others work through bowel lubrication or stimulation, saline catharsis, or bulk formation. The differences in their mechanisms of action could determine whether outcome criteria for a constipated patient are met or unmet—depending on the cause of constipation as well as on various other factors pertaining to the individual patient.

For example, most patients admitted to cardiac units receive a stool softener such as docusate sodium, an emollient laxative, to prevent constipation secondary to the inactivity of hospitalization. Docusate sodium works by reducing the surface tension of liquid bowel contents and promoting additional liquid absorption into the stool. Use of docusate sodium results in a softer stool mass that the patient can pass without straining. Unless the patient is constipated initially, administration of docusate sodium helps meet these outcome criteria: "The patient will maintain usual bowel elimination pattern while hospitalized" and "The patient will not strain during bowel movements."

If this patient had received a laxative with a different mechanism of action, the outcome criteria might not have been met. For example, a stimulant laxative such as bisacodyl would be inappropriate for the cardiac patient needing constipation prophylaxis. That is because stimulant laxatives such as bisacodyl, which work by increasing peristalsis of smooth muscle in the intestine to produce a stool within 6 to 8 hours, can cause abdominal cramping. Furthermore, frequent use can precipitate fluid and electrolyte imbalances, so these laxatives are inappropriate for the cardiac patient. Finally, the cardiac patient needs a drug that prevents constipation, not one such as bisacodyl that treats the condition.

ADVERSE DRUG REACTIONS

Adverse drug reactions, also called side effects, are physiologic reactions to a drug that are not related to the drug's therapeutic effect. They are classified as predictable and unpredictable. Predictable adverse reactions are dose-related responses to a drug that are known to occur with some patients. Unpredictable adverse reactions are those that the physician or nurse cannot foresee, such as an allergic response. Unpredictable reactions are not dose-related.

Predictable reactions

Drowsiness, a predictable reaction to the antihistamine diphenhydramine, can be detrimental if the patient needs to remain alert. However, diphenhydramine is sometimes administered specifically *for* the drowsiness it produces. For example, it may be given to patients with insomnia because the drug causes drowsiness. In this instance, the physician uses the drug's predictable adverse reaction for therapeutic effect.

The nurse, however, usually works toward preventing or minimizing the predictable adverse reactions of drugs, such as the nausea and vomiting associated with many antineoplastic drugs.

Unpredictable reactions

Unpredictable reactions may occur as allergic reactions ranging from a mild rash or pruritus to severe anaphylaxis. The initial patient history compiled by the nurse can help avoid such reactions. If the patient had a previous allergic reaction, the nurse must determine its nature by asking the patient to describe it. Information the patient provides can help the nurse if any question exists as to whether the reaction was a true allergic response or a predictable adverse reaction.

Unpredictable reactions are known as *paradoxical reactions* when drugs produce effects opposite to their designed therapeutic effects. Suppose, for example, an elderly patient takes 15 mg of the hypnotic flurazepam approximately 30 minutes before bedtime to promote sleep. If, 1 hour later, the patient is not drowsy but awake, somewhat confused, and slightly combative, the patient is experiencing a paradoxical reaction. The very young and the elderly are most likely to experience paradoxical reactions.

DRUG INTERACTIONS

A drug interaction occurs when one drug alters the pharmacokinetic or pharmacodynamic properties of another or when a drug interacts with food the patient has eaten. Most drug interactions of either type are minor and may even go unnoticed by patient and nurse; however, a few drug interactions can produce serious consequences.

Elderly patients are most likely to experience drug interactions. That is because aging alters the way the body uses drugs: the half-life of many drugs is increased, their elimination rate is diminished; and elderly patients' tissues can become more sensitive to the drug's effects, producing unexpected or undesirable responses. The nurse must be especially aware of potential drug interactions in this patient group.

Some interactions between drugs can be beneficial. These may be initiated in various situations and include interactions that reduce toxicity or increase therapeutic effect. For example, the specific receptor-blocking agent naloxone is administered to counter the toxic effects of narcotic overdose. Another type of beneficial interaction between drugs, summation, occurs when two drugs produce the same response, regardless of their mechanisms of action. Administering codeine with aspirin results in summation for pain relief, for example, even though the two drugs act by different mechanisms.

Both benefical and adverse interactions between drugs and food can occur. A beneficial interaction car occur in the patient taking supplemental doses of calcium for the treatment of osteoporosis: if the patient eats foods rich in vitamins C and D, the vitamins assist in the absorption and utilization of the calcium. The same patient may experience an adverse interaction, however, with high protein and fat intake, because protein and fat inhibit calcium absorption.

EVALUATING A DRUG'S EFFECTIVENESS

The nurse's knowledge of a drug's therapeutic effects, adverse drug reactions, and drug interactions helps the nurse evaluate whether or not the outcome criteria have been met. For example, the nurse may be administering a drug to reduce fever. One of the outcome criteria should state that the patient's temperature will be within a certain range at a certain time. If the drug given to reduce fever can produce stomach irritation, the outcome criteria should also include a measurement indicating little or no stomach irritation for the patient. In this way, specific drug information has provided the nurse with patient goals to be assessed during evaluation.

If the patient is taking several medications at a time, the nurse must assess the potential for interactions between drugs and drugs and between drugs and food and incorporate this information into the patient's outcome criteria. These outcome criteria may be related to patient teaching or compliance. For example, evaluation criteria assessing erythromycin (an antibacterial taken when the stomach is empty) may include a statement such as: "Mrs. Crawley will state why she should take erythromycin on an empty stomach."

Evaluating a drug's effectiveness also requires that the nurse: (1) know the time of the peak concentration levels, onset of action, and duration of action of the prescribed drug and (2) obtain a patient history covering any prior use of the drug and any allergic or adverse reactions that occurred. (See *Evaluation questions* for some standard questions the nurse can use.)

EVALUATING PATIENT COMPLIANCE

Patient compliance with drug therapy is critical to the drug's therapeutic effects. The nurse often lists noncompliance or potential noncompliance as a nursing diagnosis when developing the nursing care plan. A nursing diagnosis of noncompliance is intended for a patient who wishes to comply with a prescribed regimen but cannot do so because of various factors. Such a diagnosis is not made for a patient who has made an informed autonomous decision not to follow prescribed health care.

Assessing the success of patient compliance is an important part of evaluation. The following sections cover factors that help the nurse evaluate patient compliance: forms and causes of noncompliance, such as patient-related factors, drug therapy factors, the patient's relationship with caregivers; and methods for measuring patient compliance.

Evaluation questions

To evaluate the effectiveness of a patient's drug therapy, the nurse must know the answers to these questions:

• What are the intended therapeutic effects of the drug therapy?
• What is the mechanism of action by which the drug produces its therapeutic effects?
• What are the adverse reactions associated with the drug?
• What interactions between the drug and other drugs, or foods, could alter its therapeutic effect?
• What adverse reactions to drugs, if any, has the patient experienced in the past?
• How is the drug administered?
• What should the patient know about the drug? What factors might affect the patient's ability to follow the prescribed drug regimen?
• What therapeutic effect(s) has the drug produced on the patient? If none, or not enough, what drug–related, patient–related, or health care provider–related factors may be involved? What nursing interventions are needed to remove these factors' effects and achieve the original or revised outcome criteria?

FORMS AND CAUSES OF NONCOMPLIANCE

A patient may exhibit noncompliance with drug therapy by failing to take a drug, consuming an excessive amount of the drug, taking the drug at the wrong time, prematurely discontinuing the drug therapy, failing to have a prescription filled, consuming other drugs or foods that interfere with drug action, or using drugs that have not been prescribed, such as from a previous illness.

A patient may fail to take a drug because of not believing that the drug will help the problem or condition, because of not being able to afford its cost, because of a desire to avoid its adverse effects, or because of simply forgetting to take it.

A patient who takes an excessive amount of a drug may not remember when the last dose was taken. Or a patient may erroneously believe that taking more than the prescribed dose will enhance the drug's therapeutic effects.

Taking a drug at the wrong time can lead to adverse effects and can reduce or cancel its therapeutic benefit. For example, a patient who takes the diuretic furosemide in the evening rather than the morning (as prescribed) may experience sleep deprivation because of frequent urination during the night. Lack of knowledge about a drug's actions or adverse effects—as well as the patient's desire to avoid adverse reactions—can prompt a patient to alter the administration time.

Prematurely discontinuing use of a drug is a common form of noncompliance that is particularly associated with antibiotics and antihypertensives. Many patients taking antibiotics stop when they begin to feel better, not realizing that the disease may recur or that the foreshortened therapy may make the disease-producing bacteria more resistant to antibiotic therapy. Similarly, many patients stop taking antihypertensive agents when their blood pressure drops, not realizing that the drugs are required to keep the blood pressure down.

Failure to have a prescription filled may occur because the patient does not feel well enough to travel to a pharmacy, wait 10 or 15 minutes while the prescription is being filled, and then return home. As previously noted, inability to afford the drug as well as a lack of belief in its therapeutic benefit can also lead to this form of noncompliance.

Taking other drugs or eating foods that interfere with a prescribed drug's intended action can also result in patient noncompliance, cause adverse reactions, or alter the therapeutic effect. For example, a patient who consumes alcohol while taking a central nervous system depressant may have an additive depressant effect. Noncompliance can also result from a patient's knowledge deficit about the drug and its proper administration.

A patient taking a prescribed drug who also takes a drug prescribed for someone else risks altered therapeutic effects and adverse drug interactions.

Using a prescription from an earlier illness can also cause the patient harm. A patient who does not know or understand that a drug other than the prescribed one can cause harm or a patient who is troubled about the expense of health care and drugs may prompt this form of noncompliant behavior.

Patient noncompliance can be caused by various factors, which may be patient–related, drug therapy–related, or health care provider–related.

Patient-related factors

Patient-related factors include knowledge deficits, a nonsupportive environment, impaired physical abilities, and counterproductive health beliefs. Each of these factors stems from the patient's responses to the physical, psychological, and social environment.

Knowledge deficits. Noncompliance is common among patients who do not possess adequate understanding of prescribed drugs or of the diseases for which the drugs are administered. To minimize such knowledge deficits, nurses must provide the patients with concise and adequate information about the drug treatment. For example, a patient taking digoxin for the treatment of congestive heart failure must know to take the drug even when feeling well on a particular day. The patient must also understand that a resting pulse rate of more than 100 beats/minute can indicate drug toxicity rather than a need for more digoxin.

Nonsupportive environment. Nonsupportive family members and peers provide no or negative reinforcement for compliance. For example, an unemployed father or mother may refuse to pay for expensive antihypertensive drugs. Peer pressure may affect compliance in an adolescent who must adhere to insulin therapy: dietary control and vigilance in testing blood glucose levels and administering insulin make the adolescent different—at a time when fitting into the peer group is very important.

The nurse can intervene by referring the family to a social service agency that will help defray the cost of antihypertensive drugs or will suggest a peer support group for the adolescent to join.

Impaired physical abilities. Noncompliance in patients may stem from impaired physical abilities. For example, a patient with vision problems may misread the drug container and take an overdose or a subtherapeutic dose. A diminished sense of hearing can interfere with the patient's understanding of the physician's and nurse's instructions. Chronic illness can make patients feel too ill or weak even to take their drugs. The nurse can provide special aids and instructions to help combat these forms of noncompliance.

Counterproductive health beliefs. Different cultural views of illness, drugs prescribed to treat illness, and health care professionals can strongly affect compliance. Beliefs about health may also be influenced by newspapers, television, advertising, and family traditions. The nurse should assess the patient for any such beliefs that may adversely affect compliance. For example, a patient who believes that everyone must have a daily bowel movement may take regular doses of laxatives despite being told by the physician or nurse that a daily bowel movement is only one of several normal patterns. Another patient who believes only in family herbal remedies may be distrustful of packaged drugs.

Drug therapy factors

Unpleasant adverse reactions to therapy, complex or prolonged therapy, and expensive therapy can all promote noncompliance. The nurse should identify any such factors that may interfere with compliance and assist the patient in eliminating them.

Unpleasant adverse reactions. Adverse reactions to drug therapy can cause the patient to decide that the benefits of discontinuing the drug outweigh the benefits of taking it. For example, the severe nausea, vomiting, and anorexia experienced during antineoplastic therapy may lead the patient to discontinue it or take less than the prescribed dosage.

Complex or prolonged therapy. A patient whose therapy involves taking more than one drug or taking the same drug several times a day might forget a scheduled dose. Frequent dosing that interferes with activities of daily living can also cause noncompliance. Noncompliance with prolonged therapy can occur because it is expensive or tedious or because the patient does not understand its necessity. For example, patients with hypertension must take drugs for the rest of their lives. If such a patient is feeling well, continued therapy may seem unnecessary, and the patient may become noncompliant.

Expensive therapy. Some patients cannot afford the cost of drug treatments, particularly if the drugs are expensive. Elderly persons on fixed incomes are the largest consumers of drugs, yet they cannot always afford them. Recent changes in the law, making generic brands of drugs more accessible, have helped alleviate the economic burden of drug therapy.

Relationships with health care professionals

Physicians', pharmacists', and nurses' positive attitudes toward prescribed drug therapy and efforts to provide effective patient education promote compliance by establishing a therapeutic relationship. The patient who feels cared for will be more likely to care about complying with a prescribed drug regimen.

Attitudes toward prescribed therapy. What and how the nurse communicates about a prescribed drug regimen can affect the patient's attitude toward it. The nurse should provide information in a direct and honest way that gives the patient realistic hope, even when the drug prescribed may prove less than fully effective. By promoting hope, this confident attitude also promotes compliance.

Effective patient education. The quality of patient education significantly influences patient compliance. The nurse should provide the patient and family with adequate and effective education about prescribed drug therapy before they leave the hospital or clinic. A patient who has not received such information may go home unsure of when and how to take the prescribed drug and unaware of signs and symptoms of toxicity or possible adverse reactions. To avoid such problems and provide effective patient education, the nurse must carefully evaluate the drug and the patient's circumstances. (See Chapter 11, Intervention: Patient Education, for a detailed discussion of patient education.)

MEASURING PATIENT COMPLIANCE

Evaluation can help the nurse determine whether a patient is compliant with a prescribed drug regimen or not. If the patient's condition is not responding to therapy, for example, the nurse's evaluation may reveal that the patient is socially isolated and is not receiving necessary support from family members. A patient who is confused or forgetful, who expresses doubt about the drug therapy, who fails to fill a prescription, or who is involved in complex or expensive drug therapy also requires evaluation for compliance.

Current methods used to evaluate patient compliance do not always provide pure or true measurements, but they can help the nurse minimize factors that might lead to noncompliance. The methods include physiologic assessment, ratings by health care professionals, patient self-reporting, pill counts, and direct observation. Combining several methods provides more accurate measurement of compliance.

Physiologic assessment. Blood pressure and serum or urine drug levels as well as other assessments, can provide objective evidence of whether the patient is complying with the prescribed drug therapy. However, some physiologic measurements, such as for blood pressure, may be inaccurate because of alteration by other factors. The blood pressure of a patient taking antihypertensive drugs, for example, can fluctuate according to the patient's anxiety level and ingestion of certain foods. As a result, the patient may be compliant with hypertensive drug therapy but still have high blood pressure. Serum or urine levels of a drug or its metabolites may also inaccurately reflect compliance if a noncompliant patient consumes the prescribed drug dose just before the test, producing a positive impression of compliance. Body weight and heart rate also provide objective measurements of compliance, but the nurse must interpret the information carefully and in relation to other assessment data.

Ratings by health care professionals

Physicians, nurses, pharmacists, and other professionals make judgments about a patient's compliance. These judgments are often arbitrary, based on past experience. Because they are subjective, however, they should never be the only measurement used to determine patient compliance with drug therapy.

Patient self-reporting. Another type of subjective measurement of compliance, patient self-reporting sometimes requires the patient to recall complex behaviors over a long period of time. The patient is asked to recall whether or not the drug regimen was followed as prescribed, including verification that prescriptions were filled. The actual questions used to elicit the patient's information may call for objective as well as subjective responses. Researchers have shown that about half of noncompliant patients admit to noncompliance.

Pill counts. These counts also objectively measure patient compliance. The nurse compares the number of doses in the patient's prescription container to the number that should be there if the patient has been compliant. Pill counts are not entirely reliable, however: for example, if doses are missing, the patient may have spilled some of them or taken some at the wrong times. For this reason, the nurse should consider the information derived from pill counts carefully and with other compliance data.

Direct observation. Objective information about a patient's compliance can be obtained by the nurse through direct observation. Because the nurse must measure the drug dose and watch as the patient takes it, this method is practical mainly for hospital or clinical settings. It is impractical for measuring compliance when the patient takes drugs at home—unless a home health nurse visits regularly.

The nurse should remember that combining two or more measurement methods produces more accurate evaluation of patient compliance. For example, for a patient who may have difficulty affording the prescribed drugs, the nurse may use self-reporting and pill counts to measure compliance. For an elderly patient with poor vision, the nurse may measure compliance using self-reporting, occasional direct observation by a home health nurse, and pill counts.

NURSING RESPONSIBILITIES

To evaluate the effectiveness of a drug therapy and the patient's compliance accurately, the nurse must: (1) possess a thorough knowledge of each drug the patient takes, including its therapeutic effects, adverse reactions, and drug interactions; (2) assess that the patient has made an informed, autonomous decision to comply (or not comply) with the drug regimen; (3) be aware of the various forms and causes of noncompliance and use several methods to assess the patient's compliance; and (4) implement nursing interventions that promote the patient's compliance with the drug regimen. The nurse must also keep the patient's rights in mind.

Patient knowledge is the first step in promoting patient compliance. Chapter 11, Intervention: Patient Education, discusses patient teaching and its principles in detail. These are the principles and theories the nurse needs to guide the information given to all patients regarding drug therapy. The patient, who must make an informed personal decision about following a drug regimen, needs information that is accurate, clear, logical, and based on scientific rationale. Without effective patient teaching, a patient may become unintentionally noncompliant and receive little or no therapeutic benefit from the drug therapy.

The nurse, physician, pharmacist, social worker, and dietitian are all typically involved in promoting compliance. The dietitian is a resource for information about foods that may promote drug absorption or that may interact with the drug to cause adverse reactions. The social worker may help to circumvent economic factors that could lead to noncompliance.

The pharmacist also helps provide patient education. Many states now have laws that mandate pharmacists to supply prescription drug information to patients. Pharmacists are especially qualified to provide information to patients about proper administration, adverse effects, and drug interactions.

The nurse, however, has the greatest impact on compliance of any health team member. Whether in the hospital, clinic, home, or other setting, the nurse is traditionally viewed as the provider who spends the most time with the patient—time the nurse can use in part to remove barriers to compliance and encourage patients' compliance efforts. Evaluation, the last step in the nursing process, represents an optimal use of nursing time: the nurse uses evaluation to determine the need to reassess the effectiveness of prescribed drug therapy. The nurse must also document the evaluation.

DOCUMENTING THE EVALUATION

The nurse is legally required to document activities related to drug therapy, including the time of administration, the quantity administered, and the patient's reaction to the drug. To deliver the best possible patient care, the nurse should also record evaluation data. Because other nurses must be able to read the evaluation and implement appropriate nursing care, documentation must be clear, concise, and complete: it should begin with an evaluation of outcome criteria and proceed to a reassessment of specific interventions.

The format used to document the evaluation step in the nursing process can vary. Progress notes combined with flow sheets may be used; an evaluation column in the nursing care plan is another commonly used method. (See *Documenting a nursing evaluation of drug therapy* on page 254 for one method of documentation.)

CHAPTER SUMMARY

Chapter 16 covered the evaluation step of the nursing process as it relates to drug therapy. Evaluation was discussed in terms of assessing drug effectiveness and measuring patient compliance. Here are the highlights of the chapter:
● The nurse evaluates a patient's drug therapy to determine if related outcome criteria have been met. The outcome criteria serve as the basis for assessing the success (partial or total) or failure of a patient's drug therapy.

Documenting a nursing evaluation of drug therapy

The example below illustrates how a nurse may document evaluation of drug therapy. This example focuses on the potential for noncompliance; a similar method could be used to document the evaluation of therapeutic effectiveness.

	Potential noncompliance: hydrochlorothiazide (HCTZ)
S Subjective	"I HAVE THREE KIDS AND MY WIFE IS PREGNANT. SEEMS TO ME IF I COULD JUST LOSE A FEW POUNDS I WOULDN'T NEED THESE PILLS ANYWAY. I SURE CAN'T AFFORD THEM ON UNEMPLOYMENT. I CAN BARELY PAY RENT AND BUY GROCERIES. THIS MEDICATION KEEPS ME UP HALF THE NIGHT GOING TO THE BATHROOM."
O Objective	NEWLY DIAGNOSED ESSENTIAL HYPERTENSION. BLOOD PRESSURE CURRENTLY RANGING 126-148/80-94. HCTZ 50mg P.O. b.i.d. WT. CURRENTLY 210 lb. HT. 5'10". FAVORITE FOODS INCLUDE CHINESE FOODS AND SPAGHETTI. CITY BUS DRIVER, UNEMPLOYED FOR 3 MONTHS. HIGH SCHOOL EDUCATION.
A Assessment	POTENTIAL NONCOMPLIANCE: HCTZ RELATED TO: (a) LIMITED INCOME, (b) ADVERSE DRUG REACTION (INCREASED URINARY OUTPUT), (c) POSSIBLE KNOWLEDGE DEFICIT CONCERNING CHRONIC NATURE AND POTENTIAL EFFECTS OF HYPERTENSION.
P Plan	(1) CONSULT WITH PHYSICIAN CONCERNING CHANGING HCTZ TO 100mg P.O. q.d., (2) CONSULT WITH DIETITIAN—HELP PATIENT MAINTAIN LOW-SODIUM DIET AND REDUCE WEIGHT TO IDEAL, (3) CONSULT WITH SOCIAL WORKER—POTENTIAL SOURCES FOR FINANCIAL ASSISTANCE, (4) FURTHER ASSESS PATIENT'S KNOWLEDGE REGARDING PRESCRIBED DRUG AND DISEASE PROCESS.
I Intervention	(1) PHYSICIAN CHANGED HCTZ TO 100mg P.O. q.d., (2) DIETITIAN WILL SEE PATIENT AND WIFE ON 10/18 TO SUGGEST WAYS TO FOLLOW LOW-SODIUM, LOW-CALORIE DIET, (3) SOCIAL WORKER HAS SEEN PATIENT AND IS HELPING PATIENT OBTAIN HCTZ AT NO COST, (4) PATIENT DESCRIBED HYPERTENSION CORRECTLY AND EXPRESSED A DESIRE TO CONTINUE WITH PRESCRIBED REGIMEN.
E Evaluation	POTENTIAL FOR NONCOMPLIANCE STILL EXISTS, BUT CAUSES HAVE BEEN REDUCED.
R Re-evaluation	ASSESS PATIENT FOR MEDICATION (AND DIETARY) COMPLIANCE IN 2 WEEKS AT HIS NEXT CLINIC VISIT. USE PILL COUNT, BLOOD PRESSURE, WEIGHT, AND SELF-REPORTING FOR EVALUATION.

If outcome criteria are not met, the nurse must reapply appropriate steps in the nursing process to implement the effective intervention.

• The nurse evaluates drug effectiveness in terms of therapeutic effect and any occurrence of adverse reactions or drug interactions. The therapeutic effect represents the drug's actions that benefit the patient. Adverse drug reactions include predictable, dose-related reactions and unpredictable, non–dose-related reactions, such as allergic responses. Drug interactions, which occur between drugs or between a drug and a food, may be beneficial or adverse.

• The nurse also implements the evaluation step to assess patient compliance. Patients are evaluated for factors that may hinder their ability to comply with therapy. Patient-related factors include knowledge deficits, a nonsupportive environment, impaired physical abilities, and counterproductive health beliefs. Drug therapy factors include unpleasant adverse reactions, complex or prolonged therapy, and expensive therapy. The patient's relationship with health care professionals can also promote compliance. By establishing a therapeutic relationship with the patient, conveying positive attitudes about the drug therapy, and educating the patient, the nurse can intervene to remove or reduce barriers to compliance.

• The nurse should document the evaluation data in the patient record. Documentation provides a legal record and a reference for future use by the nurse or physician. The record can also be used to help determine future drug therapy.

BIBLIOGRAPHY

Atkinson, L., and Murray, M. *Understanding the Nursing Process.* New York: Macmillan Publishing Co., 1986.

Carpenito, L. *Nursing Diagnosis: Application to Clinical Practice.* Philadelphia: J.B. Lippincott Co., 1983.

Contanch, P.H. "Relaxation Training for Control of Nausea and Vomiting in Patients Receiving Chemotherapy," *Cancer Nursing.* 6:277, August 1983.

Cummings, K., et al. "Construct Validity Comparisons of Three Methods for Measuring Patient Compliance," *Health Service Research.* 19:103, April 1984.

Gillman, A.G., et al., eds. *Goodman and Gilman's The Pharmacological Basis of Therapeutics,* 7th edition. New York: Macmillan Publishing Co., 1985.

Hagen, E. "Conceptual Issues in the Appraisal of the Quality of Care." Division of Nursing, U.S. Department of Health, Education, and Welfare. Pub. No. HRA-75-40. Washington, D.C.: U.S. Government Printing Office, May 1975.

Klinger, M. "Compliance and the Post-MI Patient," *Canadian Nurse.* 80:32, August 1984.

Levine, R. *Pharmacology: Drug Actions and Reactions,* 3rd edition. Boston: Little, Brown & Co., 1983.

McCord, M. "Compliance: Self-Care or Compromise?" *Topics in Clinical Nursing.* January 1986.

McMillan, E. "Patient Compliance with Antihypertensive Drug Therapy," *Nursing.* 2:761, June 1984.

Moseley, J. "Alterations in Comfort," *Nursing Clinics of North America.* 20:427, June 1985.

Simonson, W. *Medications and the Elderly: A Guide for Promoting Proper Use.* Rockville, Md.: Aspen Systems Corp., 1984.

DRUGS AFFECTING THE AUTONOMIC NERVOUS SYSTEM

This unit focuses on drugs that influence one component of the nervous system: the efferent, or motor, limb of the peripheral nervous system. Yet the nurse must remember the interrelationship of all components of the nervous system when planning and assessing drug therapy. The nurse can achieve clinical objectives for many autonomic nervous system disorders by understanding the system, how it communicates, and how it adapts to alterations in its environment.

The nervous system, which controls and coordinates functions throughout the body, has two major divisions: the central nervous system (CNS) containing the brain and spinal cord; and the peripheral nervous system containing afferent, or sensory, neurons carrying information to the CNS, and efferent, or motor, neurons carrying information from the CNS. The peripheral nervous system, which mediates between the CNS and the external and internal environments, is subdivided into the somatic nervous system and the autonomic nervous system.

The drugs discussed in this unit affect information transmittal by the motor neurons of the somatic and the autonomic divisions of the peripheral nervous system. To implement the nursing process in patients receiving such drug therapy, the nurse needs a working knowledge of this system.

Anatomy and physiology

The somatic and autonomic nervous systems act in parallel to control and coordinate voluntary, involuntary and reflex movements and visceral functions. However, these two systems have anatomic and physiologic differences that influence drug therapy and nursing assessment.

The somatic nervous system. Efferent neurons of the somatic nervous system travel to skeletal (striated) muscles and control both reflex and voluntary movements. The cell bodies of these neurons lie within the CNS and send their axons directly to specialized synapses called neuromuscular junctions on the skeletal muscles that they innervate.

The autonomic nervous system. Efferent neurons of the autonomic nervous system innervate smooth and cardiac muscle, glands, and other viscera. Unlike the somatic nervous system, the autonomic nervous system is subdivided: the sympathetic nervous system (adrenergic) and the parasympathetic nervous system (cholinergic).

The sympathetic and parasympathetic nervous systems have two neurons (rather than one, as in the somatic nervous system) carrying information to the target sites. The cell bodies of the first neurons, like those of the somatic nervous system, originate in the CNS. The neurons of the sympathetic nervous system originate from the thoracic and lumbar regions of the spinal cord, and those of the parasympathetic nervous system originate from either the brain stem or the sacral region of the spinal cord. The two systems are referred to, respectively, as the thoracolumbar and craniosacral divisions.

Axons from these first neurons leave the CNS and travel to ganglia where they synapse with a second neuron that travels to the target site. Because of the intervening ganglia, the axons of the first neurons are called preganglionic fibers; those of the second neurons are called postganglionic fibers.

The preganglionic fibers of the sympathetic nervous system are short, terminating in ganglia that lie adjacent to the spinal cord (paravertebral chain) or a short distance from the cord (such as the celiac ganglion). The preganglionic fiber that innervates the adrenal medulla is an exception. This preganglionic fiber goes directly from the spinal cord to special cells in the adrenal medulla without synapsing. The adrenal medulla is analogous to a sympathetic postganglionic neuron (its secretory cells originate in nervous tissue) and releases norepinephrine and epinephrine directly into the circulation. Postganglionic fibers travel some distance to reach their target sites. (See *Sympathetic division activity* on page 258 for an illustration of preganglionic and postganglionic fibers and neurotransmission.)

In contrast to the sympathetic nervous system, most preganglionic fibers of the parasympathetic nervous system are long and travel to ganglia located close to or in

Glossary

Acetylcholine: reversible choline acetic acid ester, present in many parts of the body, that facilitates impulse transmission from one nerve fiber to another across a synaptic junction; also a parasympathomimetic agent.

Acetylcholinesterase: catalytic enzyme that enhances break down of acetylcholine into acetic acid and choline.

Adrenergic: activated or transmitted by epinephrine or epinephrine-like substances.

Alkaloid: organic, basic substance found in plants.

Alpha-adrenergic receptor: adrenergic receptor of the sympathetic nervous system that responds to norepinephrine and to various blocking agents.

Anticholinesterase: substance that inhibits the action of cholinesterase.

Antidyskinetic: agent used to counteract an impairment of ability to execute voluntary movement.

Antimuscarinic: agent that inhibits stimulation of muscarinic receptors.

Autonomic nervous system: that portion of the nervous system that controls the involuntary visceral functions of the body.

Beta-adrenergic receptor: adrenergic receptor of the sympathetic nervous system that responds to epinephrine and various blocking agents.

Catecholamine: class of sympathomimetic neuroregulators that includes dopamine, norepinephrine, and epinephrine.

Catechol-o-methyltransferase: enzyme diffusely present in all tissues that breaks down catecholamines.

Cholinergic: stimulated, activated, or transmitted by acetylcholine.

Cholinesterase: enzyme present in all body tissues that acts as an enzyme in the hydrolysis of acetylcholine into choline and acetic acid.

Chronotropic: altering the rate of cardiac muscle contraction.

Cycloplegic: agent that paralyzes the ciliary muscle of the eye.

Dopaminergic: stimulated, activated, or transmitted by dopamine.

Dromotropic: altering the conductivity of a nerve fiber.

Ganglion: group of nerve cell bodies located outside the CNS.

Inotropic: altering the force of muscular contraction.

Monoamine oxidase: catalytic enzyme in the nerve endings that enhances deamination or breakdown of catecholamines.

Motor end-plate: branching nerve terminals of a motor neuron of the voluntary muscles.

Muscarinic receptor: receptor located in effector cells that is stimulated by acetylcholine and muscarine.

Mydriatic: agent that dilates the pupil of the eye.

Neurohormone: hormone that stimulates the neural mechanism.

Neuromuscular junction: joining of a nerve ending and a muscle fiber at the fiber's midpoint so that action potential in the fiber travels bidirectionally.

Neuron: nerve cell; the structural unit of the nervous system.

Neurotransmitter: chemical substance secreted by the neuron at the synapse that acts on receptor proteins in the membrane of the adjacent neuron to stimulate, inhibit, or modify its activity.

Nicotinic receptor: receptor located in effector cells that is stimulated by acetylcholine and nicotine.

Parasympathetic nervous system: cholinergic division of the autonomic nervous system.

Parasympatholytic: agent that opposes the effects of impulses conveyed by the parasympathetic nervous system.

Parasympathomimetic: agent that produces effects similar to those from stimulation of the parasympathetic nerves.

Spasmolytic: agent that eliminates spasms.

Sympathetic nervous system: adrenergic division of the autonomic nervous system.

Sympatholytic: agent that opposes the impulses conveyed by the adrenergic postganglionic fibers of the sympathetic nervous system.

Sympathomimetic: agent that produces effects similar to those of impulses conveyed by the adrenergic postganglionic fibers of the sympathetic nervous system.

Synapse: area surrounding the point of contact between the processes of two adjacent neurons or between a neuron and effector organ where an impulse is transmitted through the action of a neurotransmitter.

Vasopressor: agent that stimulates the contraction of muscular tissue of capillaries and arteries.

the walls of their target sites. The postganglionic fibers of the parasympathetic nervous system are short. This dissimilarity in the pattern of distribution of preganglionic and postganglionic fibers facilitates the contrasting effects of the two systems. The characteristics of the sympathetic nervous system permit a more generalized, widespread effect whereas those of the parasympathetic nervous system permit a more discrete, localized effect. (See *Parasympathetic division activity* on page 259 for an illustration of preganglionic and postganglionic fibers and neurotransmission.)

Usually both systems send information to the same target sites. Exceptions include the adrenal medulla, sweat glands, spleen, and hair follicles, which are in-

Sympathetic division activity

The sympathetic branch of the autonomic nervous system has two neurons that carry information to effector organs. Neurons originate from within the CNS (thoracolumbar region). Preganglionic and post-ganglionic fibers transmit nerve impulses. Preganglionic fibers are short, terminating in ganglia that lie either adjacent to the spinal cord or a short distance from it. The preganglionic fiber that directly innervates the adrenal medulla without synapsing at a ganglion, causes release of norepinephrine and epinephrine directly into the circulation. Postganglionic fibers are long and travel some distance through effector cells to reach effector organs. This transmittal is carried out by chemicals (neurotransmitters). Major neurotransmitters are acetylcholine (ACh), norepinephrine, epinephrine, and to a less extent, dopamine.

Major physiologic effects are alpha and beta adrenergic: Vasoconstriction; vasodilation; heart rate, force of contraction, and conduction velocity increase; bronchial smooth muscle relaxation; GI tract smooth muscle relaxation; GI sphincter contraction; urinary system smooth muscle relaxation; sphincter contraction; pupillary dilation and ciliary muscle relaxation; sweat glands secretion increase; pancreatic secretion decrease; and thick salivary secretions.

Examples of types of drugs that influence these functions: adrenergic agonists and antagonists and ganglionic blocking agents.

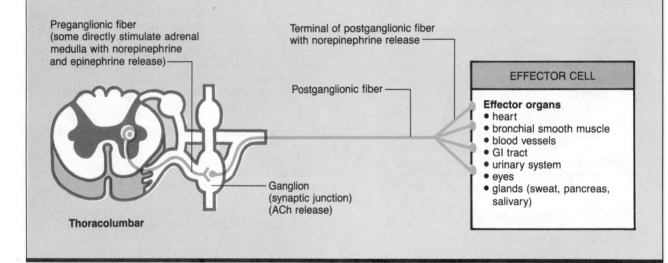

Preganglionic fiber (some directly stimulate adrenal medulla with norepinephrine and epinephrine release)

Terminal of postganglionic fiber with norepinephrine release

Postganglionic fiber

Ganglion (synaptic junction) (ACh release)

Thoracolumbar

EFFECTOR CELL

Effector organs
- heart
- bronchial smooth muscle
- blood vessels
- GI tract
- urinary system
- eyes
- glands (sweat, pancreas, salivary)

nervated by the sympathetic nervous system only. Because the physiologic functions of the two systems are usually opposite, dual innervation balances physiologic effects. Drug therapy sometimes disrupts this critical balance, as when the parasympathetic nervous system is blocked and the activity of the sympathetic nervous system is left unopposed. Knowing the physiologic effects of each system allows the nurse to predict what may happen when a given drug is used therapeutically.

Stimulation of the somatic nervous system can be viewed as initiating a single activity, skeletal muscle contraction; however, the physiologic effects of the subdivisions of the autonomic nervous system are much more complex. As a generalization, however, the sympathetic nervous system can be viewed as an activity-response system whereas the parasympathetic nervous system is a vegetative-homeostatic system.

Stimulation of the sympathetic nervous system produces heart and respiratory rate increase, pupillary dilation, smooth muscle vasoconstriction, skeletal muscle vasodilation, gastrointestinal (GI) activity decrease, fat and glycogen breakdown increase, and metabolic rate increase. These effects are sometimes called the "fight or flight" response because they prepare the individual to face or run from something threatening.

Conversely, stimulation of the parasympathetic nervous system produces heart and respiratory rate decrease, pupil constriction and enhanced accommodation, digestion and elimination increase, GI tone enhancement, and sphincter tone relaxation. These activities are considered energy conserving and homeostatic.

Neuron communication

The nervous system communicates via chemicals called neuroregulators, or neurotransmitters, that transmit neuron information between adjacent cells. In the motor limb of the peripheral nervous system, the major neurotransmitters are acetylcholine, norepinephrine, epinephrine, and, to a lesser extent, dopamine.

Acetylcholine is released from all preganglionic neurons of the autonomic nervous system, from all postganglionic neurons of the parasympathetic nervous system, from some postsynaptic neurons of the sympathetic nervous system, and at neuromuscular junctions within the somatic nervous system. Acetylcholine's duration of action is short; it is rapidly degraded by the enzyme acetylcholinesterase.

Norepinephrine and epinephrine are released from the adrenal medulla. Norepinephrine also is released from the postganglionic adrenergic fibers of the sympathetic nervous system. The epinephrine and norepinephrine released from the adrenal medulla have effects similar to direct adrenergic neuronal stimulation but can reach and stimulate target sites that do not receive direct innervation from adrenergic fibers.

The duration of action of norepinephrine released at the synapse is extremely short because it rapidly re-enters the neuron from which it was released (reuptake), diffuses from the area, or is degraded by the enzymes monoamine oxidase or catechol-o-methyltransferase. The duration of action of the epinephrine and norepinephrine released from the adrenal medulla, however, may last 10 times longer because removal from the circulation is less rapid than from neuronal synapses. This slower removal from the circulation emphasizes the potential difference between the effects of administered drugs and endogenous substances released within the body.

Parasympathetic division activity

The parasympathetic branch of the autonomic nervous system has two neurons that carry information to the cells of effector organs. Neurons originate in the CNS (craniosacral region). Preganglionic and postganglionic fibers transmit nerve impulses. Most preganglionic fibers are long and travel to ganglia located close to or in the walls of the effector organs. In contrast, the postganglionic fibers are short. The major (neurotransmitter) is acetylcholine.

Physiologic effects: vasodilation of salivary glands; heart rate, force of contraction, and conduction velocity decrease; bronchial smooth muscle constriction; GI tract tone and peristalsis increase, with sphincter relaxation; urinary system sphincter relaxation, and bladder tone increase; pupillary constriction; pancreatic, salivary, and lacrimal secretions increase.

Examples of types of drugs that influence these functions: Cholinergic agonists and antagonists and ganglionic blocking agents.

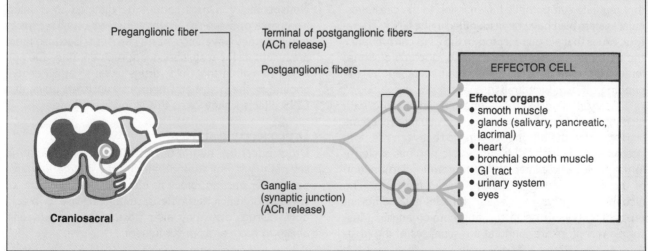

Preganglionic fiber

Terminal of postganglionic fibers (ACh release)

Postganglionic fibers

Ganglia (synaptic junction) (ACh release)

Craniosacral

EFFECTOR CELL

Effector organs
- smooth muscle
- glands (salivary, pancreatic, lacrimal)
- heart
- bronchial smooth muscle
- GI tract
- urinary system
- eyes

Dopamine is a precursor to norepinephrine and a neurotransmitter. It can interact with dopaminergic, alpha- and beta-adrenergic receptors and can stimulate the release of norepinephrine from adrenergic fibers.

Drug effects

Effects are sometimes achieved through a drug's interaction with specific receptors on a target cell. Receptors are dynamic cellular components that can be altered by many conditions. Knowledge of receptor physiology has improved drug specificity and the understanding of how the body adapts to exogenously administered drugs or an altered internal environment. The mechanisms of action for drugs discussed in this unit depend upon receptor types, presynaptic receptors, receptor regulation, and nonspecific drug effects.

Types of receptors. The major classes of receptors currently identified in the motor limb of the peripheral nervous system include alpha-adrenergic receptors, beta-adrenergic receptors, dopamine receptors, muscarinic receptors, and nicotinic receptors. Target tissues may have one or a combination of these receptors. A drug's effects are determined by the numbers of each receptor and the drug's specificity.

The catecholamines norepinephrine and epinephrine exert their effects by interacting with alpha- and beta-adrenergic receptors. Each has two subtypes: alpha$_1$ and alpha$_2$, and beta$_1$ and beta$_2$. Norepinephrine has a greater effect on alpha$_1$ and alpha$_2$, and beta$_1$ receptors than on beta$_2$ receptors, whereas epinephrine has an equal effect on alpha and beta receptors. Thus, epinephrine can exert greater metabolic, vasodilatory, and bronchodilatory effects than norepinephrine can.

Over the last decade, alpha-adrenergic receptors that regulate sympathetic transmission to the cardiovascular system also have been identifed in the CNS. Therefore, drugs that act on receptors in the CNS can influence the peripheral nervous system. Also, dopamine can interact with dopaminergic, alpha, and beta receptors, depending on its concentration.

Acetylcholine exerts its effect by interacting with nicotinic and muscarinic receptors. Nicotinic receptors are located in the autonomic ganglia (between pre- and postsynaptic fibers of the autonomic nervous system), in the motor end-plates at the neuromuscular junction of the somatic nervous system, and in the CNS. The nicotinic receptors on skeletal muscle have different properties than those in the autonomic ganglia. Muscarinic receptors are found at the synapses of the post-synaptic fibers of the parasympathetic nervous system, on some postsynaptic fibers of the sympathetic nervous system, and in the CNS.

Presynaptic receptors. The amount of a neurotransmitter released from a neuron is modulated by neuroregulators and presynaptic receptors on the neuron. Presynaptic alpha-adrenergic receptors are alpha$_2$ receptors.

Presynaptic receptors have clinical importance. For example, an adrenergic blocking agent that nonselectively blocks alpha$_1$ and alpha$_2$ receptors will block the contraction of vascular smooth muscle (alpha$_1$) and the negative feedback to adrenergic fibers (alpha$_2$). The negative feedback block will release more norepinephrine that can stimulate the heart's beta-adrenergic receptors and cause tachycardia.

Receptor regulation. Altered environmental conditions can change receptor number or density (up or down regulation) or change the affinity of a receptor for an agonist or antagonist (uncoupling). Drug effects and withdrawal effects relate to receptor number or affinity. For instance, long-term administration of a beta agonist can decrease the density of beta receptors and reduce the drug's effect. In contrast, long-term administration of a beta antagonist, or blocker, can increase the density of receptors and the response to sudden withdrawal of a beta-blocking agent.

A number of clinical conditions such as diabetes mellitus and hypothyroidism or hyperthyroidism can affect receptor concentration or affinity. Thus the patient's current clinical status must be considered when the nurse assesses drug therapy.

Nonspecificity. Drugs cannot be directed to a select body area or tissue site. Rather, they act on all receptors to which they have access and can bind. Because there are receptors for acetylcholine, norepinephrine, and epinephrine within the CNS, drugs given to affect acetylcholine in the peripheral neurons can exert unwanted CNS effects if they cross the blood-brain barrier.

Drug selection and use

Drugs affect the neural transmission of information in several ways. For example, they may imitate a neurotransmitter's action, block its effect at a receptor site, or enhance or inhibit its synthesis, storage, release, or breakdown. Drugs also may alter postsynaptic target cells' ability to recover from stimulation.

Drug selection is based on mechanism of action and clinical objectives. For example, if hypertension treatment is aimed at lowering norepinephrine levels to minimize vasoconstriction, a drug that inhibits norepinephrine's effects will be considered. Drug selection is based on specificity for a particular target tissue, efficacy, adverse effects and toxicity, and cost. The cost must be evaluated in dollars and consequence on the patient's activities and self-concept (such as impotence from antihypertensive agents).

Drugs that influence the somatic or autonomic nervous systems can be categorized according to: (1) location of their primary effect, (2) primary effect, such as facilitation or inhibition of sympathetic or parasympathetic effects, and (3) the receptor with which they interact. The drug categories discussed in this unit produce effects similar to acetylcholine, norepinephrine, or epinephrine, or inhibit the effects of those substances.

Drug categories that produce effects similar to acetylcholine include cholinergic agents, parasympathomimetic agents, cholinesterase inhibitors, muscarinic agents, and nicotinic agents. Drugs that inhibit the sympathetic nervous system also can permit acetylcholine's unopposed activity within the parasympathetic nervous system.

Drug categories that inhibit the effects of acetylcholine include cholinergic blocking agents, anticholinergic agents, parasympatholytic agents, antimuscarinic agents, ganglionic blocking agents, and neuromuscular blocking agents. Drugs that facilitate sympathetic nervous system activity can antagonize acetylcholine's effects.

Drug categories that produce effects similar to norepinephrine and epinephrine include adrenergic agents (catecholamines or noncatecholamines that are alpha, beta, dopaminergic, or nonselective); sympathomimetic agents, or monoamine oxidase inhibitors. Drugs that inhibit the parasympathetic nervous system also allow unopposed sympathetic nervous system activity.

Drug categories that inhibit the effects of norepinephrine and epinephrine include adrenergic blocking agents, sympatholytic agents, and ganglionic blocking agents—which block both the sympathetic nervous system and parasympathetic nervous system at the preganglionic level. Drugs that facilitate parasympathetic activity also can antagonize the effects of norepinephrine and epinephrine.

Adverse drug reactions

Adverse drug reactions usually relate to physiologic effects and usually can be anticipated. These reactions include unwanted drug effects, adaptive changes caused by the drug, and adaptive changes already occurring because of clinical condition, drug therapy, or the aging process.

Unwanted drug effects. These effects occur when a drug's action cannot be aimed selectively. For example, an adrenergic blocking agent used to control blood pressure affects the CNS secondarily. Drugs that penetrate the blood-brain barrier are much more likely to produce a CNS effect than those that cannot cross this barrier.

Another example is the tachycardia that may occur when a nonselective alpha-adrenergic blocking agent is used.

Adaptive changes caused by the drug. Certain changes such as the decreased density of beta receptors that can occur after long-term use of a beta agonist, pose problems of drug withdrawal and drug tolerance.

Adaptive changes already occurring. Clinical conditions such as diabetes mellitus and hypothyroidism can lead to altered receptor numbers or affinity. Aging may alter receptor responsiveness.

Nursing assessment

Drug therapy is complex, and the nurse is responsible for anticipating problems, assessing efficacy, recognizing adverse reactions, and providing appropriate information to patients who must understand the therapeutic goals and what to monitor.

To achieve these goals, the nurse must formulate a nursing diagnosis. Answers to the following questions provide data with which to formulate a nursing diagnosis:
- What kind of drug is being discussed, for example, an alpha-adrenergic agonist or a selective beta$_1$ antagonist?
- What are the drug's physiologic effects? How does stimulation or inhibition of these physiologic functions affect what is exhibited clinically?
- How does the nervous system adapt to the drug's effects? Are receptors altered, does up or down regulation occur, or is the presynaptic system affected?
- How does the patient's adaptation to the drug influence the drug's effectiveness? What are the effects of sudden withdrawal or discontinuance?
- What are the nursing implications and what needs to be monitored and discussed with the patient?

Chapter 17
Cholinergic Agents

Chapter 17 explores those agents that mimic acetylcholine's effects and stimulate the parasympathetic nervous system. The two types of acetylcholine receptor sites, muscarinic and nicotinic, are differentiated, and the basic physiologic action of acetylcholine is reviewed. The primary clinical uses for these agents as antimyasthenics and antidotes for neuromuscular blocking agents are discussed. The nursing focus of the chapter is on assisting patients in managing the effects of cholinergic agents.

Chapter 18
Cholinergic Blocking Agents

Those agents that compete with acetylcholine at receptor sites in the CNS, autonomic ganglia, autonomic effector organs, and neuromuscular junctions are discussed in Chapter 18. The clinical uses of the antimuscarinic agents, such as belladonna alkaloids, quaternary ammonium compounds, and tertiary amines, are explored in reversing bradycardia, decreasing salivary and respiratory secretions, decreasing GI motility and secretions, and decreasing urinary tract spasticity. Detailed nursing implications include rationales for intervention.

Chapter 19
Adrenergic Agents

Adrenergic agents, or catecholamines and noncatecholamines, are presented in Chapter 19. The discussion begins with a review of the physiologic actions of the catecholamines, similar to those produced by sympathetic nervous system stimulation. The discussion differentiates among alpha, beta$_1$, and beta$_2$ receptor activity effects and the clinical uses of the catecholamines. The chapter investigates alpha-active drugs to treat hypotensive states and beta-active drugs to treat respiratory diseases, hypersensitivity, bradycardia, and heart block.

Chapter 20
Adrenergic Blocking Agents

Chapter 20 explores alpha- and beta-adrenergic and ganglionic blocking agents used to inhibit sympathetic nervous system function. Alpha-adrenergic blockers that decrease blood pressure are discussed, as are adverse effects related to vasodilation. Beta-adrenergic blocking agents are looked at for their selective action on cardiospecific beta$_1$ receptors and their nonselective action on both beta$_1$ and beta$_2$ receptors. The clinical use of beta blockers in treating hypertension, cardiac dysrhythmia, and angina is detailed. Ganglionic blocking agents, which are nonselective in their blocking action, are also discussed, as is their role in hypotension.

Chapter 21
Neuromuscular Blocking Agents

In Chapter 21 the neuromuscular blocking agents are examined as muscle relaxants that facilitate surgery. The two types of neuromuscular blocking agents, nondepolarizing, or curare-like, and depolarizing, or acetylcholine-like, are explored. A major emphasis of the chapter is the nursing care required for patient safety during these agents' administration.

Nursing diagnoses

Several nursing diagnoses are appropriate for planning care for patients receiving drug therapy that affects the peripheral nervous system. Most of these diagnoses relate to the patient's physiologic and life-style changes, including:

● Potential activity intolerance related to a decreased or increased heart rate or orthostatic hypotension due to drug therapy

● Anxiety related to an increased or decreased heart rate, bronchiolar constriction, loss of voluntary movement, or change in life-style due to drug therapy

● Alteration in bowel elimination: constipation or diarrhea related to drug therapy

● Ineffective breathing pattern related to inhibition of skeletal muscle stimulation due to ganglionic blocking agents

● Potential alterations in cardiac output: decreased due to drug therapy

● Alterations in comfort: pain related to diarrhea, constipation, urinary retention or loss of voluntary movement due to drug therapy

● Alterations in family processes related to life-style changes due to drug therapy

● Fear related to loss of voluntary movement due to ganglionic blocking agents and cardiac dysfunction due to adrenergic agonists

● Potential for impaired gas exchange related to bronchiolar constriction and inhibition of skeletal muscle stimulation due to drug therapy

● Potential for injury related to orthostatic hypotension or loss of voluntary movement due to drug therapy

● Knowledge deficit related to all aspects of drug therapy

● Impaired physical mobility related to the loss of voluntary movement due to ganglionic blocking agents

● Alterations in nutrition: less than body requirements related to increased bowel motility or loss of voluntary movement due to drug therapy

● Self-care deficit related to loss of voluntary movement due to ganglionic blocking agents

- Disturbance in self-concept related to loss of voluntary movement or changes in life-style due to drug therapy
- Potential for sensory-perceptual alterations related to dysfunction in neural transmission due to drug therapy
- Sexual dysfunction related to inhibition of skeletal muscle stimulation and loss of voluntary movement due to beta blocking agents or ganglionic blocking agents
- Potential for impaired skin integrity related to loss of voluntary movement due to ganglionic blocking agents
- Impaired social interaction related to life-style changes due to drug therapy
- Impaired swallowing related to loss of voluntary movement due to ganglionic blocking agents
- Alterations in tissue perfusion related to increased vascular resistance due to drug therapy
- Potential alterations in urinary elimination patterns related to changes in urinary bladder or sphincter tone due to drug therapy.

CHAPTER 17

CHOLINERGIC AGENTS

OBJECTIVES

After reading and studying this chapter, you should be able to:
1. Describe the actions of acetylcholine and acetylcholinesterase in the parasympathetic nervous system.
2. Discuss the three major clinical indications for the cholinergic agents.
3. Explain the pharmacokinetics of the cholinergic agonists.
4. Explain the pharmacokinetics of the anticholinesterase agents.
5. Contrast the mechanisms of action of the cholinergic agonists with those of the anticholinesterase agents.
6. Describe significant adverse effects of the cholinergic agents and their associated nursing implications.

INTRODUCTION

Cholinergic agents are drugs that directly or indirectly promote the function of the neurotransmitter acetylcholine. The cholinergics are also called parasympathomimetics because they produce effects that imitate parasympathetic nerve stimulation.

Cholinergic agents have three major clinical indications. They are used to reduce intraocular pressure in patients with glaucoma or during ophthalmologic surgery, to treat atony of the gastrointestinal (GI) tract or bladder, and to diagnose and treat myasthenia gravis. Some of the cholinergic agents are important antidotes to neuromuscular blocking agents, tricyclic antidepressants, and belladonna alkaloids.

Cholinergic agents achieve their effects in one of two ways: they mimic the action of acetylcholine or inhibit its destruction at cholinergic receptor sites. Chapter 17 discusses the two main classes of drugs used as cholinergic agents: cholinergic agonists and anticholinesterase agents.

Physiology of the parasympathetic nervous system

Part of the autonomic nervous system, the parasympathetic nervous system controls the body's visceral functions: it conserves energy and maintains organ function.

The parasympathetic nervous system has two subdivisions, the cranial and the sacral. The cranial subdivision is made up of cranial nerves III (oculomotor), VII (facial), IX (glossopharyngeal), and X (vagus).

The oculomotor nerve innervates the pupillary sphincters and the ciliary muscles; the facial nerve innervates the lacrimal, sublingual, and submaxillary glands and mucous membranes of nose and palate; and the glossopharyngeal nerve innervates the parotid gland. The vagus nerve carries about 75% of all parasympathetic fibers. The organs under vagal stimulation include the lungs, heart, stomach (including the pyloric valve), liver, small intestine, and the upper two thirds of the colon and kidney. (See *The parasympathetic nervous system* for a schematic depicting the nerve–target organ relationships.)

The cranial nerves give rise to preganglionic fibers that synapse with postganglionic fibers either at ganglia near the target organs or, in the case of the vagus nerve, in the target organ itself. The postganglionic fibers innervate the target organs through autonomic effector cells, where acetylcholine is synthesized and secreted.

The sacral portion of the parasympathetic nervous system arises from the second, third, and fourth segments of the sacral spinal cord. The sacral parasympathetic fibers form the pelvic nerves, which distribute their fibers to the bladder, genitalia, sex organs, distal colon, rectum, and anal sphincter, and lower portion of the ureters.

The preganglionic and postganglionic fibers of the parasympathetic nervous system are cholinergic; that is, they synthesize and secrete the neurotransmitter acetylcholine. Acetylcholine's action lasts for a few seconds at most because most of it is quickly destroyed by the cholinesterase enzymes.

The parasympathetic nervous system

When parasympathetic nerves are stimulated, they release acetylcholine from the nerve endings. The acetylcholine binds with receptor sites on the target organs and stimulates muscle contraction. The nerves and their corresponding sites are shown below.

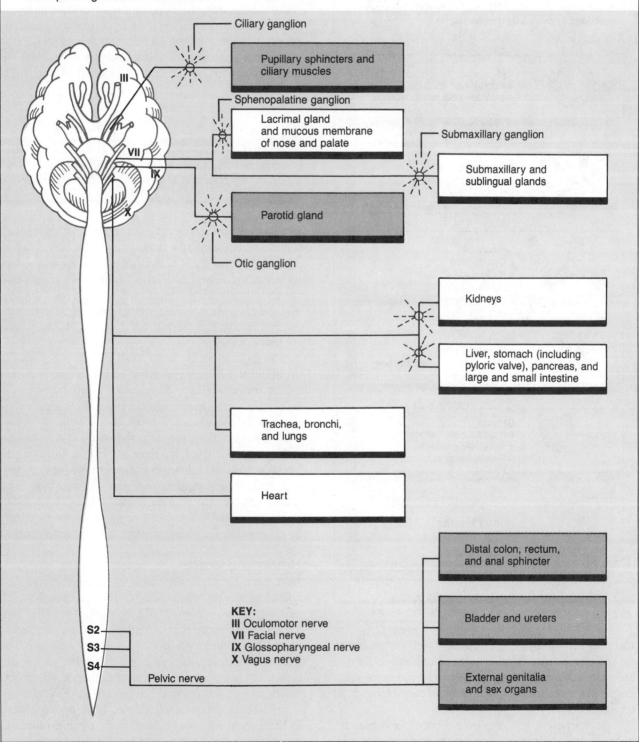

Ciliary ganglion

Pupillary sphincters and ciliary muscles

Sphenopalatine ganglion

Lacrimal gland and mucous membrane of nose and palate

Submaxillary ganglion

Submaxillary and sublingual glands

Parotid gland

Otic ganglion

Kidneys

Liver, stomach (including pyloric valve), pancreas, and large and small intestine

Trachea, bronchi, and lungs

Heart

Distal colon, rectum, and anal sphincter

Bladder and ureters

External genitalia and sex organs

Pelvic nerve

KEY:
III Oculomotor nerve
VII Facial nerve
IX Glossopharyngeal nerve
X Vagus nerve

Effects of the parasympathetic nervous system on its target organs

The representative responses that acetylcholine triggers in parasympathetic nervous system target organs are depicted in this illustration.

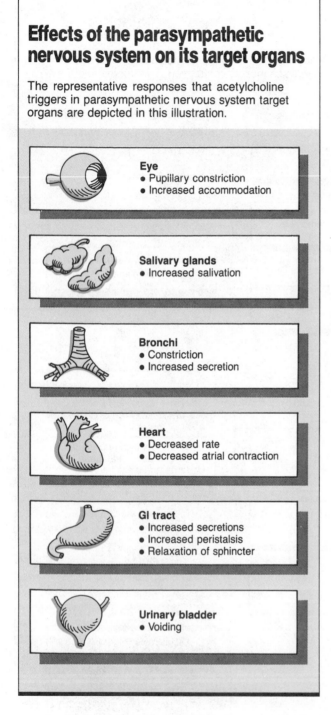

Eye
- Pupillary constriction
- Increased accommodation

Salivary glands
- Increased salivation

Bronchi
- Constriction
- Increased secretion

Heart
- Decreased rate
- Decreased atrial contraction

GI tract
- Increased secretions
- Increased peristalsis
- Relaxation of sphincter

Urinary bladder
- Voiding

Acetylcholine lasts long enough, however, to stimulate the target organ by combining with receptor sites on cell membranes. That allows calcium and sodium to enter the cells of the target organ, resulting in depolarization of the cell membrane and contraction of the target organ muscle.

Acetylcholine activates both nicotinic and muscarinic receptors. Nicotinic receptors are present in the syn-

apses between the pre-ganglionic and post-ganglionic neurons of the sympathetic and parasympathetic nervous systems, in the motor end-plates of skeletal muscle at the neuromuscular function, and in the central nervous system (CNS). Muscarinic receptors are present in all the effector cells stimulated by postganglionic neurons of the parasympathetic nervous system, the postganglionic chlorinergic neurons of the sympathetic nervous system, and in the CNS. (See *Effects of the parasympathetic nervous system on its target organs* for details.)

For a summary of representative drugs, see *Selected major drugs: Cholinergic agents* on pages 274 and 275.

CHOLINERGIC AGONISTS

Cholinergic agonists directly stimulate cholinergic receptors, thus mimicking the action of natural acetylcholine. They include synthetic acetylcholine; choline esters, such as bethanechol and carbachol; and naturally occurring cholinomimetic alkaloids such as pilocarpine. Functionally, this class also includes metoclopramide, a dopamine antagonist that may sensitize the upper GI tract to acetylcholine's effects.

Acetylcholine is rarely used clinically because its unpredictable effects can act at both nicotinic and muscarinic receptor sites and because it is rapidly destroyed by acetylcholinesterase. Although the choline esters and cholinomimetic alkaloids resist breakdown by acetylcholinesterase, they, too, lack specificity of action. Clinically, they are used for their effects on the eye, the intestine, and the urinary bladder, but, because of their widespread parasympathomimetic actions, they have many adverse effects. Metoclopramide is also resistant to acetylcholinesterase, but it has fewer adverse effects. Its cholinergic action is limited to the upper GI tract.

History and source

As a class, the cholinergic agonists are old drugs. Acetylcholine was first synthesized in 1867, although its role as a neurotransmitter was not discovered until the early 1900s. Since then, many synthetic choline derivatives have been developed, but only carbachol and bethanechol have clinical applications. (Methacholine, another synthetic cholinergic agent, has therapeutic effects, but its adverse effects make it impractical for clinical use.)

Cholinomimetic alkaloids also have a long history. In 1869, muscarine was isolated from *Amanita muscaria*, a poisonous mushroom, and played a key role in developing the receptor theory of neurohumoral transmission. Pilocarpine, named for the South American plant from which it was isolated, was discovered less than 10 years later. It stimulates salivary and sweat glands and constricts the pupils of the eyes. Arecoline is an alkaloid of the betel nut, a well-known East Indian euphoriant. Of these drugs, only pilocarpine is in clinical use today.

PHARMACOKINETICS

The action and metabolism of the cholinergic agonists vary widely, depending on their affinity for either nicotinic or muscarinic receptors and on their susceptibility to inactivation by the enzyme acetylcholinesterase.

Absorption, distribution, metabolism, excretion

With the exception of metoclopramide, the cholinergic agonists are rarely administered I.M. or I.V. because they are subject to immediate breakdown by cholinesterases in the interstitial and intravascular spaces. In addition, cholinergic agonists administered I.M. and I.V. take effect rapidly and increase the likelihood of a cholinergic crisis.

Usually, the cholinergic agonists are administered intraocularly, orally, or subcutaneously. Because these routes limit drug absorption, the number of adverse reactions is minimized. For example, when cholinergic agonists are administered in the eye, pressure applied on the inner canthus prevents their drainage through the lacrimal ducts and subsequent absorption through the nasal mucosa. This reduces systemic response to the medications. Adverse reactions with oral administration seem to be reduced when the drugs are given on an empty stomach. Subcutaneous administration may result in a more rapid and effective response.

The most useful cholinergic agonists bind primarily with muscarinic receptors and are not susceptible to cholinesterases. The most commonly used drug in this class, bethanechol, has an affinity for muscarinic receptors in the bladder and GI tract and is resistant to cholinesterases. Drugs that bind with both nicotinic and muscarinic receptors, such as carbachol, acetylcholine, and methacholine, are of limited therapeutic use because of their widespread action. Currently, they are used intraocularly, where their absorption is limited.

All cholinergic agonists are metabolized by cholinesterases at the muscarinic and nicotinic receptor sites, in the plasma, and in the liver. However, some of the cholinergic agonists are more susceptible to the enzymes than others. Drugs that are rapidly metabolized by cholinesterases (acetylcholine and methacholine) are rarely used clinically. Carbachol, bethanechol, metoclopramide, and pilocarpine are more resistant to the action of these enzymes and are therefore more useful clinically. All the drugs in this class are excreted by the kidneys.

Onset, peak, duration

When administered orally, bethanechol begins acting within 30 to 90 minutes, reaches peak concentration levels in 1 to 3 hours, and has a duration of action of 6 to 8 hours. Subcutaneously, bethanechol works much more rapidly, with an onset of action of 5 to 15 minutes, a peak concentration level in 15 to 30 minutes, and a duration of action of 2 hours.

Metoclopramide's onset of action is 30 to 60 minutes when it is administered orally; 10 to 15 minutes, intramuscularly; and 1 to 3 minutes, intravenously. It is the only drug in this class that is ever administered I.M. or I.V. Its duration of action is 1 to 2 hours, and it has a half-life of 4 to 6 hours. (See Chapter 79, Ophthalmic Agents, for a discussion of the ophthalmic cholinergic agonists carbachol and pilocarpine.)

PHARMACODYNAMICS

The cholinergic agonists combine with cholinergic receptors at organs innervated by the parasympathetic nervous system, producing effects equivalent to those of postganglionic parasympathetic nerve impulses. (See *Pharmacologic actions of the cholinergic agents* on page 268 for a summary of the quantitative and selective effects of these drugs on target organs.)

Mechanism of action

Cholinergic agonists mimic the action of acetylcholine at the autonomic effector site. They bind with receptors on the cell membrane of smooth muscles, changing the permeability of the cell membrane and permitting calcium and sodium to flow into the cells. This depolarizes the cell membrane, causing muscle contraction.

PHARMACOTHERAPEUTICS

Clinical indications for the cholinergic agonists are twofold: to treat atonic conditions of the GI tract or bladder and to reduce intraocular pressure in the anterior chamber of the eye. The latter indication is useful in patients with glaucoma and in those undergoing ophthalmologic surgery. Less commonly, cholinergic agonists are used to diagnose belladonna intoxication because belladonna derivatives such as atropine are cholinergic antagonists. Consequently, atropine is considered an antidote for the cholinergic agonists.

Pharmacologic actions of the cholinergic agents

Cholinergic agents have a differential parasympathomimetic effect on the various body systems that are quantitative and selective for a body system. The nurse should be aware of these differences in order to provide quality patient care.

DRUG	SITE OF ACTION							
	Bronchi	Cardiovascular System	Central Nervous System	Eye	Gastrointestinal System	Myoneural Junction	Salivary Glands	Urinary Bladder
Cholinergic agonists								
bethanechol	+ +	+ +	–	+ +	+ + +	–	+	+ + +
carbachol	+	+	–	+ + +	+ +	–	+	+ +
metoclopramide	+	+	+ +	+	+ + +	–	+	+
pilocarpine	+ +	+ + +	+ +	+ + +	+ +	–	+ + +	+ +
Anticholinesterase agents								
ambenonium	+	+	+	+	+	+ + +	+	+
edrophonium	+	+	–	+	+	+ +	+	+
echothiophate	+	+	?	+ + +	+	+	+	+
neostigmine	+	+	+	+	+ +	+ + +	+	+ + +
physostigmine	+	+	+ + +	+	+	+ + +	+	+
pyridostigmine	+	+	+	+	+	+ + +	+	+

KEY + minor effect
+ + moderate effect
+ + + major effect
– no effect

bethanechol chloride (Duvoid, Myotonachol, Urecholine). A choline ester, bethanechol stimulates the smooth muscle of the GI tract and urinary bladder. It is used to treat gastroesophageal reflux, postoperative abdominal distention, congenital megacolon, and urinary retention. USUAL ADULT DOSAGE: for GI atony, 10 to 20 mg P.O. t.i.d. or q.i.d., always given orally unless a complete GI obstruction is present (then the dose may be given S.C.); for urinary retention secondary to hypotonic or atonic bladder, up to 50 mg P.O. t.i.d.; for acute urinary retention, 5 mg S.C.

carbachol (Carbacel, Isopto Carbachol, Miostat). A choline ester, carbachol reduces intraocular pressure during ophthalmologic procedures. (See Chapter 79, Ophthalmic Agents, for a complete description.)

metoclopramide hydrochloride (Reglan). As a cholinergic agonist, metoclopramide promotes GI emptying and facilitates GI intubation and the transit of barium during radiologic examinations; it is also used to treat gastric stasis in diabetic patients, esophageal reflux, and nausea and vomiting secondary to chemotherapy. The drug's effectiveness as an antiemetic is most likely related to its action as a dopaminergic blocker.
USUAL ADULT DOSAGE: for gastroesophageal reflux and diabetic gastroparesis, 10 to 15 mg P.O. q.i.d. (before meals and at bedtime); to stimulate peristalsis during radiologic examinations, 10 mg I.V. as a single dose; as an antiemetic, 2 mg/kg body weight I.V. 30 minutes before chemotherapy treatment and as needed during treatment; except for use as an antidote, the daily dose should not exceed 0.5 mg/kg body weight, to prevent extrapyramidal symptoms.

pilocarpine hydrochloride (Adsorbocarpine, Akarpine, Isopto Carpine, Pilocar). A naturally occurring cholinomimetic alkaloid, pilocarpine reduces intraocular pressure in glaucoma. (See Chapter 79, Ophthalmic Agents, for a complete description.)

Drug interactions

The effect of the cholinergic agonists is intensified by the simultaneous presence of anticholinesterase agents and ganglionic blocking agents. The anticholinesterase agents inhibit the breakdown of acetylcholine at the receptor sites. The ganglionic stimulating agents, such as nicotine, initially stimulate the postganglionic neuron as acetylcholine does. Over the long term, however, these drugs have a depressant effect. The action of cholinergic agonists is limited by interaction with antimuscarinic drugs, neuromuscular blocking agents, and sympathomimetics. Antimuscarinic drugs, such as atropine and disopyramide, block the action of the cholinergic agonists on the autonomic effector, and neuromuscular blocking agents inhibit the action of acetylcholine on the skeletal muscles. The sympathomimetics produce a response opposite to that of the cholinergic agonists at muscarinic receptors. Adverse effects of the cholinergic agonists are accentuated by ganglionic blocking agents such as trimethaphan. (See *Drug interactions: Cholin-*

DRUG INTERACTIONS
Cholinergic agonists

Drug interactions involving the cholinergic agonists usually occur with drugs that also act at the autonomic effector cells.

DRUG	INTERACTING DRUGS	POSSIBLE EFFECTS	NURSING IMPLICATIONS
bethanechol, carbachol, metoclopramide, pilocarpine	other cholinergic agents, particularly anticholinesterase agents (ambenonium, echothiophate, edrophonium, neostigmine, physostigmine, pyridostigmine)	Increase potential for cholinergic toxicity	• Observe the patient for signs of a toxic response, including generalized weakness, fasciculations, dysphagia, and respiratory weakness. • Observe the patient for signs of cardiovascular dysfunction, including bradycardia and hypotension. • Have atropine on hand as an antidote. • Have respiratory support equipment available: suction, oxygen, and mechanical ventilator.
	cholinergic blocking agents (atropine, belladonna, homatropine, methantheline, methscopolamine, propantheline, scopolamine)	Antagonize effect of acetylcholine at the muscarinic receptors	• Have atropine available as the antidote for cholinergic agonists.
	ganglionic blocking agents (mecamylamine, trimethaphan)	Antagonize effect of cholinergic agonists at autonomic ganglia, producing both parasympatholytic and sympatholytic action	• Monitor the patient's blood pressure frequently. • Monitor the patient's bowel movements and urine output.
	neuromuscular blocking agents (atracurium, gallamine, metocurine, pancuronium, tubocurarine, vecuronium)	Antagonize effect of acetylcholine at neuromuscular junction	• Monitor the patient's therapeutic response and expect less muscle relaxation during intubation.
	procainamide, quinidine	Diminish vagal transmission	• Monitor the patient's cardiovascular status: heart rate, rhythm, and blood pressure.
	sympathomimetics (ephedrine, epinephrine, isoproterenol)	Antagonize effects of cholinergic agonists	• Monitor the patient's cardiovascular status: heart rate, rhythm, and blood pressure. • Monitor the patient's bowel movements and urine output. • Auscultate the patient's lungs frequently.

ergic agonists on page 269 for information on interacting drugs, their possible effects, and implications.)

ADVERSE DRUG REACTIONS

Adverse drug reactions to the cholinergic agonists result most often from their nonspecific effects throughout the parasympathetic nervous system.

Predictable reactions

The cholinergic agonists generally bind with receptors throughout the parasympathetic nervous system, creating undesirable parasympathomimetic effects outside the target organ. For example, the use of bethanechol to reduce urinary retention will also increase GI motility, which may cause nausea, belching, vomiting, intestinal cramps, and diarrhea. Effects of the drug on the eye may include blurred vision and decreased accommodation. Cardiovascular responses may follow high doses, and vasodilation, decrease in cardiac rate, and decrease in the force of cardiac contraction may cause hypotension. Salivation or sweating may increase greatly. The drug's bronchoconstrictor effect may produce shortness of breath. Even the desired effect on the urinary bladder is problematic because urinary frequency may replace retention. Usually, the greater the dose, the greater the generalized parasympathomimetic effect. Metoclopramide can also produce dose-related extrapyramidal symptoms, such as tremor and rigidity.

Unpredictable reactions

Cholinergic overstimulation can result from patient hypersensitivity, drug overdose, or, rarely, subcutaneous administration. This overstimulation may result in circulatory collapse, resulting in hypotension, shock, and cardiac arrest.

NURSING IMPLICATIONS

Most nursing implications for the cholinergic agents are aimed at reducing their adverse effects.
- Administer these drugs by the appropriate route to avoid toxic effects.
- Give cholinergic agonists 1 hour before or 2 hours after meals to reduce nausea and vomiting; however, if gastric hyperacidity is present, give the drugs with meals.
- Be aware that the patient's serum levels of amylase and lipase may rise because cholinergic agents increase pancreatic secretion and contraction of Oddi's sphincter.
- Recognize that the patient's serum glutamic-oxaloacetic transaminase (SGOT) and serum bilirubin levels may rise because the contraction of Oddi's sphincter slows bile excretion.

- Monitor the patient's cardiovascular function for adverse reactions.
- Instruct patients with orthostatic hypotension to sit up or arise slowly to minimize dizziness.
- Have intravenous atropine (0.6 mg) available as an antidote.
- Palpate or percuss the patient's bladder before you administer these drugs for urinary retention; if the patient does not void within 1 hour, notify the physician. Catheterization may be necessary.
- Monitor the patient's bowel sounds and note the presence of flatus and bowel movements when giving these drugs for hypotonicity of the GI tract.
- Change bed linens and clothing as necessary to keep the patient comfortable if diaphoresis (profuse sweating) occurs.
- Have toilet facilities available for the patient, and keep call bell within the patient's reach.
- Provide the patient with frequent oral hygiene if increased salivation occurs.

ANTICHOLINESTERASE AGENTS

Anticholinesterase agents inhibit the enzyme acetylcholinesterase, thus slowing the destruction of acetylcholine. The subsequent buildup of acetylcholine produces continued stimulation of cholinergic receptors throughout the body. This action is short term in drugs that are used therapeutically, the so-called reversible anticholinesterase agents. Other anticholinesterase agents, the organophosphates, have a long-term or irreversible action. Used primarily as toxic insecticides and pesticides, they have also been used as nerve gases in chemical warfare. Only two of them, echothiophate and isoflurophate, have therapeutic usefulness.

History and source

The first reversible anticholinesterase agent, physostigmine (or eserine), was derived from the West African Calabar bean. Used clinically in 1877 to treat glaucoma, the drug was not described chemically until 1929. Shortly thereafter, neostigmine was discovered and used to treat myasthenia gravis. Neostigmine is the most widely used anticholinesterase agent today.

Before and during World War II, irreversible anticholinesterase agents were used. These organophosphates were originally developed as insecticides, then quickly adapted to chemical warfare. Fortunately, their use during the war was limited. As insecticides, however, they continue to alter our environment because of their long duration of action and resistance to chemical decomposition, resulting in contamination of water supplies.

Lange and Krueger's research in 1932 on the organophosphates probably provided the basis for Schrader's massive research on these agents in 1952. Schrader structurally defined and synthesized about 2,000 organophosphates.

PHARMACOKINETICS

Reversible and *irreversible* refer to the duration of the anticholinesterase agents' blocking effect. With reversible anticholinesterase agents, the blocking effect lasts for minutes to hours; with the irreversible anticholinesterase agents, the effects are sustained for days or even weeks. The major difference between these agents is their pharmacokinetics.

Absorption, distribution, metabolism, excretion

Many anticholinesterase agents are readily absorbed from the GI tract, subcutaneous tissue, and mucous membranes. The exceptions are neostigmine and related quaternary ammonium compounds, which are absorbed poorly from the GI tract and are given in larger doses when administered orally. If absorption from the GI tract is enhanced, overdose may occur. The organophosphates are potentially toxic because they are absorbed through all the routes mentioned above, as well as the skin and alveolar membrane.

Theoretically, the anticholinesterase agents stimulate cholinergic receptors, primarily the muscarinic in the CNS and the autonomic effector organs, and primarily the nicotinic in the autonomic ganglia and skeletal muscle. In therapeutic doses, fortunately, their actions are more limited. Only physostigmine readily penetrates the blood-brain barrier. The quaternary ammonium compounds such as neostigmine act relatively selectively at the neuromuscular junctions, where they function both as anticholinesterase agents and as cholinergic agonists. Their effects on the autonomic ganglia and the autonomic effector organs are comparatively less. In contrast, the lipid-soluble anticholinesterase agents, such as the organophosphate di-isoprophyl phosphorofluoridate (DFP) act ubiquitously.

Most anticholinesterase agents are metabolized in the body by the plasma esterases and excreted in the urine.

Onset, peak, duration

Ambenonium begins acting in 20 to 30 minutes and continues for 3 to 8 hours. Edrophonium takes effect 2 to 10 minutes after I.M. administration and continues for 5 to 30 minutes. With I.V. administration, it has an onset of action of 30 to 60 seconds and a duration of action of 10 minutes. Oral neostigmine has a half-life of 40 to 60 minutes; its onset of action is 45 to 75 minutes, it reaches peak concentration levels in 1 to 2 hours, and its duration of action is 2 to 4 hours. Injectable neostigmine has a half-life of 50 to 90 minutes. When administered I.M., it takes effect in 20 minutes, reaches peak concentration levels in 30 minutes, and continues to act for 2 to 4 hours. With I.V. administration, onset of action is in 4 to 8 minutes and peak concentration levels are reached in 20 to 30 minutes; action continues for 2 to 4 hours. Physostigmine reaches peak concentration levels within 5 minutes of I.V. administration and has a duration of action of 30 to 60 minutes. Pyridostigmine when given I.M. takes effect in less than 15 minutes and has a duration of action of 2 to 4 hours. With I.V. administration, it has an onset of action of 2 to 5 minutes and a duration of action of 2 to 4 hours.

PHARMACODYNAMICS

The anticholinesterase agents, like the cholinergic agonists, increase the effect of acetylcholine at receptor sites in the CNS, at autonomic ganglia, at autonomic effector cells on the viscera, and at the motor end-plate. Depending on the site and the drug's duration of action, they can have both stimulant and depressant effects on the cholinergic receptors. However, in therapeutic doses, their effects are fairly predictable.

Mechanism of action

Anticholinesterase agents act at the autonomic effector sites and at the neuromuscular junction to inhibit the action of the enzyme acetylcholinesterase. Ordinarily, this enzyme inactivates acetylcholine. Thus, the effect of the anticholinesterase agents is to increase the amount of acetylcholine available at the receptor sites and to prolong its effect.

PHARMACOTHERAPEUTICS

Anticholinesterase agents are important therapeutically because of their effects upon the eye, the GI tract, and the skeletal neuromuscular junction. Their ability to reduce intraocular pressure makes them useful adjuncts to ophthalmologic surgery and in treating glaucoma. They stimulate tone and peristalsis in the GI tract in patients with gastroparesis. Probably their most important use is to promote muscle contraction in patients

DRUG INTERACTIONS

Anticholinesterase agents

Drug interactions involving the anticholinesterase agents usually occur at either nicotinic or muscarinic receptor sites.

DRUG	INTERACTING DRUGS	POSSIBLE EFFECTS	NURSING IMPLICATIONS
ambenonium, echo-thiophate, edro-phonium, neostig-mine, physostig-mine, pyridostig-mine	local, parenteral, or inha-lation anesthetics	Antagonize neuromuscular blockade effect	• Monitor and record the patient's muscle strength. • Monitor the therapeutic response in patients with myasthenia gravis because they may re-quire increased dosages of anticholinesterase agents. • Observe the patient for respiratory depression.
	antibiotics (aminoglyco-sides, capreomycin, linco-mycin, polymixin)	Antagonize neuromuscular blockade effect	• Observe the patient for respiratory depression. • Monitor the therapeutic response in patients with myasthenia gravis because they may re-quire increased dosages of anticholinesterase agents.
	other cholinergic agents, particularly cholinergic ag-onists (bethanechol, car-bachol, metoclopramide, pilocarpine)	Increase potential for tox-icity	• Observe the patient for signs of a toxic re-sponse, including generalized weakness, fas-ciculations, dysphagia, and respiratory weakness. • Observe the patient for signs of cardiovas-cular dysfunction, including bradycardia and hypotension • Have I.V. atropine on hand as an antidote. • Have respiratory support equipment on hand: suction, oxygen, and mechanical ventilator.
	cholinergic blocking agents (atropine, bella-donna, homatropine, methantheline, methsco-polamine, propantheline, scopolamine)	Antagonize effect of ace-tylcholine at muscarinic receptors; may mash early signs of cholinergic crisis	• Have I.V. atropine available as antidote for the anticholinesterase agents. • Monitor the patient for adverse reactions re-lated to the anticholinesterase agents.
	pralidoxime	Reactivates cholinester-ase after poisoning with organophosphates	• Monitor the patient for a decreased thera-peutic response to the anticholinesterase agents.
	ganglionic blocking agent (mecamylamine)	Antagonizes effect of anti-cholinesterase agents at autonomic ganglia, producing both an anti-cholinergic and a choliner-gic effect	• Monitor the patient's blood pressure closely. • Monitor the patient's muscle strength, partic-ularly respiratory strength, and swallowing ability. • Monitor the patient's bowel movements and urine output.
	neuromuscular blocking agents (atracurium, gal-lamine, metocurine, pan-curonium, tubocurarine, vecuronium)	Antagonize the effect of acetylcholine at the neuro-muscular junction	• Monitor the patient for a decreased thera-peutic response to the anticholinesterase agents.
	procainamide quinidine	Diminish vagal transmis-sion and produce neuro-muscular blockade	• Monitor the patient's cardiovascular status: heart rate, rhythm, and blood pressure. • Monitor the patient's muscle strength, partic-ularly respiratory strength.
	quinine	Increases the refractory period of skeletal muscle, reducing its response to acetylcholine	• Monitor the patient's muscle strength, partic-ularly respiratory strength.

with myasthenia gravis. (Neostigmine is also used to diagnose myasthenia gravis.) Anticholinesterase agents are also antidotes to the competitive neuromuscular blocking agents, tricyclic antidepressants, and belladonna alkaloids. They are used also to increase bladder tone.

ambenonium (Mytelase). A reversible anticholinesterase agent, ambenonium is used as an antimyasthenic. Its duration of action is longer than that of neostigmine or pyridostigmine, but its action is not as specific as that of the other agents and it produces many adverse reactions. USUAL ADULT DOSAGE: 2.5 to 5 mg P.O. t.i.d. or q.i.d.; adjust as needed.

echothiophate iodide (Echodide, Phospholine Iodide). An irreversible anticholinesterase agent, echothiophate is used as an antiglaucoma agent and an eye stimulant. (See Chapter 79, Ophthalmic Agents, for a complete description.)

edrophonium chloride (Tensilon). A reversible anticholinesterase agent, edrophonium is a parenteral medication with multiple uses. Because of its short duration of action, it is the drug of choice for the diagnosis of myasthenia gravis; it is also used to differentiate myasthenia gravis from cholinergic toxicity. Edrophonium may be used as an antidote to the nondepolarizing blocking agents, such as metocurine iodide and pancuronium bromide, but it is not as effective as neostigmine or pyridostigmine. It is used to terminate attacks of paroxysmal supraventricular tachycardia and tachydysrhythmia unresponsive to digitalis. USUAL ADULT DOSAGE: for diagnosing myasthenia gravis, initially 10 mg I.M. or 1 to 2 mg I.V., followed by 8 mg I.V. if no response occurs in 45 seconds (keep respiratory support equipment and atropine at hand to counteract toxic effects); for differentiating myasthenia gravis from cholinergic toxicity, 1 mg I.V. followed by an additional 1 mg I.V. if the patient is not further impaired; for neuromuscular block, 10 mg I.V. given over 30 to 45 seconds, repeated to a maximum of 40 mg; for paroxysmal supraventricular tachycardia, 5 to 10 mg slow I.V. push, repeated in 10 minutes if necessary.

neostigmine (Prostigmin). A reversible anticholinesterase agent, neostigmine is available in oral and injectable forms. Oral neostigmine is an antimyasthenic agent. Parenteral neostigmine is the most widely used of the anticholinesterase agents. Its clinical indications are the diagnosis and treatment of myasthenia gravis, the pre-

vention and treatment of postoperative distention and urinary retention, and as an antidote to neuromuscular blocking agents. USUAL ADULT DOSAGE: for myasthenia gravis, initially 15 mg P.O. every 3 to 4 hours or 0.5 to 2 mg I.M. or I.V. every 1 to 3 hours; for postoperative distention and urinary retention, 0.5 to 1 mg I.M. or S.C. every 4 to 6 hours; for neuromuscular blockade, 0.5 to 2 mg I.V., repeated as necessary.

physostigmine salicylate (Antilirium). A reversible anticholinesterase agent, physostigmine is used to treat tricyclic antidepressant and diazepam overdose. Its ability to cross the blood-brain barrier makes it the drug of choice for this purpose. Physostigmine is also used as an antiglaucoma agent and a miotic. (See Chapter 79, Ophthalmic Agents, for additional information.) USUAL ADULT DOSAGE: 0.5 to 2 mg I.M. or I.V.; when given I.V., administer at a rate of not more than 1 mg/ minute; repeat as necessary.

pyridostigmine (Mestinon, Regonol). A reversible anticholinesterase agent, pyridostigmine is used as an antimyasthenic agent and an antidote to the nondepolarizing neuromuscular blocking agents; it is available in oral and parenteral forms. USUAL ADULT DOSAGE: for myasthenia gravis, 60 to 120 mg P.O. every 3 to 4 hours or 2 mg I.M. or I.V. every 2 to 3 hours, adjusted as needed; as an antidote, 10 to 20 mg I.V.

Drug interactions

Interacting drugs usually alter the actions of the anticholinesterase agents at either the nicotinic or muscarinic receptor sites. Cholinergic agonists and other cholinesterase inhibitors act at both sites. Therefore, combinations of the drugs must be used with caution to avoid precipitating a toxic response. Drugs with neuromuscular blocking action antagonize the effect of the anticholinesterase agents at the muscarinic receptors in the skeletal muscle. These include selected antibiotics and anesthetics, as well as the neuromuscular blocking agents. Antimuscarinic agents such as atropine interfere with the anticholinesterase agents in both the central and peripheral nervous systems. Therefore, they may be used as antidotes. Ganglionic blocking agents antagonize the effect of these drugs at the nicotinic receptor sites only. (See *Drug interactions: Anticholinesterase agents* for more details.)

SELECTED MAJOR DRUGS

Cholinergic agents

This chart summarizes the major cholinergic agents in clinical use.

DRUG	MAJOR INDICATIONS	USUAL ADULT DOSAGES	NURSING IMPLICATIONS
Cholinergic agonists			
bethanechol	Urinary retention	10 to 50 mg P.O. b.i.d. to q.i.d. or 5 mg S.C. t.i.d. or q.i.d.	• Administer to the patient when the patient's stomach is empty unless otherwise directed by the physician.
	Postoperative abdominal distention, GI atony, and megacolon	10 to 20 mg P.O. t.i.d. or q.i.d.	• Administer this agent P.O. or S.C. only. • Administer cautiously to patients with asthma, coronary insufficiency, epilepsy, hypertension or hypotension, hyperthyroidism, inflammation of the GI tract, obstruction of the urinary tract, parkinsonism, or peptic ulcer. • Observe the patient for 30 minutes to 1 hour after subcutaneous administration; have atropine (0.6 mg) available in a syringe for use as an antidote. • Monitor the patient's heart rate, rhythm, and blood pressure frequently. • Instruct the patient who develops orthostatic hypotension to get up slowly. • Auscultate the patient's breath sounds frequently. • Monitor the patient for bowel sounds, passage of flatus, and bowel movements. • Palpate or percuss the patient's bladder before drug use for urinary retention. • When bethanechol is given for urinary retention, monitor the patient for micturition, which should occur within 1 hour; if not, urinary catheterization may be necessary.
Anticholinesterase agents			
edrophonium	Differential diagnosis of cholinergic toxicity and myasthenic crisis	1 mg I.V. followed by an additional 1 mg if patient is not further impaired.	• Administer cautiously to patients with asthma, atelectasis, cardiac dysrhythmias, intestinal or urinary tract obstruction, or pneumonia. • Have atropine (0.6 mg) available in a syringe as an antidote. • Have respiratory support equipment available: suction, oxygen, and mechanical ventilator.
	Myasthenia gravis	10 mg I.M. or 1 to 2 mg I.V., followed by 8 mg if no response in 45 seconds	• Monitor and record the patient's muscle strength because the dose will produce increased strength in patients with myasthenia gravis.
	Antidote to neuromuscular blockade	10 mg I.V. over 30 to 45 seconds; repeat if necessary	
	Supraventricular tachycardia	5 to 10 mg I.V.; repeat once if necessary	• Monitor the patient's heart rate, rhythm, and blood pressure.
neostigmine	Myasthenia gravis	15 mg P.O. every 3 to 4 hours or 0.5 to 2 mg I.V. every 1 to 3 hours	• Monitor and record changes in muscle strength. In patients with myasthenia gravis, significant improvement occurs within 1 hour.

SELECTED MAJOR DRUGS

Cholinergic agents continued

DRUG	MAJOR INDICATIONS	USUAL ADULT DOSAGES	NURSING IMPLICATIONS
neostigmine (continued)			• Observe the patient for signs of cholinergic toxicity. • Have atropine (0.6 mg) available in a syringe as an antidote.
	Postoperative distention or urinary retention	0.5 mg I.M. or S.C. every 4 to 6 hours	• Monitor the patient for bowel sounds, passage of flatus, and bowel movements. • Palpate or percuss the patient's bladder before drug administration. • Monitor the patient's therapeutic response; if the patient does not void in 1 hour, catheterization may be needed.

ADVERSE DRUG REACTIONS

Adverse reactions to the anticholinesterase agents are almost invariably secondary to the increased action of acetylcholine at parasympathetic, CNS, and motor receptors. These reactions are difficult to control, particularly at high doses.

Predictable reactions

Parasympathomimetic effects are common. In the eye, they include blurred vision and decreased accommodation; in the skin, increased sweating; in the GI system, increased salivation, belching, nausea, vomiting, intestinal cramps, and diarrhea. The bronchoconstrictor effect may occur as shortness of breath, wheezing, or tightness in the chest. Vasodilation, decreased cardiac rate, and decreased cardiac contraction can result in hypotension, although this effect is partially offset by the decreased metabolism of acetylcholine at the preganglionic receptor sites in the sympathetic nervous system. At the motor end-plate, hyperpolarization of the skeletal muscles reduces effective contractions. Adverse reactions in the CNS include irritability, anxiety or fear, and, in some cases, seizures.

Unpredictable reactions

Reaction to the anticholinesterase agents is difficult to predict in patients with myasthenia gravis. The therapeutic dose varies from day to day, and increased muscle weakness may result from either underdosage, resistance to the drug, or overdosage. Differentiating between a toxic response and a myasthenic crisis is often difficult. A physician who uses edrophonium to distinguish between the two must have respiratory support equipment (a suction machine, oxygen, and a mechanical ventilator) and emergency drugs, such as atropine and pralidoxime, available to counteract cholinergic crisis.

NURSING IMPLICATIONS

When the anticholinesterase agents are used for their parasympathomimetic effects, the nursing implications are the same as those for the cholinergic agonists. When the drugs are used to treat myasthenia gravis, the nurse's responsibilities increase. Patients taking antimyasthenic drugs may eventually learn to alter their dosage as needed, and to do so they need to know how to monitor their response to the drugs. The nursing implications include the following:

• Teach the patient how the anticholinesterase agents work at the neuromuscular junction.

• Instruct the patient to report adverse reactions to the physician.

• Describe ways in which the more frequent adverse reactions can be managed at home; for example, if nausea and vomiting occur after oral administration, tell the patient to take the medication with food or milk.

• Demonstrate how the patient should assess and record changes in muscle strength and help the patient practice the assessment.

• Help the patient develop a systematic means of keeping track of each dose daily and its effect.

CHAPTER SUMMARY

This chapter presented cholinergic agonists and anticholinesterase agents and explained their actions on the parasympathetic nervous system. Highlights include:

• Cholinergic agents directly or indirectly mimic the effects of acetylcholine in the body. Because these effects are usually similar to the effects of the parasympathetic nervous system, the cholinergic agents are also called parasympathomimetic drugs.

• Cholinergic agonists replicate the action of acetylcholine at the muscarinic receptor sites in the viscera and, to a lesser degree, at the nicotinic receptor sites in the autonomic ganglia. They have little effect on the CNS and the motor end-plate. Therapeutically, they are used for their actions on the eye, the GI tract, and the urinary bladder.

• The anticholinesterase agents facilitate the action of acetylcholine by inhibiting its destruction by the acetylcholinesterase enzyme. They act at cholinergic receptor sites in the CNS, the motor end-plates, the autonomic ganglia, and autonomic effector organs. Their primary therapeutic use is to diagnose and treat myasthenia gravis and to counteract neuromuscular blocking agents. They are occasionally used to treat glaucoma, to treat hypotonia of the GI tract or urinary bladder, and in ophthalmologic surgery.

• The adverse effects of the cholinergic agents affect the parasympathetic nervous system, peripheral nervous system, and CNS.

• Most nursing implications are directed toward managing, and teaching patients about, adverse reactions to the drugs. When anticholinesterase agents are used for long-term treatment of myasthenia gravis, the patient needs detailed instructions from the nurse.

BIBLIOGRAPHY

Abrams, A.C. *Clinical Drug Therapy.* Philadelphia: J.B. Lippincott Co., 1983.

Berne, R.M., and Levy, M.N., eds. *Physiology.* St. Louis: C.V. Mosby Co., 1983.

Craig, C.R., and Stitzel, R.E. *Modern Pharmacology,* 2nd ed. Boston: Little, Brown & Co., 1986.

FitzGerald, M.J.T. *Neuroanatomy: Basic and Applied.* Philadelphia: Bailliere Tindall, 1985.

Goodman, A.G., et al, eds. *Goodman and Gilman's The Pharmacological Basis of Therapeutics,* 7th ed. New York: Macmillan Publishing Co., 1985.

Greenblatt, D.J., and Shader, R.I. *Pharmacokinetics in Clinical Practice.* Philadelphia: W.B. Saunders Co., 1985.

Guyton, A.C. *Textbook of Medical Physiology,* 7th ed. Philadelphia: W.B. Saunders Co., 1986.

USP Dispensing Information—Vol. I. Drug Information for the Health Care Provider, 7th ed. Rockville, Md.: United States Pharmacopeial Convention, Inc., 1987.

USP Dispensing Information—Vol. II. Advice for the Patient: Drug Information in Lay Language, 7th ed. Rockville, Md.: United States Pharmacopeial Convention, Inc., 1987.

CHAPTER 18

CHOLINERGIC BLOCKING AGENTS

OBJECTIVES

After reading and studying this chapter, you should be able to:

1. Describe the mechanism of action of the cholinergic blocking agents.

2. Indicate the effect that cholinergic blocking agents have on target organs innervated by the parasympathetic nervous system.

3. Differentiate among the types of antimuscarinic cholinergic blocking agents.

4. List the major clinical indications for the cholinergic blocking agents.

5. Describe the pharmacokinetics of the cholinergic blocking agents.

6. Describe the major adverse reactions to these drugs and the nursing implications.

7. Teach the patient the safe administration of a drug having a narrow margin of safety between therapeutic and toxic dosages.

INTRODUCTION

Cholinergic blocking agents interrupt parasympathetic nerve impulses in the central and autonomic nervous systems. Their primary clinical indications include spastic conditions of the gastrointestinal (GI) and urinary tracts, cardiac dysrhythmias, motion sickness, parkinsonism, and chronic asthma. They are also used as preanesthesia medications and as relaxants for the GI tract during diagnostic procedures and for the eye and pupil during ophthalmologic surgery. They serve as antidotes to cholinergic agents, certain organophosphate pesticides, and neuromuscular blocking agents.

As a group, cholinergic blocking agents have various names. Because they oppose the effects of parasympathetic nerve impulses, they are called parasym-

patholytic drugs. Because they block the action of acetylcholine (which transmits parasympathetic nerve impulses), they are called anticholinergic drugs. Because their sites of activity are muscarinic receptors, they are also called antimuscarinic drugs.

Cholinergic blocking agents constitute two classes: ganglionic blocking agents and antimuscarinic drugs. Although ganglionic blocking agents block the transmission of adrenergic and cholinergic stimuli, their clinical use is limited to their adrenergic effects. Therefore, they are discussed in Chapter 20, Adrenergic Blocking Agents.

The antimuscarinic drugs, of which atropine sulfate is the prototype, exert their blockade effect at postganglionic cholinergic nerve endings at the muscarinic receptor sites. Chapter 18 focuses on these agents.

Physiology of the muscarinic receptor

Understanding the cholinergic blocking agents depends on understanding the physiology of the parasympathetic nervous system and the pharmacology of the cholinergic agents. (See Chapter 17, Cholinergic Agents, for a detailed discussion.)

Usually, cholinergic blocking agents compete with acetylcholine at muscarinic receptor sites in the central nervous system (CNS), the autonomic ganglia, and smooth muscle innervated by parasympathetic nerves, and at the neuromuscular junction. (See Chapter 21, Neuromuscular Blocking Agents, for a further discussion.)

The cholinergic blocking agents usually block the effects of the parasympathetic nerves, allowing the effects of the sympathetic adrenergic nervous system to predominate: the pupils of the eyes dilate and the eye muscles relax; bronchi dilate and respiratory secretions decrease; GI peristalsis decreases; and urine is retained. (See *Effects of cholinergic blocking agents* on page 278 for an illustration of specific responses.)

Some cholinergic blocking agents that can cross the blood-brain barrier have a further effect on the CNS. The brain contains two kinds of muscarinic receptors,

Effects of cholinergic blocking agents

The physiologic effects of the cholinergic blocking agents are widespread. This chart illustrates the organs affected and the physiologic responses that occur.

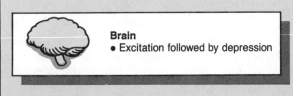

Brain
- Excitation followed by depression

Eye
- Pupillary dilation
- Decreased accommodation

Salivary glands
- Decreased salivation

Bronchi
- Dilation
- Decreased secretion

Heart
- Increased rate
- Increased contractility

GI tract
- Decreased secretions
- Decreased peristalsis

Urinary bladder
- Retention of urine

M_1 and M_2. M_1 receptors predominate in the cerebral cortex and the gray matter of the corpus striatum and the hippocampus, both of which lie in the lateral ventricle of the cerebrum. M_2 receptors are most common in the cerebellum. When cholinergic blocking agents, in low to moderate doses, combine with these receptors, the CNS is stimulated; if the dosage level increases, the CNS is depressed.

Muscarinic receptors are also present in the medulla oblongata, which controls the heart. Vagal stimulation of the heart results from muscarinic action in the CNS and in the heart muscle. The resulting cholinergic blockade can reverse life-threatening bradycardia or asystole.

For a summary of representative drugs, see *Selected major drugs: Cholinergic blocking agents* on page 284.

CHOLINERGIC BLOCKERS

The cholinergic blocking agents block the action of acetylcholine at muscarinic receptors in the parasympathetic nervous system. The major drugs in this class are the belladonna alkaloids—atropine sulfate, homatropine hydrobromide, hyoscyamine sulfate, and scopolamine hydrobromide—and their quaternary ammonium derivatives, clidinium bromide, glycopyrrolate, and propantheline bromide. More limited in their usefulness but still important are the tertiary amines, benztropine mesylate, dicyclomine hydrochloride, and oxybutynin chloride, ethopropazine hydrochloride (a phenothiazine derivative that has antimuscarinic properties), and trihexyphenidyl hydrochloride (a synthetic drug structurally similar to the belladonna alkaloids). Because benztropine, ethopropazine, and trihexyphenidyl are almost exclusively treatments for parkinsonism, they are discussed fully in Chapter 23, Antiparkinsonian Agents.

History and source

The belladonna alkaloids are widely distributed in nature. Atropine is found in such common plants as nightshade, jimsonweed, stinkweed, and thorn apple. Scopolamine and hyoscyamine are present in the shrub henbane.

Belladona preparations have been used for various purposes throughout the ages. Belladonna—the word means "beautiful lady"—was once a popular cosmetic that made the eyes shine and the pupils enlarge. During the Roman Empire and the Middle Ages, the drug was frequently used as a poison. The first documented reports of its therapeutic use stem from the ancient Hindus.

The pure alkaloid atropine was isolated in 1831 by Mein. Its action on the heart was discovered in 1867 and that on the salivary glands in 1872.

Because the belladonna alkaloids are relatively nonselective, researchers have developed and tested numerous synthetic compounds over the years. Of these, only the quaternary ammonium and tertiary amine derivatives are important clinically. Unfortunately, they provide few advantages over the natural alkaloids.

PHARMACOKINETICS

The belladonna alkaloids are more readily absorbed and widely distributed in the body than are their derivatives. Onset of action depends more on how the drug is administered than on the drug used.

Absorption, distribution, metabolism, excretion

The belladonna alkaloids are absorbed from the GI tract, the mucous membranes, the skin, and the eyes. The quaternary ammonium derivatives and dicyclomine are absorbed primarily through the GI tract, although much less readily than the alkaloids.

The belladonna alkaloids are more widely distributed than the quaternary ammonium derivatives or dicyclomine. The alkaloids readily cross the blood-brain barrier; the other drugs in this class do not. Scopolamine has a greater effect on the CNS than does atropine. It also strongly affects the eye and secretory glands. Atropine has a greater effect on the heart, the intestine, the urinary tract, and the bronchi. The quaternary ammonium derivatives have an affinity for the GI tract and, to a lesser degree, for the urinary bladder. They also have an effect on the nicotinic receptors, which affects the cardiovascular system and the neuromuscular junctions.

The belladonna alkaloids have low to moderate binding with serum proteins, are metabolized in the liver by hydrolysis (splitting by the addition of water) and are excreted by the kidneys. The metabolism of the quaternary ammonium derivatives is more complicated. Hydrolysis occurs in the GI tract and the liver; excretion is in feces and urine. Dicyclomine's metabolism is unknown, but it is excreted approximately 50% in urine and 50% in feces.

Onset, peak, duration

The route chosen to administer the cholinergic blocking agents, for the most part, determines how quickly they take effect. Administered intravenously, most have an onset of action of 1 minute; intramuscularly or subcutaneously, onset of action takes about 30 minutes; orally, about 30 to 60 minutes. Belladonna is administered orally only, and its onset of action takes 1 to 2 hours. The duration of action of the belladonna alkaloids lasts up to 6 hours, depending on the drug chosen; the elimination half-life ranges from 3½ to 24 hours, depending on the drug. The quaternary ammonium derivatives have a similar duration of action, but shorter half-lives.

PHARMACODYNAMICS

The cholinergic blocking agents compete with acetylcholine and cholinergic agonists at muscarinic receptor sites in the CNS and at the junction between the postganglionic parasympathetic nerve and the smooth muscle (neuromuscular junction). The resulting blockade of the nerve stimulus may be overcome by increasing acetylcholine concentrations at the receptor sites, accomplished by administering the anticholinesterase agent physostigmine (the antidote for cholinergic blocking agents), which blocks the enzyme that destroys acetylcholine.

Mechanism of action

The action of the cholinergic blocking agents is either stimulating or depressing, depending on the target organ. In the brain, they seem to do both: low drug levels stimulate, and high levels depress. Drug effects are also determined by the condition being treated. Parkinsonism, for example, is characterized by a dopamine deficiency that intensifies the stimulating effects of acetylcholine. Antimuscarinic agents blunt or depress this effect. In other cases, the effects of these on the CNS seem to be stimulatory.

In the bronchial tubes, cholinergic blocking agents decrease cyclic guanosine monophosphate (cGMP) levels, relaxing the bronchi. They are most effective when bronchial constriction is secondary to cholinergic agents and least effective when it is secondary to asthma.

PHARMACOTHERAPEUTICS

All the cholinergic blocking agents are used to treat spastic conditions of the GI and urinary tracts because they relax muscles and decrease GI secretions. The quaternary ammonium compounds, such as propantheline, are the drugs of choice for these conditions because they cause fewer adverse effects than the belladonna alkaloids. However, the alkaloids are used with morphine to treat biliary colic. Parenteral doses of cholinergic blocking agents are used before such diagnostic procedures as endoscopy or sigmoidoscopy to relax the GI smooth muscle.

Because cholinergic blocking agents counteract bronchospasm and reduce respiratory secretions, they are used to treat chronic asthma. As preanesthesia medications, they reduce salivation and gastric secretions and depress the respiratory system. They also block cardiac vagal inhibition during anesthesia.

The belladonna alkaloids have several therapeutic CNS effects. Scopolamine, given with morphine or meperidine, reduces excitement and produces amnesia in the preanesthesia patient. It is also the drug of choice in treating motion sickness. Although other drugs are more effective for other dyskinesias, the cholinergic blocking agents play an important role in treating extrapyramidal symptoms from drugs and in treating parkinsonism.

The belladonna alkaloids also have important therapeutic effects on the heart. Parenteral atropine is the drug of choice to treat sinus bradycardia. It blocks the vagal effects of the SA (sinoatrial) nodal pacemaker and is particularly useful when dysrhythmia results from anesthetics, choline esters, or succinylcholine.

Cholinergic blocking agents are also used as cycloplegics to paralyze the ciliary muscles of the eye, altering the shape of the lens, and as mydriatics to dilate the pupils. They make it easier to measure refractive errors during an ophthalmic examination or to perform ophthalmologic surgery. Occasionally, they are used as adjuncts to antibiotics in treating eye infections.

The belladonna alkaloids, particularly atropine and hyoscyamine, are effective antidotes to cholinergic and anticholinesterase agents. Atropine is the drug of choice to treat poisoning from organophosphate pesticides. Atropine and hyoscyamine also counteract the effects of the neuromuscular blocking agents by competing for the same receptor sites.

atropine sulfate (Arco-Lase Plus, Atropine Sulfate Injection). The prototype of the cholinergic blocking agents, atropine sulfate is a belladonna alkaloid that has the broadest clinical application of any drug in this class. Atropine stimulates or depresses the central nervous system, depending on the dose. It has a more potent action on the heart, intestine, and bronchial muscle than the other belladonna alkaloids and is used to treat bradycardia, spastic conditions of the GI tract, and, occasionally, asthma. As a preanesthesia medication, atropine reduces secretions and minimizes vagal reflexes. It is also used as an antidote to cholinergic agents and neuromuscular blocking agents. Atropine's role as an antiar-

rhythmic is discussed more fully in Chapter 35, Antiarrhythmic Agents. Atropine is available in oral and parenteral forms.

USUAL ADULT DOSAGE: to reverse dysrhythmias, bradycardia, or sinus arrest, 0.4 to 1 mg I.V. every 2 hours, as needed, up to a maximum of 2 mg; as a preanesthesia medication to reduce secretions, 0.2 to 0.6 mg I.M. given 30 to 60 minutes before surgery; and to reverse neuromuscular blockade, 0.6 to 1.2 mg I.V. before or concurrently with 0.5 to 2.5 mg of neostigmine in a separate syringe.

belladonna. A crude botanical preparation, belladonna contains atropine, hyoscyamine, scopolamine, and minor alkaloids. It is used primarily to decrease GI motility and inhibit gastric secretions in peptic ulcer, irritable bowel syndrome, and other GI disorders. Although belladonna was once used to treat vertigo and dyskinesia, more effective agents are now available. Belladonna is available as tablets and tincture.

USUAL ADULT DOSAGE: 15-mg tablet P.O. t.i.d. or q.i.d., 30 minutes before meals and h.s.; 0.18 to 0.3 mg (0.6 to 1 ml) of tincture P.O. t.i.d. or q.i.d., 30 minutes before meals and h.s.

benztropine mesylate (Cogentin). A tertiary amine, benztropine is used primarily as an antidyskinetic in treating parkinsonism. (See Chapter 23, Antiparkinsonian Agents, for more information.)

clidinium bromide (Quarzan). A quaternary ammonium derivative of the belladonna alkaloids, clidinium is used to treat peptic ulcer.

USUAL ADULT DOSAGE: 2.5 to 5 mg P.O. t.i.d. or q.i.d. before meals and h.s.

dicyclomine hydrochloride (Antispas, Bentyl, Viscerol). A tertiary amine derivative, dicyclomine is used to treat irritable bowel syndrome. It is rapidly absorbed after oral or intramuscular administration, but effects occur only with large doses.

USUAL ADULT DOSAGE: 20 mg P.O. q.i.d. initially; can be increased up to a total of 160 mg/day; 20 mg I.M. daily in 4 divided doses.

ethopropazine hydrochloride (Parsidol). A phenothiazine derivative, ethopropazine is used as a cholinergic blocking agent for its antidyskinetic properties in treating parkinsonism. (See Chapter 23, Antiparkinsonian Agents, for complete information.)

glycopyrrolate (Robinul, Robinul Forte). A quaternary ammonium derivative, glycopyrrolate is the synthetic cholinergic blocking agent that most closely approximates the action of atropine. Even so, its action on the CNS is minimal, and GI absorption is poor. Glycopyrrolate is used to treat peptic ulcer. As a preanesthesia medication, it reduces secretions, aids in preventing aspiration of gastric contents, and reduces dysrhythmias. It is currently being studied as a means of treating chronic asthma. Glycopyrrolate is also effective in reversing neuromuscular blockade when used with cholinergic drugs. It is available in oral and parenteral forms.

USUAL ADULT DOSAGE: for peptic ulcer, 1 to 2 mg P.O. b.i.d. or t.i.d., or 0.1 to 0.2 mg I.M. or I.V. t.i.d. to q.i.d.; as preanesthesia medication, 0.004 mg/kg of body weight I.M. given 30 to 60 minutes before anesthetic is to be administered; for bradycardia during surgery, 0.1 mg I.V.; as a cholinergic adjunct to reverse neuromuscular blockade, 0.2 mg I.V. for each milligram of neostigmine, in the same syringe.

homatropine hydrobromide (Homatrocel Ophthalmic, Isopto Homatropine). A quaternary ammonium derivative, homatropine is an ophthalmic solution used as a cycloplegic and a mydriatic. (See Chapter 79, Ophthalmic Agents, for further information.)

hyoscyamine sulfate (Anaspaz, Cystospaz-M, Levsin). A belladonna alkaloid, hyoscyamine's actions are similar to those of atropine, but with more potent central and peripheral effects. It is effective at half the dosage of atropine. The drug is available in oral and parenteral forms.

USUAL ADULT DOSAGE: for spastic GI disorders, 0.125 to 0.25 mg P.O. t.i.d. or q.i.d., 30 to 60 minutes before meals and h.s., or 0.25 to 0.5 mg I.M., I.V., or S.C. every 6 to 8 hours; as a cholinergic adjunct to reverse neuromuscular blockade, 0.3 to 0.6 mg I.V. for each 0.5 to 2 mg of neostigmine, in a separate syringe.

oxybutynin chloride (Ditropan). A tertiary amine, this agent produces a direct spasmolytic effect on the urinary bladder and provides some local anesthesia and mild analgesia.

USUAL ADULT DOSAGE: for neurogenic bladder, 5 mg P.O. b.i.d. or t.i.d., up to a maximum of 5 mg P.O. q.i.d.

propantheline bromide (Pro-Banthine). A quaternary ammonium derivative, propantheline is used mainly to reduce secretions and spasms in the GI tract. It provides symptomatic relief in patients with peptic ulcer, pancreatitis, gastritis, irritable bowel syndrome, diverticulitis, and colitis and also acts as a spasmolytic for the ureters and urinary bladder.

USUAL ADULT DOSAGE: 15 mg P.O. q.i.d. 30 minutes before meals and h.s.

scopolamine hydrobromide (Transderm Scop, Triptone). A belladonna alkaloid, scopolamine has a greater effect on the CNS than any other drug in this class, making it the drug of choice for motion sickness. Scopolamine is also useful as a preanesthesia medication. It not only reduces excessive salivation and respiratory tract secretions in anesthesia, but it also produces a sense of euphoria and amnesia. Scopolamine is readily absorbed from the GI tract and the mucous membranes. In treating motion sickness, scopolamine is usually administered topically via a skin patch behind the ear. One transdermal system delivers 0.5 mg of medication over a period of 3 days. The drug is also available in oral and parenteral dosage forms.

USUAL ADULT DOSAGE: for motion sickness, a 0.5–mg transdermal patch or 0.25 to 0.75 mg P.O. 1 hour before the effect is desired; as a preanesthesia medication, 0.3 to 0.6 mg I.M., I.V., or S.C. 30 to 60 minutes before surgery.

trihexyphenidyl hydrochloride (Artane, Trihexane, Trihexidyl). A synthetic drug structurally similar to the belladonna alkaloids, trihexyphenidyl is used primarily as an antidyskinetic in treating parkinsonism. (See Chapter 23, Antiparkinsonian Agents, for more information.)

Drug interactions

Cholinergic blocking agents cause two main types of interactions with other drugs. Because these drugs decrease gastric motility and delay gastric emptying, they usually decrease the absorption of other medications. The delayed gastric emptying keeps the drugs in prolonged contact with the gastrointestinal mucosa, which can increase their adverse effects. Finally, a number of antacids and antidiarrheals reduce the absorption of the cholinergic blocking agents.

Some interactions change the action of the cholinergic blocking agents. Most common is a general enhancement of the whole range of anticholinergic effects. Drugs that do this include antiarrhythmics, antidepressants, antidyskinetics, antiemetics, antihistamines, antipsychotics, antivertigo agents, CNS stimulants, and skeletal muscle relaxants. Other drugs enhance one or more of the actions of the cholinergic blocking agents. For example, when antimyasthenic agents or opiate-class analgesics are given with cholinergic blocking agents, they reduce intestinal motility further. In contrast, ganglionic blocking agents cancel the effects of cholinergic blocking agents on gastric acid secretion. Finally, cholinergic agents counteract the effects of cholinergic blocking agents. (See *Drug interactions: Cholinergic blocking agents* on page 282 for more details.)

DRUG INTERACTIONS
Cholinergic blocking agents

The nurse must be aware of the many frequently administered medications that interact with the cholinergic blocking agents.

DRUG	INTERACTING DRUGS	POSSIBLE EFFECTS	NURSING IMPLICATIONS
atropine, belladonna, clidinium, dicyclomine, glycopyrrolate, hyoscyamine, propantheline, scopolamine	carbonic anhydrase inhibitors	Enhance antimuscarinic effect from alkalinization of the urine	• Encourage the patient to ingest food and fluids that increase the acidity of the urine, such as cranberry juice. • Monitor the patient for adverse effects.
	antacids, antidiarrheals	Reduce absorption of cholinergic blockers	• Give these medications at least 1 hour before or after giving cholinergic blockers.
	antiarrhythmics (including disopyramide, procainamide, quinidine), tricyclic and tetracyclic antidepressants, antidyskinetics (including amantadine, pimozide), antiemetics and antivertigo agents (including buclizine, cyclizine, meclizine), diphenhydramine antipsychotics (including haloperidol, phenothiazines, thioxanthenes)	Enhance antimuscarinic effect	• Monitor the patient for signs of adverse reactions of cholinergic blockers. • Monitor for constipation, which may become severe or result in paralytic ileus.
	cholinergic agonists (bethanechol, metoclopramide), anticholinesterase agents (neostigmine, pyridostigmine)	Reverse antimuscarinic action	• Monitor the patient for therapeutic effects of the cholinergic blocking agents.
	digoxin	Increases serum concentration levels of digoxin by decreasing gastrointestinal motility	• Monitor the patient's apical pulse frequently. • Observe the patient for signs of digitalis toxicity.
	ganglionic blocking agents (guanadrel, guanethidine, reserpine)	Decrease anticholinergic effect in the eye and the GI tract	• Monitor the patient for constipation which may become severe or result in paralytic ileus. • Monitor the patient's bowel sounds frequently.
	opiate-like analgesics	Decrease gastrointestinal motility	• Monitor the patient for constipation which may become severe or result in paralytic ileus. • Monitor the patient's bowel sounds frequently.

ADVERSE DRUG REACTIONS

The widespread action of the cholinergic blocking agents often produces therapeutic benefits that are accompanied by undesirable effects. The use of drugs that interact with cholinergic blocking agents further increases the possibility of adverse reactions.

Predictable reactions
Predictable adverse reactions are a function of the affinity of the muscarinic receptors for specific drugs and of the drug dose. Dosage is particularly crucial: the difference between a therapeutic and a toxic dose is small with the cholinergic blocking agents. Also, some people are much more susceptible than others to these drugs' effects. These include infants, elderly patients, fair-skinned children with Down's syndrome, and children with spastic paralysis or brain damage.

Adverse reactions increase in severity as the dosage increases. Small doses are accompanied by decreases in salivation, bronchial secretions, and sweating—reducing the patient's ability to cope with heat. As the dosage increases, the pupils dilate, visual accommodation decreases, and heart rate increases. Still larger doses inhibit urination and intestinal motility, followed by a decrease in gastric secretions and motility.

With drug overdose, all these effects are exaggerated. Patients who experience cholinergic blocking agent toxicity are described in the mnemonic "Hot as a hare, blind as a bat, dry as a bone, and mad as a hatter." CNS excitation is prominent at toxic doses. The patient becomes restless, irritable, and disoriented, even hallucinatory or delirious. (Scopolamine may cause this reaction even in therapeutic doses, although the reaction is more likely if the patient has severe pain.) If the process is not reversed (physostigmine is the usual antidote), the excitatory phase is followed by CNS depression, unconsciousness, medullary paralysis, and death.

Unpredictable reactions

Cholinergic blocking agents may precipitate problems in patients with some underlying diseases. The drugs sometimes cause a dangerous rise in intraocular pressure in those with unrecognized narrow-angle glaucoma. Because aqueous humor cannot drain from the anterior chamber of the eye, severe pain and blindness result. These drugs should be administered cautiously to patients over age 40 because of the chance of undiagnosed glaucoma. The incidence of temporary drug-induced blindness has increased as the use of topical scopolamine has increased.

In patients with coronary artery disease, tachycardia secondary to the administration of cholinergic blocking agents can lead to congestive heart failure. This may be compounded by the atrial and ventricular dysrhythmias that sometimes occur with the cholinergic blocking agents.

In patients with benign prostatic hypertrophy, cholinergic blocking agents may cause urinary obstruction. The agents therefore need to be used cautiously in elderly male patients.

Heatstroke is another potential complication with these drugs because they inhibit such heat-regulating mechanisms as sweating. (The flush associated with toxic doses of the belladonna alkaloids may be the body's attempt to compensate for this effect by peripheral vasodilation.) Heatstroke occurs more frequently with strenuous activity and high environmental temperatures. Elderly patients with cardiovascular disease are most susceptible to heatstroke.

NURSING IMPLICATIONS

The nursing implications for the cholinergic blocking agents focus on four general areas: teaching patients how to reduce their need for the drugs; ensuring proper administration; alleviating adverse reactions; and knowing how to prevent and recognize toxicity.

● Because many of the clinical indications for cholinergic blocking agents are believed to have a psychosomatic component, teach the patient more effective means of handling stressors. Help the patient learn to balance the demands of home, work, and play; to practice good health habits; and to use relaxation techniques.

● Have the patient avoid substances that increase gastric acidity, including alcohol, cigarette smoke, caffeine, and aspirin.

● Advise the patient to limit milk and before-bedtime snacks because they increase gastric secretions.

● When the objective is to reduce GI acidity and motility, give cholinergic blocking agents 30 minutes before meals and at bedtime.

● Do not administer cholinergic blocking agents concurrently with antacids or antidiarrheals; give them at least 1 hour apart.

● Recommend sugarless gum, hard sugarless candies, or ice to reduce a dry mouth.

● Emphasize the need for scrupulous oral hygiene when cholinergic blocking agents are used long-term, because reduced saliva increases the likelihood of caries and periodontal disease.

● Recommend that patients wear dark glasses and have someone drive them home if they're receiving cholinergic blocking agents that produce mydriasis and cycloplegia.

● Explain that the patient may have difficulty urinating or defecating. Adequate fluid intake and a high-fiber diet may offset the tendency for constipation, but difficulty in voiding is harder to alleviate. Stroking the abdomen or using Credé's method (massaging the bladder) may help.

● Administer analgesics to patients in pain as ordered when they are receiving cholinergic blocking agents; otherwise, the likelihood of CNS excitation increases.

● Teach the patient to reduce the potential for heatstroke by moving slowly and staying in the shade in hot weather, avoiding strenuous exercise, taking frequent sponge baths, and using fans or air conditioners.

● Teach the patient to avoid drug toxicity by taking only the amount of medicine ordered. The patient who misses a dose should take it as soon as possible; if it is almost time for the next dose, the patient should wait until then and take a single dose only. Stress that patients should not double the dose without consulting the physician.

Cholinergic blocking agents

This chart summarizes the cholinergic blocking agents in clinical use.

DRUG	MAJOR INDICATIONS	USUAL ADULT DOSAGES	NURSING IMPLICATIONS
atropine	Reversal of dysrhythmias, bradycardia, and sinus arrest	0.4 to 1 mg I.V. every 2 hours, as needed, up to a maximum of 2 mg	• Administer I.V. doses slowly. • Monitor the patient's EKG. • Monitor the patient's heart rate and rhythm and blood pressure frequently.
	Preanesthesia medication	0.2 to 0.6 mg I.M. 30 to 60 minutes before surgery	• Mix in the same syringe with other preoperative drugs, unless contraindicated.
	Cholinergic adjunct to reverse neuromuscular blockade	0.6 to 1.2 mg I.V. before or concurrently with 2 to 2.5 mg of neostigmine in a separate syringe	• Provide respiratory support until the antidote becomes effective. • Monitor the patient's heart rate and rhythm and blood pressure frequently.
	Dyskenesia in parkinsonism	0.1 to 0.2 mg P.O. q.i.d.	• Monitor the patient for urinary retention and tachycardia.
dicyclomine	Irritable bowel syndrome	20 mg P.O. t.i.d. or q.i.d., up to a maximum of 160 mg/day, or 20 mg I.M. daily in 4 divided doses	• Administer with or immediately following food to lessen gastric irritation. • Do not administer parenteral form I.V. • Watch for local irritation at injection site. • Instruct the patient to avoid alcoholic beverages. • Advise the patient that the drug may cause drowsiness.
propantheline	Peptic ulcer and spastic bladder	15 mg q.i.d., 30 minutes before meals and h.s.	• Do not administer antacids or antidiarrheals within 1 hour of giving this medication. • Advise the patient to limit the ingestion of alcohol or other CNS depressants.
scopolamine	Preanesthesia medication	0.3 to 0.6 mg I.M., I.V., or S.C. 30 to 60 minutes before surgery	• Anticipate rebound need for REM sleep (patient may report nightmares). • Anticipate patient memory loss with high doses.
	Motion sickness	0.5 mg topically to postauricular skin (lasts for 3 days) or 0.25 to 0.75 mg P.O. 1 hour before effect is desired	• Assess the patient for occasional adverse reactions (restlessness, irritability, confusion, hallucinations) with therapeutic doses. • Advise the patient to limit the ingestion of alcohol and other CNS depressants.

CHAPTER SUMMARY

Chapter 18 focused on the antimuscarinic cholinergic blocking agents, which exert a blockade effect at postganglionic cholinergic nerve endings. Chapter highlights include:

• Cholinergic blocking agents interrupt parasympathetic nerve impulses in the central and autonomic nervous systems by competing with the neurotransmitter acetylcholine at muscarinic receptor sites.

• The effects of the cholinergic blocking agents are vagal stimulation of the heart, mydriasis and cycloplegia of the eye, dilation of the bronchi and an increase in respiratory secretions, a decrease in GI motility and secretions, and retention of urine.

• The antimuscarinic drugs, of which atropine is the prototype, include the belladonna alkaloids, their quaternary ammonium derivatives, and the tertiary amines.

• Clinical indications for the cholinergic blocking agents include cardiac dysrhythmia, motion sickness, parkinsonism, chronic asthma, spastic conditions of the GI and urinary tracts, poisoning by organophosphate pesticides, and toxicity from cholinergic agents or neuromuscular blocking agents. They are also used to decrease salivary and respiratory secretions during anesthesia, relax the GI tract during diagnostic procedures, and relax eye muscles and dilate the pupil during ophthalmologic examinations and surgery.

• Because of the drugs' lack of selectivity, even therapeutic doses of the cholinergic blocking agents are accompanied by multiple adverse reactions, usually extensions of the anticholinergic actions.

• Unpredictable adverse reactions include a dangerous rise in intraocular pressure in patients with unrecognized narrow-angle glaucoma, tachycardia leading to congestive heart failure in patients with coronary artery disease, urinary obstruction in patients with benign prostatic hypertrophy, and heatstroke, particularly in elderly patients with cardiovascular disease.

• The margin of safety between therapeutic and toxic doses is extremely small.

• The nurse must teach patients to minimize their need for cholinergic blocking agents; administer their daily doses safely; alleviate adverse reactions; and prevent, recognize, and obtain treatment for toxicity.

BIBLIOGRAPHY

Abrams, A.C. *Clinical Drug Therapy.* Philadelphia: J.B. Lippincott Co., 1983.

Berne, R.M., and Levy, M.N., eds. *Physiology.* St. Louis: C.V. Mosby Co., 1983.

Craig, C.R., and Stitzel, R.E. *Modern Pharmacology,* 2nd ed. Boston: Little, Brown & Co., 1986.

FitzGerald, M.J.T. *Neuroanatomy: Basic and Applied.* Philadelphia: Bailliere Tindall, 1985.

Goodman, A.G., et al., eds. *Goodman and Gilman's The Pharmacological Basis of Therapeutics,* 7th ed. New York: Macmillan Publishing Co., 1985.

Goth, A., ed. *Medical Pharmacology: Principles and Concepts.* St. Louis: C.V. Mosby Co., 1984.

Greenblatt, D.J., and Shader, R.I. *Pharmacokinetics in Clinical Practice.* Philadelphia: W.B. Saunders Co., 1985.

Greenstein, S.H., et al. "Systemic Atropine and Glaucoma," *Bulletin of the New York Academy of Medicine* 60:961, December 1984.

Guyton, Arthur C. *Textbook of Medical Physiology,* 7th ed. Philadelphia: W.B. Saunders Co., 1986.

Keepers, G.A., et al. "Initial Anticholinergic Prophylaxis for Neuroleptic-Induced Extrapyramidal Syndromes," *Archives of General Psychiatry* 10:1113, October 1983.

Mann, J.S., and George, C.F. "Anticholinergic Drugs in the Treatment of Airway Disease," *British Journal of Diseases of the Chest* 79:209, 1985.

Pullen, G.P., et al. "Anticholinergic Drug Abuse: A Common Problem?" *British Medical Journal* 289:612, September 1984.

USP Dispensing Information—Vol. I. Drug Information for the Health Care Provider, 6th ed. Rockville, Md.: United States Pharmacopeial Convention, Inc., 1985.

ADRENERGIC AGENTS

OBJECTIVES

After reading and studying this chapter, you should be able to:

1. Differentiate between the drugs that are classified as catecholamines and noncatecholamines.

2. Compare the methods of actions of adrenergic agents: direct, indirect, or dual.

3. Differentiate among the effects of alpha-, beta$_1$-, and beta$_2$-receptor stimulation.

4. Explain the relationship between an agent's therapeutic use and its receptor activity.

5. Describe clinical situations that require catecholamine use.

6. Describe clinical situations in which the noncatecholamines are useful.

7. Discuss the adverse effects and nursing implications of both the catecholamines and the noncatecholamines.

INTRODUCTION

Pharmacologically, adrenergic agents are compounds that cause biological responses similar to those produced by activation of the sympathetic nervous system (SNS). The SNS is a large part of the autonomic nervous system (ANS), which is the part of the nervous system concerned with control of involuntary bodily functions. The SNS consists of ganglia, nerves, and plexuses that supply the involuntary muscles. Most of the nerves of the SNS are motor, but some are sensory.

Adrenergic agents, which are also called sympathomimetics, include a large number of endogenous substances and synthetic drugs that have a wide range of therapeutic uses. Classifying adrenergic agents is thus difficult. The classification system used in this chapter divides adrenergic agents into two groups: catecholamines (including endogenous and synthetic agents) and noncatecholamines.

Adrenergic agents may be further divided by their method of action. Thus, they may be direct-acting (acting directly on the sympathetically innervated organ or tissue), indirect-acting (triggering the release of a neuro-transmitter, usually norepinephrine), or dual-acting (combining both direct and indirect actions).

Both endogenous catecholamines (such as epinephrine, norepinephrine, and dopamine hydrochloride) and synthetic catecholamines (such as isoproterenol hydrochloride, isoproterenol sulfate, and dobutamine hydrochloride) are direct-acting. Noncatecholamines may be direct-acting (such as albuterol, isoetharine hydrochloride, isoetharine mesylate, metaproterenol sulfate, methoxamine hydrochloride, nylidrin hydrochloride, phenylephrine hydrochloride, ritodrine hydrochloride, and terbutaline sulfate), indirect-acting (such as amphetamines), or dual-acting (such as ephedrine sulfate, mephentermine sulfate, and metaraminol bitartrate). These agents can activate the SNS alpha and beta receptors selectively, nonselectively, or in combination.

The therapeutic use of adrenergic agents depends on the receptor activity of the particular agent. (See *Adrenergic receptor sites* for location and effect of the receptor sites, and *Adrenergic drugs: Receptor activity, action, and use* on page 288 for details about catecholamines and noncatecholamines.) Most adrenergic agents stimulate alpha or beta receptors to produce their pharmacologic effects, thus mimicking the action of norepinephrine or epinephrine. Other adrenergic agents, called dominergic agents, act primarily on the SNS receptors stimulated by dopamine. Individual drugs differ in receptor activity, although in some the differences may be only quantitative.

Agents that act on alpha receptors are called alphamimetics or alpha agonists. Their most important effects therapeutically involve vasoconstriction of arterioles in the skin, kidneys, mesentery, and splanchnic area. The local effects of alpha$_1$-receptor stimulation are used for hemostasis, pupil dilation, nasal and ophthalmic decongestion, and hypotension associated with allergic reactions. The vasopressor effects of alpha$_1$-receptor stimulation are useful in clinical conditions involving hypotension, shock, and decreased cardiac and cerebral circulation. The therapeutic potential of alpha$_2$-receptor stimulants has not been fully researched, although some

Adrenergic receptor sites

This chart lists receptor types and locations and identifies the effect of an adrenergic or dopaminergic drug on the receptor.

RECEPTOR TYPE	LOCATION	EFFECT
Adrenergic		
alpha$_1$	Blood vessels • arterioles	Constriction
	Sphincters • urinary bladder	Contraction
	Muscles • eye (radial) • skin (pilomotor)	Contraction Contraction
	Glands • salivary • pancreas	Secretion Decreased insulin secretion
alpha$_2$	Adipose tissue	Inhibition of lipolysis
	Skeletal blood vessels	Constriction
beta$_1$	Heart	Increased rate, conduction, and contractility
	Adipose tissue	Lipolysis
	Kidneys	Renin release
beta$_2$	Smooth muscle • bronchial • GI tract • urinary bladder	Relaxation Relaxation Relaxation
	Skeletal blood vessels	Dilation
	Uterus	Relaxation
	Liver	Glycogenolysis
Dopaminergic		
	Coronary arteries	Dilation
	Renal blood vessels	Dilation
	Mesenteric or visceral blood vessels	Dilation

antihypertensive agents (methyldopa and clonidine) are known to have alpha$_2$-receptor activity in the central nervous system (CNS).

Agents that act on beta receptors are called beta-mimetics or beta agonists. Their most important effects therapeutically are cardiac stimulation, smooth muscle relaxation, and vasodilation of blood vessels in the brain, heart, and skeletal muscle. The cardiac stimulant effects of beta$_1$-receptor activation are used only under certain restricted conditions. The beta$_2$-receptor effects of smooth muscle relaxation have important therapeutic uses, including bronchial relaxation in asthma or chronic obstructive pulmonary disease. The beta$_2$-receptor effects of vasodilation of blood vessels are therapeutically used in conditions requiring increased blood flow to these organs. When administering catecholamines, the nurse must remember that the pharmacologic actions of these nonselective drugs may overlap, producing undesirable adverse reactions.

Agents that act on dopamine receptors are called dopaminergic agents or agonists. Dopamine receptors are found primarily in the CNS; dopaminergic agonists are most often used to treat parkinsonism. (See Chapter 23, Antiparkinsonian Agents, for more information on treating this disorder.) Dopamine, however, also stimulates beta$_1$-receptors in the heart where it increases the force of myocardial contraction (produces a positive inotropic effect). Dopamine also possesses indirect activity, stimulating the release of norepinephrine.

For a summary of representative drugs, see *Selected major drugs: Adrenergic drugs* on pages 303 to 307.

CATECHOLAMINES

Catecholamines may be endogenous or synthetic. Endogenous catecholamines share a complex pathway of synthesis: tyrosine is acted upon by tyrosine hydroxylase to become dopa; dopa is then acted upon by dopa decarboxylase to become dopamine. Dopamine, in turn, is acted upon by dopamine beta-hydroxylase to become norepinephrine, which, in the adrenal medulla, may then be acted upon by methyltransferase to become epinephrine.

Because of their common basic chemical structure, catecholamines share certain properties. Although they may produce some CNS effects, such as anxiety, headache, or tremors, they penetrate the blood-brain barrier poorly or not at all. They are ineffective when ingested

Adrenergic drugs: Receptor activity, action, and use

This chart summarizes the receptor activity, action, and use of the major catecholamines and noncatecholamines. This information forms an important knowledge base for the nurse administering these drugs.

DRUG	RECEPTOR ACTIVITY	ACTION	USE
Catecholamines			
dobutamine	Beta$_1$	Cardiac stimulation	Inotropic drug
dopamine	Dopaminergic, alpha (only at high doses), beta$_1$	Vasoconstriction (high doses) Dilates renal vessels at low doses	Shock, hypotension, inotropic drug
epinephrine	Alpha, beta$_1$, beta$_2$	Cardiac stimulation Vasoconstriction Bronchodilation	Anaphylaxis, acute hypotension, cardiac arrest, topical vasoconstriction
isoproterenol	Beta$_1$, beta$_2$	Cardiac stimulation Bronchodilation	Shock, digitalis toxicity, asthma
norepinephrine or levarterenol	Alpha, beta$_1$	Vasoconstriction	Shock, hypotension
Noncatecholamines			
Direct-acting: albuterol	Beta$_1$ < beta$_2$	Bronchodilation	Asthma, bronchitis, emphysema
isoetharine	Beta$_1$ < beta$_2$	Bronchodilation	Inhalation therapy
metaproterenol	Beta$_1$ < beta$_2$	Bronchodilation	Inhalation therapy
methoxamine	Alpha	Vasoconstriction	Hypotension, termination of paroxysmal atrial tachycardia
nylidrin	Beta$_1$, beta$_2$	Vasodilation	Peripheral vascular disorders
phenylephrine	Alpha, beta (weak)	Vasoconstriction	Shock, hypotension, nasal congestion, termination of paroxysmal atrial tachycardia
ritodrine	Beta$_1$ < beta$_2$	Smooth muscle relaxation	Preterm labor for uterine relaxation
terbutaline	Beta$_1$ < beta$_2$	Bronchodilation Uterine relaxation	Emphysema, asthma, preterm labor
Dual-acting: ephedrine	Alpha, beta, CNS	Bronchodilation Vasoconstriction	Nasal congestion, hypotension, narcolepsy
mephentermine	Alpha < beta	Vasoconstriction Appetite depression	Hypotension, appetite depression
metaraminol	Alpha > beta	Vasoconstriction	Shock, hypotension

orally because they are inactivated rapidly in the gastrointestinal (GI) tract and liver. Compared to noncatecholamines, they have a short duration of action. They are relatively unstable, especially in solution, and readily decompose.

Before receiving catecholamines, patients must be carefully assessed for a past history of conditions, such as hypertension, diabetes mellitus, and hyperthyroidism, or medications (including over-the-counter medications) that might contraindicate the use of these drugs. The physical examination and interview are important in determining the probability of therapeutic drug effects, adverse reactions to the drug, and possible drug interactions.

History and source

In 1732, Winslow, believing that the ANS controlled the body's sympathies, called the system sympathetic. In the 1800s, Bichat, convinced that the ANS, and not voluntary processes, controlled nutrition, called the ANS vegetative. Gaskell used the term *involuntary nervous system* to differentiate the ANS from the voluntary nervous system, which controlled skeletal muscle. The names *sympathetic* and *parasympathetic*, used for the two divisions of the ANS, were coined by Langley, who introduced the receptor concept in 1905.

The chemical differences between cholinergic and adrenergic fibers were demonstrated by Dale and coworkers in 1933. In the mid-1940s, a precursor of epinephrine, norepinephrine, was identified, and both substances were found to occur naturally in the body. During this time, dopamine, another precursor of epinephrine and norepinephrine, was also identified. Ahlquist helped clarify the varied actions of the catecholamines in 1948 by demonstrating that the adrenergic effector cells in the SNS contain alpha and beta receptors.

The first synthetic catecholamine to be studied was isoproterenol, in an experiment comparing the different physiologic effects elicited by epinephrine, norepinephrine, and isoproterenol. Animal studies examining the role of epinephrine in producing glycogenolysis (breakdown of glycogen to glucose) in the dog liver were performed by Sutherland in the 1950s, and the role of $3':5'$-adenosine monophosphate (cyclic AMP) was identified.

This work led to an important step in the understanding of the way adrenergic receptors function. When epinephrine occupies the beta$_2$ receptors of bronchial smooth muscle, a reaction occurs in which the receptor is first activated by epinephrine at the membrane site, then intracellular cyclic AMP is formed, producing relaxation, with resulting bronchodilation. Also, when beta$_1$ receptors in the heart are stimulated, a reaction occurs producing cyclic AMP, which leads to increased heart rate and force of contraction. Thus, catecholamines stimulate beta receptors, producing cyclic AMP, which in turn produces the pharmacologic effect. Cyclic AMP, however, is not involved in alpha-receptor response to catecholamines.

During the 1970s, proof of a second class of alpha receptors was provided. Alpha$_2$ receptor sites are primarily located presynaptically; these receptors function as a negative feedback system.

PHARMACOKINETICS

Catecholamines are rapidly inactivated by monoamine oxidase (MAO) and catechol-o-methyltransferase (COMT) in the GI tract and liver, so they must be administered parenterally or via mucous membranes. When given sublingually, a catecholamine must be completely absorbed before any saliva is swallowed to prevent this rapid metabolism.

Absorption, distribution, metabolism, excretion

Catecholamines are destroyed by the digestive enzymes, but rapidly absorbed from mucous membranes. Subcutaneous absorption is slowed by local vasoconstriction secondary to the drug's administration. Intramuscular absorption is more rapid because this route results in less local vasoconstriction.

These drugs are widely distributed in the body, with norepinephrine found primarily in the SNS nerve terminals. They either do not cross the blood-brain barrier (such as dopamine and dobutamine) or cross it poorly (such as epinephrine, isoproterenol, and norepinephrine); epinephrine and norepinephrine can cross the placenta.

Metabolism with inactivation of the drugs occurs in the GI tract, lungs, kidneys, plasma, and other tissues, but most occurs in the liver, through the action of MAO and COMT. Interference with these enzymes will prolong the drug's duration of action.

Metabolites and some unchanged drugs are primarily excreted in the urine; a small amount of isoproterenol is excreted in the feces, and some epinephrine is excreted in breast milk.

Onset, peak, duration

The route of administration largely determines the onset of action, peak concentration levels, and duration of action. (*See Catecholamines: Summary of pharmacokinetics* on page 290 for comparative information on the drugs, their routes of administration, onset, peak, duration, and half-life.) Onset of action is generally rapid

Catecholamines: Summary of pharmacokinetics

The pharmacokinetics of the catecholamines directly affect their therapeutic uses. Data are available for all properties except half-life, which is available only for dobutamine and dopamine. Their half-life is 2 minutes.

DRUG	ROUTE	ONSET	PEAK	DURATION
dobutamine	I.V. infusion	1 to 3 min	10 min or less	Short
dopamine	I.V. infusion	2 to 5 min	Immediate	5 to 10 min
epinephrine	S.C. injection	3 to 5 min	20 min	Unknown
	Parenteral suspension	5 to 10 min	Immediate upon absorption	8 to 10 hr
	Oral inhalation	1 min	Immediate upon absorption	Unknown
	Topical	1 to 60 min	4 to 8 hr	1 to 24 hr
isoproterenol	I.V.	Immediate	Immediate	Less than 1 hr
	Parenteral	Rapid	Immediate upon absorption	1 to 2 hr
	Oral inhalation	Rapid	Immediate upon absorption	1 to 2 hr
	Sublingual	Rapid	Immediate upon absorption	1 to 2 hr
	Rectal	Rapid	Immediate upon absorption	2 to 4 hr
norepinephrine	I.V. infusion	Immediate	Immediate	1 to 2 min

with all catecholamines. I.V. administration is the most rapid route; topical administration is the slowest. Subcutaneous administration involves a delay in onset of action from vasoconstriction, an effect that is lessened with I.M. injection.

Concentration levels peak early with most catecholamines, but depend largely on the drug itself and its administration route.

The duration of action also depends on the route, with drugs administered by parenteral suspension lasting longer than those administered by I.V. infusion. The half-life of catecholamines is usually short.

PHARMACODYNAMICS

Catecholamines function as adrenergic neurotransmitters. The endogenous catecholamine epinephrine is also classified as a neurohormone and functions not only as a neural activator, but also as an endocrine regulator. The effects of exogenous epinephrine may be different from the endogenous chemical because circulating levels are much higher than endogenous epinephrine levels.

Physiologic release of epinephrine, which is about 10 to 30 mcg/minute, increases heart rate and cardiac output and shunts blood from the peritoneal cavity to the skeletal muscles, myocardium, and liver. Epinephrine amounts in excess of this, as might be given exogenously, can produce a generalized alpha-type effect on blood vessels, with resulting widespread vasoconstriction.

Mechanism of action

When catecholamines combine with alpha or beta receptors, chemical or electrical events occur that produce either excitatory or inhibitory effects. In most cases, alpha-receptor activation generates an excitatory response (except for intestinal relaxation). Beta-receptor activation is mostly inhibitory (except in the myocardial cells, where norepinephrine elicits excitatory effects). (*See Adrenergic drugs: Receptor activity, action, and use* on page 288.)

To prevent prolonged effects, catecholamines are quickly inactivated by either uptake into nerve terminals, enzymatic transformation, or diffusion. The reuptake process involves active transport and is the most important mechanism for inactivation. This mechanism also results in conservation and recycling of the drug, which is not destroyed. Enzymatically, endogenous catecholamines are inactivated primarily by MAO; catecholamines that are given exogenously are inactivated primarily by COMT. The diffusion process, whereby catecholamines are absorbed into the circulation and metabolized elsewhere in the body, accounts for only a small portion of catecholamine inactivation.

Norepinephrine and epinephrine are less potent than isoproterenol in stimulating beta receptors. Dopamine has a weak, indirect action on alpha receptors, stimulating release of norepinephrine. Norepinephrine and epinephrine are equal in their alpha$_1$-stimulating abilities. This alpha$_1$ activation generally stimulates smooth muscle contraction.

Because the blood vessels that the alpha$_1$ receptors control are in the internal organs, mucosal surface, and skin, a systemic increase in blood pressure results from alpha$_1$ activation. However, alpha$_2$ receptors serve as a negative feedback system to limit norepinephrine release from the neuron. Norepinephrine also activates alpha$_2$ receptors on the nerve terminal, inhibiting further endogenous norepinephrine release.

Isoproterenol, which stimulates both beta$_1$ and beta$_2$ receptors, is a more potent beta$_1$-receptor stimulant than either epinephrine or norepinephrine. Dobutamine is also a beta$_1$ stimulant, exerting a weak, indirect effect. Beta$_1$ receptors in the conduction tissue of the heart speed cell repolarization when stimulated, leading to positive chronotropic (rate) and dromotropic (conduction) effects. Beta$_1$ stimulation in fat tissue produces fat breakdown, releasing fatty acids for heart and liver energy sources. However, this effect has no therapeutic application.

Norepinephrine, dopamine, and dobutamine are weak beta$_2$-adrenergic receptor stimulants; epinephrine and isoproterenol are equally strong in activating beta$_2$ sites. Beta$_2$ stimulants cause bronchodilation by relaxing bronchial smooth muscle via beta$_2$ activation. Additional beta$_2$ effects include vasodilation and shunting of blood to the skeletal muscles, brain, and heart. An effect of beta$_2$ stimulation not used therapeutically is liver glycogenolysis (also an alpha$_1$ effect).

The combination of alpha$_1$, beta$_1$, and beta$_2$ actions is valuable in the fight or flight response. Beta$_1$ stimulation by norepinephrine is reinforced by epinephrine, producing an increased heart rate and cardiac output, with blood shunted to muscles, brain, and heart by beta$_2$ vasodilation action. Alpha$_1$ receptors control calcium entry into cells, which leads to enzyme changes and produces alpha$_1$ effects (including vasoconstriction of the skin and abdominal organs), and epinephrine provides energy by producing glycogenolysis in the liver and lipolysis in fat cells. Alpha$_2$ receptors oppose beta-receptor action by inhibiting adenylate cyclase, an enzyme necessary for this reaction.

The clinical effects of catecholamines depend on the dose and the route of administration. In the cardiovascular system, these effects may also depend on the vascular bed. The positive inotropic action (marked increase in strength of contraction) results from the influx of calcium into cardiac fibers, producing more complete emptying of the ventricles and increasing cardiac work load and oxygen consumption. Also, the positive dromotropic action may occur with catecholamine agents as well as a positive chronotropic effect from the increased rate of membrane depolarization in the pacemaker cells of the sinus node. This produces in a more rapid attainment of the action potential threshold, so the pacemaker cells fire more often. Reflex bradycardia may occur from increased vasoconstriction and blood pressure. Catecholamines may precipitate spontaneous firing in the Purkinje's fibers, producing pacemaker activity and possibly producing premature ventricular contractions and fibrillation. Epinephrine is likelier than norepinephrine to produce this spontaneous firing.

Although the catecholamines cross the blood-brain barrier poorly, their use produces various CNS effects. Both epinephrine and isoproterenol produce alertness, tremulousness, respiratory stimulation, and anxiety; less anxiety and tremulousness are noted with the use of norepinephrine. Epinephrine and norepinephrine improve cerebral blood flow through their effect on peripheral circulation, resulting in increased systemic blood flow.

Catecholamines produce general relaxation of nonvascular smooth muscles. One effect of this is bronchodilation. Isoproterenol exerts greater effects than epinephrine, and epinephrine exerts greater effects than norepinephrine. Epinephrine may also act to decrease bronchial secretions by constricting bronchial vessels.

Catecholamines reduce peristalsis in the GI tract. Epinephrine causes the urinary bladder sphincter to contract and the detrusor muscle to relax. The physiologic effects of dopamine are primarily dose-related. With low doses of dopamine, only dopaminergic receptors are activated, with the resultant vasodilation of the renal arteries leading to increased renal blood flow and, usually, increased urine output. With high doses of dopamine, alpha and beta effects are noted.

Insulin secretion is inhibited by epinephrine. In addition, catecholamines stimulate glycogenolysis in liver and skeletal muscle, and lipolysis in adipose tissue. This results in increased circulating blood glucose and free fatty acids. Norepinephrine, epinephrine, and isoproterenol also increase oxygen consumption.

Although catecholamines usually produce decreased glandular secretions, causing such an effect as a dry mouth, epinephrine may increase saliva. Also, local sweating of the palms, axillae, and genital area may occur with some catecholamines.

PHARMACOTHERAPEUTICS

The particular receptor activity that exists alone or predominates if more than one receptor type is activated determines how the drug is used therapeutically. Of the catecholamines, norepinephrine has the most nearly pure alpha activity. Drugs with only beta-related therapeutic uses include dobutamine and isoproterenol, and epinephrine stimulates both alpha and beta receptors.

The therapeutic uses of catecholamines are related not only to their systemic effects, but also to their local effects. The local vasoconstrictive actions of the drugs make them useful as nasal decongestants to treat inflammatory and allergic conditions; as ophthalmic decongestants to treat conjunctivitis and ocular congestion; as intraocular hypotensive agents to treat simple, open-angle glaucoma; as topical hemostatics to control superficial bleeding; as local anesthetic adjuncts to prolong action by retarding absorption; and as antiallergens to treat hypersensitivity and anaphylaxis. Local application of various drugs dilates pupils without concurrent cycloplegia (paralysis of ciliary muscles) or increased intraocular pressure. These effects are beneficial primarily in ophthalmic examinations.

The alpha stimulators can be used systemically to relieve hypotension. Hypotension may be caused by numerous conditions, including sympathectomy, pheochromocytomectomy, spinal anesthesia, myocardial infarction, transfusion reaction, septicemia, drug reactions, or shock. In general, the pressor effects are used for conditions related to loss of vasomotor tone or loss of adequate circulating blood volume.

Beta$_1$-active drugs are used to treat bradycardia and heart block (as seen in Stokes-Adams syndrome and carotid sinus syndrome) and insufficient cardiac output.

They may also be used to terminate paroxysmal atrial or nodal tachycardia. Because they are believed to make the heart more responsive to defibrillation, they are used in cases of ventricular fibrillation, asystole, or cardiac arrest.

Catecholamines that exert beta$_2$ activity are used to treat acute and chronic bronchial asthma, emphysema, bronchitis, and acute hypersensitivity reactions to drugs.

The effects of drugs that are exogenously administered differ somewhat from the natural effects of endogenous catecholamines. Thus, the patient's response will also differ somewhat from the normal physiologic response to endogenous catecholamines. Also, the effects of catecholamines administered exogenously are of short duration, which may limit their therapeutic usefulness.

Isoproterenol is both longer-acting and less toxic than epinephrine. Epinephrine, dopamine, dobutamine, and isoproterenol increase cardiac output, while norepinephrine may have no effect or may lower it slightly (the potent vasoconstricting action may cause a reflex bradycardia). Epinephrine increases atrioventricular conduction and may produce more severe tachycardia than norepinephrine because epinephrine is a more potent beta stimulant. Isoproterenol usually produces tachycardia but improves cardiac output because of the drug's positive inotropic and chronotropic actions. Decreased blood pressure may result from low-dose epinephrine because of decreased total peripheral vascular resistance, or from isoproterenol because of a pure vasodilator action. Increased blood pressure may result from high-dose epinephrine, high-dose dopamine, or norepinephrine because of the increased total peripheral vascular resistance with activation of alpha receptors. Both norepinephrine and dopamine decrease blood flow in skeletal muscle, while epinephrine increases perfusion to skeletal muscle by beta$_2$-induced vasodilation.

In most cases, epinephrine is useful therapeutically for its alpha activities in allergic reactions. It is the drug of choice for anaphylactic shock because it counteracts the hypotensive effects of histamine. Alpha pressor effects are also beneficial for local vasoconstriction when prolongation of locally administered drugs is desired. Epinephrine is also used clinically for its beta effects of bronchodilation in acute asthma attacks and for its cardiac effects.

Norepinephrine, with its alpha vasopressor effects, counteracts hypotension from septicemic shock and spinal anesthesia.

Dopamine's therapeutic value is based on its dopaminergic, beta$_1$, and alpha-agonist activity. The drug is used in low doses to dilate renal arteries, preventing renal shutdown in cardiogenic or bacteremic shock. Dopamine may also be helpful in treating chronic refractory congestive heart failure because of its positive inotropic activity.

The beta effects of dobutamine are valuable clinically to increase cardiac contractility and cardiac output without an undue increase in heart rate or conductivity in patients with congestive heart failure.

Isoproterenol is useful therapeutically for its beta actions on the heart in shock or heart block. It is routinely used as a bronchodilator for patients with asthma.

dobutamine hydrochloride (Dobutrex). A synthetic direct-acting beta-active agent, dobutamine is administered only intravenously, with actions somewhat similar to those of isoproterenol and low doses of dopamine. This drug is used to increase cardiac output for patients with acute congestive heart failure and those undergoing cardiopulmonary bypass surgery.

USUAL ADULT DOSAGE: I.V. infusion only; 2.5 to 10 mcg/kg/minute. The drug is reconstituted in 10 to 20 ml of sterile water or D_5W and then further diluted in D_5W, 0.9% normal saline, or ⅙M sodium lactate solution. Infusion rates up to 40 mcg/kg/minute may be required.

dopamine hydrochloride (Intropin, Dopastat). A naturally occurring neurotransmitter, dopamine is a precursor of epinephrine and norepinephrine. Its actions are dose-dependent, with dopaminergic activity only at approximately 2 to 5 mcg/kg/minute, mixed dopaminergic and beta activity at 5 to 10 mcg/kg/minute, and predominantly alpha activity at greater than 10 mcg/kg/minute. It acts both directly and indirectly (releases norepinephrine stores) on alpha and $beta_1$ receptors. It is used to treat shock with related renal shutdown and chronic refractory congestive heart failure. Discontinue the drug gradually.

USUAL ADULT DOSAGE: I.V. infusion only, usually by an electronic infusion pump; initially, 1 to 5 mcg/kg/minute diluted in appropriate sterile solution as recommended by manufacturer. For severely ill patients, increase by 5 to 10 mcg/kg/minute increments to a total of 20 to 50 mcg/kg/minute.

epinephrine hydrochloride/epinephrine bitartrate (Parenteral: Adrenalin, Sus-Phrine), (Inhalation: AsthmaHaler, Medihaler-Epi), **epinephrine** (Inhalation: Bronkaid Mist, Primatene Mist). Epinephrine is the prototype sympathomimetic agent. Available in many forms, it is widely used for bronchodilation, pulmonary decongestion, potentiation and prolongation of anesthetic action, and topical hemostasis. It is also used to treat acute asthmatic attacks; anaphylactic, allergic, and hypersensitivity reactions; acute hypotension; and cardiac

arrest. (See Chapter 79, Ophthalmic Agents, for use in glaucoma and ocular congestion.)

USUAL ADULT DOSAGE: for cardiac arrest, 1 to 10 ml I.V. of a 1:10,000 concentration repeated at 5-minute intervals as required. If no I.V. site is available, 10 ml of 1:10,000 solution via endotracheal tube, or 1 to 10 ml of 1:10,000 solution intracardiac (no longer recommended by American Heart Association's recent ACLS guidelines). Dosage for bronchospasm, hypersensitivity reactions, and anaphylaxis is 0.1 to 0.5 ml of 1:1,000 solution intramuscularly or subcutaneously. For acute asthmatic attacks, the dosage is one inhalation of a 1:100 solution, repeated once if needed after at least 1 minute. As adjunct to local anesthesia, a concentration of 1:200,000 to 1:20,000 is used. For nasal congestion, 0.1% solution applied topically; as a hemostatic, topically applied 1:50,000 or 1:1,000 solution; for spinal anesthesia, 0.2 to 0.4 ml 1:1,000 added to anesthetic solution and administered intraspinally.

USUAL PEDIATRIC DOSAGE: for bronchospasm, 0.005 to 0.01 mg/kg of a 1:200 suspension administered subcutaneously, used only in emergency situations.

isoproterenol hydrochloride (Oral: Isuprel. Inhalation: Vaso-Iso), **isoproterenol sulfate** (Inhalation: Medihaler-Iso). A powerful, direct-acting beta-receptor stimulator, isoproterenol may have longer action and be less toxic than epinephrine. Uses include treatment of asthma; bronchospasm associated with respiratory disorders and general anesthesia; adjunct management of shock, cardiac arrest, Stokes-Adams syndrome, atrioventricular block, and carotid sinus hypersensitivity.

USUAL ADULT DOSAGE: for bronchospasm during anesthesia, 0.01 to 0.02 mg of a 1:50,000 solution in saline or 5% dextrose I.V. For shock, 0.25 to 2.5 ml/minute (0.5 to 5 mcg/minute) of a 1:500,000 solution in 5% dextrose is given intravenously. In cardiac arrest, I.V. injection of 1 to 3 ml (0.02 to 0.06 mg) of a 1:50,000 dilution, or I.V. infusion of 1.25 ml/minute (5 mcg/minute) of a 1:250,000 solution, or 1 ml (0.2 mg) undiluted I.M. or S.C. For intracardiac administration; 0.1 ml (0.02 mg) of 1:5,000 solution is administered. For heart block, initially 10 mg sublingually, with range of 5 to 50 mg, or initially 5 mg rectal administration may be given, with 5 to 15 mg maintenance. For bronchospasm, sublingual or rectal administration the dosage is 10 to 20 mg t.i.d. or q.i.d., to a maximum of 60 mg/daily, or inhalation of solution, 120 to 262 mcg (one to two inhalations) 4 to 6 times a day or aerosol, 80 to 160 mcg (one to two inhalations) 4 to 6 times a day.

DRUG INTERACTIONS

Catecholamines

Drug interactions involving catecholamines can be among the most serious. Catecholamines can produce similar and significant reactions throughout the body, including hypotension, hypertension, cardiac dysrhythmias, seizures, and hyperglycemia in diabetics. If catecholamines must be administered with other drugs, the patient must be monitored frequently. Note that all interactions may not occur between all catecholamines and drugs listed.

DRUG	INTERACTING DRUGS	POSSIBLE EFFECTS	NURSING IMPLICATIONS
dobutamine, dopamine, epinephrine, isoproterenol, norepinephrine	alpha-blockers (phentolamine, phenothiazines)	Antagonize catecholamines with alpha activity, cause hypotension	• Administer with caution. • Monitor the patient's blood pressure.
	antianginals (nitrates)	Block pressor effects	• Avoid concurrent administration. • Monitor the patient's blood pressure.
	antiarrhythmics	Increase cardiac output, lower pulmonary wedge pressure	• Monitor the patient's pulse rate and blood pressure.
	antidiabetic agents	Inhibit insulin, inducing hyperglycemia	• Administer with caution. • Monitor the patient's blood glucose level.
	beta-blockers (propranolol)	Mutually antagonize effects; may allow the domination of alpha effects of the adrenergic, causing hypertension; inhibit adrenergic stimulation of heart, bronchial tree (bronchial constriction, asthma)	• Avoid concurrent administration. • Monitor the patient's blood pressure.
	cardiac glycosides (digitalis)	Cause cardiac dysrhythmias	• Administer with caution. • Monitor the patient's pulse rate.
	diuretics (thiazide, other)	Decrease arterial response, produce mutually additive effects, caused cardiac dysrhythmias, produce hypokalemia	• Administer with caution or avoid administration. • Monitor the patient's pulse rate. • Monitor the patient's intake and output. • Monitor the patient's serum potassium level.
	sympathomimetics	Produce additive effects (hypertension, cardiac dysrhythmias), enhances adverse effect	• Alternate drugs as prescribed, or monitor closely. • Inform the patient about over-the-counter medications. • Monitor the patient's pulse rate and blood pressure.
	urine acidifiers (ascorbic acid, ammonium chloride)	Increase urine acidity, enhancing excretion of ephedrine	• Increase dose of ephedrine as prescribed. • Monitor the patient for subtherapeutic effects.

norepinephrine or levarterenol (Levophed, Noradrenaline). Norepinephrine is a direct-acting sympathomimetic amine with predominantly alpha-adrenergic activity and minor beta₁ activity in the heart. It is used for acute hypotension and shock, adjunctive treatment of cardiac arrest, myocardial infarction, and anaphylaxis.

USUAL ADULT DOSAGE: I.V. infusion only; initially 2 to 3 ml/minute (8 to 12 mcg/minute) of a 4-mg norepinephrine:1,000 ml 5% dextrose solution (4 mcg/ml dilution). Maintenance dose is 0.5 to 1 ml/minute (2 to 4 mcg/minute).

Drug interactions

Knowledge of the interactions between catecholamines and other agents is essential because of the potential for additive effects, which might lead to a hypertensive crisis or cardiac dysrhythmias. (See *Drug interactions: Catecholamines* for interacting drugs, possible effects, and nursing implications.)

Drugs that must not be used with catecholamines, or that should be used concurrently only with extreme caution, include MAO inhibitors, tricyclic antidepressants, oxytocics, furazolidone, ergot alkaloids, antihistamines, some general anesthetics (especially halothane and cyclopropane), digitalis, or other sympathomimetic agents. Beta-blockers such as propranolol reduce the effects of the catecholamines and increase total peripheral resistance by allowing uncompensated alpha stimulation with beta blockade, which may result in hypertension and reflex bradycardia. The combined use of nitroprusside (a peripheral vasodilator) and dopamine or dobutamine may increase cardiac output and lower the left ventricular filling pressure.

ADVERSE DRUG REACTIONS

Because of the widespread actions of the catecholamines, adverse reactions affect the CNS, cardiovascular system, GI tract, skeletal and smooth muscles, and all other body systems. Although the reactions vary from drug to drug, the nurse must be aware of their possibility and must carefully monitor and assess patients on catecholamine therapy.

Predictable reactions

Many CNS manifestations may be noted, including restlessness, nervousness, anxiety, fear, dizziness, vertigo, headache (throbbing to severe), and insomnia. Adverse cardiovascular reactions include pallor or flushing, palpitations, cardiac dysrhythmias, tachycardia or slow and forceful heartbeat, hypotension or hypertension, cerebrovascular accident, and angina. Skeletal muscle adverse reactions may include weakness or mild tremors. The most common GI adverse reactions noted include nausea, vomiting (which may be severe), and diarrhea.

Unpredictable reactions

With extravasation of I.V. catecholamines, necrosis can occur from local vasoconstriction. Tissue sloughing may follow.

NURSING IMPLICATIONS

Because of their varied actions and uses, catecholamine adrenergic agents have many nursing implications. (See

also *Proper preparation and administration of catecholamines* on page 296 for important points to remember when administering these drugs.)

- Administer catecholamines cautiously to elderly patients (because of possible reduced cardiac reserve and the likelihood of dysrhythmias, confusion, or cerebrovascular accident); to pregnant patients (because of possible adverse effects on the fetus); and to patients with hypertension (may cause further increase in blood pressure, cardiac output, or vasoconstriction). Also administer cautiously to patients with any of the following conditions: hyperthyroidism (may cause increase in hypermetabolic state); diabetes mellitus (may have an anti-insulin effect with unpredictable effects on diabetes control); parkinsonism (may cause exacerbation of autonomic effects of parkinsonism); circulatory or cardiovascular disease (may cause vasoconstriction, dysrhythmias, tachycardia or bradycardia, hypertension or hypotension); psychoneuroses (may cause agitation, CNS effects may exacerbate the psychoneuroses being treated); prostate hypertrophy (may cause urinary retention secondary to increased sphincter tone); or glaucoma (may cause increased intraocular pressure).
- Monitor elderly patients on intranasal catecholamines to detect systemic absorption and avoid possible adverse reactions.
- Be alert for signs of overdose, such as headache, vomiting, hypotension, hypertension, blurred vision, cardiac dysrhythmias, or chest pains. Consult the physician for dosage adjustments.
- With prolonged use be alert for the possibility of edema, oliguria, anuria, or hemorrhage.
- Instruct the patient to report if the drug seems to lose its effectiveness over time, because tolerance to the drug can occur.
- Teach the patient to rinse the mouth with water after administration to prevent dry mouth.

NONCATECHOLAMINES

Noncatecholamine adrenergic drugs have a wide variety of therapeutic uses. This wide use is related to the many physiologic effects of these drugs, including local or sys-

Proper preparation and administration of catecholamines

Besides observing other important implications, the nurse should remember these points before administering any catecholamines.

Preparation

- Do not expose solutions to heat, light, or air; they may deteriorate rapidly.
- Do not use any solution that is yellow or amber-colored, or that contains a precipitate.
- In patients dependent on catecholamines for blood pressure support, keep an additional bag of the solution available.

- Use a syringe with calibrations small enough to ensure accurate dosage measurement.
- Always have antidotal drug (phentolamine) on hand when administering I.V. drugs.

Administration

- Always aspirate with the syringe before S.C. or I.M. injection to avoid systemic effects.
- For I.V. infusion, use a large vein (preferably a central line) when possible and rotate peripheral I.V. insertion sites to minimize the risk of necrosis from infiltration.
- Never administer catecholamines for hypotension through the proximal port of a pulmonary artery catheter being used for cardiac output measurement; the patient might inadvertently receive a bolus of the drug.
- Use some type of infusion control device to ensure accurate drug delivery and prevent overdose.
- With I.V. administration, gradually titrate up dose and monitor blood pressure and pulse rate every 3 to 5 minutes until they stabilize, then every 15 minutes.
- With all catecholamines, gradually decrease infusion rate when weaning off dose. Continue monitoring vital signs every 15 minutes to ensure circulatory stability.
- With I.V. administration, observe closely for cyanosis or pallor (signs of shock or excessive peripheral vasoconstriction).
- During drug infusion, continually monitor electrocardiogram, blood pressure, cardiac rate, cardiac rhythm, and, when possible, cardiac output and pulmonary wedge pressure.
- Monitor for bradycardia; the rate of the infusion of alpha stimulants should be decreased as prescribed to return the heart rate to normal; atropine, isoproter-

enol, dopamine, or dobutamine may be ordered if necessary.
- With I.V. drugs, decrease or discontinue the drug as prescribed if the heart rate exceeds 120 to 140 beats per minute.
- Note that duration of I.V. drug action is brief, and the effects terminate shortly after discontinuation of I.V. infusion.
- Massage S.C. and I.M. injection sites to hasten absorption.
- Always dilute dopamine, dobutamine, isoproterenol, and norepinephrine as prescribed before I.V. administration.
- Do not give I.V. infusion of vasoconstrictors into leg veins, especially in elderly patients, because of the possibility of occlusive vascular diseases.
- With inhalant drugs, allow 1 to 2 minutes between inhalations to prevent systemic effects.
- Monitor urine output regularly to assess for renal perfusion and urinary retention.
- To prevent systemic effects with inhalation drugs, use the minimum number of inhalations to relieve the symptoms.
- If I.V. norepinephrine extravasates, stop the infusion immediately and infiltrate with 10 to 15 ml of saline solution containing 5 to 10 mg phentolamine as prescribed.
- Do not infuse concurrently in I.V. lines being used to administer blood products or heparin because of incompatibility.

temic vasoconstriction (mephentermine, metaraminol, methoxamine, phenylephrine), nasal and ophthalmic decongestion; bronchodilation (albuterol, ephedrine, isoetharine, metaproterenol, terbutaline), smooth muscle relaxation (nylidrin, terbutaline, ritodrine), and CNS stimulation and appetite suppression. (See Chapter 29, Cerebral Stimulating Agents.)

In this chapter, drugs will be discussed in relation to their direct- or dual-acting mechanism of action and their adrenergic receptor activity (alpha, beta$_1$, or beta$_2$).

Before receiving noncatecholamine adrenergic drugs, patients must be carefully assessed for a history of conditions or medications that might contraindicate such therapy. The physical examination and interview are essential to assess the efficacy of the drug therapy and to detect signs or symptoms of adverse reactions.

History and source

Ephedrine, obtained from *Ephedra vulgaris*, was introduced into North America in 1924. However, this drug had been used for thousands of years by primitive peoples and is known to have been in use in China for 2,000 years before its U.S. introduction. Since the discovery by Ahlquist in 1948 of two receptor types, alpha and beta, much work has been done to identify those drugs that activate one or another of the receptor types. Subsequent identification of beta$_1$ and beta$_2$ subtypes and more recent proof in the 1970s of specific alpha$_1$ and alpha$_2$ receptors have encouraged research into receptor specificity. The development of beta$_2$-specific drugs that achieve beta$_2$ effects (primarily bronchodilation, vasodilation of skeletal blood vessels, and relaxation of uterine muscle in pregnant patients) without the cardiac stimulant side effects of beta$_1$ stimulation is particularly important. Drugs with greater selectivity for beta$_2$ receptors (such as albuterol, isoetharine, metaproterenol, terbutaline, nylidrin, and ritodrine) produce fewer undesirable effects than the older, nonspecific drugs.

PHARMACOKINETICS

Unlike catecholamines, most noncatecholamine adrenergic drugs are effective orally (isoetharine, however, is degraded if swallowed). These drugs generally have a longer duration of action than catecholamines and may act directly or indirectly on the adrenergic receptors or may exert a combination of the two actions. (*See Noncatecholamines: Summary of receptor activity.*)

Absorption, distribution, metabolism, excretion

The absorption of noncatecholamine adrenergic drugs depend on the route of administration. Drugs administered by inhalation, such as albuterol, are gradually absorbed from the bronchi, causing lower systemic drug levels after the patient inhales recommended doses. Oral drugs are well absorbed from the GI tract and are widely distributed in the body fluids and tissues. Some drugs cross the blood-brain barrier (for example, ephedrine) and may be found in high concentrations in the brain and cerebrospinal fluid. Albuterol is one drug that does not cross the blood-brain barrier. Albuterol, terbutaline, ritodrine, and possibly ephedrine cross the placenta, and ephedrine and terbutaline are excreted in breast milk.

Metabolism and inactivation of the noncatecholamines occur primarily in the liver, where large concentrations of MAO are found, but also occur in the lungs, GI tract, and other tissues.

These drugs and their metabolites are excreted primarily in the urine, some, such as inhaled albuterol, within 24 hours, and others, such as oral albuterol, taking

---

Noncatecholamines: Summary of receptor activity

This table summarizes the pharmacologic activity of the noncatecholamines.

DRUG	RECEPTORS ACTIVATED
Direct-acting	
albuterol	Beta$_2$ effects greater than beta$_1$
isoetharine	Beta$_2$ effects greater than beta$_1$
metaproterenol	Beta$_2$ effects greater than beta$_1$
methoxamine	Alpha
nylidrin	Beta$_1$, beta$_2$
phenylephrine	Alpha, beta$_1$ (weak)
ritodrine	Beta$_2$ effects greater than beta$_1$
terbutaline	Beta$_2$ effects greater than beta$_1$
Dual-acting	
ephedrine	Alpha, beta
mephentermine	Beta > alpha
metaraminol	Alpha > beta

---

up to 3 days. Of clinical importance, acidic urine increases excretion of many noncatecholamine drugs; alkaline urine slows excretion of these drugs.

Onset, peak, duration

Variations in the onset of action, peak concentration level, and duration of action of noncatecholamine drugs are primarily functions of the route of administration. (*See Noncatecholamines: Summary of pharmacokinetics* on page 299 for comparative information on the drugs, their routes of administration, onset, peak, duration, and half-life.) The onset of action is generally rapid after most routes of administration, occurring between 1 and 30 minutes after inhalation, between 10 and 120 minutes after oral ingestion, between 1 and 60 minutes after I.V. infusion, and between 5 and 60 minutes after I.M., S.C., or topical application.

The peak action is usually between 5 and 15 minutes for inhalation, between 1 and 8 hours for oral administration, and between 30 and 60 minutes after parenteral administration.

The duration of action ranges from 15 minutes after I.M. administration of metaraminol to 6 hours after inhalation or oral administration of albuterol. The specific half-life of many of these drugs is unknown, but ranges between 3 and 5 hours. Nasal decongestants usually have a fairly long duration of action and therefore should be used only two to three times a day.

PHARMACODYNAMICS

Noncatecholamine adrenergic drugs may be direct-acting, indirect-acting, or dual-acting (unlike catecholamines, which are primarily direct-acting). Direct-acting noncatecholamine drugs achieve their effects by occupying receptor sites on organs and structures innervated by the SNS. Drugs that exhibit primarily alpha activity include methoxamine and phenylephrine; those that selectively exert beta$_2$ activity include albuterol, isoetharine, metaproterenol, nylidrin, ritodrine, and terbutaline.

Indirect-acting noncatecholamines exert their effects by stimulating norepinephrine release from its storage sites. Dual-acting noncatecholamine adrenergic drugs combine both actions; they include ephedrine, mephentermine, and metaraminol. Nylidrin also acts directly on smooth muscle to cause relaxation.

Mechanism of action

All of the noncatecholamine adrenergic drugs, such as albuterol, isoetharine, and metaproterenol, share a similar chemical structure with the catecholamines. In contrast to the catecholamines, most noncatecholamines are effective when given orally and may act longer. This is partly because of their resistance to the inactivating enzymes of the liver and other tissues and partly because of relatively large doses. They are, however, largely inactivated by MAO, as are catecholamines, and are therefore potentiated by MAO inhibitors. Methoxamine and metaraminol, used primarily as vasopressors, act both directly and indirectly to produce generalized vasoconstriction.

Bronchodilating drugs may be direct- or dual-acting and may nonselectively activate alpha and beta receptors or selectively activate primarily beta$_2$ receptors. Nonspecific receptor effects include tachycardia, increased blood pressure, and increased cardiac output; beta$_2$-selective receptor effects include relaxation of bronchial, uterine, and vascular smooth muscle.

Drugs used to relax smooth muscles (nylidrin, ritodrine, terbutaline, and albuterol) exert a direct, predominantly beta-specific activity. Nylidrin also exerts a direct effect on vascular smooth muscle, not affected by beta blockade.

PHARMACOTHERAPEUTICS

Because noncatecholamines stimulate the sympathetic nervous system and produce varied physiologic effects, they are used widely. The bronchodilatory effects of drugs such as albuterol, ephedrine, metaproterenol, and terbutaline are used to treat acute and chronic bronchial asthma, emphysema, pulmonary fibrosis, and chronic bronchitis.

Ephedrine, methoxamine, phenylephrine, mephentermine, and metaraminol may be used for their pressor effects with spinal anesthesia and, after sympathectomy, for hypotension, nosebleeds, and for vasoconstriction during regional anesthesia.

Metaraminol may be used (rarely) to treat hypotension in patients with septicemia, or after barbiturate overdose, myocardial infarction, or trauma.

Ephedrine is primarily used to treat nasal congestion, ophthalmic conditions, allergic disorders, bronchospasm associated with asthma, or as a CNS stimulant in narcolepsy. Rarely, it may also be administered for myasthenia gravis, enuresis, as a respiratory stimulant after CNS depressant overdose, and for its cardiac stimulant effects in patients with cardiogenic shock, heart block, Stokes-Adams syndrome, bradycardia, or cardiac arrest.

Various noncatecholamines may be used for migraine headache, certain dermatoses, low cardiac output, allergic reactions, anaphylactic reactions, paroxysmal supraventricular tachycardia (phenylephrine or methoxamine), and wide-angle glaucoma. They may also be given to produce mydriasis (pupil dilatation) with ocular examination or uveitis (phenylephrine), to reduce spasms associated with ureteral and biliary colic, for dysmenorrhea, or to delay delivery in preterm labor (terbutaline or ritodrine). Nylidrin is administered for decreased blood flow, including chronic occlusive vascular disorders such as arteriosclerosis or thromboangiitis obliterans.

Many differences exist among the drugs, making general statements difficult. The various drugs are more or less effective depending on the route of administration, the dose, and the desired therapeutic effect and patient tolerance. For example, when bronchodilation is desired, metaproterenol might be chosen over the catecholamine isoproterenol. Although the two drugs are similar chemically and pharmacologically, patients are less likely to develop a tolerance to metaproterenol. Metaproterenol is a more effective bronchodilator orally than ephedrine and is longer-acting than isoproterenol. Albuterol is only one-half to one-quarter as active as isoproterenol in producing increased heart rate in some patients and might be chosen as a bronchodilator for a patient who also has cardiac disease or hypertension.

Noncatecholamines: Summary of pharmacokinetics

The nurse administering noncatecholamines must be aware of their pharmacokinetic properties to assess the patient's therapeutic response.

DRUG	ROUTE	ONSET	PEAK	DURATION	HALF-LIFE
albuterol	Inhalation	5 to 15 min	0.5 to 2 hr	3 to 4 hr	4 to 6 hr
	Oral	30 min	2 to 3 min	4 to 6 hr	4 to 6 hr
ephedrine	Oral, nasal	15 to 60 min	*	2 to 4 hr	*
	I.V., I.M., S.C.	Rapid	Rapid	1 hr	*
isoetharine	Inhalation	1 min	5 to 15 min	1 to 4 hr	*
mephentermine	I.M.	5 to 15 min	*	1 to 4 hr	*
	I.V.	Immediate	*	30 to 45 min	*
	S.C.	5 to 15 min	*	30 to 60 min	*
metaproterenol	Oral	15 min	1 hr	3 to 4 hr	*
	Inhalation	1 to 5 min	30 min to 1 hr	1 to 5 hr	*
metaraminol	I.M.	10 min	*	20 to 60 min	*
	I.V.	1 to 2 min	*	20 to 60 min	*
	S.C.	5 to 20 min	*	20 to 60 min	*
methoxamine	I.M.	15 to 20 min	*	60 to 90 min	*
	I.V.	Immediate	0.5 to 2 min	10 to 15 min	*
nylidrin	Oral	10 min	30 to 90 min	2 hr	*
phenylephrine	I.V.	Immediate	Rapid	15 to 20 min	*
	S.C., I.M.	1 to 15 min	*	30 to 50 min	*
	Intranasal	10 to 15 min	*	3 to 4 hr	*
ritodrine	Oral	10 to 120 min	2 to 3 hr	4 to 6 hr	10 hr
	I.V.	Immediate	Rapid	1½ to 2 hr	10 hr
terbutaline	Oral	30 min	1 to 2 hr	4 to 8 hr	13 to 18 hr
	Inhalation	5 to 30 min	30 to 60 min	3 to 6 hr	13 to 18 hr
	S.C.	6 to 15 min	30 to 60 min	*	13 to 18 hr

*Information unknown or unavailable

Ephedrine is pharmacologically similar to epinephrine, but is longer-acting, less potent, and has a slower onset of action. Metaraminol is similar in overall effects to norepinephrine but is less potent and has a slower onset and a longer duration of action. Methoxamine and phenylephrine have similar pharmacologic effects.

albuterol (Proventil, Ventolin). A direct-acting drug that is comparatively long-acting and relatively selective for beta$_2$ receptors, particularly in bronchial, uterine, and vascular smooth muscle, and mast cells, albuterol is used primarily for bronchospasm associated with reversible obstructive airway disease. It may also be used to treat several conditions, including prevention of exercise-induced bronchospasm, preterm labor, and hyperkalemic familial periodic paralysis.

USUAL ADULT DOSAGE: as an inhalation (metered spray), one to two inhalations of 90 to 180 mcg every 4 to 6 hours; the initial oral dose is 2 to 4 mg t.i.d. or q.i.d.; maximum daily dose is 32 mg.

USUAL PEDIATRIC DOSAGE: for ages 6 to 12 years, 2 mg P.O. q.i.d.

ephedrine sulfate (Efedron, Vatronol). Ephedrine is a dual-acting drug that activates alpha and beta receptors. Although pharmacologically similar to epinephrine, it is longer-acting, less potent, and has a slower onset of action. It is used for its nasal decongestant effects with hay fever, allergic rhinitis, and sinusitis; for its bronchodilator effects with acute and chronic asthma; and occasionally for its CNS stimulant actions for narcolepsy. It is also rarely used for hypotension, enuresis, myasthenia gravis, dysmenorrhea, Stokes-Adams syndrome, and to produce mydriasis.

USUAL ADULT DOSAGE: 25 to 50 mg P.O., S.C., I.M., or slow I.V., as necessary, to maximum total daily dose of 150 mg; as an intranasal drug, two to three drops of a 0.5% solution or a small amount of 0.6% jelly in each nostril four or fewer times a day for 3 to 4 consecutive days; do not repeat before 2 hours.

USUAL PEDIATRIC DOSAGE: for ages 6 to 12, 6.25 to 12.5 mg every 4 to 6 hours; for ages 2 to 6, 0.3 to 0.5 mg/kg every 4 to 6 hours.

isoetharine hydrochloride (Arm-A-Med, Beta-2, Bronkosol, Dey-Lute, Dispos-a-Med), **isoetharine mesylate** (Bronkometer). Isoetharine is a direct-acting, $beta_2$-selective agent with a particular affinity for bronchial and selected arteriolar muscle receptors that produces few cardiac symptoms. It is used for its bronchodilatory effects with bronchial asthma, bronchitis, and emphysema.

USUAL ADULT DOSAGE: three to seven undiluted inhalations by hand-held nebulizer; one to two inhalations by aerosol nebulizer every 4 to 6 hours to a total of 12 per day; wait after the initial inhalation to see if a second is necessary. With intermittent positive-pressure breathing (IPPB), 0.25 to 1 ml, diluted with saline solution (1:3) or other diluent; or use 2 to 8 ml of a unit-dose vial.

mephentermine sulfate (Wyamine). Mephentermine is a dual-acting agent with predominately $beta_1$, but also alpha receptor activity. CNS effects are prominent only with large doses. It is used for its pressor effects to treat hypotension related to ganglionic blockade, spinal anesthesia, hemorrhage, and cardiogenic shock.

USUAL ADULT DOSAGE: 15 to 45 mg single dose as I.M. or I.V. injection, 30 mg supplements as needed; 1 mg/minute of 0.1% solution in 5% dextrose by I.V. infusion.

metaproterenol sulfate (Alupent, Metaprel). A direct-acting $beta_2$-selective agent, metaproterenol is used for its bronchodilatory effects to treat asthma, bronchitis, and emphysema. This drug is also under investigation for treatment and prophylaxis of heart block and for management of premature labor.

USUAL ADULT DOSAGE: 20 mg P.O. t.i.d. or q.i.d.; 10 inhalations of 5% solution by hand-held nebulizer; two to three (0.65-mg) sprays by aerosol nebulizer every 3 to 4 hours to a maximum of 12 per day; or two inhalations from a metered-dose inhaler t.i.d.

USUAL PEDIATRIC DOSAGE: for ages 6 to 9, or less than 60 pounds (27 kg), 10 mg t.i.d. or q.i.d. Not recommended for children under age 6.

metaraminol bitartrate (Aramine). A potent dual-acting synthetic agent that acts predominantly on alpha receptors, but also acts on $beta_1$ receptors, metaraminol is used for its vasopressor effects to treat shock caused by hemorrhage, medication reactions, surgical complications, cardiogenic shock, and septicemia.

USUAL ADULT DOSAGE: 2 to 10 mg S.C. or I.M., with at least 10 minutes before an additional dose is given, to prevent cumulative effects; for severe shock, I.V. injection of 0.5 to 5 mg, followed by I.V. infusion of 15 to 100 mg/500 ml of D_5W or normal saline solution (adjust rate of infusion to maintain blood pressure at desired level).

USUAL PEDIATRIC DOSAGE: 0.1 mg/kg S.C. or I.M.; I.V. injection of 0.01 mg/kg; 0.4 mg/kg I.V. infusion.

methoxamine hydrochloride (Vasoxyl). A direct-acting agent that acts on alpha receptors, methoxamine is related pharmacologically to phenylephrine. It has no direct effect on the heart, but tends to slow heart rate as a reflex action from increased peripheral vasoconstriction. It is used for its pressor effects during anesthesia and for paroxysmal atrial tachycardia.

USUAL ADULT DOSAGE: for vasopressor effects in emergencies, 3 to 5 mg slow I.V. or 10 to 15 mg I.M.; for tachycardia, 10 mg slow I.V., or 10 to 20 mg I.M., repeated if necessary, only after 15 minutes.

nylidrin hydrochloride (Arlidin). A direct-acting agent that acts predominantly on beta receptors, nylidrin also acts directly on muscle, producing relaxation that is not blocked by beta-blockers. It is used for its direct smooth muscle and arteriolar smooth muscle relaxant effects for symptomatic relief to treat peripheral vascular disorders such as diabetic vascular disease, Raynaud's disease,

DRUG INTERACTIONS

Noncatecholamines

Noncatecholamines can produce significant reactions throughout the body, including hypotension, hypertension, cardiac dysrhythmias, seizures, and hyperglycemia in diabetics. If noncatecholamines must be administered with other drugs, the patient must be monitored frequently. Note that all interactions may not occur between all noncatecholamines and the drugs listed.

DRUG	INTERACTING DRUGS	POSSIBLE EFFECTS	NURSING IMPLICATIONS
albuterol, ephedrine, isoetharine, mephentermine, metaproterenol, metaraminol, methoxamine, nylidrin, phenylephrine, ritodrine, terbutaline	anesthetics (general), cyclopropane, and halogenated hydrocarbons	Sensitize the heart to adrenergic agents, cause cardiac dysrhythmias from increased cardiac irritability, increases hypotension if used with agents having predominant beta$_2$ activity (ritodrine, terbutaline)	• Avoid, or administer with extreme caution for patients scheduled for surgery if general anesthesia is to be used. agent. • Monitor the patient's blood pressure.
	antipsychotics (lithium)	Decrease pressor effects of alpha-adrenergic agents (epinephrine, norepinephrine, phenylephrine, methoxamine)	• Increase dose of alpha stimulant as prescribed. • Monitor the patient's blood pressure.
	beta blockers (ritodrine, terbutaline)	Increase effects of agents with predominantly beta activity, can complement or antagonize agents with predominant alpha activity	• Avoid concurrent administration or administer with caution.
	MAO inhibitors (furazolidone)	Cause severe hypertension from pressor potentiation of pressor effects of both drugs	• Avoid concurrent administration. • Monitor the patient's blood pressure.
	oxytocics	Counteract oxytocic effects (terbutaline and ritodrine), cause hypertension crisis from potentiation of effects of both drugs, produce cerebrovascular accident	• Avoid concurrent use; maintain blood pressure under 130/80.
	tricyclic antidepressants	Increase pressor effects, increase hypertension from potentiation of pressor effects of both drugs, cause cardiac dysrhythmias	• Avoid concurrent administration. • If administered concurrently, reduce adrenergic dosage as prescribed. • Monitor the patient's pulse rate and blood pressure.
	urine alkalinizers (acetazolamide, sodium bicarbonate)	Cause decreased excretion, prolong action	• Reduce dose of adrenergics excreted unchanged in the urine as prescribed. • Monitor the patient for increased adverse effects.

acrocyanosis, frostbite, night leg cramps, thromboangiitis obliterans, ischemic ulcer, thrombophlebitis, Meniere's disease, and circulatory disturbances of the inner ear.
USUAL ADULT DOSAGE: 3 to 12 mg P.O. t.i.d. or q.i.d.

phenylephrine hydrochloride (Neo-Synephrine). A potent, direct-acting agent with strong alpha-receptor and weak beta-receptor actions, phenylephrine produces lit-

tle or no CNS activity. It is used for its systemic and topical vasopressor effects with anesthesia and for treating shock, paroxysmal supraventricular tachycardia, rhinitis, allergies, uveitis, and to produce mydriasis.
USUAL ADULT DOSAGE: for its pressor effects, 2 to 5 mg I.M. or S.C. initial dose, not to exceed 5 mg every 10 to 15 minutes; by I.V. injection, 0.1 to 0.5 mg, subsequent doses no more often than 10 to 15 minutes in

increments no larger than 0.2 mg; I.V. infusion of 100 to 200 drops/minute of a 1:50,000 solution of D_5W or normal saline solution until stable, then 40 to 60 drops/minute. As an intranasal drug, two to three drops, one to two sprays (0.25% to 0.5%), or a small amount of nasal jelly placed into each nostril every 3 to 4 hours. (See Chapter 79, Ophthalmic Agents, for use as an ophthalmic decongestant and mydriatic.)

USUAL PEDIATRIC DOSAGE: 0.1 mg/kg S.C. or I.M.

ritodrine hydrochloride (Yutopar). Ritodrine is a direct-acting agent that preferentially stimulates $beta_2$ receptors in uterine smooth muscle, causing reduced intensity and frequency of contractions. Other effects include bronchial relaxation and some vascular smooth muscle relaxation. This drug is used for preterm labor in selected patients, but its safety and effectiveness during advanced labor have not been established.

USUAL ADULT DOSAGE: initially 0.1 mg/minute by I.V. infusion, increased by 50 mcg/minute every 10 minutes to a maximum of 350 mcg/minute. Continue for 12 hours after labor has ceased. Oral therapy of 10 mg is begun 30 minutes before terminating I.V. infusion, then 10 mg every 2 hours for 24 hours, then 10 to 20 mg every 4 to 6 hours as long as necessary. The total dose should not exceed 120 mg/day.

terbutaline sulfate (Brethaire, Brethine, Bricanyl). A direct-acting synthetic agent with selective $beta_2$ activity, terbutaline is used for its bronchodilation effects to treat bronchial asthma, bronchitis, and emphysema. It may also be used to delay delivery in preterm labor.

USUAL ADULT DOSAGE: 10 mcg/minute by I.V. infusion with maximum dose of 80 mcg/minute for 4 hours, then oral therapy until term. Oral therapy of 2.5 to 5 mg t.i.d.; 0.25 mg S.C., repeat in 15 to 30 minutes if needed; two inhalations separated by 1 minute no more than every 6 hours.

USUAL PEDIATRIC DOSAGE: over age 12, 2.5 mg t.i.d. or q.i.d.

Drug interactions

Drugs known to interact with various noncatecholamines include MAO inhibitors, furazolidone, beta-blockers (for example, propanolol), other sympathomimetics, acetazolamide, sodium bicarbonate, ammonium chloride, ascorbic acid, barbiturates, guanethidine, phenothiazines, anesthetics (especially cyclopropane and halogenated hydrocarbons), corticosteroids, digitalis, methyldopa, rauwolfia alkaloids, oxytocics, tricyclic antidepressants, lithium, ergot alkaloids, and reserpine. All interactions vary from drug to drug, but the nurse must be aware of their potential for causing interactions. Many of these drugs are also contraindicated with catechol-

amines. (See Drug interactions: Noncatecholamines on page 301 for more details.)

ADVERSE DRUG REACTIONS

Adverse reactions to noncatecholamine adrenergic drugs primarily affect the CNS, cardiovascular system, GI and genitourinary tracts, skeletal and smooth muscles, and all other body systems. The adverse effects of any noncatecholamine drug depend on its receptor activity. Other considerations include the intended therapeutic effect of the drug and whether the drug crosses the blood-brain barrier. For example, if ephedrine given for its bronchodilation effects interferes with sleep, the insomnia is considered an adverse reaction; however, if the drug is given to treat narcolepsy, the insomnia is the desired therapeutic effect. Although adverse reactions vary from drug to drug, the nurse must know their potential and must monitor the patient closely.

Predictable reactions

Untoward CNS adverse reactions to the noncatecholamines include headache, restlessness, nervousness, anxiety or euphoria, irritability, trembling, drowsiness or insomnia, lethargy, dizziness, light-headedness, incoherence, and convulsions. Possible adverse cardiovascular reactions include hypertension or hypotension, palpitations, bradycardia or tachycardia, dysrhythmias, cardiac arrest, cerebral hemorrhage, tingling or coldness in the extremities, pallor or flushing, anginal pain, and alterations in maternal and fetal heart rates and blood pressure. Skeletal muscle reactions may include weakness, mild tremors, or muscle cramps. Other possible adverse reactions include sweating, urinary urgency or incontinence, pilomotor stimulation, stinging and burning of the nasal mucosa or eyes, blurred vision, sneezing, dryness of the orpharynx, nausea, vomiting, unusual taste, erythema, and transient elevations in blood glucose level and increased insulin requirements in diabetic patients. These drugs should not be used in diabetic patients because the vasoconstriction induced may aggravate the already compromised microcirculation.

Unpredictable reactions

Prolonged use of certain noncatecholamine drugs, such as metaraminol, may result in shock because continued vasoconstriction prevents volume expansion. Hypotension can occur after discontinuation of these drugs because of depletion of the intrinsic catecholamines in the storage granules of the nerve endings.

Although rare, overdose of nasal decongestants can cause marked somnolence, sedation, hypotension, bradycardia, and even coma. Methoxamine and other drugs

(Text continues on page 307.)

SELECTED MAJOR DRUGS

Adrenergic drugs

This chart summarizes the major adrenergic drugs currently in clinical use.

DRUG	MAJOR INDICATIONS	USUAL ADULT DOSAGES	NURSING IMPLICATIONS
Catecholamines			
dobutamine	Acute congestive heart failure, cardiopulmonary bypass surgery	I.V. infusion: 2.5 to 10 mcg/kg/min of either a 250-mcg/ml, 500-mcg/ml, or 1,000-mcg/ml solution in D_5W or normal saline solution; rates up to 40 mcg/kg/min may be required	• Correct hypovoelmia as prescribed before initiation of therapy. • Avoid extravasation by using a deep vein insertion for I.V. Use phentolamine, as prescribed for extravasation • Use microdrip and I.V. control device for flow rate accuracy. • Monitor blood pressure and pulse rate every 3 to 5 minutes until stable, then every 15 minutes. • Monitor intake and output, expect diuresis and electrolyte loss from improved cardiac output and renal perfusion. • Assess for signs of possible overdose: headache, vomiting, cardiac dysrhythmias, hypotension, hypertension, chest pain, and blurred vision. • Do not administer with alkaline solutions. • Protect drug from heat and light, and discard if discolored.
dopamine	Shock, decreased renal function	I.V. infusion: initially 1 to 5 mcg/kg/min diluted as recommended; may increase by 5- to 10-mcg/kg/min increments to 20 to 50 mcg/kg/min in critically ill patients	• Correct hypovolemia as prescribed before initiation of therapy. • Avoid extravasation by using a deep vein insertion of I.V. Use phentolamine, as prescribed for extravasation. • Use microdrip and I.V. control device for flow rate accuracy. • Monitor BP and pulse rate every 3 to 5 minutes until stable, then every 15 minutes. • Monitor intake and output, expect diuresis and electrolyte loss from improved cardiac output and renal perfusion. • Assess for peripheral ischemia, indicated by decreased peripheral pulses and cold extremities; may use topical nitroglycerin as presdribed to increase blood flow. • Assess for signs of possible overdose: headache, vomiting, cardiac dysrythmias, hypotension, hypertension, chest pain, and blurred vision. • Protect drug from heat and light, and discard if discolored.
epinephrine	Bronchospasm, asthma, nasal and ophthalmic congestion, simple open-angle glaucoma, allergic conditions, hypotension, cardiac arrest, superficial bleeding control	Cardiac arrest: 1 to 10 ml of a 1:10,000 solution I.V., repeated at 5-min intervals; 1 to 10 ml of 1:10,000 intracardiac (not recommended); 10 ml of 1:10,000 solution via endotracheal tube	• Check order, concentration of solution, dosage, and rate closely. • Protect drug from light and heat; discard if discolored. • Massage S.C. or I.M. injection site to hasten absorption. • Monitor BP and pulse rate every 3 to 5 minutes until stable, then every 15 minutes. • After I.V. administration, assess for periph-

continued

SELECTED MAJOR DRUGS

Adrenergic drugs continued

DRUG	MAJOR INDICATIONS	USUAL ADULT DOSAGES	NURSING IMPLICATIONS
epinephrine (continued)		Bronchospasm: 0.1 to 0.5 ml 1:1,000 solution S.C. or I.M., or 0.1 to 0.3 ml 1:200 S.C.; one inhalation, repeat once after at least 1 min, if needed Hemostasis: 1:50,000 to 1:1,000 topically applied Local anesthetic adjunct: 1:100,000 to 1:20,000 mixed with local anesthetic Bronchospasm in children: 0.005 to 0.01 mg/kg of a 1:200 solution S.C.	eral ischemia, indicated by decreased peripheral pulses and cold extremities; may use topical nitroglycerine as prescribed to increase blood flow. ● Avoid extravasation by using a deep vein insertion for I.V. Use phentolamine, as prescribed for extravasation. ● Monitor intake and output, expect diuresis and electrolyte loss from improved cardiac output and renal perfusion. ● Use microdrip and I.V. control device for flow rate accuracy. ● With inhalant, let 1 or 2 minutes elapse before giving additional medication to avoid overdose or adverse reactions. ● Do not administer inhaled isoproterenol concurrently; space 4 hours apart. ● Institute bronchial hygiene, postural drainage, exercises, and hydration to prevent mucous plugs and raise secretions. ● Teach patient to rinse mouth after inhalation to minimize dryness and irritation. ● Inform the patient that intranasal application might temporarily sting or burn slightly. ● Protect drug from heat and light, and discard if discolored. ● Assess diabetic patients for blood glucose levels. ● Assess for signs of possible overdose: headache, vomiting, cardiac dysrhythmias, hypotension, hypertension, chest pain, and blurred vision.
isoproterenol	Asthma, bronchospasm, shock, cardiac arrest or dysrhythmias	Bronchospasm: 10 to 20 mg sublingually or rectally t.i.d. or q.i.d. to a maximum of 60 mg/day; 120 to 262 mcg 4 to 6 times/day by hand-held nebulizer; 80 to 160 mcg 4 to 6 times/day by aerosol nebulizer	● Monitor BP and pulse rate every 3 to 5 minutes until stable, then every 15 minutes. ● Monitor intake and output, expect diuresis and electrolyte loss from improved cardiac output and renal perfusion. ● Avoid extravasation by using a deep vein insertion for I.V. Use phentolamine, as prescribed for extravasation. ● Use microdrip and I.V. control device for flow rate accuracy. ● After I.V. administration, assess for peripheral ischemia, indicated by decreased peripheral pulses and cold extremities; may use topical nitroglycerine as prescribed to increase blood flow. ● Have oxygen and emergency respiratory assistance nearby. ● Protect drug from light and heat, and discard if discolored. ● Expect transient facial flushing, palpitations, and precordial discomfort with sublingual administration. ● Monitor respiratory rate; rebound bronchospasm may occur. ● Teach patient to use lowest number of inhalations possible.

SELECTED MAJOR DRUGS

Adrenergic drugs continued

DRUG	MAJOR INDICATIONS	USUAL ADULT DOSAGES	NURSING IMPLICATIONS
isoproterenol (continued)			• Teach patient to rinse mouth after inhalation to minimize dryness and irritation. • Inform patient that sputum and saliva may become pink after inhalation—a harmless response. • Assess for signs of possible overdose: headache, vomiting, cardiac dysrhythmias, hypotension, hypertension, chest pain, and blurred vision.
norepinephrine	Acute hypotension, shock, cardiac arrest, myocardial infarction, anaphylaxis	I.V. infusion: 2 to 3 ml/min of a 4-mg norepinephrine:1,000 ml 5% dextrose solution initially; maintenance dose is 0.5 to 1 ml/min.	• Do not administer in normal saline solution. Dilute in D_5W to prevent possible oxidation and loss of potency. • Avoid extravasation by using a deep vein insertion for I.V. Use phentolamine, as prescribed for extravasation. • Use microdrip and I.V. control device for flow rate accuracy. • After I.V. administration, assess for peripheral ischemia, indicated by decreased peripheral pulses and cold extremities; may use topical nitroglycerine as prescribed to increase blood flow. • Monitor BP and pulse rate every 3 to 5 minutes until stable, then every 15 minutes. • Monitor intake and output, expect diuresis and electrolyte loss from improved cardiac output and renal perfusion. • Assess for signs of possible overdose: headache, vomiting, cardiac dysrhythmias, hypotension, hypertension, chest pain, and blurred vision. • If long-term therapy is used, change I.V. site frequently to reduce necrosis from vasoconstriction. • Protect drug from heat and light, and discard if discolored.
Noncatecholamines			
albuterol	Bronchospasm	One to two inhalations every 4 to 6 hours 2 to 4 mg P.O. t.i.d. to q.i.d., to a maximum of 32 mg/day	• Teach the patient to avoid contact of drug with the eyes. • Advise the patient of the prescribed dosage interval between inhalations (may vary from 1 to 10 minutes; check with the physician). • Discontinue drug and notify physician if wheezing or bronchospasm occur after therapy. • Evaluate pulmonary function status of the patient before and during therapy to determine progress. • Assess for improvement within 60 to 90 minutes after drug administration; notify physician if no relief occurs. • Teach the patient to rinse mouth to relieve dryness after inhalation therapy.

continued

Adrenergic drugs continued

DRUG	MAJOR INDICATIONS	USUAL ADULT DOSAGES	NURSING IMPLICATIONS
albuterol (continued)			• Teach the patient and family to avoid OTC drugs that contain sympathomimetics. • Protect drugs from light, air, cold, and heat; discard if discolored.
metaproterenol	Bronchodilation	Oral: 20 mg t.i.d. to q.i.d., initially Hand-held nebulizer: 10 inhalations of a 5% solution; aerosol nebulizer: 2 to 3 sprays every 3 to 4 hours to a maximum of 12/day Children: age 6 to 9 or less than 60 lb (27 kg), 10 mg t.i.d. to q.i.d.	• Perform respiratory assessment before and after treatment. • Teach the patient proper inhalation and assessment techniques. If no relief occurs, the patient should notify the physician. • Assess effects of drug after long-term use, because the drug may have a shorter duration. • Teach the patient to avoid contact between inhaled drug and the eyes. • Teach the patient to take drug only as prescribed because of possible adverse effects. • Teach the patient to rinse mouth after inhalation to minimize dryness and irritation. • Protect these drugs from light, air, heat, and cold. Discard if discolored.
ritodrine	Preterm labor	Initially, 0.1 mg/min, by I.V. infusion; increase by 50 mcg/min every 10 minutes to a maximum of 350 mcg/min; continue for 12 hours after labor has ceased 10 mg P.O. begun 30 minutes before terminating I.V. infusion, then 10 mg every 2 hours for 24 hours; then 10 to 20 mg every 4 to 6 hours as long as necessary	• Monitor closely for cardiovascular adverse effects, BP, and maternal and fetal heart rate. • Place the patient in left lateral recumbent position to prevent hypotension during I.V. therapy. • Evaluate for circulatory overload during I.V. therapy. • Monitor for hypokalemia with prolonged infusions.
terbutaline	Bronchodilation, preterm labor	10 mcg/min I.V. infusion with maximum dose of 80 mcg/min for 4 hours, then oral therapy until term 2.5 to 5 mg P.O. t.i.d.; 0.25 mg S.C., repeat in 15 to 30 minutes if needed Inhalation: two inhalations separated by 1 minute no more often than every 6 hours	• Administer oral medication with food to reduce GI symptoms. • Place the obstetric patient in left lateral position to improve fetal blood flow. • Administer S.C. medication in the lateral deltoid area. • Take BP and heart rate before each dose of medication to assess change from baseline value. • With prolonged I.V. infusions, monitor for hypokalemia. • Teach that rapid pulse may persist; other adverse reactions are transient. • Teach the patient pulse-taking technique and individual limits of change in rate. • Evaluate cardiovascular adverse effects, especially with S.C. medication and in patients with cardiac dysrhythmias. • Teach the patient proper inhalation and assessment techniques. If no relief occurs, the patient should notify the physician.

SELECTED MAJOR DRUGS

Adrenergic drugs continued

DRUG	MAJOR INDICATIONS	USUAL ADULT DOSAGES	NURSING IMPLICATIONS
terbutaline (continued)			• Teach the patient on inhalator therapy to use no other aerosol bronchodilator while on terbutaline. • Teach the patient to take drug only as prescribed. • Evaluate efficacy of drug, because tolerance can develop with long use. • Monitor the patient for 12 hours after drug is discontinued, because cardiovascular signs and symptoms may occur. • Observe for tachycardia and report promptly if it occurs. • Evaluate intake and output for pattern, and institute fluid restriction as prescribed. • Teach the patient to avoid OTC medications that contain sympathomimetic agents. • Protect drug from air, light, heat, or cold. Discard if discolored.

can cause severe headache and sustained, severe hypertension. In rare instances, ephedrine and other agents may cause respiratory depression.

Confusion, delirium, or even hallucinations, as well as tremors, may follow large doses of ephedrine. This drug may also produce paradoxical bronchospasm or aggravation of ketoacidosis. Enlargement of the parotid gland is a possible, although rare, result of metaproterenol administration. Care must be exercised with I.V. ritodrine and terbutaline because lactic acidosis, chest pain, dysrhythmias, dyspnea, bloating, chills, or anaphylactic shock may occur.

NURSING IMPLICATIONS

Many of the nursing implications for catecholamines are appropriate for the noncatecholamines.
• Administer noncatecholamines with caution to diabetic patients because of the possibility of hyperglycemia.
• Protect these drugs from light, excessive heat or cold, and moisture. Do not use discolored drugs.
• Do not administer mephentermine with epinephrine HCl or hydralazine HCl, because they are incompatible.
• With prolonged patient therapy, carefully monitor intake and output, blood pH, PCO_2, and bicarbonate levels.
• Infuse I.V. medications into a large vein to avoid extravasation.
• If extravasation occurs with I.V. medication, inject the area within 12 hours with 10 to 15 ml normal saline solution containing phentolamine (Regitine) as prescribed.
• Avoid subcutaneous use of metaraminol because of possible tissue necrosis and sloughing, especially in shock from poor circulation.
• Assess for and, if possible, correct hypoxia, hypercapnia, and acidosis as prescribed before administering norepinephrine or mephentermine.
• Monitor the intake and output ratio and pattern to assess renal response, which may initially decrease, then increase as blood pressure rises, and then decrease again with excessive dosage.
• Monitor electrolytes because diuresis may occur, producing an excessive loss of sodium and potassium.
• For I.V. administration, use an I.V. pump or microdrip apparatus to control flow rate.
• After I.V. administration, monitor electrocardiogram (EKG), blood pressure, and heart rate every 3 to 5 minutes until stable, then every 15 minutes.
• Monitor the serum potassium levels of patients who are on ritodrine or terbutaline to prevent hypokalemia.
• Monitor EKG, blood pressure, heart rate, and urine output during drug administration.
• Perform respiratory assessment before and after treatment to evaluate effectiveness.
• Instruct the patient to initiate inhalation therapy on arising and before meals to improve lung ventilation and to reduce fatigue accompanying eating.
• Teach the patient to avoid contact between inhaled drug and the eyes.
• Teach the patient using nasal medications to blow the

nose gently, with both nostrils open, to clear nasal passages before administration of medication.

• Teach the patient proper inhalation and assessment technique. If no relief occurs, the patient should notify the physician.

• Teach the patient to rinse the mouth after inhalation to minimize dryness and irritation.

• Advise the patient to avoid over-the-counter sympathomimetics and to be alert to their adverse effects.

CHAPTER SUMMARY

Chapter 19 covered the catecholamine and noncatecholamine adrenergic drugs. Drugs in each class were described in relation to their history and source, pharmacokinetics, pharmacodynamics, pharmacotherapeutics, adverse drug reactions, and nursing implications. Here are the highlights of the chapter:

• Adrenergic drugs produce biological responses similar to those produced by the SNS.

• Alpha activation produces primarily vasoconstrictive and smooth muscle contraction effects; beta$_1$ activation produces primarily cardiac stimulant effects; and beta$_2$ activation produces primarily smooth muscle relaxation as well as bronchodilatory and vasodilatory effects.

• The therapeutic use of a drug depends on its receptor activity.

• Catecholamines may be endogenous or synthetic.

• Catecholamines are ineffective when administered orally.

• Catecholamines function as adrenergic transmitters, causing direct action at alpha, beta$_1$, or beta$_2$ adrenergic receptor sites.

• Alpha-active drugs are used primarily to relieve hypotension.

• Beta-active drugs are used primarily for respiratory diseases, hypersensitivity conditions, and cardiac stimulation.

• Noncatecholamine adrenergic drugs may act directly, indirectly, or in both ways to exert effects on sympathetic receptor sites.

• Noncatecholamine drugs are active orally and generally have a longer duration of action than catecholamines.

• Noncatecholamine drugs primarily produce bronchodilation, vasopression, smooth muscle relaxation, and cardiac stimulation.

• Adverse reactions to adrenergic drugs can involve all body systems.

BIBLIOGRAPHY

American Heart Association. "Standards and Guidelines for Cardiopulmonary Resuscitation and Emergency Cardiac Care," *Journal of American Medical Association.* 255:2891, June 6, 1986.

Armstrong, C. "Effects of Maternal Beta Sympathomimetic Therapy on the Neonate," *Neonatal Network.* December 1985.

Brengman, S.L. "Ritodrine Hydrochloride and Preterm Labor," *American Journal of Nursing.* 83:537, April 1983.

Converse, J. "Care of the Patient Receiving Therapy with Betamimetic Agents," *Wisconsin Medical Journal.* 82:32, 1983.

DiJoseph, J.F., et al. "Alpha$_2$ Receptors in the Gastrointestinal System: A New Therapeutic Approach," *Life Sciences.* 35:1031, 1984.

Galant, S.P. "Current Status of Beta-Adrenergic Agonists in Bronchial Asthma," *Pediatric Clinics of North America.* 30:931, 1983.

Giles, T.D., et al. "Central Alpha-Adrenergic Agonists in Chronic Heart Failure and Ischemic Heart Disease," *Journal of Cardiovascular Pharmacology.* 7:S51, 1985.

Gilman, A.G., et al., eds. *Goodman and Gilman's The Pharmacologic Basis of Therapeutics,* 7th edition. New York: Macmillan Publishing Co., 1985.

Heinsimer, J.A., and Lefkowitz, R.J. "Adrenergic Receptors: Biochemistry, Regulation, Molecular Mechanism, and Clinical Implications," *Journal of Laboratory Clinical Medicine.* 100:641, November 1982.

Hussar, D.A. "New Drugs," *Nursing83.* 13:121, May 1983.

Kaplan, N.M. "Alpha$_2$-Adrenergic Agonists in the Treatment of Hypertension," *Journal of Cardiovascular Pharmacology.* 7:S64, 1985.

Kelly, W.H. "Controversies in Asthma Therapy with Theophylline and the Beta$_2$-Adrenergic Agonists," *Clinical Pharmacology.* 3:386, July/August 1984.

Ralston, S.H. "Alpha Agonist Drug Use During CPR," *Annals of Emergency Medicine.* 13:786, September 1984.

Shim, C. "Adrenergic Agonists and Bronchodilator Aerosol Therapy in Asthma," *Clinics in Chest Medicine (Philadelphia).* 5:659, December 1984.

Souney, P.F., et al. "Pharmacotherapy of Preterm Labor," *Clinical Pharmacy.* 2:29, January/February 1983.

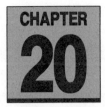

CHAPTER 20

ADRENERGIC BLOCKING AGENTS

OBJECTIVES

After reading and studying this chapter, you should be able to:

1. Distinguish among alpha-adrenergic, beta-adrenergic, and autonomic ganglionic blocking agents.
2. Identify the major drugs in each class of adrenergic blocking agents.
3. Describe the major physiologic effects of each class of drugs and their mechanisms of action.
4. Discuss therapeutic uses and contraindications for each class of adrenergic blocking agents.
5. Explain why arteriosclerosis, bronchospastic disease, congestive heart failure, hypertension, diabetes mellitus, and thyrotoxicosis require cautious administration of beta-adrenergic blocking agents.
6. Identify the major drug interactions, adverse reactions, and nursing implications for each drug class.

INTRODUCTION

Adrenergic blocking agents, or sympatholytics, are used therapeutically to disrupt sympathetic nervous system function. These agents may block impulse transmission (and thus sympathetic nervous system stimulation) at adrenergic neurons, adrenergic receptor sites, or adrenergic ganglia. This action at these sites may be exerted by interrupting the action of sympathomimetic (adrenergic) agents (see Chapter 19, Adrenergic Agents), by reducing available norepinephrine, or by preventing the action of cholinergic agents (see Chapter 17, Cholinergic Agents). Adrenergic blocking agents are classified according to their site of action as, respectively, alpha-blockers, beta-blockers, or autonomic ganglionic blockers.

For a summary of representative drugs, see *Selected major drugs: Adrenergic blocking agents* on pages 325 to 328.

ALPHA-ADRENERGIC BLOCKERS

Alpha-adrenergic blocking agents interrupt the actions of sympathomimetic agents at alpha-adrenergic receptor sites, relaxing vascular smooth muscle, increasing peripheral vasodilation, and decreasing blood pressure. Drugs in this class include ergoloid mesylates, ergotamine tartrate, phenoxybenzamine hydrochloride, phentolamine mesylate, tolazoline hydrochloride, and prazosin hydrochloride. (See Chapter 39, Peripheral Vascular Agents, for a brief discussion of tolazoline and Chapter 37, Antihypertensive Agents, for information on prazosin.)

History and source

Alpha-adrenergic blocking agents, both natural and synthetic, have been in clinical use for many years. Ergot, a fungus that grows on rye and other grains, has been known since early recorded times. Ergot alkaloids were the first known adrenergic blocking agents.

PHARMACOKINETICS

Much is unknown about the action of alpha-adrenergic blocking agents in the body. Generally, these agents are erratically absorbed when administered orally and are more rapidly and completely absorbed when administered sublingually or by inhalation. This unreliable absorption is one reason for the limited clinical use of these drugs.

Absorption, distribution, metabolism, excretion

Ergoloid mesylates are largely inactivated by the first-pass effect; only about one third of the drug reaches the systemic circulation. Ergotamine is distributed through-

How alpha-adrenergic blockers affect peripheral blood vessels

By occupying alpha-receptor sites, the alpha-adrenergic blockers cause vessel muscle-wall relaxation, vasodilatation, and reduced peripheral vascular resistance. These effects can cause orthostatic hypotension when the patient changes position from supine to standing because of altered blood flow redistribution.

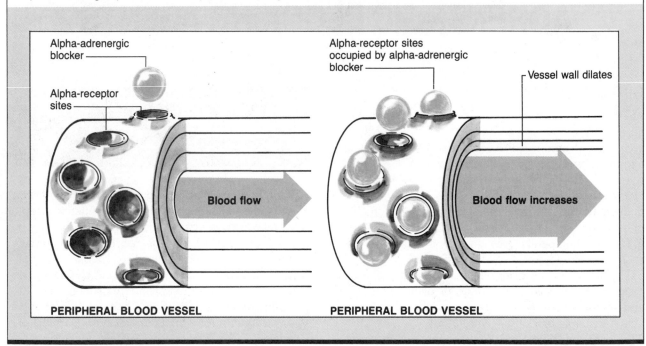

out the body and sequestered in tissues (explaining its long duration of action), then excreted in the bile after hepatic metabolism. Absorption of phenoxybenzamine is erratic, with only 20% to 30% of the drug reaching the systemic circulation. Little is known about phenoxybenzamine's distribution, metabolism, and excretion. The pharmacokinetics of phentolamine are unknown.

Onset, peak, duration

The various alpha-adrenergic blocking agents vary considerably in their onset of action, peak concentration levels, and duration of action. The onset of action varies widely: that of ergoloid mesylates is unknown; that of ergotamine is erratic or rapid (when administered by inhalation). Phentolamine has an onset of action within 2 to 20 minutes, whereas phenoxybenzamine takes 2 hours.

Peak concentration levels occur in 1 to 2 hours with ergoloid mesylates, 1 to 3 hours with ergotamine, and 4 to 6 hours with phenoxybenzamine. The time of occurrence of peak concentration levels with phentolamine

is 2 to 20 minutes. The duration of action of phentolamine is short—15 to 45 minutes, depending on route of administration; ergotamine's is 24 hours, and phenoxybenzamine's is 3 to 4 days. Ergoloid mesylate's duration of action is unknown.

PHARMACODYNAMICS

Alpha-adrenergic blockers exert three main pharmacologic actions: they interfere with or block the synthesis, storage, release, and reuptake of norepinephrine by neurons; they block acetylcholine at the preganglionic synapse; and they competitively or noncompetitively antagonize epinephrine, norepinephrine, or sympathomimetic agents at alpha-receptor sites.

Alpha-receptor sites are categorized as either alpha$_1$ or alpha$_2$. Alpha$_1$ receptors are located postsynaptically; alpha$_2$ receptors, primarily presynaptically, where they mediate a feedback system that controls norepinephrine release.

Pharmacologic classification does not recognize the specificity of alpha-receptor activity; the category of alpha-adrenergic blockers includes drugs that block the stimulation of alpha$_1$ receptors and that also may or may not block alpha$_2$ stimulation. Agents that selectively block only alpha$_2$-receptor sites are currently used only in the laboratory. They have no clinically therapeutic uses and are not commercially available at present.

Mechanism of action

The most important therapeutic action of alpha-adrenergic blockers is occupation of alpha-receptor sites on the vascular smooth muscle. (See *How alpha-adrenergic blockers affect peripheral blood vessels* for a detailed description of this process.) This action prevents the excitatory response to sympathetic stimulation or sympathomimetic agents; this response typically causes vasoconstriction in these vessels. The resultant relaxation of vascular walls and dilation of vessels result in increased local blood flow to the skin and other organs and a tendency for arterial blood pressure to decrease because of decreased peripheral vascular resistance. The degree of hypotensive effect produced depends on the sympathetic tone present before drug administration. Only a small change in blood pressure is produced with the patient in a supine position; however, orthostatic hypotension often develops with the patient in an upright position because of prevention of the vasoconstriction necessary for blood flow redistribution.

Alpha-adrenergic blockers, such as phenoxybenzamine and phentolamine, often cause tachycardia in addition to lowering blood pressure. This is because the decrease in systemic blood pressure, particularly when the patient is standing, activates baroreceptor reflexes that increase impulse activity in sympathetic cardiac nerves, producing a reflex tachycardia. If severe, this tachycardia may precipitate coronary insufficiency, angina, or even heart failure. Prazosin, which blocks alpha$_1$-receptor sites only, is less likely to cause this reflex tachycardia.

Ergotamine not only acts on receptors but also stimulates smooth muscle directly, producing vasoconstriction primarily in the uterus and blood vessels. This action causes a reduction in extracranial blood flow that produces decreased cerebral blood flow and a decline in arterial pressure.

Phenoxybenzamine acts by forming a stable bond with the alpha-receptor site. Phentolamine and tolazoline compete for alpha-receptor sites, but this blockade is short-acting, persisting only for a few hours.

PHARMACOTHERAPEUTICS

Therapeutic use of alpha-adrenergic blockers is based on their smooth muscle relaxation and vasodilation and the resultant increased local blood flow to skin and other organs and decreased blood pressure from decreased peripheral vascular resistance. Conditions in which these effects prove beneficial include hypertension and peripheral vascular disorders.

Although rarely (if ever) used to treat primary (essential) hypertension, because of the risk of rebound tachycardia, the alpha-adrenergic blockers phenoxybenzamine and phentolamine are important in treating the secondary hypertension caused by pheochromocytoma, a chromaffin-cell tumor of the adrenal gland that secretes excessive epinephrine and norepinephrine.

Certain peripheral vascular disorders—mainly those with a vasospastic component causing poor local blood flow, such as Raynaud's disease (intermittent pallor, cyanosis or redness of fingers), acrocyanosis (symmetrical mottled cyanosis of hands and feet), and aftereffects of frostbite—respond well to alpha-adrenergic therapy.

The vasodilation effect of alpha-adrenergic blockers also may prove beneficial in patients with septic shock. Ergotamine is used to treat migraine headaches, because it causes vasoconstriction of the dilated carotid artery. Ergoloid mesylates are used to enhance cerebral blood flow, particularly in elderly patients.

ergoloid mesylates (Deapril-ST, Hydergine). This combination of three hydrogenated ergot alkaloid derivatives increases cerebral vasodilation and decreases blood pressure and is thought to cause increased metabolic activity in the brain and to improve cerebral circulation. As a result, it is used to treat symptoms attributed to cerebral arteriosclerosis—decreased or impaired mental capacity and function, depression, and anxiety—especially in elderly patients.
USUAL ADULT DOSAGE: 1 mg P.O. or sublingually t.i.d.; dosage is adjusted gradually for optimal individual effect. Alleviation of symptoms is usually gradual; 3 or 4 weeks may be needed for full therapeutic effect.

ergotamine tartrate (Ergomar, Ergostat, Medihaler Ergotamine). This natural amino acid alkaloid of ergot is used to relieve the pain of vascular headaches, such as migraines. It works directly on the smooth muscle of external carotid artery branches to interrupt vasodilation and distention of cranial arterioles by causing vasocon-

DRUG INTERACTIONS

Alpha-adrenergic blockers

Drug interactions involving alpha-adrenergic blocking agents primarily affect the cardiovascular system and may include profound hypotension or vascular collapse, hypertension, and cardiac dysrhythmias.

DRUG	INTERACTING DRUGS	POSSIBLE EFFECTS	NURSING IMPLICATIONS
ergoloid mesylates, ergotamine	alcohol	May cause hypotension	• Monitor the patient's blood pressure frequently.
	caffeine	Increases ergotamine effect	• Monitor the patient for an increased therapeutic effect.
	dopamine	Increases pressor effects	• Monitor the patient's blood pressure frequently.
	nitroglycerin	May cause potential hypotension by excessive vasodilation	• Monitor the patient's blood pressure frequently.
	sympathomimetics, including many over-the-counter medications	Enhance cardiac stimulation; may cause hypotension with rebound hypertension	• Monitor the patient's blood pressure and heart rate frequently.

striction. Combining ergotamine with caffeine (in such products as Cafergot, Cafetrate, Ercatab, and Cafergot suppositories) potentiates the cranial vasoconstricting action of both substances; caffeine enhances the vasoconstrictor effects and is also reported to enhance the absorption of ergotamine. Belladonna alkaloids also are combined with ergotamine; their anticholinergic and antiemetic effects combat the excessive nausea and vomiting some patients experience during migraine attacks. Phenobarbital is added in some products (Cafergot P-B tablets and suppositories) for sedation. Another combination containing ergotamine, caffeine, and tartaric acid (Wigraine suppositories) is used when belladonna is not required.

USUAL ADULT DOSAGE: 2 mg P.O. or sublingually at onset of attack, then 2 mg every 30 minutes until resolution occurs, or maximum dose (6 mg per attack or 10 mg per week) is reached; inhalations (0.36 mg) 5 minutes apart until pain is relieved (maximum of 6 inhalations a day or 15 inhalations a week); for combination therapy, one or two tablets or suppositories every 15 minutes to 1 hour. Do not exceed six tablets or two suppositories per attack, or ten tablets or five suppositories per week.

phenoxybenzamine hydrochloride (Dibenzyline). This long-acting, noncompetitive alpha-adrenergic blocking agent can produce and maintain a state called chemical sympathectomy. It acts on both alpha$_1$- and alpha$_2$-receptor sites (although about 100 times more potently on alpha$_1$-receptor sites) to increase blood flow to the skin, mucosa, and viscera and to lower blood pressure whether the patient is supine or erect. It has no parasympathetic activity and produces no increase in cardiac output or perfusion of the liver or kidneys. Phenoxybenzamine is used to treat Raynaud's disease, postfrostbite syndrome, acrocyanosis, arteriosclerosis obliterans, and other peripheral vascular disorders. It is also used sometimes to control the hypertension and diaphoresis associated with pheochromocytoma.

USUAL ADULT DOSAGE: initially, 10 mg P.O. twice daily, increasing by 10 mg every 2 to 4 days to achieve maximum effect with minimal adverse reactions (may take several weeks to reach maximal effects); usual range is 20 to 60 mg/day.

phentolamine mesylate (Regitine). An alpha-adrenergic blocker with transient and incomplete action, phentolamine is a more potent structural analogue of tolazoline. It exerts alpha-adrenergic blocking as well as direct smooth muscle, parasympathomimetic, and some sympathomimetic and histamine-like actions. It is used to diagnose pheochromocytoma (using the Regitine-blocking test) and to control hypertension in patients with pheochromocytoma during surgical excision of the tumor. It is also used to prevent tissue necrosis and sloughing related to extravasation of I.V. vasopressor drugs such as norepinephrine or dopamine.

USUAL ADULT DOSAGE: for hypertension associated with pheochromocytoma, 5 mg I.M. or I.V. before surgery, 5 mg I.V., if needed, during surgery; for necrosis prevention, 5 to 10 mg in 10 ml normal saline solution injected into the area of extravasation.

Drug interactions

Many agents interact synergistically with alpha-adrenergic blocking agents and can potentiate or cause mutually additive effects, often with serious sequelae. The most serious include severe hypotension or vascular collapse; blockage of therapeutic blood pressure decreases, possibly leading to hypertensive crisis, cerebrovascular accident, or any of the many other complications of hypertension; and increased cardiac stimulation, causing dysrhythmias or angina. (See *Drug interactions: Alpha-adrenergic blockers* for interacting drugs and specific effects.)

ADVERSE DRUG REACTIONS

Adverse reactions caused by blockage of alpha receptors are primarily related to the drugs' vasodilation effect. However, because of the varied mechanisms of action of the alpha-adrenergic blocking agents, many adverse reactions are possible with these drugs.

Predictable reactions

Some of the reactions that can occur include such cardiovascular manifestations as orthostatic hypotension or severe hypertensive episodes, bradycardia or tachycardia, edema, dyspnea, light-headedness, flushing, dysrhythmias, angina, myocardial infarction (MI), cerebrovascular spasm, or a shocklike state. Central nervous system (CNS) manifestations that may occur include paresthesias, tingling of extremities, muscle weakness, fatigue, nervousness, depression, insomnia, drowsiness, lethargy, sedation, vertigo, syncope, confusion, headache, or CNS stimulation. The nurse may also note eye, ear, nose, and throat manifestations, such as nasal stuffiness, blurred vision, increased nasopharyngeal secretions, epistaxis, miosis (pinpoint pupils), conjunctival infection, ptosis (drooping of the eyelids),

---

Ergotism

Prolonged ergotamine use, overdose, or chronic poisoning related to diseases that increase sensitivity to the drug may induce a condition known as *ergotism*. In this condition, prolonged constriction of blood vessels causes the extremities to become cold, pale, and numb. Arterial peripheral pulses diminish and eventually disappear. Muscle pain may occur even at rest, and the patient may also experience confusion, vomiting, convulsions, or vision loss. Untreated, vasoconstriction can cause a severe lack of blood flow that could lead to tissue damage, even gangrene. Treatment includes immediate discontinuation of the drug and symptomatic therapy.

---

tinnitus, reddened sclera, or dry mouth. Gastrointestinal (GI) manifestations are common and may consist of sublingual irritation, nausea, vomiting, heartburn, diarrhea, abdominal pain, or exacerbation of peptic ulcer. Urinary frequency and impotence are among genitourinary reactions that may be noted. (See *Ergotism* for an explanation of this ergot-induced condition.)

Unpredictable reactions

With long-acting noncompetitive alpha-adrenergic blockers, such as phenoxybenzamine, the beta-adrenergic receptors are left unopposed, possibly leading to an exaggerated hypotensive response and tachycardia. Genitourinary findings may include incontinence or priapism. Hematologic manifestations are rare; however, granulocytopenia, leukopenia, thrombocytopenia, and pancytopenia have been reported with some agents. Various dermatologic manifestations may occur, including rash, allergic dermatitis, pruritus, alopecia, or lichen planus. Other unpredictable adverse reactions reported are allergic phenomena, including shock, diaphoresis, and arthralgia. Increased serum uric acid and blood urea nitrogen levels may also occur.

NURSING IMPLICATIONS

Because of their differing actions and uses, alpha-adrenergic blocking agents have many, varied nursing implications.

• Do not expect to administer alpha-adrenergic blockers to patients with congestive heart failure, angina, MI, or cerebrovascular insufficiency.

- Anticipate cautious use of these drugs with pregnant patients and patients with renal insufficiency, marked cerebral or coronary arteriosclerosis, peptic ulcer disease, or respiratory infection.
- Administer ergotamine cautiously to elderly patients and lactating women.
- During alpha-adrenergic blocker therapy, assess the patient for signs and symptoms of vascular insufficiency: numbness, coldness, and tingling or weakness in the extremities.
- Monitor the patient's blood pressure and pulse rate with the patient supine and standing (if appropriate) to assess drug efficacy.
- Administer I.V. drugs with the patient in the supine position to decrease the risk of orthostatic hypotension. During I.V. infusion, assess the patient's blood pressure and pulse frequently until stabilized.
- Administer oral drugs with milk to reduce gastric irritation.
- Store the drugs in a light-resistant, airtight container.
- Advise the patient to avoid alcohol consumption; explain that alcohol used in combination with alpha-adrenergic blocking agents may cause tachycardia and hypotension.
- Teach the patient to minimize orthostatic hypotension by arising slowly from a supine to an upright position and by dangling the legs over the side of the bed and exercising the feet for a few minutes before standing.
- Instruct the patient to assume a head-low position or to lie down if dizziness, faintness, or weakness occurs.
- Teach the patient that ergotamine is more effective for headache if taken in the early stage of an attack.
- Caution the patient not to exceed the prescribed dosage; explain that adverse reactions can result from higher doses.
- Inform the patient that drug actions may be intensified by also taking over-the-counter (OTC) allergy preparations.
- Advise the patient to lie quietly in a dark room after taking the medication, to increase its effectiveness.

BETA-ADRENERGIC BLOCKERS

Beta-adrenergic blocking agents, the most widely used adrenergic blockers, prevent sympathetic nervous system stimulation by inhibiting the action of catechol-amines and other sympathomimetic agents at beta-adrenergic receptor sites (see Chapter 36, Antianginal Agents, and Chapter 37, Antihypertensive Agents, for additional information and clinical uses for this group of drugs). Many beta-adrenergic blocking agents (including labetalol hydrochloride, nadolol, propranolol hydrochloride, and timolol maleate) are nonselective in their blocking action, affecting both beta$_1$- (located mainly in the heart) and beta$_2$- (located in bronchi, blood vessels, and the uterus) receptor sites. The newer beta-adrenergic blocking agents acebutolol hydrochloride, atenolol, and metoprolol tartrate are selective: they primarily affect beta$_1$-receptor sites. Beta-adrenergic blockers also exhibit a pharmacologic property known as intrinsic sympathetic activity (ISA). Drugs that exhibit ISA, such as pindolol, are sometimes classified as partial agonists.

Beta-adrenergic blockers are used extensively to treat hypertension, cardiac dysrhythmias, and angina pectoris as well as hyperthyroidism and other related disorders of sympathetic nervous system overstimulation.

History and source

The first beta-adrenergic blocker available for use in the United States was propranolol, introduced in 1968. Since that time, nonselective agents have been developed; nadolol was introduced in 1980, and subsequently other nonselective drugs such as timolol have become commercially available. The cardioselective agents acebutolol, atenolol, and metoprolol have become the beta-adrenergic blockers of choice for most clinical indications because they have limited pulmonary adverse effects.

PHARMACOKINETICS

Beta-adrenergic blockers are usually rapidly and well absorbed from the GI tract and are protein-bound to some extent.

Absorption, distribution, metabolism, excretion

Food does not inhibit their absorption and may actually enhance absorption of some agents. Some beta-adrenergic blockers are absorbed more completely than others; for instance, oral atenolol is only 50% absorbed, whereas oral propranolol is often 75% or more absorbed. Most agents are protein-bound to some extent. Acebutolol, atenolol, metoprolol, and timolol are weakly protein-bound; pindolol and labetalol, moderately protein-bound; and propranolol, highly protein-bound (up to 90%).

Beta-adrenergic blockers: Summary of pharmacokinetics

This chart provides a quick reference for administration routes and pharmacokinetic processes of the beta-adrenergic blocking agents. The nurse who administers these agents should be familiar with the variations.

DRUG	ROUTE	ONSET	PEAK	DURATION	HALF-LIFE
acebutolol	Oral	Unknown	2½ to 3½ hours	Unknown	3 to 4 hours
atenolol	Oral	1 hour	2 to 4 hours	24 hours	6 to 9 hours
labetalol	Oral	Rapid	1 to 2 hours	8 to 10 hours	6 to 8 hours
	I.V.	Immediate	5 minutes	Unknown	5 to 8 hours
metoprolol	Oral	10 minutes	90 minutes	Up to 6 hours	3 to 4 hours
	I.V.	Rapid	20 minutes	5 to 8 hours	3 to 4 hours
nadolol	Oral	Unknown	2 to 4 hours	24 hours	10 to 24 hours
pindolol	Oral	Rapid	1 to 2 hours	24 hours	3 to 4 hours
propranolol	Oral	30 minutes	1 to 1½ hours	6 hours	3 to 6 hours
	I.V.	2 minutes	15 minutes	3 to 6 hours	3 to 6 hours
timolol	Oral	30 minutes	1 to 2 hours	4 to 6 hours	3 to 4 hours
	Ophthalmic	15 to 30 minutes	1 to 2 hours	24 hours	Unknown

Beta-adrenergic blockers are widely distributed in body tissues, with the highest concentrations found in the heart, liver, lungs, and saliva. Some agents (such as metoprolol and timolol) cross the blood-brain barrier; timolol crosses the placental barrier.

With the exception of nadolol and atenolol, beta-adrenergic blockers are metabolized to some extent in the liver. Acebutolol, labetalol, metoprolol, propranolol, and timolol undergo extensive first-pass metabolism in the liver; 60% to 65% of pindolol is metabolized in the liver. Excretion is primarily in the urine, as metabolites or in unchanged form, with some excretion also occurring in feces and bile, and some secretion in breast milk. Nadolol is not metabolized, is excreted unchanged in the urine (about 70%) and feces, and is secreted in breast milk. Atenolol is excreted primarily unchanged in urine.

Onset, peak, duration

The onset of action of beta-adrenergic blockers is primarily dose- and drug-dependent; peak concentration levels are route-dependent. Duration of action varies according to dose and usually ranges from 4 hours for oral timolol to 24 hours for oral atenolol. Half-life varies from a low of 3 to 4 hours for timolol and pindolol to a high of 10 to 24 hours for nadolol. (See *Beta-adrenergic blockers: Summary of pharmacokinetics* for the specifics of each drug's activity.)

PHARMACODYNAMICS

Beta-adrenergic blocking agents act primarily as competitive adrenergic antagonists, preventing beta-adrenergic receptors from responding to sympathetic impulses, catecholamines, or other adrenergic agents. Physiologically, these drugs compete for the available beta-receptor sites located on the membrane of cardiac muscle (primarily beta$_1$ receptors) and smooth muscle of bronchi and blood vessels (beta$_2$ receptors). Some agents, in addition to their beta activity, also exhibit some CNS activity; acebutolol and pindolol demonstrate ISA,

Major effects of beta-adrenergic blockers

By blocking the action of endogenous catecholamines and other sympathomimetic agents at beta-receptor sites, beta-adrenergic blockers counteract the stimulating effects of these agents. The diagram below shows the effects of beta-adrenergic blockers on the pulmonary and cardiovascular systems.

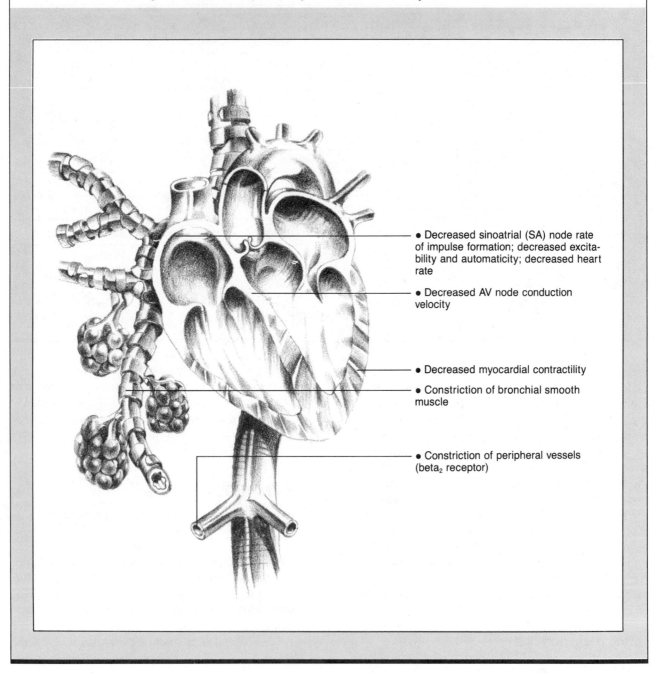

- Decreased sinoatrial (SA) node rate of impulse formation; decreased excitability and automaticity; decreased heart rate
- Decreased AV node conduction velocity
- Decreased myocardial contractility
- Constriction of bronchial smooth muscle
- Constriction of peripheral vessels (beta$_2$ receptor)

occupying a receptor site to exert a weak activation in preference to occupation of the site by a stronger stimulating agent. The minimal decrease in cardiac output and pulse rate is evidence of pindolol's ISA. This makes it a useful agent for patients with bradycardia and reduced cardiac reserve.

Mechanism of action

Beta-adrenergic blocking agents produce a competitive blocking action not only at adrenergic nerve endings but also in the adrenal medulla; that accounts for their widespread effects. Some researchers speculate that certain beta-adrenergic blockers, such as metoprolol and propranolol, produce CNS activity, with effects exerted at the vasomotor center in the brain stem to reduce tonic sympathetic nerve impulse transmission. These agents can reduce or block myocardial stimulation, vasodilation, bronchodilation, glycogenolysis (production of glucose from glycogen), and lipolysis (fat hydrolysis). The effects of this blockade include increased peripheral vascular resistance, decreased systemic blood pressure, decreased contractile force, decreased myocardial oxygen consumption, slowed atrioventricular (AV) conduction, and decreased cardiac output. Pulmonary manifestations include increased bronchial smooth muscle tone; metabolic manifestations include inhibition of the sympathetic response to hypoglycemia. CNS manifestations include weakness, lethargy, and fatigue. Other manifestations include decreased plasma renin activity (particularly in patients with high levels before beta-adrenergic blocker therapy) and decreased production of aqueous humor in the eye, not accompanied by miosis or hyperemia (increased blood).

The ophthalmic actions of beta-adrenergic blockers are of great importance; these agents are rapidly becoming the drugs of choice in the treatment of glaucoma. (See Chapter 79, Ophthalmic Agents.) The cardiovascular actions also are of great clinical significance, as is the decreased renin activity. At present, the bronchial and CNS actions are primarily viewed as causes of adverse effects, although investigations may eventually demonstrate that the CNS effects have some psychiatric or neurologic value.

Some physiologic manifestations of the various beta-adrenergic blocking agents are related to the drugs' classification as either selective or nonselective. Selective beta-adrenergic blockers, which preferentially block beta$_1$-receptor sites, produce effects primarily related to prevention of cardiac excitation. Nonselective beta-adrenergic blockers, which block both beta$_1$- and beta$_2$-receptor sites, prevent not only cardiac excitement but also bronchiolar dilation. For instance, nonselective beta-adrenergic blockers can cause bronchospasm in patients with chronic obstructive lung disorders, but this adverse effect is largely eliminated with the use of selective drugs, which have minimal beta$_2$ activity.

PHARMACOTHERAPEUTICS

Beta-adrenergic blockers are used to treat a number of conditions and are under investigation for use in many more. As mentioned earlier, their clinical usefulness is based largely (but not exclusively) on their cardiovascular effects. (See *Major effects of beta-adrenergic blockers*.) Cardiovascular indications for beta-adrenergic blockers include hypertension, angina pectoris, prevention of reinfarction after MI, supraventricular dysrhythmias, and hypertrophic cardiomyopathy. Other uses include the treatment of migraine headaches, anxiety, wide-angle glaucoma, pheochromocytoma, and the cardiovascular symptoms associated with thyrotoxicosis.

acebutolol hydrochloride (Sectral). This selective beta$_1$-adrenergic blocking agent exerts mild intrinsic sympathomimetic activity. It acts to lower heart rate, blood pressure, and cardiac output, making it useful in the treatment of hypertension and ventricular dysrhythmias. USUAL ADULT DOSAGE: initially, 200 mg P.O. b.i.d. or 400 mg P.O. daily, with the dosage gradually increased to achieve optimal response (for hypertension, the range is 400 to 800 mg/day); for ventricular dysrhythmia, 600 to 1,200 mg/day). A lower maintenance dosage is required for an elderly patient; avoid giving more than 800 mg/day.

atenolol (Tenormin). This long-acting, selective beta$_1$ blocker exhibits minimal protein binding. It decreases cardiac output and systolic and diastolic blood pressure; however, like other beta-adrenergic blocking agents, it increases peripheral vascular resistance at rest and with exercise. Atenolol is used as a first-step agent in treating hypertension, alone or in combination with other agents, and also has been used in the prophylactic management of stable angina pectoris. USUAL ADULT DOSAGE: initially, 50 mg P.O. once a day; increase to 100 mg once a day, if necessary, after 1 to 2 weeks; reduce to 50 mg on alternate days for patients with renal failure.

DRUG INTERACTIONS

Beta-adrenergic blockers

Drug interactions involving beta-adrenergic blockers primarily affect the cardiovascular and respiratory systems.

DRUG	INTERACTING DRUGS	POSSIBLE EFFECTS	NURSING IMPLICATIONS
acebutolol, atenolol, labetalol, metopro-lol, nadolol, pin-dolol, propranolol, timolol	antacids	Delay absorption of drug from GI tract	• Administer several hours apart. • Monitor the patient for a decreased thera-peutic effect.
	antiarrhythmics (lidocaine, procainamide, phenytoin, quinidine, disopyramide)	Enhance hypotensive ef-fects; increase plasma levels of lidocaine (poten-tial toxicity); may cause additive cardiac depres-sant effects	• Monitor the patient's blood pressure and pulse rate frequently.
	anticholinergics (atropine)	Enhance effects because of increased GI absorption of drug; antagonize car-diac depressant activity of some beta-adrenergic blockers	• Monitor the patient for an altered therapeutic response to these drugs.
	insulin and oral hypogly-cemic agents	Prolong duration of action of hypoglycemic agents (possible hypoglycemia); may mask tachycardia as a sign of hypoglycemia (diaphoresis and agitation still present)	• Administer these drugs cautiously. • Monitor the patient's blood glucose levels frequently.
	antihypertensives (gua-nethidine, methyldopa, hy-dralazine, clonidine, prazosin, minoxidil, capto-pril, reserpine)	May cause additive hypo-tension and bradycardia; possible pulmonary hyper-tension in uremic patients; possible rebound hyper-tension after antihyperten-sive discontinuation	• Monitor the patient's blood pressure and heart rate frequently.
	anti-inflammatories (indo-methacin, salicylates)	Decrease hypotensive ef-fects of beta-adrenergic blockers by inhibiting prostaglandin synthesis	• Monitor patient for altered beta-adrenergic blocker effects.
	antithyroid agents (me-thimazole, propylthiouracil)	Increase plasma concen-tration of propranolol	• Monitor the patient's therapeutic response.
	barbiturates	Stimulate metabolism of beta-adrenergic blockers that are extensively me-tabolized	• Monitor the patient for altered response to beta-adrenergic blockers that are metabolized by the liver (propranolol, metoprolol).
	cardiac glycosides	May cause additive brady-cardia and depression of AV conduction	• Monitor the patient's blood pressure and heart rate frequently.
	calcium channel blockers	Increase pharmacologic and toxicologic effects of both agents	• Monitor the patient for adverse effects.

DRUG INTERACTIONS

Beta-adrenergic blockers continued

DRUG	INTERACTING DRUGS	POSSIBLE EFFECTS	NURSING IMPLICATIONS
acebutolol, atenolol, labetalol, metoprolol, nadolol, pindolol, propranolol, timolol (continued)	sympathomimetics (epinephrine, dobutamine, dopamine, isoproterenol, terbutaline, metaproterenol, albuterol, ritodrine)	May cause hypertension and reflex bradycardia from unopposed alpha effects (vasoconstriction) and increased vagal tone	• Monitor the patient's blood pressure and heart rate frequently.
	cimetidine	Reduces metabolism of beta-adrenergic blockers; enhances ability of beta-adrenergic blockers to reduce pulse rate	• Monitor the patient for altered response to beta-adrenergic blockers.
	oral contraceptives	Inhibit metabolism of metoprolol	• Monitor the patient for increased therapeutic response.
	furosemide	Enhances hypotensive activity by inhibiting hepatic metabolism and increasing bioavailability of drug	• Monitor the patient's blood pressure frequently.
	phenothiazines	Inhibit hepatic metabolism and may have mutually additive hypotensive effects	• Monitor the patient for enhanced effects of both drugs.
	rifampin	Inhibits therapeutic response to metoprolol	• Monitor the patient for altered response to metoprolol.
	theophyllines	Impair bronchodilating effects of theophyllines by nonselective beta-adrenergic blockers	• Monitor the patient's therapeutic response.

labetalol hydrochloride (Trandate, Normodyne). This selective alpha$_1$- and nonselective beta-adrenergic blocking agent decreases blood pressure without reflex tachycardia or a marked decrease in heart rate; it is used to control blood pressure in severe hypertension.

USUAL ADULT DOSAGE: initially 100 mg P.O. b.i.d., alone or with diuretic therapy. After 2 or 3 days, increase by 100 mg b.i.d. to achieve the desired therapeutic effect; maintenance dose is individualized, with a usual range of 200 to 400 mg b.i.d. (Severe hypertension may require 1,200 to 2,400 mg/day.) For I.V. injection, 20 mg by slow injection over 2 minutes, repeat every 10 minutes to a maximum of 300 mg; I.V. infusion, 40 ml (two 100-mg ampules) in 160 ml of I.V. fluid (approximately 1 mg:1 ml) administered at 2 ml/minute (2 mg/minute), or 40 ml (two 100-mg ampules) in 250 ml I.V. fluid (approximately 2 mg:3 ml) administered at a rate of 3 ml/minute to deliver 2 mg/minute. Rate is adjusted according to blood pressure response. When a satisfac-

tory response is reached (usually after infusion of 50 to 200 mg), oral therapy is begun at a 200-mg initial dose, followed in 6 to 12 hours by a 200 to 400-mg dose and adjusted according to the individual's response.

metoprolol tartrate (Lopressor, Betaloc). This selective beta$_1$ blocker produces few unwanted beta$_2$ effects except at high doses. It has some CNS activity and is used alone or in combination as a second-step antihypertensive agent or for MI.

USUAL ADULT DOSAGE: for hypertension, initially, 100 mg/day P.O. in single or divided doses, increased weekly until optimal effects are obtained (usual range is 100 to 450 mg/day); for MI, 5 mg I.V., 2 minutes apart, for three doses; then 50 mg P.O. every 6 hours for 48 hours, then 100 mg P.O. every 12 hours.

nadolol (Corgard). This nonselective beta-adrenergic blocker, which does not cross the blood-brain barrier, decreases standing and supine blood pressures as well as plasma renin activity. It is used to treat hypertension and may be combined with a diuretic for enhanced effects. It is also used for long-term prophylactic management of stable angina pectoris. The drug is administered orally, in a single daily dose. Because it is excreted unchanged in the urine, dosage must be reduced in patients with impaired renal function.

USUAL ADULT DOSAGE: for hypertension, initially, 40 mg/day P.O., increased gradually in 40 to 80 mg doses to a maximum of 640 mg/day (usual range, 80 to 320 mg); for angina, initially, 40 mg P.O. once a day, increased every 3 to 7 days to achieve optimal effects (usual range is 80 to 240 mg once a day). For a patient with renal failure, dosing intervals are based on creatinine clearance levels.

pindolol (Visken). This nonselective beta-adrenergic blocking agent has significant partial beta agonist activity and some intrinsic sympathomimetic activity. As a result, it causes less reduction in cardiac contractility and heart rate and slows conduction less markedly than do other beta-adrenergic blockers. This drug is used in the first-step management of hypertension, either alone or in combination with other agents.

USUAL ADULT DOSAGE: initially, 5 mg P.O. b.i.d., increased by 10 mg every 3 to 4 weeks (to a maximum of 60 mg) until optimal effects are achieved.

propranolol hydrochloride (Inderal). This nonselective beta-adrenergic blocking agent produces some centrally mediated peripheral vasodilation and also decreases the heart rate by slowing conduction through the atria and the AV node. Propranolol increases exercise tolerance by blocking the sympathetic effects of exertion (such as increased heart rate and blood pressure) and decreases myocardial oxygen requirements in patients with angina. This drug is used in the management of many clinical conditions, including first-step management of hypertension, cardiac dysrhythmias, MI, prophylactic management of angina pectoris, hypertrophic subaortic stenosis, and migraine. It undergoes extensive first-pass metabolism in the liver—the reason for the significant difference between oral and I.V. dosages.

USUAL ADULT DOSAGE: for hypertension, initially, 40 mg P.O. b.i.d., increased until optimal effects are reached (usual range is 120 to 240 mg in two or three divided doses or 120 to 160 mg of sustained-release capsules once a day) to a maximum of 640 mg/day; for angina,

initially, 10 to 20 mg P.O. t.i.d. or q.i.d., increased every 3 to 7 days until optimal effects are obtained (usual dosage is 160 mg/day in divided doses) to a maximum of 320 mg/day; for dysrhythmias, 10 to 30 mg P.O. t.i.d. or q.i.d.; for hypertrophic subaortic stenosis, 20 to 40 mg P.O. t.i.d. or q.i.d., or 80 to 160 mg of sustained-release capsules once a day; for MI, 180 to 240 mg P.O. daily in three or four divided doses to a maximum of 240 mg/day; for migraine, 80 mg P.O. daily in divided doses, increased as necessary (usual range, 160 to 240 mg/day); for parenteral emergency use administration, 1 to 3 mg I.V. at an infusion rate of 1 mg/minute; a second dose may be given within 2 to 3 minutes.

timolol maleate (Blocadren, Timoptic). This nonselective beta-adrenergic blocking agent, although structurally similar to propranolol, is approximately 5 to 10 times more potent than propranolol and does not cross the blood-brain barrier. This drug is a valuable agent in the treatment of chronic open-angle glaucoma, aphakic glaucoma, secondary glaucoma, and ocular hypertension. (See Chapter 79, Ophthalmic Agents for a summary of the drug's ophthalmic uses.) The oral form is used as a first-step agent, alone or in combination with other agents, to manage hypertension as well as to prevent reinfarction after myocardial infarction.

USUAL ADULT DOSAGE: initially, 10 mg P.O. b.i.d.; maintenance dose, 20 to 40 mg/day in two divided doses; maximum 60 mg/day in two divided doses.

Drug interactions

Many agents can interact synergistically with beta-adrenergic blocking agents to cause potentially dangerous effects, either by potentiating or creating additive effects of one or both drugs or by inhibiting the desired effects of the drugs. Some of the most serious potential effects include cardiac depression, dysrhythmias, respiratory depression, severe bronchospasm, and severe hypotension that could lead to vascular collapse. (See *Drug interactions: Beta-adrenergic blockers* on pages 318 and 319 for more detailed information.)

ADVERSE DRUG REACTIONS

Generally, beta-adrenergic blockers have a low frequency of adverse reactions. Most that do occur are drug- or dose-dependent. Adverse reactions occur most often from I.V. rather than oral administration and in elderly patients and those with impaired renal or hepatic function.

Adverse beta-adrenergic blocker reactions in chronic disease

This table lists common chronic disorders that place affected patients at increased risk for adverse reactions to beta-adrenergic blockers, along with the potential effects and etiologic mechanisms.

DISORDERS	POSSIBLE REACTIONS	CAUSES
Arteriosclerosis	Reflex tachycardia, acute angina pectoris, cardiac failure	Lowered blood pressure from direct cardiac action of some beta-adrenergic blocking agents
Bronchospastic disease	Severe respiratory distress	Inhibition of beta$_2$ effect, resulting in bronchospasm
Congestive heart failure, hypertension	Further cardiac failure	Increased myocardial depression
Diabetes mellitus	Masking of hypoglycemic signs and symptoms	Suppression of hypoglycemic response
Thyrotoxicosis	Masking of clinical signs	Suppression of tachycardia
	Thyroid storm	Abrupt beta-adrenergic blocker withdrawal

Predictable reactions

Beta-adrenergic blocker toxicity is marked primarily by dysrhythmias, orthostatic hypotension, CNS disturbances, and GI or respiratory distress. Cardiovascular reactions include hypotension, bradycardia, peripheral vascular insufficiency (Raynaud's disease), AV block, and congestive heart failure. Beta-adrenergic blockers should be used cautiously, if at all, in patients with congestive heart failure or heart block.

The most common respiratory reaction is bronchospasm. Although selective agents are less likely than nonselective agents to cause bronchospasm, caution is nevertheless advisable when administering all beta-adrenergic blockers, particularly to patients with bronchial asthma, bronchitis, or emphysema. GI manifestations commonly include diarrhea, nausea, vomiting, constipation, abdominal discomfort, anorexia, and flatulence. CNS effects may include dizziness, insomnia, fatigue, weakness, lethargy, disorientation, memory loss, visual disturbances, sedation, hallucinations, or behavioral changes. Elderly patients, in particular, are at increased risk for CNS effects. Hematologic adverse reactions, also rare, include prevention of platelet agglutination, granulocytopenia, and thrombocytopenic purpura. Other reported adverse reactions include headache, impotence or decreased libido; nasal stuffiness; diaphoresis; tinnitus; and dry mouth, eyes, and skin.

Unpredictable reactions

Adverse reactions indicating an allergic response include rash, fever with sore throat, laryngospasm, and possibly respiratory distress. Although most patients tolerate beta-adrenergic blockers fairly well, patients with various preexisting chronic conditions are at special risk for adverse reactions to beta-adrenergic blocker therapy. (See *Adverse beta-adrenergic blocker reactions in chronic disease* for a list of these conditions and associated adverse drug reactions.)

NURSING IMPLICATIONS

Because beta-adrenergic blockers are the most widely used adrenergic blocking agents, the nurse must be familiar with the following considerations:
• Before administering a beta-adrenergic blocker, assess the patient's history for congestive heart failure, bradycardia, heart block, liver or kidney disease, thyroid disease, myasthenia gravis, use of psychotropic medication, pregnancy, or use of monoamine oxidase (MAO)

inhibitors (within the past 2 weeks); these conditions may contraindicate beta-adrenergic blocker therapy.

• In a diabetic patient, monitor blood glucose levels frequently; beta-adrenergic blockers can potentiate hypoglycemia and mask its signs and symptoms.

• Administer beta-adrenergic blockers with extreme caution to patients with respiratory conditions such as asthma, hay fever, bronchitis, emphysema, or allergic rhinitis. Severe bronchospasm may occur. (The selective agents atenolol, metoprolol, and labetalol usually have less bronchospastic activity than do nonselective agents.)

• During I.V. beta-adrenergic blocker therapy, have emergency drugs on hand: atropine for possible bradycardia, epinephrine (or another vasopressor) for possible hypotension, and isoproterenol and aminophylline for possible bronchospasm.

• Store drugs at room temperature and protect them from moisture, light, and air.

• To monitor the patient's therapeutic response, assess the patient's blood pressure, apical and radial pulses, fluid intake and output, daily weight, respirations, and circulation in the extremities before and during beta-adrenergic blocker therapy.

• Throughout I.V. therapy, monitor the patient's EKG, central venous pressure, and arterial pressure.

• During prolonged therapy, assess the patient's hematologic, renal, and hepatic function regularly.

• Give oral beta-adrenergic blockers before meals or at bedtime to facilitate absorption. Avoid late-evening dosages if insomnia occurs.

• Teach the patient and family members to assess their individual reactions to physical and psychological stress, and help them to plan appropriate life-style changes and activities to reduce stress.

• Advise the patient never to abruptly stop taking the prescribed drug; explain that abrupt withdrawal can cause MI, dysrhythmias, or other serious complications.

• Advise the patient to avoid alcohol and smoking and to consult the physician before using OTC cold, cough, or allergy preparations, because of potential adverse interactions.

• Caution the patient against driving or operating machinery until after adjusting to the CNS effects of the drug.

• Instruct the patient to sit or lie down immediately if dizziness or a fainting feeling occurs.

• Discuss potential adverse reactions with the patient and explain what to do if they develop.

• Teach the patient to measure his pulse rate and to report slowing or irregularity to the physician.

AUTONOMIC GANGLIONIC BLOCKERS

All nerve impulse transmission from preganglionic to postganglionic fibers in the autonomic nervous system (both the parasympathetic and the sympathetic branches) is mediated by the neurotransmitter acetylcholine. By inhibiting the action of acetylcholine, ganglionic blocking agents reduce or prevent the transmission of impulses in the autonomic nervous system. These drugs are classified according to their type of action as either depolarizing or nondepolarizing (antidepolarizing) agents. Depolarizing agents initially stimulate postganglionic fibers, then block further activity by continuing to occupy the receptor sites, thereby preventing postganglionic repolarization. (Nicotine, a drug that has no therapeutic use, belongs to this classification.) Nondepolarizing agents function as competitive antagonists of acetylcholine at postganglionic receptor sites and exert no initial stimulatory action. The clinically useful ganglionic blockers, such as trimethaphan camsylate and mecamylamine hydrochloride, belong to the nondepolarizing category and cause primarily sympatholytic effects: vasodilation and decreased blood pressure.

Because of their broad and somewhat unpredictable effects and because other, more specific agents are available, ganglionic blocking agents have limited clinical uses. Like alpha- and beta-adrenergic blocking agents, they exert potent hypotensive effects, but they also produce problematic parasympatholytic effects such as constipation, paralytic ileus, and decreased urinary bladder tone with urinary retention.

History and source

Ganglionic blocking agents are of the quaternary ammonium compound group, with tetraethylammonium chloride considered to be the prototype for drugs having ganglionic activity. However, problems with tetraethylammonium chloride—including a short duration of action, ineffectiveness when administered orally, and the unwanted effects of ganglionic stimulation—made it undesirable for use in treating hypertension. In 1950, methonium derivatives were introduced, and hexamethonium chloride soon became the antihypertensive drug of choice, even though its erratic absorption and duration of action and its severe adverse reactions were serious drawbacks. Since the early 1960s and the introduction of newer antihypertensives with more selective durations of action, ganglionic blocking agents have been used to produce hypotensive states only in special circumstances.

PHARMACOKINETICS

The two ganglionic blocking agents in use today, trimethaphan and mecamylamine, have similar pharmacokinetic actions, differing primarily in route of administration.

Absorption, distribution, metabolism, excretion

Administered orally, ganglionic blocking agents are well absorbed from the GI tract, but at erratic rates. Higher doses are usually required at night; lower doses in warm weather. The drugs are widely distributed throughout the body. Both trimethaphan and mecamylamine cross the placenta, and mecamylamine crosses the blood-brain barrier as well. Possibly metabolized by pseudocholinesterase, the drugs are excreted by the kidneys, largely in unchanged form. Excretion of mecamylamine is enhanced by acidic urine and slowed by alkaline urine. A small amount is excreted in the feces.

Onset, peak, duration

The onset of action of ganglionic blockers is route-dependent, beginning immediately after I.V. administration and within 30 minutes to 2 hours after oral administration. With oral therapy, peak concentration levels are reached 3 to 5 hours after administration; duration of action is 6 to 12 hours. Note, however, that full therapeutic effects may not be achieved for 2 to 3 days with oral medication. With I.V. therapy, the duration of action is 10 to 30 minutes, with rebound hypertension occurring shortly after discontinuation.

PHARMACODYNAMICS

Ganglionic blocking agents prevent nerve transmission by competing with acetylcholine at the postganglionic synapses of the autonomic nervous system. They work not only at the ganglia of the autonomic nervous system but also in the adrenal medulla, where the drugs prevent the cells from secreting epinephrine and norepinephrine into the circulation, thereby blocking sympathetic impulses to cells. Administration of ganglionic blocking agents causes vasodilation, which may be accompanied by a loss of the normal baroreceptor reflex action that serves to normalize blood pressure.

Mechanism of action

Besides blocking sympathetic stimulation of the adrenal medulla to prevent the secretion of epinephrine and norepinephrine into the systemic circulation, ganglionic blocking agents block acetylcholine at postganglionic cells by competitive inhibition. This blockage of impulse transmission and reduction of circulating catecholamines diminish vasoconstrictor tone, leading to vascular dilation and a decrease in arterial pressure. When the patient stands, the compensatory vasoconstrictor reflexes that respond to position changes by regulating blood pressure are suppressed. As a result, blood collects in the leg veins, causing decreased venous return and decreased cardiac output. Trimethaphan may also have a direct vasodilation effect on blood vessels. Along with the desired decrease in arterial pressure, decreased venous return and decreased cardiac output can lead to such undesirable effects as orthostatic hypotension and syncope. Other undesirable effects include inhibited diaphoresis, loss of body heat, and lowered body temperature from vasodilation in the skin.

PHARMACOTHERAPEUTICS

Clinical use of ganglionic blocking agents is limited by the drugs' many potential adverse reactions, including significant orthostatic hypotension, paralytic ileus, and urinary retention. The drugs are selectively used, however, to treat hypertensive emergencies, pulmonary edema resulting from pulmonary hypertension, and uncomplicated malignant hypertension; to provide controlled hypotension during surgery, such as for brain tumors, cerebral aneurysms, AV fistulas, aortic grafts and transplants, and coarctations; and to predict the effects of a sympathectomy.

mecamylamine hydrochloride (Inversine). This competitive antagonist of acetylcholine is a potent, long-acting agent that decreases blood pressure in normotensive and hypertensive patients. Tolerance to mecamylamine rarely develops, and its effects are most pronounced while the patient is standing or sitting. The drug is used to control moderate to severe essential hypertension and uncomplicated malignant hypertension.

USUAL ADULT DOSAGE: initially, 2.5 mg P.O. b.i.d., increased by 2.5-mg increments every 2 days until the optimum effects are obtained; average total daily dose, 25 mg, usually given in three divided doses.

DRUG INTERACTIONS

Autonomic ganglionic blockers

Combining certain drugs with ganglionic blocking agents can cause significant adverse reactions, including tachycardia, orthostatic hypotension, congestive heart failure, and stroke. This table summarizes the interactions that can cause these and other reactions and the appropriate nursing actions.

DRUG	INTERACTING DRUGS	POSSIBLE EFFECTS	NURSING IMPLICATIONS
trimethaphan, mecamylamine	alcohol	Increases hypotensive effects	• Monitor the patient's blood pressure frequently.
	anesthetics	Increase hypotensive effects	• Monitor the patient's blood pressure.
	anticholinergics	Increase hypotensive effects	• Monitor the patient's blood pressure frequently.
	reserpine	Increases hypotensive effects	• Monitor the patient's blood pressure frequently.
	depolarizing muscle relaxants	Increase neuromuscular blocking effects with prolonged respiratory depression	• Monitor the patient's respiratory rate and provide mechanical ventilatory support, as needed.
	MAO inhibitors	Increase hypotensive effects	• Monitor the patient's blood pressure frequently.
	nondepolarizing muscle relaxants	Increase neuromuscular blocking effects with prolonged respiratory depression	• Monitor the patient's respiratory rate and provide mechanical ventilatory support, as needed.
	sympathomimetics	Increase sympathomimetic effects	• Monitor the patient's therapeutic response to the sympathomimetics.
	thiazide diuretics	Increase hypotensive effects	• Monitor the patient's blood pressure frequently.
	urine alkalinizers	Decrease drug excretion, ganglionic blocker toxicity	• Monitor the patient for adverse effects.
	urine acidifiers	Increase drug excretion	• Monitor the patient's therapeutic response.
	vasodilators	Increase hypotensive effects	• Monitor the patient's blood pressure frequently.

trimethaphan camsylate (Arfonad). This potent, short-acting, competitive ganglionic blocking agent directly relaxes vascular smooth muscle. It can also stimulate histamine release. Tolerance to this agent can develop in 48 hours after therapy is begun. Trimethaphan is administered by continuous I.V. infusion for controlled hypotension during neurologic, ophthalmic, and plastic surgery procedures, for short-term control of blood pressure during hypertensive emergencies, and for emergency treatment of pulmonary hypertension causing pulmonary edema. It is under investigation for use in the management of a dissecting aortic aneurysm and ischemic heart disease when other agents cannot be used.

USUAL ADULT DOSAGE: initially, 3 to 4 ml/minute I.V. of a 1 mg/ml solution (500 mg, or 10 ml of drug in 500 ml of dextrose 5% in water); adjust to individual need within range of 0.3 to 6 mg/minute.

(Text continues on page 328.)

SELECTED MAJOR DRUGS

Adrenergic blocking agents

This chart summarizes the major adrenergic blockers currently in clinical use.

DRUG	MAJOR INDICATIONS	USUAL ADULT DOSAGES	NURSING IMPLICATIONS
Alpha-adrenergic blockers			
ergotamine	Migraine	2 mg P.O. or sublingually at onset of attack, then 2 mg every 30 minutes until resolution occurs or maximum dosage (6 mg per attack or 10 mg per week) is achieved; inhalations (0.36 mg) 5 minutes apart until pain is relieved (maximum six inhalations/day). For combination therapy: 1 to 2 tablets or suppositories every 15 to 60 minutes; do not exceed 6 tablets or 2 suppositories per attack, or 10 tablets or 5 suppositories per week	• Instruct the patient to initiate therapy as soon as possible in the early stage of an attack. • During therapy, assess the patient for signs and symptoms of vascular insufficiency: numbness, coldness, and tingling or weakness in the extremities. • Administer oral drugs with milk to reduce gastric irritation. • Advise the patient to lie quietly in a dark room after taking the medication, to increase its effectiveness. • Teach the patient the signs and symptoms of an adverse reaction: irregular heartbeat, nausea, vomiting, numbness or tingling in fingers or toes, or pain or weakness in the extremities. • Obtain baseline vital signs and a headache history before administering this agent.
phentolamine	Hypertension associated with pheochromocytoma Prevention of necrosis related to extravasation	5 mg I.M. or I.V. before surgery; 5 mg I.V. if needed, during surgery 5 to 10 mg in 10 ml normal saline solution injected into the area of extravasation	• Obtain the patient's baseline standing and supine blood pressure and pulse and respiratory rate before administering this agent. • With I.V. or I.M. administration, assist the patient in assuming a supine position. • If the drug is ordered before surgery, give the prescribed dose 1 to 2 hours before the procedure. • Monitor the patient for dizziness or lightheadedness, and institute safety measures, such as elevating the side rails and assisting with mobility, as appropriate. • Monitor the patient for adverse reactions such as severe hypotension, tachycardia, cardiac dysrhythmias, nausea, vomiting, and diarrhea. • Instruct the patient to avoid over-the-counter (OTC) cough, cold, allergy, or weight-loss medications, unless they have been approved by the physician.
Beta-adrenergic blockers			
atenolol	Hypertension, angina	50 mg P.O. once/day; increase to 100 mg/day after 1 to 2 weeks if necessary; reduce to 50 mg every other day for patients with renal failure	• Administer beta-adrenergic blockers with extreme caution to patients with respiratory conditions such as asthma, hay fever, bronchitis, emphysema, or allergic rhinitis. Severe bronchospasm may occur. • Monitor the patient's apical pulse rate before drug administration (especially if the patient is taking digitalis); withhold the drug and notify the physician if the pulse rate is below 60. • Teach the patient to measure the pulse rate and to report slowing or irregularity to the physician.

continued

SELECTED MAJOR DRUGS

Adrenergic blocking agents continued

DRUG	MAJOR INDICATIONS	USUAL ADULT DOSAGES	NURSING IMPLICATIONS
atenolol (continued)			• Protect the drug from light, heat, and moisture. • Advise the patient not to discontinue taking the drug abruptly, because of possible precipitation of tachycardia, angina, MI, or thyroid storm. • Advise the patient not to take any OTC preparations without first consulting the physician.
metoprolol	Hypertension Myocardial infarction	100 mg/day P.O. with weekly increase to achieve desired effects. Maintenance dose: 100 to 450 mg/day 5 mg I.V. every 2 minutes for three doses; then 50 mg P.O. every 6 hours for 48 hours; then 100 mg every 12 hours	• Monitor the patient's blood urea nitrogen (BUN), serum creatinine, serum transaminase, alkaline phosphatase, lactate dehydrogenase, and serum uric acid levels, because metoprolol may increase these values. • Assess the patient's apical pulse before drug administration; note any changes in baseline rate, rhythm, or quality, and changes in blood pressure, and report any significant changes to the physician. • Advise the patient that optimal effects of the drug may not be apparent for up to 1 week. • Advise the patient to avoid scheduling a late-evening dose if it produces insomnia or vivid, disturbing dreams. • Monitor closely for signs of potential heart failure in patients with congestive heart failure who are on digitalis or diuretics: dyspnea on exertion, orthopnea, edema, distended neck veins, night cough, crackles, and weight gain. • Assess diabetic patients for signs and symptoms of hypoglycemia: diaphoresis, fatigue, irritability, hunger, and confusion. • Assess for ocular symptoms; explain to the patient the need to notify the physician immediately if such symptoms develop. • Advise the patient not to drive or operate dangerous equipment until the CNS response to the drug has been determined. • Teach the patient not to discontinue the drug abruptly and not to alter the prescribed dose or administration schedule. • Before discharge, teach the patient to measure pulse rate and to report a slowed or irregular rate to the physician. • Advise the patient not to take any OTC preparations without first consulting the physician.
nadolol	Hypertension	40 mg P.O. once a day; increased gradually in 40 to 80 mg doses to a maximum of 640 mg/day (usual range, 80 to 320 mg). For a patient with renal failure, dosing intervals are based on creatinine clearance levels.	• Before administering the drug, assess the patient's blood pressure and apical pulse for baseline values; withhold the drug and notify the physician if the rate is less than 60. • Before discharge, teach the patient how to measure the pulse rate. • Teach the patient to report a weight gain of 3 to 4 pounds (1.4 to 1.8 kg) per day, cough, orthopnea, fatigue, tachycardia, dyspnea on exertion, edema, or anxiety.

SELECTED MAJOR DRUGS

Adrenergic blocking agents continued

DRUG	MAJOR INDICATIONS	USUAL ADULT DOSAGES	NURSING IMPLICATIONS
nadolol (continued)	Angina	40 mg P.O. once a day; increased every 3 to 7 days to desired effect (range, 80 to 240 mg/day).	• Advise the patient to lie down if dizziness occurs and to use caution while driving or operating dangerous equipment. • Teach the patient to taper the dose gradually and never to discontinue the drug abruptly or alter the dose or administration schedule without consulting the physician.
propranolol	Hypertension	40 mg P.O. b.i.d. to desired effect (usual range, 120 to 240 mg in two or three divided doses, or 120 to 160 mg of sustained-release capsules once a day)	• Administer beta-adrenergic blockers with extreme caution to patients with respiratory conditions such as asthma, hay fever, bronchitis, emphysema, or allergic rhinitis. Severe bronchospasm may occur. • Administer propranolol before meals at bedtime to stabilize absorption of the drug. • Assess baseline data—apical pulse, respirations, blood pressure, and periphral circulation—before administering the drug. • Monitor the patient for bradycardia, especially with digitalis therapy; withhold the drug if the heart rate is less than 60 and notify the physician.
	Angina	10 to 20 mg P.O. t.i.d. or q.i.d. increased every 3 to 7 days to achieve desired effects (usual dose, 160 mg/day in divided doses)	• During I.V. administration, monitor the patient's electrocardiogram (EKG) and blood pressure. • Monitor the patient for adverse effects: assess intake and output and daily weight; observe for and report dyspnea on exertion, orthopnea, night cough, crackles, edema, and distended neck veins, which may indicate congestive heart failure.
	Dysrhythmias	10 to 30 mg P.O. t.i.d. or q.i.d. Emergencies: 1 to 3 mg I.V. push (1 mg/minute) repeated in 2 to 3 minutes	• Monitor diabetic patients for hypoglycemia; teach such patients to recognize the signs and symptoms of hypoglycemia not masked by propranolol, such as fatigue, sweating, hunger, or confusion.
	Hypertrophic subaortic stenosis	20 to 40 mg P.O. t.i.d. or q.i.d. or 80 to 160 mg of sustained-release capsules once a day	• Teach the patient to measure the pulse rate, and to report slowing or irregularity to the physician.
	Myocardial infarction	180 to 240 mg P.O. daily in 3 or 4 divided doses	• Instruct the patient never to discontinue drug therapy abruptly, but rather to taper it gradually over a 1- to 2-week period, as ordered.
	Migraine	80 mg P.O. daily in divided doses, increased as necessary (usual range, 160 to 240 mg/day)	• To minimize the effects of orthostatic hypotension, instruct the patient to change position slowly, particularly when moving from a supine to an upright position, and teach the patient to dangle the legs over the bedside for a few minutes before standing. • Advise the patient to lie down if dizziness or light-headedness occurs and to avoid driving or operating dangerous machinery if these CNS effects occur. • Advise the patient to avoid alcohol or limit consumption to prevent elevation of arterial pressure. • Advise the patient not to take any OTC preparations without first consulting the physician.

continued

SELECTED MAJOR DRUGS

Adrenergic blocking agents continued

DRUG	MAJOR INDICATIONS	USUAL ADULT DOSAGES	NURSING IMPLICATIONS
Autonomic ganglionic blocker			
trimethaphan	Hypertension, controlled hypotension in surgery	3 to 4 ml/minute I.V. of a 1 mg/ml solution (500 mg or 10 ml of drug in 500 ml D_5W); adjust individually (within a 0.3 to 6 mg/minute range)	• Before giving trimethaphan, obtain a patient history; administer the drug cautiously to patients with a history of allergies. • Have equipment and supplies available to treat a possible hypotensive reaction: oxygen, resuscitation and ventilation equipment, and vasopressor medication. • Dilute the drug before use. • Do not mix any other drugs with the trimethaphan drug solution. • Use a microdrip administration set or an infusion pump for exact dosage administration. • Position the patient in a supine or head-down position to minimize cerebral anoxia; drug action is enhanced by the reverse Trendelenburg position. • Pupil dilation occurs with the drug; therefore, pupil size cannot be used to determine cerebral anoxia. • Assess the patient's intake and output and check for bladder distention if an indwelling catheter is not in place.

Drug interactions

Many agents can interact with ganglionic blocking agents to cause potentially dangerous effects, either by potentiating or creating additive effects of either or both drugs or by inhibiting the desired effects of the drugs. Perhaps the most dangerous effect is severe hypotension, which can progress to vascular collapse. (See *Drug interactions: Autonomic ganglionic blockers* on page 324 for a summary of the drugs that can interact with ganglionic blockers to produce this and other effects.)

ADVERSE DRUG REACTIONS

Adverse reactions to ganglionic blocking agents are related to their broad, nonspecific blocking effects on the parasympathetic and sympathetic nervous systems.

Predictable reactions

Mild adverse reactions are frequently associated with ganglionic blocking agents and can involve many body systems. Possible cardiovascular manifestations include either tachycardia or bradycardia and orthostatic hypotension. CNS effects may include restlessness, weakness, fatigue, sedation, cycloplegia, or mydriasis. GI and genitourinary signs and symptoms may include glossitis, nausea, vomiting, or anorexia as well as parasympathetic manifestations—dry mouth, constipation (sometimes preceded by small, frequent, liquid stools), decreased bowel sounds, loss of GI tract tone, and decreased bladder tone with urinary hesitancy. Other reactions may include suppression of diaphoresis and respiratory depression.

Severe adverse reactions—often dose-related—can include extreme hypotension, rapid pulse, cyanosis, angina-like pain, vascular collapse, abdominal distention, paralytic ileus, urinary retention, dizziness, syncope, tremors, mental disturbance, paresthesias, and impaired sexual function.

Patients who have undergone sympathectomy, have hypertensive encephalopathy, or are on low-sodium diets are particularly sensitive to these agents.

Unpredictable reactions

Allergic manifestations may include urticaria, pruritus, and a histamine-like reaction of the vein when the I.V. agent is administered.

NURSING IMPLICATIONS

The ganglionic blocking agents' ability to cause severe drug interactions and adverse reactions requires the nurse to be aware of the following considerations:

• Because it can cause histamine release, trimethaphan should be administered with extreme caution to patients with histories of allergy.

• Mecamylamine should be administered with caution to patients with renal, cerebral, or coronary hypertrophy; bladder neck or urethral obstruction; prostatic hypertrophy; or elevated serum blood urea nitrogen (BUN) levels.

• During ganglionic blocker therapy, assess the patient for constipation, abdominal distention, or decreased bowel sounds, which may indicate paralytic ileus.

• Monitor the patient for urinary retention by measuring fluid intake and output and assessing for edema.

• When administering ganglionic blockers intravenously, continuously monitor the patient's blood pressure, pulse, and respiratory rate. After administration, monitor these parameters frequently to assess the patient's therapeutic responses.

• To minimize the risk of cerebral hypoxia, I.V. medication is administered with the patient in a supine or head-down position. Drug action is enhanced by the reverse Trendelenburg position.

• Discontinue the patient's I.V. infusion gradually.

• Trimethaphan must be diluted (1 mg/1 ml of dextrose 5%) before administration.

• Do not mix trimethaphan with any other drug for I.V. administration.

• Administer trimethaphan by continuous I.V. infusion, with the dose titrated in response to the blood pressure. Use microdrip tubing or an infusion pump to facilitate accurate dosage administration.

• Give mecamylamine after meals to enhance absorption, with smaller doses in the morning, when the patient's response is usually greater.

• Monitor the patient for rebound hypertensive crisis during the withdrawal of ganglionic blocking agents.

• Remember that pupillary dilation occurs with use of the drugs; do not use this parameter during patient assessment.

• Explain to the patient that ganglionic blocker effects may be enhanced by fever, infection, exercise, salt depletion, hemorrhage, or pregnancy.

• Teach the patient to minimize orthostatic hypotension by arising slowy from the supine position and dangling the legs over the bedside for a short time before standing.

CHAPTER SUMMARY

Chapter 20 discussed adrenergic blockers as they are used therapeutically to disrupt sympathetic nervous system function. Here are the highlights of the chapter:

• Adrenergic blocking agents, also called *sympatholytics,* are used therapeutically to block sympathetic nervous system function. This drug class includes alpha-adrenergic blockers, beta-adrenergic blockers, and autonomic ganglionic blockers.

• Blockage of alpha-adrenergic receptor sites results in decreased blood pressure due to prevention of contraction of smooth muscles surrounding the arterioles. As a result, alpha-adrenergic blockers provide some therapeutic benefit in treating certain types of hypertension.

• Alpha-adrenergic blocking agents are erratically absorbed, with wide distribution and possible sequestering of the drug in various body tissues, and are usually excreted in urine.

• Adverse reactions to alpha-adrenergic blockers are mostly related to their vasodilation effect and mainly involve the cardiovascular system.

• Beta-adrenergic blockers are classified as selective or nonselective. Selective beta-adrenergic blockers, which preferentially block $beta_1$-receptor sites, produce effects primarily related to the prevention of cardiac excitation. Nonselective beta-adrenergic blockers, which block both $beta_1$- and $beta_2$-receptor sites, prevent not only cardiac excitation but also bronchodilation.

• Because of their cardiovascular effects, beta-adrenergic blockers are used extensively to treat hypertension, cardiac dysrhythmias, and angina pectoris.

• Beta-adrenergic blockers are rapidly and well absorbed, somewhat protein-bound, widely distributed in the body, and excreted primarily in the urine.

• Autonomic ganglionic blocking agents, like alpha- and beta-adrenergic blockers, exert potent hypotensive effects. They work at both the postganglionic fibers of the autonomic nervous system and the adrenal medulla to prevent ephinephrine and norepinephrine secretion.

• Autonomic ganglionic blocking agents exert a nonselective blocking action, inhibiting nerve transmission not only in the sympathetic nervous system but also in the parasympathetic nervous system. Because of their wide-ranging and other unpredictable effects, these agents have limited clinical uses.

BIBLIOGRAPHY

Frishman, W.H., and Teicher, M. "Beta-Adrenergic Blockade: An Update," *Cardiology* 72:280, November/December 1985.

Frishman, W.H., et al. "Use of Beta-Adrenergic Blocking Agents after Myocardial Infarction," *Postgraduate Medicine* 78:40, December 1985.

Kanto, J.H. "Current Status of Labetalol, the First Alpha- and Beta-Blocking Agent," *International Journal of Clinical Pharmacological Therapy and Toxicology* 23:617, November 1985.

Massie, B.M. "Antihypertensive Therapy with Calcium-Channel Blockers: Comparison with Beta-Blockers," *American Journal of Cardiology* 56:97H, December 1, 1985.

Mauro, V.F., and Zeller, F.P. "Early Use of Beta-Adrenergic-Blocking Agents in Myocardial Infarction," *Drug Intelligence and Clinical Pharmacy* 20:14, January 1986.

Pratt, C.M., et al. "The Role of Beta-Blockers in the Treatment of Patients after Infarction," *Cardiology Clinics* 2:13, February 1984.

Squire, A., and Kupersmith, J. "Beta-Adrenergic Blocking Agents: Review and Update," *Mt. Sinai Journal of Medicine* 52:553, September 1985.

Tesch, P.A. "Exercise Performance and Beta-Blockers," *Sports Medicine* 2:389, November/December 1985.

Vlietstra, R.E., and McGoon, M.D. "Beta-Adrenergic Blockers: Choosing Among Them," *Postgraduate Medicine* 76:71, September 1, 1985.

Wood, A.J.J. "How the Beta-Blockers Differ: A Pharmacologic Comparison," *Drug Therapeutics* 13:59, October 1984.

CHAPTER 21

NEUROMUSCULAR BLOCKING AGENTS

OBJECTIVES

After reading and studying this chapter, you should be able to:
1. Differentiate between the actions of nondepolarizing and depolarizing neuromuscular blocking agents.
2. Describe the physiology of the motor end-plate where neuromuscular blocking agents exert their effect.
3. List the major clinical indications for the neuromuscular blocking agents.
4. Describe the pharmacokinetics of the neuromuscular blocking agents.
5. Explain the additive effects that result when drugs interact with the neuromuscular blocking agents.
6. Identify the antidotes to the neuromuscular blocking agents, and describe their mechanisms of action.
7. Describe the nursing implications for patients receiving a neuromuscular blocking agent.

INTRODUCTION

Neuromuscular blocking agents are drugs that act to relax the skeletal muscles by disrupting the transmission of nerve impulses. Because the drugs do not cross the blood-brain barrier, the patient remains conscious and aware of pain.

Neuromuscular blocking agents have three major clinical indications: to relax skeletal muscles during surgery, to reduce the intensity of muscle spasms in drug or electrically induced convulsions, or to manage patients who are fighting mechanical ventilation. This chapter discusses the two main classes of natural and synthetic drugs used as neuromuscular blocking agents: nondepolarizing and depolarizing agents.

For a summary of representative drugs, see *Selected major drugs: Neuromuscular blocking agents* on pages 336 and 337.

The motor end plate

The motor nerve axon divides to form branching terminals called motor end plates. These are enfolded in muscle fibers but are separated from the fibers by the synaptic cleft.

A stimulus to the nerve causes the release of acetylcholine into the synaptic cleft. There, acetylcholine occupies receptor sites on the muscle cell membrane, depolarizing the membrane and causing muscle contraction. Neuromuscular blocking agents act at the motor end plate by competing with acetylcholine for the receptor sites or by blocking depolarization.

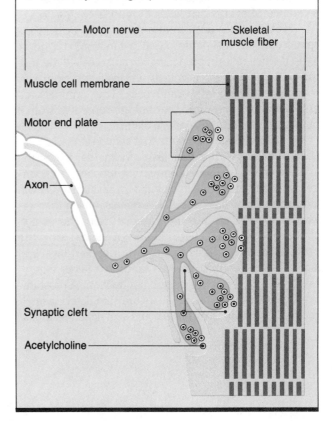

The pharmacokinetics of the nondepolarizing agents

This chart compares the onset of action, peak concentration level, and duration of action of the nondepolarizing blocking agents. Note that all have rapid onset of action and reach peak concentration level in 3 to 5 minutes. Their duration of action varies greatly.

DRUG	ONSET OF ACTION	PEAK CONCENTRATION LEVEL	DURATION OF ACTION
atracurium	2 min	3 to 5 min	20 to 70 min
gallamine	1 to 2 min	3 to 5 min	15 to 30 min
metocurine	1 to 4 min	3 to 5 min	25 to 90 min
pancuronium	less than 1 min	3 to 5 min	12 to 60 min
tubocurarine	1 to 2 min	3 to 5 min	60 min
vecuronium	1 to 2 min	3 to 5 min	20 to 30 min

The physiology of the motor end plate

Neuromuscular blocking agents act at the motor end plate of the motor unit. The motor end plate is the junction between the motor nerve and the skeletal muscle. (See *The motor end plate* on page 331 for an illustration of the physiology and a description of the sequence of events that leads to muscle contraction.)

Motor nerves arise from anterior horn cells in the spinal cord; at the neuromuscular junction, the nerve axon divides to form branching terminals called the motor end plate. These terminals are insulated from surrounding fluid by Schwann's cells. The terminals are enfolded into the muscle fiber but are separated from it by a space called the synaptic cleft.

The sequence of events that triggers muscle contraction begins with a stimulus to the nerve. When the impulse reaches the neuromuscular junction, depolarization occurs, resulting in an influx of calcium ions from the extracellular fluid into the terminals, which then release acetylcholine into the synaptic cleft. The acetylcholine combines with receptor sites on the postjunctional muscle cell membrane, depolarizing it and facilitating the entry of sodium (and, to a lesser extent, calcium). The result is a muscle contraction. Almost immediately after the muscle fibers are stimulated, acetylcholine is inactivated by the enzyme acetylcholinesterase.

NONDEPOLARIZING BLOCKING AGENTS

The nondepolarizing blocking agents, also called competitive or stabilizing agents, are derived curare alkaloids and their synthetic analogues. They produce intermediate to prolonged muscle relaxation, such as that required during surgery for intubation and ventilation.

History and source

Curare is a generic term for various South American arrow poisons derived from plants, most notably species of *Strychnos* and *Chondodendron*. Curare was first used medically by West in 1932 to treat tetanus and spasticity. In 1942, curare was used by Griffith and Johnson to promote muscle relaxation during anesthesia.

PHARMACOKINETICS

Since plasma levels of the nondepolarizing blocking agents are difficult to predict, nerve stimulators are used to assess drug effects on the patient.

Absorption, distribution, metabolism, excretion

Because nondepolarizing blocking agents are poorly absorbed from the gastrointestinal tract, they are administered parenterally. The intravenous route is preferred because the action is more predictable. The drugs, which are rapidly distributed throughout the body, act on the motor end-plates and, to a lesser degree, on the autonomic ganglia. A variable but large proportion of the nondepolarizing agents is lost, unchanged, in the urine. Some of the newer drugs, such as pancuronium, vecuronium, and atracurium, are partially metabolized in the liver.

Onset, peak, duration

Nondepolarizing blocking agents have a rapid onset of action after intravenous administration. Their half-lives vary from 20 minutes to 4 hours. The onset of action of, clinical effect of, and rate of recovery from pancuronium, vecuronium, and atracurium depend on dosage, as well as numerous other factors. Acidosis, inhalation anesthetics, renal or hepatic dysfunction, and hypothermia may prolong the action of these agents. The duration of action of metocurine and tubocurarine is related directly to the total dose and the depth of anesthesia produced by the accompanying anesthetic agent. Repeated doses of metocurine and tubocurarine result in a cumulative effect. The duration of paralysis associated with gallamine is related to total dose, the type of anesthetic, and the depth of anesthesia. (See *The pharmacokinetics of the nondepolarizing agents* for a comparison of the onset of action, peak concentration level, and duration of action of each member of this class of drugs.)

PHARMACODYNAMICS

The therapeutic action of the nondepolarizing blocking agents is based on the relaxation or paralysis of the skeletal muscles.

Mechanism of action

The nondepolarizing blocking agents compete with acetylcholine at the cholinergic receptor sites of the skeletal muscle membrane. This blocks acetycholine's transmitter action, preventing the muscle membrane from depolarizing. The effect can be counteracted clinically by anticholinesterase drugs, such as neostigmine or pyridostigmine, which inhibit the action of acetylcholinesterase, the enzyme that destroys acetylcholine.

The initial muscle weakness produced by the drugs quickly changes to a flaccid paralysis that affects the muscles in a specific sequence. The first muscles to exhibit flaccid paralysis are those innervated by the motor portions of the cranial nerves and small, rapidly moving muscles like those in the eyes, face, and neck. Next, the limb, abdomen, and trunk muscles become flaccid. Finally, the intercostal muscles and the diaphragm are paralyzed. Recovery from the paralysis usually occurs in the reverse order.

Because these drugs do not cross the blood-brain barrier, no alterations in consciousness or pain perception occur. Patients are aware of what is happening to them and may experience extreme anxiety and pain, but they cannot communicate their feelings.

Nondepolarizing blocking agents also alter the cardiovascular dynamics. First, the mild ganglionic blockade may cause hypotension and tachycardia. Second, all of these drugs except vecuronium increase histamine release to varying degrees, which may accentuate the hypotension. Pancuronium causes little or no histamine release and no ganglionic blockade. Histamine release also produces bronchial spasm and excessive bronchial or salivary secretions. These manifestations are further accentuated by decreased venous return and diminished respiratory excursion from loss of skeletal muscle tone.

PHARMACOTHERAPEUTICS

Nondepolarizing blocking agents are used for intermediate or prolonged muscle relaxation. They facilitate endotracheal intubation and are used during surgery to decrease the amount of anesthetic required and to facilitate the operative manipulations. They are also used to paralyze patients who need ventilatory support but who fight the endotracheal tube and ventilator. Nondepolarizing blocking agents also prevent muscle injury during electroshock therapy by reducing the intensity of muscle spasms. Tubocurarine has an additional use in the diagnostic testing for myasthenia gravis and nerve root compression masked by muscle spasm.

atracurium besylate (Tracrium). Atracurium is used primarily as an adjunct to anesthesia. Unlike the other drugs in this class, atracurium does not appear to have a cumulative effect on the duration of blockade, provided that recovery is allowed to begin before each maintenance dose is given. Doses may thus be administered at relatively regular intervals with predictable blocking effects.
USUAL ADULT DOSAGE: initially, 0.4 to 0.5 mg/kg of body weight I.V.; maintenance dose, usually 0.08 to 0.1 mg/kg every 20 to 45 minutes, depending on duration of action.

gallamine triethiodide (Flaxedil). Gallamine is used to manage patients undergoing mechanical ventilation. But, it is sometimes replaced by pancuronium for long-term ventilation and by succinylcholine for short intubation procedures.

DRUG INTERACTIONS
Nondepolarizing blocking agents

Most interacting drugs enhance the blocking action of the neuromuscular blocking agents and require that the patient be closely observed to prevent fatal complications.

DRUG	INTERACTING DRUGS	POSSIBLE EFFECTS	NURSING IMPLICATIONS
atracurium, gallamine, metocurine, pancuronium, tubocurarine, vecuronium	local or parenteral anesthetics	Potentiate neuromuscular blockade	• Anticipate possible prolonged apnea. • Keep equipment available to provide mechanical ventilation. • Monitor the patient's heart rate and rhythm and blood pressure for signs of cardiovascular collapse. • Be prepared to replace fluids and electrolytes, as necessary. • Keep the antidotes neostigmine and pyridostigmine available.
	inhalation anesthetics	Potentiate neuromuscular blockade by stabilizing the postjunctional membrane	
	aminoglycosides	Potentiate neuromuscular blockade by inhibiting acetylcholine release at the preganglionic terminal and by stabilizing the postjunctional membrane	
	clindamycin	Potentiates neuromuscular blockade	• Monitor the patient for adverse reactions and consult the physician regarding a dosage decrease.
	polymyxin	Potentiates neuromuscular blockade	
	cholinesterase inhibitors	Antagonize neuromuscular blockade	• These agents may be used as antidotes for the nondepolarizing agents.
	calcium channel blockers	Potentiate neuromuscular blockade	
	magnesium salts	Potentiate neuromuscular blockade	• Monitor the patient for adverse reactions and consult the physician regarding a dosage decrease.
	potassium-depleting medications (including amphotericin B, furosemide, and thiazide diuretics)	Potentiate neuromuscular blockade	• Assess potassium level before administration. • Closely monitor patients with decreased renal function.

USUAL ADULT DOSAGE: initially, 1 mg/kg of body weight I.V.; then 0.5 to 1.0 mg/kg every 30 to 40 minutes, not to exceed 100 mg per dose.

metocurine iodide (Metubine). Metocurine is used to reduce trauma during electroshock therapy and to manage patients undergoing mechanical ventilation.
USUAL ADULT DOSAGE: for endoctracheal intubation, 0.2 to 0.4 mg/kg I.V. given over 30 to 60 seconds; supplemental dosage during anesthesia is 0.5 to 1 mg I.V. For electroshock therapy, 1.75 to 5.5 mg I.V. given slowly.

pancuronium bromide (Pavulon). Used to manage patients undergoing mechanical ventilation, pancuronium has minimal histamine-releasing effects, does not block sympathetic ganglia, and therefore does not produce hypotension and bronchospasm. However, it affects the vagus nerve, resulting in an increased pulse rate, as well as increased systolic blood pressure and cardiac output.
USUAL ADULT DOSAGE: for endotracheal intubation, a bolus dosage of 0.06 to 0.1 mg/kg is recommended; for anesthesia purposes, 0.04 to 0.1 mg/kg of body weight I.V.; repeated doses of 0.01 to 0.02 mg/kg administered every 20 to 60 minutes.

tubocurarine chloride (Tubarine). Used as an adjunct in anesthesia to manage patients undergoing endotracheal intubation and mechanical ventilation. Also used to reduce the intensity of muscle spasms in drug- or electrically-induced convulsions and as a diagnostic aid for myasthenia gravis.

USUAL ADULT DOSAGE: for anesthesia purposes, initially 40 to 60 units I.V. slowly over 60 to 90 seconds, then 20 to 30 units in 3 to 5 minutes (1 unit equals .15 mg); for electroshock therapy, 1 unit/kg I.V. slowly; for diagnosis of myasthenia gravis, $\frac{1}{15}$ to $\frac{1}{5}$ the electroshock dosage.

vecuronium bromide (Norcuron). Vecuronium is used for all intermediate and long-term neuromuscular blockade in patients with heart disease or asthma because it does not cause histamine release, which results in hypotension and bronchospasm.

USUAL ADULT DOSAGE: 0.08 to 0.1 mg/kg of body weight I.V.; maintenance dose, 0.01 to 0.015 mg/kg I.V. every 12 to 15 minutes.

Drug interactions

Most drugs that interact with the nondepolarizing blocking agents have an additive effect. For example, some antibiotics and anesthetics potentiate the neuromuscular blockade. Drugs that alter the serum levels of calcium, magnesium, or potassium also alter the effects of the nondepolarizing blocking agents. The anticholinesterases (neostigmine, pyridostigmine, and edrophonium) are antagonistic to nondepolarizing blocking agents and are used as antidotes to the neuromuscular blocking agents. (See *Drug interactions: Nondepolarizing blocking agents* for details regarding these effects and important nursing implications.)

ADVERSE DRUG REACTIONS

Nondepolarizing blocking agents most commonly produce adverse reactions when given to patients who are debilitated, have fluid and electrolyte imbalances, or have respiratory, hepatic, neuromuscular, or renal disorders.

Predictable reactions

The prolonged pharmacologic effects of these drugs are responsible for most adverse reactions. The most serious adverse reaction is apnea. Ganglionic blockade and histamine release may cause a cardiovascular reaction, usually hypotension. However, histamine release may also produce skin reactions, bronchospasm, and excessive bronchial and salivary secretions. Antidotes used to restore breathing may accentuate the hypotension and bronchospasms.

Pancuronium and gallamine selectively block the vagus nerve and may result in tachycardia, cardiac dysrhythmias, and hypertension.

Unpredictable reactions

Allergic reactions to nondepolarizing blocking agents are rare.

NURSING IMPLICATIONS

Patients receiving neuromuscular blocking agents completely depend on the nurse, sometimes for their survival. Remember these special nursing implications when administering these drugs:

● Use caution when administering nondepolarizing blocking agents to patients with renal, hepatic, cardiac, or pulmonary impairment; fluid and electrolyte imbalances; or myasthenia gravis.

● When the drugs are administered for the first time, make sure personnel skilled in intubation and mechanical ventilation are available.

● Keep antidotes to neuromuscular blocking agents available.

● Be sure the mechanical ventilator is functioning properly. Do not turn off the alarm because a patient receiving one of these drugs may die if the ventilator is accidentally disconnected.

● Suction the patient whenever necessary because the cough reflex is suppressed and the patient may have increased respiratory secretions.

● Monitor the patient's vital signs, fluid intake and output, and electrolytes before and throughout the therapy.

● Since cognition is not depressed by these drugs, keep the patient fully informed to reduce anxiety. Explain all procedures in advance, and emphasize that nurses will closely monitor the patient. Post a sign at the bedside to remind all personnel to follow these guidelines.

● Medicate the patient for pain because neuromuscular blocking agents do not relieve pain.

● Use artificial tears to prevent corneal ulceration if the patient's eyes remain open. Do not tape the patient's eyes shut or you will increase patient anxiety. Eye movement is one of the first signs of recovery.

DEPOLARIZING BLOCKING AGENTS

Succinylcholine is the only therapeutic depolarizing blocking agent. Although it is similar to the nondepolarizing blocking agents in its therapeutic effect, its mechanism of action differs.

History and source

Succinylcholine was first used in 1906 by Hunt and Taveau in experiments with animals that received curare, which masked succinylcholine's effects. Forty years elapsed before succinylcholine's action at the motor endplate was recognized, and it was first used clinically around 1949.

PHARMACOKINETICS

Because succinylcholine is poorly absorbed from the gastrointestinal tract, the preferred administration route is intravenous, but the intramuscular route may be used if necessary. When given intravenously, succinylcholine has an onset of action of 30 seconds. The drug reaches a peak concentration level in 1 minute; its duration of action is 4 to 10 minutes. It is hydrolyzed in the liver and plasma by pseudocholinesterase, and a resulting metabolite, succinylmonocholine, produces a nondepolarizing blocking action. Succinylcholine is excreted via the kidneys; approximately 10% is excreted unchanged.

PHARMACODYNAMICS

Succinylcholine's therapeutic action is twofold: Phase I is a depolarizing blocker and Phase II is a nondepolar-

---

SELECTED MAJOR DRUGS

Neuromuscular blocking agents

Physicians prescribe neuromuscular blocking agents to induce short- and long-term muscle relaxation. Patients receiving these agents must be closely monitored because of drug effects. Patients may require ventilatory support.

DRUG	MAJOR INDICATIONS	USUAL ADULT DOSAGES	NURSING IMPLICATIONS
Nondepolarizing blocking agents			
pancuronium	Used as adjunct to anesthesia Used to assist in mechanical intubation and ventilation Used to prevent trauma during electroshock therapy	For endotracheal intubation a bolus dosage of 0.06 to 0.1 mg/kg of body weight is recommended. For anesthesia purposes 0.04 to 0.1 mg/kg of body weight I.V.; repeat doses of 0.01 to 0.02 mg/kg every 20 to 60 minutes as needed.	• The drug is contraindicated in patients with hypersensitivity to bromides. • Administer with caution to patients with renal, hepatic, cardiac, or pulmonary impairment; fluid and electrolyte imbalances; or myasthenia gravis. • Assess baseline vital signs. • Monitor electrolytes regularly for adverse reactions. • Keep endotracheal equipment, oxygen, suction, and mechanical ventilator available for respiratory support. • Keep antidotes (edrophonium, neostigmine, or pyridostigmine) available. • Provide emotional reassurance and support for the patient.
tubocurarine	Used as adjunct to anesthesia Used to assist in mechanical intubation and ventilation	For anesthesia purposes the dosage is initially 40 to 60 units I.V. slowly over 60 to 90 seconds then 20 to 30 units in 3 to 5 minutes (one unit equals 0.15	• Administer with caution to patients with renal, hepatic, cardiac, or pulmonary impairment; fluid and electrolyte imbalance; or myasthenia gravis. Also use caution in patients undergoing a cesarean section. • Do not mix with barbiturates.

SELECTED MAJOR DRUGS

Neuromuscular blocking agents continued

DRUG	MAJOR INDICATIONS	USUAL ADULT DOSAGES	NURSING IMPLICATIONS
tubocurarine (continued)	Used to prevent trauma during electroshock therapy Used as a diagnostic aid for myasthenia gravis	mg). For electroshock therapy the dosage is one unit/kg of body weight I.V. slowly. For diagnosis of myasthenia gravis the dosage is ⅟₁₅ to ⅕ the electroshock therapy dosage.	• Assess baseline vital signs. • Monitor electrolytes regularly for adverse reactions. • Monitor intake and output. • Keep endotracheal equipment, oxygen, suction, and mechanical ventilator available for respiratory support. • Keep antidotes (edrophonium, neostigmine, or pyridostigmine) available. • Provide emotional reassurance and support for the patient.
Depolarizing blocking agents			
succinylcholine	Used as adjunct to anesthesia Used to facilitate intubation and orthopedic manipulation Used to prevent trauma during electroshock therapy	For short surgical procedures 0.3 to 1.1 mg/kg of body weight I.V.; then 0.04 to 0.07 mg/kg of body weight as needed; for longer surgical procedures, continuous I.V. infusion of 0.1% to 0.2% solution at a rate of 0.5 to 10 mg/min for up to 1 hour.	• Administer with caution to patients with renal, pulmonary, or neuromuscular disorders; fluid and electrolyte imbalances; increased intraocular pressure; or a family history of malignant hyperthermia or low serum pseudocholinesterase levels. • Use only freshly prepared solutions. • Do not mix with barbiturates. • If given intramuscularly, inject deep into the muscle. • Administer an initial test dose of 10 mg, as prescribed, to determine the patient's sensitivity to the drug. • Assess baseline vital signs, and monitor regularly for adverse reactions. • Keep endotracheal equipment, oxygen, suction, and mechanical ventilator available for respiratory support. • Reassure the patient that muscle soreness is normal (sometimes counteracted by hexafluorenium or a nondepolarizing agent). • Provide emotional reassurance and support for the patient.

izing blocker. Initially, succinylcholine acts like acetylcholine and depolarizes the postsynaptic membrane of the muscle. However, succinylcholine is not inactivated by cholinesterase, so the depolarization lasts longer. This results in brief periods of repetitive excitation, manifested by muscle fasciculations (uncoordinated contractions of muscle fibers). These are rapidly followed by muscle paralysis and flaccidity. With subsequent doses of the drug or interactions with other drugs, this depolarizing blocking action becomes a nondepolarizing blocking action. Consequently, the antidotes for a nondepolarizing blocker may also be effective against succinylcholine.

PHARMACOTHERAPEUTICS

Succinylcholine is the drug of choice in situations requiring short-term muscle relaxation—for example, during intubation and electroshock therapy.

succinylcholine (Anectine, Quelicin, Sucostrin). Physicians use succinylcholine primarily to induce short-term muscle relaxation.
USUAL ADULT DOSAGE: for short surgical procedures, 0.3 to 1.1 mg/kg of body weight; for longer surgical procedures, continuous I.V. infusion of 0.1% to 0.2% solution at a rate of 0.5 to 10.0 mg/minute for up to 1 hour, then 0.04 to 0.07 mg/kg of body weight is recommended.

Drug interactions

The action of succinylcholine is potentiated by a number of anesthetics, antibiotics, and cholinesterase inhibitors. However, succinylcholine does not interact with the majority of drugs that alter serum electrolyte levels. Cholinesterase inhibitors antagonize Phase II of succinylcholine's blocking action.

ADVERSE DRUG REACTIONS

The primary adverse drug reactions to succinylcholine are the same as those to the nondepolarizing blocking agents: prolonged apnea and cardiovascular alterations.

Predictable reactions

Patients commonly experience muscle pain from the fasciculations that occur in Phase I. These may also cause myoglobinemia and myoglobinuria, especially in children. The concomitant rise in the serum potassium level can be dangerous to patients with renal or neuromuscular disorders. The transient elevation of intraocular pressure that occurs during Phase I may be harmful to patients with previously elevated intraocular pressure.

Unpredictable reactions

Neuromuscular blockade may be potentiated by certain genetic predispositions, such as a low pseudocholinesterase level and the tendency to develop malignant hyperthermia. A low pseudocholinesterase level is also present in liver disorders because pseudocholinesterase is synthesized in the liver. To determine the patient's sensitivity to succinylcholine, an initial test dose of 10 mg may be administered.

Tachyphylaxis (decreasing response to stimulation) may occur with repeated doses of succinylcholine.

NURSING IMPLICATIONS

The overall nursing implications for succinylcholine are the same as those for the nondepolarizing blocking agents listed on page 335 in this chapter.

CHAPTER SUMMARY

Here are the highlights of this chapter:
• Neuromuscular blocking agents relax skeletal muscles by disrupting nerve impulse transmission. They have three major uses: to relax skeletal muscles during surgery, to reduce the intensity of muscle spasms in drug or electrically induced convulsions, or to manage patients who are fighting mechanical ventilation.

• The two classes of neuromuscular blocking agents are nondepolarizing and depolarizing blocking agents.

• The nondepolarizing blocking agents are used when intermediate or prolonged duration of action is required. They compete with acetylcholine at the receptor sites on the postjunctional membrane (motor end-plate), blocking the depolarization required for muscle contraction. This class is composed of curare alkaloids and their synthetic derivatives.

• The depolarizing blocking agent acts like acetylcholine and results in depolarization of the postjunctional membrane. However, unlike acetylcholine, the depolarizing agent is not subject to breakdown by cholinesterase. Therefore, the depolarization lasts longer and the muscle temporarily loses its ability to respond. With continued drug use, the depolarizing blocking action changes to a nondepolarizing blocking action. Succinylcholine is the drug of choice for short-term muscle relaxation.

• The nurse must monitor the vital functions of any patient receiving these drugs. The maintenance of respiratory function is the top priority. However, because these drugs also alter cardiovascular function and fluid and electrolyte balance, careful monitoring is required.

BIBLIOGRAPHY

Berne, R.M., and Levy, M.N., eds. *Physiology.* St. Louis: C.V. Mosby Co., 1983.

Craig, C.R., and Stitzel, R.E. *Modern Pharmacology,* 2nd edition. Boston: Little, Brown & Co., 1986.

Engbaek, J., and Viby-Mogensen, J. "Precurarization—A Hazard to the Patient?" *Acta Anaesthesiologica Scandinavica.* 28(1):61, January 1984.

Engbaek, J., et al. "Precurarization with Vecuronium and Pancuronium in Awake, Healthy Volunteers: The Influence on Neuromuscular Transmission and Pulmonary Function," *Acta Anaesthesiologica Scandinavica,* 29(1):117, January 1985.

FitzGerald, M.J.T. *Neuroanatomy: Basic and Applied.* Philadelphia: Bailliere Tindall, 1985.

Goodman, A.G., et al, eds. *Goodman and Gilman's The Pharmacological Basis of Therapeutics,* 7th edition. New York: Macmillan Publishing Co., 1985.

Goth, A., ed. *Medical Pharmacology: Principles and Concepts,* 11th edition. St. Louis: C.V. Mosby Co., 1984.

Greenblatt, D.J., and Shader, R.I. *Pharmacokinetics in Clinical Practice.* Philadelphia: W.B. Saunders Co., 1985.

Guyton, A.C. *Textbook of Medical Physiology,* 7th edition. Philadelphia: W.B. Saunders Co., 1986.

Harper, K.W., et al. "Reversal of Neuromuscular Block," *Anaesthesia.* 39(8):772, August 1984.

Herrold, R.K. "The Drug Connection," *American Journal of Nursing.* 84(11):1389, November 1984.

Lowry, K.G., et al. "Vecuronium and Atracurium in the Elderly: A Clinical Comparison with Pancuronium," *Acta Anaesthesiologica Scandinavica,* 29(4):405, May 1985.

Mirakhur, R.K. "Antagonism of Neuromuscular Block in the Elderly," *Anaesthesia.* 40(3):254, March 1985.

Scott, R.D.F., and Basta, S.J. "Cardiovascular and Autonomic Effects of Muscle Relaxants," *Comprehensive Therapy.* 11(3):56, March 1985.

Taylor, P. "Are Neuromuscular Blocking Agents More Efficacious in Pairs?" *The Journal of Anesthesiology.* 63:1, 1985.

USPDI: Drug Information for the Health Care Provider, vol. 1, 6th edition. Rockville, Md.: United States Pharmacopeial Convention, Inc., 1985.

Ward, S., and Neill, E.A.M. "Pharmacokinetics of Atracurium in Acute Hepatic Failure (with Acute Renal Failure)," *British Journal of Anaesthesia.* 55(12):1169, December 1983.

DRUGS TO TREAT NEUROLOGIC AND NEUROMUSCULAR SYSTEM DISORDERS

Unit four discusses pharmacologic agents used to treat neurologic and neuromuscular system disorders, including skeletal muscle relaxing, antiparkinsonian, and anticonvulsant agents. An overview of the anatomy and physiology of the nervous system will assist the nurse in understanding the pharmacotherapeutics of these agents.

Anatomy of the nervous system

The nervous system is composed of the central and peripheral divisions. The central nervous system (CNS) consists of the brain and spinal cord. (See *Structures of the central nervous system* on page 343 for an illustration of the components.)

The brain is composed of the cerebrum, diencephalon, cerebellum, and brain stem. Two structurally matched hemispheres make up the cerebrum, the largest portion of the brain. Each hemisphere contains four lobes—frontal, parietal, temporal, and occipital. The surface of the cerebrum (cortex) is composed of gray matter made of neuron cell bodies, axon terminals, and dendrites. The interior of the cerebrum is composed of white matter made of basal ganglia. The corpus callosum facilitates communication between the corresponding areas in the two hemispheres.

The diencephalon, located anterior to the brain stem, includes the hypothalamus and thalamus. The cerebellum lies at the base of the brain below the occipital lobes of the cerebrum. The brain stem, composed of the midbrain, pons, and medulla oblongata, relays all messages between the upper and lower levels of the nervous system; cranial nerves III through XII originate there.

The spinal cord serves as a communication pathway between the brain and the peripheral nervous system. The spinal cord's gray matter functions as a reflex center for spinal reflexes. It joins the brain stem at the level of the foramen magnum and terminates near the second lumbar vertebra. The spinal cord comprises a central H-shaped mass of gray matter divided into dorsal (or posterior) and ventral (or anterior) horns. Cell bodies in the dorsal horn relay sensory (afferent) impulses, and those in the ventral horn relay motor (efferent) impulses. White matter surrounding these horns consists of myelinated axons of sensory and motor nerves grouped in ascending and descending tracts. (See *Cross section of the spinal cord* on page 344 for a depiction of these structures.)

The peripheral nervous system is composed of the cranial and spinal nerves, which carry sensory messages from organs and tissues to the brain and motor instructions from the brain to target organs.

The 12 pairs of cranial nerves provide for the sensory and motor needs primarily of the head but also of the neck, chest, and abdomen. Cranial nerves I and II originate in the frontal lobe, whereas III through XII originate in the brain stem.

The 31 pairs of spinal nerves originate in the spinal cord. These paired nerves include 8 cervical, 12 thoracic, 5 lumbar, 5 sacral, and 1 coccygeal. Cervical 3 to thoracic 2 supply the upper extremities, whereas thoracic 9 through 12 supply the lower extremities.

Physiology of the nervous system

The nervous system governs all movement, sensation, thought, and emotion. Two types of cells constitute the nervous system: neuroglial cells and neurons. Neuroglial cells perform specialized support functions, such as supplying nutrients to the neurons, assisting in the production of cerebrospinal fluid, and providing electrical insulation for the axons of the CNS neurons.

The neuron consists of a cell body and two types of appendages, a long one (an axon) and one or more shorter ones (dendrites). Cell bodies form the gray matter in the brain, brain stem, and spinal cord. The axon transmits impulses from the cell body to other neurons, while dendrites receive impulses from nearby cells and conduct them toward the cell body.

Neurons perform one of three roles in transmitting impulses: reception of sensory stimuli, transmission of motor responses, or integration of activities and coordination of communication between body parts. Sensory neurons carry stimuli from the peripheral sensory organs, such as the skin, to the spinal cord and brain. Motor

Glossary

Absence seizure: generalized seizure characterized by an abrupt loss of consciousness or unawareness with staring; also called petit mal seizure.

Acetylcholine: reversible choline acetic acid ester in many parts of the body that facilitates impulse transmission from one nerve fiber to another across a synaptic junction.

Actin: muscle protein in muscle filaments that acts with myosin to contract and relax muscle.

Agonist: drug that has an affinity for a receptor and enhances or stimulates the receptor's functional properties.

Akinesia: abnormal absence of movement.

Anticholinergic: agent that blocks acetylcholine release at the myoneural junction.

Areflexia: absence of reflexes.

Asthenia: lack or loss of strength and energy.

Ataxia: impaired ability to coordinate movement.

Atonic seizure: generalized seizure accompanied by akinesia and usually loss of consciousness.

Axon: cylindrical extension of a nerve cell that carries impulses away from the neuron cell body.

Cholinergic: agent that stimulates acetylcholine release at the myoneural junction; also known as parasympathomimetic.

Clonic seizure: rhythmic contraction and relaxation of muscles, characterized by loss of consciousness and marked autonomic signs and symptoms.

Decerebrate: describes behavior characterized by a lack of brain function.

Dendrite: branching process that extends from the nerve cell and carries impulses to the cell body.

Dopamine: neurotransmitter produced by the decarboxylation of dopa, an intermediate product in the synthesis of norepinephrine.

Dopaminergic: stimulated, activated, or transmitted by dopamine.

Dyskinesia: impaired power of voluntary movement resulting in fragmentary or incomplete movements.

Dystonia: disordered muscle tone.

Electroencephalogram (EEG): graphic recording of electrical currents produced in the brain.

Encephalitis: inflammation of the brain.

Epilepsy: disorder characterized by one or more of the following symptoms: paroxysmally recurring impairment or loss of consciousness, involuntary excess or cessation of muscle movements, psychic or sensory disturbances, and derangement of the autonomic nervous system.

Ganglion: group of nerve cell bodies located outside the CNS.

Generalized seizure: bilaterally symmetrical, violent, involuntary contractions of voluntary muscles involving loss of consciousness; more specifically classified as absence, myoclonic, clonic, tonic, tonic-clonic, or atonic seizure.

Hyperkinesia: abnormally increased motor function or activity.

Hyperpyrexia: highly elevated body temperature.

Hypotonia: abnormally decreased muscle tone, tension, or activity.

Interneuron: any neuron, in a chain of neurons, that is situated between the primary afferent neuron and the final motor neuron.

Monoamine oxidase inhibitor: substance that opposes the action of monoamine oxidase, an enzyme in the nerve endings that deaminates, or breaks down, catecholamines.

Myoclonic seizure: bilaterally symmetrical, involuntary lightning jerks of voluntary muscles lasting from seconds to minutes and characterized by the retention of consciousness.

Myofibril: slender, threadlike contractile element that parallels the long axis of a muscle fiber.

Myosin: abundant muscle protein that acts with actin to produce muscle contraction and relaxation.

Neuromuscular junction: joining of a nerve ending and a muscle fiber at the fiber's midpoint so that action potential in the fiber travels bidirectionally.

Neurotransmitter: chemical substance secreted by the neuron at the synapse that acts on receptor proteins in the membrane of the adjacent neuron to stimulate, inhibit, or modify the neuron's activity.

Paraplegia: motor and sensory paralysis of the legs and lower part of the body.

Parasympatholytic: agent that blocks the passage of impulses through the parasympathetic nervous system; also known as anticholinergic.

Paresthesia: abnormal burning, pricking, or tingling sensation.

Parkinson's disease: disorder characterized by muscular rigidity, immobile facies, tremors that disappear upon volitional movement, and loss of associated autonomic movement and salivation.

Partial seizure: focal or local violent, involuntary contractions of voluntary muscles; more specifically classified as simple, complex, or secondarily generalized seizure.

Quadriplegia: paralysis of all four extremities.

Relaxant: agent that reduces or lessens muscle tension.

Rigidity: abnormal muscle stiffness or inflexibility.

continued

Glossary continued

Sarcolemma: delicate elastic sheath that surrounds a striated muscle fiber.

Sarcoplasmic reticulum: network of tubular and flat vesicular structures that conduct electrical impulses and coordinate the contraction of myofibrils.

Spasm: sudden, violent, involuntary contraction of a muscle or group of muscles, accompanied by pain, dysfunction, involuntary movement, and distortion.

Spasticity: increased muscle tension resulting in continually increased resistance to stretching.

Status epilepticus: series of rapidly repeated epileptic seizures without periods of consciousness separating them.

Synapse: area of contact between the processes of two adjacent neurons where an impulse is transmitted.

Synaptic cleft: space between a nerve fiber terminal and the fiber membrane.

Tonic-clonic seizure: contraction of all skeletal muscles in rhythmic alternating tonic and clonic patterns, followed by depression of all central functions; also known as grand mal seizure.

Tonic seizure: abrupt increase in muscle tone, resulting in contraction, loss of consciousness, and marked autonomic signs and symptoms.

Tremor: involuntary trembling or quivering.

Urticaria: vascular reaction of the skin characterized by the transient appearance of smooth, slightly elevated patches that are redder or paler than surrounding skin; often accompanied by severe pruritus.

---

neurons carry impulses from the brain and spinal cord to tissues and organs. Interneurons relay impulses within the CNS.

All human functions rely on the electrical and chemical transmission of impulses from neuron to neuron. This transmission occurs across a synapse, or the contact point between two neurons. Neurotransmission is facilitated by neurotransmitters, such as acetylcholine and dopamine. (See *Neurotransmission* on page 345 for an illustration of this process.)

Chapter 22
Skeletal Muscle Relaxing Agents

Chapter 22 discusses those centrally and peripherally acting agents used to treat musculoskeletal spasms and spasticity. Beginning with an overview of normal muscle physiology, the chapter provides a clinical delineation of musculoskeletal spasms and spasticity. Then the mechanisms of action of the two types of muscle relaxing agents are detailed. The pharmacotherapeutic uses of the various agents are presented, as well as nursing implications and patient education information.

Chapter 23
Antiparkinsonian Agents

Chapter 23 describes Parkinson's disease and the agents used to treat it. The two major drug classes presented are the synthetic anticholinergic agents and the dopaminergic agents. Clinical benefits for the patient are emphasized, as are potential adverse reactions. Associated nursing implications and specific nursing interventions, including patient education, are explored.

Chapter 24
Anticonvulsant Agents

The chapter introduction discusses the four factors used to select an anticonvulsant. Then the international classification system for seizure disorders, including clinical characteristics, is presented. The classes of anticonvulsants discussed are hydantoins, barbiturates, iminostilbenes, benzodiazepines, succinimides, and valproic acid. The specific clinical uses for each drug are delineated, as well as other pharmacologic properties. Nursing implications and interventions and patient education are highlighted.

Nursing diagnoses

The nursing diagnoses that are most applicable when caring for patients receiving drugs for neurologic or neuromuscular system disorders are:

• Activity intolerance related to neurologic or neuromuscular system pathology or dysfunction

• Alterations in bowel elimination: constipation or diarrhea related to neurologic or neuromuscular system pathology or dysfunction, or drug therapy

• Alterations in comfort: pain related to spasticity or immobility

• Alterations in family processes related to neurologic or neuromuscular system pathology or dysfunction, drug therapy, or life-style changes

• Alterations in health maintenance related to neurologic or neuromuscular system pathology or dysfunction, or drug therapy

Structures of the central nervous system

The brain, brain stem, and spinal cord function synergistically to control movement, sensation, thought, and emotion. Major structures and their functions are given below.

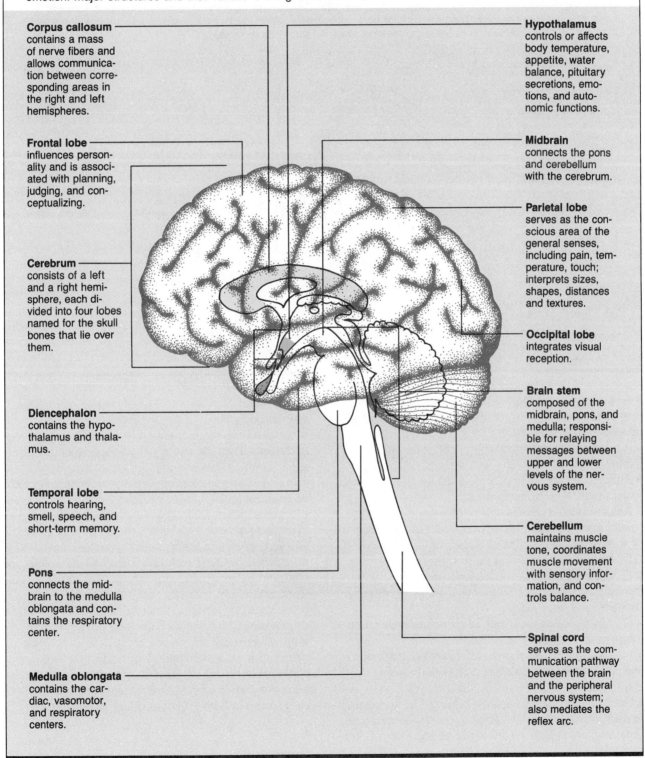

Corpus callosum contains a mass of nerve fibers and allows communication between corresponding areas in the right and left hemispheres.

Frontal lobe influences personality and is associated with planning, judging, and conceptualizing.

Cerebrum consists of a left and a right hemisphere, each divided into four lobes named for the skull bones that lie over them.

Diencephalon contains the hypothalamus and thalamus.

Temporal lobe controls hearing, smell, speech, and short-term memory.

Pons connects the midbrain to the medulla oblongata and contains the respiratory center.

Medulla oblongata contains the cardiac, vasomotor, and respiratory centers.

Hypothalamus controls or affects body temperature, appetite, water balance, pituitary secretions, emotions, and autonomic functions.

Midbrain connects the pons and cerebellum with the cerebrum.

Parietal lobe serves as the conscious area of the general senses, including pain, temperature, touch; interprets sizes, shapes, distances and textures.

Occipital lobe integrates visual reception.

Brain stem composed of the midbrain, pons, and medulla; responsible for relaying messages between upper and lower levels of the nervous system.

Cerebellum maintains muscle tone, coordinates muscle movement with sensory information, and controls balance.

Spinal cord serves as the communication pathway between the brain and the peripheral nervous system; also mediates the reflex arc.

Cross section of the spinal cord

The spinal cord consists of gray matter, including the ventral and dorsal horn, surrounded by white matter. White matter contains many nerve fiber tracts that relay messages to and from the brain. When a peripheral nerve is stimulated, the impulse travels to the dorsal root ganglion through the sensory neuron dendrite to the dorsal horn. The impulse travels to the brain via the nerve fiber tracts. Then the brain responses travel down the spinal cord and out the ventral root to the motor neuron axon. A motor response results.

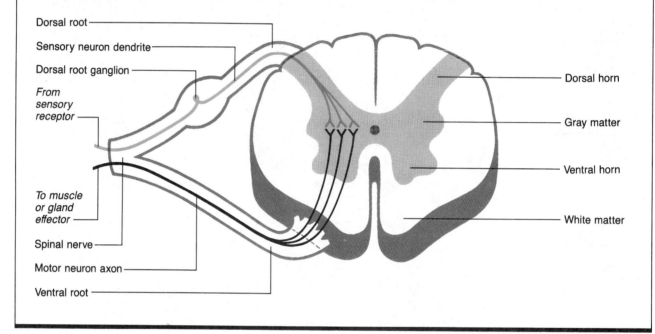

Dorsal root
Sensory neuron dendrite
Dorsal root ganglion
From sensory receptor
To muscle or gland effector
Spinal nerve
Motor neuron axon
Ventral root

Dorsal horn
Gray matter
Ventral horn
White matter

- Alterations in nutrition: less than body requirements, related to neurologic or neuromuscular system pathology or dysfunction
- Alterations in oral mucous membranes related to drug therapy
- Alterations in thought processes related to neurologic system pathology or dysfunction
- Anxiety related to all aspects of neurologic or neuromuscular system pathology or dysfunction, particularly periodically altered levels of consciousness and loss of sensory and motor function, or drug therapy
- Diversional activity deficit related to neurologic or neuromuscular system pathology or dysfunction, particularly spasticity and immobility
- Dysfunctional grieving related to neurologic or neuromuscular function
- Fear related to all aspects of neurologic or neuromuscular system pathology or dysfunction, or drug therapy
- Fluid volume deficit: potential, related to neurologic or neuromuscular system pathology or dysfunction, particularly altered levels of consciousness and loss of motor function

- Hopelessness related to loss of neurologic or neuromuscular function
- Impaired adjustment related to neurologic or neuromuscular system pathology or dysfunction, or drug therapy
- Impaired communication: verbal, related to neurologic or neuromuscular system pathology or dysfunction
- Impaired home maintenance management related to neurologic or neuromuscular system pathology or dysfunction, or drug therapy
- Impaired physical mobility related to neurologic or neuromuscular system pathology or dysfunction, particularly ataxia and spasticity, or drug therapy
- Impaired skin integrity: potential, related to neurologic or neuromuscular system pathology or dysfunction
- Impaired social interaction related to neurologic or neuromuscular system pathology or dysfunction, particularly altered levels of consciousness and spasticity
- Impaired swallowing related to neurlogic or neuromuscular system pathology or dysfunction, or drug therapy

Neurotransmission

Neurotransmission is the conduction of impulses across the synapse. It involves the transmitter neuron's presynaptic terminal, target receptor neuron (postsynaptic receptor), and the synaptic cleft between the two neurons. Numerous presynaptic terminals branch from the tips of axons. These terminals contain synaptic vesicles, which, when stimulated, release neurotransmitter substances into the synaptic cleft to excite or inhibit the target receptor neuron. On a larger scale, the interneuron synapses with the sensory neuron and the motor neuron, as shown below.

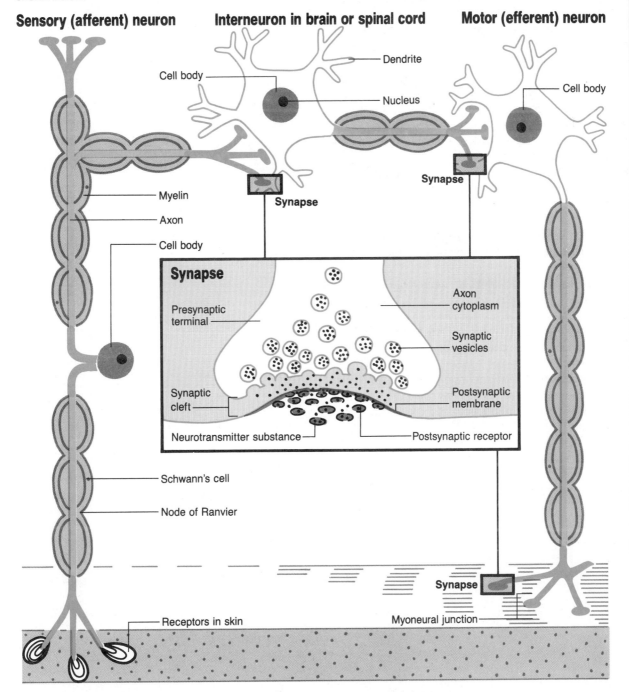

- Ineffective airway clearance related to altered levels of consciousness or to neurologic or neuromuscular system pathology or dysfunction
- Ineffective family coping: compromised, related to neurologic or neuromuscular system pathology or dysfunction, drug therapy, life-style changes, or inadequate support system
- Ineffective individual coping related to neurologic or neuromuscular system pathology or dysfunction, drug therapy, life-style changes, or inadequate support system
- Knowledge deficit related to all aspects of neurologic or neuromuscular system pathology or dysfunction, or drug therapy
- Noncompliance related to drug therapy
- Potential for injury related to neurologic or neuromuscular system pathology or dysfunction—particularly altered levels of consciousness, muscular weakness, paralysis, or ataxia—or drug therapy
- Powerlessness related to loss of neurologic or neuromuscular function
- Self-care deficit related to neurologic or neuromuscular system pathology or dysfunction, or drug therapy
- Self-concept disturbances related to loss of neurologic or neuromuscular function or life-style changes
- Sensory-perceptual alterations related to neurologic or neuromuscular system pathology or dysfunction, or drug therapy
- Sexual dysfunction related to neurologic or neuromuscular system pathology or dysfunction, or drug therapy
- Sleep pattern disturbances related to neurologic or neuromuscular system pathology or dysfunction, particularly spasticity
- Social isolation related to neurologic or neuromuscular system pathology or dysfunction, particularly altered levels of consciousness, immobility, and spasticity.

22

SKELETAL MUSCLE RELAXING AGENTS

OBJECTIVES

After reading and studying this chapter, you should be able to:
1. Differentiate among the skeletal muscle relaxing agents that act centrally and those that act peripherally.
2. Describe the mechanism of action of the centrally and peripherally acting skeletal muscle relaxing agents.
3. Discuss the physiology of skeletal muscle contraction.
4. List the therapeutic uses for the various groups of skeletal muscle relaxing agents.
5. Define spasm and spasticity.
6. Describe the adverse reactions that occur when these agents are given with central nervous system (CNS) depressants.
7. Discuss the mechanism of action of baclofen and its use with lesions of the spinal cord.

INTRODUCTION

Skeletal muscle relaxing agents relieve musculoskeletal pain or spasm and severe musculoskeletal spasticity. They are used to treat acute, painful musculoskeletal conditions and the muscle spasticity associated with multiple sclerosis, cerebral palsy, cerebrovascular accident, and spinal cord injuries. Chapter 22 discusses the two main classes of skeletal muscle relaxing agents—centrally acting and peripherally acting agents—and baclofen and diazepam, two other drugs that are used to manage musculoskeletal disorders.

The physiology of skeletal muscle contraction

Skeletal muscles are innervated by large nerve fibers containing motor neurons that originate in the anterior horns of the spinal cord, but the neurotransmitters that relay excitatory or inhibitory signals to the spinal motor neurons are not completely understood. Five have been identified— acetylcholine, norepinephrine, serotonin, glycine, and gamma-aminobutyric acid (GABA); of them, acetylcholine is an excitatory neurotransmitter, and glycine and GABA are inhibitory.

Nerve endings join muscle fiber at the neuromuscular junction. Skeletal muscles themselves are made up of muscle fibers composed of actin and myosin filaments—protein molecule compounds that are responsible for muscle contraction. These filaments are embedded in the sarcoplasm, which also holds a network of tubules, the sarcoplasmic reticulum. Skeletal muscle contraction apparently is triggered by high concentrations of sodium which trigger the release of calcium ions from the sarcoplasmic reticulum. (See Chapter 21, Neuromuscular Blocking Agents, for an illustration of this process.)

Some drugs that relieve skeletal muscle spasticity are believed to act in the spinal cord to alter neurotransmitter function, whereas others act peripherally on the skeletal muscle itself. The centrally acting skeletal muscle relaxants probably inhibit interneuron activity in the spinal cord and the brain.

Acute musculoskeletal spasms and spasticity

Severe cold, lack of blood flow to a muscle, or overexertion can elicit pain or other sensory impulses that are transmitted by the posterior sensory nerve fibers to the spinal cord and the higher levels of the CNS. These sensory impulses may cause a reflex (involuntary) muscle contraction, or spasm. The muscle contraction further stimulates the sensory receptors to a more intense contraction, establishing a cycle. The centrally acting muscle relaxants are believed to break this cycle by acting as CNS depressants.

Spasticity is a motor disorder characterized by an increase in muscle tone from hyperexcitability of the anterior motor neurons. This hyperexcitability may arise from a lack of inhibition or from excess stimulation produced by signals transmitted from the brain through the interneurons in the spinal cord to the anterior motor neurons. Spasticity is associated with a number of clinical conditions, called upper motor neuron disorders, including multiple sclerosis, cerebral palsy, cerebral vascular accident (stroke), and spinal cord injuries. The skeletal muscle relaxants vary in their efficacy; they apparently reduce spasticity by reducing hyperexcitability.

For a summary of representative drugs, see *Selected major drugs: Skeletal muscle relaxing agents* on page 356.

CENTRALLY ACTING SKELETAL MUSCLE RELAXANTS

Such conditions as trauma, inflammation, anxiety, and pain can be associated with acute muscle spasms. The following drugs have been used to try to alleviate such spasms: carisoprodol, chlorphenesin carbamate, chlorzoxazone, cyclobenzaprine hydrochloride, metaxalone, methocarbamol, and orphenadrine citrate. Lack of controlled clinical trials makes assessing these agents difficult. They are known, however, to be ineffective in treating spasticity associated with chronic neurologic disease.

History and source

Antodyne was introduced in 1910 as an analgesic and antipyretic. The drug also caused paralysis of skeletal muscles. In 1946, Berger and Bradely found that mephenesin was a potent skeletal muscle relaxant with activity similar to that of antodyne. Thus, mephenesin became the prototype muscle relaxant, although its clinical usefulness was limited by its brief duration of action.

Methocarbamol replaced mephenesin as a muscle relaxant because of its significantly longer duration of action. The other centrally acting skeletal muscle relaxants were developed in an effort to improve further on mephenesin.

PHARMACOKINETICS

The pharmacokinetic properties of the centrally acting skeletal muscle relaxants are not yet well defined. In general, these drugs are absorbed from the gastrointestinal (GI) tract, widely distributed in the body, metabolized in the liver, and excreted by the kidneys. The centrally acting muscle relaxants have an onset of action between 30 and 60 minutes; their duration of action varies from 3 to 24 hours. (See *Pharmacokinetics of the centrally acting skeletal muscle relaxants* for a comparison of the drugs in this class.)

Pharmacokinetics of the centrally acting skeletal muscle relaxants

As this chart shows, the centrally acting skeletal muscle relaxants' onset of action is 30 minutes to 1 hour. Cyclobenzaprine has the longest duration of action at 12 to 24 hours.

DRUG	ONSET OF ACTION	TIME TO PEAK CONCENTRATION	DURATION OF ACTION
carisoprodol	30 min	4 hours	4 to 6 hours
chlorphenesin	Not available	1 to 3 hours	4 to 6 hours
chlorzoxazone	1 hour	3 to 4 hours	3 to 4 hours
cyclobenzaprine	1 hour	4 to 8 hours	12 to 24 hours
metaxalone	1 hour	2 hours	4 to 6 hours
methocarbamol	30 min	1 to 2 hours	Not available
orphenadrine	1 hour	2 hours	4 to 6 hours

PHARMACODYNAMICS

The precise mechanism of action of these drugs is not known. They are known, however, to be CNS depressants.

Mechanism of action

The skeletal muscle relaxant effects of the centrally acting agents are minimal and probably related to their sedative effects. The drugs do not directly relax skeletal muscle and do not depress neuronal conduction, neuromuscular transmission, or muscle excitability.

Carisoprodol is structurally related to meprobamate, a CNS depressant. Chlorphenesin and methocarbamol are chemically related to each other, and both have sedative effects. Chlorzoxazone is a benzoxazole derivative unrelated to the other centrally acting skeletal muscle relaxants, but with similar activity. Cyclobenzaprine is structurally related to the tricyclic antidepressants, and, like them, it enhances the effects of norepinephrine and has anticholinergic effects. Metaxalone is an oxazolidinone derivative. Oxazolidinone is a cyclic carbamate of methocarbamol.

Orphenadrine is an anticholinergic agent that may reduce skeletal muscle spasm through an atropine-like central action. It also blocks the effects of the excitatory neurotransmitter acetylcholine. Although orphenadrine does not directly relax skeletal muscle, it may produce analgesic effects. Orphenadrine also produces antihistaminic effects, but it stimulates rather than depresses the CNS.

PHARMACOTHERAPEUTICS

The centrally acting skeletal muscle relaxants are used as adjuncts to rest and physical therapy in treating acute, painful musculoskeletal conditions. Their beneficial effects probably derive from their sedative properties and

---

DRUG INTERACTIONS

Centrally acting skeletal muscle relaxants

Drug interactions involving the centrally acting skeletal muscle relaxants are infrequent; they usually result from simultaneous administration of CNS depressant drugs, including alcohol.

DRUG	INTERACTING DRUGS	POSSIBLE EFFECTS	NURSING IMPLICATIONS
carisoprodol, chlorphenesin, cyclobenzaprine, metaxalone, methocarbamol, orphenadrine	CNS depressants (alcohol, narcotics, barbiturates, anticonvulsants, tricyclic antidepressants, antianxiety agents)	Increase sedative and other CNS effects, including motor skill impairment and respiratory depression	• Monitor the patient for changes in level of consciousness. • Monitor the patient for signs of respiratory depression. • Advise the patient of possible additive effects, especially with alcohol.
cyclobenzaprine	Monoamine oxidase (MAO) inhibitors	May cause hyperpyrexia, excitation, and convulsions	• Expect 14 days to elapse between the administration of the last dose of an MAO inhibitor and the first dose of cyclobenzaprine. • Monitor the patient's CNS status and body temperature frequently.
	guanethidine, clonidine	Decrease the antihypertensive effect of guanethidine and clonidine	• Be prepared to administer an increased dosage of antihypertensive agents as ordered.
	cholinergic blocking agents	Increase anticholinergic effects, including confusion and hallucinations	• Monitor the patient for signs and symptoms of an adverse reaction; be prepared to administer a reduced dosage of cholinergic blocking agent as ordered.
orphenadrine	cholinergic blocking agents	Increase anticholinergic effects, including confusion and hallucinations	• Monitor the patient for signs and symptoms of an adverse reaction; be prepared to administer a reduced dosage of cholinergic blocking agent as ordered.

they do not appear to be as effective as diazepam for treating musculoskeletal pain. They are ineffective in treating skeletal muscle hyperactivity secondary to such chronic neurologic disorders as cerebral palsy.

carisoprodol (Soma). Carisoprodol is used to treat acute, painful musculoskeletal conditions.
USUAL ADULT DOSAGE: 350 mg P.O. t.i.d. and h.s.

chlorphenesin carbamate (Maolate). Used for short-term treatment of acute, painful musculoskeletal conditions, chlorphenesin should not be given for more than 8 weeks.
USUAL ADULT DOSAGE: 800 mg P.O. t.i.d. until a beneficial response is obtained; then the dosage should be reduced to the lowest effective level, with maintenance at 400 mg P.O. q.i.d.

chlorzoxazone (Paraflex). Used to treat acute, painful musculoskeletal conditions or severe muscle spasm, chlorzoxazone should be taken with food to avoid gastric distress.
USUAL ADULT DOSAGE: for musculoskeletal conditions, 250 mg P.O. t.i.d. or q.i.d.; for spasm, initial dose is 500 mg t.i.d. or q.i.d. and may be increased up to 750 mg P.O. t.i.d. or q.i.d.; when a beneficial response is obtained, the dosage should be reduced to the lowest effective level.

cyclobenzaprine hydrochloride (Flexeril). Used for short-term treatment of muscle spasm, cyclobenzaprine should not be given for more than 3 weeks.
USUAL ADULT DOSAGE: 10 mg P.O. b.i.d. to q.i.d.; may be increased to a maximum of 60 mg daily.

metaxalone (Skelaxin). Used to treat acute, painful musculoskeletal conditions.
USUAL ADULT DOSAGE: 800 mg P.O. t.i.d. or q.i.d.

methocarbamol (Robaxin). Used to treat acute, painful musculoskeletal conditions, methocarbamol is also used as supportive therapy in tetanus management.
USUAL ADULT DOSAGE: for musculoskeletal conditions, initially 1.5 to 2 g P.O. q.i.d., for 48 to 72 hours with maintenance at 4 to 4.5 g P.O. daily in 3 to 6 divided doses, or not more than 500 mg (5 ml) I.M. into each buttock every 8 hours, or 1 to 3 g (10 to 30 ml) I.V. daily directly into I.V. tubing at 3 ml/minute or 1 g in 250 ml of dextrose 5% in water or normal saline solution—maximum dose 3 g daily; I.M. and I.V. doses should not exceed 3 g daily for 3 consecutive days; for

tetanus, 1 to 2 g into the tubing of an infusing I.V. line at a rate of 300 mg/minute or 1 to 3 g as an infusion every 6 hours.
USUAL PEDIATRIC DOSAGE: for tetanus, 15 mg/kg of body weight I.V. every 6 hours.

orphenadrine citrate (Norflex, Norgesic). Used to treat acute, painful musculoskeletal conditions, orphenadrine is highly toxic at even slight overdoses.
USUAL ADULT DOSAGE: 100-mg extended-release tablet P.O. every 12 hours, or 25- to 50-mg compound (with aspirin and caffeine) P.O. t.i.d. or q.i.d., or 60 mg I.M. or I.V. every 12 hours p.r.n. injected over 5 minutes with the patient in the supine position; switch to oral form for maintenance.

Drug interactions
The centrally acting skeletal muscle relaxants interact with few drugs, but all interact with other CNS depressants (including alcohol), causing additive depression of the CNS. Cyclobenzaprine interacts with monoamine oxidase (MAO) inhibitors: 14 days must elapse between the last dose of an MAO inhibitor and the first dose of cyclobenzaprine. Cyclobenzaprine may decrease the effects of the antihypertensive agents guanethidine and clonidine. Orphenadrine and cyclobenzaprine sometimes enhance the effects of cholinergic blocking agents. Methocarbamol may antagonize the cholinergic effects of the anticholinesterase agents used to treat myasthenia gravis. (See *Drug interactions: Centrally acting skeletal muscle relaxants* on page 349 for details about the interactions and relevant nursing implications.)

The centrally acting skeletal muscle relaxants also interfere with some laboratory tests. Metaxalone may produce false-positive results for glucose with the copper reduction method. (It does not interfere with the glucose oxidase method.) Methocarbamol may cause false-positive results for urine 5-hydroxyindoleacetic acid and for urine vanillylmandelic acid.

ADVERSE DRUG REACTIONS
The most common adverse reactions to the centrally acting skeletal muscle relaxants are extensions of their therapeutic effects on the CNS.

Predictable reactions
Drowsiness and dizziness are the most common predictable adverse reactions to drugs in this class. Occasionally, nausea, vomiting, diarrhea, constipation, heartburn, abdominal distress, or ataxia occurs. Areflexia, flaccid paralysis, respiratory depression, and hypotension are seen occasionally after oral administration

of any of these drugs except methocarbamol. With parenteral administration, reactions may include syncope, hypotension, flushing, blurred vision, asthenia, lethargy, vertigo, lack of coordination, and bradycardia.

Because orphenadrine has an anticholinergic effect, adverse reactions may include dry mouth, urinary hesitancy, blurred vision, and tachycardia. At high doses, cyclobenzaprine, which is structurally similar to the tricyclic antidepressants, shares their toxic potential; reactions include tachycardia and orthostatic hypotension. Physical and psychological dependence is a possibility after long-term use of these agents; abrupt cessation of the drug may cause severe withdrawal symptoms.

Unpredictable reactions
Rarely, parenteral orphenadrine causes an anaphylactic reaction. Chlorphenesin contains tartrazine dye, which may cause an allergic reaction.

NURSING IMPLICATIONS
Because the centrally acting skeletal muscle relaxants act on the CNS, the nurse must be aware of the following special implications for their administration:
• Do not administer these drugs to patients who have a known hypersensitivity to them or to pregnant or lactating women.
• Inform patients that these agents may impair their ability to perform activities requiring mental alertness or physical coordination, such as operating machinery or driving a motor vehicle.
• Advise patients to avoid alcohol and other CNS depressants while taking these drugs.
• Remember that metaxalone may produce false-positive results for laboratory glucose tests that are based on the copper reduction method.
• Do not administer carisoprodol to patients who have acute intermittent porphyria because it may increase porphyrin synthesis.
• Administer chlorzoxazone cautiously to patients with impaired liver function; monitor liver function in these patients frequently.
• Administer cyclobenzaprine and orphenadrine cautiously to patients who have a history of urinary retention, cardiac decompensation, or tachycardia; these drugs are contraindicated in patients who have narrow-angle glaucoma or myasthenia gravis.
• Do not give parenteral methocarbamol to patients who have convulsive disorders because it may precipitate seizures.

• Give parenteral orphenadrine over 5 minutes with the patient in the supine position; keep the patient supine for 5 to 10 more minutes, then help the patient to a sitting position.

PERIPHERALLY ACTING SKELETAL MUSCLE RELAXANTS

Dantrolene sodium is the only peripherally acting skeletal muscle relaxant. Similar to the centrally acting agents in its therapeutic effect, dantrolene differs in its mechanism of action. Because its major effect is on the muscle, dantrolene has a lower incidence of CNS adverse effects, but high therapeutic doses are hepatotoxic. Clinically, dantrolene seems most effective for spasticity of cerebral origin. Because it produces muscle weakness, dantrolene is of questionable benefit in patients with borderline strength.

History and source
The first drug used to treat spasticity was curare, but its usefulness was limited because it produced general rather than specific relaxation. Dantrolene was introduced as a peripherally acting skeletal muscle relaxant in 1974.

PHARMACOKINETICS
Dantrolene is poorly absorbed from the GI tract. It is highly plasma–protein-bound, metabolized by the liver, and excreted in the urine.

Absorption, distribution, metabolism, excretion
Only about 35% of an oral dose of dantrolene is absorbed from the GI tract, and blood concentrations vary widely among patients after oral administration—partly because dantrolene has a strong affinity for plasma–protein binding, particularly with albumin. Dantrolene undergoes significant liver metabolism to compounds that are much less active than the parent molecule; these metabolites are excreted primarily in the urine.

Onset, peak, duration
Although the peak concentration level of a single dose of dantrolene occurs about 5 hours after it is ingested, the drug's therapeutic benefit may not be evident for a

week or more. Dosage increases should not exceed two per week. Dantrolene's elimination half-life in healthy adults is 8.7 hours. Because dantrolene undergoes significant hepatic metabolism, however, its half-life may be prolonged in patients with impaired liver function.

PHARMACODYNAMICS

Dantrolene is chemically and pharmacologically unrelated to the other skeletal muscle relaxants. It probably acts directly on the muscle contractile mechanism, as opposed to affecting reflex pathways within the CNS.

Mechanism of action

Dantrolene may act by inhibiting calcium release from the sarcoplasmic reticulum in muscle cells. The sarcoplasmic reticulum stores calcium until the muscle is activated electrically by an action potential; then it releases calcium, which triggers muscle contraction.

Although dantrolene appears to affect the CNS as well, any central effect remains unproven. CNS effects, such as drowsiness, possibly result indirectly from decreased skeletal muscle activity. At therapeutic concentration levels, dantrolene has a minimal effect on cardiac or intestinal smooth muscle.

PHARMACOTHERAPEUTICS

Dantrolene helps manage all types of spasticity, regardless of where the lesion is located, but is most effective when the lesion is cerebral. Patients with multiple sclerosis, cerebral palsy, spinal cord injury, or cerebrovascular accident may all benefit from dantrolene. It is particularly useful for reducing spasticity in patients whose nursing care is impeded by severe muscle contractions. It also benefits patients whose rehabilitation program has been slowed by spasticity. If these patients

---

Malignant hyperthermic crisis

This hereditary and highly fatal defect is triggered by inhalation anesthetics, depolarizing muscle relaxants, and curare-like neuromuscular blocking agents. The drugs prolong an increase in the release of calcium from the sarcoplasmic reticulum, producing intense muscle contraction, body heat, and metabolic acidosis. Dantrolene is the drug of choice to prevent or treat malignant hyperthermic crisis because it reduces the release of calcium by the sarcoplasmic reticulum.

---

have reversible spasticity, its relief should speed restoration of residual function. The patient's gait or ability to stand or sit may also improve.

Dantrolene is also used to treat and prevent malignant hyperthermic crisis. (See *Malignant hyperthermic crisis* for additional information.)

Positive patient response to dantrolene therapy is difficult to predict, and the benefits of long-term dantrolene therapy in ambulatory patients must be weighed against the drug's adverse effects, chiefly muscle weakness and liver damage.

Dantrolene has more severe adverse effects than baclofen. Comparative studies of dantrolene and diazepam have found them to be equally effective. Dantrolene is probably preferable for elderly patients or patients with CNS lesions who may be more affected by the sedative effects of diazepam, but diazepam probably is preferable for patients with significant baseline muscle weakness. Simultaneous use of dantrolene and diazepam seems to control spasticity better than either drug alone, with smaller doses and fewer adverse effects. However, the combination has the potential to cause an additive sedative effect.

dantrolene sodium (Dantrium). Dosages must be titrated to the individual patient's response, always using the lowest dosage possible. Maintain each dosage level for 4 to 7 days to determine the patient's response. If benefits are not evident in 45 days, discontinue therapy to avoid liver damage.

USUAL ADULT DOSAGE: for spasticity, 25 mg P.O. daily, increased to 25 mg b.i.d., t.i.d., or q.i.d., and then by increments of 25 mg to a maximum of 100 mg q.i.d.; for prevention of malignant hyperthermic crisis, 4 to 8 mg/kg of body weight daily P.O. in 4 divided doses for 1 to 2 days before surgery with last dose 3 to 4 hours before surgery; for management of malignant hyperthermic crisis, 1 mg/kg of body weight by rapid I.V. infusion, which may be repeated up to a cumulative total of 10 mg/kg; for prevention of recurrence of malignant hyperthermic crisis, 4 to 8 mg/kg of body weight daily P.O. in 4 divided doses for 3 days after the crisis.

Drug interactions

CNS depressants combined with dantrolene increase CNS depression, which may lead to sedation, motor skill impairment, and respiratory depression. No other interactions are reported.

ADVERSE DRUG REACTIONS

The most common adverse reaction to dantrolene is muscle weakness. The drug may also depress liver function or cause idiosyncratic hepatitis.

Predictable reactions

Dose-related adverse reactions to dantrolene are usually transient, lasting up to 4 days after therapy begins. The most common is muscle weakness, rarely severe enough to cause slurring of speech, drooling, and enuresis. Other common reactions include drowsiness, dizziness, lightheadedness, diarrhea, nausea, malaise, and fatigue. If weakness or diarrhea is severe, the dosage may be decreased or the drug discontinued. Other adverse GI reactions that may respond to a dosage decrease include anorexia, vomiting, gastric irritation, abdominal cramps, constipation, difficulty swallowing, and GI bleeding. Constipation is sometimes severe enough to resemble bowel obstruction.

Neurologic adverse reactions include visual and speech disturbances, headache, taste alteration, depression, confusion, hallucinations, nervousness, insomnia, and seizures.

Urogenital reactions include urinary frequency, incontinence, nocturia, difficult urination, urinary retention, hematuria, crystalluria, and difficult erection.

Cardiovascular reactions, in the form of pleural effusion with pericarditis, are rare.

Unpredictable reactions

Fatal and nonfatal hepatitis from dantrolene appear to be idiosyncratic reactions. In most cases, nausea, anorexia, vomiting, and abdominal discomfort precede hepatitis, which occurs most commonly in patients receiving more than 300 mg daily for longer than 2 months. The risk of dantrolene hepatotoxicity is greatest in women over age 35 who simultaneously take estrogens and in patients with baseline liver function test abnormalities. The abnormal liver function test results induced by dantrolene may return to normal when the drug is discontinued. Other unpredictable reactions include acneiform rash, erratic blood pressure, pruritus, urticaria, excessive tearing, chills and fever, and a feeling of suffocation.

NURSING IMPLICATIONS

Dantrolene's mechanism of action and adverse effects are different from those of the centrally acting skeletal muscle relaxants. The nurse must be aware of the following implications:

● Do not administer dantrolene to patients with a known hypersensitivity, to women who are or may become pregnant or who are lactating, to patients who must use spasticity to maintain posture and balance, or to patients with active hepatic disease such as hepatitis or cirrhosis.
● Administer dantrolene cautiously to patients who have severely impaired cardiac or pulmonary function.
● Inform patients about possible weakness, drowsiness, or dizziness caused by the drug.
● Administer dantrolene cautiously to patients receiving other drugs that produce drowsiness.
● Monitor the patient's liver function at baseline and during therapy with the following tests: SGPT, SGOT, alkaline phosphatase, and total bilirubin.
● Reconstitute dantrolene with 60 ml of sterile, not bacteriostatic, water when administering it I.V.
● Empty capsules into fruit juice or another liquid immediately before administration to patients who have difficulty swallowing capsules.

Diazepam as a skeletal muscle relaxing agent

Diazepam (Valium) is a benzodiazepine with antispastic effects besides its antianxiety, hypnotic, and anticonvulsant ones. Useful in various chronic disorders in which spasticity is a component, diazepam is one of the most effective agents available for treating acute muscle spasms. It seems to work by enhancing the neurotransmitter GABA's inhibitory effect on muscle contraction.

In treating spasticity, diazepam is useful alone or in combination with other drugs, especially in patients with spinal cord lesions and occasionally in patients with cerebral palsy. It is useful in patients who have painful continuous muscle spasms and are not too susceptible to the drug's sedative effect. However, its tranquilizing properties may be helpful in depressed or anxious patients. Diazepam's use is limited by its CNS effects and the tolerance that develops with prolonged use.

Diazepam therapy is initiated with 2 mg P.O. twice daily; the dosage is increased slowly every few days until adverse reactions develop or until it reaches 10 mg t.i.d. A slow upward titration will minimize the sedation associated with diazepam. In the elderly patient, the initial dosage should not exceed 2 mg daily. For additional information on diazepam, see Chapter 32, Antianxiety Agents.

OTHER SKELETAL MUSCLE RELAXANTS

Two other drugs, diazepam and baclofen, are used as skeletal muscle relaxants. Diazepam is primarily an antianxiety agent and is discussed more fully in Chapter 32, Antianxiety Agents. Its use as a skeletal muscle relaxant is summarized in *Diazepam as a skeletal muscle relaxing agent* on page 353.

Baclofen is an analogue of the neurotransmitter GABA and probably acts in the spinal cord. Baclofen has the advantage of producing less sedation than diazepam and less peripheral muscle weakness than dantrolene. For some physicians, therefore, it is the drug of choice to treat spasticity.

History and source
Baclofen was introduced in the United States in 1977 as a muscle relaxant for the relief of spasticity. Europeans, however, have more clinical experience with baclofen.

PHARMACOKINETICS

Baclofen is rapidly absorbed from the GI tract. It is widely distributed, undergoes minimal liver metabolism, and is excreted primarily unchanged in the urine.

Absorption, distribution, metabolism, excretion
Baclofen is absorbed in varying amounts from the GI tract. The amount varies widely from patient to patient and is reduced as the dosage is increased.

Baclofen is widely distributed throughout the body, but only small amounts cross the blood-brain barrier. Although concentration levels of baclofen are therefore considerably lower in the brain and nerve tissue than in the blood, they decline more slowly there. At therapeutic blood concentration levels, baclofen is about 30% bound to serum proteins. The drug crosses the placenta, but its distribution into breast milk is uncertain.

Baclofen undergoes limited liver metabolism and is almost completely excreted within 72 hours after oral administration; 70% to 80% is excreted in the urine unchanged or as metabolites, and the remainder is excreted in the feces.

Onset, peak, duration
The beneficial effects of baclofen may or may not occur immediately—the onset of therapeutic effect ranges from hours to weeks. Peak blood concentration levels of the drug are attained in 2 to 3 hours and are sustained for 8 hours. The elimination half-life of baclofen is 2½ to 4 hours. Abrupt withdrawal of the drug may precipitate hallucinations, seizures, and acute exacerbations of spasticity.

PHARMACODYNAMICS

The exact mechanism of action of baclofen has not been established. It is believed to work in the spinal cord. Biochemically, baclofen resembles an inhibitory neurotransmitter.

Mechanism of action
Animal studies have helped to identify baclofen's site of action as the spinal cord. However, some of its adverse effects, such as respiratory depression at higher doses, enhanced electroencephalogram (EEG) activity, and sedation, suggest an additional supraspinal site of action.

Baclofen seems to depress neuron activity, decreasing the degree and frequency of muscle spasms and reducing muscle tone. Researchers question whether baclofen produces these effects by suppressing excitatory neurotransmitter release, by directly inhibiting spinal pathways, or both. Baclofen resembles the inhibitory neurotransmitter GABA. Although baclofen does not displace GABA from its receptor-binding sites, it may compete with GABA at presynaptic GABA receptors. Its overall effect reduces the frequency and severity of painful flexor or extensor muscle spasms. Baclofen also reduces protracted muscle spasms of the lower extremities in patients with spinal spasticity.

PHARMACOTHERAPEUTICS

Baclofen's principal clinical indication is for the paraplegic or quadriplegic patient with lesions of the spinal cord, most commonly caused by multiple sclerosis or trauma. Baclofen provides these patients with a significant reduction in the number and severity of painful flexor spasms. Aside from waking patients at night, these spasms are painful and unpleasant in the day and may cause sudden falls in ambulatory patients. Baclofen also improves bladder and bowel control, and it may make the patient's hygiene and nursing care more comfortable by relaxing tightly flexed legs. Aside from these benefits, however, baclofen does not improve stiff gait, increase manual dexterity, or improve residual muscle function.

DRUG INTERACTIONS

Baclofen

Drug interactions involving the skeletal muscle relaxant baclofen often cause symptoms to worsen, requiring dosage adjustments.

DRUG	INTERACTING DRUGS	POSSIBLE EFFECTS	NURSING IMPLICATIONS
baclofen	fentanyl	Prolongs fentanyl-induced analgesia	• Be prepared to administer a reduced dosage of fentanyl as ordered.
	lithium carbonate	Aggravates hyperkinetic symptoms	• Monitor the patient for worsening of spasticity.
	tricyclic antidepressants	Increase muscle relaxant effect	• Be prepared to administer a reduced dosage of baclofen as ordered.
	CNS depressant drugs (including alcohol, narcotics, barbiturates, anticonvulsants, antianxiety agents)	Increase sedative and other CNS effects, including motor skill impairment and respiratory depression	• Monitor the patient for changes in level of consciousness. • Monitor the patient for signs of respiratory depression. • Advise the patient about possible additive effects, especially with alcohol.

Baclofen and diazepam have comparable antispastic effects in patients with multiple sclerosis; however, baclofen is usually preferred because it produces a lower incidence of sedation.

Baclofen has been used experimentally to treat a number of other conditions, with limited success.

baclofen (Lioresal). Because the dosage must be individualized to produce the best response without adverse effects, baclofen should be started at low doses and titrated slowly. Full clinical benefit may require 1 to 2 months of treatment.

USUAL ADULT DOSAGE: initially, 5 mg P.O. t.i.d., increased by 15 mg daily at 3-day intervals until an optimal response is achieved, usually at 40 to 80 mg daily in 3 or 4 divided doses not to exceed 80 mg/day.

Drug interactions

Few drug interactions are reported with baclofen; the most significant is an increase in CNS depression when baclofen is administered with other CNS depressants, including alcohol. (For additional information on interacting drugs and their possible effects, see *Drug interactions: Baclofen.*)

ADVERSE DRUG REACTIONS

Baclofen has few major adverse reactions when administered appropriately to patients with spinal lesions. General CNS depression produces the most problems.

Predictable reactions

The most common adverse reaction to baclofen is transient drowsiness. Other, less frequent adverse reactions include fatigue, nausea, vertigo, hypotonia, muscle weakness, depression, and headache. These can be avoided by a slow titration of the dose.

Elderly patients or patients with strokes and brain disorders may experience psychiatric disturbances, such as hallucinations, euphoria, depression, confusion, and anxiety. Increases in dosage should be made even more slowly in these patients.

Other rare neuropsychiatric disturbances include insomnia, muscle pain, paresthesia, tinnitus, slurred speech, tremor, rigidity, ataxia, blurred vision, strabismus, nystagmus, diplopia, and dysarthria. Baclofen rarely causes adverse genitourinary reactions. Cardiovascular reactions include hypotension and, rarely, dyspnea, chest pain, and syncope. Adverse GI reactions include nausea, vomiting, constipation, and, rarely, dry mouth, anorexia, taste disorders, and diarrhea.

Skeletal muscle relaxing agents

This table summarizes the major skeletal muscle relaxing agents currently in clinical use.

DRUG	MAJOR INDICATIONS	USUAL ADULT DOSAGES	NURSING IMPLICATIONS
carisoprodol	Acute muscle spasms	350 mg P.O. t.i.d. and h.s.	• Contraindicated in known sensitivity and in pregnancy. • Advise patients not to perform activities that require mental alertness.
dantrolene	Spasticity, prevention and treatment of malignant hyperthermic crisis	25 mg daily to 100 mg P.O. q.i.d.; prevention: 4 to 8 mg/kg P.O. daily for 1 to 2 days before surgery or for 3 days after crisis; treatment: 1 mg/kg I.V. to a cumulative total of 10 mg/kg	• Contraindicated in known sensitivity, pregnancy, or hepatic disease. • Advise patients not to perform activities that require mental alertness. • Monitor the patient's liver function tests.
diazepam	Acute muscle spasms and spasticity	2 mg P.O. b.i.d. to 10 mg P.O. t.i.d.	• Contraindicated in known sensitivity and in pregnancy. • Advise patients not to perform activities that require mental alertness. • Administer cautiously to patients with narrow-angle glaucoma and underlying pulmonary, renal, or hepatic diseases.
baclofen	Spasticity	40 to 80 mg P.O. daily	• Contraindicated in known sensitivity and in pregnancy. • Advise patients not to perform activities that require mental alertness. • Be prepared to administer a reduced dosage to patients with impaired renal function. • Monitor epileptic patients for seizure activity.

Unpredictable reactions

Rash, allergic skin disorders, and pruritus have occurred with baclofen, as have ankle edema, weight gain, and excessive diaphoresis.

NURSING IMPLICATIONS

Appropriate titration with baclofen should minimize most potential problems. The nurse, however, must still be aware of the following implications:
• Do not administer baclofen to patients with a known hypersensitivity or to pregnant or lactating women unless the benefits outweigh the risks.
• Be aware that patients with impaired renal function may require a reduced dosage, since baclofen is excreted primarily unchanged in the urine.

• Monitor the EEG and clinical status of epileptic patients during therapy with baclofen because seizure control may deteriorate.
• Inform patients that baclofen may impair their ability to perform activities requiring mental alertness or physical coordination.
• Monitor the patient for increased CNS depression caused by concurrent administration of baclofen and CNS depressants, including alcohol.
• In cases of overdose, induce emesis if the patient is conscious or use gastric lavage if the patient is comatose; endotracheal intubation may be necessary to maintain adequate respiratory function, but do not use respiratory stimulants.

CHAPTER SUMMARY

Chapter 22 investigated the skeletal muscle relaxing agents, which act to relieve musculoskeletal pain or spasm and severe musculoskeletal spasticity. Here are the chapter highlights:

• Some skeletal muscle relaxing drugs act in the spinal cord to alter neurotransmitter function; these are centrally acting drugs. Others act on the skeletal muscle itself; these are peripherally acting drugs.

• Two other drugs—baclofen, which acts on the spinal cord, and diazepam, an antianxiety agent—have valuable antispasm effects.

• The centrally acting skeletal muscle relaxants probably relieve acute musculoskeletal spasms as a result of their CNS depressant activity. Drugs in this class are carisoprodol, chlorphenesin, chlorzoxazone, cyclobenzaprine, metaxalone, methocarbamol, and orphenadrine.

• Patients with multiple sclerosis, cerebral palsy, spinal cord injury, or cerebrovascular accident may all benefit from dantrolene, although some patients may not respond to the drug. If a patient does not clearly benefit from dantrolene, it should be discontinued because of its hepatotoxic potential.

• Diazepam may be the most effective skeletal muscle relaxant available for the relief of acute muscle spasms. It is also effective for the relief of spasticity associated with chronic neurologic disorders. Diazepam is as effective as baclofen or dantrolene for relieving spasticity, but it causes a higher incidence of adverse CNS effects.

• Baclofen is considered by some physicians as the drug of choice for treating muscle spasms in patients with multiple sclerosis or spinal cord lesions.

• Spasticity has no cure, but baclofen, dantrolene, and diazepam may offer relief.

BIBLIOGRAPHY

American Hospital Formulary Service. *Drug Information 87* McEvoy, G.K., et al., eds. Bethesda, Md.: American Society of Hospital Pharmacists, 1987.

American Medical Association. *AMA Drug Evaluations,* 6th ed. Philadelphia: W.B. Saunders Co., 1986.

Davidoff, R.S. "Antispasticity Drugs: Mechanisms of Action," *Annals of Neurology* 17:107-116, 1986.

Gilman, A.G., et al., eds. *Goodman and Gilman's The Pharmacological Basis of Therapeutics,* 7th ed. New York: Macmillan Publishing Co., 1985.

Mediphor Editorial Group. *Drug Interaction Facts 1987.* St. Louis: J.B. Lippincott Co., 1987.

Young, R.R., and Delwaide, P.J. "Spasticity," *New England Journal of Medicine* 204(1):28-33, 96-99, 1981.

CHAPTER 23

ANTIPARKINSONIAN AGENTS

OBJECTIVES

After reading and studying this chapter, you should be able to:

1. Describe the symptoms and effects of Parkinson's disease.

2. Explain the mechanisms of action of the anticholinergic and dopaminergic agents.

3. Identify the major adverse reactions to the anticholinergic agents and their nursing implications.

4. Describe the general pharmacokinetic processes of the anticholinergics and the dopaminergics.

5. Compare the action of levodopa to that of levodopa-carbidopa.

6. Identify the major adverse reactions to the dopaminergic agents and their nursing implications.

INTRODUCTION

Drug therapy is an important part of the treatment for Parkinson's disease, also known as parkinsonism and paralysis agitans. Parkinson's disease is a progressive neurologic disorder caused by a depletion, degeneration, or destruction of dopamine in the neurons of the brain's basal ganglia. Four cardinal features characterize this involuntary movement disorder: tremor at rest, akinesia (complete or partial loss of muscle movement), rigidity (increased muscle tone), and disturbances of posture and equilibrium. The frequency and severity of these signs increase as the disease progresses. Approximately 85% of Parkinson's cases are idiopathic: they arise spontaneously from an unknown cause. The remaining 15% result from drugs, encephalitis, neurotoxins, trauma, arteriosclerosis, or other neurologic disorders.

This chapter includes synthetic anticholinergic and dopaminergic agents used to treat Parkinson's disease.

For a summary of representataive drugs, see *Selected major drugs: Antiparkinsonian agents* on page 368.

ANTICHOLINERGIC AGENTS

Anticholinergic agents are sometimes called parasympatholytics because they antagonize functions that are controlled primarily by the parasympathetic nervous system.

Anticholinergics are classified in three chemical categories: synthetic tertiary amines, phenothiazine derivatives, and antihistamines. The synthetic tertiary amines constitute the largest group, including benztropine mesylate, biperiden hydrocholoride, biperiden lactate, procyclidine hydrochloride, and trihexyphenidyl hydrochloride. Ethopropazine (a phenothiazine derivative) and diphenhydramine hydrochloride and orphenadrine citrate (antihistamines) constitute the remainder of the anticholinergics.

History and source

In the late 19th and early 20th centuries, physicians used natural belladonna alkaloids, such as atropine and hyoscyamine, to treat Parkinson's disease. Today, physicians primarily use synthetic anticholinergics, which were developed in the 1950s.

PHARMACOKINETICS

In general, the blood absorbs anticholinergic agents from the gastrointestinal (GI) tract and delivers them to their action site in the brain. Most of these agents undergo hepatic metabolism and renal excretion.

Absorption, distribution, metabolism, excretion

Although detailed information for specific anticholinergic agents is unknown, their pharmacokinetic processes follow a general pattern.

After oral administration, nearly complete absorption occurs readily in the GI tract. (Food does not significantly reduce absorption of anticholinergic agents.) A large amount of diphenhydramine undergoes first-pass metabolism after oral administration: only 40% to 50% of a dose reaches the circulation unchanged.

The exact distribution of most of these agents is undetermined. However, most researchers believe that anticholinergics cross the blood-brain barrier and penetrate brain tissue because they affect the central nervous system (CNS).

The liver metabolizes most anticholinergic agents at least partially. Diphenhydramine is almost completely metabolized. So is orphenadrine, which is metabolized into at least eight compounds.

Anticholinergics are usually excreted in urine as metabolites and unchanged drug. Trihexyphenidyl is also believed to be excreted by the kidneys, but principally as an unchanged drug.

Onset, peak, duration

For most of the anticholinergic agents, the onset of action occurs within 1 hour, peak concentration level is reached in 2 to 4 hours, and duration of action is up to 6 hours.

Benztropine is a long-acting drug with a duration of action up to 24 hours in some patients. For most anticholinergic agents, the half-life is undetermined.

PHARMACODYNAMICS

In the brain, anticholinergic agents counteract the cholinergic activity that is believed to be present in Parkinson's disease.

Mechanism of action

Parkinson's disease results from the degeneration of dopaminergic neurons in the basal ganglia. Because dopamine helps control motor activity, a lack of it will cause problems in coordinating smooth motor movements. At the same time, an excess of acetylcholine develops, producing an excitatory effect on the CNS which may cause the parkinsonian tremor.

The mechanism of action of the anticholinergic agents is not known, but these drugs prolong dopamine's action by blocking its reuptake into presynaptic neurons in the CNS. They also suppress central cholinergic activity.

PHARMACOTHERAPEUTICS

Anticholinergic agents are used most commonly in the early stages of Parkinson's disease, when symptoms are mild and do not have a major impact on the patient's life-style. Anticholinergic agents effectively control po-

lysialia (excessive salivation) and are about 20% effective in reducing the incidence and severity of akinesia and rigidity.

Anticholinergics may be used alone or in combination with amantadine in the early stages of Parkinson's disease. They may be given with levodopa during the later stages to further relieve symptoms. No single anticholinergic is consistently superior, but a patient may respond more favorably to one agent than to another. Trihexyphenidyl is the most widely used drug of the group. Benztropine and diphenhydramine also are used commonly.

Most anticholinergics maintain their effectiveness with long-term administration and rarely require dosage adjustment after the proper dosage is reached. However, as the disease advances, anticholinergics are not effective enough by themselves. If any antiparkinsonian agent must be discontinued and replaced with another drug, this should be done gradually. Abrupt withdrawal of anticholinergics can produce confusion, exhaustion, and exacerbation of parkinsonian symptoms.

The adverse effects of the anticholinergics are usually dose-limiting; that is, they increase with the dosage. Ethopropazine has a high incidence of adverse effects that are intolerable to some patients. Because the anticholinergics are more likely to cause adverse CNS effects in elderly patients, these drugs may be more successful in younger patients.

The doses mentioned in this section are used to treat idiopathic parkinsonism, unless otherwise specified.

Diphenhydramine, benztropine, and biperiden may be administered I.V. or I.M. to treat Parkinson's disease. But these parenteral routes are usually reserved for use when the disease is acute or when oral administration is not feasible. In idiopathic Parkinson's disease, I.V. administration is not usually needed to achieve a rapid response.

benztropine mesylate (Cogentin). Used alone or with other antiparkinsonian agents, benztropine may be especially useful in treating elderly patients who cannot tolerate the CNS-stimulating properties of other anticholinergics, such as orphenadrine and trihexyphenidyl. Because the drug's effects are cumulative, benztropine may take 2 to 3 days to become fully effective. Therefore, dosage increases should be slow, allowing time for the drug to take effect.

USUAL ADULT DOSAGE: 0.5 to 1 mg P.O. daily, preferably as a single dose h.s. for the first few days, increased by 0.5 mg every few days, until the most effective dose (maximum of 6 mg/day) is reached; maintenance dose, 1 to 2 mg P.O., I.V., or I.M. daily. Some patients will achieve 24-hour symptom control with a single bedtime dose of 2 mg or more.

DRUG INTERACTIONS

Anticholinergic agents

The most common interactions occur between anticholinergic agents and drugs that have anticholinergic properties. Other interactions involving antipsychotic drugs and methotrimeprazine may produce serious problems.

DRUG	INTERACTING DRUGS	POSSIBLE EFFECTS	NURSING IMPLICATIONS
benztropine, biperiden, procyclidine, trihexyphenidyl, ethopropazine, diphenhydramine, or phenadrine	amantadine	Increases incidence of anticholinergic adverse effects	• Monitor the patient for increased complaints of minor adverse reactions, such as dry mouth, blurred vision, urinary retention, and constipation.
	levodopa	Decreases levodopa absorption, which could lead to worsening parkinsonian signs and symptoms	• Monitor the patient for increased rigidity, bradykinesia, and tremor. Instruct the patient to report any of these problems to the physician. • Expect to increase the levodopa dosage, as prescribed.
	antipsychotics (chlorpromazine, thioridazine, perphenazine, prochlorperazine, trifluoperazine, thiothixene, haloperidol, loxapine)	Decrease effectiveness of anticholinergics; decrease effectiveness of antipsychotics; increase incidence of anticholinergic adverse effects	• Avoid concomitant use of anticholinergics and antipsychotics. If an antipsychotic drug is necessary, thioridazine is generally preferred. • Observe the patient for an increase in parkinsonian signs or deterioration in mental status. Instruct the patient and family to report either of these problems to the physician. • Monitor the patient for increased anticholinergic adverse reactions.
	methotrimeprazine	Increases incidence of extrapyramidal signs and symptoms, such as tremors and rigidity	• Observe the patient closely for increased extrapyramidal signs and symptoms. • Administer these drugs together only if absolutely necessary.

biperiden hydrochloride (Akineton) **and biperiden lactate** (Akineton Lactate). This anticholinergic agent is useful for initial or adjunctive treatment of all forms of Parkinson's disease.
USUAL ADULT DOSAGE: for idiopathic Parkinson's disease, 2 mg P.O. t.i.d. or q.i.d.; for acute drug-induced parkinsonism, 2 mg I.M. or I.V. repeated every 30 minutes up to a maximum parenteral dose of 8 mg in 24 hours. The oral dosage should be adjusted according to the patient's requirements and tolerance for adverse effects. With prolonged therapy, drug tolerance may develop, requiring a dosage increase.

procyclidine hydrochloride (Kemadrin). Indications for this agent include initial or adjunctive treatment of all forms of Parkinson's disease. Procyclidine may relieve muscle rigidity more than tremor. Its dosage should be individualized according to the patient's age, therapeutic response, and form of Parkinson's disease. For instance, younger patients usually tolerate and require larger doses

than elderly patients, and drug-induced Parkinson's disease may require a larger dose than the idiopathic form of the disease.
USUAL ADULT DOSAGE: initially, 2.5 mg P.O. b.i.d. or t.i.d. after meals; if tolerated, dosage is gradually increased up to 5 mg t.i.d. or q.i.d; maintenance dose ranges from 10 to 20 mg P.O. daily, but may reach 60 mg/day in severe cases.

trihexyphenidyl hydrochloride (Artane, Hexaphen, Trihexane). This agent is used for initial or adjunctive treatment of all forms of Parkinson's disease, including idiopathic, postencephalitic, and drug-induced. About 50% to 75% of patients will respond to trihexyphenidyl, but maximum response commonly requires combining this drug with others. Trihexyphenidyl is available in regular tablets, in sustained-release capsules, and as an elixir. Sustained-release capsules are not preferred in treating Parkinson's disease because they may exacerbate symptoms and they may be ineffective. Dosages of trihexyphenidyl should be carefully adjusted to the patient's requirements and response.

USUAL ADULT DOSAGE: initially, 1 mg P.O. daily, increased by 2 mg every 3 to 5 days until a desirable response is achieved, intolerable adverse effects occur, or a daily dose of 10 mg is reached; the dosage usually ranges from 3 to 15 mg P.O. t.i.d. Patients with postencephalitic Parkinson's disease may require a higher dosage but rarely tolerate more than 20 mg/day. Concurrent administration of levodopa and trihexyphenidyl may require a dosage reduction, adjusted to individual response and tolerance. If trihexyphenidyl is replacing another anticholinergic agent, the trihexyphenidyl dosage should be gradually increased while the other agent is gradually withdrawn. Tolerance to trihexyphenidyl may develop with prolonged use.

ethopropazine (Parsidol). A phenothiazine derivative, ethopropazine is used as an adjunctive treatment of all forms of Parkinson's disease.

USUAL ADULT DOSAGE: initially, 50 mg. P.O. once or twice daily, increased gradually to the lowest possible effective dose: 100 to 400 mg P.O. daily for mild to moderate symptoms, 500 to 600 mg P.O. daily for severe symptoms. Adverse effects limit ethopropazine's usefulness.

diphenhydramine hydrochloride (Benadryl). This antihistamine's anticholinergic properties are responsible for its effectiveness in Parkinson's disease. Also a sleep aid, diphenhydramine may be useful for elderly patients who cannot tolerate more potent CNS-stimulating agents and for those with insomnia. For patients with mild Parkinson's disease, diphenhydramine may be used alone or in conjunction with other anticholinergics. Diphenhydramine may be administered orally, I.V. or I.M.; it is also available as an oral syrup and elixir containing 5% and 14% alcohol, respectively.

USUAL ADULT DOSAGE: initially, 25 mg P.O. t.i.d., increased gradually to 25 to 50 mg P.O. t.i.d. or q.i.d. at 4- to 6-hour intervals, according to the patient's response and tolerance; 10 to 100 mg I.M. or I.V. The maximum adult daily dosage is 300 mg orally or 400 mg parenterally. (See Chapter 63, Antihistaminic Agents, for more information on diphenhydramine.)

orphenadrine citrate (Norflex). This antihistamine is used in the adjunctive treatment of all forms of Parkinson's disease and for pain relief in musculoskeletal dis-

orders. Orphenadrine produces slight CNS stimulation and may cause mild euphoria. The oral sustained-release preparation is used in the treatment of Parkinson's disease.

USUAL ADULT DOSAGE: initially, 50 mg P.O. t.i.d., increased gradually up to 250 mg P.O. daily, according to the patient's tolerance and response. (See Chapter 63, Antihistaminic Agents, for additional information.)

Drug interactions

A few drugs, such as amantadine, levodopa, and the antipsychotics, produce clinically significant interactions when used with anticholinergics. (See *Drug interactions: Anticholinergic agents* for details.)

ADVERSE DRUG REACTIONS

Most of the adverse reactions of the anticholinergics are an extension of their pharmacologic effects. About 30% to 50% of patients experience mild adverse reactions that are dose-related. Typically, reactions decrease as treatment continues, but they limit the dosage that the patient can take.

Anticholinergic agents produce various predictable adverse reactions. One way to review them is to start at the head of the body and move down. (See *Predictable adverse reactions to the anticholinergics* on page 362 for more details.)

Anticholinergic agents can also produce various unpredictable reactions, including urticaria and allergic skin rashes that may lead to exfoliation. Diphenhydramine can also produce a photosensitivity reaction (abnormal reaction of the skin to sunlight), causing burning and redness with minimal exposure.

Rare adverse reactions include blood dyscrasias. Prolonged therapy with some antihistamines may precipitate narrow-angle glaucoma and psychiatric disturbances that differ from the confusion usually associated with anticholinergic therapy.

NURSING IMPLICATIONS

When monitoring a patient receiving anticholinergic drugs, the nurse must be aware of the following points.
• Do not administer anticholinergics to patients with narrow-angle glaucoma. Elderly patients and those with open-angle glaucoma should receive regular eye examinations, including intraocular pressure measurements.
• Caution a male patient with prostatic hypertrophy that he may experience severe urinary retention. Expect to discontinue anticholinergic agents for such a patient.

Predictable adverse reactions to the anticholinergics

Common predictable adverse reactions to anticholinergic agents are described below. Use this illustration as a head to toe guide when assessing a patient.

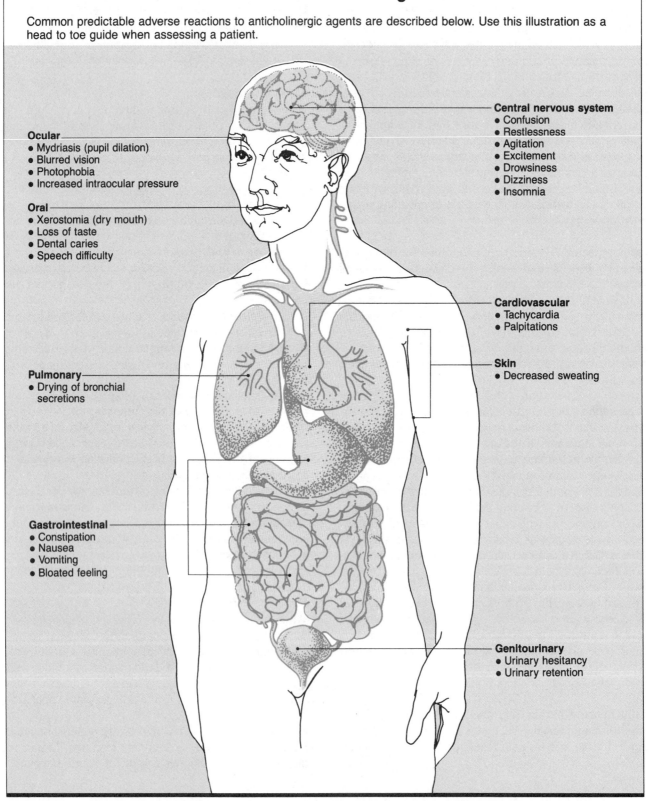

Ocular
- Mydriasis (pupil dilation)
- Blurred vision
- Photophobia
- Increased intraocular pressure

Oral
- Xerostomia (dry mouth)
- Loss of taste
- Dental caries
- Speech difficulty

Pulmonary
- Drying of bronchial secretions

Gastrointestinal
- Constipation
- Nausea
- Vomiting
- Bloated feeling

Central nervous system
- Confusion
- Restlessness
- Agitation
- Excitement
- Drowsiness
- Dizziness
- Insomnia

Cardiovascular
- Tachycardia
- Palpitations

Skin
- Decreased sweating

Genitourinary
- Urinary hesitancy
- Urinary retention

• Expect an elderly patient or a patient with dementia to experience confusion with an anticholinergic agent. In a patient with asthma or chronic obstructive pulmonary disease, anticholinergics may thicken bronchial secretions, causing increased breathing difficulty.

• Administer anticholinergic agents cautiously to patients with tachycardia, cardiac dysrhythmias, hypotension, hypertension, hyperthyroidism, coronary artery disease, or congestive heart failure.

• Administer anticholinergic agents cautiously to patients with gastric ulcer, esophageal reflux, or hiatal hernia associated with reflux esophagitis, because these drugs can prolong gastric emptying, decrease gastric motility, and decrease lower esophageal sphincter pressure.

• Exercise extreme caution when giving anticholinergics to a patient with diarrhea—a possible sign of incomplete intestinal obstruction—or to a patient with mild to moderate ulcerative colitis.

• Encourage a patient with constipation to ambulate, drink more fluids, and eat more dietary fiber, if possible. Administer a bulk-forming laxative or stool softener, if prescribed. Routinely check the patient for the presence of bowel sounds to help rule out the possibility of GI obstruction.

• Notify the physician if the patient experiences sustained tachycardia, confusion, eye pain, or a skin rash.

• Instruct the patient to take anticholinergics either during or shortly after meals to prevent adverse GI reactions.

• Instruct the patient that xerostomia (dry mouth) can be relieved by drinking cold beverages, sucking on hard candy, chewing gum, or using a nonprescription saliva substitute, such as Xero-Lube or Moi-Stir. Tell the patient that good oral hygiene is especially important because xerostomia increases susceptibility to tooth decay.

• Caution a patient taking anticholinergics not to discontinue long-term therapy before consulting the physician.

• Caution the patient about performing tasks that require alertness because these drugs may cause drowsiness and blurred vision. Remind the patient that alcohol may increase the drowsiness.

• Advise the patient to avoid prolonged exposure to high temperatures because anticholinergics increase the risk of heat stroke by reducing the ability to sweat.

• Instruct the patient not to take over-the-counter cough or cold preparations, diet aids, or analeptics (agents used to stay awake) before consulting with the physician.

• Instruct family members to report any signs of confusion or mental changes to the physician, especially if the patient is elderly.

DOPAMINERGIC AGENTS

Dopaminergics include four chemically unrelated drugs: levodopa, the metabolic precursor to dopamine; carbidopa-levodopa, a drug composed of the substance carbidopa, along with levodopa; amantadine hydrochloride, an antiviral; and bromocriptine mesylate, a semisynthetic ergot alkaloid.

History and source
In 1961, two separate investigators tested levodopa, which represented a major advancement in treating Parkinson's disease. Seven years later, researchers discovered by chance that the antiviral drug amantadine was also useful in treating this disorder. Then, in 1974, scientists reported clinical effectiveness of bromocriptine in patients with Parkinson's disease.

PHARMACOKINETICS
Like anticholinergics, dopaminergic agents are absorbed from the GI tract into the bloodstream and are delivered to their action site in the brain. The liver, kidneys, or both eliminate these drugs from the body.

Absorption, distribution, metabolism, excretion
Levodopa competes with dietary amino acids for absorption from the small intestine and is absorbed by active transport processes. Consequently, levodopa absorption is slowed when the drug is ingested with food. The body absorbs most of a levodopa, carbidopa-levodopa, or amantadine dose from the GI tract after oral administration, but it absorbs only about 28% of a bromocriptine dose. Carbidopa absorption ranges from about 40% to 70%. After absorption, bromocriptine undergoes substantial first-pass metabolism in the liver.

Levodopa is widely distributed into most body tissues, including the GI tract, liver, pancreas, kidneys, salivary glands, and skin. Carbidopa-levodopa is also widely distributed. However, levodopa penetrates the brain and CNS in small amounts, and carbidopa-levodopa does not.

Large amounts of levodopa are metabolized in the lumen of the stomach and during the first pass through the liver. After absorption, more than 95% is converted into dopamine peripherally (outside the CNS). But peripherally produced dopamine is ineffective because it cannot penetrate the CNS, where it is needed. To work, levodopa must undergo conversion to dopamine within the brain. When carbidopa is combined with levodopa, carbidopa blocks the peripheral conversion of levodopa to dopamine and allows levodopa to cross the blood-brain barrier. The levodopa is then converted in the brain to dopamine. Carbidopa also increases plasma levodopa concentration levels, which may make smaller levodopa doses effective. This, in turn, reduces the number of adverse effects from levodopa alone.

Carbidopa-levodopa is not extensively metabolized. The kidneys excrete approximately one third of it as unchanged drug within 24 hours. Levodopa is extensively metabolized to various compounds that are excreted by the kidneys.

The pharmacokinetic processes of amantadine and bromocriptine are not completely understood. Although amantadine undergoes some hepatic metabolism, about 90% of it is excreted unchanged by the kidneys. Therefore, an elderly patient or a patient with renal insufficiency will require a lower dose of amantadine based on the degree of renal impairment. In contrast, almost all of a bromocriptine dose is hepatically metabolized to pharmacologically inactive compounds. Elimination of bromocriptine and its metabolites occurs primarily in the feces, although 2% to 2.5% is excreted in the urine.

Onset, peak, duration

The onset of action, peak concentration levels, and duration of action of levodopa—with or without carbidopa—vary widely in patients. Levodopa's onset of action usually occurs in 30 to 45 minutes, and its duration of action ranges from 2 to 5 hours. Administration of levodopa with food may delay its onset of action. Levodopa produces a short-term improvement that subsides 5 hours after a dose and a long-term improvement with prolonged therapy. The half-life of carbidopa-levidopa is approximately 2 hours, or about double that of levodopa alone.

Amantadine usually produces clinical effects faster than levodopa, in 48 hours. If the patient does not respond in 2 weeks, the drug should be discontinued. Amantadine's peak concentration levels occur approximately 1 to 4 hours after administration. Its half-life varies greatly but averages 15 hours.

Bromocriptine's onset of action varies somewhat; improvement in parkinsonian signs may occur 30 to 90 minutes after a single dose. Peak concentration levels occur in approximately 2 hours, and the duration of action is 3 to 5 hours. Bromocriptine has a half-life of 6 hours.

PHARMACODYNAMICS

The dopaminergic agents act in the brain by increasing the dopamine concentration or by enhancing neuro-

transmission of dopamine. These two mechanisms help improve motor function.

Mechanism of action

Levodopa is pharmacologically inactive until it crosses the blood-brain barrier and is converted by enzymes in the brain to dopamine. Following this conversion, levodopa acts primarily by increasing dopamine concentrations in the basal ganglia. Carbidopa enhances levodopa's effectiveness.

Amantadine's mechanism of action is less clear. Amantadine may increase the amount of dopamine in the brain by increasing dopamine release or by blocking dopamine reuptake from presynaptic neurons.

Bromocriptine stimulates dopamine receptors in the brain, producing effects that are similar to dopamine's.

PHARMACOTHERAPEUTICS

Usually, dopaminergic agents are used to treat patients with severe Parkinson's disease or patients who do not respond to anticholinergics alone. Besides the drugs listed in this section, two other drugs are undergoing testing for treating Parkinson's disease. (See *New antiparkinsonian agents under investigation* for details.)

levodopa (Dopar, Larodopa, Levopa). The most effective drug for parkinsonism, levodopa is used to treat the

---

New antiparkinsonian agents under investigation

Researchers are investigating selegiline (Deprenyl), a type B monoamine oxidase (MAO) inhibitor, to determine its usefulness as an adjunct to levodopa in the later stages of Parkinson's disease. Preliminary trials have found that selegiline prolongs levodopa's therapeutic effectiveness. But they also have shown that the response to the drug varies greatly and that it has little effect on patients with long-term Parkinson's disease. Unlike other MAO inhibitors, selegiline does not interact with levodopa or tyramine-containing foods to produce a hypertensive crisis in most patients. Trials continue.

Another investigational agent, pergolide, is being tested as an adjunct to levodopa. Although this potent dopamine agonist decreases akinesia, rigidity, and gait disorders, its beneficial effects seem to decrease after 6 months of therapy. Pergolide seems as effective as bromocriptine, but with fewer cardiovascular adverse effects. Research continues.

DRUG INTERACTIONS

Dopaminergic agents

Among the dopaminergic agents, levodopa causes most of the significant interactions with other drugs and with foods. Levodopa and monoamine oxidase (MAO) inhibitors can produce a hypertensive crisis when given concomitantly. Less serious drug interactions can also occur with other dopaminergics, producing additive toxicities or decreasing the effectiveness of the dopaminergic drug.

DRUG	INTERACTING DRUGS	POSSIBLE EFFECTS	NURSING IMPLICATIONS
levodopa	pyridoxine (vitamin B_6)	Decreases effectiveness of levodopa caused by increased peripheral conversion of levodopa to dopamine by vitamin B_6	• Instruct the patient taking levodopa without carbidopa to avoid vitamin B_6 supplements or multiple vitamins containing vitamin B_6. • Be aware that this drug interaction may not occur in a patient taking carbidopa-levodopa.
levodopa, carbidopa-levodopa	MAO inhibitors	Cause hypertensive crisis; increase toxic effects of levodopa	• If this combination is given, monitor the patient for hypertension. • Document and inform the physician if a patient starting levodopa has not taken an MAO inhibitor in the past 2 weeks.
	phenytoin	Decreases effectiveness of levodopa	• Observe the patient for increased signs of parkinsonism, such as bradykinesia, rigidity, and tremor. • Tell the patient to report any worsening of parkinsonian symptoms to the physician. • Expect to increase the levodopa dose or administer an alternative anticonvulsant as prescribed.
	antipsychotics (chlorpromazine, thioridazine, perphenazine, prochlorperazine, trifluoperazine, thiothixene, haloperidol, loxapine)	Decrease effectiveness of levodopa	• Avoid concomitant use of antipsychotics. If an antipsychotic medication is required, thioridazine is generally preferred. • Observe the patient for an increase in parkinsonian signs.
levodopa, carbidopa-levodopa, bromocriptine	reserpine	Decreases therapeutic response to levodopa by depletion of dopamine stores in the brain	• Avoid administering reserpine to a patient receiving levodopa. • Monitor the patient's blood pressure, and observe for orthostatic hypotension, especially during dosage adjustments. • Instruct the patient with orthostatic hypotension to arise slowly from a lying or sitting position.
levodopa, carbidopa-levodopa, amantadine	anticholinergics	Increase anticholinergic adverse effects with amantadine, including adverse effects on mental function; decrease levodopa absorption, possibly leading to worsening of parkinsonian signs and symptoms or exacerbation of abnormal involuntary movements	• Observe the patient taking amantadine for changes in mental status, urinary retention, and dry mouth. • Expect to reduce the dose of either agent, as prescribed, if intolerable anticholinergic adverse reactions occur. • Monitor the patient taking levodopa for increased rigidity, bradykinesia, and tremor or for exacerbation of abnormal involuntary movements.

idiopathic and postencephalitic forms, especially in moderate to severe cases in advanced stages. Levodopa can be administered alone or in combination with other drugs.

USUAL ADULT DOSAGE: initially, 0.5 to 1 gram P.O. b.i.d., t.i.d., or q.i.d., increased by 100 to 750 mg every 3 to 7 days until an optimum response is achieved or the maximum dosage of 8 grams is reached. The usual optimum dosage ranges from 3 to 6 grams P.O. in 3 or more divided doses. The typical patient reaches this level in 6 to 8 weeks.

carbidopa-levodopa (Sinemet). In this combination drug, carbidopa allows more levodopa to be converted to dopamine in the brain by inhibiting peripheral conversion. Physicians use carbidopa-levodopa to treat idiopathic, postencephalitic, and symptomatic Parkinson's disease. Carbidopa-levodopa is available as combination tablets of 10 mg carbidopa/100 mg levodopa, 25 mg carbidopa/100 mg levodopa, or 25 mg carbidopa/250 mg levodopa. Carbidopa (Lodosyn) is also available by itself in a 25 mg tablet.

USUAL ADULT DOSAGE: initially, 25 mg carbidopa/-250 mg levodopa P.O.; if the patient is not currently receiving levodopa, initiate dosage with one tablet of 10 mg carbidopa/100 mg levodopa or 25 mg carbidopa/100 mg levodopa t.i.d. Increase by one tablet daily or every other day to dosage of 6 tablets per day. The usual dosage of carbidopa-levodopa ranges from 75/300 to 150/1,500 mg P.O. daily.

In a patient switching from levodopa alone to carbidopa-levodopa, discontinue levodopa at least 8 hours before initiating combination therapy. Then start carbidopa-levodopa with a daily dosage of no more than 25% of the previous levodopa dosage. Patients on combination therapy require close monitoring because therapeutic and adverse effects develop more rapidly.

amantadine hydrochloride (Symmetrel). This drug may be used by itself in the early stages of Parkinson's disease or with other drugs in the advanced stages. Available as a capsule or as syrup, amantadine is especially effective against rigidity and bradykinesia, but less effective against tremor.

USUAL ADULT DOSAGE: 100 mg P.O. b.i.d.; adjust dosage as prescribed in patients with renal insufficiency; in patients with other serious illnesses or active seizure disorders and in patients who are already receiving other antiparkinsonian agents, 100 mg P.O. daily for at least 1 week, then 100 mg b.i.d.. If amantadine must be withdrawn, do so gradually to avoid precipitating parkinsonian crisis and possible life-threatening complications.

bromocriptine mesylate (Parlodel). This drug is used primarily as an adjunct to levodopa in the later stages of idiopathic or postencephalitic Parkinson's disease. Used in combination with levodopa, bromocriptine may reduce levodopa's long-term adverse effects.

USUAL ADULT DOSAGE: initially, 1.25 mg P.O. once or twice daily with meals, increased by 1.25 to 2.5 mg every 2 to 3 days, up to 100 mg t.i.d. or q.i.d. The usual adult maintenance dose ranges from 10 to 40 mg P.O. daily. The patient's therapeutic response needs to be assessed every 2 weeks to ensure that the lowest effective dose is being used. To prevent levodopa's adverse effects, the levodopa dose may need to be reduced as the bromocriptine dose is increased. If necessary, bromocriptine should be withdrawn gradually.

Drug interactions

The most serious interaction between the dopaminergics and other drugs occurs when levodopa is combined with monoamine oxidase (MAO) inhibitors. This combination can produce hypertensive crisis. Other interactions between dopaminergics and other drugs usually decrease the effectiveness of the dopaminergic agent, especially levodopa. (See *Drug interactions: Dopaminergic agents* on page 365 for a summary.)

In some patients, levodopa may produce a significant interaction with foods. Dietary amino acids can decrease levodopa's effectiveness by competing with it for absorption from the intestine and slowing its transport to the brain. Therefore, if a patient's response deteriorates regularly after meals, the patient may need to reduce protein intake and avoid taking levodopa with meals to minimize this reaction.

ADVERSE DRUG REACTIONS

Among the dopaminergics, amantadine produces the fewest adverse reactions. Adverse reactions to bromocriptine and levodopa are mainly dose-related and can occur peripherally or in the CNS.

Predictable reactions

The adverse reactions to levodopa or carbidopa-levodopa are usually dose-dependent and reversible. Carbidopa decreases levodopa's peripheral effects but not its CNS effects. Levodopa commonly produces GI adverse reactions, such as nausea, vomiting, and anorexia. It can also cause orthostatic (postural) hypotension as well as other, less common cardiovascular adverse effects, such as palpitations, tachycardia, dysrhythmias, flushing, and hypertension. Additional adverse reactions include dark-colored urine and sweat, urinary frequency or retention, and visual difficulties.

The most distressing problem with levodopa is the drug's loss of effectiveness after 3 to 5 years. The problem takes one of two forms: the on-off phenomenon, characterized by sharp fluctuations between mobility and immobility, or the end-of-dose deterioration (also known as the wearing-off effect), a progressive decrease in the duration of beneficial effects from each levodopa dose. The use of smaller, more frequent doses of levodopa and the addition of bromocriptine to the regimen can reduce both problems.

Amantadine produces relatively few adverse reactions at usual dosages. However, long-term therapy produces livedo reticularis (diffuse, mottled reddening of the skin usually confined to the lower extremities), which is often accompanied by mild ankle edema. Other relatively common adverse reactions include urinary retention, orthostatic hypotension, anorexia, nausea, and constipation. CNS effects may include inability to concentrate, confusion, light-headedness, anxiety, irritability, dizziness, and hallucinations.

Besides cost, adverse reactions are the most important factor limiting the use of bromocriptine. Adverse reactions are more common at the start of therapy and when dosage exceeds 20 mg/day. GI adverse reactions, such as nausea, occur frequently. Other common initial adverse reactions include orthostatic hypotension, vomiting, acute anxiety, dizziness, and sedation. Erythromelalgia (intermittent burning and throbbing sensations in the extremities) may also occur. Bromocriptine can adversely affect the cardiovascular system by producing persistent orthostatic hypotension (which may result in syncope), edema in the ankles and feet, palpitations, ventricular tachycardia, bradycardia, and exacerbation of angina. Confusion, hallucinations, delusions, nightmares, and erythromelalgia are especially notable during long-term or high-dosage (100 mg or more daily) bromocriptine therapy, but they are usually reversible. The presence of CNS adverse reactions usually limits the dosage and is the main reason for discontinuation of bromocriptine therapy.

Unpredictable reactions

Amantadine may cause a skin rash, leukopenia, eczematoid dermatitis, seizures, oculogyric episodes, and lingual and facial dyskinesias (movement impairments). These reactions, however, are rare.

Bromocriptine therapy has been associated with pleuropulmonary reactions, such as pulmonary infiltrates, pleural effusions, and thickening of the pleura. Bladder dysfunction with incontinence, urinary frequency, and urinary retention have also been reported. Signs and symptoms of ergotism, including numbness and tingling of the extremities, cold feet, and muscle cramps in the legs and feet, may also occur.

Following withdrawal of levodopa, some patients experience hyperpyrexia (extreme elevation of body temperature) and neuroleptic malignant syndrome (characterized by hyperthermia, akinesia, altered consciousness, muscular rigidity, and profuse sweating). Both of these reactions can be fatal. Hematologic effects—such as leukopenia, granulocytopenia, thrombocytopenia, hemolytic anemia, and decreased hemoglobin and hematocrit levels—may also occur. When used alone, levodopa can cause transient elevations of liver enzymes, bilirubin, and blood urea nitrogen (BUN). When combined with carbidopa, levodopa may produce lower BUN, serum creatinine, and uric acid laboratory test values.

NURSING IMPLICATIONS

The nurse must be aware of the following considerations with dopaminergic agents.

• Administer amantadine cautiously to a patient with recurrent eczematoid dermatitis, seizure disorders, renal insufficiency, or recurrent psychosis.

• If a patient experiences insomnia during amantadine therapy, give the second daily dose earlier in the evening.

• Relieve the ankle edema associated with amantadine therapy by elevating the patient's legs if appropriate; this drug-induced edema is unresponsive to diuretics.

• Monitor the blood pressure periodically to detect orthostatic hypotension in a patient receiving bromocriptine.

• Be aware that elderly patients and patients with dementia are usually susceptible to CNS adverse reactions to bromocriptine.

• Expect to reduce the bromocriptine dosage for a patient with hepatic dysfunction.

• Administer bromocriptine cautiously to a patient with a history of myocardial infarction with a residual dysrhythmia.

• Caution the patient that bromocriptine may cause alcohol intolerance.

• Do not administer levodopa to patients with narrow-angle glaucoma. Use with caution in a patient with dysrhythmias following myocardial infarction; with a history of active peptic ulcer or psychosis; with bronchial asthma or emphysema; with severe cardiovascular, pulmonary, renal, hepatic, or endocrine disease; and in a patient who requires a sympathomimetic agent such as epinephrine.

• Be aware that levodopa interferes with various laboratory test results. For instance, urine glucose tests may produce false-positive (Clinitest) or false-negative (Clinistix, Tes-Tape) results; urinary ketone tests may produce false-positive results with Acetest, Ketostix, and Labstix.

• Administer levodopa (without carbidopa) and bromocriptine with meals to decrease GI adverse reactions.

Antiparkinsonian agents

This chart summarizes the most commonly used agents for treating Parkinson's disease.

DRUG	MAJOR INDICATIONS	USUAL ADULT DOSAGES	NURSING IMPLICATIONS
Anticholinergic agents			
trihexyphenidyl	Control of symptoms in the early stages of Parkinson's disease (given alone or with amantadine) and in the advanced stages (given with levodopa)	3 to 15 mg P.O. t.i.d.	• Be aware that anticholinergics may precipitate or increase urinary retention in a patient with prostatic hypertrophy.
benztropine		1 to 2 mg P.O., I.V., or I.M. daily	• Caution the patient about performing tasks that require alertness because these drugs may cause drowsiness or blurred vision. Remind the patient that alcohol may increase the drowsiness.
diphenhydramine		25 to 50 mg P.O. t.i.d. or q.i.d., or 10 to 100 mg I.M. or I.V. t.i.d. or q.i.d.	• Routinely check the patient for the presence of bowel sounds to rule out GI obstruction.
			• Administer anticholinergics either during or shortly after meals, to prevent adverse GI reactions.
			• Inform the patient that xerostomia can be relieved by drinking cold beverages, sucking hard candy, chewing gum, or using a nonprescription saliva substitute. Encourage oral hygiene.
			• Administer levodopa (without carbidopa) with meals to decrease GI adverse reactions.
Dopaminergic agents			
levodopa	Control of moderate to severe symptoms in Parkinson's disease (timing of initiation of levodopa therapy is controversial)	3 to 6 grams P.O. daily in 3 or more divided doses	• Administer carbidopa-levodopa when the patient's stomach is empty to ensure adequate absorption.
carbidopa-levodopa		75/300 to 150/1,500 mg P.O. daily	• Administer with caution to a patient with residual dysrhythmias after myocardial infarction or with a history of peptic ulcer disease or psychosis.
			• Teach the patient beginning levodopa therapy about the on-off phenomenon, and instruct the patient to report any unusual, uncontrolled body movements to the physician.

• Inform the patient that levodopa may cause harmless discoloration of the urine or sweat.

• Tell diabetic patients that levodopa can interfere with urine glucose and ketone test results and that they should report any abnormal results to the physician before changing the dosage of any hypoglycemic agents.

• Teach the patient beginning levodopa therapy about the on-off phenomenon, and instruct the patient to report any unusual, uncontrolled body movements to the physician.

• Advise the patient beginning levodopa therapy that the drug may take several weeks or months to reach its maximum efficacy.

• Instruct the patient on long-term levodopa or bro-

mocriptine therapy not to discontinue these drugs before consulting the physician.

• Administer carbidopa-levodopa when the patient's stomach is empty to ensure adequate absorption.

CHAPTER SUMMARY

This chapter concentrated on drugs for Parkinson's disease. Here are highlights:

• Two major drug classes, the anticholinergics and the dopaminergics, are used to treat Parkinson's disease. The anticholinergics include many clinically similar drugs, whereas the dopaminergics include four distinctly different drugs.

• Anticholinergic agents may be used alone or in combination with amantadine in the early stages of Parkinson's disease, and in combination with levodopa in the more advanced stages. Although trihexyphenidyl, benztropine, and diphenhydramine are used most often, no single anticholinergic agent is clinically superior to the others. Effectiveness depends on the patient.

• Although anticholinergic agents control tremor, they are not effective alone as the disease progresses. Usually, anticholinergics produce minor, troublesome adverse effects. They can, however, produce significant CNS toxicity in susceptible patients, especially in the elderly and in patients receiving other drugs that produce anticholinergic adverse effects.

• Levodopa, a dopaminergic agent, is the most effective drug used to treat Parkinson's disease. Levodopa therapy is usually begun during advanced stages, either alone or in combination with carbidopa. Carbidopa given with levodopa is preferred because it reduces the levodopa dosage, decreasing GI and cardiovascular adverse reactions.

• Levodopa presents two major therapeutic problems after 3 to 5 years of treatment: sharp fluctuations between mobility and immobility in the patient and a progressive decrease in beneficial effects. Although smaller, more frequent doses help, both problems become increasingly difficult to manage as the disease progresses.

• Bromocriptine, another dopaminergic agent, serves primarily as an adjunct to levodopa in the advanced stages of Parkinson's disease. Bromocriptine helps control the problems of long-term levodopa use. Bromocriptine's major drawbacks are its high cost and its adverse effects. Adverse CNS effects deserve special consideration, especially in elderly patients and in those who are receiving levodopa. CNS toxicity usually limits the dose that a patient can take.

• Amantadine is used alone or in combination with anticholinergics in the early stages of Parkinson's disease; in later disease stages, it may also be used with levodopa. Patients taking amantadine commonly develop a tolerance to it shortly after therapy begins. Tolerance does not develop, however, when the drug is used in combination with levodopa or bromocriptine. Amantadine produces relatively benign adverse effects, but it can produce more severe ones if its dosage is not reduced for elderly patients or patients with renal insufficiency or seizure disorders.

BIBLIOGRAPHY

American Hospital Formulary Service. *Drug Information 86.* McEvoy, G.K., et al., eds. Bethesda, Md.: American Society of Hospital Pharmacists, 1986.

Berg, M.J., et al. "Parkinsonism—Drug Treatment: Part I," *Drug Intelligence and Clinical Pharmacy* 21:10, January 1987.

Cedarbaum, J.M. "Parkinsonism: Treatment Strategies," *Drug Therapy* 15:47, November 1985.

Erwin, W.G., and Turco, T.F. "Current Concepts in Clinical Therapeutics: Parkinson's Disease," *Clinical Pharmacy* 5:742, 1986.

Feldman, R.G. "Temporary Levodopa Withdrawal," *The New England Journal of Medicine* 314:851, March 1986.

Foster, N.L., et al. "Peripheral Beta Adrenergic Blockade in the Treatment of Parkinsonian Tremor," *Annals of Neurology* 16:505, October 1984.

Friedman, J.H. "'Drug Holidays' in the Treatment of Parkinson's Disease," *Archives of Internal Medicine* 145:913, May 1985.

Friedman, J.H., et al. "A Neuroleptic Malignantlike Syndrome Due to Levodopa Therapy Withdrawal," *Journal of the American Medical Association* 254:2792, November 1985.

Gibberd, F.B. "The Management of Parkinson's Disease," *The Practitioner* 230:139, February 1986.

Goetz, C.G. "Skin Rash Associated with Sinemet 25/100," *The New England Journal of Medicine* 309:1387, December 1983.

Hunt-Fugate, A.K. "Adverse Reactions Due to Dopamine Blockade by Amoxapine," *Pharmacotherapy* 4:35, January/February 1984.

Jankovic, J. "Parkinsonian Disorders," in *Current Neurology,* vol. 5. Edited by Appel, S.H., New York: John Wiley & Sons, 1984.

Kastrup, E.K., et al., eds. *Facts and Comparisons.* St. Louis: Facts and Comparisons Division, J.B. Lippincott Co., 1986.

Kochar, A.S. "Development of Malignant Melanoma after Levodopa Therapy for Parkinson's Disease," *The American Journal of Medicine* 79:11, July 1985.

Lang, A.E. "Treatment of Parkinson's Disease with Agents Other than Levodopa and Dopamine Agonists: Controversies and New Approaches," *The Canadian Journal of Neurological Sciences* 11:210, February 1984.

Lawry, R. "A New Drug for Parkinson's Disease," *The Practitioner* 227:347, March 1983.

Maier, M.M., and Elton, R.L. "Low Dosages of Bromocriptine Added to Levodopa in Parkinson's Disease," *Neurology* 35:199, February 1985.

Mangini, R.J., ed. *Drug Interaction Facts*. Philadelphia: J.B. Lippincott Co., 1986.

Mayeux, R., et al. "Reappraisal of Temporary Levodopa Withdrawal ('Drug Holiday') in Parkinson's Disease," *The New England Journal of Medicine* 313:724, September 1985.

Melamed, E. "Initiation of Levodopa Therapy in Parkinsonian Patients Should be Delayed until the Advanced Stages of the Disease," *Archives of Neurology* 43:402, April 1986.

Miller, J.Q. "Involuntary Movements in the Elderly: Parkinson's Disease and Other Causes," *Postgraduate Medicine* 79:323, March 1986.

Morris, J.G.L. "The Treatment of Parkinson's Disease," *The Medical Journal of Australia* 143:347, October 1985.

Nutt, J.G. "The 'On-Off' Phenomenon in Parkinson's Disease: Relation to Levodopa Absorption and Transport," *The New England Journal of Medicine* 310:483, February 1984.

O'Sullivan, D.J. "Management of Parkinson's Disease," *Australian Prescriber* 9:6, 1986.

Pincus, J.H. "Rationale for Early Use of Levodopa in Parkinsonism," *The Lancet* 1:612, March 1986.

Quinn, N.P. "Anti-Parkinsonian Drugs Today," *Drugs* 28:236, 1984.

Quinn, N., and Marsden, D.C. "Lithium for Painful Dystonia in Parkinson's Disease," *The Lancet* 1:1377, June 1986.

Rajput, A.H., and Uitti, R.J. "When to Use Levodopa in Parkinsonism," *The Lancet* 1:1324, June 1986.

Rinne, U.K. "Combined Bromocriptine-Levodopa Therapy Early in Parkinson's Disease," *Neurology* 35:1196, August 1985.

Sechi, G.P., et al. "Fatal Hyperpyrexia after Withdrawal of Levodopa," *Neurology* 34:249, February 1984.

Shimomura, S.K. "Parkinson's Disease," in *Applied Therapeutics: The Clinical Use of Drugs*. Edited by Katcher, B., et al. San Francisco: Applied Therapeutics, Inc., 1983.

Staal-Schreinmachers, A.L., et al. "Low-Dose Bromocriptine Therapy in Parkinson's Disease: Double-Blind, Placebo-Controlled Study," *Neurology* 36:291, February 1986.

Still, C.N. "Involuntary Movement Disorders," *Neurologic Clinics* 2:71, February 1984.

USPDI: Drug Information for the Health Care Provider, vol. I, 6th ed. Rockville, Md.: The United States Pharmacopeial Convention, Inc., 1985.

"Drugs for Parkinsonism," *The Medical Letter* 28:62, June 1986.

CHAPTER
24

ANTICONVULSANT AGENTS

OBJECTIVES

After reading and studying this chapter, you should be able to:

1. Identify the four factors that physicians consider when choosing a specific anticonvulsant for a patient.

2. Describe the clinical characteristics of the major types of seizures as identified by the International Classification of Epileptic Seizures.

3. Describe the mechanisms of action and the types of seizures treated by the following: hydantoins, barbiturates, iminostilbenes, benzodiazepines, succinimides, and valproic acid.

4. Describe the pharmacotherapeutic differences between the free acid form and the sodium salt form of phenytoin.

5. Describe the important adverse reactions associated with each of the six major classes of anticonvulsants.

6. Identify precautions to take when administering each of the six major classes of anticonvulsants.

INTRODUCTION

Physicians prescribe anticonvulsant drugs for long-term management of chronic epilepsy (recurrent seizures) and for short-term management of acute isolated seizures not caused by epilepsy. The short-term use of anticonvulsants also provides prophylaxis after trauma or a craniotomy. Selected anticonvulsants are indicated in the emergency treatment of status epilepticus, which is characterized by a series of rapidly repeating convulsions without intervening periods of consciousness.

Seizures can be classified in various ways, but health care professionals usually use the International Classification of epileptic seizures as the standard system. (See *International classification of epileptic seizures* on page 372 for the characteristics associated with the different kinds of seizures.)

The accurate diagnosis of a seizure requires a reliable patient history, careful patient observations, and an electroencephalogram (EEG). The pharmacologic therapy used to treat seizures differs, depending on the type of seizure. The goal of anticonvulsant therapy is to control or prevent seizures. For many patients, anticonvulsant therapy is lifelong. Some patients, however, may have their drug therapy tapered and eventually discontinued, if they do not experience any seizures for a year.

Physicians determine the specific anticonvulsant drug for a patient by considering four factors:

● the accurate diagnosis of the seizure type

● the ability of the drug to control seizures while producing only minimal adverse effects

● the use of a single anticonvulsant when possible

● the appropriateness of the anticonvulsant for the patient's age and health state.

The nurse must be aware of several nursing implications concerning administration, adverse reactions, and patient teaching.

For a summary of representative drugs, see *Selected major drugs: Anticonvulsant agents* on pages 391 and 392.

HYDANTOINS

Phenytoin, the most commonly prescribed anticonvulsant agent, belongs to the hydantoin class of drugs. Mephenytoin and ethotoin are also hydantoin anticonvulsants.

History and source

Although phenytoin was synthesized in 1908, its anticonvulsant activity was not discovered until 1938 by Merritt and Putnam. The establishment of phenytoin as an anticonvulsant represented a landmark event, because it verified that anticonvulsant agents need not impair consciousness in contrast to the then commonly used bromides and phenobarbital.

International classification of epileptic seizures

Rational anticonvulsant therapy depends primarily on the accurate diagnosis of the seizure type. The following two classifications conform with the international classification scheme and reflect the current practice related to seizure types and their clinical characteristics. A third category of epileptic seizures remains unclassified because of inadequate or incomplete data. Earlier terminology appears in parentheses.

SEIZURE CLASSIFICATION	CLINICAL CHARACTERISTICS
Partial seizures—focal or local seizures	
simple partial seizures (focal; jacksonian) • sensory • motor • autonomic • psychic	Most common in older children and adults. Consciousness not impaired; an aura is a simple partial seizure.
complex partial seizures (psychomotor epilepsy) or **temporal lobe seizures**	Most common in older children and adults; brief impairment of consciousness; characterized by loss of contact with reality, automatisms (automatic behaviors such as chewing, lip smacking), and confusion that may last 1 to 2 minutes after seizure subsides.
partial seizures evolving to secondarily generalized seizures	Partial seizures may spread, or "march," and ultimately involve all other parts of the brain with subsequent loss of consciousness. A tonic-clonic seizure follows.
Generalized seizures—convulsive or nonconvulsive	
absence seizures (petit mal) • typical	Onset between 4 and 8 years; abrupt loss of consciousness, amnesia, or unawareness characterized by staring and a 3-cycle/second spike and waveform on EEG; duration of attack lasts 10 to 30 seconds; may occur as frequently as 50 to 100 times/day. No postictal or confused state follows the attack.
• atypical	Slower onset and cessation of attacks than is usually seen with absence seizures.
myoclonic seizures	Occur in older children and adults; myoclonic, lightning jerks (flexor or extensor) without loss of consciousness; last from seconds to minutes or longer and may occur daily.
clonic seizures	Rhythmic clonic contraction and relaxation of muscles, loss of consciousness, and marked autonomic signs and symptoms.
tonic seizures	Abrupt increase in muscle tone (contraction), loss of consciousness, and marked autonomic signs and symptoms.
tonic-clonic seizures (grand mal)	Can occur at any age. May be preceded by an aura or an outcry. Contraction of all skeletal muscle masses occurs in rhythmic, alternating clonic and tonic patterns, followed by depression of all central functions, a state called the postictal period. Urinary and fecal incontinence may occur. Usually lasts 2 to 5 minutes but may last much longer. The frequency of attacks varies.
atonic seizures	Seen in older children and adults. Consciousness usually lost, accompanied by loss of postural tone or akinesis. Lasts a few seconds to minutes and may occur daily.

PHARMACOKINETICS

Usually the hydantoin anticonvulsants are slowly absorbed, rapidly distributed, and extensively protein bound. These drugs are usually metabolized by hepatic microsomal enzymes and excreted unchanged as metabolites in the urine.

Absorption, distribution, metabolism, excretion

Phenytoin is slowly absorbed following oral administration and poorly absorbed after I.M. administration. Ab-

General patient-teaching tips

Regardless of the anticonvulsant prescribed, the following patient-teaching tips apply.
• Instruct the patient not to alter the prescribed drug regimen.
• Alert the patient that abrupt discontinuation of the prescribed drug could precipitate seizures or status epilepticus.
• Remind the patient to check all prescription refills to ensure that the drug preparation is the same as the prior preparation.
• Advise the patient to avoid hazardous activities until the dosage and adverse effects become stabilized.
• Teach the patient's family how to care for the patient during a seizure.
• Advise the patient not to self-medicate with over-the-counter medications.
• Advise the patient to refrain from ingesting alcohol because of its possible interactive effects with some anticonvulsants.
• Emphasize the importance of frequent follow-up care for the patient, and provide information about voluntary community organizations that provide information and support.

sorption rates, however, may vary with different phenytoin preparations. For example, Dilantin Kapseals are designed to provide extended therapy and, therefore, are absorbed more slowly; they also reach peak concentration more slowly than other preparations. Clinically, the physicians must differentiate among the various preparations and their administration routes to determine which preparation meets the therapeutic needs of a specific patient.

Phenytoin is rapidly distributed to all tissues, with highest concentrations occurring in the liver and adipose tissue; it is also extensively bound (90%) to plasma proteins, primarily albumin. Decreased protein binding occurs in neonates and in patients who are hypoalbuminemic or uremic. This decreased protein binding causes a higher free phenytoin serum concentration level that can cause toxicity, even with normal measured serum concentrations.

Phenytoin is metabolized in the liver by the hepatic microsmal enzymes. Between 60% and 70% of a single dose of phenytoin is metabolized to an inactive metabolite, a parahydroxyphenyl derivative excreted as a glucuronide in the urine. Metabolism of phenytoin also produces other inactive metabolites.

The metabolism of phenytoin is dose dependent, demonstrating saturation kinetics; that is, at a certain drug concentration, the hepatic enzymes that metabolize phenytoin become saturated. When saturation occurs, further increase in drug concentration does not result in a direct linear increment but, instead, demonstrates a disproportionate increase in plasma concentration level. Therefore, incremental increases in phenytoin dosage must be made cautiously. (See *Phenytoin saturation kinetics* on page 374 for further explanation and illustration.)

The inactive metabolites of phenytoin are excreted in bile and then reabsorbed from the gastrointestinal tract. Eventually, however, they are excreted in the urine, with an alkaline urine enhancing urinary excretion. Less than 5% of the phenytoin is excreted unchanged in the urine. Phenytoin is also excreted via lacrimation and lactation.

Mephenytoin is rapidly absorbed following oral administration. The drug then exhibits moderate protein binding (60%) in the plasma. Metabolism of mephenytoin by the liver results in 5,5-phenyl-ethyl hydantoin, an active metabolite believed to possess the therapeutic and toxic effects attributed to mephenytoin. Excretion occurs via the urine.

Ethotoin is metabolized by the hepatic microsomal enzyme system. Ethotoin, which is extensively protein bound, is excreted in the urine, primarily as metabolites.

Onset, peak, duration

When administered orally, phenytoin demonstrates a variable onset of action. The onset of action of orally administered phenytoin occurs in 30 minutes to 2 hours. The onset of action of phenytoin administered I.V. occurs within 3 to 5 minutes.

The peak plasma concentration level for prompt-acting phenytoin preparations occurs in 1½ to 3 hours, although the sustained-release preparations produce peak serum concentration levels in 4 to 12 hours.

The duration of action for phenytoin depends upon the time the drug remains in the therapeutic range. The plasma half-life after oral administration averages 22 hours, with a range of 7 to 42 hours. The range is so large because half-life changes with changes in serum concentration levels. (See *Phenytoin saturation kinetics* on page 374 for an illustration of the significance of varying phenytoin serum levels.) Steady-state serum phenytoin concentration levels are usually achieved 7 to 10 days after initiating therapy. The clinically effective serum concentration range is approximately 10 to 20 mcg/ml in patients with normal serum albumin levels and normal renal function. For a more immediate clinical effect, loading doses administered over 8 to 12 hours produce a therapeutic serum concentration level within 24 hours in most patients.

Phenytoin saturation kinetics

Phenytoin demonstrates saturation kinetics at varying serum concentrations. When saturation kinetics occur, the liver enzymes become saturated and unable to degrade any more of the drug, and the serum level rises disproportionately. The daily drug dosages necessary to reach the serum concentration level consistent with saturation vary for each individual. As illustrated on the following graph, patient A would receive 100 mg daily, while patient E would receive 500 mg to reach a therapeutic concentration. Beyond that level, saturation and rapid disproportionate increase in serum concentration occur.

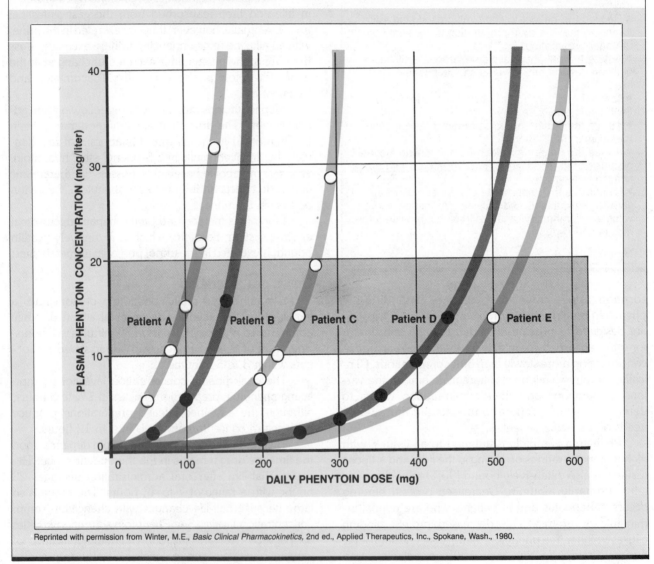

Reprinted with permission from Winter, M.E., *Basic Clinical Pharmacokinetics*, 2nd ed., Applied Therapeutics, Inc., Spokane, Wash., 1980.

Mephenytoin exhibits a rapid onset of action, achieving peak serum concentration levels in 2 to 4 hours. The duration of action of mephenytoin and its major metabolite, 5,5-phenyl-ethyl hydantoin, is longer than that of phenytoin. Half-lives of 32 to 144 hours have been reported with mephenytoin because half-life changes with changes in serum concentration levels.

Ethotoin demonstrates a rapid onset of action, achieving peak serum concentration levels in 2 to 4 hours. Ethotoin appears to undergo saturation kinetics, as does phenytoin, and its half-life ranges from 3 to 6 hours.

PHARMACODYNAMICS

The hydantoin anticonvulsants can, in most cases, stabilize nerve cells against hyperexcitability.

Mechanism of action

The primary site of action appears to be the motor cortex, where the drugs inhibit the spread of seizure activity. Specifically, phenytoin alters ion movement across cell membranes. The pharmacodynamics of mephenytoin and ethotoin are thought to mimic those of phenytoin.

Because of its general effect of stabilizing excitable cells, phenytoin also exerts significant effects on excitable tissues outside the central nervous system (CNS). Phenytoin exhibits antiarrhythmic properties similar to those of lidocaine. The drug decreases the force of myocardial contractions, suppresses ectopic pacemaker activity, improves atrioventricular (AV) conduction depressed by digitalis glycosides, and increases the effective refractory period. (See Chapter 35, Antiarrhythmic Agents, for a discussion of these effects.) Phenytoin also exerts a membrane-stabilizing effect on the pancreas and may inhibit effective insulin release.

PHARMACOTHERAPEUTICS

Because of its clinical efficacy and relatively low toxicity, phenytoin is the most commonly prescribed anticonvulsant. Phenytoin represents one of the drugs of choice to treat complex partial (also called psychomotor or temporal lobe) and tonic-clonic seizures. Physicians sometimes prescribe mephenytoin and ethotoin as adjunct therapy for partial and tonic-clonic seizures in patients who are refractory to, or intolerant of, other anticonvulsants.

phenytoin and **phenytoin sodium** (Dilantin). Phenytoin is a drug of choice to treat complex partial (psychomotor) and tonic-clonic seizures. Individualized dosage is required to achieve a therapeutic blood concentration level of 10 to 20 mcg/ml.
USUAL ADULT DOSAGE: 300 mg P.O. of a prompt-acting preparation in three divided doses daily, or sustained-release preparations in single daily dose; maintenance dose, usually 300 to 400 mg or 3 to 5 mg/kg/day with a maximum dose of 600 mg; in the acute treatment of status epilepticus, usually 15 mg/kg I.V. push at a rate not to exceed 50 mg/minute with an additional 5 mg/kg 12 hours later if required.
USUAL PEDIATRIC DOSAGE: 5 mg/kg/day administered in two to three equally divided doses; suggested maintenance dose, 4 to 7 mg/kg/day with a maximum of 300

mg/day (children over age 6 may require the minimum adult dosage of 300 mg/day); in the acute treatment of status epilepticus, 10 to 15 mg/kg administered I.V., usually at a rate not to exceed 1 to 2 mg/kg/minute in patients whose seizures are refractory to less toxic anticonvulsants.

The pediatric forms of phenytoin, both tablets and suspension, are the free acid form rather than the sodium salt used in the adult, sustained-release, and intravenous forms. The free acid form supplies about 8% more phenytoin than the sodium salt form. Therefore, the nurse must carefully monitor serum concentration levels when using different forms of preparations to manage the same patient.

mephenytoin (Mesantoin). This drug is used primarily to treat partial and tonic-clonic seizures.
USUAL ADULT DOSAGE: 50 to 100 mg P.O. daily during the first week of treatment. Subsequent weekly increases of the same amount are administered until the maintenance dose is achieved. For maintenance therapy, 200 to 600 mg P.O. daily in three equal doses, up to 800 mg or more P.O. daily.
USUAL PEDIATRIC DOSAGE: 50 to 100 mg P.O. daily during the first week of treatment. Subsequent weekly increases of the same amount are administered until the maintenance dose, 100 to 400 mg P.O. daily in three equal doses, is achieved.

ethotoin (Peganone). This drug is used for complex partial (psychomotor) and tonic-clonic seizures.
USUAL ADULT DOSAGE: 1 gram or less P.O. daily, in four to six divided doses after meals. Subsequent dosages are gradually increased over a period of several days. Maintenance therapy, 2 to 3 grams P.O. daily in four to six divided doses.
USUAL PEDIATRIC DOSAGE: usually less than 750 mg P.O. daily in four to six divided doses; maintenance dose, usually 500 mg to 1 gram P.O. daily. Occasionally, children may require larger doses for maintenance therapy.

Drug interactions

Hydantoins interact with a number of other drugs. As a result, the activities of either phenytoin, the other drug, or both are altered. (See *Drug interactions: Hydantoins* on pages 376 and 377 for a comprehensive list of interacting drugs.)

ADVERSE DRUG REACTIONS

The adverse effects of hydantoin anticonvulsants involve the central nervous, cardiovascular, gastrointestinal, and

(Text continues on page 378.)

DRUG INTERACTIONS

Hydantoins

The following drug interactions may occur with the use of phenytoin; however, these reactions may also occur when using any hydantoin anticonvulsant. Because phenytoin interacts with many drugs, this chart has been limited to interactions that have major to moderate clinical significance. Drug interactions of lesser clinical significance, involving such drugs as acetaminophen, allopurinol, antacids, and dopamine, have not been included.

DRUG	INTERACTING DRUGS	POSSIBLE EFFECTS	NURSING IMPLICATIONS
phenytoin, mephen-ytoin, ethotoin	cimetidine, disulfiram, iso-niazid, sulfonamides	Inhibit phenytoin metabo-lism, resulting in increased toxic adverse effects of phenytoin	• Monitor serum levels; phenytoin dosage may need to be decreased. • Advise the patient to report adverse reactions. • Carefully monitor complete blood count (CBC), platelet and reticulocyte counts, and liver function tests.
	phenylbutazone	Causes competitive bind-ing and inhibition of phen-ytoin metabolism, resulting in increased toxic adverse effects of pheny-toin	• Monitor serum levels; phenytoin dosage may need to be decreased. • Advise the patient to report adverse reactions. • Carefully monitor CBC, platelet and reticulo-cyte counts, and liver function tests.
	coumarin anticoagulants (dicumarol)	Produce unknown interac-tion mechanism, resulting in increased toxic adverse effects of phenytoin; phen-ytoin may also decrease the pharmacologic effect of dicumarol	• Monitor serum levels; phenytoin dosage may need to be decreased. • Advise the patient to report adverse reactions. • Carefully monitor CBC, platelet and reticulo-cyte counts, and liver function tests.
	lidocaine	Causes possible additive cardiac depressant effects	• Monitor the patient for bradycardia.
	phenobarbital	Produces variable interac-tion mechanism, resulting in either inhibition or in-duction	• Monitor phenytoin and phenobarbital serum concentration levels. • Monitor CBC, platelet and reticulocyte counts, and liver function tests. • Advise the patient to report any change in adverse reactions or seizure frequency.
	diazoxide, folic acid	Increase induction of phenytoin metabolism, re-sulting in decreased effi-cacy of phenytoin	• Monitor phenytoin serum concentration lev-els.
	levodopa	Causes unknown interac-tion mechanism, resulting in decreased efficacy of levodopa	• Observe for increased signs or symptoms of Parkinson's disease. • Advise the patient to report any change in parkinsonian signs or symptoms. • Because of decreased effect, dosage of levodopa may need to be increased.
	chloramphenicol	Inhibits phenytoin metabo-lism, resulting in increased toxic adverse effects of phenytoin; unknown inter-action mechanism, result-ing in decreased efficacy of chloramphenicol	• Monitor serum phenytoin concentration lev-els; advise patient to report adverse reactions. • Monitor CBC, platelet and reticulocyte counts, and liver function tests. • Monitor serum chloramphenicol concentra-tion levels. • Because of decreased efficacy, dosage of chloramphenicol may need to be increased.

DRUG INTERACTIONS

Hydantoins continued

DRUG	INTERACTING DRUGS	POSSIBLE EFFECTS	NURSING IMPLICATIONS
phenytoin, mepheny-toin, ethotoin (continued)	corticosteroids	Cause induction of corti-costeroid metabolism, re-sulting in decreased efficacy of corticosteroids	• Because of decreased effect, dosage of cor-ticosteroids may need to be increased. • Monitor the patient's blood pressure and weight. • Monitor serum electrolyte concentration lev-els.
	doxycycline	Causes induction of doxy-cycline metabolism, result-ing in decreased efficacy of doxycycline	• Because of decreased effect, dosage of doxycycline may need to be increased.
	methadone	Causes induction of meth-adone metabolism, result-ing in decreased efficacy of methadone	• Because of decreased efficacy, dosage of methadone may need to be increased. • Alert the patient to watch for signs of with-drawal.
	metyrapone	Causes induction of me-tyrapone metabolism, re-sulting in decreased efficacy of metyrapone	• Because of decreased effect, dosage of me-tyrapone may need to be increased.
	quinidine	Causes induction of quini-dine metabolism, resulting in decreased efficacy of quinidine	• Because of decreased effect, dosage of quinidine may need to be increased. • Advise the patient to see physician fre-quently for monitoring of cardiac status. • Alert the patient to report signs or symp-toms of dysrhythmias (palpitations, irregular pulse).
	theophylline	Produces unknown inter-action mechanism, result-ing in decreased efficacy of phenytoin; causes in-duction of metabolism, re-sulting in decreased efficacy of theophylline	• Because of decreased effects of phenytoin and theophylline, dosages of both may need to be increased. • Monitor serum concentration levels of both drugs. • Advise the patient to report increase in shortness of breath to physician. • Monitor CBC, platelet and reticulocyte counts, and liver function tests.
	thyroid hormone	Increases metabolism of thyroid hormone	• Because of increased thyroid hormone me-tabolism, the dosage requirements may be in-creased.
	oral contraceptives	Cause induction of contra-ceptive metabolism, re-sulting in decreased efficacy of contraceptives	• Because of decreased efficacy, alternate contraceptive methods may be needed.
	valproic acid	Causes displacement of phenytoin protein binding, resulting in decreased phenytoin levels; also in-hibits phenytoin metabo-lism, causing increased phenytoin levels	• Monitor phenytoin levels carefully, and be aware that breakthrough seizures may occur with use of valproic acid–phenytoin combina-tion.

hematopoietic systems, as well as cosmetic effects. The adverse reactions presented in the following discussion relate directly to phenytoin. Ethotoin produces less toxic effects than phenytoin, while mephenytoin exhibits the potential to produce more serious blood dyscrasias, including aplastic anemia.

Predictable reactions

Predictable adverse reactions of hydantoins in the CNS include slurred speech, confusion, insomnia, twitching, drowsiness, headache, blurred vision, mydriasis, hyperactive tendon reflexes, and hallucinations. In rare instances, a dose-related encephalopathy occurs. In toxic states, nystagmus, ataxia, lethargy, and diplopia occur.

The major gastrointestinal (GI) adverse reactions include nausea, vomiting, epigastric pain, and anorexia. The cardiovascular adverse reactions are depressed atrial and ventricular conduction and, in toxic states, ventricular fibrillation. With I.V. administration, the cardiovascular adverse reactions include bradycardia, hypotension, and potential cardiac arrest. The primary adverse reaction of the hematopoietic system is a folic acid deficiency that can cause macrocytic anemia.

Cosmetic toxicity includes gingival hyperplasia, hirsutism, and facial coarsening. Other adverse reactions include hyperglycemia, glycosuria, and osteomalacia. Toxic doses of phenytoin may paradoxically induce seizures.

Unpredictable reactions

Hypersensitivity reactions are often manifested as pruritis, fever, arthralgia, and a measleslike rash; exfoliative, purpuric, or bullous dermatitis; Stevens-Johnson syndrome; lymphadenopathy; acute renal failure; hepatitis; and liver necrosis. Several adverse effects also relate to the hematopoietic system, including thrombocytopenia, leukopenia, leukocytosis, agranulocytosis, pancytopenia, eosinophilia, macrocytosis, and various anemias.

NURSING IMPLICATIONS

The nurse should observe several implications important in the administration and patient teaching of the hydantoin anticonvulsants.

● Hydantoin anticonvulsants are contraindicated in patients who experience hypersensitivity to any hydantoin product. Intravenous hydantoins are contraindicated in patients with sinus bradycardia, Adams-Stokes syndrome, sinoatrial (SA) block, or second- and third-degree AV block.

● Administer cautiously in patients with impaired renal or hepatic function, alcoholism, blood dyscrasias, hypotension, myocardial insufficiency, or pancreatic disorders.

● The safe use of anticonvulsants in women of childbearing age as well as pregnant or lactating women has not been established.

● Birth defects have occurred with phenytoin use. Phenytoin can also cause fetal hydantoin syndrome, which consists of decreased prenatal growth, microcephaly, and mental deficiency in the child.

● Women taking oral contraceptives and anticonvulsants may need to use an additional contraceptive method.

● Encourage patients with gingival hyperplasia to brush meticulously and floss their teeth daily.

● Monitor the patient for signs of folic acid deficiency, including neuropathy, mental dysfunction, and psychiatric disorders.

● Neonates may need vitamin K therapy for treatment of hypoprothrombinemia if the mother received hydantoin derivatives during pregnancy.

● Monitor the patient's serum phenytoin concentration levels, because many of the drug's adverse effects are dose-related.

● Periodically monitor the patient's liver and kidney function tests as well as blood counts.

● Lower-than-usual doses are prescribed for elderly patients and for patients who are severely ill, are debilitated, or have liver damage. Lower doses help prevent adverse effects.

● Discontinue phenytoin immediately if the patient develops a skin rash and notify the physician.

● Administer I.V. phenytoin at a rate not to exceed 50 mg/minute because of its cardiotoxicity. Monitor the patient's blood pressure, pulse, and respirations every 5 minutes during administration and every 15 minutes thereafter until the patient's condition becomes stable. If the blood pressure decreases during drug administration, decrease the infusion rate.

● Have oxygen, suction, and resuscitative equipment available for immediate use if needed.

● Administer oral hydantoins with meals to minimize gastric irritation.

● Shake suspension preparations vigorously before pouring to ensure uniform distribution and exact measurement of the drug.

● Phenytoin sodium capsules are available as either prompt-acting or sustained-release preparations. Do not use prompt-acting capsules for once-a-day dosing because the drug becomes bioavailable too quickly, and toxic serum concentration levels could result. Use only sustained-release capsules (Dilantin Kapseals) for once-a-day dosing.

● The chewable tablets are not intended for once-a-day dosing. Furthermore, the chewable tablets are not dose-exchangeable with the capsules, because the free acid tablet and the sodium capsule provide different strengths of phenytoin.

- Avoid I.M. injections because phenytoin precipitates in the muscle tissue and decreases drug bioavailability.
- To avoid the precipitation of phenytoin, do not mix the I.V. form with any other drug.
- To minimize irritation, normal saline solution can be injected after I.V. phenytoin administration.
- Advise patients to report immediately drowsiness, ataxia, blurred vision, slurred speech, skin rash, sore throat, fever, mucous membrane bleeding, or glandular swelling.
- Inform the patient that phenytoin may impart a harmless pink or red to red-brown discoloration to the urine.
- Remind the patient to notify the dentist about the phenytoin therapy.
- Advise the patient to refrain from alcohol consumption because it interacts with phenytoin.

See *General patient-teaching tips* on page 373 for other guides to patient teaching.

BARBITURATES

The long-acting barbiturate phenobarbital is also one of the most widely employed anticonvulsants. Physicians use phenobarbital in long-term treatment of epilepsy and prescribe the drug selectively for acute treatment of status epilepticus. Mephobarbital, also a long-acting barbiturate, is used less frequently as an anticonvulsant. Primidone, a deoxybarbiturate that is closely related chemically to the barbiturates, is also used in the chronic treatment of epilepsy. (See Chapter 30, Sedative and Hypnotic Agents, for a discussion of barbiturates as sedatives and hypnotics.)

History and source
Phenobarbital is the oldest of the modern anticonvulsants. Hauptmann discovered the drug in 1912 through an incidental observation. Phenobarbital is a barbituric acid derivative.

Mephobarbital, which was marketed in 1935, resembles phenobarbital. Primidone was marketed in 1954 as a congener of phenobarbital.

PHARMACOKINETICS

The barbiturate anticonvulsants are metabolized in the liver. Both metabolites and unchanged drug are excreted in the urine.

Absorption, distribution, metabolism, excretion
Phenobarbital is slowly but well absorbed from the GI tract. Peak plasma concentration levels occur several hours after a single dose. The drug is 40% to 60% bound to serum proteins and to a similar extent to other tissues, including the brain.

About 75% of a phenobarbital dose is metabolized by hepatic microsomal enzymes, and 25% to 50% is excreted unchanged in the urine. Because barbiturates act as inducers of hepatic microsomal enzymes, they enhance their own metabolism as well as that of other drugs. Renal excretion can be increased by alkalinizing the urine or increasing the urinary flow rate. Phenobarbital is also excreted in breast milk.

Almost 50% of a mephobarbital dose is absorbed from the GI tract and well distributed in body tissues. The drug is bound to tissue and plasma proteins. Mephobarbital undergoes extensive metabolism by hepatic microsomal enzymes. This metabolism converts approximately 75% of a single mephobarbital dose to the major metabolite phenobarbital within 24 hours. Only 1% to 2% of a dose is excreted unchanged in the urine.

From 60% to 80% of a primidone dose is absorbed from the GI tract and distributed evenly among body tissues. The drug is to a small extent protein bound in the plasma, as is one of its active metabolites, phenylethylmalonamide (PEMA). Primidone is metabolized by hepatic microsomal enzymes to two active metabolites, phenobarbital and PEMA, which share in the anticonvulsant activity of primidone. Approximately 40% of primidone is excreted unchanged in the urine. The remaining 60% consists of unconjugated (not combined with other substances) PEMA and phenobarbital and its metabolites. Approximately 80% of PEMA is excreted in the urine. Primidone is also excreted in breast milk.

Onset, peak, duration
Phenobarbital provides an onset of action within 30 minutes after oral administration. Peak anticonvulsant effect occurs in 8 to 12 hours. The onset of action after I.V. administration occurs within 5 minutes, with the peak anticonvulsant effect within 30 minutes. Phenobarbital has an extremely long half-life of 50 to 170 hours and thus requires 10 to 35 days to reach a steady state.

Mephobarbital demonstrates a rapid onset of action, with a peak anticonvulsant effect in 6 to 8 hours. The half-life of mephobarbital is 11 to 67 hours, with a steady state in 6 to 15 days.

Primidone displays a varied onset of action, with peak anticonvulsant effect in 5 to 9 hours. The half-life of primidone also varies from 10 to 21 hours. The time needed for the drug and its metabolites to reach steady-state levels varies as follows: primidone, 2 days; PEMA, 1 week; and phenobarbital, 10 to 35 days.

PHARMACODYNAMICS

The barbiturates exhibit anticonvulsant action at sub-hypnotic dosages. For this reason, the barbiturates do not usually produce addiction when used to treat epilepsy. The anticonvulsant properties of barbiturates are attributed to both phenobarbital and other selected metabolites.

Mechanism of action

The barbiturate anticonvulsants limit seizure activity by increasing the threshold for motor cortex stimuli. This increase may be due, at least in part, to increased inhibitor action of the neurotransmitter gamma-aminobutyric acid (GABA).

PHARMACOTHERAPEUTICS

The barbiturate anticonvulsants are effective in treating partial, tonic-clonic, and febrile seizures when used alone or in combination with other anticonvulsants. I.V. phenobarbital is also used to treat status epilepticus. The major disadvantage of using phenobarbital for status epilepticus is CNS depression. Barbiturate anticonvulsants are ineffective in treating absence seizures.

Because primidone can produce significant start-up toxicity, physicians do not consider it a first choice drug. Mephobarbital is the least frequently used barbiturate anticonvulsants because of the high doses required to achieve therapeutic effect.

Therapeutic dosages of barbiturate anticonvulsants are based on serum phenobarbital levels because all of the barbiturate anticonvulsants are metabolized to phenobarbital.

phenobarbital, phenobarbital sodium (Luminal). A Schedule IV drug, phenobarbital is used for long-term treatment of partial and tonic-clonic seizures and for the acute management of status epilepticus and febrile seizures.
USUAL ADULT DOSAGE: for partial and tonic-clonic seizures, 60 to 300 mg, or 1 to 5 mg/kg P.O. daily; for status epilepticus, 5 to 10 mg/kg I.V.

USUAL PEDIATRIC DOSAGE: for partial and tonic-clonic seizures, 15 to 50 mg, or 3 to 5 mg/kg P.O. daily in two equal doses. The therapeutic plasma range for treating status epilepticus is 25 to 40 mcg/ml, whereas 15 mcg/ml is the minimum for preventing febrile seizures.

mephobarbital (Mebaral). A Schedule IV drug, mephobarbital is used to treat the same types of seizures as phenobarbital, with the exception of status epilepticus. The therapeutic serum level of phenobarbital determines the dosage adjustments of mephobarbital, because mephobarbital is metabolized to phenobarbital.
USUAL ADULT DOSAGE: 400 to 600 mg P.O. daily.
USUAL PEDIATRIC DOSAGE: 16 to 32 mg P.O. t.i.d. to q.i.d. as ordered for children under age 5; for children over age 5, 32 to 64 mg P.O. t.i.d. to q.i.d.

primidone (Mysoline). A deoxybarbiturate, primidone is used for long-term treatment of partial seizures and generalized tonic-clonic seizures. Primidone is ineffective in treating status epilepticus and absence seizures.
USUAL ADULT DOSAGE: 125 mg P.O. daily in divided doses, gradually increased by 125 mg every 3 days to tolerance or therapeutic levels of 750 to 1,500 mg P.O. daily. The therapeutic plasma concentration levels of primidone are phenobarbital, 15 to 40 mcg/ml; primidone, 5 to 12 mcg/ml; and PEMA, intermediate between phenobarbital and primidone. Primidone is given in two to four doses daily. The maximum dose is 2 grams.
USUAL PEDIATRIC DOSAGE: initially, 100 to 125 mg P.O. daily, increased weekly to therapeutic levels based on serum phenobarbital levels; for maintenance, 125 to 250 mg P.O. t.i.d., or 10 to 25 mg/kg/day in divided doses.

Drug interactions

Phenobarbital interacts with many drugs, usually altering their metabolism rate. Mephobarbital and primidone interact with the same drugs and in the same way as phenobarbital because both drugs are metabolized to phenobarbital. (See *Drug interactions: Barbiturates* for a list of the many interactions involving the barbiturate anticonvulsants.)

ADVERSE DRUG REACTIONS

The toxicity of the barbiturate anticonvulsants results primarily in adverse reactions in the CNS. Significant GI effects, blood dyscrasias, and emotional or psychiatric reactions also occur.

DRUG INTERACTIONS

Barbiturates

Most of the clinically significant interactions from barbiturates occur with phenobarbital. Mephobarbital and primidone interact with the same drugs as phenobarbital. Since primidone is converted to phenobarbital in the body, concurrent administration of primidone and phenobarbital may result in excessive phenobarbital serum levels.

DRUG	INTERACTING DRUGS	POSSIBLE EFFECTS	NURSING IMPLICATIONS
phenobarbital, mephobarbital, primidone	chloramphenicol, hydantoins, MAO inhibitors, propoxyphene, disulfiram	Inhibit phenobarbital metabolism, resulting in increased toxic effects	• Monitor serum concentration levels; phenobarbital dosage may need to be decreased. • Advise the patient to report adverse reactions. • Assess for change in level of consciousness. • Alert the patient not to drive or operate heavy machinery until the effect of the drug combination in the patient is known. • Advise the patient to avoid alcohol consumption.
	beta blockers	Cause induction of beta-blocker metabolism, resulting in decreased effectiveness of beta blockers	• Monitor desired effect in the patient (antianginal, antihypertensive, and antiarrhythmic); dosage of beta-blocker may need to be increased. • Instruct the patient to report changes in desired effect in drug therapy. • Advise the patient to report periodically for blood pressure and pulse check.
	chloramphenicol	Causes induction of chloramphenicol metabolism, resulting in decreased effectiveness of chloramphenicol; inhibits phenobarbital metabolism	• Monitor desired effect in the patient (anti-infective); dosage of chloramphenicol may need to be increased. • Monitor serum chloramphenicol and phenobarbital levels.
	corticosteroids	Cause induction of corticosteroid metabolism, resulting in decreased effectiveness of corticosteroids	• Because of decreased effect, dosage of costicosteroids may need to be increased. • Monitor the patient's weight and blood pressure. • Monitor serum electrolyte levels.
	doxycycline	Causes induction of doxycycline metabolism, resulting in decreased effectiveness of doxycycline	• Because of decreased effect, dosage of doxycycline may need to be increased.
	oral anticoagulants (dicumarol)	Produce induction of oral anticoagulant metabolism, resulting in decreased effectiveness of oral anticoagulants	• Monitor prothrombin levels; dosage of anticoagulant may need to be increased. • Advise the patient to be alert for signs and symptoms of thrombus formation: pain, tenderness, edema in the calf.
	oral contraceptives	Produce induction of oral contraceptive metabolism, resulting in decreased effectiveness of oral contraceptives	• Alert the patient that contraceptive effect may be impaired; breakthrough bleeding may occur. • Suggest alternative or additional contraceptive method.

continued

DRUG INTERACTIONS

Barbituates continued

DRUG	INTERACTING DRUGS	POSSIBLE EFFECTS	NURSING IMPLICATIONS
phenobarbital, mephobarbital, primidone (continued)	quinidine	Causes induction of quinidine metabolism, resulting in decreased effectiveness of quinidine	• Because of decreased effect, dosage of quinidine may need to be increased. • Advise the patient to see the physician frequently for monitoring of cardiac status. • Alert the patient to report any signs and symptoms of dysrhythmias (palpitations, irregular pulse).
	methoxyflurane	Causes possible induction of hepatic microsomal enzymes by barbiturates that may stimulate metabolism of methoxyflurane to nephrotoxic metabolites	• Avoid concurrent administration of phenobarbital and methoxyflurane.
	phenothiazines	Cause induction of phenothiazine metabolism, resulting in decreased effectiveness of phenothiazines	• Because of decreased effect, dosage of phenothiazine may need to be increased. • Monitor patient behavior closely. • Advise the patient and family members to report promptly to the physician any changes in behavior.
	tricyclic antidepressants	Cause induction of tricyclic antidepressant metabolism, resulting in decreased effectiveness of tricyclic antidepressants	• Because of decreased effect, dosage of tricyclic antidepressant may need to be increased. • Monitor serum levels of tricyclic antidepressants. • Advise the patient to report any change in therapeutic effect (lack of mood elevation). • Alert the family that the patient may be especially vulnerable to depression.
	CNS depressants (antianxiety agents, sedative-hypnotics, most narcotic analgesics, and alcohol)	Produce additive CNS effects, resulting in increased sedative toxicity	• Assess frequently for changes in level of consciousness and respirations. • Supervise ambulation; raise side rails, especially with elderly patients. • Alert the patient not to drive or use heavy machinery until the effects of the drug combination in the patient is known. • Alert the patient that severe respiratory and CNS depression can occur, both of which can be lethal. • Advise the patient not to drink alcohol while taking these medications.
	valproic acid	Inhibits the hepatic metabolism of phenobarbital	• Monitor for excessive phenobarbital effect, such as drowsiness. • Because of increased phenobarbital serum levels, dosage may need to be reduced.

Predictable reactions

The most frequently occurring dose-related CNS effects of phenobarbital include: drowsiness, lethargy, and dizziness; nystagmus; confusion; and ataxia with large doses.

The GI adverse effects include nausea and vomiting. Folate deficiencies and osteomalacia secondary to the induced metabolism of vitamin D may also occur. When administered I.V., phenobarbital can cause laryngospasm, respiratory depression, and hypotension secondary to decreased cardiac output. Signs of overdose include respiratory depression, pupillary constriction, oliguria, hypothermia, circulatory collapse, and pulmonary edema.

Mephobarbital exhibits adverse effects similar to phenobarbital. Primidone evokes the same CNS and GI adverse effects as phenobarbital. Primidone also has been implicated in the development of acute psychoses in patients with complex partial seizures. It may also cause alopecia, impotence, and osteomalacia.

Unpredictable reactions

Rare hematologic adverse effects of the barbiturates include agranulocytosis and thrombocytopenia leukopenia, eosinophilia, decreased serum folate levels, and megaloblastic anemia. All three barbiturate anticonvulsants can produce a hypersensitivity rash. These drugs may also produce a morbilliform rash, lupus erythematosus-like syndrome, and lymphadenopathy. Paradoxical excitement in elderly patients and children and hyperkinetic behavior in children may occur.

NURSING IMPLICATIONS

Because of the many adverse reactions and possible misuse, the nurse must observe many implications when administering barbituates.

• Barbiturate anticonvulsants are contraindicated in patients who exhibit sensitivity to barbiturates or manifest porphyria, as well as patients who have a familial history of porphyria or a history of sedative-hypnotic addiction.
• Administer barbiturate anticonvulsants cautiously to patients with severe respiratory, cardiac, or renal disease, as well as to patients with impaired hepatic function or severe anemia.
• Administer barbiturate anticonvulsants cautiously to depressed patients and those with suicidal tendencies.
• Be aware that barbiturates do not provide analgesic action and may produce restlessness when given to patients in pain.
• Elevate the bed rails for very young and very old patients because barbiturate therapy may precipitate paradoxical excitement or CNS depression.
• During prolonged therapy, monitor the patient's phenobarbital blood concentration levels, liver function tests, and serum folate levels.
• When administering oral barbiturates, be sure that the patient actually swallows the drug.
• When administering barbiturates I.V., frequently monitor vital signs, especially respirations and blood pressure.
• Do not exceed a rate of 50 mg/minute when giving an I.V. dose of barbiturates.
• Have resuscitative drugs and equipment nearby when administering barbiturates I.V.

• Remember that phenobarbital and mephobarbital are classified as Schedule IV drugs under the federal Controlled Substance Act; always keep such drugs in a locked cabinet, and handle them appropriately.
• When giving barbiturates I.M., inject the drug deep into a large muscle mass.
• When giving the drugs I.V., do not use a cloudy solution; administer a reconstituted solution within 30 minutes of preparation.
• Instruct the patient to take phenobarbital on an empty stomach.
• Instruct the patient to report to the physician the onset of fever, a sore throat, malaise, easy bruising or bleeding, jaundice, or a rash.
• Advise the patient to keep the barbiturate in a secure place to avoid taking extra doses while sedated. Safe storage can also prevent others, including children, from taking the drug.
• Reassure the patient that the barbiturate anticonvulsants are not addictive when prescribed in subhypnotic doses for epilepsy.

See *General patient-teaching tips* on page 373 for other guides to patient teaching.

IMINOSTILBENES

Carbamazepine, an iminostilbene derivative, acts as an effective anticonvulsant for partial and generalized tonic-clonic seizures, and combination of these seizures. Carbamazepine also produces sedative, anticholinergic, antidepressant, muscle-relaxant, antiarrhythmic, antidiuretic, and neuromuscular transmission-inhibiting actions. Also, carbamazepine is the only anticonvulsant compound that has a chemical structure similar to the tricyclic antidepressant drugs, such as imipramine. This similarity helps explain the observed effects of carbamazepine on behavior and emotions.

History and source

In 1957, Schindler and Blattner synthesized carbamazepine, and since the 1960s, physicians have used the drug to treat trigeminal neuralgia. The first results in epileptic patients were published in 1963. Carbamazepine has been marketed in the United States since 1974.

DRUG INTERACTIONS
Iminostilbenes

The following chart lists the drug interactions between carbamazepine, an iminostilbene derivative, and other drugs.

DRUG	INTERACTING DRUGS	POSSIBLE EFFECTS	NURSING IMPLICATIONS
carbamazepine	erythromycin, isoniazid, propoxyphene, troleando-mycin	Inhibit carbamazepine metabolism, resulting in increased toxic adverse effects	• Monitor serum carbamazepine concentration levels carefully; decreased carbamazepine dosage may be needed. • Monitor CBC and platelet and reticulocyte counts closely; hematopoietic toxicity warrants immediate withdrawal. • Advise the patient and responsible family member to notify physician immediately if the following symptoms occur: fever, sore throat or mouth, malaise, unusual fatigue, or tendency to bruise or bleed. • Toxic doses may precipitate cardiac dysrhythmias in patients with heart disease, so monitor the pulse and cardiac function carefully. • Since dizziness, drowsiness, and ataxia may occur, alert the patient to avoid hazardous tasks requiring mental alertness and physical coordination (driving, using heavy machinery).
	doxycycline	Decreases efficacy of doxycycline due to increased breakdown by the liver, resulting in decreased therapeutic effect of doxycycline	• Because of decreased effect, dosage of doxycycline may need to be increased.
	theophylline	Decreases efficacy of theophylline due to increased breakdown by the liver, resulting in decreased therapeutic effect of theophylline	• Because of decreased effect, dosage of theophylline may need to be increased.
	oral anticonvulsant (warfarin)	Decreases efficacy of warfarin due to increased breakdown by the liver, resulting in decreased therapeutic effect of warfarin	• Monitor prothrombin time carefully; dosage of warfarin may need to be increased. • Observe for signs of thrombus formation, such as Homans' sign, tenderness, or edema.
	lithium	Causes unknown interaction mechanism, resulting in neurotoxicity	• Assess for changes in level of consciousness. • Instruct the patient to report dizziness, headache, fatigue, or slurred speech immediately. • Advise the patient not to drive or operate heavy machinery until the drug combination effects on the patient are known.

PHARMACOKINETICS

Carbamazepine is absorbed slowly and erratically from the GI tract. The drug is rapidly distributed to all tissues, and 75% to 90% is bound to plasma proteins. Metabolism occurs in the liver, and carbamazepine is excreted as glucuronides in the urine.

Absorption, distribution, metabolism, excretion

The GI tract absorption of carbamazepine is slow, erratic, and possibly incomplete. After carbamazepine is widely distributed in body tissues, approximately 70% to 80% of the drug becomes protein bound. Carbamazepine is metabolized in the liver by oxidative enzyme induction to an active metabolite, 10,11-epoxide, and five other metabolites. Approximately 1% to 3% is excreted unchanged in the urine. The active metabolite 10,11-epoxide is metabolized to inactive compounds, which are excreted in urine and bile. A small amount is distributed across the placenta and excreted in breast milk.

Onset, peak, duration

The onset of action varies, with peak serum concentration levels occurring after 4 to 8 hours. The half-life also varies greatly, the result of the autoinduction of drug-metabolizing hepatic enzymes and a change in the rate of metabolism caused by other drugs.

PHARMACODYNAMICS

Carbamazepine exerts an anticonvulsant effect similar to that of phenytoin.

The anticonvulsant action of carbamazepine may occur because of the drug's ability to inhibit the spread of seizure activity or neuromuscular transmission in general. Carbamazepine also increases the discharge of noradrenergic neurons—an action that may contribute to its antiepileptic effects.

PHARMACOTHERAPEUTICS

Physicians use carbamazepine to treat generalized tonic-clonic seizures as well as both simple and complex partial seizures in adults and children. The efficacy of carbamazepine makes it a drug of choice for treating these seizures. Use of the drug also relieves pain in the treatment of trigeminal neuralgia (tic douloureux).

carbamazepine (Tegretol). This drug is used to treat both adults and children.
USUAL ADULT DOSAGE: initially, 200 mg P.O. b.i.d.; gradually increased by up to 200 mg P.O. daily, using t.i.d. regimens until desired response is obtained; for maintenance, 800 to 1,200 mg P.O. daily in children aged 12 to 15, or 1,200 mg P.O. daily in adults and children over age 15.
USUAL PEDIATRIC DOSAGE: for children age 6 to 12, 20 to 30 mg/kg, beginning with 100 mg P.O. b.i.d.; increased by 100 mg P.O. daily using at least a t.i.d. regimen. Generally, the dosage should not exceed 1 gram P.O. daily. The maintenance dose is 400 to 800 mg/day in three divided doses. Therapeutic serum concentration level is 6 to 12 mcg/ml.

Drug interactions

Carbamazepine possesses enzyme-inducing properties and generally decreases the steady-state levels of other drugs. Some anticonvulsant drugs, however, decrease the steady-state levels of carbamazepine. (See *Drug interactions: Iminostilbenes* for a list of the drugs that affect and are affected by carbamazepine.)

ADVERSE DRUG REACTIONS

Most of the adverse reactions produced by carbamazepine are tolerable and relatively minor, if the drug therapy begins slowly at a low dose and advances gradually to tolerance. Occasionally, however, serious hematologic toxicity occurs. Furthermore, because carbamazepine is structurally related to the tricyclic antidepressants, it can cause similar toxicities.

Predictable reactions

Dose-related adverse reactions include drowsiness, diplopia, ataxia, vertigo, nystagmus, headaches, tremor, and dry mouth. Because carbamazepine is related to the tricyclic antidepressants, it can produce many of the same adverse reactions, including heart failure, hypertension or hypotension, syncope, dysrhythmia, and myocardial infarction. Carbamazepine's action as a mild anticholinergic may result in urinary retention, constipation, and increased intraocular pressure. The drug can also cause water retention with long term use.

Unpredictable reactions

Urticaria and Stevens-Johnson syndrome have been reported with carbamazepine use. The occasional but significant hematologic reactions include aplastic anemia (rare), agranulocytosis, thrombocytopenia, and leukopenia. Rare instances of cholestatic and hepatocellular jaundice have also been noted. Rare psychiatric reactions have been noted, including activation of latent psychosis, mental depression with agitation, and talkativeness.

NURSING IMPLICATIONS

The nursing implications for carbamazepine center on the potential hazards of concomitant administration of contraindicated drugs and the potential for serious hematologic toxicities.

• Carbamazepine is contraindicated in patients who demonstrate hypersensitivity to carbamazepine or to tricyclic compounds.

• Carbamazepine may be contraindicated with the concomitant use of monoamine oxidase (MAO) inhibitors, because the concomitant use of MAO inhibitors and tricyclic antidepressants (closely related to carbamazepine) results in hyperpyretic crises or severe convulsions.

• Administer with extreme caution to patients with cardiac, hepatic, renal, or urinary tract disease.

• Advise the patient to take the drug with meals to decrease GI irritation and to enhance absorption.

• Instruct the patient and family members to notify the physician immediately if early signs of a hematologic problem appear. Early signs of such problems include fever, sore throat, malaise, unusual fatigue, or a tendency to bruise or bleed.

See *General patient-teaching tips* on page 373 for other guides to patient teaching.

BENZODIAZEPINES

The three drugs from the benzodiazepine class that provide anticonvulsant effects are diazepam (parenteral), clonazepam, and clorazepate dipotassium. Only clonazepam is recommended for the long-term treatment of epilepsy; diazepam is restricted to the acute treatment of status epilepticus. Physicians prescribe clorazepate as adjunctive treatment for partial seizures. (See Chapter 32, Antianxiety Agents, for the major discussion of benzodiazepines.)

History and source

Synthesized in the late 1950s and early 1960s by Sternbach, the benzodiazepines were marketed as anticonvulsants at different times: diazepam in 1968, clonazepam in 1975, and clorazepate in the late 1970s.

PHARMACOKINETICS

The benzodiazepines are metabolized in the liver to multiple metabolites, which are subsequently excreted in the urine.

Absorption, distribution, metabolism, excretion

The benzodiazepines are rapidly and almost completely absorbed from the GI tract, but are distributed at different rates. Protein binding of benzodiazepines ranges from 85% to 90%. Based on the rate of excretion or elimination, benzodiazepines are classified as long-acting, intermediate-acting, or short-acting. Metabolism of the long-acting compounds results in the formation of the major plasma metabolite N-desmethyldiazepam, which has a long half-life. The long half-life of the metabolite probably accounts for some of the pharmacologic action. The metabolites of the benzodiazepines are eventually excreted in urine. The benzodiazepines are readily distributed across the placenta and are excreted in breast milk.

Onset, peak, duration

The onset of action for the benzodiazepines is 5 to 10 minutes, with peak concentration levels reached within 60 to 90 minutes. The half-lives vary and the half-lives of the active metabolites must be considered as well as the parent compound. Diazepam and clorazepate have half-lives of 1 to 2 days, but the active metabolite, N-desmethyldiazepam, has a half-life of 30 to 200 hours. Clonazepam half-life is about 1 day. The half-lives of the benzodiazepine poorly correlate with their anticonvulsant duration of action.

PHARMACODYNAMICS

The benzodiazepines provide anticonvulsant, antianxiety, sedative-hypnotic, and muscle relaxant effects.

Mechanism of action

Although not clearly understood, benzodiazepine anticonvulsant action may increase availability of the inhibitory neurotransmitter gamma-aminobutyric acid (GABA) to brain neurons.

PHARMACOTHERAPEUTICS

Clonazepam is used to treat absence (petit mal), atypical absence (Lennox-Gastaut syndrome), atonic, and myoclonic seizures. Diazepam is not recommended for long-term treatment because of the high serum concentration levels required to control seizures and its addictive potential. Intravenously, it is routinely used as the initial control for status epilepticus. Unfortunately, because diazepam is distributed so rapidly, it provides only short-term effects of less than 1 hour. As a result, a long-acting anticonvulsant, such as phenytoin or phenobarbital, must also be given during diazepam therapy. Clorazepate is used in combination with other drugs to treat partial seizures. The therapeutic serum concentration levels for the benzodiazepines have not been well established.

clonazepam (Klonopin). A Schedule IV drug, clonazepam is used to treat absence, atypical absence, atonic, and myoclonic seizures. The dose required for seizure control is highly individualized.
USUAL ADULT DOSAGE: initially, 1.5 mg P.O. daily in three divided doses; increased by increments of 0.5 to 1 mg every 3 days until the seizures become controlled, or until adverse reactions preclude further increases. The maximum recommended dose is 20 mg P.O. daily.
USUAL PEDIATRIC DOSAGE: for children up to age 10 or weighing up to 30 kg, initially, 0.01 to 0.03 mg/kg P.O. daily in three divided doses, not to exceed 0.05 mg/kg/day; gradual increments of 0.25 to 0.5 mg P.O. may be added every 3 days; for maintenance, 0.1 to 0.2 mg/kg P.O. daily in three divided doses.

diazepam (Valium). A Schedule IV drug, diazepam is indicated to treat status epilepticus only.
USUAL ADULT DOSAGE: 5 to 10 mg I.V. at a rate not to exceed 5 mg/minute. This dose may be repeated at 10- to 15-minute intervals up to a maximum dose of 30 mg. The regimen can be repeated in 2 to 4 hours if necessary, but the total dose should not exceed 100 mg within a 24-hour period.
USUAL PEDIATRIC DOSAGE: for children older than age 5, 1 mg I.V. initially, followed by repeated doses every 2 to 5 minutes until a maximum dose of 10 mg has been given. This regimen can be repeated in 2 to 4 hours if necessary.

clorazepate dipotassium (Tranxene). A Schedule IV drug, clorazepate is recommended for adjunctive treatment of partial seizures only.
USUAL ADULT DOSAGE: 22.5 mg P.O. daily in three divided doses. Daily doses should be increased by not more than 7.5 mg per week. The maximum dose is 90 mg P.O. daily.
USUAL PEDIATRIC DOSAGE: initially, 15 mg P.O. daily in two divided doses. Daily doses should be increased by not more than 7.5 mg per week. The maximum dose for children is 60 mg/day. Clorazepate is not recommended for use in children under age 9.

Drug interactions
Drug interactions between the benzodiazepines and other CNS-active drugs can occur. (See *Drug interactions: Benzodiazepines* in Chapter 30, Sedative and Hypnotic Agents.)

ADVERSE DRUG REACTIONS

The dose-related, predictable reactions to the benzodiazepines are primarily neurologic and include drowsiness, confusion, ataxia, weakness, dizziness, nystagmus, vertigo, syncope, dysarthria, headache, tremor, and a glassy-eyed appearance. These dose-related effects diminish as therapy continues. Cardiorespiratory depression may occur with high doses and with I.V diazepam.
Idiosyncratic, unpredictable reactions to the benzodiazepines include a rash and acute hypersensitivity reactions. Hepatomegaly, leukopenia, thrombocytopenia, and eosinophilia have rarely been reported.

NURSING IMPLICATIONS
The nurse must be aware of the following implications when administering benzodiazepines:
• Benzodiazepines are contraindicated for patients with known hypersensitivity to a benzodiazepine compound, as well as for patients with liver disease, acute narrow-angle glaucoma, and in pregnant and lactating women.
• Administer benzodiazepines cautiously to patients with a history of drug abuse, shock, coma, acute alcohol intoxication, depressive neuroses, psychotic reactions, renal disease, chronic obstructive pulmonary disease, and myasthenia gravis.
• Exercise caution when administering benzodiazepines to children and to elderly or debilitated patients.
• The signs and symptoms of overdose include somnolence, confusion, diminished reflexes, and coma.
• If a patient overdoses using benzodiazepines, maintain an open airway, ventilate if necessary, monitor vital signs, and administer fluids; perform gastric lavage, and administer vasopressors as prescribed.
• Elderly and debilitated patients and those with renal or hepatic disease run a high risk of developing adverse reactions to benzodiazepines.
• Check that patients taking oral benzodiazepines do not hoard the medication.
• The oral drugs should be stored in light-resistant containers at room temperature, unless otherwise specified by the manufacturer.
• When administering diazepam I.V., do not mix it with other drugs in the same syringe. Give direct I.V. push only. *Do not* give the drug as an infusion.
• Administer I.V. diazepam no faster than 5 mg/minute in adults, and over at least a 3-minute period in children. Avoid starting I.V. in small veins. Use care to prevent extravasation.
• During I.V. administration, monitor all vital signs, and have resuscitation equipment readily available.

• The benzodiazepines are classified as Schedule IV substances under the federal Controlled Substance Act. Always handle these drugs according to legal regulations.

• Instruct the patient to notify the physician of any change in seizure control.

• Instruct patients to contact the physician if they experience nausea, vomiting, constipation, rash, restlessness, insomnia, muscle spasms, hallucinations, or persistent fatigue.

• Instruct the family members to recognize and report to the physician any signs of possible drug abuse and dependence, such as nervousness, insomnia, or diarrhea.

See *General patient-teaching tips* on page 373 for additional guides to patient teaching.

SUCCINIMIDES

Three drugs from the succinimide class that are used to treat absence (petit mal) seizures are ethosuximide, methsuximide, and phensuximide.

The succinimides evolved from a systematic search for drugs that could effectively treat absence seizures but were less toxic than the oxazolidinediones. Introduced as therapy for absence seizures in 1951, the succinimides have gradually replaced the oxazolidinediones.

PHARMACOKINETICS

The succinimides are well absorbed from the GI tract and widely distributed throughout body tissues. Plasma protein binding of the drugs is negligible. The succinimides are metabolized in the liver by microsomal enzymes. Almost 40% of ethosuximide is metabolized to its primary metabolite, the inactive hydroxyethyl derivative. This metabolite, as well as those of the other succinimides, is excreted as a glucuronide in the urine. Approximately 25% of ethosuximide is excreted unchanged in the urine.

The onset of action for the succinimides occurs rapidly. Peak serum concentration levels are reached at the following rates: methsuximide, 2 hours; phensuximide, 1 to 4 hours; ethosuximide, about 4 hours. The half-life varies from 4 to 12 hours for phensuximide, 23 to 57 hours for methsuximide and its active metabolite, to 55 hours for ethosuximide.

PHARMACODYNAMICS

The succinimides reduce frequency of absence seizures in children and adults, apparently, by depressing nerve transmission in the motor cortex and increasing the seizure threshold for stimulus.

PHARMACOTHERAPEUTICS

The succinimides are used to treat absence seizures, with ethosuximide the drug of choice. Physicians prescribe methsuximide less frequently because of the high incidence of toxicity associated with it. Methsuximide is indicated, however, for absence seizures and in combination with other anticonvulsants to treat complex partial seizures. Phensuximide is infrequently used because it is less effective. If used alone for mixed types of seizures, succinimides may increase the frequency of tonic-clonic seizures.

ethosuximide (Zarontin). This drug is used to treat absence seizures. The dosage needed to control the seizures is highly individualized.
USUAL ADULT DOSAGE: initially, 250 mg P.O. b.i.d., with dosage increases in increments of 250 mg every 4 to 7 days until seizure control is achieved with minimal adverse effects; for maintenance, 20 to 40 mg/kg P.O.; maximum dosage should usually not exceed 1.5 grams. The therapeutic serum level required to control seizures is 40 to 100 mcg/ml.
USUAL PEDIATRIC DOSAGE: initially, for children over age 6, 250 mg P.O. b.i.d.; for children aged 3 to 6, 250 mg P.O. daily; recommended dosage increment is 250 mg P.O. every 4 to 7 days until seizure control is achieved with minimal adverse effects; for maintenance, 20 mg/kg, with a maximum dosage of 1 gram for children up to age 6.

methsuximide (Celontin). This drug is used to treat absence seizures refractory to other drugs.
USUAL ADULT AND PEDIATRIC DOSAGE: initially, 300 mg P.O. daily for the first week, increased by 300 mg/day at weekly intervals if required; for maintenance, 600 to 1,200 mg; maximum dosage is 1.2 grams daily in divided doses.

phensuximide (Milontin). This drug is used to treat absence seizures. Highly individualized dosages are required to maintain seizure control.
USUAL ADULT AND PEDIATRIC DOSAGE: initially, 0.5 to 1 gram P.O. b.i.d. to t.i.d.; maximum total dosage may vary between 1 to 3 grams P.O. daily.

Drug interactions

The succinimides may inhibit the metabolism of hydantoin anticonvulsants. Carbamazepine may decrease the concentration of a succinimide by induction. Valproic acid exerts a variable effect via unknown mechanisms.

ADVERSE DRUG REACTIONS

The succinimides produce GI, neurologic, hematologic, and genitourinary adverse effects.

Predictable reactions

Adverse reactions involving the GI tract include nausea, vomiting, weight loss, abdominal pain, constipation, and diarrhea. The neurologic complaints are ataxia, dizziness, drowsiness, headache, euphoria, restlessness, irritability, lethargy, and confusion. Psychosis and suicidal ideation have occurred, but rarely.

Unpredictable reactions

The hematologic adverse reactions include eosinophilia, leukopenia, thrombocytopenia, agranulocytosis, and aplastic anemia. The genitourinary adverse reactions are urinary frequency, hematuria, and albuminuria.

Methsuximide can produce renal and hepatic damage. Other toxic reactions include increased libido, hirsutism, alopecia, and gum hypertrophy.

The following hypersensitivity reactions to succinimides can occur: Stevens-Johnson syndrome, pruritic skin eruptions, exfoliative dermatitis, and systemic lupus erythematosus.

NURSING IMPLICATIONS

Because the succinimides may produce some serious adverse reactions, the nurse must observe the following implications:
- Administer cautiously to patients with severe hepatic or renal disease.
- Administer cautiously to patients with combination types of epilepsy because succinimides may increase tonic-clonic seizures.
- Be aware that neurologic adverse effects, which occur frequently, indicate that the dosage needs to be adjusted.
- Monitor the patient for the signs of efficacy versus toxicity when adjusting dosage or when adding or terminating any other medication.
- Observe the patient for behavioral changes, which can indicate an adverse reaction. If behavioral changes occur, the drug is slowly withdrawn.
- Note that Celontin contains FD&C Yellow Dye No. 5, which can cause allergic reactions in patients with asthma or allergies to aspirin or other nonsteroidal anti-inflammatory drugs.

- Store succinimides away from the heat. Shake all suspensions well before administration.
- Inform the patient that phensuximide may change the color of the urine to pink, red, or red-brown.
- If the patient develops GI distress, instruct the patient to take the drug with meals.
- Instruct the patient to contact the physician if any of the following develop: persistent nausea, vomiting, loss of appetite, sore throat, fever, unusual bleeding or bruising, or skin rashes.

See *General patient-teaching tips* on page 373 for additional teaching points.

VALPROIC ACID

Valproic acid, a carboxylic acid with anticonvulsant activity, is not structurally related to the other anticonvulsants.

History and source

Burton synthesized valproic acid in 1882, but researchers did not discover the anticonvulsant properties of the drug until the early 1960s. Those anticonvulsant properties were discovered coincidentally when valproate was used as a vehicle for other compounds being screened for their antiepileptic properties. Clinical trials began in 1964, and the drug became available in the United States in 1978. Valproic acid had been used for about a decade in Europe before its marketing in the United States.

PHARMACOKINETICS

The two major drugs in the valproic acid class are valproate sodium and divalproex sodium. Divalproex is a pro-drug of valproic acid and becomes dissociated to valproic acid in the GI tract. Valproic acid is well absorbed when administered as valproate or divalproex. Once absorbed, it is strongly protein bound, and metabolized in the liver. Both metabolites and unchanged drug are excreted in the urine.

Absorption, distribution, metabolism, excretion

The absorption rate of valproic acid depends upon the dosage form. Valproic acid is 90% bound to plasma proteins, but that percentage decreases as the total serum concentration increases throughout the therapeutic range.

Valproic acid is metabolized in the liver to the conjugate ester of glucuronic acid. Other metabolites result from the beta oxidation by the mitochondria. The major active metabolites having anticonvulsant acitivity are 2-propyl-2-pentenoic acid and 2-propyl-3-oxopentanoic acid. These active metabolites, along with 3% of the unchanged drug, are excreted in urine. Valproic acid readily crosses the placental barrier and also appears in breast milk.

Onset, peak, duration

The onset of action of valproic acid occurs in 20 to 30 minutes. Peak serum concentration levels of valproate sodium occur in 1 to 4 hours. Serum concentration levels of divalproex sodium peak in 3 to 5 hours. The time needed to reach peak levels is longer if the patient has a full stomach or receives enteric-coated tablets. In patients not taking other drugs, the half-life is 13 to 16 hours. For patients taking other anticonvulsants, the half-life drops to 6 to 10 hours, probably as a result of hepatic enzyme induction.

PHARMACODYNAMICS

The mechanism of action for valproic acid remains unknown, but it may be related to the increased availability of the inhibitory neurotransmitter GABA to brain neurons. Valproic acid may inhibit GABA transaminase or succinic semialdehyde dehydrogenase, which would account for the increased GABA.

PHARMACOTHERAPEUTICS

Physicians prescribe valproic acid for long-term treatment of absence, myoclonic, and tonic-clonic seizures. It is also administered rectally for status epilepticus refractory to other anticonvulsants. Valproic acid must be used cautiously in young children and in patients receiving multiple anticonvulsants because of possible fatal hepatotoxicity. This risk limits the use of valproic acid as a drug of choice for seizure disorders.

valproate sodium (Depakene) and **divalproex sodium** (Depakote). A steady-state concentration level of valproate sodium is reached 1 to 4 days after initiating the dose. The effective serum concentration level for adults and children is 50 to 100 mcg/ml. Divalproex produces fewer GI adverse effects. With divalproex, a twice-daily dosing regimen is recommended.
USUAL ADULT DOSAGE: initially, 15 mg/kg P.O. daily, increased at weekly intervals by 5 to 10 mg/kg until seizures are under control or unacceptable adverse reactions develop; maximum dosage is 60 mg/kg/day, and divided doses are recommended when the total daily dose exceeds 250 mg.

Drug interactions

The most clinically significant drug interactions associated with valproic acid are inhibition of platelet aggregation, which may cause prolonged bleeding times in patients who are also receiving anticoagulants, and inhibition of the hepatic metabolism of phenobarbital. Valproic acid can also produce a false-positive result in urine ketone tests.

ADVERSE DRUG REACTIONS

Most of the adverse effects associated with valproic acid are tolerable and dose related; however, rare fatal hepatotoxicity has occurred. Physicians do not prescribe valproic acid routinely because of the possibility of hepatotoxicity.

Predictable reactions

The dose-related adverse reactions affect the GI and central nervous systems. The GI adverse reactions include nausea, vomiting, appetite changes, diarrhea, and constipation. The CNS adverse reactions include sedation, drowsiness, dizziness, ataxia, headache, decreased alertness, and muscle weakness.

Hematologic adverse reactions can occur and include inhibited platelet aggregation and prolonged bleeding time. Rare psychiatric adverse reactions include depression, hallucinations, and behavioral disorders in children.

Unpredictable reactions

The rare, fatal hepatotoxicity that has been reported is usually preceded by nonspecific symptoms such as loss of seizure control, malaise, jaundice, weakness, lethargy, facial edema, anorexia, and vomiting. The reaction may develop at any time from 3 days to 6 months after initiation of therapy, with children at the greatest risk.

A drug rash may occur, as may hyperammonemia with normal liver function. The use of valproic acid may also produce blood dyscrasias, such as anemia, leukopenia, and thrombocytopenia.

NURSING IMPLICATIONS

The nurse must be aware of some serious and potentially fatal adverse effects of valproic acid.
• Administer cautiously to patients with a history of hepatic disease. Valproic acid should not be administered to patients with liver dysfunction.
• Administer valproic acid drugs with meals to decrease the GI effects. Keep the flavorful red syrup out of the reach of children.
• Carefully monitor the serum concentration levels of anticonvulsants.

• Periodically monitor liver function studies.

• Inform the patient about the signs and symptoms of hepatotoxicity, and instruct the patient to contact the physician immediately should any of these signs develop.

• Instruct the patient to swallow each capsule whole, because the free drug can seriously irritate the GI mucosa.

• Alert the diabetic patient that the drug may produce a false-positive result on a urine ketone test.

• Remind the patient to report immediately any signs of bleeding so that platelet function can be assessed.

• Instruct the patient to inform the physician of the valproic acid therapy before any kind of surgery, including dental surgery.

See *General patient-teaching tips* on page 373 for additional guides.

OTHER ANTICONVULSANTS

The following section contains information about other drugs used less frequently to treat seizure disorders.

acetazolamide (Diamox). A carbonic anhydrase inhibitor and a sulfonamide derivative, acetazolamide is primarily used as a diuretic, but also possesses anticonvulsant properties. Physicians sometimes use acetazolamide as adjunctive or intermittent therapy in absence, partial and generalized tonic-clonic seizures.

The mechanism of action remains unknown but acetazolamide may suppress the spread of paroxysmal discharges. Hypokalemia and metabolic acidosis represent potentially serious effects associated with the use of acetazolamide. The nurse should caution patients treated with this drug to visit their physician frequently for electrolyte studies. (See Chapter 38, Diuretic Agents, for a further discussion of acetazolamide.)

trimethadione (Tridione) and **paramethadione** (Paradione). These drugs are oxazolidinediones. Since the introduction of the succinimides, physicians only occasionally use trimethadione and paramethadione as sole or adjunctive treatment for refractory absence seizures.

Both drugs are metabolized to an active metabolite, dimethadione, with a prolonged half-life of 10 days to 2 weeks. Trimethadione and paramethadione cause significant GI and CNS toxicity, and are less effective than the succinimides.

magnesium sulfate. This drug prevents or controls seizures by blocking neuromuscular transmission. Physicians use magnesium sulfate primarily as an anticonvulsant in preeclampsia or eclampsia. Magnesium sulfate is used also to treat hypomagnesemic seizures.

SELECTED MAJOR DRUGS

Anticonvulsant agents

Anticonvulsants include various agents, all possessing the ability to inhibit seizure activity. The following agents represent the various classes of agents used.

DRUG	MAJOR INDICATIONS	USUAL ADULT DOSAGES	NURSING IMPLICATIONS
Hydantoin			
phenytoin	Complex partial seizures, and tonic-clonic seizures	300 to 400 mg P.O. daily; in divided doses if a prompt-acting preparation is used; sustained-release preparations are administered as single doses	• Because of saturation kinetics, administer dose increments cautiously. • Advise the patient to practice good dental hygiene. • Instruct the patient that phenytoin preparations vary; check medication refills to verify that the same drug is dispensed. • Many drug interactions exist with phenytoin; caution the patient to report all over-the-counter and prescribed drugs; note any change in seizure control or signs of toxicity.

continued

SELECTED MAJOR DRUGS

Anticonvulsant agents continued

DRUG	MAJOR INDICATIONS	USUAL ADULT DOSAGES	NURSING IMPLICATIONS
phenytoin (continued)			• Give I.V. at no more than 50 mg/minute; monitor the blood pressure and EKG closely. • Note that the pediatric forms of the drug consist of the free acid form of phenytoin, which supplies 8% more drug than the sodium salt form. • Monitor serum concentration levels.
Barbiturate			
phenobarbital	Partial seizures, and tonic-clonic seizures	60 to 300 mg P.O. daily in divided doses	• Observe for excessive central nervous system (CNS) depression or paradoxical reactions (restlessness, agitation). • When given I.V. for status epilepticus, maintain a patent airway; monitor respiratory status closely. • Monitor serum concentration levels.
Iminostilbene			
carbamazepine	Partial seizures, and tonic-clonic seizures	200 mg P.O. daily in divided doses	• Monitor closely for blood dyscrasias. • Use of drug may result in desirable or undesirable psychotropic effects. • Monitor serum concentration levels.
Benzodiazepine			
clonazepam	Absence seizures (petit mal), atypical absence, atonic and myoclonic seizures	1.5 mg P.O. daily in three divided doses; highly individualized	• Monitor CNS effects closely. • Monitor serum concentration levels.
Succinimide			
ethosuximide	Absence seizures (petit mal)	250 mg P.O. b.i.d.; 20 to 40 mg/kg P.O. daily as maintenance dose; highly individualized	• Observe closely for neurotoxicity (ataxia, dizziness, drowsiness, headache, euphoria, restlessness, irritability, lethargy, confusion). • Monitor serum concentration levels.
Valproic acid			
valproate sodium, divalproex sodium	Absence seizures (petit mal), myoclonic, tonic-clonic seizures	15 mg/kg P.O. daily; maximum dose is 60 mg/kg P.O. daily; dosages are highly individualized and should be divided if dosages exceed 250 mg/day	• Fatal hepatotoxicity has been reported. • Drug may cause false-positive results on urine ketone tests. • Monitor serum concentration levels.

CHAPTER SUMMARY

Chapter 24 discussion centered on anticonvulsant drugs. Here are the highlights of the chapter:
• Physicians prescribe anticonvulsants for the long-term treatment of epilepsy and for short-term use in controlling acute isolated seizures not caused by epilepsy. Drug choice depends on an accurate diagnosis of the seizure type, the ability of the drug to control seizures with minimal adverse effects, the use of a single drug whenever possible, and the appropriateness of the drug for the patient's age and health state.
• The major classes of drugs used to treat patients with seizure disorders include hydantoins, barbiturates, iminostilbenes, benzodiazepines, succinimides, and valproic acid.

• The drugs of choice for partial seizures are phenytoin and carbamazepine, with phenobarbital and primidone assuming secondary importance. Physicians consider ethosuximide as the drug of choice for absence seizures.

• For most anticonvulsant drugs, physicians prescribe low initial doses and increase the dosage slowly because the drugs can produce adverse reactions even at low doses.

• Most anticonvulsants demonstrate linear kinetics; however, phenytoin exhibits saturation kinetics. Dosage increases of phenytoin must be made carefully in small increments to avoid toxicity.

• Anticonvulsants frequently interact with other drugs, sometimes producing drug toxicity. To help prevent drug interactions, the nurse should maintain an up-to-date drug history.

• Some anticonvulsants are an increased risk factor when administered to women of childbearing age or to pregnant or lactating women. Teratogenic effects have occurred in patients using anticonvulsants.

• The nurse should closely monitor anticonvulsants' serum concentration levels. Additional laboratory studies are recommended depending on the potential for toxicity.

• Anticonvulsants must never be discontinued abruptly because doing so may precipitate withdrawal seizures or status epilepticus.

BIBLIOGRAPHY

American Medical Association. *AMA Drug Evaluations,* 5th ed. Philadelphia: W.B. Saunders Co., 1983.

Delgado-Escueta, A.V., and Enrile-Bascal, F. "Combination Therapy for Status Epilepticus: Intravenous Diazepam and Phenytoin," *Advances in Neurology* 34:477, 1983.

Frey, H., and Janz, D. *Antiepileptic Drugs.* New York: Springer-Verlag, 1985.

Gram, L., and Bentsen, K.D. "Hepatic Toxicity of Antiepileptic Drugs: A Review," *Acta Neurologica Scandinavica* 68:81, 1983.

Kelly, T.E. "Teratogenicity of Anticonvulsant Drugs," *American Journal of Medical Genetics* 19:413, November 1984.

Mattson, R.H., et al. "Comparison of Carbamazepine, Phenobarbital, Phenytoin, and Primidone in Partial and Secondarily Generalized Tonic-Clonic Seizures," *The New England Journal of Medicine* 313:145, July 18, 1985.

Mattson, R.H., et al. "Use of Oral Contraceptives by Women with Epilepsy," *Journal of the American Medical Association* 256:238, July 11, 1986.

Pippenger, C.E., and Lesser, R.P. "An Overview of Therapeutic Drug Monitoring Principles," *Cleveland Clinic Quarterly* 51:241, Summer 1984.

Reynolds, E.H., and Trimble, M.R. *Drugs* 29:570, June 1985.

Whipkey, R.R., et al. "Drug Use in Pregnancy," *Annals of Emergency Medicine* 13:346, May 1984.

Woodbury, D.M., et al., eds. *Antiepileptic Drugs,* 2nd ed. New York: Raven Press, 1982.

DRUGS TO PREVENT AND TREAT PAIN

Pain, a basic protective mechanism, is a symptom of an underlying physiologic or psychological problem. Pain usually indicates that something is wrong and that health care is desirable.

Since pain is subjective, only the patient can describe it. Pain is whatever sensation the patient perceives it to be; one person's pain perceptions may vary widely from another's. Emotional states and ethnic, cultural, and religious factors all contribute to a patient's pain perception.

Pain detection and transmission

Pain sensation begins in the nociceptors, which are part of an afferent neuron. Nociceptors are free nerve endings located primarily in the skin, periosteum, joint surfaces, and arterial walls. They may be activated by mechanical, chemical, or thermal stimuli. They also are activated by chemical mediators that are released or synthesized in response to tissue damage. Regardless of the etiology, even if only minor tissue damage occurs, the chemical mediators are synthesized and stimulate the nociceptors.

Prostaglandins, histamine, bradykinin, and serotonin are chemical mediators that activate the nociceptors. Acetylsalicylic acid and other nonsteroidal anti-inflammatory drugs (NSAIDs) decrease pain by inhibiting these mediators.

Once the pain process is initiated, the impulse is communicated from the peripheral terminals of the nociceptors to the spinal cord. (See *Pain pathways* on page 396 for an illustration of the transmission pathways.) There are two types of nociceptors: the myelinated A-delta fibers and the smaller, unmyelinated, more numerous C fibers. The faster-conducting A-delta fibers signal sharp, well-localized pain, whereas the slower-conducting C fibers signal dull, poorly localized pain.

All of the nociceptors terminate in the dorsal horn of the spinal cord. The dorsal horn is essentially the control center for incoming information from the afferent neurons, for local modulation (pain impulse regulation), and for descending influences from higher centers in the central nervous system (CNS) such as emotion, attention, and memory.

Pain theory

Several theories have been suggested to define pain transmission; however, much is still unknown.

The Melzack-Wall gate control theory, the most widely accepted pain theory, states that neural mechanisms in the dorsal horn act as a regulator between the peripheral fibers and the higher processing centers in the CNS. The dorsal horn receives both pain- and non-pain-related signals from the various peripheral nerves; pain messages depend on the total information. This process, or gating effect, modulates, or regulates, afferent input before an impulse is sent to the CNS and pain is perceived. Therefore, the perception of pain may be inhibited by the simultaneous activation of sensory neurons carrying non-pain information.

At least two major and several minor ascending pathways in the spinal cord transmit messages to the brain when pain-related signals activate pain-transmission neurons in the dorsal root. The two major pathways are the spinothalamic tract and the spinoreticulothalamic tract; the former is probably the more important. Both pathways travel up the spinal cord and terminate in two separate areas of the thalamus. The two thalamic regions project to different sites in the cerebral cortex.

The thalamus is a relay station for all incoming sensory stimuli, including pain. There, a primitive awareness of pain occurs, but the sensation is not well localized or specific. From the thalamus, pain messages are directed to the cerebral cortex, where more specific localization and characterization of the pain sensation occur. The emotional aspect of pain is related partially to thalamic and limbic stimulation when incoming sensory data are relayed to the cortex.

The brain contains opiate receptors and opiate peptides (endorphins, enkephalins, and dynorphins). The endogenous peptides have a high affinity for the opiate receptors and may modulate pain sensation. These peptides, however, are not the only pain neurotransmitters. Other peptides, amino acids, and biogenic amines also are active.

Most biological systems have an autoregulation mechanism, and the pain system is no exception. This internal regulation occurs in a descending pathway of

Glossary

Analgesia: absence of sensitivity to pain.

Anesthesia: loss of feeling or sensation.

Balanced anesthesia: combination of drugs that produces a loss of feeling or sensation, with maximum beneficial drug effects and minimum adverse drug reactions.

Competitive inhibition: displacement of an agent from an opiate receptor site by an antagonist.

Endorphin: endogenous opiate in the hypothalamus and pituitary.

Enkephalin: endogenous opiate throughout the central and peripheral nervous systems.

Epidural block: loss of feeling or sensation produced by injecting an anesthetic agent between the vertebrae and beneath the ligaments into the space surrounding the dura.

Equianalgesic dose: amount of an analgesic drug that will produce the same level of pain relief as a standard agent used for comparison.

Field block: regional loss of feeling or sensation produced by using several injections of an anesthetic agent to create a pain-free area around an operative site.

Inflammation: tissue reaction to injury characterized by pain, heat, redness, edema, and sometimes loss of function.

Local infiltration: loss of feeling or sensation in a confined area produced by injecting an anesthetic agent.

Narcotic: drug derived from opium or synthetically produced that alters pain perception, induces mental changes, promotes deep sleep, depresses respirations, constricts pupils, and decreases gastrointestinal motility.

Nerve block: regional loss of feeling or sensation produced by injecting an anesthetic agent around or near a nerve to interrupt its conductivity.

Neuralgia: paroxysmal pain extending along one or more nerves.

Neuroleptanesthesia: loss of feeling or sensation produced by using a narcotic, a neuroleptic, and nitrous oxide.

Neurolysis: destruction or dissolution of nerve tissue.

Peripheral nerve block: loss of feeling or sensation produced by injecting an anesthetic agent near or around nerve fibers outside the central nervous system.

Placebo: pharmacologically inactive substance or preparation administered to a patient to achieve a "perceived" therapeutic effect.

Prostaglandins: naturally occurring fatty acids abundant in cells that affect many different cellular functions.

Regional anesthesia: loss of feeling or sensation produced by interrupting the sensory nerve conductivity from a specific body area.

Salicylism: toxic effects of excessive salicylic acid ingestion.

Spinal block: loss of feeling or sensation produced by injecting an anesthetic agent into the cerebrospinal fluid in the subarachnoid space around the spinal cord.

Sympathetic block: loss of feeling or sensation produced by the paravertebral injection of an anesthetic agent to block the sympathetic trunk.

Topical anesthesia: loss of feeling or sensation produced by direct application of a local anesthetic agent to a specified area.

---

the CNS and is responsible for maintaining the normal pain-free state.

Mechanisms of inflammation

Pain may occur alone or in combination with inflammation. Both are reactions to tissue irritation. Inflammation is an immune-mediated process characterized by redness, heat, swelling, loss of function, and pain at the site. Some of the chemical mediators of pain, including prostaglandins, bradykinin, and histamine, also mediate the inflammatory response. (See Unit Thirteen: Drugs to Control Inflammation, Allergy, and Organ Rejection, for more information on inflammation.)

Temperature regulation

The hypothalamus regulates body temperature by balancing heat production and loss. Pyrogens, secreted by toxic bacteria or released from protein breakdown as in degenerating body tissue, can cause the hypothalamic thermostat to rise. This, in turn, causes an increase in body temperature. Recent research also indicates that pyrogens may cause an increase in body temperature by causing a production of prostaglandin E_1 in the hypothalamus. Some of the drugs used to control pain inhibit prostaglandins and produce an antipyretic effect.

Chapter 25
Nonnarcotic Analgesic, Antipyretic, and Nonsteroidal Anti-Inflammatory Agents

Chapter 25 discusses the nonnarcotic, nonsteroidal agents that are used to decrease pain by inhibiting the biosynthesis of prostaglandins. It also delineates the mechanism of action of these agents and their clinical uses and toxic and adverse reactions, such as salicylism. Patient education components also are detailed.

Pain pathways

The A-delta fiber and C fiber nociceptors, when stimulated, transmit an afferent impulse through the dorsal root ganglia to the dorsal horn. Peripheral nerves also transmit information to the dorsal horn. The dorsal horn then modulates all of this information and may transmit an impulse via the spinothalamic tract to the cerebral cortex. Descending pathways carry inhibitory information from the brain to the dorsal horn to be used for further modulation.

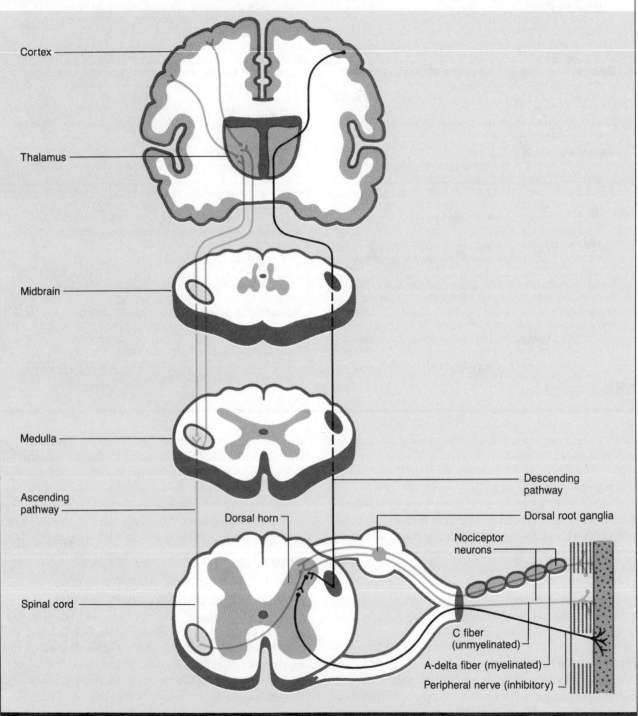

Chapter 26
Narcotic Agonist and Antagonist Agents

Opium derivatives and synthetic agents with similar pharmacologic properties are presented in Chapter 26. The pharmacotherapeutic uses for these agents in inhibiting pain impulse transmission are delineated. The other clinical uses for these agents in suppressing the cough mechanism and decreasing gastrointestinal motility also are discussed. Concepts related to narcotic administration, such as tolerance, ceiling effect, and equianalgesic dose, are explored. Nursing interventions and patient education components are highlighted.

Chapter 27
General Anesthetic Agents

Chapter 27 reviews general anesthesia and associated pharmacologic agents. It discusses various types of anesthesia, including balanced and neuroleptic, and the four stages and their clinical characteristics. The systemic effects of general anesthesia also are emphasized, including associated nursing implications.

Chapter 28
Local and Topical Anesthetic Agents

The local and topical agents used to interrupt the transmission of pain impulses from the peripheral nerves of a specific, limited body area are presented in Chapter 28. Several types of blocks are discussed, including field, spinal, epidural, peripheral, and sympathetic. The application, pharmacodynamics, and clinical uses for the topical anesthetics are detailed, and associated nursing implications are highlighted.

Nursing diagnoses

The nursing diagnoses most applicable for caring for patients receiving drugs to prevent and treat pain include:

- Activity intolerance related to pain resulting from diseases or disorders; trauma; or mechanical, chemical, or thermal stimuli
- Alterations in bowel elimination: constipation related to pain or drug therapy
- Alterations in comfort: pain related to diseases or disorders; trauma; or mechanical, chemical, or thermal stimuli
- Alterations in family processes related to pain, drug therapy, or life-style changes
- Alterations in health maintenance related to pain or drug therapy
- Alterations in oral mucous membranes related to general anesthetic agents
- Alterations in thought processes related to pain or drug therapy
- Alterations in tissue perfusion related to general anesthetic agents
- Alterations in urinary elimination patterns related to drug therapy
- Anxiety related to pain, drug therapy, or life-style changes
- Disturbances in self-concept related to pain or drug therapy
- Fear related to pain, drug therapy, or life-style changes
- Hypothermia related to general anesthetic agents
- Impaired physical mobility related to pain or drug therapy
- Impaired social interaction related to pain or drug therapy
- Ineffective airway clearance related to general anesthetic agents
- Ineffective breathing patterns related to pain or drug therapy
- Ineffective individual coping related to pain, drug therapy, or life-style changes
- Knowledge deficit related to all aspects of drug therapy and pain
- Noncompliance related to medication administration
- Potential alterations in body temperature related to inflammation or drug therapy
- Potential impairment of skin integrity related to pain or drug therapy
- Potential for infection related to drug therapy
- Potential for injury related to drug therapy
- Self-care deficit related to pain or drug therapy
- Sensory-perceptual alterations related to pain or drug therapy
- Sexual dysfunction related to pain or drug therapy
- Sleep pattern disturbances related to pain or drug therapy.

CHAPTER 25

NONNARCOTIC ANALGESIC, ANTIPYRETIC, AND NONSTEROIDAL ANTI-INFLAMMATORY AGENTS

OBJECTIVES

After reading and studying this chapter, you should be able to:

1. Describe the pharmacodynamics of the salicylates, acetaminophen—the only approved para-aminophenol derivative—and nonsteroidal anti-inflammatory drugs (NSAIDs).

2. Compare the adverse drug reactions to salicylates, acetaminophen, and the NSAIDs.

3. Explain the inflammatory process.

4. Discuss the signs, symptoms, and treatment of an acetaminophen overdose.

5. Identify the signs and symptoms of salicylate toxicity.

6. Compare the drug interactions associated with the salicylates, acetaminophen, and the NSAIDs.

INTRODUCTION

The drugs discussed in this chapter form a heterogenous collection that produce analgesic, antipyretic, and anti-inflammatory effects. Among these drugs, salicylates—especially aspirin—are the most widely used agents. This chapter will discuss the salicylates, the para-aminophenol derivative acetaminophen, NSAIDs, and a urinary tract analgesic, phenazopyridine hydrochloride.

For a summary of representative drugs, see *Selected major drugs: Nonnarcotic analgesics, antipyretic agents, and NSAIDs* on pages 412 and 413.

SALICYLATES

These agents possess analgesic, antipyretic, and anti-inflammatory properties. They usually cost less than other analgesics and most are readily available without a prescription. In fact, many over-the-counter (OTC) medications for pain, colds, and influenza contain salicylates along with other agents. Despite the recent development of new products, however, aspirin remains the cornerstone of anti-inflammatory drug therapy.

History and source

For centuries, salicylate-rich willow bark was used for its analgesic and antipyretic properties. The development of salicylate drugs began in 1829, when Leroux discovered the glycoside salicin, a compound that Piria used in 1838 to produce salicylic acid. Six years later, Cahours identified oil of wintergreen as another source of salicylic acid. The manufacture of synthetic salicylates began in 1860, and by 1875 people had begun to use sodium salicylate to treat fever and reduce the signs and symptoms of rheumatic fever. In 1879, See reported on the salicylates' uricosuric properties; later that year, Campbell used these drugs to treat gout. Finally, aspirin (acetylsalicylic acid) was introduced in 1899. Today this drug serves as the standard to which all other analgesics are compared.

PHARMACOKINETICS

Salicylates are readily absorbed and widely distributed throughout the body. They are metabolized in the liver at dose-dependent rates and excreted by the kidneys.

Absorption, distribution, metabolism, excretion

After oral administration, salicylate absorption occurs partly in the stomach but mainly in the upper part of the small intestine through passive diffusion. Absorption usually occurs within 30 minutes. The pure and buffered forms of aspirin are readily absorbed, but sustained-release and enteric-coated salicylate preparations or food or antacids in the stomach delay absorption. The rate of absorption depends on the dosage form, the gastric and intestinal pH, the presence of food or antacids in the stomach, and the gastric-emptying time.

Salicylates are widely distributed throughout the body tissues and fluids, including breast milk. They cross the placenta easily.

The liver metabolizes salicylates extensively into several metabolites. This pharmacokinetic process is dose-dependent. As the salicylate dose and serum levels increase, the metabolic pathways become saturated and cannot metabolize the drug. When this happens, metabolism shifts to alternate pathways, resulting in increased formation of toxic metabolites. Therapeutic salicylate levels range from 30 to 300 mcg/ml. Blood levels that exceed this amount may be toxic. Decreasing the salicylate dose even slightly usually decreases toxic metabolite formation. Blood levels of a salicylate can determine whether a dose has produced an adequate anti-inflammatory effect or has caused toxicity.

The kidneys excrete the salicylate metabolites and some unchanged drug. The amount of unchanged drug excreted is pH-dependent, with about 2% being excreted in acidic urine and 30% in alkaline urine.

Onset, peak, duration

The salicylates' onset of action begins about 1 hour after administration. When the drugs reach peak plasma concentration levels, in 2 hours, they are 50% to 90% serum protein-bound. The amount of protein binding, however, depends on the serum salicylate concentration level. At a low serum concentration level, such as 100 mcg/ml, protein binding nears 90%; at a higher concentration level, such as 400 mcg/ml, protein binding drops to 76%. The salicylates' half-life ranges from 3 hours for a low dose to 30 hours for a high dose.

PHARMACODYNAMICS

The salicylates produce analgesia primarily by inhibiting prostaglandin synthesis; reduce fever through hypothalamic stimulation leading to vasodilation and increased diaphoresis; and reduce inflammation through a poorly understood process that may involve their ability to inhibit prostaglandin synthesis and release during inflammation. Prostaglandins sensitize pain receptors to mechanical and chemical stimulation.

Mechanism of action

Prostaglandins play an important role in the inflammatory process, and pain impulse transmission from the periphery to the spinal cord requires prostaglandin E. Salicylates produce anti-inflammatory and analgesic effects primarily by inhibiting prostaglandin synthesis through inactivation of cyclooxygenase (prostaglandin synthetase). (See *The inflammatory process* on page 400 for more details.) Salicylates may also stabilize membranes, preventing the release of substances that cause inflammation.

These drugs' antipyretic effects, caused by prostaglandin inhibition in the brain, seem to stimulate the heat-regulating center in the hypothalamus, increasing heat elimination. The hypothalamic center then stimulates peripheral vasodilation and increases perspiration.

Aspirin inhibits platelet aggregation through irreversible pathways by interfering with the production of thromboxane A_2, which is necessary for platelet clumping. (For additional information on the use of aspirin as an antiplatelet agent, see Chapter 42, Anticoagulant Agents.)

PHARMACOTHERAPEUTICS

Salicylates are primarily used to relieve pain and reduce fever. However, they cannot effectively relieve visceral pain or severe pain from trauma.

Salicylates have little or no effect on normal body temperature but cause a marked fall if body temperature is elevated. This is especially true of aspirin. Salicylates are often the drugs of choice for relief of fever associated with common colds or influenza, because they can relieve headache and muscular ache as well.

Because salicylates inhibit prostaglandin synthesis, they suppress inflammation. Used to reduce inflammation in rheumatic fever and rheumatoid arthritis, they can provide considerable relief in 24 hours. But no matter what the clinical indication, salicylate therapy should follow one main guideline: use the lowest dose that provides relief.

aspirin (A.S.A., Bayer Timed-Release, Empirin). Aspirin is the most widely used salicylate and effectively relieves headache, neuritis, neuralgia, myalgia, rheumatoid arthritis, and dysmenorrhea.

Aspirin appears in many preparations, even in analgesic combinations with narcotics, such as Oxycodone and Codeine #3. Unlike aspirin alone, medications that contain aspirin and a narcotic require a prescription.

The inflammatory process

Anti-inflammatory drugs act by interrupting the inflammatory process. This process usually begins when tissue injury causes the release of bradykinin and histamine, which in turn cause increased capillary permeability and vasodilation. The change in capillary permeability leads to swelling and pain, and the vasodilation leads to redness and heat. Bradykinin plays a role in the formation and release of prostaglandins, which cause pain. Salicylates and nonsteroidal anti-inflammatory drugs act primarily as antiprostaglandin agents, disrupting the inflammatory process and relieving pain and inflammation.

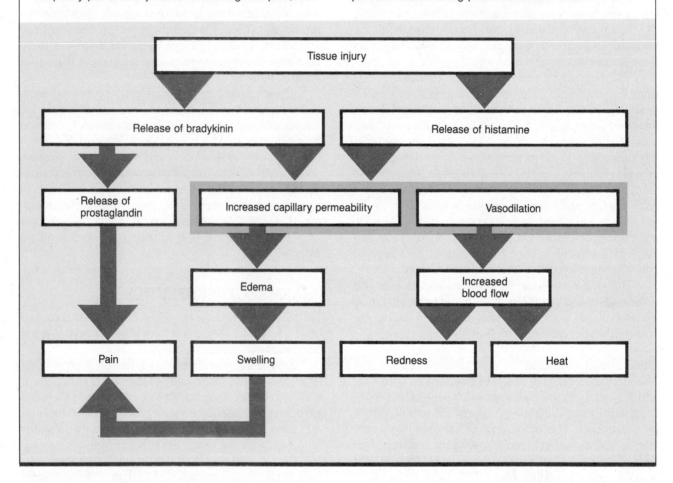

USUAL ADULT DOSAGE: for fever or mild-to-moderate pain such as headache or musculoskeletal pain, 325 to 650 mg P.O. every 3 to 4 hours p.r.n.; for dysmenorrhea, 650 mg P.O. every 4 to 6 hours, beginning 1 or 2 days before the onset of menses and continuing until the 2nd or 3rd day of menses, taken monthly for maximum effect; for rheumatic fever, 975 to 1,300 mg P.O. four to six times daily, individualized to the patient's needs, until fever and inflammation subside (about 1 week) or until the patient is asymptomatic and signs of infection have disappeared; for rheumatoid arthritis, 2.6 to 5.2 grams P.O. daily in divided doses; to prevent transient ischemic attacks (TIAs), 325 mg P.O. q.i.d. or 650 mg P.O. b.i.d. TIA prevention may sometimes occur with lower doses, such as 80 to 325 mg/day.

choline magnesium trisalicylate (Trilisate). A combination of choline salicylate and magnesium salicylate, this drug is indicated for symptomatic relief and long-term management of osteoarthritis and rheumatoid arthritis. It is also indicated in the acute phases of rheumatoid arthritis and can be used to reduce fever and relieve mild-to-moderate pain related to other disorders. Each 500 mg tablet contains the same amount of salicylate as 650 mg of aspirin.

DRUG INTERACTIONS

Salicylates

Drug interactions involving salicylates are common and sometimes severe. They frequently occur with concurrent use of other highly protein-bound or ulcerogenic agents. Because salicylates are so widely used, the nurse must obtain a thorough drug history and be alert for possible drug interactions.

DRUG	INTERACTING DRUGS	POSSIBLE EFFECTS	NURSING IMPLICATIONS
aspirin, choline magnesium trisalicylate, choline salicylate, diflunisal, salsalate, sodium salicylate	alcohol	Increases the ulcerogenic effect, leading to GI bleeding	• Monitor the patient for signs of GI bleeding, such as epigastric pain, abdominal pain or cramps, or black or tarry stools.
	oral anticoagulants and heparin	Increase the anticoagulant effect, increasing risk of bleeding	• Monitor the patient for signs of increased anticoagulant effect, such as gingival bleeding, black or tarry stools, blood in the urine, petechiae, bruises, and prolonged bleeding from cuts.
	corticosteroids	Decrease the plasma salicylate levels and increase the ulcerogenic effect	• Assess the patient for the salicylate's effectiveness after each dose. If it does not provide relief, obtain an order for a different analgesic. • Monitor the patient for epigastric pain, especially 1 to 2 hours after meals. Also assess the patient for other signs of GI bleeding, such as abdominal pain or cramps and black or tarry stools.
	nonsteroidal anti-inflammatory drugs, such as indomethacin, naproxen, and phenylbutazone	Increase the ulcerogenic effect	• Monitor the patient for epigastric pain and other signs of GI bleeding, such as abdominal pain or cramps and black or tarry stools.
	methotrexate	Increases the methotrexate effect and toxicity, causing pancytopenia	• Monitor the patient for signs of methotrexate toxicity such as diarrhea and stomatitis. • Monitor the patient for signs of severe bone marrow depression, such as fatigue, pallor, and fever. • Question any order for salicylates for a patient receiving methotrexate.
	probenecid, sulfinpyrazone	Decrease the uricosuric effect	• Be aware that even small doses of salicylates can decrease the uricosuric effects of probenecid or sulfinpyrazone. • Teach the patient not to take aspirin or other over-the-counter drugs containing salicylates unless specifically directed by the physician.
	antacids	Alkalinize urine, leading to reduced renal tubular reabsorption	• Observe the patient for signs and symptoms of reduced salicylate response, such as increased pain and inflammation. • Expect serum salicylate levels to decrease, requiring a dosage adjustment.
	oral hypoglycemics (sulfonylureas)	Increase the hypoglycemic effect	• Monitor the patient for signs and symptoms of hypoglycemia, such as fatigue, tremors, hunger, drowsiness, headache, diaphoresis, anxiety, numb mouth or tongue, and incoherent speech.
	phenytoin	Increases the phenytoin effect and toxicity	• Monitor the patient for signs and symptoms of increased phenytoin activity, such as hypotension, lethargy, and pancytopenia.

USUAL ADULT DOSAGE: for osteoarthritis, rheumatoid arthritis, fever, or mild-to-moderate pain, 2,000 to 3,000 mg P.O. once a day or 1,500 mg P.O. b.i.d.

choline salicylate (Arthropan). This nonprescription drug is used to relieve mild-to-moderate pain, reduce fever, and reduce inflammation in rheumatoid conditions. It is dispensed in liquid form—1 teaspoon (5 ml) contains 870 mg of choline salicylate—and may be mixed with fruit juice, a carbonated beverage, or water before administration.
USUAL ADULT DOSAGE: for pain or fever, 5 ml P.O. every 4 hours up to a maximum of six doses daily; for inflammation, 5 to 10 ml P.O. t.i.d. or q.i.d.

diflunisal (Dolobid). A salicylic acid derivative, diflunisal has analgesic, anti-inflammatory, and antipyretic actions, although it is not indicated for antipyretic therapy. It may be used for acute or long-term relief of mild-to-moderate pain caused by musculoskeletal problems or osteoarthritis. Diflunisal requires a prescription. Because metabolism of this drug depends on its blood concentration levels, small dosage changes may cause large changes in blood levels, leading to toxicity.
USUAL ADULT DOSAGE: for mild-to-moderate pain, initially 500 to 1,000 mg P.O. followed by 250 to 500 mg every 8 to 12 hours; for osteoarthritis, 500 to 1,000 mg/day P.O. in two divided doses; not to exceed 1,500 mg/day.

salsalate (Disalcid, Mono-Gesic). Salsalate is used for the temporary symptomatic relief of osteoarthritis, rheumatoid arthritis, and related rheumatic conditions. It is available in 750- and 1,500-mg tablets.
USUAL ADULT DOSAGE: for osteoarthritis, rheumatoid arthritis, or rheumatic conditions, 1,500 mg P.O. b.i.d. or 750 mg P.O. q.i.d., not to exceed 4,000 mg/day.

sodium salicylate (Pabalate). This salicylate is used for the temporary relief of mild-to-moderate pain. An enteric coating delays the drug's release until it reaches the alkaline environment of the intestine.
USUAL ADULT DOSAGE: for mild-to-moderate pain, 600 mg P.O. every 4 hours.

Drug interactions
Because salicylates are highly protein bound, they may interact with a large number of other protein-bound drugs by displacing them from their binding sites. This increases the serum concentration level of unbound active drug, thereby increasing the displaced drug's pharmacologic effects. Salicylates may also potentiate the effects of other drugs. Rarely, they can cause false-positive reactions in diabetic patients using the copper

---

Signs and symptoms of salicylate toxicity

Whether mild or severe, salicylate toxicity requires early detection and appropriate action to prevent more serious problems.

Mild salicylate toxicity

Mild toxicity typically affects patients taking high doses of salicylates for rheumatoid arthritis and related conditions. Its signs and symptoms may indicate that the maximum tolerable dose has been reached and that a slight dosage reduction is required. Signs and symptoms include:
- hearing loss
- dizziness
- drowsiness
- headache
- hyperventilation
- mental confusion
- nausea and vomiting
- reduced visual acuity
- diaphoresis
- thirst
- tinnitus
- diarrhea.

Severe salicylate toxicity

Severe toxicity, which occurs most frequently in infants and young children who have ingested large amounts of aspirin, requires immediate medical attention. Signs and symptoms include:
- EEG changes
- hypoglycemia
- skin eruptions
- marked changes in acid-base balance; respiratory alkalosis leading to metabolic acidosis
- central nervous system depression, seizures, coma
- hemorrhagic tendencies.

---

reduction test (Clinitest) for urine glucose, and false-negative reactions to the glucose oxidase test (Tes-Tape). (See *Drug interactions: Salicylates* on page 401 for further information.)

ADVERSE DRUG REACTIONS

The most common adverse reactions to salicylates involve the gastrointestinal (GI) system. Other reactions may include respiratory alkalosis and metabolic acidosis, hearing problems, salicylate toxicity, and hypersensitivity reactions.

Predictable reactions

Gastric distress, nausea, and vomiting frequently result from the salicylates' central action on the medulla's emetic center and their local action on the gastric mucosa secretions that protect the stomach from gastric acid. Although sodium bicarbonate may help prevent GI irritation, it also promotes salicylate excretion by the kidneys.

Large or toxic salicylate doses can cause respiratory alkalosis and increase the rate and depth of respiration. If the respiratory problem is not corrected, metabolic acidosis can occur as the body attempts to compensate for the respiratory alkalosis.

Prolonged use of salicylates sometimes results in bilateral hearing loss of 30 to 40 decibels that usually resolves within 2 weeks after therapy is discontinued. Tinnitus may occur with dosage levels used to treat arthritis, requiring a small dosage reduction. An elderly patient or a patient with impaired hearing, who may not notice the ringing sound until it is severe, should be monitored closely.

Mild salicylate toxicity, or salicylism, characteristically causes nausea, vomiting, diarrhea, thirst, diaphoresis, tinnitus, mental confusion, dizziness, impaired vision, and hyperventilation. When these signs and symptoms appear with doses used to treat rheumatic conditions, a reduction of 325 mg/day can usually reduce them to a tolerable level. Indications of severe toxicity include metabolic acidosis and related acid-base imbalances, hemorrhagic tendencies, hypoglycemia, restlessness, incoherent speech, apprehension, delirium, hallucinations, and seizures. (For further information about this adverse reaction, see *Signs and symptoms of salicylate toxicity.*)

Unpredictable reactions

Common hypersensitivity reactions include rash and, in asthmatics with nasal polyps, bronchospasm and asthma. Anaphylaxis rarely occurs.

NURSING IMPLICATIONS

Although the salicylates are commonly available in OTC preparations, the nurse should not minimize their importance and should be aware of the following implications:

• Always administer salicylates with a full glass of liquid.
• Question any order for sodium salicylate for a patient with hypertension or a patient on a sodium-restricted diet. Advise such a patient not to use effervescent aspirin products, which have a high sodium content.
• Discourage the use of salicylates—even "children's aspirin"—in a child with flulike symptoms, because they could cause Reye's syndrome, a potentially fatal disorder that causes encephalopathy and fatty infiltration of the internal organs.
• Advise an aspirin-sensitive patient to read labels carefully on OTC drugs, because many contain aspirin or other salicylates.
• Expect to discontinue aspirin 1 week before major surgery, as ordered.
• Advise the patient to discard tablets with a vinegarlike odor.
• Document a patient history of gastric ulcers or GI complaints during the nursing assessment. Salicylates frequently cause gastric distress and may reactivate a peptic ulcer.
• Assess the patient's drug history for use of an anticoagulant. Teach the patient to recognize such problem signs as gingival bleeding, prolonged bleeding from a cut, black or tarry stools, blood in the urine, petechiae, and bruises. Advise the patient to report any of these signs to the physician immediately.
• Inform the patient to keep salicylates in a cool, dry place, because exposure to heat and moisture will weaken their potency.
• Inform the patient that buffered aspirin contains too little antacid to reduce gastric irritation. Suggest that the patient take plain aspirin with food, milk, or 1 to 2 teaspoons of antacid to more effectively prevent GI distress at less expense. (If aspirin is taken with an antacid, the patient may require an increased aspirin dosage.)
• Encourage the patient to use salicylates as ordered. Because many salicylates have been available for years and can be purchased without prescriptions, some patients devalue their therapeutic effectiveness.
• Advise the patient taking sodium salicylate tablets not to crush or chew them or take them within 1 hour of ingesting milk or antacids, which may disrupt the enteric coating.
• Advise the patient taking diflunisal tablets not to crush or chew them. Expect to administer a decreased diflunisal dosage to a patient with renal failure.
• Ask a patient who reports hypersensitivity to aspirin about the actual signs and symptoms experienced. Remember that a patient may mistakenly believe that GI distress is a hypersensitivity reaction.

DRUG INTERACTIONS
Para-aminophenol derivative

When acetaminophen is given with certain drugs, its absorption may decrease; this interaction requires the nurse to space out the doses properly. Other interactions require different nursing interventions.

DRUG	INTERACTING DRUGS	POSSIBLE EFFECTS	NURSING IMPLICATIONS
acetaminophen	alcohol (chronic use)	Increases risk of hepatotoxicity	• Inform a patient with known or suspected chronic alcoholism of the increased risk of liver damage. Because acetaminophen is available over the counter, patient teaching is the only way to prevent this problem.
	barbiturates	Increase acetaminophen metabolism	• Assess the patient for a reduced therapeutic response to acetaminophen. • Expect to administer an increased acetaminophen dosage, as ordered.
	charcoal	Reduces GI absorption of acetaminophen	• Administer the charcoal and acetaminophen doses several hours apart.
	cholestyramine	Reduces GI absorption of acetaminophen	• Administer acetaminophen 1 to 2 hours before cholestyramine.

PARA-AMINOPHENOL DERIVATIVE

Although this subclass contains two substances—phenacetin and acetaminophen, only acetaminophen is available in the United States. Phenacetin was removed from all preparations in the United States because it was associated with anemia, acidosis, kidney damage, and methemoglobinemia. Acetaminophen, an analgesic and antipyretic, appears in many products to relieve pain, colds, and influenza. It has no anti-inflammatory properties. Physicians frequently choose acetaminophen over a salicylate for a patient with a history of GI bleeding, ulcers, or salicylate hypersensitivity.

History and source
Cahn and Hepp introduced acetanilid, the parent drug of this subclass, in 1886 under the name *antifebrin*. The drug's high toxicity, however, prompted a search for agents with similar therapeutic actions and fewer adverse reactions. After researchers developed para-aminophenol and it proved to be toxic, they tested its chemical derivatives. In 1887, they introduced phenacetin, which became widely used in analgesic compounds until 1979. In that year, the drug was withdrawn from the market because it was found to cause anemias and kidney damage.

Although acetaminophen, a phenacetin metabolite, was first used in 1893, it did not become popular until phenacetin's toxicity was discovered. Today, acetaminophen vies in popularity with aspirin in treating noninflammatory conditions.

PHARMACOKINETICS

Acetaminophen is rapidly and completely absorbed from the GI tract and well absorbed from the rectal mucosa. It is widely distributed in body fluids and readily crosses the placenta. After acetaminophen undergoes metabolism by hepatic enzymes, it is excreted by the kidneys and, in small amounts, in breast milk.

The drug's plasma concentration levels peak in 30 to 60 minutes, and its duration of action ranges from 3 to 5 hours. Acetaminophen's plasma protein binding varies widely—from 20% to 50%—and its half-life ranges from 1 to 3 hours.

PHARMACODYNAMICS

Acetaminophen offers significant analgesic and antipyretic actions, but unlike salicylates, does not act on inflammation or platelet function.

Although acetaminophen's mechanism of analgesic action is not fully understood, the drug may act centrally by inhibiting prostaglandin synthesis and peripherally in some unknown way. The drug's antipyretic effect results from its direct action on the heat-regulating center in the hypothalamus.

PHARMACOTHERAPEUTICS

Acetaminophen offers an alternative to patients who cannot tolerate aspirin and who do not need an analgesic with anti-inflammatory properties. A nonprescription drug, acetaminophen reduces fever and relieves headache, muscular ache, and pain in general but cannot relieve intense or visceral pain. It is the drug of choice for treating fever and flulike symptoms in children.

A patient with osteoarthritis may benefit from acetaminophen because this common form of arthritis does not result from an inflammatory process. Some physicians consider acetaminophen the drug of choice for osteoarthritis.

Besides its presence in many OTC preparations, acetaminophen is included in several combination prescription drugs, such as oxycodone hydrochloride and some codeine compounds.

acetaminophen (Datril, Panadol, Tylenol). Physicians and nurses commonly administer this drug to relieve headache, alleviate mild-to-moderate pain, and reduce fever. It is available in regular tablets, chewable tablets, caplets, elixirs, solutions, and rectal suppositories.
USUAL ADULT DOSAGE: for headache, mild-to-moderate pain, fever, or osteoarthritis, 325 to 650 mg P.O. or rectally every 3 to 4 hours p.r.n.
USUAL PEDIATRIC DOSAGE: for headache, mild-to-moderate pain, or fever, 5 to 10 mg/kg P.O. every 4 to 6 hours.

Drug interactions

Few significant interactions occur between acetaminophen and other drugs. (See *Drug interactions: Para-aminophenol derivative* for further information.) Acetaminophen may slightly increase the effects of oral anticoagulants. Antacids, anticholinergics, and narcotics may reduce acetaminophen's absorption by slowing intestinal motility; however, these interactions are not clinically significant.

ADVERSE DRUG REACTIONS

Most patients tolerate acetaminophen well. Unlike the salicylates, acetaminophen rarely causes gastric irritation or hemorrhagic tendencies.

Detection and treatment of acetaminophen-induced hepatotoxicity

Ingestion of 10 grams or more of acetaminophen may cause a severe adverse reaction: hepatotoxicity. Although hepatotoxicity signs and symptoms appear within 24 hours, they often mimic common illnesses, so the real problem goes undetected. Specific clinical and laboratory signs may not appear for 48 to 72 hours.

Signs and symptoms of acetaminophen overdose leading to hepatotoxicity typically follow this pattern:

1 to 24 hours after ingestion
• nausea
• vomiting
• diaphoresis
• malaise
• pallor

24 to 48 hours after ingestion
• decreased urine output
• abdominal pain in the right upper quadrant

2 to 6 days after ingestion
• bruises, petechiae, and bleeding caused by coagulation defects
• jaundice
• hypoglycemia
• renal failure
• encephalopathy
• cardiomyopathy
• elevated bilirubin and liver enzymes
• prolonged prothrombin and partial thromboplastin times

A patient with signs and symptoms of acetaminophen-induced hepatotoxicity requires hospitalization for close monitoring and prompt treatment. To treat acetaminophen overdose and prevent hepatic injury, the nurse can expect to immediately perform gastric lavage or induce emesis with ipecac syrup, followed by the oral administration of activated charcoal. Then the nurse should obtain blood for liver function tests and acetaminophen concentration levels. (Blood should not be obtained for acetaminophen concentration levels until at least 4 hours after ingestion.) If less than 24 hours have elapsed since ingestion, the nurse can expect to administer oral acetylcysteine (Mucomyst), an antidote that crosses liver cell membranes and inactivates acetaminophen metabolites. Because its odor and taste are unpleasant, acetylcysteine should be chilled and added to cola or to orange or grapefruit juice before administration.

Predictable reactions

Similar to an overdose, chronic use of high doses of acetaminophen can cause hypoglycemia, methemoglobinemia, leukopenia, kidney damage, renal failure, hepatotoxicity leading to coagulation defects, cyanosis, and vascular collapse. (See *Detection and treatment of acetaminophen-induced hepatotoxicity* on page 405 for detailed information.)

Unpredictable reactions

Hypersensitivity reactions to acetaminophen usually take the form of skin rashes but rarely may include fever and angioedema. Such reactions are much less common with acetaminophen than with aspirin.

NURSING IMPLICATIONS

Although acetaminophen appears in many OTC preparations, the nurse should not minimize its importance and should be aware of the following considerations:

• Be aware that the regular ingestion of acetaminophen is contraindicated in a patient with anemia or hepatic disease. Patients with renal disease should exercise caution in taking this agent.

• Inform the patient that high doses or unsupervised chronic use of this drug can cause liver damage and that excessive alcohol ingestion may increase this risk.

• Teach the patient that acetaminophen is safe and effective only when used as directed on the label. Because this drug is readily available without a prescription and is widely advertised, many patients assume that it is nontoxic. This false assumption can lead to accidental overdose when a patient attempts to relieve severe or persistent headache, fever, or pain.

• Advise the patient to read all drug labels carefully. Acetaminophen is an ingredient in many OTC drugs with brand names that do not signal its presence.

NONSTEROIDAL ANTI-INFLAMMATORY DRUGS

The search for effective anti-inflammatory drugs that would not cause the adverse reactions associated with aspirin and corticosteroids led to the development of nonsteroidal anti-inflammatory drugs (NSAIDs). These drugs, with chemical structures differing from those of corticosteroids, have anti-inflammatory, analgesic, and antipyretic properties, although they are seldom prescribed for fever. Their anti-inflammatory action equals that of aspirin.

The NSAIDs are derived from many different chemical sources. Fenoprofen calcium, ketoprofen, naproxen, and naproxen sodium are propionic acid derivatives. Meclofenamate and mefenamic acid are anthranilic acid derivatives. Phenylbutazone is a pyrazolon derivative. Piroxicam is an oxicam derivative. Indomethacin is an indoleacetic acid derivative. Tolmetin sodium is a pyrrole acetic acid derivative. Sulindac is an indeneacetic acid derivative.

NSAIDs can relieve mild-to-moderate pain from dental extractions and such conditions as soft-tissue athletic injuries and dysmenorrhea. They can also relieve the pain and inflammation of arthritis and related conditions.

History and source

Before 1949, salicylates and corticosteroids were the only available anti-inflammatory drugs. Salicylates caused severe GI irritation, however, and corticosteroids caused severe systemic complications when used to treat arthritis. So researchers began to look for safer anti-inflammatory agents. In 1949, phenylbutazone was introduced to treat rheumatoid arthritis and similar disorders. This drug, however, also caused severe adverse reactions, such as ulcers, that limited its usefulness.

Meclofenamate and mefenamic acid, discovered in the early 1950s, are indicated for short-term use only, because long-term use is associated with adverse reactions that require discontinuation.

In 1963, indomethacin was introduced to treat rheumatoid arthritis and similar disorders. Although it can cause gastric upset and dizziness, it has become the standard against which all other NSAIDs are measured.

Available since the mid-1970s, ibuprofen can now be obtained without a prescription. More recently, researchers have developed numerous related compounds, such as naproxen and ketoprofen.

In 1982, piroxicam was introduced to treat osteoarthritis and rheumatoid arthritis. Its long half-life makes once-a-day dosage possible.

There are numerous NSAIDs on the market, with new drugs appearing each year. This chapter will discuss a representative sample of those available.

PHARMACOKINETICS

The NSAIDs are absorbed in the GI tract and, for the most part, metabolized in the liver and excreted primarily by the kidneys. They differ widely, however, in their onset of action, duration of action, and half-life.

Absorption, distribution, metabolism, excretion

Afer oral administration, NSAIDs are absorbed rapidly in the GI tract. (The presence of food in the stomach can significantly delay absorption but will not affect the total amount of drug absorbed.) NSAIDs are widely distributed in the body. Most of these agents are metabolized in the liver and excreted primarily in the urine. Sulindac must be metabolized to a clinically active metabolite to be effective.

Onset, peak, duration

Onset of action varies considerably among the NSAIDs, although their analgesic effects always precede their antirheumatic effects—which may take 1 to 3 weeks to appear. Naproxen sodium, the fastest-acting NSAID, relieves pain effectively in 1 hour. Indomethacin and similar drugs reach peak plasma concentration levels in 1 to 2 hours if the stomach is empty. Their duration of action varies widely, from 2 to 85 hours, affecting the dosage frequency. Their plasma protein binding, which ranges from 90% to 99%, may contribute to potential drug interactions. Phenylbutazone has the longest half-life—78 to 85 hours—and a long duration of action. Naproxen's relatively long half-life and duration of action allow a twice-a-day dosage.

PHARMACODYNAMICS

Unlike the corticosteroids, the NSAIDs do not reduce inflammation by stimulating the pituitary-adrenal system. Instead they decrease inflammation and pain by inhibiting prostaglandin activity.

Mechanism of action

Researchers believe the NSAIDs inhibit prostaglandin synthetase, retard polymorphonuclear leukocyte motility, and affect the release and activity of lysosomal enzymes. Their ability to decrease prostaglandin concentrations in peripheral tissues may account for their anti-inflammatory effects. Fenamates may act in another way because studies have shown that they compete with prostaglandins at receptor-binding sites.

PHARMACOTHERAPEUTICS

Physicians use NSAIDs primarily to decrease inflammation and secondarily to relieve pain. Although the NSAIDs share similar indications and mechanisms of action, individual responses vary greatly: a patient may respond poorly to one drug and very well to another. Therefore, the choice of an NSAID must be made empirically. Usually, a patient receives an NSAID for a trial period of 2 to 4 weeks. If this first NSAID does not produce a therapeutic response, it is usually discontinued and replaced with a second drug for another trial period. This procedure may be repeated until relief is obtained.

Indications for NSAIDs include ankylosing spondylitis; moderate-to-severe rheumatoid arthritis; osteoarthritis in the hip, shoulder, or other large joints; osteoarthritis accompanied by inflammation; and acute gouty arthritis. The nurse may see these drugs prescribed interchangeably. For example, tolmetin is the only NSAID specifically indicated for juvenile arthritis, although naproxen, indomethacin, and ibuprofen are effective and are frequently used. Because of their toxicity, indomethacin and phenylbutazone should be used only after other drug therapy has proven ineffective.

fenoprofen calcium (Nalfon). Fenoprofen, a propionic acid derivative, is primarily used for symptomatic relief of acute and chronic forms of osteoarthritis and rheumatoid arthritis; it may also be used to relieve mild-to-moderate pain.
USUAL ADULT DOSAGE: for osteoarthritis and rheumatoid arthritis, 300 to 600 mg P.O. t.i.d. or q.i.d. up to a maximum of 3,200 mg/day; for mild-to-moderate pain, 200 mg P.O. every 4 to 6 hours.

ibuprofen (Advil, Motrin, Nuprin). The only over-the-counter NSAID, ibuprofen is used to relieve the signs and symptoms of osteoarthritis and rheumatoid arthritis, to relieve mild-to-moderate pain, and to treat dysmenorrhea. Nonprescription ibuprofen is available in 200-mg tablets. Higher dosage forms require a prescription.
USUAL ADULT DOSAGE: for mild-to-moderate pain, 200 to 400 mg P.O. every 4 to 6 hours; for dysmenorrhea, 400 mg P.O. every 4 hours, p.r.n., given as soon as pain begins; for arthritis, 400 to 800 mg P.O. t.i.d. or q.i.d. A patient with rheumatoid arthritis usually requires a higher dose than a patient with osteoarthritis.

indomethacin (Indocin). This NSAID, an indoleacetic acid derivative, is usually reserved for adults with rheumatoid arthritis or osteoarthritis who do not respond to salicylates or other treatments. It effectively controls the pain and inflammation associated with the active stages of moderate-to-severe rheumatoid arthritis; with acute flare-ups of chronic rheumatoid arthritis; and with ankylosing spondylitis, bursitis, and acute gouty arthritis. For oral administration, indomethacin is available in 25- and 50-mg capsules and in a sustained-release 75-mg capsule. For rectal administration, it is available in 50-mg suppositories.
USUAL ADULT DOSAGE: for moderate-to-severe rheumatoid arthritis or osteoarthritis and acute flare-ups of chronic rheumatoid arthritis, ankylosing spondylitis, 25 to 50 mg P.O. t.i.d. of regular indomethacin with food, increased to a maximum of 200 mg/day. For night pain

DRUG INTERACTIONS

Nonsteroidal anti-inflammatory drugs

Drug interactions with the nonsteroidal anti-inflammatory drugs are common and can be severe. They frequently require dosage adjustment, drug discontinuation, or drug substitution.

DRUG	INTERACTING DRUGS	POSSIBLE EFFECTS	NURSING IMPLICATIONS
indomethacin	corticosteroids	Increase the ulcerogenic effect	• Monitor the patient for epigastric and abdominal pain, abdominal cramps—especially 1 to 2 hours after eating—and signs of GI bleeding, such as bloody or tarry stools.
	captopril	Decreases the antihypertensive effect of captopril	• Monitor the patient for an increased blood pressure. • Expect to adjust the captopril dosage as ordered.
	furosemide	Decreases the antihypertensive and diuretic effects of furosemide	• Monitor the patient's blood pressure and fluid intake and output to detect decreased effects. • Anticipate substitution of a different NSAID, such as sulindac, for indomethacin.
	oral anticoagulants	Increase the anticoagulant effect	• Monitor the patient for gingival bleeding, black or tarry stools, blood in the urine, petechiae, bruises, or prolonged bleeding from a cut. • Monitor the patient's prothrombin time and partial thromboplastin time, and adjust the anticoagulant dosage as ordered.
sulindac	oral anticoagulants	Increase hypoprothrombinemic activity, causing bleeding	• If concurrent use is unavoidable, monitor the patient for signs of bleeding, such as blood-tinged urine, black or tarry stools, and easy bruising. • Expect to substitute ibuprofen, naproxen, or tolmetin for sulindac as ordered; these drugs are less likely to interact with anticoagulants.
piroxicam	lithium carbonate	Inhibits renal excretion of lithium, leading to toxicity	• Observe the patient for signs of lithium toxicity, such as tremors and stupor. • Monitor the patient's lithium blood levels.
phenylbutazone	anabolic steroids	Increase phenylbutazone concentration levels and the risk of adverse reactions such as nausea and vomiting	• Monitor the patient for adverse reactions.
	oral anticoagulants	Inhibit anticoagulant metabolism	• Expect to substitute ibuprofen, naproxen, or tolmetin for phenylbutazone as ordered; these drugs are less likely to interact with anticoagulants.
	oral hypoglycemics (sulfonylureas)	Increase the hypoglycemic effect	• Observe the patient for signs and symptoms of hypoglycemia, such as tremors, light-headedness, and diaphoresis. • Expect to adjust the oral hypoglycemic dosage as ordered.

DRUG INTERACTIONS

Nonsteroidal anti-inflammatory drugs continued

DRUG	INTERACTING DRUGS	POSSIBLE EFFECTS	NURSING IMPLICATIONS
phenylbutazone (continued)	digitalis glycosides	Increase digitalis metabolism, decreasing its therapeutic effect	• Monitor the patient for signs of decreased digitalis effectiveness, such as rapid heartbeat and congestive heart failure, noted by bibasilar rales, and pitting edema.
	methotrexate	Displaces methotrexate from plasma protein binding sites, causing methotrexate toxicity	• Monitor the patient for signs and symptoms of methotrexate toxicity, such as thrombocytopenia, ulcerated stomatitis, enteritis, and alopecia.
	phenytoin	Extends the half-life of phenytoin, leading to toxicity	• Monitor the patient for signs and symptoms of phenytoin toxicity, such as confusion, hypotension, and dysrhythmias.
mefenamic acid	oral anticoagulants	Increase hypothrombinemic activity, causing bleeding	• Expect to substitute ibuprofen, naproxen, or tolmetin for mefenamic acid, as ordered. • Monitor the patient for signs of hemorrhage, such as blood-tinged urine, black or tarry stools, or easy bruising, if these drugs must be administered together.

and morning stiffness associated with osteoarthritis, 100 mg P.O. of the total daily dosage may be given at bedtime. For bursitis or tendinitis, 75 to 150 mg P.O. may be given in three or four divided doses. For gouty arthritis, 50 mg P.O. t.i.d. may be given. The 75-mg sustained-release preparation can be given for all indications except gouty arthritis.

ketoprofen (Orudis). This NSAID, a propionic acid derivative, is used to treat the signs and symptoms of osteoarthritis and rheumatoid arthritis.
USUAL ADULT DOSAGE: for osteoarthritis and rheumatoid arthritis, 75 mg P.O. t.i.d. or 50 mg P.O. q.i.d. initially, given with milk or food, increased to a maximum of 300 mg/day, if needed.

meclofenamate (Meclomen). Meclofenamate, an anthranilic acid derivative, can relieve the signs and symptoms of acute and chronic rheumatoid arthritis and osteoarthritis. However, it should not be used as a first-line drug, because it can cause severe adverse reactions.
USUAL ADULT DOSAGE: for acute and chronic rheumatoid arthritis and osteoarthritis, 200 to 400 mg P.O. daily, given in three or four equal doses of 50 to 100 mg each. Therapy should begin at a low dose and increase based on the patient's response.

mefenamic acid (Ponstel). This NSAID, an anthranilic acid derivative, may be prescribed for short-term man-

agement of dysmenorrhea or acute moderate pain of less than one week duration such as that associated with insertion of an intrauterine device or postoperative pain.
USUAL ADULT DOSAGE: for dysmenorrhea and acute moderate pain of short duration, 500 mg P.O. initially, followed by 250 mg every 6 hours p.r.n., for no more than 7 days.

naproxen (Naprosyn). Naproxen, a propionic acid derivative, is used to relieve mild-to-moderate pain and to treat osteoarthritis, rheumatoid arthritis, ankylosing spondylitis, tendinitis, bursitis, acute gout, and dysmenorrhea. Its 13-hour half-life allows twice-a-day dosage.
USUAL ADULT DOSAGE: for acute tendinitis and bursitis, dysmenorrhea, and mild-to-moderate pain, 500 mg P.O. initially followed by 250 mg P.O. every 6 to 8 hours, p.r.n.; for osteoarthritis, rheumatoid arthritis, and ankylosing spondylitis, 250 to 375 mg P.O. in the morning and evening separated by about 12 hours, increased to a maximum of 1,000 mg/day, if needed. A patient who awakens with morning pain should take unequal doses, with the larger one in the evening.

naproxen sodium (Anaprox). Naproxen sodium is a propionic acid derivative. It is used for the same indications as naproxen, with one major advantage: more rapid absorption.
USUAL ADULT DOSAGE: for dysmenorrhea, acute tendinitis and bursitis, and mild-to-moderate pain, two 275-

mg tablets P.O. initially, followed by 275 mg every 6 to 8 hours, p.r.n., up to a maximum of 1,375 mg/day; for rheumatoid arthritis, osteoarthritis, and ankylosing spondylitis, two 275-mg tablets P.O. initially, morning and evening, or 275 mg in the morning and 550 mg in the evening, increased to a maximum of 1,100 mg/day.

phenylbutazone (Butazolidin). Phenylbutazone, a pyrazolon derivative, is reserved for use when other NSAIDs have proven unsatisfactory, because it can cause severe adverse reactions. It is used mainly for symptomatic relief of severe rheumatoid arthritis, ankylosing spondylitis, and osteoarthritis of the hips and knees.
USUAL ADULT DOSAGE: for rheumatoid arthritis, ankylosing spondylitis, and osteoarthritis, 300 to 600 mg P.O. daily given in three or four divided doses until condition improves, then decreased to the minimum dose needed to produce a satisfactory response—usually 100 to 200 mg, but less than 400 mg/day. If a favorable response does not occur within 7 days of therapy, the patient should receive a different drug.

piroxicam (Feldene). Piroxicam, an oxicam derivative, is indicated for symptomatic relief of acute and chronic osteoarthritis and rheumatoid arthritis. Piroxicam has a long half-life (50 hours), making a single daily dose possible. However, it does not produce maximum effects for about 2 weeks.
USUAL ADULT DOSAGE: for acute and chronic osteoarthritis and rheumatoid arthritis, 20 mg P.O. once daily or 10 mg every 12 hours.

sulindac (Clinoril). Sulindac, an indeneacetic acid derivative, is indicated for acute or long-term use. Sulindac provides symptomatic relief of osteoarthritis, rheumatoid arthritis, ankylosing spondylitis, bursitis, and acute gouty arthritis.
USUAL ADULT DOSAGE: for osteoarthritis, rheumatoid arthritis, ankylosing spondylitis, bursitis, and acute gouty arthritis, 150 to 200 mg P.O. b.i.d. with food.

tolmetin sodium (Tolectin). Tolmetin, a pyrrole acetic acid derivative, is used to relieve the signs and symptoms of osteoarthritis, rheumatoid arthritis, and juvenile rheumatoid arthritis.
USUAL ADULT DOSAGE: for osteoarthritis and rheumatoid arthritis, initially 400 mg P.O. t.i.d., including a dose upon arising and at bedtime; increase as needed. For rheumatoid arthritis, a maximum of 2,000 mg/day given in four divided doses. For osteoarthritis, a maximum of 1,600 mg/day given in four divided doses.
USUAL PEDIATRIC DOSAGE: for juvenile rheumatoid arthritis, initially 20 mg/kg/day for children over age 2; then 15 to 30 mg/kg/day.

Nonsteroidal anti-inflammatory drugs: Summary of adverse reactions

NSAIDs can produce numerous adverse reactions in four major body systems: the central nervous system, the gastrointestinal system (most common site), the renal system, and the eyes.

Central nervous system

- depression
- dizziness
- drowsiness
- headache
- mental confusion
- tinnitus
- vertigo

Eyes

- blurred vision
- decreased acuity
- corneal deposits

Gastrointestinal system

- abdominal pain
- bleeding
- anemia
- diarrhea
- nausea
- ulcerations
- perforation
- hepatotoxicity

Renal system

- cystitis
- hematuria
- kidney necrosis
- nephrotic syndrome (rare)

Drug interactions

A wide variety of drugs can interact with NSAIDs, especially with indomethacin, mefenamic acid, phenylbutazone, piroxicam, and sulindac. Because they are highly protein bound, NSAIDs are likely to interact with other protein-bound drugs, such as oral anticoagulants. They may also interfere with antihypertensive drugs, such as beta-adrenergic blockers and thiazides, decreasing their antihypertensive effects. This interaction is not fully documented, however, and may not occur with all NSAIDs. (For further information about significant interactions, see *Drug interactions: Nonsteroidal anti-inflammatory drugs* on pages 408 and 409.)

ADVERSE DRUG REACTIONS

All of the NSAIDs produce similar adverse reactions that rarely require discontinuation of therapy. In general, the NSAIDs are better tolerated than salicylates or corticosteroids.

Predictable reactions

GI tract disturbances are the most common adverse reactions to NSAIDs. Other adverse reactions affect the central nervous system, the renal system, and the eyes. (See *Nonsteroidal anti-inflammatory drugs: Summary of adverse reactions* for detailed information.)

Phenylbutazone has an unusually high incidence of adverse reactions, frequently causing nausea, vomiting, abdominal discomfort, dyspepsia, diarrhea, and skin rashes. Other reactions include gastric ulceration and hemorrhage, vertigo, insomnia, and the combination of sodium and water retention, increased plasma volume, and decreased urine volume—which may lead to peripheral edema, acute pulmonary edema, and cardiac symptoms. Phenylbutazone sometimes causes thrombocytopenia, aplastic anemia, granulocytopenia, and other blood dyscrasias. At highest risk for adverse reactions are elderly patients, especially women, and patients receiving high doses or long-term therapy. Adverse reactions limit phenylbutazone's use to short-term therapy—1 week or less for a patient over age 60.

Unpredictable reactions

NSAIDs can cause hypersensitivity reactions, evidenced by skin rashes, urticaria, angioedema, hypotension, dyspnea, and an asthmalike syndrome. With phenylbutazone, hypersensitivity reactions include pruritus, fever, arthralgia, polyarthritis, Stevens-Johnson syndrome, and anaphylaxis. With piroxicam, skin rashes and photosensitivity occur more frequently than with the other NSAIDs. With any NSAID, therapy should be discontinued at the first sign of a hypersensitivity reaction.

NURSING IMPLICATIONS

The nurse must closely monitor the patient receiving NSAIDs, especially phenylbutazone and indomethacin, and be aware of the following considerations:

• Be aware that NSAIDs are contraindicated in a patient with asthma.
• Withhold meclofenamate or mefenamic acid if diarrhea occurs, and consult the physician.
• Monitor baseline hematologic studies before phenylbutazone treatment begins.
• Monitor vision problems and expect to discontinue the NSAID until an ophthalmic examination rules out drug therapy as the cause.
• Obtain a complete drug history, because a patient with aspirin hypersensitivity may also be hypersensitive to NSAIDs.
• Teach the patient to recognize the signs and symptoms of adverse reactions and to report any reaction promptly to the physician.
• Emphasize to the patient the importance of returning for periodic blood tests as ordered.
• Advise the patient receiving indomethacin to avoid driving or operating machinery until the drug's effects are evaluated, because drowsiness and dizziness frequently occur at the beginning of therapy.
• Advise the patient that some NSAIDs, such as naproxen, ibuprofen, and fenoprofen, may take several weeks to produce the maximum therapeutic effect.

URINARY TRACT ANALGESIC

Phenazopyridine hydrochloride (Azodine, Pyridium), an azo dye, produces a local analgesic effect on the urinary tract, usually within 24 to 48 hours after therapy begins. It relieves the pain, burning, urgency, and frequency that occur with urinary tract infections.

The usual dosage ranges from 100 to 200 mg P.O. t.i.d. after meals for 2 days only. After oral administration, phenazopyridine is 35% metabolized in the liver, with the remainder excreted unchanged in the urine. The drug colors the urine orange or red, which may permanently stain fabrics it contacts. A yellow tinge to the skin or sclera may indicate drug accumulation and the need to discontinue phenazopyridine therapy. Because this drug can alter the results of some urine glucose tests, such as Tes-Tape and Clinistix, the nurse should use Clinitest for an accurate determination.

(Text continues on page 414.)

Nonnarcotic analgesics, antipyretic agents, and NSAIDs

The following chart features the most frequently used drugs in this category.

DRUG	MAJOR INDICATIONS	USUAL ADULT DOSAGES	NURSING IMPLICATIONS
Salicylates			
aspirin	Mild-to-moderate pain Fever	325 to 650 mg P.O. every 3 to 4 hours p.r.n.	• Give aspirin with a full glass (200 to 240 ml) of water or milk to minimize the risk of adverse GI reactions.
	Dysmenorrhea	650 mg P.O. every 4 to 6 hours, beginning 1 or 2 days before the onset of menses and continuing until the 2nd or 3rd day of menses	• Be aware that salicylism is sometimes used as a guide for maximum dosage in rheumatic conditions. Once the patient experiences symptoms of salicylism, the dose is reduced. • Be aware that a patient with hay fever, asthma, or nasal polyps is more likely to be hypersensitive to salicylates.
	Rheumatic fever	975 to 1,300 mg P.O. four to six times daily until fever and inflammation subside	• Advise the patient that a hypersensitivity reaction could happen at any time, even if salicylates have been tolerated for a long time. • Do not rely on tinnitus and decreased hearing as indications of toxicity in an elderly patient or a patient with impaired hearing.
	Rheumatoid arthritis	2.6 to 5.2 grams P.O. daily in divided doses	
	Transient ischemic attacks	325 mg P.O. q.i.d. or 650 mg P.O. b.i.d.	
diflunisal	Mild-to-moderate musculoskeletal pain	500 to 1,000 mg P.O. initially, followed by 500 mg every 8 to 12 hours; not to exceed 1,500 mg/day	• Give diflunisal with a full glass of water or milk or with food to minimize gastric irritation. • Advise the patient that taking higher-than-prescribed doses can produce dangerous cumulative effects.
	Osteoarthritis	500 to 1,000 mg P.O./day in two divided doses	• Advise the patient that liver and kidney function tests and ophthalmic examinations will be required periodically during therapy. • Inform the patient to immediately report signs of GI bleeding, such as severe abdominal pain, black or tarry stools, or vomiting of blood. • Be aware that responses to the drug may not occur for up to several weeks in some patients. • Advise the patient not to crush, chew, or break tablets.
Para-aminophenol derivative			
acetaminophen	Headache Fever Mild-to-moderate pain Osteoarthritis	325 to 650 mg P.O. or rectally every 3 to 4 hours, p.r.n.	• Teach the patient that overdose or chronic use can cause liver damage. • Monitor baseline liver function tests before beginning administration and periodically during therapy. • Advise the patient that self-medication to reduce fever may mask a serious illness. Explain that, if a fever lasts more than 3 days, the patient should obtain medical advice. • Advise the patient to seek medical advice if pain continues for more than 5 days. • Inform the patient that the drug should be stored in a light-resistant container, because transfer to a clear glass or plastic container may eventually affect the drug's potency.

SELECTED MAJOR DRUGS

Nonnarcotic analgesics, antipyretic agents, and NSAIDs continued

DRUG	MAJOR INDICATIONS	USUAL ADULT DOSAGES	NURSING IMPLICATIONS
Nonsteroidal anti-inflammatory drugs			
ibuprofen	Mild-to-moderate pain	200 to 400 mg P.O. every 4 to 6 hours	• Advise a patient with aspirin hypersensitivity not to take ibuprofen.
	Dysmenorrhea	400 mg P.O. every 4 hours, p.r.n. as soon as pain begins	• Be aware that fluid retention and edema may occur. Closely monitor a patient with cardiac decompensation.
	Osteoarthritis Rheumatoid arthritis	400 to 800 mg P.O. t.i.d. or q.i.d.	• Advise a patient who is not under a physician's care to discontinue the drug and consult a physician if pain lasts for more than 72 hours. • Advise the patient to avoid alcohol, aspirin, and other drugs that may cause GI irritation and bleeding.
indomethacin	Rheumatoid arthritis Osteoarthritis Ankylosing spondylitis Acute gouty arthritis Bursitis and tendinitis	25 to 50 mg P.O. t.i.d. of indomethacin with food, increased to a maximum of 200 mg/day, which may be given as mostly (up to 100 mg) P.O. or rectally h.s.; 75 mg P.O. daily of sustained-release indomethacin	• Document that the patient is not hypersensitive to aspirin. • Administer indomethacin with food or milk or immediately after meals to minimize GI irritation. • Monitor the patient's weight periodically, and assess for edema to detect sodium and water retention caused by indomethacin. • Be aware that the most frequent adverse effect is a frontal headache. • Monitor the results of the patient's baseline kidney and liver function tests, an ophthalmic examination, and blood counts before beginning long-term therapy and periodically during therapy. • Be aware that indomethacin may mask signs of infection.
naproxen	Osteoarthritis Rheumatoid arthritis Ankylosing spondylitis	250 to 375 mg P.O. morning and evening, increased to a maximum of 1,000 mg/day, if needed	• Administer naproxen with food or milk to decrease GI irritation. • Monitor the results of the patient's liver and kidney function tests, hemoglobin counts, and ophthalmic examinations periodically during prolonged therapy.
	Tendinitis Bursitis Dysmenorrhea Mild-to-moderate pain	500 mg P.O. initially, then 250 mg every 6 to 8 hours, p.r.n.	• Advise the patient to avoid alcohol, aspirin, and other drugs that may cause GI irritation and bleeding.
tolmetin	Osteoarthritis Rheumatoid arthritis	400 mg P.O. t.i.d. initially, including a dose upon arising and at bedtime, increased as needed to a maximum of 2,000 mg/day given in four divided doses for rheumatoid arthritis or 1,600 mg/day given in four divided doses for osteoarthritis	• Administer tolmetin with food or milk or after meals to decrease GI irritation. • Carefully evaluate a patient with a history of peptic ulcer: ulcer reactivation and severe gastric bleeding may occur during therapy. • Weigh the patient weekly, and observe the patient for signs of edema. • Monitor the patient's blood pressure regularly to detect any elevation that may be caused by tolmetin. • Advise the patient to report any nosebleed, black or tarry stools, bruises, itching and skin rashes, edema, recurrent headaches, abdominal pain, or diarrhea. • Monitor fluid intake and output; advise the patient to report any edema, bloating, or significant decrease in urine output.

CHAPTER SUMMARY

Chapter 25 covered nonnarcotic analgesic, antipyretic, and nonsteroidal anti-inflammatory drugs. Here are the highlights of the chapter:

• The three subclasses of nonnarcotic analgesics include: salicylates, para-aminophenol derivatives, and nonsteroidal anti-inflammatory drugs (NSAIDs).

• Aspirin, a salicylate and the most widely used analgesic, is available alone or in combination with other ingredients in OTC remedies for pain, colds, and influenza.

• Salicylates act primarily by inhibiting prostaglandin synthesis, thus reducing inflammation. They can also act as antipyretics and analgesics. Salicylates are used to treat headache, neuralgia, myalgia, dysmenorrhea, and arthritis. Their major adverse reactions include tinnitus and hearing loss, gastric distress, and ulcerogenic effects.

• Acetaminophen is currently the only para-aminophenol derivative used in the United States. Its effects are antipyretic and analgesic but not anti-inflammatory. A common ingredient in many OTC analgesics, acetaminophen causes few adverse reactions when taken in usual doses.

• The NSAID category includes many drugs that act by inhibiting prostaglandin synthesis. Physicians use these drugs primarily to provide symptomatic relief of arthritis and related conditions and for conditions that cause mild-to-moderate pain, such as dysmenorrhea. Most NSAIDs are highly protein bound, accounting for many of their drug interactions. They commonly cause adverse reactions in the GI system, such as pain and bleeding. Administering low doses of these drugs decreases GI reactions without decreasing the drugs' effectiveness.

• The only urinary analgesic, phenazopyridine, acts as a local analgesic in the urinary tract. It is used to relieve the pain, burning, and other symptoms associated with urinary tract infections.

BIBLIOGRAPHY

Alexander, D., and Spencer, R. "Over-the-Counter Analgesics, Antipyretics, and Anti-Inflammatories: The Nurse's Role in Selection and Use," *Journal of Community Health Nursing* 3:11, 1986.

Cardos-Davies, T.H. "Non-Steroidal Anti-Inflammatory Drugs, Arthritis, and Gastrointestinal Bleeding in Elderly In-Patients," *Age and Aging* 13:295, 1984.

Gilman, A.G., et al., eds. *Goodman and Gilman's The Pharmacological Basis of Therapeutics,* 7th ed. New York: Macmillan Publishing Co., 1985.

Gorman, T.K., and Marsh, M.E. "Arthritis at an Early Age," *American Journal of Nursing* 84:1472, December 1984.

Goth, A. *Medical Pharmacology: Principles and Concepts,* 11th ed. St. Louis: C.V. Mosby Co., 1984.

Griffin, J.P. "Fever: When to Leave it Alone," *Nursing86* 16:58, February 1986.

Henniz, L.M., and Burrows. S.K. "Keeping up on Arthritis Needs," *RN* 49:32, February 1986.

Lamy, P.P. "Possible Gastrotoxicity of NSAIDs in the Elderly," *Journal of Gerontological Nursing* 12:32, March 1986.

Lamy, P.P. "Possible Renal Effects of Nonsteroidal Anti-Inflammatory Drugs," *Journal of Gerontological Nursing* 11:38, December 1986.

Manoguerra, A.S. "Acetaminophen," *Emergency* 17:14, November 1985.

Newberger, G.B. "The Role of the Nurse with Arthritis Patients on Drug Therapy," *Nursing Clinics of North America* 19:593, December 1984.

Strand, C.V., and Clark, S.R. "Adult Arthritis: Drugs and Remedies," *American Journal of Nursing* 83:266, February 1983.

CHAPTER 26

NARCOTIC AGONIST AND ANTAGONIST AGENTS

OBJECTIVES

After reading and studying this chapter, you should be able to:

1. Discuss how narcotic agonists act to relieve pain.

2. Distinguish between narcotic agonists and narcotic antagonists.

3. Discuss the clinical indications for the various narcotic agents.

4. Describe the common adverse reactions to narcotic drugs.

5. Describe the pain-relieving action of the mixed narcotic agonist-antagonists.

6. Describe the action of naloxone hydrochloride and its use in treating narcotic overdose.

INTRODUCTION

Narcotic agonists (analgesics), which include opium derivatives and synthetic drugs with similar pharmacologic properties, can relieve or decrease pain without causing loss of consciousness. Most narcotic agonists also possess antitussive and antidiarrheal actions. Morphine sulfate is the narcotic agonist against which all others are compared.

Narcotic drugs can alter the patient's perception of pain and emotional response to it. These drugs alter pain perception by: (1) inhibiting the transmission of pain impulses in sensory pathways in the spinal cord, (2) reducing cortical responses to painful stimuli in the brain stem, thalamus, and limbic system, and (3) altering behavioral responses to pain as they are mediated in the frontal lobe. As a result of this threefold action, pain decreases, and the patient may become less tense and more tranquil. The patient may even become euphoric, probably as a result of the narcotic's effects on the limbic system. This euphoria, however, may lead to repeated drug use, even in the absence of pain, possibly resulting in drug dependence. (See Chapter 6, Drug Abuse, De-

pendence, and Addiction, for a discussion of the factors involved in the development of drug dependence.)

With continuous use, the patient may develop tolerance to many of the effects of narcotic drugs. Tolerance can occur even in the absence of psychological or physical dependence and is usually manifested by a decreased duration of analgesia. Thus, the patient requires larger doses to produce the analgesic effects. Another kind of tolerance occurs with continuous narcotic use, as the body adapts to such physiologic effects as respiratory depression and sedation. The smooth muscle effects of narcotic drugs develop more slowly; therefore, constipation may occur and persist.

Narcotic agonists act as analgesics to relieve pain by attaching to opiate receptor sites. Narcotic antagonists block the effects of narcotic agonists, including pain relief and adverse reactions, most notably respiratory depression. Some narcotic analgesics, called mixed narcotic agonist-antagonists, display both agonist and antagonist properties: The agonist component relieves pain, and the antagonist component decreases the risk of toxicity and drug dependence. These mixed narcotic agonist-antagonists are less likely than agonists to result in respiratory depression and drug abuse.

In recent years, researchers have isolated endogenous morphine-like compounds, endorphins and enkephalins, from subcortical brain areas. Beta-endorphin, found in largest amounts in the pituitary gland, is the principal endorphin and one of the most potent. Methionine enkephalin and leucine enkephalin are the principal enkephalins. Occurring primarily in the basal ganglia, brain stem, and spinal cord, enkephalins seem to modify pain impulse transmission in the same way as the narcotic drugs, by attaching to opiate receptor sites. Whether released in the presence of a narcotic agonist or in response to other stimuli, enkephalins may also decrease the patient's perception of pain and emotional response to it.

Neither endorphins nor enkephalins are absorbed orally, and both are degraded rapidly by enzymes. As a result, they are of little clinical value at present. However, endorphins and enkephalins may facilitate placebo-induced analgesia, which occurs in about one third of patients with anginal, arthritic, dental, or postoperative pain who receive placebos. The narcotic antagonist naloxone blocks both attachment of narcotic analgesics to opiate receptor sites and placebo-induced analgesia—leading researchers to conclude that endorphins and enkephalins act via receptor combination.

This chapter includes discussions of the narcotic agonist, the mixed narcotic agonist-antagonist, and the narcotic antagonist agents.

For a summary of representative drugs, see *Selected major drugs: Narcotic agonist and antagonist agents* on pages 429 and 430.

NARCOTIC AGONISTS

The term *narcotic* refers to any analgesic derived from active opium poppy alkaloids as well as to compounds chemically similar to the alkaloids. Because the Harrison Narcotic Act of 1914 established a legal definition of narcotics based on their habit-forming nature, however, the term *narcotic* is often inaccurately used to refer to any drug that is capable of producing dependence or restricted by the Controlled Substance Act.

Morphine serves as the standard against which the effectiveness and adverse reactions of other narcotic drugs as well as nonnarcotic analgesics are measured.

History and source
The first authoritative reference to opium is found in the third century B.C. writings of Theophrastus. By the middle of the 16th century, European physicians were thoroughly familiar with the uses of opium.

The word opium is derived from the Greek word for juice. Opium is the exudate from *Papaver somniferum*, a species of poppy. Powdered opium (dried exudate) contains three active alkaloid derivatives—morphine, codeine, and papaverine hydrochloride. Morphine and codeine provide analgesic action; papaverine, a smooth muscle relaxant, is used to treat peripheral vascular disease. (See Chapter 39, Peripheral Vascular Agents, for more information on this use of papaverine.) The principal alkaloid, morphine, which constitutes al-

most 10% of opium, was isolated by the German pharmacist Sertürner in the early 19th century. Researchers isolated codeine in 1832 and papaverine in 1848.

Adverse reactions to the opium derivatives, and their high potential for causing dependence and abuse, eventually led to the development of synthetic narcotic agonists. In 1939, Eisleb and Schaumann introduced meperidine hydrochloride, originally thought to be an atropine-like agent but soon recognized as a strong analgesic. Methadone was introduced for use shortly after World War II but did not gain widespread use in narcotic maintenance programs for a number of years.

PHARMACOKINETICS
Narcotic agonists are well absorbed from the gastrointestinal (GI) tract and the rectal mucosa and are distributed to most body tissues. Parenteral administration produces the most rapid onset of action. The duration of action varies, depending on the drug and the route of administration used.

Absorption, distribution, metabolism, excretion
The narcotic agonists are administered by the oral, intravenous (I.V.), subcutaneous (S.C.), intramuscular (I.M.), epidural, intrathecal, sublingual, and rectal routes. Opium derivatives are well absorbed from the nasal mucosa and lung surface; oral doses are readily absorbed from the GI tract. I.V. administration produces the most rapid (almost immediate) and reliable analgesic effects. Absorption from S.C. and I.M. injections depends on the lipid solubility of the narcotic drug administered and the amount of the patient's fatty tissue. The S.C. and I.M. routes may result in delayed absorption and peak concentration levels of the drug, especially in patients with impaired tissue perfusion.

Until recently, parenteral routes were preferred for morphine administration, because the first-pass effect causes rapid metabolism and inactivation of oral doses. However, a concentrated oral solution and a sustained-release tablet have recently become available for use in cancer patients and others with severe chronic pain. Although these new dosage forms do not avoid the first-pass effect, they enable the patient to receive morphine in smaller solution volumes or in sustained-release tablets, thereby avoiding the need for previous injections or I.V. lines. The oral form allows the patient and the patient's family more mobility.

Narcotic agonists are widely distributed throughout body tissues, displaying relatively low plasma protein-binding capacity (30% to 35%). The drugs are extensively metabolized in the liver, and the metabolites are excreted by the kidneys. A minor amount, 7% to 10% of the dose, is excreted in feces via the biliary tract.

Pharmacokinetics of selected narcotic agonists

All narcotic agonists have a rapid onset of action when administered I.V. and reach peak concentration levels in 20 to 40 minutes; duration of action varies primarily according to the drug administered. This chart outlines the pharmacokinetics of narcotic agonists administered I.M.

DRUG	ONSET OF ACTION (MINUTES)	PEAK CONCENTRATION LEVEL (MINUTES)	DURATION OF ACTION (HOURS)
codeine	15 to 30	60 to 90	4 to 6
morphine	5 to 20	30 to 90	4 to 6
hydromorphone hydrochloride	15 to 30	30 to 90	3 to 5
levorphanol tartrate	15 to 45	60 to 90	4 to 8
meperidine	15 to 30	30 to 60	2 to 4
methadone hydrochloride	10 to 15	60 to 120	4 to 6; 12 to 15 with chronic therapy
oxymorphone hydrochloride	5 to 10	30 to 60	3 to 6

Meperidine is metabolized to normeperidine, a toxic metabolite with a longer half-life than meperidine. With chronic administration or high doses of meperidine (especially by the oral route), normeperidine may accumulate and cause seizures. Normeperidine accumulation also occurs commonly in patients with renal failure or sickle-cell disease. Normeperidine is also excreted by the kidneys.

Onset, peak, duration
After parenteral administration of a narcotic agonist, onset of action usually occurs within 30 minutes. Duration of action varies, depending on the drug administered. Peak drug concentration levels occur within 20 to 40 minutes after I.V. administration and 60 to 120 minutes after S.C. or I.M. injection, depending on the drug administered. Narcotic agonist half-life varies, depending on the drug administered and the route of administration. (See *Pharmacokinetics of selected narcotic agonists* for a comparison of the drugs in this class.)

PHARMACODYNAMICS

Narcotic agonists act primarily at opiate receptor sites, binding to the receptors centrally and peripherally and activating the endogenous pain relief system. This receptor-site binding produces the therapeutic effects of analgesia and cough suppression along with narcotic adverse reactions, including respiratory depression and constipation.

Mechanism of action
The opiate receptors that narcotic agonists occupy in the central and peripheral nervous systems are most numerous in the hypothalamus, the limbic system, the midbrain, the thalamus, and the substantia gelatinosa of the spinal cord. In sensory neurons, pure narcotic analgesics alter the release of neurotransmitters, including acetylcholine, dopamine, norepinephrine, and substance P.

The existence of five types of opiate receptors (mu, kappa, sigma, delta, and epsilon) has been postulated but not proved; pure narcotic agonists appear to act primarily at the mu receptors. Researchers have observed that when a narcotic occupies the presumed mu, kappa, and sigma receptors, identifiable clinical effects occur. This is not the case with the delta and epsilon receptors (which may be related to either enkephalins or beta-endorphin): their narcotic-related clinical effects have not yet been determined. (See *Opiate receptors and their effects* on page 418 for a discussion of the physiologic effects of these receptors.)

The mechanism of action and therapeutic uses of the synthetic narcotic agonists are similar to those of the opium derivatives. A notable exception is the antitussive effect of the opium derivatives, which is lacking in some of the synthetic narcotic agonists.

Opiate receptors and their effects

Narcotic agonists stimulate five types of opiate receptors: mu, kappa, sigma, delta, and epsilon. The following chart lists three receptors and the physiologic effects that can occur when a narcotic agonist binds to each. Clinical effects for delta and epsilon are unknown.

TYPE OF OPIATE RECEPTOR	CLINICAL EFFECT
mu	• Euphoria • Physical dependence • Respiratory depression • Supraspinal analgesia
kappa	• Miosis • Sedation • Spinal analgesia • Respiratory depression
sigma	• Dysphoria • Hallucinations • Respiratory stimulation • Vasomotor stimulation

Narcotic agonists, especially morphine, affect the smooth muscle of the GI and genitourinary tracts, causing contraction of the bladder and ureters and decreased intestinal peristalsis. The narcotic agonists also cause blood vessel dilation, especially in the face, head and neck. Narcotic agonists also depress the cough center in the brain, thereby producing antitussive effects and causing constriction of the bronchial musculature. Any of these effects can become adverse reactions.(See *Narcotic sites of action* for an illustration of narcotic agonists' various sites and effects.)

PHARMACOTHERAPEUTICS

Narcotic agonists are used to relieve severe pain in both acute, chronic, and terminal illnesses and to reduce preanesthesia patient anxiety. They also have antidiarrheal and antitussive effects. Morphine reduces the dyspnea of pulmonary edema and left ventricular failure by reducing anxiety and by producing peripheral vasodilation, which decreases cardiac work load. Physicians sometimes use opium derivatives in obstetric analgesia, but only with extreme caution, because these drugs cross the placenta and can compromise respirations in the newborn.

An equianalgesic dose of a narcotic drug is a dose that produces the same level of analgesia as an agent and dose selected as a standard, usually 10 mg of morphine I.M. Occasionally, a patient must be changed from one narcotic drug to another (for example, when the postoperative patient is allowed to take drugs orally.) When this is necessary, referring to the equianalgesic dose decreases the risk of toxicity and inadequate pain relief. (See *Narcotic agonists: Equianalgesic doses* on page 420 for the various narcotic agonist doses equianalgesic to 10 mg of morphine I.M.)

codeine. A Schedule II drug, codeine is used for relief of mild to moderate pain and as an antitussive. Codeine, which possesses good oral potency, is often combined with 650 mg of aspirin or acetaminophen for an additive analgesic effect. Such a combination places the medication in Schedule III because the potential for abuse is further diminished. However, the combination increases the potential for adverse reactions and drug interactions, because both aspirin and acetaminophen are potent medications. Codeine is not used frequently for chronic severe pain, because it exhibits an analgesic ceiling effect—as the oral or parenteral codeine dose is increased, the level of analgesia increases only slightly after a dose of 60 to 120 mg (P.O.) is reached, but adverse reactions (most notably GI upset and constipation) become more pronounced. As a result, the patient cannot tolerate the codeine. For cough suppression in adult patients, the low potential for abuse, good oral potency, and relatively low dose required to suppress the cough make codeine a preferred agent.
USUAL ADULT DOSAGE: for analgesia, 30 to 60 mg P.O. every 3 to 4 hours, or 15 to 60 mg S.C. or I.M. every 3 to 4 hours (a 30-mg oral dose of codeine is equianalgesic to about a 15-mg dose of codeine by S.C. or I.M. injection); for cough suppression, 10 to 15 mg P.O., usually in liquid form.

fentanyl citrate (Sublimaze). A Schedule II drug, fentanyl is a potent synthetic narcotic agonist available for parenteral use. Fentanyl is administered I.V. before, during, and immediately after surgery. The drug is also used as an anesthetic agent with oxygen in selected high-risk surgical patients and for obstetric analgesic—a use not approved by the Food and Drug Administration (FDA). Fentanyl can be given by continuous infusion and via the epidural route.
USUAL ADULT DOSAGE: except for anesthesia maintenance during surgery, 0.05 to 0.1 mg I.M. or I.V.; for anesthesia maintenance during surgery, 0.025 to 0.05 mg I.V., 100 mcg (0.1 mg) is equianalgesic to 10 mg of morphine I.M. or 75 mg of meperidine I.M.

hydrocodone bitartrate and acetaminophen (Vicodin). This combination product is used to relieve mild to moderate pain. Each tablet contains 5 mg hydrocodone and 500 mg acetaminophen.

USUAL ADULT DOSAGE: starting dose, one to two tablets every 4 to 6 hours for pain relief.

hydrocodone and phenyltoloxamine (Tussionex). A long-acting antitussive combination, hydrocodone and phenyltoloxamine is available in capsule, liquid, and tablet form. The usual dose contains 5 mg of hydrocodone and 10 mg of phenyltoloxamine. Children over age 5 can be given the drug at 12-hour intervals; however, the antitussive agent of choice for children is dextromethorphan. Because hydrocodone and phenyltoloxamine has a high potential for abuse, it should be prescribed only when dextromethorphan or codeine is undesirable or ineffective.

USUAL ADULT DOSAGE: one capsule or tablet or 1 teaspoonful (5 ml) every 8 to 12 hours.

Narcotic sites of action

As this anatomic illustration shows, narcotics act at many different sites, producing effects that generally are therapeutic but that occasionally may be adverse.

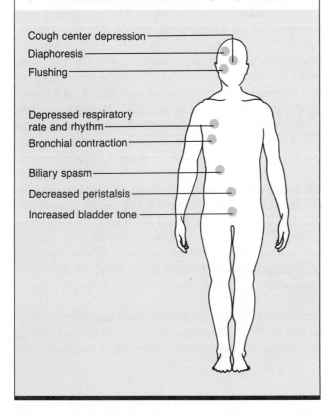

Cough center depression
Diaphoresis
Flushing

Depressed respiratory rate and rhythm
Bronchial contraction

Biliary spasm
Decreased peristalsis
Increased bladder tone

hydromorphone hydrochloride (Dilaudid). A Schedule II drug, hydromorphone is a potent synthetic narcotic agonist that is a related to morphine. Used to relieve moderate to severe pain, hydromorphone can be administered orally, rectally, or parenterally. Continuous I.V. infusions of hydromorphone are used to relieve severe pain.

Unlike codeine, hydromorphone does not exhibit a ceiling effect: as the dose of hydromorphone increases, so does the level of analgesia. Hydromorphone is therefore very useful in treating chronic severe pain. Hydromorphone is highly soluble in water, and a highly concentrated solution for parenteral use is available for patients requiring high doses. Hydromorphone powder can also be used to make highly concentrated parenteral solutions, if needed.

USUAL ADULT DOSAGE: for parenteral use, a starting dose of 1 to 2 mg S.C., I.V., or I.M. every 4 to 6 hours to control pain; for oral administration, a starting dose of 2 mg every 4 to 6 hours, which may be increased to 12 to 15 mg every 4 hours in patients with severe pain; for rectal administration, one 3-mg suppository every 6 to 8 hours.

levorphanol tartrate (Levo-Dromoran). A Schedule II drug, levorphanol is a synthetic narcotic agonist possessing good oral potency. It is indicated for relief of moderate or severe pain; relief of pain from myocardial infarction (MI), severe trauma, or renal or biliary colic; relief of postoperative pain; and relief of intractable pain from cancer or other causes. Levorphanol is available in oral tablets and in parenteral solution.

USUAL ADULT DOSAGE: 2 to 3 mg P.O. or S.C. every 3 to 4 hours.

meperidine hydrochloride (Demerol). A Schedule II drug, meperidine is a synthetic narcotic agonist most commonly prescribed for postoperative pain. Meperidine can be administered orally, I.M., S.C., or I.V. Meperidine is available as a tablet, parenteral liquid, or oral syrup. Parenteral meperidine is especially effective for the relief of moderate to severe visceral pain, for obstetric analgesia, and as a preoperative medication.

USUAL ADULT DOSAGE: for moderate to severe pain, 50 to 150 mg parenterally or P.O. every 3 to 4 hours; for preoperative or obstetric analgesia, 50 to 100 mg I.M. or S.C.; for obstetric analgesia, sometimes combined with scopolamine and repeated at 1- to 3-hour intervals.

methadone hydrochloride (Dolophine). A Schedule II drug, methadone is a synthetic narcotic agonist indicated for the relief of severe pain, for detoxification treatment of narcotic addiction, and for the management of nar-

Narcotic agonists: Equianalgesic doses

The so-called standard narcotic agonist dose, 10 mg of morphine sulfate I.M., is used to calculate equally effective (equianalgesic) doses of the various narcotic agonists. This method is particularly useful when a patient must be switched from one narcotic agonist to another with no change in dose effectiveness. In this chart, which lists equianalgesic doses of selected narcotic agonists, all doses are I.M. except for codeine, which is administered orally.

NARCOTIC AGONIST	EQUIANALGESIC DOSE
codeine	120 mg
morphine	10 mg
hydromorphone	1.5 mg
levorphanol	2 mg
meperidine	75 to 100 mg
methadone	8 to 10 mg
fentanyl	0.1 to 0.2 mg
oxymorphone	1.0 to 1.5 mg

cotic dependence—although the drug produces tolerance and physical and psychological dependence. Methadone is used for analgesia in terminal illness on a scheduled basis (every 6 to 12 hours around the clock). Methadone has good oral potency; 20 mg P.O. are equianalgesic to 10 mg of morphine sulfate I.M. The drug can accumulate in patients with impaired hepatic or renal function and in elderly patients, sometimes causing respiratory depression. Methadone should be administered I.V. only with extreme caution.

Methadone is dispensed daily only by hospitals, pharmacies, FDA-approved community agencies, and designated state authorities with maintenance or detoxification programs. Detoxification programs administer smaller and smaller doses until the physiological dependence is reduced and the drug can be stopped. Maintenance programs provide enough methadone to replace the amount of illegal narcotic taken. Some physicians feel that methadone maintenance therapy administered once daily allows psychosocial rehabilitation of the participant. Symptoms of anxiety or stress do not necessarily reflect withdrawal and should not form the basis for dosage increase.

USUAL ADULT DOSAGE: for pain relief, 2.5 to 10 mg I.M. or S.C. every 3 to 4 hours, as needed, or 5 to 15 mg P.O.; for detoxification, 15 to 50 mg P.O. daily in liquid form, with additional doses if withdrawal symptoms do not subside or if symptoms recur. Maintenance doses vary depending on the amount of narcotic taken to maintain the habit.

morphine sulfate (Duramorph, Rouxanol). A Schedule II drug, naturally occurring morphine is considered the best narcotic agonist for relief of severe pain. Among its many indications, morphine is used to relieve postoperative pain, pain from MI, and terminal cancer pain. Morphine sulfate is available in oral tablets, solutions, rectal suppositories, sustained-release tablets, and parenteral forms. It can be administered by a multitude of routes—oral, rectal, sublingual, S.C., I.M., I.V., epidural, and intrathecal—and by implantable pumps. Because morphine does not exhibit a ceiling effect, as the dose is increased, the level of analgesia also increases. Morphine is frequently used as a continuous infusion in patients with severe pain.
USUAL ADULT DOSAGE: initially, 10 mg per 70 kg of body weight when given parenterally (a 60-mg oral dose of morphine is equianalgesic to a 10-mg parenteral dose). Reportedly, some patients can tolerate doses of 8 grams or more per day.

morphine sulfate sustained-release tablets (MS Contin, Roxanol SR). Each tablet of this Schedule II drug contains 30 mg of morphine sulfate in a wax matrix, which allows the morphine to be released slowly and continuously as the matrix melts in the GI tract. This helps the patient remain pain-free for a longer time (6 to 12 hours) than with rapid-release tablets, which provide pain relief for 3 to 4 hours. Morphine sulfate sustained-release tablets are indicated for prolonged relief of chronic, severe pain. They should not be administered as needed, because the release of medication is slowed and the products are not indicated for mild or intermittent pain.
USUAL ADULT DOSAGE: variable (titrated to the patient's individual needs); a starting dose of one tablet (30 mg) every 12 hours may be used when the narcotic need is not known. Some patients may need to take the drug at 8-hour intervals. Dosage more frequent than four times a day (at equal intervals) is not recommended.

morphine sulfate intensified oral solution (Roxanol). A Schedule II drug dispensed in bottles of 30 and 120 ml containing 20 mg/ml, morphine sulfate intensified solution is indicated for the relief of severe acute pain and for relief of chronic pain in patients unable to swallow tablets. These solutions are also indicated for patients with high narcotic requirements who are unable to tolerate the large volume of solution required with regular morphine sulfate solution (5 mg/5 ml). Intensified oral solutions and sustained-release tablets are often used for terminally ill patients who require medication on a regularly scheduled basis to achieve effective relief. Once

pain is relieved, the patient may sleep for a number of hours after each dose. The nurse should be careful not to interpret this reaction as indicating a need for a dosage decrease. Such patients may be experiencing rebound sleep because the previously uncontrolled pain had deprived them of sleep. The dose should be maintained for at least 2 days before reduction, as long as the patient's respiratory and cardiovascular status remains adequate.

DRUG INTERACTIONS

Narcotic agonists

Drug interactions involving the narcotic agonists commonly lead to increased (and possibly lethal) respiratory and central nervous system (CNS) depression.

DRUG	INTERACTING DRUGS	POSSIBLE EFFECTS	NURSING IMPLICATIONS
codeine, morphine, hydromorphone, levorphanol, meperidine, methadone, fentanyl, oxymorphone	alcohol	Increases CNS depression, especially respiratory depression	• Advise the patient to avoid concomitant alcohol ingestion. Teach the patient outside the hospital to read labels on all over-the-counter cough syrups and cold remedies for possible alcohol content. • If alcohol ingestion occurs, monitor the patient's respirations every 30 minutes for 2 hours and report any change to the physician.
	monoamine oxidase (MAO) inhibitors	Increase effects of the drug; cause rigidity, hypotension, excitation	• Avoid administering a narcotic agonist to a patient within 10 days after administration of an MAO inhibitor.
	barbiturates	Cause additive CNS effects; increase sedation	• To avoid extreme patient drowsiness or deep sleep, administer doses at least 2 hours apart, as ordered. • Respiratory depression may occur, so monitor the patient every 20 to 30 minutes for 2 hours after concomitant administration.
	phenothiazines	Cause sedation; may enhance respiratory depression, hypotension, or orthostatic hypotension; cause enhanced anticholinergic effects	• Because the patient may become drowsy or go into a deep sleep, still experiencing pain but too tired to complain about it, administer doses at least 2 hours apart, as ordered. • Respiratory depression may occur, so monitor the patient every 20 to 30 minutes for 2 hours after concomitant administration. • Monitor the patient's blood pressure and have the patient change position slowly.
	skeletal muscle relaxants used during surgery	Increase neuromuscular blocking action	• Monitor the patient for apnea. • Have emergency resuscitation equipment available, because respiratory paralysis may occur. • Monitor the patient's arterial blood gas levels.
	cimetidine	May inhibit narcotic metabolism, leading to increased respiratory and CNS depression	• Monitor the patient for any increase in sedation. • Monitor the patient's respiratory rate every 20 to 30 minutes for 2 hours after concomitant administration.

⌐DULT DOSAGE: initially, 10 to 30 mg every 4
⌐lowever, dosage is variable, depending on pa-
⌐sponse, and should be titrated to pain relief.

oxycodone hydrochloride (Roxicodone). A Schedule II
drug, oxycodone is a semisynthetic oral narcotic analgesic structurally similar to codeine. Oxycodone is available in 5-mg tablets and in a 5 mg/5 ml suspension and
is most frequently prescribed in combination with aspirin
or acetaminophen.
USUAL ADULT DOSAGE: for pain relief, a starting dose
of 5 mg P.O. every 3 to 6 hours.

✓**oxycodone hydrochloride and acetaminophen** (Percocet, Tylox). Each Schedule II Percocet tablet contains 5
mg of oxycodone and 325 mg of acetaminophen; each
Tylox tablet contains 5 mg of oxycodone and 500 mg
of acetaminophen. These combination products are indicated for the relief of moderate to moderately severe
pain. Nurses should be aware of Percocet's antipyretic
effect when assessing the vital signs of a patient taking
this drug.
USUAL ADULT DOSAGE: one to two tablets every 6 hours
for pain relief; increases in dosage for patients with severe
pain are limited by the amount of acetaminophen contained in the tablets. The maximum recommended daily
dose of acetaminophen is 4 to 6 grams.

✓**oxycodone hydrochloride and aspirin** (Percodan). Each
Schedule II Percodan tablet contains 4.8 mg of oxycodone and 325 mg of aspirin. Percodan is indicated
for moderate to moderately severe pain. Because it contains aspirin, this combination product produces numerous drug interactions and may cause bleeding.
Percodan is also an antipyretic.
USUAL ADULT DOSAGE: one to two tablets P.O. every
6 hours for pain relief.

oxymorphone hydrochloride (Numorphan). A Schedule II drug, oxymorphone is a potent synthetic narcotic
analgesic effective for moderate to severe pain. Clinical
indications for oxymorphone include preoperative and
obstetric analgesia, as well as the treatment of patients
with pain from pulmonary edema or left ventricular failure. One milligram of oxymorphone administered parenterally is equianalgesic to 10 mg I.M. of morphine
sulfate.
USUAL ADULT DOSAGE: for obstetric analgesia, 0.5 to
1 mg I.M.; for other indications, 1 to 1.5 mg S.C. or
I.M. every 4 to 6 hours; when administered I.V., the
initial dose is 0.5 mg.

propoxyphene hydrochloride (Darvon). A Schedule IV
drug, propoxyphene is a weak synthetic narcotic agonist
used for relief of mild pain. The drug is frequently used
in combination with aspirin (Darvon Compound). Propoxyphene is available as 32- or 65-mg capsules. Darvon Compound contains 389 mg of aspirin in addition
to propoxyphene.
USUAL ADULT DOSAGE: one 65-mg capsule every 4
hours, as needed

propoxyphene napsylate (Darvon-N). A Schedule IV
drug, propoxyphene napsylate is a more stable salt of
propoxyphene than propoxyphene hydrochloride and
is available in liquid and tablet form. A 100-mg dose of
the napsylate salt is equianalgesic to 65 mg of the hydrochloride, the difference being molecular weight. Darvon-N contains 100 mg of propoxyphene napsylate.
Doses of 50 and 100 mg are combined with 325 and
650 mg of acetaminophen, respectively, in Darvocet-N
50 and Darvocet-N 100. Darvon-N with A.S.A. contains
100 mg of propoxyphene napsylate and 325 mg of
aspirin.
USUAL ADULT DOSAGE: one capsule every 4 hours, as
needed.

Drug interactions
The use of narcotic agonists with any other drugs known
to decrease respiration, including alcohol, sedatives,
hypnotics, and anesthetics, increases the patient's risk
of severe respiratory depression. Concomitant therapy
with tricyclic antidepressants, phenothiazines, or anticholinergics may cause severe constipation and urinary
retention. (See *Drug interactions: Narcotic agonists* on
page 421 for a detailed list of possible interactions and
nursing implications.)

ADVERSE DRUG REACTIONS
Narcotic agonists produce numerous adverse reactions
that affect most body systems. Central nervous system
(CNS) reactions, the most common, usually affect the
respiratory and GI tracts.

Predictable reactions
One of the most predictable adverse reactions to the
opium derivatives is decreased rate and depth of respiration that worsens as the dosage is increased. This
may cause periodic, irregular breathing or precipitate
asthmatic attacks in susceptible patients. Narcotic agonists' effect of suppressing cough is usually considered
therapeutic; however, as these adverse reactions indicate, it may sometimes be undesirable.

Dilation of peripheral arteries and veins from narcotic agonists leads to flushing and orthostatic hypoten-

sion; the extremities may feel warm and heavy. (Little change in blood pressure or pulse rate occurs when the patient is recumbent.) Increased respirations may be from a medullary effect of the drug.

Adverse reactions in the GI tract include nausea, vomiting, biliary colic, and constipation. Nausea and vomiting are more likely to occur in ambulatory patients; however, this reaction differs with specific narcotic agonists, even in the same patient. Biliary colic is most likely to occur with morphine; meperidine is least likely to produce or exacerbate this condition. Narcotic agonists may cause constipation through sedation that reduces response to the defecation impulse, through significant reduction in peristalsis and through increased water absorption from intestinal contents.

Some patients receiving these drugs, especially males with prostatic hypertrophy, experience urinary retention. Narcotic agonists may also prolong obstetric labor and produce respiratory depression in the neonate.

Pupil constriction (miosis) also occurs with narcotic agonists and persists throughout long-term therapy.

Narcotic agonists are contraindicated in patients with head injury or increased intracranial pressure, because the drugs may mask changes in level of consciousness. These changes, which may be subtle, are early signs that the patient is developing CNS problems.

The incidence and severity of adverse reactions associated with narcotic agonists may increase as the dose increases. For example, euphoria and mood elevation may become heightened, and depressed respirations may become slower and more shallow. When toxic levels are reached, blood pressure and pulse decline, and bronchoconstriction may develop. The patient may also experience seizures. Death from narcotic overdose usually results from respiratory failure.

Physicians and nurses must always be alert for the development of patient tolerance to the effects of narcotic drugs. (See "Introduction" on page 415.) When a patient who has become tolerant to a narcotic drug suddenly stops receiving it, withdrawal symptoms may occur, including increased sensory perceptions (especially those of pain and touch), tactile hallucinations, increased GI secretions, nasopharyngeal secretions, diarrhea, dilated pupils, and photophobia.

Responses to a narcotic agonist vary from patient to patient and even in the same patient over the course of the therapy. Although the presence of pain increases the patient's tolerance to the narcotic agonist, the severity of adverse reactions does not usually increase. Patients with hypothyroidism, multiple sclerosis, or myasthenia gravis are particularly sensitive to opiates. Renal or hepatic dysfunction interferes with the elimi-

nation of these drugs, prolongs their duration of action, and may increase the risk of accumulation—especially with meperidine and methadone. Infants and patients with compromised respiratory function (for example, cor pulmonale or obstructive lung disease) can be particularly sensitive to the respiratory effects of opiates.

Meperidine frequently produces tremors, palpitations, tachycardia, and delirium.

Unpredictable reactions

Severe hypersensitivity reactions to narcotic agonists are rare and usually occur as urticaria or a skin rash; even I.V. administration rarely causes anaphylaxis. Some patients may experience itching or wheal formation at the injection site, but this is usually a local, histamine-mediated response not indicating hypersensitivity. When patients with decreased renal function are given meperidine, accumulation of normeperidine may cause CNS stimulation and possibly seizures.

NURSING IMPLICATIONS

The therapeutic effects of the narcotic agonists can easily become adverse reactions. It is necessary for the nurse to monitor dosage effects and the patient's vital signs.

• Because narcotic agonists can cause respiratory depression and may increase cerebrospinal fluid (CSF) pressure, administer these drugs with extreme caution to patients with head injuries, brain tumors, increased intracranial pressure, or intracranial lesions.

• Withhold a repeat dose and consult the physician if the patient's respiratory rate is 8 to 10 breaths/minute or less. Note and document the rate and depth of respirations.

• Advise the patient not to ambulate without assistance immediately after a dose or until the patient's response to the narcotic is determined. Vomiting, orthostatic hypotension, and dizziness are more likely to occur in ambulatory than in recumbent patients.

• Physicians and nurses are particularly at risk for developing narcotic dependence. Learn to recognize signs and symptoms of dependence and the proper way to report cases of possible dependence. Some state nurses' associations have committees and other agencies to assist the nurse who has a problem with substance abuse, including abuse of narcotics and alcohol. (For additional information see Chapter 6, Drug Abuse, Dependence, and Addiction.)

• Elderly patients may become restless after narcotic agonist administration, so be sure the bed rails are up and the bed is in the low position.

• Before administering the initial dose of a narcotic agonist, obtain the patient's baseline blood pressure, pulse, and respiration data.

• Measure and record the patient's fluid intake and output to assess for urinary retention.

• Assess the patient for decreased peristalsis, abdominal distention, and constipation. If constipation develops, consult the physician for an order for a laxative or stool softener.

• Assess the patient's pain before each dose; determine and record the pain's onset, duration, location, intensity, and quality.

• Be aware that narcotic agonists are most effective when administered before pain becomes severe.

• Consider the routine scheduling of narcotic doses for patients with terminal illness.

• Pain control can sometimes be improved by adding a nonnarcotic analgesic agent, such as aspirin, acetaminophen, or a nonsteroidal anti-inflammatory drug to the narcotic regimen or by alternating doses of the narcotic and nonnarcotic drugs. As appropriate, discuss this option with the patient's physician.

• Note and record the patient's response to each dose, including the degree of pain relief and occurrence of any adverse reactions. If the therapeutic response is inadequate or adverse reactions occur, consult the physician.

• Be familiar with federal, state, and institutional regulations concerning narcotic drugs. For example, they are usually kept in a double-locked, secure place in hospitals and certain other health agencies. Doses of such drugs are usually written on a special narcotics sheet, and narcotic supplies are counted at every shift change. Some facilities may require one or more nurses' signatures on the narcotic sheet for each dose administered.

• Instruct the patient taking morphine sulfate sustained-release tablets not to crush or break them, because this will negate the sustained-release effect.

MIXED NARCOTIC AGONIST-ANTAGONISTS

The mixed narcotic agonist-antagonists—pentazocine, butorphanol tartrate, nalbuphine hydrochloride, and buprenorphine hydrochloride—originally appeared to have less abuse potential than the pure narcotic agonists. However, both butorphanol and pentazocine have reportedly caused dependence.

History and source

The discovery and use of mixed narcotic agonist-antagonists arose out of the search for "ideal" analgesics, those with little or no potential for abuse. Research on the narcotic antagonist nalorphine suggested that such analgesics might possess both agonist and antagonist properties. Pentazocine was the first mixed narcotic agonist-antagonist introduced, followed almost 15 years later by butorphanol and nalbuphine. In 1985, buprenorphine was marketed in the United States after several years of availability in Europe.

PHARMACOKINETICS

The pharmacokinetics of the mixed narcotic agonist-antagonists closely resemble those of morphine, with some differences in onset of action and duration of action.

Absorption, distribution, metabolism, excretion

The mixed narcotic agonist-antagonists can be administered orally or by the S.C., I.M., or I.V. route, but pentazocine is the only drug in this category available in oral form. Absorption occurs rapidly from parenteral sites. These drugs are distributed to most body tissues and also cross the placenta. They are metabolized in the liver and excreted primarily by the kidneys, although over 10% of a butorphanol dose and a small amount of a pentazocine dose are excreted in the feces.

Onset, peak, duration

Slight variations exist among the onset of action, peak concentration level, and duration of action of parenterally administered mixed narcotic agonist-antagonists. The onset of action of butorphanol occurs within 10 to 30 minutes, peak concentration levels occur within 30 to 60 minutes, and the drug's duration of action is 3 to 4 hours. The onset of action of buprenorphine is 15 minutes, the drug's peak concentration level is reached in 60 minutes, and its duration of action is 5 to 6 hours. Nalbuphine has an onset of action of less than 15 minutes, reaches peak concentration levels in 20 to 45 minutes, and has a duration of action of 3 to 6 hours. Orally administered pentazocine has an onset of action of 15 to 30 minutes, reaches peak concentration levels in less than an hour, and has a duration of action of 3 to 4 hours. The plasma half-life of butorphanol after I.V. administration is 3 to 4 hours. The plasma half-life of buprenorphine is approximately 2 hours after I.V. injection. The half-life of nalbuphine is 5 hours. The half-life of pentazocine is 2 to 3 hours.

PHARMACODYNAMICS

Although the mixed narcotic agonist-antagonists occupy the same opiate receptor sites as the narcotic agonists, they have few or no antitussive or GI effects.

Mechanism of action

The exact mechanism of action of the mixed narcotic agonist-antagonists has not been established. The site of action of butorphanol may be opiate receptors in the limbic system. Like pentazocine, butorphanol also acts on pulmonary circulation, increasing pulmonary artery and pulmonary capillary wedge pressures and pulmonary vascular resistance. Both drugs also increase systemic arterial pressure and the overall cardiac work load. Buprenorphine seems to dissociate slowly from binding sites and, therefore, has a longer duration of action than the other drugs in this class.

PHARMACOTHERAPEUTICS

Physicians prescribe the mixed narcotic agonist-antagonists primarily for the relief of moderate to severe pain, for obstetric analgesia in selected cases, and for preoperative medication to reduce anxiety and the perception of pain. (See *Mixed narcotic agonist-antagonists: Equianalgesic doses* for equianalgesic doses comparable to 10 mg of morphine sulfate I.M.)

Some physicians prefer to use mixed narcotic agonist-antagonists because the risk of drug dependence is lower with them than with the narcotic agonists. Mixed narcotic agonist-antagonists are also less likely to cause respiratory depression.

butorphanol tartrate (Stadol). A potent analgesic, butorphanol is indicated for moderate to severe pain, for obstetric analgesia during labor, and for preoperative medication.
USUAL ADULT DOSAGE: 2 mg I.M. every 3 to 4 hours, with a dosage range of 1 to 4 mg (higher doses are not recommended); or 1 mg I.V. every 3 to 4 hours, with a dosage range of 0.5 to 2 mg.

buprenorphine hydrochloride (Buprenex). A Schedule IV drug and a semisynthetic opioid, buprenorphine has an analgesic effect approximately 30 times as potent as that of morphine sulfate. Buprenorphine is used for relief of moderate to severe pain.
USUAL ADULT DOSAGE: for adults and children over age 13, 1 ml (0.3 mg) I.M. or by slow I.V. injection at up to 6-hour intervals, as needed. Doses up to 2 ml (0.6 mg) may be given depending on patient response and pain severity. Higher doses are not recommended.

Mixed narcotic agonist-antagonists: Equianalgesic doses

This chart lists the equianalgesic I.M. doses (based on the standard dose of 10 mg of morphine sulfate I.M.) for the mixed narcotic agonist-antagonist drugs.

MIXED NARCOTIC AGONIST-ANTAGONISTS	EQUIANALGESIC DOSE
butorphanol (Stadol)	2 mg
buprenorphine (Buprenex)	0.3 mg
nalbuphine (Nubain)	10 mg
pentazocine (Talwin)	30 mg

nalbuphine hydrochloride (Nubain). Equianalgesic to morphine sulfate on a milligram-to-milligram basis, nalbuphine is indicated for relief of moderate to severe pain and for preoperative and obstetric analgesia. No oral form of the drug is available.
USUAL ADULT DOSAGE: 10 mg per 70 kg of body weight I.V., I.M., or S.C. every 3 to 6 hours, as necessary, not to exceed 160 mg/day.

pentazocine hydrochloride and **pentazocine lactate** (Talwin). A Schedule IV drug, pentazocine is used for the relief of moderate pain, as a preoperative medication, and as a supplement to surgical anesthesia. The S.C. route should be used only when necessary, because severe tissue damage can result. Pentazocine may cause psychotomimetic effects, such as dysphoria, especially with chronic administration; this limits its usefulness in patients with chronic or severe pain.
USUAL ADULT DOSAGE: for pain relief, 30 mg of pentazocine lactate I.M., I.V., or S.C., repeated every 3 to 4 hours; doses should not exceed 30 mg I.V. or 60 mg I.M. or S.C.; or 50 to 100 mg of pentazocine hydrochloride P.O. every 3 to 4 hours.

pentazocine hydrochloride and **naloxone hydrochloride** (Talwin-Nx). In this product, 50 mg of oral pentazocine is combined with 0.5 mg of naloxone. The naloxone was added following reports that narcotic addicts were injecting themselves with a solution made from crushing the tablets.

USUAL ADULT DOSAGE: 50 to 100 mg P.O. every 3 to 4 hours.

pentazocine hydrochloride and **aspirin** (Talwin Compound). Each tablet of Talwin Compound contains 12.5 mg of pentazocine and 325 mg of aspirin. Two tablets produce an additive analgesic effect of pentazocine and aspirin as well as the anti-inflammatory and antipyretic action of aspirin. Talwin Compound is used for the relief of moderate pain.
USUAL ADULT DOSAGE: two tablets P.O. t.i.d. or q.i.d.

pentazocine hydrochloride and **acetaminophen** (Talacen). Each caplet of Talacen contains 25 mg of pentazocine and 650 mg of acetaminophen. Talacen is used for the relief of moderate pain.
USUAL ADULT DOSAGE: one caplet P.O. every 3 to 4 hours.

Drug interactions

Patients who have become dependent on narcotic agonists will almost always experience withdrawal symptoms if they are given mixed narcotic agonist-antagonists. The exception is nalbuphine, which can be administered just before, together with, or just after an injection of a narcotic agonist without antagonizing it. Patients with a known or suspected history of narcotic abuse should not receive any of the mixed narcotic agonist-antagonists. Supportive measures should be readily available in the event that one of these drugs is inadvertently administered to a narcotic-dependent patient.

Increased CNS depression and an additive decrease in respiratory rate and depth may result if mixed narcotic agonist-antagonists are administered to patients taking or using other CNS depressants, such as barbiturates or alcohol. If concomitant administration is necessary, the dosage of one or the other drug should be reduced.

ADVERSE DRUG REACTIONS

Adverse reactions to the mixed narcotic agonist-antagonists occur less frequently than reactions to narcotic agonists and usually affect the CNS and the GI tract.

The most common predictable adverse reactions to these drugs include nausea and vomiting, light-headedness, sedation, and euphoria. Dysphoria, visual hallucinations, confusion, and disorientation may also occur (especially in elderly patients). These effects limit the chronic use of these agents in patients with severe pain. Respiration may be depressed with initial doses but does not worsen with increased dosage. Insomnia and disturbed dreams may occur, especially with pentazocine and nalbuphine, and anticholinergic effects (dry mouth,

constipation, and urinary retention) are common. The patient may experience changes in blood pressure, primarily hypertension, especially with nalbuphine. The mixed narcotic agonist-antagonists can also cause hypersensitivity reactions.

NURSING IMPLICATIONS

The mixed narcotic agonist-antagonists were originally welcomed as safe, useful analgesics. However, they have proven to have adverse reactions and abuse potential. The nurse should be aware of the following:
• The mixed narcotic agonist-antagonists may increase intracranial pressure; administer these drugs cautiously to patients with head injuries or intracranial lesions. These drugs may also obscure signs of increasing intracranial pressure, such as confusion or changes in level of consciousness.
• Do not administer these drugs to patients with asthma, obstructive pulmonary disease, or any disorder causing decreased pulmonary reserve from respiratory depression.
• Because butorphanol and pentazocine may increase cardiac work load, carefully monitor patients with MI or angina who are receiving these drugs.
• Because mixed narcotic agonist-antagonists may increase pressure in the biliary tract, administer these agents cautiously to patients with known or suspected gallbladder disease.
• If dependence on buprenorphine occurs, expect the patient to experience withdrawal symptoms for up to 14 days after the drug is stopped.
• Be aware that respiratory depression does not appear with increased doses of butorphanol.
• Be aware that nalbuphine causes respiratory depression equal to morphine.
• Advise the patient taking nalbuphine to avoid activities that require alertness until response to the drug has been determined.
• Do not mix pentazocine in the same syringe as a barbiturate.
• The narcotic antagonist naloxone can reverse the effects of pentazocine and nalbuphine, but it will not totally reverse the effects of buprenorphine. Be aware that mechanical ventilation of the patient may be necessary.
• Pentazocine causes subcutaneous nodules, induration, and severe tissue sclerosis, particularly when administered by S.C. injection. Record and inspect injection sites so they can be rotated and observed.
• Be aware that the mixed narcotic agonist-antagonists have some usefulness during labor but usually are not recommended for use during pregnancy or lactation.

- Do not administer a mixed agonist-antagonist to a narcotic-dependent patient, because it may precipitate withdrawal symptoms.

NARCOTIC ANTAGONISTS

The pure narcotic antagonists naloxone hydrochloride and naltrexone hydrochloride have an affinity for the opiate receptors but do not stimulate them. Instead, these drugs attach to the receptors and prevent narcotic drugs, enkephalins, and endorphins from producing their effects. Physicians use naloxone to treat narcotic overdose. Naltrexone is used as an adjunct therapy to keep detoxified patients drug-free, similar to the use of disulfiram (Antabuse) to prevent resumption of alcohol abuse.

History and source

As early as 1915, drug researchers had some indication that the substance N-allylnorcodeine prevented or abolished the respiratory depression induced by heroin and opium. In 1941, Hart and McCawley described nalorphine as having an antagonistic effect on morphine. Ten years later, Echenhoff and associates reported the use of nalorphine as a morphine antidote in humans. In 1953, researchers discovered that the administration of nalorphine precipitated acute withdrawal symptoms in former addicts who had recently taken narcotic drugs. In nonaddicted patients, nalorphine was noted to produce anxiety and dysphoria rather than euphoria. Further research led to the discovery of naloxone and other drugs with full or partial antagonist properties.

PHARMACOKINETICS

Naloxone is administered I.M. or I.V.; naltrexone is administered orally in tablet or liquid form. Both drugs are metabolized by the liver and excreted by the kidneys.

Absorption, distribution, metabolism, excretion

Naloxone is usually administered I.V. even though it is readily absorbed from I.M. injection sites. Naltrexone is administered orally. Both drugs occupy opiate receptor sites without initiating any response (in the absence of narcotic drugs); both are also rapidly deactivated by first-pass metabolism in the liver and are excreted by the kidneys. A small portion of a naltrexone dose is excreted in the feces.

Onset, peak, duration

Naloxone has an immediate onset of action and a duration of action of only 2 to 3 minutes. The nurse must monitor the patient carefully, because the effects of the narcotic overdose often last longer than the effects of the antagonist, and repeated doses may be necessary. Onset of action of naltrexone occurs within 20 to 30 minutes; peak concentration levels occur in 1 hour. The plasma half-life of naloxone is 60 to 90 minutes. The half-life of naltrexone is 13 hours.

PHARMACODYNAMICS

Narcotic antagonists block the effects of narcotics by occupying the opiate receptor sites, displacing any narcotic molecules already present, and blocking further narcotic binding at these sites: this is known as competitive inhibition. Both naloxone and naltrexone seem to have the highest affinity for the mu opiate receptors.

PHARMACOTHERAPEUTICS

Naloxone is the drug of choice for managing a narcotic overdose because, within seconds after administration, it reverses the respiratory depression and sedation and helps stabilize the patient's vital signs. Naloxone administration also reverses the analgesic effects of narcotic drugs, so a patient who was given a narcotic drug for pain relief may complain of pain or even experience withdrawal symptoms. These symptoms' severity depends on the narcotic used and the amount.

Naloxone challenge test

Planned use of naltrexone commonly requires that a negative naloxone challenge test be obtained before administration of the first naltrexone dose.

For an I.V. naloxone challenge, 0.8 mg (2 ml) is drawn up into a sterile syringe and 0.2 mg (0.5 ml) is injected. While the needle is still in place, observe the patient for 30 seconds for signs and symptoms of withdrawal. If no evidence of withdrawal appears, inject the remaining 0.6 mg (1.5 ml) and observe the patient for an additional 20 minutes.

For an S.C. naloxone challenge, 0.8 mg (2 ml) is administered S.C., and the patient is observed for 45 minutes for withdrawal symptoms.

With either form of the test, occurrence of withdrawal symptoms indicates a potential risk to the patient, and naltrexone therapy should *not* be initiated. The naloxone challenge test can be repeated in 24 hours. If no withdrawal symptoms occur, naltrexone therapy may begin.

Naltrexone: Summary of adverse reactions

Adverse reactions to naltrexone can appear in almost all body symptoms, as this chart demonstrates. (Hepatoxicity may occur in a small number of patients.)

Central nervous system

- Anxiety
- Nervousness
- Dizziness
- Headache
- Depression
- Disorientation

Gastrointestinal

- Anorexia
- Nausea
- Vomiting
- Diarrhea
  or constipation
- Thirst

Skin

- Acne
- Alopecia
- Rash
- Itching

Eye, ear, nose, and throat

- Cough
- Nasal congestion
- Shortness of breath
- Blurred vision
- Tinnitus

Cardiovascular

- Hypertension
- Edema
- Palpitations
- Phlebitis
- Epistaxis

Genitourinary

- Changes in libido
- Delayed ejaculation
- Urinary frequency

If repeated injections of naloxone are needed, but the patient does not improve after receiving three doses or 10 mg, supportive methods such as mechanical ventilation should be instituted; lingering depressant effects may be from nonnarcotic drugs or a mixed overdose.

Naltrexone is used only as an adjunct to psychotherapy or counseling for patients who have been detoxified from narcotic drugs and wish to remain so. Before naltrexone treatment is initiated, a naloxone challenge test may be obtained after the patient has been without narcotics for 7 to 10 days. (See *Naloxone challenge test* on page 427 for details.)

naloxone hydrochloride (Narcan). A narcotic antagonist related to oxymorphone, naloxone is the drug of choice for complete or partial reversal of respiratory depression caused by narcotic overdose. Physicians also use naloxone to diagnose suspected narcotic overdose.
USUAL ADULT DOSAGE: initially, 0.4 to 2 mg I.V., I.M., or S.C., repeated every 2 to 3 minutes as needed, depending on the degree of counteraction achieved. If the patient does not respond after 10 mg have been administered, the diagnosis of narcotic overdose should be reevaluated; the patient may have ingested a nonnarcotic drug or a combination of drugs.

naltrexone hydrochloride (Trexan). Naltrexone is used as an adjunct to psychotherapy or counseling for detoxified addicts who have been narcotic-free for 7 to 10 days, as verified by urinalysis. The patient should also be free of withdrawal symptoms before starting naltrexone treatment. A naloxone challenge test may be obtained before naltrexone treatment is initiated.
USUAL ADULT DOSAGE: 50 mg P.O. every 24 hours; other dosage schedules include 50 mg on weekdays, 100 mg on Saturday, and no dose on Sunday; 100 mg every other day; or 150 mg every third day. The total weekly dose should be 350 mg given in at least three doses.

Drug interactions

There are no significant drug interactions with naloxone or naltrexone except that, if given to a patient receiving a narcotic agonist or to a narcotic addict, naltrexone will cause withdrawal symptoms.

ADVERSE DRUG REACTIONS

Naloxone may cause nausea and vomiting and, occasionally, hypertension and tachycardia. An unconscious patient returned to consciousness abruptly after naloxone administration may hyperventilate and experience tremors.

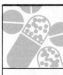

SELECTED MAJOR DRUGS

Narcotic agonist and antagonist agents

This chart summarizes narcotic agonists, mixed narcotic agonist-antagonists, and narcotic antagonists in clinical use.

DRUG	MAJOR INDICATIONS	USUAL ADULT DOSAGES	NURSING IMPLICATIONS
Narcotic agonists			
morphine	Severe pain from myocardial infarction, cancer, major surgery, pulmonary edema	10 mg/70 kg of body weight I.M., I.V., or S.C., titrated to pain relief	• Before administration, note the rate, depth, and rhythm of the patient's respirations. If the respiratory rate is less than 10 breaths/minute, withhold the drug.
morphine, sustained-release	Terminal cancer pain or other conditions in which prolonged pain relief is desirable	30 mg P.O. every 8 to 12 hours, titrated to pain relief	• Suppression of cough by narcotic drugs can lead to atelectasis and hypostatic pneumonia in postoperative patients. Encourage regularly scheduled deep breathing, coughing, and turning.
morphine, oral concentrate	Severe acute pain, chronic pain	10 to 30 mg P.O. every 4 hours; dosage varies with patient response	• Monitor the patient's fluid intake and output, because urinary retention may occur. • Monitor the patient's bowel elimination pattern to detect possible constipation early. • Be aware that institutional policy dictates the valid time limit for narcotic orders—most commonly, 48 to 72 hours. • Record the location, onset, duration, intensity, and quality of pain and the results of analgesic administration, especially its onset of action and duration of action. • Be aware that nonverbal clues, such as restlessness, a drawn or pained facial expression, anorexia, and increased pulse or respirations, may indicate a patient's need for pain relief. • Advise the patient not to smoke or ambulate after the drug is given because of its sedative effect.
meperidine	Moderate to severe visceral pain, obstetric analgesia	50 to 150 mg parenterally or P.O. every 3 to 4 hours, as needed	• Before administration, note the rate, depth, and rhythm of the patient's respirations. • Monitor the patient's vital signs frequently for hypotension and increased pulse rate.
	Preoperative medication	50 to 100 mg I.M. or S.C.	• Advise the patient not to smoke or ambulate after receiving the drug because of its sedative effect. • Be aware that institutional policy dictates the valid time limit for narcotic orders—most commonly, 48 to 72 hours. • The I.M. route is the preferred parenteral route; S.C. injection is painful and can cause local irritation. The I.V. route can cause tachycardia and syncope. • Record the location, onset, duration, intensity, and quality of pain and the results of analgesic administration.
propoxyphene	Mild to moderate pain	65 mg P.O. every 4 hours, as needed	• Advise the patient to avoid alcohol or other CNS depressants, which may cause excessive sedation and respiratory depression. • Adverse reactions are most common in ambulatory patients. Instruct the patient to lie down if drowsiness, nausea, or lightheadedness occurs.

continued

SELECTED MAJOR DRUGS

Narcotic agonist and antagonist agents continued

DRUG	MAJOR INDICATIONS	USUAL ADULT DOSAGES	NURSING IMPLICATIONS
Mixed narcotic agonist-antagonists			
butorphanol	Moderate to severe pain, obstetric analgesia, preoperative medication	2 mg I.M. every 3 to 4 hours or 1 mg I.V. every 3 to 4 hours, as needed	• During obstetric analgesia, monitor the neonate for signs of respiratory depression. • Obtain a complete drug history before administration, because acute withdrawal symptoms may occur in opiate-dependent patients.
nalbuphine	Moderate to severe pain, obstetric analgesia, preoperative medication	10 mg/70 kg of body weight I.M., S.C., or I.V. every 3 to 6 hours; not to exceed 160 mg/day	• Advise the patient that the use of this drug together with alcohol and other CNS depressants may cause excessive sedation.
Narcotic antagonist			
naloxone	Narcotic overdose	0.4 to 2 mg I.V. every 2 to 3 minutes depending on patient response; may also be given I.M. or S.C.	• Monitor and record the patient's vital signs before and after administration. (Respirations may become very rapid.) • With drug-related respiratory depression of unknown cause, try to obtain a history of the possible cause from family or friends, because naloxone is not useful in treating toxicity from nonnarcotic CNS depressants. • Have emergency measures readily available: ventilation equipment, oxygen, and I.V. fluids.

Naltrexone produces numerous adverse reactions affecting a number of body systems. (*See Naltrexone: Summary of adverse reactions* on page 428 for a discussion of these reactions.) The variety and number of adverse reactions to this drug have delayed its full acceptance in maintaining narcotic abstinence. Patients should be carefully monitored, even if they receive the drug on an outpatient basis.

NURSING IMPLICATIONS

The narcotic antagonists are commonly administered in emergencies. To care for these patients safely, the nurse should be aware of the following considerations:
• Administer naloxone cautiously to patients with cardiac irritability or narcotic addiction.
• Be aware that naloxone is the safest drug to use when the drug causing a patient's respiratory depression is unknown.
• The duration of action of the narcotic may exceed the duration of action of naloxone: observe the patient for a relapse into respiratory depression, and be prepared to administer another dose when ordered.

• Monitor the patient's respiratory rate and depth, and be prepared to provide oxygen, ventilation, and other resuscitation measures, as needed.
• Be aware that naloxone does not reverse respiratory depression produced by diazepam.
• Do not give naltrexone to patients receiving narcotic drugs, those addicted to narcotic drugs, or those in the acute phase of narcotic withdrawal.
• Do not administer naltrexone until a naloxone challenge test is performed.
• Administer narcotic antagonists cautiously to patients with mild liver disease or a recent history of liver disease.
• Advise the patient receiving naltrexone to carry a medication alert card and to notify medical personnel about the drug before accepting any medical treatment.

CHAPTER SUMMARY

Chapter 26 included discussions of narcotic agonists, mixed narcotic agonist-antagonists, and narcotic antagonists. Here are the highlights of the chapter:

• Narcotic drugs—both narcotic agonists and mixed narcotic agonist-antagonists—modify the sensation of pain by inhibiting the transmission of pain impulses, reducing cortical responses to painful stimuli, and altering behavioral responses to pain.

• Narcotic agonists include the opium derivatives and the synthetic narcotics used to relieve pain. Oral, rectal, and parenteral forms are available.

• Adverse reactions to narcotic agonists include respiratory depression, constipation, and urinary retention. Tolerance as well as psychological and physiologic dependence may occur with long-term narcotic use.

• Morphine is considered the narcotic standard; all narcotic drugs are compared with it.

• Oxycodone with acetaminophen or aspirin (Percocet or Percodan) is a combination drug that exemplifies the additive effect of nonnarcotic-narcotic combination analgesics. Concentrated oral solutions of morphine and a sustained-release tablet have recently been marketed for use in treating cancer pain and chronic intractable pain. Among the synthetic narcotic agonists, meperidine (Demerol) is the most frequently used.

• Mixed narcotic agonist-antagonists produce analgesic effects similar to those of morphine but have less potential for abuse and dependence. They have little or no antitussive effect.

• Mixed narcotic agonist-antagonists cause fewer adverse reactions in the GI tract compared with narcotic agonists, and the respiratory depression they cause does not worsen with higher doses.

• Pentazocine, the oldest mixed narcotic agonist-antagonist, is an effective analgesic for moderate pain. An oral dosage form (Talwin) combines pentazocine with aspirin, providing an additive analgesic effect and anti-inflammatory and antipyretic actions.

• Buprenorphine and nalbuphine, also mixed narcotic agonist-antagonists, have a longer duration of action than pentazocine, up to 6 hours. Both effectively relieve moderate to severe pain.

• The narcotic antagonists naloxone and naltrexone work by competitive inhibition at the opiate receptor sites, displacing narcotic molecules and thereby preventing them from exerting their effects.

• Naloxone is used to diagnose and treat narcotic overdose.

• Naltrexone is used as an adjunct treatment with detoxified addicts who are highly motivated to remain drug-free.

BIBLIOGRAPHY

Bast, C., and Hayes, P. "Patient Controlled Analgesia," *Nursing86* 16:25, January 1986.

Baumann, T.J., et al. "Patient-Controlled Analgesia in the Terminally Ill Cancer Patient," *Drug Intelligence and Clinical Pharmacy* 20:297, April 1986.

Crabtree, B.L. "Review of Naltrexone, A Long-Acting Opiate Antagonist," *Clinical Pharmacy* 3:273, May/June 1984.

Friedman, F.B. "PRN Analgesics: Controlling the Pain or Controlling the Patient?," *RN* 46:67, March 1983.

Gilman, A.G., et al., eds. *Goodman and Gilman's The Pharmacological Basis of Therapeutics,* 7th ed. New York: Macmillan Publishing Co., 1985.

Goth, A. *Medical Pharmacology: Principles and Concepts,* 11th ed. St. Louis: C.V. Mosby Co., 1984.

Katzung, B.G., ed. *Basic and Clinical Pharmacology.* Los Altos, Calif.: Lange Medical Pubs., 1982.

McGuire, L., and Wright, A. "Continuous Narcotic Infusion: It's Not Just for Cancer Patients," *Nursing84* 14:50, December 1984.

Miller, K. "Naltrexone," *Emergency* 18:12, May 1986.

Newman, R.G. "The Need to Redefine 'Addiction,'" *New England Journal of Medicine* 308:1096, May 1983.

Pageau, M.G., and Coombs, D.W. "New Analgesic Therapy Relieves Cancer Pain Without Oversedation," *Nursing85* 15:47, April 1985.

Paice, J.A. "Intrathecal Morphine Infusion for Intractable Cancer Pain: A New Use for Implanted Pumps," *Oncology Nursing Forum* 13:41, May/June 1986.

Portenoy, R.K. "Continuous Infusion of Opioids," *American Journal of Nursing* 86:318, March 1986.

Smith, K.A. "Teaching Family Members Intrathecal Morphine Administration," *Journal of Neuroscience Nursing* 18:95, April 1986.

Stuart, G.J., et al. "Continuous Intravenous Morphine Infusions for Terminal Pain Control: A Retrospective Review," *Drug Intelligence and Clinical Pharmacy* 20, December 1986.

Todd, B. "Narcotic Analgesia for Chronic Pain," *Geriatric Nursing* 7:53, January/February 1986

Zola, E.M., and McLeod, D.C. "Comparative Effects and Analgesic Efficacy of the Agonist-Antagonist Opioids," *Drug Intelligence and Clinical Pharmacy* 17:411, June 1983.

CHAPTER 27

GENERAL ANESTHETIC AGENTS

OBJECTIVES

After reading and studying this chapter, you should be able to:

1. Explain the differences between balanced anesthesia and neuroleptanesthesia.

2. Explain the stages of anesthesia.

3. Define and distinguish between inhalation and injection anesthetic agents.

4. Describe the pharmacokinetics and mechanism of action of inhalation anesthetic agents.

5. Describe the adverse effects of inhalation anesthetic agents and the appropriate nursing implications of those effects.

6. Describe the mechanism of action, adverse effects, and nursing implications of injection anesthetics.

INTRODUCTION

General anesthetic agents depress the central nervous system (CNS) to produce loss of consciousness, loss of responsiveness to sensory stimulation including pain, and relaxation of muscles. General anesthesia may result from one or a combination of drugs.

These drugs are either volatile liquids or gases vaporized in oxygen and administered by inhalation or nonvolatile solutions administered by injection.

Often, combinations of drugs are used to produce anesthesia. One kind of anesthesia, neuroleptanesthesia, is produced by administering a neuroleptic drug (a tranquilizer or an antipsychotic) combined with an opiate analgesic and nitrous oxide. The patient can be aroused almost immediately from this anesthesia if necessary. Another kind of anesthesia, balanced anesthesia, is produced by administering a barbiturate, an opiate analgesic, and a cholinergic blocking agent, then inducing anesthesia with another barbituate and maintaining it with a combination of inhalation and injection anesthetics plus a neuromuscular blocking agent. When properly administered, balanced anesthesia minimizes

cardiovascular effects, allows an early return to consciousness, and reduces postoperative nausea, vomiting, and excitement.

The practice of anesthesia includes more than proper administration of anesthetic agents. Monitoring and maintenance of vital signs, fluids, electrolytes, acid-base balance, body temperatures, and positioning, and assurance of the patient's well-being from before surgery through recovery are vital components of anesthesia practice.

The choice of a particular anesthetic for a patient involves several considerations, including the physiologic state of the patient, the medical history, the type of surgical procedure, and the anticipated postoperative course.

Chapter 27 will discuss the two main classes of general anesthetics—inhalation and injection—and their use singly and in combination.

Anesthesia administration

Anesthesia administration is divided into three stages: induction, maintenance, and emergence.

Induction is the initiation of anesthesia and is often accomplished with an intravenous agent that has a rapid onset of action and a short duration of action. Its purpose is to produce a rapid, pleasant, and stressless transition from consciousness to sleep. Induction agents include the ultra-short-acting barbiturates (thiopental sodium, thiamylal sodium, or methohexital sodium); the benzodiazepine sedatives (diazepam, lorazepam, and midazolam); or the rapid-acting hypnotic etomidate.

Administration of the primary anesthetic—the maintenance stage—begins during induction. The transition to maintenance anesthesia is completed as the induction stage effects diminish. Maintenance levels of anesthesia can be continued for many hours if necessary, until surgery is completed.

Emergence follows the withdrawal of anesthetic agents. Drugs are administered to reverse the effects, and the patient exhales or otherwise excretes the anesthetic agents. The anesthesia process is completed after the patient is observed postoperatively.

Selected preoperative medications

The nurse often administers preoperative medications. Many combinations of drugs are used, but the most common one is a narcotic combined with an antianxiety agent and a cholinergic blocking agent. The following are commonly administered preoperative medications, their action, and dosages. Before administration, the nurse should explain the drug effects to the patient, provide privacy by closing the curtains, and ensure safety by pulling up the bed side rails.

DRUG	DOSAGE	ACTION
Narcotics		
meperidine	50 to 100 mg I.M. or S.C. 30 to 90 minutes before surgery	Alter perception and emotional response to pain
morphine	8 to 12 mg I.M. 30 to 90 minutes before surgery	Alter perception and emotional response to pain
Barbiturates		
pentobarbital	150 to 200 mg I.M. 40 to 60 minutes after surgery	Sedates the patient
secobarbital	200 to 300 mg P.O. 1 to 2 hours before surgery	Sedates the patient
Cholinergic blocking agents		
atropine	0.4 to 0.6 mg I.M. 45 to 60 minutes before surgery	Reduces secretions, vomiting, and laryngospasm
scopolamine	0.4 to 0.6 mg S.C. 45 to 60 minutes before surgery	Reduces secretions, vomiting, and laryngospasm
Antianxiety agents		
diazepam	5 to 10 mg I.V. immediately before surgery	Sedates the patient
hydroxyzine	25 to 100 mg I.M. 30 to 60 minutes before surgery	Reduces anxiety

During surgery, the anesthesiologist or nurse anesthetist continuously monitors and adjusts the depth of anesthesia—the degree of depression of CNS function.

Stages of anesthesia

The depth of anesthesia is gauged in four stages, originally described for ether anesthesia in the 1920s.

Stage 1—Analgesia. This stage begins with onset of anesthesia and ends with loss of consciousness. Smell and pain sensations are lost before unconsciousness ensues. The patient may experience hallucinations and dreams. Inhalation anesthetics may cause coughing or choking at this stage if other anesthetic agents are not used.

Stage 2—Excitement. This stage begins with loss of consciousness. Reflexes become more prominent and respirations irregular; autonomic activity increases. Complications of anesthesia are most frequently noted in this stage. Stages 1 and 2 correspond to induction of anesthesia.

Stage 3—Surgical anesthesia. This stage reaches the degree of anesthesia under which the procedure may be performed safely. Respirations normalize. Surgical anesthesia extends across four planes that represent increasing depth of anesthesia and diminution of reflexes and muscle tone. Precise maintenance of anesthesia depth is necessary for successful completion of a surgical procedure.

Stage 4—Medullary paralysis. Also referred to as the toxic stage, stage 4 signifies the loss of respirations and collapse of the circulatory system, requiring mechanical ventilation and perfusion.

Apart from the general anesthesic agents, other drugs are used before, during, and after anesthesia to assist in patient management. Before surgery, the nurse anesthetist has two concerns: to allay the patient's anxiety over the procedure and to control secretions that could complicate the anesthesia. Other preoperative needs include producing amnesia for the period of the operation and combating postoperative nausea. Various drugs are used as preoperative medications, including antihistamines, opiates, sedatives, neuroleptics, and anticholinergics. (For a list of these medications, their usual dosages, and their effects, see *Selected preoperative medications* on page 433.)

Drugs used during surgery include neuromuscular blocking agents, which permit mechanical ventilation or allow access to areas guarded by large muscle groups, such as the abdomen. Other seemingly unrelated drugs, such as vasodilators, alpha-adrenergic blocking agents, ganglionic blocking agents, corticosteroids, vasopressors, and cardiac agents, are used during surgery to prevent or rectify various problems as well as to compensate for the effects of coexisting medical conditions.

Postoperative drugs are given to reverse the effects of drugs given before or during surgery. For example, atropine, neostigmine, or pyridostigmine antagonizes neuromuscular blocking agents; naloxone reverses the effects of opiates; antiemetic antihistamines and major tranquilizers counteract the nausea from potent inhalation anesthetic agents; and opiates and other analgesics combat pain.

For a summary of representative drugs, see *Selected major drugs: General anesthetic agents* on pages 443 and 444.

INHALATION ANESTHETICS

Five inhalation anesthetics are used frequently: enflurane, halothane, isoflurane, methoxyflurane, and nitrous oxide. Methoxyflurane's use is limited because it produces renal toxicity at high doses.

History and source

Wells, a Boston dentist, observed that patients receiving "laughing gas" (nitrous oxide) felt little or no pain during tooth extraction. An attempt in 1845 to demonstrate the surgical use of nitrous oxide failed. Thus, the discovery of surgical anesthesia is generally credited to Morton, another Boston dentist and medical student who, in 1846, conducted the first successful demonstration of surgical anesthesia using diethyl ether. Chloroform (now recognized to be hepatotoxic) was introduced in 1847, and nitrous oxide was reintroduced in dental and surgical practice in 1863. Cyclopropane, discovered in 1929, was used widely for 30 years but was as highly flammable as ether. Then in 1956, halothane was introduced as the first potent, nonflammable anesthetic, and it quickly achieved widespread use. Halothane was the first of a group known as the halogenated anesthetics because each anesthetic compound contains one or more of the halogens (bromine, chlorine, fluorine, and iodine); others include methoxyflurane, introduced in the 1960s; enflurane, 1970s; and isoflurane, 1980s. Enflurane and isoflurane, discovered by Terrell, are the most widely used inhalation anesthetic agents.

PHARMACOKINETICS

Inhalation anesthetics are administered as gases, so dosages are not expressed in weight, as with other drugs. Because the amount of anesthetic in the lungs is known to be proportional to the amount in the brain at equilibrium, the quantity of anesthetic agent needed can be determined by a measurement called the minimum alveolar concentration (MAC). MAC is defined as the alveolar anesthetic concentration level at which 50% of patients do not move during a surgical incision.

Absorption, distribution, metabolism, excretion

The absorption and elimination rates of an anesthetic are governed by the anesthetic's solubility in blood. Basically, the lower the solubility of the anesthetic in blood, the faster its absorption and elimination. Nitrous oxide, with the lowest solubility, is absorbed and eliminated the fastest, followed by isoflurane, enflurane, halothane, and methoxyflurane.

Absorption is also affected by alveolar ventilation—the provision of air or gas to the alveoli—and perfusion—the amount of blood passing through the alveoli. Diseases, such as emphysema or congestive heart failure, can increase or decrease the absorption of inhalation anesthetics by changing ventilation or perfusion.

Inhalation anesthetics enter the blood from the lungs and are distributed to other tissues. Distribution is most rapid to organs with high blood flow: brain, liver, kidneys, and heart. All the inhalation anesthetics cross the blood-brain barrier, some at greater concentrations than others. This characteristic determines the agent's potency. Methoxyflurane is the most potent inhalation anesthetic. Halothane, isoflurane, enflurane, and nitrous oxide follow in order of potency.

The inhalation anesthetics are eliminated primarily by the lungs, but also by the liver in the case of enflurane, halothane, and methoxyflurane. Metabolites are excreted in the urine.

Onset, peak, duration

Onset of action and peak concentration levels of the inhalation anesthetics vary greatly, depending on therapeutic and patient factors. Therapeutic variables include concentration of the anesthetic and the presence of other CNS-depressant drugs in the bloodstream. Patient variables include age, pregnancy, respiratory and circulatory status, hypotension, and hypothermia.

The duration of action for each inhalation anesthetic is determined by the rate at which the anesthetic leaves the brain.

PHARMACODYNAMICS

Inhalation anesthetics are general depressants of the CNS, although they affect other organ systems.

DRUG INTERACTIONS

Inhalation anesthetics

The most significant drug interactions involving inhalation anesthetics are caused by other CNS depressants.

DRUG	INTERACTING DRUGS	POSSIBLE EFFECTS	NURSING IMPLICATIONS
enflurane, halothane, isoflurane, methoxyflurane, nitrous oxide	alcohol	Increases anesthetic requirement	• Check anesthesia record for the amount administered. • Monitor the patient's respirations, blood pressure, pulse rate, and level of consciousness.
	amiodarone	Causes hypotension and increases risk of bradycardia	• Monitor the patient's blood pressure and pulse frequently postoperatively.
	anticoagulants	Increase anticoagulant effect	• Observe the patient for hematuria, melena, bruising, and petechiae. • Monitor bleeding times.
	antihypertensives, chlorpromazine, diuretics, other hypotensive agents	Increase hypotensive effects	• Monitor the patient's blood pressure frequently.
	CNS depressants	Increase CNS and respiratory depression and cause hypotension	• Monitor the patient's rate and rhythm of respirations, level of consciousness, and blood pressure.
	magnesium sulfate	Increases CNS depression	• Monitor the patient's level of consciousness.
	methyldopa	Decreases anesthetic requirement	• Monitor the patient's respiratory rate, blood pressure, pulse rate, and level of consciousness.
	xanthines (caffeine, theophylline)	Increase risk of dysrhythmias	• Monitor the patient's pulse rate, blood pressure, and respirations. • Prepare the patient for a cardiac monitor, as ordered.

continued

DRUG INTERACTIONS

Inhalation anesthetics continued

DRUG	INTERACTING DRUGS	POSSIBLE EFFECTS	NURSING IMPLICATIONS
enflurane, halothane, isoflurane, methoxyflurane	aminoglycoside antibiotics, capreomycin, citrate-anticoagulated blood, clindamycin, lincomycin, neuromuscular blocking agents, polymyxin	Increase neuromuscular blockage	• Monitor the patient's respirations. • Monitor the patient's ability to move limbs as anesthesia diminishes.
	beta-adrenergic blocking agents	Produce prolonged, severe hypotension	• Monitor the patient's blood pressure frequently.
	catecholamines (dopamine, epinephrine, norepinephrine), doxapram, ephedrine, metaraminol, methoxamine; other sympathomimetics	Increase risk of dysrhythmias	• Monitor the patient's pulse rate and blood pressure. • Prepare the patient for a cardiac monitor, as ordered.
	ketamine	Prolongs recovery from ketamine	• Monitor the patient's vital signs and level of consciousness. • Maintain a quiet environment with minimal stimulation to prevent hallucinations and excitement.
	ritodrine	Increases risk of hypotension, dysrhythmias	• Monitor the patient's vital signs frequently.
	succinylcholine	Increases risk of malignant hyperthermia and neuromuscular blockade; repeated use increases risk of bradycardia	• Monitor the patient's vital signs, including temperature. • Monitor the patient's airway and his ability to move extremities.
enflurane, halothane, methoxyflurane	agents that induce production of hepatic enzymes (such as isoniazid, barbiturates, and cimetidine)	Increase anesthetic metabolism	• Monitor the patient's urine output, blood urea nitrogen (BUN), and serum creatinine. • Monitor the patient's liver enzymes.
enflurane	isoniazid	Increases release of nephrotoxic fluorine from enflurane	• Monitor the patient's urine output, BUN, and serum creatinine.
enflurane, halothane, isoflurane	oxytocic agents	Decrease uterine contractions	• Monitor fetal heart rate and the patient's contractions.
halothane	phenytoin	Increases risk of hepatotoxicity and phenytoin toxicity	• Monitor the patient's liver enzymes. • Observe the patient for signs of phenytoin toxicity, such as hypotension and ventricular fibrillation.
methoxyflurane	nephrotoxic agents	Increase risk of anesthetic toxicity	• Observe whether the patient rouses normally as anesthesia diminishes.
nitrous oxide	alfentanil, fentanyl, sufentanil	Increase respiratory and CNS depression and hypotension; decrease heart rate and cardiac output	• Monitor the patient's vital signs frequently.

Mechanism of action

The ability of an inhalation anesthetic to enter the brain depends on its degree of lipid solubility. Movement of the inhalation anesthetics throughout the brain and spinal cord is rapid and efficient, but little more is known about their mechanism of action.

Usually, inhalation anesthetics depress the CNS, but paradoxically some seem to increase the potential for seizure activity. Outside the CNS, the halogenated anesthetics affect other organ systems. They interfere with the transmission of nerve impulses, relax skeletal and uterine smooth muscles, reduce arterial blood pressure and redirect blood flow (which may endanger circulation in the brain and kidneys), decrease respirations, increase the fraction of carbon dioxide in the blood, depress the exchange of oxygen and carbon dioxide in the lungs, and decrease renal and hepatic blood flow and hepatic enzyme activity (which may cause nausea and vomiting).

Nitrous oxide counteracts the cardiovascular effects of the halogenated anesthetics while increasing their anesthetic effects. It appears to have little effect on respiratory function alone but adds to respiratory depression when used with one of the halogenated agents. It has no effect on the musculature, liver, or gastrointestinal (GI) tract; long-term use may cause changes in red and white blood cell production.

PHARMACOTHERAPEUTICS

Inhalation anesthetics are used for surgery because they offer more precise and rapid control of depth of anesthesia than injection anesthetics. Of the inhalation anesthetics available, the most often used are halothane, enflurane, and isoflurane, often with nitrous oxide. Which anesthetic is used depends on a careful evaluation of the patient's physical condition, medical history, and medication profile; the type of surgical procedure; and an assessment of anticipated postoperative needs.

enflurane (Ethrane). During induction, enflurane causes marked CNS excitation, and grand mal–like seizures have been reported when high concentrations were administered to hypocapnic patients.
USUAL ADULT DOSAGE: dosages are individualized and continuously monitored and altered throughout surgery.

halothane (Fluothane). Halothane relaxes the bronchial smooth muscle, making it useful for anesthesia during surgery on patients with asthma. Because halothane sensitizes the heart to the action of catecholamines, which may lead to cardiac dysrhythmias, catecholamine dosages should be reduced in patients receiving halothane.

USUAL ADULT DOSAGE: dosages are individualized and continuously monitored and altered throughout surgery.

isoflurane (Forane). Isoflurane produces the greatest degree of skeletal muscle relaxation of all the inhalation anesthetics.
USUAL ADULT DOSAGE: dosages are individualized and continuously monitored and altered throughout surgery.

methoxyflurane (Penthrane). Because methoxyflurane can produce renal toxicity at high doses, it is used only occasionally, for relief of labor pains.
USUAL ADULT DOSAGE: dosages are individualized and continuously monitored and altered throughout labor.

nitrous oxide. A rapidly acting anesthetic agent, nitrous oxide produces little or no toxicity in clinically useful concentration levels. Much less potent than the halogenated anesthetics, it is used primarily as an adjunct to them or to the injection anesthetics.
USUAL ADULT DOSAGE: dosages are individualized and continuously monitored and altered throughout surgery.

Drug interactions

The most important drug interactions involving inhalation anesthetics are with other CNS, cardiac, or respiratory depressant drugs. The potent anesthetics greatly enhance the depressant effects of normally safe levels of these drugs. (See *Drug interactions: Inhalation anesthetics* on pages 435 and 436 for details.)

ADVERSE DRUG REACTIONS

Many of the predictable adverse reactions can be planned for when the anesthesiologist or nurse anesthetist collects data preoperatively.

Predictable reactions

The most common adverse reaction associated with inhalation anesthetics is an exaggerated patient response to a normal dose. Surgical patients often are debilitated, predisposing them to an exaggerated response, and even smaller-than-normal doses may result in hypotension, prolonged respiratory depression, and prolonged recovery. These effects can be avoided by using a detailed medical history before surgery to plan anesthesia. In elderly patients, confusion, agitation, and memory loss may accompany a prolonged recovery from the anesthesia and may be mistaken for signs of dementia.

The postoperative reactions are much the same as those seen with other CNS depressant drugs: cardiopulmonary depression, confusion, sedation, nausea and vomiting, ataxia, and hypothermia.

Methoxyflurane sometimes causes dose-related nephrotoxicity. Called high-output renal failure, the syndrome begins 2 to 4 days postoperatively as the patient suddenly produces massive amounts of dilute urine. Treatment involves aggressive maintenance of fluid and electrolyte balance; mortality has been reported as high as 50%, which accounts for the limited use of this drug.

Unpredictable reactions

Malignant hyperthermia, characterized by a sudden and often lethal increase in body temperature, is a serious and unexpected reaction to inhalation anesthetic agents. It occurs in genetically susceptible patients only and may result from a failure in calcium uptake by muscle cells. The skeletal muscle relaxant dantrolene is used to treat this condition.

Rarely (approximately 1 in 10,000 cases), liver necrosis develops several days after halothane use. Although it is not infective in origin, the necrosis resembles hepatitis clinically, so it is called halothane hepatitis. Symptoms include rash, fever, jaundice, nausea and vomiting, eosinophilia, and alterations in liver function. This often-fatal syndrome occurs most frequently with multiple exposures to the drug. An immunologic or chemical response to a toxic metabolite may explain this phenomenon. Treatment is symptomatic.

NURSING IMPLICATIONS

Although the nurse does not administer inhalation anesthetics, when they are given, the nurse must be aware of the following implications for patient care:

• Be aware that halogenated anesthetics are contraindicated in patients whose history suggests a genetic predisposition to malignant hyperthermia; in patients with a head injury or any disorder that would increase intracranial pressure; and in patients with myasthenia gravis. Halothane is contraindicated after use of metabolized halogenated agents and in patients with cardiac dysrhythmias or pheochromocytoma. Methoxyflurane is contraindicated in patients with renal impairment. Nitrous oxide is contraindicated in patients with hepatic disorders.

• Document an accurate and complete patient history, including details about difficulties relatives had with surgery, which could reflect tendencies toward malignant hyperthermia.

• Advise the patient not to eat for 8 hours before surgery to allow the stomach to empty and prevent the aspiration of stomach contents into the lungs during anesthesia.

• Monitor the patient's vital signs frequently to detect potential problems. Assess the adequacy, rate, and depth of the patient's ventilations. Maintain a patent airway.

Assess the patient's level of consciousness, arousal, and orientation.

• Keep in mind that treatment of predictable adverse reactions, such as cardiovascular and respiratory depression, prolonged sedation, and nausea and vomiting, is symptomatic and that these conditions are usually reversible. Inform the anesthesiologist of severe adverse reactions.

• Exercise extreme caution when giving additional analgesics before recovery from anesthesia is complete. The dose of analgesic will vary, depending on the residual analgesic effect of the inhalation anesthetic agent. Monitor patients closely for signs of respiratory depression if they receive narcotic analgesics for pain control within 8 hours of surgery.

• Be aware that the patient may be unsteady and need assistance during early ambulation after surgery.

• Tell patients that their psychomotor functions may be impaired for 24 hours or longer after inhalation anesthesia.

INJECTION ANESTHETICS

Injection anesthetics are used usually in situations requiring a short duration of anesthesia, such as outpatient surgery. The injection anesthetics also are used to promote rapid induction of anesthesia or to supplement inhalation anesthetics.

Three agents in this class—droperidol, etomidate, and ketamine hydrochloride—are used solely as injected general anesthetics. The others are drawn from other chemical categories—barbiturates (thiopental sodium) and benzodiazepines (diazepam), for example—and are used secondarily as anesthetics. Detailed considerations of their primary uses appear in Chapter 30, Sedative and Hypnotic Agents, and Chapter 32, Antianxiety Agents.

History and source

Barbiturates were the first injection anesthetics in general use. Hexobarbital was used as a general anesthetic in 1932, followed by methohexital sodium in 1935.

Droperidol is a butyrophenone tranquilizer introduced in 1960 for use in anesthesia. It is similar to haloperidol, which is an antipsychotic agent. Ketamine, introduced in 1970, is a phencyclidine derivative similar to LSD. Etomidate was introduced in 1982 and is not related to any class of sedative-hypnotic agents.

PHARMACOKINETICS

All injection anesthetics bypass the mechanisms that reduce bioavailability, distributing rapidly into the CNS.

Absorption, distribution, metabolism, excretion

Effects of the injection anesthetics appear quickly, beginning 15 seconds to a few minutes after administration. Intramuscular injection of the opiates may delay absorption and decrease peak effect when compared to intravenous administration.

The barbiturates depend on hepatic transformation for elimination, as do the benzodiazepine and opiate agents and the hypnotic etomidate.

Onset, peak, duration

All the injection anesthetics have a rapid onset of action and are short-acting. Etomidate, the opiates, and the barbiturates begin to act within 60 seconds; the benzodiazepines act within 1 to 15 minutes. The opiates reach peak concentration levels in 3 to 20 minutes. Rapid redistribution of barbiturates from the brain to other tissues ends anesthetic action; therefore, their duration of action is much shorter than would be anticipated from their half-lives.

PHARMACODYNAMICS

Because the injection anesthetics come from different chemical classes, their mechanisms of action differ.

Mechanism of action

Barbiturates seem to enhance responses to the CNS neurotransmitter gamma-aminobutyric acid (GABA) and to depress the excitability of CNS neurons. The benzodiazepines also stimulate responses to GABA, thus inhibiting the brain's response to stimulation of the reticular activating system (RAS), the area of the brain stem that controls alertness. Etomidate, too, may have GABA-like effects, including direct inhibition of the RAS. Droperidol induces neurolepsis by blocking postsynaptic dopamine receptors in sections of the brain. The opiates occupy sites on specialized receptors scattered throughout the CNS and modify the release of neurotransmitters from sensory nerves entering the CNS.

PHARMACOTHERAPEUTICS

The short duration of action of these agents is an advantage in shorter surgical procedures—including outpatient surgery.

The subcategories of injection anesthetics have various pharmacologic characteristics. The barbiturates are used alone in surgery that is not expected to be painful and as adjuncts to other agents in more extensive procedures. The benzodiazepines produce sedation and amnesia, but not analgesia. Etomidate is used to induce anesthesia and to supplement low-potency inhalation anesthetics such as nitrous oxide. The opiates provide analgesia and supplement other anesthetic agents. Droperidol is almost never used alone, but in conjunction with analgesics.

alfentanil (Alfenta). An ultra-short-acting drug, alfentanil may be used with nitrous oxide or with a barbiturate and nitrous oxide, or as the primary anesthetic in surgery where ventilatory assistance is maintained.
USUAL ADULT DOSAGE: for induction of anesthesia, 130 to 245 mcg/kg of body weight I.V., followed by an infusion of 0.5 to 1.5 mcg/kg/minute; for analgesia, 8 to 20 mcg/kg of body weight I.V., followed by 3 to 5 mcg/kg or a continuous infusion of 0.5 to 1 mcg/kg/minute in patients who will breathe unassisted; dose in ventilator patients is 20 to 50 mcg/kg I.V., followed by incremental doses of 5 to 15 mcg/kg.

diazepam (Valium). The most widely used benzodiazepine, diazepam is used to increase the sedative and amnesic effects of other anesthetic agents.
USUAL ADULT DOSAGE: 10 to 20 mg I.M. or I.V. before surgery.

droperidol (Inapsine). Droperidol is the only neuroleptic agent used for general anesthesia.
USUAL ADULT DOSAGE: for induction, 2.5 mg/9 to 11 kg I.V. with an analgesic or a general anesthetic; for maintenance, 1.25 to 2.5 mg I.V.

etomidate (Amidate). Etomidate is used to induce anesthesia rapidly or to augment another anesthetic agent during maintenance anesthesia.
USUAL ADULT DOSAGE: for induction, 0.2 to 0.6 mg/kg of body weight I.V., administered over 30 to 60 seconds; for maintenance, smaller individual I.V. doses or a continuous I.V. infusion.

fentanyl citrate (Sublimaze). A narcotic analgesic, fentanyl is one of a series of compounds with potent but brief opiate-like activity. Fentanyl is used as an adjunct

DRUG INTERACTIONS

Injection anesthetics

Because drug interactions involving the injection anesthetics can cause increased CNS depression and hypotension, the nurse must assess the patient's vital signs and level of consciousness frequently.

DRUG	INTERACTING DRUGS	POSSIBLE EFFECTS	NURSING IMPLICATIONS
droperidol	CNS depressants	Increase CNS depressant effects	• Monitor the patient's vital signs, level of consciousness, and ability to move limbs.
	hypotensive agents	Increase hypotensive effects	• Monitor the patient's blood pressure frequently.
	neuroleptics, metoclopramide	Increase risk of extrapyramidal effects	• Monitor the patient for tremors. • Monitor the patient's vital signs.
etomidate	antidepressants, antihypertensives with CNS depressant effects, magnesium sulfate, monoamine oxidase inhibitors	Increase CNS depressant effects	• Monitor the patient's vital signs, level of consciousness, and ability to move limbs.
	hypotensive agents	Increase hypotensive effects	• Monitor the patient's blood pressure frequently.
	ketamine	Increases risk of hypotension and respiratory depression	• Monitor the patient's blood pressure and respirations frequently.
ketamine	inhalation anesthetics	Prolong anesthetic effects	• Monitor the patient's vital signs, level of consciousness, and ability to move limbs.
	antihypertensives with CNS depressant effects (reserpine, clonidine, and methyldopa)	Increase risk of hypotension and respiratory depression	• Monitor the patient's blood pressure and respirations frequently.
	thyroid hormones	Increase risk of hypertension and tachycardia	• Monitor the patient's blood pressure and pulse rate frequently.

to general anesthesia, in balanced anesthesia, as a primary drug for induction of anesthesia, and as a preoperative and postoperative analgesic.
USUAL ADULT DOSAGE: for induction, 0.05 to 0.1 mg/kg of body weight by slow I.V.; as an adjunct to general anesthesia, 0.002 to 0.05 mg/kg of body weight I.V., depending on the procedure and on other agents used. In balanced anesthesia, 0.05 to 0.1 mg/kg of body weight I.V. is administered. For preoperative analgesia, 0.05 to 0.1 mg I.M. is administered 30 to 60 minutes before surgery. For postoperative analgesia, 0.05 to 0.1 mg I.M. is administered, repeated in 1 to 2 hours if necessary.

ketamine hydrochloride (Ketalar). Used as an anesthetic in minor surgical or diagnostic procedures, ketamine is also used for induction or as the sole anesthetic agent in high-risk patients for whom cardiac or respiratory depressant drugs are contraindicated.
USUAL ADULT DOSAGE: for induction, 1 to 2 mg/kg of body weight I.V. or 5 to 10 mg/kg of body weight I.M.; for maintenance, adjusted according to the patient's vital signs and response.

lorazepam (Ativan). A benzodiazepine, lorazepam is used mainly to induce anterograde amnesia.
USUAL ADULT DOSAGE: 0.05 mg/kg of body weight (to a maximum of 4 mg) I.M. at least 2 hours before surgery or 0.044 mg/kg of body weight (to a maximum of 2 mg) I.V. at least 15 minutes before anesthesia.

methohexital sodium (Brevital). Methohexital is a barbiturate used where a short duration of action is either tolerable or desirable, as in anesthesia for electroshock therapy.

USUAL ADULT DOSAGE: for induction, 5 to 12 ml (50 to 120 mg) I.V. as a 1% solution (some sources recommend a 2-ml test dose before the induction dose); for maintenance, 2 to 4 ml (20 to 40 mg) I.V. as a 1% solution for 5 to 7 minutes of anesthesia. Some anesthesiologists prefer a continuous infusion of a 0.2% solution with the rate modulated to the patient's response.

thiamylal sodium (Surital). Thiamylal is an ultra-short-acting barbiturate used where a short duration of action is either tolerable or desirable, as in anesthesia for electroshock therapy.
USUAL ADULT DOSAGE: for induction of anesthesia, 3 to 5 mg/kg of body weight I.V. as a 2.5% solution (a 2-ml test dose is sometimes recommended). For maintenance, 2 to 4 ml (50 to 100 mg) I.V. as a 2.5% solution every 30 to 40 seconds until the desired effect is obtained; for use as a preoperative medication, 1 to 3 mg I.V. 30 minutes before surgery.

thiopental sodium (Pentothal Sodium). Thiopental is an ultra-short-acting barbiturate used where a short duration of action is either tolerable or desirable, as in anesthesia for electroshock therapy.
USUAL ADULT DOSAGE: for induction, 3 to 4 mg/kg of body weight I.V. or 2 to 3 ml (50 to 75 mg) every 30 to 40 seconds until the desired effect is obtained, as a 2.5% solution (a 1- to 3-ml test dose is sometimes given). For maintenance, 2 to 4 ml (50 to 100 mg), as required. Some anesthesiologists use continuous infusions of 0.2% to 0.4% solutions; the dose is adjusted by altering the infusion rate.

chlordiazepoxide hydrochloride (Librium). The original injectable benzodiazepine, chlordiazepoxide is used to increase the effects of other anesthetic agents.
USUAL ADULT DOSAGE: 50 to 100 mg I.M. 1 hour before surgery.

midazolam hydrochloride (Versed). Midazolam is a benzodiazepine used for preoperative sedation, induction of anesthesia, or maintenance of anesthesia in short procedures.
USUAL ADULT DOSAGE: for preoperative sedation, 0.07 to 0.08 mg/kg I.M. 1 hour before surgery. For induction, the dosage is titrated according to the patient's age and clinical status.

meperidine hydrochloride (Demerol). An opiate, meperidine is used as an adjunct to general anesthesia, as an obstetric anesthetic, and as a preoperative analgesic.
USUAL ADULT DOSAGE: as an adjunct, dose is dependent on patient response, delivered I.V. by repeated slow injection or continuous infusion; for obstetric anesthesia,

50 to 100 mg I.M. or S.C. at 1- to 3-hour intervals when contractions are regular; as a preoperative analgesic, 50 to 100 mg I.M. 30 to 90 minutes before surgery.

morphine sulfate. Like meperidine, the opiate morphine is used as an adjunct to general anesthesia, as an obstetric anesthetic, and as a preoperative analgesic.
USUAL ADULT DOSAGE: as an adjunct, dose is dependent on patient response, delivered I.V. by continuous infusion; for obstetric anesthesia, 10 mg I.M. or S.C.; as a preoperative analgesic, 5 to 12 mg I.M. or S.C.

sufentanil citrate (Sufenta). A derivative of fentanyl, sufentanil is approximately eight times as potent as its parent drug, but somewhat shorter-acting. Sufentanil is used as an adjunct to other anesthetics and in balanced anesthesia.
USUAL ADULT DOSAGE: as an adjunct, initially 1 to 2 mcg/kg of body weight I.V., depending on the procedure and other agents used, with supplemental doses of 10 to 25 mcg/kg of body weight I.V., as necessary; in balanced anesthesia, initially 8 to 30 mcg/kg of body weight I.V., with supplemental doses of 25 to 50 mcg/kg of body weight I.V., as necessary.

Drug interactions

Injection anesthetics interact with many other drugs. As with the inhalation anesthetics, the majority of these interactions require the nurse to monitor the patient's vital signs, airway, and level of consciousness. The opiates, barbiturates, and benzodiazepines and their interactions are covered in Chapter 26, Narcotic Agonist and Antagonist Agents; Chapter 30, Sedative and Hypnotic Agents; and Chapter 32, Antianxiety Agents. (For additional information on drugs that interact with droperidol, etomidate, and ketamine, see *Drug interactions: Injection anesthetics*.)

ADVERSE DRUG REACTIONS

Adverse reactions to the injection anesthetics are frequently extensions of their therapeutic effects.

Predictable reactions

CNS adverse reactions are most common after ketamine anesthesia; they include prolonged recovery, unpleasant dreams, irrational behavior, excitement, disorientation, delirium, and hallucinations.

Predictably, the barbiturates and ketamine cause respiratory depression. Airway reflex hyperactivity with hiccoughs, coughing, and muscle twitching and jerking is seen with thiopental and etomidate. Thiopental also depresses cardiac function and causes peripheral vasodilation, whereas ketamine increases heart rate, cardiac output, and blood pressure in patients who are not severely ill. The opiates sometimes cause changes in heart rate, including dysrhythmias. The rare circulatory failure and respiratory arrest seen with the benzodiazepines appear to be associated with too-rapid drug administration or concomitant narcotic administration. Phlebitis has been reported with diazepam administration.

Muscle rigidity and spasms follow administration of several of the injection anesthetics, including ketamine and the opiates; the reaction seems to be directly proportional to the rate of infusion. Fentanyl and ketamine may cause convulsions. Extrapyramidal manifestations are the most prominent adverse reactions to droperidol.

Etomidate and ketamine can cause nausea and vomiting. Excess salivation, tearing, shivering, and increased cerebrospinal fluid and intraocular pressure also are noted with ketamine. The only other major adverse reaction to etomidate is pain on administration, which can be avoided by rapid administration into a large vein or with use of a preoperative analgesic.

When the benzodiazepines and ketamine are given to pregnant women, fetal depression is often noted.

Unpredictable reactions

Rash and hypersensitivity reactions are infrequent with etomidate, the opiates, and the barbiturates; anaphylaxis has been reported with the barbiturates only. Extravasation of the barbiturates may cause neuritis and vasospasm. No unpredictable reactions have been reported for the benzodiazepines, ketamine, or droperidol.

NURSING IMPLICATIONS

Because the injection anesthetics vary greatly in their precautions, contraindications, and other considerations, the nurse must be aware of the following implications:

• Keep intravenous fluids and vasopressors available to treat hypotension as prescribed.
• Monitor the patient's vital signs frequently; advise the physician of changes immediately.
• Remember that barbiturate anesthetics are contraindicated when the patient's history includes porphyria, anemia, asthma or other respiratory disease, diabetes, drug use or dependence, hepatic impairment, hyperkinesis, hyperthyroidism, hypoadrenalism, depressive or suicidal tendencies, acute or chronic pain, renal impairment, cardiac disease, hypertension, or a debilitated state.

• Use dextrose 5% in water or normal saline solution to administer methohexital because it is incompatible with lactated Ringer's solution or acid drug solutions such as atropine.
• Note that benzodiazepine anesthetics are contraindicated in alcohol intoxication, coma or shock, myasthenia gravis, narrow-angle glaucoma, porphyria, and pulmonary impairment.
• Note that droperidol is contraindicated in patients with renal or hepatic impairment and in elderly or debilitated patients.
• Assess for extrapyramidal reactions to droperidol; call the physician if symptoms appear.
• Avoid Trendelenburg's position for patients who have received droperidol anesthesia because it may cause deeper anesthesia and respiratory arrest.
• Note that etomidate is contraindicated in patients who are pregnant, taking immunosuppressive drugs, experiencing sepsis, or having transplants.
• Note that ketamine is contraindicated in conditions in which blood pressure increases would be dangerous (heart failure, history of stroke, head trauma, or intracerebral mass or bleeding), alcohol abuse, cardiac failure, eye injuries that open the eye, hypertension, increased cerebrospinal fluid pressure, increased intraocular pressure, certain psychiatric disorders, and hyperthyroidism.
• Physically support the patient during administration of ketamine because the onset of action is rapid.
• Do not mix barbiturates and ketamine in the same syringe; they are chemically incompatible.
• Keep environmental stimulation to a minimum to prevent emergence reactions.
• Note that opiates are contraindicated in a patient with respiratory depression or diarrhea caused by antibiotic-associated colitis or poisoning. They should be used cautiously in a patient with asthma or respiratory impairment, cardiac dysrhythmias, a history of seizures, drug abuse or dependence, emotional instability or suicidal tendencies, gallbladder disease, recent GI surgery, head injury, increased intracranial pressure, intracranial lesions, hepatic impairment, hypothyroidism, prostatic hypertrophy, urethral stricture, recent urinary tract surgery, impaired renal function, and in patients who are extremely young, old, or debilitated.

SELECTED MAJOR DRUGS

General anesthetic agents

This chart summarizes the major inhalation and injection anesthetics currently in clinical use.

DRUG	MAJOR INDICATIONS	USUAL ADULT DOSAGES	NURSING IMPLICATIONS
Inhalation anesthetics			
enflurane	General anesthesia	Individualized and continuously monitored and altered throughout surgery	• Monitor the patient's postoperative pain because this drug has no residual analgesic effect. • Monitor the patient's blood pressure, heart rate and rhythm, and body temperature after surgery. • Caution the patient about residual psychomotor impairment lasting about 24 hours. • Advise the patient not to drink alcohol or use any other CNS depressants for 24 hours after anesthesia.
halothane	General anesthesia	Individualized and continuously monitored and altered throughout surgery	• Monitor the patient's postoperative pain because recovery and analgesia are brief. • Advise the patient to change positions cautiously because halothane causes vasodilation. • Monitor the patient's blood pressure, heart rate and rhythm, and body temperature after surgery. • Caution the patient about residual psychomotor impairment lasting about 24 hours. • Advise the patient not to drink alcohol or use any other CNS depressants for 24 hours after anesthesia. • Have atropine available to reverse bradycardia if prescribed. • Be aware that shivering is common during the recovery phase.
nitrous oxide	General anesthesia	Individualized and continuously monitored and altered throughout surgery	• Monitor the patient's blood pressure, heart rate and rhythm, and body temperature after surgery. • Caution the patient about residual psychomotor impairment lasting about 24 hours. • Advise the patient not to drink alcohol or use any other CNS depressants for 24 hours after anesthesia.
Injection anesthetics			
thiopental sodium	General anesthesia induction and maintenance	For induction, 3 to 4 mg/kg of body weight I.V. as a 2.5% solution; for maintenance, 50 to 100 mg I.V., as required	• Contraindicated in patients with severe hepatic dysfunction, hypersensitivity to barbiturates, porphyria, shock, or impending shock, and in patients for whom general anesthetics would be hazardous. • Administer with caution to debilitated patients and in those with asthma, respiratory obstruction, severe hypertension or hypotension, myocardial disease, congestive heart failure, severe anemia, or extreme obesity.

continued

General anesthetic agents continued

DRUG	MAJOR INDICATIONS	USUAL ADULT DOSAGES	NURSING IMPLICATIONS
thiopental sodium (continued)			• Monitor the patient's vital signs before, during, and after anesthesia. • Have resuscitative equipment and emergency drugs available. • Reduce postoperative nausea by having the patient fast before drug administration. • Advise the patient not to drink alcohol or use any other CNS depressants for 24 hours after anesthesia.
etomidate	General anesthesia induction and maintenance	For induction, 0.2 to 0.6 mg/kg of body weight I.V. over 30 to 60 seconds; for maintenance, smaller individual I.V. doses or a continuous I.V. infusion	• Contraindicated in labor and delivery, including cesarean sections. • Monitor the patient's vital signs before, during, and after anesthesia. • Have resuscitative equipment and drugs available.
ketamine	General anesthesia induction and maintenance	For induction, 1 to 2 mg/kg of body weight I.V. or 5 to 10 mg/kg of body weight I.M.; for maintenance, adjusted according to the patient's vital signs and response	• Contraindicated in patients with a history of stroke; in patients who would be endangered by a significant rise in blood pressure; in patients with significant hypertension or severe cardiac decompensation; and in surgery of the pharynx, larynx, or bronchial tree (unless used with muscle relaxants). • Administer with caution to chronic alcoholic patients, alcohol-intoxicated patients, and patients with elevated cerebrospinal fluid pressure. • Advise the patient to refrain from oral intake of food for at least 6 hours before elective surgery. • Because of rapid onset of action, physically support the patient during administration. • Do not mix barbiturates and ketamine in the same syringe; they are chemically incompatible. • Monitor the patient's vital signs before, during, and after anesthesia. • Assess cardiac function in patients with hypertension or cardiac depression. • Maintain a patent airway and have resuscitation equipment available. • Start supportive respirations if respiratory depression occurs; use mechanical support if possible rather than administering analeptics. • Keep verbal, tactile, and visual stimulation at a minimum to reduce emergence reactions.
fentanyl	Preoperative analgesia	0.05 to 0.1 mg I.M. 30 to 60 minutes before surgery	• Monitor the patient's vital signs frequently. • Assess the patient for respiratory depression. • Have narcotic antagonist drugs and resuscitation equipment available.
	Adjunct to general anesthesia	0.002 to 0.05 mg/kg of body weight I.V.	

COMBINATION ANESTHETICS

Two or more anesthetics used together to produce a desired anesthesia state constitute a combination anesthetic. The two types of combination anesthetics are neuroleptanesthesia and balanced anesthesia.

Neuroleptanalgesia is a state of altered consciousness free of pain, from administration of an opiate analgesic and a neuroleptic drug (an antipsychotic drug without hypnotic effects, such as a tranquilizer). When nitrous oxide is added, neuroleptanesthesia results: the patient is unconscious but can be roused easily if necessary. Neuroleptanesthesia is valuable when the patient's cooperation is necessary during surgery.

The drugs most frequently used in neuroleptanesthesia are droperidol and fentanyl, although diazepam and ketamine also have been combined with other opiates such as meperidine, morphine, and pentazocine.

Balanced anesthesia combines nitrous oxide with a more potent general anesthetic such as a barbiturate, an opiate analgesic, and a neuromuscular blocking agent. The opiate is given as premedication; the barbiturate and nitrous oxide induce anesthesia. The opiate is given again in small doses after induction to provide the desired level of analgesia. The neuromuscular blocking agent makes surgical manipulation easier, but it requires assisted ventilation.

A common balanced anesthesia combination includes fentanyl (opiate) and thiopental (barbiturate) with atropine (cholinergic blocking agent), nitrous oxide, and a neuromuscular blocking agent such as succinylcholine. Morphine may be used instead of fentanyl in patients for whom minimal cardiovascular effects are desired.

Naloxone, which reverses the effects of opiates, is used frequently at the end of surgery to reduce postoperative analgesia. The patient must be observed frequently until the analgesic is eliminated from the body.

When properly administered, balanced anesthesia minimizes cardiovascular effects, allows an early return of consciousness, and prevents postoperative nausea, vomiting, excitement, and pain.

Balanced anesthesia is contraindicated in patients who cannot tolerate FIO_2 of 25% to 40% or whose anemia limits the blood's oxygen-carrying capacity.

CHAPTER SUMMARY

This chapter explained the types of anesthesia and presented the inhalation and injection general anesthetics that produce them. Highlights include:

• General anesthesia may be induced with one or combined agents. These drugs are either volatile liquids or gases vaporized in oxygen and administered by inhalation or nonvolatile solutions administered by injection.

• The four stages of anesthesia encompass loss of consciousness, irregular respiration and increased autonomic activity, normal respiration and decreased reflexes and muscle tone, and loss of respiration and collapse of the circulatory system. Depth of anesthesia must be precisely controlled to permit successful surgery.

• Medications may be administered before surgery to sedate the patient, cause amnesia, or prevent undesirable conditions during surgery.

• Enflurane, halothane, isoflurane, methoxyflurane, and nitrous oxide are the inhalation anesthetics in current use.

• Three agents—droperidol, etomidate, and ketamine—are used solely as injection anesthetics. Other drugs used as injection anesthetics include the barbiturates and the benzodiazepines.

• Many drugs interact with inhalation and injection anesthetics; thus, caution is needed when medicating a patient after anesthesia.

• Anesthetics can be combined to produce balanced anesthesia or neuroleptanesthesia. Balanced anesthesia minimizes cardiovascular effects, allows an early return to consciousness, and prevents certain postoperative adverse effects. Neuroleptanesthesia produces an unconscious patient who can be roused easily.

• For all general anesthetics, the nurse must closely monitor the patient's vital signs, maintain airway patency, and observe the return to consciousness.

BIBLIOGRAPHY

Bennett, D.R., ed. *AMA Drug Evaluations*. Chicago: American Medical Association, 1983.

Cullen, D.J. "Anesthetic Depth and MAC," in *Anesthesia*. Miller, R.D., ed. New York: Churchill Livingstone, 1986.

Drug Information for the Health Care Provider, vol. 1. Bethesda, Md.: United States Pharmacopeial Convention, 1987.

Eger, E.I., II. "Uptake and Distribution of Inhaled Anesthetics," in *Anesthesia.* Miller, R.D., ed. New York: Churchill Livingstone, 1986.

Hansten, P.D. *Drug Interactions.* Philadelphia: Lea & Febiger, 1985.

Koblin, D.D., and Eger, E.I., II. "How Do Inhaled Anesthetics Work?" in *Anesthesia.* Miller, R.D., ed. New York: Churchill Livingstone, 1986.

Marshall, B.E., and Wollman, H. "General Anesthetics," in *Goodman and Gilman's The Pharmacological Basis of Therapeutics.* Gilman, A.G., et al., eds. New York: Macmillan Publishing Co., 1985.

Newberg, L.A. "Induction of General Anesthesia," in *Clinical Anesthesia Procedures of the Massachusetts General Hospital.* Labowitz, P.W., et al., eds. Boston: Little, Brown & Co., 1982.

Nursing88 Drug Handbook. Springhouse, Pa.: Springhouse Corp., 1988.

Smith, T.C., and Wollman, H. "History and Principles of Anesthesiology," in *Goodman and Gilman's The Pharmacological Basis of Therapeutics.* Gilman, A.G., et al., eds. New York: Macmillan Publishing Co., 1985.

CHAPTER 28

LOCAL AND TOPICAL ANESTHETIC AGENTS

OBJECTIVES

After reading and studying this chapter, you should be able to:

1. Differentiate between local and topical anesthetics.

2. Explain how a nerve block works.

3. Describe how pain impulses are conducted in the body.

4. Explain the mechanism of action of a local and a topical anesthetic.

5. Identify the major drug interactions, adverse reactions, and nursing implications for local and topical anesthetics.

6. Explain why vasoconstrictors are sometimes used with local anesthetics.

7. Explain why local anesthestics without preservatives must be used in certain nerve block procedures.

INTRODUCTION

Local and topical anesthetics are used to interrupt the transmission of pain impulses from peripheral nerves by causing a temporary loss of sensation in a limited area of the body. Local anesthetics must be injected to produce anesthesia, whereas topical anesthetics are applied directly to the skin or mucous membranes. Some local anesthetics can be used topically.

The physiology of pain

Pain is one of the brain's interpretations of signals sent from nerve endings in the skin and other tissues. These signals are transmitted by the peripheral and central nervous systems. Researchers are unclear about the characteristics of the stimuli that produce the cerebral interpretation of pain.

Nerve cells transmit an electrical impulse that results from differences in the intracellular and extracellular fluids and the semipermeable cell membrane that separates them. The cell membrane's surface normally carries a positive electrical charge produced by extracellular

sodium concentrations. Its interior carries a negative charge produced by potassium concentrations. When a painful stimulus activates the free nerve endings, the cell membrane's permeability temporarily changes, allowing sodium to enter the cell and potassium to leave. This shift in the content of intracellular and extracellular fluids, called depolarization, changes the cell membrane's electrical charge, allowing an electrical impulse to be transmitted.

The electrical current from one stimulated nerve cell is transmitted to adjoining cells, causing similar shifts in fluid content and electrical charge. These shifts continue toward the spinal cord, travel through the cord, and enter the brain.

After a nerve cell transmits the current, it pumps sodium out through the membrane and returns to its original condition, ready to send another impulse; this is repolarization.

Different types of nerves exist in different parts of the body. Large nerves, coated with a protein called myelin, relay pain messages in the spinal nerves of the central nervous system (CNS) and proximal parts of the autonomic nervous system. These myelinated nerves transmit information much faster than the smaller, uncoated nerves found in the autonomic nervous system. Both types of nerves may relay pain messages at the same time, but the patient will feel the two types of pain at slightly different times. The first sensation—a sharp, penetrating pain—occurs immediately after the stimulus and comes from the large, myelinated fibers. The second sensation—a burning pain—appears shortly after the first and is probably transmitted by small, nonmyelinated nerves.

Controlling pain

Some pain, such as that from a surgical or dental procedure, may be prevented. Other pain, such as that from a disease or injury, can be relieved only after it occurs. In either case, physicians can use local and topical anesthetics to manage the pain.

Blocking the pain pathway

Nerve endings transmit pain signals through the peripheral and central nervous systems to the brain. Administering an anesthetic at any point on this pain pathway can block the signal transmission and relieve pain. The illustration below shows several points where an anesthetic may be administered.

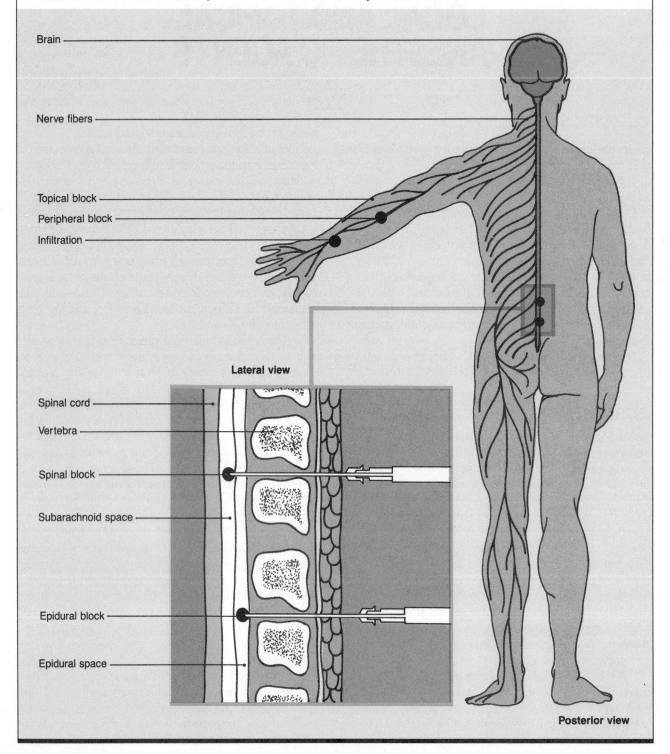

Brain

Nerve fibers

Topical block

Peripheral block

Infiltration

Lateral view

Spinal cord

Vertebra

Spinal block

Subarachnoid space

Epidural block

Epidural space

Posterior view

The field block

To produce a wall of anesthesia around a lesion or an incision, the physician can use a field block. Injections must be given to delineate the anesthetized area, or field. In the field block illustrated below, the arrows show the direction of the injections.

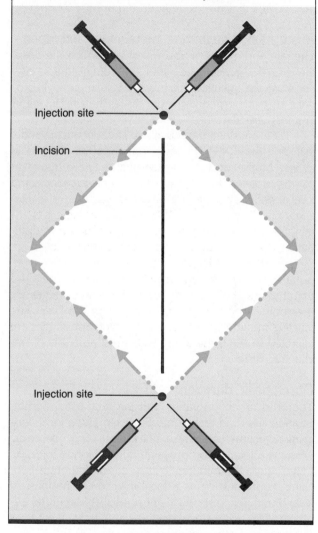

Injection site

Incision

Injection site

Local—and some topical—agents cause anesthesia by blocking a nerve, causing a temporary interruption in the transmission of impulses through nerves that come in contact with the anesthetic. When local anesthetics block large nerves that carry impulses from large areas of skin and tissue, they produce a wide field of anesthesia. This makes possible diagnostic procedures or treatments that otherwise would be intolerable.

For a summary of representative drugs, see *Selected major drugs: Local and topical anesthetic agents* on pages 459 and 460.

LOCAL ANESTHETICS

Many clinical situations require local anesthetics to prevent or relieve pain. These agents also offer a safe alternative to general anesthesia for elderly or debilitated patients.

The physician can administer local anesthetics in various places to block different groups of nerves. Local anesthetics can be used for local effects of course, but they also can be administered to function as central, peripheral, intravenous, regional, retrobulbar, or transtracheal nerve blocks. (See *Blocking the pain pathway* for an illustration of some of these areas.)

Local infiltration involves injecting a local anesthetic into an area that has been injured or that will undergo surgery. One particularly useful type of local infiltration is the field block, which uses several injections to produce a wall of anesthetic around a lesion or an incision. (See *The field block* for an illustration of this technique.)

A *central nerve block* can be given in the spinal, perineal, epidural, caudal, or lumbar area to produce anesthesia in the CNS. A *spinal* (or subarachnoid) *block* requires penetrating the second layer of the spinal cord (the arachnoid membrane at the base of the spine) and injecting a local anesthetic into the cerebrospinal fluid (CSF). A *saddle block* is a type of spinal anesthetic administered near the lower end of the spinal column in which the block is confined to the perineal or saddle area. An *epidural block* places the local anethestic next to the spinal cord's outermost covering, the dura mater. A *caudal block,* a special type of epidural block, is administered near the sacrum. A *lumbar block* is a type of epidural block administered low in the spinal column, near the lumbar vertebrae.

A *peripheral nerve block* places a local anesthetic next to nerve fibers in the peripheral nervous system. Paracervical and pudendal blocks are types of peripheral nerve blocks used in obstetric procedures. *Sympathetic block* is a peripheal nerve block of sympathetic nerve trunks that is used to relieve pain resulting from injury to the arms or legs and injury or disease of the internal organs. *Intercostal block* is a type of peripheral nerve block produced by injection of anesthetic near the intercostal nerves.

An *intravenous regional nerve block* is reserved for specific surgical procedures, such as hand or foot surgery. To prepare the patient for this type of anesthesia, the physician applies a tourniquet to the proximal end of the patient's arm or leg and then applies a pressure

Distribution of spinal anesthesia

In spinal anesthesia, the type of solution injected helps direct the anesthesia to the part of the spinal cord where it is needed. Hypobaric solutions—less dense than the cerebrospinal fluid (CSF)—rise above the point of injection. Isobaric solutions—of equal density as the CSF—remain near the injection site. Hyperbaric solutions—more dense than the CSF—tend to fall with gravity below the injection site.

The direction the drug travels also depends on the patient's position, movement, spine curvature, amount of subarachnoid space, and the drug dose and the drug solution's specific gravity and volume.

bandage to force blood away from the area to be anesthetized. Then, a local anesthetic solution is infused into the limb to provide anesthesia during the procedure.

A *retrobulbar nerve block* involves injecting a local anesthetic into nerves behind the eyeball in preparation for ocular surgery.

A *transtracheal nerve block* eliminates reflex activity that occurs from contact with mucous membranes during upper airway surgery. It requires inserting a needle through the cricoid cartilage into the larynx so that an anesthetic solution can be sprayed on the laryngeal mucosa.

History and source
Researchers discovered the local anesthetic properties of cocaine hydrochloride in 1880. They also found that an ester (a compound of alcohol and one or more organic acids) was an essential contributing agent to cocaine's local anesthetic action. Within 5 years, cocaine became widely used in ophthalmology, dentistry, and surgery that required nerve blocks. Although cocaine proved effective, it was short-acting, prone to cause tissue irritation and hypersensitivity reactions, unstable in solutions, and addictive. So in 1892, chemists began to search for a synthetic cocaine that would promote anesthesia without causing these problems. Their efforts produced procaine hydrochloride in 1906 and tetracaine hydrochloride in 1931. These compounds were useful but unstable, and they caused patient hypersensitivity and easily produced toxicity.

In 1946, the introduction of lidocaine hydrochloride marked the first use of an anesthetic with an amide (a compound containing radical NH_2 and radical CO)—rather than an ester—structure. This structure provided greater stability in solution, lengthened the duration of

action, and produced far fewer hypersensitivity reactions. As a result, amides soon became the most widely used local anesthetics.

PHARMACOKINETICS
Absorption of local anesthetics varies widely, yet distribution occurs throughout the body. Esters and amides undergo different types of metabolism, but both yield metabolites that are excreted in the urine.

Absorption, distribution, metabolism, excretion
The rate and extent of absorption varies with the dose, the drug's characteristics, and the administration site. For example, injection in a highly vascular area will produce faster absorption by more tissues than will injection in a less vascular area.

Local anesthetics are distributed throughout the body, including the CNS. They also can cross the placenta in inverse proportion to the extent that they are bound to plasma proteins. In other words, a highly protein-bound local anesthetic reaches the fetus in smaller quantities than a less protein-bound one. When a local anesthetic is administered in the spine, several factors influence its distribution. (See *Distribution of spinal anesthesia* for details.)

Ester anesthetics are metabolized into inactive components by esterase enzymes in the plasma. They also undergo metabolism in the liver. Amide anesthetics are metabolized by microsomal enzymes in the liver. The inactive metabolites of ester and amide anesthetics are excreted in the urine along with small amounts of unchanged drug.

Onset, peak, duration
The onset of action varies with the drug used, administration site, and technique. For example, a local lidocaine injection can cause anesthesia in 30 seconds, whereas a local chloroprocaine hydrochloride injection may require 10 minutes to take effect. Although lidocaine works quickly as a local injection, it requires at least 5 minutes to produce anesthesia with epidural administration. (See *Local anesthetics: Onset, peak, and duration* for further information.)

PHARMACODYNAMICS
Researchers believe that local anesthetics block the transmission of impulses across the nerve cell membranes.

Mechanism of action

Local anesthetics block nerve impulses at the point of contact in all kinds of nerves. They apparently accumulate and cause the nerve cell membrane to expand. As the membrane expands, the cell loses its ability to depolarize, which is necessary for transmission of impulses. Small nerves and nerves without myelin sheaths exhibit anesthetic effects before large, myelinated nerves.

Local anesthetics: Onset, peak, and duration

The onset of action, peak concentration levels, and duration of action of a local anesthetic varies with the drug used. The nurse can use the data below to predict when a drug's effect will wear off and to anticipate the patient's need for more medication.

DRUG	ONSET OF ACTION	DURATION OF ACTION
bupivacaine for dental anesthesia	2 to 10 minutes	2.7 to 3.5 hours
bupivacaine for epidural anesthesia	4 to 17 minutes	3 to 9 hours
bupivacaine for spinal anesthesia	1 minute	2 hours
chloroprocaine	6 to 12 minutes	30 to 60 minutes
dibucaine for spinal anesthesia	10 to 15 minutes	6 hours
etidocaine	2 to 8 minutes	4.5 to 13 hours
lidocaine	30 seconds to 5 minutes	75 to 140 minutes
mepivacaine	7 to 15 minutes	115 to 150 minutes
prilocaine	less than 2 minutes	1 to 2 hours
procaine	2 to 5 minutes	1 hour
propoxycaine	2 to 5 minutes	2 to 3 hours
tetracaine	15 minutes	1.5 to 3 hours

PHARMACOTHERAPEUTICS

Clinical indications for local anesthetics include preventing and relieving pain from a medical procedure, disease, or injury. Local anesthetics are used for severe pain that topical anesthetics or analgesics cannot relieve. Also, they are often preferred to general anesthetics for surgery in an elderly or debilitated patient or a patient with a disorder that affects respiratory function, such as chronic obstructive pulmonary disease or myasthenia gravis.

For some procedures, a local anesthetic with epinephrine should be used. (See *Local anesthetics and vasoconstrictors* on page 452 for additional information.) For some patients, an anesthetic that contains a preservative (for example, multidose mepivacaine hydrochloride) is used; however, this type of anesthetic would not be used for subarachnoid or epidural anesthesia because it can cause chronic inflammation of the arachnoid membrane.

bupivacaine hydrochloride (Marcaine). An amide anesthetic, bupivacaine is used in infiltration, spinal and epidural (caudal and lumbar) anesthesia, and peripheral and sympathetic nerve blocks. It is highly bound to plasma proteins, making its placental transfer the lowest of the local anesthetics. A single bupivacaine dose should not exceed 175 mg when administered alone or 225 mg when administered with epinephrine (1:200,000). The total daily dosage should not exceed 400 mg of solution without preservatives. Doses should usually not be repeated more than once every 3 hours. With long-acting bupivacaine, the dose should not need to be repeated for 12 hours when it is given with epinephrine. USUAL ADULT DOSAGE: for caudal anesthesia, 37.5 to 75 mg in 15 to 30 ml of a 0.25% solution or 75 to 150 mg in 15 to 30 ml of a 0.5% solution; for lumbar anesthesia, 25 to 50 mg in 10 to 20 ml of a 0.25% solution, 50 to 100 mg in 10 to 20 ml of a 0.5% solution, or 75 to 100 mg in 10 to 20 ml of a 0.75% solution; for infiltration, up to 175 mg in 70 ml of a 0.25% solution; for peripheral block in dental procedures, 9 to 18 mg in 1.8 to 3.6 ml of a 0.5% solution with 1:200,000 epinephrine; for a sympathetic block, 50 to 125 mg in 20 to 50 ml of a 0.25% solution; for peripheral block in other procedures, 12.5 to 25 mg in 5 to 70 ml of a 0.25% solution or 25 to 75 mg in 5 to 35 ml of a 0.5% solution; for retrobulbar block, 15 to 30 mg in 2 to 4 ml of a 0.75% solution; for spinal block in cesarean section, 7.5 to 10 mg in 1 to 1.4 ml of a 0.75% solution;

for spinal block in vaginal delivery, 6 mg in 0.8 ml of a 0.75% solution; for spinal block in lower extremity or perineal surgery, 7.5 mg in 1 ml of a 0.75% solution; for spinal block in lower abdominal surgery, 12 mg in 1.6 ml of a 0.75% solution.

chloroprocaine hydrochloride (Nesacaine, Nesacaine-CE). An ester anesthetic, chloroprocaine is used for infiltration anesthesia as well as for peripheral, sympathetic, and epidural blocks. A chloroprocaine dose should not exceed 800 mg when administered alone or 1 gram when administered with epinephrine.

USUAL ADULT DOSAGE: for caudal anesthesia, 300 to 500 mg in 15 to 25 ml of a 2% solution or 450 to 750 mg in 15 to 25 ml of a 3% solution repeated every 40 to 60 minutes; for lumbar and sacral epidural anesthesia, 40 to 50 mg per segment in 2 to 2.5 ml per segment of a 2% solution or 60 to 75 mg in 2 to 2.5 ml of a 3% solution repeated every 40 to 50 minutes using 40 to 120 mg less than initial dose of the 2% solution or 60 to 180 mg less of the 3% solution; for peripheral block at the brachial plexus, 600 to 800 mg in 30 to 40 ml of a 2% solution; for peripheral block in the digits, 30 to 80 mg in 3 to 4 ml of a 1% to 2% solution; for peripheral block in the retrobulbar area, 10 to 20 mg in 0.5 to 1 ml of a 2% solution; for peripheral block in the mandibular area, 40 to 60 mg in 2 to 3 ml of a 2% solution; for peripheral block in the paracervical area, 30 mg in 3 ml of a 1% solution at four sites; for peripheral block in the pudendal area, 200 mg in 10 ml of a 2% solution on each side. The dose for infiltration anesthesia varies with the clinical indication.

Local anesthetics and vasoconstrictors

Some local anesthetics are combined with vasoconstrictors, primarily epinephrine, to produce local vasoconstriction that controls local bleeding and reduces anesthetic absorption. Reduced absorption prolongs the anesthetic's action at the site and limits its distribution and CNS effects.

However, the use of epinephrine with local anesthetics is contraindicated in patients with cardiovascular disease and in elderly patients, because systemic absorption of this vasoconstrictor can cause tachycardia, palpitations, and chest pain. Epinephrine should also be avoided when anesthetizing an area with small vessels, such as the fingers, toes, nose, and ears, because ischemia and necrosis could result.

dibucaine hydrochloride (Nupercainal). An amide anesthetic, dibucaine is used primarily for spinal anesthesia. This extremely potent drug has a high risk of toxicity and must be used with caution.

USUAL ADULT DOSAGE: for subarachnoid anesthesia in the perineum and lower limbs, 2.5 to 5 mg in 0.5 to 1 ml of a 0.5% isobaric solution; for subarachnoid anesthesia in the lower abdomen, 5 to 7.5 mg in 1 to 1.5 ml of a 0.5% isobaric solution, or 6.7 to 10 mg in 10 to 15 ml of a 0.067% hypobaric solution; for subarachnoid anesthesia in the upper abdomen, 10 mg in 2 ml of a 0.5% isobaric solution, or 10 to 12 mg in 15 to 18 ml of a 0.067% hypobaric solution; for subarachnoid anesthesia in the legs, 4 mg in 6 ml of a 0.067% hypobaric solution; for subarachnoid anesthesia in the perineal area, 2.5 mg in 1 ml of a 0.25% hyperbaric solution with dextrose 5%, for subarachnoid anestheia in the pelvic structures, 5 mg in 2 ml of a 0.25% hyperbaric solution with dextrose 5%; for obstetric procedures, 2.5 mg in 1 to 2 ml of a 0.25% hyperbaric solution with dextrose 5%.

etidocaine hydrochloride (Duranest). An amide anesthetic, etidocaine is used for peripheral, sympathetic, and epidural anesthesia. Other uses include intravenous regional anesthesia, paracervical block in obstetrics, and intercostal nerve block. Highly protein-bound, etidocaine is less likely to cross the placenta than other agents. It is long-acting and potent with a high risk of toxicity. A dose of etidocaine should not exceed 300 mg when administered alone or 400 mg when administered with epinephrine.

USUAL ADULT DOSAGE: for caudal anesthesia, 50 to 150 mg in 10 to 30 ml of a 0.5% solution or 100 to 300 mg in 10 to 30 ml of a 1% solution; for lumbar anesthesia in cesarean section or intraabdominal, pelvic, or lower limb surgery, 100 to 300 mg in 10 to 30 ml of a 1% solution or 150 to 300 mg in 10 to 20 ml of a 1.5% solution repeated every 2 to 3 hours; for lumbar anesthesia in vaginal procedures, 50 to 150 mg in 10 to 30 ml of a 0.5% solution or 50 to 200 mg in 5 to 20 ml of a 1% solution repeated every 2 to 3 hours; for infiltration anesthesia, 5 to 400 mg in 1 to 80 ml of a 0.5% solution; for peripheral block, 25 to 400 mg in 5 to 80 ml of a 0.5% solution or 50 to 400 mg in 5 to 40 ml of a 1% solution repeated every 2 to 3 hours.

lidocaine hydrochloride [lignocaine] (Xylocaine Hydrochloride). An amide anesthetic, lidocaine may be used for infiltration anesthesia or for peripheral, sympathetic, epidural, or spinal blocks. It has also been used intra-

DRUG INTERACTIONS

Local anesthetic agents

Anesthetics with vasoconstrictors can interact with other drugs to produce serious adverse effects. The nursing implications for these and other local anesthetics are detailed below.

DRUG	INTERACTING DRUGS	POSSIBLE EFFECTS	NURSING IMPLICATIONS
bupivacaine, chloroprocaine, dibucaine, etidocaine, lidocaine, mepivacaine, prilocaine, procaine, propoxycaine, tetracaine	antimyasthenics	Worsen myasthenic symptoms	• Obtain a complete patient drug history to avoid interactions. • Monitor the patient for exacerbation of myasthenic symptoms, such as skeletal muscle weakness and fatigue.
	CNS depressants	Cause additive CNS depression	• Monitor the patient's vital signs and level of consciousness.
	guanadrel, guanethidine, mecamylamine	Cause severe hypotension and bradycardia	• Monitor the patient's blood pressure and pulse rate.
	monoamine oxidase inhibitors	Cause severe hypertension	• Monitor the patient's blood pressure.
	neuromuscular blocking agents	Increase or prolong blocking effects	• Expect the physician to reduce the dose of the neuromuscular blocking agent.
	opioid anesthetics	Decrease blood pressure, heart rate, and respiratory rate	• Observe the patient's vital signs closely.
ester anesthetics (chloroprocaine, procaine, propoxycaine, tetracaine)	cholinesterase inhibitors	Increase risk of toxicity	• Monitor the patient for signs of toxicity, such as increased heart rate.
	sulfonamides	Decrease antibacterial effects	• Expect the physician to increase the sulfonamide dose.
lidocaine	beta-adrenergic blocking agents, cimetidine	Increase risk of lidocaine toxicity	• Monitor for signs of lidocaine toxicity, such as confusion, restlessness, and tremors.
anesthetics with vasoconstrictors	inhalation anesthetics	Cause dysrhythmias	• Continuously monitor the EKG while the patient is receiving an inhalation anesthetic.
	tricyclic antidepressants, monoamine oxidase inhibitors, ergot oxytocics	Cause severe hypertension	• Monitor the patient's blood pressure, and alert the physician to any changes.
	phenothiazines, haloperidol, droperidol	Cause severe hypotension	• Monitor the patient's blood pressure, and alert the physician to any changes.

peritoneally to anesthetize the peritoneum and pelvic organs. A rapid-acting agent, lidocaine is somewhat toxic. In addition to its use as a local anesthetic, lidocaine is also effective as a topical anesthetic (see page 460) and as an antiarrhythmic (see Chapter 35, Antiarrhythmic Agents). A single adult dose of lidocaine should not exceed 4 to 5 mg/kg or 300 mg—whichever is lower. When given with epinephrine, lidocaine should not exceed 7 mg/kg or 500 mg.

USUAL ADULT DOSAGE: for caudal anesthesia in obstetric procedures, 200 to 300 mg in 20 to 30 ml of a 1% solution; for caudal anesthesia in surgical procedures, 225 to 300 mg in 15 to 20 ml of 1.5% solution; for lumbar analgesia, 250 to 300 mg in 25 to 30 ml of a 1% solution; for lumbar anesthesia, 225 to 300 mg in

15 to 20 ml of a 1.5% solution or 200 to 300 mg in 10 to 15 ml of a 2% solution; for thoracic anesthesia, 200 to 300 mg in 20 to 30 ml of a 1% solution; for infiltration percutaneous anesthesia, 5 to 300 mg in 1 to 60 ml of a 0.5% to 1% solution; for intravenous regional anesthesia, 50 to 300 mg in 10 to 60 ml of a 0.5% solution; for peripheral block in brachial areas, 225 to 300 mg in 15 to 20 ml of a 1.5% solution; for peripheral block in dental procedures, 20 to 100 mg in 1 to 5 ml of a 2% solution, possibly with epinephrine 1:100,000; for peripheral block in intercostal areas, 30 mg in 3 ml of a 1% solution; for peripheral block in paracervical areas, 100 mg in 10 ml of a 1% solution per side, repeated every 90 minutes as needed; for peripheral block in paravertebral areas, 30 to 50 mg in 3 to 5 ml of a 1% solution; for peripheral block in pudendal areas, 100 mg in 10 ml of a 1% solution per side; for sympathetic block in cervical areas, 50 mg in 5 ml of a 1% solution; for sympathetic block in lumbar areas, 50 to 100 mg in 5 to 10 ml of a 1% solution; for retrobulbar block, 120 to 200 mg in 3 to 5 ml of a 4% solution; for spinal block in vaginal delivery, 9 to 15 mg in 0.6 to 1 ml of a 1.5% solution with dextrose or 1 ml of a 5% solution with dextrose; for spinal block in cesarean section and deliveries requiring intrauterine manipulation, 75 mg in 1.5 ml of a 5% solution with dextrose; for spinal block in abdominal surgery, 75 to 100 mg in 1.5 to 2 ml of a 5% solution with dextrose; for transtracheal anesthesia, 80 to 120 mg in 2 to 3 ml of a 4% solution; the patient may also require topical administration to achieve anesthesia.

mepivacaine hydrochloride (Carbocaine, Isocaine). An amide anesthetic, mepivacaine is used for infiltration and epidural anesthesia, and for peripheral and sympathetic nerve blocks. Its toxicity resembles that of lidocaine. Because it is effective without a vasoconstrictor, mepivacaine is especially useful for elderly patients or those with cardiovascular disease. Ordinarily, a single dose or a series of doses used for one procedure should not exceed 400 mg. The total 24-hour dosage should not exceed 1 gram.

USUAL ADULT DOSAGE: for caudal anesthesia, 150 to 400 mg in 15 to 40 ml of a 1% solution, 150 to 375 mg in 10 to 27.5 ml of a 1.5% solution, or 200 to 400 mg in 10 to 20 ml of a 2% solution; for infiltration anesthesia, up to 400 mg in 40 ml of a 1% solution or 80 ml of a 0.5% solution; for peripheral block in brachial, cervical, intercostal, or pudendal areas, 50 to 400 mg in 5 to 40 ml of a 1% solution or 100 to 400 mg in 5 to 20 ml of a 2% solution; for peripheral block in a single dental site, 54 mg in 1.8 ml of a 3% solution or 36 mg in 1.8 ml of a 2% solution with levonordefrin 1:20,000; for peripheral block in the entire oral cavity, 270 mg in

9 ml of a 2% solution or 180 mg in 9 ml of a 3% solution with levonordefrin 1:20,000; for peripheral block in pain management, 10 to 50 mg in 1 to 5 ml of a 1% solution or 20 to 100 mg in 1 to 5 ml of a 2% solution; for peripheral block in the paracervical area, up to 100 mg in up to 10 ml of a 1% solution per side, repeated every 90 minutes, as needed; for peripheral block in the paracervical and pudendal (transvaginal) area, up to 150 mg in up to 15 ml of a 1% solution per side.

prilocaine hydrochloride (Citanest). An amide anesthetic, prilocaine is used for infiltration and nerve block anesthesia in dental procedures. Its use as a spinal anesthetic is declining because it can produce methemoglobinemia. The total amount given over 2 hours should not exceed 400 mg.

USUAL ADULT DOSAGE: for peripheral block in dental procedures, 40 to 80 mg in 1 to 2 ml of a 4% solution. Solution may contain 1:200,000 epinephrine; for infiltration anesthesia, 300 to 600 mg in 30 ml of a 1% or 2% solution; for caudal block, 200 to 300 mg in 20 to 30 ml of a 1% solution; for vaginal delivery, 400 to 600 mg in 20 to 30 ml of a 2% solution; for lumbar epidural, 150 to 500 mg in 15 to 25 ml of 1% or 2% solution.

procaine hydrochloride (Novocain). An ester anesthetic, procaine can produce infiltration and spinal anesthesia, and peripheral and sympathetic nerve block. In dental procedures, this drug is used for infiltration and nerve block. In other settings, it is administered I.V. to manage intractable pain. It is the least toxic local anesthetic.

USUAL ADULT DOSAGE: for infiltration anesthesia, 350 to 600 mg in 70 to 120 ml of 0.5% solution, or 140 to 280 mg in 50 to 100 ml of a 0.25% solution; for peripheral block, 500 mg in up to 100 ml of a 0.5% solution, 200 ml of a 0.5% solution, 100 ml of a 1% solution, or 50 ml of a 2% solution; for spinal block in the perineal area, 50 mg in 0.5 ml of a 10% solution; for spinal block in the perineum and legs, 100 mg in 1 ml of a 10% solution; for spinal block up to the costal margin, 200 mg in 2 ml of a 10% solution.

propoxycaine hydrochloride (Ravocaine). An ester anesthetic, propoxycaine is used in combination with procaine and levonordefrin, a vasoconstrictor. Its primary uses include infiltration and nerve block in dental procedures. During a procedure, the total dosage should not exceed 0.275 ml/kg.

USUAL ADULT DOSAGE: for peripheral block in a single dental site, 1.8 ml of a 0.4% solution with procaine 2% and levonordefrin 1:20,000 or norepinephrine 1:30,000 (43.2 mg total anesthetic); for peripheral block in the entire oral cavity, 9 ml of a 0.4% solution with procaine 2% and levonordefrin 1:20,000 or norepinephrine 1:30,000 (216 mg total anesthetic).

tetracaine hydrochloride (Pontocaine). An ester anesthetic, tetracaine is the most widely used spinal anesthetic. Its high lipid solubility allows it to be rapidly absorbed throughout the body.
USUAL ADULT DOSAGE: for low spinal or saddle block anesthesia and for obstetric procedures, 2 to 5 mg in 0.2 to 0.5 ml of a 1% solution with dextrose 10% or 2 to 4 mg in 1 to 2 ml of a 0.2% solution with dextrose; for spinal block in the perineal area, 5 mg in 0.5 ml of a 1% solution with CSF or dextrose 10% or 3 to 6 mg in 1 to 2 ml of a 0.3% solution with dextrose; for spinal block in the perineum and legs, 10 mg in 1 ml of a 1% solution with CSF or dextrose 10%; for spinal block up to the costal margin, 15 to 20 mg in 1.5 to 2 ml of a 1% solution with CSF; for spinal block in the lower abdomen, 9 to 12 mg in 3 to 4 ml of a 0.3% solution with dextrose; for spinal block in the upper abdomen, 15 mg in 5 ml of a 0.3% solution with dextrose.

Drug interactions

Local anesthetics produce few significant interactions with other drugs. Severe interactions can occur, however, when anesthetics with vasoconstrictors are given concurrently with certain other drugs. (See *Drug interactions: Local anesthetic agents* on page 453.) No interactions between local anesthetics and food occur.

ADVERSE DRUG REACTIONS

Adverse reactions to local anesthetics usually result from three main causes: overdose, hypersensitivity, and improper injection technique.

Predictable reactions

High plasma concentration levels of the local anesthetics can cause CNS and cardiovascular reactions. The dose-related CNS reactions to stimulation include anxiety, apprehension, restlessness, nervousness, disorientation, confusion, dizziness, blurred vision, tremors, twitching, shivering, and seizures. CNS depression follows, with drowsiness, unconsciousness, and respiratory arrest. The stimulatory phase may not occur, however, if the patient has received lidocaine or another amide anesthetic. Other CNS reactions may include nausea, vomiting, chills, miosis, and tinnitus. Cardiovascular reactions are also usually dose-related and typically occur with high plasma concentration levels of local anesthetics. These effects may include myocardial depression, bradycardia, cardiac dysrhythmias, hypotension, cardiovascular collapse, and cardiac arrest.

Local anesthetic solutions that contain vasoconstrictors such as epinephrine can also produce CNS and cardiovascular reactions, such as anxiety, dizziness, headache, restlessness, tremors, palpitations, tachycardia, anginal pain, and hypertension. Extreme reactions include pulmonary edema and ventricular fibrillation. Norepinephrine may be less likely to cause cardiac dysrhythmias, but it may cause reflex bradycardia. A burning sensation at the injection site also occurs commonly with these drugs. In rare cases, this reaction may be severe, producing pain, skin discoloration, tissue irritation, swelling, neuritis, neurolysis, and tissue necrosis and sloughing.

Unpredictable reactions

Ester anesthetics and preservatives in amide anesthetics can cause hypersensitivity reactions, with dermatologic symptoms, edema, status asthmaticus, or anaphylaxis. A patient who is hypersensitive to an *ester* anesthetic will probably not be sensitive to an *amide* agent, although the patient may be sensitive to other *ester* anesthetics. A local anesthetic solution with a preservative such as paraben, phenol, or bisulfite may produce chronic inflammation of the arachnoid membrane if it is used for subarachnoid or epidural anesthesia.

Local anesthetics may produce methemoglobinemia (the presence in the blood of oxidized hemoglobin that cannot combine irreversibly with oxygen). Although this reaction is rare, it occurs most frequently with prilocaine. Cyanosis may be the only symptom, but if it is severe, oxygen and methylene blue may be needed.

NURSING IMPLICATIONS

Although the physician or anesthetist will administer a local anesthetic, the nurse must prepare and closely observe the patient receiving it. (See *Typical reactions to local anesthetics* on page 456.) The nurse must be aware of these considerations:
• Keep drugs and resuscitation equipment on hand when a local anesthetic is administered parenterally.
• Expect to see a local anesthetic administered slowly and aspirated frequently to avoid intravascular injection.
• Position the patient properly for a subarachnoid block to prevent CSF leakage and headache and to ensure proper anesthetic distribution. Afterward, ensure that the patient stays flat in bed with the bed rails up for the time ordered by the physician.
• Be aware that spinal and epidural anesthesia are contraindicated in a patient with a serious CNS or spinal cord disease. Expect to use a peripheral nerve block for such a patient.
• Be aware that a central nerve block is also contraindicated in a patient with spinal deformities, bleeding from

Typical reactions to local anesthetics

After a local anesthetic is administered, a patient's sensory reactions usually diminish in the order shown in this chart. Sensory functions usually return in reverse order. But after epidural or spinal anesthesia, sympathetic activity does not necessarily return simultaneously with sensation.

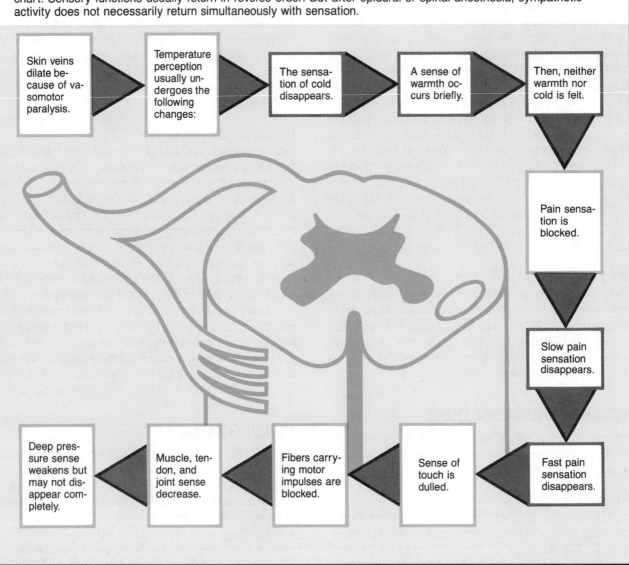

Skin veins dilate because of vasomotor paralysis.

Temperature perception usually undergoes the following changes:

The sensation of cold disappears.

A sense of warmth occurs briefly.

Then, neither warmth nor cold is felt.

Pain sensation is blocked.

Slow pain sensation disappears.

Fast pain sensation disappears.

Sense of touch is dulled.

Fibers carrying motor impulses are blocked.

Muscle, tendon, and joint sense decrease.

Deep pressure sense weakens but may not disappear completely.

a traumatic lumbar puncture, occlusive arterial disease, pernicious anemia with spinal cord involvement, severe anemia, cachexia, septicemia, bowel obstruction, chronic backache, chronic headache, a history of migraine, extreme youth or advanced age, high or low blood pressure, emotional instability, hysteria, nervous tension, bleeding tendencies, or hypofibrinogenemia.

• Anticipate the cautious use of an anesthetic with a vasoconstrictor in an elderly patient or a patient with cardiovascular disease.

• Be aware that anesthetics with vascoconstrictors are contraindicated in a patient undergoing anesthesia of the fingers, toes, ears, nose, or penis.

• Remember that a local anesthetic with a vasoconstrictor should not be used if a halogenated inhalation anesthetic may be used later.

• Observe the extremity that has undergone regional anesthesia. Check its peripheral pulse, color, and temperature, and compare it to the unaffected extremity.

• Do not pemit a patient taking a monoamine oxidase inhibitor or a tricyclic antidepressant to receive a local anesthetic with a vasoconstrictor, because severe hypertension may result.

• Help prevent maternal hypotension by elevating the patient's legs and positioning her on her left side after peripheral or epidural anesthesia.

• Expect to monitor the fetus, especially during paracervical block, to detect any fetal bradycardia and acidosis.

• Expect that anesthesia for an obstetric procedure will not be injected during a contraction or when the patient is bearing down, because excess absorption could result.

• Be aware that an anesthetic containing a vasoconstrictor may decrease the intensity of uterine contractions and prolong labor. It may also interact with an ergot-type oxytocic agent, causing severe hypertension.

• Remember that the effects of local anesthetics on fetal development have not yet been determined.

• Be aware that peripheral anesthesia may alter the dynamics of childbirth, increasing the need for forceps-assisted delivery.

• Remember that low spinal (saddle block) and caudal anesthesia are contraindicated in a psychologically unsuited patient who is unable to remain quiet or maintain the position and in a patient with pelvic disproportion, abruptio placentae, unengaged fetal head, or placenta previa, unless a cesarean section will be done.

• Anticipate avoidance of a central nerve block when intrauterine manipulations are necessary.

• Ensure that the gag reflex has returned before feeding a patient whose throat has been anesthetized.

• Discard partially used vials of local anesthetics that do not contain preservatives.

• Expect to see a test dose given for an ester anesthetic used for an epidural block before the full dose is administered.

• Anticipate cautious use of an amide anesthetic in a patient with hepatic impairment, because the agent must be metabolized in the liver.

• Teach the patient who has received a spinal anesthetic about the importance of remaining in a supine position.

• Teach all patients who have received local anesthetics to protect numb areas until sensation returns.

TOPICAL ANESTHETICS

Topical anesthetics are applied directly to the skin or mucous membranes. Some of the injectable local an-

esthetics, such as dibucaine, lidocaine, and tetracaine, are also effective topically. All these agents may be used to prevent or relieve minor pain.

Tetracaine and proparacaine hydrochloride are used as topical ophthalmic anesthetics. (See Chapter 79, Ophthalmic Agents, for information about their uses in ophthalmology.) Benzocaine is used in combination with other agents in several otic preparations. (See Chapter 80, Otic Agents, for further information.)

History and source

Benzyl alcohol, clove oil, and menthol are among the oldest topical anesthetics. Benzocaine and butacaine sulfate are newer agents that are closely related to the local anesthetics. With a slightly different chemical structure, butamben picrate, dyclonine hydrochloride, and pramoxine hydrochloride also share the local anesthetics' mechanism of action.

Dichlorotetrafluoroethane and ethyl chloride provide anesthesia by temporarily freezing the skin.

PHARMACOKINETICS

Topical application of these anesthetics does not produce significant systemic absorption, except for mucosal application of cocaine. However, systemic absorption may occur with frequent or high-dose application to the eye or large areas of burned or injured skin. Tetracaine and other esters are extensively metabolized in the blood and, to a lesser extent, in the liver. Dibucaine, lidocaine, and other amides are primarily metabolized in the liver. Both types of topical anesthetics are excreted in the urine.

Topical anesthetics have a rapid onset of action, producing anesthesia in a few minutes. However, the peak concentration levels and duration of action vary with the drug used. For example, the effects of cocaine peak in 2 to 5 minutes and last for 30 minutes to 2 hours, but dibucaine's activity peaks in less than 15 minutes and lasts for 2 to 4 hours. Dyclonine reaches peak effectiveness in less than 10 minutes and has a duration of action of less than 1 hour. With lidocaine administration, peak effects occur in 2 to 5 minutes, and the anesthetic action lasts for 30 minutes to 1 hour. Pramoxine's activity peaks in 3 to 5 minutes. Tetracaine's activity peaks in 3 to 8 minutes and lasts for 30 minutes to 1 hour.

PHARMACODYNAMICS

Benzocaine, butacaine, butamben, cocaine, dyclonine, and pramoxine produce topical anesthesia by blocking transmission of nerve impulses. They accumulate in the nerve cell membrane, causing it to expand and lose its ability to depolarize, thus blocking transmission of impulses.

The aromatic compounds, such as benzyl alcohol and clove oil, appear to stimulate the nerve endings. Clove oil may stimulate the nerve endings by counter-irritation that interferes with pain perception.

Ethyl chloride and dichlorotetrafluoroethane superficially freeze the tissue, stimulating the cold sensation receptors and blocking the nerve endings in the frozen area.

PHARMACOTHERAPEUTICS

Topical anesthetics relieve or prevent pain—especially minor burn pain—and itching and irritation. They are also used to anesthetize an area before an injection is given and to numb mucosal surfaces before a tube, such as an indwelling (Foley) catheter, is inserted. In a spray or solution, a topical anesthetic is also used to alleviate sore throat or mouth pain.

benzocaine (Americaine, Anbesol, Ora-Jel, Solarcaine). An ester anesthetic, benzocaine is active topically only. Available in ointments, creams, and sprays in concentrations of 0.5% to 20%, it is used to treat sunburn pain, pruritus, and hemorrhoidal itching and pain. Benzocaine is also available as a jelly, syrup, or lozenge for toothache or mouth sores.
USUAL ADULT DOSAGE: apply locally b.i.d. or t.i.d.

benzyl alcohol. Derived from balsam, this clear, colorless, oily liquid is the base of ester local anesthetics. It is used topically to relieve itching.
USUAL ADULT DOSAGE: 5% gel apply locally t.i.d. or q.i.d.

butacaine sulfate. An ester anesthetic, butacaine is used topically as a 4% ointment to relieve pain associated with dental appliances, such as braces.
USUAL ADULT DOSAGE: apply as needed for temporary relief of dental pain.

butamben picrate (Butesin Picrate). Butamben is available as a 1% anesthetic ointment for skin irritations and minor burns.

USUAL ADULT DOSAGE: apply thinly on painful or denuded lesions.

clove oil. An aromatic oil distilled from clover, clove oil's major active ingredient is eugenol; it is used in dentistry to decrease the sensation of pain.
USUAL ADULT DOSAGE: apply as needed for temporary relief of dental pain.

cocaine hydrochloride. This Controlled Substance, Schedule II drug, the original ester anesthetic, may be applied to the mucosa to provide topical anesthesia during head and throat surgery. It also acts as a vasoconstrictor.
USUAL ADULT DOSAGE: A typical concentration is the 4% solution applied locally.

dibucaine hydrochloride (Nupercainal). This topical anesthetic may be used to treat painful skin and mucosal conditions, such as sunburn, abrasions, and hemorrhoids.
USUAL ADULT DOSAGE: 0.5% to 1% lotion, cream, or ointment applied locally several times a day.

dichlorotetrafluoroethane (Freon 114, Frigiderm). A clear, colorless gas, this topical agent anesthetizes by freezing. It may be used during minor surgical procedures or dermabrasion.
USUAL ADULT DOSAGE: apply as needed during procedure to produce satisfactory skin freezing.

dyclonine hydrochloride (Dyclone). A ketone anesthetic, dyclonine may be useful for a patient who is hypersensitive to ester or amide anesthetics. This topical anesthetic may be used to relieve surface pain and itching and to anesthetize mucous membranes in endoscopic or cystoscopic procedures.
USUAL ADULT DOSAGE: 0.5% or 1% solution applied locally as needed.

ethyl chloride. Like dichlorotetrafluoroethane, ethyl chloride freezes the skin to produce anesthesia. It can reduce skin irritation, produce local anesthesia for minor operative procedures, and relieve the pain of insect stings, burns, and myofascial and visceral pain syndromes.
USUAL ADULT DOSAGE: for skin irritation, spray affected area once or twice from a distance of 24 inches (61 cm) and repeat as needed; for local anesthesia, apply a fine spray from a distance of 12 inches (30 cm); for other indications, apply the smallest dosage possible to produce the desired effect.

Local and topical anesthetic agents

This chart summarizes the major local and topical anesthetics currently in clinical use.

DRUG	MAJOR INDICATIONS	USUAL ADULT DOSAGES	NURSING IMPLICATIONS
Local anesthetics			
bupivacaine	Caudal anesthesia	37.5 to 150 mg	• Keep drugs and equipment for resuscitation on hand during anesthetic administration.
	Infiltration anesthesia	Up to 175 mg	• Anticipate frequent aspiration to avoid intravascular administration.
	Peripheral anesthesia	12.5 to 25 mg	• Prevent maternal hypotension in peripheral or epidural block by elevating the patient's legs and positioning her on her left side.
	Retrobulbar anesthesia	15 to 30 mg	• Expect to see cautious use of an anesthetic with a vasoconstrictor in an elderly patient or a patient with cardiovascular disease.
	Spinal anesthesia	6 to 12 mg	• Liver disease may prolong the half-life of bupivacaine. • Do not use a solution with preservatives for epidural or spinal block. • Discard partially used vials of anesthetic without preservatives. • The 0.75% bupivacaine solution is no longer recommended in obstetric anesthesia.
chloroprocaine	Caudal anesthesia	300 to 500 mg	• Anticipate hypersensitivity testing before chloroprocaine administration.
	Epidural anesthesia	40 to 75 mg/segment	• Chloroprocaine is contraindicated for a patient who is hypersensitive to any other ester anesthetics.
	Infiltration anesthesia	Variable	
	Peripheral anesthesia	10 to 800 mg	
lidocaine	Caudal anesthesia	200 to 300 mg	• Liver disease may prolong the half-life of lidocaine.
	Infiltration anesthesia	5 to 300 mg	• Solutions with epinephrine should be used cautiously in patients with cardiovascular disease.
	Peripheral anesthesia	20 to 300 mg	• Keep drugs and equipment for resuscitation on hand during anesthetic administration.
	Spinal anesthesia	9 to 120 mg	
procaine	Infiltration anesthesia	350 to 600 mg	• Anticipate hypersensitivity testing before procaine administration.
	Peripheral anesthesia	500 mg	• Procaine is contraindicated for a patient who is hypersensitive to any other ester anesthetic.
	Spinal anesthesia	50 to 200 mg	
Topical anesthetics			
benzocaine	Dermal anesthesia, mucosal anesthesia	Apply locally b.i.d. or t.i.d.	• Benzocaine is contraindicated for any patient who is allergic to procaine or PABA (an ingredient in many sunscreens). • Use the smallest dose necessary for relief. • Discontinue use if a rash or irritation occurs. • Clean and dry the rectal area before applying benzocaine. • Avoid contact with the eyes.
cocaine	Mucosal anesthesia	4% solution applied locally	• Cocaine is contraindicated for a patient who is hypersensitive to any other ester anesthetic.

continued

SELECTED MAJOR DRUGS

Local and topical anesthetics continued

DRUG	MAJOR INDICATIONS	USUAL ADULT DOSAGES	NURSING IMPLICATIONS
cocaine (continued)			• Cocaine is used intraoperatively on oral, laryngeal, and nasal mucosa. • Administer cocaine cautiously to a patient with hypertension, cardiovascular disease, or hyperthyroidism.
dibucaine	Dermal anesthesia, mucosal anesthesia	Apply 0.5% to 1% lotion, cream, or ointment locally several times a day	• Keep dibucaine out of the reach of children to prevent accidental poisoning. • Clean and dry the rectal area before applying dibucaine.
ethyl chloride	Dermal anesthesia	Spray affected area once or twice from a distance of 12 to 24 inches (30 to 61 cm)	• Do not apply ethyl chloride to broken skin or mucosa. • Avoid inhalation of ethyl chloride. • Ethyl chloride is highly flammable.
lidocaine	Dermal anesthesia, mucosal anesthesia	Apply as 2% to 5% gel or ointment, or 15 ml viscous liquid as needed	• Administer lidocaine with caution in an elderly patient or a patient with large areas of broken skin or mucous membranes. • After anesthetizing the mouth or pharynx with lidocaine, have the patient wait 1 hour before eating.
tetracaine	Dermal anesthesia, mucosal anesthesia	Apply 0.5% ointment or 1% cream, as needed, up to maximum of 28 grams/day	• Tetracaine is contraindicated for a patient who is allergic to procaine or PABA. • Clean and dry the rectal area before applying tetracaine. • Tetracaine is contraindicated for a patient with hypersensitivity to any other ester anesthetic.

lidocaine (Xylocaine). Available as lidocaine or lidocaine hydrochloride, this anesthetic is usually used on mucous membranes as a gel or viscous liquid to ease the discomfort caused by instruments used during urethral catheterization or gastroscopy. It is also used in cancer patients to relieve stomatitis, although it decreases the gag reflex and the sense of taste.
USUAL ADULT DOSAGE: apply 2% to 5% gel or ointment or 15 ml of viscous liquid as needed.

menthol. A benzyl alcohol derivative, menthol's anesthetic action is used to relieve pruritus. It is available in creams and lotions in varying concentrations.
USUAL ADULT DOSAGE: apply 0.25% or 2% lotion or cream as needed for a total of 750 mg/day for pain relief or 600 mg in 6 hours for procedural preparation.

pramoxine hydrochloride (Tronothane). This topically administered local anesthetic is used as a 1% cream or lotion to ease minor irritations of the skin and mucous membranes.
USUAL ADULT DOSAGE: apply 1% cream or jelly every 3 to 4 hours as needed.

tetracaine (Pontocaine). This anesthetic is available as tetracaine or tetracaine hydrochloride in ointment (0.5%) and cream (1%) forms. It is usually used to relieve minor skin and mucous membrane irritation.
USUAL ADULT DOSAGE: apply 0.5% ointment or 1% cream as needed up to a maximum of 28 grams/day.

Drug interactions
Few interactions with other drugs occur with topical anesthetics because they are not well absorbed systemically. The ester derivatives, such as tetracaine, can interact with cholinesterase inhibitors, increasing the risk of anesthetic toxicity. They may also interact with sulfonamide agents, impairing their effectiveness. To avoid these interactions, the nurse must obtain a complete patient drug history. When used topically, lidocaine can interact with beta-adrenergic blocking agents and cimetidine, increasing the risk of lidocaine toxicity. When these medications must be given concurrently, the nurse must monitor the patient for signs of toxicity, such as confusion, restlessness, and tremors.

No interactions between the topical anesthetics and food have been described.

ADVERSE DRUG REACTIONS

Predictable reactions to topical anesthetics vary with the chemical class. Agents that are used as local anesthetics may produce CNS and cardiovascular reactions. (See the section on adverse drug reactions under local anesthetics in this chapter on page 455.) Benzyl alcohol can cause topical reactions, such as skin irritation. Refrigerants such as ethyl chloride and dichlorotetrafluoroethane may produce frostbite in the application area.

Any topical anesthetic can cause a hypersensitivity reaction that may include a rash, itching, hives, swelling of the mouth and throat, and breathing difficulty.

NURSING IMPLICATIONS

Topical anesthetics are widely used and require the nurse's attention to these considerations:
• Discourage prolonged use of topical anesthetics without medical supervision.
• Use the lowest dose necessary for relief of symptoms.
• Be aware that a child or elderly patient may require a smaller dose.
• Use benzocaine with caution in a child because it can cause methemoglobinemia.
• Be aware that benzocaine and tetracaine are contraindicated in a patient who is allergic to procaine or para-aminobenzoic acid (PABA), an ingredient in many sunscreen products.
• Before applying an anesthetic rectally, clean and dry the area thoroughly.
• Avoid contact with eyes.
• Discontinue use if a rash develops.
• Keep dibucaine out of the reach of children to prevent ingestion and accidental poisoning.
• Be aware that dyclonine is contraindicated in cystoscopy after an intravenous pyelogram. Dyclonine will produce a precipitate with the iodine in the contrast material.
• Do not apply a refrigerant to broken skin or mucous membranes.
• Advise the patient whose oropharyngeal mucosa has been anesthetized to delay eating until sensation returns.

CHAPTER SUMMARY

Local and topical anesthetics can interrupt pain impulses at their point of contact with nerves. Local anesthetics are usually injected, but some are applied topically; topical anesthetics are applied directly to skin or mucous membranes. Here are the chapter highlights:
• Local anesthetics produce their effect in a limited body area, but they are distributed throughout the body.
• When applied to the skin or mucous membranes, topical anesthetics can relieve minor irritation or prevent discomfort during diagnostic testing or other procedures.
• When injected near nerves, local anesthetics can produce nerve block anesthesia for pain relief or surgery.
• Most topical anesthetics are applied to the surface of the skin or mucous membranes. In special formulations, they may also be used in the eyes and ears.
• Hypersensitivity reactions may occur with local and topical anesthetic agents, especially with ester anesthetics.

BIBLIOGRAPHY

American Hospital Formulary Service. *Drug Information 87*. McEvoy, G.K., et al., eds. Bethesda, Md.: American Society of Hospital Pharmacists, 1987.

American Medical Association. *Drug Evaluations*, 6th ed. Philadelphia: W.B. Saunders Co., 1986.

Foye, W.O., ed. *Principles of Medical Chemistry*. Philadelphia: Lea & Febiger, 1974.

Gilman, A.G., et al., eds. *Goodman and Gilman's The Pharmacological Basis of Therapeutics*, 7th ed. New York: Macmillan Publishing Co., 1985.

Guyton, A.C. *Textbook of Medical Physiology*. Philadelphia: W.B. Saunders Co., 1976.

Hansten, P.D. *Drug Interactions*. Philadelphia: Lea & Febiger, 1985.

Kastrup, E.K., ed. *Facts and Comparisons*. St. Louis: Facts and Comparisons Division, J.B. Lippincott Co., 1986.

Labat, A.J. *Regional Anesthesia*. St. Louis: Warren H. Green, Inc., 1985.

Mangini, R.J., ed. *Drug Interaction Facts*. St. Louis: J.B. Lippincott Co., 1987.

Nursing88 Drug Handbook. Springhouse, Pa.: Springhouse Corp., 1988.

Swinyard, E.A. "Local Anesthetics." In *Remington's Pharmaceutical Sciences*, 17th ed. Easton, Pa.: Mack Publishing Co., 1985.

USPDI. *Drug Information for the Health Care Provider*, Vol. 1. Bethesda, Md.: United States Pharmacopeial Convention, 1987.

DRUGS TO ALTER PSYCHOGENIC BEHAVIOR AND PROMOTE SLEEP

The pharmacologic treatment of psychiatric disorders is relatively new. The discovery of chlorpromazine and its value in treating schizophrenia did not occur until the 1950s. Before this, the psychiatric hospital stay was lengthy, with little to offer the patient but custodial care. With the discovery of phenothiazines, the prognosis for schizophrenia improved dramatically. Patients were able to leave hospitals sooner, live in the community, and take part in other therapies previously unavailable to them. The role of the nurse as patient custodian was redefined; emphasis was placed instead on the therapeutic nurse-patient relationship.

In the past 30 years, newer drugs have become available for various psychiatric disorders. Antianxiety agents, such as diazepam, and antidepressant agents, such as amitriptyline, are prescribed commonly. Although these medications sometimes are used alone, psychiatric drugs usually are intended to be used with other therapeutic modalities, such as the combination of pharmacotherapy with psychotherapy.

Chapter 29
Cerebral Stimulating Agents
Chapter 29 discusses agents that stimulate the central nervous system (CNS), including amphetamines, anorexiants, psychotherapeutic stimulants, cocaine, and CNS and respiratory stimulants. The clinical uses of these agents in treating narcolepsy, attention deficit disorder, obesity, and pain are detailed.

Chapter 30
Sedative and Hyponotic Agents
Three main classes of sedative and hypnotic agents are explored in Chapter 30. The chapter begins with an overview of the physiology of sleep, the four major categories of sleep disorders, and the process for assessing sleep and rest habits. Then the clinical uses of these agents are described. The numerous nonpharmacologic nursing interventions that are adjuncts to drug therapy in treating sleep disorders also are presented. Two dietary sources that promote relaxation and sleep are explored.

Chapter 31
Antidepressant and Antimanic Agents
Chapter 31 presents the characteristics and pathophysiology of such affective disorders as depression and mania. It then discusses the major classes of agents used to treat those disorders, including tricyclic antidepressants, second-generation antidepressants, monamine oxidase inhibitors, and lithium. The rationales for the specific selection of one drug over another drug also are discussed, as are nursing implications and patient education needs.

Chapter 32
Antianxiety Agents
The huge degree to which the population suffers anxiety is discussed in the introduction to Chapter 32. The symptoms and classifications of anxiety also are reviewed. Then the major drug classes used to treat anxiety are presented, including benzodiazepines, buspirone, barbiturates, antihistamines, and beta blockers. Rationales for the selection of specific drugs and their major adverse reactions are detailed. The nursing implications related to drug administration and patient education are also included.

Chapter 33
Antipsychotic Agents
Chapter 33 discusses antipsychotic, or neuroleptic, agents and their clinical uses. The chapter begins with a brief review of the anatomy and physiology of some areas of the CNS, including the pyramidal and extrapyramidal tracts and the limbic system. Then the major classes of neuroleptic drugs are discussed in terms of their pharmacokinetic, pharmacodynamic, and pharmacotherapeutic properties. Major emphasis is placed on early recognition of neurologic adverse reactions, such as extrapyramidal symptoms and tardive dyskinesia, that may accompany the use of these agents. Nursing assessment information is also detailed.

Glossary

Affective disorder: mood disturbance in the presence of an elated or depressive state.

Akathisia: condition characterized by restlessness and agitation; feelings range from inner disquiet to inability to sleep or sit still.

Amnesia: loss of memory.

Anorexiant: agent that produces a decrease in appetite; also called anorexigenic.

Anticonvulsant: agent that prevents or relieves convulsions.

Antidepressant: agent that prevents or relieves depression.

Antiemetic: agent that prevents or alleviates nausea and vomiting.

Antimanic: agent that prevents or diminishes mania.

Antipsychotic: agent that prevents or diminishes psychosis.

Anxiety: feeling of apprehension, uncertainty, and fear.

Anxiolytic: agent that prevents or diminishes anxiety.

Ataxia: impaired ability to coordinate movement.

Attention deficit disorder (ADD): state of minimal brain dysfunction characterized by hyperkinesis, lack of concentration, and decreased learning ability.

Autism: mental disorder characterized by extreme withdrawal and abnormal absorption in fantasy.

Deamination: chemical removal of an amino group, NH_2, from an organic molecule.

Delirium: acute alteration in consciousness characterized by confusion, disorientation, physical restlessness, incoherence, and, often, delusions or hallucinations.

Dementia: progressive mental or intellectual decline.

Depression: emotional dejection characterized by an absence of cheerfulness and hope disproportionate to circumstances.

Dyskinesia: impaired power of voluntary movement causing fragmentary or incomplete movements.

Dystonia: disordered muscle tone.

Euphoria: exaggerated sense of well-being.

Gamma-aminobutyric acid (GABA): inhibitory neurotransmitter secreted by nerve terminals in the spinal cord, the cerebellum, the basal ganglia, and many areas of the cerebral cortex.

Gilles de la Tourette's syndrome: disease characterized by motor incoordination, the meaningless repetition of words, and the use of obscene language.

Glucuronic acid conjugation: combination of glucuronic acid with a dry molecule to produce a more water-soluble, less active, or less toxic substance.

Hydroxylation: oxidative reaction between a hydroxyl (OH) radical and another substance to form a more water-soluble substance.

Hyperkinesis: abnormally increased motor function or activity.

Hypersomnia: uncontrollable drowsiness; condition characterized by periods of deep, long sleep.

Hypnotic: agent that induces sleep.

Hypochondriasis: morbid anxiety about health, often associated with a simulated disease.

Insomnia: inability to sleep; abnormal wakefulness.

Limbic system: entire basal system of the brain responsible for controlling an individual's emotional behavior and drive.

Mania: mood disorder characterized by an expansive emotional state, elation, hyperirritability, overtalkativeness, a flight of ideas, and increased motor activity.

Manic-depressive: bipolar mental disorder characterized by fluctuations between mania and depression.

Monoamine oxidase: enzyme in the nerve endings that breaks down catecholamines.

Narcolepsy: condition characterized by an uncontrollable desire to sleep or by sudden attacks of sleep.

Narcoleptic: agent that acts to produce narcolepsy.

Narcosis: reversible condition characterized by stupor or insensibility produced by drugs.

Obsessive-compulsive: mental disorder characterized by the need to perform certain acts repetitively or to carry out certain rituals.

Panic: extreme, unreasoned anxiety or fear.

Parasomnia: state of no response to stimuli, verbal or mental; dysfunction usually associated with sleep.

Phobia: persistent, abnormal dread or fear.

Pseudoparkinsonism: state resembling Parkinson's syndrome and characterized by muscular rigidity, immobile facies, tremor that disappears with volitional movement, shuffling gait, and salivation.

Psychosis: mental disorder characterized by loss of contact with reality and derangement of personality.

Schizophrenia: group of severe emotional disorders characterized by delusions, hallucinations, loss of contact with reality, and bizarre or regressive behavior.

Sedative: agent that allays excitement and produces drowsiness.

continued

Glossary continued

Serotonin: neurotransmitter secreted by the raphe nuclei that inhibits pain pathways and helps control an individual's mood; it may induce sleep.

Substantia nigra: layer of pigmented gray matter; area for the secretion of gamma-aminobutyric acid.

Tachyphylaxsis: decreasing responses to consecutive injections of medication made at short intervals.

Tardive dyskinesia: neurologic syndrome characterized by involuntary movements, such as sucking and smacking of the lips, lateral jaw movements, and darting of the tongue; athetoid movements and postures of the extremities, trunk, and neck may be present also.

Nursing diagnoses

Several nursing diagnoses are appropriate for planning care for patients being treated with the drugs discussed in Unit Six. Those nursing diagnoses include:

- Alterations in family process related to psychogenic pathology or drug therapy
- Alterations in health maintenance related to psychogenic pathology or drug therapy
- Alterations in nutrition: less than body requirements, related to psychogenic pathology or drug therapy
- Alterations in nutrition: more than body requirements, related to psychogenic pathology
- Alterations in thought processes related to psychogenic pathology or drug therapy
- Anxiety related to psychogenic pathology, drug therapy, or life-style changes
- Disturbance in self-concept related to psychogenic pathology, drug therapy, or life-style changes
- Diversional activity deficit related to psychogenic pathology or drug therapy
- Dysfunctional grieving related to psychogenic pathology, drug therapy, or life-style changes
- Fear related to psychogenic pathology or drug therapy
- Hopelessness related to psychogenic pathology
- Impaired adjustment related to psychogenic pathology or drug therapy
- Impaired home maintenance management related to psychogenic pathology or drug therapy
- Impaired physical mobility related to psychogenic pathology or drug therapy
- Impaired social interaction related to psychogenic pathology or drug therapy
- Impaired verbal communication related to psychogenic pathology or drug therapy
- Ineffective family coping: compromised, related to psychogenic pathology, drug therapy, or life-style changes

- Ineffective individual coping related to psychogenic pathology, drug therapy, or life-style changes
- Knowledge deficit related to all facets of drug therapy
- Noncompliance related to drug therapy
- Potential for injury related to psychogenic pathology or drug therapy
- Potential for violence related to psychogenic pathology
- Powerlessness related to psychogenic pathology or drug therapy
- Self-care deficit related to psychogenic pathology or drug therapy
- Sensory-perceptual alterations related to psychogenic pathology or drug therapy
- Sleep-pattern disturbance related to psychogenic pathology or drug therapy
- Spiritual distress related to psychogenic pathology.

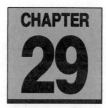

CHAPTER 29

CEREBRAL STIMULATING AGENTS

OBJECTIVES

After reading and studying this chapter, you should be able to:

1. Explain the uses of amphetamines and their pharmacokinetics.

2. Describe the significant interactions between amphetamines and other drugs.

3. Explain the use of nonamphetamine anorexigenic agents and their pharmacokinetics.

4. Describe the interactions between the nonamphetamine anorexigenics and other drugs.

5. Explain the uses and contraindications for the psychotherapeutic central nervous system (CNS) stimulants.

6. Describe the clinical use of cocaine hydrochloride.

INTRODUCTION

Many natural and synthetic substances can stimulate the central nervous system, but only a few are used therapeutically. This chapter will describe only those therapeutic drugs which cause prominent CNS stimulation as their primary action. Because of this action, cerebral stimulating agents may be used to treat an attention deficit disorder (ADD), narcolepsy (a disorder marked by an uncontrollable desire for sleep or sudden, unpredictable attacks of sleep), obesity, and some types of respiratory depression. Based on their clinical uses and pharmacologic effects, these drugs have four categories: amphetamines and amphetamine-like agents, nonamphetamine anorexigenic agents, psychotherapeutic CNS stimulants, and other CNS stimulants, including respiratory stimulants and cocaine. Many cerebral stimulating agents have a high abuse potential and are classified as controlled substances. Schedule I substances have the highest abuse potential; Schedule V drugs have the lowest. (See *Schedules of controlled drugs* in Chapter 1, Introduction to Pharmacology, for further information.)

The subjective effects of CNS stimulants depend on the user, the environment, the drug dose, and the route of administration. As the dose increases, and the route of adminsitration exert an increasing influence on subjective effects.

For a summary of representative drugs, see *Selected major drugs: Cerebral stimulating agents* on page 473.

AMPHETAMINES

This group of cerebral stimulating agents includes amphetamine sulfate, dextroamphetamine sulfate, and methamphetamine hydrochloride as well as benzphetamine hydrochloride, diethylpropion hydrochloride, and phentermine hydrochloride, which are not amphetamines, but amphetamine-like agents that produce similiar pharmacologic actions. These drugs act as powerful CNS stimulants. They also act on alpha- and beta-adrenergic receptors, indirectly stimulating the sympathetic nervous system, which in turn helps regulate various homeostatic functions, including the heart rate, force of cardiac contraction, vasomotor tone, and carbohydrate and fatty acid metabolism.

History and source

Although researchers first synthesized amphetamine in 1887, it was not introduced into medical practice until 1936. For the next 20 years, physicians used amphetamine extensively and considered it a relatively safe agent, although some toxic effects and dependence were reported in the medical literature. In 1963, the American Medical Association (AMA) Council on Drugs recognized the amphetamines' abuse potential but considered it "a small problem." By 1966, however, the AMA had reversed its position.

PHARMACOKINETICS

Amphetamines are completely absorbed, widely distributed, metabolized in the liver, and excreted in the urine.

Absorption, distribution, metabolism, excretion

After oral administration, amphetamines are completely absorbed from the gastrointestinal (GI) tract in 3 hours. They are widely distributed throughout the body and reach high concentration levels in the brain and cerebrospinal fluid.

Metabolism takes place in the liver and involves hydroxylation (addition of a hydroxide) and deamination (removal of an amine). The accumulation of hydroxylated metabolites may lead to amphetamine psychosis.

Amphetamine excretion depends on urine pH. The kidneys excrete these agents more rapidly in acidic urine than in alkaline urine. A patient with alkaline urine—from sodium bicarbonate or other urinary alkalizing agents, can develop intense amphetamine psychosis that lasts for more than 3 days after the amphetamine is discontinued, because excretion does not occur promptly.

Onset, peak, duration

The onset of action usually occurs in 1 hour, although it can be delayed if a sustained-release preparation is administered. Peak concentration levels and duration of action vary among individuals and depend on the dosage form. Also, an amphetamine's duration of action depends on urine pH. Acidic urine with a pH of less than 5.6 yields a plasma half-life of 7 to 8 hours; alkaline urine increases the half-life up to 33 hours. For every unit increase in urine pH, the plasma half-life increases by about 7 hours.

PHARMACODYNAMICS

Although the exact sites and mechanisms of action are not fully understood, amphetamines seem to release norepinephrine from stores in adrenergic nerve terminals and directly affect the alpha- and beta-receptor sites. In the CNS, the main sites of action appear to be the cerebral cortex and the reticular activating system (RAS).

Mechanism of action

Like other sympathomimetics, amphetamines act by releasing norepinephrine from storage sites in the sympathetic nerves. Amphetamine effects, therefore, resemble those of norepinephrine but have a slower onset of action and usually a longer duration of action. Unlike norepinephrine, amphetamines cause tachyphylaxis (decrease in drug effectiveness with repeated administration).

The amphetamines' pharmacologic actions include CNS and sympathomimetic activity, increased blood pressure, mydriasis, bronchodilation, and urinary bladder sphincter contraction. They can also increase motor activity and mental alertness, reduce fatigue, and cause mild euphoria followed by depression and fatigue. Their effects on the GI tract are varied and unpredictable. When a patient's breathing is depressed by another CNS drug, an amphetamine can stimulate respiration.

PHARMACOTHERAPEUTICS

Amphetamines are used to treat narcolepsy. They may also be used as adjuncts in treating ADD in children, such as hyperkinetic syndrome and minimal brain dysfunction, and in the short-term treatment of exogenous obesity. Their anorexigenic effects seldom last for more than a few weeks, however, and the patient may develop tolerance. Prolonged administration for exogenous obesity or combating fatigue is not recommended.

amphetamine sulfate (Benzedrine). A Schedule II drug, amphetamine may be used to treat narcolepsy, ADD, or exogenous obesity.
USUAL ADULT DOSAGE: for narcolepsy, 5 mg P.O. daily initially, increased by 10 mg/day every week up to a maximum of 60 mg daily, in divided doses or one sustained-release dose daily; for exogenous obesity, 5 to 30 mg P.O. daily in divided doses 30 to 60 minutes before meals, or one sustained-release dose of 10 to 15 mg daily in the morning.
USUAL PEDIATRIC DOSAGE: for narcolepsy in children age 6 to 12, 5 mg P.O. daily initially; increased by 5 mg/day every week, if necessary, to control attacks. For narcolepsy in children age 12 or older, 10 mg P.O. daily, with 10-mg increments weekly p.r.n. For ADD in children age 3 to 5, 2.5 mg P.O. daily, increased by 2.5 mg/day every week, as needed. For children age 6 or older, 5 mg P.O. once or twice daily, increased by 5 mg/day every week, as needed. The pediatric dosage will rarely exceed 40 mg/day.

benzphetamine hydrochloride (Didrex). A Schedule III drug, benzphetamine is an amphetamine-like anorexigenic used as an adjunct in treating exogenous obesity.
USUAL ADULT DOSAGE: 25 to 50 mg P.O. once daily; increased, if needed, up to 25 to 50 mg b.i.d. or t.i.d.

DRUG INTERACTIONS

Amphetamines

Drug interactions involving amphetamines can occur with many agents and may be serious. Interactions with MAO inhibitors may be life-threatening.

DRUG	INTERACTING DRUGS	POSSIBLE EFFECTS	NURSING IMPLICATIONS
amphetamine, benzphetamine, dextroamphetamine, diethylpropion, methamphetamine	MAO inhibitors	Increase the amount of norepinephrine present in adrenergic storage sites, causing release of large amounts of norepinephrine to react with a receptor for up to several weeks after MAO inhibitors are discontinued; as a result, may produce headache, hyperpyrexia, hypertension—possibly leading to hypertensive crisis, intracranial hemorrhage, and bradycardia	• Obtain a complete patient drug history to see if MAO inhibitors were used in the past 2 to 3 weeks. If so, notify the physician. • Monitor the patient's temperature, blood pressure, and pulse carefully. • Assess for signs of drug abuse, such as abnormal pupil size, exhaustion, or altered mental status, which may make the patient an unreliable historian of drug use. • Concurrent use should be avoided.
	guanethidine	Decreases antihypertensive effect of guanethidine	• Monitor the blood pressure closely. • Concurrent use should be avoided. If an amphetamine is necessary, expect to use another antihypertensive that will not interact with it.
	phenothiazines	Decrease the effect of both drugs	• Watch for a worsening of symptoms in a patient who begins amphetamine therapy and receives a phenothiazine for a psychotic disorder, such as schizophrenia. • Expect to see a reduction in the anorexigenic effects of an amphetamine during phenothiazine therapy. • Concurrent use should be avoided.
	urinary alkalinizers (such as potassium citrate, sodium acetate, sodium bicarbonate, sodium citrate, sodium lactate, tromethamine)	Decrease amphetamine excretion	• Monitor the patient for increased—possibly toxic—amphetamine effects, such as excess CNS stimulation or cardiovascular effects. • Expect to decrease the amphetamine dosage, as prescribed.
	urinary acidifiers (such as ammonium chloride, potassium phosphate, sodium acid phosphate)	Increase amphetamine excretion	• Monitor the patient for reduced amphetamine effectiveness. • Expect to increase the amphetamine dosage, as prescribed.

dextroamphetamine sulfate (Dexampex, Dexedrine, Spancap). A Schedule II drug, dextroamphetamine is used to treat narcolepsy, exogenous obesity, and ADD. Its CNS-stimulating effect is about twice that of amphetamine, and it is sometimes given with amphetamine in the combination product Biphetamine.
USUAL ADULT DOSAGE: for narcolepsy, 5 to 10 mg P.O. daily initially, increased by 10 mg every week up to a maximum of 60 mg/day in divided doses; or one sustained-release dose daily. The extended-release capsules should not be used for initial doses. For exogenous obesity, 5 to 30 mg P.O. daily in divided doses 30 to 60 minutes before meals, or one sustained-release dose of 10 to 15 mg daily in the morning.
USUAL PEDIATRIC DOSAGE: for narcolepsy in children age 6 to 12, 5 mg P.O. daily, initially; increased by 5 mg/day every week, as necessary, to control attacks. For

narcolepsy in children age 12 and older, 10 mg P.O. daily, increased by 10-mg/day at weekly increments, as needed. For ADD in children age 3 to 5, 2.5 mg P.O. daily; increased by 2.5 mg/day every week, as needed. For children age 6 or older, 5 mg P.O. once or twice daily, increased by 5 mg /day every week, as needed. The pediatric dosage will rarely exceed 40 mg/day.

diethylpropion hydrochloride (Tenuate, Tepanil). This schedule IV drug is used as an anorexigenic.
USUAL ADULT DOSAGE: 25 mg P.O. t.i.d. 1 hour before meals; or one 75-mg sustained-release dose midmorning.

methamphetamine hydrochloride (Desoxyn, Methampex). A Schedule II drug, methamphetamine is used to treat exogenous obesity in adults and ADD in children. When possible, its administration should be interrupted to assess the child's behavior and determine if therapy should continue.
USUAL ADULT DOSAGE: for short-term adjunct therapy in exogenous obesity, 2.5 to 5 mg P.O. b.i.d. or t.i.d. 30 minutes before meals; or one long-acting 10- to 15-mg tablet daily before breakfast.
USUAL PEDIATRIC DOSAGE: for ADD in children age 6 and older, 2.5 to 5 mg P.O. once or twice daily; increased by 5 mg/day every week, as necessary, to control behavior (usual effective dosage ranges from 20 to 25 mg P.O. daily).

phentermine hydrochloride (Anoxine, Fastin, Ionamin). A Schedule IV drug, phentermine is an amphetamine-like agent used as an adjunct in the short-term treatment of exogenous obesity.
USUAL ADULT DOSAGE: 8 mg P.O. t.i.d. 30 minutes before meals, or 15 to 37.5 mg P.O. once daily in the morning.

Drug interactions
The most significant interactions with amphetamines involve monoamine oxidase (MAO) inhibitors, guanethidine monosulfate, and urinary alkalinizers, such as sodium bicarbonate or carbonic anhydrase inhibitors. (See *Drug interactions: Amphetamines* on page 467 for significant interactions.)

ADVERSE DRUG REACTIONS

Amphetamines can produce adverse reactions in the cardiovascular system that may be serious and require close monitoring of vital signs. They can also produce CNS, GI, endocrine, and allergic reactions. Safety for use in pregnant or lactating women has not been established.

Predictable reactions
Cardiovascular reactions to amphetamines may include palpitations, tachycardia, and hypertension. In the CNS, they can produce restlessness, hyperactivity, talkativeness, and insomnia. Long-term use can cause depression, psychosis, and addiction. In the GI system, these drugs can produce dry mouth, an unpleasant taste, diarrhea or constipation, as well as anorexia and weight loss, which are undesirable reactions when the drugs are not used as anorexigenics. In the endocrine system, reactions can include impotence and changes in libido. With heavy amphetamine use, reversible elevations in serum thyroxine levels may occur.

Unpredictable reactions
Allergic reactions to amphetamines are rare and usually mild, typically producing rash and urticaria. Patients who are allergic to aspirin may also be allergic to amphetamines that contain the dye tartrazine.

NURSING IMPLICATIONS

The nurse must closely monitor patients receiving amphetamine and be aware of these implications.
• Amphetamines are contraindicated in patients with advanced arteriosclerosis, cardiovascular disease, moderate to severe hypertension, hypersensitivity to sympathomimetic amines, glaucoma, agitation, or a history of drug abuse. They are also contraindicated during MAO inhibitor therapy and for 14 days after discontinuation of this therapy.
• Be aware that amphetamines are not indicated in all cases of ADD. For example, they are not usually indicated when symptoms are related to an acute stress reaction.
• The drug is usually discontinued when tolerance to its anorexigenic effects develops.
• Be aware that, because tolerance and extreme psychological dependence are likely to develop with these abused drugs, a patient may take much more than the prescribed dose. Chronic intoxication can cause amphetamine psychosis, which is often clinically indistinguishable from paranoid schizophrenia.
• Monitor the patient for signs of Gilles de la Tourette's syndrome, such as progressive muscular jerks of the face, shoulders, and arms, which may be precipitated or exacerbated in children.
• Closely monitor the blood pressure of a patient receiving an antihypertensive drug; an amphetamine may reverse its beneficial effects.

• Be aware that abrupt cessation after prolonged high dosage causes extreme fatigue, mental depression, and changes on the sleep electroencephalogram.
• Advise the patient to avoid other stimulants, such as caffeine-rich colas, coffee, and the over-the-counter (OTC) drug No-Doz; they may intensify the anorexigenics' adverse effects.
• Explain the drug's adverse reactions, and instruct the patient to contact the physician if any occur.
• Instruct the patient to take the drug 1 hour before meals, if used for obesity, and emphasize the importance of adhering to the weight-reduction program.
• Advise the patient to avoid activities that require alertness or good psychomotor coordination until the CNS response to the drug is determined.
• Instruct a lactating patient to alert the physician if she is taking an amphetamine.

NONAMPHETAMINE ANOREXIGENIC AGENTS

Also known as anorectics or anorexiants, the nonamphetamine anorexigenics are indirect-acting sympathomimetic amines. This class of drugs includes fenfluramine hydrochloride, mazindol, phendimetrazine tartrate, phenmetrazine hydrochloride, and phenylpropanolamine hydrochloride. These drugs are synthetic preparations that became available relatively recently. Their abuse potential, which is similar to that of the amphetamines, was quickly recognized.

PHARMACOKINETICS

All nonamphetamine anorexigenic agents are readily absorbed. Their other pharmacokinetic processes, however, are incompletely known.

Absorption, distribution, metabolism, excretion
After oral administration, these drugs are readily absorbed from the GI tract. Although researchers have not yet determined distribution patterns for all of the agents, they do know that fenfluramine is widely distributed in body tissues.

Most of a fenfluramine dose is metabolized in the liver to inactive compounds, whereas mazindol is not metabolized appreciably. The metabolism of phendi-

metrazine and phenmetrazine is unknown. Only about 10% to 20% of phenylpropanolamine is metabolized in the liver to active hydroxylated metabolites.

Patient variations, urinary flow rate, and pH affect the rate of fenfluramine elimination. Fenfluramine is excreted principally as inactive metabolites, mazindol and phenylpropanolamine are excreted primarily as unchanged drug. The exact excretion of phendimetrazine and phenmetrazine is unknown.

Onset, peak, duration
Fenfluramine's onset of action ranges from 1 to 2 hours. Peak concentration levels are reached in 2 to 4 hours; duration of action is 4 to 6 hours. The usual half-life—about 20 hours—can drop to 11 hours if the urine pH is less than 5.

Mazindol's onset of action is 30 to 60 minutes; its duration of action is 8 to 15 hours, and its half-life is unknown.

Immediate-release forms of the other nonamphetamine anorexigenic drugs produce initial effects in less than an hour; peak concentration levels are reached in 1 to 2 hours; duration of action is 4 to 6 hours. Phendimetrazine's half-life ranges from 2 to 10 hours and phenylpropanolamine's half-life ranges from 3 to 4 hours. Phenmetrazine's half-life is unknown.

PHARMACODYNAMICS

Fenfluramine may inhibit the appetite by acting on the hypothalamus. Its cardiovascular and CNS effects appear to resemble those of the amphetamines, but its pressor effects are 10 to 20 times less potent than dextroamphetamine's. Unlike the other drugs in this class, fenfluramine produces a CNS depression similar to that of the sedative psychotherapeutic drugs.

Mazindol produces CNS and cardiac stimulation; however, its mechanism of action as an appetite suppressant is undefined.

Although phenmetrazine, phendimetrazine, and phenylpropanolamine seem to show no primary effect on appetite, they may produce anorexigenic effects secondary to CNS stimulation.

PHARMACOTHERAPEUTICS

Anorexigenic agents are used primarily as short-term (8 to 12 weeks) adjuncts in treating exogenous obesity, which should include a total weight-reduction program.

fenfluramine hydrochloride (Pondimin). A Schedule IV drug, fenfluramine is commonly used to treat exogenous obesity. It also may be helpful in treating autistic children

DRUG INTERACTIONS

Nonamphetamine anorexigenic agents

The anorexigenic agents listed below can interact with many other drugs and may produce severe reactions, especially hypertension.

DRUG	INTERACTING DRUGS	POSSIBLE EFFECTS	NURSING IMPLICATIONS
fenfluramine, mazindol, phendimetrazine, phenmetrazine, phenylpropanolamine	MAO inhibitors	Increase norepinephrine storage in adrenergic neurons, causing a release of larger amounts of norepinephrine to react with the receptor sites for up to several weeks after MAO inhibitors are discontinued; as a result, may produce headache, hyperpyrexia, or hypertension, possibly leading to hypertensive crisis, intracranial hemorrhage, and bradycardia	• Avoid concurrent use of phenylpropanolamine and MAO inhibitors. • Obtain a complete patient drug history to see if MAO inhibitors were used in the past 2 to 3 weeks. If so, notify the physician. • Monitor the patient's temperature, blood pressure, and pulse carefully. • Assess the patient for signs of drug abuse, such as abnormal pupil size, exhaustion, or altered mental status, which may make the patient an unreliable historian of drug use. • Remember that phenylpropanolamine is available to patients over the counter.
	phenothiazines	Decrease the effect of both drugs	• Concurrent use of these drugs should be avoided. • Assess for a worsening of symptoms in a patient who begins anorexigenic therapy and receives a phenothiazine for a psychotic disorder, such as schizophrenia. • Expect to see a reduction in the anorexigenic agent's effects during phenothiazine therapy.
	insulin, oral hypoglycemic agents	Cause additive hypoglycemic activity	• Be aware that the hypoglycemic agent's dosage may need to be reduced. • Monitor the patient's blood and glucose levels closely.
phenylpropanolamine, fenfluramine	beta-adrenergic blocking agents, alcohol, tricyclic antidepressants, CNS depressants, indomethacin	Cause hypertension and possible severe CNS depression	• Concurrent use of these drugs should be avoided. • Monitor the patient's blood pressure closely.

with elevated serotonin levels, although it has not yet received Food and Drug Administration (FDA) approval for this use.

USUAL ADULT DOSAGE: 20 mg P.O. t.i.d. 30 to 60 minutes before meals, gradually increased by 20 mg/day at weekly intervals to a maximum of 120 mg/day in divided doses. If extended-release capsules are ordered: 60 mg daily to a maximum of 120 mg/day, if tolerated.

mazindol (Mazanor, Sanorex). A Schedule IV drug, mazindol is used only as a short-term adjunct in treating exogenous obesity.

USUAL ADULT DOSAGE: 1 mg P.O. t.i.d. 1 hour before meals or 2 mg P.O. once daily 1 hour before lunch.

phendimetrazine tartrate (Bontril, Phenazine, Plegine). A Schedule IV drug, phendimetrazine can be a useful adjunct in the short-term management of exogenous obesity.

USUAL ADULT DOSAGE: 35 mg P.O. b.i.d. or t.i.d. 1 hour before meals, or 105 mg P.O. of a sustained-release form once daily in the morning.

phenmetrazine hydrochloride (Preludin). A Schedule II drug, this anorexigenic is also used as an adjunct in treating obesity.

USUAL ADULT DOSAGE: 25 mg P.O. b.i.d. or t.i.d. 1 hour before meals, or 75 mg P.O. of a sustained-release form once daily.

phenylpropanolamine hydrochloride (Acutrim, Dexatrim, Prolamine). Sold over the counter, phenylpropanolamine is used in appetite-suppressing products as well as many cold and influenza preparations.

USUAL ADULT DOSAGE: 25 mg P.O. t.i.d. 1 hour before meals, or 75 mg P.O. of a sustained-release form once daily.

Drug interactions

Because these drugs (except for fenfluramine) stimulate the CNS, do not administer them with other CNS stimulants, to avoid additive effects. (See *Drug interactions: Nonamphetamine anorexigenic agents* for specific information.)

ADVERSE DRUG REACTIONS

Nonamphetamine anorexigenics may produce adverse reactions in the cardiovascular, CNS, GI, and genitourinary systems as well as various other effects. Safety for use in pregnant or lactating patients has not been established.

Predictable reactions

Cardiovascular reactions to anorexigenics may include palpitations, tachycardia, dysrhythmias, hypertension or hypotension, fainting, dyspnea, precordial pain, and pulmonary hypertension. Phenylpropanolamine may cause hypertensive crisis and renal failure.

In the CNS, adverse reactions may include overstimulation, nervousness, restlessness, dizziness, insomnia, weakness, fatigue, malaise, anxiety, euphoria or dysphoria, drowsiness, depression, tremor, dyskinesia, dysarthria, confusion, headache, and, rarely, psychotic episodes. An epileptic patient may experience more convulsive episodes. Serious CNS reactions, such as seizures or stroke, can occur; fenfluramine may produce CNS depression, drowsiness, or impotence. Discontinuation of fenfluramine after only 1 month at 60 mg/day can produce withdrawal symptoms, including ataxia, tremors, disturbed concentration, loss of sense of reality, hallucinations, visual field inversion, depression, and suicidal feelings.

In the GI system, anorexigenics can cause dry mouth, an unpleasant taste, nausea, vomiting, diarrhea, constipation, or abdominal pain. In the genitourinary system, adverse reactions may include dysuria, polyuria, or urinary frequency as well as impotence, libido changes, menstrual upset, gynecomastia, or—with mazindol—testicular pain. Ocular reactions may include mydriasis, eye irritation, or blurred vision.

Unpredictable reactions

Although rare, unpredictable reactions may include hair loss, nasal dryness, excessive sweating, chills, flushing, fever, bone marrow depression, granulocytopenia, and leukopenia. Allergic reactions, also rare, produce such reactions as rash and urticaria.

NURSING IMPLICATIONS

The nurse must be alert for signs of anorexigenic abuse and should also pay particular attention to the following:
- Nonamphetamine anorexigenic agents are contraindicated in patients with advanced arteriosclerosis, cardiovascular disease, moderate to severe hypertension, known hypersensitivity to sympathomimetics, glaucoma, agitation, or a history of drug abuse. They are also contraindicated during CNS-stimulant or MAO inhibitor therapy and for 14 days after discontinuation of MAO inhibitor therapy.
- Anticipate the development of tolerance and tachyphylaxis to the anorexigenic agent in a few weeks. Be aware that cross-tolerance (tolerance to other drugs in the same class) usually develops.
- Assess the patient for signs of drug abuse, because intense psychological or physical dependence may occur with long-term therapy.
- Monitor a diabetic patient's blood and urine glucose levels closely and expect to alter the hypoglycemic dosage as prescribed.
- Be aware that abrupt discontinuation of long-term, high-dose therapy can cause dizziness, extreme fatigue, and depression.
- Teach the patient to take the drug 1 hour before meals, if used to treat obesity, and emphasize the importance of adhering to a weight-reduction program.
- Advise the patient to avoid other stimulants, such as caffeine-rich colas, coffee, and No-Doz; they may intensify the anorexigenics' adverse effects.
- Advise the patient to use caution while driving or performing other tasks that require alertness.
- Advise the patient who is pregnant or attempting to conceive to inform the physician, because these drugs may be harmful to the fetus.
- Advise a lactating patient to alert the physician if she is taking an anorexigenic.
- Remind the patient not to chew extended-release capsules.

PSYCHOTHERAPEUTIC C.N.S. STIMULANTS

Methylphenidate hydrochloride and pemoline constitute this group. Structurally related to amphetamines, these drugs are synthetic preparations. Methylphenidate was introduced in the early 1970s; pemoline followed a few years later. Their abuse potential, similar to the amphetamines', was recognized shortly after their introduction. Today, psychotherapeutic CNS stimulants are used to treat ADD; methylphenidate is also used to treat narcolepsy.

PHARMACOKINETICS

After oral administration, methylphenidate and pemoline are rapidly and well absorbed from the GI tract; however, their distribution is not fully known. About 80% of a methylphenidate dose is metabolized to ritalinic acid, and more than 50% of a pemoline dose is transformed into various metabolites, at least one of which has CNS activity. About 95% of a methylphenidate dose and about 75% of a pemoline dose is excreted in the urine in 24 hours.

Onset, peak, duration

With immediate-release methylphenidate, the onset of action occurs in less than 1 hour. The drug reaches peak blood concentration level in 1 to 3 hours. Although its plasma half-life is 1 to 3 hours, the drug's duration of action is 3 to 6 hours. With the sustained-release form, effects last for at least 8 hours.

Pemoline begins to take effect in 1 to 2 hours and achieves peak blood concentration level in 2 to 4 hours. In adults, the plasma half-life ranges from 9 to 14 hours; in children, from 2 to 12 hours. When pemoline is administered to a child with ADD, the drug's onset of action occurs gradually, and therapeutic effects may take 2 to 3 weeks.

PHARMACODYNAMICS

Although their mechanisms of action are not fully understood, methylphenidate and pemoline seem to work in similar ways. The main sites of activity appear to be the cerebral cortex and the subcortical structures, including the thalamus and the RAS. To stimulate the CNS, they may promote nerve impulse transmission by releasing stored norepinephrine from nerve terminals in the brain. They exert a paradoxical calming effect in ADD.

PHARMACOTHERAPEUTICS

These drugs are used as adjuncts in treating the symptoms of ADD including moderate to severe distractability, short attention span, hyperactivity, emotional lability, and impulsiveness in children over age 6. They can improve behavior, concentration, and learning ability in 70% to 80% of all children with ADD but should not be the sole form of therapy for or be used indiscriminately with undisciplined or hyperactive children. Methylphenidate is also used to treat narcolepsy.

methylphenidate hydrochloride (Ritalin). A Schedule II drug, methylphenidate is used to treat narcolepsy in adults and ADD in children.
USUAL ADULT DOSAGE: 10 mg P.O. b.i.d. or t.i.d. ½ to 1 hour before meals. The dosage should be individualized and may range from 10 to 60 mg/day.
USUAL PEDIATRIC DOSAGE: initially, 5 mg P.O. b.i.d. before meals initially, with 5- to 10-mg increments weekly as needed, up to 60 mg/day. If improvement does not occur after 1 month, the drug is discontinued. If symptoms become worse or the patient experiences adverse reactions, the dose is reduced or the drug discontinued.

pemoline (Cylert). A Schedule IV drug, pemoline is used as an adjunct in ADD therapy; however, its beneficial effects may not appear until the third or fourth week.
USUAL PEDIATRIC DOSAGE: for children age 6 and older, initially 37.5 mg P.O. daily, given in the morning, and increased by 18.75 mg daily every week until the desired clinical response is achieved or a maximum of 112.5 mg/day is administered. The effective dosage usually ranges from 56.25 to 75 mg/day. Dosage has not been established for children under age 6.

Drug interactions

Methylphenidate may decrease the hypotensive effects of guanethidine monosulfate and may lead to amphetamine-like interaction with MAO inhibitors, producing fever and hypertensive crisis. Although these interactions may be severe, they rarely occur.

Pemoline produces no known interactions; however, the nurse should exercise caution if other CNS stimulants are administered concomitantly.

SELECTED MAJOR DRUGS

Cerebral stimulating agents

The chart below summarizes the major cerebral stimulating drugs currently in clinical use.

DRUG	MAJOR INDICATIONS	USUAL ADULT DOSAGES	NURSING IMPLICATIONS
Amphetamines			
amphetamine	Narcolepsy	5 to 60 mg P.O. daily in divided doses	• Amphetamines are contraindicated in advanced arteriosclerosis, cardiovascular disease, known sensitivity, hypertension, and glaucoma or during MAO-inhibitor therapy or for 14 days thereafter. • Assess the patient for symptoms of drug abuse and tolerance. • Expect to discontinue the drug after a few weeks if used to treat obesity. • Administer amphetamines 6 hours before bedtime to prevent insomnia. • Advise the patient that over-the-counter products, such as caffeine and antacids, can exaggerate the drug's effects.
	Adjunct treatment of exogenous obesity	5 to 30 mg P.O. daily in divided doses before meals	
Nonamphetamine anorexigenic agents			
fenfluramine	Adjunct treatment for exogenous obesity	20 mg P.O. t.i.d. to maximum 120 mg/day in divided doses before meals	• Anorexigenics are contraindicated in advanced arteriosclerosis, cardiovascular disease, known sensitivity, hypertension, and glaucoma or during MAO inhibitor therapy or for 14 days thereafter. • Expect to discontinue the drug after a few weeks. • Administer fenfluramine 6 hours before bedtime to prevent insomnia. • Advise the patient that over-the-counter antacids and products containing caffeine, such as No-Doz, can exaggerate the drug's effects. • Remind the patient not to chew extended-release capsules.
Psychotherapeutic CNS stimulants			
methylphenidate	Narcolepsy	10 to 60 mg P.O. daily in divided doses	• Methylphenidate is contraindicated in patients with known sensitivity to the drug and in those with marked anxiety or glaucoma.

ADVERSE DRUG REACTIONS

Adverse reactions to methylphenidate and pemoline may affect not only the CNS but also the cardiovascular and GI systems. Safety for use in pregnant or lactating patients has not been established.

Predictable reactions

With methylphenidate, CNS reactions—especially nervousness and insomnia—are most common and can usually be controlled by lowering the dosage or taking the last daily dose at least 6 hours before bedtime. Other CNS reactions include dizziness, headache, dyskinesia, chorea, drowsiness, Gilles de la Tourette's syndrome, and toxic psychosis. Cardiovascular reactions include increased or decreased blood pressure and pulse, tachycardia, palpitations, angina, and cardiac dysrhythmias. GI reactions may include anorexia, weight loss, nausea, and abdominal pain.

With pemoline, the most common CNS reaction is insomnia, a transient effect that usually occurs early in therapy. Dyskinetic movements of the tongue, lips, face, and extremities can also occur, along with Gilles de la Tourette's syndrome, nystagmus, seizures, increased irritability, depression, dizziness, headache, drowsiness, and hallucinations. Common GI reactions can include anorexia with weight loss—although this is usually transient—nausea, stomachache, and diarrhea. Pemoline may also elevate the liver enzymes—serum glutamic-oxaloacetic transaminase (SGOT), serum glutamic-pyruvic transaminase (SGPT) (also known as AST and ALT respectively), and alkaline phosphatase—and cause reversible hepatitis and jaundice.

Unpredictable reactions

In some patients, methylphenidate can produce various hypersensitivity reactions, including rash, urticaria, fever, arthralgia, exfoliative dermatitis, and erythema multiforme. Pemoline may cause a rash. Both drugs may suppress a child's normal weight and height, although studies have not yet proven the cause.

NURSING IMPLICATIONS

During treatment with these easily abused drugs, the nurse must ensure the following:
• Be aware that methylphenidate and pemoline are contraindicated in patients who are sensitive to them and should not be used in children younger than age 6. Methylphenidate is contraindicated in patients with glaucoma or those with marked anxiety, tension, or agitation.
• Assess the patient for signs of Gilles de la Tourette's syndrome, such as facial or vocal tics and jerking movements. Both drugs can precipitate this disorder.
• Closely monitor the heart rate and rhythm and blood pressure in a patient receiving methylphenidate.
• Monitor the complete blood count with differential and platelet count periodically for a patient receiving prolonged methylphenidate therapy.
• Monitor the SGOT, SGPT, and alkaline phosphatase levels periodically for a patient receiving pemoline.
• Administer pemoline with caution, and expect to alter the dosage in a patient with impaired hepatic or renal function.
• Assess the patient for signs of drug abuse, tolerance, and physical and psychological dependence.
• Advise the patient to avoid activities that require good psychomotor coordination until the CNS response to these drugs is determined.
• Administer these drugs with or after meals to help avoid appetite suppression in a child.
• Administer the last daily dose at least 6 hours before bedtime if either drug interferes with sleep.

• Monitor the height and weight of a child receiving long-term therapy, to detect growth suppression. Expect the drug to be temporarily discontinued if growth suppression is detected.

OTHER CEREBRAL STIMULATING AGENTS

Doxapram hydrochloride and nikethamide are used to treat respiratory depression. They seem to work by selectively stimulating the depressed central respiratory centers. However, in most cases, they are not as useful as direct, supportive measures, such as mechanical ventilation and maintenance of cardiovascular functions.

I.V. caffeine sodium benzoate may be used as a CNS and respiratory stimulant. Today, however, more effective agents have replaced caffeine in many of these applications. (See Chapter 44, Methylxanthine Agents, for detailed information on using caffeine to treat respiratory problems.)

Doxapram and nikethamide stimulate all levels of the CNS. Doxapram produces respiratory stimulation by acting on the carotid chemoreceptors. Nikethamide transiently increases respiratory rate by directly stimulating the medullary respiratory center. It may also stimulate respiration through reflex activation of carotid chemoreceptors. Because doxapram is more potent and safer than nikethamide in stimulating depressed respiratory function, it is more commonly used.

One other drug, cocaine hydrochloride, may be used as a CNS stimulant, although it is more commonly used as a topical anesthetic in head and throat surgery. (See Chapter 28, Local and Topical Anesthetic Agents, for information about this use.)

doxapram hydrochloride (Dopram). A potent drug, doxapram may be used with supportive measures to hasten arousal and treat respiratory depression associated with overdose of CNS depressants, such as barbiturates, opiates, or general anesthetics. It may play a part in the short-term management of chronic obstructive pulmonary disease (COPD) associated with acute hypercapnia and in postanesthesia respiratory depression not caused by a skeletal muscle relaxant. An adequate airway and oxygenation should be established before administering the drug. Doxapram is contraindicated in patients with a history of convulsive disorders, epilepsy, head injury pulmonary embolism, pneumothorax, acute asthma, pulmonary fibrosis, extreme dyspnea, certain pulmonary disorders, uncompensated heart failure, severe hypertension, or cerebrovascular accident. The safe use of doxapram during pregnancy has not been established. An adequate airway must be maintained and oxygenation assured during doxapram therapy.

The usual adult dosage for drug-induced CNS depression is 0.5 to 2 mg/kg I.V. p.r.n. or 1 to 3 mg/minute by I.V. infusion, up to a maximum of 3 grams daily.

nikethamide (Coramine). Another potent drug, nikethamide may be used with supportive measures to treat CNS depression, respiratory depression, and circulatory failure associated with an overdose of a CNS depressant, cholinesterase inhibitor, or carbon monoxide; CNS depression in acute alcoholism; neonatal asphyxia; electroshock therapy; shock; cardiac decompensation and coronary occlusion; and respiratory failure caused by COPD. However, this drug's transient action and high toxicity may prohibit its use in these conditions.

cocaine hydrochloride. Used for centuries as a CNS stimulant, this Schedule II drug is used today only as a CNS stimulant in Brompton's cocktail, an oral analgesic containing morphine or heroin used to manage chronic and severe cancer pain. A dose of Brompton's mixture contains 10 mg of cocaine hydrochloride. However, recent clinical studies have shown that the cocaine in this mixture offers no significant advantages, and most institutions have stopped using it.

When cocaine hydrochloride is given orally, it is well absorbed, metabolized in the liver, and excreted in the urine. It causes the following CNS stimulating reactions: euphoria, stimulation, reduced fatigue, loquacity, sexual stimulation, increased mental ability, alertness, and increased sociability. It is likely to cause physical and psychological dependence and may cause adverse reactions, including vomiting, tremors, tonic-clonic convulsions, nervousness, restlessness, excitement, hallucinations, tachypnea, tachycardia, and hypertension.

CHAPTER SUMMARY

Chapter 29 investigated the cerebral stimulating agents, which, despite their relatively great abuse potential, have legitimate clinical indications, often in situations where no other safe, effective treatment exists. Here are chapter highlights:

• The amphetamine agents—amphetamine, dextroamphetamine, and methamphetamine—and the amphetamine-like agents—benzphetamine, diethylpropion, and phentermine—are used to treat narcolepsy and exogenous obesity.

• The amphetamines and amphetamine-like agents are controlled substances that can cause amphetamine psychosis with prolonged use and withdrawal symptoms with abrupt discontinuation.

• These agents can cause some serious interactions with such drugs as MAO inhibitors, guanethidine, and urinary alkalinizers. They may cause adverse reactions in the CNS as well as the cardiovascular, GI, endocrine, and other body systems.

• Nonamphetamine anorexigenic agents include fenfluramine, mazindol, phendimetrazine, phenmetrazine, and the OTC drug phenylpropanolamine. These indirect-acting sympathomimetic amines are generally used to treat exogenous obesity.

• Except for phenylpropanolamine, the anorexigenics are controlled substances with a fairly high abuse potential. However, they can all produce severe adverse reactions in the CNS and the cardiovascular, GI, genitourinary, and other body systems. They interact with many of the same drugs as the amphetamines.

• Methylphenidate and pemoline are psychotherapeutic CNS stimulants. Both are used to treat ADD, and methylphenidate may be used to manage narcolepsy as well. Both are contraindicated in patients sensitive to them; neither drug is used in children younger than age 6. Methylphenidate is contraindicated in patients with glaucoma, marked anxiety, tension, or agitation.

• Psychotherapeutic CNS stimulants are also controlled substances but interact with far fewer drugs than the amphetamines do. They may produce adverse reactions in the CNS and the cardiovascular and GI systems.

• Because of their selective CNS effects, doxapram and nikethamide are used with supportive measures to treat respiratory depression.

• Although the CNS and respiratory stimulants are not controlled substances, they are potent, fast-acting drugs with a narrow margin of safety. They can produce serious—possibly life-threatening—reactions, especially in the CNS and cardiovascular system.

• Cocaine may be used in Brompton's mixture as a CNS stimulant. However, clinical use of this controlled substance is rare because of its abuse and addiction potential.

BIBLIOGRAPHY

American Hospital Formulary Service. *Drug Information 87.* McEvoy, G.K., et al., eds. Bethesda, Md.: American Society of Hospital Pharmacists, 1987.

American Medical Association. *AMA Drug Evaluations,* 6th ed. Philadelphia: W.B. Saunders Co., 1986.

Geffner, E.S. *Compendium of Drug Therapy 1986-1987.* New York: Biomedical Information Corp., 1986.

Gilman, A.G., et al., eds. *Goodman and Gilman's The Pharmacological Basis of Therapeutics,* 7th ed. New York: Macmillan Publishing Co., 1985.

Hansten, P.D. *Drug Interactions,* 5th ed. Philadelphia: Lea & Febiger, 1985.

Kastrup, E.K., et al., eds. *Facts and Comparisons.* St. Louis: Facts and Comparisons Division, J.B. Lippincott Co., 1986.

Katzung, B.G. *Basic and Clinical Pharmacology,* 3rd ed. Los Altos, Calif.: Appleton & Lange, 1987.

Mangini, R.I., ed. *Drug Interaction Facts.* Philadelphia: J.B. Lippincott Co., 1987.

Nursing88 Drug Handbook. Springhouse, Pa.: Springhouse Corp., 1988.

CHAPTER 30

SEDATIVE AND HYPNOTIC AGENTS

OBJECTIVES

After reading and studying this chapter, you should be able to:

1. Differentiate between a sedative and a hypnotic.

2. Describe a typical sleep cycle from stage 1 sleep through stage 5.

3. Describe the four major categories of sleep disorders.

4. Explain why health care practitioners prescribe the benzodiazepines as sedatives and hypnotics rather than the barbiturates.

5. Describe the pharmacokinetic properties of the benzodiazepines, barbiturates, and the nonbenzodiazepines-nonbarbiturates.

6. Discuss the clinical indications for each of the three major groups of sedative and hypnotic drugs.

7. Describe significant adverse reactions and nursing implications associated with each of the three major classes of sedative and hypnotic drugs.

8. Describe how alcohol and over-the-counter (OTC) products function as sleep aids.

INTRODUCTION

Sedatives are drugs that act to reduce activity or excitement, calming a patient. Some degree of drowsiness often accompanies the use of sedatives. When administered in large doses, sedatives are considered hypnotics, which induce a state resembling natural sleep. Chapter 30 discusses three main classes of synthetic drugs used as sedatives and hypnotics: the benzodiazepines, the barbiturates, and the nonbenzodiazepine-nonbarbiturate drugs. The chapter also discusses alcohol and OTC sleep aids, and two dietary sources that may have some sedative effects (herbs and L-tryptophan).

The physiology of sleep

Sleep represents an active state of unconsciousness from which a person can be awakened with an appropriate stimulus. A naturally occurring state, sleep occupies about one third of an adult's life. Though researchers know that a lack of sleep causes physical and psychological symptoms and generally believe that the body requires sleep for restoration, they have not yet identified the precise relationship between sleep and cellular renewal.

While sleeping, a person passes through several cycles, each cycle involving five stages. The first four stages, characterized by non-rapid eye movement (NREM), account for 75% to 80% of a typical period of sleep. The stages progress from light sleep, stages 1 and 2, to deep sleep, stages 3 and 4. NREM, especially stage 4, helps maintain physical health and well-being and represents what some people refer to as obligatory sleep. After completing stage 4, the sleeper regresses through stages 3 and 2 to reach the fifth and last stage, called rapid eye movement (REM) sleep. REM sleep accounts for the remaining 20% to 25% of a normal period of sleep. REM sleep, a physiologically active period characterized by rapid eye movements, is essential for physiologic and mental restoration. During REM sleep, the person integrates new learning and experiences into the memory.

Following REM sleep, the sleeper begins a second cycle, proceeding through stages 2 to 4, then back through stages 3 and 2, and finally into a longer period of REM sleep. Changes in body position usually mark the transition from one stage of sleep to another. A typical cycle averages 90 minutes, with the duration of stage 4 decreasing and the REM stage lengthening with each cycle. Each time a person awakens, a new cycle begins. (See *NREM and REM sleep* on page 478 for a summary of the major characteristics, including similarities and differences, of the different stages of sleep.)

Sleep disorders

The four major categories of sleep disorders are: (1) insomnias, or disorders of initiating and maintaining sleep, (2) hypersomnias, or disorders of excessive som-

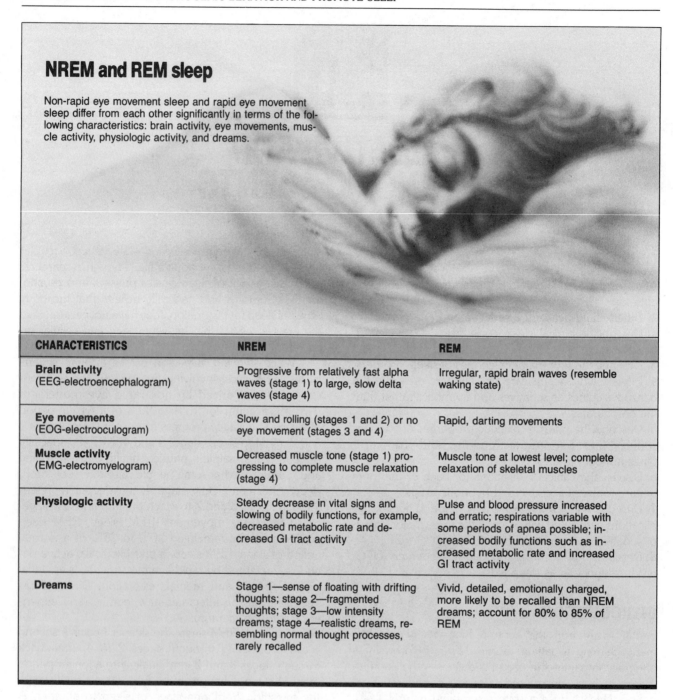

NREM and REM sleep

Non-rapid eye movement sleep and rapid eye movement sleep differ from each other significantly in terms of the following characteristics: brain activity, eye movements, muscle activity, physiologic activity, and dreams.

CHARACTERISTICS	NREM	REM
Brain activity (EEG-electroencephalogram)	Progressive from relatively fast alpha waves (stage 1) to large, slow delta waves (stage 4)	Irregular, rapid brain waves (resemble waking state)
Eye movements (EOG-electrooculogram)	Slow and rolling (stages 1 and 2) or no eye movement (stages 3 and 4)	Rapid, darting movements
Muscle activity (EMG-electromyelogram)	Decreased muscle tone (stage 1) progressing to complete muscle relaxation (stage 4)	Muscle tone at lowest level; complete relaxation of skeletal muscles
Physiologic activity	Steady decrease in vital signs and slowing of bodily functions, for example, decreased metabolic rate and decreased GI tract activity	Pulse and blood pressure increased and erratic; respirations variable with some periods of apnea possible; increased bodily functions such as increased metabolic rate and increased GI tract activity
Dreams	Stage 1—sense of floating with drifting thoughts; stage 2—fragmented thoughts; stage 3—low intensity dreams; stage 4—realistic dreams, resembling normal thought processes, rarely recalled	Vivid, detailed, emotionally charged, more likely to be recalled than NREM dreams; account for 80% to 85% of REM

nolence, (3) parasomnias, or dysfunctions associated with sleep, sleep stages, or partial arousals, and (4) disorders of the sleep-wake schedule.

Insomnias represent the most common sleep problems in our society. Hypersomnias may occur as difficulties in arousing from sleep, excessive daytime sleeping and napping, and actual "sleep attacks," such as falling asleep while driving or eating. Narcolepsy ("sleep attacks") accounts for about 60% of all hypersomnias;

sleep apnea accounts for another 20% to 25%. Sleep apnea, a condition characterized by the cessation of respirations, occurs intermittently during the sleep cycle and may last anywhere from a few seconds to over a minute. Parasomnias, which occur during normal sleep periods, include sleepwalking (somnambulism), night terrors, nocturnal enuresis (bed-wetting), and nightmares. Disorders of the sleep-wake schedule often accompany sudden time changes. Workers changing shifts at their jobs and travelers flying across several time zones typically experience disorders of the sleep-wake schedule.

Assessment of sleep and rest habits

Because physicians often order sedatives and hypnotics p.r.n., a comprehensive nursing assessment of the need for the drugs is especially important. The nurse must assess the patient's sleep and rest habits before identifying any present or potential sleep and rest problems. Assessing the sleep and rest habits of hospitalized patients also helps the nurse develop a plan to minimize any disruption of established patterns. A sleep history documents the patient's usual pattern of sleep and rest. If a patient identifies insomnia as a problem, the nurse must obtain a thorough sleep history and assess the signs and symptoms that indicate a lack of sleep. (See *Assessing sleep and rest habits* for the factors that the nurse should address when obtaining a patient's sleep history.) The nurse should also identify the amount of sleep that the patient considers necessary in 24 hours for optimal functioning. Considering all the factors as well as the patient's perception of the quality of sleep in the past month helps the nurse to identify the potential or actual

sleep problem. Once the sleep problem has been defined, the nurse can determine the appropriate nursing interventions.

See *Selected major drugs: Sedative and hypnotic agents* on pages 494 to 497 for a summary of the drugs discussed in this chapter.

BENZODIAZEPINES

Benzodiazepines produce many actions, including daytime and preanesthetic sedation, sleep induction, relief of anxiety and tension, skeletal muscle relaxation, and anticonvulsant activity. The benzodiazepines discussed here are mainly used for their sedative or hypnotic effects. Such benzodiazepines include flurazepam hydrochloride, lorazepam, temazepam, and triazolam. When other benzodiazepines are used clinically, they secondarily exert a sedative or hypnotic effect. Discussions of the other benzodiazepines appear in the appropriate chapters related to their primary clinical use.

History and source

In 1957, Sternbach synthesized the first benzodiazepine compound, chlordiazepoxide, but this drug was not used clinically until 1961. Until then, physicians most commonly used barbiturates as sedatives and hypnotics, but the barbiturates caused many toxic effects. The new benzodiazepine class of drugs largely replaced the barbiturates, since the new class possessed many of the same features as the barbiturates yet appeared to be safer.

In the 1960s and 1970s, researchers synthesized many new benzodiazepine compounds, which eventually reached the market as sedatives or hypnotics. The popularity of benzodiazepines grew steadily. At present, health care practitioners generally regard benzodiazepines as the sedative and hypnotic drugs of choice for clinical use.

PHARMACOKINETICS

Benzodiazepines are well absorbed and widely distributed in the body. All benzodiazepines are metabolized in the liver and are primarily excreted in the urine.

Absorption, distribution, metabolism, excretion

When taken orally, benzodiazepines are absorbed from

Assessing sleep and rest habits

When obtaining a sleep history, the nurse should focus questions on the patient's usual sleep habits to determine if they have changed over the last month. The nurse should address the following topics.

- History: personal history of allergies; past and present medical conditions; complete drug history including all prescription and OTC sleep aids; caffeine intake including coffee, tea, soda; family history; general emotional state and affect
- Number of hours of sleep per day
- Sleep pattern: usual time of retiring and arising
- Usual length of time to fall asleep; any difficulties associated with falling asleep
- Usual number of awakenings during the sleep period; reasons for awakenings (bladder tension, dreams, feeling of anxiety or depression); difficulty falling back to sleep after awakening
- Feeling upon awakening (rested, groggy, tired, disoriented)
- Usual sleep environment: type of bed, number of pillows, blankets, amount of light, noise, ventilation
- Prebedtime routines: exercise habits, use of beverages such as warm milk or tea, warm bath or shower, reading, watching TV, other relaxation measures
- Number, time of day, and length of daytime naps

the GI tract, with peak concentrations occurring at any time between 30 minutes and 8 hours, but usually within 1 to 3 hours. An intramuscular injection of a benzodiazepine results in erratic absorption, with the exception of lorazepam, which is readily absorbed to peak concentration levels in 60 to 90 minutes.

These drugs are widely distributed into body tissues; they also cross the blood-brain barrier and placenta. The lipid solubility of benzodiazepines increases their distribution and potential for redistribution; the redistribution of the drugs enhances their duration of action. Conversely, protein binding decreases the distribution of benzodiazepines. Most benzodiazepines and their active metabolites bind to plasma proteins. For example, flurazepam becomes 97% protein bound, lorazepam 91%, temazepam 98%, and triazolam 91%.

The benzodiazepines are extensively metabolized in the liver. Metabolism of flurazepam occurs via hydroxylation, which produces active metabolites with long half-lives, while metabolism of lorazepam and temazepam occurs via glucuronic acid conjugation. Triazolam is metabolized by hydroxylation to form a very active metabolite that is rapidly conjugated to an inactive metabolite. Metabolized benzodiazepines are excreted in the urine.

Onset, peak, duration

Most benzodiazepines register a relatively rapid onset of action: under 30 minutes. However, flurazepam and lorazepam have a slower onset of action, from 1 to 2 hours in some patients, because of slow absorption. The peak concentration level and duration of action vary among patients, as well as among the specific drugs. For example, triazolam reaches a peak concentration level in just over 1 hour but has a short duration of action and an elimination half-life of 2 to 3 hours. By comparison, flurazepam takes 1 to 3 hours to reach a peak concentration level but has a duration of action of up to 18 hours, including a half-life of 47 to 100 hours. Flurazepam becomes more effective after two consecutive uses because the active metabolite accumulates in the body. Because of age-related factors, flurazepam used by elderly patients exhibits a significantly prolonged half-life, with a mean half-life of 120 hours in females and 160 hours in males. In patients suffering severe liver dysfunction, the half-life of flurazepam is also prolonged because the liver, which metabolizes the drug, cannot work efficiently. Other sedatives and hypnotics (lorazepam, temazepam, and triazolam) do not form long-acting active metabolites, and, as a result, the actions of the drugs are not as significantly prolonged in elderly patients and in patients with significant liver dysfunction.

PHARMACODYNAMICS

Researchers have not established the locations of drug action or the mechanisms of action for the benzodiazepines. Though the drug action sites remain unknown, researchers believe the principal sites are the cerebral cortex and the limbic, thalamic, and hypothalamic levels of the central nervous system (CNS).

Mechanism of action

Researchers believe that benzodiazepines act at several sites in the CNS. One theory suggests that the drugs enhance the effects of the inhibitory neurotransmitter gamma-aminobutyric acid (GABA). Since GABA is inhibitory, receptor stimulation increases inhibition and blocks both limbic and cortical arousal. Another theory suggests that because benzodiazepine receptors are found in various structures of the CNS but not outside it, the drugs have little effect on other body systems.

When administered at low therapeutic doses, benzodiazepines decrease anxiety by acting on the limbic system and related brain areas that help regulate emotional activity. The drugs can usually calm or sedate the patient without causing drowsiness. (See Chapter 32, Antianxiety Agents, for a detailed discussion of benzodiazepines used to treat anxiety.) At higher doses, benzodiazepines exhibit sleep-producing properties, probably because the drugs depress the activating system located in the reticular formation of the midbrain.

The clinical use of benzodiazepines results in a net increase in total sleep time and produces a deep, refreshing sleep. Many experts hypothesize that the benzodiazepines improve the quality of sleep because of their effect on REM sleep. In most cases, benzodiazepines decrease the frequency of eyeball movement and the time spent in REM sleep. Flurazepam (in low doses) and temazepam, however, shorten stages 3 and 4 of NREM sleep and do not significantly diminish REM sleep. If temazepam has any effect on REM sleep, the effect resembles that of triazolam, which decreases REM sleep in the early hours but allows the sleeper to make up the lost REM time later in the sleep period. Benzodiazepines that do decrease total REM sleep time also allow for more frequent REM cycles later in the sleep period.

PHARMACOTHERAPEUTICS

Clinical indications for the benzodiazepines include relaxing and calming a patient during the day or before surgery and treating insomnia characterized by difficulty falling or staying asleep or early-morning awakenings.

Other clinical indications include producing I.V. anesthesia, treating alcohol withdrawal, treating anxiety and seizure disorders, and producing skeletal muscle relaxation. More information regarding these clinical indications for the benzodiazepines appears in the appropriate chapters of this book.

In most cases, physicians prefer benzodiazepines to barbiturates because of the effectiveness and safety of the former. Benzodiazepines offer many advantages, including fewer adverse effects and abuse, few drug interactions, a wide margin of safety between therapeutic and toxic doses that makes overdose less likely, and a rare incidence of physical and psychological dependence with therapeutic doses.

Despite their many advantages, benzodiazepines do have disadvantages. Abuse of the drugs can cause overdose, but with much less frequency than barbiturates. The potential for physical and psychological dependence exists with high doses and long-term use. Lorazepam, temazepam, and triazolam display minimal accumulation with multiple doses, while multiple doses of flurazepam can cause accumulation because of the long half-life of the drug. Furthermore, benzodiazepines can produce a synergistic action with other CNS depressants, further enhancing the depressant effects of the other drugs. If combined, such drugs can be lethal.

flurazepam hydrochloride (Dalmane). A Schedule IV drug, flurazepam is used as a hypnotic in patients with insomnia, such as those with poor sleep habits, and in acute or chronic medical situations requiring restful sleep. It is only for short-term and intermittent use.
USUAL ADULT DOSAGE: 15 to 30 mg P.O. at bedtime. Elderly and debilitated patients receive 15 mg P.O. at bedtime.

lorazepam (Ativan). A Schedule IV drug, lorazepam is used for sedation before surgery, insomnia from anxiety or transient situational stress, the management of anxiety disorders, and short-term relief of anxiety, or anxiety associated with depressive symptoms. This drug is for short-term and intermittent use only.
USUAL ADULT DOSAGE: for preoperative sedation, 0.05 mg/kg up to 4 mg I.M. 2 hours prior to the procedure; and as a hypnotic, 2 to 4 mg P.O. at bedtime. For elderly and debilitated, patients, 1 to 2 mg is given at bedtime for sleep.

temazepam (Restoril). A Schedule IV drug, temazepam is used only as a hypnotic to relieve insomnia associated with complaints of difficulty falling asleep, frequent nocturnal awakenings, or early-morning awakenings.

USUAL ADULT DOSAGE: as a hypnotic, 15 to 30 mg P.O. at bedtime; for elderly and debilitated patients, the initial dose is 15 mg P.O. Decreased bioavailability may result from the first-pass effect (8%) or because 96% of the drug is bound by plasma proteins.

triazolam (Halcion). A Schedule IV drug, triazolam is used to treat insomnia from various physical or psychological states. It is very short-acting and therefore has less tendency to cause morning drowsiness ("hangover" effect). This drug should not be used for longer than 1 month for managing insomnia.
USUAL ADULT DOSAGE: 0.25 to 0.5 mg P.O. at bedtime; and for elderly and debilitated patients, 0.125 to 0.25 mg P.O. at bedtime.

Drug interactions

Few interactions between drugs involve benzodiazepines, and those relate mainly to the use of benzodiazepines with other CNS depressant drugs. (See *Drug interactions: Benzodiazepines* on page 482 for details about interactions between drugs.) No interactions between drugs and food involving benzodiazepines have been documented.

ADVERSE DRUG REACTIONS

Benzodiazepines exhibit few adverse effects. Some mild allergic reactions as well as some idiosyncratic effects have been reported.

Predictable reactions

Common adverse reactions, such as daytime sedation and "hangover" effect, can occur with clinically effective doses of benzodiazepines, but the adverse reactions occur less frequently than those accompanying barbiturates. Dose-related dizziness and ataxia may also occur. Rebound insomnia may occur, especially with short-acting drugs such as triazolam. Elderly patients, debilitated patients, and patients with liver disease are more likely to experience predictable adverse reactions to benzodiazepines.

Fatigue, muscle weakness, mouth dryness, nausea, and vomiting result occasionally from benzodiazepine use. Though rare, respiratory depression may follow I.V. administration. Respiratory depression more frequently occurs with elderly or debilitated patients, patients with limited ventilatory reserve, and patients receiving other CNS depressants. Signs and symptoms of psychological and physical dependence occur with prolonged use and

DRUG INTERACTIONS

Benzodiazepines

Drug interactions involving the benzodiazepines discussed in this chapter occur infrequently. However, when interactions occur, they are more frequently seen with the concurrent use of other CNS depressant drugs, including alcohol. The additive effects of CNS drugs with benzodiazepines can be lethal.

DRUG	INTERACTING DRUGS	POSSIBLE EFFECTS	NURSING IMPLICATIONS
flurazepam, lorazepam, temazepam, triazolam	CNS depressants (including alcohol, narcotics, barbiturates, anticonvulsants, tricyclic antidepressants)	Enhance sedative and other CNS depressant effects. Effects may be supra-additive, causing impairment of motor skills and respiratory depression. Possible lethal effect especially with high doses. Combination with anticonvulsant drugs can cause changes in seizures, especially in frequency or severity.	• Monitor for changes in level of consciousness and muscle coordination. • Monitor for signs of respiratory depression. • Advise about possible additive effects of other CNS depressant drugs. • Warn patient that alcohol increases the effect of drug and can cause serious depression of CNS. • Supervise ambulation; raise side rails, especially with elderly patients. • Advise against driving and use of heavy machinery because of possible impaired motor skills. • Observe for changes in frequency and severity of seizures when these drugs are used with anticonvulsant drugs.
flurazepam, triazolam	cimetidine (Tagamet)	May cause benzodiazepine effects with resulting excessive sedation and increasing CNS depression	• Monitor for signs of increasing CNS depressant effects; notify physician if any changes noted. • Advise against driving and use of heavy machinery because increased sedation is possible. • Supervise ambulation; raise side rails, especially with elderly patients.
	cigarettes	May lessen benzodiazepine effects	• Warn patients that cigarette smoking when using these drugs may decrease the drug's effectiveness.
	levodopa	Decreases levodopa effects, resulting in decreased jerk-control of parkinsonism symptoms	• Monitor patient for increasing symptoms of parkinsonism such as increased tremors and muscle twitching. • Instruct the patient or family to notify the physician if parkinsonism symptoms change.

high doses, but rarely with usual doses. If a patient becomes physically dependent, sudden withdrawal may cause weakness, delirium, and tonic-clonic seizures.

Unpredictable reactions
Rare and usually mild allergic reactions to benzodiazepines include skin rash, pruritus, urticaria, burning eyes, and photosensitivity. Rare idiosyncractic reactions, which occur primarily in elderly patients, include nervousness, restlessness, talkativeness, apprehension, euphoria, and excitement.

NURSING IMPLICATIONS

Although the benzodiazepines are generally more desirable for nighttime sedation than barbiturates, the nurse must still be aware of the following implications.
• Benzodiazepines are contraindicated in patients with known sensitivity, acute narrow-angle glaucoma, and liver disease; and in pregnant women and nursing women.
• Use benzodiazepines cautiously in patients with chronic pulmonary insufficiency, psychoses, and in lactation, shock, and coma.

• Use caution when administering benzodiazepines to children and to patients who may become pregnant, are addiction-prone, have impaired renal function, are elderly or debilitated, or have anxiety states associated with depression.

• Conduct a general patient assessment, especially for signs of CNS and respiratory depression.

• Dosages of benzodiazepines may need to be reduced for patients who are also taking other drugs with CNS depressant effects.

• Benzodiazepines may have to be discontinued in patients who become irritable and restless; the patients may hallucinate or behave violently.

• Assist with any necessary gastric lavage, respiratory assistance, and general physiologic supportive measures if overdose occurs. Carefully monitor vital signs and intake and output (I and O).

• Be prepared to administer drugs such as epinephrine and corticosteroids in hypersensitivity reactions.

• The majority of sedatives and hypnotics are subject to the Controlled Substance Act of 1970 and its five schedules. This classification of drugs reflects their potential for causing physical or psychological dependence and their potential for abuse. In a hospital setting, the nurse administering sedatives and hypnotics must assume specific responsibilities according to the Controlled Substance Act. Chapter 1, Introduction To Pharmacology, provides more information on those responsibilities.

• A patient should take the drugs as prescribed and should not change the dosage without checking with a physician.

• If a patient takes the drugs over an extended period of time, the patient should not suddenly discontinue use, because withdrawal symptoms may occur.

• The use of other CNS depressant drugs may result in additive effects.

• A patient should read the labels and avoid OTC drugs that contain antihistamines, which are CNS depressants.

• Using alcohol while taking benzodiazepines may result in respiratory depression.

• A patient should not drive or use heavy machinery, at least until the patient knows the drug's effects because benzodiazepines decrease mental alertness.

• A patient should know the possible adverse effects of the drugs. The nurse should instruct the patient to notify a physician if adverse reactions occur.

• Benzodiazepine containers should not be left on the bedside stand. The patient may forget how many pills have been taken and accidentally take an overdose. Drugs should be kept out of the reach of children.

• Prescribed drugs should not be given to oth members or friends.

• For a patient having difficulty sleeping or who is complaining of insomnia, consider several different measures before resorting to the p.r.n. hypnotic ordered by the physician. Suggest a warm bath or shower or a glass of warm milk before the patient retires, encourage moderate daily exercise several hours before sleeping, advise the patient to eliminate daytime naps, and encourage reading and the use of other relaxation techniques.

• Consider the hospitalized patient's daily routines and bedtime rituals in planning care and administering drugs. Do not awaken a patient to administer a sedative or hypnotic. When administering a hypnotic orally, observe and make sure that the patient actually takes the drug and does not hoard it for possible later use. After administering the drug, implement safety measures, such as siderails and assistance with ambulation since the patient could become confused or unsteady when upright. Give special assistance to elderly patients during ambulation.

• If a patient awakens confused and excited, do not apply restraints but attempt to calm the patient, orient the patient to the surroundings, and talk quietly until the patient relaxes. Unless necessary, do not awaken the patient during the night. Allow the patient at least 90 minutes of uninterrupted rest or sleep whenever possible and use times when the patient awakens spontaneously to make necessary checks or to administer required treatments. Question the rationale for routines that require waking the patient, especially during the night.

• Use nursing judgments when deciding whether to administer a second p.r.n. sedative or hypnotic during the night. Try to find out why the patient cannot sleep, use comfort measures such as back rubs, and administer analgesics for pain. Remember, hypnotics are *not* analgesics. The "hangover" effect, sometimes seen the day after administration of a hypnotic, often occurs from nonjudicious use of hypnotics during the night.

BARBITURATES

The major pharmacologic action of the barbiturates reduces overall CNS alertness. The actions of barbiturates include daytime and preoperative sedation, a hypnotic effect for patients complaining of insomnia, for anesthesia, relief of anxiety, and anticonvulsant activity. The following section discusses the barbiturates used primarily as sedatives and hypnotics, including amobarbital, aprobarbital, butabarbital, mephobarbital, pentobarbital, phenobarbital, secobarbital, and talbutal.

History and source

In 1864, the German chemist Adolf von Baeyer synthesized barbituric acid. In 1903, the chemist Emil Fischer and the physician Josef von Mehring introduced barbital, a derivative of barbituric acid, into the field of medicine. Unlike the parent compound barbituric acid, barbital possessed hypnotic activity.

Health care practitioners widely used barbital for about a decade until the introduction of phenobarbital in 1912. Both barbital and phenobarbital represented technologic improvements over the bromides, which at that time were the most frequently prescribed sedatives. Since 1912, over 2,000 derivatives of barbituric acid have been synthesized. Health care practitioners currently use about one dozen barbiturates as sedatives, hypnotics, anesthetics, or anticonvulsants. The introduction of the first benzodiazepine, chlordiazepoxide, into the market in 1961 began the decline in the use of barbiturates.

PHARMACOKINETICS

Barbiturates are well absorbed, rapidly distributed, metabolized by the liver, and excreted via the metabolic processes as well as in the urine.

Absorption, distribution, metabolism, excretion

Barbiturates are well absorbed following both oral and I.M. administration. The I.M. route is usually avoided, however, because the alkalinity of the soluble preparations causes pain and necrosis at the injection site.

Barbiturates, which are weak acids, are rapidly distributed to all body tissues and fluids. The highest concentrations go to the brain, liver, and kidneys. Barbiturates also cross the placental barrier and can depress neonatal respirations and the CNS. Lipid solubility is the dominant factor in the distribution of barbiturates within the body. The more lipid-soluble the barbiturate, the more rapidly the drug penetrates all tissues of the body. Secobarbital displays the highest lipid solubility, and phenobarbital has the lowest.

Barbiturates are primarily metabolized by the microsomal enzymes in the liver. Longer-acting barbiturates metabolize more slowly than short-acting ones.

Barbiturates are excreted primarily by the kidneys. Some, such as mephobarbital and metharbital, undergo metabolic changes in the liver before they are excreted by the kidneys. Others, such as aprobarbital and phenobarbital, are excreted partly in an altered form and partly in their unchanged forms. Still others, such as butabarbital, secobarbital, and pentobarbital, are excreted in a completely altered form. The more slowly the system metabolizes or excretes a barbiturate, the more prolonged the drug's action.

Onset, peak, duration

The duration of drug action represents the main difference among barbiturates. The duration may be ultrashort-acting, short-acting, intermediate-acting, or long-acting. Peak concentration levels also vary, depending on the onset of action. (See *The different actions of barbiturates* for the onset, peak, and duration of short-acting, intermediate-acting, and long-acting barbiturates.)

The duration of action of a barbiturate depends in part upon the rate of drug metabolism and the rate of drug redistribution throughout the body. The duration of action varies among patients and even in the same patient from time to time. The half-lives of barbiturates vary from drug to drug. For example, secobarbital has a half-life of 15 to 40 hours, mephobarbital 11 to 67 hours, and phenobarbital 50 to 170 hours. Note, however, that because of the rapid distribution of some barbiturates, no correlation exists between duration of action and half-life. When used over extended periods of time, all barbiturates will accumulate.

PHARMACODYNAMICS

Researchers do not know the primary sites of drug action and the mechanisms of action of barbiturates. Researchers believe the primary action sites to be the neuronal fibers and synapses that integrate the wake-sleep centers of the brain, primarily at the level of the thalamus and the ascending reticular formation.

Mechanism of action

Barbiturates are considered to be nonspecific CNS depressants, similar to benzodiazepines in that they facilitate neurotransmission in the CNS. The sites of barbiturate action appear to be less selective than the sites of benzodiazepine action. As sedative-hypnotics, barbiturates depress the sensory cortex, decrease motor activity, alter cerebral function, and produce drowsiness, sedation, and hypnosis. Barbiturates appear to act at the level of the thalamus where they inhibit the ascending

The different actions of barbiturates

The onset of action, peak concentration level, and duration of action vary significantly depending upon the specific barbiturates. The following graph illustrates the comparison of short-acting, intermediate-acting, and long-acting barbiturates.

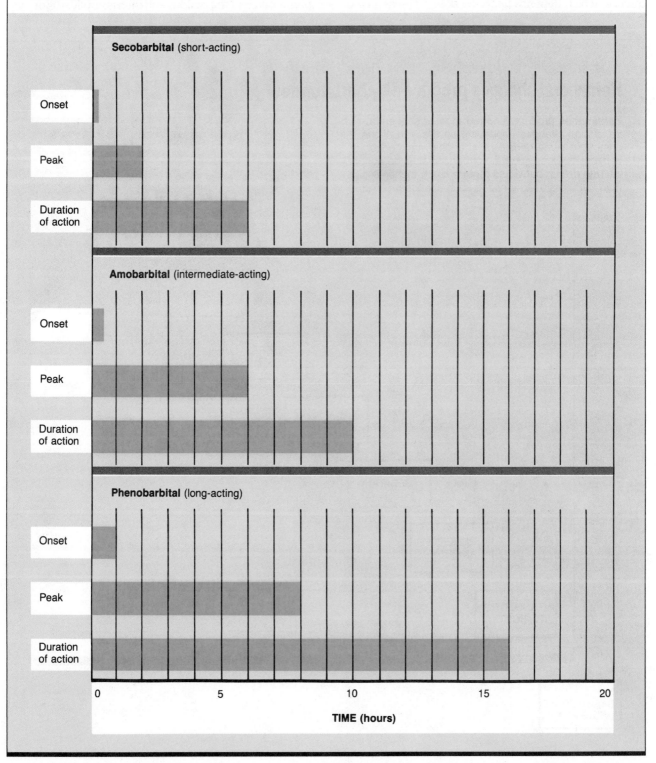

conduction in the reticular formation, thus interfering with the transmission of impulses to the cortex.

Barbiturates produce a sequence of CNS depressant effects ranging from mild sedation and relief of anxiety to anesthesia and coma. (See *Behavioral changes produced by barbiturates* for an illustration of the sequence, which depends upon the dose.) The degree of CNS depression also depends on other factors such as the person's age, emotional state, and the drug administration route.

Barbiturates decrease stages 3 and 4 of NREM sleep. The drugs also reduce the amount of time a person spends in REM sleep, or dream sleep. If barbiturates are prescribed for long periods and then abruptly withdrawn,

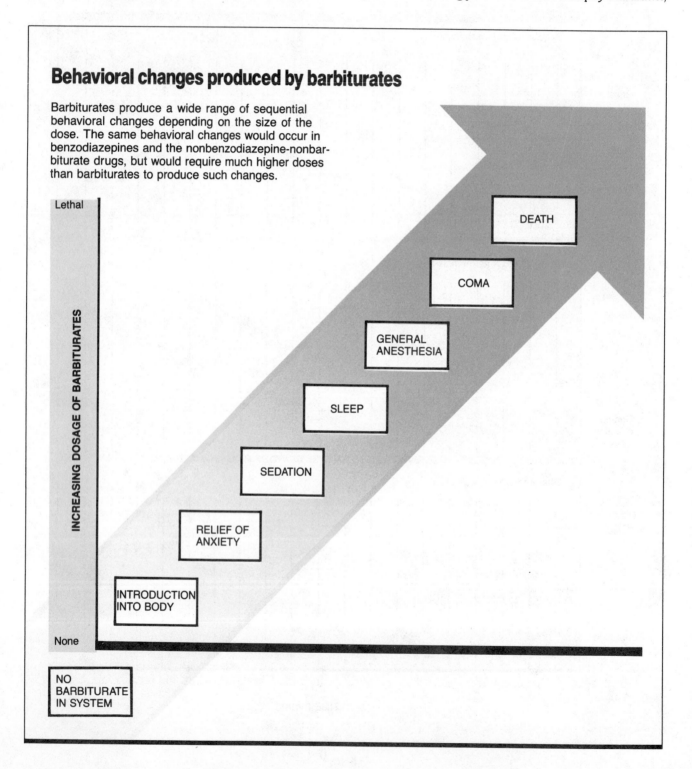

Behavioral changes produced by barbiturates

Barbiturates produce a wide range of sequential behavioral changes depending on the size of the dose. The same behavioral changes would occur in benzodiazepines and the nonbenzodiazepine-nonbarbiturate drugs, but would require much higher doses than barbiturates to produce such changes.

INCREASING DOSAGE OF BARBITURATES

Lethal

None

DEATH

COMA

GENERAL ANESTHESIA

SLEEP

SEDATION

RELIEF OF ANXIETY

INTRODUCTION INTO BODY

NO BARBITURATE IN SYSTEM

the patient may experience REM sleep rebound, with a marked increase in dreaming, nightmares, or insomnia.

Patients can also develop a tolerance for barbiturates, which decreases the sedative, hypnotic, and mood-altering effects of the drugs. Also, as tolerance increases, the therapeutic index decreases and the drugs become less safe. Tolerance can occur after only weeks or after a few months of therapy.

PHARMACOTHERAPEUTICS

Barbiturates have many clinical indications including daytime sedation, hypnotic effects, anesthesia, and anticonvulsant effects. Chapter 24, Anticonvulsant Agents, details the use of barbiturates as anticonvulsant agents. Barbiturates are not frequently used for daytime sedation. When used, they are usually given for short time periods, usually less than 2 weeks. If alcohol or other CNS depressants are used concurrently with barbiturates, the combination may produce additive CNS depressant effects, which can be lethal. The use of barbiturates as sedatives and hypnotics is declining, because physicians now regard the benzodiazepines as the sedatives and hypnotics of choice.

Barbiturates offer no real advantages over the benzodiazepines as sedatives and hypnotics and, in fact, present many disadvantages, including a greater probability of causing drug tolerance, a high potential for physical and/or psychological dependence, a high liability for abuse, severe withdrawal symptoms when drug use is discontinued suddenly after chronic use, life-threatening toxicity resulting from overdose, and depression of the respiratory center after large doses. More toxic than the benzodiazepines, barbiturates, especially long-acting forms, are more prone to accumulate in the system.

The use of barbiturates with those over age 60 is not recommended.

amobarbital, amobarbital sodium (Amytal). A Schedule II drug, amobarbital is used for conditions that require degrees of sedation. Minimal doses are used to relieve anxiety and tension, and hypnotic doses to treat insomnia and acute psychotic disorders.
USUAL ADULT DOSAGE: for sedation, 30 to 50 mg P.O. or I.M. b.i.d. or t.i.d.; for hypnotic effect, 65 to 200 mg P.O. or I.M. at bedtime.

aprobarbital (Alurate). A Schedule III drug, aprobarbital is used for daytime sedation and the induction of sleep, on a short-term basis.
USUAL ADULT DOSAGE: for sedation, 40 mg P.O. t.i.d.; as a hypnotic agent, 40 to 160 mg P.O. at bedtime.

butabarbital sodium (Butisol, Buticaps). A Schedule III drug, butabarbital is used as a daytime mild sedative for anxiety, as a preoperative sedative, and for insomnia for use up to 2 weeks.
USUAL ADULT DOSAGE: for sedation, 15 to 30 mg P.O. t.i.d. or q.i.d.; for preoperative sedation, 50 to 100 mg P.O. 60 to 90 minutes before surgery; and as a hypnotic agent, 50 to 100 mg P.O. at bedtime.

mephobarbital (Mebaral). A Schedule IV drug, mephobarbital is used for daytime sedation to relieve anxiety, tension, and apprehension, and as adjunct therapy for grand mal and petit mal epilepsy.
USUAL ADULT DOSAGE: for daytime sedation, 32 to 100 mg P.O. t.i.d. or q.i.d.

pentobarbital sodium (Nembutal). A Schedule II drug, pentobarbital is used as a daytime sedative to reduce nervous tension in patients with various medical and psychiatric conditions; as a preoperative sedation for minor diagnostic or surgical procedures; for short-term treatment of insomnia, for a period of up to 2 weeks; and for the emergency control of convulsions.
USUAL ADULT DOSAGE: for daytime sedation, 20 to 40 mg P.O. b.i.d. to q.i.d.; for preanesthetic sedation, 150 to 200 mg P.O. or I.M.; and for a hypnotic effect, 100 mg P.O., 120 to 200 mg rectal, or 100 to 200 mg I.M.

phenobarbital, phenobarbital sodium (Luminal). A Schedule IV drug, phenobarbital is used as a sedative to relieve mild to moderate anxiety or tension, as a preoperative sedative, as treatment for insomnia, and as an anticonvulsant.
USUAL ADULT DOSAGE: for daytime sedation, 15 to 30 mg P.O. b.i.d. to q.i.d.; for preoperative sedation, 100 to 200 mg I.M. 60 to 90 minutes before surgery; and for its hypnotic effect, 100 to 320 mg P.O. or I.M. at bedtime.

secobarbital sodium (Seconal). A Schedule II drug, secobarbital is used as a mild sedative; as a short-acting hypnotic for insomnia, especially in patients with difficulty falling asleep; and as treatment for acute convulsive disorders, such as local anesthetic reactions, tetanus, and status epilepticus.
USUAL ADULT DOSAGE: for daytime sedation, 30 to 50 mg P.O. t.i.d. to q.i.d. and 120 to 200 mg rectal suppository; for preoperative sedation, 200 to 300 mg P.O. 1 to 2 hours before surgery; and as a hypnotic, 100 to 200 mg P.O., 120 to 200 mg rectally, and 100 to 200 mg I.M. at bedtime.

talbutal (Lotusate). A Schedule III drug, talbutal is used as a daytime sedative and to relieve insomnia short-term.

USUAL ADULT DOSAGE: for sedation, 30 to 60 mg P.O. b.i.d. to t.i.d.; and for its hypnotic effect, 120 mg P.O. 15 to 30 minutes before bedtime.

Drug interactions

Barbiturates cause many interactions between drugs. (See *Drug Interactions: Barbiturates* and *Phenobarbital* in Chapter 24, Anticonvulsants.) An interaction between the drug and food can occur with a protein-deficient diet and is characterized by increased duration of action. This

---

DRUG INTERACTIONS

Barbiturates

Drug interactions involving barbiturates are frequent and can be very serious. Interactions often occur with concurrent use of other CNS depressant drugs, including alcohol. The additive effects can be lethal.

DRUG	INTERACTING DRUGS	POSSIBLE EFFECTS	NURSING IMPLICATIONS
amobarbital, aprobarbital, butabarbital, mephobarbital, pentobarbital, phenobarbital, secobarbital, talbutal	CNS depressants (alcohol, anticonvulsants, narcotics, antihistamines, tricyclic antidepressants).	Increase CNS depression; potentiate of CNS depressant effects; may lead to drowsiness, lethargy, stupor, coma, respiratory depression	• Assess frequently for changes in level of consciousness and respirations. • Supervise ambulation; raise side rails, especially with elderly patients. • Inform the patient not to drive or use heavy machinery until the drug effects are known. • Warn that the potentiation resulting from combining the drugs can cause respiratory and CNS depression, both of which can be lethal. • Inform the patient that alcohol may enhance the depressant effect of prescribed drugs. Ideally, patient should not drink alcohol; if the patient will not abstain completely, urge the patient to drink in moderation, especially at start of therapy.
	oral anticoagulants	Decrease anticoagulant effect; as a result, the blood may clot despite anticoagulant treatment	• Monitor prothrombin time carefully; dosage of anticoagulant may need adjustment. • Observe for signs of thrombus (clot) formation such as Homans' sign (calf pain with dorsiflexion of the foot), tenderness, and edema.
	corticosteroids	Decrease effect of corticosteroids from increased breakdown by liver, resulting in decreased therapeutic effect	• Because of decreased effect, dosage may need to be increased. • Monitor the patient's weight and blood pressure. • Monitor serum electrolytes.
	phenytoin	May decrease effect of phenytoin; as a result, seizures may not be properly controlled	• Perform frequent neurologic assessments to note CNS changes. • Observe for increased seizures or a change in seizure activity.
	oral contraceptives	May decrease effect of contraceptive, resulting in an increased risk of pregnancy unless an alternative method of contraception is used	• Inform the patient that oral birth control measures may not be completely effective and that increased risk of pregnancy may exist. • Suggest an alternative method of contraception to patients using barbiturates.
	MAO inhibitors	May enhance depressant effect of barbiturates	• Assess frequently for changes in mental alertness and for increased CNS and respiratory depression.

is caused by an inhibition of an enzyme that degrades barbiturates.

ADVERSE DRUG REACTIONS

Barbiturates cause many adverse drug reactions, some of which are minor. Other more serious drug reactions include severe CNS and respiratory depression.

Predictable reactions

The most frequently reported adverse reactions relate to the CNS and include drowsiness, lethargy, headache, mental depression, and vertigo. After hypnotic doses, the "hangover" effect frequently occurs, accompanied by an impairment both of judgment and motor skills, which can last for many hours. When hypnotic doses are discontinued, the patient may experience REM sleep rebound, as well as a decrease in stage 2 NREM sleep. Patients, especially elderly ones, may exhibit excitement and confusion, particularly when taking short-acting compounds such as secobarbital.

The respiratory system can suffer serious adverse reactions including hypoventilation, laryngospasm, bronchospasm, and severe respiratory depression, specifically when large doses are administered intravenously and too rapidly. Large doses of barbiturates suppress the hypoxic and chemoreceptor drive of the respiratory system, resulting in a decrease in the rate and rhythm of the respirations.

The cardiovascular system can also suffer adverse reactions such as mild bradycardia and hypotension. Infrequently, adverse reactions to barbiturates affect the GI tract, resulting in nausea, vomiting, diarrhea, and epigastric pain.

Acute barbiturate toxicity causes overdose symptoms, which can be severe. The symptoms are characterized by CNS and respiratory depression, and death can result from respiratory failure followed by cardiac arrest.

With prolonged use, the patient can develop drug tolerance as well as psychological and physical dependence upon the barbiturate. Withdrawal symptoms resemble those associated with chronic alcoholism and occur after sudden discontinuation after chronic use.

Unpredictable reactions

Allergic reactions mainly involve the skin and mucous membranes and occur more commonly in patients with past allergies or asthma. Allergic reactions include these signs and symptoms: skin rashes of various kinds, urticaria, angioedema, and fever. Rare occurrences of photosensitivity have also been reported. Other signs and symptoms of allergic reactions to barbiturates include rare blood dyscrasias, such as pancytopenia, leukopenia, granulocytopenia, thrombocytopenia, and megaloblastic anemia secondary to folic acid depletion.

Idiosyncratic reactions include paradoxical anxiety, agitation, restlessness, and rage or paradoxical excitement (delirium rather than sedation). The idiosyncratic reactions occur most frequently among elderly patients and patients with severe uncontrolled pain.

NURSING IMPLICATIONS

Barbiturates are no longer considered the drugs of choice as sedatives or hypnotics because of the high risk of barbiturate toxicity and dependence. However, when barbiturates are given, the nurse must be aware of the following implications.

• Barbiturates are contraindicated for patients with a personal or family history of porphyria, hypersensitivity to barbiturates, pulmonary insufficiency, severe cardiac or renal disease, mentally depressed individuals with suicidal tendencies or with a history of drug abuse, and in pregnancy and lactation.

• An elderly or debilitated patient may require lower than recommended doses. Discontinue the drug slowly after long-term therapy.

• Carefully monitor a patient who is taking anticoagulants and stops taking a barbiturate, because serious bleeding may occur.

• Rotate the amobarbital ampule (do not shake); mix the solution with sterile water only; discard solutions that do not clear within 5 minutes; use the solution within 30 minutes after opening to minimize deterioration; and when using the I.M. route of administration, inject the solution slowly and deeply into a large muscle mass. Remember, the I.M. route is a poor route for administering barbiturates.

• Do not use a cloudy pentobarbital, phenobarbital, or secobarbital solution or mix the solution with other medications; use the solution within 30 minutes after opening to minimize deterioration; and when administering I.M., inject the solution into a large muscle mass.

Patient teaching is essential when a patient is receiving barbiturates because of the high risk of toxicity and dependence that accompany this class of drug. (See *Patient-teaching tips* on page 490 for some general instructions for the patient who is going to take barbiturates at home.)

Patient-teaching tips

The patient taking a barbiturate as a hypnotic at home requires general and drug-specific instructions. The nurse can also use the same instructions with benzodiazepines and nonbenzodiazepine-nonbarbiturate drugs, giving oral instructions first, then written ones to take home.

MEDICATION NAME _____

DOSAGE AND TIME SCHEDULE _____

WHAT KIND OF DRUG IS IT?
The drug you will take is called a hypnotic drug. It will help you relax and fall asleep. It may also prevent you from awakening frequently during the night and early morning.

GENERAL INSTRUCTIONS TO FOLLOW
● Follow the instructions on the prescription precisely. Do NOT increase or decrease the drug dosage or the number of times prescribed. Also, do NOT discontinue the drug without consulting with your physician.
● The drug may cause you to be drowsy or less alert upon arising. Until you learn how the drug affects you, do NOT drive or operate dangerous machinery or put yourself in situations where decreased mental alertness may be dangerous.
● The drug will add to the effect of alcohol and other drugs that slow down the nervous system such as antihistamines, tranquilizers, narcotics, or other prescription pain relievers. Before taking any of the drugs just mentioned, consult with your physician.
● Your drug has been prescribed especially for you. Do not share the drug with your relatives or friends.
● Notify the nurse or physician if you start or stop taking any other drug while taking your hypnotic drug.
● Keep the drug and all other medications out of the reach of children.

NONBENZODIAZEPINES-NONBARBITURATES

Like the barbiturates, the nonbenzodiazepine-nonbarbiturate drugs act as hypnotics to treat simple insomnia short-term, but lose their effectiveness by the end of the second week. The drugs also provide preoperative sedation and sedation before EEG studies. The following section discusses nonbenzodiazepine-nonbarbiturate drugs including chloral hydrate, ethchlorvynol, ethinamate, glutethimide, methyprylon, and paraldehyde.

History and source
Chloral hydrate and paraldehyde were introduced in the late 19th century for use in promoting sedation and sleep. The popularity of the drugs decreased after the introduction of the barbiturates, but interest resurfaced when the barbiturates were found to cause dependence.

More recent nonbenzodiazepine-nonbarbiturate drugs offer few advantages, if any, over the barbiturates they were meant to replace. Though still in use, the nonbenzodiazepine-nonbarbiturate drugs have practically been replaced by the benzodiazepines.

PHARMACOKINETICS

Nonbenzodiazepine-nonbarbiturate drugs are rapidly absorbed from the GI tract, metabolized in the liver, and excreted in the urine.

Absorption, distribution, metabolism, excretion
Rapid absorption from the GI tract occurs after oral administration, with the exception of glutethimide, which is erratically absorbed. The drugs are generally distributed to the cerebrospinal fluid (CSF), milk, and fetal blood. The distribution pattern of ethinamate remains unknown, though the drug is rapidly destroyed in the tissues.

The nonbenzodiazepine-nonbarbiturate drugs are primarily metabolized in the endoplasmic reticulum of the liver. Glutethimide and ethchlorvynol both undergo extensive enterohepatic recirculation, with the liver destroying 80% to 90% of the drugs. Excretion occurs primarily through the urine via the kidneys and to a small degree in the feces via bile. Following therapeutic doses, clinically insignificant amounts are excreted in human milk.

Onset, peak, duration

The onset of action for nonbenzodiazepine-nonbarbiturate drugs is rapid in most cases, with chloral hydrate displaying an onset of action within 10 to 15 minutes. The other drugs have an onset of action of 15 to 45 minutes. Drug action usually reaches a peak concentration level at 1 to 2 hours, with the exception of glutethimide, which reaches peak concentration at 1 to 6 hours from erratic absorption from the GI tract.

The duration of action, including half-life, varies among the drugs. Generally, however, the duration lasts 4 to 8 hours. Ethchlorvynol has a duration of action and half-life of 10 to 25 hours, the longest among the nonbenzodiazepine-nonbarbiturate drugs.

PHARMACODYNAMICS

The mechanisms of action for the nonbenzodiazepine-nonbarbiturate drugs are not completely known, but the drugs produce depressant effects similar to the barbiturates. At high doses, the drugs can produce CNS depression of the respiratory center, causing respiratory failure and death.

PHARMACOTHERAPEUTICS

Nonbenzodiazepine-nonbarbiturate drugs are most often used to treat simple insomnia short-term and for sedation before surgery. The drugs offer no special advantages over other sedatives and hypnotics and, in fact, are quite similar to the barbiturates. Many physicians believe that chloral hydrate produces less excitement in elderly patients than the barbiturates, but this has not been confirmed. The disadvantages of the drugs include being habit-forming, causing physical dependence, and being subject to abuse.

chloral hydrate (Noctec, SK-Chloral Hydrate). A Schedule IV drug, chloral hydrate is used as a daytime sedative and as a hypnotic to relieve insomnia.
USUAL ADULT DOSAGE: for sedation, 250 mg P.O. or 325 mg rectally t.i.d. after meals; and for a hypnotic effect, 0.5 to 1 gram P.O. or rectally 15 to 30 minutes before bedtime. The dose of chloral hydrate should not exceed 2 grams daily.

ethchlorvynol (Placidyl). A Schedule IV drug, ethchlorvynol is used as a daytime sedative and for short-term hypnotic therapy of insomnia (not to exceed 1 week).
USUAL ADULT DOSAGE: for sedation, 200 mg P.O. b.i.d. or t.i.d.; and for a hypnotic effect, 0.5 to 1 gram P.O. at bedtime. The dose should be adjusted carefully in elderly and debilitated patients.

ethinamate (Valmid). A Schedule IV drug, ethinamate is used as a hypnotic for the short-term treatment of insomnia (not to exceed 1 week).
USUAL ADULT DOSAGE: 0.5 to 1 gram P.O. 20 minutes before bedtime. The usual dose for elderly and debilitated patients is 500 mg P.O.

glutethimide (Doriden). A Schedule III drug, glutethimide is used as a daytime and preoperative sedative and for the short-term treatment of insomnia (not to exceed 1 week).
USUAL ADULT DOSAGE: for its hypnotic effects, 250 to 500 mg P.O. at bedtime. The daily dose should not exceed 1 gram for adults, and in elderly or debilitated patients the daily dose should not exceed 0.5 gram.

methyprylon (Noludar). A Schedule III drug, methyprylon is used as a hypnotic for transient or intermittent insomnia.
USUAL ADULT DOSAGE: 200 to 400 mg P.O. before bedtime.

paraldehyde (Paral). A Schedule IV drug, paraldehyde is used infrequently but sometimes for sedation, as a hypnotic for insomnia, to treat alcohol withdrawal syndrome, and to control seizures caused by tetanus. Its most frequent use is for alcohol withdrawal.
USUAL ADULT DOSAGE: for sedation, 5 to 10 ml P.O. or rectal; for its hypnotic effect, 10 to 30 ml P.O. or rectal at bedtime. Anticonvulsant dosage is 5 to 10 ml I.M. or 5 ml I.V. diluted in normal saline solution. For alcohol withdrawal, 5 to 10 ml P.O. or 5 ml I.M. every 4 to 6 hours up to a maximum of 60 ml P.O. or 30 ml I.M. during the first 24 hours, then 5 to 10 ml P.O. or 5 ml I.M. every 6 hours to a maximum of 40 ml/day P.O. or 30 ml I.M. until desired response is achieved. I.V. dosages are rarely administered and are reserved for emergencies.

Drug interactions

The main interaction between nonbenzodiazepine and nonbarbiturate drugs occurs when the drugs are used

DRUG INTERACTIONS

Nonbenzodiazepines-Nonbarbiturates

Drug interactions that occur with this class of drug are mainly from nonbenzodiazepines-nonbarbiturates used with other CNS depressants.

DRUG	INTERACTING DRUGS	POSSIBLE EFFECTS	NURSING IMPLICATIONS
chloral hydrate, ethchlorvynol, ethinamate, glutethimide, methyprylon, paraldehyde	CNS depressant drugs (alcohol, tranquilizers, antihistamines, barbiturates, narcotics)	Cause drowsiness, respiratory depression, stupor, coma, or death	• Assess for CNS and respiratory changes. • Advise the patient to prohibit or sharply curtail alcohol use during administration. (Combination of alcohol with chloral hydrate is called a "Mickey Finn.") • Supervise ambulation; use side rails, especially with elderly patients. • Caution patient not to drive or use heavy machinery until the drug effects are known.
	oral anticoagulants	Increase effect of anticoagulant by decreasing plasma protein binding, resulting in the increased risk of bleeding	• Monitor prothrombin levels; dosage may need to be adjusted. • Observe for symptoms of increased bleeding, such as bruising or bleeding anywhere on the body. • Observe for black or tarry stools.
paraldehyde	disulfiram (Antabuse)	Increases paraldehyde blood levels causing increased CNS depression; possibly toxic disulfiram reaction (respiratory depression, cardiac dysrhythmias, convulsions, unconsciousness)	• Monitor for increased signs of CNS and respiratory depression. • Warn the patient not to use alcohol because doing so can be lethal.

with other CNS depressants, causing additive depression of the CNS. (See *Drug Interactions: Nonbenzodiazepines-Nonbarbiturates*.) No interactions between the drugs and food occur.

ADVERSE DRUG REACTIONS

The most frequent adverse predictable reactions involving nonbenzodiazepine-nonbarbiturate drugs include GI symptoms and some "hangover" effects. Respiratory depression can also occur. Hypersensitivity and idiosyncratic reactions are rare.

Predictable reactions

Drug reactions affect the GI system, resulting in nausea, vomiting, and some gastric irritation. The affected CNS, which occurs especially with hypnotic doses, can produce the "hangover" effect. Compared to the "hang-

over" produced by barbiturates and benzodiazepines, the nonbenzodiazepine-nonbarbiturate "hangover" occurs less frequently, especially in elderly patients. Habitual use can cause tolerance and dependence. Chronic and acute toxicity can occur, and abrupt withdrawal from large doses may cause dangerous withdrawal symptoms similar to those seen with withdrawal from barbiturates.

Unpredictable reactions

Rare and mild hypersensitivity reactions include skin rashes and urticaria. Also rare, idiosyncratic reactions can include marked excitement, hysteria, prolonged hypnosis, profound muscular weakness, and syncope without marked hypotension.

NURSING IMPLICATIONS

The nonbenzodiazepine-nonbarbiturate drugs closely resemble the barbiturates in their potential to cause toxicity and dependence. The nurse must be aware of some special implications when administering these drugs.

• Nonbenzodiazepines-nonbarbiturates are contraindicated in patients with markedly impaired renal and hepatic function, hypersensitivity, a history of drug abuse, and suicidal tendencies; do not give chloral hydrate in liquid form to patients with gastritis or ulcers; do not give glutethimide to patients with glaucoma, prostatic hypertrophy, stenosing peptic ulcer, pyloroduodenal or bladder neck obstruction, or cardiac dysrhythmias because of the anticholinergic effect; do not give paraldehyde to patients with gastroenteritis or bronchopulmonary disease.

• Elderly and debilitated patients should receive lower doses than those recommended for other adults.

• Exercise caution when using the drugs with patients who are mentally depressed, have other emotional disorders, or are in labor.

• Chloral hydrate has a disagreeable taste and causes gastric irritation. Minimize the unpleasant taste and gastric irritation by giving the drug after meals and diluting it or administering it with a liquid, such as juice or soda. Store chloral hydrate in a dark container and refrigerate suppositories.

• Minimize transient dizziness or ataxia associated with ethchlorvynol by giving the drug with milk or food. Store ethchlorvynol and glutethimide in a tight, light-resistant container to avoid possible deterioration; a slight darkening of the liquid from exposure to light and air will not affect safety or potency.

• Use paraldehyde from containers that have been opened for less than 24 hours because the drug decomposes upon exposure to light; do not give the drug if it is brown or has an acetic acid odor. The oral liquid form must be diluted in iced milk, syrup, or fruit juice to disguise the taste and odor and reduce gastric distress. Because the drug reacts with some plastics, use glass syringes and metal needles. When administering I.M., inject deep into a large muscle mass and massage the site. For rectal administration, minimize irritation by diluting the drug with vegetable oil (one part drug to two parts diluent); then administer the drug as a retention enema.

Other implications for nonbenzodiazepine-nonbarbiturate drugs have been previously discussed in relation to the benzodiazepines.

OTHER SEDATIVES

Alcohol and many over-the-counter products, especially those containing antihistamines, are often used as nonprescription sedatives. Two dietary sources, herbs and L-tryptophan, may have some usefulness as sleep aids.

Alcohol is the most widely used and abused drug in the United States. Alcohol is a CNS depressant and can be considered a nonprescription sleep aid, a purpose it has served since ancient times. After rapid absorption from an empty stomach, alcohol enters the bloodstream and quickly travels to the CNS where it diffuses past the blood-brain barrier. Metabolism occurs primarily in the liver, where most of the absorbed alcohol is broken down for the production of energy, with the unchanged remainder leaving the body in the urine and breath. Alcohol has been used to improve appetite and digestion and, in elderly patients, to promote sleep. Alcohol causes many adverse reactions in the body, and continuous consumption of large amounts can cause serious effects on gastric and hepatic function. Alcohol use with other CNS depressants can be lethal. Nurses need to be prepared to educate patients about alcohol and its effects on the body. For a more complete discussion, refer to Chapter 6, Drug Abuse, Dependence and Addiction.

Over-the-counter (OTC) sleep aids are readily available for purchase in the United States. These OTC drugs usually contain an antihistamine (diphenhydramine, doxylamine, or pyrilamine), which has some sedative properties. The common antihistamines pyrilamine maleate and diphenhydramine are found in Nevine, Nytol, Sleep-eze, and Sominex. The antihistamines, being CNS depressants, affect sleep; however, researchers have not studied the effect extensively. Chapter 63, Antihistaminic Agents, presents further discussion of the antihistamines. Minor atropine-like adverse effects, such as dry mouth, can result from use of OTC drugs. Confusion and disorientation can also occur, especially in elderly patients.

Two dietary sources, herbs and L-tryptophan, also promote relaxation and sleep. Herbs, found in many products such as tea, have a quieting, relaxing effect and can help a person fall asleep. L-tryptophan, an essential amino acid found in a variety of high-protein foods, increases the brain levels of serotonin. Serotonin acts as a neurotransmitter and helps induce and promote sleep. The well-known sleepiness that occurs after eating a large meal, particularly one containing meat, may be related to the L-tryptophan content of the meal.

Current research seems to indicate that people who ordinarily have trouble falling asleep may benefit from a dose of L-tryptophan. However, the Food and Drug Administration has not approved L-tryptophan as a sleep aid in the United States; health food stores sell L-tryptophan as a dietary supplement.

SELECTED MAJOR DRUGS

Sedative and hypnotic agents

This chart summarizes the major sedative and hypnotic drugs currently in clinical use.

DRUG	MAJOR INDICATIONS	USUAL ADULT DOSAGES	NURSING IMPLICATIONS
Benzodiazepines			
flurazepam	Hypnotic for insomnia	15 to 30 mg P.O. h.s.	• Contraindicated in known sensitivity and in pregnancy. • Supervise ambulation; raise side rails, especially for elderly patients. • In elderly patients and those with severe liver disease, the half-life is even more prolonged; monitor for adverse reactions. • The low end of dosage range should be used for elderly and debilitated patients. • Multiple doses can cause accumulation because of a long half-life; observe for adverse reactions. • Warn patient not to perform activities that require mental alertness, such as driving or using heavy machinery, until the drug's effects on the patient are known.
lorazepam	Sedative before surgery	0.5 mg/kg up to 4 mg I.M. 2 hours before operative procedure	• Contraindicated in known sensitivity and in pregnancy. • Supervise ambulation; raise side rails, especially for elderly patients. • Monitor for dependence with long-term use. • The low end of dosage range should be used for elderly and debilitated patients. • Warn patient not to perform activities that require mental alertness, such as driving or using heavy machinery, until the drug's effects on the patient are known.
	Hypnotic for insomnia due to anxiety or transient situational stress, anxiety disorders	2 to 4 mg P.O. h.s.	
temazepam	Hypnotic for insomnia	15 to 30 mg P.O. h.s.	• Contraindicated in known sensitivity and in pregnancy. • Supervise ambulation; raise side rails, especially for elderly patients. • Drug has less tendency to cause "hangover" effect, so patient is more alert and active. • The low end of dosage range should be used for elderly and debilitated patients.
triazolam	Hypnotic for insomnia	0.25 to 0.5 mg P.O. h.s.	• Contraindicated in known sensitivity and in pregnancy. • Supervise ambulation; raise side rails, especially for elderly patients. • The low end of dosage range should be used for elderly and debilitated patients. • Drug has less tendency to cause "hangover" effect, so patient is more alert and active.

SELECTED MAJOR DRUGS

Sedative and hypnotic agents continued

DRUG	MAJOR INDICATIONS	USUAL ADULT DOSAGES	NURSING IMPLICATIONS
Barbiturates			
amobarbital	Sedative for anxiety and tension Hypnotic for insomnia, acute convulsive disorders, manic disorders	30 to 50 mg P.O. or I.M. b.i.d. or t.i.d. 65 to 200 mg P.O. or I.M. h.s.	• Contraindicated in patients with known sensitivity, porphyria, severe cardiac or renal disease, severe depression, pregnancy, or history of drug abuse. • I.M. injections are painful and may cause tissue necrosis; avoid the I.M. route if possible. • Supervise ambulation. • Do not use with patients over age 60.
aprobarbital	Daytime sedative Hypnotic for insomnia	40 mg P.O. t.i.d. 40 to 160 mg P.O. h.s.	• Contraindicated in patients with known sensitivity, porphyria, severe cardiac or renal disease, severe depression, pregnancy, or history of drug abuse. • Supervise ambulation; raise side rails, especially for elderly patients. • Advise patient not to perform activities that require mental alertness until response to drug is known.
mephobarbital	Daytime sedative, adjunct treatment of grand mal and petit mal epilepsy	32 to 100 mg P.O. t.i.d. or q.i.d.	• Contraindicated in patients with known sensitivity, porphyria, severe cardiac or renal disease, severe depression, pregnancy, or history of drug abuse. • Supervise ambulation. • Observe for signs of toxicity. • When used as an anticonvulsant, observe seizure frequency and severity. • Advise patient not to perform activities that require mental alertness until response to drug is known.
pentobarbital	Daytime sedative Sedative before surgery Hypnotic for insomnia, emergency control of convulsions	20 to 40 mg P.O. b.i.d. to q.i.d. 150 to 200 mg P.O. or I.M. in two divided doses 100 mg P.O., 120 to 200 mg rectal, 100 to 200 mg I.M.	• Contraindicated in patients with known sensitivity, porphyria, severe cardiac or renal disease, severe depression, pregnancy, or history of drug abuse. • Do not mix with other medications. • May cause restlessness or delirium in presence of pain; monitor the patient closely. • Supervise ambulation; raise side rails, especially for elderly patients. • Observe for signs of barbiturate toxicity; overdose can be fatal. • Monitor prothrombin times when a patient on pentobarbital starts or ends anticoagulant therapy; dosage may need adjustment.
phenobarbital	Daytime sedative Sedative before surgery Hypnotic for insomnia, anticonvulsant	15 to 30 mg P.O. b.i.d. to q.i.d. 100 to 200 mg I.M. 60 to 90 minutes before surgery 100 to 320 mg P.O. or I.M. h.s.	• Contraindicated in patients with known sensitivity, porphyria, severe cardiac or renal disease, severe depression, pregnancy, or history of drug abuse. • Supervise ambulation; raise side rails, especially for elderly patients. • Long-term use of high dosage may cause drug dependence and severe withdrawal symptoms; withdraw gradually. • Observe for signs of barbiturate toxicity; overdose can be fatal.

continued

SELECTED MAJOR DRUGS

Sedative and hypnotic agents continued

DRUG	MAJOR INDICATIONS	USUAL ADULT DOSAGES	NURSING IMPLICATIONS
phenobarbital (continued)			• Depression of respiratory center of CNS can occur with high doses; monitor respirations. • Careful monitoring of prothrombin time is necessary if the patient is on an anticoagulant. Abrupt withdrawal of barbiturate may cause serious bleeding.
secobarbital	Daytime sedative	30 to 50 mg P.O. t.i.d. or q.i.d., 120 to 200 mg rectal	• Contraindicated in patients with known sensitivity, porphyria, severe cardiac or renal disease, severe depression, pregnancy, or history of drug abuse. • Supervise ambulation; raise side rails, especially for elderly patients. • Long-term use with high dosage may cause drug dependence and severe withdrawal symptoms; withdraw gradually. • Observe for barbiturate toxicity; overdose can be fatal. • Depression of respiratory center of CNS can occur with high doses; monitor respirations.
	Sedative before surgery	200 mg P.O. 1 to 2 hours before surgery	
	Hypnotic for insomnia, acute convulsive disorders	100 to 200 mg P.O., 120 to 200 mg rectal, 100 to 200 mg I.M.	
Nonbenzodiazepines-Nonbarbiturates			
chloral hydrate	Daytime sedative	250 mg P.O. or 325 mg rectal t.i.d. after meals	• Contraindicated in patients with marked hepatic or renal impairment, hypersensitivity, gastritis, or ulcers. Use with caution in severe cardiac disease and mental depression and in patients with suicidal tendencies. • Give after meals; dilute or administer with liquids such as juice or soda to decrease unpleasant taste and gastric irritation. • Oral administration is contraindicated in gastric disorders. • Supervise ambulation; raise side rails, especially for elderly patients.
	Hypnotic for insomnia	0.5 to 1 g P.O. or rectal 15 to 30 minutes before bedtime	
ethchlorvynol	Daytime sedative	100 to 200 mg P.O. b.i.d. or t.i.d.	• Contraindicated in patients with markedly impaired renal and hepatic function, hypersensitivity, history of drug abuse, or suicidal tendencies. • Give with milk or food to decrease dizziness or ataxia (transient) caused by rapid absorption. • Supervise ambulation.
	Hypnotic for insomnia	0.5 to 1 g P.O. h.s.	
glutethimide	Hypnotic for insomnia	250 to 500 mg P.O. h.s.	• Contraindicated in patients with severe renal impairment, porphyria; use cautiously in patients with mental depression, suicidal tendencies, history of drug abuse, prostatic hypertrophy, stenosing peptic ulcer, pyloroduodenal or bladder neck obstruction, narrow-angle glaucoma, or cardiac dysrhythmias. • Drug is effective for short-term use only. • Supervise ambulation; raise side rails, especially for elderly patients. • Withdraw the drug gradually to decrease possible withdrawal symptoms. • Observe for signs of toxicity; overdose can be fatal. • Dependence is possible with long-term use; monitor for signs and symptoms of toxicity.

SELECTED MAJOR DRUGS

Sedative and hypnotic agents continued

DRUG	MAJOR INDICATIONS	USUAL ADULT DOSAGES	NURSING IMPLICATIONS
methyprylon	Hypnotic for insomnia	200 to 400 mg P.O. h.s.	• Contraindicated in intermittent porphyria; use cautiously in patients with renal or hepatic impairment. • Supervise ambulation; raise side rails, especially for elderly patients. • Long-term use may cause drug dependence and life-threatening withdrawal symptoms, so withdraw drug gradually and monitor the patient closely.
paraldehyde	Sedative Hypnotic for insomnia	5 to 10 ml P.O. or rectal 10 to 30 ml P.O. or rectal	• Contraindicated in gastroenteritis with ulceration; use cautiously in patients with impaired hepatic function or in asthma or other pulmonary diseases. • Oral liquid must be diluted in iced milk, syrup, or fruit juice to disguise the taste and odor and reduce gastric distress. • Drug reacts with some plastics, so use glass syringe and metal needles. • For rectal administration, dilute with vegetable oil to minimize irritation (1:2 or 1 part medication to 2 parts diluent); give as a retention enema. • Supervise ambulation. • Depression of respiratory center of CNS can occur with high doses, so monitor respirations. • Ventilate room to remove exhaled paraldehyde. • Use with caution in patients with hepatic disease.

CHAPTER SUMMARY

The highlights of this chapter:
• Sedatives act to reduce activity or excitement and calm a patient. Drowsiness often accompanies the use of sedatives. Administered in large doses, sedatives are considered to be hypnotics, inducing a state resembling natural sleep.
• The three main classes of sedative and hypnotic drugs are benzodiazepines, barbiturates, and nonbenzodiazepine-nonbarbiturate drugs. Two dietary sources, herbs and L-tryptophan, as well as alcohol and over-the-counter drugs, have also been used to promote sleep.
• Sleep defines an active state of unconsciousness from which a person can be awakened with appropriate stimulus. During a period of sleep, a person passes through several cycles. Each cycle consists of four stages of NREM (non-rapid eye movement) sleep and one stage of REM (rapid eye movement) sleep.
• The four major sleep disorders include insomnia, hypersomnia, parasomnia, and disorders of the sleep-wake schedule.
• The benzodiazepines include four primary sedative and hypnotic drugs: flurazepam, lorazepam, temazepam, and triazolam. Most physicians prefer the benzodiazepines because of their effectiveness and safety. Adverse reactions involving benzodiazepines are rare and usually occur in the CNS. Few adverse reactions occur outside the CNS, because the benzodiazepine receptors are primarily there.
• Flurazepam has an intermediate onset of action because of slow absorption and a long half-life. The drug's long half-life results from a long-acting active metabolite produced during drug metabolism. Flurazepam becomes more effective after one to two uses, but after

several doses, the drug accumulates because of the long half-life. On the other hand, the short-acting triazolam has a rapid onset of action. Triazolam has less tendency to accumulate and cause morning drowsiness. Drug interactions with the benzodiazepines are rare and mainly occur with the use of other CNS depressant drugs, causing an additive effect that can be lethal.

• The use of barbiturates is declining because of their severe toxic effects. Barbiturates include amobarbital, aprobarbital, butabarbital, mephobarbital, pentobarbital, phenobarbital, secobarbital, and talbutal. Like benzodiazepines, barbiturates are CNS depressants capable of producing a wide range of effects, from sedation to hypnosis to anesthesia to coma.

• Barbiturates exhibit a high potential for physical and psychological dependence, high abuse level, and life-threatening toxicity with overdose, causing severe CNS and respiratory depression. Several drug-drug interactions involving barbiturates can occur, including the additive effects when combined with other CNS depressants, including alcohol. Adverse reactions are common and include depression of the CNS and respiratory systems.

• Nonbenzodiazepine-nonbarbiturate drugs include the following: chloral hydrate, ethchlorvynol, ethinamate, glutethimide, methyprylon, and paraldehyde. The most frequent adverse reactions involving the drugs are GI symptoms, especially with chloral hydrate and paraldehyde. The benzodiazepines have practically replaced the nonbenzodiazepine-nonbarbiturate drugs, though the latter are still used.

• Other sources of sedative and hypnotic effects include alcohol, OTC drugs, herbs, and L-tryptophan. OTC sleep aids contain antihistamines, primarily diphenhydramine, doxylamine, and pyrilamine.

BIBLIOGRAPHY

AHFS (American Hospital Formulary Service). *Drug Information '86.* Bethesda, Md.: American Society of Hospital Pharmacists, 1986.

AMA Division of Drugs. *AMA Drug Evaluation,* 6th ed. Philadelphia: W.B. Saunders Co., 1986.

Dukes, M.N.G., ed. *Side Effects of Drugs Annual 10.* Amsterdam: Elsevier Science Publications, 1986.

Goth, A. *Medical Pharmacology: Principles and Concepts,* 11th ed. St. Louis: C.V. Mosby Co., 1984.

Griffith, H. *Complete Guide to Prescription and Non-Prescription Drugs.* Tucson, Ariz.: HP Books, 1985.

Harkness, R. *Drug Interactions Handbook.* Englewood Cliffs, N.J.: Prentice-Hall, 1984.

Nursing87 Drug Handbook. Springhouse, Pa.: Springhouse Corp., 1987.

Patterson, H.R. *Current Drug Handbook 1984-85.* Philadelphia: W.B. Saunders Co., 1984.

Rosenberg, J., and Rosenberg-Rosen, M. *Drug Interactions,* 2nd ed. Oradell, N.J.: Medical Economics Books, 1984.

CHAPTER

31

ANTIDEPRESSANT AND ANTIMANIC AGENTS

OBJECTIVES

After reading and studying this chapter, you should be able to:

1. Discuss the clinical indications for antidepressant and antimanic agents.

2. Explain the mechanism of action of the monoamine oxidase (MAO) inhibitors.

3. Teach the patient which drugs and foods to avoid during MAO inhibitor therapy.

4. Describe the major adverse effects of MAO inhibitors.

5. Describe the major adverse effects of tricyclic antidepressants.

6. Compare the pharmacokinetic, pharmacodynamic, and pharmacotherapeutic properties of the tricyclic antidepressants with those of the second-generation antidepressants.

7. Describe the major adverse effects of lithium.

8. Identify the major drugs that interact with lithium.

INTRODUCTION

Antidepressant and antimanic agents are used to treat affective disorders. MAO inhibitors, tricyclic antidepressants, and second-generation antidepressants are used to treat unipolar disorders, characterized by periods of clinical depression. Lithium is used to treat bipolar disorders, characterized by alternating periods of manic behavior and clinical depression.

Affective disorders

Depression and mania are the most common affective disorders—or syndromes—producing mood disturbances not related to any other physical or psychiatric conditions. These disorders affect twice as many women as men, with unipolar depressions accounting for 90%

of the cases. This type of depression typically has a gradual onset of vague complaints, making it difficult to diagnose.

Diagnosis requires a prominent and persistent mood disturbance and the presence of several of the following signs and symptoms for at least 2 weeks: poor appetite, weight loss, sleep disturbances, agitation, loss of interest in activities, fatigue, feelings of worthlessness, slowed thinking or the inability to concentrate, and thoughts of death.

For 30% to 50% of these patients, depression occurs as a single episode; for the remainder, depression recurs. All these patients may require treatment with drugs such as tricyclic antidepressants, second-generation antidepressants, MAO inhibitors, or (occasionally) lithium.

Unlike depression, mania produces periods of euphoria, rapid speech, flight of ideas, lack of need for sleep, and overactivity. Mania may occur alone or it may alternate with depression, resulting in manic-depressive illness, a bipolar disorder. Manic-depressive illness occurs much less frequently than depression. Lithium is the drug of choice in treating mania and manic-depressive illness.

Because diminished concentration levels of one or both of the neurotransmitters norepinephrine and serotonin occur in depression, and because excessive neurotransmitter concentration levels occur in mania, many theorists believed that depletion of norepinephrine or serotonin was the biological cause of depression. This belief led to the discovery of agents to treat depression that could increase neurotransmitter availability in the brain.

Researchers were puzzled when antidepressant and antimanic drugs took weeks to produce a therapeutic response. Later, the receptor-sensitivity theory explained this phenomenon: in depression, the receptor site for norephinephrine and serotonin is hyposensitive to stimulation of the alpha-adrenergic receptor that releases the neurotransmitters, norepinephrine and serotonin; in mania, the receptor site is hypersensitive; antidepressant agents produce adaptive changes over several weeks that return the receptor to normal sensitivity.

For a summary of representative drugs, see *Selected major drugs: Antidepressant and antimanic agents* on pages 510 to 512.

M.A.O. INHIBITORS

MAO inhibitors are divided into two classifications based on chemical structure: the hydrazines, which include isocarboxazid and phenelzine sulfate, and the single non-hydrazine tranylcypromine sulfate. All of these drugs nonselectively inhibit the monoamine oxidase,which metabolizes neurotransmitters at receptor sites. Researchers have subdivided this enzyme into type A, which can produce hypertensive crisis in a patient who eats food containing tyramine, and type B, which is sensitive to different amines and not associated with hypertensive reactions. Currently available MAO inhibitors affect both type A and type B enzymes; however, research continues for agents that will selectively affect type A and type B enzymes. In the future, administering a type B MAO inhibitor may allow the patient to eat tyramine-rich foods without fear of hypertensive crisis, a severe interaction between a drug and a food. (See *Foods that may interact with MAO inhibitors* on page 502 for more details.)

History and source
MAO inhibitors were discovered in the 1950s when antituberculosis testing of isoniazid derivatives produced iproniazid. This prototype MAO inhibitor had no effect on tuberculosis—but it produced euphoria and reversed symptoms of depression. Although the drug is no longer available because of its hepatotoxicity, its discovery initiated the search for other MAO inhibitors.

PHARMACOKINETICS
Little information exists regarding the pharmacokinetics of these agents.

Absorption, distribution, metabolism, excretion
MAO inhibitors are rapidly and completely absorbed from the gastrointestinal (GI) tract and are metabolized in the liver to inactive metabolites. These metabolites are excreted mainly by the GI tract, and to a lesser degree, by the kidneys.

Onset, peak, duration
The onset of action of an MAO inhibitor ranges from 1 to 2 weeks, and a full clinical response may be delayed for 3 to 4 weeks. The therapeutic effects may continue for 1 to 2 weeks after discontinuation. Several factors account for the delayed onset of action of these drugs. The MAO inhibitors have relatively short half-lives (measured in hours), but the half-life of the enzyme they inhibit is about 12 days. Thus, the drugs can inhibit enzyme production within a short time, but they cannot affect the circulating enzyme.

No correlation exists between plasma MAO inhibition and plasma levels of MAO inhibitors. However, a direct correlation has been demonstrated between platelet MAO inhibition and therapeutic response.

PHARMACODYNAMICS
Administering these agents inhibits the monoamine oxidase synthesis and action, thus increasing the concentration levels of the neurotransmitters norepinephrine and serotonin.

Mechanism of action
Although their exact mechanism of action is unclear, the MAO inhibitors appear to work by inhibiting monoamine oxidase, the enzyme that normally metabolizes the neurotransmitters (norepinephrine and serotonin), because they inhibit neurotransmitter intracellular metabolism. This action makes more norepinephrine and serotonin available to the receptors, relieving the symptoms of depression.

PHARMACOTHERAPEUTICS
MAO inhibitors are used to treat psychiatric conditions, especially atypical depression. This disorder produces the signs opposite to those of typical depression. For example, the patient gains weight, lacks suicidal ten-

dencies, and has an increased libido. In treating atypical depression, MAO inhibitors are more effective than tricyclic antidepressants and have a shorter onset of action than usual—approximately 3 to 5 days.

MAO inhibitors may be used to treat typical depression when it is resistant to other therapies or when other therapies are contraindicated.

Other clinical uses include depression accompanied by anxiety, phobic anxieties, neurodermatitis, hypochondriasis, and refractory narcoleptic states. The safety and effectiveness of MAO inhibitors in patients under age 16 have not been established.

isocarboxazid (Marplan). This MAO inhibitor exerts its effects within 1 week in patients who are depressed because of weight gain or overeating. Its therapeutic use is declining, however, because of its lack of consistent effectiveness.

USUAL ADULT DOSAGE: 30 mg P.O. daily as a single dose or in divided doses, decreased to 10 to 20 mg/day when a therapeutic response occurs. Doses that exceed 30 mg/day can increase adverse effects and are not recommended.

phenelzine sulfate (Nardil). Phenelzine is less potent than other MAO inhibitors, less likely to produce hypertensive crisis, and produces fewer adverse reactions than tranylcypromine. It may be most effective in treating panic or phobic disorders.

USUAL ADULT DOSAGE: 15 mg P.O. t.i.d. or approximately 1 mg/kg/day, increased rapidly to 60 to 90 mg depending on the patient's tolerance and therapeutic response. In 2 to 6 weeks after the maximum response occurs, the dose is slowly decreased to a maintenance level as low as 15 mg/day.

tranylcypromine sulfate (Parnate). This nonhydrazine compound acts more rapidly than phenelzine, but produces more adverse reactions. Its mild central nervous system (CNS) stimulant effects preclude administering an evening dose.

USUAL ADULT DOSAGE: 10 mg P.O. b.i.d., increased to 20 mg in the morning and 10 mg in the afternoon if the response is inadequate after 2 to 3 weeks. If a therapeutic response does not appear after 1 week at this dosage, it is unlikely to occur. Doses in excess of 30 mg/day are more likely to produce adverse effects.

DRUG INTERACTIONS

MAO inhibitors

MAO inhibitors can interact with several frequently used drugs, causing potentially severe effects.

DRUG	INTERACTING DRUGS	POSSIBLE EFFECTS	NURSING IMPLICATIONS
isocarboxazid, phenelzine, tranylcypromine	amphetamines	Increase catecholamine release and hypertension	• Do not administer amphetamines with an MAO inhibitor.
	tricyclic antidepressants	Cause hyperpyrexia, excitation, seizures	• Monitor the patient's temperature and level of consciousness.
	barbiturates	Inhibit barbiturate metabolism	• Question a barbituate order for a patient receiving an MAO inhibitor. • Monitor the patient's level of consciousness if these drugs must be given concurrently.
	doxapram	Causes hypertension and dysrhythmias; potentiates the adverse effects of doxapram	• Monitor the patient's vital signs frequently.
	sympathomimetics	Increase catecholamine release and hypertension	• Avoid giving sympathomimetics to a patient receiving an MAO inhibitor.
	levodopa	Increases storage and release of dopamine, norepinephrine, or both, leading to hypertension	• Avoid giving levodopa to a patient receiving an MAO inhibitor.

Foods that may interact with MAO inhibitors

Many foods contain tyramine, a substance that can produce a hypertensive crisis in a patient receiving an MAO inhibitor. To avoid this severe interaction between a drug and a food, inform the patient about which foods to avoid during treatment. Foods with a high tyramine content should be avoided completely, those with a moderate content may be eaten occasionally, and those with low tyramine levels are allowable in limited quantities.

Foods with a high tyramine content

- Red wines, such as Chianti and burgundy
- Beer
- Aged cheeses, such as bleu, Swiss, and cheddar
- Aged or smoked meats, such as herring, sausage, and corned beef
- Liver, such as chicken or beef liver
- Yeast extracts, such as brewer's yeast
- Fava or broad beans, such as Italian green beans

Foods with a moderate tyramine content

- Sour cream
- Ripe avocados
- Yogurt
- Ripe bananas
- Meat extracts, such as bouillon

Foods with a low tyramine content

- Chocolate
- Figs
- American, mozzarella, cottage, and cream cheeses
- Distilled spirits, such as gin, vodka, and scotch
- White wines

Drug interactions

Certain foods and drugs can interact with MAO inhibitors and may produce severe reactions. The most serious reactions involve tyramine-rich foods and sympathomimetic agents. (See *Drug interactions: MAO inhibitors* on page 501 for information about interactions between MAO inhibitors and drugs, and see *Foods that may interact with MAO inhibitors* for information about interactions between MAO inhibitors and foods.)

ADVERSE DRUG REACTIONS

Although MAO inhibitors can produce a significant number of adverse reactions, they may produce fewer adverse reactions than tricyclic antidepressants do.

Predictable reactions

The most common adverse reaction is orthostatic hypotension, which can lead to syncope. This reaction occurs most often with tranylcypromine therapy. Impotence and edema may also occur, especially with phenelzine therapy.

Other adverse reactions vary according to the drug used and may diminish with time or require dose reduction. If an adverse reaction persists, the patient may receive a different MAO inhibitor. If sedation or insomnia occurs, administration can be changed to the early evening or the morning to lessen the effect. Other adverse reactions may include urinary retention, dry mouth, and paresthesias.

Abrupt withdrawal of an MAO inhibitor can induce nightmares, tremors, headache, and muscle aches. To avoid withdrawal reactions, the drug dosage must be tapered over 17 days.

Unpredictable reactions

Infrequently, MAO inhibitors produce rashes, mostly maculopapular. These drugs may also result in hepatotoxicity, although this is rare.

NURSING IMPLICATIONS

Because MAO inhibitor therapy can result in potentially severe interactions with other drugs and foods, the nurse must emphasize patient education.

- Teach the patient about the drugs and foods to avoid during MAO inhibitor therapy.
- Teach the patient how to recognize the signs of a hypertensive crisis.
- Instruct the patient to inform other physicians about the MAO inhibitor therapy. For example, if elective surgery is planned, the drug must be discontinued 10 to 14 days before surgery.
- Caution the patient not to stop taking the MAO inhibitor abruptly and explain that the therapy should be tapered as prescribed by the physician.
- Instruct the patient to take the drug at bedtime if it produces sedation.

• Instruct the patient to take the last daily dose in the afternoon to avoid insomnia, if the drug causes stimulation.

TRICYCLIC ANTIDEPRESSANTS

The tricyclic antidepressants include seven drugs that produce similar effects in the treatment of depression but differ in their abilities to increase neurotransmitter concentration levels.

History and source
Researchers synthesized imipramine hydrochloride, the first tricyclic antidepressant, in 1948 while searching for drugs with neuropsychiatric properties. In 1958, studies revealed that imipramine hydrochloride could relieve depression effectively. Further research demonstrated the usefulness of amitriptyline hydrochloride, its metabolites, and the metabolites of imipramine in treating depression. During the 1960s, additional modification of the basic structure of the tricyclic antidepressants yielded additional agents.

PHARMACOKINETICS
After oral administration, the tricyclic antidepressants undergo extensive hepatic metabolism that varies considerably among individuals.

Absorption, distribution, metabolism, excretion
Tricyclic antidepressants are completely absorbed after oral administration, but their bioavailability ranges from 30% to 70% because of the first-pass effect. The extreme fat solubility of these drugs accounts for their wide distribution throughout the body (the highest concentration levels appear in the brain and heart), slow excretion, and long half-life.

The tricyclic antidepressants are extensively metabolized in the liver. All of the tricyclic antidepressants are pharmacologically active, and some of their metabolites

DRUG INTERACTIONS
Tricyclic antidepressants

Tricyclic antidepressants can interact with several frequently used drugs, causing potentially severe effects.

DRUG	INTERACTING DRUGS	POSSIBLE EFFECTS	NURSING IMPLICATIONS
amitriptyline, desipramine, doxepin, imipramine, nortriptyline, protriptyline, trimipramine	amphetamines	Increase catecholamine effects, leading to hypertension	• Administer amphetamines cautiously to a patient receiving tricyclic antidepressants. • Monitor the patient's blood pressure.
	barbiturates	Increase metabolism and decrease blood levels of tricyclic antidepressants	• Monitor the patient for a decreased therapeutic effect.
	cimetidine	Impairs hepatic metabolism of tricyclic antidepressants, leading to toxicity	• If these drugs must be given together, monitor the patient for signs of toxicity such as dry mouth, blurred vision, orthostatic hypotension, urinary retention, and tachycardia.
	MAO inhibitors	Cause hyperpyrexia, excitation, seizures	• Monitor the patient's body temperature and level of consciousness.
	sympathomimetics	Increase catecholamine effects, leading to hypertension	• If these drugs must be given together, monitor the patient's blood pressure and heart rate frequently.

are also active. Eventually, the metabolites are hydroxylated and then conjugated to form inactive compounds that are excreted in the urine. Only small amounts of active drug are excreted.

Onset, peak, duration
The tricyclic antidepressants' half-lives vary from 8 to 120 hours and average 24 hours, except for that of protriptyline hydrochloride, which is 3 to 4 days. Because the tricyclic antidepressants have long half-lives, a noticeable response may not occur for 10 to 14 days; a full response, for up to 30 days.

Plasma tricyclic antidepressant levels vary widely because of individual differences in metabolism. Subtherapeutic or toxic concentration levels may reflect a patient's metabolic status.

PHARMACODYNAMICS
Tricyclic antidepressant administration increases neurotransmitter concentration levels, reducing the signs and symptoms of depression.

Mechanism of action
Researchers hypothesize that tricyclic antidepressants increase the amount of norepinephrine or serotonin or of both, normalizing the hyposensitive receptor site associated with depression. This normalization process takes up to several weeks, slowing the onset of antidepressant action.

PHARMACOTHERAPEUTICS
The drugs of choice for episodes of major depression, tricyclic antidepressants are especially effective in treating depression of insidious onset accompanied by weight loss, anorexia, and/or insomnia. Physical signs and symptoms may respond after 1 to 2 weeks of therapy; psychological symptoms, after 2 to 4 weeks. Tricyclic antidepressants are much less effective in patients with hypochondriasis, atypical depression, or depression accompanied by delusions. They may, however, be helpful in treating acute episodes of depression, producing a response in about two thirds of these patients. After a patient's acute depressive episode, the dosage is reduced to the lowest level that will relieve symptoms. This maintenance therapy is continued for 6 to 12 months, and then the dosage is decreased every 3 to 7 days until the drug is discontinued. A patient who experiences two acute episodic relapses in 2 years may require long-term tricyclic antidepressant therapy, which may last for several years.

These agents are also being investigated for use in preventing migraine headaches and in treating phobias, enuresis, attention deficit disorders, duodenal or peptic ulcer disease, and diabetic neuropathies.

The relative effectiveness of the tricyclic antidepressants has not been established; therefore, a patient who fails to respond to one tricyclic antidepressant may respond to a different one, to a combination of lithium and a tricyclic antidepressant, or to a combination of an MAO inhibitor and a tricyclic antidepressant (if special precautions are taken). Although a single daily dose is possible because of the tricyclic antidepressants' long half-life, dosages are divided to decrease the risk of adverse effects or to allow the patient to adjust to them before changing to a once-daily dosage. Dosages should be reduced for elderly patients.

amitriptyline hydrochloride (Elavil, Emitrip, Endep). This tricyclic antidepressant is used primarily to treat depression. It is as potent as desipramine, doxepin hydrochloride, imipramine, and trimipramine maleate, but produces greater sedative and anticholinergic effects.
USUAL ADULT DOSAGE: initially, 50 to 75 mg P.O. increased by 25 to 50 mg every 1 to 2 days as tolerated, to 200 mg; if no response occurs after 1 week, the dosage is increased by 25 mg daily, as tolerated, to a maximum of 300 mg daily. Amitriptyline may be given I.M. at 20 to 30 mg q.i.d. or as a single dose h.s. Elderly or adolescent patients may require an initial dosage of 30 mg P.O. daily in divided doses, increased to 100 mg as tolerated.

desipramine hydrochloride (Norpramin, Pertofrane). Used to treat depression, desipramine is a metabolite of imipramine, but produces fewer sedative and anticholinergic effects.
USUAL ADULT DOSAGE: initially, 50 to 75 mg P.O., increased to a maximum of 300 mg daily; for an elderly patient, 25 to 50 mg P.O. daily, increased to 150 mg. Higher dosages may be prescribed with caution.

doxepin hydrochloride (Adapin, Sinequan). Doxepin is used to treat depression.
USUAL ADULT DOSAGE: initially, 25 to 50 mg P.O. daily in divided doses or as a single dose h.s., gradually increased to 150 mg with a maximum of 300 mg daily, if necessary; for an elderly patient, initially 25 to 50 mg P.O. daily, gradually increased to a maximum of 100 mg, if needed.

imipramine hydrochloride (Janimine, SK-Pramine, Tofranil). Imipramine shares amitriptyline's dosage schedule for treating depression. It is used also to treat enuresis in children age 6 and over.
USUAL ADULT DOSAGE: initially, 50 to 75 mg P.O. daily increased to a maximum of 300 mg, or 30 to 40 mg daily increased to 100 mg in an elderly or debilitated patient.
USUAL PEDIATRIC DOSAGE: for enuresis in children age 6 and over, 25 mg 1 hour before bedtime, up to a maximum of 50 mg daily in children under 12 and 75 mg daily in children over 12. Imipramine is also available in injectable form for administration using the same dosage schedule up to a maximum of 100 mg/day.

nortriptyline hydrochloride (Aventyl, Pamelor). This drug is twice as potent as most of the other tricyclic antidepressants. As a result, the dosages are much lower for treating depression.
USUAL ADULT DOSAGE: initially, 25 mg. P.O. t.i.d. or q.i.d., increased every 1 to 2 days by 10 to 25 mg, as tolerated. If the response is inadequate after 1 week, the dosage can be increased by 10 mg daily to a maximum of 150 mg. The dosage for elderly patients should not exceed 100 mg/day.

protriptyline hydrochloride (Vivactil). The most potent tricyclic antidepressant, protriptyline is about five times more potent than amitriptyline. Usually, this agent is used to treat depression; it produces the mildest sedative effects of all the tricyclic antidepressants.
USUAL ADULT DOSAGE: initially, 10 to 15 mg P.O. daily increased by 5 mg every 1 to 2 days, as tolerated, to 30 mg/day. If the response is inadequate after 1 week, the dosage can be increased by 5 mg/day, as tolerated, to a maximum of 60 mg/day. Elderly patients usually receive smaller dosages.

trimipramine maleate (Surmontil). Trimipramine is used to treat depression and is under investigation for treating duodenal ulcers.
USUAL ADULT DOSAGE: for depression, initially, 50 to 75 mg P.O./day, increased to a maximum of 300 mg/day; for duodenal ulcers, 50 mg P.O. daily. A patient receiving more than 200 mg/day will require close observation because of the increased incidence of adverse effects. Elderly patients rarely receive more than 100 mg/day.

Drug interactions

Tricyclic antidepressants can interact with numerous drugs, especially MAO inhibitors and sympathomimetics. (See *Drug interactions: Tricyclic antidepressants* on page 503 for further information.)

ADVERSE DRUG REACTIONS

Reactions to tricyclic antidepressants frequently include anticholinergic effects, sedation, orthostatic hypotension, and cardiovascular effects. Because adverse reactions can differ markedly among agents and because no one agent is more effective than the others, the patient's therapy can be changed from one tricyclic antidepressant to another to eliminate intolerable adverse reactions.

Predictable reactions

Orthostatic hypotension often occurs with tricyclic antidepressant therapy. In these cases, the dosage may be reduced or nortriptyline may be prescribed because it is less likely to cause this problem.

A conduction delay, demonstrated by a widening Q-T interval, may also occur with tricyclic antidepressant therapy. This adverse reaction can exacerbate congestive heart failure or an existing bundle branch block. A patient taking a tricyclic antidepressant will need to be monitored for palpitations, tachycardia, and electrocardiogram (EKG) changes. In therapeutic concentrations, these agents can act as antiarrhythmics, but in toxic concentrations, they can induce dysrhythmias.

Anticholinergic adverse reactions frequently occur with tricyclic antidepressant therapy, but may diminish or disappear as treatment continues. Reactions include blurred vision, urinary retention, dry mouth, and constipation.

At high doses, tricyclic antidepressants can cause seizures. Other adverse reactions include sedation, jaundice, a fine resting tremor, decreased libido, inhibited ejaculation, transient eosinophilia and leukopenia, and, rarely, granulocytopenia (agranulocytosis).

Unpredictable reactions

Rashes may occur during the first 2 months of therapy, particularly with amitriptyline and imipramine. They are usually mild and do not require discontinuation of therapy. Photosensitivities may also occur.

NURSING IMPLICATIONS

Patient education is particularly important because of the tricyclic antidepressants' potential for drug interactions and adverse reactions. The nurse should also be aware of the following implications.

• Monitor a suicidal patient very closely until the drug takes full effect.

• Alert the patient not to stop taking a tricyclic antidepressant abruptly after long-term use because abrupt withdrawal can produce nausea, headache, and malaise.

• Advise the patient not to drive or operate dangerous machinery if blurred vision or sedation occurs.

• Inform the patient that urinary retention can occur.

• Teach the patient which food sources will increase dietary bulk to prevent constipation.

• Instruct the patient to arise from a supine position slowly and gradually to decrease the effects of the orthostatic hypotension.

• Alert the patient that a full therapeutic response may take 2 to 3 weeks.

• Instruct the patient to take the entire drug dose at bedtime to avoid sedation and anticholinergic effects, unless otherwise prescribed.

• Warn the patient that the use of alcohol or other central nervous system (CNS) depressants may increase sedation.

• Monitor the patient's blood pressure and heart rate frequently.

• Warn the patient to keep tricyclic antidepressants out of the reach of children, because an overdose could be fatal.

SECOND-GENERATION ANTIDEPRESSANTS

Developed recently to treat depression with fewer adverse reactions, these antidepressants are chemically different from each other and from tricyclic antidepressants and MAO inhibitors. Three second-generation antidepressants are currently available: amoxapine, maprotiline hydrochloride, and trazodone hydrochloride.

History and source

Introduced in 1980, amoxapine—a metabolite of the antipsychotic loxapine succinate—was the first of the second-generation antidepressants. Maprotiline, a structurally modified tricyclic antidepressant, was recognized in 1981. Trazodone, which has an entirely different structure from the tricyclic antidepressants, was introduced in the United States in 1982.

PHARMACOKINETICS

The second-generation antidepressants are chemically distinct from one another and differ somewhat in their pharmacokinetic properties.

Absorption, distribution, metabolism, excretion

All of these agents are completely absorbed after oral administration and widely distributed throughout the body, except for cardiac tissue.

Amoxapine undergoes extensive metabolism in the liver, producing some active metabolites. Only 3% of it is excreted unchanged by the kidneys; the rest is excreted as glucuronides.

Maprotiline is also metabolized in the liver, producing some active metabolites. Most of the drug is excreted in the urine, but 30% leaves the body in the feces.

Although trazodone is extensively metabolized in the liver, the therapeutic activity of its metabolites is unknown. The kidneys excrete most of this drug.

Onset, peak, duration

Some of these drugs have shorter half-lives than other antidepressants. Amoxapine achieves peak concentration levels in 1 to 2 hours and has a half-life of 8 hours. Some of its metabolites have half-lives of up to 30 hours. Steady-state concentration levels can be attained in 2 to 7 days.

Maprotiline reaches peak concentration levels in 8 to 24 hours. Its half-life is about 43 hours, and steady-state levels are attained in 8 to 10 days.

The concentration levels of trazodone peak in 1 to 2 hours. This drug has a relatively short half-life of 4 to 12 hours and can achieve steady-state concentration levels in 2 days.

PHARMACODYNAMICS

The biochemical activity of second-generation antidepressants resembles that of the tricyclic antidepressants.

Mechanism of action

Like the tricyclic antidepressants, second-generation antidepressants inhibit reuptake of the neurotransmitters norepinephrine or serotonin, or both, thus restoring hyposensitive receptor sites to normal so that increased neurotransmitter concentration levels can exert a therapeutic effect. Amoxapine and maprotiline primarily inhibit the reuptake of norepinephrine, inhibiting serotonin reuptake to a lesser extent. Trazodone inhibits reuptake of serotonin only.

PHARMACOTHERAPEUTICS

Second-generation antidepressants are used to treat the same major depressive episodes as the tricyclic antidepressants, and have the same degree of effectiveness.

amoxapine (Asendin). A loxapine derivative, amoxapine possesses some antipsychotic effects besides its antidepressant effects.
USUAL ADULT DOSAGE: initially, 50 mg P.O. t.i.d., increased to 300 mg/day after 3 days, if tolerated; after 2 weeks, increased to a maximum of 400 mg/day, if necessary; for an elderly patient initial dose is 25 mg P.O. t.i.d.

maprotiline hydrochloride (Ludiomil). Maprotiline has significant sedative properties and is used to treat depression.
USUAL ADULT DOSAGE: initially, 50 to 100 mg P.O. daily, given in two divided doses or as a single dose; increased after 2 weeks, as needed and tolerated, by 25-mg increments to 150 to 200 mg daily, up to a maximum of 300 mg, if necessary; an elderly patient may require an initial dosage of 25 mg P.O. daily.

trazodone hydrochloride (Desyrel). This second-generation agent is used to treat depression. It has the least anticholinergic activity of the second-generation antidepressants and may be somewhat less effective.
USUAL ADULT DOSAGE: initially, 150 mg P.O. daily in divided doses, increased by 50 mg every 3 to 4 days up to a maximum of 400 mg/day (600 mg/day for a severely ill hospitalized patient); for an elderly patient, initially, 50 mg P.O. daily.

Drug interactions

Few interactions have been documented between amoxapine or maprotiline and other drugs. Patients receiving drugs that interact with tricyclic antidepressants, however, should be observed for similar interactions with the second-generation antidepressants.

Trazodone may produce additive effects when combined with other drugs. For instance, it can increase sedation when combined with a CNS depressant and may produce an additive hypotensive effect when used with a hypotensive agent. It can also increase digoxin and phenytoin levels during concomitant therapy.

ADVERSE DRUG REACTIONS

Second-generation antidepressants produce fewer adverse reactions than tricyclic antidepressants do. Seizures may occur with all three of these antidepressants, particularly maprotiline, especially at high dosages. To prevent seizures, dosages should be prescribed below the maximum. Trazodone sometimes produces sedation and dizziness, but rarely produces anticholinergic effects; to minimize these adverse reactions, give the drug before bedtime or with food. Amoxapine and maprotiline may cause anticholinergic effects, orthostatic hypotension, and tachycardia.

Trazodone can also produce the unpredictable adverse reaction of priapism.

NURSING IMPLICATIONS

The nurse should include the following in patient education.
• Tell the patient not to stop the drug abruptly, because abrupt withdrawal can produce adverse reactions.
• Advise the patient to avoid driving or operating dangerous machinery, because drowsiness can occur.
• Teach the patient to take most of the dosage at bedtime if sedation is a problem.
• Instruct the patient to take trazodone with meals or a snack to enhance absorption and decrease dizziness.

LITHIUM

Lithium is the drug of choice to prevent or treat mania. Its discovery was a milestone in treating mania and bipolar disorders.

History and source

Since the 1800s the alkali metal lithium has served as a gout treatment and as a salt substitute, among other uses. Then, in the 1940s, researchers discovered that lithium produced lethargy in animals. This finding led to successful testing of lithium with manic patients.

PHARMACOKINETICS

An active drug, lithium is not metabolized and is excreted from the body unchanged.

Absorption, distribution, metabolism, excretion

After oral administration, lithium is rapidly and completely absorbed and is distributed to body tissues, with highest concentration levels occurring in the kidneys, thyroid gland, and bone. The kidneys excrete lithium unchanged at a rate that parallels the glomerular filtration rate (GFR). Because 80% of the lithium is reabsorbed at the renal tubules, the renal clearance rate is 20% of the GFR.

Lithium crosses the placenta and is detectable in the fetus. It also is excreted in breast milk.

Onset, peak, duration

Serum concentration levels of lithium peak 2 to 3 hours after administration. Initially, the half-life is 2 hours, but it increases to 20 hours as therapy continues. Steady-state concentration levels are reached in 6 days with fixed-dose administration.

PHARMACODYNAMICS

Although the exact mechanism of action is unknown, lithium diminishes the excessive catecholamine response in mania.

Mechanism of action

In mania, the patient experiences excessive catecholamine stimulation. In a bipolar disorder, the patient is affected by swings between the excessive catecholamine stimulation of mania and the diminished catecholamine stimulation of depression. Lithium may normalize the catecholamine receptors by increasing norepinephrine and serotonin uptake, reducing the release of norepinephrine from the synaptic vesicles, and inhibiting norepinephrine's postsynaptic action.

PHARMACOTHERAPEUTICS

Lithium is used primarily to treat acute episodes of mania and to prevent relapses of bipolar disorders. It can produce 70% to 80% improvement in manic patients within 1 to 2 weeks and can reduce the 2-year relapse incidence to 50%. After an acute manic episode, lithium therapy is typically continued for 3 to 6 months and then tapered off. A patient who experiences a relapse every 1 to 2 years, however, may require long-term prophylactic therapy.

Other uses of lithium under investigation include preventing unipolar depression and migraine headaches and treating resistant depression, alcohol dependence, anorexia nervosa, inappropriate secretion of antidiuretic hormone, and neutropenia.

lithium carbonate and **lithium citrate** (Eskalith, Lithane, Lithobid). Lithium's two salts have identical effects and dosage schedules. The only difference: lithium citrate is more soluble. Because lithium's therapeutic dosage range is narrow, dosages require regular adjustment. Blood levels drawn 12 hours after the last daily dose serve as an adjustment guide.
USUAL ADULT DOSAGE: to treat acute mania, 300 to 600 mg P.O. up to q.i.d., adjusted to achieve a blood level of 1 to 1.5 mEq/liter; to prevent a relapse of a bipolar disorder, 0.6 to 1.2 mEq/liter, and 2 mEq/liter as a maximum dose.

Drug interactions

Serious interactions with other drugs can occur because of lithium's narrow therapeutic range. These interactions may occur in the kidneys, where the clearance can increase or decrease, or at the receptor site, where potentiation takes place. (See *Drug interactions: Lithium* for further information.)

ADVERSE DRUG REACTIONS

Adverse reactions to lithium affect various body systems and may occur in any phase of therapy; most are dose-related. Because GI complaints are associated with increasing blood levels of lithium, they are most frequent during the initial phase of therapy and after dosage adjustments. About 50% of patients experience a fine tremor that may diminish with dosage reduction and worsen with dosage increase. Polyuria of 2 to 3 liters/

DRUG INTERACTIONS
Lithium

Lithium can interact with several drugs; most interactions affect lithium excretion and can be managed with dosage adjustments.

DRUG	INTERACTING DRUGS	POSSIBLE EFFECTS	NURSING IMPLICATIONS
lithium	thiazide diuretics	Increase lithium reabsorption in the kidneys	• Monitor the patient's serum lithium levels and renal function.
	piroxicam	Inhibits lithium excretion	• Monitor the patient's serum lithium levels.
	potassium iodide	Increases hypothyroid activity	• Avoid concomitant use. If these drugs must be given together, observe the patient for signs and symptoms of hypothyroidism such as fatigue, cold sensitivity, and a decreased pulse rate.
	sodium bicarbonate	Increases lithium excretion	• Monitor the patient's serum lithium levels.
	sodium chloride	Alters lithium excretion in proprotion to sodium chloride intake	• Be aware that a patient on a severe salt-restricted diet is susceptible to lithium toxicity. • Advise the patient that increased salt intake will decrease lithium's therapeutic effects.

day may appear, accompanied by polydipsia. When blood levels exceed 1.5 mEq/liter, toxicity may occur, producing confusion, lethargy, slurred speech, hyperreflexia, and convulsions.

Long-term lithium therapy may result in distal tubule atrophy and a decrease in GFR. A diabetes insipidus syndrome can occur, producing a daily urine output exceeding 3 liters and a low urine specific gravity. Hypothyroidism and nontoxic goiters may affect about 4% of patients. Other adverse reactions include weight gain, skin eruptions, alopecia, and leukocytosis.

NURSING IMPLICATIONS

Safe administration of lithium requires patient teaching and an awareness of the following implications.
• Monitor the patient's lithium concentration levels regularly during therapy and after dosage adjustments.
• Administer lithium with food to reduce GI irritation.
• Monitor the patient's urine output.
• Obtain baseline tests of the patient's thyroid and renal functions and an EKG reading.
• Advise the patient that lithium may take 1 to 2 weeks to produce a therapeutic response.

CHAPTER SUMMARY

Chapter 31 discussed the antimanic and antidepressant agents. Here are the highlights of the chapter:
• Various agents are used to treat depression, mania, and bipolar disorders such as manic-depressive illness.
• Although MAO inhibitors can interact with many drugs and foods, they remain the treatment of choice for atypical depression. They may also be used to treat other types of depression, but they are not drugs of choice except when depression is resistant or when other therapies are contraindicated.
• The tricyclic antidepressants are preferred for treating major depressive episodes. They can produce many adverse effects, however.
• The second-generation antidepressants were recently developed to replace the tricyclic antidepressants, which they have not done. Although they produce fewer adverse effects, none are more effective than the tricyclic antidepressants.

(Text continues on page 513.)

SELECTED MAJOR DRUGS

Antidepressant and antimanic agents

This chart summarizes the major antidepressant and antimanic drugs currently in clinical use.

DRUG	MAJOR INDICATIONS	USUAL ADULT DOSAGES	NURSING IMPLICATIONS
MAO inhibitors			
isocarboxazid	Atypical depression	30 mg P.O. daily in a single dose or divided doses, reduced to 10 to 20 mg/day when condition improves	• Be aware that isocarboxazid is contraindicated in elderly or debilitated patients and in patients with severe hepatic or renal impairment; congestive heart failure; pheochromocytoma; hypertensive, cardiovascular, or cerebrovascular disease; or severe or frequent headaches. It is also contraindicated within 10 days of elective surgery requiring general anesthesia, cocaine, or local anesthetic containing sympathomimetic vasoconstrictors. • Administer cautiously to hyperactive, agitated, schizophrenic, or suicidal patients and to patients with diabetes or epilepsy. • Withhold the drug and notify the physician if the patient develops signs or symptoms of an overdose, such as palpitations, frequent headaches, and/or severe hypertension. • Advise the patient to avoid consuming large amounts of caffeine and any over-the-counter (OTC) preparations for colds, hay fever, or diets. • Tell the patient to sit up for 1 minute before getting slowly out of bed, to reduce the effects of orthostatic hypotension. Supervise the patient's ambulation. • Continue patient monitoring for 10 days after the drug is discontinued, because its effects are long lasting. • Advise the patient to expect a time lag of 1 to 4 weeks before noticeable therapeutic effects occur.
tranylcypromine	Atypical depression	10 mg P.O. b.i.d., increased to a maximum of 30 mg/day after 2 to 3 weeks, if necessary	• Withhold the drug and notify the physician if the patient develops signs of an overdose, such as palpitations and severe orthostatic hypotension. • Observe the patient for suicidal tendencies. • Continue patient monitoring for 7 days after the drug is discontinued because its effects are long lasting. • Advise the patient to expect a time lag of 1 to 3 weeks before noticeable therapeutic effects occur. • Advise the patient to avoid consuming OTC preparations for colds, hay fever, or diets. • Tell the patient to sit up for 1 minute before getting slowly out of bed, to reduce the effects of orthostatic hypotension.

SELECTED MAJOR DRUGS

Antidepressant and antimanic agents continued

DRUG	MAJOR INDICATIONS	USUAL ADULT DOSAGES	NURSING IMPLICATIONS
Tricyclic antidepressants			
amitriptyline	Depression	50 to 75 mg P.O. h.s. increased to 200 mg/day, then to a maximum of 300 mg daily, if needed; or 20 to 30 mg I.M. q.i.d. or as a single dose h.s.	• Be aware that amitriptyline is contraindicated in a patient during the acute recovery phase of myocardial infarction and in patients with prostatic hypertrophy or a history of seizure disorders. • Administer cautiously to patients with suicidal tendencies, urinary retention, narrow-angle glaucoma, increased intraocular pressure, cardiovascular disease, or impaired hepatic function and in patients receiving hyperthyroid medication or electroshock therapy or undergoing elective surgery. • Monitor the patient's mood changes, and observe the patient for suicidal tendencies. • Monitor the patient for urinary retention and constipation. Increase fluids and consult the physician regarding a stool softener to relieve constipation. • Advise the patient not to combine this drug with alcoholic beverages or other depressants, to avoid increased sedation. • Advise the patient to expect a time lag of 10 to 14 days before noticeable therapeutic effects occur and a time lag of 30 days for full effects. • Advise the patient not to take any other prescription or OTC drugs before consulting the physician. • Tell the patient to avoid activities that require alertness and coordination until the central nervous system (CNS) response to the drug is determined. • Advise the patient to take the full dose at bedtime whenever possible.
doxepin	Depression	25 to 50 mg P.O. daily initially, increased to a maximum of 300 mg daily, if necessary	• Be aware that doxepin is contraindicated in patients with urinary retention, narrow-angle glaucoma, or prostatic hypertrophy. • Monitor the patient's mood changes, and observe for suicidal tendencies. • Monitor the patient for urinary retention and constipation. Increase fluids and consult the physician regarding a stool softener to relieve constipation. • Advise the patient to expect a time lag of 10 to 14 days before noticeable therapeutic effects occur and a time lag of 30 days for full effects. • Advise the patient not to take any other prescription or OTC drugs before consulting the physician. • Tell the patient to avoid activities that require alertness and coordination until the CNS response to the drug is determined.

continued

SELECTED MAJOR DRUGS

Antidepressant and antimanic agents continued

DRUG	MAJOR INDICATIONS	USUAL ADULT DOSAGES	NURSING IMPLICATIONS
Second-generation antidepressants			
trazodone	Depression	150 mg P.O. daily in divided doses, increased by 50 mg/day every 3 to 4 days up to a maximum of 400 mg/day; (600 mg/day for severely ill)	• Administer cautiously to a patient with cardiac disease. • Note the patient's complaints of prolonged and painful erections, which may indicate priapism. • Observe the patient for suicidal tendencies and mood changes. • Administer the drug after meals or snacks to increase absorption and decrease dizziness. • Advise the patient to expect a time lag of 10 to 14 days before noticeable therapeutic effects occur and of a time lag of 30 days for full effects.
Lithium			
lithium	Mania and bipolar disorder relapse	300 to 600 mg P.O. up to q.i.d., adjusted to achieve lithium blood level of 1 to 1.5 mEq/liter for acute mania, 0.6 to 1.2 mEq/liter to prevent bipolar disorder relapses, and 2 mEq/liter as a maximum dose	• Be aware that lithium is contraindicated in elderly or debilitated patients or those who cannot be closely monitored, and in patients with thyroid disease, epilepsy, renal or cardiovascular disease, brain damage, severe dehydration, or sodium depletion. • Obtain the patient's baseline EKG, electrolyte levels, and thyroid and renal function studies. • Monitor the patient's lithium blood concentration levels 8 to 12 hours after the first dose (usually before the morning dose) two or three times weekly for the first month, then once a week or monthly during maintenance. • Advise the patient to expect a time lag of 1 to 3 weeks before noticeable therapeutic effects occur. • Weigh the patient daily to detect sudden weight gain caused by edema. • Monitor follow-up thyroid and renal function tests every 6 to 12 months. • Administer this agent after meals with plenty of water to minimize GI upset. • Monitor the patient's urine specific gravity, and report levels below 1.015, which may indicate diabetes insipidus. • Monitor the patient's blood glucose levels. • Advise the patient not to switch brands of lithium or take other prescription or OTC drugs before consulting the physician. • Advise the patient to carry an identification card that describes the drug's toxicity and provides emergency information. • Advise an ambulatory patient to avoid activities that require alertness and coordination. • Monitor the patient for transient nausea, polyuria, thirst, and discomfort, which may occur in the first few days. • Tell the patient and family members to watch for signs and symptoms of toxicity, such as diarrhea, vomiting, drowsiness, muscular weakness, and ataxia. If these signs or symptoms appear, they should withhold one dose and call the physician.

• Lithium effectively treats manic episodes and prevents relapses of bipolar disorders. This drug has a narrow therapeutic range and a high incidence of adverse effects, however, so lithium therapy requires close patient monitoring.

BIBLIOGRAPHY

Bryant, S.G., and Brown, C.S. "Current Concepts in Clinical Therapeutics: Major Affective Disorders, Part 1," *Clinical Pharmacy* 5:304, April 1986.

Bryant, S.G., and Brown, C.S. "Current Concepts in Clinical Therapeutics: Major Affective Disorders, Part 2," *Clinical Pharmacy* 5:385, May 1986.

Davidson, J. "When and How to Use MAO Inhibitors," *Drug Therapy* 197, January 1983.

Feighner, J.P. "The New Generation of Antidepressants," *Journal of Clinical Psychiatry* 44:49, May 1983.

Lader, M. "Combined Use of Tricyclic Antidepressants and Monoamine Oxidase Inhibitors," *Journal of Clinical Psychiatry* 33:20, September 1983.

Leasar, T.S., and Tollefson, G. "Lithium Therapy: Careful Workup, Close Follow-up to Avoid Toxicity," *Postgraduate Medicine* 75:269, January 1984.

Pare, C.M.B. "The Present Status of Monoamine Oxidase Inhibitors," *British Journal of Psychiatry* 146:576, June 1985.

Quitkin, P.M. "The Importance of Dosage in Prescribing Antidepressants," *British Journal of Psychiatry* 147:593, December 1985.

Rabkin, J., et al. "Adverse Reactions to Monoamine Oxidase Inhibitors. Part I. A Comparative Study," *Journal of Clinical Psychopharmacology* 4:270-8, October 1984.

Rabkin, J., et al. "Adverse Reactions to Monoamine Oxidase Inhibitors. Part II. Treatment Correlates and Clinical Management," *Journal of Clinical Psychopharmacology* 5:2, February 1985.

Richardson, J.W., and Richelson, E. "Antidepressants: A Clinical Update for Medical Practitioners," *Mayo Clinic Proceedings* 59:330, May 1984.

Tollefson, G.D. "Monoamine Oxidase Inhibitors: A Review," *Journal of Clinical Psychiatry* 44:280, August 1983.

White, K., and Simpson, G. "The Combined Use of MAOIs and Tricyclics," *Journal of Clinical Psychiatry* 45:67, July 1984.

Zisook, S. "A Clinical Overview of Monoamine Oxidase Inhibitors," *Psychosomatics* 26:240, March 1985.

ANTIANXIETY AGENTS

OBJECTIVES

After reading and studying this chapter, you should be able to:

1. Describe the three major types of antianxiety agents.
2. Explain why the benzodiazepines are the drugs of choice for treating anxiety.
3. Compare the mechanism of action of the benzodiazepines with that of the barbiturates, and describe how each type of drug produces different adverse reactions.
4. Explain why the new agent buspirone hydrochloride is so promising in treating anxiety.
5. Explain why physicians tend to prescribe the benzodiazepines as antianxiety agents more often than the barbiturates.

INTRODUCTION

Antianxiety agents, also called anxiolytics, include some of the most frequently prescribed drugs in the United States. They are used primarily to treat anxiety disorders, which affect 7% to 18% of the American population.

This chapter presents the three main types of drugs used to treat anxiety disorders: the commonly prescribed benzodiazepines; the new drug buspirone; and the former drugs of choice, the barbiturates. It will also discuss meprobamate and several other drugs that are used (rarely) to treat anxiety.

Anxiety disorders

The American Psychiatric Association divides anxiety disorders into two main types: nonphobic and phobic. Nonphobic anxieties can be subdivided into generalized anxiety disorders (the most common), obsessive-compulsive disorders, and panic disorders. Phobic anxieties can take many forms, such as phobias of crowds or heights. An anxiety disorder may be a primary medical condition or may occur secondary to another medical or social problem.

Whatever its type, anxiety disorder symptoms include nervousness and tension as well as tremors, tachy-cardia, bowel and urinary complaints, diaphoresis, and palpitations.

Neither the etiologies of anxiety disorders nor the actions of the drugs used to treat them are fully understood. However, researchers have discovered that antianxiety agents relieve the symptoms of anxiety by mediating neurotransmitters in the midbrain. Today, medical specialists in many different fields (only one fourth of them psychiatrists) treat these common disorders with antianxiety agents.

For a summary of representative drugs, *see Selected major drugs: Antianxiety agents* on page 520.

BENZODIAZEPINES

Currently, the benzodiazepines are the drugs of choice to treat anxiety disorders. Although 12 benzodiazepines are marketed in the United States, one of them is used solely as an anticonvulsant, and three others as hypnotics. The remaining benzodiazepines are all used as antianxiety agents. Diazepam is also used as a muscle relaxant. However, with dosage adjustment, almost any benzodiazepine can be used as an antianxiety, hypnotic, or anticonvulsant agent.

History and source

In 1957, Sternbach synthesized the first benzodiazepine. When chlordiazepoxide hydrochloride was studied, one investigator noted that it produced "taming" effects without causing significant ataxia or hypnosis. In 1960, it became the first benzodiazepine marketed in the United States. To date, more than 2,000 benzodiazepine compounds have been synthesized.

PHARMACOKINETICS

Benzodiazepines are well absorbed and widely distributed in the body. In the liver, long-acting agents are broken down into active metabolites that may have even longer half-lives than the parent compounds. Short-acting agents are metabolized to inactive metabolites. (However, alprazolam is a short-to-intermediate–acting agent that is metabolized to an active compound.) All benzodiazepines are primarily excreted in the urine.

Absorption, distribution, metabolism, excretion

After oral administration, benzodiazepines are rapidly and completely absorbed from the gastrointestinal (GI) tract. Even clorazepate dipotassium, an inactive compound, is rapidly absorbed after decarboxylation (splitting off of carbon dioxide molecules) in the GI tract. Its active metabolite desmethyldiazepam is also rapidly absorbed. Prazepam and oxazepam undergo much slower absorption. After I.M. injection, chlordiazepoxide and diazepam are absorbed slowly and erratically, but lorazepam is absorbed rapidly and completely.

Benzodiazepines and their metabolites are well distributed throughout the body. Because long-acting agents are more lipophilic (have a greater affinity for fat) than short-acting agents, they can accumulate in fatty tissue with continued therapy. All benzodiazepines and their metabolites cross the placenta: fetal concentrations of diazepam may even equal those of the mother.

Metabolism occurs in one of two ways. For lorazepam, oxazepam, and certain other benzodiazepines, metabolism involves hepatic conjugation with glucuronic acid. This produces water-soluble inactive compounds that are excreted in the urine. For alprazolam, chlordiazepoxide, diazepam, clorazepate, halazepam, and prazepam, metabolism involves hepatic oxidation to active compounds with half-lives that may be longer than those of the parent compounds. These metabolites are then conjugated to inactive compounds that are excreted in the urine.

Onset, peak, duration

After oral administration, most benzodiazepines reach peak concentration levels in 1 to 2 hours. Prazepam and oxazepam typically peak later, however. Peak concentration levels of prazepam's active metabolite occur about 6 hours after administration; oxazepam concentration levels peak between 2½ and 8 hours after administration.

Benzodiazepines produce antianxiety, muscle relaxant, and anticonvulsant effects after the first dose. These effects will increase until steady-state concentration levels are reached. Long-acting agents accumulate with repeated doses to reach steady-state concentration levels and produce a full therapeutic response in 5 to 10 days. After steady-state levels are attained, these agents can be given once or twice daily; the therapeutic response will persist for days after discontinuation.

Prolonged half-lives of the long-acting agents, such as diazepam, may occur in elderly patients and in patients with liver disease because these patients have an increased percentage of fatty tissue in their bodies. Short-acting benzodiazepines with no active metabolites will accumulate more rapidly and reach steady-state concentration levels in 2 to 4 days. These agents require multiple doses every day. If the patient misses 1 day of therapy, the blood level—and the therapeutic response—will decline rapidly.

PHARMACODYNAMICS

Although researchers have not established the exact mechanism of action of benzodiazepines, most believe that these drugs inhibit excitation. The principal sites are the cerebral cortex and the limbic, thalamic, and hypothalamic levels of the central nervous system (CNS).

Mechanism of action

Current theories suggest that the benzodiazepines enhance the effects of gamma-aminobutyric acid (GABA). A natural inhibitor of excitatory stimulation, GABA affects the limbic system and helps control emotions. Enhancement of GABA activity is responsible for the action of benzodiazepines.

Unlike barbiturates, which can depress the CNS directly, benzodiazepines work indirectly by enhancing GABA activity. This synergistic action may explain the safer adverse reaction profile of the benzodiazepines, especially in overdoses.

PHARMACOTHERAPEUTICS

Benzodiazepines are used in the short-term treatment of generalized anxiety. Other clinical uses include producing sedative and hypnotic effects, treating seizure disorders, producing skeletal muscle relaxation, treating insomnia, providing light anesthesia, and managing alcohol withdrawal. (More information about these other clinical indications appears in the appropriate chapters of this book.)

Currently, the benzodiazepines are the drugs of choice for treating anxiety. They have replaced the barbiturates because they produce fewer adverse reactions, less respiratory depression, and fewer drug interactions, and because they are less addicting and habit-forming and have milder withdrawal symptoms. They are, however, more expensive than barbiturates.

alprazolam (Xanax). A Schedule IV drug, alprazolam is the only benzodiazepine that also seems to have anti-

depressant activity. Although not as effective as the tricyclic antidepressants, it may be useful in treating anxiety associated with depression.
USUAL ADULT DOSAGE: initially, 0.25 to 0.5 mg P.O. t.i.d., increased, as tolerated, to a maximum of 4 mg/day; for elderly patients, initially, 0.25 mg P.O. b.i.d. or t.i.d., increased gradually.

chlordiazepoxide hydrochloride (A-poxide, Librium). A Schedule IV drug, chlordiazepoxide can be used to treat anxiety and alcohol withdrawal. This drug is available in oral or injectable form. I.M. injections, not recommended for children under age 12, must be prepared with the diluent provided and must be administered deep I.M.
USUAL ADULT DOSAGE: for anxiety, 5 to 10 mg P.O. t.i.d., increased to 25 mg t.i.d. or q.i.d., as needed: for anxiety in an elderly patient, 5 mg P.O. b.i.d. to q.i.d. increased as needed; for alcohol withdrawal, 50 to 100 mg P.O., I.M., or I.V. to a maximum of 300 mg/day.

clorazepate dipotassium (Tranxene). A Schedule IV drug, clorazepate is used to treat anxiety and alcohol withdrawal and can be used as an adjunct in managing partial seizures. (For seizure dosage information, see Chapter 24, Anticonvulsant Agents.)
USUAL ADULT DOSAGE: for anxiety, 7.5 mg P.O. t.i.d., or 15 mg P.O. h.s., increased as tolerated and as needed, to a maximum of 60 mg/day; for anxiety in an elderly patient, 7.5 to 15 mg P.O. daily, increased as needed; for acute alcohol withdrawal: Day 1—30 mg P.O. initially, followed by 30 to 60 mg P.O. in divided doses; Day 2—45 to 90 mg P.O. in divided doses; Day 3—22.5 to 45 mg P.O. in divided doses; Day 4—15 to 30 mg P.O. in divided doses; gradually reduce daily dosage to 7.5 to 15 mg P.O.

diazepam (Valium, Valrelease). A Schedule IV drug, diazepam is used to treat anxiety, alcohol withdrawal, skeletal muscle spasms, and status epilepticus. Besides the standard oral form, diazepam is available in I.V., I.M., and sustained-release oral forms.
USUAL ADULT DOSAGE: for anxiety, 2 to 10 mg P.O. b.i.d. to q.i.d. (initially, 1 to 2 mg P.O. b.i.d. for an elderly patient) or 15 to 30 mg P.O. of sustained-release capsule once daily; for alcohol withdrawal, 10 mg P.O. t.i.d. or q.i.d. for the first 24 hours, decreased to 5 mg t.i.d. or q.i.d., as needed; for skeletal muscle spasms, 2 to 10 mg P.O. t.i.d. or q.i.d.; for status epilepticus, 5 to 10 mg slow I.V. push at no more than 5 mg/minute, repeated, as needed, every 10 to 15 minutes to a maximum of 30 mg.

halazepam (Paxipam). A Schedule IV drug, halazepam is used to treat anxiety.

USUAL ADULT DOSAGE: for anxiety, 20 to 40 mg P.O. t.i.d. or q.i.d.; for anxiety in an elderly patient, 20 mg P.O. once a day or b.i.d. The optimal daily dosage ranges from 80 to 160 mg.

lorazepam (Ativan). A Schedule IV drug, lorazepam is used to treat anxiety and to provide preoperative sedation.
USUAL ADULT DOSAGE: for anxiety, 2 to 3 mg P.O. b.i.d. or t.i.d., increased to a maximum of 6 mg/day; for anxiety in an elderly patient, 1 to 2 mg P.O. b.i.d. or t.i.d., increased as needed; for preoperative sedation, 2 to 4 mg I.M. or I.V.

oxazepam (Serax). A Schedule IV drug, oxazepam is used to treat anxiety, especially in patients with hepatic disease. It is safe for these patients because it does not accumulate the way long-acting benzodiazepines with active metabolites do.
USUAL ADULT DOSAGE: for anxiety, 10 to 15 mg P.O. t.i.d. or q.i.d., increased as needed to 15 to 30 mg t.i.d. or q.i.d.; for anxiety in an elderly patient, 10 mg P.O. t.i.d., increased to 15 mg t.i.d. or q.i.d. as needed.

prazepam (Centrax). A Schedule IV drug, prazepam is also used to treat anxiety disorders.
USUAL ADULT DOSAGE: for anxiety, 10 mg P.O. t.i.d., increased to a maximum of 60 mg/day, as needed; for anxiety in an elderly patient, 10 to 15 mg P.O. daily, in divided doses increased as needed.

Drug interactions

Fewer, less severe drug interactions occur with the benzodiazepines than with the barbiturates. The major interactions relate to the use of benzodiazepines with other CNS depressants, producing additive effects. (See *Drug interactions: Benzodiazepines* in Chapter 30, Sedative and Hypnotic Agents, for more on interactions.)

ADVERSE DRUG REACTIONS

Most adverse reactions to the benzodiazepines affect the CNS; less than 1% affect other body systems.

Predictable reactions

The most predictable reactions are neurologic. Sedation is the most common, affecting 4% to 12% of all patients taking chlordiazepoxide or diazepam. A dosage reduction may eliminate this adverse effect. Benzodiazepines can also impair motor coordination, reaction time, and cognitive reasoning. Although these reactions usually affect driving skills, some anxious patients actually drive better because their anxieties are relieved. Diazepam, alprazolam, and lorazepam can also cause dosage-related amnesia.

The benzodiazepines have a potential for abuse, tolerance, and physical dependence. As a result, abrupt discontinuation of long-term, high-dosage therapy can cause a withdrawal reaction. Because some benzodiazepines have long half-lives, withdrawal symptoms may take a week to appear. This reaction may occur less frequently with benzodiazepines than with other antianxiety agents, although its true incidence is unknown.

Unpredictable reactions

Benzodiazepines may rarely cause unpredictable reactions, including mild allergic reactions such as skin rash, pruritus, and urticaria. They may also cause paradoxical excitation in elderly patients.

NURSING IMPLICATIONS

Although the benzodiazepines produce fewer drug interactions and adverse reactions than many other antianxiety agents, the nurse must be aware of several important points.
- Do not administer benzodiazepines to a pregnant patient, because they may cause birth defects.
- Do not administer these agents to breast-feeding women, because they may cause pharmacologic effects in the newborn.
- Expect to reduce the dosage for an elderly patient, especially if the agent has active metabolites.
- Avoid I.M. administration, if possible; absorption after I.M. injection is slow and erratic.
- Administer I.V. preparations slowly to reduce the risk of phlebitis and cardiovascular collapse.
- Inform the patient that drowsiness may occur.
- Advise the patient not to drive or operate dangerous machinery.
- Tell the patient not to stop taking the medication without consulting the physician, because a withdrawal reaction can occur if therapy is discontinued abruptly.
- Warn the patient not to combine benzodiazepines with other CNS depressants, including alcohol.

BUSPIRONE

The first anxiolytic in a new class of agents, buspirone hydrochloride's structure and mechanism of action differ from those of other antianxiety agents. Research on the antianxiety effects of buspirone began in the late 1970s, but the drug was not marketed until 1986.

PHARMACOKINETICS

Buspirone is rapidly absorbed and metabolized by the liver. Few other details about its metabolism are known.

Absorption, distribution, metabolism, excretion

After oral administration, buspirone is rapidly absorbed. Its bioavailability is decreased, however, because of a large first-pass effect. Although the distribution of buspirone has not been fully explained, researchers have found that, in the brain, some of its metabolites accumulate at higher levels than the parent compound does. Buspirone's metabolism also remains largely unknown. After administration, 40% of a dose appears in the urine as metabolites, less than 1% is excreted unchanged, and nearly 60% is unaccounted for.

Onset, peak, duration

Plasma levels peak 1 hour after oral administration. The half-life averages 2½ hours and ranges from 0.9 to 9.4 hours. However, buspirone's onset of action ranges from 1 to 2 weeks.

PHARMACODYNAMICS

Researchers have not yet identified buspirone's site and mechanism of action, but they know that, in contrast to theories about the benzodiazepines, buspirone does not affect GABA receptors. Rather, it seems to produce various effects in the midbrain and acts as a midbrain modulator.

PHARMACOTHERAPEUTICS

Currently, buspirone is indicated to treat generalized anxiety states. Few clinical trials have compared buspirone to other agents, but patients who have not previously been exposed to benzodiazepines seem to respond better to buspirone. This drug's slow onset of action, however, makes it ineffective for p.r.n. use.

buspirone hydrochloride (Buspar). So far, five clinical trials have demonstrated that buspirone is as effective as diazepam or clorazepate in relieving anxiety. Milligram for milligram, buspirone equals diazepam in potency.
USUAL ADULT DOSAGE: 5 mg P.O. t.i.d., increased by 5 mg daily every 2 to 3 days, as needed, to a maximum dose of 60 mg/day. For most patients, the maintenance dose is 20 to 30 mg/day.

Drug interactions

To date, researchers have discovered no interactions between buspirone and other drugs. Unlike other antianxiety agents, buspirone does not interact with alcohol or other CNS depressants.

ADVERSE DRUG REACTIONS

Buspirone produces far fewer adverse reactions than the benzodiazepines. Researchers have found that the most common reactions include dizziness, light-headedness, insomnia, and headache.

At this time, no data exist regarding buspirone overdose, and the drug does not appear to have an abuse potential.

NURSING IMPLICATIONS

Although buspirone appears to cause minimal adverse reactions and drug interactions, it should be used with caution, because clinical trials have not yet determined the consequences of long-term buspirone therapy.
• Monitor the patient carefully for adverse drug reactions or interactions as soon as buspirone therapy begins.
• Be aware that patients are not switched from long-term benzodiazepine therapy to buspirone without tapering off the benzodiazepine to avoid a benzodiazepine withdrawal reaction.

BARBITURATES

Until the benzodiazepines were introduced about 25 years ago, the barbiturates were the most frequently prescribed antianxiety agents. Although no longer the drugs of choice, barbiturates are still used for their antianxiety, anticonvulsant, preanesthetic, sedative, and hypnotic effects.

This chapter presents two barbiturates as examples: phenobarbital sodium, a long-acting agent commonly used for its anticonvulsant and sedative effects, and pentobarbital sodium, a short-to intermediate-acting agent principally used for its hypnotic and sedative properties. (See Chapter 30, Sedative and Hypnotic Agents, for further information about barbiturates.)

History and source

Von Baeyer synthesized the prototype barbiturate, barbituric acid, in 1864. Nearly 40 years later, the first hypnotic barbiturate, barbital, was introduced. Because barbital's onset of action was about 22 hours, however, it was eventually replaced by drugs with shorter onsets of action. In 1912, phenobarbital was introduced; it remains one of the most frequently prescribed barbiturates. Although more than 2,500 barbiturates have been synthesized, only 12 are marketed today.

PHARMACOKINETICS

Barbiturates are well absorbed, rapidly distributed, metabolized in the liver, and excreted in the urine. Barbiturates fall into four classifications based on duration of action: long-acting agents, intermediate-acting agents, short-acting agents, and ultrashort–acting agents. The ultrashort–acting agents are used to induce and maintain anesthesia.

Absorption, distribution, metabolism, excretion

The barbiturates are well absorbed after oral, intramuscular, or rectal administration. For oral administration, the sodium salt form is absorbed more rapidly than the acid form.

Because barbiturates are lipophilic, they are distributed throughout the body and highly concentrated in the fatty tissue of the liver and brain. Phenobarbital, which has a reduced lipophilic effect, enters and exits the brain more slowly, so it has an extended duration of action. Barbiturates also cross the placenta.

Slowly metabolized by the microsomal enzymes in the liver, barbiturates produce inactive metabolites. The kidneys eliminate most barbiturates as metabolites, except for phenobarbital: 25% to 50% of phenobarbital is excreted unchanged in the urine.

Onset, peak, duration

After oral administration, phenobarbital reaches peak plasma concentration levels in 8 to 12 hours and steady-state concentration levels in 3 to 4 weeks if a loading dose is not given. Its half-life ranges from 50 to 170 hours.

Pentobarbital demonstrates onset of action in 15 to 60 minutes after oral administration and achieves peak concentration levels in 30 to 60 minutes. The half-life of pentobarbital averages 15 to 48 hours.

PHARMACODYNAMICS

The neurotransmitter GABA appears to mediate the actions of the barbiturates. A powerful inhibitor of excitatory stimulation, GABA appears in 40% of the brain synapses.

Mechanism of action

The barbiturates depress all excitable body tissues through an unknown mechanism of action apparently mediated by GABA. In therapeutic concentrations, barbiturates enhance the effects of GABA, but at higher concentrations, they directly depress all neurons. Enhancement of GABA blocks excitatory activity such as anxiety, convulsions, and spinal cord stimulation. GABA activity at higher concentrations explains the sedative, anticonvulsant, and other effects of the barbiturates.

PHARMACOTHERAPEUTICS

In treating anxiety, barbiturates are more effective than meprobamate and equally as effective as the benzodiazepines. But because barbiturates cause many adverse reactions, including severe respiratory depression, they have been largely replaced by the benzodiazepines as antianxiety agents. Physicians most commonly prescribe the barbiturates as anticonvulsant, anesthetic, sedative, and hypnotic agents. (See Chapter 24, Anticonvulsant Agents; Chapter 27, General Anesthetic Agents; and Chapter 30, Sedative and Hypnotic Agents.) Phenobarbital is also used to manage barbiturate or nonbarbiturate withdrawal in dependent patients and is under investigation for use in treating congenital biliary defects and hyperbilirubinemia in neonates.

pentobarbital sodium (Nembutal Sodium). A Schedule II drug, pentobarbital is usually used as a hypnotic but can be used as a sedative or antianxiety agent.
USUAL ADULT DOSAGE: for sedation or to relieve anxiety, 20 mg P.O. t.i.d. or q.i.d. The dose must be individualized for each patient and reduced for an elderly patient.

phenobarbital sodium (Luminal Sodium). A Schedule IV drug, phenobarbital can be used as an antianxiety agent.
USUAL ADULT DOSAGE: 30 to 120 mg P.O. daily in two or three divided doses. The dose must be individualized for each patient and reduced for an elderly patient.

Drug interactions
When administered with other CNS depressants, the barbiturates can produce additive depressant effects. Other drug interactions are also likely to occur, because barbiturates can stimulate the enzymes that degrade other drugs, thereby decreasing their duration of action. (See *Drug interactions: Barbiturates* in Chapter 30, Sedative and Hypnotic Agents.)

ADVERSE DRUG REACTIONS

The most serious adverse reactions involve the CNS and the respiratory system. Other, less serious, reactions can occur, including allergic reactions and GI complaints.

Predictable reactions
The most common predictable adverse reactions involve the CNS and include sedation, lethargy, ataxia, headache, mental depression, and impaired motor coordination and reaction time. When used as hypnotics, these drugs can produce a hangover effect or confused state the next day, especially in elderly patients.

In an otherwise healthy person, barbiturates produce respiratory depression equal to that produced by sleep. In a patient with a pulmonary disease, respiratory depressant effects are more pronounced. Even low doses of phenobarbital can produce severe changes in the blood oxygen saturation and blood pH levels: respiratory effects are more drastic in a patient who has taken an overdose.

Long-term use can lead to tolerance and physical or psychological dependence on the barbiturate. Then if therapy is abruptly discontinued, a withdrawal reaction can occur in 8 to 12 hours. Withdrawal symptoms include anxiety, insomnia, nausea, vomiting, hallucinations, muscular irritability, and seizures. To avoid a potentially fatal withdrawal reaction, long-term therapy should be tapered over a period of 1 to 2 weeks.

Unpredictable reactions
These reactions include dermatologic and allergic manifestations, paradoxical excitation, blood dyscrasias, and local reactions to parenteral administration.

NURSING IMPLICATIONS

Barbiturates are infrequently used as antianxiety agents because of their high risk of adverse reactions and dependence. But when these drugs are given, the nurse must be aware of the following considerations.
• Administer barbiturates with caution in a patient who is taking other CNS depressants, including alcohol.
• Administer only with extreme caution in a patient with a pulmonary disease.
• Assess for ataxia, confused states, paradoxical excitation, and agitation, especially in an elderly patient. Raise the bed rails and supervise the patient's walks, if necessary.
• Be alert for depression, suicidal thoughts, or hoarding of medication (a barbiturate overdose can be fatal).
• Do not administer an I.V. barbiturate faster than 60 mg/minute.
• Give injections deep I.M. to avoid sterile abscesses and tissue sloughing.
• Monitor the patient's blood counts before therapy begins.
• Alert the patient about the possible effects of sedation, and advise the patient to avoid driving or operating dangerous machinery while taking the drug.
• Advise the patient not to stop taking the medications without first consulting the physician because a withdrawal reaction can occur with abrupt discontinuation of barbiturates.
• Instruct the patient to report a sore throat, easy bruising, or fever.

SELECTED MAJOR DRUGS

Antianxiety agents

This chart summarizes the most common antianxiety agents currently in clinical use.

DRUG	MAJOR INDICATIONS	USUAL ADULT DOSAGES	NURSING IMPLICATIONS
Benzodiazepines			
clorazepate	Anxiety	7.5 mg P.O. t.i.d. increased to 60 mg/day	• Be aware that clorazepate is contraindicated in patients with acute narrow-angle glaucoma, depressive neuroses, psychotic reactions, and in children under age 18.
	Alcohol withdrawal	Day 1—30 mg P.O. followed by 30 to 60 mg P.O. in divided doses; Day 2—45 to 90 mg P.O. in divided doses; Day 3—22.5 to 45 mg P.O. in divided doses; Day 4—15 to 30 mg P.O. in divided doses; gradually reduced to 7.5 to 15 mg P.O. daily	• Expect to reduce the dose for an elderly patient. • Assess for signs of drug abuse.
diazepam	Anxiety	2 to 10 mg P.O. b.i.d. to q.i.d.	• Be aware that diazepam is contraindicated in patients with shock, coma, and acute alcohol intoxication.
	Alcohol withdrawal	10 mg P.O. t.i.d. or q.i.d. for 24 hours, decreased to 5 mg t.i.d. or q.i.d.	• Assess for signs of drug abuse. • Alert the patient to avoid activities that require mental alertness.
	Skeletal muscle spasms	2 to 10 mg P.O. t.i.d. or q.i.d.	• Inject at a rate of no more than 5 mg/minute for I.V. administration to prevent adverse reactions.
	Status epilepticus	5 to 10 mg slow I.V. push repeated every 10 to 15 minutes to a maximum of 30 mg	
Miscellaneous			
buspirone	Anxiety	5 mg P.O. t.i.d., increased by 5 mg q 2 to 3 days, as needed, to a maximum of 60 mg/day	• Monitor the patient closely, because expected reactions to this relatively new drug are unknown.

OTHER ANTIANXIETY AGENTS

Although benzodiazepines, buspirone, and barbiturates are commonly used to treat anxiety disorders, meprobamate, beta blockers, and antihistamines may also be used as antianxiety agents.

meprobamate (Equanil, Meprocon, Miltown, SK-Bamate). This drug was widely used in the past to treat anxiety. It is rarely used today, however, because of its low degree of effectiveness, the severity of its adverse effects, and the advent of safer, more effective agents. A carbamate derivative, meprobamate is the only drug of its class to be used as an antianxiety agent rather than a muscle relaxant. After oral administration, meprobamate is well absorbed from the intestines and distributed uniformly throughout the body. It is partially metabolized in the liver to inactive metabolites and is excreted by the kidneys. Although meprobamate is a CNS depressant, its exact site and mechanism of action in anxiety relief is unknown. When meprobamate is prescribed for the short-term management of anxiety, the usual adult dosage is 1,200 to 1,600 mg P.O. in three or four divided doses and may be increased to a maximum of 2,400 mg/day. It is sometimes used for preoperative sedation and for hypnotic effects in insomnia. When administered with other CNS depressant drugs, meprobamate usually causes additive depressant effects. Meprobamate's CNS depressant action accounts for its adverse reactions, which commonly include sedation, ataxia, and hypotension. Dependence can develop, and severe withdrawal reactions have occurred after abrupt discontinuation of high doses given for several weeks. Unpredictable reactions may also occur, including allergic reactions, paradoxical excitement, and congenital heart defects, if given during the first 6 weeks of pregnancy. Although meprobamate usage is rare, the nurse must be prepared to instruct the patient about this drug's adverse reactions and drug interactions.

Beta blockers. These drugs can relieve the somatic symptoms associated with anxiety. Although most studies show that benzodiazepines are more effective in treating anxiety disorders, beta blockers are useful in treating acute situational anxiety that causes somatic symptoms. The usual adult dosage is 40 to 60 mg P.O. (of propranolol hydrochloride or an equivalent beta blocker) given 1 to 2 hours before the patient enters the stressful situation.

antihistamines. These drugs, particularly hydroxyzine hydrochloride and diphenhydramine hydrochloride, may be used to treat anxiety. Their use is rare, however, and most studies indicate that they are not effective antianxiety agents.

CHAPTER SUMMARY

Here are the highlights of this chapter:
• Benzodiazepines have replaced barbiturates as the drugs of choice to treat anxiety. They offer a safer adverse reaction profile and produce no respiratory depression even in overdoses. And unlike the barbiturates, benzodiazepines do not cause major drug interactions. Benzodiazepines typically produce mild CNS effects—drowsiness, motor incoordination, and decreased reaction time. Other adverse reactions rarely occur.
• Buspirone is the newest antianxiety agent. Preliminary data indicate that it causes no drug interactions, no drug dependence, almost no sedation, and only minor adverse effects such as dizziness and headache. Nevertheless, a patient receiving buspirone must be closely monitored until researchers discover more about its effects.

• Although barbiturates are effective in treating anxiety, they have been largely replaced by the benzodiazepines for a number of reasons. Barbiturates interact with many drugs, because they inhibit the hepatic enzymes that degrade those drugs. They also cause many adverse effects, including respiratory depression, which is especially dangerous in a patient who has a pulmonary disease or an overdose. They are also associated with many allergic reactions.
• Meprobamate seems less effective than other antianxiety agents and is rarely used today to treat anxiety disorders. Other drugs that are used rarely to treat anxiety include beta blockers and antihistamines.

BIBLIOGRAPHY

Allen, R.M. "Tranquilizers and Sedative/Hypnotics: Appropriate Use in the Elderly," *Geriatrics* 41:75, 1986.

Ballenger, J.C. "Psychopharmacology of the Anxiety Disorders," *Psychiatric Clinics of North America.* 7:757, 1984.

Dominugez, R.A., and Goldstein, B.J. "25 Years of Benzodiazepine Experience: Clinical Commentary on Use, Abuse, and Withdrawal," *Hospital Formulary* 20:1000, 1985.

Dommisse, C.S., and DeVane, C.L. "Buspirone: A New Type of Anxiolytic," *Drug Intelligence and Clinical Pharmacy* 19:624, 1985.

Eison, M.A., and Temple, D.L. "Buspirone: Review of Its Pharmacology and Current Perspectives on Its Mechanism of Action," *American Journal of Medicine* 80:1, 1986.

Greenblatt, D.J., et al. "Drug Therapy. Current Status of Benzodiazepines, Part I," *New England Journal of Medicine* 309(6):354, August 11, 1983.

Greenblatt, D.J., et al. "Current Status of Benzodiazepines, Part 2," *New England Journal of Medicine* 309(7):410, August 18, 1983.

Newton, R.E., et al. "Review of the Side-Effect Profile of Buspirone," *American Journal of Medicine* 80:17, 1986.

Shehi, G.M., and Patterson, W.M. "Interactions of Benzodiazepines and Other Commonly Used Drugs," *Internal Medicine* 6:95, 1985.

CHAPTER
33

ANTIPSYCHOTIC AGENTS

OBJECTIVES

After reading and studying this chapter, you should be able to:

1. Identify medications that are frequently prescribed as antipsychotic agents.

2. Discuss the clinical indications for the antipsychotic agents.

3. Describe the mechanism of action of the antipsychotic agents.

4. Identify common adverse reactions to the antipsychotic agents, and describe appropriate nursing interventions.

5. Assess a patient receiving an antipsychotic agent for therapeutic and adverse effects.

6. Explain the importance of early detection of symptoms of tardive dyskinesia.

7. Explain the drug regimen and adverse effects of an antipsychotic agent to the patient.

INTRODUCTION

Widely used in psychiatric hospitals and many settings, antipsychotic agents can control psychotic symptoms, such as delusions, hallucinations, and thought disorders, that can occur with schizophrenia, mania, and other psychoses. They can help treat organic psychiatric disorders, such as dementia, delirium, and stimulant-induced psychoses, and can sedate agitated patients. They are also used to treat the movement disorders Gilles de la Tourette's syndrome and Huntington's disease; to augment the effects of analgesics and anesthetics preoperatively to control pain; and to treat nausea, vomiting, intractable hiccups, and pruritus.

Antipsychotic agents are also called major tranquilizers or neuroleptics: *antipsychotic* because they can eliminate signs and symptoms of psychoses; *major tranquilizer* because they can calm an agitated patient; *neuroleptic* because they have a neurobiological adverse effect, abnormal body movements. Many people prefer *neuroleptic* because it accurately describes the drugs' broader use in nonpsychiatric settings.

No matter what they are called, all antipsychotic agents belong to one of two major groups: phenothiazines and nonphenothiazines. This chapter will discuss both groups.

An understanding of the effects of antipsychotic drugs requires a knowledge of the anatomy and physiology of the central nervous system (CNS), including the functions of the pyramidal and extrapyramidal tracts, and the limbic system and related structures in the brain.

An area of the brain's cerebral cortex, known as the primary motor, or pyramidal, area, controls voluntary motor functions. Motor signals are transmitted from this area to the anterior motor neurons through the pyramidal tract. The extrapyramidal tracts primarily control involuntary motor functions by transmitting motor signals from the cortex and spinal cord to the brain. Some extrapyramidal pathways pass through the substantia nigra, one of the lower basal ganglia composed of neurons that connect with other associated areas of the extrapyramidal system. The limbic system of the brain includes all of the basal ganglia and controls emotional behavior and drive. The basal ganglia work with the motor cortex and cerebellum to provide motor control in the body. Although stimulation of certain parts of the basal ganglia can produce muscle contractions or complex movements, the ganglia usually inhibit excessive muscle tone and prevent rigidity or spasticity. This action requires dopamine at synaptic receptor sites. Dopamine, a neurotransmitter substance, is released by the substantia nigra.

One theory suggests that schizophrenia results from excess dopamine in the limbic system. This theory is based on evidence that dissociated thought patterns and drives, hallucinations, and delusions tend to disappear when psychotic patients receive antipsychotic drugs inhibiting dopamine action.

For a summary of representative drugs, see *Selected major drugs: Antipsychotic agents* on page 531.

PHENOTHIAZINES

Antipsychotics can be classified on the basis of chemical structure. Many clinicians believe that one of these groups, the phenothiazines, should be treated as three distinct drug classes because of their differences in adverse effects. The three classes include aliphatics (which may cause sedation and anticholinergic effects), piperidines (which may cause sedation), and piperazines (which may cause extrapyramidal reactions).

The phenothiazines include chlorpromazine hydrochloride, promazine hydrochloride, and triflupromazine hydrochloride of the aliphatic subgroup; acetophenazine maleate, carphenazine maleate, fluphenazine decanoate, perphenazine, and trifluoperazine hydrochloride of the piperazine subgroup; and mesoridazine besylate and thioridazine hydrochloride of the piperidine subgroup. Prochlorperazine, also a phenothiazine, is used almost exclusively for nausea and vomiting control. (See Chapter 49, Emetic and Antiemetic Agents, for a discussion of prochlorperazine.) Because their chemical structures vary, each subgroup produces slightly different actions and adverse reactions, but all are equally effective in treating the symptoms of psychoses. The choice of a drug must be based on its therapeutic and adverse effects in a particular patient.

History and source

When chlorpromazine was first given to French surgical patients as an antihistamine, it caused a marked tranquilizing effect. This led Delay and Deniker to test the drug with schizophrenic patients in France in 1952. Their success marked a major breakthrough in treating the mentally ill. Because the medication made patients more manageable, physicians and nurses could emphasize positive treatments, including psychosocial, occupational, and milieu therapy (providing a supportive, nonthreatening, stable environment). Use of the drug and other new treatments enabled many patients who would otherwise have been institutionalized to live in communities.

Although drugs with fewer adverse effects have largely replaced chlorpromazine, this prototype antipsychotic drug remains in use.

PHARMACOKINETICS

Although the phenothiazines are absorbed erratically, they are distributed to many tissues and are highly con-

centrated in the brain. All phenothiazines are metabolized in the liver and are excreted in urine and bile.

Absorption, distribution, metabolism, excretion

After oral administration, phenothiazines are absorbed erratically, although liquid preparations tend to be better absorbed than tablets or capsules. After intramuscular (I.M.) administration, the drugs are absorbed more completely.

The drugs are distributed to most body tissues and are highly concentrated in the CNS. They are 91% to 99% bound to plasma proteins and are highly lipophilic (having a high affinity for fatty tissue). The unchanged drug and its metabolites are stored in tissues with a good blood supply, such as the brain and lungs. Phenothiazines can also enter fetal circulation.

The phenothiazines are extensively metabolized in the liver by hepatic enzymes. Active metabolites accumulate in fatty tissues and prolong drug activity up to 3 months after discontinuation.

Metabolized phenothiazines are excreted by the kidneys in urine and to a smaller degree in the bile, although elderly patients exhibit a decreased capacity to eliminate them. Metabolites may appear in the urine up to 3 months after the last dose.

Onset, peak, duration

The onset of action varies with the type of preparation. A liquid preparation will produce effects in 2 to 4 hours. The onset of action with tablets is unpredictable. An I.M. injection usually produces effects in 15 to 30 minutes. Although the onset of action and tranquilizing effects usually occur in a few hours, the antipsychotic effects (the normalizing of thoughts, moods, and actions) may take several weeks to appear.

The duration of action for a single dose is up to 24 hours. This long action permits once-daily dosing after the optimum therapeutic dose has been determined. The half-life ranges from 10 to 30 hours for an oral phenothiazine and up to 9 days for some long-acting preparations. And because fatty tissues slowly release accumulated phenothiazine metabolites into the plasma, the phenothiazines may produce effects up to 3 months after their discontinuation.

PHARMACODYNAMICS

Although the phenothiazines' mechanism of action is not fully understood, researchers believe that these drugs depress the reticular activating system, the hypothalamus, the chemoreceptor trigger zone (CTZ), and to some extent, the vomiting center. Phenothiazines also stimulate the extrapyramidal system.

Mechanism of action

Researchers believe that the phenothiazines cause a reduction of stimuli to the brain stem reticular activating system, which produces a sedative action. They further postulate that these drugs block postsynaptic dopamine receptors in the limbic system and hypothalamus to produce an antipsychotic action. At the same time, the phenothiazines may interfere with the transmitter function of dopamine in the extrapyramidal tract, causing extrapyramidal symptoms (abnormal body movements).

Researchers also theorize that phenothiazines inhibit the medullary CTZ, thereby producing an antiemetic effect on chemically induced nausea and vomiting, as after an operation. (The drugs, however, cannot reduce nausea and vomiting related to gastric irritants or vestibular disorders, such as motion sickness.) Additional actions include alpha-adrenergic blocking effects and anticholinergic effects, which account for some of the adverse drug reactions.

PHARMACOTHERAPEUTICS

Phenothiazines are used primarily to treat schizophrenia, calm anxious or agitated patients, improve thought processes, and alleviate delusions and hallucinations. These agents may be used to treat other psychiatric disorders, such as brief reactive psychosis, atypical psychosis, schizoaffective psychosis, pervasive development disorder (autism), bipolar affective disorder (manic-depressive disorder), and major depression with psychosis. In manic-depressive patients, the phenothiazines are administered with lithium until the slower-acting lithium becomes effective. The phenothiazines can be used to quiet mentally retarded children and agitated elderly patients, particularly those with organic brain syndrome. However, they may cause extrapyramidal symptoms, especially in elderly women.

Shortly after phenothiazine administration, a quieting and calming effect occurs, but this sedation differs from that produced by CNS depressants; with the phenothiazines, the patient is easily aroused, alert, responsive, and has good motor coordination. After several days of phenothiazine therapy, affective changes occur: formerly fearful schizophrenic patients are no longer bothered by delusions and hallucinations; autistic and withdrawn patients become more responsive and open

to communication. After several weeks of therapy, the patient becomes more coherent, and hallucinations and delusions frequently disappear. Unfortunately, symptoms usually return when medication is discontinued.

The phenothiazines are also used to augment the preoperative effects of analgesics and to manage pain, anxiety, and nausea in cancer patients. Additional indications vary with the specific phenothiazine. Chlorpromazine is used to treat intractable hiccups and shivering associated with CNS damage. It also serves as an effective antiemetic, as does prochlorperazine. (See Chapter 49, Emetic and Antiemetic Agents, for further information about these uses.) Physical dependence does not result from these drugs, but psychological dependence can.

Initial dosing with phenothiazines can be rapid or slow, depending on the severity of symptoms and the patient's age and physical condition. In acute psychosis, the patient receives a loading dose; a patient receiving high doses must be hospitalized so that the drug's effectiveness and adverse reactions can be monitored. When the symptoms are under control, the patient receives a low maintenance dose. Because phenothiazines have long half-lives, the maintenance dose may consist of a single bedtime dose. If severe orthostatic hypotension occurs in the morning, the patient may require divided doses.

Unlike other adults, an elderly or debilitated patient will receive a small initial dose that is increased gradually until a favorable response is achieved. After the patient has taken that dose for about 2 weeks, it is gradually reduced to the lowest effective maintenance dose.

This section will describe the typical dosages for the phenothiazines. Higher dosages may be used, however, particularly in institutional settings.

chlorpromazine hydrochloride (Thorazine). An aliphatic phenothiazine, chlorpromazine was the prototype for all the phenothiazines and was the first antipsychotic agent marketed. It is used to treat schizophrenia and other psychoses, intractable hiccups, and nausea or vomiting. Most patients develop a tolerance to its sedative effects. Patients over age 40 who do not tolerate chlorpromazine well will have increased incidence of dizziness, hypotension, ocular changes, and dyskinesia.
USUAL ADULT DOSAGE: for psychosis, 200 to 600 mg P.O. in divided doses initially, increased to a maintenance dose of 500 to 1,000 mg P.O. daily in divided

DRUG INTERACTIONS
Phenothiazines

Drug interactions involving phenothiazines can be serious. Interactions occur frequently with concurrent use of alcohol or other CNS depressants.

DRUG	INTERACTING DRUGS	POSSIBLE EFFECTS	NURSING IMPLICATIONS
carphenazine, fluphenazine, mesoridazine, perphenazine, promazine, thioridazine, trifluoperazine, triflupromazine	propranolol	Inhibits metabolism of both drugs; increases hypertensive effects	• Monitor the patient closely, and expect to reduce the dosage of one of the drugs. • Frequently monitor the patient's blood pressure.
	guanethidine	Inhibits uptake of guanethidine with chlorpromazine administration	• Frequently monitor the patient's blood pressure. • Expect to increase the guanethidine dose, or replace guanethidine with another antihypertensive agent as prescribed.
	amphetamines	Inhibit amphetamine effects	• Do not administer these drugs concurrently.
	antacids and antidiarrheals	Inhibit absorption of oral phenothiazine	• Separate antacid or antidiarrheal doses from phenothiazine doses by at least 2 hours.
	anticholinergics	Increase anticholinergic effects; decrease antipsychotic effects	• Do not administer together routinely. If the drugs must be given concurrently, assess the patient for signs of reduced phenothiazine effects, such as increased psychotic behavior or agitation. • Perform abdominal assessments to monitor the patient for diminished or absent bowel sounds, abdominal pain, constipation, and other abdominal problems.
	barbiturates	Inhibit metabolism of phenothiazines or CNS depressants; increase CNS depressant effects; increase metabolism of chlorpromazine	• Observe the patient for erratic therapeutic effects by behavior changes, such as increased psychotic behavior or agitation, and for increased depressant effect, such as stupor.
	levodopa	Reduces antiparkinsonian effects of levodopa when phenothiazines block dopamine receptors in the CNS	• Avoid concurrent administration, if possible. • Monitor the patient for an increase in Parkinson's symptoms.
	lithium	Increases chance of neurotoxicity, seizures, delirium, and encephalopathy in manic patients; can produce respiratory depression and hypotension	• Monitor the patient for reduced phenothiazine response and changes in neurologic status. • Monitor the patient's vital signs frequently.

doses, although some adults may receive up to 2 grams/day, or 25 mg I.M. initially, repeated with additional 25 to 50 mg in 1 hour if needed and tolerated, then 3 to 12 hours p.r.n. For nausea and vomiting, 50 to 100 mg rectally every 6 to 8 hours p.r.n., 10 to 25 mg P.O. every 4 to 6 hours p.r.n., or 25 to 50 mg I.M. every 3 to 4 hours p.r.n; for intractable hiccups, 25 to 50 mg P.O. or I.M. t.i.d. or q.i.d.

promazine hydrochloride (Sparine). An aliphatic phenothiazine, promazine is used as a sedative because it lacks antipsychotic properties.
USUAL ADULT DOSAGE: for sedation in mild-to-moderate agitation, 10 to 200 mg P.O. or I.M. every 4 to 6 hours; for sedation in severe agitation, 50 to 150 mg I.M., may repeat in 30 minutes up to a maximum of 300 mg.

triflupromazine hydrochloride (Vesprin). An aliphatic phenothiazine, this drug is used to treat psychoses.
USUAL ADULT DOSAGE: as a sedative in severe agitation in psychoses, 60 to 150 mg I.M. or 50 to 150 mg P.O. daily in two to three divided doses.

acetophenazine maleate (Tindal). A piperazine phenothiazine, this drug is used solely to treat psychotic disorders.
USUAL ADULT DOSAGE: initially, 20 mg P.O. t.i.d. or q.i.d. adjusted to 40 to 80 mg/day for outpatients or 80 to 120 mg/day for inpatients. Hospitalized patients with severe schizophrenia may receive doses from 400 to 600 mg/day.

carphenazine maleate (Proketazine). A piperazine phenothiazine, carphenazine can relieve the symptoms of psychoses.
USUAL ADULT DOSAGE: 12.5 to 50 mg P.O. b.i.d. or t.i.d., increased gradually to a maximum of 120 mg/day.

fluphenazine decanoate (Prolixin), **fluphenazine enanthate** (Prolixin Enanthate), and **fluphenazine hydrochloride** (Permitil Hydrochloride). A piperazine phenothiazine, fluphenazine is available in several forms to treat psychotic symptoms. The decanoate salt and the enanthate salt are depot forms of injection. They are stored in the fat and released slowly into the blood to provide extended action. Because their effects last for up to 6 weeks, they are frequently used with chronically ill patients when compliance is a problem. After the maintenance dose has been established, these drugs can be given on an outpatient basis. Most physicians prefer the decanoate form because it has a longer duration of

action than the enanthate form. The hydrochloride salt is available in two forms: a nondepot injection and an oral preparation.
USUAL ADULT DOSAGE: initially, 12.5 to 25 mg I.M. or S.C. every 1 to 6 weeks, then 25 to 100 mg p.r.n. for maintenance with fluphenazine decanoate or enanthate; with fluphenazine hydrochloride injection, 1.25 to 2.5 mg I.M. every 6 to 8 hours; with fluphenazine hydrochloride oral preparations, 0.5 to 10 mg daily in divided doses every 6 to 8 hours, increased up to 20 mg/day. The shorter-acting fluphenazine hydrocloride is usually prescribed for the patient who has never taken phenothiazines, to determine response.

perphenazine (Trilafon). A piperazine phenothiazine, perphenazine is used to treat psychoses.
USUAL ADULT DOSAGE: for control of psychotic symptoms in hospitalized patients, initially, 8 to 16 mg P.O. b.i.d., t.i.d., or q.i.d., increased to 64 mg/day; in nonhospitalized patients, 4 to 8 mg P.O. t.i.d.

trifluoperazine hydrochloride (Stelazine). A piperazine phenothiazine, this agent is used to control the manifestations of psychoses.
USUAL ADULT DOSAGE: 1 to 5 mg P.O. b.i.d., possibly increased gradually up to 40 mg/day, or 1 to 2 mg I.M. every 4 to 6 hours p.r.n. If I.M. dose exceeds 10 mg/24 hours, the injections should not be given more frequently than 4-hour intervals because of cumulative effect.

mesoridazine besylate (Serentil). A piperidine phenothiazine, this antipsychotic is also an effective sedative.
USUAL ADULT DOSAGE: for antipsychotic effects, 10 to 50 mg P.O. b.i.d. or t.i.d., or 25 mg I.M. repeated in 30 to 60 minutes p.r.n.; for schizophrenia, adults may receive up to 400 mg P.O. daily; for anxiety, 10 mg P.O. t.i.d. up to 150 mg/day.

thioridazine hydrochloride (Mellaril). A piperidine phenothiazine, thioridazine is used to treat the symptoms of psychoses. It is also an effective sedative and is used for dementia (in elderly patients) and depressive neurosis and for alcohol withdrawal, although it cannot correct the nausea and vomiting associated with it.
USUAL ADULT DOSAGE: to control psychotic symptoms, 50 to 100 mg P.O. t.i.d., gradually increased up to 800 mg/day in divided doses, if needed. Usual maintenance dose is 200 to 800 mg/day. Dosage must not exceed

Neurologic effects of antipsychotic agents

Phenothiazines and other antipsychotic drugs commonly produce adverse neurologic reactions ranging from extrapyramidal effects, such as dystonia, akathisia, and pseudoparkinsonism, to tardive dyskinesia.

Dystonia
In the first week of antipsychotic therapy, the patient may exhibit an acute dystonic reaction, an extrapyramidal effect manifested by spasms in the tongue, face, neck, back, and sometimes lower extremities that may resemble a seizure. Spasms sometimes affect certain groups of muscles only. Contracted cervical muscles can result in torticollis, an unnatural or twisted position of the neck. Opisthotonos, grimacing, perioral spasms, or pharyngeal or laryngeal spasms with dysphagia or dyspnea can also occur. Eye muscle spasms can cause oculogyrations—abnormal eye movements. Frequently accompanied by excessive salivation, these dystonic spasms typically occur when a patient receives large doses of antipsychotic agents that are likely to produce extrapyramidal symptoms. They usually disappear with a dosage reduction or administration of 25 to 50 mg I.M. of diphenhydramine (Benadryl) or 1 to 2 mg I.M. or I.V. of benztropine (Cogentin).

Pseudoparkinsonism
Later in the course of treatment, pseudoparkinsonism may occur. This extrapyramidal effect produces muscle tremors, cogwheel rigidity (muscle rigidity that gives way in little jerks when the muscle is passively stretched), shuffling gait, drooling, and a decrease in arm swing and associative movements when walking. Bradykinesia (slow movement) and akinesia (immobility) may also occur. Pseudoparkinsonism results from a direct blockade of dopamine receptors by antipsychotic agents. This reaction may be controlled with the use of antiparkinsonian agents such as amantadine.

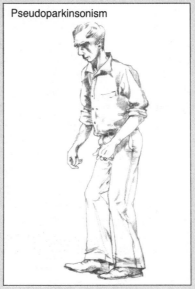
Pseudoparkinsonism

Tardive dyskinesia
Tardive dyskinesia may appear after several months or years of treatment with antipsychotic drugs. Tardive dyskinesia is characterized by abnormal muscle movement, primarily around the mouth, such as lip smacking, rhythmic darting of the tongue, and constant chewing movements. Slow, aimless involuntary movements of the arms or legs may also occur. Although the exact mechanism of tardive dyskinesia is not clear, researchers believe that it may differ from that of the other extrapyramidal symptoms. Tardive dyskinesia usually affects elderly women, but can occur in younger patients as well, even after short-term antipsychotic therapy. If the medication is discontinued when first signs, such as fine wormlike tongue movements, are detected, tardive dyskinesia can sometimes be prevented.

Prevention of this adverse reaction is vital because no effective treatment is available and the reaction is usually irreversible.

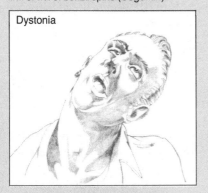
Dystonia

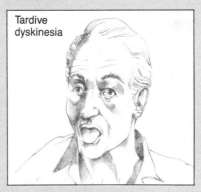
Tardive dyskinesia

Akathisia
Another extrapyramidal effect, akathisia (a continuous restlessness or inability to sit or stand still) may occur in the first 90 days of therapy. The patient attempts to relieve the discomfort of remaining quiet by tapping a foot, moving about in a chair, or pacing constantly. This symptom can easily be mistaken for agitation, which requires treatment with a higher dose of antipsychotic. However, akathisia should be managed by decreasing the antipsychotic dose or by giving an antiparkinsonian agent, such as benztropine.

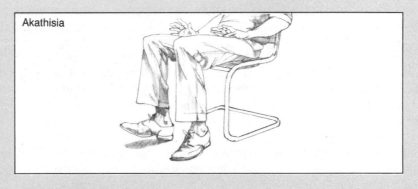
Akathisia

800 mg/day because retinal pigmentation may result. For dementia, 10 to 25 mg b.i.d. or at bedtime. For its nonpsychotic uses, 25 mg P.O. t.i.d., increased to 200 mg/day in divided doses.

Drug interactions

The use of phenothiazines with alcohol and CNS depressants, such as barbiturates and narcotics, may enhance depressant effects, causing hypotension, respiratory depression, or coma. Phenothiazines may also enhance the effects of antihypertensives by increasing the alpha-adrenergic blocking action. They may also increase adverse reactions, such as dry mouth or blurred vision, when taken with anticholinergics, such as atropine. They can interact with other drugs as well. (See *Drug interactions: Phenothiazines* on page 525 for other possible effects.)

ADVERSE DRUG REACTIONS

Phenothiazines produce various adverse reactions ranging from mild, such as dry mouth, to severe, such as tardive dyskinesia. A suitable drug produces minimal adverse reactions, but a physician cannot always predict a specific agent's effects on a given patient and may not obtain reliable information from a mentally ill patient. To monitor phenothiazine therapy properly, the nurse must have a thorough knowledge of the potential adverse reactions for these drugs.

Predictable reactions

Neurologic reactions are the most common and serious adverse reactions to phenothiazine therapy. They include extrapyramidal effects, which may appear any time after the first few days of therapy, and tardive dyskinesia, which usually occurs after several years of treatment. (See *Neurologic effects of antipsychotic agents* on page 527 for details about these adverse reactions.)

Phenothiazines can cause severe—possibly irreversible—tardive dyskinesia, but their actions sometimes mask it. So a "drug holiday" may be ordered for a long-term phenothiazine patient to unmask this adverse reaction. The patient receives no antipsychotic drugs for 4 or more weeks, and during this drug holiday, the physician or nurse observes the patient for adverse reactions. A drug holiday is also used to delay the appearance of tardive dyskinesia, which is related to the total accumulated dose of a phenothiazine.

Phenothiazines may also produce adverse reactions in the autonomic nervous and endocrine systems. (See *Adverse reaction potential of phenothiazines* for additional information.)

Unpredictable reactions

Hypersensitivity to phenothiazines can cause unpredictable reactions. For example, photosensitive skin reactions frequently occur and can be serious enough to warrant instructing all patients to stay out of the sun or use a suncreen with a skin protection factor of 15 or more. Other skin reactions, such as urticaria and dermatitis, occur less frequently.

Although they are less common, more serious adverse reactions can occur, including blood dyscrasias, jaundice, and neuroleptic malignant syndrome (NMS), which produces muscle rigidity, hyperpyrexia, and cardiovascular collapse. When these reactions occur, the phenothiazine should be discontinued or, if the patient is psychiatrically unstable, the dosage should be reduced.

NURSING IMPLICATIONS

Because the phenothiazines are powerful drugs that can produce serious adverse reactions, they are usually reserved for use in patients with psychoses and other situations where their use is strongly indicated. When they are used, however, the nurse must be aware of the following considerations:

• Use caution when administering phenothiazines in combination with alcohol, narcotics, or other CNS depressants, because they can augment the depressant effects.

• Be aware that the antiemetic action of phenothiazines may mask nausea and suppress vomiting that might otherwise serve as signs of an underlying disease.

• Administer phenothiazines cautiously to a patient with a seizure disorder, prostate disorder, liver disease, or cardiac disorder.

• Carefully observe and report patient behavior because the response to treatment can vary widely among individuals.

• Document the effects of the therapy so that the patient may receive the lowest effective dose. Note, in particular, whether the patient is sedated, stimulated, agitated, or overactive, and describe any changes in thought patterns and speech that might indicate hallucinations or delusions.

• Observe the patient for extrapyramidal symptoms. Notify the physician immediately if an acute dystonic reaction occurs, particularly if face or neck spasms interfere with swallowing or breathing.

• Assess the patient for early signs of tardive dyskinesia, such as wormlike movements of the tongue, and if these signs appear, suggest a change in the medication regimen.

Adverse reaction potential of phenothiazines

The chart below indicates the relative potential of phenothiazines to produce specific adverse reactions.

PHENOTHIAZINES	SEDATION	EXTRAPYRAMIDAL SYMPTOMS	HYPOTENSION	ANTICHOLINERGIC EFFECTS
Aliphatic subgroup				
chlorpromazine	High	Moderate	High	High
promazine	Moderate	Moderate	Moderate	High
triflupromazine	Moderate	Moderate	Moderate	High
Piperazine subgroup				
acetophenazine	Moderate	Moderate	Low	Moderate
carphenazine	Moderate	High	Low	Moderate
fluphenazine	Low	High	Low	Low
perphenazine	Moderate	Moderate	Low	Low
trifluoperazine	Low	High	Low	Low
Piperidine subgroup				
mesoridazine	High	Low	Moderate	Moderate
thioridazine	High	Low	Moderate	Very high

● Notify the physician immediately if symptoms of serious conditions develop, such as hypotension, urinary retention or hesitancy, dermatitis, unexplained sore throat and fever, jaundice, or opaque deposits in the lens and cornea of the eye.

● Report any anticholinergic effects, such as dry mouth, blurred vision, decreased sweating, and constipation, and try to relieve them. For example, offer the patient sugarless gum or chipped ice to relieve dry mouth, and increase the patient's fluid and fiber intake to prevent constipation.

● Inform the patient about other troublesome adverse effects that may occur, such as photosensitivity, nasal congestion, tachycardia, decreased sexual ability, menstrual changes, and breast swelling.

NONPHENOTHIAZINES

Based on their chemical structures, nonphenothiazine antipsychotics can be divided into several drug classes, including the butyrophenones, such as haloperidol and haloperidol decanoate; dibenzoxazepines, such as loxapine succinate; dihydroindolones, such as molindone hydrochloride; diphenyl-butylpiperidines, such as pimozide; and thioxanthenes, such as chlorprothixene and thiothixene.

Although chemically different from the phenothiazines, the nonphenothiazines are used to treat psychotic symptoms with equal effectiveness and produce similar actions and adverse reactions. Individual reactions to nonphenothiazines can vary. Therefore, a physician usually prescribes the nonphenothiazine that produces the greatest therapeutic action and fewest adverse reactions for each patient.

PHARMACOKINETICS

Nonphenothiazines are absorbed, distributed, metabolized, and excreted in the same manner as the phenothiazines. Their onset of action, peak concentration levels, and duration of action are similar to those of the phenothiazines.

PHARMACODYNAMICS

The mechanism of action of nonphenothiazines resembles that of the phenothiazines.

Adverse reaction potential of nonphenothiazines

The chart below indicates the relative potential of nonphenothiazines to produce specific adverse reactions.

NONPHENOTHIAZINES	SEDATION	EXTRAPYRAMIDAL SYMPTOMS	HYPOTENSION	ANTICHOLINERGIC EFFECTS
Butyrophenone subgroup				
haloperidol	Low	Very high	Low	Very low
Dibenzoxazepine subgroup				
loxapine	Low	Moderate	Low	Low
Dihydroindolone subgroup				
molindone	Moderate	Moderate	Low	Low
Thioxanthene subgroup				
chlorprothixene	High	Moderate	Moderate	Moderate
thiothixene	Low	Moderate	Moderate	Low
Diphenyl-butylpiperidine subgroup				
pimozide	Low	Very high	Low	Moderate

PHARMACOTHERAPEUTICS

As a group, nonphenothiazines are used to treat psychotic disorders. Specific drugs in this group may serve additional functions. For example, thiothixene is also used to control acute agitation. Haloperidol and pimozide may be used to treat Gilles de la Tourette's syndrome.

droperidol (Inapsine). This butyrophenone nonphenothiazine acts as a tranquilizer and antiemetic during surgical and diagnostic procedures. As a preoperative medication, it may be used alone or in conjunction with a narcotic analgesic. Because it enhances the effects of CNS depressants, it may produce hypotension and respiratory depression after surgery.
USUAL ADULT DOSAGE: preoperatively, 2.5 to 10 mg I.M. 30 to 60 minutes before procedure. Elderly or debilitated patients or those receiving other CNS depressants may require dosage modification. Patients undergoing surgery will require individualized doses.

haloperidol (Haldol), haloperidol decanoate (Haldol Decanoate). A butyrophenone nonphenothiazine, this antipsychotic agent is available in short-acting form and in long-acting form (the decanoate form). Both are used to treat dyskinesia in Gilles de la Tourette's syndrome and symptoms of psychoses. In elderly patients, they may be used to treat the symptoms of dementia.
USUAL ADULT DOSAGE: 0.5 to 5 mg (0.5 to 2 mg for an elderly patient) P.O. b.i.d. or t.i.d. of the short-acting form, increased p.r.n. up to 100 mg/day for a limited period in a hospital setting; 2 to 5 mg I.M. of the short-acting form repeated every hour p.r.n. until symptoms are controlled and then repeated at 4- to 8-hour intervals; up to 100 mg I.M. initially of the long-acting form repeated at monthly intervals in doses of up to 300 mg. Haloperidol decanoate is not to be administered I.V.

loxapine succinate (Loxitane). A dibenzoxazepine nonphenothiazine, loxapine is used to treat the manifestations of psychoses.
USUAL ADULT DOSAGE: 10 mg P.O. b.i.d. to q.i.d., increased to 60 to 100 mg/day; for severe agitation 12.5 to 50 mg I.M. every 4 to 6 hours.

molindone hydrochloride (Moban). A dihydroindolone nonphenothiazine, molindone is used to control psychotic symptoms.
USUAL ADULT DOSAGE: 50 to 75 mg P.O. daily, increased to 225 mg P.O. daily in 3 or 4 divided doses.

SELECTED MAJOR DRUGS

Antipsychotic agents

This chart summarizes the major antipsychotic agents in clinical use.

DRUG	MAJOR INDICATIONS	USUAL ADULT DOSAGES	NURSING IMPLICATIONS
Phenothiazines			
chlorpromazine	Symptomatic relief of psychoses	200 to 600 mg P.O. initially, increased to a maintenance dose of 500 to 1,000 mg P.O. daily in divided doses	• Use precaution with liquid form, which can irritate skin. • Do not give within 2 hours of administering an antacid or antidiarrheal. • Observe the patient for and report adverse reactions: sedation, extrapyramidal symptoms, tardive dyskinesia, and anticholinergic effects. • Dilute liquid concentrate with water, fruit juice, noncola beverages, soup, or pudding. • Instruct the patient to avoid alcohol and other CNS depressants. • Teach the patient to take chlorpromazine exactly as prescribed, even when symptoms have been relieved.
fluphenazine decanoate	Symptomatic relief of psychoses when compliance is a problem	Initially, 12.5 to 25 mg I.M. or S.C. every 1 to 6 weeks, then 25 to 100 mg p.r.n. for maintenance	• Inform the patient that the effects of fluphenazine decanoate may last up to 6 weeks. Adverse reactions may occur during this time.
Nonphenothiazines			
haloperidol haloperidol decanoate	Symptomatic relief of psychosis, relief of dyskinesia in Gilles de la Tourette's syndrome	0.5 to 5 mg/day P.O. b.i.d. or t.i.d., increased p.r.n. up to 100 mg/day	• Use precautions with liquid form, which can irritate the skin. • Do not give within 2 hours of administering an antacid or antidiarrheal. • Observe the patient for and report adverse reactions: sedation, extrapyramidal symptoms, tardive dyskinesia, and anticholinergic effects. • Dilute liquid concentrate with water, fruit juice, noncola beverages, soup, or pudding. • Instruct the patient to avoid alcohol and other CNS depressants. • Teach the patient to take haloperidol exactly as prescribed, even when symptoms have been relieved. • Inform the patient that the effects of haloperidol decanoate may last about a month. Adverse reactions may occur during this time.

pimozide (Orap). This diphenyl-butylpiperidine nonphenothiazine suppresses severe motor and phonic tics in patients with Gilles de la Tourette's syndrome when these symptoms do not respond to other treatments.
USUAL ADULT DOSAGE: 1 to 2 mg P.O. daily in divided doses, increased to a maintenance dose from 7 to 16 mg P.O. daily, not to exceed 0.3 mg/kg/day.

chlorprothixene (Taractan). A thioxanthene nonphenothiazine, this antipsychotic agent is also effective as a sedative for agitation in patients with severe neurosis and depression.
USUAL ADULT DOSAGE: for psychotic disorders, 25 to 50 mg P.O. t.i.d. or q.i.d., increased gradually up to 600 mg/day; for sedation of an agitated patient, 25 to 50 mg I.M. t.i.d. or q.i.d., increased as needed up to 600 mg/day. Transfer to oral doses may be accomplished by alternating I.M. and P.O. routes of administration as prescribed.

thiothixene (Navane). A thioxanthene nonphenothiazine, this agent is used to treat acute psychosis.
USUAL ADULT DOSAGE: initially, 4 mg I.M. b.i.d. or q.i.d., increased gradually until symptoms are controlled; then 6 to 10 mg/day P.O. in divided doses; may be increased gradually to optimal dose of 20 to 30 mg/day or, if indicated, up to doses of 60 mg/day until symptoms are controlled, then decreased gradually. For elderly patients, one half to one third of the I.M. or oral dosage is prescribed.

Drug interactions

Nonphenothiazines interact with fewer drugs than the phenothiazines do. However, their dopamine-blocking activity can inhibit levodopa and may cause disorientation in patients receiving both medications. Haloperidol may also augment the effects of lithium, producing encephalopathy. When given concurrently with lithium, haloperidol should be used initially to control acute symptoms and then decreased as lithium is added to the regimen.

ADVERSE DRUG REACTIONS

The nonphenothiazines cause the same adverse reactions as the phenothiazines. (See *Adverse reaction potential of nonphenothiazines* on page 530 for details.)

NURSING IMPLICATIONS

Because nonphenothiazines can produce a wide range of adverse effects, the nurse must thoroughly understand the following considerations:
• Be aware that nonphenothiazines are contraindicated in coma or CNS depression and should be used with caution in an elderly or debilitated patient or in one with a severe cardiovascular disorder, allergy, glaucoma, liver disease, or urinary retention.
• Expect to administer a low initial dose to an elderly patient and to increase the dose gradually.
• Advise the patient to avoid activities that require alertness and good psychomotor coordination until the CNS response to the drug is determined. Inform the patient that drowsiness and dizziness usually subside after a few weeks.
• Monitor the patient for hypotension after initial I.M. administration of nonphenothiazines.
• Tell the patient to avoid combining nonphenothiazines with alcohol or other CNS depressants.
• Protect haloperidol from exposure to light. Haloperidol may be administered if it becomes slightly yellow, but must be discarded if the solution is markedly discolored, because its potency will have decreased.

• Be aware that a nonphenothiazine should not be withdrawn abruptly unless severe adverse effects make discontinuation necessary.
• Suggest that the patient chew sugarless gum or hard candy, or use mouthwash to relieve dry mouth.
• Be aware that pimozide is recommended only for treatment of tics associated with Gilles de la Tourette's syndrome. It is contraindicated for drug-induced motor and phonic tics.
• Avoid concurrent administration of pimozide and other drugs that prolong the Q-T interval, such as antiarrhythmic agents. Be sure to monitor the patient's electrocardiogram before and after treatment, particularly the Q-T interval.
• Inform the patient and family about the serious adverse effects of pimozide before they decide to proceed with pimozide therapy. This drug is indicated only in a patient who has failed to respond to standard treatment.
• Tell the patient taking an antipsychotic agent to use a sunscreen and to wear protective clothing to avoid a possible photosensitivity reaction.
• Assess for an allergic reaction in a patient taking chlorprothixene, because it contains tartrazine.

CHAPTER SUMMARY

This chapter presents antipsychotic agents, or neuroleptics, used to control the symptoms of psychoses, especially schizophrenia. Although they cannot cure mental illness, they can improve the quality of life for many mentally ill patients and their families. They allow patients who might otherwise be institutionalized for life to function independently in the community. Here are the highlights of this chapter:
• Antipsychotic agents are also used to calm or sedate agitated or disturbed patients with psychotic symptoms, alleviate nausea and vomiting, and enhance the effects of analgesics and anesthetics.
• Because antipsychotic agents can cause serious neurologic adverse reactions, such as extrapyramidal symptoms and tardive dyskinesia, the nurse must carefully assess a patient for these and report them to the physician.
• Other serious adverse reactions may include hypotension, skin rashes, eye changes, difficulty urinating,

jaundice, an unexplained sore throat, and fever. Less serious reactions include dry mouth, decreased sweating, constipation, blurred vision, photosensitivity, nasal congestion, tachycardia, menstrual changes, and breast swelling.

• Phenothiazines and nonphenothiazines produce similar actions and adverse reactions, but the response to these drugs varies widely from patient to patient. That is why effective antipsychotic therapy requires the nurse to observe accurately and report the patient's behavior and the drug's effects.

• With antipsychotic therapy, the nurse must also monitor and promote compliance. The nurse should teach the patient about the drug, its regimen, its therapeutic and adverse effects, and other considerations.

BIBLIOGRAPHY

Baldessarini, R.J. "Drugs and the Treatment of Psychotic Disorders." In *Goodman and Gilman's The Pharmacological Basis of Therapeutics*, 7th ed. Goodman, A.G., et al., eds. New York: Macmillan Publishing Co., 1985.

Coyle, J.T., and Enna, S.J. *Neuroleptics: Neurochemical, Behavioral, and Clinical Perspectives*. New York: Raven Press, 1983.

Davidhizer, R.E., et al. "Attitudes of Patients with Schizophrenia Toward Taking Medication," *Research in Nursing and Health* 9:139, June 1986.

Engle, V.F., et al. "Tardive Dyskinesia: Are Your Older Clients at Risk?" *Journal of Gerontological Nursing* 11:25, 1985.

Field, W.E. "Hearing Voices," *Journal of Psychosocial Nursing* 23:9, 1985.

Guyton, A.T. *Textbook of Medical Physiology*, 7th ed. Philadelphia: W.B. Saunders Co., 1985.

Haber, J., et al. *Comprehensive Psychiatric Nursing*, 2nd ed. New York: McGraw-Hill Book Co., 1982.

Kerr, L.E. "Oral Liquid Neuroleptics," *Journal of Psychosocial Nursing* 24:33, 1986.

McGill, C.W., and Lee, E. "Family Psychoeducational Intervention in the Treatment of Schizophrenia," *Bulletin of the Menninger Clinic* 50:269, 1986.

Neizo, B., and Murphy, M.K. "Medication Groups on an Acute Psychiatric Unit," *Perspectives in Psychiatric Care* 21:70, 1983.

Scrak, B.M., and Greenstein, R.A. "Tardive Dyskinesia: Evaluation in a Nurse-Managed Prolixin Program," *Journal of Psychosocial Nursing and Mental Health Services* 24:10, 1986.

Selander, J.M., and Miller, W.C. "Prolixin Group: A Recidivism Rate Study Using Mirror Image Controls," *Journal of Psychosocial Nursing and Mental Health Services* 23:16, 1985.

USPD1 Vol. 1: Drug Information for the Health Care Provider, 6th ed. Rockville, Md.: United States Pharmacopeial Convention, 1986.

USPD1 Vol.2: Advice for the Patient, 6th ed. Rockville, Md.: United States Pharmacopeial Convention, 1986.

DRUGS TO IMPROVE CARDIOVASCULAR FUNCTION

The circulatory system includes the heart and blood vessels. In this system, arteries generally carry oxygen and nutrients to the cells, and veins carry away the unoxygenated blood and the waste products of cellular metabolism. Because this system represents a vital function, a dysfunction in the blood flow, heart, kidneys, and/or circulation can seriously affect an individual's health.

Blood flow. Blood flow results from pressure differences in the circulatory system, which are caused by the force of the blood flow through the vessels and the force or resistance to that blood flow.

Blood pressure refers to the force exerted by the blood against the vessel walls. Arterial blood pressure is determined by cardiac output and peripheral resistance. Usually, an increase or decrease in cardiac output or peripheral resistance will increase or decrease blood pressure correspondingly. Similarly, increases or decreases in blood flow and tissue perfusion will accompany blood pressure changes. Cardiac output is a function of the heart rate and stroke volume.

The heart. Coronary arteries supply blood to the myocardium; coronary veins carry away the waste products of metabolism. (See *Coronary circulation* on page 536 for an illustration.) The coronary arteries arise from the aorta and fill during diastole.

Cardiac function depends on conduction of electrical impulses throughout the myocardium. When recorded by an electrocardiogram (EKG), the heart's electrical activity appears as deflection points designated by the letters P, Q, R, S, T, and U. This electrical activity results in the heart's contraction and ejection of blood. (See *Electrical activity and the EKG* on page 537 for an illustration of this activity.)

The kidneys. The kidneys regulate the body's fluid and electrolyte balance and dispose of waste products. Blood enters the kidneys through the renal arteries and is filtered at the glomerulus. Then the filtrate enters the renal tubular system, where it is altered and concentrated or diluted. Then the concentrate or diluted urine leaves the kidneys through the renal pelvis and ureters to the bladder for excretion. Blood leaves the kidneys through the renal veins.

The kidneys also help regulate blood pressure through the renin-angiotensin system. They release the hormone renin in response to a decrease in renal blood flow or, more specifically, to a decrease in the glomerular filtration rate. Renin acts on angiotensinogen (a plasma protein) to form angiotensin I. Angiotensin I is converted to angiotensin II as it circulates through the lungs. Angiotensin II, a potent vasoconstrictor, increases peripheral resistance and sodium and water reabsorption, contributing to an increase in blood pressure.

Circulation. Peripheral circulation refers to blood ejected from the left side of the heart; pulmonary circulation, to blood ejected from the right side. In peripheral circulation, the heart pumps blood to all body tissues and organs except the lungs. Arteries and arterioles carry the blood away from the heart; capillaries allow the exchange of nutrients for cellular waste products; then the venules and veins return the blood to the right side of the heart. In pulmonary circulation, the heart pumps blood to the lungs via the pulmonary arteries, and the pulmonary veins return the blood to the left side of the heart. Unlike peripheral circulation, pulmonary circulation uses the veins to carry oxygen-rich blood and the arteries to carry unoxygenated blood and waste products.

Chapter 34
Cardiac Glycoside Agents and Bipyridines
Chapter 34 explores inotropic agents used to treat congestive heart failure and supraventricular dysrhythmias by decreasing contractility. It discusses digoxin, digitoxin, and the nonglycoside amrinone. These agents can produce significant adverse reactions, and the chapter details them and their associated nursing implications.

Chapter 35
Antiarrhythmic Agents
Chapter 35 examines the drugs used to treat abnormalities of cardiac electrical activity. It begins with an overview of the heart's conduction system, and then

Glossary

Afterload: pressure in the arteries leading from the ventricle that must be overcome for ejection to occur.

Atrioventricular (AV) block: obstructed transmission of electrical impulses from the atria to the ventricles caused by AV node damage or depression.

Automaticity: ability to independently generate an electrical impulse.

Cardiac output: amount of blood pumped by the heart per unit of time, normally about 5 liters/minute.

Chronotropic: altering the rate of cardiac muscle contraction.

Conductivity: capacity of cells to conduct current.

Contractility: capacity for shortening or contracting in response to a stimulus.

Depolarization: neutralization of electrical polarity in cardiac cells caused by an influx of sodium ions.

Diastole: period of ventricular dilation that occurs between the second and first heart sounds.

Diastolic blood pressure: pressure exerted in the vessels when the ventricles are at rest.

Dysrhythmia: abnormal variation in cardiac conduction, rhythm, or rate.

Ectopy: generation of electrical impulses by cardiac cells outside the normal conduction pathways.

Excitability: readiness of a cell to respond to a stimulus.

Fibrillation: twitching movements of cardiac muscle resulting from so rapid a transmission of independent impulses that coordinated contractions cannot occur.

Frank-Starling law of the heart: principle that, within physiologic limits, the heart pumps all the blood that comes to it without allowing excessive damming of blood in the veins.

Glomerular filtration rate: quantity of blood filtered by the glomeruli per unit of time, usually about 120 ml/minute.

Hypertension: peristently high arterial blood pressure.

Infarction: formation of a localized area of tissue necrosis caused by hypoxia resulting from inadequate blood flow to the area.

Inotropic: affecting the force of cardiac muscle contraction.

Ischemia: decreased blood supply to an area caused by vascular constriction or obstruction.

Mean arterial pressure: average blood pressure throughout each cardiac cycle, usually about 96 mm Hg.

Orthostatic hypotension: decrease in blood pressure that occurs when a person stands erect. Also called postural hypotension.

Peripheral vascular resistance: pressure that blood must overcome as it flows in a vessel.

Preload: blood volume in the ventricle at the end of diastole.

Pulse pressure: difference between systolic and diastolic blood pressures, usually about 40 mm Hg.

Reentry or **circus movement:** abnormal transmission of an electrical impulse around and around in cardiac muscle without stopping.

Refractory period: period of depolarization after excitation, during which cardiac muscle cannot respond to another normal cardiac impulse.

Repolarization: restoration of electrical polarity in cardiac cells caused by an outflow of potassium ions from the cells.

Stroke volume: blood output from the ventricle during systole, usually about 70 ml.

Systole: period of ventricular contraction that occurs between the first and second heart sounds.

Systolic blood pressure: pressure exerted in the vessels when the ventricles contract.

---

presents the six classes of antiarrhythmic agents. It also describes the mechanisms of action of these agents, which primarily block three cardiac mechanisms: the fast sodium channel, the slow calcium channel, and the autonomic innervation of myocardial cells.

Chapter 36
Antianginal Agents

Chapter 36 presents the drugs used to treat angina: nitrates, beta blockers, and calcium channel blockers. In this chapter, an overview of coronary blood flow and oxygen consumption precedes a survey of abnormalities that produce angina. The discussion also differentiates among the pharmacokinetic processes of the various classes of antianginal agents.

Chapter 37
Antihypertensive Agents

Chapter 37 focuses on the agents used to treat hypertension, a disease that affects millions of Americans. Beginning with a brief review of the physiology of blood pressure, the chapter next provides clinical definitions of the various types of hypertension. Then it discusses clinical assessments, nonpharmacologic therapies, and the stepped-care approach to hypertension manage-

(Text continues on page 538.)

Coronary circulation

Coronary arteries arise from the aorta and supply blood to the myocardium. The coronary veins carry blood from the myocardium via the coronary sinus. The illustration below shows the location of the major structures of the coronary circulation.

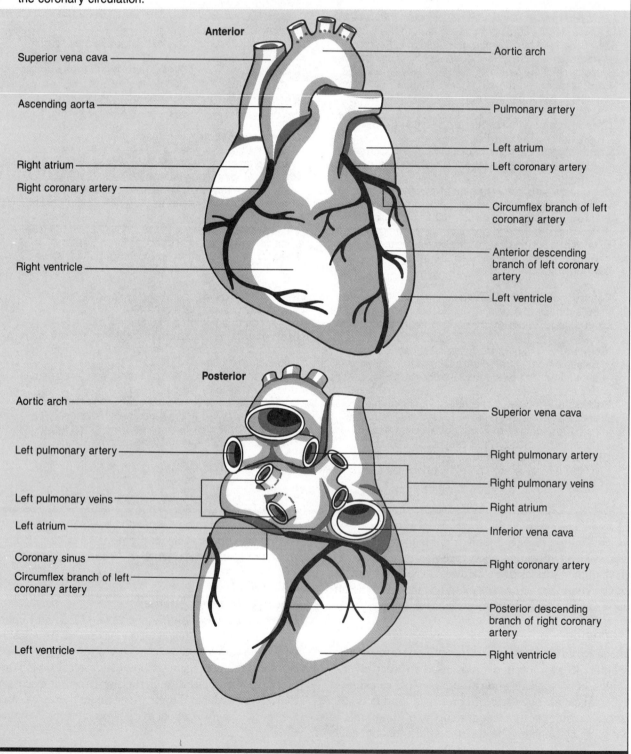

Electrical activity and the EKG

On an EKG tracing, electrical activity in the myocardium appears as a series of deflection points. Each deflection point—P, Q, R, S, T—corresponds to a specific area where electrical activity occurs. (Note: A U wave may also occur.)

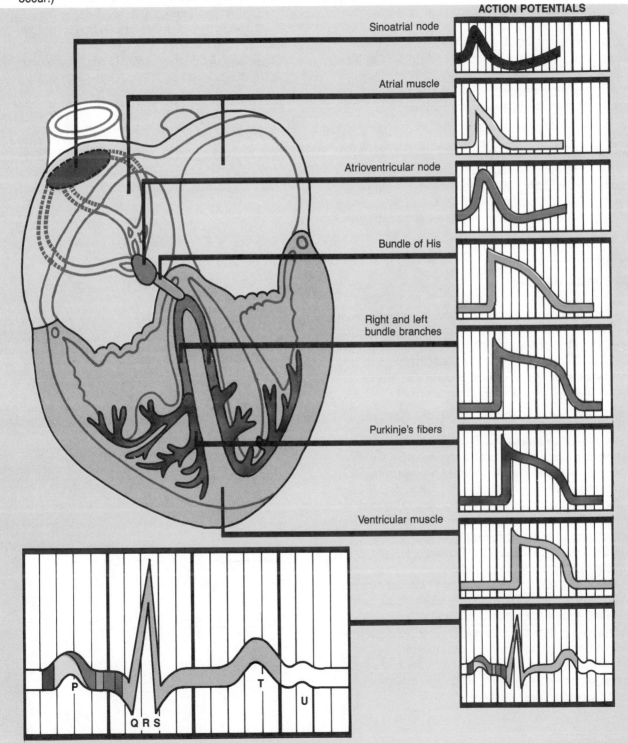

ment. The chapter presents the many types of sympatholytic, vasodilating, and angiotensin antagonist agents.

Chapter 38
Diuretic Agents

Chapter 38 explores those agents used to increase the renal excretion of water and electrolytes from the body. It presents the diuretic agents according to their classification: thiazide and thiazide-like diuretics, loop diuretics, potassium-sparing diuretics, carbonic anhydrase inhibitor diuretics, osmotic diuretics, and mercurial diuretics. It also investigates the adverse reactions to these agents and associated nursing implications.

Chapter 39
Peripheral Vascular Agents

Chapter 39 describes the agents used to produce peripheral vasodilation, which include beta-adrenergic stimulators, direct-acting vasodilators, and hemorrheologics. It also discusses their mechanisms of action and clinical indications.

Chapter 40
Antilipemic Agents

Chapter 40 examines the antilipemic agents used to lower abnormally high lipid blood levels. It begins with an overview of the lipids' composition and role in the body. Then it describes the clinical conditions managed with bile sequestering agents, fibric acid derivatives, and cholesterol synthesis inhibitors. It concludes with a discussion of associated nursing implications.

Nursing diagnoses

A thorough assessment will help the nurse formulate nursing diagnoses. The nursing assessment for a patient with cardiovascular disease includes a history, physical examination, and laboratory and diagnostic data. Based on the assessment, several nursing diagnoses may be developed to apply to patients with cardiovascular dysfunction and include the following:

• Alteration in cardiac output: decreased, related to alterations in myocardial oxygenation
• Alteration in comfort: pain related to cellular hypoxia
• Alteration in fluid volume: excess, related to decreased renal perfusion and cardiac dysfunction
• Alteration in thought processes related to decreased cerebral perfusion from cardiac dysfunction
• Disturbance in self-concept, self-esteem, role performance, and personal identity related to limitations imposed by cardiac dysfunction

• Fear related to alterations in cardiac function
• Impaired gas exchange related to decreased pulmonary circulation and cardiac dysfunction
• Knowledge deficit related to cardiovascular disorders
• Knowledge deficit related to drugs used to improve cardiovascular function
• Noncompliance with the medication regimen related to the duration of therapy
• Sexual dysfunction related to cardiovascular dysfunction and adverse drug reactions
• Sleep pattern disturbance related to cardiac dysfunction.

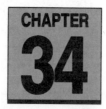

CHAPTER 34

CARDIAC GLYCOSIDE AGENTS AND BIPYRIDINES

OBJECTIVES

After reading and studying this chapter, you should be able to:

1. Describe the clinical indications of the cardiac glycosides, digoxin and digitoxin, and the bipyridine amrinone lactate.

2. Differentiate between the pharmacokinetic properties of digoxin and digitoxin.

3. Describe the physiologic effects of the cardiac glycosides and bipyridines in treating congestive heart failure.

4. Describe clinical conditions in which the cardiac glycosides or bipyridines are contraindicated or must be used cautiously.

5. Explain why digitalis toxicity frequently occurs, and describe its signs and symptoms.

6. Identify factors the nurse should monitor in assessing patients receiving cardiac glycoside or bipyridine therapy.

7. Explain the components the nurse should include in patient teaching regarding digoxin, digitoxin, or amrinone.

INTRODUCTION

Cardiac glycosides and bipyridines increase the force of cardiac contraction; that is, they exert a positive inotropic effect. For this reason, they are also called inotropic agents. Cardiac glycosides also slow the heart rate, a negative chronotropic effect.

Cardiac output represents the amount of blood pumped from the heart in one minute. It equals the heart rate multiplied by the stroke volume (amount of blood ejected by the left ventricle at each beat). Heart rate is affected by the autonomic nervous system, the conduction system, and various drugs. Stroke volume is affected by contractility, preload (the stretch of the myofibrils as the contraction begins), and afterload (the

arterial pressure against which the ventricles must contract). The Frank-Starling law of the heart states that although the volume of blood flowing into the heart varies, the myofibrils alter to keep the blood volume within the heart constant. This means that within physiologic limits, the heart pumps all the blood that comes to it without allowing excessive backing up of blood in the veins. To improve cardiac output, alterations in heart rate, contractility, preload, and afterload must occur.

For a summary of representative drugs, see *Selected Major Drugs: Cardiac glycoside agents and bipyridines* on page 546.

CARDIAC GLYCOSIDES

Digoxin and digitoxin, both digitalis preparations, are the two therapeutic cardiac glycoside agents most frequently used.

History and source

In 1785, Withering first described the use of cardiac glycosides to treat dropsy (edema). Since then, physicians have prescribed these drugs to treat cardiac disease. Today, cardiac glycosides in the form of digitalis preparations continue to be prescribed frequently for patients with congestive heart failure and supraventricular dysrhythmias.

Chemically, the cardiac glycosides are closely related; each consists of a sugar, a steroid, and a lactone. Digitalis substances occur naturally in many plants. *Digitalis lanata* (white foxglove) is the plant source for digoxin and digitoxin.

Onset of action and peak concentration levels of cardiac glycosides

Both the oral and intravenous forms of digoxin and digitoxin vary in onset of action and peak concentration levels.

DRUG	ONSET OF ACTION	PEAK CONCENTRATION LEVELS
digoxin		
P.O.	1½ to 6 hours	4 to 6 hours
I.V.	5 to 30 minutes	1½ to 3 hours
digitoxin		
P.O.	3 to 6 hours	6 to 12 hours
I.V.	30 minutes to 2 hours	4 to 8 hours

PHARMACOKINETICS

The pharmacologic properties of digoxin and digitoxin are basically the same; however, the absorption, metabolism, rate of elimination, onset of action, and duration of action differ.

Absorption, distribution, metabolism, excretion

Cardiac glycosides are usually administered orally. Absorption of digoxin from the gastrointestinal (GI) tract varies between 40% and 90%, depending on the dose form (liquid, capsule, or tablet) and preparation. Absorption variations are most pronounced among digoxin preparations from different manufacturers. The variations result from the different rate or extent of drug dissolution, rather than from the actual amount of drug contained in the preparation.

Absorption of digitoxin from the GI tract is almost complete (90% to 100%) because the drug is more lipid soluble than digoxin. Food in the GI tract and delayed gastric emptying can retard the absorption rate, but not its extent. Various malabsorption syndromes, a high-fiber diet, or certain drugs can decrease GI absorption.

Intramuscular injection of cardiac glycosides is rarely used because the drugs result in severe pain and possible injection site necrosis. The bioavailability of I.M. digoxin is 83%.

The distribution of cardiac glycosides throughout body tissues is slow and extensive. Congestive heart failure can affect the rate of steady-state distribution. The drugs are distributed to most body tissues, with concentrations in cardiac tissue 15 to 30 times those in the plasma. About 25% of digoxin is protein-bound, and about 90% or more of digitoxin becomes protein-bound.

Thirty percent of digoxin is eliminated by hepatic metabolism, and 60% is excreted by the kidneys, excretion being directly proportional to creatinine clearance. Small amounts are also excreted in the feces. When renal function is adequate, 37% of the total dose is eliminated daily. A small percentage of patients metabolize and inactivate greater amounts of digoxin; these patients may require higher-than-normal doses. Many elderly patients with age-related decreases in renal function excrete smaller amounts of digoxin via the kidneys.

Digitoxin is metabolized primarily by hepatic microsomal enzymes to inactive metabolites (92%) and to digoxin and other active metabolites (8%). Both inactive and active metabolites are then eliminated by the kidneys. Small amounts of inactive metabolites are excreted in bile and feces. Active metabolites may appear in the urine for 4 to 12 weeks. Only 11% of the total body amount is eliminated daily, and excretion is affected by renal function.

Onset, peak, duration

The onset of action and peak concentration levels for both digoxin and digitoxin vary with oral and I.V. administration. (See *Onset of action and peak concentration levels of cardiac glycosides* for these figures.) The duration of action for oral and I.V. digoxin is 2 to 6 days, with a half-life of 36 hours. The duration of action for oral and I.V. digitoxin is 2 to 3 weeks, with a half-life of 5 to 7 days. The therapeutic plasma concentration level is 0.5 to 2.5 ng/ml for digoxin and 10 to 35 ng/ml for digitoxin. The lower concentration levels are sufficient to treat patients with congestive heart failure, and the higher concentration levels are required to treat patients with atrial fibrillation.

PHARMACODYNAMICS

The cardiac glycosides provide their primary benefit by increasing contractility, which directly increases cardiac output. The secondary effects include decreases in heart size, venous return, and peripheral vascular resistance.

Mechanism of action

Cardiac glycosides act directly on the myocardium to increase the force of contraction by two mechanisms. First, they promote the calcium movement from extracellular to intracellular cytoplasm. The force of contraction is directly related to the calcium concentration in the myocardial cytoplasm. Second, the cardiac glycosides inhibit adenosine triphosphatase (ATPase), the enzyme that regulates potassium and sodium concentration in myocardial cells. Inhibition of ATPase increases the intracellular sodium concentration, which increases the force of contraction. The cardiac glycosides also decrease conduction velocity through the atrioventricular (AV) node to slow heart rate. They prolong the effective refractory period of the AV node by direct and sympatholytic effects on the sinoatrial (SA) node, thus reducing the heart rate.

Though digoxin and digitoxin produce no ventricular antiarrhythmic effects, they may correct dysrhythmias by improving myocardial size, perfusion, and electrolyte balance.

Cardiac glycosides produce mixed effects on myocardial oxygen consumption—the amount of oxygen needed for electrical and mechanical heart functions. Myocardial oxygen consumption is determined by heart rate, contractility, preload, and afterload. Although these drugs increase myocardial contractility and myocardial oxygen consumption in a normal heart, they reduce cardiac size and increase wall tension in heart failure, which results in a net decrease in myocardial oxygen consumption. The slower heart rate and more complete diastolic filling decrease venous pressure and pulmonary and systemic congestion. The mild diuretic effect of cardiac glycosides is related to the increase in contractility and the resultant increase in glomerular filtration rate.

PHARMACOTHERAPEUTICS

Physicians prescribe cardiac glycosides primarily to treat congestive heart failure and atrial dysrhythmias. The choice of drug and its route of administration depend on the disorder and the desired onset of action.

The cardiac glycosides remain the only inotropic drugs used for the long-term management of congestive heart failure. Therapy for congestive heart failure may include diuretics and venous vasodilators to decrease venous return and preload, and arterial vasodilators to decrease afterload.

The cardiac glycosides are usually useful in treating congestive heart failure associated with low cardiac output, such as that caused by ischemic, hypertensive, rheumatic, or congenital heart disease. These drugs are most beneficial in left ventricular and biventricular failure; they are usually not beneficial in congestive heart failure associated with high cardiac output, such as that caused by thyrotoxicosis or anemia. Nor are the drugs effective in congestive heart failure caused by obstructive lesions, such as idiopathic hypertrophic subaortic stenosis (IHSS). Cardiac glycosides have limited usefulness in treating patients with isolated right ventricular failure.

Cardiac glycosides are administered cautiously in patients with acute myocardial infarction because of their unpredictable effects on myocardial oxygen consump-

tion. The drugs may compromise the ischemic and injured tissues around the infarct.

Physicians sometimes prescribe cardiac glycosides to treat sinus tachycardia by slowing the rate of SA node firing. Cardiac glycosides are beneficial in atrial tachycardia and fibrillation because they increase the refractoriness of the AV node, thereby slowing the ventricular response rate. In chronic atrial fibrillation, the treatment goal is to reduce the ventricular rate rather than restore normal sinus rhythm. In treating acute atrial dysrhythmias, these drugs also restore normal sinus rhythm.

To achieve a full therapeutic effect rapidly, a large initial dose, called the digitalizing, or loading dose, is administered. The digoxin loading dose is usually 10 mcg/kg of ideal body weight. The loading dose saturates the nonspecific myocardial receptor sites. When estimating the loading dose, the patient's condition must be considered. The loading dose may be divided into two doses given 3 to 4 hours apart, possibly given I.V. if the need is urgent.

Because chronic therapy is required to establish and maintain a patient's body store of digoxin and an adequate concentration of digitalis in the heart, a maintenance dose, which can be administered orally, is given each day. The usual digoxin maintenance dose in patients with normal renal function is 1.5 mcg/kg of ideal body weight to replace daily loss. Maintenance doses are frequently adjusted to achieve optimal effect.

Because cardiac glycosides are distributed primarily in lean tissue, dose calculations for obese patients should be based on ideal body weight. Elderly patients receive decreased doses because of their diminished lean body mass and decreased renal and hepatic blood flow. A full loading dose should not be given to a patient who has received a cardiac glycoside during the previous week.

digoxin (Lanoxicaps, Lanoxin). If Lanoxicaps (digoxin solution in soft capsules) are used, smaller doses may be given because of the increased GI absorption of the preparation.
USUAL ADULT DOSAGE: 0.75 to 1.25 mg P.O. or 0.5 to 1 mg I.V. as a loading dose; usual daily maintenance dose, 0.125 to 0.5 mg P.O. or 0.25 mg I.V. Slightly higher initial doses may be used for patients with atrial dysrhythmias than for those with congestive heart failure.
USUAL PEDIATRIC DOSAGE: 20 to 60 mcg/kg P.O. of the elixir as a loading dose, then 20% to 30% of the loading dose daily as a maintenance dose.

digitoxin (Crystodigin, Purodigin). As with digoxin, maintenance doses of digitoxin may be given orally or I.V.

DRUG INTERACTIONS
Cardiac glycosides

Digoxin and digitoxin interact with several drugs. The interactions may result in decreased absorption, decreased effect, increased effect (digitalis toxicity), or dysrhythmias.

DRUG	INTERACTING DRUGS	POSSIBLE EFFECTS	NURSING IMPLICATIONS
digoxin, digitoxin	barbiturates (digitoxin only), phenylbutazone (digitoxin only), phenytoin (digitoxin only), cholestyramine resin, neomycin, antacids, kaolin-pectin, neomycin	Decrease digitalis effect	• Monitor the patient for indications of effectiveness: decrease in edema and jugular venous distention, weight loss, elimination of S₃ and basilar rales; increase in urine output, improvement in oxygenation and pulse rate and rhythm, and increase in sense of well-being. • Higher digitalis doses may be necessary.
	calcium preparations, propantheline, quinidine, verapamil	Cause digitalis toxicity	• Monitor the patient for signs and symptoms of digitalis toxicity: gastrointestinal, visual, neurologic, and cardiac disturbances. • Monitor the patient's EKG for dysrhythmia or AV block.
	amphotericin B, potassium-wasting diuretics, steroids, broad-spectrum penicillins	Cause hypokalemia, digitalis toxicity	• Monitor the patient for signs and symptoms of hypokalemia: drowsiness, hypoperistalsis, mental depression, paresthesia, muscle weakness, anorexia ,depressed reflexes, orthostatic hypotension, and polyuria. • Monitor the patient's serum digoxin or digitoxin levels. • Monitor the patient's serum potassium level and replace as prescribed; encourage the ingestion of dietary potassium
	beta-adrenergic blockers, reserpine	Produce excessive bradycardia and dysrhythmias, especially in patients with atrial fibrillation	• Monitor the patient's pulse rate frequently. • Monitor the patient's EKG as indicated. • Have resuscitation equipment available.
	succinylcholine, thyroid preparations	Cause dysrhythmias	• Monitor the patient's pulse rate frequently. • Monitor the patient's EKG as ordered.

USUAL ADULT DOSAGE: 0.8 to 1.2 mg P.O. or I.V. as a loading dose; usual daily maintenance dose, 0.05 to 0.2 mg P.O. or 0.10 mg I.V.
USUAL PEDIATRIC DOSAGE: 33 mcg/kg P.O. as a loading dose, then 10% of the loading dose daily as a maintenance dose.

Drug interactions
Cardiac glycosides interact with several drugs and some foods. Interactions with other drugs may cause decreased absorption leading to decreased effect, increased effect (digitalis toxicity), or dysrhythmias. Decreased dietary potassium increases the chance of digitalis toxicity, especially if the patient is taking potassium-wasting diuretics. Taking cardiac glycosides on a full stomach slows GI absorption. (See *Drug Interactions: Cardiac glycosides* for a list of interacting drugs and their possible effects and associated nursing implications.)

ADVERSE DRUG REACTIONS

Because of the narrow range for therapeutic doses of cardiac glycosides, digitalis toxicity occurs in 8% to 35% of all hospitalized patients and in 18% of those on cardiac glycoside therapy in extended-care facilities. The mortality from digitalis toxicity ranges from 3% to 21%.

Predictable reactions
Therapeutic concentration levels usually range from 0.5 to 2.5 ng/ml for digoxin and from 10 to 35 ng/ml for digitoxin. However, toxic plasma levels and therapeutic ranges vary for individuals.

Other factors can also lead to digitalis toxicity. Accidental or intentional overdose as well as an increased amount or bioavailability of drug in the dose form can produce toxicity. Reduced drug distribution to other body tissues may result from ventricular failure, shock, hypothyroidism, or drug interactions. Renal disease, reduced renal blood flow, or decreased metabolism can reduce drug excretion. Electrolyte imbalance, excess sympathetic activity, acute hypoxia, acid-base abnormalities, myocardial ischemia and fibrosis, or advanced age can increase patient sensitivity to the drug.

Treatment factors that can predispose patients to digitalis toxicity include cardioversion and concurrent administration of amphotericin B, I.V. calcium, I.V. glucose, potassium-wasting diuretics, propantheline, quinidine, and broad-spectrum penicillins.

The signs and symptoms of digitalis toxicity involve several body systems. (See *Signs and symptoms of digitalis toxicity* for a complete list.) Anorexia is the earliest complaint in most patients experiencing digitalis toxicity. In those with normal renal function, the toxic symptoms should subside within 36 hours after discontinuation of digoxin. Patients taking digitoxin may require 5 to 7 days for the symptoms to subside. Many physicians prefer digoxin over digitoxin because of the shorter time needed for the reparation of toxic symptoms. Digibind [digoxin-immune FAB], a newly approved therapy for digitalis toxicity, consists of fragment antigen-binding antibodies that reverse toxicity by binding with the digitalis.

Unpredictable reactions

Cardiac glycosides irritate the mucous membranes and stimulate the vomiting center, which may result in self-limiting nausea and vomiting. Although these reactions disappear as the patient adjusts to the drug, the nurse should urge reporting of these symptoms because they may also indicate toxicity. Gynecomastia occasionally occurs.

Because cardiac glycosides may increase myocardial oxygen consumption, patients with ischemic heart disease may experience anginal pain. Hypersensitivity reactions may occur 5 to 7 days after therapy begins, and include such signs and symptoms as rash, fever, eosinophilia, urticaria, pruritus, and facial and angioneurotic edema. If any of these occur, the drug should be discontinued.

NURSING IMPLICATIONS

The nurse must be aware of the following implications when caring for a patient on cardiac glycoside therapy.
• Contraindications to cardiac glycoside therapy include hypersensitivity to digitalis preparations, digitalis toxicity, AV block with a history of Stokes-Adams attacks, ventricular tachycardia if secondary to digitalis toxicity, severe myocarditis, and severe heart failure.
• Administer cardiac glycosides with extreme caution to patients with hypothyroidism, renal or liver failure, hy-

---

Signs and symptoms of digitalis toxicity

Digitalis toxicity affects several body systems, most frequently the gastrointestinal tract. The most common early symptoms are anorexia, nausea, vomiting, and diarrhea.

Gastrointestinal

- anorexia
- nausea
- vomiting
- diarrhea
- abdominal pain

Neurologic

- headache
- restlessness
- irritability
- depression
- personality change
- lassitude
- confusion
- disorientation
- insomnia
- psychosis
- convulsions
- coma

Cardiac

- onset of bradycardia
- onset of tachycardia
- onset of regularity
- onset of irregularity
- regular irregularities
- atrial tachycardia with varying AV block
- ventricular bigeminy
- ventricular tachycardia
- second-degree AV block (Wenckebach)
- complete AV block

Visual

- blurred or yellow vision
- flickering lights
- white borders on dark objects
- colored dots

---

pokalemia, hypercalcemia, hypomagnesemia, acute myocardial infarction, hypersensitive carotid sinus, chronic constrictive pericarditis, IHSS, Wolff-Parkinson-White syndrome, severe pulmonary disease, and to elderly or debilitated patients, pregnant or lactating women, premature and immature infants, and children with rheumatic carditis.
• Assess the patient's baseline apical heart rate and rhythm before starting cardiac glycoside therapy; there-

after, take the apical rate before administering each dose. Assess the apical pulse because weak or irregular beats may not be palpable at the radial pulse. Withhold the drug and notify the physician if the pulse rate is below 60 or the minimum specified in the physician's order.

• Monitor serum electrolyte and creatinine levels, especially for the patient on digoxin. Monitor liver function studies for the patient on digitoxin.

• Monitor the patient's serum digoxin or digitoxin levels as prescribed. Assess these levels for at least 8 hours after the last oral dose.

• Monitor the patient for signs and symptoms of digitalis toxicity. Check the patient's electrocardiogram (EKG) for changes that might indicate digitalis toxicity, such as lengthening of the PR interval and fluctuations in rhythm.

• Monitor the patient for signs and symptoms of hypokalemia, including anorexia, vomiting, abdominal distention, hypoperistalsis, drowsiness, apathy, fatigue, muscle weakness or cramps, diminished reflexes, paresthesia, tetany, confusion, orthostatic hypotension, bradycardia, and cardiac arrest. Instruct the patient to report vomiting or diarrhea because they increase potassium loss.

• Encourage the patient to eat foods high in potassium (orange juice, bananas, spinach, cantaloupe, watermelon, dates, raisins, soybeans, apples, prunes, beans, potatoes, molasses, squash). If the patient is taking a potassium-sparing diuretic, angiotensin-converting enzyme (ACE) inhibitor (such as captopril or enalapril), or a potassium supplement, increased dietary potassium is not indicated.

• During cardiac glycoside therapy, patients have a decreased threshold for ventricular dysrhythmia. Administer antiarrhythmics as prescribed to treat digitalis-induced ventricular dysrhythmias, including phenytoin (Dilantin), lidocaine (Xylocaine), propranolol (Inderal), verapamil (Isoptin), and atropine.

• Effective congestive heart failure therapy should produce decreased edema and jugular venous distention, weight loss, elimination of S_3 and basilar rales, increased urine output, improved oxygenation, improved heart rate and rhythm, and an increased sense of well-being. Measure the patient's daily fluid intake and output. Monitor for signs of fluid retention, including decreased urine output, distended neck veins, edema, and weight gain. Weigh the patient daily before breakfast. Remember that 1 liter of fluid weighs approximately 1 kg.

• Oral administration of cardiac glycosides is the safest and most economical route. Avoid I.M. and subcutaneous injections because of their locally irritating effects and uncertain absorption.

• When speed is essential, as in treating pulmonary edema, or when oral administration is impossible, as with vomiting or coma, administer cardiac glycosides I.V., as ordered, but slowly, taking care to avoid extravasation because irritation, necrosis, and sloughing may occur.

• Explain to the patient why the drug was prescribed, and emphasize the importance of taking it exactly as prescribed, even when the patient feels well. Instruct the patient not to take an extra dose if one dose is missed, but to notify the physician.

• Teach the patient to recognize and report a pulse rate below 60 or a change in the pulse's regularity, or the signs and symptoms of digitalis toxicity.

• Instruct the patient to recognize and report the following signs of congestive heart failure: persistent cough; shortness of breath; weight gain of 1 to 2 pounds (0.45 to 0.90 kg) in 1 day or 5 pounds (2.25 kg) in a week; swelling of ankles, legs, or hands; anorexia; nausea; and the sensation of abdominal fullness.

• Inform the patient about foods high in any prescribed potassium or sodium, inform him of calorie restrictions, and arrange for the patient to receive dietary counseling.

• Instruct the patient to store the drug in a tightly covered, light-resistant container and to consult the physician before taking any other drugs, including over-the-counter ones.

• Refer elderly or debilitated patients without adequate home supervision to a home health agency. Take periodic pill counts to evaluate compliance and detect accidental overdose.

BIPYRIDINES

The bipyridines, a new class of positive inotropic agents, are nonglycoside, noncatecholamine agents used to manage heart failure. Presently, amrinone lactate (Inocor) is the only bipyridine approved by the Food and Drug Administration (FDA), though milrinone may soon be approved.

History and source
Amrinone was originally prepared and tested as a bronchodilator for treating asthma. Researchers then tested the drug as an inotropic agent because of its effects on heart rate and smooth muscle activity.

PHARMACOKINETICS

Amrinone is administered I.V., rapidly distributed, and metabolized by the liver. The drug is excreted by the kidneys as amrinone (10% to 40%) and several other derivatives, including N-acetyl-amrinone and N-glycolyl-amrinone.

Amrinone is rapid acting, but with a short duration of action. After a single I.V. bolus dose of 0.5 to 1.5 mg/kg, cardiac output increases within 5 minutes. The peak concentration occurs in about 10 minutes, decreasing by about half in 30 to 40 minutes. Residual effects continue for about 2 hours. Amrinone's half-life is 3.6 hours in stable patients and 6 hours in patients with congestive heart failure. The normal therapeutic plasma level of amrinone is approximately 3 to 5 mcg/ml.

PHARMACODYNAMICS

Amrinone improves cardiac output by increasing contractility and decreasing systemic vascular resistance (afterload) and venous return (preload). Though the mechanism of action has not been fully determined, amrinone probably increases intracellular cyclic adenosine 3':5'-monophosphate (cAMP) levels, which facilitates calcium entry. It also relaxes the vascular smooth muscle. With increased cardiac output, renal blood flow improves and urine output increases. Amrinone's only effect on the conduction system is to facilitate AV nodal conduction. It does not increase myocardial oxygen consumption.

PHARMACOTHERAPEUTICS

Amrinone is indicated for the short-term management of congestive heart failure in patients who have not responded adequately to treatment with digitalis preparations, diuretics, and vasodilators. The nurse should closely monitor the patient hemodynamically.

amrinone lactate (Inocor). The only bipyridine available, amrinone is administered I.V.
USUAL ADULT DOSAGE: 0.75 mg/kg I.V. over 2 to 3 minutes initially; maintenance dosage, 5 to 10 mcg/kg/minute I.V. An additional bolus of 0.75 mg/kg may be administered 30 minutes after therapy begins. The rate of administration and duration of therapy depend upon the patient's therapeutic responses and adverse reactions.

Drug interactions

Patients receiving cardiac glycosides can receive amrinone since the combination may increase ventricular response rates due to enhancement of atrioventricular (AV) conduction. Amrinone interacts negatively with disopyramide (Norpace). Concurrent administration of the two drugs results in hypotension and dysrhythmias.

ADVERSE DRUG REACTIONS

Adverse drug reactions occur infrequently and usually only in patients receiving prolonged therapy. Amrinone can produce dysrhythmias, thrombocytopenia, nausea, vomiting, abdominal pain, anorexia, hypotension, fever, liver enzyme alterations, chest pain, and burning at the injection site. Mild increases in heart rate have also occurred. These effects, however, occur in only a small percentage of patients. Excessive vasodilation may occur with amrinone therapy, producing hypotension, which necessitates a dose reduction or discontinuation.

Patients on prolonged amrinone therapy have experienced hypersensitivity reactions. Signs and symptoms include pericarditis, pleuritis, and hypoxemia.

NURSING IMPLICATIONS

Amrinone may be administered I.V. as an alternative to cardiac glycoside therapy. The nurse must be aware of the following implications.
• Amrinone is contraindicated in patients who are sensitive to the drug or to bisulfite (a preservative used in amrinone solution), in patients with severe aortic or pulmonic valvular disease, and in those with IHSS. Amrinone is not recommended for patients during the acute phase of myocardial infarction.
• During amrinone therapy, a cardiac glycoside may be administered to patients with atrial fibrillation or flutter to control the enhanced AV conduction.
• Obtain baseline patient platelet counts, liver enzyme levels, electrolyte levels, blood urea nitrogen, and creatinine levels before starting amrinone therapy. Monitor these values throughout therapy.
• Frequently monitor the patient's heart rate and blood pressure to detect tachycardia or hypotension.
• Observe bleeding precautions for patients with thrombocytopenia. This adverse reaction can be reversed by decreasing the amrinone dose or discontinuing the drug.
• Before amirone therapy, administer potassium replacements as prescribed to patients with hypokalemia.
• To determine the effectiveness of amrinone therapy, monitor the patient for increased blood pressure; decreased pulmonary venous congestion, pulmonary ar-

Cardiac glycoside agents and bipyridines

This table summarizes the major cardiac glycosides and bipyridines discussed in this chapter.

DRUG	MAJOR INDICATIONS	USUAL ADULT DOSAGES	NURSING IMPLICATIONS
Cardiac glycosides			
digoxin	Congestive heart failure, supraventricular dysrhythmias	Loading: 0.75 to 1.25 mg P.O., 0.5 to 2 mg I.V. Maintenance: 0.125 to 0.5 mg P.O., 0.25 mg I.V.	• Digoxin is contraindicated for administration to patients hypersensitive to digitalis, and to patients experiencing digitalis toxicity, AV block with Stokes-Adams attacks, ventricular tachycardia, severe myocarditis, severe heart failure, and myocardial infarction (MI). • Monitor the patient for signs of effectiveness. • Monitor the patient for signs of digitalis toxicity. • Monitor the patient for signs and symptoms of hypokalemia that potentiates digitalis toxicity. • Monitor the patient's pulse rate and rhythm. • Monitor the patient's renal function.
digitoxin	Congestive heart failure, supraventricular dysrhythmias	Loading: 0.8 to 1.2 mg P.O. or I.V. Maintenance: 0.05 to 0.2 mg P.O., 0.10 mg I.V.	• Digitoxin is contraindicated for administration to patients hypersensitive to digitalis, and to patients experiencing digitalis toxicity, AV block with Stokes-Adams attacks, ventricular tachycardia, severe myocarditis, severe heart failure, and acute MI. • Monitor the patient for signs of effectiveness. • Monitor the patient for signs of digitalis toxicity. • Monitor the patient for signs and symptoms of hypokalemia that potentiates digitalis toxicity. • Monitor the patient's pulse rate and rhythm. • Monitor the patient's liver function.
Bipyridines			
amrinone	Congestive heart failure not responding to digitalis preparations, diuretics, or vasodilators	Loading: 0.75 mg/kg I.V. over 2 to 3 minutes Maintenance: 5 to 10 mcg/kg/minute I.V.	• Contraindicated for adminsitration with disopyramide (Norpace). • Monitor the patient for signs of effectiveness. • Monitor the patient's blood pressure because hypotension may indicate overdose. • Monitor the patient's EKG and hemodynamic values. • Monitor the patient's platelet counts and liver function studies.

tery pressure, and pulmonary capillary wedge pressure; decreased systemic venous congestion and central venous pressure; increased urine output; decreased weight, peripheral edema, and dyspnea; and elimination of S_3 and basilar rales.

• Monitor the patient's EKG.

• Dilute amrinone in normal saline solution before administration. Do not mix amrinone with dextrose because amrinone-dextrose solutions result in 11% to 13% activity loss after 24 hours. Use diluted solutions within 24 hours.

• Administer I.V. infusions with an infusion pump. Amrinone produces burning but not tissue sloughing at injection sites; inject the drug using central or peripheral lines.

• Instruct the patient to report any dyspnea, chest pain, palpitations, burning at injection site, nausea, vomiting, abdominal pain, or anorexia.

CHAPTER SUMMARY

Chapter 34 included discussions of the cardiac glycosides and bipyridines used to increase cardiac output in congestive heart failure. Here are the highlights of the chapter:

• Cardiac glycosides are positive inotropic agents with electrophysiologic effects; these drugs (digoxin and digitoxin) are also used to treat supraventricular dysrhythmias. Cardiac glycosides are administered orally or I.V.

• Amrinone, the only FDA-approved bipyridine, is administered I.V. for short-term treatment of congestive heart failure in patients who do not respond to digitalis preparations, diuretics, and vasodilators.

• Digoxin is excreted unchanged primarily by the kidneys; digitoxin is metabolized primarily by the liver. Amrinone is metabolized by the liver and excreted by the kidneys.

• Cardiac glycosides and bipyridines are used cautiously, if at all, in patients with acute myocardial infarction. Unpredictable effects on myocardial oxygen consumption may compromise ischemic and injured tissues. Hypokalemia predisposes patients to digitalis toxicity.

• The first indications of digitalis toxicity usually include anorexia, nausea, vomiting, and abdominal pain. Other indications are changes in heart rate and rhythm.

• Treating digitalis toxicity includes discontinuing the cardiac glycoside, correcting predisposing factors, and treating dysrhythmias.

• Cardiac glycosides and bipyridines result in these improvements in the patient with congestive heart failure: decreased edema and jugular venous distention, weight loss, elimination of S_3 and basilar rales, increased urine output, improved oxygenation, improved pulse rate and rhythm, and an increased sense of well-being.

• The patient receiving cardiac glycosides should be taught how to measure his pulse rate, how to recognize the signs and symptoms of digitalis toxicity and those of congestive heart failure and hypokalemia, and how to identify foods high in potassium.

• Though no definitive signs of bipyridine overdose have been identified, excessive hypotension can occur, which necessitates dose reduction or discontinuation.

• The patient on bipyridines must receive EKG monitoring and should receive hemodynamic monitoring.

BIBLIOGRAPHY

Barr, S. "Inocor (Amrinone Lactate)," *Critical Care Nurse.* 5:64, 1985.

Braunwald, E. "Effects of Digitalis on the Normal and the Failing Heart," *Journal of the American College of Cardiology.* 5:51A, 1985.

Braunwald, E. "Newer Positive Inotropic Agents," *Circulation.* 73:III-1, 1986.

Farah, A. "Historical Perspectives on Inotropic Agents," *Circulation.* 73:III-4, 1986.

Gilman, A.G., et al., eds. *Goodman and Gilman's The Pharmacological Basis of Therapeutics,* 7th edition. New York: Macmillan Publishing Co., 1985.

Mancini, D., et al. "Intravenous Use of Amrinone for the Treatment of the Failing Heart," *American Journal of Cardiology.* 56:8B, 1985.

McCauley, K., and Burke, K. "Your Detailed Guide to Drugs for CHF," *Nursing84.* 14:47, May 1984.

Norsen, L., and Fox, G. "Understanding Cardiac Output and the Drugs that Affect It," *Nursing85.* 15:34, April 1985.

CHAPTER 35

ANTIARRHYTHMIC AGENTS

OBJECTIVES

After reading and studying this chapter, you should be able to:

1. Differentiate between the action potential of a myocardial pacemaker cell and that of a myocardial muscle cell.

2. Explain the concepts of automaticity, excitability, contractility, and conductivity as they relate to myocardial pacemaker and muscle cells.

3. Describe the course of a normally conducted impulse from the sinus node to the ventricular myocardium.

4. Describe the mechanism of action for each of the six classes of antiarrhythmics.

5. Identify the clinical indications for treatment with each of the six classes of antiarrhythmics.

6. Identify important pharmacokinetic differences among each of the agents in the six classes of antiarrhythmics.

7. Identify the predictable and unpredictable adverse effects of the agents in the six classes of antiarrhythmics.

8. Describe nursing implications associated with each of the agents in the six classes of antiarrhythmics.

INTRODUCTION

Antiarrhythmic drugs are used to treat abnormal electrical activity of the heart. The drugs discussed in this chapter limit cardiac electrical activity to normal conduction pathways and decrease abnormally fast heart rates. (See Chapter 18, Cholinergic Blocking Agents, and Chapter 19, Adrenergic Agents, for drugs used to increase abnormally slow heart rates; see also Chapter 34, Cardiac Glycoside Agents and Bipyridines, for a discussion of the negative chronotropic action of digitalis.)

An overview of the normal electrophysiology and conduction system in the heart will help the nurse understand the action of antiarrhythmic drugs. Abnormalities of cardiac electrical activity can be diagnosed by electrocardiogram (EKG). (The following discussion includes occasional references to EKG patterns; when these are mentioned, referring to the Unit Seven Introduction can provide helpful background information.)

Cardiac muscle, or myocardium, is made up of specialized cells. These cells have certain inherent characteristics that make them different from all other body cells. Myocardial cells exhibit *automaticity*, the ability to initiate or propagate an action potential; *excitability*, the ability to respond to an electrical impulse; *conductivity*, the ability to transmit electrical impulses to the next cell; and *contractility*, the ability to shorten (contract) when stimulated.

Although all myocardial cells share the same characteristics, certain specialized cells generate electrical impulses. These pacemaker cells are located in the sinoatrial (SA) node, intranodal pathways, the atrioventricular (AV) node, the bundle of His, the right and left bundle branches, and the Purkinje fibers. Changes in the concentrations of ions within the cell are responsible for initiating electrical stimulation that depolarizes and repolarizes the myocardial cell.

Myocardial contraction occurs when myocardial cells depolarize. Immediately before depolarization, the concentration of sodium ions (Na^+) outside the cell is greater than that inside it. The myocardial intracellular charge changes when Na^+ and calcium ions (Ca^{++}) flow into the cell, while potassium ions (K^+) flow out. This change is called the *action potential*.

The mechanism that initiates the stimulus for rapid change in cell membrane permeability remains unknown. Theories suggest that certain channels (fast and slow) allow Ca^{++} and Na^+ to enter the cell in large concentrations. When intracellular concentrations of Na^+ and Ca^{++} reach threshold levels, depolarization (contraction) occurs. Immediately after depolarization, Na^+ and Ca^{++} move slowly into the cell—the plateau phase. The concentration of K^+ remains unchanged. Repolarization occurs when K^+ flows out of the cell. The cell returns to its resting state through the action of an ion-transport system called the sodium-potassium pump.

The depolarization of the cell causes the myocardial cell to contract; repolarization causes relaxation. Since the specialized pacemaker cells have the greatest action potential, electrical stimulation of the heart originates in the SA node. The impulses then spread throughout both atria and collect in the AV node, which delays the impulses slightly to allow the ventricles to fill with blood from the atria. From the AV node, the impulses travel along the bundle of His, both bundle branches, and upward through the Purkinje fibers to stimulate the ventricles to contract, ejecting blood into the pulmonary artery and aorta.

In both the atria and the ventricles, pacemaker cells also conduct impulses to the other type of myocardial cells—muscle cells that relax and contract to move blood through the heart. When impulses activate the muscle cells, the cells contract in a synchronized manner, producing atrial and ventricular contractions. The EKG records atrial depolarization (contraction) as P waves, ventricular depolarization (contraction) as QRS complexes, and ventricular repolarization (relaxation) as T waves.

When stimulated, sympathetic fibers enhance excitability (bathmotropic effect), pacemaker firing rate (chronotropic effect), conduction speed (dromotropic ef-fect), and contractility (inotropic effect). Parasympathetic stimulation depresses these effects.

Although both the sympathetic and the parasympathetic branches of the autonomic nervous system stimulate myocardial cells, the SA node itself can generate an impulse. The SA node generates 60 to 100 impulses/minute, the normal pulse rate. Other myocardial pacemaker cells exhibit automaticity at rates slower than 60 impulses/minute; myocardial muscle cells do not exhibit automaticity, unless they are damaged. Damage to myocardial cells can cause abnormalities in the conduction of electrical impulses necessary for the heart to pump blood efficiently. In coronary artery disease, for example, blood flow to the myocardium is reduced. If it is significantly reduced, insufficient oxygen will be available for the cells to survive. An area of myocardium receiving less than an adequate oxygen supply is ischemic. When an area of myocardium dies, the result is called an infarction.

Ischemic cells behave in at least two abnormal ways. First, they may have increased automaticity. For example, in the atria the SA node may fire at a rapid rate. This firing may also occur in several other cells in the atria (ectopic beats) until no effective or synchronized

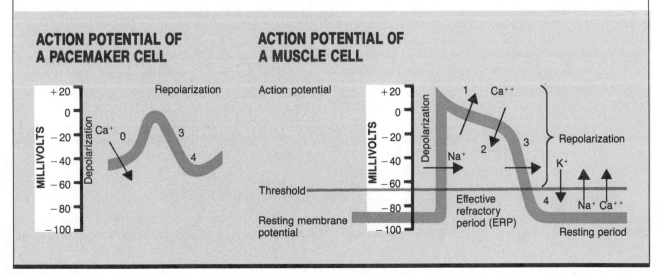

Action potentials of myocardial pacemaker and muscle cells

The intracellular charge of a myocardial cell is changed when Na^+ and Ca^{++} flow into the cell while K^+ flows out. This change in intracellular charge is referred to as *action potential*. Depolarization occurs as the usual negative resting state of the cell changes to zero in the electrical cell or to slightly positive in the muscle cell. Repolarization occurs when the cell returns to its usual negative charge. This diagram shows the different action potentials of electrical and muscle cells. The electrical cell undergoes more gradual excitation, whereas the muscle cell has a steeper slope of depolarization and rapid excitation (phase 0). The electrical cell also does not have an early rapid repolarization (phase 1) or a plateau (phase 2) and exhibits final rapid repolarization (phase 3) and spontaneous depolarization at rest (phase 4).

Once a muscle cell has been depolarized, it is not susceptible to a second depolarization until a certain time period has elapsed. This time period is the effective refractory period (ERP), roughly equal to the action potential duration (APD).

ACTION POTENTIAL OF A PACEMAKER CELL

MILLIVOLTS
+20
0
−20
−40
−60
−80
−100

Depolarization
Ca^+
Repolarization
0
3
4

ACTION POTENTIAL OF A MUSCLE CELL

Action potential

MILLIVOLTS
+20
0
−20
−40
−60
−80
−100

Depolarization
1 Ca^{++}
Na^+
2
3
Repolarization
K^+
4
Na^+ Ca^{++}

Threshold

Resting membrane potential

Effective refractory period (ERP)

Resting period

pattern exists. This chaotic electrical pattern, called *atrial fibrillation,* appears on the EKG as an irregular atrial pattern and loss of definitive P waves. In this state, the atrial muscle cells do not contract; they quiver. Although the AV node screens out some of these rapid impulses, many reach the ventricles, possibly causing the heart rate to exceed 200 beats/minute. At this rate, the ventricles do not fill sufficiently before contraction.

Damaged myocardial cells in the ventricles can initiate a stimulus to contract on their own. Whether they contract singly or in pairs, they are referred to as *premature ventricular contractions.* More than four ventricular stimulated contractions is referred to as ventricular tachycardia. This conduction pattern indicates an irritable area (foci) in the ventricle that can progress to ventricular fibrillation, similar to atrial fibrillation.

Since no pulse or circulation is generated in ventricular fibrillation, the patient will die without treatment.

Ischemic pacemaker cells can also greatly decrease conductivity. For example, an ischemic cell in the Purkinje fibers may block normally conducted impulses. If this block is complete, the cell will not excite or conduct an impulse. If the block is incomplete, the cell will not excite an impulse from the normal pathway. The cell will excite from the opposite side and may even conduct the impulse backward, resulting in dysrhythmia. These blocks are called *unidirectional.* Some of the antiarrhythmic agents can convert them to bidirectional blocks, preventing retrograde (backward) impulse and ectopic beats, which originate in ischemic myocardial muscle cells. (See *Normal conduction and unidirectional block* for an illustration.) Unidirectional block often sets up a circular impulse pattern, known as *reentry,* by which the impulse passes around the unidirectional block, travels back through the ischemic cell, and reenters the normal pathway.

Although ischemia is the most common cause of dysrhythmias, other contributing factors occur singly or together with ischemia. These factors include congenital cardiac conditions, cardiac trauma or surgery, cardiomyopathy, electrolyte or acid-base imbalances, adverse drug reactions, emboli, invasive cardiac diagnostic procedures, cardiac valvular diseases, alcoholism, respiratory diseases, and viral infections. Thus, while an antiarrhythmic is used to treat a dysrhythmia, the physician also attempts to correct the underlying condition, because doing so may eliminate the need for continued antiarrhythmic therapy.

Antiarrhythmics are categorized into six classes. Class IA contains quinidine sulfate, gluconate, or polygalacturonate; procainamide hydrochloride; and diso-

pyramide phosphate. Class IB contains lidocaine hydrochloride, mexiletine hydrochloride, and tocainide hydrochloride. Class IC contains flecainide acetate and encainide. Class II contains the beta-adrenergic blockers propranolol hydrochloride and acebutolol hydrochloride. Class III contains bretylium tosylate and amiodarone hydrochloride. Class IV contains the calcium channel blocker verapamil hydrochloride. The mechanisms of action of these drugs vary widely, but a few drugs exhibit properties common to more than one class.

The drugs discussed in this chapter are used to treat, suppress, or prevent three major mechanisms of dysrhythmias: increased automaticity, decreased conduction, and re-entry. Although mainly prescribed for adults, these drugs are occasionally prescribed for children.

For a summary of representative drugs, see *Selected major drugs: Antiarrhythmic agents* on pages 565 and 566.

CLASS IA ANTIARRHYTHMICS

Class IA antiarrhythmics include quinidine sulfate, gluconate or polygalacturonate; procainamide; and disopyramide phosphate. Physicians use class IA antiarrhythmics to treat various dysrhythmias, both atrial and ventricular. Frequently given orally, the class IA drugs are fairly safe; however, some gastrointestinal (GI) and cardiovascular adverse effects may result.

History and source
For several centuries, chemicals from the bark of the cinchona tree were used to treat malaria. At some point, a chance discovery revealed that one of these chemicals, quinine, helped regulate an irregular pulse. In the mid-1800s, Pasteur and van Heyningen described quinidine, an isomer of quinine that, by the early 1900s, Wenckebach and Frey were using regularly to treat atrial fibrillation. Quinidine thus became the prototypical antiarrhythmic, followed by the more recently discovered class IA antiarrhythmics procainamide and disopyramide.

PHARMACOKINETICS
After oral administration, class IA drugs undergo fairly rapid absorption and metabolism. Because of this, re-

searchers have developed sustained-release forms of these drugs to help maintain therapeutic levels. The nurse should closely monitor the patient's serum drug levels during therapy with the class IA drugs.

Absorption, distribution, metabolism, excretion

When administered orally, quinidine is almost completely absorbed, and procainamide and disopyramide are about 90% absorbed from the GI tract. Food and extremes in gastric pH hasten or delay absorption; delay also occurs from use of sustained-release forms of these three drugs. Quinidine's rate of absorption also depends upon the salt with which it is combined: quinidine polygalacturonate and quinidine gluconate, although not sustained-release forms, are absorbed more slowly than quinidine sulfate.

Quinidine is rarely given intramuscularly or intravenously. Procainamide, which is available in I.V. form, is rarely given intramuscularly. Disopyramide is available only in oral form.

The three drugs are distributed through all body tissues except, in the case of quinidine, the brain. Quinidine and disopyramide also enter red blood cells. Plasma protein binding is 90% for quinidine, 20% for procainamide, and 30% to 65% for disopyramide, depending upon the concentration.

All class IA antiarrhythmics are metabolized in the liver. The metabolites of these drugs provide some antiarrhythmic activity—especially the procainamide metabolite N-acetylprocainamide (NAPA), which researchers are investigating as a separate antiarrhythmic. The amount of procainamide metabolized to NAPA varies, depending upon the patient's rate of acetylation (the metabolic process by which an acetyl group is introduced into a molecule of an organic compound). All three drugs are excreted unchanged by the kidneys in the following amounts: 10% to 50% of quinidine, the percentage decreasing as urine pH increases; 40% to 70% of procainamide, depending upon the patient's rate of acetylation; and 50% of disopyramide. The metabolites of each drug are also excreted in the urine. A small percentage of disopyramide is excreted in the feces.

Onset, peak, duration

Each class IA drug has an onset of action of 30 minutes to 3 hours after oral administration, depending in part on the dose given. Sustained-release forms may have a later onset of action. Intramuscular (I.M.) procainamide produces effects in 10 to 30 minutes, and the onset of action of intravenous (I.V.) procainamide is immediate. The immediate onset of action from the I.V. route makes it the practical choice in acute situations.

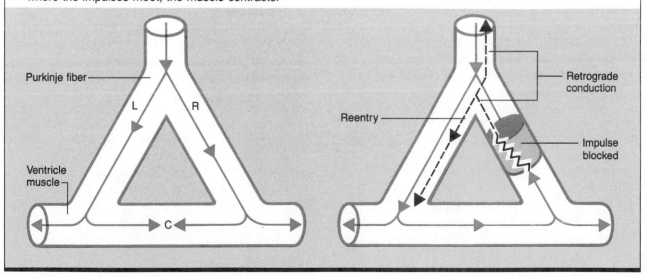

Normal conduction and unidirectional block

NORMAL CONDUCTION

Normal electrical impulse conduction flows through both left (L) and right (R) branches of the Purkinje fibers to the connecting branch (C). At the point where the impulses meet, the muscle contracts.

UNIDIRECTIONAL BLOCK

An ischemic area of conductive tissue blocks forward conduction. The impulse travels retrograde and re-enters the fiber before the next normal beat.

Purkinje fiber

L   R

Ventricle muscle

C

Retrograde conduction

Reentry

Impulse blocked

Quinidine and oral procainamide capsules attain peak concentrations in 60 to 90 minutes. Disopyramide reaches peak concentrations in 1 to 2 hours. The sustained-release forms of these agents reach peak concentrations as follows: quinidine in 3 to 4 hours, procainamide in 4 hours, and disopyramide in 5 hours. I.M. procainamide reaches peak concentrations in 15 to 60 minutes —one reason it is not used frequently.

The nurse must closely monitor the patient's serum concentration levels during therapy with class IA drugs to prevent toxicity. Normal therapeutic ranges are as follows: quinidine, 2 to 6 mcg/ml; procainamide, 4 to 10 mcg/ml; and disopyramide, 2 to 6 mcg/ml. NAPA levels resulting from procainamide metabolism range from 2 to 8 mcg/ml.

The half-life of quinidine is 6 to 8 hours; that of procainamide is 3 hours. The half-life of disopyramide is from 5 to 12 hours, and the half-life of NAPA is 7 hours.

PHARMACODYNAMICS

Class IA antiarrhythmics exert their effects by altering the myocardial cell membrane and interfering with autonomic nervous system control of pacemaker cells. The drugs partially block the fast channel in the myocardial cell membrane, reducing the influx of Na^+. This reduction alters the action potential by depressing the rate of depolarization, prolonging the plateau and repolarization and depressing the slope of the resting period. These changes reduce the rate of automaticity in ectopic foci, reduce the speed of conductivity, and increase the ERP. See *Action potentials of myocardial pacemaker and muscle cells* on page 549 for an illustration of these effects.

All three drugs (especially quinidine) also block parasympathetic nervous system discharges to the SA and AV nodes, thereby increasing the conduction rate of the AV node. This anticholinergic effect can produce dangerous increases in the ventricular heart rate if rapid atrial activity, as in atrial fibrillation, is present. The increased ventricular heart rate can, in turn, offset the capability of the antiarrhythmics to convert atrial dysrhythmias to a regular rhythm.

Class IA antiarrhythmics also slightly depress contractility: quinidine and procainamide decrease peripheral vascular resistance (afterload), and disopyramide produces peripheral vasoconstriction. Disopyramide also depresses contractility more than either quinidine or procainamide.

PHARMACOTHERAPEUTICS

Keeping in mind their differing therapeutic and adverse effects, physicians prescribe class IA antiarrhythmics to treat a variety of atrial and ventricular dysrhythmias. The drugs (especially quinidine) are synergistic with digoxin. Thus, having decreased AV conduction time with digoxin, the physician can add quinidine to convert atrial fibrillation to regular rhythm.

disopyramide phosphate (Norpace, Norpace CR). Used only to treat ventricular dysrhythmias, disopyramide suppresses the frequency of ectopic ventricular beats as well as the frequency and duration of self-limiting bursts of ventricular tachycardia. Available only in oral form, disopyramide is not useful in acute situations, which require parenteral administration.
USUAL ADULT DOSAGE: for the immediate-release form, 100 to 200 mg P.O. every 6 hours; for the sustained-release form, 300 mg P.O. every 12 hours.
USUAL PEDIATRIC DOSAGE: for infants less than 1 year old, 10 to 30 mg/kg/day P.O. in equally divided doses every 6 hours; for children 1 to 4 years old, 10 to 20 mg/kg in equally divided doses every 6 hours; for children 4 to 12 years old, 10 to 15 mg/kg in equally divided doses every 6 hours; for children 12 to 18 years old, 6 to 15 mg/kg in equally divided doses every 6 hours.

procainamide hydrochloride (Procan SR, Pronestyl). Used to prevent the recurrence of atrial fibrillation and other atrial dysrhythmias, procainamide is only moderately effective in converting these dysrhythmias to regular rhythm. Procainamide suppresses the frequency and duration of self-limiting bursts of atrial and ventricular tachycardia; it also suppresses ventricular ectopic beats. Parenteral procainamide is used to treat persistent ventricular tachycardia. Dosage is carefully adjusted to the patient's response.
USUAL ADULT DOSAGE: to convert atrial fibrillation, 1.25 grams P.O., if necessary 750 mg 1 hour later, then 500 mg to 1 gram every 2 hours until conversion or toxic signs appear; to prevent recurrence, 500 mg to 1 gram every 4 hours, or up to 1 gram of the sustained-release form every 6 hours; for ventricular ectopic, a 1-gram loading dose followed by 500 mg every 3 to 4 hours or 500 mg to 1 gram of sustained-release form every 6 hours; for frequent ventricular ectopic beats or ventricular tachycardia, 500 mg I.V. at a rate of 25 to 50 mg/minute. After the loading dose, the infusion is continued at 1 to 3 mg/minute.

USUAL PEDIATRIC DOSAGE: 50 mg/kg or 1.5 grams/m^2 P.O. daily divided into four to six doses, or 2 to 5 mg/kg (not to exceed 100 mg) I.V. over 5 minutes, every 15 minutes; or 3 to 6 mg/kg I.V. over 5 minutes followed by continuous infusion at 0.02 to 0.08 mg/kg/minute. Total dosage should not exceed 1 gram.

quinidine sulfate (CinQuin, Quinidex, Quinora), **quinidine gluconate** (Duraquin, Quinaglute), and **quinidine polygalacturonate** (Cardioquin). After converting atrial fibrillation to regular rhythm, quinidine prevents recurrence of the atrial fibrillation. It also suppresses atrial and ventricular ectopic beats as well as suppressing the frequency and duration of self-limiting bursts of atrial and ventricular tachycardia. Quinidine gluconate 267 mg or quinidine polygalacturonate 275 mg is equivalent to quinidine sulfate 200 mg.

USUAL ADULT DOSAGE: to convert atrial fibrillation, 300 to 400 mg P.O. of immediate-release quinidine sulfate every 6 hours, then 200 to 400 mg every 6 hours to maintain regular rhythm; to suppress atrial or ventricular ectopic beats, 200 to 300 mg quinidine sulfate P.O. every 6 to 8 hours or 300 to 600 mg of sustained-release quinidine sulfate every 8 to 12 hours; for maintenance of regular rhythm, 324 to 660 mg of sustained-release quinidine gluconate or 275 mg of quinidine polygalacturonate every 8 to 12 hours.

USUAL PEDIATRIC DOSAGE: 30 mg/kg or 900 mg/m^2 P.O. daily, divided into five doses.

Drug interactions

Class IA antiarrhythmics may exhibit additive or antagonistic effects with other antiarrhythmics as well as with anticholinergic and antihypertensive drugs. Quinidine used with coumarin anticoagulants can cause hypoprothrombinemia. Anticonvulsants and alkalinizing agents may affect the metabolism and excretion of quinidine. Digoxin and quinidine also interact. (See *Drug interactions: Class IA antiarrhythmics* on page 554 for further information.)

ADVERSE DRUG REACTIONS

Adverse reactions to class IA antiarrhythmics include anticholinergic effects, GI changes, and reactions unique to quinidine's source, cinchona. Also, antiarrhythmic drugs can themselves produce dysrhythmias.

Predictable reactions

Cinchonism, a reaction to the cinchona alkaloids, describes a set of quinidine-related reactions consisting of tinnitus, headache, vertigo, fever, light-headedness, and

vision disturbances. Cinchonism may appear after the first dose or with quinidine toxicity. Quinidine syncope may also occur and is probably from transient ventricular tachycardia or ectopy.

The anticholinergic property of disopyramide often produces dry mouth, blurred vision, constipation, and urinary hesitancy and retention. The negative inotropic effect of the drug combined with increased peripheral vasoconstriction sometimes results in heart failure, hypotension, chest pain, edema, and dyspnea.

Procainamide, especially the I.V. form, can produce hypotension. The drug's negative inotropic effect less frequently leads to heart failure. Because I.V. quinidine may lead to cardiovascular collapse, the drug is rarely administered by this route.

All class IA antiarrhythmics can *induce* dysrhythmias, especially conduction delays that may compound existing heart blocks. Apparent conduction through the AV node may be increased, precipitating a dangerously high ventricular rate. As the ERP and the APD increase, the EKG reflects a prolonged Q-T interval. This is a precursor to a special form of ventricular tachycardia known as Torsades de Pointes. (See *Action potentials of myocardial pacemaker and muscle cells* on page 549 for an explanation of action potential duration.)

The class IA antiarrhythmics, especially quinidine, frequently produce diarrhea and other GI symptoms, such as cramping, nausea, vomiting, anorexia, and bitter taste.

Unpredictable reactions

Up to 30% of patients using procainamide experience an adverse reaction that mimics systemic lupus erythematosus. Signs and symptoms include pain in small joints, pleuritic pain, dyspnea, fever, headache, and pericardial effusion, blood dyscrasias, and positive serum antinuclear antibody (ANA) titers. This reaction, called *drug-induced systemic lupus*, is not dose-dependent and resolves when procainamide is discontinued. Quinidine can also, rarely, cause lupuslike symptoms and hypersensitivity reactions manifested by fever, blood dyscrasias, skin eruptions, liver disorders, and anaphylaxis. All three of the class IA antiarrhythmics can precipitate congestive heart failure and can produce confusion in elderly patients.

NURSING IMPLICATIONS

To assess the effectiveness of class IA antiarrhythmics, the nurse must closely monitor the patient's vital signs and be aware that many patients requiring these drugs

DRUG INTERACTIONS

Class IA antiarrhythmics

Class IA antiarrhythmics interact with several commonly administered drugs. The nurse must be aware of these interactions to implement appropriate assessment and intervention strategies.

DRUG	INTERACTING DRUGS	POSSIBLE EFFECTS	NURSING IMPLICATIONS
quinidine, procainamide, disopyramide	neuromuscular blockers	Increase skeletal muscle relaxation	• Observe the patient for hypoventilation when administering class IA antiarrhythmics in the immediate postoperative period.
	cholinergic drugs	Decrease effect of cholinergics such as neostigmine and pyridostigmine	• Administer class IA antiarrhythmics cautiously to patients with myasthenia gravis or to patients receiving antiparkinsonian, antimuscarinic, or antispasmodic drugs.
	anticholinergic drugs	Produce additive anticholinergic effect	• Observe the patient for adverse reactions, such as dry mouth, wheezing, urinary retention, and orthostatic hypotension.
	antihypertensives	Produce additive hypotension and cardiac depression	• Monitor the patient's blood pressure frequently, and observe for signs of heart failure, such as shortness of breath and edema.
	pimodize	Potentiates cardiac dysrhythmias	• Monitor patient's EKG for prolongation of Q-T interval.
quinidine	coumarin anticoagulants	Produce hypoprothrombinemia	• Observe the patient for increased bruising, bleeding, or I.V. site oozing; monitor the patient's prothrombin time.
	digoxin	Increases serum digoxin level	• Monitor the patient's serum digoxin levels; assess for signs of digitalis toxicity: anorexia, nausea, vomiting, headache, malaise, visual disturbances, or changes in pulse rate or regularity.
	urine-alkalinizing agents	Increase serum quinidine levels	• Assess the patient for signs of quinidine toxicity, such as dysrhythmias, hypotension, and syncope.
	nifedipine	Decreases serum quinidine levels	• Monitor for cardiac arrhythmias indicating decrease in quinidine action.
	cimetidine	Increases serum quinidine levels	• Assess the patient for signs of quinidine toxicity, such as dysrhythmias, hypotension, and syncope.
quinidine, disopyramide	anticonvulsants	Increase metabolism of quinidine and disopyramide	• Monitor the patient's pulse rate and EKG for signs of decreased therapeutic effect.
procainamide	cimetidine	Increases serum procainamide levels	• Monitor therapeutic plasma levels of procainamide. • Assess patient for signs and symptoms of procainamide overdose, such as tachycardia, confusion, drowsiness, nausea, and vomiting.

have other problems, such as congestive heart failure or renal insufficiency, that enhance their risk of developing toxicity.

• Administer class IA antiarrhythmics cautiously to patients with congestive heart failure, heart block, hypotension, myasthenia gravis, urinary retention, or hepatic or renal insufficiency. These drugs are contraindicated in patients with congenital prolonged Q-T interval.

• Monitor the patient's EKG for increased ventricular rate, a Q-T interval 50% greater than normal, and conduction disturbances.

• Administer the loading dose of digoxin, if prescribed, before the first dose of class IA antiarrhythmics for the patient starting treatment for atrial tachycardia or fibrillation.

• When sending a serum sample to the laboratory for therapeutic plasma level analysis, note on a laboratory slip the time of the last dose given.

• To maintain therapeutic plasma levels, give around-the-clock dosages (when appropriate) rather than following the traditional t.i.d. or q.i.d. schedule.

• Electrolyte abnormalities, especially hypokalemia, predispose patients to dysrhythmias. Monitor electrolyte levels closely at the beginning of therapy and when administering diuretics with class IA agents.

• When administering procainamide intravenously, use an infusion pump and monitor the patient's EKG and blood pressure frequently. When switching from the I.V. to the oral route, continue the infusion for 2 hours, or as prescribed, after the first oral dose.

• Reassure the patient receiving a sustained-release form of an antiarrhythmic that what may look like tablets or capsules in the stool are just the wax matrix of the preparation and are not cause for alarm: All of the medicine has been extracted in the intestines.

CLASS IB ANTIARRHYTHMICS

Class IB antiarrhythmics include lidocaine hydrochloride, tocainide hydrochloride, and mexiletine hydrochloride. Lidocaine is one of the most widely used antiarrhythmics in acute care. Both tocainide and mexiletine were recently developed. Although they have fewer clinical indications than class IA antiarrhythmics, the class IB antiarrhythmics, especially lidocaine, are more effective and cause fewer adverse reactions. Phenytoin, which resembles the class IB antiarrhythmics, may also be used to treat dysrhythmias. (See *Phenytoin for digitalis toxicity* on page 557 for a discussion of phenytoin.)

History and source

In 1943, Lofgren synthesized lidocaine for use as a local anesthetic—a use that continues today. Lidocaine was first used in 1949 to treat dysrhythmias occurring during cardiac catheterization; its effectiveness was established by the 1960s. Tocainide, a congener of lidocaine, was developed in the late 1970s, as was mexiletine; the Food and Drug Administration (FDA) approved tocainide in 1985 and mexiletine in 1986.

PHARMACOKINETICS

The class IB antiarrhythmics exhibit considerable variation in their metabolism. These differences have important implications for their use.

Absorption, distribution, metabolism, excretion

All class IB antiarrhythmics are well absorbed from the GI tract after oral administration; however, lidocaine is not available in oral form, because most of an absorbed dose undergoes first-pass metabolism in the liver. When given intramuscularly, lidocaine is best absorbed from the deltoid muscle. Lidocaine is widely distributed throughout the body, including the brain. Distribution data for tocainide and mexiletine are incomplete, but distribution of these drugs may resemble that of lidocaine. Class IB antiarrhythmics are bound to plasma proteins in the following amounts: lidocaine, 65%; tocainide, 15%; and mexiletine, 55%.

Lidocaine is metabolized by deethylation to various metabolites, some with mild antiarrhythmic properties.

Tocainide undergoes minimal first-pass metabolism: oxidative deamination converts tocainide into inactive metabolites. After minimal first-pass metabolism, mexiletine is methylated to several metabolites with minor antiarrhythmic properties.

Less than 10% of a lidocaine dose, about 10% of a mexiletine dose, and about 50% of a tocainide dose is excreted in the urine. Metabolites of each drug also appear in the urine. Mexiletine is also secreted in breast milk.

Onset, peak, duration

Lidocaine exerts its antiarrhythmic effect in 1 to 2 minutes after I.V. bolus administration. Onset of action for tocainide is less than 30 minutes, and for mexiletine it is 30 minutes to 2 hours. Lidocaine peak concentration levels occur 10 minutes after I.M. injection. After oral administration, peak concentration levels for tocainide occur in 30 minutes to 2 hours; for mexiletine, in 2 to 3 hours. The therapeutic plasma levels are as follows: lidocaine, 1.2 to 5 mcg/ml; tocainide, 4 to 10 mcg/ml; and mexiletine, 0.5 to 2 mcg/ml.

Lidocaine provides antiarrhythmic effects for only 15 minutes after the I.V. infusion is stopped, although its half-life is 90 minutes. The durations of action for tocainide and mexiletine remain undetermined. The half-life of tocainide is 11 to 15 hours; that of mexiletine is 10 to 12 hours.

PHARMACODYNAMICS

Physicians use class IB antiarrhythmics only to treat ventricular dysrhythmias. These drugs slightly depress depolarization in myocardial cells. Like their class IA counterparts, class IB antiarrhythmics are cell membrane stabilizers and do not affect the automaticity or conductivity of the SA and AV nodes.

As their major action, class IB antiarrhythmics decrease the APD and to a lesser extent the ERP. The drugs especially affect the Purkinje fibers and myocardial cells in the ventricles. By shortening the ERP, class IB antiarrhythmics eliminate unidirectional block, which can trigger a reentry dysrhythmia. The drugs also decrease ventricular ectopy by blocking the slow influx of sodium during plateau (phase 2) and by decreasing the slope of phase 4 depolarization. Class IB antiarrhythmics neither block nor mimic autonomic control of the heart.

PHARMACOTHERAPEUTICS

Class IB antiarrhythmics are used to treat ventricular ectopic beats, ventricular tachycardia, and ventricular fibrillation. Because class IB antiarrhythmics infrequently produce serious adverse reactions, they are the drugs of choice in the acute care setting.

lidocaine hydrochloride (Xylocaine). Used to suppress frequent ventricular ectopic beats in acute ischemia, lidocaine is also used to treat ventricular dysrhythmias related to digitalis toxicity and other acute conditions, to convert ventricular tachycardia in the absence of cardiovascular collapse, and to reduce the frequency and duration of abrupt, self-limiting ventricular tachycardia. Physicians also use the drug to maintain sinus rhythm once ventricular fibrillation has been electrically defibrillated. Controversy exists over prophylactic use of lidocaine to prevent ventricular dysrhythmias in patients with suspected MI. Usually given intravenously, lidocaine may be given intramuscularly, but the resultant striated muscle damage interferes with the measurement of cardiac enzymes during diagnosis of acute MI.

USUAL ADULT DOSAGE: an initial I.V. bolus of 50 to 100 mg, followed by a second bolus of 50 to 100 mg given 5 minutes after the first; then continuous I.V. infusion at 1 to 4 mg/minute for up to 24 hours. No more than 300 mg should be given per hour. Lidocaine can be given as a 300 mg dose I.M. and repeated in 60 to 90 minutes if necessary. If continuous administration is needed, I.V. infusion is the preferred route.

USUAL PEDIATRIC DOSAGE: 0.5 to 1 mg/kg I.V. bolus, which may be repeated but should not exceed 5 mg/kg; then a continuous infusion at 10 to 50 mcg/kg/minute.

tocainide hydrochloride (Tonocard). Considered by some physicians to be the oral equivalent of lidocaine, tocainide is used to suppress frequent ventricular ectopy and to reduce the frequency and duration of abrupt self-limiting ventricular tachycardia. Physicians sometimes use tocainide when switching a patient from I.V. lidocaine to an oral antiarrhythmic.

USUAL ADULT DOSAGE: 400 to 600 mg P.O. every 8 hours; the total daily dosage may be divided into two doses. No data for pediatric dosages are available.

mexiletine hydrochloride (Mexitil). Physicians use mexiletine to treat the same clinical conditions as tocainide.

USUAL ADULT DOSAGE: 200 to 300 mg P.O. every 8 hours; the total daily dosage may be divided into two doses. Sometimes a loading dose of 400 mg P.O. is required to initiate therapy. No data for pediatric dosages are available.

Drug interactions

Class IB antiarrhythmics may exhibit additive or antagonistic effects when administered with other antiarrhythmics, such as phenytoin, propranolol, procainamide, and quinidine. Lidocaine toxicity may result from concurrent administration of propranolol or cimetidine.

ADVERSE DRUG REACTIONS

All class IB antiarrhythmics have a relatively high incidence of predictable central nervous system (CNS) disturbances, especially drowsiness, confusion, lightheadedness, paresthesias, slurred speech, vision and hearing disturbances, tremors, seizures, and coma. Lowering the dose or stopping the drug reverses these reactions. Hypotension and bradycardia sometimes occur. Up to 40% of patients taking tocainide or mexiletine experience upper GI distress, which is usually relieved by taking the drug with food or antacids.

Tocainide can lead to two rare but serious unpredictable reactions: blood dyscrasias and pulmonary fibrosis. These disappear upon discontinuation of the drug. Drug fever and hepatitis have occurred after tocainide therapy.

NURSING IMPLICATIONS

Besides having a clear understanding of the mechanisms of action of the class IB antiarrhythmics, the nurse must monitor the patient closely. The nurse must also be aware of other implications concerning these drugs.

• Class IB antiarrhythmics are contraindicated in patients with second- or third-degree heart block. Lidocaine and tocainide are contraindicated in patients with hypersensitivity to local anesthetics.

• Administer class IB antiarrhythmics cautiously to patients with hepatic or renal disease, congestive heart failure, bradycardia, or markedly altered urine pH; to elderly patients; and to patients who weigh less than 50 kg (111 pounds).

• Monitor the patient's serum potassium levels because hypokalemia exacerbates dysrhythmias.

• Lidocaine is available in prefilled syringes in two different concentrations. Use the 100-mg syringe for an I.V. push bolus. Use the 1- or 2-gram syringe for mixing in 250 or 500 ml dextrose 5% in water (D_5W).

• Administer continuous I.V. infusions using an infusion pump, with constant EKG monitoring of the patient.

• Do not use lidocaine solutions containing ephinephrine to treat dysrhythmias because these mixtures are for local anesthesia only.

• Observe for signs and symptoms of toxicity, such as CNS disturbances, especially confusion, or seizures.

• Administer tocainide and mexiletine with food or antacids to reduce upper GI tract symptoms.

CLASS IC ANTIARRHYTHMICS

The FDA has approved two class IC antiarrhythmics, flecainide acetate and encainide, which are indicated for certain types of ventricular dysrhythmias. Like the antiarrhythmics in classes IA and IB, flecainide (approved in 1985) and encainide (approved in 1987) are local anesthetics that act to stabilize the cell membrane.

Phenytoin for digitalis toxicity

Phenytoin is sometimes given intravenously to correct acute dysrhythmias caused by digitalis toxicity. (See Chapter 34, Cardiac Glycoside Agents and Bipyridines, for further details.)

Phenytoin is distributed throughout the body, and is 95% protein-bound. The drug is metabolized in the liver by oxidation to an inactive metabolite, which is then excreted in the urine. Onset of action occurs within 5 minutes of I.V. administration. (Peak or therapeutic serum concentrations are usually not important when phenytoin is used to treat dysrhythmias.) The duration of action is 4 to 6 hours, although the half-life of phenytoin is usually about 22 hours.

The mechanism of action of phenytoin in treating digitalis-induced dysrhythmias resembles that of the class IB antiarrhythmics. The drug shortens the ERP of the AV node and depresses the automaticity of ectopic myocardial cells. Phenytoin is used to shorten prolonged AV conduction time and to suppress premature ventricular beats.

USUAL ADULT DOSAGE: 100 mg I.V. push, repeated every 5 minutes until the dysrhythmia disappears; if the total dosage reaches 1 gram without effect, another antiarrhythmic should be used.

Predictable adverse reactions include pain at the infusion site, hypotension with cardiovascular collapse, a decreased level of consciousness, and ventricular fibrillation. Unpredictable reactions include rash and fever.

When administering phenytoin, the nurse should observe the following implications:

• Infuse the drug through a central line to avoid pain and phlebitis. If a peripheral site must be used, inject the drug into an I.V. line infusing normal saline solution.

• Do not dilute phenytoin; administer by I.V. push only at a rate not exceeding 50 mg/minute.

• Closely monitor the patient's heart rate and rhythm and blood pressure.

• Have emergency equipment or a code cart available.

PHARMACOKINETICS

After oral administration, flecainide and encainide are both well absorbed, probably metabolized by the liver, and excreted primarily by the kidneys.

Absorption, distribution, metabolism, excretion

Flecainide is rapidly and almost completely absorbed from the GI tract after oral administration, and absorption is not substantially affected by food or antacids. Absorption of encainide from the GI tract varies from

76% to 85%. Available data indicate that flecainide is widely distributed, with about 50% bound to plasma protein. Encainide is 90% bound to plasma protein.

Flecainide does not undergo significant first-pass metabolism. In fact, the actual site of metabolism has not been determined. Dealkylation forms two major metabolites, which exert only minor antiarrhythmic effects. The kidneys excrete about 30% of the unchanged drug and all of the metabolites: less than 5% of the drug is excreted in the feces. Encainide is rapidly demethylated in the liver to form at least two active metabolites, which are excreted in the urine.

Onset, peak, duration

Onset of action data are incomplete for flecainide, which reaches peak concentration levels in 30 minutes to 6 hours, with 2 to 3 hours the average. The therapeutic plasma level ranges from 0.2 to 1 mcg/ml. Its duration of action is undetermined, but the drug's half-life ranges from 7 to 25 hours, with 13 to 16 hours as the average.

Encainide begins to act in 1 to 2 hours when given orally. Data are incomplete, but its half-life is known to be 3 to 4 hours, and that of its metabolites, much longer. Its duration of action is 14 hours or longer.

PHARMACODYNAMICS

Flecainide primarily blocks influx of sodium in the cell membrane fast channel, thereby decreasing depolarization (phase 0 of the action potential). The drug produces no effect on resting membrane levels and little effect on ERP or APD. However, encainide shortens APD and depresses spontaneous phase 4 depolarization. Both drugs significantly delay intracardiac conduction, especially in the ventricles. This action converts unidirectional block into bidirectional block, thus interrupting reentry patterns. Flecainide has little effect on the SA or AV nodes or normal atrial cells, but it depresses function and conduction in abnormal cells. Chronic use of oral encainide therapy prolongs AV node and atrial muscle conduction, which reflects on the EKG as a wider QRS complex and a longer P-R interval.

Flecainide also increases endocardial pacing thresholds and exerts some negative inotropic effect. It does not interfere with sympathetic or parasympathetic nervous system control of the heart.

PHARMACOTHERAPEUTICS

Like class IB antiarrhythmics, class IC drugs are used to treat ventricular dysrhythmias. Some dysrhythmias respond better to class IC agents than to the class IB drugs; however, flecainide and encainide produce a greater number of serious adverse reactions.

flecainide acetate (Tambocor). Used to suppress frequent ventricular ectopic beats and to decrease the frequency and duration of the abrupt onset of self-limiting ventricular tachycardia, flecainide is also used to prevent sustained ventricular tachycardia. The drug is not useful in treating atrial dysrhythmias.
USUAL ADULT DOSAGE: 100 to 200 mg P.O. every 12 hours; dividing the daily dose into three doses given at 8-hour intervals is sometimes necessary. No data for pediatric dosages are available.

encainide hydrochloride (Enkaid). Indications for this class IC antiarrhythmic are the same as for flecainide.
USUAL ADULT DOSAGE: initially, 25 mg P.O. every 8 hours, increasing to 35 mg, then to 50 mg, and finally to a maximum of 50 mg P.O. every 6 hours to control the dysrhythmia. A 3- to 5-day interval between dosage increments is recommended. No data for pediatric dosages are available.

Drug interactions

Concurrent administration of flecainide and digoxin may increase the serum digoxin level, leading to digitalis toxicity. Concurrent administration of flecainide and alkalinizing drugs—such as carbonic anhydrase inhibitors and sodium bicarbonate—decreases the urinary excretion of flecainide. Interaction between flecainide and cimetidine decreases flecainide metabolism. The interactions of flecainide with alkalinizing drugs and cimetidine may also produce increased adverse reactions to flecainide, even at low doses.

Encainide does not interact with other antiarrhythmics or with digoxin. Cimetidine decreases the hepatic metabolism of encainide.

ADVERSE DRUG REACTIONS

Several serious reactions have been noted with class IC antiarrythmics that may limit their use.

Dose-related predictable reactions usually appear as CNS symptoms, especially dizziness, headache, and vision disturbances. Dyspnea is also frequently seen. Encainide may also be associated with abdominal and leg pain and dry mouth.

Paradoxically, as with most antiarrhythmics, class IC antiarrythmics can aggravate existing dysrhythmias and cause new ones. The physician or nurse must take care not to mistake these arrhythmogenic effects for the recurrence or spontaneous worsening of the original dysrhythmia. These effects usually occur 1 to 4 weeks after starting therapy.

Flecainide produces a negative inotropic effect and may worsen congestive heart failure (encainide does not do this). Other predictable reactions include nausea, anorexia, vomiting, dyspepsia, diarrhea, isolated numbness, chest pain, and edema. Unpredictable allergic reactions include fever, rash, and dermatitis.

NURSING IMPLICATIONS

• Flecainide and encainide are contraindicated in patients with second- or third-degree heart block, cardiogenic shock, or hypokalemia.
• Administer flecainide and encainide with caution or at lower dosages in the patient with severe renal or hepatic disease, prolonged Q-T interval, blood dyscrasias, or congestive heart failure.
• Continuously monitor the patient's EKG while initiating or adjusting class IC drug therapy.

CLASS II ANTIARRHYTHMICS

Class II antiarrhythmics are the beta-adrenergic blockers. Propranolol and acebutolol are FDA-approved antiarrhythmics. (See Chapter 36, Antianginal Agents, for their antianginal effects; Chapter 20, Adrenergic Blocking Agents, for the overall effects of propranolol and acebutolol; and Chapter 37, Antihypertensive Agents, for their antihypertensive effects.)

Beta-adrenergic blockers represent a relatively new drug class. In 1958, Powell and Slater reported the use of a beta-adrenergic blocker to selectively inhibit beta-receptor stimulation by epinephrine and norepinephrine. (See *Esmolol hydrochloride* on page 560 for details about a new class II antiarrhythmic.)

PHARMACOKINETICS

The pharmacokinetic properties of propranolol and acebutolol exhibit some similarities and some differences.

Absorption, distribution, metabolism, excretion
Both propranolol and acebutolol are almost entirely absorbed from the GI tract after oral administration. Although food may slightly delay absorption, it does not significantly affect peak concentration levels. Propranolol, which is widely distributed, crosses the blood-brain barrier; acebutolol, with low lipid solubility, does not. Propranolol is 90% protein-bound in plasma; acebutolol is 26% protein-bound.

Both drugs significantly bind to hepatic binding sites during first-pass metabolism. Propranolol is almost completely metabolized in the liver, and at least one metabolite is active. The major acebutolol metabolite of hepatic acetylation is also very active. Propranolol's metabolites are excreted in the urine. About 35% of an acebutolol dose is excreted in the urine and 55% in the feces.

Onset, peak, duration
After oral administration, the antiarrhythmic effects of propranolol begin in 30 minutes; the onset of action of acebutolol occurs after 90 minutes. Propranolol's peak concentration levels occur in 60 to 90 minutes, whereas acebutolol reaches peak concentration levels after 3 to 8 hours. Serum concentration assays have not been useful in monitoring the antiarrhythmic or toxic effects of propranolol or acebutolol.

The duration of action of propranolol is 4 to 6 hours for tablets and up to 24 hours for long-acting capsules. Acebutolol exerts some blocking capacity 24 to 30 hours after administration. The half-life of propranolol is 3.4 to 6 hours; that of acebutolol, 3 to 4 hours.

PHARMACODYNAMICS

Propranolol and acebutolol suppress dysrhythmias by several different mechanisms of action. The drugs block receptor sites in the conduction system of the heart, thereby slowing SA node automaticity and the conductivity of the AV node and other cells. These effects probably convert unidirectional block to bidirectional block. The class II antiarrhythmics also exert a significant negative inotropic effect. By decreasing myocardial oxygen demand, this action may also decrease myocardial ischemia. As ischemia abates, myocardial cells lose their automaticity, and this effect suppresses atrial and ventricular ectopy.

PHARMACOTHERAPEUTICS

Physicians do not usually use the class II drugs as their first choice to treat dysrhythmias, in part because of the multiple effects of the drugs and because of possible breakthrough ectopy. The use of these agents in combination with other antiarrhythmics remains to be evaluated.

propranolol hydrochloride (Inderal, Inderal LA). Possibly effective in a variety of dysrhythmias, including atrial and ventricular ectopy, propranolol may also effectively treat the sudden onset of self-limiting atrial or ventricular tachycardia. Propranolol is not used to terminate acute ventricular tachycardia. The drug is best used in patients with dysrhythmias associated with excess catecholamines, digitalis toxicity, or Wolff-Parkinson-White syndrome.

USUAL ADULT DOSAGE: for dysrhythmias, 10 to 30 mg P.O. every 6 to 8 hours; 0.5 to 3 mg I.V. is given for life-threatening dysrhythmias. Because of insufficient data, propranolol is not recommended for use in pediatric patients.

acebutolol hydrochloride (Sectral). In addition to its antihypertensive uses, acebutolol is indicated for the suppression of frequent ventricular ectopic beats.

USUAL ADULT DOSAGE: 200 to 600 mg P.O. every 12 hours. No data for pediatric dosages are available.

Drug interactions

Class II antiarrhythmics interact with phenothiazines and antihypertensive drugs, which potentiate hypotension. Interactions with anticholinergics and cimetidine alter the effects of Class II antiarrhythmic drugs. (See *Drug interactions: Class II antiarrhythmics* for more details about these interactions.)

ADVERSE DRUG REACTIONS

The most frequently occurring adverse reactions associated with class II antiarrhythmics involve the cardiovascular system and usually occur when the class II drug is first given.

Predictable reactions

Because they inhibit sinus node stimulation, beta-adrenergic blockers may produce bradycardia, a heart rate less than 60 beats/minute. Hypotension with peripheral vascular insufficiency may also occur. Syncope, angina, and shock may accompany these reactions. Occasionally, fluid retention and peripheral edema occur.

Because class II antiarrhythmics reduce the force of myocardial contraction and increase preload, they may exacerbate or precipitate congestive heart failure. Dysrhythmias, especially AV block, may also occur. Adverse CNS reactions include dizziness, confusion, fatigue, lassitude, and decreased libido. Typical GI reactions, such as nausea, vomiting, mild diarrhea, or constipation, are usually transient.

Propranolol and acebutolol block bronchial beta receptors that otherwise dilate bronchioles: this action

can lead to significant bronchoconstriction. Propranolol is more likely to cause this adverse reaction because it is a nonselective beta-adrenergic blocker.

Unpredictable reactions

Unpredictable reactions include rashes, blood dyscrasias, mental depression, and vivid dreams. These reactions, however, are rare.

NURSING IMPLICATIONS

When administering the class II antiarrhythmics, the nurse should remember the following implications:

• Propranolol and acebutolol are usually contraindicated for patients with asthma, sinus bradycardia, second- or third-degree heart block, diabetes mellitus, or peripheral vascular disease. They are also administered cautiously to patients with congestive heart failure or chronic obstructive pulmonary disease.

• Withhold the dose and notify the physician if the patient's pulse is less than 60 beats/minute or the systolic blood pressure is less than 90 mm Hg.

• Monitor the patient for signs of heart failure, including edema, crackles, weight gain, and shortness of breath.

Esmolol hydrochloride

The newest class II antiarrhythmic on the market is esmolol hydrochloride (Brevibloc). It inhibits adrenergic stimulation by blocking beta$_1$ receptors in the myocardium, reducing heart rate and blood pressure. It is approved for use to treat supraventricular tachycardia, atrial flutter, atrial fibrillation, paroxysmal supraventricular tachycardia, and supraventricular dysrhythmias associated with Wolff-Parkinson-White syndrome.

USUAL ADULT DOSAGE: initially, a loading dose of 500 mcg/kg/minute I.V. over 1 minute followed by a 4-minute maintenance infusion of 50 mcg/kg/minute. The heart rate and blood pressure must be closely monitored. The initial dose may be repeated within 5 minutes if the rate has not slowed satisfactorily. The maintenance infusion is titrated up to 300 mcg/kg/minute at 50-mcg/kg/minute increments every 5 to 10 minutes until the desired response occurs. Because esmolol has a very short half-life and duration of action compared to the other beta-adrenergic blockers, it may be used to treat critically ill patients who require a beta-adrenergic blocker but cannot tolerate its prolonged adverse effects.

DRUG INTERACTIONS

Class II antiarrhythmics

The interactions between class II antiarrhythmics and other drugs can be hazardous to the patient's well-being. The nurse must be aware of such interactions to provide quality patient care.

DRUG	INTERACTING DRUGS	POSSIBLE EFFECTS	NURSING IMPLICATIONS
propranolol, acebutolol	phenothiazines	Increase hypotension	• Monitor the patient for dizziness and orthostatic hypotension.
	sympathomimetics	Decrease effect of sympathomimetics	• Monitor the patient for decreased therapeutic effect.
	anticholinergics	Potentiate pressor effects, causing hypertension; reduce efficacy of the class II antiarrhythmics	• Monitor the patient's therapeutic response and heart rate and rhythm.
	antihypertensives	Increase hypotension	• Monitor the patient for dizziness and orthostatic hypotension.
	neuromuscular blockers	Enhance skeletal muscle relaxation	• Monitor the patient for hypoventilation when administering class II antiarrhythmics in the immediate postoperative period.
	verapamil	Increases cardiac depression	• Monitor the patient for decreased heart rate.
propranolol	cimetidine	Decreases propanolol metabolism	• Observe the patient for adverse reactions even at low doses of the class II antiarrhythmic.

CLASS III ANTIARRHYTHMICS

The class III antiarrhythmics bretylium and amiodarone are used to treat ventricular dysrhythmias. Both drugs significantly affect APD to produce their antidysrhythmic effect.

History and source

Bretylium was originally developed in the 1950s as an antihypertensive but was then withdrawn for that use. In the late 1970s, it was approved by the FDA for antiarrhythmic therapy. Although used for some time in Europe, amiodarone was not approved for use in the United States until 1986.

PHARMACOKINETICS

The two class III antiarrhythmics have quite different pharmacokinetic properties.

Absorption, distribution, metabolism, excretion

Bretylium's erratic GI absorption mandates parenteral administration. After oral administration, amiodarone is slowly absorbed at widely varying rates. Data about the distribution and protein binding of bretylium are lacking. Amiodarone accumulates in many sites, especially in highly vascular organs and adipose tissue. Amiodarone is 96% protein bound in plasma, but only after tissue sites are saturated.

Bretylium is excreted unchanged by the kidneys over several days. Amiodarone is metabolized in an uncertain pathway to metabolites of uncertain activity, then excreted by the liver in bile and feces.

Onset, peak, duration

In a patient with ventricular fibrillation, bretylium's onset of action begins within minutes of I.V. infusion. When the drug is given for suppression of ventricular ectopy and ventricular tachycardia, however, onset of action takes 20 minutes to 6 hours. Amiodarone's onset of action occurs within 1 to 3 weeks.

Peak concentration levels of bretylium occur 6 to 9 hours after I.M. or I.V. administration. Peak concentration levels of amiodarone may occur 3 to 7 hours after the first dose; however, they may not occur for a few weeks. The therapeutic serum level of bretylium is 0.5 to 1.5 mcg/ml; that of amiodarone is uncertain.

The duration of action of bretylium is 6 to 24 hours; its half-life is 5 to 10 hours. Effects of amiodarone may persist for weeks or even months after discontinuation. Amiodarone has an initial half-life of 2½ to 10 days and an average terminal half-life of 53 days.

PHARMACODYNAMICS

Class III antiarrhythmics greatly prolong the APD and ERP of myocardial cells, thus decreasing the rate of automaticity of ventricular ectopic beats. The drugs may convert unidirectional block to bidirectional block, but they have little or no effect on depolarization. Bretylium and amiodarone inhibit sympathetic nervous system innervation of the heart; however, they increase circulating catecholamines. Bretylium exerts a positive inotropic effect. Both drugs produce some peripheral and coronary vasodilation. The exact mechanism of action of class III antiarrhythmics that is most responsible for the antiarrhythmic effects remains uncertain.

PHARMACOTHERAPEUTICS

In part because of their adverse reactions, class III antiarrhythmics are not the first choices for antiarrhythmic therapy. The drugs produce synergistic effects when combined with any of several other antiarrhythmics.

bretylium tosylate (Bretylol). Useful in preventing and treating ventricular fibrillation and ventricular tachycardia that are unresponsive to other treatment, bretylium is used only for short-term therapy in immediately life-threatening conditions.
USUAL ADULT DOSAGE: 5 mg/kg I.V. push over 1 minute, increased to 10 mg/kg I.V. push over 1 minute if necessary. Doses may be repeated every 1 to 2 hours, or a continuous I.V. infusion of 1 to 2 mg/minute can be used. Bretylium may be given 5 to 10 mg/kg I.M. and repeated every 1 to 2 hours.

amiodarone hydrochloride (Cordarone). Indicated for preventing ventricular ectopy, amiodarone is also used to reduce the frequency and duration of persistent ventricular tachycardia unresponsive to other antiarrhythmics. Because large amounts of the drug are sequestered in various tissues, physicians usually order

loading doses. Without the loading dose, steady-state plasma levels would take months to achieve. The dose must be titrated to the patient's requirements under close EKG monitoring.
USUAL ADULT DOSAGE: loading dose, 800 to 1,600 mg/day P.O. for 1 to 3 weeks or until a response occurs; dosage is reduced gradually to a maintenance dose of 400 mg/day.

Drug interactions

Significant interactions with other cardiovascular drugs such as digoxin and antihypertensives vary. Interactions are more serious with amiodarone than with short-term bretylium therapy. (See *Drug interactions: Class III antiarrhythmics* for more information.)

ADVERSE DRUG REACTIONS

Adverse reactions to class III antiarrhythmics, especially amiodarone, vary widely and often lead to discontinuation of the drug.

Predictable reactions

Upon initial bretylium administration, orthostatic and supine hypotension commonly occur, producing dizziness. Nausea and vomiting frequently accompany rapid I.V. administration.

Like most antiarrhythmics, bretylium and amiodarone can aggravate dysrhythmias, especially bradycardia, and increase ventricular ectopic beats.

Amiodarone may precipitate hypotension in addition to nausea, anorexia, and various CNS symptoms such as fatigue, tremors, and malaise.

Unpredictable reactions

Amiodarone causes several non-dose-related reactions. Pulmonary toxicity consisting of interstitial pneumonia and alveolitis occurs in 15% of patients and can be fatal; signs and symptoms include dyspnea, cough, and X-ray changes. Corneal microdeposits occur in almost all patients, but only 10% experience vision disturbances. The deposits disappear upon dosage reduction or discontinuation of the drug. Skin photosensitivity occurs, sometimes producing a blue-gray discoloration of exposed skin. The high iodine content of amiodarone can produce hypothyroidism or hyperthyroidism.

NURSING IMPLICATIONS

When administering a class III antiarrhythmic, the nurse should remember the following implications:
• Administer amiodarone cautiously to patients with pre-existing bradycardia, sinus node disease, conduction dis-

DRUG INTERACTIONS

Class III antiarrhythmics

The interactions between class III antiarrhythmics and other drugs may cause serious consequences for the patient. The nurse must be prepared to institute appropriate assessment and intervention strategies in response to these interactions.

DRUG	INTERACTING DRUGS	POSSIBLE EFFECTS	NURSING IMPLICATIONS
bretylium, amiodarone	antihypertensives	Produce profound hypotension	• Monitor the patient for dizziness, orthostatic hypotension, and mental status changes.
	warfarin	Increase hypoprothrombinemia	• Monitor the patient for increased bruising, bleeding, and I.V. site oozing; monitor the patient's prothrombin time.
	digoxin	Increase serum digoxin level	• Monitor the patient for signs of digitalis toxicity (anorexia, nausea, vomiting, diarrhea, visual disturbances, and dysrhythmias).

turbances, severely depressed ventricular function, or marked cardiomegaly.

• Administer bretylium cautiously to patients with digitalis-induced dysrhythmias, aortic stenosis, or pulmonary hypertension.

• Monitor the patient's blood pressure and EKG continuously during bretylium therapy.

• Keep emergency resuscitation equipment available during therapy.

• Continuously monitor the patient's EKG when initiating or altering amiodarone therapy.

• Monitor the patient for hypothyroidism during amiodarone therapy. Signs and symptoms include lethargy; weight gain; cool, dry skin; bradycardia; hypotension; and cold intolerance. Also monitor the patient for hyperthyroidism; signs and symptoms include nervousness, weight loss, warm and moist skin, tachycardia, and palpitations.

• Teach patients taking amiodarone to use sunscreen products to protect themselves from photosensitivity. Instruct patients to report tingling skin followed by erythema and blistering.

CLASS IV ANTIARRHYTHMICS

Among the class IV antiarrhythmics, or calcium channel blockers, only verapamil is FDA-approved.

History and source

In the early 1960s, Hass and Hartfelder found that verapamil, a derivative of papaverine, dilated blood vessels differently than the nitrates. Then, in 1967, Fleckenstein suggested that the dilation action was caused by inhibition of calcium ion movement into cells. Later, the French investigators Rougier and Coraboeuf demonstrated that cardiac cells were depolarized not only by the rapid influx of sodium ions, but also by a slower influx of calcium ions. Thus, calcium channel blockers are also known as *slow channel blockers* or *calcium agonists.*

PHARMACOKINETICS

Verapamil, which is only given intravenously to treat dysrhythmias, is 90% protein-bound. The drug is rapidly and almost completely metabolized in the liver, and some metabolites are active. Verapamil metabolites are excreted primarily in the urine and to a lesser extent in the feces.

The antiarrhythmic effects of verapamil begin within minutes of I.V. administration. Peak concentration levels occur within 10 minutes. Serum concentration levels are not used to monitor verapamil therapy.

The drug's duration of action may be up to 6 hours but usually is less. The half-life of verapamil is 3 to 7 hours.

PHARMACODYNAMICS

Verapamil blocks the influx of calcium across the slow channels of myocardial electrical cells during the plateau (phase 2) and depolarization (phase 4) of the action potential. This blockade greatly increases the ERP of the AV node and slows the conduction rate between the atria and the ventricles.

PHARMACOTHERAPEUTICS

Verapamil is used to treat supraventricular dysrhythmias with rapid ventricular response rates.

verapamil hydrochloride (Calan, Isoptin). Physicians use I.V. verapamil to correct a rapid heart rate caused by reentry into the atria or the AV node. This rapid heart rate, called *paroxysmal supraventricular tachycardia (PSVT),* has an abrupt onset and is usually self-limiting. Physicians also use verapamil when physical vagal stimulation is unsuccessful. The drug does not affect atrial ectopic beats. I.V. verapamil also decreases the ventricular response in patients with atrial flutter and atrial fibrillation by blocking AV conduction or converting the atrial rhythm—although the latter action is rare. USUAL ADULT DOSAGE: 5 to 10 mg I.V. push over 2 minutes; if the patient tolerates but does not respond, a second I.V. dose of 10 mg, 15 to 30 minutes after the initial dose.
USUAL PEDIATRIC DOSAGE: in children under 1 year old, 0.75 to 2 mg I.V.; in children over 1 year old, 2 to 5 mg I.V.

Drug interactions

Verapamil interacts with other antiarrhythmics. Interactions with antihypertensives potentiate hypotension and heart failure; with digoxin, an increased serum digoxin level and digitalis toxicity may result. Verapamil interactions with other highly protein-bound drugs such as hydantoins, salicylates, sulfonamides, and sulfonylureas can cause adverse reactions associated with either verapamil or the other drugs.

ADVERSE DRUG REACTIONS

Verapamil commonly causes serious alterations in the cardiovascular system. The drug sometimes causes hypotension, particularly orthostatic hypotension. Verapamil's effect on the SA and AV nodes causes dysrhythmias, such as bradycardia, sinus block, and AV block. The drug also depresses myocardial contraction force, which may precipitate or exacerbate congestive heart failure.

Vasodilation produced by verapamil occasionally causes dizziness, headache, flushing, weakness, and persistent peripheral edema. Other predictable reactions include constipation and other GI disturbances, leg fatigue, and muscle cramps.

Unpredictable reactions include worsening of angina; skin eruptions; photosensitivity; pruritus; nasal congestion; and mood changes.

NURSING IMPLICATIONS

The nurse administering verapamil must be aware of the following implications:
- Administer verapamil cautiously to patients with hypotension, congestive heart failure, sick sinus syndrome, AV conduction disturbances, or hepatic impairment.
- Administer as a slow I.V. bolus over a 2-minute period. Administer I.V. verapamil over a 3-minute period to minimize adverse effects in elderly patients.
- Provide continuous EKG monitoring and frequent blood pressure assessment of the patient while giving I.V. verapamil.
- Avoid administering I.V. verapamil and an I.V. beta-adrenergic blocker concomitantly (within a few hours).

CHAPTER SUMMARY

Chapter 35 discussed antiarrhythmics. These drugs are used to treat abnormal electrical activity in the heart by limiting cardiac electrical activity to normal conduction pathways and decreasing abnormally fast heart rates. Here are the highlights of the chapter:
- Action potentials of myocardial muscle cells include rapid depolarization caused by rapid influx of Na^+ into the cell while potassium ions leave the cell. The influx of calcium ions occurs through the slow channel in the cell membrane. Repolarization occurs when potassium ions reenter the cell, while sodium ions leave the cell.
- Antiarrhythmic drugs block the fast sodium channel, the slow calcium channel, autonomic innervation of myocardial cells, or a combination of such actions.
- The normal conduction system of the heart consists of the SA node, atrial pathways, the AV node, the bundle of His, the right and left bundle branches, and the Purkinje fibers. Impulses travel along this system, leading

Antiarrhythmic agents

The following chart summarizes selected antiarrhythmics discussed in this chapter.

DRUG	MAJOR INDICATIONS	USUAL ADULT DOSAGES	NURSING IMPLICATIONS
Class IA			
quinidine	Conversion of atrial fibrillation to normal sinus rhythm	300 to 400 mg quinidine sulfate P.O. every 6 hours, then 200 to 400 mg every 6 hours to maintain regular rhythm	• Administer cautiously to patients with congestive heart failure (CHF), heart block, hypotension, myasthenia gravis, urinary retention, hepatic or renal insufficiency, or prolonged Q-T interval.
	Suppression of atrial and ventricular ectopic beats	200 to 300 mg quinidine sulfate P.O. every 6 to 8 hours	• Observe the patient's EKG for a lengthening Q-T interval, a precursor to ventricular tachycardia. Also observe for an increased ventricular rate and conduction disturbances. • Monitor the patient's serum drug levels.
Class IB			
lidocaine	Suppression of ventricular ectopic beats; conversion and prevention of ventricular tachycardia	50 to 100 mg initial I.V. bolus, followed by a second bolus of 50 to 100 mg in 5 minutes, then continuous I.V. infusion at 1 to 4 mg/minute for up to 24 hours; or 300 mg I.M., repeated in 60 to 90 minutes, if necessary	• Administer cautiously to patients with hepatic or renal disease, CHF, bradycardia, or markedly altered urine pH, and to elderly patients. • Be aware that 100-mg I.V. bolus syringes and 1- to 2-gram syringes for dilution in D_5W look alike. • Observe the patient for signs of toxicity such as CNS disturbances. • Maintain constant EKG monitoring.
Class IC			
flecainide	Suppression of frequent ventricular ectopy and acute self-limiting ventricular tachycardia; prevention of sustained ventricular tachycardia	100 to 200 mg P.O. every 12 hours	• This drug is contraindicated in patients with second- or third-degree heart block, cardiogenic shock, or hypokalemia. • Administer cautiously to patients with severe renal or hepatic disease, a prolonged Q-T interval, blood dyscrasias, or CHF. • Monitor the patient's EKG continuously while therapy is initiated or adjusted.
Class II			
propranolol	Atrial and ventricular ectopy and the sudden onset of self-limiting atrial or ventricular tachycardia	10 to 30 mg P.O. every 6 to 8 hours; 0.5 to 3 mg I.V. for life-threatening dysrhythmias	• This drug is contraindicated in patients with asthma, sinus bradycardia, second- or third-degree heart block, diabetes mellitus, or peripheral vascular disease. • Administer cautiously to patients with CHF or chronic obstructive pulmonary disease. • Withhold the dose and notify the physician about a pulse rate lower than 60 beats/minute or a systolic blood pressure less than 90 mm Hg.

continued

Antiarrhythmic agents continued

DRUG	MAJOR INDICATIONS	USUAL ADULT DOSAGES	NURSING IMPLICATIONS
Class III			
amiodarone	Ventricular dysrhythmias unresponsive to other antiarrhythmics	800 to 1,600 mg/day P.O. for 1 to 3 weeks as loading dose, reduced gradually to a maintenance dosage of 400 mg/day P.O.	• Maintain constant EKG monitoring. • Assess the patient for dyspnea and cough, subtle signs of pulmonary toxicity. • Teach the patient to use sunscreen products, and to avoid long exposure to the sun. • Monitor the patient for alterations in thyroid function.
Class IV			
verapamil	Paroxysmal supraventricular tachycardia	5 to 10 mg I.V. push, over 2 minutes, followed by a second dose of 10 mg I.V. push after 15 to 30 minutes if the patient tolerates but does not respond to the first dose	• Maintain continuous EKG montoring. • Monitor the patient's blood pressure for hypotension and heart rate for excessive bradycardia. • Administer cautiously to patients with CHF, sinus block, or conduction defects. • Do not infuse intravenously an I.V. beta-adrenergic blocker concomitantly (within a few hours).

to myocardial cell excitation and, eventually, ventricular filling and contraction.

• Myocardial cells have the properties of automaticity, excitability, contractility, and conductivity.

• The six different classes of antiarrhythmics have widely varying mechanisms of action but also share some pharmacologic properties: they possess different pharmacokinetics and pharmacodynamics and are used to treat different dysrhythmias. Class IA antiarrhythmics include quinidine sulfate, gluconate, or polygalacturonate; procainamide hydrochloride; and disopyramide phosphate. Class IB includes lidocaine hydrochloride, tocainide hydrochloride, and mexiletine hydrochloride. Class IC includes flecainide acetate and encainide hydrochloride. Class II contains the beta-adrenergic blockers propranolol hydrochloride and acebutolol hydrochloride. Class III includes bretylium tosylate and amiodarone hydrochloride. Class IV includes only verapamil hydrochloride.

• Administering antiarrhythmics requires the nurse to closely monitor such patient data as heart rate and rhythm, blood pressure, serum drug level, and interactions with other medications.

BIBLIOGRAPHY

American Hospital Formulary Service. *Drug Information 87.* McEvoy, G.K., et al., eds. Bethesda, Md.: American Society of Hospital Pharmacists, 1987.

American Medical Association. *Drug Evaluations,* 6th ed. Philadelphia: W.B. Saunders Co., 1986.

Amsterdam, E.A., et al. *Progress in Cardiology: An Update on the Management of Ventricular Arrhythmias.* Richmond, Va.: A.H. Robbins Co., 1985.

Contemporary Antiarrhythmic Therapy: Focus on Quinidine. Richmond, Va.: A.H. Robbins Co., 1986.

Cordarone. Philadelphia: Wyeth Laboratories, 1986.

Craig, C.R., et al., eds. *Modern Pharmacology,* 2nd ed. Boston: Little, Brown & Co., 1986.

Gilman, A.G., et al., eds. *Goodman and Gilman's The Pharmacological Basis of Therapeutics,* 7th ed. New York: Macmillan Publishing Co., 1985.

Kastrup, E.K., et al., eds. *Facts and Comparisons.* St. Louis: Facts and Comparisons Division, J.B. Lippincott Co., 1986.

Miura, D.S. *Clinical Pharmacology and Differentiation of Conventional and Investigational Antiarrhythmic Agents.* New York: Berlex Laboratories, Inc., 1985.

CHAPTER 36

ANTIANGINAL AGENTS

OBJECTIVES

After reading and studying this chapter, you should be able to:
1. Discuss the physiology of myocardial ischemia, which results in angina.
2. Differentiate between angina caused by atherosclerosis and coronary artery spasm.
3. Identify the mechanisms of actions and clinical indications for the antianginal agents: nitrates, beta-adrenergic blockers, and calcium channel blockers.
4. Explain how heart rate, force of myocardial contraction, preload, and afterload affect myocardial oxygen demand.
5. Explain how routes of administration influence the onset of action and clinical uses of the different nitrates.
6. List the most significant adverse reactions and drug interactions associated with the various antianginal agents.

INTRODUCTION

To pump effectively, the heart needs its own blood supply, which the coronary arteries provide. These arteries originate from the aorta at the ostia situated above the cusps of the aortic valve (the sinus of Valsalva). From there, the arteries branch out to cover and penetrate all parts of the cardiac muscle, or myocardium. After delivering oxygen and nutrients throughout the myocardium, the blood moves through large coronary veins and returns to the right atrium via the coronary sinus. The myocardium cannot extract oxygen from blood inside the chambers of the heart; instead, it depends on blood from the coronary arteries for its supply of oxygen and nutrients.

Even when the body is at rest, the percentage of oxygen extracted from coronary arterial blood by the myocardium is high, approximately 80%. During exercise or other exertion, the amount of blood flowing through the coronary arteries must increase significantly to meet the increased myocardial demand for oxygen.

Combination antianginal therapy

Combination therapy with drugs from different classes of antianginal agents is indicated for symptoms that persist despite therapy with one or more drugs from a single class. Combining drugs from different classes provides antianginal effects from different mechanisms of action and reduces the risk of adverse reactions from high doses of any one drug.

Combination therapy is also used to control different types of angina occurring in one patient. For example, a patient might take a beta-adrenergic blocker or a calcium channel blocker for long-term control and supplement this therapy with rapid-acting nitrates for unusual exertional demands. Beta-adrenergic blockers prevent the reflex tachycardia sometimes reported with nitrates; nitrates, in turn, prevent the increased preload from beta-adrenergic blockers. Calcium channel blockers and beta-adrenergic blockers together more effectively treat Prinzmetal's angina that is unresponsive to beta-adrenergic blockers alone.

During combination therapy, the nurse should monitor the patient for adverse reactions, such as severe bradycardia, congestive heart failure, or excessive hypotension.

This additional oxygen is provided normally by an increase in aortic blood pressure and by local factors that dilate the coronary arteries during a process called *autoregulation.*

Exertion increases heart rate. At rest, the heart is in systole about one-third of the time and in diastole about two-thirds of the time. This is when the majority of blood flows through the coronary arteries. As heart rate increases, time in diastole shortens; thus, exertion increases oxygen demand while decreasing the time available for the coronary arteries to supply it. The coronary arteries help maintain the balance between oxygen supply and demand usually by dilating, allowing more blood to circulate to the myocardium.

In coronary artery disease, specifically atherosclerosis, the arteries may be unable to accommodate an increased blood flow such as that caused by exertion or be unable to dilate. Atherosclerosis may result from deposits of cholesterol, platelets, or other proteins and blood components in the interior, or lumen, of the artery, causing narrowing of the lumen.

When the myocardial oxygen demand exceeds the myocardial oxygen supply, areas become ischemic, causing chest pain. When the patient experiences symptoms from this myocardial ischemia, the condition is known as *angina* or *angina pectoris*. The patient may report a crushing sensation or a feeling of pressure behind the sternum, sometimes radiating into the neck, the jaw, and the shoulders and down the arms. Initially, symptoms may be mild: the patient may confuse the angina with indigestion, heartburn, chest muscle strain, or pain referred from other organs.

Angina's painful symptoms may result from decreased coronary artery blood flow, as from atherosclerosis or eating a heavy meal; decreased oxygen-carrying capacity of the blood, as from severe anemia; or increased myocardial work load, as from exertion.

Angina usually takes one of three main forms:
• Stable angina (also called predictable or chronic angina), in which pain occurs at a predictable level of physical or emotional stress, builds gradually, and reaches maximum intensity quickly.
• Unstable angina (also called preinfarction or crescendo angina, acute coronary insufficiency, or impending myocardial infarction [MI]), in which pain takes an unpredictable course and is more severe than in stable angina.
• Prinzmetal's angina (also called variant angina), in which pain usually occurs while the patient is at rest and resembles that of unstable angina. Occasionally, a patient may have both stable and Prinzmetal's angina.

Although angina's cardinal symptom is chest pain, the drugs used to treat angina are not analgesics. The antianginal agents discussed in this chapter are used to treat angina by reducing myocardial oxygen demand, by increasing myocardial oxygen supply, or by both mechanisms. The antianginal agents are classified into the following groups: nitrates, including erythrityl tetranitrate, isosorbide dinitrate, nitroglycerin, and pentaerythritol tetranitrate; beta-adrenergic blockers, especially metoprolol tartrate, nadolol, atenolol, and propranolol hydrochloride; and calcium channel blockers, including diltiazem hydrochloride, nifedipine, and verapamil hydrochloride. Other unclassified antianginals

include dipyridamole. (See *How antianginal agents relieve angina* on page 570 for a summary of how these antianginal agents function.)

These agents are often used in combination for best results. (See *Combination antianginal therapy* on page 567 for more details.)

For a summary of representative drugs, see *Selected major drugs: Antianginal agents* on page 579.

NITRATES

Nitrates include erythrityl tetranitrate, isosorbide dinitrate, nitroglycerin, and pentaerythritol tetranitrate. Used for many years to relieve angina, these drugs are available in multiple forms with several routes of administration. Nitrates act primarily as vasodilators, working directly on vascular smooth muscle to reduce the degree of vasoconstriction. Nitrates act primarily on venous but also on arterial smooth muscle.

History and source
In 1857, an English physician named Brunton used amyl nitrite to relieve angina in his patients, theorizing that it produced its effect by reducing blood pressure. Amyl nitrite is no longer used for this purpose, partly because of its high incidence of adverse reactions and partly because of its potential for abuse.

Nitroglycerin, first synthesized in 1846, was used by Murrell in 1879 to relieve and prevent angina. In 1933, Lewis proposed that nitroglycerin produced its effects by dilating the coronary arteries. In 1959, Gorlin found that coronary artery blood flow was little changed by nitroglycerin and suggested that the drug acted primarily on systemic blood vessels. Researchers now know that both these mechanisms contribute to the effectiveness of nitroglycerin.

The development of the other organic nitrates paralleled that of nitroglycerin.

PHARMACOKINETICS

The many routes for administering nitrates account, in part, for the pharmacokinetic differences among these drugs.

Absorption, distribution, metabolism, excretion
Sublingual, buccal, and chewable tablets and lingual aerosols are almost completely absorbed through the richly vascularized oral mucosa. This vascularization en-

Pharmacokinetics of nitrates

When administering a nitrate, remember that the route of administration determines the extent of absorption and the rapidity of action.

ROUTE OF ADMINISTRATION	EXTENT OF ABSORPTION	ONSET OF ACTION
Sublingual, buccal, or lingual	Almost 100% is absorbed through the richly vascularized oral mucous membranes.	2 to 5 minutes
Oral	About 50% to 60% is absorbed through the intestines.	20 to 60 minutes
Transdermal	Absorption rate varies among patients and types and sites of application.	30 to 60 minutes
I.V.	No absorption is necessary.	2 to 5 minutes

hances the direct absorption and transportation of nitrates through the internal jugular vein and superior vena cava into the right atrium. In a patient whose mouth is dry, absorption may take longer, and some of the drug may return to the heart via the lymphatic circulation.

Nitrate capsules or tablets that are swallowed are absorbed through the gastric and intestinal mucosa. Orally administered nitrates are only about 50% to 60% absorbed.

Transdermal nitrates are absorbed slowly. The quantity of drug applied, the location and area of skin used for administration, and the amount of cutaneous circulation affect the percentage absorbed, which varies. I.V. nitroglycerin, which does not require absorption, is delivered directly into the circulation.

Once in the body, nitrates are widely distributed, especially to the liver, heart, lungs, kidneys, spleen, and blood vessel walls. Nitroglycerin is approximately 60% bound to plasma proteins.

Nitrate metabolism occurs partly in the blood but mainly in the liver. The enzyme glutathione–organic nitrate reductase converts nitrates to metabolites that are much less active. This rapid conversion in the liver explains why higher doses are needed for oral nitrates, which undergo significant first-pass metabolism after absorption into the portal vein. Erythrityl is converted faster than nitroglycerin; however, isosorbide and pentaerythritol are converted more slowly than nitroglycerin.

Metabolite excretion occurs via the kidneys.

Onset, peak, duration

Onset of the antianginal action of nitrates begins within 2 to 5 minutes of I.V., sublingual, buccal, or lingual administration. The onset of action of the nitrate forms that are swallowed occurs in 20 to 60 minutes. The onset of action of transdermal nitroglycerin occurs in 30 to 60 minutes, with hemodynamic effects occurring within 1 hour. (See *Pharmacokinetics of nitrates* for a summary of how the route of administration affects absorption and onset of action.)

Peak concentration levels of the nitrates occur almost simultaneously with their onset of action. Peak hemodynamic effects of the transdermal and oral forms occur 1 to 2 hours after administration.

The rapidly acting nitrates absorbed in the mouth have the shortest duration of action: sublingual nitroglycerin is 20 to 30 minutes; sublingual erythrityl and isosorbide, up to 2 hours. Oral forms of the nitrates produce antianginal effects for up to 5 hours for erythrityl, isosorbide, and nitroglycerin and for up to 4 hours for pentaerythritol. The half-life of isosorbide is 45 minutes; however, the half-life of one of its active metabolites is 2 to 5 hours, prolonging its duration of action. The duration of action of sustained-release oral forms may persist for up to 12 hours.

For the various formulations of transdermal nitroglycerin, duration of action varies considerably. Nitroglycerin ointment exerts antianginal effects for 3 hours and hemodynamic effects for up to 6 hours. Longer-acting transdermal patches are replaced daily, although their actual duration of action may be somewhat less than 24 hours.

With a plasma half-life of only 1 to 4 minutes, I.V. nitroglycerin is active for only a short time after discontinuation of the infusion.

PHARMACODYNAMICS

Nitrates decrease preload and myocardial oxygen demand by dilating veins. They decrease afterload and may also increase myocardial oxygen supply by dilating arteries. In the coronary circulation, nitrates redistribute circulating blood flow, improving myocardial perfusion.

Mechanism of action

Nitrates act directly on vascular smooth muscle, producing relaxation and vessel dilation. These actions are independent of autonomic nervous system innervation of smooth muscle. Although veins have much less smooth muscle tissue than arteries have, nitrates dilate the veins considerably. Because the veins dilate, less blood is returned to the heart, decreasing the volume of blood in the ventricles at the end of diastole, when the ventricles are full. (This blood volume and resultant stretch in the ventricles is called *preload*.) By decreasing

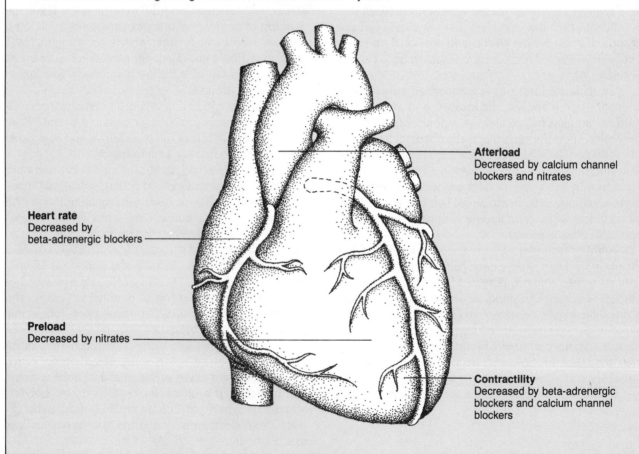

How antianginal agents relieve angina

Angina occurs when the coronary arteries, the heart's primary source of oxygen, supply insufficient oxygen to the myocardium. This increases the work load of the heart, increasing heart rate, preload, afterload, and force of myocardial contractility. The antianginal agents (nitrates, beta-adrenergic blockers, and calcium channel blockers) relieve angina by *decreasing* these four factors. Depending on the class of drug administered, myocardial oxygen demand may decrease or the myocardial blood supply may increase, or both. Also, nitrates and calcium channel blockers increase myocardial oxygen supply by producing coronary artery dilation. This diagram summarizes how antianginal agents affect the cardiovascular system.

Afterload
Decreased by calcium channel blockers and nitrates

Heart rate
Decreased by beta-adrenergic blockers

Preload
Decreased by nitrates

Contractility
Decreased by beta-adrenergic blockers and calcium channel blockers

Applying nitroglycerin ointment

The supplies for administration are a tube of nitroglycerin ointment and a sheet of nitroglycerin measurement paper.

1. After identifying the patient and explaining the procedure and medication, squeeze the prescribed amount of nitroglycerin ointment from the tube onto the special paper. Nitroglycerin is ordered and dispensed in inches. When squeezing the ointment onto the paper, allow it to flow freely from the tube. The diameter of the ointment on the paper should approximate the diameter of the tube opening.

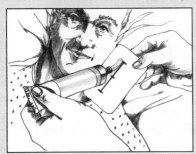

2. Place the paper on the skin medication-side-down against the skin. Spread the ointment evenly under the measurement paper. Do not rub the ointment into the skin.

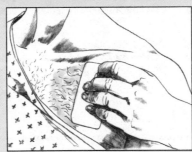

3. The chest, upper arm, and upper back are common administration sites. Other sites such as the lower leg or abdomen are also acceptable if cutaneous circulation is adequate. Administration sites should be rotated to decrease cutaneous irritation. The sheet of plastic placed over the nitroglycerin ointment increases the absorption of the medication.

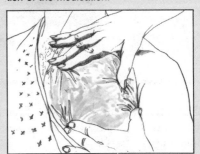

preload, nitrates reduce the myocardial demand for oxygen needed to pump blood out of the ventricles.

Nitrates also dilate arteries by direct action on arterial smooth muscle, independent of autonomic nervous system innervation. In the arterial system, most resistance to ejection of blood from the left ventricle occurs in the arterioles. The more the arterioles constrict, the more they resist left ventricular ejection. The amount of resistance is called *afterload*. Nitrates decrease afterload by dilating the arterioles, thereby decreasing the energy required for the heart to pump blood and reducing myocardial oxygen demand.

Besides decreasing myocardial oxygen demand, nitrates also promote coronary artery autoregulation to improve blood flow to ischemic areas of the myocardium and to decrease blood flow to unaffected areas. This combined effect may explain the nitrates' antianginal action. Nitrates' dilation of coronary arteries explains their effectiveness in relieving Prinzmetal's angina, which is caused by arterial spasm. Overall, their ability to decrease oxygen demand is usually more important than their ability to increase oxygen supply.

PHARMACOTHERAPEUTICS

Nitrates are indicated for immediate relief of angina, prevention of angina when an attack can be expected, and long-term prevention of chronic angina. These drugs are synergistic with certain beta-adrenergic blockers and with calcium channel blockers.

The rapidly absorbed nitrates, such as nitroglycerin, are the drugs of choice for relief of acute angina because of their rapid onset of action, ease of administration, and low cost. Daily application of the inconspicuous, long-acting nitroglycerin transdermal patch is convenient and effective for preventing chronic angina, especially for the patient who may have difficulty complying with a regimen requiring frequent doses. Oral nitrates have the advantage of seldom producing serious adverse reactions. I.V. nitroglycerin is most effective for relieving severe, acute angina because of its rapid onset of action and short half-life.

Most of the controversy associated with the use of nitrates concerns the best route of administration rather than which nitrate to administer. Of the following nitrates, the efficacy of nitroglycerin is the best established.

Most drug interactions with nitrates adversely affect the cardiovascular system and necessitate close patient monitoring by the nurse.

DRUG	INTERACTING DRUGS	POSSIBLE EFFECTS	NURSING IMPLICATIONS
erythrityl, isosorbide, nitroglycerin, pentaerythritol	alcohol	Causes severe hypotension	• Instruct the patient taking nitrates to avoid ingesting alcohol, and explain why.
	anticholinergics	Delay sublingual absorption because of dry mouth	• Offer the patient sips of water or a mouth rinse before administering a sublingual or buccal nitrate.
	antihypertensives (such as beta-adrenergic blockers, calcium channel blockers, diuretics, and vasodilators) and phenothiazines	Cause hypotension produced by additive effects on hemodynamics	• Monitor the patient closely for hypotension, especially after the first dose of a nitrate or an interacting drug.

erythrityl tetranitrate (Cardilate). Erythrityl is not used to relieve acute angina but to prevent expected and chronic angina attacks.

USUAL ADULT DOSAGE: for expected angina attacks, 10-mg chewable, sublingual, or buccal tablets; for long-term angina prevention, up to 100 mg/day in four or five doses.

isosorbide dinitrate (Isordil, Sorbitrate). Used to relieve acute angina and to prevent expected angina, isosorbide is taken as sublingual, buccal, or chewable tablets or as sustained-release capsules.

USUAL ADULT DOSAGE: for acute angina or prevention of attacks, 2.5 to 10 mg sublingually or buccally or as a chewable tablet, repeated twice at 5- to 10-minute intervals if relief is not obtained. For angina prevention, the dosage may be repeated every 2 to 3 hours, but initial dosage of the chewable tablet should be no more than 5 mg. For long-term prevention, 10 to 20 mg P.O. 3 or 4 times daily, or 20 to 40 mg of sustained-release capsules every 6 to 12 hours, or 80 mg every 8 to 12 hours.

nitroglycerin (Nitro-Bid, Nitrostat). Used for relieving acute and persistent angina, nitroglycerin is also used for long-term angina prevention.

USUAL ADULT DOSAGE: for acute angina attacks, 0.15 to 0.6 mg sublingually, or 0.4 mg of a metered-dose aerosol spray onto or under the tongue, repeated up to three times (this route is also used to prevent expected angina). For persistent angina, especially accompanying an acute MI, continuous I.V. infusion of 5 mcg/minute,

increased by 5 mcg every 3 to 5 minutes until pain is relieved. At higher doses, 10- to 20-mcg increases can be made at a time. Maximum dosage has not been established, and rates of up to 400 mcg/minute are sometimes used. For long-term prevention of angina, 1 to 3 mg of sustained-release tablets placed between the patient's upper gum and lips t.i.d. or q.i.d.; 2.5 to 9 mg of sustained-release capsules or tablets P.O. b.i.d. to q.i.d. Long-term prevention may also be accomplished with nitroglycerin 2% ointment applied to the skin in ½″ to 3″ doses or unit-dose equivalents every 3 to 4 hours. Alternatively, sustained-release transdermal patches that release 2.5 to 15 mg over 24 hours are used daily.

pentaerythritol tetranitrate (Duotrate, Peritrate). Used only for long-term prevention of angina, pentaerythritol is taken orally.

USUAL ADULT DOSAGE: for long-term prevention of angina, 10 mg P.O. q.i.d. increased to 40 mg q.i.d., as necessary; alternatively, sustained-release capsules or 30- to 80-mg tablets b.i.d.

Drug interactions

Hypotension results when nitrates interact with other antianginal and antihypertensive drugs, such as beta-adrenergic blockers, calcium channel blockers, diuretics, and vasodilators, or with phenothiazines or alcohol. Delayed absorption across the oral membrane may occur when the patient's mouth is dry from using a drug with anticholinergic effects, such as an antimuscarinic, a tricyclic antidepressant, a phenothiazine, or an antiparkinsonian drug. (See *Drug interactions: Nitrates* for a summary.)

ADVERSE DRUG REACTIONS

Most adverse reactions to nitrates are attributable to changes in the cardiovascular system. The reactions usually disappear when the dosage is reduced.

Predictable reactions

The decreased afterload produced by arteriolar dilation can cause hypotension that may be compounded by the reduced cardiac output after decreased preload. Hypotension is most noticeable when the patient assumes an upright position (orthostatic hypotension), because blood pressure is insufficient to perfuse the brain adequately. Besides a systolic blood pressure of less than 90 mm Hg, signs and symptoms of hypotension include syncope, dizziness, weakness, clammy skin, and nausea and vomiting. To compensate for the hypotension, the heart rate may increase to 150 or more beats per minute. However, this tachycardia may be counterproductive because the shortened diastolic time that results does not allow for adequate filling of the ventricles; therefore, cardiac output is further reduced.

Headache, the most common adverse reaction, is probably caused by blood vessel dilation in the meningeal layers between the brain and the skull. The pain may be severe and persistent but usually disappears after several days of nitrate administration. Headache may be relieved by acetaminophen. For patients receiving transdermal patch therapy, the application site does not affect the incidence of headache.

Transdermally applied nitrates occasionally cause local skin irritation. A generalized rash after any route of administration is uncommon, however, usually occurring only with pentaerythritol. Many patients report a stinging sensation from the sublingual tablets, but the effect is not objectionable and may even indicate that the tablets are fresh. A few patients taking nitrates experience transient flushing of the face and neck.

Tolerance to nitrates may develop over time, especially with high-dose, long-term therapy. Patients appear to develop tolerance not just to specific nitrates but to the entire class.

I.V. nitroglycerin can produce alcohol intoxication when large doses are administered for long periods. This reaction results from the alcohol used to preserve nitroglycerin in ampules or vials from which I.V. infusions are prepared. The most prominent alcohol intoxication signs are an additive hypotensive effect and depression of myocardial contractility.

Unpredictable reactions

Although rare, complete collapse of the cardiovascular system can occur even with normal doses. Signs of complete cardiovascular collapse include thready or absent peripheral pulses, loss of blood pressure, loss of consciousness, and urine and fecal incontinence.

Other unpredictable reactions include blurred vision, dry mouth, and increased peripheral edema.

NURSING IMPLICATIONS

Because nitrates are frequently prescribed, the nurse should be familiar with all aspects of their use. Patient teaching is an important element in nitrate therapy for angina.

• Be aware that nitrates are contraindicated for patients with angina from hypertrophic cardiomyopathy: the drugs may actually aggravate this type of angina. Nitrates are also contraindicated for patients with head trauma or increased intracranial pressure.
• Administer nitrates cautiously to patients with depleted intravascular fluid volume produced by dehydration, diuretic therapy, or limited fluid intake.
• Administer a patient's first nitrate dose as follows: Have the patient sit or lie down; take the patient's pulse and blood pressure before administration and again at the onset of action. If the patient becomes hypotensive, position the patient to facilitate venous return, such as in a supine or legs-elevated position, and recheck the blood pressure. If hypotension persists, remove the ointment or slow the I.V. infusion rate, notify the physician, and continue to monitor the patient's heart rate and blood pressure every 5 to 15 minutes.
• If the patient has a dry mouth, offer sips of water for swallowing or rinsing before administration of sublingual or buccal tablets because a dry mouth can inhibit absorption.
• When applying a subsequent dose of nitroglycerin ointment, remove the ointment remaining from the preceding dose and select a new administration site to avoid skin irritation. (See *Applying nitroglycerin ointment* on page 571 for more detailed information.) Remove a transdermal patch before electrical cardioversion.
• Prepare I.V. infusions of nitroglycerin cautiously. Mix the drug with dextrose 5% in water or normal saline solution in a glass bottle. Use administration tubing supplied by the manufacturer, if available, because nitroglycerin readily migrates into standard polyvinyl chloride (PVC) tubing, greatly reducing the amount actually administered. (Some manufacturers add chemicals to the ampules to prevent such migration.)

• With any patient receiving I.V. nitroglycerin, monitor the blood pressure and pulse every 5 to 15 minutes while titrating the dosage and every hour thereafter. Use an infusion pump and calculate the dose in mcg/minute in addition to ml/hour, using the tables supplied by the manufacturer.

• Instruct the patient to store sublingual nitroglycerin tablets away from heat sources, including the body; explain that the tablets maintain potency longer when kept in the original container. Also explain that, after opening the container, the patient should discard the cotton filler, because it may absorb some of the drug. Instruct the patient to replace the tablets with fresh ones every 3 months, even if many are left, and to discard the unused tablets.

• Instruct the patient to go to the nearest emergency room if angina is not relieved by three tablets taken 5 minutes apart and while resting. Explain that the pain may indicate an acute MI.

• Inform the patient using a lingual aerosol not to inhale the spray.

• Explain to the patient that nitroglycerin ointment may stain clothing and that plastic wrap can be used to cover the patch.

• Instruct the patient using long-acting patches to change them at the same time every day—right after showering, for example.

• Encourage the patient to avoid drinking alcoholic beverages while on nitrate therapy.

• Instruct the patient on oral nitrate therapy to take the tablets or capsules ½ hour before or 1 hour after meals, for better absorption.

• Instruct the patient not to stop taking nitrate medication without consulting the physician because vasospasm may follow abrupt discontinuation.

• Instruct the patient on sublingual nitrate therapy to take a dose a few minutes before engaging in activities known or expected to induce angina.

BETA-ADRENERGIC BLOCKERS

Also called *beta-adrenergic antagonists*, beta-adrenergic blockers are used for long-term prevention of angina. Propranolol hydrochloride, metoprolol tartrate, nadolol, and atenolol are the Food and Drug Administration (FDA)–approved antianginal agents. (See Chapter 20, Adrenergic Blocking Agents, for more information on beta-adrenergic blockers.)

History and source
The beta-adrenergic blockers are a relatively new drug class. In 1958, Powell and Slater reported the use of a beta-adrenergic blocker to selectively inhibit beta-receptor stimulation by epinephrine and norepinephrine.

PHARMACOKINETICS

Only oral preparations of beta-adrenergic blockers are used to treat angina. These agents display varying pharmacokinetic properties.

Absorption, distribution, metabolism, excretion
Propranolol and metoprolol, having moderate to high lipid solubility, are almost entirely absorbed from the gastrointestinal (GI) tract. Because atenolol and nadolol have a low lipid solubility, less than 50% of a dose of either drug is absorbed.

All these beta-adrenergic blockers are widely distributed, but only propranolol and metoprolol cross the blood-brain barrier. The liver extracts and binds a large portion of propranolol and metoprolol doses. Each of the beta-adrenergic blockers is plasma protein-bound as follows: propranolol, 90%; metoprolol, 12%; nadolol, 30%; and atenolol, 16%.

Propranolol is hydroxylated in the liver to form mildly active metabolites. Metoprolol is also hydroxylated but its metabolites are inactive. Nadolol and atenolol are unmetabolized.

Metabolites of propranolol and metoprolol are excreted in the urine. Unchanged, nadolol and atenolol are excreted in the urine and feces.

Onset, peak, duration
Because beta-adrenergic blockers are not used for relief of acute angina, their onset of action is difficult to measure. Propranolol usually appears in the plasma within 30 minutes; however, long-acting forms take longer. Metoprolol is present in the plasma within 10 minutes after oral administration. Corresponding data for nadolol are unavailable.

Peak concentration levels of propranolol occur within 60 to 90 minutes for tablets and within 6 hours for long-acting capsules; if the drug is taken with food, peak concentration levels are delayed but not reduced. Peak concentration levels of metoprolol occur within 90 minutes and are increased when the drug is taken with food. Nadolol and atenolol both reach peak concentration levels in 2 to 4 hours, regardless of food intake.

The duration of action of propranolol tablets is 4 to 6 hours; the duration of the long-acting capsules, up to 24 hours. The half-life of propranolol ranges from about 3 to 6 hours. The duration of action of metoprolol is about 6 hours; its half-life varies up to 4 hours. The duration of action of nadolol is also about 24 hours and its half-life ranges from 10 to 24 hours. The duration of action of atenolol is about 24 hours and its half-life is 6 to 9 hours.

Serum levels are not reliable for monitoring the effectiveness or toxicity of beta-adrenergic blockers.

PHARMACODYNAMICS

Beta-adrenergic blockers decrease blood pressure through one or more of several different mechanisms. (See Chapter 37, Antihypertensive Agents, for more information.) These drugs also block beta-receptor sites in the myocardium and in the electrical conduction system of the heart. Subsequently, decreased heart rate and diminshed force of myocardial contraction considerably reduce the heart's oxygen requirements.

Beta-adrenergic blockers do not dilate veins. In fact, the heart rate becomes slower and weaker, allowing more blood to collect in the ventricles at the end of diastole. This process actually causes a slight increase in both preload and myocardial oxygen demand. However, the combined actions of beta-adrenergic blockers decrease oxygen demand with little or no change in supply. The drugs also increase the patient's maximal exercise tolerance, because they prevent the angina that often accompanies exertion.

PHARMACOTHERAPEUTICS

Beta-adrenergic blockers are indicated for long-term prevention of angina, not for immediate relief of an angina attack or prevention of an imminent one. The drugs act synergistically with other antianginal agents. For example, because they decrease heart rate, the beta-adrenergic blockers are particularly useful for limiting the reflex tachycardia accompanying nitrate administration. However, because beta-adrenergic blockers also block peripheral vascular beta-receptors and allow some unopposed alpha constriction, they are of limited use in treating Prinzmetal's angina. Propranolol is twice as potent as nadolol.

propranolol hydrochloride (Inderal, Inderal LA). Used for the long-term prevention of angina, propranolol is also available in a long-acting form.

USUAL ADULT DOSAGE: 10 to 20 mg P.O. t.i.d. or q.i.d.; if needed, the dosage may be increased over several days up to 320 mg divided into four doses; alternatively, 80 to 160 mg of the long-acting form is administered once daily.

metoprolol tartrate (Lopressor). Used for long-term prevention of angina, the effects of metoprolol vary considerably among patients.
USUAL ADULT DOSAGE: 50 to 100 mg P.O. b.i.d. or t.i.d.

nadolol (Corgard). Used for long-term prevention of angina, nadolol has a long half-life.
USUAL ADULT DOSAGE: 40 mg P.O. once daily as an initial dose; if needed, the dosage is increased over several days up to 240 mg daily.

atenolol (Tenormin). This drug is used for the long-term prevention of angina.
USUAL ADULT DOSAGE: 50 mg P.O. once daily; after 1 week, the dose may be increased to 100 mg/day or even 200 mg/day in some patients.

Drug interactions
Beta-adrenergic blockers alter insulin and oral hypoglycemic agent requirements, and their effect of slowing the heart rate is additive when administered concurrently with digoxin. Increased hypotension may result from administering beta-adrenergic blockers with antiarrhythmics, antihypertensives, or phenothiazines. Aminophylline antagonizes beta-adrenergic blockers, and cimetidine inhibits the metabolism of propranolol. (See *Drug interactions: Beta-adrenergic blockers* on page 576 for a summary of the possible effects of concurrent administration.)

ADVERSE DRUG REACTIONS

The most common adverse reactions to beta-adrenergic blockers involve the cardiovascular system and occur when the drug is first administered.

Predictable reactions
Because they inhibit sinus node stimulation, beta-adrenergic blockers can cause bradycardia and hypotension with peripheral vascular insufficiency. Angina, syncope, or shock may accompany these reactions. Fluid retention and peripheral edema also may occur.

Because of decreased force of myocardial contractility and increased preload, congestive heart failure may be exacerbated or precipitated. Dysrhythmias, especially atrioventricular (AV) block, also can occur.

DRUG INTERACTIONS
Beta-adrenergic blockers

Beta-adrenergic blocking agents can interact with several types of frequently administered drugs, resulting in serious implications for the patient. The nurse should be aware of these interactions to provide quality patient care.

DRUG	INTERACTING DRUGS	POSSIBLE EFFECTS	NURSING IMPLICATIONS
propranolol, meto-prolol, atenolol, na-dolol	antiarrhythmics	Cause hypotension	• Monitor the patient's blood pressure when initiating or adjusting the dose as prescribed.
	anticholinergics, antimuscarinics	Cause mutual inhibition of effects; dysrhythmias	• Monitor the patient's heart rate for irregularities.
	oral hypoglycemics, insulin	Cause hyperglycemia or masking of heart-rate and blood-pressure signs of hypoglycemia	• Monitor the patient's blood glucose level more frequently when initiating beta-adrenergic blocker therapy. Beta-adrenergic blockers do not mask diaphoresis or the decreased level of consciousness that can accompany hypoglycemia; monitor the patient carefully for these adverse reactions.
	antihypertensives	Cause hypotension	• Monitor the patient's blood pressure when initiating or adjusting a dose as prescribed.
	cimetidine	Decreases metabolism of propranolol and metoprolol	• Monitor the patient for adverse reactions, which may occur more frequently.
	clonidine	Impairs blood pressure control; clonidine-withdrawal hypertension	• Monitor the patient's blood pressure; adjust clonidine as ordered, and slowly taper off the beta-adrenergic blocker before slowly tapering off clonidine, as ordered.
	digoxin	Causes bradycardia (heart rate less than 60 beats per minute)	• Monitor the patient's pulse frequently when initiating or adjusting a dose.
	phenothiazines	Cause hypotension	• Monitor the patient's blood pressure when initiating or adjusting a dose.
	sympathomimetics	Cause mutual inhibition of effects	• Monitor the patient for therapeutic effects of both agents.
	xanthines	Cause mutual inhibition of effects	• Monitor the patient's theophylline level.

Adverse central nervous system (CNS) reactions include dizziness, fatigue, lethargy, and decreased libido. Occasional GI reactions, such as nausea, vomiting, and diarrhea, are usually transient.

Significant bronchoconstriction can result from bronchial beta-receptor blockade, which otherwise dilates bronchioles. This adverse reaction is more likely to occur with propranolol and nadolol, which are nonselective beta-adrenergic blockers, but also can occur with high doses of atenolol and metoprolol.

Unpredictable reactions

Rashes, blood dyscrasias, mental depression, and vivid dreams may occur but are rare. CNS reactions occur most frequently with propranolol therapy.

NURSING IMPLICATIONS

The nurse should carefully assess the patient's condition before administering a beta-adrenergic blocker, because these drugs have several significant contraindications.
• Be aware that beta-adrenergic blockers are usually contraindicated for patients with asthma, sinus bradycardia, second- or third-degree heart block, cardiogenic

shock, right ventricular failure secondary to pulmonary hypertension, or peripheral vascular disease.

• Administer beta-adrenergic blockers cautiously to patients with diabetes mellitus, congestive heart failure, or chronic obstructive pulmonary disease.

• Withhold the dose and notify the physician if the patient's apical pulse is less than 60 beats per minute or the systolic blood pressure is less than 90 mm Hg.

• Instruct the patient taking propranolol or metoprolol to take the drug at the same time each day in relation to meals, to prevent changes in absorption. Explain to the patient taking nadolol or atenolol that the drug can be taken regardless of mealtimes.

• Instruct patients never to discontinue beta-adrenergic blocking agents abruptly. Rather, the drugs should be tapered off over several days, according to the physician's prescription. Rapid discontinuation may precipitate angina, hypertension, dysrhythmias, or an acute MI.

CALCIUM CHANNEL BLOCKERS

A class of drugs consisting of diltiazem hydrochloride, nifedipine, and verapamil hydrochloride, calcium channel blockers produce antianginal effects by mechanisms different from those of the nitrates or the beta-adrenergic blockers. For this reason, these drugs are often used to prevent angina that is unresponsive to drugs in either of the other antianginal classes.

History and source
In the early 1960s, Hass and Hartfelder noted that verapamil dilated blood vessels via mechanisms different from those of the nitrates. Other investigators discovered that diltiazem and nifedipine—although quite different in chemical structure—demonstrated effects similar to those of verapamil. In 1967, Fleckenstein suggested that verapamil produced its effect by inhibiting calcium ion movement into cells. Later, the French investigators Rougier and Coraboeuf documented that cardiac cells were depolarized not only by rapid influx of sodium ions but also by a slower influx of calcium ions. Thus, calcium channel blockers are also known as *slow channel blockers* or *calcium antagonists*.

PHARMACOKINETICS

Although they produce similar effects, the various calcium channel blockers have very different chemical structures. These structural differences may explain the pharmacokinetic differences among these drugs.

Absorption, distribution, metabolism, excretion
When administered sublingually, nifedipine is quickly and almost completely absorbed. After oral administration, 80% of diltiazem and 90% of nifedipine and verapamil is absorbed from the GI tract. Because of the first-pass effect, however, the bioavailability of these agents is much lower—only 20% for verapamil, 65% to 70% for nifedipine, and 40% for diltiazem. The calcium channel blockers are highly bound to plasma proteins in the following amounts: diltiazem, 80%; nifedipine and verapamil, over 90%.

All calcium channel blockers are rapidly and almost completely metabolized in the liver. Some metabolites of diltiazem and verapamil are active, but those of nifedipine are inactive. The metabolites of all of these agents are excreted mostly in the urine and also in the feces. Only 2% to 4% of the drug is excreted unchanged in the urine.

Onset, peak, duration
Antianginal effects begin within 30 minutes after an oral dose of diltiazem. The onset of action of oral nifedipine is 10 minutes; of verapamil, 30 to 60 minutes. Peak concentration levels of oral diltiazem occur within 2 to 3 hours; of nifedipine, within 30 minutes; and of verapamil, 30 to 60 minutes after an oral dose.

In the absence of significant hepatic disease, the half-lives of the calcium channel blockers are as follows: diltiazem and nifedipine, 3 to 4 hours; verapamil, 5 to 7 hours. The half life of verapamil increases with prolonged administration. Norverapamil, a metabolite of verapamil with less vasodilator properties, has a half-life of 8 to 12 hours.

PHARMACODYNAMICS

By blocking the flow of calcium ions into myocardial muscle cells and myocardial pacemaker cells, calcium channel blockers produce several effects in the heart. (See the section on calcium channel blockers in Chapter 35, Antiarrhythmic Agents, for more information about these effects.) Calcium channel blockers also act on vascular smooth muscle cells.

Mechanism of action

By preventing the influx of calcium ions into myocardial and vascular smooth muscle cells, calcium channel blockers inhibit the intracellular release of additional stores of calcium ions. These intracellular calcium ions would otherwise bind to the troponin-tropomyosin complex and allow actin and myosin to interact. The sliding of actin and myosin filaments past each other produces the contraction of a myocardial cell and ultimately of the whole ventricle. Thus, by inhibiting the release of intracellular calcium ions, calcium channel blockers decrease the force of myocardial contractility, thereby decreasing the oxygen demand.

Calcium channel blockers also prevent entry of calcium ions into arteriolar smooth muscle cells. This action decreases arteriolar constriction and so decreases systemic vascular resistance, or afterload. Decreasing afterload also decreases myocardial oxygen demand.

Decreased myocardial oxygen demand also results when calcium channel blockers are used to slow the heart rate, regulated by the sinus node, and to decrease conduction velocity in the heart's conducting pathways, regulated by the AV node. This mechanism is probably significant only for patients with rapid heart rates.

Beside decreasing myocardial oxygen demand, calcium channel blockers increase the oxygen supply to the myocardium by dilating the coronary arteries. Because calcium channel blockers do not appreciably induce venous dilation, they have little effect on preload.

PHARMACOTHERAPEUTICS

Calcium channel blockers are indicated only for the long-term prevention of angina. They are not routinely used to relieve acute attacks or to prevent expected ones. Calcium channel blockers are particularly effective in the

---

DRUG INTERACTIONS

Calcium channel blockers

Most drug interactions associated with calcium channel blockers result in adverse effects on the cardiovascular system. The nurse must be aware of these interactions to monitor for these effects and to intervene appropriately.

DRUG	INTERACTING DRUGS	POSSIBLE EFFECTS	NURSING IMPLICATIONS
diltiazem, nifedipine, verapamil	antihypertensives	Cause hypotension	• Monitor the patient's blood pressure frequently when initiating or adjusting the dose.
	cimetidine	Decreases hepatic clearance of the calcium channel blocker	• Monitor the patient for adverse reactions, which may occur more frequently. • Monitor the patient for orthostatic hypotension and for heart rate and rhythm changes.
	digoxin	Increases serum digoxin level	• Monitor the patient for bradycardia and nausea and vomiting. • Monitor the patient's serum digoxin levels.
	highly protein-bound drugs (oral anticoagulants, oral hypoglycemics, anti-inflammatory agents, quinidine, sulfinpyrazone)	Alter serum levels of either drug	• Monitor the patient for increased therapeutic effects and adverse reactions.
verapamil	disopyramide phosphate	Causes myocardial depression	• Do not administer these drugs within 24 hours of each other; if concurrent administration is necessary, monitor the patient for signs of congestive heart failure or decreased peripheral perfusion.
	calcium salts, vitamin D	Decrease effects of verapamil	• Do not administer concurrently; if necessary to do so, monitor the patient for effectiveness of verapamil therapy and for signs of hypercalcemia.

SELECTED MAJOR DRUGS

Antianginal agents

This chart summarizes the major antianginal agents currently in clinical use.

DRUG	MAJOR INDICATIONS	USUAL ADULT DOSAGES	NURSING IMPLICATIONS
Nitrate			
nitroglycerin	Relief of acute angina attack	0.15 to 0.6 mg sublingually for three doses, or 5 to 400 mcg/min I.V. until relief is obtained	• This drug is contraindicated in patients with hypertrophic cardiomyopathy, head trauma, or increased intracranial pressure.
	Prevention of expected attack	0.15 to 0.6 mg sublingually for three doses	• Administer the drug cautiously if the patient has a depleted intravascular fluid volume.
	Long-term prevention of angina	1 to 3 ml/g of a sustained-release tablet between the upper lip and gum t.i.d. or q.i.d., or a sustained-release transdermal patch 2.5 to 15 mg over 24 hours	• Monitor the patient's pulse and blood pressure before and after the first dose. • If the patient experiences delayed absorption from dry mouth, offer sips of water before administration. • Rotate administration sites for ointment and patches to avoid irritation. • Mix the I.V. solution in a glass bottle, using special tubing, if available. Monitor the patient's blood pressure at least every 15 minutes while adjusting the infusion rate. • Teach the patient the proper self-administration of several forms of nitroglycerin, as prescribed.
Beta-adrenergic blocker			
propranolol	Long-term prevention of angina	10 to 20 mg P.O. t.i.d. or q.i.d., increased up to 80 mg q.i.d., or 80 to 160 mg of the long-acting form P.O. daily.	• This drug is contraindicated in patients with asthma, sinus bradycardia, second- or third-degree heart block, diabetes mellitus, or peripheral vascular disease. • Administer the drug cautiously to the patients with congestive heart failure (CHF) or chronic obstructive pulmonary disease. • Withhold the dose and notify the physician if the patient's pulse is less than 60 beats per minute or if the systolic blood pressure is less than 90 mm Hg. • Teach the patient to take the drug at the same time each day.
Calcium blocker			
nifedipine	Long-term prevention of angina, especially if Prinzmetal's angina also is present	10 to 40 mg P.O. t.i.d., gradually increased to 40 mg P.O. q.i.d.	• Administer the drug cautiously to patients with hypotension, CHF, conduction abnormalities, or hepatic impairment. • Withhold the dose and notify the physician if the patient's pulse is less than 60 beats per minute or if the systolic blood pressure is less than 90 mm Hg.

prevention of Prinzmetal's angina, for which they are the drug of choice. Nifedipine produces the greatest arteriolar dilation, followed by verapamil and then diltiazem. Nifedipine also has little or no effect on the sinus and AV nodes. Calcium channel blockers do not promote bronchoconstriction and do not exacerbate peripheral vascular disease. They act synergistically with other antianginal agents.

diltiazem hydrochloride (Cardizem). This drug is used for the long-term prevention of angina.
USUAL ADULT DOSAGE: initially, 30 mg P.O. before meals q.i.d.; if necessary, gradually increase to 60 mg q.i.d.

nifedipine (Adalat, Procardia). This drug is used for the long-term prevention of angina.
USUAL ADULT DOSAGE: 10 mg P.O. t.i.d., gradually increasing up to 40 mg q.i.d., if needed.

verapamil hydrochloride (Calan, Isoptin). Verapamil is used for the long-term prevention of angina.
USUAL ADULT DOSAGE: 240 to 480 mg P.O., divided into three or four doses daily.

Drug interactions
Calcium channel blockers may interact with beta-adrenergic blockers, causing heart block or even congestive heart failure. They also may displace protein-bound digoxin, resulting in digoxin toxicity. Similar interactions (especially with verapamil) may occur between the calcium channel blockers and such other highly protein-bound drugs as warfarin sodium, phenytoin, salicylates, sulfonamides, and sulfonylureas. Calcium channel blockers also enhance the effects of antihypertensives. Interaction with dietary calcium is possible; however this has not been established. (See *Drug interactions: Calcium channel blockers* on page 578 for a summary of these interactions.)

ADVERSE DRUG REACTIONS

Calcium channel blockers frequently produce adverse cardiovascular reactions. They may also affect the GI tract and other body systems.

Predictable reactions
Undesirable alterations in the cardiovascular system are the most common and serious adverse reactions to the calcium channel blockers. Because they decrease after-

load and the force of ventricular contraction, calcium channel blockers sometimes predictably cause hypotension, including orthostatic hypotension. Dysrhythmias such as bradycardia, sinus block, and AV block result from inhibition of the sinus and AV nodes, especially by diltiazem and verapamil. The depressant action on myocardial contractility may account for the onset or worsening of congestive heart failure.

Vasodilation can produce dizziness, headache, flushing, weakness, and persistent peripheral edema. Other possible adverse reactions include GI disturbances, such as nausea, vomiting, and diarrhea, and muscle fatigue and cramps.

Unpredictable reactions
Calcium channel blockers also cause several unpredictable reactions. These include worsening of angina and skin eruptions, photosensitivity, pruritus, nasal congestion, and mood changes.

NURSING IMPLICATIONS

The nurse must be aware of the following considerations when administering calcium channel blockers.
• Administer calcium channel blockers cautiously to patients with hypotension, congestive heart failure, sick sinus syndrome, or AV conduction disturbances.
• Administer diltiazem cautiously to patients with renal or hepatic impairment.
• Withhold the dose and notify the physician if the patient's heart rate is less than 60 beats per minute or if the systolic blood pressure is less than 90 mm Hg.

OTHER ANTIANGINALS

Another drug sometimes used as an antianginal agent is dipyridamole (Persantine). In theory, dipyridamole dilates coronary arteries, thereby increasing the myocardial oxygen supply. In several studies, however, the drug did not significantly relieve angina. Possible adverse reactions include worsening angina, dizziness, headache, and GI upset. Dipyridamole is best absorbed on an empty stomach. The usual adult dosage is 50 mg P.O. t.i.d.

CHAPTER SUMMARY

Chapter 36 discussed nitrates, beta-adrenergic blockers, and calcium channel blockers as they are used to prevent or relieve angina. Here are the highlights of the chapter:

• The coronary arteries supply the heart with the blood it needs for nutrition and oxygen.

• Angina is a symptom of myocardial ischemia. Angina may result from atherosclerosis, which causes narrowing of the coronary arteries. Sometimes coronary artery spasm (associated with Prinzmetal's angina) also contributes to angina.

• Antianginal agents prevent or relieve this ischemia by decreasing myocardial oxygen demand, increasing myocardial oxygen supply, or both.

• Factors affecting oxygen demand include heart rate, force of myocardial contractility, preload, and afterload.

• Nitrates are used for the immediate relief of angina, prevention of an expected angina attack, and long-term prevention of chronic angina.

• Nitrates dilate veins, thereby decreasing preload. To a lesser extent, nitrates also dilate arteries, thereby decreasing afterload. Although they may be administered by multiple routes, nitrates provide the fastest relief when given sublingually or buccally. Nitrates include erythrityl tetranitrate, isosorbide dinitrate, nitroglycerin, and pentaerythritol tetranitrate.

• Beta-adrenergic blockers, which include propranolol hydrochloride, metoprolol tartrate, nadolol, and atenolol, are used for the long-term prevention of angina.

• Beta-adrenergic blockers depress myocardial contractility and heart rate, thereby decreasing myocardial oxygen demand. They also may cause hypotension.

• Calcium channel blockers include diltiazem hydrochloride, nifedipine, and verapamil hydrochloride. These drugs, which dilate arteries and depress myocardial contractility, are especially useful in preventing Prinzmetal's angina. They may produce adverse reactions in the cardiovascular system.

• Combination antianginal therapy is often the most effective means of relieving angina.

BIBLIOGRAPHY

American Hospital Formulary Service. *Drug Information 87.* McEvoy, G.K., et al., eds. Bethesda, Md.: American Society of Hospital Pharmacists, 1987.

American Medical Association. *Drug Evaluations,* 6th ed. Philadelphia: W.B. Saunders Co., 1986.

Craig, C.R., et al., eds. *Modern Pharmacology,* 2nd ed. Boston: Little, Brown & Co., 1986.

Gilman, A.G., et al., eds. *Goodman and Gilman's The Pharmacological Basis of Therapeutics,* 7th ed. New York: Macmillan Publishing Co., 1985.

Kastrap, E.K., et al., eds. *Facts and Comparisons.* St. Louis: Facts and Comparisons Division, J.B. Lippincott Co., 1987.

CHAPTER 37

ANTIHYPERTENSIVE AGENTS

OBJECTIVES

After reading and studying this chapter, you should be able to:

1. Differentiate between essential and secondary hypertension and describe the various stages of hypertension.

2. Describe the physiologic processes involved in homeostatic blood pressure regulation.

3. Explain the use of antihypertensive agents in the stepped-care approach to antihypertensive therapy.

4. Identify the major adverse reactions that occur with sympatholytic, vasodilating, and angiotensin antagonist agents.

5. List at least three examples of drugs in each of the three major classes of antihypertensive agents.

6. Compare the mechanisms of action of drugs in the three classes of antihypertensive agents.

7. Identify at least three general nursing implications related to antihypertensive therapy.

8. List at least three specific nursing implications related to each class of antihypertensive agents.

INTRODUCTION

Antihypertensive agents, which act to reduce blood pressure, are used to treat hypertension, a vascular disorder characterized by elevation in systolic pressure, diastolic pressure, or both.

Affecting about 60 million Americans, hypertension is closely associated with certain risk factors, such as age-, gender-, and race-related factors, obesity, a positive family history, high sodium intake, stress, diabetes mellitus, cigarette smoking, and hypercholesterolemia. For example, more men than women under age 50 develop hypertension, but men and women over age 50 have an approximately equal incidence. Hypertension also affects more blacks (27%) than whites (15%), with men and blacks developing cardiovascular complications more frequently than women and whites.

Early detection, effective treatment, and regular follow-up are critical in preventing the serious consequences of uncontrolled hypertension. Although hypertension produces few symptoms at first, the constant elevated pressure on the vessel walls can lead to cardiovascular complications that may affect the heart, eyes, kidneys, and central nervous system (CNS). Hemorrhagic and thrombotic stroke, ischemic heart disease including angina and myocardial infarction (MI), congestive heart failure (CHF), and chronic renal failure can result.

Homeostatic blood pressure regulation

Several homeostatic mechanisms regulate blood pressure. Cardiac output (CO) primarily determines the systolic blood pressure; total peripheral resistance (TPR) chiefly determines the diastolic pressure (DP); and together, the cardiac output and total peripheral resistance determine the mean arterial pressure (MAP), which is expressed by the formula:

$$MAP = CO \times TPR$$

MAP can also be expressed in terms of pulse pressure (PP), which is calculated by subtracting the diastolic from the systolic pressure. The following formula expresses this method of MAP determination:

$$MAP = DP + \frac{1}{3} PP$$

Short-term regulation of blood pressure involves the nervous and endocrine systems. A decrease in blood pressure stimulates the sympathetic nervous system, promoting the secretion of the hormones epinephrine and norepinephrine. In the sympathetic nervous system, epinephrine and norepinephrine increase the blood pressure by stimulating the beta$_1$ receptors in the heart to increase cardiac output. They also stimulate the alpha$_1$ receptors in the blood vessels, constricting and increasing their resistance to blood flow. (In the CNS, norepinephrine decreases blood pressure.) Sympathetic nervous system stimulation also involves medullary

The stepped-care approach to antihypertensive therapy

In this approach, a single, mild antihypertensive drug is initially prescribed, followed by an increased dose of the same drug. Then the physician adds or substitutes one drug after another in gradually increasing doses, as needed, until the patient achieves a predetermined blood pressure goal, experiences intolerable adverse reactions, or reaches the maximum dose of each drug.

The patient on stepped-care therapy requires blood pressure monitoring. Depending on the results, the physician may adjust the patient's therapy, as appropriate, by stepping the regimen up or down. With some exceptions, therapy usually continues for life. After the patient has maintained good blood pressure control for more than 3 months, the physician will step his therapy down as long as this does not compromise control. If the patient is on a single drug and the diastolic pressure remains continuously below 80 mm Hg, the physician will probably stop the medication temporarily to see if the patient can maintain normal pressure.

SUMMARY OF THE STEPPED-CARE APPROACH

Step 1
The patient receives a thiazide-like diuretic (or, in some cases, a beta blocker) as the initial therapy. In most paients with mild hypertension, a diuretic or a beta blocker alone controls blood pressure. Most thiazide-like diuretics and many beta blockers prove effective when taken once daily. The physician will probably choose a diuretic if the patient is over age 50 or black or has peripheral vascular disease, asthma, or chronic pulmonary disease. Using the smallest effective diuretic dose minimizes adverse reactions. If the patient is under age 50 or has ischemic heart disease, the physician may choose a beta blocker initially. Beta blockers usually reduce blood pressure to the level achieved with diuretics.

If these drugs do not control the patient's blood pressure (or if adverse reactions limit the use of other drugs), the physician may add an angiotensin-converting enzyme inhibitor at this point or at Steps 2, 3, or 4.

Step 2
If the patient does not respond to diuretic therapy, the physician will add small doses of a sympatholytic (adrenergic-inhibitor) agent, such as a beta blocker. Similarly, if the patient began therapy with a beta blocker but did not respond, the physician will add a diuretic or substitute a diuretic for the beta blocker. If these measures do not control blood pressure, the physician may order full doses of the step-2 drug or may substitute another sympatholitic. Or, instead of increasing the step-2 drug dose to the maximum, a direct vasodilator or calcium channel blocker may be added. Smaller doses of two drugs with different mechanisms of action may prove more effective than larger doses of a single drug. This approach frequently minimizes adverse reactions without significantly reducing effectiveness.

Step 3
If a third drug is needed, a vasodilating agent may be added. Hydralazine and oxidil are most frequently given, but a calcium channel blocker may be used instead. The drug chosen is administered in combination with a sympatholytic agent (step 2) and a diuretic (step 1).

Step 4
If the first three steps of therapy are ineffective and reasons other than drug failure have been ruled out, guanethidine may be added in increasing doses, as needed, or substituted for one of the step-2 or step-3 drugs.

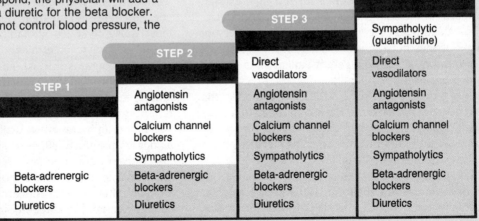

vasomotor center control of blood pressure. With a decrease in blood volume, baroreceptors in the aorta and the carotid sinuses adjust the heart rate and blood vessel resistance, thus restoring normal blood pressure.

Long-term regulation of blood pressure involves the renin-angiotensin-aldosterone system. When the blood pressure is decreased, the kidneys secrete renin, which acts on plasma protein to produce angiotensin I. The enzyme peptidyl dipeptidase then converts angiotensin I to angiotensin II, a potent vasoconstrictor. Aldosterone, a mineralocorticoid released in response to angiotensin II, acts on the kidneys to decrease sodium and water excretion. That increases the blood volume and blood pressure, at which point the renin-angiotensin-aldosterone system is inhibited, and the kidneys excrete more fluid. That reduces the blood volume, decreasing blood pressure.

Types of hypertension

When homeostatic mechanisms fail to regulate blood pressure, essential (primary), or secondary hypertension may develop. In the early phases of essential hypertension, which affects about 95% of all hypertensive patients, CO may be normal or mildly elevated. But as hypertension progresses, peripheral resistance increases and CO decreases, possibly resulting in left ventricular hypertrophy and congestive heart failure.

Secondary hypertension affects about 5% of hypertensive patients and results from such underlying disorders as aortic regurgitation, renal stenosis, pheochromocytoma, and neurologic diseases. Treatment of the underlying disorder can sometimes cure secondary hypertension.

Either form of hypertension can occur to varying degrees. According to the World Health Organization's Expert Committee on Hypertension, hypertension is present when the systolic pressure is 160 mm Hg or higher and the diastolic pressure is 95 mm Hg or higher. The Report of the Joint National Committee on Detection, Evaluation, and Treatment of High Blood Pressure further classifies hypertension based on an average of two or more readings on different patient visits.

Mild hypertension refers to a diastolic pressure between 90 and 104 mm Hg. Usually asymptomatic, the patient may not need medication but will need to reduce risk factors, such as excessive sodium intake, obesity, or smoking. If the blood pressure remains elevated, however, drug therapy may be initiated.

Moderate hypertension refers to a consistently elevated diastolic pressure, between 105 and 114 mm Hg. If it remains uncontrolled, this degree of hypertension will cause organ damage. Therefore, the patient will probably require therapy with an antihypertensive agent and a diuretic. Moderate hypertension may cause a few minor symptoms, including headache, dizziness, and epistaxis.

Severe hypertension refers to a diastolic pressure of 115 mm Hg or more. The patient is symptomatic and may experience damage to the heart, kidneys, and other organs as well as to the retinas. A patient with severe hypertension will require therapy with a potent antihypertensive agent and a diuretic.

Hypertensive crisis is a medical emergency manifested by a diastolic pressure above 140 mm Hg. Untreated, it is likely to result in severe tissue and organ damage—such as retinopathy, heart failure, renal failure, and encephalopathy. Hypertensive crisis requires aggressive parenteral treatment with a fast-acting vasodilator to reduce the diastolic pressure to 100 mm Hg or less.

Malignant hypertension also constitutes a medical emergency. It is characeirzed by a diastolic blood pressure greater than 140 mm Hg and eye ground changes, including papilledema. It also requires aggressive parenterant therapy with a potent, rapid-acting vasodilator.

Isolated systolic hypertension is characterized by a systolic blood pressure greater than 160 mm Hg and a diastolic pressure less than 90 mm Hg. Antihypertensive therapy to treat this condition is very individualized.

Assessment and treatment

While documenting the patient's history, the nurse should identify all existing risk factors, such as high sodium intake, cigarette smoking, or a family history of hypertension or early cardiac mortality. The nurse should also ask about previous antihypertensive therapy and symptoms of possible complications, such as chest pain, dyspnea, edema, or altered neurologic or renal function.

During the physical examination, the nurse should focus on the cardiovascular and target organ systems, monitoring the vital signs, examining the fundus of each eye, and assessing the heart, lungs, and neurologic system. Finally, the nurse should obtain baseline data from serum electrolyte determinations, renal function tests, electrocardiograms (EKGs), and chest X-rays.

After the diagnosis of hypertension has been confirmed, the nurse assists in implementing the prescribed nondrug or drug therapy.

Nondrug treatments—which should begin as soon as hypertension is diagnosed and continue throughout the course of antihypertensive treatment—include various life-style modifications. For example, through biofeedback, the patient can learn to relax to help control blood pressure. Regular aerobic exercise can also lower blood pressure and may help protect against coronary artery disease by elevating blood levels of high-density lipoproteins (HDL), conjugated proteins that help protect the heart. Regular exercise can also help the patient maintain a normal weight or lose excess weight. Dietary modifications can help control hypertension in several ways. A well-balanced reducing diet can help an obese patient lose excess weight—a very significant risk factor. A low-sodium diet can help control fluid volume. Paradoxically, alcohol consumption may help control hypertension—or promote it. A diet that includes one to two alcoholic drinks per day can increase the cardiac-protective HDL levels. However, when the alcohol intake reaches five or more drinks per day, hypertension may occur. The hypertensive patient should drink only in moderation.

Many patients require antihypertensive drug therapy. Antihypertensive agents do not cure hypertension; they only decrease the blood pressure. That is why some patients need long-term antihypertensive therapy.

Antihypertensive agents may be sympatholytics, vasodilators, angiotensin antagonists, or diuretics. (See Chapter 38, Diuretic Agents, for further information about these drugs.) Antihypertensive agents share the same therapeutic objective: to decrease the diastolic blood pressure below 90 mm Hg without producing undesirable adverse reactions.

The American Heart Association advocates the stepped-care approach to antihypertensive therapy. With this approach, the physician uses, as the first step in therapy, the drug or combination of drugs least likely to produce adverse reactions. Subsequent steps involve adding to the initial drug (or drugs), or substituting another drug or drug combination, until the desired blood pressure or maximum effective dose is reached, or intolerable adverse reactions are detected. (See *The stepped-care approach to antihypertensive therapy* on page 583 for further information.) In nonemergency circumstances, stepped-care therapy can reduce the blood pressure to an acceptable level in most patients within 6 months.

For a summary of representative drugs, see *Selected major drugs: Antihypertensive agents* on pages 602 and 603.

SYMPATHOLYTIC AGENTS

The sympatholytics include various groups of drugs that reduce blood pressure by inhibiting or blocking motor and secretory action in the sympathetic nervous system.

They are classified by their site or mechanism of action and include central-acting sympathetic nervous system inhibitors, ganglionic blocking agents, beta-adrenergic blocking agents, alpha-adrenergic blocking agents, mixed alpha- and beta-adrenergic blocking agents, and norepinephrine depletors.

Central-acting sympathetic nervous system inhibitors act in the CNS to reduce sympathetic activity and thus decrease arteriolar vasoconstriction. This group of sympatholytics includes methyldopa, clonidine hydrochloride, guanabenz acetate, and guanfacine.

Ganglionic blocking agents interfere with the transmission of sympathetic and parasympathetic nerve impulses through the ganglia, producing vasodilation and decreasing the blood pressure. Drugs in this group include mecamylamine hydrochloride and trimethaphan camsylate.

Beta-adrenergic blocking agents—propranolol hydrochloride, metoprolol tartrate, nadolol, atenolol, pindolol, and timolol maleate—compete with epinephrine for beta-receptor sites, antagonizing the effect of epinephrine, a sympathetic neurotransmitter, and blocking sympathetic stimulation, resulting in a decreased cardiac output.

Alpha-adrenergic blocking agents act on the sympathetic nervous system alpha receptors, preventing norepinephrine and epinephrine from occupying and activating them. With sympathetic stimulation blocked, vasodilation occurs. This class of drugs includes phentolamine, prazosin hydrochloride, and terazosin.

Labetalol is a mixed alpha- and beta-adrenergic blocking agent. This new type of antihypertensive agent nonselectively blocks beta-adrenergic receptors and selectively blocks alpha$_1$ receptors.

Norepinephrine depletors interfere with the synthesis, storage, and release of norepinephrine from the nerve terminals. This interference leads to a loss of peripheral sympathetic tone, decreasing peripheral resistance and leading to a reduction in blood pressure. Norepinephrine depletors include reserpine, guanethidine sulfate, and guanadrel sulfate. (They are sometimes referred to as *peripheral-acting sympatholytic agents*.)

History and source

In the 1940s, researchers demonstrated that excision of the thoracic sympathetic chain reduced blood pressure. That finding led to the investigation of chemical sympatholytics as antihypertensive agents. A phenylalanine derivative, methyldopa, was one of the first drugs tested and remains one of the most widely used antihypertensive agents.

First used as a nasal decongestant, the imidazole derivative clonidine was noted to have hypotensive effects as well. The new drugs, guanabenz and guanfacine, offer pharmacologic properties similar to those of clonidine.

The ganglionic blocking agents mecamylamine and trimethaphan were developed primarily from a quarternary ammonium compound, tetraethylammonium chloride. Since 1961, researchers have developed more potent and selective drugs that produce fewer adverse reactions. In 1964, Prichard and Gillman discovered the ability of the beta-adrenergic blocking agents to decrease blood pressure, propranolol being the first to be approved and used in the United States. Now many other beta-blocking agents are available with differing potency, selectivity, and pharmacokinetic properties and are widely used to treat cardiovascular diseases.

An imidazole derivative, phentolamine was one of the first nonselective alpha-adrenergic blockers used to treat hypertension. Its adverse effects limit its use, however. Prazosin was later derived from quinazoline. This alpha-adrenergic blocking agent selectively blocks alpha$_1$ receptors, producing fewer adverse reactions as it reduces blood pressure. Terazosin, introduced in 1986-1987, is chemically related to prazosin and produces even fewer adverse reactions.

Labetalol was introduced in Europe in 1975. Clinical use of this mixed alpha- and beta-adrenergic blocker in the United States began in 1984.

Some of the norepinephrine depletors are natural medications extracted from *Rauwolfia serpentina*, a tropical plant. For centuries, Indians used *Rauwolfia serpentina* as a tranquilizer. In 1953, researchers demonstrated the plant's antihypertensive qualities. Development of reserpine, an alkaloid isolated from the plant's roots and the first norepinephrine depletor, followed.

PHARMACOKINETICS

The sympatholytics are well absorbed from the gastrointestinal (GI) tract, widely distributed, metabolized in the liver, and excreted primarily in the urine.

Absorption

After oral administration, the central-acting nervous system inhibitors and the ganglionic blocking agents are well absorbed from the GI tract. The central-acting agent methyldopa undergoes first-pass metabolism after rapid absorption. The ganglionic blocking agent trimethaphan must be administered I.V., thus it is absorbed immediately and completely.

The beta-adrenergic blocking agents are well absorbed from the GI tract except for atenolol and nadolol, which are rapidly but incompletely absorbed; the presence of food may increase nadolol absorption. Alpha-adrenergic blocking agents such as prazosin and phen-

tolamine are well absorbed from the GI tract. Labetalol, the mixed alpha- and beta-adrenergic blocking agent, is also well absorbed and its absorption may be increased by ingestion of cimetidine or food or by chronic hepatic disease.

The absorption of norepinephrine depletors varies with each drug. Reserpine is slowly absorbed from the GI tract. The absorption of guanethidine is usually incomplete; guanadrel, however, is rapidly and almost completely absorbed.

Distribution

The central-acting agents are widely distributed to body tissues. Methyldopa and clonidine are less than 20% bound to plasma proteins. Guanabenz, guanfacine, and methyldopa are distributed into the CNS, and clonidine passes into the cerebrospinal fluid and the CNS.

Ganglionic blocking agents are also widely distributed. Mecamylamine crosses the blood-brain barrier and reaches high concentrations in the liver, spleen, heart, and lungs. Because its ganglionic-blocking effects may decrease GI motility in the fetus, its use is contraindicated during pregnancy. It may also be secreted in breast milk.

All alpha- and beta-adrenergic blocking agents seem to achieve wide distribution. The beta-adrenergic blocking agents propranolol and metoprolol cross the blood-brain barrier and also appear in breast milk; propranolol is about 90% bound to plasma proteins. Protein binding is much lower with the other beta-adrenergic blocking agents: 40% to 60% with pindolol, 30% with nadolol, 16% with atenolol, 12% with metoprolol, and less than 10% with timolol. The alpha-adrenergic blocking agent prazosin is also highly protein bound. Labetalol, the mixed alpha- and beta-adrenergic blocking agent, has a 25% bioavailability after oral ingestion from first pass effect, is rapidly distributed, and is about 50% protein bound. It crosses the placenta and is secreted in breast milk.

Norepinephrine depletors are widely distributed. Reserpine is particularly well distributed in adipose tissue, accounting for its long serum half-life in obese patients. It crosses the blood-brain barrier and the placenta and is secreted in breast milk. Unlike reserpine, guanethidine does not cross the blood-brain barrier. It is rapidly distributed to storage sites in the liver, kidney, and lungs. Guanadrel is widely distributed and about 20% protein bound.

Metabolism

As a rule, the central-acting, ganglionic-blocking, beta-adrenergic blocking, and mixed alpha- and beta-adrenergic blocking agents are extensively metabolized in the liver. However, some exceptions to this rule exist. For example, the ganglionic blocker trimethaphan is metabolized by pseudocholinesterase, and the metabolism

Onset, peak, and duration of sympatholytic agents

The pharmacokinetic properties of the major sympatholytic agents are summarized below.

DRUG	ROUTE	ONSET OF ACTION	PEAK CONCENTRATIONS	DURATION OF ACTION
Central-acting agents				
clonidine	P.O.	30 to 60 minutes	2 to 5 hours	Up to 8 hours (24 to 36 hours in some patients)
guanfacine	P.O.	1 to 2 hours	3 hours	15 to 20 hours
guanabenz	P.O.	1 hour	2 to 5 hours	10 to 12 hours
methyldopa	P.O. / I.V.	3 to 6 hours / Immediate	3 to 6 hours / 4 to 6 hours	24 hours / 10 to 16 hours
Ganglionic blocking agents				
mecamylamine	P.O.	30 minutes to 2 hours	3 to 5 hours	6 to 12 hours or more
trimethaphan	I.V. infusion	Immediate	Immediate	10 to 30 minutes after infusion stops
Beta-adrenergic blocking agents				
atenolol	P.O.	1 hour	2 to 4 hours	24 hours
metoprolol	P.O.	10 minutes	90 minutes	Up to 6 hours
nadolol	P.O.	Unknown	2 to 4 hours	24 hours
pindolol	P.O.	Rapid	1 to 2 hours	24 hours
propranolol	P.O.	30 minutes	60 to 90 minutes	6 hours
timolol	P.O.	30 minutes	1 to 2 hours	4 to 6 hours
Alpha-adrenergic blocking agents				
phentolamine	I.M. / I.V.	Immediate / Immediate	20 minutes / 2 minutes	30 to 45 minutes / 15 to 30 minutes
prazosin	P.O.	1 to 2 hours	2 to 4 hours	6 to 24 hours
terazosin	P.O.	2 to 4 hours		18 to 24 hours
Mixed alpha- and beta-adrenergic blocking agent				
labetalol	P.O.	20 minutes to 2 hours	1 to 4 hours	Dose dependent: 8 to 12 hours (200 mg); 10 to 24 hours (300 mg)
	I.V. infusion or bolus	2 to 5 minutes	5 to 15 minutes	2 to 4 hours
Norepinephrine depletor				
guanadrel	P.O.	60 to 90 minutes	4 to 6 hours	4 to 14 hours

of some beta-adrenergic blockers varies. Atenolol is not metabolized in the liver, for example, but about 95% of metoprolol is. Also, the liver's capacity to metabolize propranolol varies greatly from patient to patient.

Metabolism of prazosin occurs in the liver, primarily by demethylation and conjugation. Metabolism of the other alpha-adrenergic blocking agents, phentolamine and terazosin, is unknown. The norepinephrine depletor reserpine also undergoes metabolism in the liver.

Excretion

Most antihypertensive agents are primarily excreted in the urine. Among the central-acting agents, from 60% to 75% of methyldopa and clonidine is excreted this way, although methyldopa is also excreted in the feces, and is excreted in bile. Guanfacine is excreted 30% to 40% unchanged in the urine. The ganglionic blocker mecamylamine is excreted slowly by the kidneys as unchanged drug, and its rate of excretion increases in acidic urine and decreases in alkaline urine.

The amount of unchanged drug excreted varies among the beta-adrenergic blocking agents. Atenolol and nadolol are excreted 100% unchanged; pindolol, 40%. Only 6% to 10% of prazosin is excreted in the urine; the rest of this alpha-adrenergic blocking agent is excreted primarily in bile and the feces. (Its excretion may be decreased in a patient with CHF.) Labetalol metabolites are excreted in the bile and urine.

The norepinephrine depletor reserpine is primarily excreted in the feces (60%) and also in the urine. Guanethidine's excretion also occurs primarily in urine and feces.

Onset, peak, duration

The onset of action, peak concentration levels, and duration of action vary greatly among the sympatholytics. (For detailed information, see *Onset, peak, and duration of sympatholytic agents* on page 587.)

PHARMACODYNAMICS

All of the sympatholytic agents inhibit stimulation of the sympathetic nervous system. They perform this function in different ways, but they all produce the same result: decreased blood pressure from peripheral vasodilation or decreased cardiac output.

Mechanism of action

Methyldopa, a central-acting agent structurally related to the catecholamines, acts as a false neurotransmitter. Its central action involves its metabolism to the active compound L-methylnorepinephrine. In the CNS, this compound stimulates the alpha-adrenergic receptors that inhibit sympathetic output. Output inhibition decreases vascular peripheral tone and arteriolar vasoconstriction. In this way, methyldopa lowers standing and supine blood pressures and reduces renal vascular resistance. Its action has little effect on cardiac output, however, and it produces less orthostatic hypotension than peripherally acting agents.

The other central-acting agents, clonidine, guanabenz, and guanfacine, reduce hypertension through a central mechanism different from methyldopa's. They stimulate presynaptic (inhibitory) alpha-adrenergic receptors in the medulla. This stimulation decreases the sympathetic tone and resistance in the peripheral arterioles, lowering the standing and supine blood pressures and decreasing the heart rate and cardiac output. (Long-term guanabenz therapy, however, leaves the cardiac output unchanged.) These drugs also produce peripheral vasodilation, and they produce less orthostatic hypotension than peripherally acting agents. They do not alter the glomerular filtration rate.

The ganglionic blocking agents mecamylamine and trimethaphan compete with acetylcholine to occupy cholinergic receptors on the autonomic ganglia. By thus interacting with the cholinergic receptors, these drugs interrupt transmission of sympathetic impulses. The resulting reduction in sympathetic tone and cardiac output increases vasodilation and lowers the blood pressure.

Beta-adrenergic blocking agents act by competing with epinephrine for beta-adrenergic receptor sites. By thus inhibiting or blocking sympathetic stimulation, they decrease heart rate and cardiac output and reduce the blood pressure. Propranolol, nadolol, and timolol are nonselective, blocking $beta_1$ (cardiac) and $beta_2$ (noncardiac) receptors. Pindolol, atenolol, and metoprolol are selective, blocking primarily $beta_1$ receptors. By blocking the $beta_1$ receptors in the heart, these drugs decrease heart rate and myocardial contractility and ultimately lower cardiac output. Their mechanisms of action also include decreasing the effect of the renin-angiotensin-aldosterone system.

The alpha-adrenegic blocking agents prazosin and terazosin selectively block $alpha_1$ receptors, interfering with sympathetic stimulation and directly relaxing arteriolar smooth muscle. This interference reduces peripheral vascular resistance and produces vasodilation without producing tachycardia or reducing cardiac output; maximum antihypertensive effects appear when the patient is upright. Prazosin produces little or no increase in serum renin levels, cardiac output, renal blood flow, or glomerular filtration rate.

The nonselective alpha-adrenergic blocker phentolamine produces vasodilation in a slightly different way, by competitively blocking all alpha-adrenergic receptor sites and circulating epinephrine. This also increases gastric secretions, however, and may result in nausea, vomiting and diarrhea. In addition, it produces reflex tachycardia as a result of direct cardiac stimulation and orthostatic hypotension from vasodilation.

Labetalol, the mixed alpha- and beta-adrenergic blocking agent, decreases total peripheral resistance, and reduces plasma renin and aldosterone levels as well as renal vascular resistance, and may decrease cardiac output. Unlike nonselective alpha-adrenergic blockers, labetalol does not produce marked orthostatic hypotension or reflex tachycardia. In comparison with beta-adrenergic blocking agents, labetalol produces less bradycardia and reduction in blood flow as it decreases peripheral vascular resistance. It decreases standing, more than supine, blood pressure. Besides its adrenergic activity, labetalol decreases plasma angiotensin II and aldosterone levels.

The norepinephrine depletor reserpine, guanethidine, and guanadrel exert antihypertensive effects by depleting the catecholamine stores in the sympathetic nerve endings and may also inhibit norepinephrine transport to storage sites. These actions reduce the sympathetic output, thus reducing vasomotor tone. The drugs also reduce total peripheral resistance, decrease cardiac output, and result in bradycardia; these effects contribute to blood pressure reduction.

The norepinephrine depletor guanethidine selectively blocks the efferent peripheral sympathetic pathways, causing vasodilation with decreased peripheral resistance and leading to a prolonged decrease in the blood pressure. This drug reduces systolic blood pressure more than diastolic pressure and more effectively lowers standing blood pressure than supine pressure. Besides decreasing blood pressure, vasodilation may decrease renal, coronary, and cerebral blood flow as well as plasma renin activity.

Another norepinephrine depletor, guanadrel, exerts its strongest antihypertensive effects when the patient is standing. It does not decrease cardiac output or renal blood flow, but it can decrease heart rate and may result in fluid retention.

PHARMACOTHERAPEUTICS

Physicians typically use sympatholytics to lower the blood pressure of patients with mild-to-severe essential hypertension. Using the stepped-care approach to antihypertensive therapy, the physician can change the type of drug used and alter the dosage to achieve effective therapeutic effects with the fewest adverse reactions.

clonidine hydrochloride (Catapres). A central-acting nervous system inhibitor, clonidine is used as a step-2 drug in the treatment of mild to moderate hypertension. It lowers the supine and standing blood pressures and is frequently given with a diuretic or another antihypertensive agent to achieve the maximum blood pressure reduction.
USUAL ADULT DOSAGE: initially, 0.1 mg P.O. b.i.d., increased by 0.1 to 0.2 mg/day every 2 to 4 days until the desired response is achieved ; for maintenance, 0.1 to 0.2 mg b.i.d. to q.i.d. or up to a maximum of 2.4 mg/day.

guanabenz acetate (Wytensin). A central-acting agent administered orally, guanabenz is usually considered a step-2 drug. Because it does not produce orthostatic hypotension, guanabenz may be a useful substitute for guanethidine or adrenergic blocking agents when these drugs produce severe orthostatic hypotension.
USUAL ADULT DOSAGE: initially, 4 mg P.O. b.i.d., increased by 4 to 8 mg/day every 1 to 2 weeks as needed, up to a maximum of 32 mg b.i.d., although a dose this high is rarely needed.

guanfacine (Tenex). A central-acting agent, guanfacine is also considered a step-2 drug and is used to treat mild to moderate hypertension. It does not affect cardiac output but decreases total peripheral resistance. It is usually prescribed with a diuretic agent.
USUAL ADULT DOSAGE: 1 mg P.O. at bedtime may be increased to a maximum of 3 mg/day. Dosage adjustments may be required for renally impaired and elderly patients.

methyldopa (Aldomet). A central-acting agent, methyldopa is usually administered orally to control mild to moderate hypertension. It is frequently combined with a diuretic, because it can produce sodium and water retention. Usually used as a step-2 drug, methyldopa is useful for treating patients with impaired renal function. It may be administered I.V. to treat hypertensive crisis.
USUAL ADULT DOSAGE: initially, for mild to moderate hypertension, 250 mg P.O. b.i.d. or t.i.d., increased biweekly to a maintenance dosage of 500 mg to 2 grams/day in two to four divided doses or up to a maximum of 3 grams/day; for hypertensive crisis, 250 to 500 mg I.V. in 100 ml of dextrose 5% in water infused over 30 to 60 minutes, repeated every 6 hours, if necessary.

mecamylamine hydrochloride (Inversine). A potent, long-acting ganglionic blocking agent, mecamylamine is used to treat moderate to severe hypertension. As an adjunct, rather than a primary agent, it is usually used as a step-4 drug. The required dosage varies widely

DRUG INTERACTIONS

Sympatholytic agents

The sympatholytic agents can interact with many drugs to produce blood pressure changes as well as other severe reactions. For drug interactions involving the beta-adrenergic blocking agents, see Chapter 36, Antianginal Agents.

DRUG	INTERACTING DRUGS	POSSIBLE EFFECTS	NURSING IMPLICATIONS
clonidine, guan-abenz, methyl-dopa	tricyclic antidepressants, amphetamines	Increase blood pressure	• Avoid concomitant administration.
	diuretics	Increase antihypertensive effects	• Monitor the patient for hypotension.
clonidine	beta-adrenergic blocking agents	Promote a paradoxical hypertensive response	• Monitor the patient's blood pressure frequently.
methyldopa	haloperidol	Inhibits dopamine	• Observe the patient for adverse reactions, such as disorientation.
	levarterenol	Prolongs pressor response	• Monitor the patient's blood pressure frequently.
	lithium	Increases lithium toxicity	• Avoid concomitant administration.
	methotrimeprazine	Induces hypotension	• Do not administer methotrimeprazine to a patient receiving methyldopa.
mecamylamine	sodium bicarbonate	Alkalinizes urine-slowing mecamylamine, excreting and increasing its effects	• Monitor the patient for increased antihypertensive effects and toxicity.
trimethaphan	anesthetic agents, especially spinal anesthetics	Enhance hypotensive effects	• Monitor the patient's blood pressure frequently.
terazosin	beta-adrenergic blocking agents and other antihypertensive agents	Increase antihypertensive effects	• Monitor the patient's blood pressure frequently.
labetalol	cimetidine	Increases antihypertensive effects	• Monitor the patient's blood pressure frequently.
	halothane anesthesia	Enhances the hypotensive effects	• Monitor the patient's blood pressure frequently.
guanadrel	sympathomimetic agents	Inhibit antihypertensive effects	• Monitor the patient's blood pressure frequently.
	MAO inhibitors	Inhibit antihypertensive effects	• Do not give condomitantly or within 1 week of MAO-inhibitor therapy. • Monitor the patient's blood pressure to determine an effective therapeutic response.
guanethidine	amphetamines, ephedrine, levarterenol, methylphenidate, tricyclic antidepressants, phenothiazines	Inhibit antihypertensive effects	• Avoid concomitant administration. • Monitor the patient's blood pressure frequently.

DRUG INTERACTIONS

Sympatholytic agents continued

DRUG	INTERACTING DRUGS	POSSIBLE EFFECTS	NURSING IMPLICATIONS
guanethidine (continued)	ethyl alcohol	Causes vasodilation leading to orthostatic hypotension	• Instruct the patient to change positions slowly.
	methotrimeprazine	Causes orthostatic hypotension	• Avoid concurrent use. • If used together, instruct the patient to change position slowly.
	oral hypoglycemic agents	Increase hypoglycemic effect	• Monitor the patient for signs and symptoms of hypoglycemia.
	oral contraceptives	Antagonize antihypertensive effect	• Monitor the patient's blood pressure to determine a therapeutic effect.
	anticholinergic agents	Reduce anticholinergic effects	• Monitor the patient for decreased therapeutic effects.
reserpine	levodopa	Depletes dopamine, inhibiting levodopa's effect	• Avoid giving reserpine to a patient receiving levodopa for Parkinson's disease.
	methotrimeprazine	Causes hypotension	• Monitor the patient's blood pressure frequently.
	MAO inhibitors	Cause excitation and hypertension	• Avoid concomitant use.

according to patient factors, the time of day, and the season. Higher doses are usually required at night and in cold weather.

USUAL ADULT DOSAGE: initially, 2.5 mg P.O. b.i.d., increased by 2.5 mg every 2 or more days until the desired response is achieved. The average maintenance dosage is 25 mg/day given in three divided doses.

trimethaphan camsylate (Arfonad). A potent, short-acting ganglionic blocking agent, trimethaphan is administered I.V. to manage hypertensive crisis associated with pulmonary edema. Elderly patients may be unusually sensitive to its effects, necessitating dosage adjustments.

USUAL ADULT DOSAGE: 3 to 4 mg/minute I.V. of 500 mg diluted in 500 ml of dextrose 5% in water, adjusted according to the patient's response.

atenolol (Tenormin). A selective beta-adrenergic blocking agent, atenolol produces maximum effects up to 3 days after the initial oral dose. It is used as a step-2 or a step-1 agent or sometimes with other drugs and can be given safely to a patient with chronic obstructive

pulmonary disease (COPD), asthma, peripheral vascular disease (PVD), or diabetes.

USUAL ADULT DOSAGE: 50 to 100 mg P.O. once daily.

metoprolol tartrate (Lopressor). This cardioselective beta-adrenergic blocking agent may be used alone or with other antihypertensives as a step-1 or step-2 agent. It can be given safely to a patient with COPD but should be used cautiously in a patient with a hepatic or renal disease.

USUAL ADULT DOSAGE: initially, 100 mg P.O. daily in single or divided doses, increased by 50 mg/day every week up to a maximum of 450 mg/day.

nadolol (Corgard). A beta-adrenergic blocking agent, nadolol is administered orally. Because of its long half-life, however, this step-2 agent may not reach therapeutic antihypertensive levels for up to 5 days after therapy begins.

USUAL ADULT DOSAGE: initially, 40 to 80 mg P.O. daily, increased by 40 to 80 mg every week, as needed and tolerated, up to a maximum of 320 mg/day. A patient with impaired renal function may require a lower dose.

pindolol (Visken). A beta-adrenergic blocking agent, pindolol is a step-1 or step-2 agent administered orally either alone or in combination with other antihypertensive agents.
USUAL ADULT DOSAGE: initially, 5 mg P.O. b.i.d., increased by 10 mg/day every 3 to 4 weeks up to a maximum dosage of 60 mg/day.

propranolol hydrochloride (Inderal). A beta-adrenergic blocking agent, propranolol is indicated for the treatment of mild to moderate hypertension. Administered orally, this step-1 or step-2 agent may be used alone, but it is frequently given in combination with other antihypertensive agents, such as hydralazine or minoxidil, to reduce their adverse reactions.
USUAL ADULT DOSAGE: 40 mg P.O. b.i.d., increased gradually, as needed, up to a maximum of 640 mg/day.

timolol maleate (Blocadren). A beta-adrenergic blocking agent, timolol is a step-1 or step-2 drug used in the treatment of mild to moderate hypertension. Administered orally, it may be used alone or in combination with other antihypertensive agents.
USUAL ADULT DOSAGE: initially, 10 mg P.O. b.i.d., increased every week, as needed and tolerated, up to 30 mg b.i.d.; for maintenance, 20 to 40 mg/day.

phentolamine (Regitine). This alpha-adrenergic blocking agent is available as phentolamine hydrochloride and phentolamine mesylate and can be administered I.V. or I.M. It was first used to treat hypertension but is now used to prevent or control hypertensive crisis associated with pheochromocytoma surgery and to aid in the diagnosis of pheochromocytoma.
USUAL ADULT DOSAGE: to diagnose pheochromocytoma, 5 mg I.V.; 1 to 2 hours before surgical removal of pheochromocytoma, 5 mg I.M. or I.V.; during surgery, 5 mg I.V.

prazosin hydrochloride (Minipress). An alpha-adrenergic blocking agent, prazosin is usually considered a step-2 drug. Administered orally, it is most effective in reduced dosages given with a thiazide diuretic or a beta-adrenergic blocking agent. This drug may produce first-dose syncope.
USUAL ADULT DOSAGE: initially, 0.5 to 1 mg P.O. b.i.d to t.i.d., increased gradually to a maintenance dosage that meets the patient's requirements; for maintenance, 6 to 15 mg/day in divided doses when given alone or 1 to 2 mg P.O. t.i.d. when given with a diuretic or another antihypertensive agent. Dosages exceeding 20 mg/day usually do not produce increased effects.

terazosin (Vasocard). An alpha-adrenergic blocking agent, terazosin is administered orally and indicated for treatment of patients with mild to moderate hypertension. This step-2 drug may be useful in a patient who cannot tolerate diuretics or beta-adrenergic blocking agents, but it is more widely used as an adjunct to these drugs. Unlike prazosin, it does not produce first-dose syncope or lead to tolerance.
USUAL ADULT DOSAGE: 1 to 40 mg P.O. daily in one or two doses, titrated according to the patient's response.

labetalol (Normodyne). A mixed alpha- and beta-adrenergic blocking agent, labetalol is effective when used alone to treat mild to severe hypertension. It is frequently administered orally as a step-2 antihypertensive agent, but may also be used as a step-1 drug. I.V. labetalol is also effective for treating hypertensive crisis.
Labetalol is especially useful for the treatment of hypertension in patients who are resistant to other forms of antihypertensive therapy and in those who have renal or cardiac diseases, COPD, or arterial insufficiency.
USUAL ADULT DOSAGE: for hypertension, 100 mg P.O. b.i.d., increased as needed up to 400 mg b.i.d.; for hypertensive crisis, 20 to 80 mg slow I.V. bolus every 10 minutes or 2 mg/minute by continuous I.V. infusion up to a maximum of 300 mg.

guanadrel sulfate (Hylorel). A norepinephrine depletor, guanadrel is a step-2 drug administered orally to treat hypertension that has not responded sufficiently to thiazide diuretics alone.
USUAL ADULT DOSAGE: initially, 5 mg P.O. b.i.d., increased every week as needed to a maintenance dosage of 20 to 75 mg/day given in two to four divided doses.

guanethidine sulfate (Ismelin). A norepinephrine depletor administered orally, guanethidine can be used to treat moderate to severe hypertension but is not considered a primary agent. It is usually used as a step-4 drug, almost always in combination with another drug.
USUAL ADULT DOSAGE: initially, 10 to 12.5 mg P.O. once daily, increased by 10 to 12.5 mg every 5 to 7 days, as needed; for maintenance, 25 to 50 mg/day.

reserpine (Serpasil). A norepinephrine depletor, reserpine is used to treat mild to moderate hypertension. Not considered a primary agent in antihypertensive therapy, it is often combined with a diuretic or other antihypertensive agent as a step-2 drug. Its effects may not appear for up to several weeks.
USUAL ADULT DOSAGE: initially, 0.1 to 0.5 mg P.O. in a single daily dose or divided into two doses daily; for maintenance, a maximum of 0.25 mg daily.

Drug interactions

Many different drugs can interact with sympatholytic agents, frequently producing blood pressure changes and other effects. (See *Drug interactions: Sympatholytic agents* on page 590 for detailed information.)

ADVERSE DRUG REACTIONS

Many of the sympatholytic agents cause adverse reactions in the CNS and the cardiovascular system. Additional reactions affecting other body systems vary with each drug.

Predictable reactions

Central-acting and ganglionic blocking agents typically produce CNS effects, such as sedation, drowsiness, and depression. Other common reactions include forgetfulness, inability to concentrate, and vivid dreams, that usually diminish after 2 to 3 weeks of therapy. Additional adverse reactions include sodium and water accumulation, edema, hepatic dysfunction, vertigo, paresthesias, weakness, fever, nasal congestion, and dry mouth. These drugs may decrease the libido and result in impotence, limiting their usefulness in young adults. They may also produce lactation in women and men.

Other adverse reactions vary according to the specific drug used. For example, clonidine is especially likely to cause dry mouth, because it decreases salivary flow. When the drug is discontinued, rebound hypertension to pretreatment levels may result.

Guanabenz may produce cardiovascular adverse reactions, such dysrhythmias, chest pain, edema, and palpitations. Its other effects may include anxiety, ataxia, blurred vision, and nasal congestion. Like clonidine, guanabenz can produce rebound hypertension if it is discontinued suddenly. Because of its potential for producing serious adverse reactions, this drug requires cautious use in a patient with a recent MI or with cerebrovascular disease, severe coronary insufficiency, or hepatic or renal failure.

Shortness of breath, respiratory depression, and tachycardia can develop with mecamylamine therapy. The other ganglionic blocking agent, trimethaphan, can produce similar effects and may decrease serum potassium levels. Both of these agents should be used with extreme caution in a patient with prostatic hypertrophy, cardiovascular insufficiency, MI, fever or infection, hemorrhage, sodium depletion, glaucoma, or renal impairment. They should also be used cautiously in elderly patients, who may be more sensitive to the antihypertensive effects. In addition, trimethaphan requires cautious use in a patient with Addison's disease,

cerebrovascular insufficiency, diabetes mellitus, hepatic impairment, or respiratory insufficiency.

Because of their ability to penetrate the blood-brain barrier, beta-adrenergic blocking agents can produce the same CNS reactions as the central-acting and ganglionic blocking agents. (Atenolol, the least lipid-soluble beta-adrenergic blocking agent, produces the fewest CNS effects.) Cardiovascular adverse reactions may include bradycardia, hypotension, congestive heart failure, and PVD. The beta-adrenergic blocking agents may also reduce HDL cholesterol levels and increase serum triglyceride levels.

Other adverse reactions to beta-adrenergic blocking agents include nausea, vomiting, diarrhea, nightmares, depression, insomnia, and hallucinations as well as dry eyes, paresthesias, transient thrombocytopenia, agranulocytosis, sore throat, fever, and breathing difficulty. Because of these adverse reactions, beta-adrenergic blocking agents are contraindicated for use with patients with asthma or emphysema and must be used with extreme caution in patients with heart failure or hepatic or renal impairment.

In a patient with intermittent claudication or PVD, beta-adrenergic blocking agents may produce further symptoms of arterial insufficiency. In an insulin-dependent diabetic patient beta-adrenergic blocking agents can mask the early warning signs of hypoglycemia, and rarely, produce hyperglycemia. They may also alter test results for alkaline phosphatase, blood urea nitrogen (BUN), low-density lipoproteins (LDL), serum creatinine, serum potassium, serum transaminase, serum triglycerides, serum uric acid, and serum glucose.

Alpha-adrenergic blocking agents tend to produce different adverse reactions than the beta-adrenergic blocking agents. For example, prazosin produces orthostatic hypotension more frequently than the beta-adrenergic blocking agents. It also produces first-dose syncope. Overall, prazosin produces adverse reactions that are more severe than those seen with other sympatholytics. Its use should be carefully considered in a patient with angina pectoris, cardiac disease, depression, or renal impairment. Terazosin produces a few mild adverse reactions, including orthostatic hypotension and dizziness. It should be used cautiously in a patient with angina pectoris, because a decrease in blood pressure may precipitate an anginal attack. Phentolamine can also precipitate anginal attacks from rebound tachycardia and may produce hypotension as well as dizziness, weakness, flushing, palpitations, diarrhea, nausea, vomiting, and nasal congestion.

Adverse reactions to the mixed alpha- and beta-adrenergic blocking agent, labetalol, resemble those of the beta-adrenergic blocking agents. Other reactions may include scalp tingling, alopecia, orthostatic hypotension, intermittent claudication, bronchospasm, drug-induced systemic lupus erythematosus (SLE), eye irritation, myalgia, and rash. A patient with heart failure who is receiving digitalis may be given labetalol with caution, but the drug is contraindicated in patients with second- or third-degree heart block and in patients with cardiogenic shock.

Norepinephrine depletors produce a wide range of adverse reactions. Frequent adverse reactions to reserpine include drowsiness, sleep alterations, weight gain, and nasal congestion. Increased GI motility, abdominal cramps, and diarrhea may also occur along with nightmares, depression, uterine contractions, and bronchoconstriction (in a patient with bronchitis). Reserpine may also increase the risk of breast cancer. When given to a lactating woman, it may result in increased respiratory secretions, nasal congestion, and cyanosis in the infant. Reserpine may also interfere with serum glucose and urine glucose test results, producing low urine catecholamine, 17-hydroxy-corticosteroid, and 17-ketosteroid levels.

Despite these adverse reactions, reserpine remains useful because of its low cost. However, it is contraindicated in patients with acute peptic ulcer disease and acute ulcerative colitis, because it produces gastric and intestinal irritation. It must be given cautiously to a patient with renal or hepatic insufficiency, cardiac damage, or dysrhythmias, because it decreases peripheral vascular resistance and cardiac output.

The most clinically relevant adverse reaction to guanethidine and guanadrel is orthostatic hypotension, occurring primarily on awakening. Many patients also experience generalized weakness, especially early in therapy. Guanethidine can produce explosive diarrhea; failure to ejaculate; decreased myocardial contractility; fluid retention; increased BUN, serum glutamic-oxaloacetic transaminase (SGOT), and serum glutamic-pyruvate transaminase (SGPT) levels; and decreased prothrombin time and serum glucose and urine catecholamine levels. Because of the risk of these reactions, guanethidine is contraindicated in a patient with pheochromocytoma or congestive heart failure and must be used carefully in a patient with diarrhea, hepatic impairment, or bronchial asthma. (Catecholamine depletion can aggravate asthma.)

A patient receiving guanadrel may faint upon exertion or standing and may develop nocturia and dyspnea especially druing the first 8 weeks of treatment. This drug is contraindicated for a patient with congestive heart failure and should be used cautiously in a patient with peptic ulcer disease.

Unpredictable reactions

Rare reactions to central-acting agents include anorexia, vomiting, parotid pain, and rash. Pruritus, abdominal discomfort, constipation, diarrhea, nausea, vomiting, and aches in the extremities may also occur. Guanabenz may result in headaches and sexual dysfunction. In rare instances, terazosin may produce diminished hearing, chest pain, insomnia, and GI distress. The norepinephrine depletor reserpine may produce angina, bradycardia, blurred vision, impotence, and decreased libido.

NURSING IMPLICATIONS

Because antihypertensive therapy may be prolonged, patient teaching is an important factor in the success of the therapy. (See *Patient-teaching tips* on page 599.) The nurse must also be aware of the following considerations.

• Inform the patient taking clonidine that vivid dreams may occur.

• Advise the patient taking methyldopa that the drug may darken the urine.

• Give a central-acting agent between meals. If sedation occurs, give the drug in the evening. If the dosage is increased, start with an evening dose to minimize sedative effects.

• Administer a central-acting nervous system inhibitor cautiously to a patient with coronary insufficiency, recent MI, cerebrovascular disease, or severe hepatic or renal impairment because of the risks of adverse reactions.

• Monitor cardiac function when administering antihypertensive agents to a patient with angina or coronary insufficiency.

• Assist the patient with position changes and ambulation to prevent injury from orthostatic hypotension.

• Closely supervise a patient on antihypertensive therapy who has a history of depression, because it may recur.

• Monitor an elderly patient receiving a sympatholytic agent for signs of cerebral ischemia, such as syncope.

• Advise the patient that the dry mouth will usually decrease over time, and provide relief by offering cool drinks, gum, sour hard candies, or frequent oral hygiene.

• If constipation occurs, administer a laxative to the patient as prescribed and encourage an increased fluid intake.

• To prevent hypotension during therapy, administer mecamylamine with meals and make the morning dose, if used, the smallest dose of the day.

• Administer mecamylamine cautiously to a patient with prostatic hypertrophy, cardiovascular insufficiency, MI, fever or infection, hemorrhage, sodium depletion, glaucoma, or impaired renal function.

• Administer I.V. trimethaphan as a secondary or piggyback solution in a primary I.V. line. Use an infusion pump or a microdrip regulator to allow precise adjustments to the flow rate. Do not mix trimethaphan with other medications. The patient should be closely monitored during therapy to adjust the I.V. rate according to blood pressure response and should remain supine during trimethaphan administration.

• Discontinue trimethaphan immediately if excessive hypotension occurs and consult the physician. Blood pressure is usually restored within 10 minutes.

• Monitor the fluid intake and output for a patient receiving a ganglionic blocking agent, because oliguria may occur with excessive hypotension.

• Monitor the patient's blood pressure and pulse every 15 to 30 minutes for at least 2 hours during administration of an alpha-adrenergic blocking agent.

• Administer phentolamine cautiously to a patient with peptic ulcer disease, because the drug increases gastric secretions.

• To prevent severe first-dose orthostatic hypotension, instruct the patient to take the first dose of prazosin at bedtime or to remain lying down for at least 3 hours after taking it.

• Obtain a history of mental, cardiovascular, cerebral, renal, and GI diseases before initiating norepinephrine-depletor therapy. Also assess the heart rate and the EKG results.

• Monitor serum electrolyte levels, and correct any imbalances as prescribed before administering norepinephrine-depletor agents.

• Guanethidine and guanadrel are contraindicated in a patient with pheochromocytoma because they can produce severe hypertensive reactions.

• Discontinue guanethidine for 72 hours before elective surgery, as prescribed.

• Teach the patient on reserpine therapy to take the drug with food, milk, or a full glass of water to minimize the risk of GI upset.

• Administer reserpine cautiously to a patient with epilepsy because this agent may lower the threshold for seizures.

• Expect to discontinue monoamine oxidase (MAO) inhibitors as prescribed for at least 1 week before norepinephrine-depletor therapy begins to decrease the risk of interactive effects resulting in excessive sympathetic stimulation and hypertension.

• Monitor the patient receiving guanethidine or reserpine for bradycardia or dysrhythmias.

• Monitor the patient receiving reserpine, guanethidine, or guanadrel therapy for diarrhea because these agents increase gastric motility.

• Administer reserpine and guanethidine cautiously to a patient receiving digitalis or quinidine because of the risk of dysrhythmia due to additive effects.

• Obtain baseline data before beginning norepinephrine-depletor therapy. Assess the patient's sitting, standing, and supine blood pressures and pulses. Monitor and record the patient's blood pressure and pulse when starting drug therapy, before administering each dose, and during peak concentration level times.

• Monitor and record the patient's intake, output, and daily weight while the patient is receiving norepinephrine-depletor therapy. During antihypertensive therapy, sodium and fluid retention may expand the plasma volume, decreasing the therapeutic effect.

• Be aware that beta-adrenergic blocking agents may mask signs of hypoglycemia; monitor a diabetic patient's serum glucose level carefully.

• Assess the patient's hepatic and renal function before therapy with beta-adrenergic blocking agents begins and at regular intervals. If the BUN or serum creatinine level is elevated, notify the physician.

• Administer propranolol or metoprolol with food to promote its absorption. Other oral beta-adrenergic blocking agents may be administered with food or on an empty stomach.

• Anticipate gradual discontinuation of a beta-adrenergic blocking agent over 3 to 14 days. During this time, the patient should avoid vigorous physical activity.

• Instruct the patient and family about possible adverse reactions. Describe the early signs of depression, which may not occur for 6 months after therapy begins, and the risk of suicide if severe mental depression occurs.

• Alert the patient on a sodium-restricted diet that noncompliance may result in fluid retention and edema.

• Before discharge, emphasize the patient's need to consult the physician before taking over-the-counter drugs, especially sympathomimetics and decongestants.

• Instruct the patient to store these drugs in a tightly sealed container that will keep them dry and protect them from light.

VASODILATING AGENTS

Two types of vasodilating agents exist: direct vasodilators and calcium channel blockers. Both types decrease systolic and diastolic blood pressure by relaxing arteriolar smooth muscle, leading to arteriolar dilation and decreasing peripheral resistance.

Direct vasodilators act on arteries, veins, or both. They include diazoxide, hydralazine hydrochloride, minoxidil, and sodium nitroprusside. Hydralazine and minoxidil are usually used to treat resistant or refractory hypertension as step-3 and step-4 agents, respectively. Diazoxide and nitroprusside are reserved for use in hypertensive crisis.

Calcium channel blockers produce vasodilation by preventing the entry of calcium into the cells, thus reducing the mechanical activity of vascular smooth muscle. They include diltiazem hydrochloride, nifedipine, and verapamil hydrochloride and may be used as step-2 and step-3 antihypertensive drugs.

History and source
Hydralazine has been used to treat hypertension since 1951. At first, it was administered singly, but its rebound effects—such as increased cardiac output, tachycardia, and sodium and water retention—limited its use. Later, hydralazine was administered in combination with beta-adrenergic blocking agents and diuretics, with adverse reactions. Today, this direct vasodilator is widely and effectively used to manage moderate to severe hypertension.

In 1973, diazoxide was introduced for I.V. treatment of hypertensive emergencies. The introduction of minoxidil followed in 1980. This potent arterial vasodilator is now used to treat patients with severe or malignant hypertension who fail to respond to other oral agents.

Nitroprusside was used as a chemical color indicator in 1850, then in 1929 it was noted to lower blood pressure. In 1974, 45 years later, it was approved for use as an antihypertensive agent. Calcium channel blockers were introduced in Europe in the early 1970s and in the United States in the 1980s for the treatment of angina and dysrhythmias. Because of their peripheral vasodilating action, however, they have become widely used to treat hypertension.

PHARMACOKINETICS

Most of these drugs are rapidly absorbed and well distributed. They are all metabolized in the liver, and most are excreted by the kidneys.

Absorption, distribution, metabolism, excretion
I.V. diazoxide, which bypasses absorption, is 90% bound to plasma albumin, although the extent of binding is decreased in a patient with renal failure. It also crosses the placenta and is secreted in breast milk. The drug is metabolized in the liver to inactive metabolites and about one third of it is excreted unchanged by the kidneys.

After oral administration, hydralazine is readily absorbed from the GI tract, and administration with food can increase absorption. About 87% of a dose binds with plasma proteins. Hepatic metabolism occurs through acetylation, but the rate of acetylation varies widely among individuals. Less than 15% of a hydralazine dose is excreted unchanged by the kidneys.

Minoxidol is rapidly and completely absorbed from the GI tract. It undergoes extensive metabolism in the liver to less active metabolites and is excreted by the kidneys.

After I.V. administration, nitroprusside bypasses absorption and is rapidly distributed. The ferrous ion in nitroprusside reacts with compounds in the red blood cells to produce cyanide. The cyanide is metabolized in the liver and excreted by the kidneys.

About 80% of a diltiazem dose is absorbed after oral administration. Extensive first-pass metabolism occurs with this drug, making it about 40% bioavailable. Diltiazem is 80% protein bound. It then undergoes extensive metabolism to active metabolites and is excreted in the bile (65%) and the urine (35%). Only 2% to 4% of the unchanged drug appears in the urine.

After oral administration, nifedipine is rapidly and completely absorbed. It undergoes first-pass metabolism to a free acid, reducing its bioavailability to 65% to 70%, and is then 90% protein bound. All metabolites are pharmacologically inactive and most are excreted in the urine; about 10% are excreted in the feces.

Verapamil is 90% absorbed from the GI tract after oral administration, but first-pass effect yields a bioavailability of only 20% to 35%. The drug is approximately 90% protein bound. About 70% of the drug and its active metabolites are excreted in the urine, 16% in the feces.

Onset, peak, duration
Vasodilating agents vary widely in their pharmacokinetic processes. (See *Onset, peak, and duration of vasodilating agents* for detailed information.)

PHARMACODYNAMICS

The direct vasodilators relax peripheral vascular smooth muscles, lowering blood pressure by increasing blood vessel caliber and reducing total peripheral resistance. Calcium channel blockers prevent calcium transport across the cell membrane, reducing the activity of the vascular smooth muscle, thus producing vasodilation and lowering the blood pressure.

Onset, peak, and duration of vasodilating agents

The major pharmacokinetic properties of the direct vasodilators and the calcium channel blockers are summarized below.

DRUG	ROUTE	ONSET OF ACTION	PEAK CONCENTRATIONS	DURATION OF ACTION
Direct vasodilators				
diazoxide	I.V.	1 to 3 minutes	2 to 5 minutes	Usually 3 to 12 hours, but ranges from 1 to 72 hours
hydralazine	P.O. I.V. I.M.	20 to 30 minutes 5 to 20 minutes 10 to 30 minutes	2 hours 10 to 80 minutes 1 hour	2 to 8 hours 2 to 6 hours 2 to 6 hours
minoxidil	P.O.	30 minutes	2 to 8 hours	2 to 5 days
nitroprusside	I.V. infusion	Immediate	Immediate	1 to 10 minutes after infusion stops
Calcium channel blockers				
diltiazem	P.O.	30 to 60 minutes	2 to 3 hours	4 to 9 hours
nifedipine	P.O.	10 minutes	30 minutes	6 to 8 hours
verapamil	P.O.	30 to 60 minutes	30 to 60 minutes	6 to 12 hours

Mechanism of action

A thiazide derivative, diazoxide directly affects the arteries, but its action remains unclear. Hydralazine dilates arterioles directly and promotes an increase in cardiac output and cerebral and renal blood flow. Minoxidil and hydralazine act in the same way. They appear to alter cellular calcium metabolism and interfere with calcium movement. They do not decrease the glomerular filtration rate, but they seem to increase renin secretion. Nitroprusside directly relaxes arterial and venous smooth muscle.

Calcium channel blockers may act to relieve hypertension in several different ways. They all inhibit transport of calcium ions during cell membrane depolarization in cardiac and vascular smooth muscle. This inhibition reduces peripheral vascular resistance, decreasing the blood pressure. The same action dilates the coronary arteries, improving myocardial perfusion. Calcium channel blockers may also block norepinephrine-mediated vasoconstriction and inhibit renin release, suppressing the renin-angiotensin-aldosterone system.

PHARMACOTHERAPEUTICS

Vasodilating agents are usually used as adjuncts in the treatment of moderate to severe hypertension. They are seldom used as primary agents.

diazoxide (Hyperstat). This potent vasodilator is administered I.V., usually with a diuretic, to treat hypertensive crisis. It can decrease the blood pressure in 1 to 5 minutes. It can also be used to treat malignant hypertension. Its advantages include rapid action and a decreased tendency to produce sedation or extreme hypotension. It is contraindicated for use in a patient with MI, aortic aneurysm, or pulmonary edema, because it increases the cardiac work load by reflex stimulation of the sympathetic nervous system.
USUAL ADULT DOSAGE: for hypertensive crisis and malignant hypertension, 1 to 3 mg/kg, up to a maximum of 150 mg I.V. bolus; may be repeated at 5- to 15-minute intervals until an adequate reduction in blood pressure is achieved.

hydralazine hydrochloride (Apresoline). This direct vasodilator, which may be administered orally or parenterally, is primarily used as a step-3 drug and is frequently given with a thiazide diuretic or a beta-adrenergic blocking agent. It is indicated as an adjunct to treat malignant hypertension complicated by renal insufficiency or congestive heart failure. I.V. or I.M. hydralazine may be used to treat hypertensive crisis. Because it results in increased tachycardia and cardiac output, hydralazine should be used cautiously in an elderly patient or a patient with ischemic heart disease. In these individuals, the drug may produce anginal attacks, myocardial ischemia, cerebrovascular disease, or renal impairment.
USUAL ADULT DOSAGE: 40 mg P.O. daily for the first 2 to 4 days, increased to 100 mg/day for the rest of the week, then to 200 mg/day and up to a maximum of 300 mg/day, given in two to four doses; 10 to 40 mg I.V. or I.M., repeated as needed.

minoxidil (Loniten). A potent oral vasodilator, minoxidil is reserved for patients with target organ damage who have not responded to other drugs. This step-4 drug is best used with a beta-adrenergic blocking agent to control tachycardia and a diuretic to counteract fluid retention.
USUAL ADULT DOSAGE: 5 to 40 mg P.O. daily in one or two equal doses, increased up to a maximum of 100 mg/day.

sodium nitroprusside (Nipride). A potent I.V. vasodilator, nitroprusside is used in hypertensive crises for rapid reduction of blood pressure. It is preferred over diazoxide in patients with congestive heart failure because, unlike diazoxide, it does not produce water and sodium retention. Nitroprusside therapy requires blood pressure monitoring every 5 minutes.
USUAL ADULT DOSAGE: 0.5 to 10 mcg/kg/minute by I.V. infusion; average dosage is 3 mcg/kg/minute.

diltiazem hydrochloride (Cardizem). A calcium channel blocker, diltiazem may be administered orally as a step-2 or step-3 agent for controlling hypertension.
USUAL ADULT DOSAGE: 30 mg P.O. t.i.d. or q.i.d., increased gradually, as needed, up to a maximum of 360 mg/day.

nifedipine (Procardia). This calcium channel blocker is given orally to treat hypertension. It may be a part of step-2 or step-3 therapy.
USUAL ADULT DOSAGE: initially, 10 mg P.O. t.i.d., increased to a maintenance dosage of 10 to 20 mg P.O. t.i.d., or up to a maximum of 180 mg/day.

verapamil hydrochloride (Isoptin). An effective calcium channel blocker, verapamil may be administered orally as a part of step-2 or step-3 therapy for hypertension.
USUAL ADULT DOSAGE: initially, 80 mg P.O. t.i.d., up to a maximum of 480 mg/day in divided doses; or 240 mg of sustained-release verapamil once daily.

Drug interactions

Hydralazine and minoxidil produce additive effects when given with other antihypertensive drugs, such as methyldopa and reserpine. They may also produce additive effects when given with nitrates, such as isosorbide or nitroglycerin. Few other drug interactions occur with the vasodilating agents. However, when given with digitalis, nifedipine may promote digitalis toxicity. Diltiazem also may interact with drugs that affect the hepatic microsomal system.

ADVERSE DRUG REACTIONS

Direct vasodilators frequently produce adverse reactions related to reflex activation of the sympathetic nervous system: palpitations, angina, tachycardia, increased myocardial work load, EKG changes, edema, breast tenderness, fatigue, headache, and rash. Severe pericardial effusions may develop. Alkaline phosphatase, BUN, and creatinine levels may increase. Unlike the other vasodilators, calcium channel blockers do not produce rebound tachycardia or significant edema. Other adverse reactions depend on the specific drug used.

Predictable reactions

Frequent adverse reactions to diazoxide include headache, anorexia, nausea, and diaphoresis. The following adverse reactions may also occur and usually require discontinuation of therapy: rash, drug fever, urticaria, polyneuritis, GI hemorrhage, anemia, and pancytopenia. Diazoxide is also especially likely to result in excessive hypotension and reflex sympathetic stimulation. It may also produce hyperglycemia in a diabetic patient. Because of these adverse reactions, the drug should be used cautiously in a patient with heart disease or renal failure.

Hydralazine frequently produces adverse reactions, such as headache, diarrhea, constipation, dizziness or light-headedness, orthostatic hypotension, facial flushing, shortness of breath, nasal congestion, urinary hesitation, lacrimation, conjunctivitis, paresthesias, edema, tremors, and muscle cramps.

When hydralazine dosage exceeds 200 mg/day, the patient may develop SLE. Initial symptoms of SLE include myalgias, arthralgias, and pleuritis. Later symptoms may include chest pain; generalized discomfort or weakness; blood dyscrasias (rare); joint pain; paresthesias, pain, or weakness in the hands or feet; skin rash or itching; sore throat; fever; swelling of the feet or lower legs; and lymphadenopathy.

Minoxidil frequently produces hypertrichosis (hair growth), especially on the face, arms, and back, 3 to 6 weeks after therapy begins. Minoxidil is also particularly likely to produce reflex tachycardia and fluid retention. Nitroprusside produces headache, dizziness, nausea, vomiting, and abdominal pain.

Diltiazem's most serious adverse reactions, hypotension and bradycardia, may be extensions of the drug's therapeutic effect. Other reactions may include flushing, palpitations, somnolence, tremors, insomnia, headache, edema, nausea, rash, and transient elevation of liver enzymes. Diltiazem is contraindicated in a patient with second- or third-degree heart block or impaired renal function. It should be used cautiously in a patient with impaired hepatic function.

Nifedipine can produce the same reactions as diltiazem, along with peripheral edema and dizziness or light-headedness.

The most frequent adverse reaction to verapamil is constipation; other reactions include those listed for diltiazem along with atrioventricular heart block, peripheral edema, dizziness, light-headedness, fatigue, and peripheral edema.

Unpredictable reactions

Hypersensitivity reactions (urticaria, rash, pruritus, fever, chills, arthralgia, eosinophilia, and rarely, obstructive jaundice and hepatitis), and blood dyscrasias (leukopenia, agranulocytosis, thrombocytopenia) are some unpredictable reactions that may occur with some of the antihypertensive vasodilators.

NURSING IMPLICATIONS

Because antihypertensive therapy is long-term, patient teaching is an important nursing responsibility. (See *Patient-teaching tips* for more information.) The nurse must also be aware of the following considerations.
• Be aware that direct vasodilators are contraindicated in a patient with pheochromocytoma, congestive heart failure, or MI.
• During vasodilator antihypertensive therapy monitor the patient's standing, sitting, and supine blood pressures, and assess the other vital signs. Monitor the blood pressure and pulse during peak concentration level times.

Patient-teaching tips

The patient who will be taking an antihypertensive agent at home requires some general instructions. The nurse should provide these instructions orally and in writing so that the patient can take them home. The nurse should also provide more detailed information about the specific drug or drugs that the patient will be taking. Including the patient's family in the teaching sessions can help improve patient compliance.

MEDICATION NAME _____

DOSAGE AND SCHEDULE _____

The patient taking an antihypertensive agent should know that its general action is to lower blood pressure.

Instruct the patient to:
• Take the drug exactly as prescribed and to not stop taking it abruptly even if the patient feels well or has a normal blood pressure reading. Abrupt discontinuation may cause serious problems, such as severe hypertension, angina, or heart failure.
• Avoid delays in refilling prescriptions, and be prepared with enough medication for weekends and holidays. If a dose is accidentally missed, take it as soon as possible, but do not take a double dose or take the missed dose close to the time of the next scheduled dose.
• Avoid sudden changes in position to prevent dizziness, light-headedness, or fainting. If faintness occurs, lie down immediately.
• Avoid driving or operating potentially dangerous machinery until the drug's effects are known. (Some people become drowsy, light-headed, and dizzy.)

• Avoid physical exertion, especially in hot weather. It could cause dehydration and increase the risk of dizziness or fainting. Standing for a long period of time or taking a hot shower or bath can cause similar problems and should be avoided.
• Prevent complications and uncomfortable symptoms by avoiding excessive use of stimulants, such as coffee, tea, and cola drinks, and depressants, such as alcohol.
• Consult the physician before taking any over-the-counter medication.
• Return for follow-up visits as directed.
• Store these drugs in tightly sealed containers away from light and moisture.
• Try to reduce the factors that tend to increase blood pressure, such as smoking, obesity, lack of exercise, stress, and excess salt intake. Overuse of salt can also cause excess fluid retention.

- Weigh the patient daily and monitor fluid intake and output.
- Administer oral hydralazine doses with meals to promote absorption.
- When administering hydralazine, monitor the patient's cardiac function to detect dysrhythmias. Monitor the patient's blood pressure and pulse before administering the drug. During administration, monitor the blood pressure and pulse every 5 minutes for the first 30 minutes, then every 15 minutes for about 2 hours until the blood pressure stabilizes.
- Expect to give minoxidil with a beta-adrenergic blocking agent to control tachycardia and a diuretic to counteract fluid retention.
- If rapid reduction in blood pressure occurs, it can produce cerebral ischemia with symptoms including sensory disturbances, anxiety, and slowed mental processes, and impaired renal blood flow, indicated by decreased urine output. If any such sign or symptom appears, assist the patient into a supine position, elevate the patient's legs, and notify the physician immediately.
- Advise a patient taking minoxidil that hypertrichosis is likely to occur 3 to 6 weeks after treatment begins. Reassure the patient that the extra hair growth should disappear 1 to 6 months after the drug is discontinued.
- With diazoxide administration, obtain baseline blood pressure and pulse rates. Then monitor the blood pressure and pulse rate at least every 15 minutes for 2 hours after the dose is given.
- Administer diazoxide via a peripheral vein to prevent cardiac dysrhythmias, and give it with a diuretic to prevent congestive heart failure from fluid retention.
- Prevent orthostatic hypotension after diazoxide administration by maintaining the patient in a supine position for 15 to 30 minutes after administration.
- Monitor the patient receiving diazoxide therapy for increases in serum glucose levels for up to 1 week after administration.
- Be aware that diazoxide is administered cautiously to a patient with impaired ventricular function, congestive heart failure, impaired hepatic function, conduction abnormalities, or impaired renal function.
- Advise the patient taking nifedipine to swallow the capsules whole.
- Instruct the patient receiving oral verapamil to take the doses 1 hour before or 2 hours after meals.

ANGIOTENSIN ANTAGONIST AGENTS

Another class of antihypertensive agents, angiotensin antagonist agents, reduce blood pressure by interrupting the renin-angiotensin-aldosterone system. Two antagonist agents, captopril and enalapril, block the conversion of angiotensin I to angiotensin II, a potent vasoconstrictor. A third agent, saralasin, competes with angiotensin II at tissue receptors, blocking its vascular, renal, adrenal, cardiac, and CNS effects.

Captopril or enalapril may be used to treat hypertension in a patient who does not respond to the usual step-2 drugs. These agents are particularly useful in treating hypertension associated with high renin levels. The pharmacologic use of saralasin is almost exclusively limited to testing for angiotensin II–dependent hypertension associated with renal vascular disease. Because of its limited use, it is not included in the following discussion of angiotensin antagonist antihypertensive agents.

History and source

In the 1970s, researchers discovered two types of renin-angiotensin system inhibitors: angiotensin II antagonists and angiotensin converting-enzyme (ACE) inhibitors. This discovery led to the introduction of a new category of antihypertensive drugs, the angiotensin antagonist agents. Captopril was introduced in 1981 and has been effective in a broad range of patients with essential hypertension. Enalapril is the newest angiotensin antagonist agent.

PHARMACOKINETICS

Both captopril and enalapril are absorbed from the GI tract, distributed to most body tissues, metabolized in the liver, and excreted by the kidneys.

Absorption, distribution, metabolism, excretion

Captopril is well absorbed from the GI tract, although the presence of food reduces absorption. This drug is distributed to most body tissues, but does not cross the blood-brain barrier. It is secreted in breast milk. About 25% to 30% of the circulating drug is bound to plasma protein. Captopril is metabolized in the liver and more than 95% of it is excreted in the urine.

After oral administration, about 60% of enalapril is absorbed. It undergoes metabolism in the liver and rapid excretion by the kidneys and is almost completely excreted within 4 hours.

Onset, peak, duration

Captopril reaches peak concentration levels in 60 to 90 minutes and full therapeutic effectiveness in weeks. Its half-life is probably less than 3 hours, and its duration of action ranges from 6 to 12 hours.

Enalapril's onset of action occurs in 1 hour and the peak blood pressure reduction occurs in 4 to 6 hours. This drug's half-life is 11 hours, and its duration of action is 24 hours.

PHARMACODYNAMICS

The ACE inhibitors captopril and enalapril act by interfering with the renin-angiotensin-aldosterone system. They do so by inhibiting the enzyme that converts angiotensin I to angiotensin II. This inhibition decreases aldosterone release by the adrenal cortex, preventing sodium and water retention. It also reduces peripheral arterial resistance without affecting the heart rate and cardiac output. The result, in a patient with hypertension, is a decreased blood pressure.

PHARMACOTHERAPEUTICS

Angiotensin antagonist agents are recommended to treat hypertension in patients who have failed to respond adequately, or who have developed severe adverse reactions to other antihypertensive agents. They are not usually considered primary agents.

captopril (Capoten). This agent is effective in treating hypertension associated with high or normal renin levels. It is also used to treat hypertension accompanied by low renin levels, but requires adjunctive diuretic therapy. It can be used alone, but is usually given with thiazide diuretics as a step-4 drug.
USUAL ADULT DOSAGE: for hypertension, initially, 12.5 to 25 mg P.O. t.i.d., increased to 50 mg t.i.d. after 1 to 2 weeks up to a maximum of 450 mg/day.

enalapril maleate (Vasotec). A step-1 and step-2 drug, enalapril is administered orally to treat mild to moderate hypertension. If used in conjunction with a diuretic, it may produce pronounced hypotension.

USUAL ADULT DOSAGE: initially, 5 mg P.O. once daily, increased to 10 to 40 mg/day, as needed, once a day or in divided doses.

Drug interactions

Captopril enhances the hypotensive effects of diuretics and other antihypertensives, such as beta-adrenergic blocking agents, and it may be less effective when administered with indomethacin. No significant drug interactions occur with enalapril.

ADVERSE DRUG REACTIONS

Angiotensin antagonists can produce a wide range of mild to severe adverse reactions.

Predictable reactions

Severe adverse reactions can occur with captopril and may limit its use. These may include proteinuria, neutropenia, agranulocytosis, rash, pruritus, fever, flushing or pallor, hypotension, orthostatic hypotension, tachycardia, chest pain, and loss of taste sensation. These reactions may be dose related and may disappear during the first few weeks of therapy without the need for discontinuing the drug. But if the reactions persist, enalapril may be prescribed because it produces similar reactions far less frequently. Captopril may also elevate liver enzyme, BUN, serum creatinine, and serum potassium. Mouth sores and sore throat can also occur with use of either angiotensin antagonist agent.

Unpredictable reactions

Although infrequent, acute renal failure may occur with captopril. It may be reversible with discontinuation of the drug.

Enalapril may produce angioedema in some patients. When this reaction affects the face, tongue, or glottis or causes laryngeal stridor, the drug must be discontinued.

NURSING IMPLICATIONS

The nurse must provide a great deal of information for a patient receiving an antihypertensive agent. (See *Patient-teaching tips* on page 599 for more details.) The nurse must also be aware of the following considerations.

SELECTED MAJOR DRUGS

Antihypertensive agents

This chart summarizes the major antihypertensive drugs currently in use.

DRUG	MAJOR INDICATIONS	USUAL ADULT DOSAGES	NURSING IMPLICATIONS
Sympatholytic agents			
clonidine	Mild to moderate hypertension, as a step-2 drug	Initially, 0.1 mg P.O. b.i.d., increased by 0.1 or 0.2 mg/day every 2 to 4 days; maintenance dose, 0.1 to 0.2 mg b.i.d. to q.i.d. up to a maximum of 2.4 mg/day	• Inform the patient taking clonidine that vivid dreams may occur. • Closely monitor a patient with a history of depression, because it may recur. • Give this central-acting agent between meals. If sedation occurs, give the drug in the evening.
methyldopa	Mild to moderate hypertension, as a step-2 drug	Initially, 250 mg P.O. b.i.d. or t.i.d. increased biweekly to a maintenance dose of 500 mg to 2 grams/day in two to four divided doses or up to a maximum of 3 grams/day	• Monitor the patient's blood pressure at regular intervals with the patient supine, sitting, and standing. • Advise the patient that orthostatic hypotension may occur, producing dizziness and light-headedness. • Monitor the patient for signs of depression, such as anorexia, insomnia, and withdrawal. • Advise the patient taking methyldopa that the drug may darken the urine. • Give this central-acting agent between meals. If sedation occurs, give the drug in the evening.
	Hypertensive crisis	250 to 500 mg I.V. in 100 ml of dextrose 5% in water infused over 30 to 60 minutes, repeated q6h, as needed	
metoprolol	Hypertension, alone or with other antihypertensives, as a step-1 or step-2 drug	Initially, 100 mg P.O. daily in single or divided doses, increased by 50 mg/day every week up to a maximum of 450 mg/day	• Administer metoprolol with food to promote its absorption. • Anticipate gradual discontinuation of this drug over 3 to 14 days. During this time, the patient should avoid vigorous physical activity.
propranolol	Mild to moderate hypertension, alone or with other antihypertensives, as a step-1 or step-2 drug	40 mg P.O. b.i.d. increased gradually to a maximum of 640 mg/day	• Be aware that propranolol may mask signs of hypoglycemia. • Administer propranolol with food to promote its absorption.
prazosin	Hypertension, alone or with other antihypertensives, as a step-2 drug	Initially, 0.5 to 1 mg b.i.d. to t.i.d. increased gradually to a maintenance dose that meets the patient's needs; maintenance dose, 6 to 15 mg/day when given alone or 1 to 2 mg P.O. t.i.d. when given with a diuretic or another antihypertensive agent	• Be aware that syncope may occur with the first dose or a rapid dose increase. • Instruct the patient to take the first dose or the first increased dose at bedtime and to avoid rapid position changes. • Instruct the patient not to take over-the-counter medications that contain sympathomimetics without consulting the physician first.
labetalol	Mild to severe hypertension, alone or with other agents, as a step-1 or step-2 drug	100 mg P.O. b.i.d. increased, as needed, up to 400 mg b.i.d.	• Maintain the patient in a supine position during I.V. administration, and monitor the blood pressure and pulse after injection. • Instruct the patient to avoid rapid position changes because orthostatic hypoten-

SELECTED MAJOR DRUGS

Antihypertensive agents continued

DRUG	MAJOR INDICATIONS	USUAL ADULT DOSAGES	NURSING IMPLICATIONS
labetalol (continued)	Hypertensive crisis	20 to 80 mg I.V. bolus every 10 minutes or 2 mg/minute by continuous I.V. infusion up to a maximum of 300 mg	sion is likely to occur after administration.
Vasodilating agents			
diazoxide	Hypertensive crisis and malignant hypertension	1 to 3 mg/kg up to a maximum of 150 mg I.V. bolus, may be repeated at 5- to 15-minute intervals until an adequate reduction in blood pressure is achieved	• Monitor the patient's blood glucose levels for increases for up to 1 week after administration. • Maintain the patient in a supine position during administration and for 15 to 30 minutes afterward. • Monitor the patient's blood pressure and pulse at least every 15 minutes for 2 hours.
nifedipine	Hypertension, as a step-2 or step-3 drug	Initially, 10 mg P.O. t.i.d., increased to a maintenance dose of 10 to 20 mg P.O. t.i.d or up to a maximum of 180 mg/day	• Monitor the patient's standing, sitting, and supine blood pressures during therapy. • Advise the patient taking nifedipine to swallow the capsules whole.
Angiotensin antagonist agent			
captopril	Hypertension, alone or with a diuretic, as a step-4 drug	Initially, 12.5 to 25 mg P.O. t.i.d., increased to 50 mg P.O. t.i.d. after 1 to 2 weeks and up to a maximum of 450 mg/day	• Administer captopril 1 hour before meals to promote absorption. • Monitor baseline and periodic urine protein levels and WBC and differential counts. • Monitor the patient's supine and standing blood pressures during therapy.

• Assess the patient for a history of impaired renal function, autoimmune disease, or exposure to a drug that affects the white blood cell (WBC) count or the immune system before initiating therapy as prescribed.

• Be aware that an angiotensin antagonist is more effective when given with a thiazide, thiazidelike, or loop diuretic, and that captopril may counteract the potassium-depleting effects of the diuretics.

• Administer captopril cautiously to a patient with a renal disease, a serious autoimmune disease (particularly SLE), hyperkalemia, or a history of exposure to drugs that affect the bone marrow. Also administer captopril cautiously to an elderly patient who may be hypersensitive to the drug and to a patient with severe coronary insufficiency, a recent MI, or cerebrovascular disease.

• Specifically ask the patient taking an angiotensin antagonist agent about taste impairment, because the patient may not associate it with drug therapy and so may not report it.

• Before beginning angiotensin antagonist therapy, obtain a baseline blood pressure and pulse rate to use in continuous monitoring of the patient.

• Monitor the patient's fluid intake and output and daily weight in order to assess renal function.

• Monitor the patient's WBC and differential counts before starting angiotension antagonist therapy, every 2 weeks during the first 3 months of therapy, and periodically thereafter.

• Monitor the patient for proteinuria every 2 to 4 weeks for the first 3 months of therapy.

• Monitor the patient's liver function tests and serum BUN, creatinine, and potassium levels before treatment begins and monthly during the first 3 months of therapy.

• During therapy, monitor supine and standing blood pressures to detect orthostatic hypotension.

• Advise the patient taking an angiotensin antagonist agent to take it on an empty stomach, preferably 1 hour before meals, for optimum effectiveness.

CHAPTER SUMMARY

Chapter 37 discussed sympatholytic agents, vasodilating agents, and angiotensin antagonist agents as they are used in the treatment of hypertension. Here are the highlights of the chapter:

• Hypertension is a frequently occurring disease that can be successfully controlled with drug and nondrug therapy.

• Nondrug therapy should begin as soon as hypertension is diagnosed and should continue throughout the course of treatment. Nondrug interventions include a sodium-restricted diet that is also low in saturated fat, weight reduction (if the patient is obese), regular physical exercise, discontinuation of cigarette smoking, and moderate or no alcohol ingestion.

• When necessary, drug treatment using the stepped-care approach is instituted to manage hypertension. This cumulative systematic approach to antihypertensive therapy begins with agents that are least likely to produce adverse reactions and adds to or substitutes for these agents, as needed, to achieve optimum blood pressure control.

• Many types of drugs can be used singly or in combination to treat hypertension, including sympatholytic agents, vasodilating agents, and angiotensin antagonist agents.

• Sympatholytic agents reduce blood pressure by inhibiting or blocking motor and secretory action in the sympathetic nervous system. They are classified by their site or mechanism of action and include central-acting sympathetic nervous system inhibitors, ganglionic blocking agents, beta-adrenergic blocking agents, alpha-adrenergic blocking agents, mixed alpha- and beta-adrenergic blocking agents, and norepinephrine depletors.

• Direct vasodilators act on arteries, veins, or both to reduce blood pressure. They include diazoxide, hydralazine, minoxidil, and nitroprusside. These drugs act by directly relaxing arterial or venous smooth muscle. Calcium channel blockers represent a type of vasodilator that blocks the transport of calcium into cells, which is necessary for the arterial smooth muscle to maintain tone and ability to contract. Calcium channel blockers include diltiazem, nifedipine, and verapamil.

• Angiotensin antagonist agents reduce blood pressure by interfering with the renin-angiotensin-aldosterone system. They inhibit the enzyme that converts angiotensin I to angiotensin II, a potent vasoconstrictor. Angiotensin inhibition also decreases aldosterone release, preventing sodium and water retention.

BIBLIOGRAPHY

AHFS (American Hospital Formulary Service). *Drug Information.* McEvoy, G.K., et al., eds. Bethesda, Md.: American Society of Hospital Pharmacists, 1987.

Becker, P.M., and Warshae, G.A. "Managing Hypertension in Elderly Patients," *Drug Therapy* 13:61, 1983.

Beevers, D.G. et al. "Guanfacine: A New Central Acting Antihypertensive," *Pharmacotherapeutics* 2(8):513, 1981.

Bruno, H.C., et al. "Fever Induced by Labetalol," *Journal of the American Medical Association* 256:619, 1986.

Butler, J.D., and Harrison, B.L. "Keeping Pace with Calcium Channel Blockers," *Nursing83* 13:38, July 1983.

Chobanian, A. "Hypertension," *Ciba Clinical Symposia* 34:3, 1982.

Epstein, M. *Hypertension: A Practical Approach.* Philadelphia: W.B. Saunders Co., 1984.

Erfurt, J.C. *Development and Dissemination of Model Systems for Hypertension Control in Organizational Settings.* Ann Arbor, Mich.: Institute of Labor and Industrial Relations, 1974.

Frohlich, E.D. "Pharmacology and Clinical Potential of the Newer Antihypertensive Drugs," *Practical Cardiology* 9:81, 1983.

Genest, J., et al. *Hypertension: Pathophysiology and Treatment,* 2nd ed. New York: McGraw-Hill Book Co., 1983.

Gilfont, B. "Hypertension Protocol," *Nurse Practitioner* 8:25, 1983.

Gilman, A.G., et al., eds. *Goodman and Gilman's The Pharmacological Basis of Theapeutics,* 7th ed. New York: Macmillan Publishing Co., 1985.

Guazzi, M.D. "The Role of Calcium Antagonists in the Management of Hypertension," *Practical Cardiology* 8:39, 1982.

Hedner, et al. "Guanfacine in Essential Hypertension," *Clinical Pharmacy and Therapeutics* 35:604, 1984.

Kaplan, N.M. *Clinical Hypertension,* 2nd ed. Baltimore: Williams & Wilkins Co., 1982.

Kaplan, N.M. "New Approaches to the Therapy of Mild Hypertension," *The American Journal of Cardiology* 51:621, 1983.

McMahon, F.G. *Management of Essential Hypertension: The New Low-Dose Era,* 2nd ed. Mount Kisco, N.Y.: Futura Publishing Co., 1984.

"The 1984 Report of the Joint National Committee on Detection, Evaluation, and Treatment of High Blood Pressure," *Nurse Practitioner* 10:9, 1985.

Oren, A., et al. "Low-dose Captopril: An Alternative After β-blocker Reaction," *American Heart Journal* 109:554, 1985.

Schirger, A., et al. "Pindolol: A New Beta-Adrenergic Blocking Agent with Intrinsic Sympathomimetic Activity in the Management of Mild and Moderate Hypertension," *Mayo Clinic Proceedings* 58:315, 1983.

U.S. Pharmacopeial Convention. *USPDI: Drug Information for the Health Care Provider.* St. Louis: C.V. Mosby Co., 1986.

CHAPTER 38

DIURETIC AGENTS

OBJECTIVES

After reading and studying this chapter, you should be able to:

1. Differentiate among the various mechanisms of action of thiazide and thiazide-like, loop, and potassium-sparing diuretics and those of carbonic anhydrase inhibitors and osmotic diuretics.

2. Describe the absorption, distribution, metabolism, and excretion of the various types of diuretics.

3. Identify the major clinical indications for the various types of diuretics.

4. Describe the major drug interactions that can occur with the various types of diuretics.

5. Describe the fluid and electrolyte imbalances that frequently occur as a result of diuretic therapy.

6. Identify the specific nursing implications related to diuretic therapy.

INTRODUCTION

Most diuretic agents promote renal excretion of water and electrolytes by increasing the glomerular filtration rate (GFR), decreasing sodium reabsorption, or increasing the rate of sodium excretion. Physicians use diuretics clinically to increase urine volume and the net excretion of solutes and water. These agents act at different sites within the nephrons (structural and functional units of the kidney) to produce diuresis. (See *Principal sites of diuretic action* for a depiction of a nephron and the various sites of diuretic activity.) The diuretics discussed in this chapter are classified as thiazide and thiazide-like diuretics, loop and potassium-sparing diuretics, carbonic anhydrase inhibitors, and osmotic and mercurial diuretics.

For a summary of representative drugs, see *Selected major drugs: Diuretic agents* on pages 624 to 628.

THIAZIDE AND THIAZIDE-LIKE DIURETICS

Thiazide and thiazide-like diuretics are sulfonamide derivatives that inhibit sodium reabsorption, thereby increasing sodium and water excretion. Thiazide and thiazide-like diuretics may induce a hypersensitivity reaction similar to sulfonamide's; they also increase the excretion of chloride, potassium, and bicarbonate ions, which can result in electrolyte imbalances, particularly hypokalemia. The thiazide diuretics include bendroflumethiazide, benzthiazide, chlorothiazide, cyclothiazide, hydrochlorothiazide, hydroflumethiazide, methyclothiazide, polythiazide, and trichlormethiazide. The thiazide-like diuretics include chlorthalidone, metolazone, and quinethazone.

History and source

The thiazides are synthesized agents developed as a result of research on carbonic anhydrase inhibitors. The discovery of thiazides occurred in 1957 when chlorothiazide was synthesized by Novello and clinically introduced by Beyer. After extensive clinical trials, chlorothiazide was approved by the Food and Drug Administration (FDA) in 1958; FDA approval of hydrochlorothiazide followed a year later.

PHARMACOKINETICS

Thiazide diuretics are rapidly but incompletely absorbed after oral administration and are excreted in the urine. These drugs are particularly useful because of their rapid action.

Principal sites of diuretic action

Diuretics increase the urinary excretion of water and sodium, primarily by decreasing sodium chloride reabsorption in the renal tubules. Different diuretics act at different sites in the nephron, as illustrated below.

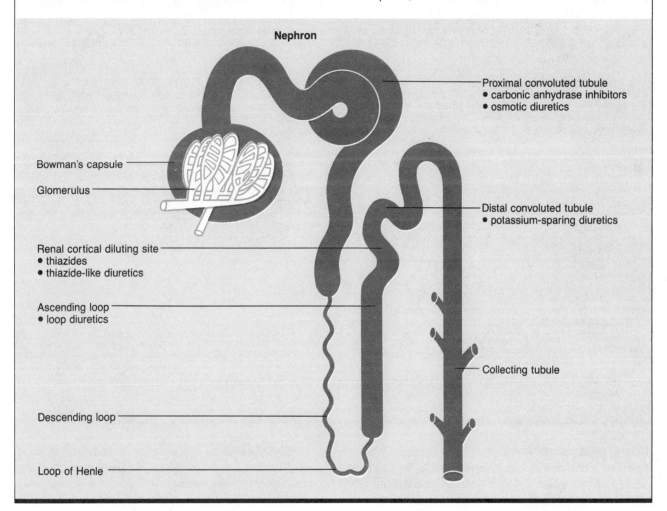

Nephron

Proximal convoluted tubule
- carbonic anhydrase inhibitors
- osmotic diuretics

Bowman's capsule

Glomerulus

Distal convoluted tubule
- potassium-sparing diuretics

Renal cortical diluting site
- thiazides
- thiazide-like diuretics

Ascending loop
- loop diuretics

Collecting tubule

Descending loop

Loop of Henle

Absorption, distribution, metabolism, excretion

Thiazide diuretics are rapidly but incompletely absorbed from the gastrointestinal (GI) tract after oral administration. Oral chlorothiazide is the most poorly absorbed (10%) thiazide diuretic. The protein binding of thiazide diuretics varies, ranging from 65% for hydrochlorothiazide to 95% for chlorothiazide. Thiazide diuretics cross the placenta and appear in breast milk. These agents differ in their degree of metabolism. Some agents, such as hydrochlorothiazide, are excreted basically unchanged in the urine, whereas others, such as polythiazide, are extensively metabolized.

The thiazides are rapidly eliminated by the kidneys because they are actively secreted by the proximal tubules. Minute quantities of these drugs usually appear in bile, but metolazone, which undergoes some enterohepatic metabolism, is present in higher quantities. Excretion of the thiazide diuretics is delayed in patients with congestive heart failure (CHF), impaired renal function, or any other disorder that reduces renal blood flow. (Thiazide diuretics are not effective in patients with renal impairment whose GFR is less than 20 ml/minute.)

Onset, peak, and duration of thiazide and thiazide-like diuretics

The onset of action, peak concentration levels, and duration of action of the thiazide and thiazide-like diuretics vary significantly. These differences will influence the nurse's plan of care for a specific patient.

DRUG	ONSET OF ACTION	PEAK CONCENTRATIONS	DURATION OF ACTION
Thiazide diuretics			
bendroflumethiazide	1 hour	4 hours	6 to 12 hours
benzthiazide	1 hour	4 to 6 hours	6 to 12 hours
chlorothiazide I.V.	15 minutes	30 minutes	2 hours
chlorothiazide P.O.	1 hour	4 hours	6 to 12 hours
cyclothiazide	6 hours	7 to 12 hours	18 to 24 hours
hydrochlorothiazide	1 hour	4 to 6 hours	6 to 12 hours
hydroflumethiazide	1 hour	4 hours	6 to 12 hours
methyclothiazide	1 hour	6 hours	24 hours
polythiazide	1 hour	6 hours	24 to 48 hours
trichlormethiazide	1 hour	6 hours	24 hours
Thiazide-like diuretics			
chlorthalidone	2 hours	4 to 6 hours	24 to 72 hours
metolazone	1 hour	2 hours	12 to 24 hours
quinethazone	1 hour	6 hours	18 to 24 hours

Onset, peak, duration

Onset of action of the thiazide and thiazide-like diuretics usually occurs within 1 hour of oral administration. Cyclothiazide is an exception: Its diuretic effects do not begin until 6 hours after oral administration. In addition, intravenous (I.V.) chlorothiazide will begin to act within 15 minutes of administration. Optimal antihypertensive effects of these agents, however, usually do not appear for 3 to 4 weeks after initiation of therapy—but they may appear within 3 or 4 days.

Peak concentration levels of thiazide and thiazide-like diuretics usually occur within 4 to 6 hours. Specifically, bendroflumethiazide, chlorothiazide, and hydroflumethiazide peak in 4 hours; benzthiazide and hydrochlorothiazide peak in 4 to 6 hours; and methyclothiazide, polythiazide, quinethazone, and trichlormethiazide peak in 6 hours. I.V. chlorothiazide and cyclothiazide are the exceptions: I.V. chlorothiazide reaches peak concentration levels within 30 minutes, but I.V. cyclothiazide takes from 7 to 12 hours.

The duration of action of the thiazide and thiazide-like diuretics is 6 to 24 hours, depending on the drug excretion rate. Specifically, I.V. chlorothiazide has a duration of action of only 2 hours; bendroflumethiazide, benzthiazide, chlorothiazide, hydrochlorothiazide, and hydroflumethiazide have a short duration of action of 6 to 12 hours; cyclothiazide and quinethazone have a duration of action of 18 to 24 hours; methyclothiazide and trichlormethiazide have a long duration of action of 24 hours; and polythiazide's duration of action may be from 24 to 48 hours. (See *Onset, peak, and duration of thiazide and thiazide-like diuretics* for a summary of these actions.)

PHARMACODYNAMICS

The thiazide and thiazide-like diuretics increase the excretion of sodium, chloride, and water by inhibiting the reabsorption of sodium. These drugs also increase the excretion of potassium ions.

Mechanism of action

Thiazide and thiazide-like diuretics interfere with the transport of sodium ions across the renal tubular epithelium at the cortical-diluting, or distal, segments of the nephrons. Like the sulfonamides, thiazides create some minor carbonic anhydrase inhibition. These effects result in increased sodium, chloride, and water excretion with excretion of sodium and chloride in approximately equal amounts and concomitant excretion of magnesium, phosphate, bromide, and iodide. At the same time, the excretion of ammonium, urates, and calcium is decreased. Thiazide diuretics may also decrease the GFR.

Researchers currently believe that the action of the thiazide and thiazide-like diuretics is primarily linked to the increased excretion of sodium. Initially, these drugs result in a decrease in circulating blood volume, thus decreasing cardiac output. If the therapy is maintained, the cardiac output stabilizes, but extracellular fluid and plasma volume decrease. Direct dilation of the arterioles and decreased peripheral vascular resistance also seem to occur.

PHARMACOTHERAPEUTICS

Thiazide and thiazide-like diuretics may be used alone or in combination with other drugs; they are primarily used to treat hypertension and edema from mild or moderate CHF. Physicians also use these drugs alone or in combination with other drugs to prevent the development and recurrence of calcium nephrolithiasis in hypercalciuric and normal calciuric patients.

Thiazides are also used to reduce urine volume in patients with diabetes insipidus and to treat the edema associated not only with CHF, but also with hepatic disease, renal disease, and corticosteroid and estrogen therapy. Although the thiazide and thiazide-like diuretics are not usually effective if the GFR is less than 20 ml/ minute, one exception exists: metolazone, which remains effective even with a decreased GFR.

Thiazides may be used alone or in combination with other drugs to treat hypertension. Although their antihypertensive effects may begin within 3 to 4 days after initiation of therapy, the drugs are most effective after 3 to 4 weeks of continued therapy. The thiazides are frequently used in combination with other drugs for the long-term control of hypertension.

bendroflumethiazide (Naturetin). This thiazide diuretic is used to treat edema and hypertension.

USUAL ADULT DOSAGE: initially, 5 to 20 mg P.O. daily or in two divided doses; for maintenance, 2.5 to 5 mg P.O. daily.
USUAL PEDIATRIC DOSAGE: initially, 0.1 to 0.4 mg/kg/ day in one or two doses; for maintenance, 0.05 to 0.1 mg/kg/day in one or two doses.

benzthiazide (Aquapres, Aquatag, Exna, Marazide, Proaqua, Urazide). Physicians use this thiazide diuretic to treat edema and hypertension.
USUAL ADULT DOSAGE: for edema, 50 to 200 mg P.O. daily or in divided doses; for hypertension, 50 mg P.O. daily to q.i.d., depending on the patient's response.
USUAL PEDIATRIC DOSAGE: 1 to 4 mg/kg P.O. daily in three divided doses.

chlorothiazide (Diuril). A thiazide diuretic, chlorothiazide is used to treat edema and hypertension. Chlorothiazide may be administered I.V. but not I.M. or S.C.
USUAL ADULT DOSAGE: for edema, 500 mg to 2 grams P.O. or I.V. daily or in two divided doses; for hypertension, 500 mg to 1 gram P.O. or I.V. daily or in divided doses.
USUAL PEDIATRIC DOSAGE: over age 6 months, 20 mg/ kg P.O. or I.V. daily in divided doses; under age 6 months, up to 30 mg/kg P.O. or I.V. daily in divided doses.

cyclothiazide (Anhydron). This thiazide diuretic is used to treat edema and hypertension.
USUAL ADULT DOSAGE: for edema, 1 to 2 mg P.O. daily or on alternate days; for hypertension, 2 mg P.O. daily to t.i.d.
USUAL PEDIATRIC DOSAGE: for edema, 0.02 to 0.04 mg/kg P.O. daily.

hydrochlorothiazide (Esidrix, HydroDiuril, Oretic). This thiazide diuretic is used to treat edema and hypertension.
USUAL ADULT DOSAGE: for edema, 25 to 100 mg P.O. daily or intermittently; for hypertension, 25 to 100 mg P.O. daily or in divided doses; dosages are increased or decreased according to the patient's response.
USUAL PEDIATRIC DOSAGE: over age 6 months, 2.2 mg/ kg P.O. daily divided in two doses; under age 6 months, 3.3 mg/kg P.O. daily divided in two doses.

hydroflumethiazide (Diucardin, Saluron). This thiazide diuretic is used to treat edema and hypertension.
USUAL ADULT DOSAGE: for edema, initially 25 to 100 mg P.O. daily, in divided doses, then maintenance with 25 to 200 mg P.O. intermittently or on alternate days; for hypertension, 50 to 100 mg P.O. once or twice a day up to a maximum of 200 mg/day.
USUAL PEDIATRIC DOSAGE: 1 mg/kg P.O. daily.

DRUG INTERACTIONS

Thiazide and thiazide-like diuretics

Drug interactions related to thiazide and thiazide-like diuretics may cause severe fluid and electrolyte imbalances and other potentially serious problems. The nurse needs to be aware of these interactions to plan appropriate nursing care.

DRUG	INTERACTING DRUGS	POSSIBLE EFFECTS	NURSING IMPLICATIONS
all thiazides and thiazide-like diuretics	oral hypoglycemic agents	May cause hyponatremia, thiazide resistance, hyperglycemia	• Monitor the patient's serum sodium and glucose levels. • Monitor the patient for signs and symptoms of hyponatremia and hyperglycemia.
	corticosteroids, ACTH, amphotericin B, extended-spectrum penicillins (carbenicillin, azocillin, mezlocillin)	May cause hypokalemia	• Monitor the patient's serum potassium levels. • Monitor the patient for the signs and symptoms of hypokalemia, such as weakness and flattened T wave on EKG.
	lithium carbonate	May cause lithium toxicity	• Monitor the patient for the signs and symptoms of lithium toxicity, such as ataxia. • Monitor the patient's serum lithium levels.
	skeletal muscle relaxants, tubocurarine, gallamine	Increase responsiveness to tubocurarine and gallamine	• Monitor the patient for the therapeutic effects of skeletal muscle relaxants.
	tetracyclines	Elevate BUN levels	• Monitor the patient's renal function.
	antihypertensive drugs	May cause orthostatic hypotension	• Monitor the patient's fluid intake and output. • Monitor the patient's serum electrolyte levels. • Weigh the patient daily. • Instruct the patient to avoid standing quickly. • Monitor the patient's sitting and standing blood pressures.
	alcohol	May cause orthostatic hypotension	• Advise the patient to stand slowly, limit alcohol intake, and avoid strenuous exercise in hot weather.
	digitalis	May cause digitalis toxicity	• Monitor the patient for the signs and symptoms of digitalis toxicity. • Monitor the patient's serum digitalis levels. • Monitor the patient's serum electrolyte levels.
	probenecid	Decreases renal excretion	• Monitor the patient's fluid intake and output. • Monitor the patient's serum electrolyte levels.
hydrochlorothiazide, chlorothiazide	cholestyramine, colestipol	Decrease therapeutic effect of diuretic	• Administer thiazide or thiazide-like diuretics 2 hours before drug administration. • Monitor the patient for the therapeutic effects of the diuretic.

methyclothiazide (Aquatensen, Enduron). This long-acting thiazide diuretic is used to treat edema and hypertension.

USUAL ADULT DOSAGE: 2.5 to 10 mg P.O. daily.

polythiazide (Lotense, Renese). A long-acting thiazide diuretic, polythiazide is used to treat hypertension and edema from cardiac failure or renal failure.

USUAL ADULT DOSAGE: for hypertension, 2 to 4 mg P.O. daily; for edema, 1 to 4 mg P.O. daily.

trichlormethiazide (Metahydrin, Naqua). This long-acting thiazide diuretic is used to treat edema and hypertension.

USUAL ADULT DOSAGE: for edema, 1 to 4 mg P.O. daily or in two divided doses; for hypertension, 2 to 4 mg P.O. daily.

chlorthalidone (Hygroton). This long-acting thiazide-like diuretic is used to treat edema and hypertension.

USUAL ADULT DOSAGE: for edema, 50 to 100 mg P.O. daily or 100 mg on alternate days (up to 200 mg/day may be necessary for therapeutic effect); for hypertension, 25 to 50 mg P.O. daily, or 100 mg three times weekly or on alternate days (up to 200 mg/day may be necessary for therapeutic effect).

USUAL PEDIATRIC DOSAGE: 2 mg/kg P.O. three times weekly.

metolazone (Diulo, Zaraxolyn). This thiazide-like diuretic is used to treat hypertension and the edema secondary to CHF, hepatic disease, or renal disease. It is occasionally used with other thiazides or furosemide. Unlike other thiazide and thiazide-like diuretics, metolazone is effective even when the patient's GFR is less than 20 ml/minute.

USUAL ADULT DOSAGE: for edema from CHF, 5 to 10 mg P.O. daily; for edema from renal or hepatic disease, 5 to 20 mg P.O. daily; for hypertension, 2.5 to 5 mg P.O. daily; the dosage may be increased or decreased to maintain the therapeutic effect.

quinethazone (Aquamox, Hydromox). This thiazide-like diuretic is used to treat edema.

USUAL ADULT DOSAGE: 50 to 100 mg P.O. daily, as needed; dosage may be increased up to 200 mg/day.

Drug interactions

Drug interactions related to the thiazide and thiazide-like diuretics result in altered fluid volume, blood pressure, and serum electrolyte levels. (See *Drug interactions: Thiazide and thiazide-like diuretics* for details of specific drug interactions.)

ADVERSE DRUG REACTIONS

Numerous adverse reactions are associated with the use of thiazide and thiazide-like diuretics. The most common are blood volume depletion, orthostatic hypotension, and hypokalemia.

Predictable reactions

Besides blood volume depletion, orthostatic hypotension, and hypokalemia, predictable adverse reactions to thiazide and thiazide-like diuretics include glucose intolerance, hypercalcemia, and hypophosphatemia, which may occur with prolonged therapy; hyperuricemia, especially in patients with a history of gout; and GI reactions, such as anorexia, nausea, and pancreatitis.

Unpredictable reactions

Hypersensitivity reactions may occur in the form of purpura, photosensitivity, rash, urticaria, necrotizing vasculitis, or blood abnormalities, which may include leukopenia, thrombocytopenia, aplastic anemia, or agranulocytosis.

NURSING IMPLICATIONS

The nursing implications related to thiazide and thiazide-like diuretics focus on these drugs' potential to affect the patient's fluid and electrolyte balance. Preventing or monitoring hypokalemia and volume depletion is essential. Also, the nurse should be aware of the following considerations:

• Thiazide and thiazide-like diuretics are contraindicated in patients who are hypersensitive to the thiazides or the sulfonamides. Monitor such patients closely for signs and symptoms of hypersensitivity reactions.

• These drugs are also contraindicated in anuric patients; administer these drugs cautiously to patients with renal disease or impaired hepatic function.

• Monitor the patient's serum potassium levels, and observe for the signs and symptoms of hypokalemia: drowsiness, confusion, apathy, coma, irritability, muscle weakness, paresthesias, muscle pain, muscle cramps, muscle tenderness, hyporeflexia, tetany, paralysis, weak pulse, bradycardia, hypoventilation, nausea and vomiting, anorexia, abdominal cramps, paralytic ileus, polydipsia, hyperglycemia, polyuria, and nocturia.

• Administer potassium supplements as ordered to maintain acceptable serum potassium levels, and encourage the patient to eat potassium-rich foods. (See *Guide to potassium-rich foods* on page 612 for a list of these foods.)

Guide to potassium-rich foods

The nurse should encourage the patient on diuretic therapy to eat potassium-rich foods. This chart can help the nurse provide information on foods the patient can include in the diet.

JUICES	mg per 100 grams
Tomato	227
Orange, fresh	200
Orange, reconstituted	186

VEGETABLES	mg per 100 grams
Potatoes	407
Lima beans	394
Carrots	341
Spinach	324
Radishes	322
Sweet potatoes	300
Brussels sprouts	295
Endive	294
Asparagus	238
Cabbage	233
Peppers	213

FRUITS	mg per 100 grams
Dates	648
Bananas	370
Raisins	355
Plums	299
Nectarines	294
Apricots	281
Prunes	262
Peaches	202
Oranges	200
Figs	152

FISH	mg per 100 grams
Sardines, canned	590
Halibut	525
Scallops	476
Salmon	421
Haddock	348
Flounder	342
Tuna	301
Perch	284
Bass	256
Oysters	203

MEATS	mg per 100 grams
Veal	500
Chicken	411
Turkey	411
Liver	380
Beef	370
Pork	326
Lamb	290

MISCELLANEOUS	mg per 100 grams
Milk, dry (nonfat solids)	1,745
Molasses (light)	917
Peanuts	674
Peanut butter	670
Gingersnaps	462
Graham crackers	384
Oatmeal cookies (with raisins)	370
Ice milk	195

• Patients receiving digitalis and thiazide therapy run an increased risk of developing digitalis toxicity from potassium depletion; monitor the patient's serum digitalis levels and pulse frequently.

• Monitor blood glucose levels in a diabetic patient who is receiving thiazide therapy.

• To monitor edema, weigh the patient daily under controlled conditions (at the same time each morning, after the patient voids, before the patient eats, with the patient wearing similar clothing at each weigh-in, and with the same scale).

• Monitor the patient's fluid intake and output carefully to detect any fluctuations.

• Monitor the patient's serum electrolyte, creatinine, and blood urea nitrogen (BUN) levels to detect any imbalances.

• Monitor serum uric acid levels in a patient with a history of gout.

• Monitor the patient for signs and symptoms of metabolic alkalosis: hypoventilation, dysrhythmias, irritability, tetany, belligerence, confusion, stupor, nausea and vomiting, and diarrhea.

• Consult with the physician about discontinuing thiazide therapy before parathyroid studies are done, because thiazides can alter the results of these tests.

LOOP DIURETICS

Loop, or high-ceiling, diuretics are highly potent agents. Very effective in treating edema, hypertension, and hypercalcemia, they are also valuable in treating patients who are resistant to less potent diuretics or who have decreased GFRs. Because of their potency, loop diuretics may produce profound diuresis, with water and electrolyte depletion. The loop diuretics include bumetanide, ethacrynate sodium and ethacrynic acid, furosemide, and indapamide.

History and source

The development of loop diuretics began around 1950 with studies of inorganic ion transport inhibitors. One inhibitor studied was a sulfhydryl-containing enzyme that was antagonized by mercurial diuretics. Study of this enzyme led to the development of ethacrynic acid. The development of other loop diuretics followed, with the introduction of furosemide in 1960, bumetanide in 1971, and indapamide in 1983.

PHARMACOKINETICS

Loop diuretics are usually well absorbed and rapidly distributed. Extensively protein-bound, these agents undergo partial or complete metabolism in the liver except for furosemide, which is excreted primarily unchanged. Loop diuretics are primarily excreted by the kidneys.

Besides their greater potency, these diuretics have a more rapid onset of action and produce a much greater volume of diuresis than other types of diuretics.

Absorption, distribution, metabolism, excretion

Bumetanide is almost completely absorbed after oral or I.M. administration. Also available for I.V. administration, it is more than 95% protein-bound. Ethacrynic acid is rapidly absorbed from the GI tract after oral administration; available for I.V. administration as well, it is also about 95% protein-bound. After oral administration, furosemide is 60% to 70% absorbed from the GI tract; taking the drug with food slows the absorption rate but has little effect on the total amount absorbed. Also available for I.V. administration, furosemide is 99% protein-bound. Indapamide is rapidly absorbed after oral administration; it is 80% protein-bound.

Bumetanide is partially metabolized in the liver. About 80% of a dose is excreted in the urine, 50% as unchanged drug and the remainder as conjugates and metabolites. About 15% is eliminated in the feces.

As ethacrynic acid accumulates in the liver, it is metabolized to active cysteine conjugate. Approximately two thirds of a dose is excreted in the urine, the remainder in the bile.

Furosemide is excreted primarily unchanged in the urine, accompanied by small amounts of a glucuronide. Amounts up to 30% may be excreted in the feces.

Indapamide is extensively metabolized in the liver, and its metabolites are detectable for more than a week after oral administration. Sixty percent of indapamide is excreted in the urine as metabolites, 20% in the feces as metabolites, and 5% in the urine as unchanged drug. Both bumetanide and furosemide cross the placenta and appear in breast milk.

Onset, peak, duration

Bumetanide's onset of diuretic action occurs within 30 minutes after oral administration, within 40 minutes after I.M. administration, and within a few minutes after I.V. administration. Peak concentration levels of bumetanide are reached within 1.5 to 2 hours after oral administration and within minutes after I.V. administration. The duration of action of bumetanide is from 3.5 to 4 hours, although it may increase to 6 hours with higher doses. Bumetanide's half-life is 1 to 1.5 hours.

Onset of diuretic action with ethacrynic acid occurs 30 minutes after oral administration and 5 minutes after I.V. administration. The duration of action is 6 to 8 hours after oral administration and 2 hours after I.V. administration. As with bumetanide, the duration of action of ethacrynic acid may increase with higher doses. Ethacrynic acid's half-life is 30 to 70 minutes.

Onset of action of furosemide occurs within 30 to 60 minutes after oral administration and 5 minutes after I.V. administration. Peak concentration levels occur within 20 to 60 minutes; the drug's duration of action is about 2 hours after an I.V. dose and 6 hours after an oral dose. The half-life of furosemide is usually 30 to 60 minutes but may increase to 75 to 155 minutes in a patient with renal or hepatic insufficiency and to 20 hours in a patient with renal system dysfunction.

Onset of action of indapamide occurs 1 hour after oral administration, and the drug reaches peak concentration levels within 2 hours. Indapamide's half-life is 14 hours.

PHARMACODYNAMICS

The loop diuretics are the most potent diuretics available, producing the greatest volume of diuresis and having a high potential for causing severe adverse reactions. Producing maximal sodium excretion of 20% to 25% of the filtered load, loop diuretics inhibit sodium and chloride reabsorption in the renal tubules by direct action on the thick ascending limb of the loop of Henle. These drugs may also inhibit sodium, chloride, and water reabsorption in the proximal tubule while increasing the excretion of ammonium and titratable acids in the distal tubule. Increased excretion of potassium from the distal tubule may result from the accelerated exchange with sodium ions caused by the increased volume of sodium delivered

DRUG INTERACTIONS

Loop diuretics

Drug interactions with loop diuretics can alter renal function, cause fluid and electrolyte imbalances, and enhance certain effects of the drug.

DRUG	INTERACTING DRUGS	POSSIBLE EFFECTS	NURSING IMPLICATIONS
bumetanide, ethacrynic acid, furosemide, indapamide	antihypertensives	Decrease blood pressure	• Monitor the patient's blood pressure, and observe for orthostatic hypotension.
	oral hypoglycemic agents	May cause hyperglycemia	• Monitor the patient's serum glucose levels. • Monitor the patient for signs and symptoms of hyperglycemia, such as thirst and lethargy.
	alcohol, barbiturates, narcotic drugs	May cause orthostatic hypotension	• Monitor the patient's blood pressure. • Observe the patient for orthostatic hypotension.
	salicylates	May cause salicylate toxicity	• Monitor the patient's serum salicylate levels.
	aminoglycosides	May cause ototoxicity	• When administering these drugs together, exercise extreme caution. • Monitor the patient's auditory acuity.
	digitalis	Potassium depletion enhances chance of digitalis toxicity	• Monitor serum potassium levels. • Monitor for signs and symptoms of digitalis toxicity.
ethacrynic acid, furosemide	oral anticoagulants	May cause hypoprothrombinemia, GI bleeding	• Monitor the patient for bleeding. • Monitor the patient's prothrombin time.
	corticosteroids	May cause hypokalemia	• Monitor the patient's serum potassium levels. • Monitor the patient for signs and symptoms of hypokalemia.
	lithium carbonate	Decreases excretion, resulting in lithium toxicity	• Monitor the patient for signs and symptoms of lithium toxicity, such as ataxia. • Monitor the patient's serum lithium levels.
	clofibrate	Causes muscular symptoms (pain and stiffness, marked diuresis	• Monitor the patient for muscular symptoms. • Monitor the patient's fluid intake and output, daily weights, blood pressure, and serum electrolyte levels.
furosemide, bumetanide	indomethacin	Inhibits antihypertensive and diuretic effects of furosemide and bumetanide	• Monitor the patient's fluid intake and output, daily weight, and blood pressure.
furosemide	neuromuscular blocking agents	Enhance neuromuscular blockade	• Monitor the therapeutic effects of neuromuscular blocking agents.
	probenecid	Inhibits furosemide excretion	• Monitor the patient's fluid intake and output, blood pressure, daily weights, and serum electrolyte levels.
	chloral hydrate	May cause diaphoresis, flushed skin, blood pressure variations, and uneasiness	• Administer furosemide with caution if the patient received chloral hydrate within the previous 24 hours.

to the distal tubule. Ethacrynic acid binds to sulfhydryl groups in renal cellular protein. Bumetanide, the shorter-acting agent, is 40 times more potent than furosemide. Indapamide also relaxes the vascular bed.

PHARMACOTHERAPEUTICS

Physicians use loop diuretics primarily to treat edema associated with CHF, hepatic or renal disease, or nephrotic syndrome. Loop diuretics are also used to treat mild hypertension, usually in combination with a potassium-sparing diuretic or a potassium supplement to prevent hypokalemia. Bumetanide has also been used to treat edema related to menstruation and lymphedema. Ethacrynic acid is also used to treat cancer-related ascites, lymphedema, acute pulmonary edema, nephrogenic diabetes insipidus, and hypercalcemia. Furosemide is also used in combination with mannitol to treat severe cerebral edema.

bumetanide (Bumex). Used to treat edema and hypertension, bumetanide may be substituted for furosemide in patients hypersensitive to that drug.
USUAL ADULT DOSAGE: 0.5 to 2 mg P.O. in a single daily dose or repeated at 4- to 5-hour intervals up to a total of 10 mg/day; maintenance doses are usually given intermittently with 1- to 2-day rest periods; 0.5 to 1 mg I.M. or I.V., injected or infused slowly over 1 to 2 minutes; I.V. doses may be repeated every 2 to 3 hours up to a total of 10 mg/day.

ethacrynate sodium (Sodium Edecrin) and **ethacrynic acid** (Edecrin). Physicians use these loop diuretics to treat acute pulmonary edema and other forms of edema.
USUAL ADULT DOSAGE: for acute pulmonary edema, 50 to 100 mg of ethacrynate sodium I.V., infused slowly over several minutes; for other forms of edema, 50 to 200 mg of ethacrynic acid P.O. once daily, after meals or on alternate days, or up to 200 mg b.i.d. if needed to obtain a therapeutic effect.
USUAL PEDIATRIC DOSAGE: for edema, initially, 25 mg of ethacrynic acid P.O. daily, gradually increased, if needed, in 25-mg increments until the therapeutic effect is obtained.

furosemide (Lasix). Used primarily to treat acute pulmonary edema and other forms of edema, furosemide is also used to treat hypertensive crisis, acute and chronic renal failure, hypertension, and hypercalcemia (because it promotes urinary calcium excretion). Furosemide can cause profound water and electrolyte depletion.

USUAL ADULT DOSAGE: for acute pulmonary edema, 40 mg I.V. injected slowly, then repeated every 2 hours as needed; for edema, 20 to 80 mg P.O. daily or b.i.d., up to 600 mg/day, or 20 to 40 mg I.M. or I.V. with repeated doses of 20 mg every 2 hours until the therapeutic effect is achieved; for hypertensive crisis and acute renal failure, 100 to 200 mg I.V. over 1 to 2 minutes; for chronic renal failure, initially, 80 mg P.O. daily, increased up to 120 mg/day until the therapeutic effect is achieved; for hypertension, 20 to 80 mg P.O. daily.
USUAL PEDIATRIC DOSAGE: for edema, 2 mg/kg P.O. daily with an increase of 1 to 2 mg/kg in 6 to 8 hours if needed, up to 6 mg/kg/day; or 1 mg/kg I.V. or I.M., titrated as needed to a maximum of 6 mg/kg/day.

indapamide (Lozol). This loop diuretic is used to treat edema and hypertension.
USUAL ADULT DOSAGE: for edema and hypertension, 2.5 mg P.O. as a single daily dose; may be increased to 5 mg P.O. as a single daily dose if needed.

Drug interactions
A variety of drugs—including aminoglycosides, oral anticoagulants, and corticosteroids—interact with the loop diuretics, causing altered renal function, fluid and electrolyte imbalances, and specific enhanced drug effects. (See *Drug interactions: Loop diuretics* for details.)

ADVERSE DRUG REACTIONS

The adverse drug reactions to loop diuretics may be severe because of these drugs' potent effects. The most severe reactions involve frequently occurring fluid and electrolyte imbalances.

Predictable reactions
Common adverse reactions to the loop diuretics include volume depletion (especially in elderly patients), orthostatic hypotension, hypokalemia, hypochloremic alkalosis, asymptomatic hyperuricemia, hyponatremia, hypochloremia, hypocalcemia, and hypomagnesemia. Transient deafness, abdominal discomfort or pain, diarrhea, impaired glucose tolerance, dermatitis, paresthesias, hepatic dysfunction, and thrombocytopenia can also occur.

Unpredictable reactions
Hypersensitivity reactions include purpura, photosensitivity, rash, pruritus, urticaria, necrotizing angiitis, exfoliative dermatitis, allergic interstitial nephritis, and erythema multiforme. Agranulocytosis can also occur.

NURSING IMPLICATIONS

The nursing implications associated with loop diuretics focus on these drugs' potential to cause fluid and electrolyte imbalances. Also, the nurse must take specific precautions regarding storage and administration of these drugs, as outlined in the following considerations:
• Be aware that loop diuretics are contraindicated in anuric patients.
• Be aware that furosemide and bumetanide are contraindicated for patients hypersensitive to sulfonamides, because such patients will have corresponding hypersensitivity to the two loop diuretics.
• Administer loop diuretics cautiously to patients with electrolyte imbalances.
• Monitor patients who are also receiving digitalis for digitalis toxicity, which may result from the potassium-depleting effect of the loop diuretics.
• Monitor patients who are also receiving oral anticoagulant therapy for bleeding and other adverse reactions, because the loop diuretics may potentiate anticoagulant effects.
• Monitor the patient's weight daily under controlled conditions (at the same time in the morning, after the patient voids, before the patient eats, with the patient wearing similar clothing at each weigh-in, and with the same scale).
• Monitor the patient's fluid intake and output carefully, noting increases and decreases.
• Monitor the patient's serum electrolyte levels frequently.
• Monitor the patient for signs and symptoms of hypokalemia, such as drowsiness, muscle cramps, hyporeflexia, and paresthesias.
• Monitor uric acid levels for a patient who has a history of gout.
• Monitor a diabetic patient's blood glucose levels carefully.
• Do not administer ethacrynate sodium or ethacrynic acid by I.M. or S.C. injection, which can cause tissue irritation.
• Administer I.M. injections of furosemide using the Z-track method to minimize tissue irritation.
• Administer furosemide I.V. infusions slowly, over 1 to 2 minutes.
• Store oral furosemide tablets and injectable furosemide in light-resistant containers to prevent discoloration.
• Refrigerate oral furosemide solution to ensure stability. Do not use discolored (yellow) injectable furosemide solutions.
• Advise the patient to decrease the risk of orthostatic hypotension by standing slowly, limiting alcohol intake, and avoiding strenuous exercise in hot weather.

• Instruct the patient taking furosemide to report to the physician any signs or symptoms of furosemide toxicity, such as tinnitus, abdominal pain, sore throat, and fever.
• Instruct the patient to include potassium-rich foods such as citrus fruits, tomatoes, bananas, dates, and apricots, in the daily diet.

POTASSIUM-SPARING DIURETICS

Potassium-sparing diuretics have weaker diuretic and antihypertensive effects than other diuretics, but they have the advantage of conserving potassium. For this reason, physicians frequently use potassium-sparing diuretics with other antihypertensive agents. Whenever these diuretics are administered, however, the nurse must closely monitor the patient for hyperkalemia. The potassium-sparing diuretics include spironolactone, triamterene, and amiloride.

History and source
Spironolactone, a 17-spirolactone steroid and competitive aldosterone antagonist, was the first potassium-sparing diuretic introduced, by Kagawa and Liddle in 1958. In 1961, triamterene, originally synthesized as a folic acid antagonist, was found to be an effective diuretic. Triamterene was derived from pteridine, which was originally isolated from butterfly wings and mammalian urine. Amiloride, the newest of the potassium-sparing diuretics, is a pyrazine derivative similar to triamterene.

PHARMACOKINETICS

Potassium-sparing diuretics are administered orally and are absorbed in the GI tract. They are metabolized in the liver with the exception of amiloride, which is not metabolized, and are excreted primarily in the urine and bile. These diuretics have a rapid onset of action, and their duration of action increases with multiple doses.

Absorption, distribution, metabolism, excretion
After oral administration, absorption of the potassium-sparing diuretics varies from 70% for spironolactone to 50% for triamterene and 20% for amiloride. Triamterene is erratically absorbed, depending on the dosage form, and has a variable bioavailability. The drugs are widely

distributed in body fluids and tissues. Spironolactone is more than 90% bound to plasma proteins; triamterene is 60% protein-bound, and amiloride is not bound at all.

After extensive first-pass metabolism, spironolactone enters the hepatic circulation. Triamterene is also extensively metabolized by the liver, but amiloride is not metabolized at all.

Spironolactone and triamterene are excreted as metabolites via the urine and feces, with very little of either drug being excreted unchanged. From 20% to 50% of amiloride is excreted unchanged in the urine, and 40% is excreted unchanged in the feces.

Onset, peak, duration

Onset of action occurs in 2 to 4 hours for spironolactone and triamterene; in 2 hours for amiloride. Spironolactone and triamterene reach peak concentration levels in 3 to 5 hours, and amiloride in 6 to 10 hours. The duration of action of spironolactone is 12 to 96 hours. Triamterene has the shortest duration of action, only 7 to 9 hours. The duration of action of amiloride is 24 hours. For all three drugs, the duration of action may be increased with multiple doses and prolonged therapy.

The half-life of spironolactone is directly related to its metabolite, canrenone, with a half-life of 3 to 12 hours. The half-life of triamterene is 90 to 120 minutes; and of amiloride, 6 to 9 hours.

PHARMACODYNAMICS

The potassium-sparing diuretics act in the distal renal tubules. Water and sodium are excreted, and potassium is retained.

Mechanism of action

The direct action of the potassium-sparing diuretics on the distal renal tubules produces mild diuretic and antihypertensive effects that increase the urinary excretion of sodium, chloride, and calcium ions and reduce the excretion of potassium and hydrogen ions. These effects lead to increased serum potassium levels and urine pH. Spironolactone does not depress the GFR, but both triamterene and amiloride do.

Amiloride and triamterene do not inhibit aldosterone or carbonic anhydrase, but spironolactone is an aldosterone antagonist. When hypovolemia, hyponatremia, hyperkalemia, or the release of renin leads to aldosterone secretion, metabolic alkalosis and potassium depletion may occur. Spironolactone counteracts these effects by competing with aldosterone for receptor sites and blocking the action of aldosterone on the distal tubules. As a result, sodium, chloride, and water are excreted and potassium is retained.

PHARMACOTHERAPEUTICS

Physicians often use potassium-sparing diuretics with other diuretics to potentiate their action or to counteract their potassium-wasting effects. Potassium-sparing diuretics are used primarily to treat edema (including refractory edema) and diuretic-induced hypokalemia in patients with CHF, cirrhosis, nephrotic syndrome, or hypertension. These drugs are also used to treat hyperaldosteronism and hirsutism, including hirsutism associated with polycystic ovary syndrome.

amiloride hydrochloride (Midamor, Moduretic). Physicians use amiloride to treat hypertension or edema associated with CHF and to assist in restoring normal serum potassium levels in patients with hypokalemia. Amiloride is usually administered in combination with other diuretics, such as the thiazide or loop diuretics.
USUAL ADULT DOSAGE: initially, 5 to 10 mg P.O. daily, increased up to 20 mg/day, if needed.

spironolactone (Aldactone). This diuretic is used to treat primary aldosteronism, essential hypertension, refractory edema, cirrhosis, nephrotic syndrome, and idiopathic edema. Spironolactone may be used in combination with other drugs to potentiate their action or to decrease potassium loss. This drug has also been used investigationally to treat hirsutism in women with polycystic ovary syndrome or idiopathic hirsutism.
USUAL ADULT DOSAGE: for essential hypertension, initially, 50 to 100 mg P.O. daily in divided doses; for edema, initially, 25 to 200 mg P.O. daily in divided doses; the total dosage is adjusted according to the patient's response.
USUAL PEDIATRIC DOSAGE: for edema, initially, 3.3 mg/kg P.O. daily in divided doses.

triamterene (Diazide, Dyrenium, Maxzide). Physicians usually use this potassium-sparing diuretic in combination with other diuretics to treat hypertension. Triamterene is also used to treat the edema associated with CHF, cirrhosis, and nephrotic syndrome as well as idiopathic edema, steroid-induced edema, and edema from hyperaldosteronism.
USUAL ADULT DOSAGE: initially, 100 mg P.O. b.i.d. after meals; the dosage may be adjusted for therapeutic effect but must not exceed 300 mg/day.

Drug interactions

Few drug interactions are associated with the use of spironolactone, triamterene, and amiloride. Those that

DRUG INTERACTIONS

Potassium-sparing diuretics

The drug interactions that occur with these diuretics may be related to their potassium-sparing effects. The nurse must observe patients receiving potassium-sparing diuretics for signs and symptoms of hyperkalemia.

DRUG	INTERACTING DRUGS	POSSIBLE EFFECTS	NURSING IMPLICATIONS
spironolactone, triamterene, amiloride	norepinephrine	Increases vasopressor effects	• Monitor the patient's blood pressure and urine output.
	potassium supplements or other potassium-sparing diuretics	May cause hyperkalemia	• Monitor the patient for signs and symptoms of hyperkalemia. Advise the patient not to use potassium-based salt substitutes.
spironolactone	ammonium chloride (acidifying doses)	May cause metabolic acidosis	• Monitor the patient for signs and symptoms of metabolic acidosis, such as restlessness and disorientation. • Monitor the patient's serum potassium levels. • Monitor the patient's blood gas values, serum CO_2 level, and urine pH.
	antipyrine	Reduces antipyrine's effect	• Monitor the patient for signs and symptoms of an inflammatory response. • Monitor the patient's white blood cell count.
	carbenoxolone	Inhibits adverse reactions and ulcer healing of carbenoxolone	• Do not administer these agents concurrently.
	lithium	May cause lithium toxicity	• Monitor the patient for signs and symptoms of lithium toxicity, such as ataxia. • Monitor the patient's serum lithium levels.
	digitalis	Decreases renal excretion	• Monitor the patient for signs and symptoms of digitalis toxicity, such as nausea and yellow vision. • Monitor the patient's serum digitalis levels.
	salicylates	Reduce clinical effects of spironolactone	• Monitor the patient's fluid intake and output and serum potassium levels.
triamterene	indomethacin	May cause nephrotoxicity	• Monitor the patient's BUN and serum creatinine levels, daily weight, and urine output.

do occur are related to the potassium-sparing effects. (See *Drug interactions: Potassium-sparing diuretics* for details.)

ADVERSE DRUG REACTIONS

Few adverse drug reactions occur with the potassium-sparing diuretics. However, their potassium-sparing effects can lead to hyperkalemia.

Predictable reactions

Hyperkalemia is the major risk, especially if a potassium-sparing diuretic is given with a potassium supplement or a high-potassium diet. Other predictable reactions to potassium-sparing diuretics include megaloblastic anemia (especially with triamterene), dizziness, hypotension, sore throat, dry mouth, nausea, and vomiting.

Spironolactone may produce headache, abdominal cramps, diarrhea, gynecomastia in men, breast soreness and menstrual abnormalities in women, and rarely, agranulocytosis. Amiloride may produce headache, nausea and vomiting, anorexia, diarrhea, muscle cramps, abdominal pain, constipation, impotence, and metabolic disturbances, including volume depletion, hyponatremia, a transient rise in the BUN level, and acidosis.

Unpredictable reactions

Hypersensitivity reactions to potassium-sparing diuretics include urticaria, pruritus, erythematous eruptions, rash, photosensitivity, and anaphylaxis.

NURSING IMPLICATIONS

The nursing implications associated with the potassium-sparing diuretics center on the capacity of these agents to cause fluid and electrolyte imbalances, especially hyperkalemia. When administering these drugs, the nurse should be aware of the following considerations:

• The potassium-sparing diuretics are contraindicated in patients with anuria or renal impairment, severe hepatic disease, or hyperkalemia. Administer these drugs cautiously to patients with impaired hepatic function or diabetes mellitus as well as to pregnant or lactating patients.

• Because of the drugs' potassium-sparing effects, monitor the patient for the signs and symptoms of hyperkalemia: confusion, hyperexcitability, muscle weakness, paresthesias, flaccid paralysis, dysrhythmias, abdominal distention, diarrhea, and intestinal colic.

• Monitor the patient's serum laboratory values for potential blood dyscrasias, especially during triamterene therapy.

• Monitor the patient's serum electrolyte levels for abnormalities.

• Monitor the patient's weight daily under controlled conditions (at the same time each morning, after the patient voids, before the patient eats, with the patient wearing similar clothing at each weigh-in, and with the same scale).

• Monitor the patient's fluid intake and output, noting increases and decreases.

• Monitor the patient's supine and standing blood pressures, and assess for orthostatic hypotension.

• Store spironolactone in a dark container away from light.

• Advise the patient to avoid eating potassium-rich foods, because these drugs conserve potassium.

• Advise the patient to decrease the risk of orthostatic hypotension by standing slowly, limiting alcohol intake, and avoiding strenuous exercise in hot weather.

CARBONIC ANHYDRASE INHIBITORS

Carbonic anhydrase inhibitors act as enzymatic blocking agents that reverse the hydration of carbon dioxide, producing a bicarbonate diuresis that promotes the excretion of sodium, potassium, and water. Physicians usually do not use carbonic anhydrase inhibitors to treat edema because of their limited diuretic effect. Instead, the carbonic anhydrase inhibitors acetazolamide, dichlorphenamide, ethoxzolamide, and methazolamide are used primarily to decrease intraocular pressure, alkalinize the urine, manage periodic paralysis, and treat acute mountain sickness.

History and source

The development of carbonic anhydrase inhibitors began with the identification of the enzyme carbonic anhydrase by Roughton in 1933 and the identification of sulfanilamide as a carbonic anhydrase inhibitor by Mann and Keilin in 1940. Initially, these discoveries were of little use, because sulfanilamide produced a diuretic effect only with high doses, making it impractical for therapy. Development of the thiadiazole sulfonamides by Roblin, however, led to the introduction of acetazolamide in 1950.

PHARMACOKINETICS

In most cases, carbonic anhydrase inhibitors are rapidly absorbed in the GI tract and distributed to specific body tissues after oral administration. (Acetazolamide may also be administered I.M. or I.V.) The drugs are primarily excreted unchanged in the urine.

Absorption, distribution, metabolism, excretion

Acetazolamide and dichlorphenamide are rapidly absorbed in the GI tract after oral administration; methazolamide is absorbed more slowly. These agents are rapidly distributed in the tissues via the plasma. Because the carbonic anhydrase inhibitors bind to the enzyme carbonic anhydrase, they are distributed to tissues with high concentrations of this enzyme—erythrocytes and the renal cortex, stomach, pancreas, eyes, and central nervous system. These drugs are not metabolized, so they are excreted primarily unchanged by the kidneys within 24 hours. The renal excretion occurs by active tubular secretion and passive reabsorption.

Indefinite pharmacokinetic information exists regarding ethoxzolamide.

Onset, peak, duration

Onset of action of the oral carbonic anhydrase inhibitors occurs in 1 to 4 hours. Acetazolamide sodium is administered parenterally, with an onset of action of 2 minutes, whereas the onset of action of oral acetazolamide occurs in 60 to 90 minutes. Onset of action of dichlorphenamide and ethoxzolamide occurs in 30 minutes to 1 hour; of methazolamide, in 2 to 4 hours.

Peak concentration levels are achieved in 15 minutes with parenteral acetazolamide sodium and in 8 to 12 hours with sustained-release oral acetazolamide. Dichlorphenamide and regular oral acetazolamide peak within 2 to 4 hours, and ethoxzolamide peaks in 2 to 6 hours. Peak concentration levels of methazolamide are reached in 6 to 8 hours.

The duration of action of dichlorphenamide, ethoxzolamide, and regular oral acetazolamide can be up to 12 hours. Parenteral acetazolamide sodium has the shortest duration of action, only 4 to 5 hours. The two longest-acting drugs are methazolamide (10 to 18 hours) and sustained-release acetazolamide (18 to 24 hours). Methazolamide has a relatively long half-life of 7.5 hours; the half-lives of the other carbonic anhydrase inhibitors are shorter.

PHARMACODYNAMICS

Carbonic anhydrase inhibitors block the action of the enzyme carbonic anhydrase, reversing the hydration of carbon dioxide and producing a bicarbonate diuresis that promotes the excretion of sodium, potassium, and water. These effects also decrease the formation of aqueous humor, thus reducing intraocular pressure.

Mechanism of action

Carbonic anhydrase inhibitors block the action of the enzyme carbonic anhydrase, which acts as a catalyst in the conversion of carbon dioxide and water to carbonic acid, which in turn dissociates to form bicarbonate and hydrogen ions. Blocking this action of carbonic anhydrase produces diuresis by reducing the available hydrogen and bicarbonate ions and depressing sodium and bicarbonate reabsorption mechanisms. These effects al-

DRUG INTERACTIONS

Carbonic anhydrase inhibitors

The carbonic anhydrase inhibitors produce few drug interactions. Most that do occur alter the reabsorption of other drugs.

DRUG	INTERACTING DRUGS	POSSIBLE EFFECTS	NURSING IMPLICATIONS
acetazolamide	amphetamines	Alter metabolism of amphetamines, enhancing their effects	• Monitor the patient for the signs and symptoms of enhanced response to amphetamines: increased blood pressure, decreased heart rate, urinary retention, central nervous system stimulation, euphoria, wakefulness, and decreased appetite.
	ephedrine	Increases reabsorption of ephedrine	• Monitor the patient for signs and symptoms of ephedrine toxicity: nervousness, insomnia, and excitability.
	salicylates	May cause salicylate intoxication	• Monitor the patient's serum salicylate levels.
acetazolamide, dichlorphenamide, ethoxzolamide, methazolamide	phenytoin	May cause osteomalacia	• Observe the patient for early signs and symptoms of osteomalacia: pain in the limbs, spine, thorax, and pelvis, and anemia.
	quinidine	Delay quinidine excretion	• Monitor the patient for signs and symptoms of quinidine toxicity: dysrhythmias, decreased blood pressure, nausea, vomiting, and diarrhea.
	methenamine	Decrease methenamine effectiveness	• Monitor the patient for the signs and symptoms of a continuing urinary tract infection: dysuria, frequency, and urgency.

kalinize the urine, increase potassium and bicarbonate excretion, and decrease citrate, ammonium, and chloride excretion. Thus, prolonged treatment with carbonic anhydrase inhibitors can lead to metabolic acidosis.

These drugs decrease intraocular pressure by decreasing the formation of aqueous humor.

PHARMACOTHERAPEUTICS

Physicians use carbonic anhydrase inhibitors—sometimes in combination with miotics—primarily to decrease the formation of aqueous humor by the ciliary body and, thereby, to control the excessive intraocular pressure associated with glaucoma. These drugs are also used, however, to treat edema related to cardiac disorders, periodic paralysis, and acute mountain sickness.

acetazolamide (Diamox) **and acetazolamide sodium** (Diamox Parenteral). Acetazolamide is used primarily to treat open-angle glaucoma that is unresponsive to miotics alone. Also, it may be used to lower intraocular pressure before eye surgery. Acetazolamide sodium is administered parenterally.
USUAL ADULT DOSAGE: for edema, 250 to 500 mg P.O., I.V., or I.M. daily or every other day; for glaucoma, 250 mg P.O. daily to q.i.d. For rapid lowering of intraocular pressure, 500 mg I.V. or I.M., repeated in 2 to 4 hours if necessary (I.M. administration is usually avoided because of the alkalinity of the solution).
USUAL PEDIATRIC DOSAGE: for edema, 5 mg/kg P.O., I.M., or I.V. daily.

dichlorphenamide (Daranide, Oratrol). This carbonic anhydrase inhibitor is used primarily to treat glaucoma.
USUAL ADULT DOSAGE: initially, 100 to 200 mg P.O., followed by 100 mg P.O. every 12 hours until the therapeutic effect is reached; for maintenance, 25 to 50 mg one to three times daily.

ethoxzolamide (Cardrase, Ethamide). This drug is used primarily to treat edema and glaucoma.
USUAL ADULT DOSAGE: for edema, 62.5 to 125 mg P.O. daily after breakfast for up to 3 consecutive days, or every other day; for glaucoma, 62.5 to 250 mg P.O. b.i.d. to q.i.d.

methazolamide (Neptazane). This diuretic is used primarily to treat glaucoma.
USUAL ADULT DOSAGE: 50 to 100 mg P.O. b.i.d. to t.i.d.

Drug interactions
The carbonic anhydrase inhibitors are associated with few significant drug interactions. Those that do occur usually affect the reabsorption of other drugs. (See *Drug interactions: Carbonic anhydrase inhibitors* for further information.)

ADVERSE DRUG REACTIONS

The major predictable adverse reactions to the carbonic anhydrase inhibitors are fluid and electrolyte imbalances, especially potassium and bicarbonate depletion. Other reactions may include drowsiness, hyperchloremic acidosis, hemolytic anemia, leukopenia, paresthesias, transient myopia, nausea and vomiting, anorexia, crystalluria, renal calculi, and asymptomatic hyperuricemia. Other predictable but less common adverse reactions include dry mouth, irritability, diarrhea, tinnitus, disorientation, dysuria, ataxia, and weight loss.

Hypersensitivity reactions, including rash, urticaria, purpura, and anaphylaxis may also occur as unpredictable reactions to these agents.

NURSING IMPLICATIONS

The nursing implications for carbonic anhydrase inhibitors mainly involve their potential to cause electrolyte imbalances. To administer these drugs safely, the nurse must be aware of the following considerations:
• These drugs are contraindicated for patients with narrow-angle (acute) glaucoma, hypersensitivity to carbonic anhydrase inhibitors or sulfonamides, chronic pulmonary disease, renal failure, hepatic insufficiency, Addison's disease or adrenocortical insufficiency, hyponatremia, hypokalemia, or hyperchloremic acidosis. They are also contraindicated during pregnancy, especially during the first trimester.
• Administer these agents cautiously to diabetic patients, because carbonic anhydrase inhibitors may increase blood glucose levels.
• Administer these drugs cautiously to patients with a history of hypercalciuria or gout.
• Monitor the patient for signs and symptoms of hypokalemia, and administer potassium supplements as prescribed.
• Monitor the patient for signs and symptoms of metabolic acidosis, including headache, drowsiness, decreased mentation, confusion, seizures, coma, fatigue, hypotension, hypoxia, dysrhythmias, Kussmaul's respirations, anorexia, nausea and vomiting, and tissue hypoxia.
• Monitor the patient's complete blood count and serum electrolyte values.
• Monitor the patient's fluid intake and output, noting increases and decreases.

- Monitor the patient's weight daily under controlled conditions (at the same time each morning, after the patient voids, before the patient eats, with the patient wearing similar clothing for each weigh-in, and with the same scale).
- Disguise the bitter taste of these drugs by softening the tablets in hot water and adding honey or syrup. Do not, however, alter the sustained-release forms of the drugs, and do not mix the tablets with fruit juices, because these drugs are unstable in acidic solutions.
- Administer a carbonic anhydrase inhibitor in the morning when possible to avoid disturbing the patient's sleep patterns because of night voiding.
- If possible, avoid I.M. injections, which cause intense pain at the injection site because of the alkaline pH of the solution.
- Do not use parenteral solutions more than 24 hours after reconstitution, because they do not contain preservatives. Suspensions, however, usually remain stable for 1 week.
- Store tablets in a tightly closed, light-resistant container.
- If the drug is administered to treat glaucoma, advise the patient to report eye pain, which may indicate that the drug is not effectively lowering intraocular pressure.
- Instruct the patient to report any adverse reactions.

OSMOTIC DIURETICS

Osmotic diuretics are low-molecular-weight substances that increase the osmolality of the plasma, glomerular filtrate, and tubular fluid by remaining in high concentrations in the renal tubules. This action decreases sodium, chloride, and water reabsorption, thereby increasing their excretion. (Potassium excretion is slightly increased.)

Physicians use the osmotic diuretics primarily to prevent oliguria and acute renal failure but also to reduce increased intracranial and intraocular pressure and to treat certain forms of drug intoxication. Because they remain effective in patients with compromised renal circulation, mannitol and urea are the primary osmotic diuretics used clinically today.

PHARMACOKINETICS

After I.V. administration, mannitol and urea are rapidly distributed and are excreted primarily unchanged in the urine.

Absorption, distribution, metabolism, excretion

Mannitol and urea are rapidly distributed to the extracellular fluid after I.V. administration. Only 7% to 10% of a mannitol dose is metabolized. Approximately 7% of a mannitol dose and 50% of a urea dose are reabsorbed by the renal tubules. They are filtered primarily by the glomeruli, and excreted largely unchanged in the urine. In a patient with severe renal insufficiency, the rate of excretion is reduced; the resulting retention of the osmotic diuretic increases extracellular tonicity, expanding the extracellular fluid and inducing hyponatremia.

Onset, peak, duration

When administered in the dosages used to decrease intraocular pressure, the onset of action of mannitol and urea is within 15 minutes. The peak concentration level for mannitol is reached in about 30 minutes to 1 hour; the peak concentration level of urea is reached in 1 to 2 hours. The duration of action of mannitol is 4 to 8 hours; of urea, 5 to 6 hours.

Diuresis occurs in 1 to 3 hours after mannitol administration and in 6 to 12 hours after urea administration. When administered in the dosages used to reduce intracranial pressure, the duration of action of mannitol is 3 to 8 hours; of urea, 3 to 10 hours. The half-life of mannitol is from 15 to 100 minutes; of urea, about 70 minutes.

PHARMACODYNAMICS

Osmotic diuretics act by increasing the osmolality of the plasma, glomerular filtrate, and tubular fluid. That decreases the reabsorption of fluid and electrolytes, increasing the excretion of water, chloride, and sodium and slightly increasing the excretion of potassium.

Osmotic diuretics are therapeutically effective because they are freely filtered at the glomeruli and are somewhat reabsorbed by the renal tubules, thus maintaining high concentration levels there. The drugs are also pharmacologically inert and resistant to extensive metabolism.

PHARMACOTHERAPEUTICS

Mannitol and urea primarily are used to reduce intracranial pressure and to prevent acute renal failure. They are effective even in a patient with compromised renal circulation.

mannitol (Osmitrol). Used primarily to prevent oliguria and acute renal failure, mannitol is also used to treat oliguria, increased intracranial pressure, increased intraocular pressure, and drug intoxication from secobarbital, imipramine, aspirin, or carbon tetrachloride. Physicians also use mannitol in combination with sorbitol as a urogenital irrigation for patients experiencing a transurethral prostatic resection; this combination minimizes the hemolytic effects of water. (For additional information on the use of mannitol for increased intraocular pressure, see Chapter 79, Ophthalmic Agents.)

USUAL ADULT DOSAGE: for oliguria and prevention of acute renal failure, 50 to 100 grams I.V. of 5% to 25% solution; to reduce intracranial or intraocular pressure, 1.5 to 2 grams/kg I.V. of 15% to 20% solution infused over 30 to 60 minutes; for preoperative intraocular medication, give 1 to 1½ hours before surgery; for drug intoxication, maximum dose of 200 grams I.V. of 5% to 10% solution over a 24-hour period; for urogenital irrigation in combination with sorbitol, a test dose of 200 mg/kg I.V. infused over 3 to 5 minutes to elicit a urine flow of 30 to 50 ml/hour, may be repeated once.

urea (Aquacara, Carbamide, Ureaphil, Ureuert). Urea is used primarily to reduce increased intracranial and intraocular pressure and to prevent acute renal failure during prolonged surgery or trauma.

USUAL ADULT DOSAGE: 1 to 1.5 grams/kg I.V. of 30% solution, infused over 1½ to 2 hours, up to a maximum dose of 120 grams/day.

USUAL PEDIATRIC DOSAGE: over age 2, 0.5 to 1.5 grams/ kg I.V. of a 30% solution infused over 1½ to 2 hours; under age 2, 0.1 to 0.5 gram/kg I.V. of a 30% solution infused over 1½ to 2 hours.

Drug interactions

No significant drug interactions occur with the use of mannitol or urea.

ADVERSE DRUG REACTIONS

Common predictable adverse reactions to the osmotic diuretics include transient expansion of plasma volume during infusion, resulting in circulatory overload and tachycardia, electrolyte imbalances, volume depletion, cellular dehydration, headache, and nausea and vomiting. Mannitol may cause rebound increased intracranial pressure 8 to 12 hours after diuresis and anginalike chest pain, blurred vision, rhinitis, thirst, and urinary retention. Urea can produce local irritation at the infusion site that may progress to necrotic sloughing if extravasation occurs.

Unpredictable adverse reactions to the osmotic diuretics include hypersensitivity reactions and thrombophlebitis.

NURSING IMPLICATIONS

Besides understanding some specific contraindications associated with the osmotic diuretics, the nurse must administer these drugs with care and closely monitor their effectiveness—as detailed in the following nursing considerations:

• Be aware that osmotic diuretics are contraindicated in patients with diagnosed acute renal failure, cardiac dysfunction, CHF, active intracranial hemorrhage, or severe dehydration.

• Weigh the patient daily under controlled conditions (at the same time each morning, after the patient voids, before the patient eats, with the patient wearing similar clothing at each weigh-in, and with the same scale).

• Monitor the patient's fluid intake and output hourly, because the therapy is based on the hourly urine flow rate.

• Monitor the patient for circulatory overload if the urine output is less than 30 to 50 ml/hour.

• Monitor the patient for serum electrolyte imbalances, particularly sodium, potassium, and chloride.

• Monitor the patient's vital signs hourly during osmotic diuretic therapy.

• Observe I.V. administration sites for local irritation, extravasation, or signs of thrombophlebitis.

• Assist the patient in maintaining adequate fluid intake to promote renal function.

• Promote mouth care, and offer ice chips and hard candies to relieve the patient's thirst.

• Parenteral mannitol crystallizes at low temperatures. To redissolve it, warm it in a hot-water bath and shake the container vigorously, then let the solution return to room temperature before administration. Do not administer crystallized medication.

• Administer mannitol using an in-line I.V. filter.

• Do not add blood products to I.V. lines used for mannitol administration, because pseudoagglutination will occur.

• Store mannitol at 59° to 86° F. (15° to 30° C.) unless otherwise ordered, and do not allow it to freeze.

MERCURIAL DIURETICS

Mercurial diuretics are fast-acting, effective diuretics that served as the major high-ceiling diuretics until the de-

(Text continues on page 628.)

SELECTED MAJOR DRUGS

Diuretic agents

This chart summarizes the actions, dosages, and nursing implications of the various diuretic agents.

DRUG	MAJOR INDICATIONS	USUAL ADULT DOSAGES	NURSING IMPLICATIONS
Thiazide and thiazide-like diuretics			
benzthiazide	Edema	50 to 200 mg P.O. daily or in divided doses	• Monitor patients also receiving digitalis therapy for signs and symptoms of digitalis toxicity.
	Hypertension	50 mg P.O. daily to q.i.d., depending on patient's response	• Monitor the patient's BUN, serum creatinine, serum electrolyte, and blood glucose levels.
			• Monitor the patient's fluid intake and output, weight, and vital signs.
			• Advise the patient to stand slowly, limit alcohol intake, and avoid strenuous exercise in hot weather, to decrease orthostatic hypotension.
			• Monitor the patient for signs and symptoms of hypokalemia or hyperglycemia.
			• Administer diuretics in the morning to avoid interference with the patient's sleep patterns.
			• Instruct the patient to eat potassium-rich foods daily.
			• Monitor the patient for hypersensitivity reactions: urticaria, rash, purpura, photosensitivity, and anaphylaxis.
			• Monitor the serum uric acid level if the patient has a history of gout.
chlorothiazide	Edema	500 mg to 2 grams P.O. or I.V. daily or in two divided doses	• Monitor patients also receiving digitalis therapy for signs and symptoms of digitalis toxicity.
	Hypertension	500 mg to 1 gram P.O. or I.V. daily or in divided doses	• Monitor the patient's BUN, serum creatinine, serum electrolyte, and blood glucose levels.
			• Monitor the patient's fluid intake and output, weight, and vital signs.
			• Advise the patient to stand slowly, limit alcohol intake, and avoid strenuous exercise in hot weather, to decrease orthostatic hypotension.
			• Monitor the patient for signs and symptoms of hypokalemia or hyperglycemia.
			• Administer diuretics in the morning to avoid interference with the patient's sleep patterns.
			• Monitor the patient receiving I.V. chlorothiazide for extravasation.
hydrochlorothiazide	Edema	25 to 100 mg P.O. daily or intermittently	• Monitor patients also receiving digitalis therapy for signs and symptoms of digitalis toxicity.
	Hypertension	25 to 100 mg P.O. daily or in divided doses	• Monitor the patient's BUN, serum creatinine, serum electrolyte, and blood glucose levels.
			• Monitor the patient's fluid intake and output, weight, and vital signs.
			• Advise the patient to stand slowly, limit alcohol intake, and avoid strenuous exercise in hot weather, to decrease orthostatic hypotension.
			• Monitor the patient for signs and symptoms of hypokalemia or hyperglycemia.
			• Administer diuretics in the morning to avoid interference with the patient's sleep patterns.

SELECTED MAJOR DRUGS

Diuretic agents continued

DRUG	MAJOR INDICATIONS	USUAL ADULT DOSAGES	NURSING IMPLICATIONS
metolazone	Edema from CHF	5 to 10 mg P.O. daily	• Monitor patients also receiving digitalis therapy for signs and symptoms of digitalis toxicity.
	Edema from renal or hepatic disease	5 to 20 mg P.O. daily	• Monitor the patient's BUN, serum creatinine, serum electrolyte, and blood glucose levels.
	Hypertension	2.5 to 5 mg P.O. daily	• Monitor the patient's fluid intake and output, weight, and vital signs.
			• Advise the patient to stand slowly, limit alcohol intake, and avoid strenuous exercise in hot weather, to decrease orthostatic hypotension.
			• Monitor the patient for signs and symptoms of hypokalemia or hyperglycemia.
			• Administer diuretics in the morning to avoid interference with the patient's sleep patterns.

Loop diuretics

DRUG	MAJOR INDICATIONS	USUAL ADULT DOSAGES	NURSING IMPLICATIONS
bumetanide	Edema and hypertension	0.5 to 2 mg P.O. in a single daily dose or repeated at 4- to 5-hour intervals up to a total of 10 mg/day; maintenance doses, usually given intermittently with 1- to 2-day rest periods, 0.5 to 1 mg I.M. or I.V. given over 1 to 2 minutes; I.V. doses may be repeated every 2 to 3 hours up to a total of 10 mg/day	• Monitor patients also receiving digitalis therapy for signs and symptoms of digitalis toxicity. • Monitor the patient's BUN, serum creatinine, serum electrolyte, and blood glucose levels. • Monitor the patient's fluid intake and output, weight, and vital signs. • Advise the patient to stand slowly, limit alcohol intake, and avoid strenuous exercise in hot weather, to decrease orthostatic hypotension. • Monitor the patient for signs and symptoms of hypokalemia or hyperglycemia. • Administer diuretics in the morning to avoid interference with the patient's sleep patterns. • Monitor the patient also taking oral anticoagulants for increased bruising and other adverse reactions, because loop diuretics potentiate the effect of oral anticoagulants. • Monitor the patient for the signs and symptoms of a hypersensitivity reaction. • Instruct the patient to include potassium-rich foods in the daily diet.
ethacrynate sodium ethacrynic acid	Acute pulmonary edema	50 to 100 mg of ethacrynate sodium I.V., infused slowly over several minutes	• Monitor patients also receiving digitalis therapy for signs and symptoms of digitalis toxicity. • Monitor the patient's BUN, serum creatinine, serum electrolyte, and blood glucose levels. • Monitor the patient's fluid intake and output, weight, and vital signs.
	Other forms of edema	50 to 200 mg of ethacrynic acid P.O., once daily, after meals or on alternate days; or up to 200 mg b.i.d. to obtain a therapeutic effect	• Advise the patient to stand slowly, limit alcohol intake, and avoid strenuous exercise in hot weather, to decrease orthostatic hypotension. • Monitor the patient for signs and symptoms of hypokalemia or hyperglycemia. • Administer diuretics in the morning to avoid interference with the patient's sleep patterns. • Do not administer I.M. or S.C. injections of ethacrynate sodium or ethacrynic acid because of the potential for tissue irritation.
furosemide	Acute pulmonary edema	40 mg I.V. injected slowly, then repeated every 2 hours as needed	• Monitor patients also receiving digitalis therapy for signs and symptoms of digitalis toxicity.

continued

SELECTED MAJOR DRUGS

Diuretic agents continued

DRUG	MAJOR INDICATIONS	USUAL ADULT DOSAGES	NURSING IMPLICATIONS
furosemide (continued)	Other forms of edema	20 to 80 mg P.O. once or twice a day up to 600 mg/day, or 20 to 40 mg I.M. or I.V. with repeated doses of 20 mg every 2 hours until the therapeutic effect is reached	• Monitor the patient's BUN, serum creatinine, serum electrolyte, and blood glucose levels. • Monitor the patient's fluid intake and output, weight, and vital signs. • Advise the patient to stand slowly, limit alcohol intake, and avoid strenuous exercise in hot weather, to decrease orthostatic hypotension. • Monitor the patient for signs and symptoms of hypokalemia or hyperglycemia.
	Hypertensive crisis and acute renal failure	100 to 200 mg I.V. over 1 to 2 minutes	• Administer diuretics in the morning to avoid interference with the patient's sleep patterns. • Store furosemide tablets and injectable solutions in light-resistant containers to prevent discoloration.
	Chronic renal failure	Initially, 80 mg P.O. daily, increased up to 120 mg/day until the therapeutic effect is reached	• Refrigerate oral furosemide solution to ensure stability. • Do not use discolored (yellow) injectable furosemide solution.
	Hypertension	20 to 80 mg P.O. daily	• Administer I.M. injections of furosemide using the Z-track method to limit tissue irritation. • Instruct the patient to report to the physician signs and symptoms of furosemide toxicity: tinnitus, abdominal pain, sore throat, or fever.

Potassium-sparing diuretics

DRUG	MAJOR INDICATIONS	USUAL ADULT DOSAGES	NURSING IMPLICATIONS
amiloride	Hypertension or edema associated with CHF	Initially, 5 to 10 mg P.O. daily, increased up to 20 mg/day if needed	• Monitor patients also receiving digitalis therapy for signs and symptoms of digitalis toxicity. • Monitor the patient's BUN, serum creatinine, serum electrolyte, and blood glucose levels. • Monitor the patient's fluid intake and output, weight, and vital signs. • Advise the patient to stand slowly, limit alcohol intake, and avoid strenuous exercise in hot weather, to decrease orthostatic hypotension. • Monitor the patient for signs and symptoms of hyperkalemia. • Administer diuretics in the morning to avoid interference with the patient's sleep patterns. • Administer amiloride cautiously to patients with impaired hepatic function or diabetes mellitus; administer cautiously to pregnant or lactating patients. • Instruct the patient to avoid eating potassium-rich foods.
spironolactone	Essential hypertension	Initially, 50 to 100 mg P.O. daily in divided doses	• Monitor patients also receiving digitalis therapy for signs and symptoms of digitalis toxicity. • Monitor the patient's BUN, serum creatinine, serum electrolyte, and blood glucose levels. • Monitor the patient's fluid intake and output, weight, and vital signs.
	Edema	Initially, 25 to 200 mg P.O. daily in divided doses	• Advise the patient to stand slowly, limit alcohol intake, and avoid strenuous exercise in hot weather, to decrease orthostatic hypotension. • Monitor the patient for signs and symptoms of hyperkalemia.

SELECTED MAJOR DRUGS

Diuretic agents continued

DRUG	MAJOR INDICATIONS	USUAL ADULT DOSAGES	NURSING IMPLICATIONS
spironolactone (continued)			• Administer diuretics in the morning to avoid interference with the patient's sleep patterns. • Store spironolactone in a light-resistant container.

Carbonic anhydrase inhibitors

DRUG	MAJOR INDICATIONS	USUAL ADULT DOSAGES	NURSING IMPLICATIONS
acetazolamide, acetazolamide sodium	Edema	250 to 500 mg P.O., I.V., or I.M. daily or every other day	• Monitor patients also receiving digitalis therapy for signs and symptoms of digitalis toxicity. • Monitor the patient's BUN, serum creatinine, serum electrolyte, and blood glucose levels. • Monitor the patient's fluid intake and output, weight, and vital signs. • Advise the patient to stand slowly, limit alcohol intake, and avoid strenuous exercise in hot weather, to decrease orthostatic hypotension. • Monitor the patient for signs and symptoms of hypokalemia. • Administer diuretics in the morning to avoid interference with the patient's sleep patterns. • These agents are contraindicated in patients with narrow-angle glaucoma, sensitivity to sulfonamides, chronic pulmonary disease, renal failure, hepatic insufficiency, Addison's disease or adrenocortical insufficiency, hyponatremia, hypokalemia, hyperchloremic acidosis; they are also contraindicated during pregnancy, especially during the first trimester. • Administer cautiously to patients with a history of hypercalciuria, diabetes mellitus, or gout. • Administer potassium supplements to the patient as ordered. • Monitor the patient for signs and symptoms of metabolic acidosis, including headache, drowsiness, decreased mentation, confusion, seizures, coma, fatigue, hypotension, hypoxia, dysrhythmias, Kussmaul's respirations, anorexia, nausea, vomiting, and tissue hypoxia. • Disguise the bitter taste of these drugs by softening the tablets in hot water and adding honey or syrup. • If the drug is being given to treat glaucoma, advise the patient to report eye pain, which could indicate the drug is ineffective in lowering intraocular pressure.
	Glaucoma	250 mg P.O. daily to q.i.d. For rapid lowering of intraocular pressure, 500 mg I.V. or I.M., repeated in 2 to 4 hours if necessary.	
dichlorphenamide	Glaucoma	Initially, 100 to 200 mg P.O., followed by 100 mg P.O. every 12 hours until the therapeutic effect is reached; for maintenance, 25 to 50 mg one to three times daily	• Monitor patients also receiving digitalis therapy for signs and symptoms of digitalis toxicity. • Monitor the patient's BUN, serum creatinine, serum electrolyte, and blood glucose levels. • Monitor the patient's fluid intake and output, weight, and vital signs. • Advise the patient to stand slowly, limit alcohol intake, and avoid strenuous exercise in hot weather, to decrease orthostatic hypotension. • Monitor the patient for signs and symptoms of hypokalemia.

continued

Diuretic agents continued

DRUG	MAJOR INDICATIONS	USUAL ADULT DOSAGES	NURSING IMPLICATIONS
dichlorphenamide (continued)			• Administer diuretics in the morning to avoid interference with the patient's sleep patterns. • Avoid I.M. injections of these drugs, when possible, because the alkaline pH of the solution produces intense pain at the injection site. • Do not use parenteral solutions more than 24 hours after reconstitution because they are made without preservatives. Suspensions usually remain stable for 1 week. Store tablets in a tightly closed, light-resistant container.
Osmotic diuretics			
mannitol	Oliguria or prevention of acute renal failure Increased intracranial or intraocular pressure Drug intoxication from secobarbital, imipramine, aspirin, or carbon tetrachloride	50 to 100 grams I.V. of 5% to 25% solution 1.5 to 2 grams/kg I.V. of 15% to 20% solution infused over 30 to 60 minutes; if preoperative medication, give 1 to 1½ hours before surgery Maximum dose of 200 grams I.V. of 5% to 10% solution over a 24-hour period	• Monitor patients also receiving digitalis therapy for signs and symptoms of digitalis toxicity. • Monitor the patient's BUN, serum creatinine, serum electrolyte, and blood glucose levels. • Monitor the patient's fluid intake and output, weight, and vital signs. • Advise the patient to stand slowly, limit alcohol intake, and avoid strenuous exercise in hot weather, to decrease orthostatic hypotension. • Administer diuretics in the morning to avoid interference with the patient's sleep patterns. • Osmotic diuretics are contraindicated in patients with diagnosed acute renal failure, cardiac dysfunction, CHF, active intracranial bleeding, or severe dehydration. • Monitor the patient for circulatory overload if the urine output is less than 30 to 50 ml/hour. • Monitor the patient's vital signs hourly during osmotic diuretic therapy. • Observe I.V. administration sites for local irritation, extravasation, or signs of thrombophlebitis. • Assist the patient in maintaining an adequate fluid intake to promote renal function. Provide mouth care for the patient, and offer ice chips and hard candies to relieve thirst. • Parenteral mannitol crystallizes at low temperatures. To dissolve, warm it in a hot-water bath and then shake the container vigorously; allow the solution to return to room temperature before administration. • Administer mannitol using an in-line I.V. filter. • Do not add blood products to I.V. lines used for mannitol administration, because pseudoagglutination will occur. • Store mannitol between 15° to 30° C. (59° to 88° F.), unless otherwise directed, and avoid freezing.

velopment of the less toxic, more effective loop diuretics in the 1960s. Although used as early as the 15th century, mercurial diuretics did not become clinically popular until 1920, after Saxl and Heilig developed clinically useful drugs. Because mercurial diuretics become inactive in an alkaline environment, acidifying agents were often used with them to enhance diuresis. After administration of a mercurial diuretic, sodium and chloride excretion and bicarbonate retention increase, leading to systemic alkalosis.

Mercurial diuretics are no longer frequently used because of their erratic oral absorption, which necessitates parenteral (usually I.M.) administration. As new diuretics have been introduced, they have gradually replaced the mercurial diuretics.

CHAPTER SUMMARY

The development of diuretic drugs has been dramatic during the mid- to late 20th century. Therapy has advanced from the more toxic mercurial diuretics to the less dangerous carbonic anhydrase inhibitors, which gave rise to the more powerful thiazide and thiazide-like diuretics. Loop diuretics are the most recently developed and the most potent diuretics available today.

Chapter 38 discussed all these agents as they are used for therapeutic diuresis. Here are the highlights of the chapter:

• Thiazide and thiazide-like diuretics are sulfonamide derivatives that inhibit sodium reabsorption, thereby increasing the excretion of water, chloride, sodium, potassium, and bicarbonate ions. They are most commonly used to treat hypertension and CHF-induced edema.

• Thiazides are ineffective if the patient's GFR is less than 20 ml/minute and are, therefore, usually ineffective in patients with renal insufficiency. Metolazone, the exception, is effective in patients with mild renal insufficiency.

• Loop diuretics, the most potent diuretics, are effective in the treatment of edema, hypertension, and hypercalcemia and for patients who are resistant to less potent diuretics or who have decreased GFRs. They act directly on the thick ascending loop of Henle, inhibiting sodium and chloride reabsorption.

• Because of the powerful diuretic qualities associated with the loop diuretics, the risk of hypokalemia is great. These diuretics are ototoxic and may produce hearing impairment at high doses.

• Potassium-sparing diuretics are less potent than the other diuretics but have the advantage of conserving potassium. Physicians usually use potassium-sparing diuretics in combination with other diuretic or antihypertensive agents.

• Because the patient may develop hyperkalemia during therapy with potassium-sparing diuretics, the nurse must monitor the patent's serum potassium levels; the patient may need a low-potassium diet.

• Carbonic anhydrase inhibitors cause a bicarbonate diuresis of moderate potency. These drugs are used primarily to treat glaucoma. However, with prolonged use, they create a metabolic acidosis that can inhibit their diuretic action. Although carbonic anhydrase inhibitors are rarely used as diuretics today, they were important landmarks in the development of diuretic therapy.

• The osmotic diuretics inhibit tubular fluid and sodium reabsorption, thereby producing diuresis. Osmotic diuretics are used to prevent acute renal failure and to reduce increased intracranial or intraocular pressure. Patients receiving osmotic diuretics should be monitored closely for signs and symptoms of fluid and electrolyte imbalances.

• Mercurial diuretics, widely used for several decades in the first half of the 20th century, are obsolete today—replaced by safer, more potent diuretics.

BIBLIOGRAPHY

American Hospital Formulary Service. *Drug Information 87.* McEvoy, G.K., et al., eds. Bethesda, Md.: American Society of Hospital Pharmacists, 1987.

Eknoyan, G., and Martinez-Maldonado, M. *The Physiological Basis of Diuretic Therapy in Clinical Medicine.* Orlando, Fla: Grune & Stratton, 1986.

Gilman, G., et al., eds. *Goodman and Gilman's The Pharmacological Basis of Therapeutics,* 7th ed. New York: Macmillan Publishing Co., 1985.

Hansten, P. *Drug Interactions,* 5th ed. Philadelphia: Lea & Febiger, 1985.

Kastrup, E.K., et al., eds. *Facts and Comparisons.* St. Louis: Facts and Comparisons Division, J.B. Lippincott Co., 1987.

Patterson, H.R., et al. *Current Drug Handbook 1984-1986.* Philadelphia: W.B. Saunders Co., 1986.

Puschett, J.B., and Greenberg, A. *Diuretics: Chemistry, Pharmacology, and Clinical Applications.* New York: Elsevier Science Publishers, 1984.

Puschett, J.B., and Greenberg, A. *The Diuretic Manual.* New York: Elsevier Science Publishers, 1985.

Shinn, A.F., and Shrewsbury R.P. *Evaluations of Drug Interactions.* St. Louis: C.V. Mosby Co., 1985.

USPDI. *Advice for the Patient, Vol. 2.* 6th ed. Rockville, Md.: United States Pharmacopeial Convention, Inc., 1985.

USPDI. *Drug Information for the Health Care Provider, Vol. 1,* 6th ed. Rockville, Md.: United States Pharmacopeial Convention, Inc., 1985.

CHAPTER
39
PERIPHERAL VASCULAR AGENTS

OBJECTIVES

After reading and studying this chapter, you should be able to:

1. Discuss what the peripheral vascular agents can and cannot do to treat peripheral vascular disease.

2. Describe the mechanism of action for direct-acting vasodilators, beta-adrenergic stimulants, hemorrheologic agents, and other peripheral vascular agents.

3. Identify the adverse reactions that can occur with each type of peripheral vascular agent.

4. Identify groups of patients to whom each type of peripheral vascular agent should not be administered.

INTRODUCTION

Peripheral vascular agents include drugs that increase blood flow by direct action (direct-acting vasodilators), or by indirect action (beta-adrenergic stimulants and hemorrheologic agents). Although these agents have been used to treat peripheral vascular diseases, their effectiveness depends on the disease.

A peripheral vascular disease can result from a vasospasm (blood vessel spasm that decreases the vessel's lumen) or an occlusion (vessel blockage). A vasospastic disease may be more responsive to drug therapy than an occlusive disease. For example, the most common vasospastic disorder is Raynaud's disease, which decreases blood flow to the skin, but this disorder may be reversible with a drug that dilates blood vessels. In arteriosclerosis obliterans, a common occlusive disorder, an organic arterial obstruction reduces the blood flow. In this disorder, a drug that dilates blood vessels in the skeletal muscles or skin cannot improve blood flow.

Effective treatment of peripheral vascular disease has not been established, and no well-controlled clinical studies have demonstrated the usefulness of peripheral vascular agents in treating these disorders. However, several types of drugs have been used in an attempt to increase peripheral blood flow to areas where a vasospastic or occlusive disorder has compromised perfusion (adequate blood flow to tissues). They include direct-acting vasodilators, beta-adrenergic stimulants, hemorrheologic agents (agents that alter the blood's viscosity), and other peripheral vascular agents.

For a summary of representative drugs, see *Selected major drugs: Peripheral vascular agents* on page 634.

DIRECT-ACTING VASODILATORS

Direct-acting vasodilators (cyclandelate, ethaverine hydrochloride, isoxsuprine hydrochloride, niacin, and papaverine hydrochloride) can increase the blood flow in normal skeletal muscle and relieve ischemia (decreased blood supply to a body organ or part) from vasospasm. In occlusive vascular disease, they have limited therapeutic value and may even be harmful. For example, autoregulatory mechanisms in skeletal muscles produce vasodilation in response to ischemia from an occlusion. Vasodilators will increase blood flow primarily to nonischemic areas adjacent to the occlusion, shifting the blood flow from diseased areas, where it is much needed, to nondiseased areas. This is known as the steal syndrome.

PHARMACOKINETICS

Direct-acting vasodilators are readily absorbed from the gastrointestinal (GI) tract and well distributed to body tissues, except for papaverine, which is up to 90% bound to plasma proteins. One drug in this class, isoxsuprine, crosses the placenta. The liver metabolizes these vasodilators, and the metabolites are excreted in the urine.

These drugs directly relax vascular smooth muscles in 1 hour. Their effects usually peak in 3 hours and last for approximately 6 hours. Oral administration of papaverine at 6-hour intervals can maintain fairly constant plasma concentrations; the sustained-release form can maintain plasma concentrations when given at 12-hour intervals.

PHARMACODYNAMICS

Direct-acting vasodilators interfere with the normal biochemical reactions of vascular smooth muscle contraction, thereby inhibiting normal muscle contraction and causing blood vessel dilation.

Mechanism of action

The spasmolytic, or muscle relaxant, action of the direct-acting vasodilators primarily affects coronary, cerebral, pulmonary, and peripheral arteries. It can also affect the smooth muscles of the bronchi, GI tract, ureters, and biliary system. As muscles relax, blood vessels dilate, increasing blood flow. Papaverine relaxes the cardiac muscle directly by depressing myocardial excitability, thus prolonging the refractory period, and depressing conduction. This direct action is unrelated to muscle innervation. In a vascular occlusion, papaverine may act by overcoming reflex vasoconstriction in collateral vessels. Papaverine produces little central nervous system (CNS) action, although large doses may depress the CNS in some patients.

Ethaverine, a synthetic papaverine derivative, provides about twice as much muscle relaxant activity but has not been studied extensively in peripheral vascular disease. It directly relaxes vascular smooth muscle and works predominantly by inhibiting phosphorylation (the process of converting phosphoric acid into a compound with alcohol, an ester).

PHARMACOTHERAPEUTICS

Because direct-acting vasodilators produce a spasmolytic effect on smooth muscles, they are principally used to relieve cerebral and peripheral ischemia from vasospasm.

cyclandelate (Cyclospasmol). Cyclandelate acts directly on vascular smooth muscles. It may be used as an adjunct to treat various peripheral vascular diseases. In animal experiments, cyclandelate has produced about three times the spasmolytic activity of papaverine, but its effectiveness in vasospastic or occlusive peripheral vascular disease in humans has not been confirmed.

USUAL ADULT DOSAGE: Initial dosage: 1.2 to 1.6 g P.O. daily in divided doses before meals and h.s. Maintenance dosage: 400 to 800 mg P.O. daily.

ethaverine hydrochloride (Ethatab). Previously used to treat peripheral vascular insufficiency, ethaverine is rarely used today because of its questionable effectiveness. This drug may be used for spastic conditions of the GI and genitourinary (GU) tracts.
USUAL ADULT DOSAGE: 100 to 200 mg P.O. t.i.d.

isoxsuprine hydrochloride (Vasodilan). Isoxsuprine is used to relieve the symptoms of cerebrovascular insufficiency and as an adjunct in the treatment of peripheral vascular diseases, such as arteriosclerosis obliterans, thromboangiitis obliterans (Buerger's disease), and Raynaud's disease.
USUAL ADULT DOSAGE: for peripheral vascular and cerebrovascular disorders, 10 to 20 mg P.O. t.i.d. or q.i.d.

niacin. Also known as nicotinic acid, niacin and its derivative nicotinyl alcohol act as weak vasodilators primarily in the blush area, which includes the ears, face, and neck. They have little effect on blood vessels in the lower extremities. Although niacin and nicotinyl alcohol are used as adjunct therapy, no evidence shows that they can effectively treat peripheral vascular disease. (See Chapter 51, Vitamin and Mineral Agents, for more information on niacin.)
USUAL ADULT DOSAGE: 100 to 150 mg P.O. three to five times daily; 300 to 400 mg P.O. every 12 hours of sustained-release niacin.

papaverine hydrochloride (Cerespan, Pavabid). Although sometimes used to treat acute and chronic vascular occlusion, this drug is primarily used to relieve ischemia from an arterial spasm. Despite its many years of use, no objective study has proved its effectiveness.
USUAL ADULT DOSAGE: 100 to 300 mg P.O. three to five times daily; 150 mg every 8 to 12 hours or 300 mg q12h of sustained-release papaverine.

Drug interactions

These drugs can interact with other vasodilators, such as antihypertensives, nitrates, and alcohol, and may cause excessive vasodilation that leads to hypotension and cerebral hypoperfusion. Papaverine may decrease the effect of levodopa in a patient with Parkinson's disease, but no other significant drug interactions are known.

ADVERSE DRUG REACTIONS

The direct-acting vasodilators produce predictable adverse reactions in many body systems, including the cardiovascular, autonomic nervous, central nervous, and GI systems. They may also cause unpredictable reactions.

Predictable reactions

In the cardiovascular system, direct-acting vasodilators may cause hypotension, tachycardia, transient palpitations, and chest pain. In the autonomic nervous system, they may produce flushing, sweating, and dry mouth. Their effects on the CNS include trembling, nervousness, weakness, dizziness, depression, vertigo, headache, and sedation. Effects on the GI system may include abdominal distress, nausea, vomiting, diarrhea, abdominal distention, and constipation. Papaverine commonly produces anticholinergic effects, such as dry mouth, constipation, and urinary retention.

Unpredictable reactions

Hypersensitivity to papaverine may produce hepatotoxicity indicated by jaundice, eosinophilia, and abnormal liver function tests. In some patients, isoxsuprine may produce a severe rash.

NURSING IMPLICATIONS

Because direct-acting vasodilators can cause severe adverse reactions, the nurse must carefully monitor patients and be aware of the following considerations:
• Do not administer isoxsuprine to a patient immediately postpartum or to a patient with arterial bleeding, hypotension, or tachycardia.
• Avoid administering these drugs to a pregnant patient, because their safety during pregnancy has not been established.
• Use with caution in a patient with severe coronary artery or cerebrovascular disease.
• Administer these drugs with food or antacids to prevent GI adverse effects.
• Watch for signs of hepatotoxicity, such as jaundice, eosinophilia, and abnormal liver function tests. Discontinue the drug if these signs are detected.
• Instruct the patient to avoid sudden posture changes if dizziness occurs.
• Advise the patient to use caution when driving or performing other tasks that require alertness.

BETA-ADRENERGIC STIMULANTS

The only beta-adrenergic stimulant used as a peripheral vascular agent is nylidrin hydrochloride. It improves skeletal muscle blood flow primarily by stimulating beta-adrenergic receptors.

A synthetic agent, nylidrin is chemically related to isoxsuprine. Although it is used primarily to treat peripheral vascular diseases, its effectiveness has not been established.

PHARMACOKINETICS

Nylidrin is rapidly and almost completely absorbed from the GI tract. Although its metabolic fate is unknown, it is excreted in the urine.

After oral administration, nylidrin's therapeutic effects begin in 10 minutes, peak in 30 minutes, and last for 2 hours.

PHARMACODYNAMICS

Nylidrin causes vasodilation, primarily in skeletal muscles, by stimulating beta-adrenergic receptors and directly relaxing vascular smooth muscle. It decreases peripheral vascular resistance, and, in normal subjects, leaves skeletal muscle blood flow unchanged. This drug increases the heart rate and cardiac output, as well as gastric acid secretion and gastric juice volume.

PHARMACOTHERAPEUTICS

Nylidrin serves as a therapeutic adjunct in treating peripheral vascular conditions, such as arteriosclerosis obliterans, thromboangiitis obliterans, diabetic vascular disease, night leg cramps, Raynaud's phenomenon and disease, ischemic ulcer, frostbite, acrocyanosis, acroparesthesia, thrombophlebitis, and chronic cold feet and hands. However, studies have not proved its effectiveness in treating these disorders.

nylidrin hydrochloride (Arlidin). This beta-adrenergic stimulant is administered orally to treat various peripheral vascular diseases.
USUAL ADULT DOSAGE: 3 to 12 mg P.O. t.i.d. or q.i.d.

Drug interactions

In patients taking other vasodilators, such as antihypertensives, nitrates, or alcohol, nylidrin can produce excessive vasodilation that may result in hypotension and cerebral hypoperfusion. No other significant drug interactions are known.

ADVERSE DRUG REACTIONS

Most adverse drug reactions to beta-adrenergic stimulants are dose-related and typically affect the nervous, cardiovascular, and GI systems.

Autonomic nervous system reactions cause flushing, sweating, and dry mouth; CNS reactions cause trembling, nervousness, weakness, dizziness, depression, vertigo, headache, and sedation. Cardiovascular reactions may include hypotension, tachycardia, transient palpitations, and chest pain. In the GI system, nylidrin may produce abdominal distress, nausea, vomiting, diarrhea, abdominal distention, and constipation.

Hypersensitivity reactions to nylidrin are rare; however, some patients may develop a rash.

NURSING IMPLICATIONS

The nurse must consider several important factors when caring for a patient receiving nylidrin:
• Avoid administering nylidrin to a pregnant or lactating patient because its safety for these patients has not been established.
• Be aware that nylidrin is contraindicated in patients with acute myocardial infarction, paroxysmal tachycardia, angina pectoris, or thyrotoxicosis.
• Use nylidrin with caution in a patient with uncompensated (uncontrolled) congestive heart failure because the condition may worsen.
• Administer nylidrin with caution to a patient with peptic ulcers because the drug increases gastric acid secretion.
• Check the patient's heart rate and blood pressure 30 minutes after administration, when the drug reaches its peak activity.
• Advise the patient to use caution when driving or performing other tasks that require alertness.
• Instruct the patient to avoid sudden posture changes if dizziness occurs.

HEMORRHEOLOGIC AGENTS

Pentoxifylline, a hemorrheologic agent, has Food and Drug Administration approval for treating intermittent claudication caused by chronic occlusive peripheral vascular disease. This xanthine derivative offers a new approach to correction of peripheral vasoconstriction. Instead of dilating the arteries, it increases erythrocyte flexibility, reduces blood viscosity, and increases microcirculatory flow and tissue perfusion.

PHARMACOKINETICS

After oral administration, pentoxifylline is well absorbed, although food in the stomach can delay the absorption rate. The drug undergoes extensive first-pass metabolism as well as metabolism in the liver. Distribution of pentoxifylline and its metabolites has not been clearly defined, but some evidence exists that binding to red blood cells occurs. The parent drug and its metabolites are excreted in the urine and feces.

Pentoxifylline and its active metabolites reach peak plasma levels in 1 hour. Their duration of action is approximately 6 to 8 hours. Because their half-life is short, a sustained-release preparation can maintain adequate plasma levels and therapeutic effects.

PHARMACODYNAMICS

Researchers believe that pentoxifylline improves oxygen supply to ischemic tissues by decreasing blood viscosity, allowing more blood to get through to the tissues. Several mechanisms may account for this action, including reduction in plasma fibrinogen levels, inhibition of platelet aggregation, and increases in erythrocyte flexibility.

PHARMACOTHERAPEUTICS

The major clinical indication for pentoxifylline is the treatment of intermittent claudication from chronic occlusive peripheral vascular disease. By enhancing tissue oxygenation, the drug allows the patient with intermittent claudication to walk greater distances without severe pain. However, it is not recommended in acute occlusive peripheral vascular disease, which produces ischemic skin ulcers, pain at rest, and gangrene.

Peripheral vascular agents

This chart summarizes the agents currently in clinical use to treat peripheral vascular disease.

DRUG	MAJOR INDICATIONS	USUAL ADULT DOSAGES	NURSING IMPLICATIONS
Direct-acting vasodilators			
cyclandelate	Adjunct in treating various peripheral vascular diseases	100 to 200 mg P.O. q.i.d. or up to a maximum of 400 mg q.i.d.	• Use with caution in a patient with severe coronary artery or cerebrovascular disease. • Administer with food or antacids to prevent GI adverse effects.
isoxsuprine	Adjunct in treating peripheral vascular disease; symptomatic relief in cerebrovascular insufficiency	10 to 20 mg P.O. t.i.d. or q.i.d.	• Do not give isoxsuprine to a patient immediately postpartum or to a patient with arterial bleeding, hypotension, or tachycardia. • Instruct the patient to avoid sudden posture changes if dizziness occurs.
niacin and nicotinyl alcohol	Adjunct in treating conditions associated with deficient circulation, such as arteriosclerosis obliterans	100 to 150 mg P.O. three to five times daily; 300 to 400 mg P.O. every 12 hours of sustained-release niacin	• Advise the patient that large doses may cause flushing of the face and neck. • Instruct the patient to avoid sudden posture changes if dizziness occurs.
papaverine	Relief of cerebral and peripheral ischemia caused by an arterial spasm	100 to 300 mg P.O. three to five times daily; 150 mg every 8 to 12 hours or 300 mg q12h of sustained-release papaverine	• Observe for signs of hepatotoxicity, such as jaundice, eosinophilia, and abnormal liver function tests. • Advise the patient to use caution when driving or performing other tasks that require alertness. • Instruct the patient to avoid sudden posture changes if dizziness occurs.
Beta-adrenergic stimulants			
nylidrin	Adjunct in treating various peripheral vascular diseases, such as arteriosclerosis obliterans and thromboangiitis obliterans	3 to 12 mg P.O. t.i.d. or q.i.d.	• Advise the patient to use caution when driving or performing other tasks that require alertness. • Instruct the patient to avoid sudden posture changes if dizziness occurs.
Hemorrheologic agents			
pentoxifylline	Symptomatic relief of intermittent claudication caused by chronic occlusive peripheral vascular disease	400 mg P.O. t.i.d. with meals for at least 8 weeks	• Do not administer to a patient who is allergic to xanthines, such as caffeine, theophylline, and theobromine. • Routinely monitor the blood pressure of a patient who is receiving pentoxifylline and an antihypertensive drug.

pentoxifylline (Trental). Although pentoxifylline has been approved only to treat intermittent claudication related to chronic occlusive peripheral vascular disease, research continues in its effectiveness with other conditions, such as coronary artery disease, cerebrovascular disease, and sickle-cell anemia.

USUAL ADULT DOSAGE: 400 mg P.O. t.i.d. with meals for at least 8 weeks.

Drug interactions
Bleeding and a prolonged prothrombin time may occur in a patient receiving pentoxifylline with an anticoagulant or another drug that inhibits platelet aggregation. No

clinically significant interactions have been noted with other drugs.

ADVERSE DRUG REACTIONS

Most patients tolerate pentoxifylline well, although some experience mild GI or CNS adverse reactions. Cardiovascular effects rarely occur but may include palpitations, angina, dysrhythmias, and hypotension.

NURSING IMPLICATIONS

Although drug interactions are not clinically significant, and adverse reactions are few, the nurse should be aware of the following considerations when administering pentoxifylline:
• Remember that pentoxifylline is a xanthine derivative and should not be administered to a patient who is allergic to xanthines, such as caffeine, theophylline, and theobromine.
• Monitor the blood pressure routinely for a patient receiving an antihypertensive drug and pentoxifylline concurrently because of the increased risk of severe hypotension.
• Advise the patient to take pentoxifylline with meals to minimize any GI disturbance.
• Advise the patient to report signs and symptoms of adverse reactions in the GI system, such as dyspepsia, nausea, and vomiting, or in the CNS, such as headaches and dizziness.

OTHER PERIPHERAL VASCULAR AGENTS

Various drugs that affect the sympathetic nervous system have been used to treat peripheral vascular disorders.

antiadrenergic drugs. Alpha-adrenergic blocking agents, such as phenoxybenzamine and tolazoline, block the response to sympathetic nerve impulses and circulating catecholamine. Their use is limited because they produce severe GI and cardiovascular adverse effects. Other drugs that block the sympathetic nervous system, such as reserpine, methyldopa, and guanethidine, can decrease vasoconstriction. But like the alpha-adrenergic blockers, severe adverse effects, especially hypotension, limit their usefulness. (See Chapter 37, Antihypertensive Agents, for more information on these drugs.)

CHAPTER SUMMARY

This chapter has described drugs that increase blood flow and may treat peripheral vascular diseases, although their effectiveness is not certain. Highlights include:
• Peripheral vascular diseases generally result from a vasospasm or an occlusion. Vasospasm is reversible and may respond to dilation of blood vessels. Because occlusion involves vessel obstruction, dilation cannot improve blood flow.
• Direct-acting vasodilators, beta-adrenergic stimulants, hemorrheologic agents, and other peripheral vascular agents have all been used in an attempt to treat these disorders.
• Although direct-acting vasodilators, beta-adrenergic stimulants, or miscellaneous peripheral vascular agents may not effectively treat peripheral vascular diseases, they may cause significant adverse reactions.
• Pentoxifylline, a hemorrheologic agent, effectively relieves some symptoms of intermittent claudication but does not alter the course of the disease.

BIBLIOGRAPHY

Aviado, D.M., and Porter, J. "Pentoxifylline: A New Drug for the Treatment of Intermittent Claudication," *Pharmacotherapy* 4:297, November/December 1984.

Baker, D., and Campbell, R.K. "Pentoxifylline: A New Agent for Intermittent Claudication," *Drug Intelligence and Clinical Pharmacy* 19:345, May 1985.

Dettelbach, H.R., and Aviado, D.M. "Clinical Pharmacology of Pentoxifylline with Special Reference to Its Hemorrheologic Effect for the Treatment of Intermittent Claudication," *The Journal of Clinical Pharmacology* 25:8, 1985.

Nursing86 Drug Handbook. Springhouse, Pa.: Springhouse Corp., 1986.

Skotnicki, S.H., et al. *Angiology* 35:685, 1984.

Trainer, F., et al. "Effects of Ethaverine Hydrochloride on the Walking Tolerance of Patients with Intermittent Claudication," *Angiology* 343, 1986.

Vyden, J.K., et al. "Lack of Effect of Cyclandelate in Peripheral Arterial Disease," 35:1, 1984.

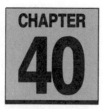
ANTILIPEMIC AGENTS

OBJECTIVES

After reading and studying this chapter, you should be able to:

1. Use the following terms correctly: lipid, lipoprotein, phospholipid, hyperlipoproteinemia, lipolysis, anabolism, catabolism.

2. Describe the blood lipid components and their fractions.

3. Identify the three major classes of antilipemic drugs and give an example of a drug found in each class.

4. Explain the mechanisms of action for each of the three major classes of antilipemic agents: bile-sequestering agents, fibric acid derivatives, and cholesterol synthesis inhibitors.

5. Identify the major drug interactions, adverse reactions, and nursing implications for each of the three major classes of antilipemic drugs.

6. Describe how niacin acts as an antilipemic agent, and identify its major adverse reactions.

7. Describe how the bile-sequestering agents and fibric acid derivatives interact with other drugs.

INTRODUCTION

Physicians use antilipemic agents to lower abnormally high blood levels of lipids (fatty substances). In normal amounts, lipids help produce energy, maintain body temperature, and provide the chemical precursors of certain body constituents. In abnormally high amounts, lipids allow excess cholesterol to form and deposit in the blood vessels as atherosclerotic plaques. These plaques help cause hypertension, slow the flow of oxygenated blood to the heart and other body organs, and increase the risk of coronary artery disease (CAD), which kills more than 500,000 people in the United States each year.

Lipids are composed of several different chemicals: free fatty acids (FFA), triglycerides (glycerol esters of FFA), sterols (cholesterol and cholesterol esters), and phospholipids (phosphoric acid esters of lipid substances). Lipids can be exogenous (derived from the diet) or endogenous (produced by the liver from the end products of lipid and carbohydrate breakdown, or catabolism). The body also produces endogenous lipids through anabolism, a constructive metabolic process that combines substances, such as cholesterol, with other substances.

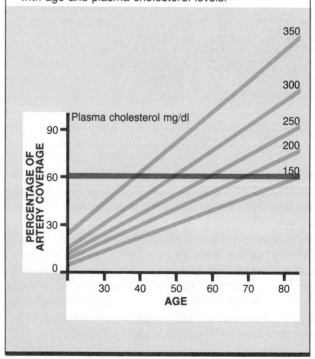

Cholesterol and coronary artery disease

When atherosclerotic plaque occludes 60% or more of the coronary arteries, the risk of coronary artery disease increases dramatically. The graph below shows how artery coverage with plaque increases with age and plasma cholesterol levels.

Types of hyperlipoproteinemia

The causes, incidence, and diagnostic findings vary with the type of hyperlipoproteinemia, as shown in the chart below.

TYPE	CAUSES AND INCIDENCE	DIAGNOSTIC FINDINGS
I (Frederickson's, exogenous hyperlipemia, idiopathic familial hyperlipoproteinemia)	• Deficient or abnormal lipoprotein lipase, resulting in decreased or absent post-heparin lipolytic activity • Relatively rare	• Increased chylomicrons, decreased very-low-density lipoproteins (VLDL), low-density lipoproteins (LDL), high-density lipoproteins (HDL) • High serum chylomicrons and triglycerides levels; slightly elevated serum cholesterol level; lower serum lipoprotein lipase level • Leukocytosis
IIa (familial hyperbetalipoproteinemia, essential familial hypercholesterolemia)	• Deficient cell surface receptor that regulates LDL degradation and cholesterol synthesis, resulting in increased levels of plasma LDL over joints and pressure points • Onset between ages 10 and 30	• Increased plasma concentrations of LDL • Increased serum cholesterol and triglycerides levels • Amniocentesis shows increased LDL level
IIb (familial combined lipidemia)	• Severe forms are like IIa; milder forms associated with obesity or diabetes • Relatively common	• Elevated LDL and VLDL levels
III (familial broad beta disease, xanthoma tuberosum)	• Unknown underlying defect results in deficient conversion of triglyceride-rich VLDL to LDL • Uncommon; usually occurs after age 20 but can occur earlier in men	• Abnormal serum betalipoprotein level • Elevated cholesterol and triglycerides levels • Slightly elevated glucose tolerance • Hyperuricemia
IV (endogenous hypertriglyceridemia, hyperbetalipoproteinemia)	• Usually occurs secondary to obesity, alcoholism, diabetes, or emotional disorders • Relatively common, especially in middle-aged men	• Elevated VLDL level • Abnormal levels of triglycerides in plasma; variable increase in serum • Normal or slightly elevated serum cholesterol level • Mildly abnormal glucose tolerance • Positive family history • Early coronary artery disease
V (mixed hypertriglyceridemia, mixed hyperlipidemia)	• Defective triglyceride clearance causes pancreatitis; usually secondary to another disorder, such as obesity or nephrosis • Uncommon; onset usually occurs in late adolescence or early adulthood	• Increased chylomicrons in plasma • Elevated plasma VLDL level • Elevated serum cholesterol and triglycerides levels

Combinations of these lipids form various lipoproteins that transport lipids throughout the body: chylomicrons, chylomicron fragments, very-low-density lipoproteins (VLDL), low-density lipoproteins (LDL), intermediate-density lipoproteins (IDL), and high-density lipoproteins (HDL). HDL, unlike other lipoproteins, may serve a protective role, clearing cholesterol from body tissues. Chylomicrons are minute lipid particles produced in the small intestine through emulsification with bile salts. Lipoproteins are larger lipid particles that have combined with proteins.

Excess of any type of lipid in the blood is known as hyperlipidemia. Hyperlipoproteinemia is excess of lipoproteins in the blood. Excess cholesterol and its derivatives is known as hypercholesterolemia, whereas excess triglycerides is hypertriglyceridemia. Any of these conditions may exist alone or in combination. All of them can be familial (hereditary) and exist from early child-

Lipoprotein synthesis and metabolism

Lipoprotein formation can be exogenous or endogenous. During exogenous formation, lipids enter the circulation from the intestine. During endogenous formation, lipids enter the circulation from the liver. The diagram below illustrates the other differences between exogenous and endogenous lipoprotein formation.

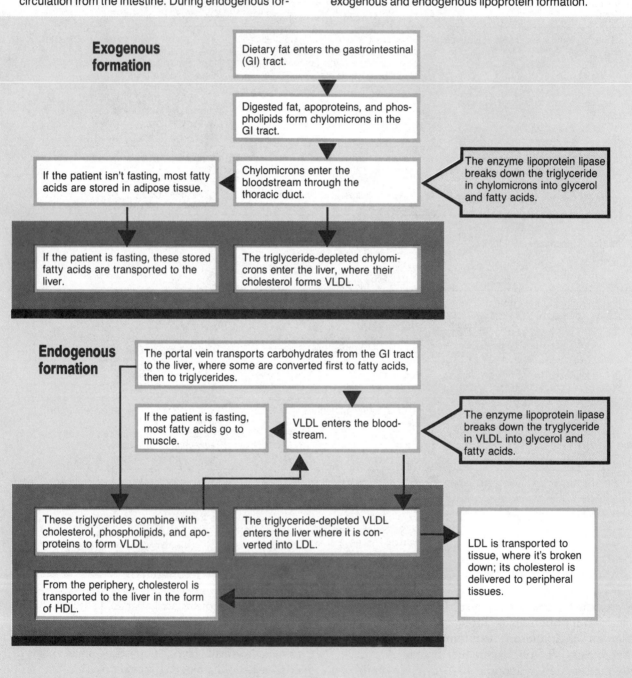

Exogenous formation

Dietary fat enters the gastrointestinal (GI) tract.

Digested fat, apoproteins, and phospholipids form chylomicrons in the GI tract.

If the patient isn't fasting, most fatty acids are stored in adipose tissue.

Chylomicrons enter the bloodstream through the thoracic duct.

The enzyme lipoprotein lipase breaks down the triglyceride in chylomicrons into glycerol and fatty acids.

If the patient is fasting, these stored fatty acids are transported to the liver.

The triglyceride-depleted chylomicrons enter the liver, where their cholesterol forms VLDL.

Endogenous formation

The portal vein transports carbohydrates from the GI tract to the liver, where some are converted first to fatty acids, then to triglycerides.

If the patient is fasting, most fatty acids go to muscle.

VLDL enters the bloodstream.

The enzyme lipoprotein lipase breaks down the tryglyceride in VLDL into glycerol and fatty acids.

These triglycerides combine with cholesterol, phospholipids, and apoproteins to form VLDL.

The triglyceride-depleted VLDL enters the liver where it is converted into LDL.

LDL is transported to tissue, where it's broken down; its cholesterol is delivered to peripheral tissues.

From the periphery, cholesterol is transported to the liver in the form of HDL.

hood or can be nonfamilial, producing higher blood lipid levels with age. The normal blood levels for cholesterol and triglycerides vary for men and women of different ages, so the nurse must consider the patient's age and gender when interpreting blood lipid levels.

The risk of CAD directly increases with the blood cholesterol level. (See *Cholesterol and coronary artery disease* on page 636.) Fortunately, reduced cholesterol levels can also reduce the risk of CAD. One national study of more than 3,000 men with Type II primary hypercholesterolemia showed that a 1% reduction in the cholesterol level produced a 2% reduction in the incidence of CAD.

Drug therapy can reduce cholesterol and other lipid levels, but is not the first treatment of choice. Experts agree that a patient should follow an initial regimen that combines proper diet, weight loss, appropriate antihypertensive therapy, and exercise. Then, if this regimen does not lower blood lipid levels sufficiently, therapy with antilipemic agents may begin.

The antilipemic agents discussed in this chapter include bile-sequestering agents (cholestyramine and colestipol hydrochloride), fibric acid derivatives (clofibrate and gemfibrozil), cholesterol synthesis inhibitors (lovostatin and probucol), and miscellaneous drugs, such as niacin.

For a summary of representative drugs, see *Selected major drugs: Antilipemic agents* on page 646.

BILE-SEQUESTERING AGENTS

Cholestyramine and colestipol are large polymers (combinations of many small molecules) containing negative (anionic) groups. These bile-sequestering agents are anion-exchange resins, because they exchange their anionic groups for similar groups from other molecules that contain carboxylic acid and phenolic acid groups. This chemical activity allows the bile-sequestering agents to remove excess bile acids in the fat depots under the skin.

The first bile-sequestering agent, cholestyramine was developed in 1959. Cholestyramine is still in use and has been joined by colestipol.

PHARMACOKINETICS

Because bile-sequestering agents have a high molecular weight, they are not absorbed from the gastrointestinal (GI) tract. Instead, they remain in the GI tract where they combine with bile acids, for about 5 hours. They are eventually excreted in the feces.

PHARMACODYNAMICS

The bile-sequestering agents lower blood levels of LDL. As these agents form insoluble complexes with the bile acids in the GI tract, the gallbladder's bile acid levels decrease. This triggers the liver to synthesize more bile acids from their precursor, cholesterol. As cholesterol leaves the bloodstream and other storage areas to replace the lost bile acids, blood cholesterol levels decrease. Because the small intestine needs bile acids to emulsify lipids and form chylomicrons, absorption of all lipids and lipid-soluble drugs decreases until the bile acids are replaced.

PHARMACOTHERAPEUTICS

Bile-sequestering agents are the drugs of choice for treating Type IIa hyperlipoproteinemia (familial hypercholesterolemia) in patients who do not respond to dietary management. A patient whose blood cholesterol levels indicate a severe risk of CAD is most likely to require one of these agents to supplement the diet.

Cholestyramine does not appear to offer any advantages over colestipol in treating hypercholesterolemia. Although some reports show that it is more effective in heterozygotes (those who inherit the trait from one parent) than in homozygotes (those who inherit the trait from both parents), other reports show variable effects.

cholestyramine (Questran). Cholestyramine is used to treat Type IIa hyperlipoproteinemia (hypercholesterolemia) when dietary changes fail to produce the desired response. Available in powder form, each 9-gram scoop or packet contains 4 grams of cholestyramine resin. It must be mixed with 120 to 180 ml of liquid, such as water, carbonated beverage, soup, cereal, or a pulpy fruit with a high moisture content, such as applesauce, pineapples, or peaches. It must not be taken in dry form because the patient may inhale the powder accidentally. USUAL ADULT DOSAGE: 9 grams of powder P.O. one to six times daily mixed with liquid.

colestipol hydrochloride (Colestid). To treat hypercholesterolemia that is unresponsive to diet, granulated co-

DRUG INTERACTIONS

Bile-sequestering agents

When given concomitantly, bile-sequestering agents will counteract the effects of acidic substances. But beta-adrenergic blocking agents will counteract the effects of the bile-sequestering agents, decreasing their effectiveness and increasing blood lipid levels.

DRUG	INTERACTING DRUGS	POSSIBLE EFFECTS	NURSING IMPLICATIONS
cholestyramine, colestipol	coumarin anticoagulants	Decrease anticoagulant effect; as a result, the blood may clot despite anticoagulant therapy	• Administer a coumarin anticoagulant 1 hour before or 6 hours after administering a bile-sequestering agent. • Monitor the patient's prothrombin time carefully, and expect to increase the anticoagulant dosage, as needed. • Monitor the patient for signs of blood clot formation, such as Homans' sign (calf pain on dorsiflexion of the foot), tenderness, and edema.
	corticosteroids	Decrease effect of corticosteroids by decreasing absorption from the GI tract	• Administer a corticosteroid 1 hour before or 6 hours after administering a bile-sequestering agent. • Monitor the patient carefully for therapeutic effects of these drugs and expect to increase the corticosteroid dosage, as needed. • Assess the patient's weight and blood pressure regularly. • Monitor the patient's serum electrolyte levels.
	acetaminophen	Lessens pain relief by decreasing absorption from the GI tract	• Administer acetaminophen 1 hour before or 6 hours after administering a bile-sequestering agent. • Monitor the patient carefully for therapeutic effects of these drugs, and expect to increase the acetaminophen dosage, as needed.
	cardiac glycosides	Decrease effect of glycosides by decreasing absorption from the GI tract	• Administer cardiac glycosides 1 hour before or 6 hours after administering a bile-sequestering agent. • Monitor the patient's cardiac glycoside levels carefully, and expect to increase the cardiac glycoside dosage, as needed. • Assess the patient for signs of congestive heart failure, such as tachycardia, edema in the feet and ankles, and hypotension.
	iron preparations	Reduce serum iron levels by decreasing absorption from the GI tract	• Administer an iron preparation 1 hour before or 6 hours after administering a bile-sequestering agent. • Monitor the patient's serum iron and hemoglobin levels, and expect to increase the iron dosage, as needed. • Inform the patient that his stools may become black.
	thiazide diuretics	Reduce diuretic effect by decreasing absorption from the GI tract	• Administer a thiazide diuretic 1 hour before or 6 hours after administering a bile-sequestering agent. • Monitor the patient carefully for therapeutic effects of these drugs, and expect to increase the thiazide diuretic dosage, as needed. • Assess the patient for edema in the feet and ankles.

DRUG INTERACTIONS

Bile-sequestering agents continued

DRUG	INTERACTING DRUGS	POSSIBLE EFFECTS	NURSING IMPLICATIONS
cholestyramine, colestipol (continued)			• Monitor the patient's serum electrolyte levels.
	thyroid hormones	Reduce T_3 and T_4 levels by decreasing absorption from the GI tract	• Administer a thyroid hormone preparation 1 hour before or 6 hours after administering a bile-sequestering agent. • Monitor the patient's T_3 and T_4 levels, and expect to increase thyroid hormone dosages, as needed.
	beta-adrenergic blocking agents	Decrease effect of bile-sequestering agent from counteraction of beta-blockers; as a result, blood lipid levels remain high	• Monitor the patient's blood lipid levels, and discuss the use of an alternative antihypertensive with the physician.

lestipol is available in 5-gram packets. It must not, however, be taken in its dry form, because accidental inhalation or esophageal distress could result. Instead, colestipol should be dissolved in liquid, such as water, milk, fruit juice, or in a highly fluid soup or a pulpy fruit with a high moisture content, such as applesauce, pineapples, or peaches. It can even be baked in cookies for the patient who finds other forms of administration unpalatable.

USUAL ADULT DOSAGE: 15 to 30 grams P.O. daily in two to four divided doses.

Drug interactions

Because bile-sequestering agents are anion-exchange resins, they may bind with acidic drugs in the GI tract, decreasing their absorption and effectiveness. (See *Drug interactions: Bile-sequestering agents* for information about drugs that commonly interact with these agents.) Other acidic drugs that are likely to be affected include barbiturates, phenytoin, penicillins, cephalosporins, thyroid hormones, thyroid derivatives, chenodiol, digitoxin, and digoxin. They may also reduce absorption of lipid-soluble vitamins, such as vitamins A, D, E, and K; poor absorption of vitamin K can significantly affect prothrombin times. Many other drugs that are normally absorbed from the GI tract—including tetracyclines—may also have decreased absorption and may need supplemental dosing during therapy with bile-sequestering agents.

ADVERSE DRUG REACTIONS

Short-term adverse reactions to these drugs are relatively mild. More severe reactions can result from long-term use. Because of this, the nurse should carefully monitor a patient receiving a bile-sequestering agent.

These drugs frequently produce GI reactions with long-term therapy. Patients who are over age 60 or who take more than 24 grams per day of cholestyramine are particularly likely to develop these reactions. Constipation affects 1 patient in 10, but is usually not serious. Severe fecal impaction, however, may occur. In 1 patient in 30, GI adverse reactions may include abdominal pain, distention, flatulence, belching, nausea, vomiting, diarrhea, or hemorrhoid irritation. Peptic ulceration and bleeding, cholelithiasis, and cholecystitis occur much less frequently, affecting only 1 patient in 100.

Miscellaneous reactions to bile-sequestering agents include headache, dizziness, anorexia, weakness, and fatigue.

NURSING IMPLICATIONS

Because bile-sequestering agents frequently produce drug interactions and adverse reactions, the nurse should pay particular attention to the following considerations:
• Advise the patient not to take the drug in its powder or granule form. Show how to mix the agent in a suitable liquid, fruit, or other food to prevent accidental inhalation or esophageal distress.
• Monitor prothrombin times regularly for a patient who is also receiving a coumarin anticoagulant.
• After withdrawing a bile-sequestering agent, observe for increased effects and possible overdose of acidic drugs that are being given concurrently.
• Monitor the patient on long-term therapy for signs of vitamin A and D deficiencies, such as night blindness and rickets.

• Assess blood cholesterol levels every 3 to 6 months for a patient receiving long-term therapy.
• Administer drugs that bind with bile-sequestering agents 1 hour before or 6 hours after giving the agent.
• Monitor bowel movements for each patient to detect constipation, diarrhea, or other adverse reactions.
• Encourage the patient to follow the prescribed diet to increase the effectiveness of antilipemic therapy.

FIBRIC ACID DERIVATIVES

Fibric acid, a branched-chain propionic acid with a phenyl group, is produced by several fungi. Derivatives of this acid are used to reduce high triglyceride levels and, to a lesser extent, high cholesterol levels. Currently, two fibric acid derivatives are available for clinical use: clofibrate and gemfibrozil.

History and source
In 1962, Thorp and Waring discovered the fibric acid derivatives. They synthesized these agents after they noted that other branched unsaturated acids had reduced cholesterol levels in animals.

PHARMACOKINETICS
Clofibrate and gemfibrozil are readily absorbed from the GI tract. After absorption, both drugs are 95% bound to plasma proteins. Then, clofibrate is hydrolyzed to free carboxylic acid derivative, the active ingredient. Gemfibrozil undergoes extensive metabolism in the liver, producing active and inactive metabolites. Both agents are excreted in the urine as unchanged drugs and as conjugates of glucuronic acid. A higher percentage of clofibrate is excreted as conjugate.

Onset, peak, duration
Both of these antilipemic agents begin to reduce VLDL levels in 2 to 5 days. Clofibrate's action peaks in 4 weeks, and its duration of action in unknown. Gemfibrozil's action peaks in 3 weeks and has a 3-week duration of action. Clofibrate's half-life is 4 to 6 hours, whereas gemfibrozil's is 1.5 hours.

PHARMACODYNAMICS
Researchers have not yet established the exact mechanism of action for these drugs. They believe that the drugs may reduce cholesterol formation early in the biosynthetic process, mobilize cholesterol from the tissues, increase sterol excretion, decrease lipoprotein synthesis and secretion, and decrease triglyceride synthesis. The decreased triglyceride synthesis probably results from inhibition of lipolysis in adipose tissue.

Gemfibrozil produces two other effects. It increases HDL levels in the blood by increasing the synthesis of certain apoproteins (substances derived from proteins), and it increases the serum's capacity to dissolve additional cholesterol.

PHARMACOTHERAPEUTICS
Physicians primarily use these drugs to reduce triglyceride levels—especially very-low-density triglycerides—and secondarily to reduce blood cholesterol levels. Therefore, they should be used primarily in patients with Types II, III, IV, and mild Type V hyperlipoproteinemia. However, these agents should be used only in patients at severe risk of CAD who have not responded adequately to diet changes, who have premature CAD or a family member with the disease, who are hypercholesterolemic or have a family member with the disease, who have marked hypertriglyceridemia, or who smoke or exhibit other risk factors, such as hypertension or overweight. Fibric acid derivatives are best indicated for patients with no previous history of CAD or angina.

In patients with Types IIa, IIb, and IV hyperlipoproteinemia, niacin is used as adjunct therapy. Fibric acid derivatives are used with these patients when niacin does not produce an adequate response, is poorly tolerated, or is contraindicated. They may also be added to combined niacin and bile-sequestering agent therapy, if these two agents do not produce an adequate response.

clofibrate (Atromid-S). Available in 500-mg capsules, clofibrate is primarily used to treat Type V hyperlipoproteinemia (mixed hyperlipidemia, mixed hypertriglyceridemia) and sometimes used to treat Types II and IV.
USUAL ADULT DOSAGE: 500 mg P.O. q.i.d.

gemfibrozil (Lopid). Available in 300-mg capsules, gemfibrozil is used to treat Type III hyperlipoproteinemia as well as Types II, IV, and V.
USUAL ADULT DOSAGE: 1,200 mg P.O. daily in two divided doses 30 minutes before the morning and evening meal. (Patient response can vary widely, so the actual dose may range from 900 to 1,500 mg/day.)

DRUG INTERACTIONS
Fibric acid derivatives

Drug interactions with fibric acid derivatives usually involve acidic drugs, such as coumarin anticoagulants, sulfonylurea antidiabetic agents, oral contraceptives, and rifampin.

DRUG	INTERACTING DRUGS	POSSIBLE EFFECTS	NURSING IMPLICATIONS
clofibrate, gemfibrozil	coumarin anticoagulants	Increase anticoagulant effect by displacing coumarin from binding sites in the serum albumin	• Monitor the patient's prothrombin time closely, and expect to adjust the anticoagulant dosage, as needed. • Assess the patient for signs of internal bleeding, such as hematuria and easy bruising. • Monitor the patient for signs of GI bleeding, such as hematemesis and melena.
	sulfonylureas	Increase hypoglycemic effect by displacing sulfonylurea from serum albumin sites, increasing insulin secretion, and competing for renal secretion	• Monitor the patient's blood glucose level, and expect to adjust the sulfonylurea dosage, as needed.
	oral contraceptives	Antagonize clofibrate action; as a result, blood lipid levels remain high	• Monitor the patient's blood lipid levels, and expect to increase the fibric acid derivative dosage, as needed.
	furosemide	Increase diuresis by displacing furosemide at plasma albumin binding sites, especially in a patient with low serum albumin levels	• Monitor the patient's urine output, and expect to decrease the furosemide dosage, as needed. • Assess the patient for signs and symptoms of low serum electrolyte levels, such as muscle pain, hypotension, and nausea.
	rifampin	Antagonizes clofibrate action with long-term rifampin dosing; as a result, blood lipid levels remain high	• Monitor the patient's blood lipid levels, and expect to increase the fibric acid derivative dosage, as needed.

Drug interactions

Because clofibrate and gemfibrozil bind strongly with plasma proteins, they can displace anticoagulants in the plasma when given concurrently. This usually requires an anticoagulant dosage reduction and close monitoring of prothrombin times to prevent an anticoagulant overdose. Although no studies have shown that these antilipemic agents displace other acidic drugs, such as barbiturates, phenytoin, thyroid derivatives, and cardiac glycosides, the possibility of displacement exists when these drugs are administered concurrently. (See *Drug interactions: Fibric acid derivatives* for additional information.)

ADVERSE DRUG REACTIONS

The most common reactions to fibric acid derivatives are GI effects, which resemble those of the bile-sequestering agents.

Predictable reactions

Several studies show that clofibrate increases the incidence of cholelithiasis and the need for cholecystectomy. The drug is associated with benign and malignant liver tumors in rodents and malignant tumors in humans. Because of these potential reactions, clofibrate is not recommended for long-term use. This antilipemic can cause other adverse reactions, including pancreatitis, cardiac dysrhythmias, intermittent claudication, thromboembolic events, and angina. It may also produce flu-like symptoms and increased creatinine phosphokinase (CPK) levels.

Like clofibrate, gemfibrozil produces cholelithiasis. It does not seem to cause the other reactions related to clofibrate, but its use should be monitored closely because of the chemical similarities of the two agents.

Unpredictable reactions

Fibric acid derivatives may produce a wide range of unpredictable reactions. These may include skin rash, alopecia, urticaria, dry skin, brittle hair, hepatomegaly, impotence, decreased libido, leukopenia, weight gain, muscle pain, and abnormal liver function test results.

NURSING IMPLICATIONS

The nurse must obtain a complete history and perform a physical assessment to determine information that is vital to safe drug administration. The nurse must also be aware of these considerations:
• Document any patient history of ulcers, diabetes, jaundice, gallstones, or liver disease before administering the first antilipemic dose. Also determine if the patient is receiving an anticoagulant.
• Determine if the patient has a history of CAD or angina.
• For a patient who must receive an anticoagulant and a fibric acid derivative, expect to reduce the anticoagulant dose by one half, and monitor the prothrombin time until it stabilizes.
• Assess the patient for dysrhythmias.
• Observe bowel movements for steatorrhea (greasy stools) or other signs of bile duct obstruction, such as right upper quadrant pain.
• Encourage the patient to follow the prescribed diet to increase the effectiveness of antilipemic therapy.

CHOLESTEROL SYNTHESIS INHIBITORS

This section will present two other antilipemic agents: probucol and lovostatin. These drugs lower lipid levels by interfering with cholesterol synthesis.

PHARMACOKINETICS

Only 2% to 8% of probucol is absorbed from the GI tract. Absorption improves somewhat if probucol is given with food. This highly lipid-soluble drug is mainly distributed in the body's fatty acid depots. Although its method of metabolism is unknown, probucol passes through the bile duct for elimination in the feces.

Probucol begins to produce effects 2 to 4 weeks after therapy begins. The effects peak in 20 to 50 days. The half-life of the drug is 24 hours. When therapy ends, some probucol remains in the body for up to 6 months.

Lovostatin is readily absorbed from the GI tract and distributed throughout the body. Little is known about its other pharmacokinetic processes.

PHARMACODYNAMICS

Although probucol's exact mechanism of action is unknown, researchers believe that it acts in one or more ways by inhibiting cholesterol transport from the intestine, inhibiting cholesterol synthesis, and increasing the secretion of cholesterol and bile acid. Probucol primarily reduces blood cholesterol levels, but it also lowers LDL levels.

Lovostatin lowers LDL levels and increases HDL levels. Its mechanism of action is not well understood, but it may function by inhibiting the enzyme that catalyzes the conversion of cholesterol's precursors. It may also stimulate the LDL receptor in the liver, reducing hepatocytic cholesterol synthesis. It may even reduce blood cholesterol levels by increasing excretion.

PHARMACOTHERAPEUTICS

The cholesterol synthesis inhibitors are used to treat various types of hyperlipoproteinemia.

probucol (Lorelco). Primarily used to treat Type 'Ia hyperlipoproteinemia (hypercholesterolemia), this agent is often used to augment colestipol therapy when colestipol alone fails to reduce cholesterol levels.
USUAL ADULT DOSAGE: 500 mg P.O. b.i.d. with morning and evening meals.

lovostatin (Mevacor). This drug may become the drug of choice for treating all types of hypercholesterolemia. It may cause fewer adverse reactions than other drugs that block cholesterol synthesis, which could allow lovostatin to be used for long-term as well as short-term therapy. Its true effectiveness, however, can be determined only after it is more extensively used in the general population.
USUAL ADULT DOSAGE: 20 to 80 mg P.O. daily in single or divided doses, preferably at the evening meal.

Drug interactions

Unlike the bile-sequestering agents and fibric acid derivatives, these antilipemic agents tend not to interact with other drugs. Probucol, however, can produce additive effects when given with clofibrate. This interaction markedly reduces HDL levels and prohibits the combined use of these agents.

ADVERSE DRUG REACTIONS

In animals, probucol has affected cardiac nerve conduction. It has also prolonged the Q-T interval of the cardiac cycle. Because the drug is intended for long-term use, an electrocardiogram (EKG) should be taken when treatment begins and after 6 months and 12 months of treatment to detect any cardiac effects. Additional adverse reactions to probucol, especially the GI effects, resemble those of the other antilipemic agents. Although the drug's teratogenic effects have not been established, a woman receiving probucol should avoid becoming pregnant for at least 6 months after treatment ends.

Lovostatin seems to be well tolerated, producing only transient GI effects. Its complete range of adverse reactions, especially long-term reactions, has not been documented. Earlier drugs that blocked cholesterol synthesis produced cataracts, alopecia, and other serious adverse reactions that caused their removal from the market. Lovostatin has already produced cataracts in one patient. Because this drug blocks the synthesis of cholesterol, a precursor of corticosteroids, it may decrease the levels of male and female sex hormones and vitamin D. However, no such adverse reactions have been reported with short-term use, and the results of long-term use are unknown.

NURSING IMPLICATIONS

The nurse must be aware of different considerations for each of the cholesterol synthesis inhibitors:
- Advise a female patient to avoid becoming pregnant for at least 6 months after probucol therapy is discontinued.
- Avoid combining probucol therapy with clofibrate therapy.
- Monitor blood cholesterol levels continuously for a patient receiving probucol.
- Monitor the EKG periodically for a patient receiving prolonged probucol therapy.
- Follow the procedures for lovostatin exactly as described in the manufacturer's instructions.

- Monitor the patient receiving lovostatin for low blood levels of male and female sex hormones, corticosteroids, and vitamin D. Assess the patient for signs of reduced levels of these agents, such as amenorrhea or impotence.
- Monitor the patient receiving lovostatin for hair loss and cataract development.
- Encourage the patient receiving probucol or lovostatin to follow the prescribed diet and exercise regimen.

OTHER ANTILIPEMIC AGENTS

Several other drugs are occasionally used to treat hyperlipoproteinemia. However, they have not received approval from the Food and Drug Administration (FDA) for this indication, so their frequency of use is low. These drugs include ethinyl estradiol, norethindrone acetate, nandrolone and other anabolic agents, and neomycin. (See Chapter 59, Androgenic and Anabolic Steroid Agents; Chapter 60, Estrogens, Progestins, and Oral Contraceptive Agents; and Chapter 66, Antibacterial Agents, for information about these drugs.) Dextrothyroxine sodium, another antilipemic agent, has been approved to treat hypercholesterolemia. Its serious cardiovascular effects, however, limit its use to pediatric patients with no history of CAD. One additional agent, niacin, may be used to treat certain kinds of hyperlipoproteinemia.

niacin [nicotinic acid] (Nicolar). A vitamin, niacin reduces blood levels of LDL, VLDL, and phospholipids, especially in Types II, III, IV, and V hyperlipoproteinemia. Its adverse reactions, however, limit its usefulness. After oral administration, it is readily absorbed and distributed throughout the body. In doses required to reduce cholesterol levels, it is excreted unchanged in the urine. Niacin's antilipemic effects normally begin in 7 to 14 days, peak in 6 to 8 weeks, and last 6 to 8 weeks after therapy ends. Although researchers have not discovered niacin's exact mechanism of action, they theorize that it inhibits the release of FFA from lipid tissues. The usual adult dosage ranges from 1 to 2 grams P.O. t.i.d., not to exceed 6 grams/day.

Niacin commonly produces skin flushing that may be reduced if the drug is administered with antacids, aspirin, or food. It may also produce GI effects similar to those of the other antilipemic agents. The flushing and GI symptoms usually disappear in 2 to 6 weeks.

Antilipemic agents

This chart summarizes the major antilipemic agents currently in clinical use.

DRUG	MAJOR INDICATIONS	USUAL ADULT DOSAGES	NURSING IMPLICATIONS
Bile-sequestering agent			
cholestyramine	Type IIa hyperlipoproteinemia (hypercholesterolemia)	9 grams of powder P.O. one to six times daily mixed with 120 to 180 ml of fluid, soups, cereal, or pulpy fruits	• Monitor the patient's serum electrolyte levels, especially calcium, for a possible decrease in concentration. • Monitor the patient's bowel movements to detect fecal impaction. • Instruct the patient not to ingest the powder without mixing it in a liquid. • Monitor the patient receiving long-term therapy for signs of vitamin A, D, E, and K deficiencies. • Assess the patient's blood cholesterol levels every 3 to 6 months. • Encourage the patient to follow the prescribed exercise, antihypertensive, and diet regimens. • Monitor the patient closely after therapy is stopped if acidic drugs were administered concurrently. Dosage adjustments of the acidic drugs may be needed.
Fibric acid derivative			
clofibrate	Type V hyperlipoproteinemia (mixed hypertriglyceridemia, mixed hyperlipidemia), Type III and Type IV hyperlipoproteinemia (secondary uses)	500 mg P.O. q.i.d.	• Monitor the patient's liver function tests (SGOT, SGPT) for increased levels, indicating hepatotoxicity. • Monitor the patient for steatorrhea (greasy stools). • If clofibrate must be given with a coumarin anticoagulant, expect to reduce the anticoagulant dose by half, and monitor the prothrombin time until it stabilizes. • Assess the patient for dysrhythmias. • Determine if the patient has an ulcer, diabetes, jaundice, or liver disease, or is taking an anticoagulant, before giving the first dose. • Determine if the patient has a history of CAD or angina before giving the first dose. • Monitor the patient on long-term therapy for signs of stomach, liver, or other carcinomas, such as changes in food tolerances or bowel habits and abdominal pain. • Encourage the patient to follow the prescribed exercise, antihypertensive, and diet regimens. • Assess the patient for flulike symptoms and increased CPK levels.

This agent can cause other adverse reactions, including abnormal liver function test results, jaundice, abnormal prothrombin times, hypoalbuminemia, hyperglycemia, and hyperuricemia. For these reasons, it is contraindicated in a patient with arterial hemorrhage or severe hypotension, liver disease, or active peptic ulcer disease, and should be administered with caution to a patient with gallbladder disease or a history of jaundice, diabetes, gout, or allergy. (See Chapter 51, Vitamin and Mineral Agents, for further information.)

CHAPTER SUMMARY

Chapter 40 discussed the antilipemic agents. Here are the highlights of this chapter:

• Blood lipids consist of free fatty acids (FFA), triglycerides, cholesterol, cholesterol esters, and phospholipids.

• These blood lipids form various fractions, including chylomicrons, chylomicron fragments, very-low-density lipoproteins (VLDL), low-density lipoproteins (LDL), intermediate-density lipoproteins (IDL), and high-density lipoproteins (HDL).

• Hyperlipoproteinemia, or excess blood lipids, is a major cause of coronary artery disease (CAD) and death in the United States. Reduction of the blood lipoprotein levels greatly reduces the risk of CAD.

• Drugs that lower the blood LDL levels and raise the blood HDL levels are effective antilipemic agents. However, these agents should not be used until a low-lipid diet has failed to reduce blood lipid levels significantly.

• The three major classes of antilipemic agents are bile-sequestering agents, fibric acid derivatives, and cholesterol synthesis inhibitors. The bile-sequestering agents include cholestyramine and colestipol. Drug interactions with these agents primarily involve lipid-soluble substances, such as certain vitamins and anticoagulants that cannot be absorbed from the GI tract when bile-sequestering agents decrease lipids.

• The fibric acid derivatives include clofibrate and gemfibrozil. These agents commonly interact with acidic drugs such as phenytoin, barbiturates, anticoagulants, thyroid hormones, thyroid derivatives, and cardiac glycosides. Because clofibrate may produce cholelithiasis and some types of cancer, it is not indicated for long-term use.

• Drugs that inhibit cholesterol synthesis include probucol and lovostatin. These agents produce no significant drug interactions. However, they have not been administered for long periods. It is important to monitor the patient closely to determine if normal levels of cholesterol-based body constituents, such as corticosteroids and sex hormones, decrease.

• Niacin also acts as an antilipemic agent. Its most common adverse reaction is flushing, but it can produce more severe adverse reactions that can limit its usefulness.

BIBLIOGRAPHY

American Hospital Formulary Service. *Drug Information 87.* McEvoy, G.K., et al., eds. Bethesda, Md.: American Society of Hospital Pharmacists, 1987.

American Medical Association. *Drug Evaluations,* 6th ed. Philadelphia: W.B. Saunders Co., 1986.

Current Medical Diagnosis and Treatment. Los Altos, Calif.: Lange Medical Publications, 1986.

Goodman, A.G., et al., eds. *Goodman and Gilman's The Pharmacological Basis of Therapeutics,* 7th ed. New York: Macmillan Publishing Co., 1985.

Lipids Research Clinics Program. "The Lipid Research Clinics Coronary Primary Prevention Trial Results," *Journal of the American Medical Association* 251: 351, January 20, 1984.

Orten, J.M., and Neuhas, O.U. *Human Biochemistry.* Toronto: C.V. Mosby Co., 1982.

Physician's Desk Reference, 40th ed. Oradell, N.J.: Medical Economics Books, 1986.

USPDI. *Drug Information for the Health Care Provider.* Rockville, Md.: U.S. Pharmacopeial Convention, 1986.

DRUGS AFFECTING THE HEMATOLOGIC SYSTEM

The drugs discussed in Unit Eight include those that affect red blood cell formation, or erythropoiesis (hematinic agents), alter the coagulation properties of the blood (anticoagulant agents), and dissolve thrombi, or blood clots (thrombolytic agents) in acute situations. Brief overviews of drugs used to control bleeding and blood derivatives are also presented in Unit Eight.

Erythropoiesis

Blood is composed of plasma, which is the liquid component, and blood cells, which are formed elements including the red blood cells, white blood cells, and platelets. A red blood cell, or erythrocyte, transports oxygen to tissues. A white blood cell, or leukocyte, defends the body against invading organisms. Platelets aid in hemostasis, stopping bleeding.

Hematinic agents provide essential building blocks for red blood cell production (erythropoiesis) by increasing hemoglobin, the necessary element for oxygen transportation.

A red blood cell is normally small, about 7 microns in diameter. Shaped like a tiny biconcave disk, the red blood cell has a large surface area relative to its volume. It can change shape as it moves through narrow blood vessels and can withstand the turbulence in small capillaries. Red blood cells are the most numerous of the formed elements of the blood. Normal red blood cell count is approximately 5,500,000 per cubic millimeter of blood.

Red blood cells carry oxygen to cells and exchange it for carbon dioxide. They carry most of these gases in combination with hemoglobin. Each red blood cell contains 200 to 300 million molecules of hemoglobin. One hemoglobin molecule contains four iron atoms, enabling the molecule to combine with four oxygen molecules and form oxyhemoglobin. The globin (protein) part of the hemoglobin molecule combines with carbon dioxide to form carbaminohemoglobin.

Red blood cell maturation occurs in red bone marrow and involves nucleated cells called hemocytoblasts, or stem cells. The stem cells divide by mitosis and evolve through several stages to a mature erythrocyte. When a red blood cell leaves the bone marrow and enters the blood, it contains hemoglobin.

The life span of a red blood cell is 105 to 120 days, after which time the blood cell breaks down—usually in the capillaries and in the reticuloendothelial cells in the lining of the hepatic blood vessels. Phagocytes in the spleen and bone marrow envelop and destroy the fragments of the red blood cell, a process known as phagocytosis. During phagocytosis, iron is released from hemoglobin and a pigment called bilirubin is formed. The iron and bilirubin are transported to the liver, where the iron is stored and the bilirubin is excreted in bile.

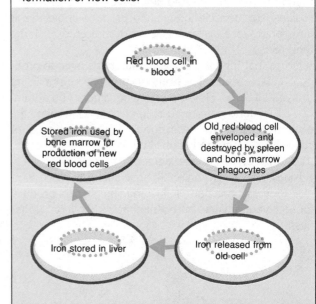

Life cycle of a red blood cell

Red blood cells are involved in a cyclic life of 105 to 120 days, which enables old cells to contribute to the formation of new cells.

Red blood cell in blood

Old red blood cell enveloped and destroyed by spleen and bone marrow phagocytes

Iron released from old cell

Iron stored in liver

Stored iron used by bone marrow for production of new red blood cells

Glossary

Anemia: deficiency in the number of red blood cells.

Anticoagulant: substance that suppresses, delays, or negates blood coagulation.

Antiplatelet: substance that interferes with activity of blood platelets.

Antithrombin III: alpha globulin that neutralizes the thrombin action and thus inhibits blood coagulation.

Blood derivatives: constituents of whole blood.

Coagulation: conversion of blood from a liquid, free-flowing state to a semisolid gel. Although coagulation, or clotting, can occur within an intact vessel, the process usually starts with tissue damage and exposure of the blood to air.

Cytopenia: deficiency in the cellular elements of the blood.

Embolus: clot or other plug, totally or partially dislodged from its site of origin and moved by blood flow to a more distant narrow site within the circulatory system, where it causes a flow obstruction.

Erythropoiesis: production of red blood cells.

Erythropoietin: glycoprotein produced by the kidneys that stimulates red blood cell production.

Ferritin: one of the complexes in which iron is stored in the body.

Fibrin: insoluble protein formed from fibrinogen by thrombin action; fibrin is the major element of a blood clot.

Fibrin split or degradation products (FSP or FDP): substances that result from plasmin action on fibrin.

Fibrinogen: high-molecular-weight plasma protein that is converted to fibrin through thrombin action; also called coagulation Factor I.

Fibrinolysis: breakdown of fibrin by the proteolytic enzyme, plasmin.

Hematinic: agent that improves blood quality by increasing hemoglobin level and number of erythrocytes.

Hemochromatosis: genetic disorder of iron metabolism characterized by iron deposits in tissues.

Hemoglobin: oxygen-carrying pigment of the erythrocytes.

Hemolytic anemia: disorder characterized by the premature destruction of red blood cells. Anemia may be minimal if the bone marrow is able to increase production of red blood cells.

Hemosiderin: microscopically visible insoluble form of iron stored in tissues.

Hemosiderosis: abnormal increase in tissue iron stores without associated tissue damage.

Hemostasis: termination of bleeding by mechanical or chemical means or by the body's complex coagulation process, which consists of vasoconstriction, platelet aggregation, and thrombin and fibrin synthesis.

Hypercoagulability: state of abnormally increased coagulation.

Hypochromic anemia: characterized by decreased hemoglobin in the red blood cells.

Macrocytic anemia: characterized by abnormally large, fragile red blood cells, usually from vitamin B_{12} or folic acid deficiency.

Megaloblastic anemia: characterized by immature, large, dysfunctional red blood cells in the bone marrow.

Microcytic anemia: characterized by abnormally small, incompletely hemoglobinized red blood cells in the bone marrow.

Myoglobin: ferrous globin complex, present in muscle tissue, that stores oxygen and contributes to muscle color.

Partial thromboplastin time (activated) (PTT or APTT): screening test to evaluate the intrinsic coagulation pathway (except Factor VII and Factor XIII) and the common pathway and to monitor heparin therapy.

Plasmin: highly specific proteolytic enzyme that dissolves fibrin clots.

Plasminogen: inactive precursor of plasmin.

Prothrombin: glycoprotein converted to thrombin by extrinsic thromboplastin during the second stage of blood coagulation; also called coagulation Factor II.

Prothrombin time (PT): screening test to evaluate the extrinsic coagulation and common pathways, and to monitor oral anticoagulant therapy.

Thrombin: enzyme derived from prothrombin that converts fibrinogen to fibrin.

Thrombin time (TT): qualitative test to measure the functional fibrinogen level.

Thrombocytopenia: decrease in the number of platelets.

Thromboembolism: obstruction of a blood vessel by a thrombus dislodged from its site of origin.

Thrombolysis: breakdown of preformed thrombin by local plasmin action.

Thromboplastin: factor necessary for thrombin production.

Thrombosis: the process of forming or developing a thrombus.

Thromboxane A_2: prostaglandin that increases the stickiness of platelets and fosters aggregation.

Thrombus: solid mass, clot, or plug formed in the circulatory system from the coagulation of blood constituents.

Tissue plasminogen activator (TPA): substance that converts inactive plasminogen to plasmin.

Tissue thromboplastin: lipoprotein peptidase released from injured tissues that stimulates coagulation; also called coagulation Factor III.

Transferrin: serum beta globulin that binds and transports iron.

The bone marrow then reuses the stored iron to produce new red blood cells. (See *Life cycle of a red blood cell* on page 648 for an illustration.) In healthy individuals, the number of red blood cells remains constant, with red blood cell production balancing destruction.

Erythropoiesis becomes more rapid when more red blood cells are needed. For example, cell production increases when red blood cells are lost in hemorrhage, and when tissue hypoxia exists. Hemorrhage and hypoxia stimulate the kidneys to produce the hormone erythropoietin, which accelerates red blood cell production in the bone marrow.

The bone marrow requires adequate supplies of iron, vitamin B_{12}, amino acids, copper, and cobalt to produce erythrocytes.

Anemia represents a significant decrease in either red blood cell or hemoglobin concentration in the circulating blood. While many types of anemia exist, the two major types are microcytic anemia, from iron deficiency, and macrocytic anemia, from vitamin B_{12} or folic acid deficiency.

Blood coagulation

The pathways involved in blood coagulation include the intrinsic (intravascular) and the extrinsic (extravascular). The intrinsic pathway is activated by injury to the endothelial layer of the blood vessel, disrupting blood flow. The disrupted blood flow initiates a chain of events that forms a thrombus, or clot. Atherosclerotic plaque is an example of this type of clotting.

The extrinsic pathway is activated by injury to tissues and vessels, such as surgical wounds or burns, releasing tissue thromboplastin into the circulation. The thromboplastin, a powerful procoagulant, stimulates a chain of events that forms a thrombus. (See *Coagulation pathways* for detailed information.)

The body also produces blood clots to repair damage in blood vessel walls from normal wear and tear. Platelets adhere to the damaged vessel area and release adenosine diphosphate, which produces platelet stickiness that helps a clot form. Vasoconstriction in the damaged blood vessel reduces blood flow and produces a stasis of blood, allowing time for the clot to form.

The body maintains a delicate balance between the formation of clots (coagulation) and the destruction of clots (fibrinolysis). Coagulation is inhibited by: (1) the liver and reticuloendothelial system, which remove clotting factors from the blood; (2) antithrombins, which neutralize thrombin; (3) adequate blood flow, which dilutes clotting factors; and (4) the fibrinolytic system, which interferes with the action of thrombin on fibrinogen.

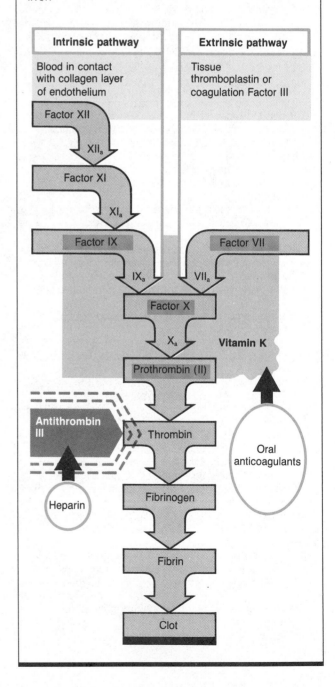

Coagulation pathways

Coagulation results from the activation of factors leading to thrombin inhibition that significantly affect coagulation. A naturally occurring protein, antithrombin III, neutralizes thrombin. Heparin increases the thrombin-neutralizing action of antithrombin III, so its effect on coagulation is *multiple*. Oral anticoagulants diminish the action of vitamin K, which is responsible for the formation of Factors II, VII, IX, and X in the liver.

Certain diseases are characterized by abnormal coagulation. Thrombus formation can occur in the venous system, causing venothrombosis (such as a pulmonary embolus), or in the arterial system, causing arterial thrombosis (such as a cerebrovascular thrombosis from a diseased mitral valve). Drugs that are used to treat or prevent thrombotic disorders are known as anticoagulant and antiplatelet drugs. They act by inhibiting formation of thrombin and of Factors II, VII, IX, and X in the liver or by interfering with platelet aggregation. (See *Coagulation factors* for details.)

Fibrinolysis

Conditions such as blood stagnation or damage to a blood vessel trigger the coagulation mechanism and activate the fibrinolytic system. The fibrinolytic system restricts clot propagation in the general circulation, breaks down the thrombus (fibrinolysis), and removes the fibrin networks as the injured area heals.

When the fibrinolytic system is activated, tissue plasminogen activator (TPA) is released from stored areas in the endothelium. TPA is released during stress reactions, vigorous exercise, hypoglycemia, and anabolic steroid use. TPA binds to fibrin and converts inactive circulating plasminogen to plasmin, the proteolytic enzyme that digests fibrin threads, fibrinogen, Factor V, Factor VIII, Factor XII, and prothrombin. The plasmin then can cause clot lysis.

Plasmin normally is inactivated in the circulation by alpha$_2$-antiplasmin, a physiologic inhibitor that prevents too much circulating plasmin, which can cause blood hypocoagulability. However, plasmin bound to fibrin is resistant to alpha$_2$-antiplasmin. Normally, fibrinolysis is restricted to a thrombus area, preventing a generalized fibrinolysis and bleeding.

Fibrinolysis of a thrombus produces fibrin degradation products (FDPs). FDPs, which are not normally present in the bloodstream, interfere with platelet aggregation and produce an anticoagulant effect.

Agents to control bleeding

Because bleeding is the major adverse effect of anticoagulant and thrombolytic agents, the nurse must be aware of the appropriate hemostatic agents. If bleeding results from a deficiency in the body's clotting factors, as in hemophilia, prescribed hemostatic agents, such as antihemophilic factor (Factor VIII) and Factor IX complex, would be administered. If the patient's bleeding is caused by fibrinolytic therapy, aminocaproic acid (Amicar) might be administered systemically. Excessive bleeding from heparin or oral anticoagulant therapy is treated with protamine sulfate or vitamin K, respectively. Additionally, several agents can be applied locally to a wound or puncture site to control bleeding and capillary oozing. (See *Agents to control bleeding* on pages 652 and 653 for some specific agents and their use.)

Blood derivatives

Whole blood or one of its component fractions may be administered to replace blood volume lost in hemorrhage or to control bleeding. Some components of whole blood that can be separated are packed red cells, plasma, normal serum albumin, plasma protein fraction, and platelets. Using component transfusions provides therapy for specific deficiencies, expands the usefulness of a single blood donation, eases chronic shortages of blood supplies, and reduces the patient's risks of viral hepatitis and exposure to sensitizing agents and drugs.

Physicians use blood derivatives primarily to provide plasma expanders in patients with hypovolemic shock and to treat hypoproteinemia associated with malnutrition, and for other conditions. (See *Whole blood and blood derivatives* on pages 654 and 655 for more details.)

Coagulation factors

With blood platelets, coagulation factors control clotting. The following lists the factors by number, name, and location.

FACTOR	SYNONYM	LOCATION
Factor I	Fibrinogen	Plasma
Factor II	Prothrombin	Plasma
Factor III	Tissue thromboplastin	Tissue cells
Factor IV	Calcium ion	Plasma
Factor V	Labile factor	Plasma
Factor VII	Stable factor	Plasma
Factor VIII	Antihemophilic globulin (AHG) or antihemophilic factor (AHF)	Plasma
Factor IX	Plasma thromboplastin component (PTC)	Plasma
Factor X	Stuart-Prower factor	Plasma
Factor XI	Plasma thromboplastin antecedent (PTA)	Plasma
Factor XII	Hageman factor	Plasma
Factor XIII	Fibrin stabilizing factor	Plasma

Agents to control bleeding

Bleeding is a major adverse reaction to anticoagulant therapy. When bleeding occurs, the nurse must be prepared to administer the prescribed controlling agents. Aminocaproic acid interacts with oral contraceptives. The other agents listed here have no significant interactions with other drugs.

DRUG	INDICATIONS AND DOSAGES	ADVERSE REACTIONS	NURSING IMPLICATIONS
aminocaproic acid (Amicar)	Excessive bleeding resulting from hyperfibrinolysis Adults: initially 5 grams P.O. or slow I.V. infusion followed by 1 to 1.25 grams/hour; maximum dose, 30 grams/day	Generalized thrombosis, dizziness, malaise, headache, hypotension, bradycardia, dysrhythmias, tinnitus, nasal stuffiness, nausea, cramps, diarrhea, skin rash	• Dilute with sterile water, normal saline, D₅W, or Ringer's solution. Monitor coagulation study results. • Drug is contraindicated in conditions associated with active intravascular clotting.
antihemophilic factor (AHF)	Bleeding from Factor VIII deficiency Adults and children: 10 to 20 IU/kg I.V. push or infusion every 8 to 24 hours	Headache, paresthesia, altered consciousness, tachycardia, hypotension, disturbed vision, nausea, vomiting, erythema, urticaria, hypersensitivity	• Ensure that the patient's blood is typed and crossmatched as prescribed for possible transfusion. • Monitor the patient's vital signs frequently. If tachycardia develops, reduce the flow rate or stop administration, and notify the physician. • Monitor the patient for allergic reactions. • Use only a plastic syringe to administer I.V. Drug may interact with a glass syringe. • Monitor coagulation study results before and during therapy. • Refrigerate concentrate until use but not after reconstitution. Before reconstituting, bring concentrate and diluent bottles to room temperature. Use the reconstituted solution within 3 hours. • Do not mix with other I.V. solutions.
Factor IX complex (Konyne, Profilnine, Proplex)	Bleeding caused by Factor IX deficiency Adults and children: Usual dosage 10 to 20 IU/kg/day; for anticoagulant overdose, 15 IU/kg	Headache, thromboembolic reactions, hypersensitivity	• Ensure that the patient's blood is typed and crossmatched as prescribed to treat possible hemorrhage. • Observe the patient for allergic reactions. • Monitor the patient's vital signs frequently. • Avoid rapid infusion that may cause adverse reactions, such as tingling sensations, fever, chills, or headache. • If hypersensitivity reaction occurs, slow the infusion and notify the physician. • Reconstitute with 20 ml sterile water. Keep refrigerated until ready to use but warm to room temperature before reconstituting. Use within 3 hours of reconstituting. • Do not administer with other I.V. solutions.
carbazochrome salicylate (Adrenosem Salicylate)	Surgery with excessive capillary bleeding or oozing Adults and children over age 12: 10 mg I.M. the night before surgery and with on-call medication; 5 mg P.O. or I.M. postoperative every 2 to 4 hours; children under age 12: 5 mg I.M. the night before surgery and with on-call	Pain at I.M. injection sites	• Drug is contraindicated in patients with sensitivity to salicylates. Obtain drug sensitivity history from the patient.

Agents to control bleeding continued

DRUG	INDICATIONS AND DOSAGES	ADVERSE REACTIONS	NURSING IMPLICATIONS
carbazochrome salicylate (continued)	medication; 5 mg P.O. or I.M. postoperative every 2 to 4 hours		
absorbable gelatin sponge (Gelfoam)	Decubitus ulcers: apply aseptically to wound. Adjunct to hemostasis in surgery: saturate with normal saline solution injection or thrombin solution, hold in place 10 to 15 seconds; when bleeding is controlled, leave in place	None reported	• Use is contraindicated in patients with active infection. • Avoid overpacking. • Sponge is systemically absorbed in 4 to 6 weeks; no need to remove.
microfibrillar collagen hemostat (Avitene)	Adjunct to hemostasis in surgery: apply drug directly to bleeding site for 1 to 5 minutes, gently remove excess, and reapply as needed	Hematoma, exacerbation of wound dehiscence, abscess formation, foreign body reaction, adhesion formation, enhanced infection in contaminated wounds, mediastinitis, hypersensitivity	• Drug is contraindicated for closure of skin incisions. • The drug is not for injection. • Do not dilute; apply dry. • Handle with smooth, dry forceps and avoid contact with nonbleeding sites, because the subtance adheres to any wet surface. • Apply directly to bleeding site.
negatol (Negatan)	Cervical bleeding: apply 1-inch gauze dipped in 1:10 dilution of drug, insert into vagina for 24 hours; increase to full strength if tolerated. Oral ulcers: apply to dried lesion with applicator, leave for 1 minute, and neutralize with large amounts of water	Local burning sensation, erythema, superficial skin desquamation	• Vaginal membrane turns grayish after negatol use. • Instruct the patient to wear perineal pad to avoid staining clothing. • When the drug is used for oral ulcers, a topical anesthetic should be applied first to prevent burning sensation. • Always clean and dry the area to be treated. • Administer this astringent, styptic, and protein denaturant, which is highly acidic, with caution.
oxidized cellulose (Oxycel, Surgicel)	Adjunct for surgical hemostasis and to control external bleeding at tumor sites: apply using sterile technique, as needed	Headache after nasal packing or application to surface wounds, sneezing, epistaxis or burning, nasal membrane necrosis or septal perforation after packing for rhinologic procedures, encapsulation of fluid, foreign body reaction, burning or stinging, possible prolongation of drainage in cholecystectomies	• Drug is contraindicated in controlling hemorrhage from large arteries, in treating serious oozing surfaces, and in implantation for bone defects. • Apply loosely against the bleeding site. • Apply dry for best hemostatic effect. • Apply sparingly to area and remove excess. • Do not use as permanent packing because cyst formation may result.

Chapter 41
Hematinic Agents
Chapter 41, Hematinic Agents, covers agents used to improve blood quality: iron, vitamin B_{12}, and folic acid. The clinical uses of hematinics in treating the various anemias are emphasized; nursing assessment techniques and patient education tips are highlighted also.

Chapter 42
Anticoagulant Agents
Chapter 42, Anticoagulant Agents, includes discussions of heparin, oral anticoagulants, and antiplatelet agents. Clinical situations that necessitate using anticoagulants

(Text continues on page 656.)

Whole blood and blood derivatives

DESCRIPTION	INDICATIONS	CONTRAINDICATIONS	CROSS MATCHING
Whole blood			
Blood complete with all plasma and cell constituents	Inadequate blood volume in hemorrhaging, trauma, or burn patients	The patient does not need blood volume increase, and a specific component is available.	Necessary
Red blood cells (packed, frozen)			
Whole blood with 80% of the plasma removed	Red blood cell deficiency; inadequate oxygen-carrying capacity of blood. Organ transplant; repeated febrile transfusion reactions (frozen red blood cells)	The patient's anemia results from a deficiency of the hematopoietic nutrients; for example, iron, vitamin B_{12}, or folic acid.	Necessary
White blood cells (leukocyte concentrate)			
Whole blood with red blood cells and 80% of plasma removed	Life-threatening granulocytopenia from intensive chemotherapy, especially infections that do not respond to antibiotics	The patient's health depends on the recovery of bone marrow functions.	Must be ABO compatible
Plasma (fresh, fresh-frozen)			
Uncoagulated plasma separated from whole blood	Clotting factor deficiency, hypovolemia, or severe hepatic disease in a patient with limited synthesis of plasma coagulation factors; prevention of dilutional hypocoagulability	Blood coagulation can be corrected with available specific therapy; the patient needs albumin only.	Unnecessary
Platelets			
Platelet sediment from platelet-rich plasma, resuspended in 30 to 50 ml of plasma	Thrombocytopenia when bleeding is caused by decreased platelet production, increased platelet destruction, functionally abnormal platelets, or massive transfusions of stored blood (dilutional thrombocytopenia)	Bleeding is unrelated to decreased number of platelets or abnormal function of platelets; the patient experiences post-transfusion purpura or thrombotic thrombocytopenic purpura.	Unnecessary (donor plasma and recipient's red blood cells should be ABO compatible)
Plasma protein fraction			
5% selected proteins solution, pooled plasma in buffered, stabilized saline diluent	Hypovolemic shock or hypoproteinemia. Shock in infants; dehydration or electrolyte deficiencies in children	The patient has severe anemia or heart failure, or has had cardiac bypass surgery.	Unnecessary
Normal serum albumin 5%, normal serum albumin 25%			
Heat-treated, aqueous, chemically processed fraction of pooled plasma	Shock; prevention of marked hemoconcentration; maintenance of electrolyte balance; hypoproteinemia; hyperbilirubinemia in infants	The patient has severe anemia or heart failure.	Unnecessary

SHELF LIFE	ADMINISTRATION TECHNIQUES	SPECIAL CONSIDERATIONS
21 days at 5° C. (41° F.)	Straight line set, Y-set, or microaggregate recipient set	• Whole blood is seldom transfused: components are extracted from it. • Plasma protein fraction or normal serum albumin is usually given as volume expander until component needs are known.
For stored fresh-packed cells, 21 days; 24 hours after opening For stored frozen cells, 3 years; 24 hours after thawing	Straight line set, Y-set, or microaggregate recipient set	• Red blood cells have the same oxygen-carrying capacity as whole blood without the volume overload hazards. Their use prevents the potassium and ammonia buildup that can occur in stored plasma. Frozen red blood cells are expensive.
24 hours after collection at 5° C. (41° F.)	Straight line set with standard in-line filter. Dose: one unit daily until infection clears (usually within 5 days)	• Infusion induces fever and can cause mild hypertension, severe chills, disorientation, and hallucinations.
For fresh plasma, within 6 hours after collection For fresh-frozen plasma, 12 months at −18° C. (−0.4° F.); 2 hours after thawing	Any straight line set; administer as rapidly as possible	• Normal saline solution not needed for Y-set because the component contains no red blood cells that otherwise would be damaged by nonisotonic solutions.
Up to 72 hours after whole blood collection	Syringe or component drip set only; administer as rapidly as possible (uninterrupted) Must use a nonwettable filter Dose: 2 units/kg of body weight to raise platelet count, at least 50,000/mm³	• Usually given when platelet count is below 10,000/mm³. • Give antihistamines before transfusion if the patient has a history of adverse reactions. Slow administration may prevent overload. • Platelets are least hazardous when given fresh.
5 years if refrigerated; 3 years at room temperature	Any straight line set; rate and volume depend on the patient's condition and response.	• Do not mix in same line with protein hydrolysates and alcohol solutions. • Frequently used as a volume expander while cross matching is done.
5 years at 2° C. (35.6° F.); 3 years at room temperature	Give undiluted, or diluted with saline solution or D₅W. In hypoproteinemia: administer slowly (1 to 3 ml/minute) to prevent rapid volume expansion. In shock: give as rapidly as possible.	• Cannot transmit hepatitis because it is heat-treated at 60° C. (140° F.) for 10 hours. • Frequently used as a volume expander while cross matching is done.

are presented, and laboratory values that the nurse uses to monitor the various therapies are discussed. Proper administration techniques and the appropriate therapeutic dosages of the drugs for various clinical conditions are emphasized. Interventions related to the adverse reaction of bleeding are detailed also.

Chapter 43
Thrombolytic Agents

Agents used to dissolve clots are the focus of Chapter 43, Thrombolytic Agents. The chapter begins with a discussion of the clinical consequences of thromboembolic conditions for patients. The various thrombolytic agents, including streptokinase, urokinase, and the experimental tissue plasminogen activators, are then discussed, as are the adverse effects of thrombolytic therapy. The protocol for using these agents for intracoronary therapy also is explained. The chapter concludes with the associated nursing implications, emphasizing appropriate laboratory values for monitoring the therapy and interventions for treating adverse reactions in the patient.

Nursing diagnoses

The most applicable nursing diagnoses for patients receiving the drugs discussed in this unit include:
- Activity intolerance related to anemia
- Alteration in bowel elimination: constipation or diarrhea, related to the adverse effects of hematinic, anticoagulant, or thrombolytic agents
- Alteration in comfort: pain, related to anemia and the adverse effects of hematinic, anticoagulant, or thrombolytic agents
- Alteration in nutrition: less than body requirements, related to nausea, vomiting, and gastrointestinal distress from the use of hematinic or anticoagulant agents
- Alteration in oral mucous membranes related to anemia and the adverse effects of hematinic, anticoagulant, or thrombolytic agents
- Alteration in tissue perfusion related to anemia or thromboembolism
- Anxiety related to the adverse effects of hematinic, anticoagulant, or thrombolytic agents
- Disturbance in self-concept related to the effects of anemia
- Fear related to the illness and the adverse effects of hematinic, anticoagulant, or thrombolytic agents
- Impaired physical mobility related to thromboembolism

- Knowledge deficit related to hematinic, anticoagulant, or thrombolytic therapy
- Potential for injury: bleeding, related to the use of anticoagulant and thrombolytic agents
- Potential for injury: gastric irritation, related to the use of hematinic or anticoagulant agents
- Potential impairment of skin integrity related to the immobility associated with thromboembolism
- Self-care deficit related to anemia
- Sexual dysfunction related to the effects of anemia.

CHAPTER 41

HEMATINIC AGENTS

OBJECTIVES

After reading and studying this chapter, you should be able to:

1. Discuss the function of iron, vitamin B_{12}, and folic acid in normal red blood cell (RBC) production.
2. Identify the symptoms of iron-deficiency anemia.
3. Identify the therapy for iron-deficiency anemia, including preparations, goals, and length of treatment.
4. Describe the process for administering iron dextran.
5. Explain the relationship between megaloblastic anemias and DNA.
6. Identify the therapy for vitamin B_{12}-deficiency anemia from malabsorption syndrome, including preparations, goals, and length of treatment.
7. Explain the role of folic acid in megaloblastic anemias.
8. Identify the treatment for folic acid deficiency.
9. Identify the nurse's role in preventing microcytic and megaloblastic anemias.

INTRODUCTION

This chapter discusses the hematinic agents that are used to treat microcytic and macrocytic anemias. Microcytic hypochromic (iron-deficiency) anemia, characterized by small, incompletely hemoglobinized erythrocytes (RBCs), results from inadequate dietary sources of iron or excessive blood loss. Iron-deficiency anemia occurs worldwide and is a health problem, particularly for women. Treatment focuses on replacing depleted iron.

Macrocytic (megaloblastic) anemia, characterized by abnormally large RBCs, results from vitamin B_{12} or folic acid deficiency. Both vitamin B_{12} and folic acid are essential elements for normal erythropoiesis (RBC production).

The symptoms of microcytic and macrocytic anemia include pallor, fatigue, rapid pulse, shortness of breath, mental irritability, and cardiac irregularities. Iron is used to treat iron-deficiency anemia; vitamin B_{12} or folic acid, or both, are used to treat macrocytic anemia.

An adequate, well-balanced diet usually provides sufficient amounts of these vitamins and minerals for normal RBC production. Meats, legumes, and green vegetables provide iron. Fish and meat supply vitamin B_{12}, and fresh green vegetables supply folic acid primarily as folate.

Some patients will develop anemia from inadequate dietary intake or from insufficient gastrointestinal (GI) tract absorption.

For a summary of representative drugs, see *Selected Major Drugs: Hematinic agents* on page 666.

IRON

Iron preparations are used to treat the most common form of anemia—iron-deficiency anemia—which results from inadequate iron ingestion, absorption, or utilization;

Daily iron requirement

Infants age 6 months to 2 years and pregnant women have the highest daily iron requirements, necessitating plenty of iron-rich foods in their diet.

Infants age 6 months to 2 years	67 mcg
Children age 2 to 12	22 mcg
Adolescents age 12 to 18 • male • female	21 mcg 20 mcg
Adult females • pregnant • nonpregnant	73 mcg 21 mcg
Adult males	13 mcg

increased iron requirement or excretion; or metabolic destruction of iron. (See *Daily iron requirement* on page 657.)

History and source

In the 16th century, the cause of chlorosis, or green sickness, in adolescent girls was recognized as an iron deficiency. In the late 1600s, Sydenham identified iron as a specific remedy for chlorosis, which replaced therapies such as bleedings and purgings. In the 1700s, Lemery and Geoffry showed that iron was present in the blood. Treatment of anemia with iron followed the principles of Sydenham and Blaud until the late 1800s, and the amount of iron prescribed was similar to modern medical practice. Additional research led to dose decreases. These doses, however, proved ineffective and discredited this anemia treatment. Researchers worked for 30 years more before they proved that the original treatment was correct.

Iron metabolism was not clearly understood until the 20th century. In 1937, McCane and Widdowson reported that iron had a limited daily absorption and excretion. At the same time, the discovery of how to measure iron concentration in plasma was made. In the early 1940s, Hahn used radioactive isotopes of iron to quantify absorption and demonstrated the intestinal mucosa's ability to regulate absorption. In the last 25 years, practical clinical measurements have been developed that permit accurate detection of iron-deficient erythropoiesis. Methods are also now available to evaluate how much iron is absorbed from food.

PHARMACOKINETICS

Iron mineral, an essential, is a component of hemoglobin, myoglobin, and certain enzymes. Although 80% of the iron in the body is used for RBC production, iron is also important in muscle metabolism and in cognitive functions of children.

Absorption, distribution, metabolism, excretion

Iron is absorbed primarily from the duodenum and upper jejunum by an active transport mechanism that moves the iron into plasma as heme or into storage as ferritin. The amount of iron absorbed depends partially on the body stores of iron; when body stores are low or erythropoiesis is accelerated, iron absorption may be increased by 20% to 30%. When total iron stores are large, only about 5% to 10% of iron is absorbed. The ferrous salt form is absorbed three times more readily than the ferric form. Ferrous sulfate, ferrous gluconate, and ferrous fumarate are absorbed almost equally although they contain different amounts of elemental iron. Enteric-coated preparations decrease iron absorption

because the iron is released past the duodenum. Larger doses of iron will result in increased amounts being absorbed but by a reduced percentage. The lymphatic system absorbs the parenteral form of iron from intramuscular sites, which results in 60% absorption in 3 days and 90% absorption after 1 to 3 weeks.

Iron is transported by the blood and bound to transferrin, the plasma iron-transport protein. About 30% of the iron is stored primarily as hemosiderin or ferritin in the reticuloendothelial cells of the liver, spleen, and bone marrow. About two thirds of the total body iron is found in hemoglobin.

Iron is excreted in feces, sweat, urine, breast milk, and through intestinal cell sloughing. The daily loss amounts to 0.5 to 1 mg in a normal male and up to 2 mg in a menstruating female.

Onset, peak, duration

Within 3 days after the patient starts oral iron therapy, the reticulocyte count will rise and hemoglobin and hematocrit levels will increase after 1 week of therapy. The peak concentration level effect will be seen in about 4 weeks. When iron is given parenterally (I.V. or I.M.), the hemoglobin level will rise approximately 1 gram/ week, with the peak concentration level occurring in 4 to 8 weeks.

PHARMACODYNAMICS

Iron is utilized by the body in erythropoiesis and is transported to intracellular sites by the protein transferrin.

Mechanism of action

Although iron serves as a component of myoglobin and various intracellular enzymes (such as cytochrome oxidase, peroxidase, and catalase), its most important role is in the normal production of hemoglobin. About 80% of iron in plasma goes to the erythroid marrow, where it is used for erythropoiesis. Erythrocytes normally circulate for about 120 days; then they are catabolized by the reticuloendothelium. Part of the iron from the destroyed erythrocyte is then bound to transferrin; part is incorporated into ferritin stores in the reticuloendothelial cells.

Iron is absorbed as heme or inorganic iron from food in the intestine. After absorption, iron immediately combines with apotransferrin, a beta globulin, to form transferrin. Transferrin transports iron to all tissues, but especially to hepatic tissue. There it is stored as ferritin (a water-soluble complex) and hemosiderin (an insoluble complex). Transferrin also transports iron directly

DRUG INTERACTIONS
Iron

A complete drug and food history must be obtained to maximize benefits of iron therapy and to decrease possible drug and food interactions.

DRUG	INTERACTING DRUGS	POSSIBLE EFFECTS	NURSING IMPLICATIONS
ferrous sulfate, ferrous gluconate, ferrous fumarate	tetracycline	Decreases tetracycline absorption	• Instruct the patient to take these drugs at least 2 hours apart.
	chloramphenicol	Delays iron incorporation into red blood cells and delays erythropoiesis	• Teach the patient not to take iron and chloramphenicol concomitantly.
	antacids	Decrease iron absorption	• Teach the patient to use food, not antacids, to buffer gastric discomfort with iron dose.
	ascorbic acid (vitamin C)	Enhances iron absorption	• Monitor the patient for signs and symptoms of adverse effects, such as nausea and constipation.
	penicillamine	Decreases penicillamine absorption	• Instruct the patient not to take these drugs together.
	coffee, tea	Inhibit iron absorption	• Teach the patient to avoid drinking coffee or tea for at least 1 hour after iron dose.
	eggs, milk	Inhibit iron absorption	• Teach the patient not to use eggs or milk to buffer the gastric effects of iron therapy.

to the mitochondria of erythroblasts (immature RBCs) in the bone marrow, where it is used to synthesize hemoglobin.

PHARMACOTHERAPEUTICS

Iron therapy is used to prevent and treat iron-deficiency anemia. Iron-deficiency anemia is confirmed by peripheral blood smears, which contain hypochromic (pale), microcytic (small) erythrocytes. Two common causes of iron deficiency are slow, insidious GI bleeding and heavy menstrual bleeding.

Iron therapy is used to prevent anemias in infants aged 6 months to 2 years—periods of rapid growth. Pregnant women need iron therapy to replace the iron used by the developing fetus.

Iron-deficiency anemias can be successfully treated in most individuals with oral drug therapy. Hundreds of iron preparations are commercially available, ranging from simple water-soluble iron salts to sustained-release enteric-coated preparations to multivitamins with iron.

These products vary in their iron content, absorption rate, adverse effects, and cost.

Parenteral drug therapy is indicated for patients who cannot absorb oral preparations, are noncompliant with oral therapy, or have bowel disorders such as ulcerative colitis. The only currently available parenteral iron is iron dextran, which builds up iron stores more rapidly than oral preparations but does not correct anemia any faster.

The length of iron therapy varies. The goal is to restore normal hemoglobin levels and replenish iron stores. The rate of repair of hemoglobin is 0.2 grams/day per deciliter of whole blood, so the RBC mass is usually reconstituted in 1 to 2 months. The replenishment of iron stores may take several months. The individual with an inadequate diet may require continued low-dose therapy, whereas the individual with an adequate diet will not require further treatment when the hemoglobin is restored to normal. The average length of treatment with iron for deficiency anemias is 6 months.

ferrous sulfate (Feosol, Fer-In-Sol, Fer-Iron). Ferrous sulfate contains 20% elemental iron (percentage of pure iron in the compound), or 65 mg of elemental iron per 325-mg tablet. The most widely used form of iron and the most economical, it is indicated to prevent and treat iron-deficiency anemia and is available as tablet, elixir, capsule, and sustained-release preparations.

USUAL ADULT DOSAGE: 300 mg to 1.2 grams P.O. daily depending on the severity of the anemia.

USUAL PEDIATRIC DOSAGE: 150 to 600 mg P.O. daily for a child who weighs 33 to 66 lb (15 to 30 kg); 5 mg/kg P.O. daily for a child who weighs less than 33 lb.

ferrous gluconate (Fergon). Ferrous gluconate contains 11.6% elemental iron and comes in tablets, capsules, and elixir preparations. The indications for use are the same as for ferrous sulfate and it is tolerated as well as ferrous sulfate.

USUAL ADULT DOSAGE: 325 to 650 mg P.O. q.i.d.

USUAL PEDIATRIC DOSAGE: for iron deficiency anemia, 100 to 300 mg P.O. t.i.d.

ferrous fumarate (Feostat, Fumerin). Ferrous fumarate contains 33% elemental iron and comes in tablets, sustained-release tablets, and suspension forms. The indications are the same as for ferrous sulfate.

USUAL ADULT DOSAGE: for iron-deficiency anemia, 100 to 400 mg P.O. daily to q.i.d.

iron dextran (Imferon). One milliliter of iron dextran contains 50 mg of elemental iron. Iron dextran is used to treat iron-deficiency anemia in patients who cannot tolerate oral therapy.

USUAL ADULT DOSAGE: 0.5 ml I.M. or I.V. initially as a test dose, then 2 ml (100 mg) I.M. daily for a patient under 110 lb (50 kg) or 5 ml (250 mg) I.M. daily for a patient over 110 lb; or 2 ml I.V. daily at a rate of 1 ml/minute infused slowly. No single dose should exceed 100 mg I.V.

USUAL PEDIATRIC DOSAGE: 0.5 ml I.M. or I.V. initially as a test dose, then 0.5 ml (25 mg) for an infant under 11 lb (5 kg); or 1 ml (50 mg) for a child under 20 lb (9 kg).

Drug interactions

Few drugs interact with iron, but some antibiotics, antacids, and vitamin preparations such as ascorbic acid may alter iron's absorption rate. Similarly, a few foods may interfere with iron absorption. (See *Drug Interactions: Iron* on page 659 for the specifics of each interaction.)

ADVERSE DRUG REACTIONS

The major adverse reaction to iron therapy is gastric irritation. Accidental iron poisoning may be a danger when children have access to iron preparations, because iron tablets that are red and sugarcoated can be mistaken for candy. Parenteral iron dextran may elicit an acute allergic reaction that can be fatal.

Predictable reactions

Iron preparations often cause GI discomfort due to the irritating effect of the iron salts on the gastric mucosa. Symptoms of GI discomfort are typically anorexia, nausea, vomiting, constipation, and diarrhea. Iron preparations will make the stool darker in color, and liquid preparations can stain the teeth. When iron dextran is given by I.M. injection, the patient may experience soreness, inflammation, and skin discoloration at the injection site. The nurse can use the Z-track administration technique to prevent skin discoloration. Rapid I.V. administration may result in lymphadenopathy (local phlebitis at the infusion site) and peripheral vascular reddening (flushing).

Unpredictable reactions

Iron dextran injection may cause acute hypersensitivity reactions, including anaphylaxis, dyspnea, urticaria and other rashes, pruritus, arthralgia and myalgia, febrile episodes, sweating, and allergic purpura. A test dose of iron dextran should be administered before initiating therapy. Hypotension, convulsions, arthritic reactiva-

Foods high in iron

Instruct your patients that the foods listed below are high in iron.

IRON-RICH FOODS	
• liver	• dried apricots
• beef	• peaches
• veal	• prunes
• lamb	• figs
• pork	• dates
• turkey	• raisins
• chicken	• molasses
• oysters	• dried navy and
• eggs	lima beans
• peanut butter	• enriched breads
• soybeans	and cereals

tion, leukocytosis, headache, backache, dizziness, malaise, transitory paresthesias, and shivering have also been reported.

NURSING IMPLICATIONS

The nurse needs to know the contraindications, precautions, and cautions for iron therapy, as well as how to prepare and administer the drug properly, how to prevent and treat adverse reactions, and what to teach patients and families about iron.

• Iron therapy is usually contraindicated in patients with hemochromatosis, hemosiderosis, hemolytic anemias, or known hypersensitivity to any ingredient, as well as in patients with peptic ulcers, regional enteritis, or ulcerative colitis.

• Some of the oral iron preparations contain tartrazine yellow, which may produce allergic reactions, including bronchospasm. This response is particularly demonstrated by individuals with aspirin hypersensitivity. Check the preparation's product listing for tartrazine.

• To prevent GI discomfort, advise the patient to take iron with meals, to avoid taking a bedtime dose, and to take the preparation separate from coffee, milk, eggs, tea, or antacids.

• Before initiating therapy, a test dose of 0.5 ml I.V. or I.M. of iron dextran may be given to assess the patient's response. If no adverse reactions are evident up to 1 hour after the test dose, give the total dose.

• Assess the patient carefully for signs of allergic response during I.V. infusion of iron dextran. Use only single-dose vials for I.V. therapy because multidose vials contain the preservative phenol, which can cause serious adverse reactions.

• For I.V. infusion, dilute the calculated dose of iron dextran in 200 to 250 ml of normal saline solution and administer over several hours.

• Administer iron dextran I.M. by the Z-track technique to avoid leakage into subcutaneous tissue.

• Help the patient explore possible explanations for the anemia (for example, an inadequate diet, overuse of aspirin, symptoms of GI or uterine bleeding) to prevent recurrence. (See *Foods high in iron* for information that should be included in patient teaching.)

• Teach the patient to prevent accidental poisoning in small children; to take liquid preparations with a straw to prevent tooth stains; to understand the special iron requirements of infants, adolescents, and pregnant women; and to recognize the signs and symptoms of anemia (fatigue, weakness, shortness of breath, intermittent glossitis, and pallor).

Accidental iron poisoning in children

Signs and symptoms of accidental iron poisoning include nausea, vomiting, and abdominal pain leading to shock. Shock is caused by GI hemorrhage and high concentrations of unbound ionic iron in the plasma. Death may result from cardiovascular collapse in a few hours to 2 days. A child who survives the poisoning episode may have end-organ damage, including pyloric and antral stenosis, hepatic cirrhosis, and central nervous system damage. Accidental iron poisoning is treated with vasopressor drugs, oxygen, and systemic alkalinizing agents. A specific antidote, deferoxamine, may be given if serum iron levels are greater than 300 mg/dl. Deferoxamine converts both free and tissue-bound iron to a harmless chelate complex, which is excreted by the kidneys. It can be given via nasogastric tube or I.V. If the I.V. route is used, the infusion rate should not exceed 15 mg/kg of body weight per hour.

See also *Accidental iron poisoning in children* for information about this drug-related emergency.

VITAMIN B$_{12}$

Megaloblastic anemias result from defective deoxyribonucleic acid (DNA) synthesis. Defective DNA synthesis is usually from a vitamin B$_{12}$ or folic acid deficiency. The anemia results from decreased erythrocyte formation and the immaturity, fragility, and early destruction of these cells. As a result, the bone marrow contains large erythroid precursors with immature nuclei and mature hemoglobin-containing cytoplasm (megaloblasts). Large oval erythrocytes and neutrophils with six or more lobes appear in a peripheral blood smear. This chapter will discuss vitamin B$_{12}$ and folic acid separately. (See also Chapter 51, Vitamin and Mineral Agents, for more information on folic acid.)

History and source

Vitamin B$_{12}$ was discovered after almost a century of research on the use of liver extract in treating pernicious anemia. By 1924, Minot had begun to feed liver to a few patients with pernicious anemia, an incurable disease at the time. After the patients' conditions improved, clinical trials to test liver efficacy were run on 45 patients. The trials, completed in 1926, demonstrated that the RBC count was restored to normal within 2 months. A few years later, Castle demonstrated that an extrinsic vitaminlike substance was needed for erythropoiesis.

In the early 1940s, Rickes, Smith, and Parker isolated and crystallized vitamin B_{12}. The vitamin was then isolated in a strain of *Streptomyces griseus,* a cheap source that facilitated commercial production of vitamin B_{12} by 1949. Since it turned out to be a cobalt-containing molecule, vitamin B_{12} was named cyanocobalamin. Hodgkin then defined the vitamin's crystal structure by X-ray diffraction and received the Nobel prize in 1964 for these efforts.

PHARMACOKINETICS

Vitamin B_{12} (cyanocobalamin) is available in oral and injectable forms. Vitamin B_{12} absorption depends on an intrinsic factor in the gastric mucosa, and most cases of vitamin B_{12}-deficiency megaloblastic anemia are from the patient's inability to absorb vitamin B_{12}. Therefore,

the injectable form is most frequently used to treat this form of anemia.

Absorption, distribution, metabolism, excretion

Absorption of vitamin B_{12} depends on an intrinsic factor secreted by parietal cells in the body of the stomach. Vitamin B_{12} binds with intrinsic factor, a glycoprotein, and is absorbed in the ileum. Vitamin B_{12} is abundant in a diet of normal protein sources (for example, meat, seafood, milk, eggs, and liver). It even appears in a strict vegetarian diet, which usually includes legumes contaminated with bacteria that synthesize vitamin B_{12}, so most cases of this anemia result from malabsorption. The intrinsic factor is secreted by the same cells that secrete hydrochloric acid (HCl). Since parietal cells are stimulated to produce HCl and intrinsic factor by histamine, histamine analogues, and gastrin, an increase in stimulation by any of these will produce an increase in intrinsic factor. Approximately 500 to 1,000 units of intrinsic factor are required for maximal absorption of 1 mcg of vitamin B_{12}.

When cyanocobalamin is injected either intramuscularly or subcutaneously, it is absorbed and binds to transcobalamin II for transport to the tissues. Vitamin

Response of blood to vitamin B_{12} therapy

After administration, vitamin B_{12} increases erythropoiesis almost immediately. It affects the hematocrit and reticulocyte count within days, as shown in the graphs below.

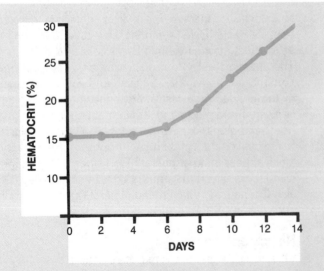

Hematocrit begins to rise by day 7 or 8.

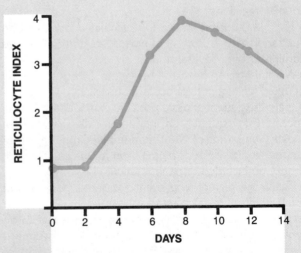

Increased reticulocyte production occurs about day 2 or 3 and reaches a peak by day 6 or 8.

DRUG INTERACTIONS
Vitamin B$_{12}$

A small number of drugs may interfere with vitamin B$_{12}$ absorption or delay a therapeutic response.

DRUG	INTERACTING DRUGS	POSSIBLE EFFECTS	NURSING IMPLICATIONS
vitamin B$_{12}$	neomycin, colchicine, para-aminosalicylic acid, excessive alcohol consumption (longer than 2 week duration)	Cause vitamin B$_{12}$ malabsorption	• Monitor the patient's drug regimen, and report any interactions to the physician. • Monitor the patient for signs and symptoms of a decreased therapeutic response.
	chloramphenicol	Interferes with erythrocyte maturation, thus delaying therapeutic response to vitamin B$_{12}$	• Be aware of possible delayed therapeutic response when assessing B$_{12}$ therapy.
	methotrexate, pyrimethamine, most antibiotics	Invalidate diagnostic microbiological blood assays of B$_{12}$ levels	• Be aware of this effect when reviewing laboratory results.

B$_{12}$ is transported in the bloodstream to the liver, where 90% of the body's supply is stored. The liver slowly releases vitamin B$_{12}$ as needed for cellular metabolic functions. It is excreted in breast milk during lactation. Approximately 3 to 8 mcg of vitamin B$_{12}$ are secreted in bile each day and then reabsorbed in the ileum. Within 48 hours after injection of 100 to 1,000 mcg of vitamin B$_{12}$, 50% to 98% of the dose appears in urine. The major portion is excreted within the first 8 hours.

Onset, peak, duration

The onset of action is quite fast; mature erythrocytes appear in a blood smear within 3 days. Patients usually feel better within 24 hours of therapy. The first objective change is the disappearance of the megaloblastic morphology of the bone marrow. The plasma iron concentration level dramatically decreases, and the reticulocyte count increases on the 2nd or 3rd day and peaks 6 to 8 days later. By the 10th day, the platelet count is higher than normal, and the granulocyte count reverts to normal within 2 weeks. (See *Response of blood to vitamin B$_{12}$ therapy* for further details.)

PHARMACODYNAMICS

The following are some of the known and speculated functions of vitamin B$_{12}$ in the body.

Mechanism of action

When vitamin B$_{12}$ is taken orally or by injection, it replaces vitamin B$_{12}$ that the body would normally absorb from the diet. This vitamin is essential for cell growth and replication and for the maintenance of normal myelin throughout the nervous system. When the vitamin B$_{12}$ supply is inadequate, folate becomes trapped as methyltetrahydrofolate and thus results in a functional deficiency of other intracellular forms of folic acid.

Vitamin B$_{12}$ may also be involved in the metabolism of lipids and carbohydrates. Impairment of this metabolism may interfere with synthesis of the lipid portion of the myelin sheath and contribute to the neurologic damage that is seen in patients with vitamin B$_{12}$ deficiency. Neurologic deficits may also be from the concurrent abnormality in folate metabolism.

PHARMACOTHERAPEUTICS

Two vitamin B$_{12}$ drugs, cyanocobalamin and hydroxocobalamin, are used to treat vitamin B$_{12}$-deficiency anemia. Vitamin B$_{12}$ is usually administered by the I.M. route, because vitamin B$_{12}$-deficiency anemia is often related to an inability to absorb dietary sources. A vitamin B$_{12}$ deficiency is diagnosed by determination of plasma concentrations of vitamin B$_{12}$ and gastric function tests. Measurement of gastric acidity can be an indirect measure of gastric function since the same cell secretes HCl and intrinsic factor. The Schilling test quantifies ileal absorption of vitamin B$_{12}$. (See *Causes of vitamin B$_{12}$ and folic acid deficiencies* on page 665.)

cyanocobalamin [vitamin B₁₂] (Betalin-12, Rubramin PC). Cyanacobalamin is indicated for vitamin B_{12} deficiency caused by malabsorption syndrome, as seen in pernicious anemia; GI pathology, dysfunction, or surgery; or inadequate dietary intake. Cyanacobalamin is usually given I.M. since in many cases the lack of intrinsic factor prevents absorption in the stomach. For patients with pernicious anemia, parenteral therapy is recommended and required for life.

USUAL ADULT DOSAGE: 100 to 1,000 mcg as a nutritional supplement, 15 mcg in an oral multivitamin preparation; 100 mcg I.M. or S.C. daily for 10 to 30 days or 100 mcg daily for 14 days followed by 100 mcg monthly. Considerably higher doses may be required for critically ill patients with neurologic or infectious diseases or hyperthyroidism.

hydroxocobalamin [vitamin B₁₂] (Alphamin, Alpha Redisol). Hydroxocobalamin is indicated for the same conditions as cyanocobalamin. Administer hydroxocobalamin I.M. only. Hydroxocobalamin is absorbed more slowly than cyanocobalamin and produces higher blood levels. Hydroxocobalamin has resulted in antibody formation to the transcobalamin II–vitamin B_{12} complex and thus is not recommended.

USUAL ADULT DOSAGE: 30 mcg I.M. daily for 5 to 10 days followed by 100 to 200 mcg monthly.

Drug interactions

Only a few drugs interfere with gastric absorption of vitamin B_{12}. Drugs that suppress bone marrow may produce a lack of responsiveness to vitamin B_{12}. Some drugs will invalidate vitamin B_{12} diagnostic microbiological blood assays. (See *Drug Interactions: Vitamin B_{12}* on page 663.)

ADVERSE DRUG REACTIONS

No predictable adverse reactions occur with vitamin B_{12} therapy. However, some unpredictable reactions may occur when vitamin B_{12} is administered parenterally. These include hypersensitivity reactions that could result in anaphylaxis and death, cardiovascular reactions (pulmonary edema, congestive heart failure, and peripheral vascular thrombosis), hematologic reactions (polycythemia vera), dermatologic reactions (itching, transient exanthema, and urticaria), and GI reactions (mild diarrhea). Severe, swift optic nerve atrophy has been reported in patients with hereditary optic nerve atrophy. Some patients report a feeling of swelling throughout the entire body.

NURSING IMPLICATIONS

The nurse will administer vitamin B_{12} to inpatients and outpatients and must be aware of several implications.

● Do not administer vitamin B_{12} to any patient with a hypersensitivity to cobalt, vitamin B_{12}, or any component of the medication. If a patient with cobalt sensitivity requires vitamin B_{12}, then an intradermal test dose is recommended.

● Do not administer vitamin B_{12} to patients with Leber's disease (hereditary optic nerve atrophy).

● Administer vitamin B_{12} cautiously and only if necessary to a pregnant or lactating patient.

● Monitor blood folate levels for a patient who is receiving large doses of vitamin B_{12} (more than 10 mcg/day) because such doses can mask a folate deficiency. In these cases, the hematologic picture becomes normal and may mask the true cause of a megaloblastic anemia.

● During treatment of severe megaloblastic anemia, the patient may develop hypokalemia from increased erythrocyte potassium requirement during erythropoiesis. Monitor the patient's serum potassium levels for 48 hours, and replace potassium as prescribed.

● Store the parenteral form of the drug in a light-resistant container at room temperature.

● Stress the importance of monthly vitamin B_{12} injections to the patient with pernicious anemia.

● Teach the patient that a well-balanced diet can eliminate vitamin deficiencies.

● Stress the importance of therapy to the patient receiving permanent I.M. injections because neurologic damage can occur (degenerative spinal cord lesions, for example) as soon as 3 months after a vitamin B_{12} deficiency develops.

FOLIC ACID

The second cause of megaloblastic anemia is folic acid deficiency. Like vitamin B_{12}, folic acid, as folate, is available in sufficient quantities in the average diet. Fresh green vegetables, liver, yeast, and some fruits are particularly rich in folates. Since most of the folate is absorbed in the proximal portion of the GI tract, folic acid deficiency may accompany pathology in the jejunum. Nontropical and tropical sprue are also causes of folic acid deficiency and megaloblastic anemias.

History and source

In the 1930s, some women in India developed a form of anemia similar to pernicious anemia, but without the neurologic deficits. This deficiency responded well to treatment with crude liver extract, but not to purified liver extract. Evidently, the purification of liver extract removed some factor that was different from that in vitamin B_{12}. This factor was first named Wills factor after its discoverer and later became known as vitamin M.

In 1941, Mitchell isolated the factor from leafy green vegetables and called it folic acid. In 1945, the synthesis of folic acid was completed by a team from Lederle Laboratories.

PHARMACOKINETICS

Folate is required for nucleoprotein synthesis and the maintenance of normal erythropoiesis. Present in many foods, it must undergo hydrolysis, reduction, and methylation in the GI tract before it can be absorbed.

Absorption, distribution, metabolism, excretion

Folates present in food are mostly in the form of reduced polyglutamates. Folate absorption requires transport and the action of an enzyme in the mucosal cell membranes. The mucosa of the duodenum and upper jejunum are rich in dihydrofolate reductase and can methylate most of the reduced folate.

Once absorbed, folate is rapidly transported to the tissues. It is distributed to all body tissues, but the largest amounts are found in the cerebrospinal fluid. Folate supplies are maintained from food and by the enterohepatic cycle. The liver actively reduces and methylates the folate components, transports them to bile for reabsorption by the gut, and subsequently delivers them to the tissues. This pathway may provide as much as 200 mcg of folate daily for recirculation to the tissues.

Folates are excreted in urine and feces and secreted in breast milk.

Adults need 50 to 100 mcg of folic acid daily from food to balance the normal daily losses. However, since about 5 to 10 mg of folic acid are stored in the liver and other tissues, an unreplenished body supply could last for 3 to 6 months.

Onset, peak, duration

Within 48 hours after the patient starts folic acid therapy, megaloblastic erythropoiesis disappears, the plasma iron level falls, and erythropoiesis becomes more efficient. The reticulocyte count begins to rise by the 2nd day and reaches a peak concentration level by the 5th or 7th day. The hematocrit begins to rise by the 2nd week.

Causes of vitamin B_{12} and folic acid deficiencies

Folic acid deficiencies are common during pregnancy, but vitamin B_{12} deficiencies are uncommon then because patients with pernicious anemia are usually sterile.

VITAMIN B_{12} DEFICIENCY	FOLIC ACID DEFICIENCY
Common causes	**Common causes**
• Partial gastrectomy • Pernicious anemia • Sprue	• Alcoholism • Cancer chemotherapy with folic acid antagonists • Hemolytic anemia • Liver disease • Myeloproliferative disease • Overcooking folate-containing foods • Pregnancy • Sprue and malabsorption syndromes
Uncommon causes	**Uncommon causes**
• Blind loop syndrome • Cancer • Congenital or family deficiency of folate • Drugs • Fish tapeworm • Poor diet • Pregnancy • Regional ileitis • Selective malabsorption of vitamin B_{12} • Severe chronic pancreatitis • Thyroid disease	• Anticonvulsants and oral contraceptives • Dialysis • Infiltrative lesions of small intestine • Skin diseases, such as psoriasis and exfoliative dermatitis • Vitamin C deficiency

Hematinic agents

This chart summarizes drugs used to treat iron-deficiency anemia and megaloblastic anemia.

DRUG	MAJOR INDICATIONS	USUAL ADULT DOSAGES	NURSING IMPLICATIONS
Iron preparations			
ferrous sulfate (20% elemental iron)	To prevent and treat iron-deficiency anemia	300 mg to 1.2 grams P.O. daily	• Instruct the patient to use food to buffer gastric discomfort. • Teach the patient proper medication storage to protect children in the household. • Teach the patient about adequate dietary sources of iron. • Teach families about the need for additional iron during infancy, adolescence, and pregnancy.
iron dextran	To treat iron-deficiency anemia in patients who cannot tolerate oral therapy	0.5 ml I.M. or I.V. initially as a test dose, then 2 ml I.M. daily for a patient under 110 lb (50 kg) or 5 ml I.M. daily for a patient over 110 lb; or 2 ml I.V. daily at a rate of 1 ml/minute infused slowly	• Test dose of 0.5 ml I.M. or I.V. administered before therapy to assess for hypersensitivity. • Use Z-track injection technique when giving medication I.M. • Use single-dose vials without preservatives.
Vitamin B$_{12}$			
cyanocobalamin	To treat vitamin B$_{12}$-deficiency anemia caused by malabsorption as seen in pernicious anemia or in GI pathology, dysfunction, or surgery	100 mcg I.M. or S.C. daily for 10 to 30 days, or 100 mcg daily for 14 days followed by 100 mcg monthly	• Assess the patient for cobalt sensitivity. • Administer intradermal test dose for patients with history of sensitivity to cobalt. • Monitor the patient's serum potassium levels for the first 48 hours of treatment of severe megaloblastic anemia. • Store the drug in a light-resistant container at room temperature. • Teach the patient about the importance of a well-balanced diet.
Folic acid			
folic acid	To treat megaloblastic anemia from folic acid deficiency Prophylactic treatment in pregnancy, liver disease, hemolytic anemia, alcoholism, skin disease, and renal failure	100 to 400 mcg P.O. daily; 1 mg P.O. 1 to 3 times daily for severe malabsorption	• Assess the patient's dietary patterns, and teach the patient sources of folic acid (meat, eggs, green leafy vegetables). • Teach the patient the correct way of cooking vegetables to preserve the folic acid content. • Teach the female patient about increased need for folic acid during pregnancy.

PHARMACODYNAMICS

The role of folic acid in the body has been fairly well defined since its synthesis in the 1940s.

Mechanism of action
Folic acid is an essential component for normal erythrocyte production and growth. A deficiency results in megaloblastic anemia and low serum and RBC folic acid levels. Neurologic abnormalities do not result from folic acid deprivation but frequently accompany it in patients suffering from alcoholism or liver disease.

PHARMACOTHERAPEUTICS

Folic acid deficiency has many causes. (See *Causes of vitamin B$_{12}$ and folic acid deficiencies* on page 665 for a list of common and uncommon causes of deficiency.)

Parenteral folic acid is seldom required except to reverse the effect of antifolates during cancer chemotherapy or during a therapeutic trial to determine the hematopoietic response before oral therapy begins. Patients who are pregnant or undergoing treatment for liver disease, hemolytic anemia, alcoholism, skin disease, or renal failure will need prophylactic folic acid therapy.

folic acid [folate, vitamin B$_9$] (Folvite). Folic acid is used to treat megaloblastic anemia from folic acid deficiency as seen in sprue, nutritional anemias, pregnancy, alcoholism, and liver disease. Folic acid is available in many multivitamin and iron preparations in doses of 100 mcg to 1 mg. Doses of folic acid above 400 mcg require a prescription.
USUAL ADULT DOSAGE: 100 to 400 mcg/day P.O.; 1 mg P.O. 1 to 3 times daily for severe malabsorption, I.M., I.V., or S.C.

leucovorin calcium (Wellcovorin). Leucovorin calcium is given as an I.M. injection to prevent and treat the undesired hematopoietic effects of folic acid antagonists, such as methotrexate, used in cancer chemotherapy. Dosage varies with the chemotherapeutic agent being used. Leucovorin calcium may also be given P.O. or I.V. (See Chapter 74, Antimetabolite Agents, for additional information on leucovorin calcium.)

Drug interactions
Antifolates that inhibit dihydrofolate reductase include methotrexate, antimalarial agents, triamterene (diuretic), pentamidine (antiparasite), and trimethoprim (urinary tract infection agent). These antifolates may cause a deficiency of active folate compounds, which can lead to megaloblastic anemia. Leucovorin calcium may be required to minimize interference.

In large doses, folic acid may increase seizure activity because it counteracts the effects of anticonvulsant agents, such as phenytoin, phenobarbital, and primidone. Drugs such as glutethimide, isoniazid, cycloserine, and oral contraceptives may interfere with folic acid absorption. Folic acid may interfere with the antimicrobial action of pyrimethamine.

ADVERSE DRUG REACTIONS

Allergic responses (erythema, rash, itching) have been reported after leucovorin calcium and folic acid administration.

NURSING IMPLICATIONS

The greatest nursing emphasis during folic acid administration is on patient assessment and teaching.
• Assess the patient's drug history and remember that antifolates, some anticonvulsants, and oral contraceptives may decrease folate metabolism.
• Assess the patient's dietary habits. Elderly, chronic alcoholic, and indigent patients may have diets that lack vegetables, eggs, and meat.
• Teach the patient the dietary sources of folate: eggs, vegetables, and meats. Instruct the patient not to overcook vegetables because this may destroy folic acid compounds.
• Teach the female patient about the increased need for folic acid during pregnancy.
• Be aware that folic acid therapy can mask a vitamin B$_{12}$ deficiency by improving hematologic abnormalities but allowing neurologic damage to progress.

CHAPTER SUMMARY

Chapter 41 discussed two major types of anemias: microcytic hypochromic anemia, or iron-deficiency anemia, and macrocytic (megaloblastic) anemia caused by vitamin B$_{12}$ or folic acid deficiencies. Both anemias can generally be prevented with adequate dietary intake and may result from conditions that produce inadequate absorption or utilization. Here are the highlights of the chapter:
• Iron, vitamin B$_{12}$, and folic acid are all important for normal RBC production, and all three elements are present in a diet that includes sufficient meat and green leafy vegetables.

- Iron-deficiency anemia results from excessive blood loss, inadequate dietary iron intake, or increased iron requirements during such rapid growth stages as pregnancy and infancy.
- Iron-deficiency anemia is correctable with oral administration of an iron preparation such as ferrous sulfate or ferrous gluconate. The course of therapy is approximately 6 months. Iron treatment restores normal hemoglobin levels and creates iron stores in the body.
- The patient should receive a test dose of iron dextran before full therapy to detect any adverse reactions.
- Malabsorption in the GI tract usually causes megaloblastic anemia. For proper absorption of vitamin B_{12}, the body requires an intrinsic factor secreted by gastric cells.
- Patients who cannot absorb vitamin B_{12} from their diet will require monthly I.M. injections for life to ensure proper cellular metabolic functioning. Cyanocobalamin and hydroxocobalamin are used in vitamin B_{12} therapy.
- Folic acid therapy can mask a vitamin B_{12} deficiency, which can cause neurologic damage if left untreated. Large doses of vitamin B_{12} can mask a folic acid deficiency.
- Folic acid deficiencies are most commonly seen in patients with liver disease, sprue, alcoholism, or malabsorption syndrome.
- Treating a folic acid deficiency with 1 mg of oral folic acid daily will successfully reverse the anemia.

BIBLIOGRAPHY

Anthony, C.P., and Thibodeau, G.A. *Anatomy and Physiology,* 11th edition. St. Louis: C.V. Mosby Co., 1983.

Christensen, D.J. "Differentiation of Iron Deficiency and the Anemia of Chronic Disease," *Journal of Family Practice* 20:35, January 1985.

Fochi, F., et al. "Efficacy of Iron Therapy: A Comparative Evaluation of Four Iron Preparations Administered to Anemic Pregnant Women," *Journal of International Medical Research* 13:1, January 1985.

Gilman, A.G., et al., eds. *Goodman and Gilman's The Pharmacological Basis of Therapeutics,* 7th edition. New York: Macmillan Publishing Co., 1985.

Kastrup, E.K., et al., eds. *Facts and Comparisons.* St. Louis: Facts and Comparisons Division, J.B. Lippincott Co., 1985.

Nicolle, L.S. "Anemia of Chronic Disorders," *Nurse Practitioner* 9:19, November 1984.

Reich, P.R. *Hematology: Physiological Basis for Clinical Practice,* 2nd edition. Boston: Little, Brown & Co., 1984.

Sneader, W. *Drug Discovery: The Evolution of Modern Medicine.* New York: John Wiley & Sons, 1985.

Steinberg, D. *Anemia.* Philadelphia: W.B. Saunders Co., 1982.

Williams, S.R. *Mowry's Basic Nutrition and Diet Therapy.* St. Louis: Times Mirror/C.V. Mosby Co., 1984.

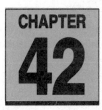

CHAPTER 42

ANTICOAGULANT AGENTS

OBJECTIVES

After reading and studying this chapter, you should be able to:

1. Describe the indications for heparin sodium, the oral anticoagulants, and the antiplatelet drugs.

2. Describe specific monitoring of heparin and warfarin, and state the normal values for each.

3. Describe how heparin and the oral anticoagulants produce their effects.

4. Discuss the effects and nursing implications of drug interactions associated with heparin, the oral anticoagulants, and the antiplatelet drugs.

5. Explain how the nurse should assess for potential bleeding complications in patients receiving heparin, the oral anticoagulants, or the antiplatelet drugs.

6. Explain important points the nurse should include in patient teaching concerning therapy with heparin, the oral anticoagulants, and the antiplatelet drugs.

INTRODUCTION

A delicate balance exists in the body between blood clotting and breakdown (lysis) of clots. Under normal physiologic conditions, little or no clotting occurs. However, certain diseases, such as thromboembolism, cause

Laboratory tests to monitor anticoagulants

The following chart provides the laboratory tests and valves that are appropriate for the different types of anticoagulant. Therapeutic ranges are also given.

DRUG CLASS	APPROPRIATE LABORATORY TEST	NORMAL VALUES	THERAPEUTIC RANGE* DURING ANTICOAGULANT THERAPY
heparin	Activated partial thrombo-plastin time (APTT)	16 to 25 seconds	1½ to 2½ times control
	Partial thromboplastin time (PTT)	30 to 45 seconds	
coumarin compounds	Prothrombin time (PT)	12 seconds	PT ratio of 1.2 to 1.5; PT ranges from 14 to 18** seconds.
antiplatelet drugs	Bleeding time test	3 to 10 minutes	Bleeding time may be 2 times control in 95% of patients. May increase to 10 times control in hyperresponsive patients.

*Each hospital determines its own therapeutic range to reflect its laboratory's specific reagents, instrumentation, and personnel.

**New reduced ranges as recommended by The American College of Chest Physicians and the National Heart, Lung & Blood Institute, 1986, for selected conditions such as venous clots. May need to be in range of 1.5 to 1.8 for other conditions such as mechanical heart valves or rheumatic mitral valve disease.

an abnormal tendency toward clotting. The resultant clots, or thrombi, may obstruct venous or arterial circulation severely. Physicians prescribe anticoagulant drugs to reduce clotting and thereby prevent further coagulation in high-risk patients. Three types of anticoagulants are discussed in this chapter: heparin, the oral anticoagulants, and the antiplatelet drugs. Heparin combined with dihydroergotamine mesylate (Embolex) sometimes is used to prevent postoperative deep vein thrombosis and pulmonary embolism. (See *Embolex* for more on this drug.)

Heparin, a naturally occurring substance, is administered parenterally to prevent a clot from enlarging during an acute thromboembolic event. The drug also is used to prevent thromboembolism in selected high-risk patients, such as those undergoing hip surgery. Heparin most frequently is used in inpatient settings but may be used in well-supervised home care settings.

The oral anticoagulants include the coumarin compounds and the indanedione compounds, represented in this chapter by anisindione. These drugs are used prophylactically in patients at high risk for developing venous thromboembolism and are taken orally most frequently by outpatients requiring prolonged therapy.

Antiplatelet drugs currently used clinically include aspirin, dipyridamole, and sulfinpyrazone (the uses of ticlopidine are under investigation). Other drugs with antiplatelet activity include dextrans, clofibrate, and indomethacin. They may be used alone or in combination with an oral anticoagulant to disrupt platelet aggregation, reducing arterial thromboembolism. The antiplatelet drugs currently are receiving extensive clinical trials to document their usefulness in preventing arterial clotting.

For a summary of representative drugs, see *Selected major drugs: Anticoagulant agents* on page 683.

Embolex

The physician may prescribe Embolex—heparin sodium combined with dihydroergotamine mesylate—to prevent postoperative deep vein thrombosis and pulmonary embolism after major abdominal, thoracic, or pelvic surgery.

Heparin accelerates formation of an antithrombin III–thrombin complex. It inactivates thrombin and prevents fibrinogen's conversion to fibrin. Dihydroergotamine (a semisynthetic ergot alkaloid) is an alpha-adrenergic blocking agent that has a direct effect on the smooth muscle of peripheral blood vessels. It speeds venous return and therefore inhibits venostasis.

When administering Embolex, keep the following important points in mind:
• Avoid administering the drug to a patient with uncontrollable active bleeding.
• Monitor platelet counts, hematocrit, and occult blood in stool. Notify the physician of signs of bleeding.
• Before administering Embolex, check the patient's history for allergy to lidocaine (Embolex contains lidocaine, which acts as a local anesthetic at the injection site to reduce irritation). Also, ask the patient about allergies to heparin or ergot alkaloids.
• Administer Embolex by deep subcutaneous injection into an anterior abdominal wall fold above the iliac crest. To avoid hematoma at the injection site, avoid administering the drug I.M.
• Be aware of adverse reactions, such as bleeding, nausea, vomiting, mild local pain, itching, and numbness and tingling of the fingers and toes.

HEPARIN

Found naturally in body tissues, heparin also is prepared commercially from animal tissue for use in preventing clot formation and treating thromboembolism. Heparin impairs blood coagulation both inside the body (in vivo) and outside it (in vitro)—such as in a test tube—but does not affect the synthesis of clotting factors. Thus, the drug cannot dissolve clots, an action performed by the body's own fibrinolytic system or hastened by thrombolytic agents, which are discussed in the following chapter.

History and source
In 1916, a medical student discovered a phospholipid anticoagulant while researching an ether-soluble anticoagulant precursor. In 1922, Howell discovered a water-soluble mucopolysaccharide that was named *heparin* because of its abundance in the liver. Heparin initially was used to prevent blood clotting in laboratory specimens. Then in 1938, with the improved purification of tissue extracts, clinical trials of heparin began. It was used clinically in exchange transfusions between donors and patients, a technique that saved many lives during World War II. Since that time, heparin has been used widely to treat venous thrombosis. In 1948, Best suggested that low-dose heparin might be useful clinically to keep the blood fluid, but the usefulness of low-dose prophylactic heparin treatment was not proven until the 1970s.

Heparin exists intracellularly in mammalian tissues containing mast cells and abundantly in the liver, lungs, and intestines. The physiologic function of this naturally occurring heparin is unknown. It has only 10% to 20% of the anticoagulant activity of commercially prepared heparin, because when it is released from mast cells, macrophages ingest and destroy it. Thus, naturally occurring heparin cannot be found in circulating blood. Furthermore, heparin in mast cells is inactive.

Heparin is prepared commercially from extractions of bovine lung and porcine intestinal mucosa; it also can be extracted from sheep and whales. Alhough all forms of heparins are biologically equivalent, porcine mucosal heparin produces a lower incidence of heparin-induced thrombocytopenia.

PHARMACOKINETICS

Heparin must be administered parenterally to achieve distribution to the intravascular compartments. It is metabolized in the liver, and its metabolites are excreted in the urine. Its onset of action and peak concentration levels vary according to the route of administration. Although I.V. administration allows immediate distribution, the subcutaneous (S.C.) route is used in low doses to prevent thromboembolism in high-risk patients.

Absorption, distribution, metabolism, excretion

Because of its polarity and large molecular size, heparin is not well absorbed from the gastrointestinal (GI) tract, so it must be administered parenterally. The I.V. route is preferred for high-dose treatment of acute thrombotic episodes, with the S.C. route preferred for low-dose prophylactic therapy. Distribution is immediate after I.V. administration, using either I.V. bolus or continuous I.V. infusion, but it is much less predictable with an S.C. injection. The I.M. route should be avoided because of the danger of local bleeding.

After I.V. administration, heparin is distributed to the intravascular compartments with little of the drug reaching the tissues. It then is taken up by the endothelium of the vascular and lymphatic system and by the cells of the reticuloendothelial system. After administration, heparin concentration levels in the epithelium can be 1,000 times greater than in the plasma, demonstrating a highly specific uptake by the endothelium. Heparin does not cross the placenta or pass into breast milk. The enzyme heparinase metabolizes heparin in the liver. Half-life, approximately 1 to 1½ hours, is dose-related. The anticoagulant effect is measured by the activated partial thromboplastin time (APTT) test and the partial thromboplastin time (PTT) test.

Metabolites are excreted in the urine. (With a large dose, heparin itself appears in the urine.) Patients with hepatic or renal disease excrete heparin more slowly, prolonging its half-life and, thus, its anticoagulant effect. Patients with pulmonary embolism display rapid heparin excretion and may require increased doses.

Onset, peak, duration

With I.V. administration, heparin onset of action is almost immediate, and peak concentration levels occur within minutes. The patient's clotting time will return to normal within 2 to 6 hours after administration of a one-time I.V. bolus. With S.C. administration, onset is delayed for about 2 hours. Serum half-life of heparin is dose-related; that is, the duration of action is extended with higher doses.

PHARMACODYNAMICS

Heparin interferes with clotting and reduces the concentration levels of triglycerides in the plasma. Heparin also has anticomplement properties and a slight antihistaminic effect.

Mechanism of action

Heparin indirectly inactivates thrombin by accelerating the interaction between thrombin and antithrombin III, a thrombin-inactivating glycoprotein found in the blood. Factors XIIa, IXa, XIa, and Xa are inactivated also. (See *Coagulation pathways* on page 650 in the Unit Eight Introduction.) Low heparin doses increase the activity of antithrombin III against Factor Xa and thrombin and can inhibit the initiation of clotting, whereas much larger doses are necessary to inhibit fibrin formation once a clot has been formed. This relationship between dose and effect is the rationale for using low-dose heparin to prevent clotting. Whole blood clotting time, thrombin time, PTT, and APTT are all prolonged during heparin therapy. However, these times may be prolonged only slightly with low or ultra-low prophylactic doses.

Heparin's effect on triglycerides and platelets may impede development of atherosclerotic plaques in blood vessels. For example, heparin has been shown to reduce triglyceride levels by releasing lipid-hydrolyzing enzymes from tissues into blood. These enzymes break down the triglycerides of chylomicrons and very-low-density lipoproteins bound to capillary endothelial cells. Extrahepatic tissues then metabolize the hydrolyzed fatty acids and partial glycerides.

DRUG INTERACTIONS

Heparin

Many interactions involving heparin increase the risk of bleeding or clot formation.

DRUG	INTERACTING DRUGS	POSSIBLE EFFECTS	NURSING IMPLICATIONS
heparin	oral anticoagulants (warfarin, dicumarol, phenprocouman)	Increase risk of bleeding	• Monitor the patient's activated partial thromboplastin time (APTT) carefully. • Assess the patient for signs of bleeding (gums, urine, I.V. and injection sites, nasogastric drainage, and wounds).
	antiplatelet agents (aspirin, dipyridamole)	Increase risk of bleeding	• Educate the patient about the dangers of taking aspirin-containing drugs while on heparin therapy. • Assess the patient for signs of bleeding.
	oral contraceptives	Increase risk of clot formation	• Monitor the patient's APTT; it may not be in the therapeutic range due to the oral contraceptive.
	digitalis, quinidine, tetracycline, neomycin, penicillin, phenothiazines, antihistamines	Increase risk of clot formation	• Do not add any of these drugs to heparin solutions. • Administer I.V. forms through separate or flushed I.V. lines.
	solutions with pH< 6.0 (dextrose solutions)	Increase risk of clot formation	• Use normal saline solution for heparin infusions.

By maintaining the electronegativity of the blood vessel surface, heparin also decreases platelet adhesiveness and release of platelet-derived growth factor. Heparin demonstrates many immune-mediating effects in laboratory experiments. It activates macrophages, increases the migration of B lymphocytes, and inhibits T and B lymphocytes. It also inhibits sensitivity reactions, such as anaphylaxis and antigen-antibody reactions.

PHARMACOTHERAPEUTICS

Physicians prescribe heparin to prevent and treat venous thromboembolisms, characterized by inappropriate or excessive intravascular activation of blood clotting. Venous thromboembolism results from venous stasis (slow blood flow). The clot consists of a fibrin network enmeshed with erythrocytes and platelets. It also has a long tail that can detach and travel to distant sites, such as the lungs, and cause pulmonary embolism. Immediate I.V. heparin administration is indicated for treating acute thromboembolism.

Heparin also is used whenever the patient's blood must circulate outside the body through a machine. Thus, the patient undergoing open-heart surgery receives heparin so that the blood does not clot while the patient is on the cardiopulmonary bypass machine. Similarly, the patient undergoing hemodialysis receives heparin during each treatment.

The physician may order heparin for a patient with disseminated intravascular coagulation (DIC) when massive clotting is the primary manifestation of the disorder. In this situation, the heparin halts further clotting, allowing the body to restore its clotting factors and prevent bleeding. Heparin also is used to treat arterial clotting and atrial fibrillation with embolization. (During atrial fibrillation, the inefficient and inadequate pumping of the atria may cause clots to form that can detach and travel to the lungs or brain.)

Heparin is used in prostatic and orthopedic surgery, which in many cases activates the coagulation mechanisms excessively. A patient undergoing total hip or knee replacement may receive a postoperative heparin dose of 15,000 to 20,000 units/day to prevent venous thromboembolism.

Heparin is the drug of choice to treat thromboembolism and to prevent clot formation in the venous system because of its immediate anticoagulant effect after I.V. administration. The nurse can monitor the anticoagulant effect by monitoring the patient's APTT and PTT. The APTT is more sensitive than the PTT and more common for monitoring heparin therapy and screening for clotting factor deficiencies in the intrinsic coagulation system. When the APTT is maintained at 1½ times the control, the risk of recurrent venous thromboembolism is about 3%. (See *Laboratory tests to monitor anticoagulants* on page 669 for a summary of appropriate tests.)

The effects of heparin can be reversed easily by administering protamine sulfate, which has a specific affinity for heparin and forms a stable nondissociable salt with it. (See *Protamine sulfate* on page 674 for more information on this drug.) Heparin produces relatively few adverse reactions when the APTT is maintained within the therapeutic range.

heparin sodium. Used to treat thromboembolism, heparin also is used to prevent clot formation in the venous system. Low-dose S.C. heparin is used to prevent thromboembolism in high-risk patients, including patients immobilized on bed rest for long periods, those undergoing pelvic surgery, and those with a preoperative history of clot formation.

USUAL ADULT DOSAGE: to treat pulmonary embolism or thromboembolism, 5,000 to 10,000 units as a bolus, followed by continuous I.V. infusion of 1,000 to 2,000 units/hour. For intermittent I.V. treatment, 5,000 to 10,000 units every 6 hours; for S.C. administration to prevent thromboembolism in high-risk patients, 10,000 to 12,000 units every 8 hours, or 14,000 to 20,000 units every 12 hours. For low-dose S.C. therapy, 5,000 units 2 hours before surgery, then 5,000 units every 8 to 12 hours for 7 days or until the patient is fully ambulatory. Hip surgery patients may receive as much as 30,000 units/day to maintain the APTT at the upper end of the normal range.

USUAL PEDIATRIC DOSAGE: for continuous I.V. infusion, 50 units/kg I.V. bolus, followed by infusion of 100 units/kg over 4 hours; for intermittent I.V. treatment, 50 to 100 units/kg every 4 hours.

Drug interactions

Because heparin acts synergistically with all the oral anticoagulants, the risk of patient bleeding increases when both types of drugs are administered. The prothrombin time (PT), used to monitor the effects of oral anticoagulants, may be prolonged if the patient also takes heparin. Similarly, the risk of bleeding increases when the patient takes an antiplatelet drug, such as aspirin or dipyridamole, while receiving heparin. Oral contraceptives may decrease antithrombin III, increasing the potential for clot formation. Drugs that antagonize or inactivate heparin include antihistamines, digitalis, nicotine, phenothiazine, tetracycline hydrochloride, quinidine, quinine sulfate, neomycin sulfate, and I.V. penicillin. Some of these drugs are incompatible with highly acidic heparin and should not be mixed in the same solution. Heparin is inactivated rapidly in solutions with a pH below 6. Therefore, normal saline solution rather than dextrose solutions should be used with heparin. (See *Drug interactions: Heparin* for a summary.)

ADVERSE DRUG REACTIONS

One of the clinical advantages of heparin is that it produces relatively few adverse reactions, of which the most predictable is bleeding. The nurse usually can prevent

---

Heparin: Summary of adverse reactions

Heparin interferes with the normal human clotting cascade. Although this effect has therapeutic uses, it also has dangerous potential to cause bleeding.

ADVERSE REACTION	NURSING IMPLICATIONS
Predictable	
Bleeding	• Monitor the patient's APTT or PTT daily. • Assess the patient for bleeding. • Monitor the patient's platelet count regularly.
Unpredictable	
Hypersensitivity response—rash, hives, chills, fever	• Question the patient about an allergy history. • Monitor the patient's response to a test dose of heparin before initiating therapy. • Assess the patient for signs of hypersensitivity during treatment.
Alopecia	• Explain to the patient that hair loss is reversible. • Support the patient's efforts to maintain body image (for example, suggest wearing an attractive scarf, hat, or wig.
Osteoporosis, bone fractures	• Use safety precautions for elderly patients on long-term heparin therapy (for example, use bed rails, assist with ambulation).

Protamine sulfate

Protamine sulfate is a strong base that neutralizes acidic heparin by binding with it to form a stable compound with no anticoagulant effect. However, protamine sulfate administered in the absence of heparin can produce an anticoagulant effect.

Protamine sulfate is available in a 1% solution or a 50-mg powder form. One mg will neutralize approximately 100 units of heparin. The calculated dose should equal that required to neutralize half the previous heparin dose.

Administer protamine sulfate by I.V. only and slowly (not more than 50 mg per single injection, unless additional monitoring of clotting times is performed). Rapid injection can cause complications such as dyspnea, flushing, bradycardia, and hypotension. Because protamines are proteins that occur in the sperm of salmon and some other fish, hypersensitivity reactions may occur in patients with allergies to fish.

bleeding by closely monitoring the patient's APTT to maintain it within the therapeutic range (1½ to 2½ times the control). The drug may cause hypersensitivity reactions in some patients.

Predictable reactions

The potential for bleeding exists in all patients receiving high doses of heparin to treat thromboembolism. The nurse should monitor the patient's urine, stool, and emesis for blood and watch for bleeding from the gingiva or nose, at injection sites, and in subcutaneous tissue (hematoma).

Bleeding leads to more serious consequences if it occurs in the brain (subdural hematoma), at arterial puncture sites, or in or behind the peritoneum (intraperitoneal or retroperitoneal hemorrhage). The severity of this bleeding can be reduced by omitting or decreasing the heparin dose, and the risk of bleeding usually can be reduced by carefully monitoring the APTT. The hemoglobin (Hb) and hematocrit (Hct) should be routinely monitored for indications of bleeding. The risk of bleeding is low in patients on low-dose heparin, so monitoring their bleeding times is unnecessary usually.

Heparin may depress the platelet count, resulting in thrombocytopenia, depending on the type of heparin used: porcine heparin may have a greater tendency than bovine heparin to produce thrombocytopenia. The nurse should monitor the patient's platelet count regularly during heparin therapy. If thrombocytopenia occurs, heparin should be discontinued as ordered to return the platelet count to normal.

Unpredictable reactions

Because heparin is procured from animal sources, it can produce hypersensitivity reactions. Although such reactions occur rarely, heparin should be administered cautiously to a patient with a history of allergies. Administering a trial dose of 1,000 units can determine the patient's allergic potential. Hypersensitivity reactions can produce such signs and symptoms as chills, fever, urticaria, rash, anaphylaxis, and alopecia, which are reversible upon discontinuation of treatment. Osteoporosis and spontaneous fractures may occur in patients who have been on long-term heparin therapy. (See *Heparin: Summary of adverse reactions* on page 673 for the nursing implications associated with both predictable and unpredictable adverse reactions to this drug.)

NURSING IMPLICATIONS

The nurse must know the contraindication to heparin therapy, the proper routes and methods of administration, and how to prevent adverse reactions. The nurse must know these implications:

• Do not administer heparin to patients who demonstrate hypersensitivity reactions, who are bleeding actively, or who have bleeding disorders such as hemophilia. It is contraindicated also in patients with severe hypertension, alcoholism, or a history of GI ulcers, or in patients undergoing brain, spinal cord, or eye surgery.
• Administer heparin cautiously to patients with hepatic or renal disease, because the liver and kidneys are involved in the metabolism and excretion of the drug.
• Administer heparin cautiously to elderly women, because they seem to have the highest incidence of adverse reactions to it.
• Administer heparin cautiously in pregnant patients, even though it does not cross the placenta.
• Do not administer heparin to a pregnant patient with a threatening abortion.
• Monitor the patient's APTT, PTT, and platelet count daily; notify the patient's physician if the therapeutic range is exceeded.
• Assess the patient for early signs of bleeding (gingiva, epistaxis, hematuria, hematemesis, injection-site oozing).
• Assess wound, drainage tube, and I.V. sites carefully for signs of bleeding.
• Have the antidote protamine sulfate readily available in case of severe bleeding. (See *Protamine sulfate* for its use in counteracting the effects of heparin.)

• Monitor the patient's APTT before each heparin dose during the early stages of intermittent dose therapy until the therapeutic level is reached. Then monitor the APTT every 12 hours for 3 days.

• Monitor the patient's APTT every 4 hours during early stages of treatment using continuous I.V. infusion; once the therapeutic range ($1\frac{1}{2}$ to $2\frac{1}{2}$ times that of the control) is achieved, monitor the APTT every 12 hours for 3 days.

• Never administer heparin I.M., and avoid other I.M. injections if possible.

• Avoid aspirating and massaging after administering an S.C. injection of heparin to prevent risk of subcutaneous bleeding.

• Use a flowchart to record the time and results of pertinent laboratory studies such as PT, APTT, hemoglobin, and platelet count, and the administration time, dose, and injection site of heparin.

• Check the patient's urine, stool, and emesis regularly for occult blood.

• Monitor the patient's vital signs, Hb, and Hct for indications of bleeding.

• Assess the patient with hepatic or renal disease carefully for signs of bleeding.

• Assess the patient with a history of peptic ulcers or ulcerative colitis for signs of bleeding such as melena.

• Observe for purpura (subcutaneous bleeding).

• Use normal saline solution, which has a low pH, for continuous or intermittent I.V. infusion, to avoid the risk of a higher pH solution causing clotting.

• Use an infusion pump for continuous I.V. infusion to ensure correct dosage, as prescribed.

• Check the drug label carefully before administering, because heparin is available in different strengths.

• Remember that heparin is prescribed in units or international units (IU) rather than in milligrams.

• Do not mix any other drug with a heparin infusion because heparin is highly acidic and a drug interaction may occur.

• Be aware that heparin is stable at room temperature.

• Protect heparin from freezing and inspect all vials for particulate matter or discoloration; if either is present, discard the vial.

• Teach the patient and family about home care heparin therapy, including how to properly administer the drug and how to observe for signs of bleeding.

• Teach hospitalized patients the signs and symptoms of bleeding and precautions to take after venipuncture.

• Help the home care patient make any provisions necessary for regular monitoring of the APTT; be aware that this may not be necessary if the APTT is maintained at the lower end of the therapeutic range ($1\frac{1}{2}$ times the control).

• Advise the patient that all normal activities of daily living may be performed if the platelet count is normal.

• Reassure the patient and his family that alopecia is reversible.

• Advise the patient to avoid drinking alcohol and smoking, because either can alter the response to heparin.

• Encourage the patient to use an electric razor and a soft toothbrush to avoid the risk of bleeding from cuts or irritated gums.

• Advise the patient to avoid all over-the-counter aspirin preparations and antihistamines, unless the physician is consulted first.

ORAL ANTICOAGULANTS

Two kinds of oral anticoagulants currently are available: the coumarin compounds, widely used in the United States, and the indanedione compounds, less frequently used because of their toxic effects. Both the coumarin and indanedione compounds inhibit liver synthesis of the vitamin K–dependent clotting factors prothrombin (Factor II) and Factors VII, IX, and X. The drugs are used to prevent recurrence of thromboembolism in patients requiring long-term management. They also are prescribed for patients at high risk for developing thromboembolism, such as a patient with prosthetic heart valves. The coumarin compounds discussed in this chapter are warfarin sodium and potassium, dicumarol, and phenprocoumon. The indanedione compound discussed is anisindione.

History and source
During the 1920s in North Dakota and Alberta, Canada, researchers determined that cattle were dying of hemorrhagic septicemia after eating hay prepared from spoiled sweet clover. Based on this finding, Link and colleagues worked for many years to isolate the bleeding factor. Then, in 1939, Campbell finally isolated the first crystals of an anticoagulant agent; clinical trials began at the Mayo Clinic during the 1940s. In 1942, the new anticoagulant dicumarol was marketed. Since then, hundreds of coumarin compounds, varying in potency, onset of action, and duration of action, have proved clinically useful.

PHARMACOKINETICS

The oral anticoagulants produce their effect only in vivo, as opposed to heparin, which also produces in vitro. Therefore, they are referred to as *indirect anticoagulants*.

Warfarin sodium is the major coumarin compound and the oral anticoagulant most frequently used in the United States. The indanedione drug anisindione is infrequently used because of its severe toxic effects.

Absorption, distribution, metabolism, excretion

Warfarin is absorbed rapidly and almost completely after oral administration; food decreases the rate of absorption but not the total amount absorbed. Toxicity may occur from repeated absorption of warfarin-containing rodenticides via the skin or from accidental ingestion by children. Dicumarol, another coumarin compound, is absorbed more slowly and erratically. Because of water solubility, the indanedione compound anisindione is absorbed rapidly and completely. (The coumarin and indanedione compounds usually are found in the plasma about 1 hour after administration.)

Warfarin, dicumarol, and anisindione are bound extensively to plasma albumin.

Because warfarin is 99% plasma protein-bound, it does not diffuse into erythrocytes, cerebrospinal fluid, or urine. Warfarin is secreted into breast milk, so breastfeeding is not recommended, although it usually does not change the PT of infants. The coumarin and indanedione compounds can cross the placenta and may cause fetal deformities and hemorrhagic diseases.

The coumarin and indanedione compounds are converted to inactivated metabolites in the liver (first-pass effect). These metabolites are secreted in bile, then into the duodenum, where they are reabsorbed partially before being excreted in urine. Warfarin, dicumarol, anisindione and phenprocoumon are excreted in breast milk. Unabsorbed dicumarol may be excreted unchanged in feces.

Onset, peak, duration

Onset of action of the coumarin compounds occurs within 24 to 72 hours. Onset of action of anisindione occurs within 48 to 72 hours. Peak concentration levels of all the oral anticoagulants are measured by the PT. Among the coumarin compounds, warfarin has the shortest period of peak concentration level, ½ to 3 days; phenprocoumon, 2 to 3 days; and dicumarol, 3 to 5 days. Anisindione takes 2 to 3 days to achieve peak concentration levels.

Although the oral anticoagulants appear quickly in the plasma after administration, therapeutic anticoagulation does not occur until the blood has been depleted of clotting factors. Factor VII, with the shortest half-life, is the first clotting factor to be depleted. Significant depletion of Factor X and prothrombin (Factor II) may take 2 to 3 days. Thus, maximum anticoagulation and antithrombotic effects may not be achieved for 3 to 5 days after initiation of therapy.

The duration of action of warfarin is 2 to 5 days; of dicumarol, 2 to 10 days; of anisindione, 1 to 3 days. The half-life of the coumarin compounds varies from ½ to 2 days for warfarin and 1 to 2 days for dicumarol, up to 6½ days for phenprocoumon, and 3 to 5 days for anisindione.

PHARMACODYNAMICS

The oral anticoagulant agents are vitamin K antagonists. Their administration results in the production of biologically inactive precursor coagulation proteins.

Mechanism of action

The oral anticoagulants alter the synthesis of vitamin K–dependent clotting factors, including prothrombin, Factor VII, Factor IX, and Factor X. The alteration does not impede the synthesis of these factors (which remain immunologically detectable); instead, it makes them dysfunctional. The resulting therapeutic anticoagulant effect does not occur until the already circulating clotting factors are depleted; this takes from several hours for Factor VII to 2 to 3 days for prothrombin. Thus, optimal PT response is achieved in 1 to 4 days.

The anticoagulant effects of the coumarin compounds and anisindione are enhanced in patients with inadequate dietary intake of vitamin K or fat, and in patients with deficient vitamin K absorption. The anticoagulant effects are decreased in patients with increased intake of vitamin K. Patients with hepatic disease experience an increased anticoagulant effect because the disease causes impaired hepatic synthesis of clotting factors. Hypermetabolic states, such as fever and hyperthyroidism, also increase the response to oral anticoagulants, whereas hypometabolic states reduce it.

Pregnancy appears to decrease response to the anticoagulants because of the increased activity of Factors VII, VIII, IX, and X. The oral anticoagulants can cross the placenta and seriously damage the fetus; thus, heparin, because it does not cross the placenta, is the anticoagulant of choice during pregnancy.

PHARMACOTHERAPEUTICS

Physicians prescribe the oral anticoagulants to treat thromboembolism after initial treatment with heparin. Warfarin, however, may be started without heparin in outpatients at high risk for thromboembolism. The oral anticoagulants are the drugs of choice for the prophylactic therapy of deep vein thrombosis and for patients with prosthetic heart valves or diseased mitral valves. They sometimes are combined with an antiplatelet drug, such as dipyridamole, to decrease risk of arterial clotting.

The oral anticoagulants offer several advantages. They can be taken on an outpatient basis, and they can be easily monitored using the patient's PT. (See *Laboratory tests to monitor anticoagulants* on page 669 for appropriate tests.) Their major disadvantage is that they interact with numerous drugs, producing an increased risk of bleeding or clotting. Overall, the coumarin compounds are the drugs of choice, because they produce relatively few adverse reactions except for bleeding, which occurs in 20% to 30% of patients. Warfarin is the most commonly prescribed coumarin compound. Anisindione, the most toxic oral anticoagulant, is used rarely in the United States. The effects of the oral anticoagulants can be reversed with adequate doses of phytonadione (vitamin K_1).

warfarin sodium (Coumadin). Warfarin sodium is the only coumarin compound that can be administered orally and by I.M. or I.V. injection; however, parenteral injection offers no clinical advantage, so warfarin usually is administered orally. It is used to treat thromboembolism after initial treatment with heparin. Long-term prophylactic warfarin therapy is used for patients with artificial heart valves and frequently is combined with antiplatelet drugs such as dipyridamole to prevent thromboembolism resulting from mitral stenosis and atrial fibrillation. It may be used after heparin therapy in patients with anterior or apical myocardial infarction (MI) accompanied by mural endocardial thrombosis.

Warfarin may be used instead of S.C. heparin to prevent venous thromboembolism in patients undergoing total hip and knee replacement surgery.
USUAL ADULT DOSAGE: for venous thrombosis, 10 mg P.O. daily for the first 2 to 3 days, adjusted to PT results, then a maintenance dose of 2 to 10 mg P.O. daily; the dose for other conditions is less clear, but patients with prosthetic heart valves, recurrent embolism, and rheumatic mitral valve disease may require higher PT ratios of 1.5 to 2.

warfarin potassium (Athrombin-K). Available in oral form only, warfarin potassium is used for the same conditions as warfarin sodium.
USUAL ADULT DOSAGE: Same as warfarin sodium.

dicumarol (Dicumarol Pulvules). Available for oral administration, dicumarol is difficult to use clinically be-

cause of slow and incomplete absorption. Dicumarol is used for the same clinical indications as warfarin.
USUAL ADULT DOSAGE: 200 to 300 mg P.O. the first day, then 25 to 200 mg/day, depending on PT results.

phenprocoumon (Liquamar). Phenprocoumon is available in oral form only. It is a long-acting coumarin compound with a long half-life and duration of action; thus, the drug is difficult to control clinically.
USUAL ADULT DOSAGE: initially, 24 mg P.O. on the first day; as maintenance dose, 0.75 to 6 mg P.O. daily, depending on PT results.

anisindione (Miradon). Used for the same clinical indications as warfarin, anisindione is a relatively short-acting indanedione compound.
USUAL ADULT DOSAGE: initially, 300 mg P.O. on the first day, 200 mg P.O. on the second day, 100 mg P.O. on the 3rd day, then 25 to 250 mg P.O. daily as maintenance dose.

Drug interactions
Many patients on oral anticoagulant therapy are treated with other drugs. The hazards of serious interactions between anticoagulants and other drugs are ever present, and many clinically significant interactions occur. The most frequently prescribed drugs that interact with the oral anticoagulants include barbiturates, salicylates, and phenylbutazone. Many foods, especially those high in vitamin K, also interact with the oral anticoagulants. However, only a diet containing high amounts of vitamin K is likely to cause problems.

The PT of a patient taking oral anticoagulants must be reevaluated whenever a drug is added or deleted from the drug regimen. Reevaluating the PT helps monitor the many possible interactions involving drugs. The mechanisms underlying these interactions include inhibition of vitamin K production or absorption, displacement of the anticoagulant from its albumin-binding sites, inhibition or induction of enzymes responsible for metabolizing warfarin, and other mechanisms that are less well understood. (See *Drug interactions: Oral anticoagulants* on page 678 for a list of some interacting drugs and related nursing implications.)

ADVERSE DRUG REACTIONS

The use of oral anticoagulants may produce bleeding complications from inadequate monitoring of PT, from drug interactions that increase the anticoagulant effect

DRUG INTERACTIONS

Oral anticoagulants

This chart illustrates the wide range of potential interactions between oral anticoagulants and other drugs and between oral anticoagulants and food.

DRUG	INTERACTING DRUGS OR FOODS	POSSIBLE EFFECTS	NURSING IMPLICATIONS
warfarin	salicylates, phenylbutazone, oxyphenbutazone, sulfinpyrazone, indomethacin, dipyridamole, quinidine, quinine, clofibrate, alkalyzing agents, anabolic and androgenic steroids, potassium products, chloral hydrate, chloramphenicol, disulfiram, heparin	Increase bleeding tendency	• Monitor the patient's prothrombin time (PT) frequently after any new drug is added to the patient's drug regimen. • Assess the patient for signs of bleeding (epistaxis, bleeding gums, hematuria, or bruising). • Advise the patient to avoid using any over-the-counter product containing aspirin.
	barbiturates, glutethimide, ethchlorvynol, griseofulvin, carbamazepine, rifampin, estrogen, oral contraceptives, vitamin K, cholestyramine, colestipol	Increase clotting	• Assess the patient for thromboembolism (increased pain, swelling, redness in calf, any symptoms of pulmonary embolism, increased shortness of breath, chest pain, or fever). • Monitor the patient's PT frequently after any of these drugs is administered.
	phenytoin	Increases danger of phenytoin toxicity; may increase anticoagulant effect of dicumarol	• Monitor the patient carefully for any sign of phenytoin toxicity (nystagmus, ataxia, slurred speech, or confusion).
	foods high in vitamin K (cabbage, cauliflower, broccoli, asparagus)	Increase clotting	• Obtain a dietary history from the patient to learn the amount of vitamin K–rich foods in the daily diet. • Caution the patient against sudden increases in ingestion of vitamin K–rich foods.
	mineral laxatives, aluminum hydroxide	Decrease absorption and effectiveness; increase clotting	• Assess the patient's use of laxatives and aluminum hydroxide–containing antacids. • Instruct the patient to follow a high-fiber, high-bulk diet for good elimination instead of using laxatives.
	alcohol	Increases risk of clotting with chronic abuse; acute intoxication increases risk of bleeding	• Obtain a history from the patient and family about the extent of alcohol use. • Monitor the patient for bleeding. • Monitor the patient's PT frequently.

of the drugs, or from the patient's noncompliance. Elderly patients who respond more sensitively to oral anticoagulants are at increased risk of bleeding.

Other common causes of bleeding include peptic ulcers and occult GI tumors. Bleeding from these causes may only be apparent when the patient's urine, stool, or emesis is tested for occult blood. More obvious bleeding may appear as epistaxis, gingiva, or ecchymoses.

Predictable reactions

Minor bleeding, the primary predictable reaction to oral anticoagulant therapy, usually can be controlled by reducing the dosage of the anticoagulant. Severe bleeding may occur in the GI or urinary tract, or in the uterus. Ecchymosis and hematoma formation may occur at arterial puncture sites (for example, after a blood gas sample is taken). Severe bleeding may occur as intraperitoneal hemorrhage from a ruptured corpus luteum, retroperitoneal hemorrhage, hemopericardium and intracranial hemorrhage, and adrenal hemorrhage.

Patients receiving oral anticoagulants must be assessed carefully for minor and major bleeding, and their PT responses must be monitored carefully. Bleeding can occur, however, even when the patient's PT falls within the therapeutic range.

Treating minor bleeding includes immediately discontinuing the oral anticoagulant and, if necessary, administering oral or parenteral vitamin K as prescribed. Several hours will elapse before vitamin K returns the PT time to normal. Severe bleeding requires vitamin K therapy and administering plasma or fresh whole blood to replace the vitamin K–dependent clotting factors.

Vitamin K should be used cautiously to reverse anticoagulant therapy, because it can produce a rebound hypercoagulable state that is a threat to patients with artificial heart valves who are prone to clot formation. The patient with the artificial valve is best treated with fresh frozen plasma to provide clotting factors.

Red-orange urine, nausea, vomiting and diarrhea, abdominal cramping, priapism, mouth ulcers, and nephropathy may rarely occur.

Unpredictable reactions

Unpredictable and rare adverse reactions to the coumarin compounds include alopecia, urticaria, dermatitis, skin necrosis, hepatitis, and jaundice. Other rare adverse reactions include fever, hypersensitivity reactions, agranulocytosis, leukopenia, and eosinophilia.

NURSING IMPLICATIONS

The nurse must consider the numerous contraindications and precautions before administering oral anticoagulants.

• Know that oral anticoagulants are contraindicated in patients with active or past intestinal bleeding; thrombocytopenia; malignant hypertension; recent neurologic or eye surgery; subacute bacterial endocarditis; chronic alcoholism; or hepatic or renal disease (the liver and kidneys are involved in metabolism and excretion of these drugs).

• Know that oral anticoagulants usually are contraindicated during pregnancy and lactation, but they can be administered cautiously in the second and early third trimester. If warfarin must be given during lactation, alert the mother to the potential risks.

• Know that oral anticoagulants are contraindicated in patients with conditions requiring intensive salicylate therapy, such as arthritis.

• Expect to use oral anticoagulants in long-term outpatient treatment only when the patient is compliant and and is aware of the drug's potential adverse effects.

• Monitor PT responses daily for inpatients and every 1 to 4 weeks for outpatients; be aware that for venous thromboembolism, the therapeutic range established by the American College of Chest Physicians and the National Heart, Lung, and Blood Institute is a PT ratio of 1.2 to 1.5 times the control.

• Assess for signs of occult bleeding even when the PT is within the therapeutic range.

• Have vitamin K readily available to treat bleeding, as prescribed.

• Treating minor bleeding involves omitting one or more doses as ordered until the PT returns to therapeutic range. If minor bleeding continues, administer vitamin K_1 (phytonadione) 1 to 10 mg P.O. as prescribed.

• If frank bleeding occurs, administer 5 to 50 mg of vitamin K parenterally as prescribed. Small doses (1 to 15 mg) are recommended to prevent a hypercoagulable state that may occur after rapid reversal of prolonged PT.

• If severe bleeding occurs, administer 250 to 500 ml of fresh frozen plasma or give commercial Factor IX complex as prescribed. Be aware that plasma concentrates are associated with a high risk of hepatitis and are used cautiously when no alternative exists.

• Check and record the PT daily and before administering an oral anticoagulant. When the patient initially receiving heparin is switched to warfarin, expect heparin therapy to continue until the therapeutic effects of warfarin begin; this may take several days.

• Notify the physician immediately if the therapeutic range is exceeded, and withhold the next dose as prescribed.

• Test urine, stool, and nasogastric drainage for occult blood.

• Assess the patient regularly for signs of clot formation, such as thrombophlebitis (calf pain, tenderness, and redness).

• Immediately report any sign of pulmonary embolism to the physician (shortness of breath, chest pain, decreased arterial oxygen as noted in arterial blood gas results, fever, tachypnea).

• Monitor the patient's vital signs carefully for any indications of severe internal bleeding; use extra care in assessing elderly patients for signs of bleeding.

• The dosage should be individualized for each patient according to the PT; the dosage may change daily.

• Administer low-dose S.C. heparin into the anterior abdominal wall fold above the iliac crest to avoid the risk of bleeding.

- Inform the patient to follow the written instructions for dosage; encourage the patient to keep a daily log to reinforce taking the correct dosage.
- Instruct the patient receiving warfarin to take it in the evening and to have PT drawn in the morning for accurate results. Teach the patient the importance of having blood drawn for PT (usually monthly after stabilization).
- Instruct the patient not to take any prescription or over-the-counter drug without first contacting the physician who ordered the anticoagulant therapy. Provide the patient and family members with written information about the interactions between oral anticoagulants and other drugs or food.
- Instruct the patient to avoid alcohol intake, increased amounts of green leafy vegetables, and all medications containing aspirin.
- Teach the patient the importance of reporting immediately to the physician any blood in stool or urine, and any bruising.
- Encourage the patient to wear a medical identification bracelet to alert medical personnel in case of trauma or sudden illness.
- Encourage the patient to avoid activities with high risk of physical injury.

ANTIPLATELET DRUGS

The antiplatelet drugs have shown some potential for preventing arterial thromboembolism, particularly in patients at risk for MI and cerebrovascular accidents from arteriosclerosis. These drugs, with varying mechanisms of action, are presently the subject of many clinical research trials. The antiplatelet drugs include aspirin, dipyridamole, and sulfinpyrazone. Dextrans, clofibrate, and indomethacin show some antiplatelet activity. (See *Other drugs with antiplatelet activity.*) Ticlopidine, available in Europe, is under investigation but not commercially available in the United States.

These drugs' potential to prevent arterial thromboembolism is under study; they may interfere with platelet aggregation in atherosclerotic plaque development. When damage occurs to the endothelial lining of an artery, platelets adhere to the site of injury. Circulating platelets converge on the wound site, first touching and then adhering to the collagen fibers of the torn vessel lining (endothelium). This contact of platelets with col-

Other drugs with antiplatelet activity

The drugs discussed here have shown some clinical usefulness because of their antiplatelet activity. Dextrans are partially hydrolyzed polymers of glucose and are usually used as plasma expanders. Although they do not alter platelet aggregation in vitro, dextrans may alter bleeding time and polymerization of fibrin, thus exerting antiplatelet action in vivo. Dextrans reduce platelet adhesiveness by coating platelets and the blood vessel endothelium. They also lower the level of circulating von Willebrand factor, increase the susceptibility of clots to fibrinolysis, and reduce erythrocyte aggregation, blood viscosity, and venous stasis. Dextrans may also dilute clotting factors through their oncotic effect.

Clofibrate, a hypolipidemic drug, may reduce platelet adhesiveness in vitro and increase abnormally short survival of platelets in some patients with coronary artery disease.

Indomethacin, an anti-inflammatory analgesic often used to treat rheumatoid arthritis, inhibits platelet aggregation but has a shorter duration of action than aspirin.

Other drugs that interfere with platelet function are tricyclic antidepressants, penicillin and related antibiotics, nitroprusside, chloroquine, and alcohol. However, these drugs are not used clinically as antiplatelet agents.

lagen stimulates the platelets to secrete adenosine diphosphate (ADP), which causes them to break down and become adhesive, sticking together in clumps. Additional ADP activates greater numbers of platelets, which also collect at the site. This aggregation loosely plugs the wound to prevent further blood loss. Serotonin, also secreted by platelets, causes smooth muscle contraction, which facilitates vascular constriction and hemostasis. Thus, platelet adhesion rather than fibrin formation is the predominant hemostatic reaction.

History and source
Aspirin, dipyridamole, and sulfinpyrazone are well-known drugs that have been widely available for many uses. Aspirin is well known for its analgesic, antipyretic, and anti-inflammatory properties; dipyridamole for its possible vasodilating effects; and sulfinpyrazone for its antigout action. Now, these drugs are being studied for their potential antithrombotic effects.

PHARMACOKINETICS

The pharmacokinetic properties of aspirin, dipyridamole, and sulfinpyrazone vary, although all three are administered orally.

Absorption, distribution, metabolism, excretion
Aspirin is absorbed rapidly in the stomach and upper intestine (absorption is delayed with enteric-coated preparations and by food), then is distributed quickly into the bloodstream. Following metabolism in the liver, aspirin is eliminated by the excretion of salicylic acid in the kidneys and by the oxidation and conjugation of metabolites.

Dipyridamole is absorbed from the GI tract; it is almost completely plasma protein-bound (91% to 97%). The drug is distributed widely in body tissues and is capable of crossing the placenta in small amounts. Di-

pyridamole is metabolized in the liver and excreted in bile. This drug may undergo enterohepatic cycling before partial excretion in the feces. Small amounts may be excreted in the urine.

Sulfinpyrazone is well absorbed after oral administration and is 98% to 99% protein-bound. After rapid but incomplete metabolism in the liver, yielding active and inactive metabolites, about 45% of the drug is excreted unchanged in the urine.

Onset, peak, duration
Aspirin's onset of action and peak concentration level as an antiplatelet drug are still being investigated. The duration of action of aspirin's platelet-inhibitor effect is the life span of the platelet, approximately 10 days. The half-life of aspirin is approximately 15 minutes.

The peak plasma concentration level of dipyridamole occurs 2 to 2½ hours after oral administration.

DRUG INTERACTIONS

Antiplatelet drugs

The antiplatelet drugs cause clinically significant interactions with any drugs that may cause bleeding. Some of the more clinically significant drugs are discussed here.

DRUG	INTERACTING DRUGS	POSSIBLE EFFECTS	NURSING IMPLICATIONS
aspirin	heparin, oral anticoagulants	Increase risk of bleeding	• Monitor the patient's activated partial thromboplasm time (APTT), prothrombin time (PT), and bleeding times daily. Report any prolonged results to the physician. • Assess the patient for signs of minor or major bleeding.
	sulfinpyrazone	Antagonizes uricosuric properties of sulfinpyrazone	• Assess the patient for increased signs and symptoms of gout.
dipyridamole	oral anticoagulants	May enhance action of oral anticoagulant, increasing risk of bleeding	• Monitor the patient's PT to assess that it remains in the therapeutic range after administering dipyridamole. Advise the patient to report any bleeding to the physician.
	aspirin	May enhance antiplatelet action, increasing risk of bleeding	• Assess the patient's bleeding times daily. • Assess the patient's PT for risk of bleeding.
sulfinpyrazone	aspirin, oral anticoagulants	May decrease uricosuric properties Enhance effect of oral anticoagulant, increasing risk of bleeding	• Assess the patient's PT for increased signs and symptoms of gout. Report any such signs or symptoms to the physician. Concurrent administration should be avoided. • Monitor the patient's PT daily. • Assess the patient for signs of minor and major bleeding. Teach the patient the signs of minor bleeding, such as melena and bleeding gums, and advise the patient to report any such findings to the physician.

Sulfinpyrazone's onset of action, peak concentration level, and duration of action as an antiplatelet drug are still being investigated. The drug may require several days of administration; some effects persist after withdrawal.

PHARMACODYNAMICS

The antiplatelet drugs interfere with platelet activity in different drug-specific and dose-related ways. The antithrombotic effects of these drugs have not been proven but have been suggested by tests of platelet function in patients receiving the drugs.

Mechanism of action

Low doses of aspirin (325 mg per day) appear to inhibit clot formation by blocking prostaglandin synthetase action, which in turn prevents formation of the platelet-aggregating substance thromboxane A_2. In vitro studies of dipyridamole have shown that this drug can inhibit platelet aggregation. However, in vivo studies have not shown the same effects.

Sulfinpyrazone appears to inhibit several platelet functions. At doses of 400 to 800 mg/day, sulfinpyrazone lengthens platelet survival; doses of more than 600 mg/day prolong the patency of arteriovenous shunts used for hemodialysis. A single dose produces rapid inhibition of platelet aggregation, suggesting that the drug directly affects circulating platelets.

PHARMACOTHERAPEUTICS

The antiplatelet drugs are under investigation today because evidence exists that platelet aggregation significantly promotes atherosclerotic plaque development. For example, at injured endothelial sites, platelet aggregation and subsequent fibrin formation can create arterial clots. Also, certain patient-related factors, such as a history of gout, diabetes, hypertension, hyperlipidemia, or cigarette smoking, may contribute to plaque development by promoting platelet aggregation.

The antiplatelet drugs, especially aspirin, act synergistically with heparin and the oral anticoagulants, thus increasing the risk of bleeding when these drugs are used in combination. The adverse reactions some of these drugs cause may limit their usefulness in preventing arterial clotting.

The patient's bleeding time and platelet aggregation studies can measure the effectiveness of the antiplatelet ability of these agents. (See *Platelet activity tests* on page 684 for information on these two tests.)

aspirin. Although varying studies have evaluated dosages of aspirin to prevent arterial clotting, no convincing evidence exists that one dosage is more effective than another. Although no dosages have been established, low dosages of aspirin have shown some effectiveness in preventing aortocoronary bypass shunt thrombosis. Aspirin also has shown some effectiveness in reducing clot formation in arteriovenous shunts in patients on hemodialysis and in patients with unstable angina. In some studies with male patients, aspirin has been effective in reducing the risk of recurring transient ischemic attacks. Aspirin also may be used to help prevent reinfarction and sudden death in men with acute MI and possibly to prevent postoperative venous thrombosis in patients who undergo elective hip and knee surgery.
USUAL ADULT DOSAGE: to prevent clot formation in arteriovenous shunts in hemodialysis patients, 160 mg P.O. daily. To prevent clot formation in patients with unstable angina, 325 mg P.O. daily. To help prevent reinfarction and sudden death in men with acute MI, 300 to 1,500 mg P.O. daily. For men with cerebral ischemic disease, 325 mg P.O. q.i.d. or 650 mg P.O. b.i.d. Lower dosages, such as 80 to 325 mg P.O. daily, may help prevent cerebral ischemic disease.

dipyridamole (Persantine). In combination with warfarin, dipyridamole may help prevent thromboembolism in patients with prosthetic heart valves. Combined with aspirin, the drug may be effective in patients with cerebral ischemic attacks and in patients who undergo coronary bypass graft surgery. Controversy concerning these combination therapies still exists, however. Some physicians advocate giving dipyridamole and aspirin 2 days preoperatively to decrease platelet adhesiveness at the site of aorta–saphenous vein anastomoses. Physicians seem to agree that dipyridamole should be used in combination with warfarin in patients with prosthetic heart valves who develop thromboembolic complications while receiving therapeutic dosages of warfarin.
USUAL ADULT DOSAGE: for graft patency after coronary artery bypass surgery, 300 to 400 mg P.O. daily in divided doses (at this dosage, the drug may act as a vasodilator rather than as an antiplatelet agent); for patients with prosthetic heart valves who develop complications while on warfarin, 225 mg P.O. daily.

sulfinpyrazone (Anturane). This uricosuric drug may correct shortened platelet survival and may prolong the patency of arteriovenous shunts used in hemodialysis. One study reported its effectiveness in helping to prevent MI.
USUAL ADULT DOSAGE: trial dosages to correct shortened platelet survival, 400 to 800 mg P.O. daily; to

DRUG INTERACTIONS

Anticoagulant agents

The drugs listed in this chart, representative of the different types of anticoagulants, are considered major anticoagulant agents and have many significant nursing implications.

DRUG	MAJOR INDICATIONS	USUAL ADULT DOSAGES	NURSING IMPLICATIONS
Parenteral anticoagulant			
heparin	Venous thromboembolic disease	Continuous I.V. infusion: 5,000- to 10,000-unit bolus followed by 1,000 to 2,000 units/hour Intermittent I.V. therapy: 5,000 to 10,000 units every 6 hours. Low-dose S.C. therapy: 5,000 units every 8 to 12 hours	• Heparin is contraindicated in patients with hypersensitivity reactions to this drug, hemorrhagic disorders, severe hypertension, alcoholism, or GI ulcers. • Administer cautiously in patients with hepatic or renal diseases and in elderly or pregnant patients. • Use an infusion pump for a continuous I.V. infusion as prescribed. • Monitor the patient's APTT before each intermittent I.V. dose early in treatment and then daily. • Assess the patient for signs of bleeding. • Monitor the patient's platelet count, hemoglobin level, and hematocrit daily. • Avoid I.M. injections. • Have the antidote protamine sulfate readily available. • Use a flowchart to record coagulation studies. • Monitor the patient's urine, stool, and emesis for occult blood.
Oral anticoagulants			
warfarin	Thromboembolic disease after initial treatment with heparin; drug of choice to prevent deep vein thrombosis in patients with prosthetic heart valves or diseased mitral valves	10 mg P.O. daily for 2 to 3 days, then adjusted according to PT results; maintenance dose, 2 to 10 mg P.O. daily	• Warfarin is contraindicated in patients with a history of GI bleeding, thrombocytopenia, renal or hepatic disease, malignant hypertension, recent neurologic or eye surgery, or alcoholism. • Warfarin is contraindicated in patients who need intensive salicylate therapy. • Assess the patient for possible interactions with other drugs, especially barbiturates, salicylates, and phenylbutazone. • Monitor the patient's PT daily. • Assess the patient for signs of bleeding. • Have vitamin K readily available to treat bleeding, as prescribed.
dicumarol	Same indications as warfarin	200 to 300 mg P.O. the first day, then 25 to 200 mg daily depending on PT results	• Same nursing implications as warfarin.
Antiplatelet agents			
aspirin	Clot formation prevention in shunts in hemodialysis patients	160 mg P.O. daily	• Aspirin is contraindicated in patients with aspirin hypersensitivity. • Administer with extreme caution to patients on heparin or oral anticoagulant therapy and those with hemorrhagic disorders or gastric ulcers.
	Clot formation prevention in patients with unstable angina	325 mg P.O. daily	

Platelet activity tests

Two of the platelet activity tests used to monitor antiplatelet therapy are bleeding time and platelet aggregation studies.

The *bleeding time* test measures the duration of bleeding after a standardized skin incision. Bleeding time depends on the elasticity of the blood vessel wall and on the number and functional capacity of platelets. Bleeding time may be measured by one of four methods: Duke, Ivy, template, or modified template. The template methods are the most frequently used and the most accurate.

After vascular injury, platelets gather at the injury site and clump together to form an aggregate—a plug—that helps maintain hemostasis and promotes healing. The *platelet aggregation* test, an in vitro procedure, measures the rate at which the platelets in a sample of citrated platelet-rich plasma form a clump after the addition of an aggregating reagent (adenosine diphosphate, epinephrine, thrombin, collagen, or ristocetin). Since evenly suspended platelets aggregate and fall to the bottom of the tube, the greater the aggregation, the less turbid the sample. A spectrophotometer measures changes in turbidity and prints a graphic record of the results.

---

prolong the patency of arteriovenous shunts in patients on hemodialysis, 600 mg P.O. daily; to help prevent MI, 800 mg P.O. daily.

Drug interactions

Low doses of aspirin prescribed for its antiplatelet activity should produce few adverse reactions. (See Chapter 25 for more information on aspirin interactions.) The risk of bleeding increases in patients receiving both heparin and large doses of aspirin because aspirin's effect on platelets increases bleeding time. Aspirin can also antagonize the uricosuric effect of sulfinpyrazone.

The additive effect of dipyridamole with aspirin and of dipyridamole with warfarin has been used to prevent thromboembolic disorders in patients with aortocoronary bypass grafts or prosthetic heart valves. Sulfinpyrazone administered concurrently with many other drugs can cause some serious adverse reactions. (See Chapter 65, Uricosurics, Other Antigout Agents, and Gold Salts, for additional sulfinpyrazone drug interactions.) One significant sulfinpyrazone drug interaction is potentiation of the action of the oral anticoagulants by displacing the coumarin compounds from their albumin-binding sites. As a result, prothrombin activity is further depressed,

increasing the risk of bleeding. (See *Drug interactions: Antiplatelet drugs* on page 681 for some interactions and related nursing implications.)

ADVERSE DRUG REACTIONS

The adverse drug reactions to aspirin, dipyridamole, and sulfinpyrazone are discussed below.

Predictable reactions

GI tract signs and symptoms are the most frequent adverse reactions associated with the aspirin dosage prescribed to prevent arterial clotting. These signs and symptoms include stomach pain, heartburn, nausea, constipation, hematemesis, melena, and slight gastric blood loss—rarely, a patient may experience significant GI bleeding or peptic ulcer disease.

Aspirin produces its principal predictable reaction by damaging the gastric mucosa. Because this damage requires acid in the stomach, it can be minimized by large dosages of antacids. The gastric damage may also be minimized by using enteric-coated tablets. Although aspirin usually is administered in fairly low dosages as an antiplatelet agent, repeated administration of large dosages of aspirin may cause salicylism, with symptoms including dizziness, tinnitus, difficulty hearing, nausea, vomiting, diarrhea, mental confusion and lethargy. An overdose of aspirin may result in respiratory alkalosis from hyperpnea and tachypnea.

Dipyridamole, usually well tolerated, produces minimal adverse reactions that may include headache, dizziness, nausea, flushing, weakness, syncope, and mild GI distress. These disappear when the drug is discontinued.

The major adverse reaction to sulfinpyrazone is epigastric discomfort, which may aggravate or reactivate peptic ulcer disease. Taking the drug with food, milk, or an antacid usually reduces this discomfort.

Unpredictable reactions

Hypersensitivity reactions to the antiplatelet drugs, particularly anaphylaxis, can occur; the most common is the induction of bronchospasm with asthma-like symptoms. Dipyridamole may cause a skin rash. Unpredictable reactions to sulfinpyrazone may include skin rash, blood dyscrasias (anemia, leukopenia, agranulocytosis, thrombocytopenia, or aplastic anemia), and bronchoconstriction. Some patients have experienced reversible renal dysfunction following sulfinpyrazone therapy.

NURSING IMPLICATIONS

The nurse should obtain a history from all patients who are to receive antiplatelet drugs. Doing so will help the nurse identify hypersensitive patients, those taking anticoagulants, and those at risk because of diseases or disorders. Recognizing these factors helps the nurse prevent adverse reactions.

• Antiplatelet drugs are contraindicated in patients with aspirin hypersensitivity.

• Administer aspirin cautiously to patients who report hypersensitivity to other nonsteroidal anti-inflammatory drugs. Administer with extreme caution to patients taking heparin or oral anticoagulants because of the increased risk of bleeding. Be aware that the potential benefits of preventing clotting may be outweighed by the risk of bleeding in patients with hemophilia, gastric ulcers, or hemorrhagic disorders.

• Obtain a careful drug history before administering any antiplatelet drug, to help prevent adverse reactions. Also obtain a careful history of any previous peptic ulcer disease, and assess the patient for signs of gastric hemorrhage.

• Know that dosages of coumarin compounds may need to be reduced as prescribed if aspirin is being added to the patient's drug regimen.

• Administer aspirin or sulfinpyrazone with milk, food, or an antacid because these drugs frequently produce gastric discomfort.

• Instruct the patient taking aspirin or sulfinpyrazone at home to take it with milk, food, or antacid and to report any severe gastric pain to the physician.

• Do not administer aspirin if it has a strong vinegarlike odor, which indicates deterioration of the drug. Give dipyridamole 1 hour before meals with a full glass of water.

• Monitor the patient's bleeding times and platelet aggregation studies; they are the best indicators of the effectiveness of antiplatelet therapy.

• Monitor the APTT, PTT, or PT if the patient is receiving heparin or a coumarin compound.

• Assess the patient for any signs of minor or major bleeding (minor: epistaxis, gingival bleeding, hematuria, hematemesis, or melena; major: frank bleeding from the stomach or a wound, hematoma formation, hypotension, or tachycardia).

• Teach the patient and family how to recognize the signs of bleeding, and advise them to report any such signs to the physician.

• Instruct the patient taking aspirin not to take additional aspirin-containing over-the-counter products without consulting the physician.

• Teach the patient to avoid contact sports where the chance of injury that could lead to bleeding is high.

CHAPTER SUMMARY

Chapter 42 focused on heparin, the oral anticoagulants, and the investigational use of the antiplatelet drugs in anticoagulant therapy. Here are the highlights of the chapter:

• Heparin is the drug of choice to treat and prevent venous thromboembolism because of its immediate anticoagulant effect when administered I.V. Heparin is also excreted rapidly.

• Low-dose S.C. heparin is often used to prevent thromboembolism in high-risk patients.

• Heparin arrests clot formation by accelerating the interaction between antithrombin III and thrombin. It does not, however, dissolve existing clots.

• The anticoagulant effect of heparin is best monitored by the APTT or PTT, which should be maintained at 1½ to 2½ times the control.

• Patients on high-dose continuous or intermittent heparin therapy need frequent nursing assessment for signs of minor and major hemorrhage.

• Patients who are on home therapy need to have laboratory access for monitoring APTT or PTT values.

• Because heparin is synergistic with all oral anticoagulants, the risk of bleeding is increased in patients receiving both drugs.

• In patients with severe bleeding, protamine sulfate is used to neutralize heparin.

• The coumarin compounds, the most commonly used oral anticoagulants in the United States, are the drugs of choice for long-term management of patients with thromboembolism and patients at high risk, such as those with prosthetic heart valves. The oral anticoagulants alter the synthesis of the vitamin K–dependent clotting factors—Factors II, VII, IX, and X.

• The oral anticoagulants are monitored using the patient's PT; new lower recommended values have been established for some disorders to minimize hemorrhagic complications.

• The major adverse reactions to oral anticoagulants are hemorrhagic complications. Treatment includes discontinuing the drug and administering oral or parenteral vitamin K as ordered.

• The nurse should teach patients receiving oral anticoagulants (and their families) about how the drugs interact with other drugs and with food, how to check for signs of bleeding, and the necessity of having blood drawn for PT results as prescribed.

• Researchers are studying antiplatelet drugs as possible therapies for preventing arterial clotting, especially in patients with MI and those with cerebral ischemic disease. Aspirin is currently the most widely researched antiplatelet drug; dipyridamole and sulfinpyrazone are also under investigation.

• Although many drugs are known to alter platelet function, the clinical efficacy of these drugs in preventing arterial clotting remains the subject of intense clinical trials.

• Bleeding times and platelet aggregation studies are the best indicators of the effectiveness of antiplatelet therapy.

BIBLIOGRAPHY

American Hospital Formulary Service. *Drug Information 87.* McEvoy, G.K., et al., eds. Bethesda, Md.: American Society of Hospital Pharmacists, 1987.

Bertelé, V., and Salzman, E.W. "Anthrombotic Therapy in Coronary Artery Disease," *Arteriosclerosis* 5:119, March/April 1985.

Craig, C.R., and Stitzel, R.E. *Modern Pharmacology,* 2nd ed. Boston: Little, Brown & Co., 1986.

Elwood, P.C. "Aspirin in the Prevention of Myocardial Infarction: Current Status," *Drugs* 28(1):1, July 1984.

Hermelin, L.I., and Eichenberger, J.W. "Monitoring Thrombolytic Therapy: The New Laboratory Challenge," *Journal of Medical Technology* 2(2):89, February 1985.

Hirsh, J., et al. "Dose Antiplatelet Agents: The Relationship Among Side Effect and Antithrombotic Effectiveness," *Chest* 89(2):45, February 1986.

Hirsh, J., et al. " 'Therapeutic Range' for Oral Anticoagulant Therapy," *Chest* 89(2):115, February 1986.

Hudak, C.M., et al. *Critical Care Nursing,* 4th ed. Philadelphia: J.B. Lippincott Co., 1986.

Huerta, B.J., and Limberg, L. "Anticoagulation in Atrial Fibrillation," *Heart & Lung* 14(5):521, September 1985.

Jaques, L.B. "The New Understanding of the Drug Heparin," *Chest* 88(5):751, November 1985.

Kastrup, E.K., et al., eds. *Facts and Comparisons.* St. Louis: Facts and Comparisons Division, J.B. Lippincott Co., 1987.

Moake, J.L., and Levin, J.D. "Thrombotic Disorders," *Clinical Symposia 1985 Annual.* Summit, N.J.: CIBA-GEIGY, 1985.

Palkuti, H.S. "Laboratory Monitoring of Anticoagulant Therapy," *Journal of Medical Technology* 2:81, 1985.

Pauker, S.G., et al. "A Decision Analytic View of Anticoagulant Prophylaxis for Thromboembolism in Heart Disease," *Chest* 89(2):995, February 1986.

Quick, D., and Trowbridge, A.A. "Heparin Applications and Future Prospects," *Chest* 88(5):755, November 1985.

Sneader, W. *Drug Discovery: The Evolution of Modern Medicines.* New York: John Wiley & Sons, 1985.

Valladores, B.K., and Lemberg, L. "Platelet Aggregation and Atherosclerosis," *Heart & Lung* 15(2):211, March 1986.

CHAPTER
43

THROMBOLYTIC AGENTS

OBJECTIVES

After reading and studying this chapter, you should be able to:
1. Identify the approved clinical indications for streptokinase and urokinase therapy.
2. Describe the mechanisms of action by which these drugs dissolve thrombi.
3. Explain why patients undergoing thrombolytic therapy are at increased risk for bleeding.
4. Identify the drug interactions that occur when streptokinase or urokinase is used with heparin, oral anticoagulants, antiplatelet drugs, or aminocaproic acid.
5. Identify the adverse reactions to streptokinase and urokinase.
6. Describe the nursing assessments and interventions required during thrombolytic therapy.
7. Discuss representative experimental thrombolytic agents.

INTRODUCTION

Thromboembolic occlusion of an artery may result in the necrosis (death) of tissue distal to the obstruction, and the patient may lose the function of part or all of the affected organ. Though thrombi will disintegrate in 7 to 10 days by the action of the fibrinolytic system, tissue death can occur in hours.

If emboli that acutely occlude the major artery or vein are dissolved quickly, blood flow may be reestablished to distal tissues, and necrosis may be minimized or prevented. Thrombolytic therapy may be indicated for a pulmonary embolus or a deep vein thrombosis to dissolve the thrombus and reestablish circulation. Thrombolytic agents convert plasminogen to plasmin, allowing the hydrolysis (chemical alteration of a compound with water) of the fibrin that forms the clot. The use of thrombolytic therapy immediately after acute myocardial infarction is currently under investigation.

Thrombolytic therapy is not commonly accepted in medicine today. In the last decade, researchers have conducted many clinical trials to determine the indica-

tions for therapy, the benefits and risks, and the appropriate route and dosage. In the trials, serious, unpredictable bleeding from the therapy has overwhelmed all other issues, and subsequent research is directed toward developing thrombolytic agents that are more selective in their actions.

For a summary of representative drugs, see *Selected major drugs: Thrombolytic agents* on page 693.

STREPTOKINASE AND UROKINASE

The major thrombolytic drugs discussed in this chapter include streptokinase and urokinase. The chapter also includes information about more experimental agents, such as tissue-type plasminogen activator (t-PA), acylated streptokinase-plasminogen complex, and single-chain urokinase-type plasminogen activator. (See *Experimental thrombolytic agents* on page 689 for a further discussion of t-PA and single-chain urokinase-type plasminogen activator.)

History and source

Streptokinase, derived from group C beta-hemolytic streptococci, was discovered in 1933. Urokinase, derived from human renal cells grown in culture, was discovered in 1951. Since 1959, clinical studies using both these agents have tested the efficacy of systemic thrombolysis in patients with myocardial infarction, pulmonary embolism, and deep vein thrombosis. In 1977, the Food and Drug Administration (FDA) approved streptokinase to treat deep vein thrombosis and pulmonary embolism and approved urokinase to treat pulmonary embolism.

Since 1979, clinical studies have evaluated the efficacy of thrombolytic agents in patients with acute myocardial infarction. In 1980, an FDA and National Institutes of Health–sponsored conference on the thrombolytic agents recommended that physicians use streptokinase and urokinase to manage deep vein thrombosis and severe pulmonary embolism.

PHARMACOKINETICS

Both streptokinase and urokinase produce a systemic thrombolytic state (in which fibrin is loosened or dissolved) characterized by depletion of plasminogen, the presence of free plasmin in the plasma, decreased alpha$_2$-antiplasmin levels, decreased fibrinogen levels, increased levels of fibrin degradation products (FDPs), and prolonged thrombin time.

Absorption, distribution, metabolism, excretion

After intravenous (I.V.) or intracoronary administration, both streptokinase and urokinase are distributed immediately throughout the circulation, quickly activating plasminogen. Streptokinase is rapidly removed from the circulation by antibodies and the mononuclear phagocytic system (reticuloendothelial system). It does not ap-

pear to cross the placenta. Urokinase is rapidly metabolized by the liver, and small amounts are excreted in bile and urine. Research has not yet determined if it crosses the placenta.

Onset, peak, duration

The onset of action of both streptokinase and urokinase is almost immediate, with rapid plasminogen activation after I.V. or intracoronary administration.

In clinical studies, streptokinase serum half-life decreases in two phases: first, a half-life of 18 minutes, then 83 minutes. The serum half-life of urokinase is 20 minutes.

After therapy is discontinued, the thrombolytic effects of both streptokinase and urokinase disappear within a few hours, but the systemic effect on coagulation and the risk of bleeding may persist for 12 to 24 hours. The effect of these drugs on systemic coagulation is noted by decreased plasma levels of fibrinogen and plasminogen and increased levels of circulating FDPs. (See the Unit Eight Introduction for a discussion of normal coagulation.) For 4 hours, thrombin time is decreased to less than twice the normal control value.

Fibrinolytic actions of streptokinase and urokinase

These thrombolytic agents act on plasminogen to dissolve fibrin. Streptokinase acts indirectly to form a plasminogen activator complex. This complex converts residual plasminogen to the enzyme plasmin, which then lyses the clot's fibrin and other plasma components. As the clot breaks up, it releases fibrin degradation products (FDPs) into the bloodstream. Urokinase works differently at the start of the process by acting directly on plasminogen to form plasmin.

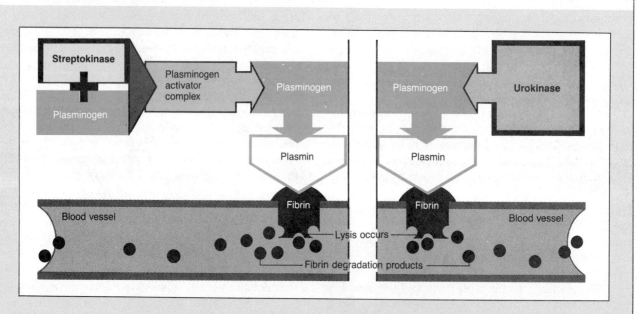

PHARMACODYNAMICS

Both streptokinase and urokinase convert plasminogen to the enzyme plasmin, which lyses (dissolves) thrombi, fibrinogen, and other plasma proteins.

Mechanism of action

Streptokinase indirectly activates plasminogen by forming an activator complex that later converts residual plasminogen into the proteolytic (protein-splitting) enzyme plasmin. Therapeutic doses of streptokinase introduce a high level of activator into the bloodstream but relatively little plasmin. As the circulating activator diffuses into the thrombus, it activates adsorbed preplasmin II, which hydrolyzes fibrin. This action leads to endogenous lysis (dissolution). Plasmin generated in the circulation binds to antiplasmin and is released at the thrombus site, resulting in the external lysis of the clot.

During the first few hours of treatment, rapidly activated plasminogen can produce hyperplasminemia (excessive plasmin in the blood) and possible coagulation defects from increased hydrolysis and depleted fibrinogen and coagulation Factors V and VII. These changes, combined with the dissolution of fibrin, increase the risk of bleeding.

Streptokinase also decreases blood and plasma viscosity as well as the tendency for erythrocytes and platelets to aggregate. These actions increase blood flow and produce a perfusion of collateral blood vessels. Because streptokinase is highly antigenic, repeated administration produces antibodies that diminish the drug's effect and may promote allergic reactions.

Experimental thrombolytic agents

Three thrombolytic agents have shown promise in experimental trials; however, they have not been approved for clinical use.

Tissue-type plasminogen activator (t-PA)

Originally extracted from human melanoma cells grown in tissue culture, t-PA is now made by recombinant DNA techniques. The drug remains the focus of extensive clinical research.

Tissue-type plasminogen activator, using fibrin as a cofactor, activates the conversion of plasminogen to plasmin. When t-PA is released into the circulation, it alters coagulation only at the thrombus and not systemically. Bleeding and complications—bleeding at puncture sites and hematoma formation at catheter sites, associated with streptokinase and urokinase—are reduced in t-PA therapy. Because t-PA is a human protein, it usually does not produce an allergic response.

Patients receiving t-PA have significant differences in drug metabolism and clearance from those receiving streptokinase or urokinase. Significant differences that do not appear to be dose-related also occur in the plasma drug levels at midinfusion. The liver, which plays a crucial role in the clearance of t-PA, may influence the plasma drug levels.

The half-life of t-PA is 3 to 7 minutes. Because the drug spares circulating plasminogen, the hazards of bleeding are reduced in the early phase of acute myocardial infarction. Plasminogen levels return to baseline shortly after t-PA therapy is discontinued.

Not yet available for clinical use, t-PA is being investigated for the same clinical indications as streptokinase and urokinase: deep vein thrombosis, pulmonary embolism, and coronary thrombosis.

Results in patients with acute coronary thrombosis indicate recanalization of the affected vessel. A recent study also has noted I.V. t-PA to be as effective as intracoronary streptokinase. Because the dosage of t-PA required for the rapid lysis of coronary thrombi activates plasma plasminogen sufficiently to break down large amounts of fibrinogen, t-PA will probably interact with heparin, oral anticoagulants, and the antiplatelet drugs and increase the risk of bleeding.

Acylated streptokinase-plasminogen complex

This thrombolytic agent circulates in the bloodstream without reacting with either plasma inhibitors or plasminogen. It binds directly to fibrin and has a prolonged fibrinolytic effect. These two properties make it a potentially useful thrombolytic agent. Animal studies show acylated streptokinase-plasminogen complex to be significantly more thrombolytic than streptokinase. A clinical advantage is that acylated streptokinase-plasminogen complex can be given as a single I.V. bolus.

Single-chain urokinase-type plasminogen activator or pro-urokinase

Animal studies demonstrate an increased fibrinolytic effect for this agent and less derangement of systemic hemostatic mechanisms than with urokinase. One clinical study of six patients with myocardial infarction demonstrated rapid recanalization of occluded coronary arteries without systemic activation of the fibrinolytic system.

Urokinase, an active protease, directly converts plasminogen to plasmin within and on the surface of thrombi and emboli. The plasmin breaks down fibrin, fibrinogen, and other procoagulant plasma proteins. Urokinase also produces an anticoagulant effect by dissolving fibrinogen and increasing the level of FDPs. With a greater affinity than streptokinase for fibrin-bound plasminogen, urokinase produces a milder systemic coagulation defect. Urokinase is nonantigenic and does not produce allergic reactions. (See *Fibrinolytic actions of streptokinase and urokinase* on page 688 for an illustration of how these drugs work.)

PHARMACOTHERAPEUTICS

The FDA has approved the plasminogen activators streptokinase and urokinase for treating certain thromboembolic disorders. These drugs have also been used to dissolve thrombi in arteriovenous cannulas to reestablish blood flow. The thrombolytic agents are the drugs of choice to break down newly formed thrombi; they seem most effective when administered immediately after thrombosis. Because streptokinase and urokinase act synergistically with heparin, the risk of bleeding is compounded if heparin is used concurrently. Streptokinase and urokinase may not be effective drugs for treating acute myocardial infarction (MI).

streptokinase (Kabikinase, Streptase). The first thrombolytic agent introduced, streptokinase is used to treat deep vein thrombosis, pulmonary embolism, arterial thrombosis and embolism, and coronary thrombosis and to dissolve thrombi in arteriovenous cannulas. Patients who have had previous streptococcal infections will have antistreptokinase antibodies in their systems. To overcome these antibodies, large loading doses are usually administered. An initial loading dose of 250,000 units overcomes the antibody level in 90% to 95% of the patients and initiates fibrinolysis.

USUAL ADULT DOSAGE: for deep vein thrombosis, an I.V. loading dose of 250,000 units given over 30 minutes, followed by an I.V. infusion of 100,000 units/hour for up to 72 hours, depending on clinical results. For pulmonary embolus, the dosage is same as for deep vein thrombosis, but the infusion continues for only 24 hours. For arterial thrombosis and emboli, dosages have not been established but usually range between 5,000 and 50,000 units/hour; treatment may be used in conjunction with surgery (arterial embolectomy). (See *Streptokinase therapy for acute myocardial infarction* for additional uses for this drug.)

urokinase (Abbokinase). Approved by the FDA for dissolving acute pulmonary emboli and coronary thromboses as well as for clearing clotted arteriovenous catheters, urokinase provides some advantages over streptokinase. Because it is nonantigenic, urokinase does not cause allergic reactions, and it has a greater affinity for fibrin-bound plasminogen than for plasma plasminogen—limiting its effect on systemic plasminogen. Despite these advantages, urokinase does not have greater clinical efficacy or cause less bleeding than streptokinase. Urokinase is much more expensive. It is indicated for patients who cannot tolerate streptokinase.

USUAL ADULT DOSAGE: for pulmonary embolism, 4,400 units/kg/hour I.V. for 10 minutes as a loading dose; then 4,400 units/kg/hour as a constant infusion over 12 to 24 hours. For coronary thrombosis, a bolus of 2,500 to

DRUG INTERACTIONS

Thrombolytic agents

Because of their anticoagulant effects, the thrombolytic agents are extremely dangerous when used with heparin, oral anticoagulants, and antiplatelet drugs.

DRUG	INTERACTING DRUGS	POSSIBLE EFFECTS	NURSING IMPLICATIONS
streptokinase, urokinase	heparin, oral anticoagulants, antiplatelet drugs (aspirin and dipyridamole)	Increase risk of bleeding	• Monitor the patient's thrombin time after therapy; do not administer heparin or oral anticoagulants until the patient's thrombin time is less than twice that of control. • Assess the patient for signs of bleeding, especially at puncture sites and invasive line insertion sites. • Assess the patient's vital signs for indication of hemorrhage.

Streptokinase therapy for acute myocardial infarction

Most researchers agree that prompt reperfusion of the coronary circulation by thrombolytic therapy improves left ventricular function and ejection fraction, thereby promoting immediate and long-term survival. As a result, thrombolytic therapy has become an accepted experimental treatment in certain patients with acute myocardial infarction.

Streptokinase can be administered intravenously or directly into the affected coronary artery via cardiac catheterization. Research results indicate higher reperfusion rates with the direct intracoronary route. Intracoronary thrombi have been dissolved in approximately 75% to 80% of patients when the intracoronary route was used, as opposed to 50% to 60% with the I.V. route. Better results have occurred when therapy is begun within 4 hours of the onset of acute chest pain and when the total dose of streptokinase is more than 200,000 units.

The protocol for intracoronary thrombolytic therapy includes:
• routine hematologic laboratory and coagulation studies
• pretreatment with an antihistamine and a corticosteroid to prevent allergic reactions
• 325 mg of aspirin P.O. and 10 mg of nifedipine sublingually (aspirin decreases platelet aggregation; nifedipine decreases coronary artery spasm)
• right and left ventricular catheterization
• localization of affected coronary artery
• nitroglycerin infusion to rule out coronary artery spasm
• for total occlusion, a bolus dose of 10,000 to 50,000 units over 1 to 2 hours, followed by continuous infusion of 2,000 to 5,000 units/minute until angiography confirms thrombolysis
• repeated coronary angiography every 15 minutes or until a maximum dose of 400,000 units
• streptokinase infusion continued for an additional 15 to 30 minutes.

The average streptokinase dose for intracoronary reperfusion is 200,000 to 400,000 units, and the average time is 30 to 45 minutes. If used to treat arteriovenous cannula occlusion or shunts, the usual dosage is 250,000 units in 2 ml of I.V. solution. This solution is injected into each limb of the catheter and clamped for 2 hours, after which the contents of each catheter are aspirated.

Streptokinase has also been used to dissolve thrombi in the axillary and subclavian veins after advancement of a catheter to the site of obstruction.

At the end of streptokinase therapy, heparin and oral anticoagulants are begun. Heparin, however, should not be given before the patient's thrombin time is less than twice the control.

Aminocaproic acid (Amicar)

Although its effectiveness is not well documented, aminocaproic acid is used as an antidote to the thrombolytic agents.

Action

• Inhibits plasminogen activator substances and, to a lesser degree, plasminic activity, thereby inhibiting thrombolysis

Administration and dosage

• Oral or I.V. loading dose of 5 grams followed by 1 gram/hour for the next 2 to 4 hours to a maximum of 30 grams in 24 hours
• For I.V. infusion, 4 to 5 grams diluted in 250 ml of diluent (normal saline solution, D_5W, or lactated Ringer's solution) for the first hour of treatment, followed by a continuous infusion of 1 gram/hour in 50 ml of diluent

Adverse reactions

• GI: nausea, cramps, diarrhea
• Cardiovascular: hypotension, especially if infused undiluted
• CNS: dizziness, tinnitus, headache, delirium, seizures
• Miscellaneous: conjunctival suffusion, nasal stuffiness, acute renal failure, thrombophlebitis, prolongation of menstruation

10,000 units of heparin I.V. followed with urokinase at 6,000 units/minute for up to 2 hours via intracoronary catheter. For a clot in a central catheter or shunt, 5,000 units/ml of I.V. fluid equal to the volume of the catheter is inserted and kept in the catheter for 5 to 60 minutes before being aspirated. If the clot cannot be dislodged, try again in 5 minutes. If the catheter still is not clear after 30 minutes, cap it and allow the urokinase to remain in the catheter for up to 1 hour. Then try to aspirate the clot again.

After the patient completes urokinase therapy, infuse heparin and an oral anticoagulant to prevent rethrombosis. Before starting the heparin infusion, verify the patient's thrombin time, the best indicator of thrombolytic therapy; it should be less than twice the normal control (usually about 4 hours after the cessation of urokinase).

Drug interactions

Streptokinase and urokinase interact with heparin, the oral anticoagulants, and the antiplatelet drugs to increase the patient's risk of bleeding. Heparin and the oral anticoagulants are often instituted after the therapy, but not until the patient's thrombin time is less than twice the control. Aminocaproic acid (Amicar) inhibits streptokinase and can be used to reverse its fibrinolytic effects. (See *Drug interactions: Thrombolytic agents* on page 690 for a summary of the drug interactions involving streptokinase and urokinase.)

ADVERSE DRUG REACTIONS

The major reactions associated with the thrombolytic agents are bleeding and allergic responses, especially with streptokinase. When administered via intracoronary catheter, the thrombolytic agents can produce hemorrhagic infarction at the site of myocardial necrosis, as well as reperfusion dysrhythmias.

Predictable reactions

Both during and after treatment, the nurse must closely assess the patient for signs of bleeding, which occurs frequently with thrombolytic therapy. Streptokinase and urokinase dissolve fibrin deposits at all sites, not just at the arterial thrombus obstructing coronary or pulmonary circulation. Thus, bleeding can occur at a sutured wound or any puncture site, such as an arterial line or central line catheter site. Pressure dressings applied to the oozing areas will usually control bleeding so that the dose does not have to be reduced.

Major bleeding may occur in some patients, resulting from a systemic bleeding disturbance. Hemorrhaging may occur intracranially, in the gastrointestinal (GI) or urinary tract, in the vagina, or retroperitoneally. The infusion of streptokinase or urokinase may be discontinued and blood replacement begun, as ordered, in such instances.

Allergic reactions to streptokinase are common, because most patients possess circulating streptococcal antibodies. Symptoms include urticaria, itching, flushing, nausea, headache, or musculoskeletal pain. The reperfusion dysrhythmias that occur are usually premature ventricular contractions requiring no treatment. Occasionally, more serious dysrhythmias, such as complex or grouped premature ventricular contractions, ventricular tachycardia, and fibrillation occur and may require emergency antiarrhythmic therapy or defibrillation. Bradycardia after intracoronary thrombolytic therapy may warrant treatment with atropine or a pacemaker.

Some patients experience fever (an average of 1.5 F. degrees [0.8 C. degrees] increase) after therapy, par-

Contraindications of thrombolytic agents

Careful patient selection reduces the probability of serious bleeding.

Absolute contraindications

Patients who:
• have had a prior allergic response to streptokinase (urokinase may be substituted)
• have active bleeding lesions
• have had an intracranial disorder (cerebrovascular accident, transient ischemic attacks, or neoplasm within last 2 months
• have had recent cardiopulmonary resuscitation
• have bleeding disorders such as hemophilia
• have had recent GI bleeding
• have severe uncontrolled hypertension

Relative contraindications

Patients who:
• are over age 70
• have a history of multiple MIs or previous coronary artery bypass surgery (because of the difficulty in identifying the vessel involved in the MI)
• have had large abrasive wounds, fractures, major surgery, or deep organ biopsies within last 10 days
• have severe hepatic failure
• have uremia
• are pregnant
• have diabetic hemorrhagic retinopathy
• have mitral stenosis with atrial fibrillation (because of the high likelihood of left ventricular thrombus)

ticularly after receiving streptokinase. The cause of this response has not been established.

Unpredictable reactions

An anaphylactic response to streptokinase, although rare, represents a serious unpredictable reaction. Symptoms range from minor breathing difficulties to bronchospasm, periorbital swelling, or angioneurotic edema. Some patients have experienced hemorrhagic infarction at the site of the myocardial damage after thrombolytic therapy. This reaction does not seem to have any clinical significance.

NURSING IMPLICATIONS

The careful selection of patients for thrombolytic therapy is the best method for preventing adverse reactions, particularly bleeding. Patients with active bleeding, especially in the GI tract, those with intracerebral pathology, and those who have had recent surgery, obstetrical delivery, deep organ biopsies, or cardiopulmonary resuscitation are at high risk for bleeding complications. Any patient on heparin therapy must be treated cautiously because of the synergistic effect between heparin and the thrombolytic agents. (See *Contraindications of thrombolytic agents* for a more comprehensive list.) The nurse also should be aware of these nursing implications:

SELECTED MAJOR DRUGS

Thrombolytic agents

Thrombolytic agents are used to dissolve thrombi in deep vein thrombosis, pulmonary embolism, arterial thrombosis and emboli, and coronary thrombosis. They are also used to dissolve clots in arteriovenous catheters.

DRUG	MAJOR INDICATIONS	USUAL ADULT DOSAGES	NURSING IMPLICATIONS
streptokinase	Deep vein thrombosis	250,000 units as a loading dose, then 100,000 units/hour I.V. for up to 72 hours	• The drug is contraindicated in patients with GI bleeding or intracerebral disorders and in patients who have had recent surgery, obstetrical delivery, deep organ biopsy, or cardiopulmonary resuscitation.
	Pulmonary embolism	A loading dose plus 100,000 units/hour I.V. for 24 hours	• Assess the patient for minor bleeding at puncture and wound sites. Apply pressure dressings to control bleeding, as ordered.
	Arterial thrombosis and embolism	5,000 to 50,000 units/hour	• Assess the patient's vital signs frequently for signs of bleeding.
	Coronary thrombosis	200,000 to 400,000 units I.V. over 30 to 45 minutes	• Assess the patient for allergic reactions to streptokinase. • Assess the patient for dysrhythmias during intracoronary perfusion.
	Dissolving clots in arteriovenous cannula	2 ml (250,000 units) injected into a cannula; clamp the cannula and wait 2 hours; then aspirate the drug and clot	• Immobilize the patient's leg for 24 hours after femoral coronary cannulation and perfusion and assess the pedal pulses for adequate circulation. • When reconstituting streptokinase, direct the flow of diluent against the side of the vial, then roll and tilt the vial gently to mix. Do not shake the vial because foaming and flocculation will occur.
urokinase	Pulmonary embolism	4,400 units/kg/hour I.V. as a loading dose, then 4,400 units/kg/hour I.V. for 12 to 24 hours	• The drug is contraindicated in patients with GI bleeding or intracerebral disorders and in patients who have had recent surgery, obstetrical delivery, deep organ biopsy, or recent cardiopulmonary resuscitation.
	Coronary thrombosis	A bolus of 2,500 to 10,000 units I.V. of heparin, followed by 6,000 units/minute for up to 2 hours	• Use the drug cautiously in patients on heparin therapy. • Reconstitute the drug immediately before use.
	I.V. catheter clearance	5,000 units/ml of I.V. fluid equal to the volume of the catheter injected into catheter; clamp the catheter and wait 5 minutes; then aspirate the drug and clot	

- Premedicate the patient with antihistamines and corticosteroids, as ordered, to decrease the allergic response to streptokinase.
- Monitor the patient's coagulation studies during thrombolytic therapy. Coagulation studies are recommended before and 4 hours after the systemic administration of streptokinase or urokinase. These studies should demonstrate a prolongation of partial thromboplastin time, a reduction in fibrinogen levels, and the appearance of FDPs. If these effects do not occur, the patient is probably resistant to the drug, and fibrinolysis of the thrombus is not occurring. Prothrombin time, thrombin time, activated partial thromboplastin time, quantitative fibrinogen, euglobulin clot lysis, and plasminogen levels can be used. Each of these studies measures different factors and times along the coagulation cascade. The partial thromboplastin time measures how quickly a clot forms after thrombin is added to a patient's plasma sample. Thrombin converts fibrinogen to a fibrin clot, and the time that elapses until clot formation provides an estimation of plasma fibrinogen levels.
- Treat severe bleeding complications by stopping the infusion and infusing fresh whole blood, packed red cells, or fresh frozen plasma, as ordered. The physician may order aminocaproic acid as an antidote. (See *Aminocaproic acid [Amicar]* on page 691 for more information about this substance.)
- Monitor the patient closely for signs of bleeding during thrombolytic therapy, especially at puncture and wound sites.
- Monitor the patient's vital signs frequently to assess for internal bleeding.
- Assess the patient's chest pain if the intracoronary route is used: a decrease may signal myocardial reperfusion. Also, evaluate the patient's electrocardiogram (EKG) pattern, especially the ST segment and any ventricular dysrhythmias. Monitor the patient's thrombin time 4 hours after the beginning of therapy. The thrombin time should be prolonged, indicating fibrinolysis. Report any excessive prolongation to the physician.
- Continue to assess the patient for bleeding complications for 24 hours after thrombolytic therapy.
- Leave the femoral venous and arterial sheaths in place for 24 hours after intracoronary thrombolytic therapy. Immobilize the patient's entire leg for 24 hours to prevent bleeding. If bleeding occurs at the femoral insertion site, apply direct pressure with a pressure dressing or Amicar-soaked sponges. Monitor the patient's color, temperature, and femoral, popliteal, and dorsalis pedis pulses every 15 minutes for 1 hour, then every 30 minutes for 8 hours, and then once each shift.
- Do not administer intramuscular (I.M.) injections or insert new arterial lines during therapy or for 24 hours after therapy.

- Administer medications through existing I.V. sites, orally, or by nasogastric tube, as ordered.
- Observe the patient for signs of microembolism, such as skin mottling, pallor, or cyanosis.
- Observe the patient's EKG for dysrhythmias, particularly premature ventricular contractions, ventricular tachycardia, or fibrillation.
- Keep antiarrhythmic drugs, such as lidocaine, and a defibrillator easily accessible at all times.
- Have aminocaproic acid available as an antidote.
- Observe the patient for signs of an allergic reaction to streptokinase: nausea, pruritus, flushing, fever, musculoskeletal pain, dyspnea, bronchospasm, and angioneurotic edema.
- Monitor the patient's thrombin time after thrombolytic therapy is stopped; it should be less than twice the control before instituting heparin therapy.
- Administer acetaminophen rather than aspirin, as ordered for a febrile response, to decrease the patient's risk of bleeding.
- Explain the treatment to the patient and family. Also explain that the patient may receive oral anticoagulant therapy to prevent rethrombosis after the critical phase has passed. (See Chapter 42, Anticoagulant Agents, for points to be included in patient teaching.)

CHAPTER SUMMARY

Chapter 43 presented the thrombolytic agents. These drugs activate and convert plasminogen to plasmin, which dissolves thrombi. The major disadvantage of streptokinase and urokinase is lack of specificity: they activate not only the plasminogen bound to the fibrin clot but also plasma plasminogen, creating a generalized systemic thrombolytic state that increases the risk of bleeding at puncture and wound sites. Here are the chapter highlights:

- The thrombolytic agents are used to dissolve thrombi in deep vein thrombosis, pulmonary embolism, arterial thrombosis and emboli, and coronary thrombosis and to clear clotted arteriovenous cannulas. These drugs are infused parenterally either into the general circulation or directly into the thrombosed blood vessel.
- The thrombolytic drugs are being studied for reperfusing coronary arteries after acute myocardial infarction. The intracoronary perfusion of the thrombolytic drugs has dissolved coronary thrombi in approximately 75%

to 80% of patients. However, the unpredictable outcomes make the widespread application of thrombolytic therapy risky.

• Researchers are presently developing a tissue-type plasminogen activator (t-PA). Theoretically, t-PA activates only fibrin-bound plasminogen and does not induce a systemic thrombolysis.

• In administering the thrombolytics, the nurse must control the infusion rate and carefully assess the patient for signs of bleeding and allergic reactions. Complications such as dysrhythmias and peripheral circulation disturbances after intracoronary reperfusion must be closely assessed. The nurse must be prepared to intervene quickly in hemorrhagic or cardiac dysrhythmic complications and should have appropriate emergency drugs and equipment available.

• Patients must be carefully selected for thrombolytic therapy, which should begin as soon as possible after thrombosis. Bleeding complications are significantly reduced if patients are free of blood dyscrasias, fresh surgical wounds, and intracerebral and GI pathology.

• If bleeding occurs, the nurse may have to stop the thrombolytic infusion and administer fresh whole blood, packed red cells, or fresh frozen plasma, as ordered.

• Aminocaproic acid (Amicar) may be used as an antidote, although this use is not well documented.

BIBLIOGRAPHY

Alter, B.R., et al. "Interventional Therapy for the Treatment of Acute Myocardial Infarction: Thrombolysis With and Without Angioplasty," *Cardiology Clinics* 3(1):29, February 1985.

Bertelé, V., and Salzman, E.W. "Antithrombotic Therapy in Coronary Artery Disease," *Arteriosclerosis* 5(2):119, March/April 1985.

Craig, C.R., and Stitzel, R.E. *Modern Pharmacology*, 2nd ed. Boston: Little, Brown & Co., 1986.

Dewood, M.A., and Amsterdam, E.E. "Value and Limitations of Thrombolytic Therapy in Early Acute Transmural Myocardial Infarction," *Cardiology* 72:255, September-December 1985.

Druy, E.M., et al. "Lytic Therapy in the Treatment of Axillary and Subclavian Vein Thrombosis," *Journal of Vascular Surgery* 2(6):821, November 1985.

Goodman, A.G., et al., eds. *Goodman and Gilman's The Pharmacological Basis of Therapeutics*, 7th ed. New York: Macmillan Publishing Co., 1985.

Kastrup, E.K., et al., eds. *Facts and Comparisons*. St. Louis: Facts and Comparisons Division, J.B. Lippincott Co., 1987.

Kleehammer, P.S., and Henson, B. "Intracoronary Streptokinase: Direct Attack on Acute MI," *RN* 46:26, December 1983.

Moake, J.L., and Levine, J.D. "Thrombotic Disorders," *Clinical Symposia* 37:4, 1985.

Palkuti, H.S. "Laboratory Monitoring of Anticoagulant Therapy," *Journal of Medical Technology* 2:81, 1985.

Rentrop, K.P. "Thrombotic Therapy in Patients with Acute Myocardial Infarction," *Circulation* 71(4):627, April 1985.

Sherry, S. "Tissue Plasminogen Activator (t-PA). Will It Fulfill Its Promise?" *New England Journal of Medicine* 313(16):1014, October 17, 1985.

Sherry, S., and Gustafson, E.R. "The Current and Future Use of Thrombolytic Therapy," *Annual Review of Pharmacology and Toxicology* 25:413, 1985.

Statland, B.E., and Ito, R.K. "Thrombolytic Therapy: Minimizing the Risks," *Diagnostic Medicine* 7(1):24, January 1984.

Topol, E., et al. "Coronary Thrombolysis with Recombinant Tissue-Type Plasminogen Activator," *Annals of Internal Medicine* 103(16):837, December 1985.

Verstraete, M., and Collen, D. "Thrombolytic Therapy in the Eighties," *Blood* 67(6):1529, June 1986.

DRUGS TO IMPROVE RESPIRATORY FUNCTION

The pharmacologic agents used to improve respiratory function that are discussed in this unit include methylxanthines, expectorants, antitussives, mucolytics, and decongestants. These drugs are used to relieve constricted airways, mucosal edema, cough, abnormally viscid secretions, and nasal congestion. Cromolyn sodium, an agent that prevents acute asthmatic attacks by stabilizing mast cells and inhibiting histamine, is also discussed. (See *Cromolyn sodium* for more on the use of this unique drug.)

Respiratory function
The respiratory system extends from the nose to the pulmonary capillaries. It oxygenates tissue, removes carbon dioxide, regulates acid-base balance, and provides defense against infection.

Glossary

Antitussive: agent that suppresses or inhibits cough.

Bronchoconstriction: narrowing of the bronchi, resulting in increased airway resistance and decreased airflow in conducting airways.

Bronchodilatation: state of relaxed bronchiolar smooth muscle cells, resulting in a widened lumen of the bronchi and bronchioles.

Bronchodilator: substance that relaxes the bronchioles.

Bronchorrhea: excessive secretions from the bronchial mucous membrane.

Bronchospasm: paroxysmal bronchoconstriction from smooth muscle constriction.

Cilia: minute, vibrating, hairlike projections attached to the free surface of cells.

Coryza: profuse discharge from the nasal mucosa.

Cough (tussis): sudden noisy expulsion of air from the lungs.

Decongestant: agent that reduces swelling of mucous membranes and relieves congestion.

Demulcent: agent that soothes inflamed mucous membranes.

Expectorant: agent that promotes the expulsion of respiratory secretions.

Goblet cells: unicellular mucous glands found especially in respiratory and gastrointestinal epithelium.

Inspissated: thickened or dried out; used to describe mucus.

Methylxanthines: drug classification that includes caffeine and theophylline, whose actions include central nervous system stimulation, smooth muscle relaxation, vasodilation, diuresis, and cardiac stimulation.

Minute ventilation: amount of air breathed in during a 1-minute period; can be calculated by multiplying the exhaled tidal volume by the respiratory rate. Also called total ventilation.

Mucin: mucopolysaccharide or glycoprotein that is the chief constituent of mucus.

Mucociliary clearance, or **escalator, mechanism:** defense mechanism of the respiratory tract, consisting of ciliated epithelial cells and mucous secretions that trap debris and bacteria and facilitate their removal.

Mucokinesis: movement of mucus in the respiratory tract.

Mucokinetic agents: agents that facilitate mucokinesis.

Mucolytic: having the ability to break down the composition of mucus.

Mucus: coating of the mucous membranes containing glandular secretions, various inorganic salts, desquamated cells, and leukocytes.

Respiratory insufficiency: impaired ability to oxygenate and remove carbon dioxide from the blood.

Rhinitis: inflammation of the nasal mucosa.

Sympathomimetics: agents that mimic the sympathetic nervous system by producing the same or similar effects on the end organ.

Vasoconstrictor: agent that constricts or narrows the lumen of blood vessels.

Viscid: sticky.

Cromolyn sodium

Cromolyn sodium was synthesized to enhance the bronchodilator properties of the chromone drug khellin. Structural modification of khellin yielded cromolyn, which lacks bronchodilator activity but prevents allergic bronchospasm.

Cromolyn sodium prevents the release of histamine and slow-reacting substance of anaphylaxis by stabilizing the mast cells membrane, thereby preventing further degranulation of the cells. This reduces the stimulus for bronchospasm and bronchoconstriction.

Cromolyn sodium is used clinically primarily as prophylactic treatment of bronchial asthma. It is not useful, however, in treating acute asthmatic attacks or status asthmaticus.

Cromolyn sodium is usually well tolerated by patients, even with prolonged continuous therapy. Adverse reactions are infrequent and minor. The most frequently seen adverse reactions are bronchospasm, sneezing, wheezing, cough, nasal congestion, and pharyngeal irritation. Dizziness, dysuria, joint swelling, joint pain, nausea, headache, and skin rash may also occur.

Cromolyn sodium is administered by inhalation because it is poorly absorbed after oral administration. The drug is not metabolized and is excreted unchanged, 50% in urine and 50% in bile.

Cromolyn sodium is available for inhalation in two forms, a metered-dose aerosol inhaler and a turbo inhaler. The aerosol delivers a small dose in a fine white mist. The turbo inhaler delivers a larger dose of dry white powder. Clinical trials have shown both delivery systems to be of equal efficacy. The aerosol requires the patient to synchronize his breathing with dose delivery. The turbo inhaler is less likely to be confused with the bronchodilators that are available and used for acute asthmatic attacks. The two types of devices are illustrated below.

When administering cromolyn sodium for bronchial asthma, monitor the patient's respiratory patterns and the integrity of the patient's nasal and oral passages before and after therapy. Also inform the patient that throat irritation and cough may be decreased by gargling and/or drinking after each treatment.

Metered-dose aerosol inhaler

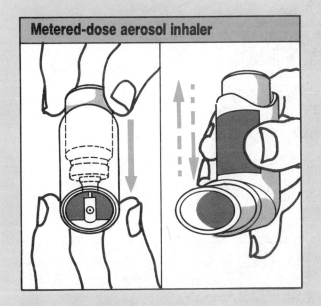

Turbo inhaler

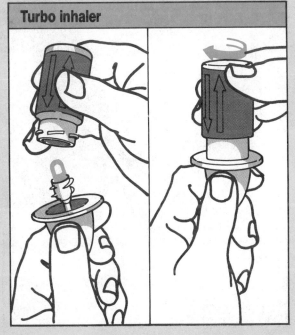

Oxygen–carbon dioxide exchange. Air flows into the lungs via the conducting airways (nose to bronchioles) and reaches the alveoli, where gas exchange occurs. Oxygen diffuses from the alveoli into the pulmonary capillaries, where most of the oxygen is bound to the hemoglobin in the red blood cells (RBCs). Only a small percentage is dissolved in the plasma. The RBCs are then transported to all tissues, where oxygen is diffused from the blood into the cell to be used for cellular metabolism. Carbon dioxide, a by-product of cellular me-

Normal respiratory anatomy and physiology

A knowledge of intrapulmonary blood circulation and gas exchange will help the nurse understand the actions of the drugs discussed in this unit. The respiratory system's major structures are illustrated below. The insert below right, shows intrapulmonary blood circulation around the alveolus; the insert below left, shows the partial pressures of the carbon dioxide and oxygen exchanged.

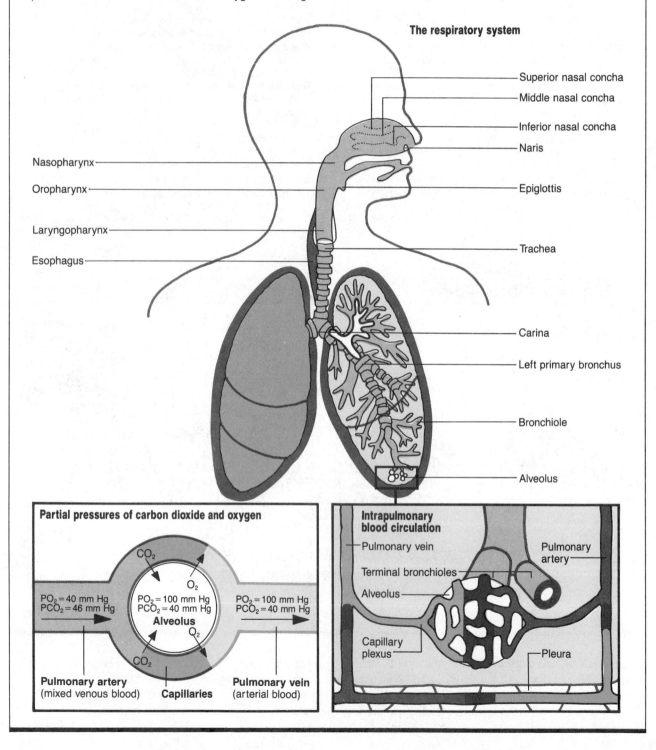

The respiratory system

- Superior nasal concha
- Middle nasal concha
- Inferior nasal concha
- Naris
- Epiglottis
- Trachea
- Carina
- Left primary bronchus
- Bronchiole
- Alveolus

Nasopharynx
Oropharynx
Laryngopharynx
Esophagus

Partial pressures of carbon dioxide and oxygen

CO_2
O_2

$PO_2 = 40$ mm Hg
$PCO_2 = 46$ mm Hg

$PO_2 = 100$ mm Hg
$PCO_2 = 40$ mm Hg
Alveolus

$PO_2 = 100$ mm Hg
$PCO_2 = 40$ mm Hg

O_2
CO_2

Pulmonary artery
(mixed venous blood)

Capillaries

Pulmonary vein
(arterial blood)

Intrapulmonary blood circulation

- Pulmonary vein
- Terminal bronchioles
- Alveolus
- Capillary plexus

Pulmonary artery

Pleura

Tissue lining respiratory tract

The cilia and acidic mucus produced by the goblet cells lining the respiratory tract are part of the respiratory system's defense mechanism.

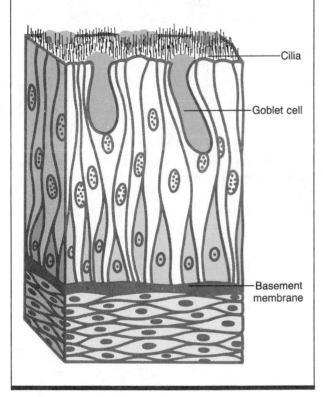

— Cilia

— Goblet cell

— Basement membrane

tabolism. Carbon dioxide, a by-product of cellular metabolism, is returned to the lungs to be eliminated. After diffusing from the blood into the alveoli, the carbon dioxide is exhaled from the lungs. (See *Normal respiratory anatomy and physiology* for an illustration of this process.) Such conditions as mucosal edema, alveolar damage, bronchoconstriction, or a disrupted mucociliary clearance mechanism affect the integrity of the respiratory structures and can alter oxygen–carbon dioxide gas exchange.

Acid-base balance. The respiratory system is a major regulator of acid-base balance; the blood-buffer system and the kidneys are the other regulators. Normal arterial blood pH ranges between 7.35 to 7.45; blood pH can be lowered or raised by the retention or excretion of hydrogen ions and bicarbonate ions. Carbon dioxide and water combine in the presence of carbonic anhydrase (a catalyst) to form carbonic acid, as follows:

$$CO_2 + H_2O \rightleftharpoons H_2CO_3 \rightleftharpoons H + HCO_3$$

This reaction, which is reversible, is affected by respiratory and renal function. In respiratory function, the retention of carbon dioxide increases hydrogen ion levels in the blood, thereby decreasing the blood pH; this process is known as respiratory acidosis. Similarly, the elimination of carbon dioxide by the respiratory system causes the blood to become more alkaline; this is known as respiratory alkalosis. The alterations in carbon dioxide levels are regulated by breathing frequency and the depth of the breaths, which is measured as minute ventilation. The respiratory system can restore normal arterial blood pH in minutes; however, dysfunction of the system can be the primary cause of an acid-base imbalance.

Defense mechanism. The nose filters, humidifies, and warms air during inhalation. It also traps particles in the mucosa to prevent their deposition lower in the respiratory tract. Both the mucosa and its secretions are influenced by the parasympathetic and sympathetic nervous systems. Sympathetic stimulation causes vasoconstriction of the nasal vascular structures and decreased mucus production. Parasympathetic stimulation has the opposite effect: it narrows the airway by vascular engorgement of mucosal tissues and increases mucus production.

Cilia are hairlike projections from the columnar epithelial cells that line the nasal and tracheal passageways. Ciliary undulations project respiratory secretions and particles toward the oropharynx to be coughed out or swallowed. The respiratory tract mucus, produced by the goblet cells, contains lysosomes and other elements that fight invading bacteria. The mucus also clears particles via the "mechanical" mucociliary escalator. (See *Tissue lining respiratory tract,* which depicts the action of cilia and mucus.)

The cough is a protective mechanism that rapidly expels air and particles from the airways. The sneeze clears the nasal passageway. Should particles evade the mucociliary defense mechanism and reach the lower respiratory tract, alveolar macrophages are present to phagocytize and detoxify them.

Chapter 44
Methylxanthine Agents

Methylxanthine agents are used to relax constricted airways (bronchospasm) and to treat bronchial asthma. The patient's response to methylxanthine therapy depends partially on the predominant problem—whether it is accumulated mucous or bronchial smooth muscle spasm. Many methylxanthine preparations are available; the parenteral route is used to treat acute bronchoconstriction, and the oral route is used for chronic maintenance therapy. The maintenance doses of methylxanthine agents are always individualized. Adrenergic bronchodilators, such as isoproterenol, albuterol, and metaproterenol, also are commonly used with methylxanthines to treat asthma; they are discussed in Unit Three.

Chapter 45
Expectorant, Antitussive, and Mucolytic Agents

Expectorant agents purportedly facilitate removal of the viscid mucus associated with various respiratory conditions, but their efficacy is doubtful. The most widely used expectorant agent is guaifenesin, an ingredient found in many over-the-counter cough and cold preparations. Patients with chronic respiratory diseases and associated mucus accumulation (such as bronchitis and emphysema) may receive expectorant and mucolytic agents as well as bronchodilators. Retained secretions can impair gas exchange and predispose the patient's lung tissue to bacterial growth. Therefore, the respiratory tract must be kept clear of excessive viscid secretions. Postural drainage and deep coughing, both important adjuncts to pharmacologic therapy, facilitate removal of respiratory secretions.

Antitussive agents are used to suppress cough. Both narcotic and nonnarcotic agents are used to help relieve an annoying, dry, hacking cough that interferes with the ability to talk or sleep. However, antitussive agents should be avoided in treating a patient with a productive cough, which is necessary and beneficial in clearing the airways.

Acetylcysteine is the only mucolytic agent used to treat patients with abnormally viscid, inspissated mucous secretions. It also is used orally to treat acetaminophen overdose.

Chapter 46
Decongestant Agents

Various sympathomimetic amines and local vasoconstrictors are available to treat nasal congestion associated with colds or allergic rhinitis. Systemic or topical decongestants can be administered to improve nasal airway patency by shrinking the respiratory mucosa. The agents differ in their duration of action, intensity of vasoconstriction, and potential for rebound congestion.

Nursing diagnoses

The nursing diagnoses that are most applicable to patients receiving drugs to improve respiratory function are:
- Activity intolerance related to impaired oxygenation
- Alterations in comfort related to pain from coughing or pleuritic irritation
- Alterations in nutrition related to coughing, accumulated secretions, and altered respiratory function
- Altered oral mucous membranes related to mouth breathing, coughing, and expectorating
- Altered thought processes related to impaired oxygenation
- Anxiety related to compromised respiratory function
- Fear related to altered respiratory function
- Impaired gas exchange related to altered respiratory function and an accumulation of secretions
- Impaired verbal communication related to coughing and altered respiratory function
- Ineffective airway clearance related to the accumulation of copious, tenacious secretions
- Ineffective breathing pattern related to bronchoconstriction, accumulated secretions, and coughing
- Knowledge deficit related to the etiology of altered respiratory function, drug therapy, or other interventions to facilitate improved respiratory function
- Potential for infection related to the accumulation of copious, tenacious secretions and altered respiratory function
- Potential increase in body temperature related to an accumulation of secretions
- Sensory-perceptual alteration related to altered respiratory function, coughing, and an accumulation of secretions
- Sleep pattern disturbance related to coughing and altered respiratory function.

CHAPTER 44

METHYLXANTHINE AGENTS

OBJECTIVES

After reading and studying this chapter, you should be able to:

1. Explain the clinical indications for theophylline, its derivatives, and caffeine.

2. Explain the actions of methylxanthine agents when they are used to treat asthma, chronic bronchitis, emphysema, and neonatal apnea.

3. Describe the pharmacokinetic properties of the various methlyxanthine agents, and explain their effects on drug administration.

4. Discuss the interactions associated with the methylxanthine agents and other drugs.

5. Describe the predictable and unpredictable adverse reactions to methylxanthine therapy and the nursing implications related to them.

6. Describe the signs and symptoms of methylxanthine toxicity.

INTRODUCTION

The methylxanthine agents (also called xanthines) are used extensively to treat asthma, chronic bronchitis, emphysema, and neonatal apnea. Theophylline and its derivatives and caffeine are the agents used to treat these disorders. Theophylline is also used for its diuretic effect in treating congestive heart failure (CHF) and Cheyne-Stokes respiration; however, this chapter does not cover these uses. Chapter 44 focuses on the methylxanthine agents as they are used to treat respiratory diseases.

For a summary of representative drugs, see *Selected major drugs: Methylxanthine agents* on pages 710 and 711.

THEOPHYLLINE, THEOPHYLLINE DERIVATIVES, AND CAFFEINE

The methylxanthine agents are used primarily to treat asthma, chronic bronchitis, emphysema, and neonatal apnea. The nurse should be aware, however, that some controversy exists regarding certain clinical uses for these agents.

History and source

The methylxanthine derivative agents are plant alkaloids easily obtained all over the world. Primarily methylated forms of xanthine, which is structurally related to uric acid, these agents have been consumed for centuries for their ability to elevate mood, decrease fatigue, and increase work capacity. Examples of some of the commonly consumed beverages are tea brewed from the leaves of *Thea sinensis*, which contains caffeine and small amounts of theophylline; coffee from *Coffea arabica* fruit; cola from *Cola acuminata* nuts; and chocolate and cocoa from *Theobroma cacao* seeds, which contain theobromine and some caffeine.

Introduced in 1946, dyphylline was developed in an attempt to find a methylxanthine agent that could act as a bronchodilator but be more soluble and less toxic than theophylline. Today, theophylline and its derivatives and caffeine are manufactured synthetically.

PHARMACOKINETICS

The methylxanthine agents vary pharmacokinetically according to the agent administered, its dosage form, and the route of administration. The pharmacokinetic dif-

Theophylline salts

Theophylline is only slightly water-soluble. Its solubility can be increased by mixing it with other elements, to form theophylline salts.

THEOPHYLLINE FORMULATION	PERCENTAGE OF THEOPHYLLINE CONTENT	EQUIVALENT DOSE FOR A 100-MG DOSE OF THEOPHYLLINE
anhydrous theophylline (Slo-bid Gyrocaps, Theo-Dur, Theo-24)	100%	100 mg
anhydrous aminophylline (Aminophyllin Injection, Somophyllin-DF Oral Liquid, Somophyllin Rectal Solution)	85%	118 mg
oxtriphylline (Brondecon, Choledyl)	64%	156 mg
theophylline sodium glycinate (Asbron G, Synophylate)	46%	217 mg

ferences are particularly significant with the theophylline salts (aminophylline, oxtriphylline, and theophylline sodium glycinate), developed to increase the solubility of theophylline, which is only slightly water-soluble. When administered orally or parenterally, the salts appear as theophylline in the blood. (See *Theophylline salts* for the amount of theophylline contained in the various products.) Dyphylline is freely water-soluble, and is not dissociated to theophylline in blood. Caffeine is more soluble than theophylline in water and lipids and, because caffeine is a weak base, its solubility can be increased in the presence of citric and benzoic acids.

Absorption

Theophylline's rate and extent of absorption depend on the dosage form administered. When theophylline is given as an oral liquid, a rapid-release tablet, or a retention enema, it is rapidly and completely absorbed. However, rectal suppositories are erratically absorbed and less commonly used. Absorption of some of the slow-release products (Theolair-SR and Theo-24) de-

pends on gastric pH, which affects the rate of dissolution and extent of absorption. Administering other slow-release products (Theo-Dur Sprinkle, Uniphyl) with meals can significantly alter absorption. Because of these factors, slow-release theophylline products should be administered with a small amount of food or when the patient's stomach is empty. Also, substituting one slow-release theophylline product for another is inadvisable, because their rate and extent of absorption may vary.

Dyphylline is incompletely absorbed after oral or I.M. administration and is approximately 75% bioavailable.

Caffeine is well absorbed after oral administration; however, rectal preparations may be absorbed slowly and erratically. Caffeine should not be given I.M. because of the irritating effect of the solution.

Distribution

The volume of distribution for theophylline ranges from 0.3 liter/kg to 0.7 liter/kg of body weight, averaging 0.5 liter/kg. These values remain relatively constant from infants to adults, even in the presence of other disease states. Theophylline is not distributed well into adipose tissue, so theophylline dosage should be based on the patient's ideal or actual body weight, whichever is less. Theophylline is approximately 60% protein-bound in adults but only about 36% protein-bound in the neonate. It readily crosses the placenta, producing similar serum concentration levels in the mother and fetus. Theophylline also crosses into breast milk.

No information on dyphylline's distribution and protein-binding capacity is available.

Caffeine is distributed rapidly and widely. The volume of distribution is approximately 0.5 liter/kg in adults and 0.8 liter/kg in neonates. Less than 20% of a caffeine dose is protein-bound in the plasma. Caffeine readily crosses the blood-brain barrier and the placenta, and small amounts appear in breast milk.

Metabolism and excretion

Theophylline is metabolized primarily in the liver. Because theophylline's rate of metabolism varies greatly among patients, dosages need to be individualized and serum concentration levels monitored. Liver disease, CHF, cor pulmonale, pulmonary edema, and prolonged high fever can decrease theophylline's metabolism and prolong half-life. Certain drugs can also increase or decrease theophylline's elimination. (See *Drug interactions: Theophylline*, on page 708.) Also, smoking and high-protein diets increase the theophylline excretion rate, whereas high-carbohydrate diets decrease it. In children and adults, about 10% of a dose is excreted unchanged in the urine; in neonates and infants, as much as 50% of a dose may be excreted unchanged in the urine because the immature liver has limited metabolizing ability. The major metabolites are also excreted in the urine.

Dyphylline is unmetabolized. Approximately 83% of a dose is excreted unchanged in the urine. Because dyphylline is not converted to theophylline, the nurse cannot use theophylline serum concentration levels to monitor therapy. Dyphylline should not be used in neonates because information concerning such use is lacking.

Although caffeine can be a significant metabolite of theophylline in neonates, it is not a major metabolite in older infants or adults.

Like theophylline, caffeine is extensively metabolized by the liver. In an adult, about 2% of a dose is excreted unchanged in the urine; in the neonate, however, about 85% of a dose is excreted this way.

Onset, peak, duration

Theophylline's onset and duration of action are related to the patient's serum theophylline concentration level, which in turn depends on the drug's absorption and excretion rates. The excretion rate varies significantly from patient to patient. (See *Theophylline half-life* for averages among different patient groups.) To treat respiratory disease, a serum concentration level of 10 to 20 mcg/ml is considered therapeutic. To treat neonatal apnea, a serum concentration level of 5 to 10 mcg/ml is required.

To achieve a therapeutic serum concentration level of theophylline rapidly, physicians often order a loading dose to be administered as a rapid-release tablet or liquid or an aminophylline I.V. injection. Using these preparations and administration routes produces theophylline's onset of action within 1 hour. Subsequently, a maintenance dose is started to keep theophylline's serum concentration level within the therapeutic range. If no loading dose is administered, the maximum benefit from theophylline therapy occurs when the amount of drug excreted and the amount of drug absorbed is the same (steady state). For example, the average half-life of theophylline administered to a child age 2 is 4 hours. Steady state occurs after the patient has begun maintenance therapy and five half-lives have passed—that is, in 20 hours (5 × 4 hours) or approximately 1 day. At this time, the serum peak and serum trough concentration levels are approximately the same after each dose.

The nurse should monitor peak serum concentration levels because they correlate with both peak effectiveness and drug toxicity. (See "Predictable reactions"

Theophylline half-life

The half-life of theophylline can vary greatly from patient to patient. For this reason, theophylline blood concentration levels should be monitored to provide useful clinical information for proper dosage and patient monitoring.

PATIENT POPULATION	AVERAGE HALF-LIFE*
Neonate	20 to 30 hours
Children age 1 to 12	3 to 4 hours
Nonsmoking adults	7 to 8 hours
Nonsmoking elderly adults	9 to 10 hours
Smoking adults	4 to 5 hours

*In patients without diseases that can alter theophylline pharmacokinetics.

---

on page 709.) When an oral rapid-release tablet or liquid is administered, peak concentration level is achieved about 1 to 2 hours after a dose. (See *Maintaining serum theophylline concentration levels* on page 704 for further information.) As theophylline concentration levels decrease to below the therapeutic range, the drug effects also decrease. Duration of action is influenced by the half-life of the product used. In general, the half-life averages 3½ hours for young children and 8 to 9 hours for adults.

Dyphylline's half-life is 2 to 2½ hours. In anuric patients, the half-life may increase to 3 to 4 times the normal range. After oral or I.M. administration, peak serum concentration levels occur in about 1 hour. Dyphylline's onset and duration of action remain unknown because therapeutic serum concentration levels have not been determined.

Caffeine's onset of action usually occurs within 30 minutes after administration and peak concentration levels within 1 to 2 hours. Caffeine's duration of action depends on the patient's serum concentration levels. In treating neonatal apnea, serum caffeine concentration levels of 5 to 20 mcg/ml are considered therapeutic. Caffeine's half-life in the neonate ranges from 31 to 144 hours, averaging greater than 60 hours. The half-life decreases with age, averaging 3 to 6 hours in adults.

PHARMACODYNAMICS

The methylxanthine agents display similar pharmacologic activity but may differ in the intensity of their effects on the target organs.

Because most methylxanthine agents are powerful central nervous system (CNS) stimulants, they decrease drowsiness and fatigue and stimulate more rapid thinking. These agents also increase awareness of sensory stimuli while decreasing reaction time. In the medulla, these agents stimulate the respiratory center; in the spinal cord, they increase reflex excitability. After CNS excitation by methylxanthine agents, the patient usually experiences a slight depression.

The methylxanthine agents also act on the cardiovascular system, directly stimulating the myocardium and increasing myocardial contractility. By directly relaxing vascular smooth muscle, these agents dilate coronary, pulmonary, and systemic blood vessels. They also strengthen skeletal muscle contractions and reduce muscle fatigability. Methylxanthine agents also cause diuresis, partly the result of improved cardiac function from increased renal blood flow and glomerular filtration rate. These agents appear to have a direct action at the renal tubules, increasing sodium and chloride excretion.

Of all the methylxanthine agents, theophylline provides potent cardiac stimulation, smooth muscle relaxation, and diuresis. Caffeine provides the most potent CNS and skeletal muscle stimulation.

Methylxanthine agents stimulate gastric acid secretion; this may partly explain the adverse gastrointestinal (GI) reactions they can cause.

Mechanisms of action

Although methylxanthine agents decrease nonspecific airway reactivity and, in the presence of bronchospasm, relax bronchial smooth muscle, their specific mechanism of action in reversible obstructive airway disease, such as asthma, is incompletely understood. Researchers believe that these agents inhibit the enzyme phosphodiesterase, causing decreased degradation of cyclic AMP (adenosine $3',5'$ monophosphate), an apparent bronchodilator. However, theophylline inhibits this enzyme at in vitro concentration levels considerably higher than are considered clinically safe. Thus, this enzyme-inhibiting action does not account for the actions of these agents. A more likely explanation for the action of the methylxanthine agents is the inhibition of adenosine receptors. Other proposed mechanisms of action include the antagonism of prostaglandins and the effects on the translocations of intracellular calcium.

In nonreversible obstructive airway disease (chronic bronchitis, emphysema, and apnea), the methylxanthine agents appear to increase the central respiratory center's sensitivity to carbon dioxide while also stimulating respiratory drive. In chronic bronchitis and emphysema, these agents decrease diaphragmatic fatigue and improve cardiac ventricular function.

Maintaining serum theophylline concentration levels

This chart provides suggested theophylline dosage changes for maintaining a therapeutic serum concentration level based on peak serum concentration levels drawn with the patient at a steady-state level.

SERUM CONCENTRATION LEVELS	SUGGESTED DOSAGE CHANGES
<7.5 mcg/ml	Increase daily dosage by up to 25%; recheck serum concentration levels during steady state before further dosage changes.
7.5 to 10 mcg/ml	Increase daily dosage by up to 25%; recheck serum concentration levels within at least 6 months.
10 to 20 mcg/ml	No dosage change; if patient is on long-term oral treatment, recheck serum concentration levels every 6 to 12 months or if adverse reactions to theophylline occur; if steady-state levels are in the upper therapeutic range, a 10% dosage decrease may be ordered if adverse reactions occur.
20 to 25 mcg/ml	Decrease the daily dosage by 10%, as ordered, even if no adverse reactions occur; recheck serum theophylline concentration levels within at least 6 months.
25 to 30 mcg/ml	Omit the next dose and decrease daily dosage by 25%, as ordered; recheck serum theophylline concentration levels during steady state.
> 30 mcg/ml	Omit the next two doses and decrease the dosage by 50%, as ordered; recheck serum theophylline concentration levels during steady state.

To ensure the patient is at a steady-state level, theophylline doses should be administered at regular intervals, with no doses missed for 48 to 72 hours.

Reprinted with permission from Weinberger, M. "Slow-Release Theophylline Rational and Basis for Product Selection," *New England Journal of Medicine* 308(13):760–64, March 31, 1983.

PHARMACOTHERAPEUTICS

Theophylline, its salts (aminophylline, oxtriphylline, and theophylline sodium glycinate), and dyphylline are indicated to treat asthma, chronic bronchitis, and emphysema. Caffeine is used primarily as a CNS stimulant and may be found in many OTC preparations, prescription antihistamines, and barbituates (to offset the sedative effects of these drugs), and with ergot alkaloids to produce cerebrovascular constriction in the treatment of migraine headaches. Theophylline and caffeine are also used to treat neonatal apnea, although their use for this condition is unapproved by the Food and Drug Administration (FDA).

Theophylline acts as a bronchodilator, assists in ventricular emptying, decreases diaphragmatic fatigue, and increases mucociliary clearance. Theophylline relieves the bronchospasm associated with asthma better than dyphylline does. On a milligram-for-milligram basis, theophylline appears to have approximately 5 to 10 times the potency of dyphylline; however, it also causes

Guidelines for suggested theophylline dosage for infants

Because the theophylline half-life is longer in infants compared with older children and adults, theophylline dosing must be conservative. Guidelines suggest theophylline be given 1 to 3 mg/kg every 6 to 12 hours as listed below.

INFANT (UP TO AGE 6 MONTHS)	MAINTENANCE DOSAGE
Preterm (younger than 40 weeks postconception)	1 mg/kg every 12 hours
Term (birth or 40 weeks postconception) Up to 4 weeks postnatal	1 to 2 mg/kg every 12 hours
Age 4 to 8 weeks	1 to 2 mg/kg every 8 hours
Age 8 weeks and older	1 to 3 mg/kg every 6 hours
Postconception age = gestational age at birth + postnatal age	

Long-term oral theophylline dosing

The theophylline dose is based on ideal body weight or actual body weight, whichever is less. (Actual weight up to 25% over ideal weight is also safe.) To determine the effects of a particular dosage on serum concentration levels, obtain peak concentration serum levels after no doses have been missed for 48 to 72 hours.

When changing dosages based on serum concentration levels, the total daily dose is divided into an appropriate dosage interval for the product used. For patients age 1 or older, start at 16 mg/kg/day or a maximum of 400 mg/day, whichever is less. After 3 days with no adverse reactions, increase to 20 mg/kg/day for ages 1 to 9 and 16 mg/kg/day for ages 9 and older, but no more than 600 mg/day. After an additional 3 days without adverse reactions, increase the dosage to the following.

AGE	DOSAGE
1 to 9 years	22 mg/kg/day
9 to 12 years	20 mg/kg/day
12 to 16 years	18 mg/kg/day
16 years and older	13 mg/kg/day

The maximum daily dosage should not exceed 800 mg/day without theophylline serum concentration level monitoring.

Reprinted with permission from Weinberger, M. "Slow-Release Theophylline Rationale and Basis for Product Selection," *New England Journal of Medicine* 308(13):760-64, March 31, 1983.

more adverse reactions. Concomitant use of beta$_2$-adrenergic stimulants, such as albuterol, terbutaline, and metaproterenol, with theophylline or dyphylline produces additive bronchodilation in patients with chronic stable asthma but is controversial as therapy for patients with acute asthma. Beta$_2$-adrenergic agents relieve acute bronchospasm better than theophylline does. Combined use of these drugs to treat acute asthma is still common, although it does not appear to produce additive effects.

Treating chronic bronchitis and emphysema with theophylline or dyphylline is also controversial because bronchospasm is not a major component of these diseases: thus, the methylxanthine agents' activity is related to their effects on nonspecific airway reactivity, the diaphragm, ventricular function, and mucus clearance. To date, theophylline has produced subjective improvements—for example, the patient claims to feel less breathless—but researchers have not substantiated them objectively. Anticholinergic agents (atropine and ipratropium), beta$_2$-adrenergics, and theophylline are used to provide symptomatic relief for patients with chronic bronchitis and emphysema.

In patients with neonatal apnea (with or without bradycardia), theophylline and caffeine are equally effective. Theophylline is more readily available, but caf-

Dosage intervals for theophylline

Each type of theophylline product has its own recommended dosage interval that should be maintained to ensure optimum efficacy. If the total daily theophylline dosage is divided by the number of dosage intervals in a 24-hour period, the dosage can be determined.

DRUG	PATIENT POPULATION	
	Children and smoking adults	Nonsmoking adolescents and adults
Anhydrous theophylline		
Slow-release tablets		
Constant-T	q 8 hr	q 12 hr
LABID	q 8 hr	q 12 hr
Quibron-T/SR	q 8 hr	q 12 hr
*Respbid	q 8 hr	q 12 hr
Sustaire	q 12 hr	q 12 hr
Theo-Dur	q 12 hr	q 12 to 24 hr
*Theolair-SR	q 8 hr	q 12 hr
*Uniphyl	—	q 12 to 24 hr
Slow-release capsules		
Bronkodyl S-R	q 8 hr	q 12 hr
Elixophyllin SR	q 8 hr	q 12 hr
Slo-bid Gyrocaps	q 12 hr	q 12 hr
Slo-Phyllin Gyrocaps	q 8 hr	q 12 hr
Somophyllin-CRT	q 8 hr	q 12 hr
*Theo-24	—	q 12 to 24 hr
Theobid Duracaps	q 8 hr	q 12 hr
Theoclear L.A.	q 8 hr	q 12 hr
*Theo-Dur Sprinkle	q 12 hr	q 12 hr

DRUG	PATIENT POPULATION	
	Children and smoking adults	Nonsmoking adolescents and adults
Slow-release capsules (continued)		
Theophyl-SR	q 8 hr	q 12 hr
Theospan-SR	q 8 hr	q 12 hr
Theovent	q 8 hr	q 12 hr
Rapid-release oral liquids, tablets		
regardless of brand used	q 4 to 6 hr	q 6 to 8 hr
Aminophylline		
Rapid-release oral tablets, liquids, or rectal solutions		
regardless of brand used	q 4 to 6 hr	q 6 to 8 hr
Slow-release tablets		
Phyllocontin	q 8 hr	q 12 hr
Oxtriphylline		
Rapid-release tablet or liquids		
Choledyl	q 6 hr	q 6 to 8 hr
Slow-release tablets		
Choledyl SA	q 8 hr	q 12 hr
Theophylline sodium glycinate		
Rapid-release liquid		
Synophylate	q 6 hr	q 6 to 8 hr

*The rate and extent of absorption can be significantly affected when theophylline is given with food.

feine has a longer half-life, making a once-daily dosage possible. Caffeine may also have a wider therapeutic index.

anhydrous theophylline (Slo-bid Gyrocaps, Theo-24, Theo-Dur). Available in a variety of oral formulations, anhydrous theophylline is used to treat asthma, chronic bronchitis, and emphysema. Therapy should be guided by monitoring serum theophylline levels, patient response, and the occurrence of adverse reactions.

USUAL ADULT DOSAGE: for asthma, chronic bronchitis, and emphysema, dosage varies and is calculated based on actual or ideal body weight, whichever is less. Usually the initial maximum dosage for adults is 13 mg/kg/day or a total of 800 mg/day, whichever is less. (See *Long-*

term oral theophylline dosing on page 705 for suggested amounts.) For instituting oral therapy after administering I.V. aminophylline, the total daily dosage of oral theophylline should equal the aminophylline hourly infusion rate multiplied by 24 hours × 0.8 (aminophylline is 80% theophylline). When switching a patient from I.V. to oral therapy, the I.V. administration should be discontinued when the oral administration begins. (See *Dosage intervals for theophylline* for suggested intervals for different preparations.)

For neonatal apnea, the therapeutic serum concentration level is 5 to 10 mcg/ml; loading dose, 5 mg/kg P.O. or I.V. (if I.V., administer over 20 to 30 minutes); maintenance dose, 2 mg/kg every 12 hours; final dosage is determined by serum theophylline concentration levels and patient response.

aminophylline (Aminophylline, Somophyllin). Available in an oral liquid, a rectal solution, an injectable solution, tablets, and suppositories, aminophylline is used to treat asthma, chronic bronchitis, and emphysema. Dosage should be based on the theophylline content of the preparation.

USUAL ADULT DOSAGE: a loading dose may be given first. If the patient has received no aminophylline or theophylline in the previous 24 hours, the loading dose is 5 to 6 mg/kg I.V. over 20 to 30 minutes to avoid cardiac toxicity. If the patient has received aminophylline or theophylline in the previous 24 hours, the serum theophylline concentration level should be determined before giving any additional aminophylline. This serum concentration level serves as the basis for calculating the loading dose. If the serum theophylline concentration level cannot be determined quickly, some physicians elect to give half the normal loading dose, or 2.5 to 3 mg/kg. After the loading dose, a maintenance dose of 0.4 to 0.7 mg/kg/hr is administered I.V. or the patient is switched to the oral dosage form.

Aminophylline should be given as a constant infusion with the use of an infusion pump. If the patient has been on oral theophylline long-term in therapeutic dosages, the hourly infusion rate can be determined by dividing the daily dose by 24 hours. For example, a patient who has been receiving 600 mg/day of theophylline should be given an infusion of 25 mg/hr (600 mg ÷ 24 hr = 25 mg/hr ÷ 0.8 = 31 mg/hr of aminophylline). For oral administration, calculate the long-term oral dose of theophylline and divide by 0.8. (See *Long-term oral theophylline dosing* on page 705; *Guidelines for suggested theophylline dosage for infants* on page 705; and *Dosage intervals for theophylline* for adult and pediatric dosage schedules.) Some aminophylline products state the amount of theophylline in each dosage unit.

Rectal administration of theophylline may be accomplished using aminophylline rectal solutions; however, because of erratic and incomplete absorption, rectal suppositories are not recommended. Retention enemas have limited patient acceptability because of the retention volume required. Dosages and dosage intervals are the same as those for rapid-release oral theophylline products.

oxtriphylline (Brondecon, Choledyl). This agent is used to treat asthma, chronic bronchitis, emphysema, and similar chronic obstructive pulmonary diseases. To calculate the oxtriphylline dosage, divide the anhydrous theophylline dose by 0.64 because oxtriphylline is about 64% anhydrous theophylline.

USUAL ADULT DOSAGE: 200 mg P.O. every 6 to 8 hours.
USUAL PEDIATRIC DOSAGE: for ages 2 to 12, 3.7 mg/kg P.O. every 6 hours. (See *Dosage intervals for theophylline* for appropriate dosage intervals for the product used.)

theophylline sodium glycinate (Asbron G, Synophylate). This theophylline salt, containing approximately 46% theophylline, is used to treat asthma, chronic bronchitis, and emphysema.

USUAL ADULT DOSAGE: 330 to 600 mg P.O. every 6 to 8 hours.
USUAL PEDIATRIC DOSAGE: for ages 6 to 12, 220 to 330 mg P.O. every 6 to 8 hours; for ages 3 to 6, 110 to 165 mg P.O. every 6 to 8 hours; for ages 1 to 3, 55 to 110 mg P.O. every 6 to 8 hours.

dyphylline (Dylline, Lufyllin). Dyphylline is used to treat acute and chronic bronchial asthma and reversible bronchospasms associated with chronic bronchitis and emphysema.

USUAL ADULT DOSAGE: up to 15 mg/kg P.O. every 6 hours, or 250 to 500 mg I.M. up to a maximum of 15 mg/kg every 6 hours.
USUAL PEDIATRIC DOSAGE: 4.4 to 6.6. mg/kg/day in divided doses.

caffeine. Physicians usually prescribe caffeine as caffeine citrate, which contains a 50% caffeine base. This preparation must be compounded extemporaneously, because it is unavailable commercially. The I.V. caffeine and sodium benzoate solution available commercially should not be used in neonates, because the benzoate will displace bound bilirubin.

USUAL PEDIATRIC DOSAGE: in neonatal apnea, a loading dose of 10 mg/kg P.O. of caffeine base; for maintenance, 2.5 mg/kg/day P.O. of caffeine base started 24 hours after the initial loading dose.

DRUG INTERACTIONS
Theophylline

Interactions between theophylline and other drugs often increase the risk of toxicity or subtherapeutic levels.

DRUG	INTERACTING DRUGS	POSSIBLE EFFECTS	NURSING IMPLICATIONS
theophylline	cimetidine	Increases theophylline concentration levels by inhibiting theophylline's rate of metabolism, resulting in potentially toxic levels	● Avoid concomitant cimetidine administration. If an H_2-antagonist is desired, ranitidine or famotidine can be used instead, because they do not significantly alter theophylline's metabolism.
	erythromycin	Increases theophylline concentration levels by altering theophylline's rate of metabolism	● If administered concomitantly, decrease the theophylline dosage by 25%, as ordered, and monitor the patient for theophylline's adverse reactions.
	troleandomycin	Increases theophylline concentration levels by altering theophylline's rate of metabolism	● Avoid concomitant administration with theophylline.
	allopurinol (high dose)	Increases theophylline concentration levels, probably by altering theophylline's rate of metabolism	● Observe the patient for signs and symptoms of theophylline toxicity, such as palpitations and restlessness.
	oral contraceptives	Possibly increase serum theophylline concentration levels, probably by inhibiting the cytochrome P-450 system	● Encourage the patient to use an alternative contraception method, if possible.
	propranolol	Increases theophylline concentration levels by altering theophylline's rate of metabolism	● Because propranolol can cause bronchospasm, do not administer it to patients with pulmonary disease.
	phenobarbital, phenytoin, rifampin, carbamazepine	Possibly decrease serum theophylline concentration levels, probably by increasing theophylline's rate of metabolism	● Monitor the patient's serum theophylline concentration levels and expect the dosage to be adjusted.
	halothane	Increases cardiac toxicity	● Administer concomitantly with extreme caution.
	lithium	Increases lithium clearance	● Monitor serum lithium levels and expect the dosage to be adjusted.

Drug interactions

Some interactions that can occur between theophylline or its salts and food or other drugs can result in dangerously elevated or subtherapeutic drug levels and subsequent loss of effectiveness.

Drugs that frequently cause excessive serum theophylline concentration levels when given with theophylline include cimetidine, troleandomycin, erythromycin, propranolol, oral contraceptives, and high doses of allopurinol. Other agents that can increase theophylline concentration levels are vidarabine, verapamil, thiabendazole, furosemide, quinolone antibiotics such as ciprofloxacin, and influenza vaccines.

Drugs that increase theophylline excretion and thereby decrease serum concentration levels include phenobarbital, phenytoin, carbamazepine, and rifampin. Smoking cigarettes or marijuana also increases theophylline elimination. Taking some theophylline products near mealtimes can decrease their rate and extent of absorption. As discussed previously, diet can also affect the rate of theophylline excretion from the body.

Probenecid inhibits renal excretion of dyphylline, increasing its half-life and prolonging its action. Drugs that alter theophylline's metabolism and excretion do not affect dyphylline; however, drugs that affect theophylline's excretion may also affect caffeine's excretion. Concomitant administration of adrenergic agonists or consumption of caffeinated beverages may result in additive adverse reactions or signs and symptoms of methylxanthine toxicity. (See *Drug interactions: Theophylline* for a summary of the interactions between this and other drugs.)

ADVERSE DRUG REACTIONS

The adverse reactions to the methylxanthine agents can be transient or symptomatic of toxicity. These reactions commonly affect the central nervous, cardiac, and gastrointestinal systems.

Predictable reactions

Administering methylxanthine agents, particularly theophylline, may first produce toxicity and other adverse reactions rather than therapeutic effects. These transient adverse reactions can occur (1) when a patient who has not previously taken the drug begins methylxanthine therapy; (2) when a patient who has previously taken the drug, but not recently, restarts the therapy; or (3) when the dosage is increased for a patient who is already taking the drug and is experiencing a change in health status or altered dietary intake. These adverse reactions, which usually occur shortly after administration of the first dose, can affect the GI tract and the central nervous system (CNS). Irritation of the GI tract and increased gastric acid secretion may cause nausea, vomiting, abdominal cramping, epigastric pain, anorexia, or diarrhea. CNS adverse reactions include headache, irritability, restlessness, anxiety, insomnia, and dizziness (rarely).

Methylxanthine agents can also produce adverse reactions when a dose results in a high serum concentration level. (For theophylline and caffeine, this level is usually above 20 mcg/ml.) After administration of a rapid-release product, such adverse reactions can occur within 1 to 2 hours; after an I.V. loading dose, they can occur shortly after the infusion is completed, usually within 1 hour. With slow-release theophylline preparations, adverse reactions can occur 3 to 8 hours after administration. The adverse reactions that may occur include nausea, vomiting, diarrhea, and such CNS symptoms as irritability, insomnia, anxiety, headache, and seizures (with very high drug concentration levels).

Although theophylline crosses into breast milk, its use is not contraindicated in a lactating patient. The nurse, however, should be aware that the neonate may experience tachycardia or vomiting. Monitoring the patient for these adverse reactions is important. Methylxanthine agents can also irritate the myocardium, producing such cardiovascular symptoms as tachycardia, palpitations, extrasystoles, or dysrhythmias. Also, these drugs can cause peripheral vasodilation and hypotension.

Unpredictable reactions

Although hypersensitivity reactions to methylxanthine can occur, they are extremely rare and are typically associated with the base of the theophylline salt formulations. For example, the ethylenediamine component of aminophylline can produce a type of contact dermatitis. Some patients may not tolerate methylxanthine agents very well; usually less than 1% of children and 4% of adults receiving theophylline will develop these severe reactions. These unpredictable reactions can occur even with a dose too low to achieve a therapeutic effect. Shortly after receiving the drug, the hypersensitive patient displays severe signs and symptoms of theophylline toxicity, which may include nausea, vomiting, diarrhea, headache, and occasionally anxiety and dizziness.

NURSING IMPLICATIONS

When administering methylxanthine agents, the nurse must observe numerous precautions:
- Be aware that methylxanthine agents are contraindicated in patients with a history of hypersensitivity to them. Such a patient may display cross-sensitivity to all these agents.
- Do not administer rectal methylxanthine solutions or suppositories if rectal irritation or infection is present.
- Be aware that dyphylline injection is for I.M. use only.
- Aminophylline given I.M. produces severe pain at the injection site.
- Administer methylxanthine products cautiously in patients with seizure disorders, migraine headaches, dysrhythmias, acute myocardial infarction, or other cardiac diseases. These agents can worsen cardiac problems by causing cardiac irritation.
- Administer dyphylline cautiously in a patient with impaired renal function because the drug undergoes renal excretion after limited metabolism and may accumulate in such a patient.

Methylxanthine agents

This chart summarizes the major methylxanthine derivative agents currently in clinical use.

DRUG	MAJOR INDICATIONS	USUAL ADULT DOSAGES	NURSING IMPLICATIONS
theophylline	Asthma, bronchitis, and emphysema. The rapid-release oral liquids are used to treat neonatal apnea.	The specific dosage is based on theophylline serum concentration levels, the drug's effectiveness, and occurrence of adverse reactions. The daily dosage is divided into 6- or 8-hour doses for rapid-release products and 8- or 12-hour doses for slow-release products. Initial maximum dosage in adults is 13 mg/kg/day of theophylline or a total of 800 mg/day, whichever is less.	• Theophylline is contraindicated in patients sensitive to methylxanthine derivative agents. • Monitor the patient's theophylline serum concentration levels for safe and optimal use. • Inform the patient about theophylline's adverse reactions and the importance of reporting any that occur. • Monitor theophylline serum concentration levels and expect to make dosage adjustments. • Administer cautiously to a patient with liver or cardiac impairment. Both can alter theophylline excretion. • Monitor for significant interactions that occur between theophylline and other drugs.
aminophylline	Asthma, chronic bronchitis, and emphysema. The rapid-release oral liquids are used to treat neonatal apnea.	Adult dosage should be based on theophylline content. The specific dosage is based on theophylline serum concentration levels, the drug's effectiveness, and occurrence of adverse reactions. The daily dosage is divided into 6- or 8-hour doses for rapid-release products and 8- or 12-hour doses for slow-release products. I.V. loading dose, 5 to 6 mg/kg; maintenance for the next 12 hours, 0.6 to 0.7 mg/kg/hr; then 0.3 to 0.5 mg/kg/hr. Initial maximum adult dosage is 13 mg/kg/day of theophylline or 800 mg/day total, whichever is less.	• Aminophylline is contraindicated in patients sensitive to methylxanthine or ethylenediamine. • Monitor the patient's theophylline serum concentration levels for safe and optimal use. • Inform the patient about theophylline's adverse reactions and the importance of reporting any that occur. • Monitor theophylline serum concentration levels and expect to make dosage adjustments. • Administer cautiously to patients with liver or cardiac impairment because either will alter theophylline excretion. • Monitor the patient for drug interactions that can occur between theophylline salts and other drugs.
oxtriphylline	Asthma, chronic bronchitis, and emphysema	200 mg P.O. every 6 to 8 hours. The daily dosage using the slow release product should be divided into 8- or 12-hour doses. The specific dosage is based on theophylline serum concentration, patient response, and occurrence of adverse reactions. The initial dose should not exceed 13 mg/kg/day theophylline or a total of 800 mg/day, whichever is less.	• Oxtriphylline is contraindicated in patients sensitive to methylxanthines or choline derivative agents. • For safe and optimal use, theophylline serum concentration levels must be monitored. • Instruct patient to recognize adverse reactions and report them if they occur. • Use oxtriphylline cautiously in patients with liver or cardiac impairment because both alter theophylline's excretion. • Significant drug interactions occur with theophylline salts and need to be monitored.

SELECTED MAJOR DRUGS

Methylxanthine agents continued

DRUG	MAJOR INDICATIONS	USUAL ADULT DOSAGES	NURSING IMPLICATIONS
dyphylline	Asthma, chronic bronchitis, and emphysema	Up to 15 mg/kg P.O. every 6 hours, or 250 mg to 500 mg (up to 15 mg/kg) I.M.	• Dyphylline is contraindicated in patients sensitive to methylxanthine derivative agents. • Administer dyphylline cautiously to patients with renal disease, which may cause accumulation of the drug. Administer the drug cautiously to patients with heart disease because of its cardiac stimulant effect. • Inform patients about dyphylline's adverse reactions and the importance of reporting any that occur.

• Acute gastric and peptic ulcer disease can be aggravated by I.V. or oral administration of methylxanthine derivative agents.

• For theophylline and its salts, alter the dosage as ordered if hepatic disease, CHF, cor pulmonale, severe hypoxia, prolonged fever, or pulmonary edema is present. These problems decrease theophylline's metabolism and can lead to excessive serum concentration levels of the drug.

• When theophylline is administered with such drugs as cimetidine or erythromycin, monitor the patient's serum concentration levels and observe for toxic and adverse reactions.

• With all the methylxanthine agents, monitor the patient for adverse reactions that may indicate excessive serum concentration levels, such as nausea, vomiting, diarrhea, irritability, insomnia, cardiac dysrhythmias, and seizures. If any adverse reactions occur, discontinue the drug, as ordered, and consult the physician about altering the dosage.

• Monitor the patient's serum theophylline level when theophylline products are used or the caffeine serum level when caffeine products are used. When theophylline is used in a neonate, both theophylline and caffeine serum levels should be monitored because theophylline is metabolized to caffeine in the neonate.

• To treat an acute overdose of oral preparations, induce emesis unless seizures are present or the patient is comatose. Giving activated charcoal binds methylxanthine preparations in the GI tract, and repeating the charcoal dose draws theophylline out of the systemic circulation. A saline cathartic or sorbitol can be added to the charcoal to prevent charcoal-induced constipation; as a last resort, dialysis with a charcoal filter may be used.

• Monitor the patient's serum theophylline concentration levels to ensure maximum safety and effectiveness of the therapy. For patients with asthma, emphysema,

or chronic bronchitis, therapeutic serum concentration levels range from 10 to 20 mcg/ml. For treating neonatal apnea, concentration levels range from 5 to 10 mcg/ml.

• When administering caffeine to treat neonatal apnea, monitor the patient's serum caffeine concentration level to ensure safety and effectiveness. Therapeutic serum concentration levels of caffeine range from 5 to 20 mcg/ml.

• Mix the loading dose for I.V. aminophylline in dextrose 5% or in normal saline solution. Administer this dose over 20 to 30 minutes.

• Administer I.V. maintenance doses by constant infusion, using an infusion pump. Use a standard concentration level, and vary the volume administered except when the patient is volume-restricted. Dosages are best expressed in mg/hr and ml/hr, using a standard concentration level for accuracy and safety.

• When switching a patient from I.V. to oral theophylline or dyphylline, stop the infusion when starting the oral drug.

• Administer adjusted dosages of drugs cautiously; always be alert for signs and symptoms of toxicity associated with these drugs.

• When administering theophylline salt, use serum theophylline concentration levels to monitor the patient's response.

• Because dyphylline is not metabolized to theophylline *in vivo*, do not use theophylline concentration levels to monitor dyphylline therapy.

• Use peak serum concentration levels to monitor therapy with oral methylxanthine preparations. Peak concentration levels of rapid-release products occur 1 to 2 hours after administration; of slow-release products, about 4 hours after administration. If no adverse reactions occur, measure peak serum concentration levels when the steady-state level has been reached. Reaching the steady-state level requires that the patient receive the drug at regular intervals for 48 to 72 hours.

• If vomiting occurs shortly after administration of an oral methylxanthine preparation, consult the physician before repeating the dose. If the patient misses a dose, do not increase or double subsequent doses without first consulting the physician.

• Encourage the patient receiving a theophylline enema or rectal solution to retain it as long as possible.

• Administer a methylxanthine oral preparation with a full glass of water and a small amount of food. Bead-filled capsules may be taken apart and their contents scattered on small amounts of soft food for administration to patients unable to swallow tablets. Slow-release products should not be chewed or crushed.

• Advise the patient not to ignore theophylline's adverse reactions but to contact the physician as soon as possible if any adverse reaction occurs.

• Advise the patient to avoid using products that contain methylxanthine while on methylxanthine therapy. The additional agents may not contribute to the therapy's effectiveness and may cause adverse reactions.

CHAPTER SUMMARY

Chapter 44 covered the methylxanthine agents used clinically in the United States, including theophylline and its salts, dyphylline, and caffeine. Here are the highlights of the chapter:

• Physicians use theophylline, its salts, and dyphylline to treat asthma, chronic bronchitis, and emphysema. Theophylline, its salts, and caffeine are used to treat neonatal apnea.

• The therapeutic response of asthma patients to methylxanthine agents is bronchodilation. Theophylline and its salts are more potent bronchodilators than dyphylline. Bronchodilation is not a significant pharmacologic response to these agents in patients with chronic bronchitis and emphysema.

• In patients with chronic bronchitis and emphysema, the methylxanthine agents improve cardiac function and ventilation, decrease diaphragmatic fatigue, and promote the elimination of mucus.

• Theophylline, administered as an oral liquid, a rapid-release tablet, or a rectal solution, is rapidly and completely absorbed. Slow-release preparations are absorbed at varying rates and degrees. Caffeine is well absorbed after oral administration. Dyphylline is incompletely absorbed.

• Dosages of methylxanthine agents should be individualized using serum concentration levels, patient responses, and occurrence of adverse reactions as guides.

• Drug interactions involving methylxanthine agents can result in toxicity or reduced effectiveness.

• Adverse reactions to methylxanthine include nausea and vomiting, abdominal cramping, anorexia, diarrhea, and CNS adverse reactions, including headache, anxiety, irritability, restlessness, and dizziness. Seizures may occur rarely.

BIBLIOGRAPHY

American Hospital Formulatory Service. *Drug Information 87*. McEvoy, G.K., et al., eds. Bethesda, Md.: American Society of Hospital Pharmacists, 1987.

American Medical Association. *Drug Evaluations,* 6th ed. Philadelphia: W.B. Saunders Co., 1986.

Gisclon, L.G., et al. "Pharmacokinetics of Orally Administered Dyphylline," *American Journal of Hospital Pharmacy* 36:1179, September 1979.

Hendeles, L., et al. "Theophylline," in *Applied Pharmacokinetics—The Principles of Therapeutic Drug Monitoring,* 2nd ed. Evans, W.E., ed. Spokane, Wash.: Applied Therapeutics, 1986.

Kastrup, E.K., ed. *Facts and Comparisons*. St. Louis: J.B. Lippincott Co., Facts and Comparisons Division, 1987.

Rall, T.W. "The Methylxanthines," in *Goodman and Gilman's The Pharmacological Basis of Therapeutics,* 7th ed. Gilman, A.G., ed. New York: Macmillan Publishing Co., 1985.

Roberts, R.J. *Drug Therapy in Infants—Pharmacologic Principles and Clinical Experience*. Philadelphia: W.B. Saunders Co., 1984.

USPDI. *Drug Information for the Health Care Provider,* vol. 1, 7th ed. Rockville, Md.: United States Pharmacopeial Convention, 1987.

Weinberger, M. "Slow-Release Theophylline Rationale and Basis for Product Selection," *New England Journal of Medicine* 308(13):760-64, March 31, 1983.

CHAPTER 45

EXPECTORANT, ANTITUSSIVE, AND MUCOLYTIC AGENTS

OBJECTIVES

After reading and studying this chapter, you should be able to:

1. Describe the physiology of the cough mechanism.

2. Differentiate among the different actions of expectorants, antitussives, and mucolytics.

3. Describe the purported mechanisms of action for the expectorants, including the iodides and guaifenesin.

4. Identify the predictable and unpredictable adverse reactions associated with the iodides.

5. Explain the difference between centrally acting and peripherally acting antitussives.

6. Identify the potential risks involved for the patient when using antitussives.

7. Explain why acetylcysteine is the one mucolytic used clinically in the United States.

8. Describe the most important components of patient teaching for acetylcysteine.

9. Explain the use of acetylcysteine in acetaminophen overdose.

INTRODUCTION

Secretions of the respiratory tract, which originate from goblet cells and bronchial glands, combine to form mucus. Approximately 100 ml of mucus is produced daily; the mucus is composed of water, lipids, glycoproteins, carbohydrates, and deoxyribonucleic acid (DNA). Mainly protective in nature, mucus acts as a barrier to prevent water loss from the epithelium. Mucus also plays an important role in the mucociliary clearance mechanism, protecting the epithelium from mechanical irritants, noxious agents, and microorganisms. (See *Tissue lining respiratory tract*, in Unit Nine Introduction for an illustration of these defense mechanisms.) Inhaled particles are trapped in the mucus, and the debris is propelled to the oropharynx via the mucociliary escalator mechanism to be swallowed or expectorated.

The mucociliary clearance mechanism is compromised by inhibited ciliary function. Ciliary inhibition can result from chronic exposure to cigarette smoke or from a change in the viscosity or amount of mucus, which occurs in bronchitis and cystic fibrosis. Expectorants may assist clearance by increasing mucous output or altering the composition of mucus. Although the efficacy of expectorants is unsubstantiated, they are found in many over-the-counter preparations and are widely advertised. The mucolytic acetylcysteine liquefies tenacious secretions in the airway.

Besides the mucociliary clearance mechanism, the cough also facilitates removal of respiratory secretions. The cough is triggered by stimulating nerve receptors that are sensitive to chemicals and other irritants. These cough receptors are located throughout the respiratory tract as well as in the stomach, pleura, and diaphragm. Once the receptors are stimulated, the impulse travels via the afferent pathway, mainly via the vagus nerve, to the cough center in the medulla. The cough reflex is then processed and coordinated in the brain stem.

The muscular contractions that constitute the cough are initiated via the efferent nervous pathways. The cough mechanism consists of three phases: inspiratory phase, compressive phase, and expiratory phase. After the deep inhalation of the inspiratory phase, the glottis closes and the expiratory muscles contract against the closed glottis. The compressive phase ends with the sudden opening of the glottis, producing a flow rate necessary for an effective cough by releasing the high intrathoracic pressure. The expiratory phase allows for the removal of debris from the respiratory tract.

Expiratory muscles contract even further during this phase, compressing the tracheobronchial tree. This compression contributes to an effective cough by decreasing the diameters of the airways, thus increasing the velocity and shearing forces of the gas in the airways. The cough serves as an important protective mechanism when the cilia prove ineffective against abnormal quantities or types of materials in the respiratory tract.

The numerous causes of the cough include congenital anomalies, infections, diseases such as cystic fibrosis, foreign body aspiration, reactive airway disease, irritants, and psychogenic reactions. A condition frequently associated with a transient cough is the common cold. Coughs can be productive or nonproductive of sputum. They may also be described as chronic, paroxysmal, or recurrent.

Although coughing is useful, protective, and beneficial, it can be irritating and exhaustive and can interfere with an individual's activities of daily living. Coughing can also cause further complications. The intrathoracic pressures generated during the compressive phase can lead to rib fractures, ruptured rectus abdominis muscles, a pneumothorax, bradycardia, and syncope.

Treatment of a cough depends upon its cause. The cessation of smoking often improves the cough associated with chronic bronchitis. Bronchodilators relieve the chronic cough of asthmatics. If the cough is disruptive to an individual's sleep or activities of daily living, antitussives, which suppress the cough mechanism, may be an acceptable risk. Antitussives, however, are contraindicated in suppurative lung disease or a condition in which sputum is increased because they might promote atelectasis or pneumonia.

This chapter discusses the expectorant and mucolytic agents, which purport to enhance mucokinesis (the removal of mucus), and drugs that act to suppress coughing, the narcotic and nonnarcotic antitussives.

For a summary of representative drugs, see *Selected major drugs: Expectorant, antitussive, and mucolytic agents* on page 723.

EXPECTORANTS

Expectorants facilitate mucokinesis. Most drugs purported to remove mucus liquefy viscid secretions and thereby aid in mobilizing and evacuating secretions.

Providing adequate hydration of 2 or 3 liters of fluid per day also enhances mucokinesis. Overhydration, however, does not thin mucus and may actually impair its clearance. Deep-breathing exercises and frequent position changes may also help to increase mucokinesis.

Some frequently used expectorants that are discussed in this chapter include iodinated glycerol, potassium iodide, guaifenesin, and terpin hydrate.

History and source

The use of expectorants dates back centuries to the days of folk medicine, when individuals were exposed to aromatic vapors, incenses, and steaming water. Oral expectorants eventually surpassed inhalation methods in popularity. Today, the oral ingredients frequently appear in over-the-counter (OTC) preparations. A number of OTC cough and cold products contain both a cough suppressant and an expectorant.

PHARMACOKINETICS

Because expectorants have not been thoroughly researched, data on peak concentration levels, duration of action, and half-life remains unavailable.

Absorption, distribution, metabolism, excretion

Iodinated glycerol, potassium iodide, guaifenesin, and terpin hydrate are absorbed via the gastrointestinal tract and distributed to the bronchial glands. The iodides are also distributed to the salivary, lacrimal, and thyroid glands, as well as across the placenta. Guaifenesin is metabolized by the liver. The metabolic fate of iodinated glycerol is unknown. Excretion of the expectorants is primarily renal, though the iodides are also excreted in breast milk.

Onset, peak, duration

The onset of action for expectorants is immediate to 30 minutes. Data remains unavailable on the peak concentration levels, duration of action, and half-life of the expectorants.

PHARMACODYNAMICS

Expectorants are thought to increase mucus by acting on the bronchial glands or by reducing the adhesiveness and surface tension of the mucus. Expectorants may also provide a soothing demulcent effect on respiratory tract mucosa. The use of expectorants remains controversial because their efficacy has not been clearly established.

Mechanism of action

The iodides, iodinated glycerol and potassium iodide, are thought to enter the bronchial glands of the tracheobronchial mucosa via the bloodstream and stimulate gland cells to secrete a watery mucus. The iodides also appear to stimulate ciliary activity and the salivary glands, causing rhinorrhea and salivation. Potassium iodide may have a direct mucolytic effect.

Guaifenesin and terpin hydrate supposedly increase the secretion of mucus by reducing adhesiveness and surface tension. The increased flow of less viscid secretions promotes ciliary action, thus facilitating the removal of mucus.

PHARMACOTHERAPEUTICS

Expectorants are used for the symptomatic relief of cough from colds, as well as for minor bronchial irritations, bronchitis, influenza, sinusitis, bronchial asthma, emphysema, and other respiratory disorders. Physicians prescribe the iodides less frequently because of the potential for toxic effects (especially on the thyroid) if taken in excessive amounts or used in prolonged therapy. Patients may better tolerate iodinated glycerol than the inorganic iodide because the iodine and glycerol are organically bound; as a result, no iodine is free to cause gastrointestinal irritation.

Potassium iodide is most frequently used when preparing patients for thyroidectomy. When given preoperatively, potassium iodide reduces vascularity, firms glandular tissue, and shrinks cells in the thyroid gland; these effects facilitate thyroidectomy. (See Chapter 56 for further discussions of thyroid and antithyroid agents.) Guaifenesin, the most popular expectorant, is safe if taken as directed. It can be used alone or in combination with antitussives, analgesics, and antihistamines. (See

Combination products for some commonly prescribed combination products.) Researchers have not clearly established the efficacy of terpin hydrate. The elixir has a high alcohol content, which can cross the placenta, causing congenital abnormalities in the fetus.

potassium iodide (Pima, SSKI). Potassium iodide is used to liquefy tenacious mucus in such conditions as chronic bronchiectasis and bronchial asthma.
USUAL ADULT DOSAGE: for expectorant action, 300 to 650 mg P.O. t.i.d. to q.i.d. The patient may begin with 300 to 600 mg q2h initially until the desired effect occurs. Potassium iodide is also available in saturated solution with 1 gram potassium iodide per ml. The solution dose is 0.3 to 0.6 ml using a calibrated dropper.

iodinated glycerol (Organidin). This drug serves as adjunctive therapy in respiratory conditions such as bronchial asthma, bronchitis, and emphysema.
USUAL ADULT DOSAGE: 60 mg P.O. q.i.d.

guaifenesin (Breonesin, Robitussin). Guaifenesin relieves the dry hacking cough associated with the common cold as well as with other upper respiratory infections such as bronchitis, laryngitis, pharyngitis, and influenza.

Combination products

Combination products contain varying amounts of different ingredients. The nurse must be aware of these ingredients to understand their potential effects upon the therapeutic regimen. This chart is only a sampling. Other combinations such as Benylin DM combine antitussives and decongestants. The following chart lists readily available combination products that the nurse should know about.

DRUG	EXPECTORANT	ANTITUSSIVE	OTHER INGREDIENTS
Cheracol	guaifenesin, 20 mg/ml	codeine phosphate, 2 mg/ml	alcohol, 4.75%
Conar Expectorant Syrup	guaifenesin, 20 mg/ml	dextromethorphan hydrobromide, 3 mg/ml	phenylephrine hydrochloride, 2 mg/ml
Formula 44D	guaifenesin, 13 mg/ml	dextromethorphan hydrobromide, 2 mg/ml	phenylpropanolamine hydrochloride, 2.4 mg/ml alcohol, 20%
Robitussin-DM	guaifenesin, 20 mg/ml	dextromethorphan hydrobromide, 3 mg/ml	alcohol, 1.4%
Vicks Cough Syrup	guaifenesin, 5 mg/ml	dextromethorphan hydrobromide, 0.7 mg/ml	alcohol, 5% sodium citrate, 40 mg/ml

USUAL ADULT DOSAGE: 200 to 400 mg P.O. q4h, not to exceed 2.4 grams/day.

terpin hydrate. This drug increases mucus production. The increased mucus helps liquefy and reduce the viscosity of thick secretions.
USUAL ADULT DOSAGE: 5 to 10 ml P.O. of the elixir every 4 to 6 hours. The elixir is not recommended for pediatric use because of its high alcohol content.

Many of the expectorant ingredients are found in nonprescription OTC preparations. Therefore, the nurse must be aware of all the ingredients in combination cough and cold products and the usual dosage range for children. Pediatric doses for these products vary, but the nurse can usually rely on the following general guidelines: children ages 6 to 12, give one-half the adult dosage; children ages 2 to 6, give one-fourth the adult dosage. No recommended dosage has been established for children under age 2.

Drug interactions

Few interactions between drugs or between drugs and food occur with the expectorants. Iodinated glycerol and potassium iodide administered with lithium or the antithyroid drugs may potentiate the hypothyroid and goitrogenic effects. Potassium iodide combined with potassium-sparing diuretics or potassium-containing drugs may increase serum potassium levels and lead to cardiac dysrhythmias and cardiac arrest. Guaifenesin administered with anticoagulants may increase the risk of bleeding. Terpin hydrate should not be administered to patients taking disulfiram because they may experience an alcohol-disulfiram reaction. (See Chapter 6, Drug Abuse, Dependence, and Addiction, for more information about disulfiram.)

ADVERSE DRUG REACTIONS

Of the expectorants, the iodides produce the most potentially toxic adverse reactions. Adverse reactions, usually nausea or vomiting, from guaifenesin rarely or infrequently occur. Terpin hydrate often causes drowsiness.

Predictable reactions

The prolonged use of large doses of iodides can cause thyroid gland hyperplasia, hypothyroidism, goiter, thyroid adenoma, skin eruptions, and iodism. Gastric irritation commonly occurs; however, iodinated glycerol is less irritating to the gastrointestinal tract than the inorganic iodide. Patients with cystic fibrosis may experience an increased susceptibility to the goitrogenic effect of iodine, and adolescents with acne may find their con-

dition aggravated. Potassium toxicity may occur in some patients taking potassium iodide.

Guaifenesin may produce emesis if taken in doses larger than necessary for the expectorant action. Diarrhea, drowsiness, nausea, vomiting, and abdominal pain may also occur. Nausea and vomiting are predictable reactions occurring with terpin hydrate use.

Unpredictable reactions

Patients with iodide sensitivity may experience the following: angioedema (submucosal swelling), laryngeal edema (swelling of the larynx), cutaneous and mucosal hemorrhage, and signs and symptoms of serum sickness, including fever, arthralgia (joint pain), lymph node enlargement, and eosinophilia (increase of eosinophils). Other manifestations attributed to iodide hypersensitivity include urticaria (pruritic skin eruptions), thrombocytopenic purpura (a bleeding disorder), and fatal periarteritis (an inflammatory condition of the arteries).

NURSING IMPLICATIONS

Although the efficacy of expectorants remains uncertain, they are readily available in OTC preparations. Therefore, the nurse needs to know about them.
● Iodinated glycerol and potassium iodide are contraindicated in patients with iodide sensitivity. Pregnant and lactating women should not receive iodides because abnormal thyroid function or goiter may occur in the neonate. The iodides are also contraindicated in patients with thyroid disease, tuberculosis, or acute bronchitis.
● Patients with renal disease or hyperkalemia and patients taking potassium supplements should not take potassium iodide because increased serum potassium levels can cause cardiac dysrhythmias and death.
● Enteric-coated potassium iodide has been associated with lesions in the small intestine, which may cause hemorrhage and death.
● Prolonged iodide therapy may alter thyroid function tests results.
● Guaifenesin is safe when used as directed. No problems have been documented in lactating or pregnant women taking guaifenesin.
● Guaifenesin interferes with both urinary 5-hydroxyindoleacetic acid (5-HIAA) and urinary vanillylmandelic acid (VMA) tests, resulting in falsely increased determinations.
● Because of its high alcohol content, terpin hydrate is contraindicated in patients with peptic ulcer or severe diabetes mellitus.
● Obtaining the patient's history of allergies can decrease the risk of adverse reactions to the iodides. The signs and symptoms of iodism include unpleasant brassy taste,

burning in the mouth and throat, soreness of gums and teeth, increased salivation, coryza, sneezing, and eye irritation. Mild iodism can simulate a head cold.

• Patients taking iodides should be monitored for hypothyroidism.

• Debilitated patients, as well as patients with ineffective coughs or with respiratory insufficiency, may experience difficulty handling their mucous secretions and may require suctioning.

• Suctioning equipment should always be available for patients receiving expectorants.

• The patient's respiratory rate, rhythm, and characteristics should be assessed. Adventitious breath sounds, such as rales, may occur.

• Any adverse effects, including any increase in temperature and sputum viscosity, change in sputum color, increased cough frequency, chills, sweating, prolonged headache, rash, or dyspnea, should be reported to the physician immediately.

• Potassium iodide solution can be mixed with a glass of water, fruit juice, or other liquid. Taking the solution after meals or at bedtime with food may minimize gastric irritation.

• Diluting potassium iodide well and using a glass drinking straw can help prevent injury to the teeth.

• Potassium iodide solutions that have turned brown, indicating decomposition, should be discarded.

• If crystallization of potassium iodide occurs, the solution should be warmed and gently shaken.

• Iodinated glycerol is frequently used with other drugs such as theophylline, codeine, and dextromethorphan.

• Patients taking expectorants should increase their fluid intake to 2 to 3 liters per day; doing so should help thin and mobilize respiratory secretions. Patients should avoid fluid overload.

• Patients should notify a physician if they become short of breath or begin to wheeze.

• The patient should know the signs and symptoms of iodism and report these symptoms to the physician.

• The patient should learn to cough effectively.

• The patient taking terpin hydrate should know about the expectorant's high alcohol content.

ANTITUSSIVES

An antitussive is any agent that suppresses or inhibits coughing. Centrally acting antitussives suppress cough by depressing the cough center in the medulla. Narcotics are centrally acting antitussives that effectively suppress cough. Peripherally acting antitussives act on the cough receptors located throughout the airway. A number of peripherally acting antitussives, such as local anesthetics, bronchodilators, and mucokinetic drugs, can alleviate many types of cough. Home remedies, such as honey and whiskey, cough drops, and rock candy, may also relieve cough.

Because the cough acts as a protective mechanism by removing accumulated mucus and irritants, it should not under normal circumstances be suppressed. However, a persistent cough can itself begin to act as an irritant and can lead to a cough-irritant-cough cycle. Such a cycle can prove exhaustive and even interrupt an individual's ability to sleep or talk.

The major antitussives include codeine, hydrocodone bitartrate, dextromethorphan hydrobromide, and benzonatate. Other drugs that provide antitussive activity include diphenhydramine hydrochloride and lidocaine.

History and source

The narcotic antitussives are made from opium alkaloids and their derivatives. Codeine, isolated in 1832, remains one of the most frequently used narcotic antitussives and serves as the standard of comparison for all other cough suppressants. Codeine provides an antitussive activity and produces a drying effect on the respiratory tract mucosa.

Hydrocodone bitartrate is a codeine derivative that provides an antitussive activity greater than codeine. The sedative properties and dependence liability of hydrocodone bitartrate are also greater than that of codeine. Dextromethorphan, a methylated dextro isomer of levorphanol, equals codeine in its ability to suppress cough. Dextromethorphan is nonaddictive and nonanalgesic. Benzonatate is a peripherally acting antitussive with anesthetic properties. Benzonatate is thought to be as effective as codeine for cough suppression.

PHARMACOKINETICS

The antitussives are well absorbed through the gastrointestinal tract, metabolized in the liver, and excreted in the urine.

Absorption, distribution, metabolism, excretion

The narcotic antitussives are absorbed via the gastrointestinal tract, metabolized in the liver, and excreted in the urine. Codeine and other narcotic antitussives are distributed across the placenta in pregnant women and are excreted in the breast milk of lactating women. No such data is available for dextromethorphan. Pharmacokinetic information on benzonatate is also unavailable.

Onset, peak, duration

The onset of action for codeine occurs in 30 minutes. Both codeine and hydrocodone bitartrate reach peak concentration levels in about 1 hour. Duration of action varies: codeine lasts about 4 hours, and hydrocodone bitartrate lasts between 4 and 6 hours. Codeine has a half-life of 2½ to 3 hours, while the half-life of hydrocodone bitartrate is 4 hours.

Dextromethorphan and benzonatate provide an onset of action in about 15 to 30 minutes. The duration of action for dextromethorphan and benzonatate varies, ranging from 3 to 8 hours.

PHARMACODYNAMICS

The narcotic antitussives, chemically classified as phenanthrenes (codeine, hydrocodone bitartrate), are opium alkaloids. These antitussives suppress the cough reflex by a direct effect on the cough center in the medulla. They also exert a drying effect on the respiratory tract mucosa, which increases the viscosity of bronchial secretions. Both codeine and hydrocodone bitartrate produce sedative and constipating effects. (See Chapter 26, Narcotic Agonist and Antagonist Agents, for a detailed discussion of these drugs.)

Dextromethorphan is a methylated dextro isomer of levorphanol (an opiate analgesic) that acts centrally to suppress cough. Dextromethorphan, unlike codeine and hydrocodone bitartrate, produces no analgesia, addiction, or central nervous system depression.

Mechanism of action

Codeine, hydrocodone bitartrate, and dextromethorphan suppress the cough reflex by directly affecting the sensitivity of the cough center in the medulla to incoming stimuli. Benzonatate, the peripherally acting antitussive, acts by anesthetizing cough receptors of vagal afferent fibers throughout the bronchi, alveoli, and pleura. (See *Location of action: Antitussives.*)

PHARMACOTHERAPEUTICS

The treatment of a cough should be directed at the cause. Treatment may include removing an irritant, such as cigarette smoke; administering antihistamines for postnasal drip; administering a bronchodilator to relieve bronchospasm; or administering an antitussive. Antitussives are used to treat a serious, nonproductive cough that interferes with a patient's ability to rest or carry out activities of daily living.

The narcotic antitussives effectively suppress cough; however, they act centrally and can cause respiratory depression, which may be detrimental in patients with pulmonary disease. Narcotics also possess the potential for abuse; however, if the narcotic is used in antitussive dosages and for a short time, addiction liability is low. Potent narcotics are reserved for treating intractable cough, usually associated with cancer of the lung. Opiates taken with other central nervous system (CNS) depressants can be fatal.

The nonnarcotic antitussive dextromethorphan is the most widely used cough suppressant in the United States. Some data suggest that dextromethorphan may provide better antitussive activity than codeine. The popularity of dextromethorphan may also stem from the fact that the drug produces few adverse reactions and is nonaddictive.

Benzonatate, another nonnarcotic antitussive, relieves cough associated with respiratory conditions such as pneumonia, bronchitis, and the common cold, as well as with chronic pulmonary diseases such as emphysema. At recommended doses, benzonatate does not depress

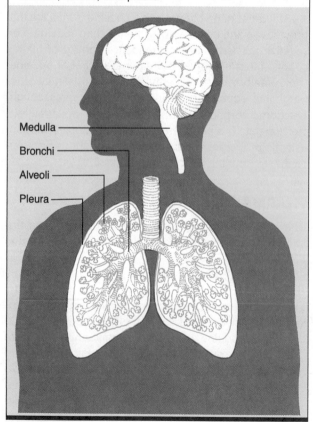

Location of action: Antitussives

Codeine, hydrocodone bitartrate, and dextromethorphan act directly on the cough center in the medulla. The peripherally acting benzonatate acts on the bronchi, alveoli, and pleura.

Medulla
Bronchi
Alveoli
Pleura

Characteristics of antitussives

The following chart compares four antitussives. The nurse must know these comparisons to plan appropriate follow-up care for the patient.

DRUG	MECHANISM OF ACTION	EFFECTIVENESS	DEPENDENCE POTENTIAL	C.N.S. DEPRESSION	OTHER EFFECTS
codeine	Centrally acting	Less than morphine	Yes	Sedation	Drying effect on respiratory mucosa
hydrocodone bitartrate	Centrally acting	Greater than codeine	Yes	Sedation	Physical dependence potential is greater than that for codeine
dextromethorphan	Centrally acting	Equal to codeine	No	Not at recommended dose	No analgesia
benzonatate	Peripherally acting	Equal to codeine	No	Sedation	None

respiration. It can also be used as adjunctive treatment during bronchial diagnostic tests, such as bronchoscopy, when the patient must avoid coughing during the procedure. Benzonatate does not present the risk of addiction that codeine does. (See *Characteristics of antitussives* for a comparison of the drugs discussed in this section.)

codeine. A Schedule II drug, codeine is used to suppress the nonproductive cough that interferes with the patient's activities or leads to exhaustion.
USUAL ADULT DOSAGE: 10 to 30 mg P.O. every 4 to 6 hours, not to exceed 120 mg/day.

dextromethorphan hydrobromide (Robitussin-DM). This drug is used to treat nonproductive cough from minor throat and bronchial irritation.
USUAL ADULT DOSAGE: 10 to 20 mg P.O. q4h, or 30 mg every 6 to 8 hours, not to exceed 120 mg/day. The long-acting preparation (60 mg) can be taken every 12 hours.

hydrocodone bitartrate (Hycodan). A Schedule II drug, hydrocodone bitartrate is used in combination with other antitussives or expectorants to relieve nonproductive cough.
USUAL ADULT DOSAGE: 5 to 10 mg P.O. every 4 to 6 hours. Initiate therapy with a 5-mg dose; a single adult dose should not exceed 15 mg.

benzonatate (Tessalon). This drug provides symptomatic relief of cough associated with respiratory conditions.

Benzonatate can be administered before bronchial diagnostic tests to suppress cough during the procedure.
USUAL ADULT DOSAGE: 100 mg P.O. every 4 to 6 hours, not to exceed 600 mg/day.

Drug interactions
The narcotic antitussives potentiate the depressant effects of monoamine oxidase (MAO) inhibitors, alcohol, and other CNS depressants. Dextromethorphan may cause excitation and hyperpyrexia when taken with MAO inhibitors. Benzonatate produces no significant drug interactions. (See *Drug interactions: Antitussives* on page 720 for a list of interacting drugs, their effects, and the nursing implications associated with each interaction.)

ADVERSE DRUG REACTIONS

Toxic doses of the narcotic antitussives can produce miosis, bradycardia, tachycardia, hypotension, narcosis, seizures, and circulatory collapse or respiratory arrest.

Overdose of dextromethorphan can result in euphoria, hyperactivity, a sense of intoxication, nystagmus, staggering gait, lethargy, uncoordinated movements, stupor, and shallow breathing.

Benzonatate can cause dizziness, drowsiness, headache, nasal congestion, burning eyes, nausea, constipation, and skin rash.

Predictable reactions
Antitussive doses of codeine seldom cause respiratory depression. The patient may, however, experience an

DRUG INTERACTIONS

Antitussives

Drug interactions involving narcotic antitussives can be serious. The nurse must give special attention to patient teaching to prevent problems.

DRUG	INTERACTING DRUGS	POSSIBLE EFFECTS	NURSING IMPLICATIONS
codeine	MAO inhibitors (isocarboxazid, phenelzine, tranylcypromine)	Cause excitation, hypertension or hypotension, coma	• Instruct the patient to avoid concomitant use of these drugs.
	CNS depressants (alcohol, barbiturates, sedative-hypnotics)	May increase CNS depressant effects (drowsiness, lethargy, stupor, respiratory depression, coma, death)	• Monitor the patient closely for CNS depression. • Instruct the patient to avoid concomitant use of these drugs.
dextromethorphan	MAO inhibitors (isocarboxazid, phenelzine, tranylcypromine)	Cause excitation, hyperpyrexia, hypotension, coma	• Instruct the patient to avoid concomitant use of these drugs. • These drugs are contraindicated within 2 weeks of stopping MAO inhibitors.
hydrocodone bitartrate	MAO inhibitors	Cause excitation, hypertension or hypotension, coma	• Instruct the patient to avoid concomitant use of these drugs.

impaired ability to perform activities that require mental alertness or coordination. Repeated doses of codeine increase the chance for nausea, vomiting, constipation, dizziness, sedation, palpitations, pruritus, excessive perspiration, and agitation. Prolonged ingestion of codeine may result in physical dependence.

Usual oral antitussive doses of hydrocodone bitartrate do not usually produce adverse reactions. Ambulatory patients, however, may experience dizziness, sedation, nausea, and vomiting more so than nonambulatory patients. Rash, pruritus, constipation, euphoria, and dysphoria can also occur with hydrocodone bitartrate use.

Central nervous system depression may occur with extremely high doses of dextromethorphan. At recommended doses, adverse reactions rarely occur. Patients most frequently complain of drowsiness and gastrointestinal upset.

When taking benzonatate, patients can experience sedation, headache, dizziness, nasal congestion, nausea, gastrointestinal upset, and constipation. "Chilly" sensations, skin eruptions, pruritus, and numbness in the chest have also been reported.

Unpredictable reactions
Hypersensitivity reactions to codeine rarely occur; however, hives, itching, rash, and swelling of the face can

result from codeine use. Physical dependence can also occur. Hypersensitivity reactions to hydrocodone bitartrate can occur, but hypersensitivity reactions to dextromethorphan and benzonatate are rare.

NURSING IMPLICATIONS
The central and peripheral actions of different antitussives have important implications for nurses.
• Antitussives are contraindicated in patients with known hypersensitivity to any of the ingredients in the antitussive and in women who are pregnant or lactating. Dextromethorphan is contraindicated in patients taking MAO inhibitors.
• Asthmatic or debilitated patients, and patients with emphysema should not take narcotic antitussives because these drugs produce a drying effect on respiratory secretions that may increase the viscosity of secretions and suppress the cough reflex. Both effects may lead to respiratory insufficiency.
• Because narcotics are addicting, prolonged use may lead to physical dependence. Narcotic antitussives are also contraindicated in patients with a history of drug abuse.
• Patients should understand that their ability to perform activities requiring mental alertness, such as driving a car, may be impaired.

- The patient should avoid ingesting alcohol because of potential CNS depression.
- Antitussives should not be used by a patient with a productive cough or by a patient for whom coughing is beneficial, such as a postoperative patient.
- Antitussives should be used with caution by a patient who is also taking CNS depressants.
- The patient's allergy and drug history can help decrease the risk of adverse reactions from the narcotic and nonnarcotic antitussives. Carefully monitoring high-risk patients, such as the elderly and debilitated, also helps. An overdose is treated by giving a narcotic antagonist such as naloxone and instituting resuscitative measures.
- Because coughing can exhaust a patient, nursing measures should promote comfort and adequate rest.
- Antitussives are available in combination preparations, with analgesics, antipyretics, antihistamines, and decongestants. Antitussives also come as tablets, capsules, lozenges, and elixirs or syrups.
- The patient should swallow benzonatate capsules whole; the patient should not chew these capsules because the release of benzonatate in the mouth can anesthetize the oral mucosa.
- The patient should report persistent cough (lasting longer than 7 days) or a cough that changes from nonproductive to productive.
- The patient should keep the antitussive out of the reach of children.
- The patient should not exceed the prescribed or recommended dose.
- The patient should know about the additive effect of CNS depressants with the antitussives.

OTHER ANTITUSSIVES

diphenhydramine hydrochloride (Benadryl, Benylin). This drug is effective in suppressing cough. Though an antihistamine, diphenhydramine is thought to have both a central and peripheral mechanism of action. Adverse reactions include the typical reactions to other antihistamines, including sedation and anticholinergic effects. (See Chapter 63, Antihistaminic Agents, for a discussion of antihistamines.) The nurse should administer diphenhydramine cautiously in patients taking sedatives or tranquilizers because of the additive CNS depressant effect. Ingesting alcohol requires caution, too.

lidocaine hydrochloride (Xylocaine). This drug is a local anesthetic that physicians can prescribe to suppress the cough reflex associated with tracheal intubation. Lidocaine is also administered topically for diagnostic procedures such as bronchoscopy. (See Chapter 28, Local and Topical Anesthetic Agents, for further discussion.)

MUCOLYTICS

The epithelial tissues and bronchial glands of the respiratory tract continuously produce mucus, which the mucociliary escalator removes. If the mucus becomes excessive or so viscid that it interferes with the ciliary action, it can obstruct the airways. Mucolytics are drugs that purportedly alter mucus composition and thereby reduce its viscosity. The two types of mucolytics include thiol compounds and proteolytic enzymes. Many thiol compounds have been studied for their mucolytic activity. Though some may provide mucolytic activity, they are toxic for use *in vivo*.

Health care professionals rarely use the proteolytic enzymes because the expense and toxicity of these enzymes outweigh the minor therapeutic benefits. Proteolytic enzymes include deoxyribonuclease, trypsin, chymotrypsin, and leucine aminopeptidase.

Acetylcysteine is the only thiol compound used clinically in the United States. This thiol mucolytic is used to treat patients with abnormal, viscid, or inspissated (thick, hard) mucus.

History and source
Acetylcysteine was introduced in the early 1960s after researchers learned that the amino acid L-cysteine possessed mucolytic properties. Acetylcysteine is a derivative of L-cysteine.

PHARMACOKINETICS
Acetylcysteine is absorbed from the pulmonary epithelium and metabolized in the liver.

Absorption, distribution, metabolism, excretion
Acetylcysteine acts directly on the mucus. After the drug-mucus reaction, the remaining acetylcysteine is absorbed from the pulmonary epithelium and metabolized in the liver. Researchers do not know if acetylcysteine is ex-

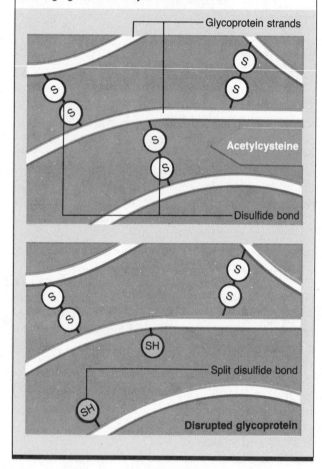

Action of acetylcysteine

Acetylcysteine's free sulfhydryl group splits the disulfide bridge between glycoprotein molecular complexes, disrupting the glycoprotein strands and changing the viscosity of the mucus.

Glycoprotein strands

Acetylcysteine

Disulfide bond

Split disulfide bond

Disrupted glycoprotein

creted in the breast milk of lactating women; controlled studies of the use of acetylcysteine in pregnant women are unavailable.

Onset, peak, duration

The onset of action of acetylcysteine occurs 1 minute after inhalation and immediately after direct application or instillation. Maximal effect occurs in 5 to 10 minutes after inhalation. Additional data about peak concentration levels, duration of action, and half-life remain unavailable.

PHARMACODYNAMICS

Acetylcysteine decreases the viscosity of respiratory tract secretions by altering the molecular composition of mu-

cus. Deoxyribonucleic acid (DNA) and glycoproteins contribute to the mucus viscosity. The glycoprotein molecular complexes are bridged by disulfide bonds. When acetylcysteine splits these disulfide bonds, mucus viscosity decreases.

Mechanism of action

The mechanism of action of acetylcysteine depends upon the sulfhydryl group in the drug. Drugs such as acetylcysteine that contain a free sulfhydryl group split the disulfide bridges between glycoprotein molecular complexes. The action alters the molecular composition of mucus and decreases mucus viscosity. (See *Action of acetylcysteine.*)

The mechanism of action when acetylcysteine is used for acetaminophen (acetylcysteine metabolite) overdose has not been fully determined. Evidence suggests that a sulfhydryl-containing compound inactivates the hepatotoxic metabolite.

PHARMACOTHERAPEUTICS

Mucolytics are used as adjunctive therapy to treat patients with abnormal, viscid, or inspissated mucous secretions. Patients who develop atelectasis secondary to mucous obstruction, as well as patients with bronchitis, emphysema, or pulmonary complications of cystic fibrosis, may benefit from mucolytic therapy. Mucolytics may also be used to prepare patients for bronchograms and other bronchial studies. Acetylcysteine is the antidote for acetaminophen overdosage; however, it does not protect all patients from hepatic damage caused by the overdose.

acetylcysteine (Mucomyst). This agent reduces mucus viscosity. Acetylcysteine can be used for lung disorders in which an overproduction of mucus in the respiratory tract causes an accumulation of secretions. This accumulation may interfere with gas exchange and provide a medium for infection. Acetylcysteine is also available as a combination product with isoproterenol, a bronchodilator. Acetylcysteine is usually administered via a nebulizer.

USUAL ADULT DOSAGE: via the nebulizer, 3 to 5 ml of a 20% solution, t.i.d. to q.i.d., or 6 to 10 ml of a 10% solution, t.i.d. to q.i.d.; for direct instillation, 1 to 2 ml of a 20% solution, which can be administered every hour via the tracheal tube or a percutaneous transtracheal catheter.

For tracheostomy care, 1 to 2 ml of a 10% to 20% solution should be given every 1 to 4 hours; for diagnostic procedures, 1 to 2 ml of a 20% solution or 2 to 4 ml of a 10% solution—two to three doses should be given prior to the procedure.

Expectorant, antitussive, and mucolytic agents

The following chart summarizes the major expectorant, antitussive, and mucolytic agents currently in clinical use.

DRUG	MAJOR INDICATIONS	USUAL ADULT DOSAGES	NURSING IMPLICATIONS
Expectorant			
guaifenesin	Cough associated with common cold and upper respiratory infection	200 to 400 mg every 2 to 4 hours, not to exceed 2.4 grams/day	• Guaifenesin interferes with urinary 5-hydroxyindoleacetic acid and vanillylmandelic acid tests. • Monitor cough and respiratory status. • Guaifenesin is found in many over-the-counter cough and cold preparations.
Narcotic antitussive			
codeine	Nonproductive cough	10 to 30 mg every 4 to 6 hours, not to exceed 120 mg/day	• Avoid administering to pregnant or lactating women. • Administer cautiously to patients who need to perform activities requiring mental alertness. • Tolerance and physical dependence is possible. • Drug is contraindicated in patients with productive cough.
Nonnarcotic antitussive			
dextromethorphan	Nonproductive cough	10 to 20 mg every 4 hours or 30 mg every 6 to 8 hours; long-acting preparations, 60 mg every 12 hours	• Do not administer dextromethorphan to patients taking monoamine oxidase inhibitors. • Drug is available in many over-the-counter preparations. • Monitor cough.
Mucolytic			
acetylcysteine	Bronchopulmonary diseases (chronic bronchitis, emphysema, bronchiectasis, pneumonia, atelectasis, cystic fibrosis)	Nebulization: 3 to 5 ml (20% solution) t.i.d. to q.i.d. or 6 to 10 ml (10% solution) t.i.d. to q.i.d. Direct instillation: 1 to 2 ml (20% solution) every hour	• Instruct patient to cough before and after treatment to clear airways. • Carefully monitor high-risk patients (those with respiratory insufficiency, asthmatics, elderly, debilitated) for increased respiratory difficulties. • Suction patients who cannot expectorate secretions. • Use plastic, glass, aluminum, or stainless steel nebulizer equipment. • Refrigerate unused solution; discard solution after 96 hours. • Dilute solution with sterile water when three fourths of the original volume has been used. • Reduce unpleasant effects by washing the patient's face and encouraging the patient to rinse the mouth after treatments.

To treat acetaminophen overdose, a 5% solution should be used, with a loading dose of 140 mg/kg P.O. followed by 70 mg/kg P.O. q4h for 17 doses. If the patient vomits within an hour of a dose of acetylcysteine, the dose should be repeated.

Drug interactions

Acetylcysteine is incompatible with the following drugs: amphotericin B, chlortetracycline hydrochloride, erythromycin lactobionate, oxytetracycline hydrochloride, ampicillin sodium, tetracycline hydrochloride, iodized oil, hydrogen peroxide, chymotrypsin, and trypsin. Activated charcoal decreases acetylcysteine's effectiveness. Therefore, in acetaminophen overdose, activated charcoal should be removed by gastric lavage before the oral administration of acetylcysteine.

ADVERSE DRUG REACTIONS

Acetylcysteine provides a wide margin of safety; however, its "rotten egg" odor during administration may lead to nausea.

Predictable reactions

With prolonged or persistent use, acetylcysteine may produce stomatitis, nausea, vomiting, drowsiness, and severe rhinorrhea. Asthmatic patients may have difficulty breathing; the frequency of this adverse reaction increases with the 20% solution.

Unpredictable reactions

Hypersensitivity rarely occurs; however, a rash can develop with prolonged or frequent exposure to acetylcysteine. Patients may have bronchorrhea, which may cause increased airway obstruction for those who cannot expectorate effectively. Because bronchospasm can occur unpredictably, the nurse must monitor patients during inhalation therapy.

NURSING IMPLICATIONS

Although acetylcysteine is usually administered via inhalation by a respiratory therapist, the nurse performs important functions in patient assessment and safety and should be aware of the following implications:

• Administer acetylcysteine cautiously to patients who have asthma or respiratory insufficiency because they can develop increased airway obstruction.

• To decrease the risk of adverse reactions, obtain a history from the patient, especially noting any respiratory problems and allergies.

• Assess the patient's respiratory status before and after each treatment for any breathing difficulty, poor cough, or dyspnea. The patient may need to be suctioned.

• Be prepared to administer a beta$_2$ bronchodilator by aerosol should the patient experience bronchospasm.

• Administer acetylcysteine via a nebulizer. Since acetylcysteine reacts with iron, copper, and rubber, frequently monitor the patient's nebulizer equipment for reactive effects. The drug does not react with glass, plastic, aluminum, or stainless steel.

• Because acetylcysteine does not contain an antimicrobial agent, avoid contamination of the solution and refrigerate an opened vial. Discard opened vials after 96 hours.

• Know that acetylcysteine may discolor to a light purple, which does not significantly affect the drug's mucolytic efficacy or safety.

• Note that both 10% and 20% acetylcysteine solutions may be used undiluted. However, after the patient nebulizes three fourths of the initial volume of solution, dilute the remaining solution with an equal volume of sterile water for injection USP.

• When administering acetylcysteine to treat acetaminophen overdose, remove previously administered activated charcoal by gastric lavage before acetylcysteine administration. Should the patient vomit within 1 hour of acetylcysteine administration, the dose should be repeated.

• Follow acetylcysteine administration with chest physiotherapy and postural drainage if ordered, and encourage coughing and deep breathing to facilitate removal of respiratory secretions.

• Have the patient gargle after the respiratory treatments to relieve the unpleasant odor and dryness; wash the patient's face to eliminate the stickiness caused by the drug.

• Clean the equipment after use since any drug residue may clog or corrode the equipment parts.

• Teach the patient the proper use and maintenance of the nebulizer.

• Inform the patient of the importance of gargling posttreatment to relieve odor; also inform the patient about effective coughing before and after each treatment.

• Instruct the patient to seek medical help if the condition becomes progressively worse.

CHAPTER SUMMARY

Chapter 45 discussion centered on expectorants, antitussives, and mucolytics. The chapter began with a discussion of mucus production in the respiratory tract, the mucociliary clearance mechanism, and cough. Here are the highlights of the chapter:

• Expectorants are administered to patients who experience difficulty expectorating sputum or who retain respiratory tract secretions. Though expectorants may enhance clearance of secretions from the tracheobronchial tree, the efficacy of these agents remains doubtful.

• Guaifenesin, the most frequently used expectorant, is safe when given in recommended dosages. Many combination products that include expectorants are available over the counter. The iodides, iodinated glycerol and potassium iodide, are less frequently used because of their potential for toxicity.

• Narcotic and nonnarcotic antitussives are used to treat a nonproductive cough that is irritating and exhausting.

• The narcotic antitussives act centrally, but codeine and hydrocodone bitartrate differ in their sedative properties and dependence liability.

• Dextromethorphan, the most widely used antitussive in the United States, is effective and rarely causes adverse reactions. Benzonatate, a nonnarcotic antitussive, is as effective as codeine in suppressing cough and does not cause dependence.

• The antihistamine diphenhydramine has shown effective antitussive action. The local anesthetic lidocaine is also useful in suppressing cough associated with intubation procedures.

• If used in recommended dosages, antitussives are safe. However, the nurse must use caution when administering centrally acting antitussives with other central nervous system depressants. The nurse should carefully monitor elderly and debilitated patients and patients with pulmonary disease.

• Antitussive agents should not be used in patients with a productive cough or in situations where coughing is beneficial.

• Mucolytics reduce the mucus viscosity and elasticity. They are used to facilitate sputum expectoration and to unblock airways that are plugged with mucus.

• Acetylcysteine is the only thiol compound mucolytic clinically used in the United States.

• Aerosol administration of acetylcysteine can produce bronchospasm; therefore, bronchodilators may be given in combination with acetylcysteine.

• Acetylcysteine is relatively safe; however, the drug should be administered cautiously to patients who are unable to cough effectively because they may develop increased airway obstruction.

• Acetylcysteine is the antidote for acetaminophen overdose.

BIBLIOGRAPHY

American Hospital Formulary Service. *Drug Information 1986.* McEvoy, G.K., et al., eds. Bethesda, Md.: American Society of Hospital Pharmacists, 1986.

American Medical Association. *AMA Drug Evaluations.* New York: John Wiley & Sons, 1983.

Barberi, E. "Mucolytics," *American Family Physician* 28:175, August 1983.

Bryant, B., and Cormier, J. "Cold and Allergy Products," in *Handbook of Nonprescription Drugs,* 8th ed. Washington, D.C.: American Pharmaceutical Association, 1986.

"Cough Medicine," *Drug and Therapeutics Bulletin* 23:85, November 4, 1985.

"Do Mucolytics Help in Chronic Bronchitis and Asthma?" *Drug and Therapeutics Bulletin* 23:29, April 20, 1984.

Ferguson, J.A. "Progress in the Treatment of Cough," *American Pharmacy* 23:48, September 1983.

Gilman, A.G., et al., eds. *Goodman and Gilman's The Pharmacological Basis of Therapeutics,* 7th ed. New York: Macmillan Publishing Co., 1985.

Hollinger, M. *Respiratory Pharmacology and Toxicology.* Philadelphia: W.B. Saunders Co., 1985.

Irwin, R., et al. "Cough: A Comprehensive Review," *Archives of Internal Medicine* 137:1186, September 1977.

Katona, B., and Wason, S. "Dextromethorphan Danger," *The New England Journal of Medicine* 1314:993, April 10, 1986.

Minette, A. "Background of Mucolytic Treatment in Chronic Bronchitis," *European Journal of Respiratory Disease* 64:401, August 1983.

Pavia, D. "Effects of Pharmacologic Agents on the Clearance of Airway Secretions," *Seminars in Respiratory Medicine* 5:345, 1984.

Selcow, J. "Ancillary Medical Therapy: Help or Hindrance?" *The Journal of Asthma* 20:369, 1983.

United States Pharmacopeial Convention. *Drug Information for the Health Care Provider, vol. I, USPDI,* 6th ed. Easton, Pa.: Mack Publishing Co., 1986.

Yurkioka, H., et al. "Intravenous Lidocaine as a Suppressant of Coughing during Tracheal Intubation," *Anesthesia and Analgesia* 64:1189, December 1985.

Zanjanian, M.H. "Expectorants and Antitussive Agents: Are They Helpful?" *Annals of Allergy* 44:290, May 1980.

Ziment, I. *Respiratory Pharmacology and Therapeutics.* Philadelphia: W.B. Saunders Co., 1978.

CHAPTER 46

DECONGESTANT AGENTS

OBJECTIVES

After reading and studying this chapter, you should be able to:

1. Describe the physiologic mechanisms that contribute to the development of upper respiratory tract signs and symptoms.

2. Explain the mechanism of action of systemic and topical decongestants in relieving upper respiratory tract signs and symptoms.

3. Differentiate between the pharmacokinetic properties of the systemic and topical decongestants.

4. Describe the physiologic mechanisms that produce rebound nasal congestion, and explain why this phenomenon may preclude the use of ephedrine.

5. Identify the major drug interactions that can occur if systemic decongestants are administered with other sympathomimetic amines or local vasoconstrictors.

6. Identify the important points to be included during patient teaching of decongestants, and explain their importance.

INTRODUCTION

Decongestants provide their major benefit by helping to relieve upper respiratory signs and symptoms associated with the common cold. Reviewing the physiologic mechanisms by which these respiratory signs and symptoms develop will assist in understanding the use of the decongestants discussed in this chapter.

The respiratory system serves as one of the first lines of defense against microbial invasion of the body. Hairs located in the nasal turbinates filter out the largest invading particles. Smaller particles become trapped in the nasal mucus or mix with acidic nasal secretions. The cilia in the epithelium lining the nose move the trapped particles toward the pharynx, where they are either swallowed or coughed to the exterior. Particles that manage to reach the lower respiratory tract become trapped in

mucus secreted by the goblet cells and bronchial glands. Cilia in the lower respiratory passages then sweep the mucus up toward the pharynx where it and the trapped particles are swallowed or expectorated. (See *Tissue lining respiratory tract* in Unit Nine Introduction for an illustration of these defense mechanisms.) Particles or microorganisms not removed in this manner are carried lower into the alveoli where macrophages ingest them.

Organisms entering the mouth come in contact with saliva, which acts as a cleanser of the oral cavity. Saliva contains IgA antibodies and, even more important, lysozyme, which breaks down the cell walls of bacteria. Swallowed saliva as well as swallowed mucous secretions from the respiratory passages force the trapped organism into contact with gastric acids, enzymes, and bile.

When invading organisms elude the respiratory and oropharyngeal barriers, infection results. As the infecting organism acts on invaded structures, cellular disruption and neutrophil migration occur. Histamine, released from circulating basophils, connective tissue, mast cells, and platelets, causes local vasodilation and increased permeability to protein. The neutrophils release active kallikrein, which passes through the permeable capillaries, splitting kininogen into kinins. The kinins, being potent vasodilators, cause further vasodilation and permeability to protein. As these changes occur, fluid leaks from capillaries into the surrounding tissues, resulting in edema and swelling of the nasal passages. The use of decongestants relieves the swelling in clogged nasal passages associated with the common cold. Primarily synthetic versions of epinephrine, most decongestants are termed sympathomimetic in action and are used either systemically or topically.

For a summary of representative drugs, see *Selected major drugs: Decongestant agents* on page 734.

SYSTEMIC DECONGESTANTS

The systemic decongestants, as sympathomimetic amines, activate the sympathetic division of the autonomic nervous system. The three major systemic decongestants are ephedrine, pseudoephedrine, and phenylpropanolamine. These three drugs stimulate alpha receptors in vascular smooth muscle, thereby constricting arterioles of the nasal mucosa while reducing blood flow and edema. These actions open the nasal passages, increase airflow, and promote sinus drainage.

History and source
The work of Oliver and Schäfer in 1895 provided the foundation for the study of naturally occurring catecholamines and for the subsequent work of Barger and Dale in 1910. Studying the relationship between synthetic amines and epinephrine, Barger and Dale coined the term "sympathomimetic" to describe the synthetic derivatives that acted like sympathetic amines. The work of Tainter, Chang, and Burn in the late 1920s and early 1930s clarified differences between the sympathomimetic amines, suggesting that qualitative as well as quantitative differences existed. In 1948, Ahlquist attributed at least a portion of the differences in sympathomimetic action to a specificity for alpha or beta receptor sites. In 1958, Burn and Rand identified another reason for the differences in sympathomimetic action, namely that some sympathomimetic derivatives caused a release of norepinephrine. Subsequently, many investigations have attempted to define and describe further the drug action of sympathomimetic amines.

Ephedrine, the oldest of the systemic decongestants, occurs naturally as a plant alkaloid, and its use dates to 2000 B.C. in Chinese medicine. Today, ephedrine as well as phenylpropanolamine and pseudoephedrine are synthetically produced.

PHARMACOKINETICS
The systemic decongestants prove clinically effective when taken orally. The drugs are widely distributed throughout the body and are excreted primarily unchanged in the urine.

Absorption, distribution, metabolism, excretion
The systemic decongestants discussed in this chapter are readily absorbed from the GI tract after oral intake. The drugs are widely distributed throughout the body into various tissues and fluids, including the cerebrospinal fluid, placenta, and breast milk. Slowly and incompletely metabolized by the liver, the drugs are excreted largely unchanged in the urine within 24 hours after oral administration.

For ephedrine and pseudoephedrine, 55% to 75% of the drug is excreted unchanged, whereas 80% to 90% of phenylpropanolamine is similarly excreted. The process of excreting ephedrine and pseudoephedrine is accelerated by acidic urine. Conversely, in alkalinized urine with a pH of about 8.0, the rate of excretion decreases, increasing reabsorption in the renal tubules.

Onset, peak, duration
After oral administration of the systemic decongestants, the onset of nasal decongestion is 15 to 30 minutes, peaking within 60 to 90 minutes. The duration of action is 3 to 6 hours for tablets and syrups, and 8 to 12 hours for sustained-release capsules and tablets.

Phenylpropanolamine has a half-life of 3 to 4 hours. For ephedrine and pseudoephedrine, the half-life is 3 hours with a urine pH of 5.0, and about 6 hours with a pH of 6.3.

PHARMACODYNAMICS
The systemic decongestants are used for their vasoconstrictor effects in reducing nasal congestion associated with the common cold and other upper respiratory disorders. Drug effects result from direct or indirect action on target receptors.

Mechanism of action
Ephedrine, pseudoephedrine, and phenylpropanolamine act both directly and indirectly. When taken orally, the drugs act directly on alpha-adrenergic receptors in the nasal mucosa and elsewhere, causing contraction of urinary and gastrointestinal sphincters, mydriasis, and decreased pancreatic beta cell secretion. The major activity of these drugs, however, occurs indirectly and results in the release of norepinephrine from storage sites. The release of norepinephrine, a catecholamine, together with the direct action on receptors, produces subsequent vasoconstriction and nasal decongestion.

Additional effects of the drugs result primarily from stimulation of beta-adrenergic receptors. The effects of this indirect drug action include increased heart rate, force of myocardial contraction, and cardiac output, as well as relaxation of bronchial smooth muscle.

PHARMACOTHERAPEUTICS
Systemic decongestants are indicated for the symptomatic relief of swollen nasal membranes resulting from hay fever, allergic rhinitis, vasomotor rhinitis, acute coryza,

sinusitis, and the common cold. Ephedrine, pseudo-ephedrine, and phenylpropanolamine are administered orally, frequently in combination with other drugs, such as antihistamines, antimuscarinics, antipyretic-analgesics, caffeine, and antitussives.

The systemic decongestants offer the advantages of lengthy symptom relief and over-the-counter availability. The major disadvantage is the systemic stimulation that occurs primarily as a result of beta-receptor stimulation combined with norepinephrine release from the indirect action. The topical decongestants serve as alternatives to these systemic drugs. While the topical drugs produce fewer systemic adverse effects, equally distressing effects do occur. (See "Adverse Drug Reactions" on pages 732 and 733 for details about reactions to topical decongestants.)

ephedrine sulfate. Physicians rarely prescribe ephedrine because of rebound hyperemia of the nasal mucosa, central nervous system (CNS) stimulation, transient hypertension, and palpitations associated with the drug's use. Effective orally, ephedrine is available in capsules and syrup.
USUAL ADULT DOSAGE: 25 to 50 mg P.O. every 3 to 4 hours.

pseudoephedrine hydrochloride (Neo-Synephrinol Day Relief, Novafed, Sudafed), **pseudoephedrine sulfate** (Afrinol Repetabs). Similar to ephedrine in its uses and properties, pseudoephedrine is more frequently used because of the infrequent occurrence of CNS stimulation and hypertension associated with its use. Associated rebound congestion is minimal to absent. Available without a prescription, pseudoephedrine is used to treat nasal congestion and serous otitis media accompanied by eustachian tube congestion.
USUAL ADULT DOSAGE: 60 mg P.O. every 4 to 6 hours; with sustained-release preparation, 120 mg P.O. every 12 hours.

phenylpropanolamine (Propagest, Rhindecon, Sucrets Cold Decongestant Formula). The most frequently used oral nasal decongestant, phenylpropanolamine resembles ephedrine pharmacologically while producing fewer adverse effects. The use of phenylpropanolamine can relieve nasal congestion associated with acute and chronic rhinitis, sinusitis, and the common cold. Available as a single-ingredient decongestant and in combination with other products, phenylpropanolamine is available over the counter.
USUAL ADULT DOSAGE: 25 mg P.O. every 4 hours, or 75 mg of the sustained-release preparation every 12 hours. Dosage should not exceed 150 mg P.O. daily.

Drug interactions

When given concurrently with other drugs, systemic decongestants may result in one of three different types of drug interactions. The first type of interaction may occur with the simultaneous administration of two or more drugs having opposing effects. Under these circumstances, the effects of one drug override the intended effects of the second.

DRUG INTERACTIONS
Systemic decongestants

Systemic decongestants potentiate the effect of sympathetic nervous system stimulating drugs, interfere with the action of adrenergic blocking drugs, and interact with monoamine oxidase (MAO) inhibitors, releasing large amounts of stored norepinephrine. The following combinations of sympathomimetics and systemic decongestants can produce life-threatening interactions.

DRUG	INTERACTING DRUGS	POSSIBLE EFFECTS	NURSING IMPLICATIONS
ephedrine, phenyl-propanolamine, pseudoephedrine	other sympathomimetics, including epinephrine, norepinephrine, dopamine, dobutamine, isoproterenol, metaproterenol, terbutaline, phenylephrine, tyramine	Increased CNS stimulation	• Do not administer drugs concurrently.
	MAO inhibitors	May cause severe hypertension, or hypertensive crisis	• Do not administer drugs concurrently.

A second type of interaction between drugs occurs when systemic decongestants are administered with other sympathomimetic amines. This interaction causes additive or cumulative drug effects, and potentiates the adverse effects of both drugs.

The third type of drug interaction occurs with the concurrent administration of drugs that interfere with the excretion of sympathomimetic amines. Because the excretion of systemic decongestants depends on the acidity of the urine, the nurse needs to monitor drugs that alter urine pH. In the presence of alkaline urine, renal tubular reabsorption of sympathomimetic amines increases. (See *Drug interactions: Systemic decongestants* for a summary of the drug interactions associated with these drugs.)

ADVERSE DRUG REACTIONS

The systemic decongestants produce primarily predictable, dose-related adverse effects associated with norepinephrine action; however, not all of the reactions are predictable. The unpredictable reactions associated with systemic decongestants include drug sensitivity and teratogenic effects.

Predictable reactions

The incidence and severity of adverse reactions depend on the patient's sensitivity to systemic decongestants. Patients who are sensitive to other sympathomimetic amines may also be sensitive to the systemic decongestants. The nurse should discourage the use of systemic decongestants by patients exhibiting this kind of drug sensitivity.

For nonsensitive patients, the incidence of adverse reactions is low. The most frequent adverse reactions result from CNS stimulation and include nervousness, restlessness, and insomnia. Nausea, palpitations, increased difficulty in urinating, and dose-related elevations in blood pressure occasionally occur.

Unpredictable reactions

Less predictable reactions to systemic decongestants include first-time drug sensitivity reactions, teratogenic effects, and effects in breast-feeding infants. Other reactions include irregular or unusually slow heartbeat, feeling of tightness in the chest, hallucinations, seizures, headache, and greatly elevated blood pressure.

Because of the unpredictable and unknown effects of systemic decongestants on the fetus, a pregnant patient should avoid these drugs. Furthermore, these decongestants distribute to breast milk and result in high risk to the breast-feeding infant.

NURSING IMPLICATIONS

The nurse must carefully note the patient's condition and age because these factors can affect the action of systemic decongestants. Because systemic decongestants are available over the counter, the nurse must emphasize patient teaching.

● Systemic decongestants are contraindicated in patients with porphyria, severe coronary artery disease, cardiac dysrhythmias, closed-angle glaucoma, and psychoneurosis, as well as in patients on MAO inhibitor therapy. Administer systemic decongestants cautiously in elderly patients and patients with hypertension, hyperthyroidism, cardiovascular disease, or prostatic hypertrophy.

● Instruct the patient how to use systemic decongestants correctly. Teach the patient how to identify and deal with predictable adverse reactions, and review CNS stimulation and other effects with the patient. Tell the patient to report any adverse reactions to the physician, since a change in dosage may be indicated.

● Instruct the patient not to use systemic decongestants during pregnancy and lactation or if the patient has a history of any of the following problems: cardiovascular disease, diabetes mellitus, closed-angle glaucoma, hypertension, hyperthyroidism, and prostatic hypertrophy.

● Tell the patient that systemic decongestants may interfere with sleep, and suggest taking the drug a few hours before bedtime to minimize the possibility of insomnia. Also, remind the patient not to take more than the recommended amount and to consult with the physician before taking over-the-counter products.

● Instruct the patient to use the drug in its complete form when taking timed-release capsules or long-acting tablets. The patient should not break, cut, crush, or chew the capsule or tablet.

TOPICAL DECONGESTANTS

Selected sympathomimetic amine decongestants provide immediate relief from nasal congestion and swollen mucous membranes when applied directly to the nasal mucosa. Because these drugs, referred to as topical decongestants, are only applied directly to the mucous

Instilling drops to treat nasal and sinus congestion

Obtain a box of tissues and the ordered medication. After identifying the patient and explaining the procedure and medication, help the patient assume the appropriate position. For drops, place the patient in the head low or supine position with the head supported by a pillow. With incorrect patient positioning, the drops will run down the back of the throat and be ineffective. When instilling sprays, the patient should be upright. For drops, place the dropper ⅓ to ½ inch inside the nostril, being careful to avoid touching the dropper to the nostril. Squeeze the dropper bulb to deliver the prescribed number of drops. Instruct the patient to remain in this position for 5 minutes to prevent the medication from running out of the nostrils. Repeat on opposite side if necessary.

To relieve clogged eustacian tubes, have the patient turn the head laterally to the affected side.

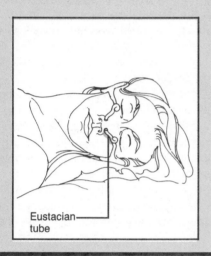

Eustacian tube

To relieve sphenoid and/or ethmoid sinus congestion, have the patient hyperextend the neck over a pillow.

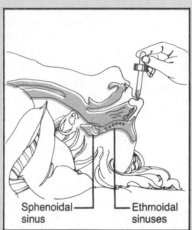

Sphenoidal sinus — Ethmoidal sinuses

To relieve maxillary and frontal sinus congestion, have the patient rotate the head laterally after hyperextension.

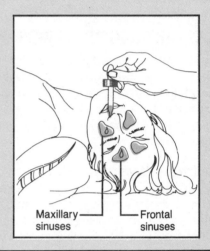

Maxillary sinuses — Frontal sinuses

membranes and are not administered orally, they are discussed separately.

The mechanism of action of topical decongestants resembles that of the systemic decongestants; however, the topical decongestants display more receptor specificity and usually provide a faster onset of action, shorter duration, and fewer systemic effects. Topical decongestants include imidazoline derivatives (naphazoline, oxymetazoline, tetrahydrozoline, xylometazoline) and sympathomimetic amines (epinephrine, ephedrine, phenylephrine, and propylhexedrine).

History and source

The work of Oliver and Schäfer provided the foundation for the discovery of the topical decongestants. (See "History and source" on page 727 for a discussion of the development of systemic and topical decongestants.)

The topical decongestants that are synthetically derived sympathomimetic amines (epinephrine, ephedrine, phenylephrine, and propylhexedrine) provide a fairly potent sympathetic stimulating effect if taken internally. All the sympathomimetic amine decongestants closely resemble epinephrine in structure. Phenylephrine was one of the drugs studied by Barger and Dale in 1910, while ephedrine was introduced into Western medicine by Chen and Schmidt in 1924.

Structurally unrelated to epinephrine, imidazoline derivatives were discovered in 1894 by Ladenburg. Since 1894, the imidazoline group has undergone many structural revisions, with several of the resulting derivatives acting like sympathomimetic amines.

PHARMACOKINETICS

Topical application of the sympathomimetic amines and imidazoline derivatives provides immediate relief of nasal congestion and restricts drug absorption. The duration of symptom relief, however, is usually short.

Absorption, distribution, metabolism, excretion

Topical decongestants act directly on the alpha receptors of the nasal vascular smooth muscle, thereby constricting arterioles and reducing blood flow in the edematous membranes. As a result of this direct vasoconstriction, vascular absorption becomes negligible.

If topical decongestants are accidentally administered in greater than therapeutic levels or are administered so that a large amount of the drug enters the nasopharynx and is swallowed, drug absorption will occur and systemic sympathetic stimulation will follow. When swallowed, both epinephrine and phenylephrine are irregularly absorbed from the GI tract and metabolized in the liver by the enzymes catechol-o-methyltransferase (COMT) and monoamine oxidase (MAO). By-products of the metabolism are excreted in the urine. Furthermore, epinephrine is distributed to the placenta and breast milk. Information on the absorption, distribution, metabolism, and excretion of other topical decongestants is not available.

Onset, peak, duration

Onset of action rapidly follows the application of topical decongestants. Drug action then peaks quickly. Epinephrine, phenylephrine, and propylhexedrine provide symptomatic relief within seconds, peaking in 2 to 4 minutes with a 30-minute to 2-hour duration of action. The imidazoline derivatives provide relief from nasal congestion within 5 to 10 minutes following application, and duration is 3 to 10 hours depending on the preparation.

PHARMACODYNAMICS

Topical decongestants act locally and directly to stimulate alpha-adrenergic receptors in nasal vascular smooth muscle. These drugs provide rapid relief of nasal congestion.

Mechanism of action

The stimulation of alpha-adrenergic receptors in nasal vascular smooth muscle results in increased alpha-adrenergic activity and vasoconstriction. The subsequent reduced nasal mucosal blood flow, together with decreased capillary permeability, decreases the edema associated with inflammation. The action of topical decongestants also helps drain sinuses, clear nasal passages, and open eustachian tubes, temporarily improving aeration.

PHARMACOTHERAPEUTICS

The fact that topical decongestants act directly on the alpha-adrenergic receptors in the nose helps explain their narrow scope of use, in contrast to the systemic decongestants, which act on alpha-adrenergic receptors throughout the body. The topical decongestants provide two major advantages: minimal adverse reactions and rapid relief of symptoms.

The rebound nasal congestion that occurs with frequent or long-term use of these drugs is their main disadvantage. This rebound congestion results from an alteration of the vasomotor stability of the nasal mucous membranes caused by repeated and prolonged sympathetic stimulation from the vasoconstrictors. Compensatory parasympathetic activation produces vasodilation and increased secretion. Temporary relief of rebound congestion occurs with even more frequent use of the drugs. When rebound congestion occurs, the patient should discontinue the drug treatment.

ephedrine (Efedron Nasal, Vatronol Nose Drops). This drug is infrequently used because of rebound hyperemia or congestion of the nasal mucosa and tachyphylaxis. Ephedrine is available in 0.5% to 0.6% drops, jelly, and syrup.

USUAL ADULT DOSAGE: 2 to 3 drops or a small amount of jelly in each nostril every 3 to 4 hours. Duration of therapy should not exceed 4 days.

epinephrine 0.1% (Adrenalin). This endogenously occurring catecholamine is available in drops or spray. Epinephrine drops are usually applied by physicians, who use the drug to control epistaxis or to control bleeding during nasal surgery. Because of the systemic sympathetic stimulating effects of epinephrine, use of the drug as a decongestant is limited.

USUAL ADULT DOSAGE: as a decongestant, 1 to 2 drops every 4 to 6 hours; when used to control epistaxis, not to exceed 1 ml over a 15-minute period.

naphazoline (Privine). An imidazoline derivative, naphazoline is topically applied to the nasal mucosa to relieve nasal congestion associated with the common cold, acute or chronic rhinitis, sinusitis, hay fever, and other allergies.

USUAL ADULT DOSAGE: 2 drops or sprays of 0.05% solution in each nostril, repeated every 3 to 6 hours. Duration of therapy should not exceed 5 days because longer use may cause rebound nasal congestion.

oxymetazoline (Afrin, Duration, Dristan Long Lasting). This drug is topically applied to the nasal mucosa to relieve nasal congestion associated with the common cold, acute or chronic rhinitis, sinusitis, hay fever, and other allergies. The duration of action for oxymetazoline, an imidazoline derivative sympathomimetic amine, is longer than that of the other imidazoline derivatives.

USUAL ADULT DOSAGE: 2 to 3 drops or 1 to 2 sprays of 0.05% solution in each nostril b.i.d., morning and evening. As with other topical decongestants, use oxymetazoline for short-term relief of symptoms because long-term use of the drug can lead to rebound congestion.

phenylephrine (Coricidin Nasal Mist, Neo-Synephrine, Sinarest Nasal Spray). One of the most widely prescribed topical nasal decongestants, phenylephrine provides effects less potent than those of epinephrine but of longer duration. Phenylephrine is recommended for use in patients with otic inflammation or infection because application to the nasal mucosa can open obstructed eustachian tubes. Phenylephrine also helps shrink swollen nasal and pharyngeal membranes, thus increasing visualization of the membranes, which makes the drug useful before surgery. Available in 0.25% to 1% solution and in 0.5% jelly, phenylephrine is applied to each nostril and inhaled.
USUAL ADULT DOSAGE: 1 to 2 sprays or a small amount of jelly in each nostril every 3 to 4 hours. Rebound congestion is less likely to occur with a dosage interval of 4 hours or greater.

propylhexedrine (Benzedrex, Vicks Inhaler). Available in inhalers, propylhexedrine is used topically to relieve nasal congestion associated with the common cold, acute or chronic rhinitis, sinusitis, hay fever, and other allergies. Because propylhexedrine provides a wider margin of safety than ephedrine or epinephrine, it can be used when an increased pressor effect is undesirable. As with other topical decongestants, use propylhexedrine for short-term relief of symptoms because prolonged use can cause rebound congestion.
USUAL ADULT DOSAGE: 2 inhalations in each nostril from the 250-mg inhaler.

tetrahydrozoline (Tyzine). An imidazoline derivative sympathomimetic amine like oxymetazoline, tetrahydrozoline is topically applied to the nasal mucosa to relieve nasal congestion associated with the common cold, acute or chronic rhinitis, sinusitis, hay fever, and other allergies.
USUAL ADULT DOSAGE: 2 to 4 drops or sprays of 0.1% solution in each nostril. Doses may be repeated every 3 hours. Long-term use can cause rebound congestion.

xylometazoline (Neo-Synephrine II Long Acting, Otrivin). Another imidazoline derivative sympathomimetic amine, xylometazoline is topically applied to the nasal mucosa to relieve nasal congestion associated with the common cold, acute or chronic rhinitis, sinusitis, hay fever, and other allergies.
USUAL ADULT DOSAGE: 2 or 3 drops or sprays of 0.1% solution in each nostril every 8 to 10 hours, not to exceed three times in 24 hours. Long-term use can lead to rebound congestion.

Drug interactions
Because of the topical drug route and vasoconstrictor action, which decrease drug absorption, drug interactions involving topical decongestants seldom occur. Nonetheless, if topical decongestants are swallowed, they can cause drug interactions.

One type of interaction may occur after the simultaneous administration of topical decongestants and other drugs having opposing effects. This interaction causes the effects of one drug to override the intended effects of the second.

A second type of interaction between drugs occurs when topical decongestants are administered with similarly acting drugs. This interaction causes additive or cumulative drug effects and may potentiate the adverse effects of both drugs. (See *Drug interactions: Topical decongestants* for a summary of interactions.)

ADVERSE DRUG REACTIONS
The topical decongestants cause primarily predictable adverse reactions associated with drug dosage and duration of use. Some unpredictable adverse reactions can occur, however, including drug sensitivity and teratogenic effects.

Predictable reactions
The incidence and severity of adverse reactions depends on the patient's sensitivity to topical decongestants and on the duration of action and frequency of drug use. Patients who display sensitivity to sympathomimetics may also be sensitive to the topical decongestants; the nurse should discourage use of these drugs by these patients.

The most frequently reported adverse reaction associated with the use of topical decongestants is the development of rebound nasal congestion. The disorder is characterized by hyperemia of the nasal mucosa, which appears red, boggy, and swollen. The rebound nasal congestion usually resolves spontaneously within a few days after discontinuation of the topical decongestant. Upon discontinuation of the drug, however, some patients may require supportive therapy using an oral decongestant and a normal saline spray.

The second most frequent adverse reaction is a transient burning and stinging of the nasal mucosa on application. Patients also report sneezing and dryness or ulceration of the mucosa.

DRUG INTERACTIONS

Topical decongestants

Drug interactions associated with topical decongestants are few but can cause major problems for the patient.

DRUG	INTERACTING DRUGS	POSSIBLE EFFECTS	NURSING IMPLICATIONS
ephedrine, epinephrine, naphazoline, oxymetazoline, phenylephrine, propylhexedrine, tetrahydrozoline, xylometazoline	MAO inhibitors	Increased CNS stimulation, increased hypertension, and possibly hypertensive crisis	• Do not administer drugs concurrently.
	beta-adrenergic blocking agents, methyldopa, reserpine, guanethidine, tricyclic antidepressants	Decrease hypotensive drug action, increase pressor effect, increase hypertension	• Do not administer drugs concurrently.
	digitalis glycosides	Increase risk of cardiac dysrhythmias	• Do not administer drugs concurrently.
	acetazolamide and sodium bicarbonate	Increase CNS stimulation, hypertension, cardiac dysrhythmias, insomnia from toxic drug levels	• Do not administer drugs concurrently.

Less frequently occurring adverse reactions result from CNS stimulation and include nervousness, restlessness, and insomnia. Occasionally, nausea, palpitations, increased difficulty in urinating, and dose-related elevations in blood pressure occur. Similar to the systemic effects caused by an overdose of most adrenergic drugs, these effects are more commonly associated with the administration of epinephrine, ephedrine, phenylephrine, and propylhexedrine. As a result, physicians carefully evaluate the use of topical vasoconstrictor decongestants for patients with cardiovascular disease, diabetes mellitus, increased intraocular pressure, hypertension, hyperthyroidism, or prostatic hypertrophy.

Unpredictable reactions

Less predictable adverse reactions include first-time drug sensitivity reactions, teratogenic effects, and effects in breast-feeding infants. Other reactions are irregular or unusually slow heartbeat, feeling of tightness in the chest, hallucinations, seizures, headache, and greatly elevated blood pressure.

Safe use of topical decongestants during pregnancy and lactation has not been determined. Because of the unpredictable or unknown effect of decongestants on the fetus, pregnant patients should carefully consider the risk versus the benefit of these drugs. Use these decongestants cautiously in lactating mothers because of the drugs' distribution in breast milk and the unknown risk to the infant.

NURSING IMPLICATIONS

The nurse should administer topical decongestants cautiously, noting any problems the patient may have. Furthermore, because topical decongestants are frequently used, the implications for patient care and patient teaching are extremely important.

• Topical decongestants are contraindicated in narrow-angle glaucoma. Administer these drugs cautiously if the patient has a history of cardiovascular disease, diabetes mellitus, hypertension, hyperthyroidism, or prostatic hypertrophy.

• When educating the patient about local vasoconstrictors, first review CNS stimulation and other effects of the drugs. Instruct the patient to report any adverse reactions to the physician, explaining that a change in dosage may be indicated.

• Remind the patient not to exceed the recommended amount, frequency, and duration of use. Duration of therapy should not exceed 4 days. Caution the patient about taking other over-the-counter products that may interact with these drugs. Warn the patient not to take these agents during pregnancy and lactation.

• To minimize the CNS stimulating effects of topical decongestants, instruct the patient in proper methods of administration, that is, the lateral head low position for drops, the upright head position for sprays. Instruct the patient who is using decongestants to relieve blocked eustachian tubes to instill the drops by lying supine with the head turned 15 degrees toward the affected ear. Explain to the patient that the drops instilled in the affected nasal passage should be allowed to flow along

---

SELECTED MAJOR DRUGS

Decongestant agents

The drugs summarized in this chart are frequently used (and representative) decongestants.

DRUG	MAJOR INDICATIONS	USUAL ADULT DOSAGES	NURSING IMPLICATIONS
Systemic decongestants (sympathomimetic amines)			
phenylpropanol-amine	Nasal congestion associated with acute or chronic rhinitis, sinusitis, the common cold, hay fever, and other allergies	25 mg P.O. every 4 hours or 75 mg of the sustained-release preparation every 12 hours, not to exceed 150 mg in 24 hours	• Contraindicated in patients with porphyria, severe coronary artery disease, cardiac dysrhythmias, narrow-angle glaucoma, psychoneurosis, and in patients on MAO inhibitor therapy.
pseudoephedrine		60 mg P.O. every 4 to 6 hours or 120 mg sustained-release preparation P.O. every 12 hours	• Administer cautiously to elderly patients and those with hypertension, hyperthyroidism, cardiovascular disease, or prostatic hypertrophy. • To minimize the possibility of insomnia, have the patient take the last dose of the day a few hours before bedtime. • Do not administer to pregnant or lactating patients. • Administer sustained-release capsules or tablets whole; remind patient not to break, crush, or chew medication. • Caution patient about taking other over-the-counter drugs because of possible interactions.
Topical decongestants (local vasoconstrictors)			
naphazoline	Nasal congestion associated with acute or chronic rhinitis, sinusitis, the common cold, hay fever, and other allergies	2 drops or sprays of 0.05% solution in each nostril, repeated every 3 to 6 hours	• Drug is contraindicated in patients with narrow-angle glaucoma. • Administer cautiously to patients with hypertension, diabetes mellitus, or advanced arteriosclerosis. • Drug may cause rebound congestion; advise patient to take in accordance with recommendations for frequency and duration.
phenylephrine		1 to 2 sprays or small amount of jelly into each nostril, repeated every 3 to 4 hours	• Duration of therapy should not exceed 4 days. • Review with patient proper administration procedure, which helps prevent CNS effects: lateral head low position for drops, upright head position for sprays.
oxymetazoline		2 or 3 drops or 1 to 2 sprays of 0.05% solution in each nostril b.i.d.	• Not recommended for use during pregnancy or lactation. • Caution patient about taking other over-the-counter drugs because of possible interactions.
tetrahydrozoline		2 or 4 drops or sprays of 0.1% solution in each nostril every 4 to 6 hours, no more frequently than every 3 hours	
xylometazoline		2 or 3 drops or sprays of 0.1% solution in each nostril every 8 to 10 hours, not to exceed 3 times in 24 hours	

the floor of the nose to the low point, where they will collect. The low point marks the entrance of the eustachian tube. Instruct the patient to remain in this position for 5 minutes. When both sides require treatment, the patient should repeat the procedure on the second side after the 5-minute wait.

rarely occurs when recommended dosages and frequencies of administration are followed. More prominent and bothersome is the frequent occurrence of rebound nasal congestion, which prompts drug dependence. Limiting drug use to 3 to 4 days assists in preventing the rebound-dependence phenomenon.

CHAPTER SUMMARY

Chapter 46 presented decongestants and their use in relieving nasal congestion, rhinitis, and eustachian tube occlusion associated with sinusitis, the common cold, hay fever, and other allergies. The chapter included discussions that explained how the sympathomimetic action of decongestants, acting primarily on alpha-adrenergic receptors, promotes vasoconstriction of the nasal mucosa, thereby decreasing inflammation, congestion, and edema. Here are the highlights of the chapter:

• Decongestants are discussed in this chapter according to their route of administration because the distinction helps in discriminating between the pharmacokinetics, observed adverse effects, and nursing implications for the different drugs. Orally administered decongestants, known for their sympathomimetic effects, are discussed as systemic decongestants. Ephedrine, the oldest sympathomimetic amine, represents the systemic decongestants. Topically administered decongestants are powerful vasoconstrictors. The topical decongestants include the imidazoline derivatives and sympathomimetic amines.

• Systemic decongestants promote nasal decongestion through stimulation of alpha-adrenergic receptors in the nasal mucosa (direct action) and stimulation of norepinephrine release (indirect action). Systemic decongestants include ephedrine, phenylpropanolamine, and pseudoephedrine. The mild adverse reactions that occur resemble those resulting from sympathetic nervous system stimulation. Administered orally, systemic decongestants provide a longer duration of action than the topical decongestants.

• Topical decongestants promote nasal decongestion through direct stimulation of the alpha-adrenergic receptors in the nasal mucosa vascular smooth muscle. Topical decongestants include ephedrine, epinephrine, naphazoline, phenylephrine, propylhexedrine, tetrahydrozoline, and xylometazoline.

• Topical decongestants provide almost immediate relief of symptoms. Sympathetic nervous system stimulation

BIBLIOGRAPHY

American Hospital Formulary Service. *Drug Information 1986.* McEvoy, G.K., et al., eds. Bethesda, Md.: American Society of Hospital Pharmacists, 1986.

"Decongestant, Cough, and Cold Preparations," in *AMA Drug Evaluations,* 5th ed. Chicago: American Medical Association, 1983.

Findlay, J.W.A., et al. "Pseudoephedrine and Triprolidine in Plasma and Breast Milk of Nursing Mothers," *British Journal of Pharmacology* 18:901, December 1984.

Guyton, A.C. *Textbook of Medical Physiology,* 7th ed. Philadelphia: W.B. Saunders Co., 1986.

Hansten, P.D. *Drug Interactions,* 5th ed. Philadelphia: Lea & Febiger, 1985.

Hughes, S.C., et al. "Placental Transfer of Ephedrine Does Not Affect Neonatal Outcome," *Anesthesiology* 63:217, August 1985.

Huzulakova, I., and Dukes, M.N.G. "Drugs Affecting Autonomic Functions of the Extrapyramidal System," in *Meyler's Side Effects of Drugs,* 10th ed. Dukes, M.N.G., ed. New York: Elsevier Science Publishing Co., 1984.

Kastrup, E.K., et al., eds. *Facts and Comparisons, 1986.* St. Louis: Facts and Comparisons Division, J.B. Lippincott Co., 1985.

Sneader, W. *Drug Discovery: The Evolution of Modern Medicine.* Chichester, Great Britain: John Wiley & Sons, 1985.

United States Pharmacopeial Convention. *Advice for the Patient, vol. II, USPDI.* Kingsport, Tenn.: Kingsport Press, 1983.

United States Pharmacopeial Convention. *Drug Information for the Health Care Provider, vol. I, USPDI* Kingsport, Tenn.: Kingsport Press, 1983.

Weiner, N. "Norepinephrine, Epinephrine, and the Sympathomimetic Amines," in *Goodman and Gilman's The Pharmacological Basis of Therapeutics,* 7th ed. Gilman, A.G., et al., eds. New York: Macmillan Publishing Co., 1985.

DRUGS TO IMPROVE GASTROINTESTINAL FUNCTION

The gastrointestinal (GI) tract has three major functions: digestion of foods and fluids, absorption of foods and fluids, and excretion of metabolic waste. In the GI tract, various hormones and enzymes break down food into particles that are small enough to permeate cell membranes and be used for cellular energy. The GI tract itself helps prevent infection by maintaining mucous membrane integrity, secreting immunoglobulins, and destroying pathogens.

GI disorders frequently disrupt activities of daily living, interrupt work schedules, and lead to hospital admissions. Many are pathologic, such as benign or malignant tumors, peptic ulcer disease, gastroesophageal reflux, regional ileitis (Crohn's disease) and ulcerative colitis, malabsorption, intestinal obstruction, and diverticulosis. Others are psychophysiologic disorders. Whether the cause is pathologic or psychophysiologic, however, GI disorders frequently produce similar signs and symptoms that are typically so vague and nonspecific that many patients delay seeking treatment.

Signs and symptoms
Common signs and symptoms of GI tract disorders include anorexia, dysphagia, nausea, vomiting, dyspepsia, epigastric or abdominal pain, abdominal distention, flatulence, diarrhea, constipation, and rectal bleeding. These findings may indicate many possible causes. GI tract disorders may cause fluid and electrolyte imbalances with resultant cardiac dysrhythmias and hypovolemia, extended areas of inflammation or infection, abscesses or fistulas, malnutrition, perforated structures with resultant peritonitis, and altered body image. Medical management of GI disorders is usually conservative, symptomatic, and supportive. Initial treatment usually consists of diet therapy, rest, and stress management. If these measures prove ineffective, drug therapy or surgery may be used.

Clinical indications
Unit Ten discusses drugs that are used to manage GI tract disorders. It presents the major drug categories, including adsorbents, antiflatulents, digestive agents, antidiarrheals, laxatives and cathartics, emetics, antiemet-

ics, antacids, histamine antagonists, and sucralfate. Because many of the drugs in these categories are available over the counter, self-medication is common.

This unit also presents two general categories of drug therapy: (1) treatment of specific diseases such as digestive enzyme deficiencies, portal-systemic encephalopathy, acute toxic poisoning, peptic ulcer disease, and esophageal reflux; and (2) control of symptoms of specific diseases such as nausea, vomiting, epigastric pain, dyspepsia, flatulence, diarrhea, and constipation.

Chapter 47
Adsorbent, Antiflatulent, and Digestive Agents
Chapter 47 reviews normal GI tract function before exploring activated charcoal, an adsorbent agent used to treat acute poisoning. It also discusses simethicone, an antiflatulent used to treat conditions that promote excess gas formation, and the digestive agents hydrochloric acid, pepsin, bile acids and salts, and pancreatic enzymes.

Chapter 48
Antidiarrheal and Laxative Agents
Chapter 48 discusses diarrhea and constipation and reviews the drugs used to treat them. It explores antidiarrheal agents, including opium tincture, loperamide, diphenoxylate, and kaolin-pectin mixtures, as well as various laxatives, including lactulose, glycerin, hyperosmolar laxatives, dietary fiber and bulk-forming agents, emollient laxatives, and stimulant laxatives. The chapter also discusses the clinical use of stool softeners.

Chapter 49
Emetic and Antiemetic Agents
Chapter 49 examines the physiology of nausea and vomiting and the conditions that stimulate them. Next, it explains the use of emetics, such as apomorphine and ipecac syrup, to induce vomiting after ingestion of toxic substances. Then it discusses the various antiemetic agents including antihistamines, phenothiazines, benzquinamide, scopolamine, metoclopramide, nabilone, and dronabinol.

Glossary

Adsorbent: drug that inhibits the GI absorption of various drugs, toxins, and chemicals by attracting and holding them to its surface.

Antacid: drug that neutralizes gastric acids.

Antidiarrheal: drug that decreases both the frequency of defecation and water content of the stools.

Antiemetic: drug that relieves nausea and vomiting.

Antiflatulent: drug that decreases gastrointestinal gas.

Bile: golden brown to greenish yellow fluid, secreted by the liver into the intestine, that assists in fat emulsification and absorption.

Cathartic: agent that promotes evacuation of the bowels.

Constipation: decreased movement of fecal matter through the large intestine.

Diarrhea: increased frequency or weight and liquidity of stools produced by the rapid movement of fecal matter through the large intestine.

Digestant: drug that enhances digestion in the GI tract.

Emetic: drug that induces vomiting.

Emollient: drug that softens the stool by increasing water content of fecal material by reduction in surface tension of bowel contents.

Gastrin: hormone secreted by the pyloric mucosa that increases the flow of gastric juices.

Histamine antagonist: drug that decreases gastric acid secretion by inhibiting gastric histamine (H_2) release.

Laxative: drug that stimulates defecation by forming bulk, stimulating peristalsis, or providing lubrication or chemical irritation.

Nausea: unpleasant epigastric or abdominal sensation that, in many cases, leads to vomiting.

Pepsin: proteolytic enzyme in gastric juice that acts as a catalyst in protein hydrolysis.

Ulcer: cutaneous or mucosal lesion caused by gradual erosion, disintegration, and necrosis of underlying tissue.

Vomiting: forcible expulsion of gastric contents through the mouth.

Chapter 50
Peptic Ulcer Agents

Chapter 50 begins with the pathophysiology of peptic, duodenal, and gastric ulcers. It then examines antacids, histamine₂-receptor antagonists, and sucralfate for treating ulcers, emphasizing their clinical use, safety, and effectiveness. The chapter concludes with a brief discussion of five types of drugs under investigation for use in ulcer therapy.

Nursing diagnoses

For a patient with a GI tract disorder, nursing diagnoses based on history data and a complete physical examination can facilitate nursing care. When assessing the patient, the nurse should remember that many drugs can cause GI symptoms as adverse reactions. A comprehensive assessment may lead to any of the following nursing diagnoses:

• Activity intolerance related to fluid and electrolyte imbalances and fatigue

• Alteration in bowel elimination: constipation, related to decreased activity level and inadequate fluid intake

• Alteration in bowel elimination: diarrhea, related to hypermotility

• Alteration in comfort: pain, related to abdominal distention and abdominal pain

• Alteration in nutrition: less than body requirement, related to decreased food intake

• Alteration in oral mucous membranes related to vomiting

• Disturbance in self-concept related to chronic GI tract disorder

• Fluid volume deficit related to upper or lower GI bleeding, severe diarrhea, or severe vomiting

• Ineffective airway clearance related to vomiting

• Ineffective breathing pattern related to abdominal distention and abdominal pain

• Knowledge deficit related to the therapeutic regimen

• Potential for injury related to the ingestion of toxic substances

• Sleep pattern disturbance related to nausea, vomiting, or altered bowel elimination

ADSORBENT, ANTIFLATULENT, AND DIGESTIVE AGENTS

OBJECTIVES

After reading and studying this chapter, you should be able to:

1. Describe the physiology of digestion from the stomach to the large intestine, explaining how enzymes and hormones from the stomach, liver, pancreas, and duodenum aid digestion.

2. Explain how an adsorbent works to treat an acute poisoning.

3. Describe the mechanism of action by which antiflatulents work in the gastrointestinal tract.

4. Identify the purpose of each of the three major groups of digestants.

5. Delineate the pharmacokinetic properties of hydrochloric acid (dilute), bile salts, and pancreatic enzymes.

6. Identify predictable and unpredictable adverse reactions associated with digestants.

INTRODUCTION

The alimentary tract's primary function is to provide the human body with fluids and nutrients. Before the cells can use these fluids and nutrients, various absorptive, peristaltic, and digestive functions must occur.

The stomach mucosa consists of two sets of tubular glands: gastric glands and pyloric glands. The gastric glands secrete hydrochloric acid, pepsinogen, intrinsic

Major digestive hormones

Understanding the major digestive hormones in terms of their sources, activating substances, and actions assists the nurse in analyzing the relationship between these substances and the physiology of digestion.

HORMONE	SOURCE	ACTIVATING SUBSTANCES	ACTION
gastrin	Gastric mucosa of the pylorus	Partially digested proteins in the pylorus	• Stimulates release of gastric juice rich in pepsinogen and hydrochloric acid
secretin	Duodenal mucosa	Partially digested proteins, fats, and acids in the duodenum	• Stimulates secretion of low-enzyme, high-bicarbonate pancreatic juice • Stimulates secretion of bile by liver • May enhance cholecystokinin activity in producing pancreatic enzymes; may inhibit gastric motility, acid secretion, and pyloric sphincter contraction
cholecystokinin	Duodenal mucosa	Partially digested proteins, fats, and acids in the duodenum	• Stimulates secretion of high-enzyme pancreatic juice • Inhibits gastric emptying and secretion and intestinal motility • Stimulates gallbladder contractions leading to a release of bile

Major digestive substances

Digestive substances are essential for the body to use ingested foods. Each digestive substance functions in a specific way on specific food components to produce usable nutrients.

SUBSTANCE	SOURCE	FOOD COMPONENT	PRODUCT
pepsin	Gastric glands	Proteins	Polypeptides, peptides, proteoses (partially digested proteins)
gastric acid	Gastric juice	Emulsified fats	Fatty acids, glycerol
bile	Liver (stored in and released from gallbladder)	Unemulsified fats	Emulsified fats
trypsin	Pancreatic juice	Proteins, polypeptides	Proteoses, peptides, amino acids
chymotrypsin	Pancreatic juice	Proteins, polypeptides	Polypeptides, amino acids
lipase	Pancreatic juice	Bile-emulsified fats	Fatty acids, glycerol
amylase	Pancreatic juice	Starch	Maltose, isomaltose
ribonuclease	Pancreatic juice	Nucleic acids	Nucleotides
deoxyribonuclease	Pancreatic juice	Nucleic acids	Nucleotides
carboxypolypeptidase	Pancreatic juice	Polypeptides	Smaller polypeptides

factor, and mucus; the pyloric glands secrete mucus, pepsinogen, and the hormone gastrin. At a pH of approximately 0.8, hydrochloric acid is extremely acidic. When pepsinogen comes in contact with the hydrochloric acid, active pepsin, a proteolytic enzyme, is formed. This pepsin digests protein when the pH of the pepsin is less than 3.5.

As food enters the antrum of the stomach, the pyloric glands secrete gastrin, which aids digestion by stimulating: (1) secretion of hydrochloric acid and pepsin, (2) secretion of intrinsic factor and pancreatic enzymes, (3) release of insulin and flow of hepatic bile, and (4) gastric and intestinal motility.

Hepatocytes (cells within the liver) continually produce bile, which is ultimately secreted into the common bile duct. From the common bile duct, bile is either emptied directly into the duodenum or concentrated and stored in the gallbladder. Substances secreted in the bile include bile salts, bilirubin, cholesterol, lecithin, and electrolytes. As bile is concentrated in the gallbladder, the mucosa reabsorbs large amounts of fluid and electrolytes. In the intestines, bile salts serve two major functions: they act as a detergent on fat particles, thereby decreasing the surface tension of the fat particles and converting them into smaller sizes (emulsification); and

they help absorb cholesterol, fatty acids, monoglycerides, and other lipids from the intestinal tract. As fats are absorbed in the intestines, the fat-soluble vitamins A, D, E, and K are also absorbed.

The major functions of the pancreas include insulin production by the beta islet cells and the production of pancreatic juice, which is released into the duodenum. Pancreatic juice includes specific enzymes that aid in the digestion of proteins, carbohydrates, and fats. The major proteolytic enzymes include trypsin (the most abundant), chymotrypsin, carboxypolypeptidase, ribonuclease, and deoxyribonuclease. Pancreatic amylase is the major digestive enzyme for carbohydrates, while pancreatic lipase is the major digestive enzyme for fats. Secretin and cholecystokinin are hormones that increase pancreatic enzyme secretion. The acid content of the stomach releases secretin from the duodenum, whereas food content stimulates the release of cholecystokinin. (See *Major digestive substances* for a summary of some digestive secretions.)

Parasympathetic stimulation via the vagus nerve also increases enzyme release into the acinar cells of the pancreas. The combined result of these hormonal and neuronal actions is the increased secretion of pancreatic fluid, bicarbonate, and enzymes (trypsin, amylase, and lipase) into the small intestine to aid digestion. (See *Major digestive hormones* on page 738 for a summary of these important digestives.)

Adsorbent agents are used when toxins have been ingested. Toxins ingested through the GI tract that cause poisoning or overdose include drugs, such as amphetamines, aspirin, barbiturates, cocaine, morphine, opium, and tricyclic antidepressants. Ingested poisonous mushrooms also produce toxins.

Two major disturbances of digestion in the gastrointestinal tract include gastric bloating with or without flatulence, and inadequate or incomplete digestion. Antiflatulents are commonly indicated for patients with functional gastric bloating. Under normal physiologic conditions, gases collect in the gastrointestinal tract from swallowed air, bacterial action, and gas diffusion from the blood into the lumen. Nitrogen and oxygen are the primary gases found in the stomach. Approximately 10 liters of gas enter or are formed daily in the large intestine. This gastrointestinal gas may be absorbed or expelled either through belching or flatus.

Physicians use digestive agents (digestants) in these clinical situations involving incomplete digestion: hydrochloric acid for hypochlorhydria and achlorhydria, bile salts as replacement therapy for conditions that cause bile salt deficiencies in the upper intestines, and pancreatic enzymes for conditions that cause decreased production of pancreatic juice (pancreatitis or cystic fibrosis).

This chapter covers both natural and synthetic adsorbents, antiflatulents, and digestants.

For a summary of representative drugs, see *Selected Major Drugs: Adsorbent, antiflatulent, and digestive agents* on page 745.

ADSORBENTS

An adsorbent is an agent that attracts molecules of a liquid, gas, or dissolved substance to its surface. The attracted molecules concentrate in a thin layer over the surface of the adsorbent. Physicians prescribe adsorbents in acute situations to prevent the absorption of drugs or toxins from the gastrointestinal tract. The major adsorbent used clinically is activated charcoal, a black powder residue obtained from the distillation of various organic materials.

PHARMACOKINETICS

Adsorbent agents belong to the class of drugs known as protective agents of the gastrointestinal mucosa, which are designed to prevent contact with possible irritants.

Absorption, distribution, metabolism, excretion
Adsorbents are chemically inert powders that attract dissolved or suspended substances, such as gases, toxins, and bacteria, thereby preventing the absorption of these substances in the gastrointestinal tract. Adsorbents, which are neither absorbed nor metabolized by the body, are excreted unchanged in the feces.

Onset, peak, duration
The adsorbent activated charcoal must be administered soon after ingestion of a poison because it can only bind drugs or toxins that have not yet been absorbed from the gastrointestinal tract. Duration of action depends upon the agent's transit time through the bowel and the resultant contact time for adsorption to occur. The particle size of the charcoal also influences duration of action. Activated charcoals composed of small particles prove the most effective because the small particles provide a larger total surface area for the toxin to adhere to.

PHARMACODYNAMICS

Adsorbents are general-purpose antidotes used for acute episodes of oral poisoning. The adsorbent's effectiveness depends upon its quick administration after toxin ingestion and the adsorbent's total surface area, which is determined by particle size.

Mechanism of action
Adsorbents attract and bind toxins in the intestinal lumen, thus inhibiting absorption of the toxins from the gastrointestinal tract. No one adsorbent is useful for all toxins; instead, specific adsorbents work with specific toxins.

PHARMACOTHERAPEUTICS

No one adsorbent is effective for all toxins. Activated charcoal is indicated in many situations of acute oral poisoning, but it is not indicated in acute poisoning from cyanide, ethanol, methanol, iron, sodium chloride alkalies, inorganic acids, or organic solvents. (See *Common toxins treated by activated charcoal*.)

activated charcoal (Charcocaps, Digestalin). Activated charcoal is an odorless, tasteless black powder obtained from the destructive distillation of several organic substances treated to increase their adsorptive power.

Common toxins treated by activated charcoal

Activated charcoal is used to treat numerous toxins. Knowing which toxins are susceptible to activated charcoal assists the nurse in planning patient care and teaching strategies.

- amphetamines
- antimony
- aspirin
- atropine
- barbiturates
- camphor
- carbon tetrachloride
- cardiotoxic glycosides
- cocaine
- phenothiazines
- potassium permanganate
- propoxyphene
- quinine
- sulfonamides
- tricyclic antidepressants

USUAL ADULT DOSAGE: 5 to 10 times the estimated weight of the drug or chemical ingested, or a minimum dose of 30 grams, mixed in 250 ml of water. Give activated charcoal P.O. within 30 minutes of the poisoning. The dose may be repeated every 2 hours when used for drugs that undergo enterohepatic circulation (such as phenobarbital) or for drugs that are resecreted into the stomach (such as tricyclic antidepressants).

Drug interactions

Do not administer activated charcoal simultaneously with ipecac syrup; the activated charcoal will adsorb the ipecac, rendering it inactive. Give emetics, such as ipecac, and allow emesis to occur before administering activated charcoal because emesis enhances the effectiveness of the activated charcoal by decreasing the amount of toxin in the GI tract to be adsorbed. The result is a more complete removal of the toxin.

ADVERSE DRUG REACTIONS

A predictable adverse reaction to activated charcoal administration is black stools. No known unpredictable adverse reactions exist. Furthermore, toxicity does not occur with activated charcoal, even at the maximum dose.

NURSING IMPLICATIONS

Adsorbents are administered in emergencies to treat acute oral poisoning. Be aware of the following nursing implications:
- Alert the patient to avoid eating ice cream after administration of activated charcoal because ice cream decreases the drug's adsorbent capacity.
- Give activated charcoal after emesis and not simultaneously with ipecac syrup.
- Be aware that large doses of activated charcoal may be needed to treat the toxic state if food is present in the patient's stomach.
- Add fruit juice to the mixture of activated charcoal and water to make it more palatable.
- Caution the patient to anticipate black stools from the activated charcoal.

ANTIFLATULENTS

Antiflatulents are mixtures of liquid dimethylpolysiloxanes and silica gel that possess antifoaming and water-repellent properties. Antiflatulents disperse gas pockets in the GI tract. Antiflatulents are available either alone or in combination with antacids.

PHARMACOKINETICS

Antiflatulents are physiologically inactive and are not absorbed in the gastrointestinal tract. Because antiflatulents are not absorbed, they do not interfere with gastric secretion or nutrient absorption. Antiflatulents are distributed only in the intestinal lumen and are eliminated intact in the feces. Antiflatulents provide an immediate onset of action, with duration of action lasting approximately 3 hours.

PHARMACODYNAMICS

Antiflatulents are physiologically inactive substances that provide defoaming action in the GI tract. Simethicone, a pale gray transparent liquid, is a mixture of liquid dimethylpolysiloxanes and silica gel that displays specific defoaming and water-repellent properties. By producing a film in the intestines that can collapse gas bubbles, simethicone disperses and helps prevent the formation of mucus-enclosed gas pockets.

PHARMACOTHERAPEUTICS

Physicians prescribe antiflatulents to treat conditions in which excess gas is a problem. These conditions typically include functional gastric bloating, postoperative gaseous bloating, diverticulitis, spastic or irritable colon, air swallowing, and peptic ulcer. Although simethicone has been frequently employed to decrease gas shadows during bowel radiography and to improve visualization during gastroscopy, clinical research trials have not supported this use.

simethicone (Mylicon). Simethicone is available in drops as an oral suspension (40 mg in 0.6 ml), in chewable tablets (40 to 125 mg), in tablets (50 to 95 mg), or in capsules (125 mg).
USUAL ADULT DOSAGE: 160 to 500 mg P.O. daily in divided doses, given after each meal and at bedtime.

Drug interactions

Antiflatulents do not produce any significant drug interactions.

ADVERSE DRUG REACTIONS

The predictable reaction involving antiflatulents is the expulsion of excessive gas via rectal flatus or belching. The antiflatulents do not cause any known unpredictable adverse reactions.

NURSING IMPLICATIONS

Observe the following implications when administering antiflatulents:
• Before administering antiflatulents, obtain a complete history and physical examination of the patient to rule out pathologic abdominal problems.
• Monitor the patient for the effectiveness of the antiflatulent.
• Teach the patient to shake the antiflatulent suspension before pouring the dose.
• Caution the patient to chew tablets well before swallowing.
• Caution the patient to use antiflatulents only when necessary and to avoid long-term use.
• If clinically advisable, encourage patients with functional gastric bloating to increase activity and exercise.

DIGESTIVES

Digestive agents (digestants) aid digestion in patients who lack one or more of the specific substances that naturally digest food. This section discusses digestants that function in the gastrointestinal tract, liver, and pancreas.

Dilute hydrochloric acid and glutamic acid hydrochloride replace natural gastric acids and are used to treat gastric hypochlorhydria (diminished hydrochloric acid in gastric juice), achlorhydria (absence of hydrochloric acid in gastric juice), and gastric achylia (absence of proteolytic enzymes and hydrochloric acid).

Bile salts (sodium salts of bile acids) and bile acids, such as dehydrocholic acid, are used to initiate bile flow from the liver. The precursor of bile salts is cholesterol, which is supplied in the diet or produced by the liver. Bile salts are converted to cholic acid and chenodeoxycholic acid. These acids conjugate with glycerine and taurine to form bile acids. The salts of the bile acids are then secreted in the bile.

Pancreatin and pancrelipase are used either to supplement or replace exocrine pancreatic secretions. These digestants aid the digestion of proteins, carbohydrates, and fats. (See *Sites of enzyme and hormone formation* for an illustration of the organs that contribute digestive secretions.)

PHARMACOKINETICS

The digestants are natural body substances. As such, they are absorbed, distributed, metabolized, and excreted as they would be if they were produced by the patient rather than taken therapeutically.

Absorption, distribution, metabolism, excretion

Hydrochloric acid and glutamic acid hydrochloride are distributed in the distal portion of the stomach and are absorbed in the gastrointestinal tract. These digestants are excreted as a part of the normal gastrointestinal tract elimination.

Approximately 80% of the bile salts are reabsorbed from the terminal ileum of the small intestine where they enter the enterohepatic circulation. Bile salts and bile acids are eventually excreted through the gastrointestinal tract as bile end products in the feces.

Pancreatic enzymes are absorbed within the gastrointestinal tract. They are distributed in the intestinal lumen and excreted as part of the normal gastrointestinal elimination.

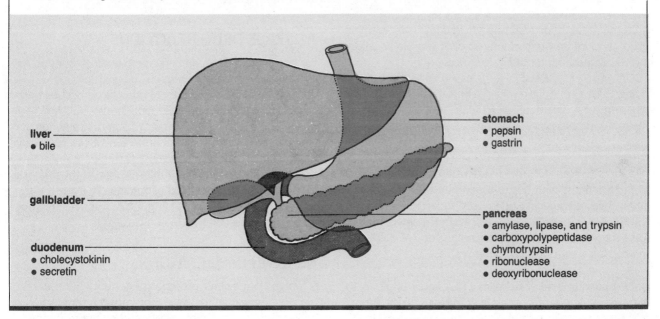

Sites of enzyme and hormone formation

This anatomic illustration shows where various enzymes and hormones are produced in the gastrointestinal tract. Most digestive enzymes and hormones are formed at sites near their locus of physiologic action.

liver
- bile

gallbladder

duodenum
- cholecystokinin
- secretin

stomach
- pepsin
- gastrin

pancreas
- amylase, lipase, and trypsin
- carboxypolypeptidase
- chymotrypsin
- ribonuclease
- deoxyribonuclease

Onset, peak, duration

The onset of action, peak concentration level, and duration of action of the digestants resemble those of the bodily produced substances they replace. Onset and duration of action depend on the type and amount of food ingested.

PHARMACODYNAMICS

The action of digestants resembles the action of the body substances they replace. When administered, both dilute hydrochloric acid and glutamic acid hydrochloride convert pepsinogen in the stomach into pepsin. The hydrochloric acid and pepsin initiate the digestion of the stomach contents by beginning the digestion of protein within the lower third of the stomach.

Bile acids, referred to as choleretic drugs, stimulate the bile production in the liver. Bile salts, however, provide little choleretic action. Bile salts emulsify fats, causing them to break into small pieces. These salts also help in the absorption of fatty acids, fat-soluble vitamins, cholesterol, and other lipids from the intestinal tract, thereby promoting normal digestion.

Pancreatic enzymes replace the normal exocrine pancreatic enzymes. Pancreatic enzymes act to digest proteins via trypsin, digest carbohydrates via amylase, and digest fats via lipase.

PHARMACOTHERAPEUTICS

Clinical indications for using the gastric digestants include those conditions in which the patient produces none or insufficient amounts of the normally occurring gastric acids. For example, dilute hydrochloric acid is indicated for patients with hypochlorhydria or achlorhydria.

Bile acids and bile salts may be administered to: (1) increase cholesterol solubility, thereby preventing accumulation of recurrent biliary calculi, (2) replace the natural substances in patients with pathologic conditions in which the concentration of bile components in the small intestine is low, and (3) facilitate drainage of the common bile duct via a T-tube in postcholecystectomy patients.

Pancreatic enzymes are used in clinical situations characterized by an insufficiency of pancreatic enzymes (specifically, pancreatitis and cystic fibrosis). Pancreatic enzymes are also used to treat steatorrhea, a disorder of fat metabolism.

hydrochloric acid, dilute. This agent is used to treat hypochlorhydria, achlorhydria, and gastric achylia.
USUAL ADULT DOSAGE: diluted form (10% solution), 5 to 10 ml in 125 to 250 ml of water in several divided doses at 15-minute intervals. The patient must sip the solution through a glass straw to prevent damage to tooth enamel.

glutamic acid hydrochloride (Acidulin). This agent is used, as is dilute hydrochloric acid, to treat hypochlorhydria, achlorhydria, and gastric achylia.
USUAL ADULT DOSAGE: 1 to 3 capsules (340 mg to 1 gram) P.O. t.i.d. before meals. The capsule form of this digestant prevents damage to teeth, but glutamic acid hydrochloride is not as effective as dilute hydrochloric acid.

bile salts (Bilron, Ox-Bile Extract Enseals). Once used to treat patients with biliary fistula and resection of the ileum, bile salts are not often used today.
USUAL ADULT DOSAGE: 1 to 2 enteric-coated tablets (324 mg each) P.O. t.i.d. after meals, or 150- to 600-mg capsules with or after meals.

dehydrocholic acid (Decholin). This agent is given to stimulate bile flow from the liver. The hydrocholeretic activity of this bile acid also stimulates T-tube drainage in postcholecystectomy patients.
USUAL ADULT DOSAGE: 250 to 750 mg P.O. t.i.d. after meals.

pancreatin (Dizymes). A natural substance obtained from fresh porcine or bovine pancreas, pancreatin is a combination of the enzymes amylase, trypsin, and lipase. Pancreatin replaces endogenous exocrine pancreatic enzymes and aids in digestion of starches, fats, and protein.
USUAL ADULT DOSAGE: 1 to 3 tablets P.O. after meals.

pancrelipase (Cotazym, Ilozyme, Pancrease, Viokase). Pancrelipase is derived from porcine pancreas. The lipase activity of pancrelipase is greater than that of pancreatin, making pancrelipase useful in treating steatorrhea and exocrine pancreatic secretion insufficiency associated with diseases such as cystic fibrosis.
USUAL ADULT DOSAGE: 1 to 3 capsules or tablets P.O. before or with meals, and 1 capsule or tablet P.O. with snacks, or 0.7 g powder P.O. before meals or snacks.

Drug interactions

No significant drug interactions occur with the administration of hydrochloric acid, glutamic acid hydrochloride, bile salts, or the bile acid dehydrocholic acid. However, antacids negate the effects of pancreatin and pancrelipase. Because of this, avoid administering antacids with pancreatin or pancrelipase.

ADVERSE DRUG REACTIONS

Hydrochloric acid can damage tooth enamel. For this reason, always administer hydrochloric acid through a glass straw. A massive overdose of hydrochloric acid can also cause acid-base abnormalities (specifically, metabolic acidosis). The bile salts and bile acids can produce abdominal cramping and diarrhea. Administration of the pancreatic enzymes often causes nausea and diarrhea.

Bile salts may reduce the resistance of the mucosal barrier of the stomach and esophagus to acid. If a dislodged gallstone is obstructing a biliary duct, the choleretic bile acids can produce biliary colic.

NURSING IMPLICATIONS

Although physicians prescribe digestants infrequently, the nurse must still be aware of important implications concerning their administration and contraindications.
• Hydrochloric acid is contraindicated in peptic ulcer disease.
• Inform the patient that the number of bowel movements will decrease during digestant therapy and that the stool consistency will improve when replacement therapy reaches an adequate therapeutic level.
• Instruct the patient to store digestants in tight containers at room temperature to prevent their deterioration.
• Bile salts are contraindicated in marked hepatic dysfunction and biliary obstruction.
• The bile acid dehydrocholic acid is contraindicated in the presence of biliary obstruction, nausea, vomiting, or abdominal pain.
• Pancreatic enzymes are contraindicated in patients sensitive to porcine or bovine products.
• Inform the patient that hydrochloric acid tastes sour.
• Administer dilute hydrochloric acid through a glass straw to prevent damage to tooth enamel.
• Instruct the patient taking pancreatic enzyme products to balance fat, protein, and carbohydrate intake to avoid indigestion.

Adsorbent, antiflatulent, and digestive agents

The following chart summarizes selected adsorbents, antiflatulents, and digestants discussed in this chapter.

DRUG	MAJOR INDICATIONS	USUAL ADULT DOSAGES	NURSING IMPLICATIONS
Adsorbent			
activated charcoal	Acute toxic poisoning	5 to 10 times the estimated weight of the drug or chemical toxin ingested, or a minimum dose of 30 grams in a mixture with 250 ml of water, P.O.	• Caution the patient to avoid ice cream since it decreases the adsorbent capacity. • Give after emesis; do not give simultaneously with ipecac syrup. • Inform the patient to anticipate black stools. • May need to give larger doses if food is in the stomach. • Add fruit juice to the mixture of activated charcoal and water to make it more palatable.
Antiflatulent			
simethicone	Excess GI tract gas	160 to 480 mg P.O. daily in divided doses, given after each meal and at bedtime	• Advise the patient to chew tablets well and not to swallow the tablet whole. • Obtain a complete history and physical examination before administration to rule out pathologic abdominal problems. • Caution the patient to avoid long-term use. • If clinically advisable, encourage the patient to increase activity and exercise. • Monitor for the effectiveness of this agent.
Digestants			
hydrochloric acid (dilute)	Hypochlorhydria and achlorhydria	5 to 10 ml in 125 to 250 ml of water P.O. in divided doses at 15-minute intervals	• Advise patient to sip hydrochloric acid through a glass straw during meals to prevent damage to tooth enamel.
glutamic acid hydrochloride	Hypochlorhydria and achlorhydria	1 to 3 capsules P.O. t.i.d. before meals (340 mg to 1 g)	• Do not give in presence of gastric hyperacidity or peptic ulcer disease. • Monitor the patient's response to these agents.
bile salts	Insufficient bile production	1 to 2 tablets P.O. t.i.d. after meals; or 150 to 600 mg P.O. with or after meals	• Do not administer when the patient is nauseated or vomiting, or has abdominal pain.
dehydrocholic acid	Insufficient bile production	250 to 750 mg P.O. b.i.d. or t.i.d. after meals for 4 to 6 weeks	• Do not administer when the patient is nauseated or vomiting, or has abdominal pain. • Frequent use may result in dependence on laxatives.
pancreatin	Insufficient pancreatic enzymes	1 to 3 tablets P.O. after meals	• Contraindicated in patients who are sensitive to porcine or bovine products. • Administer pancreatin in enteric capsules to prevent its destruction by pepsin.
pancrelipase	Insufficient pancreatic enzymes and steatorrhea	1 to 3 capsules P.O. before or with meals and 1 capsule P.O. with any snack	• Teach the patient to balance dietary intake carefully to avoid abdominal discomfort and indigestion. • Inform the patient that replacement agents will decrease the number of bowel movements. • Teach the patient to store drugs in tight containers at room temperature. • Monitor the patient's response to these agents.

CHAPTER SUMMARY

Chapter 47 began with a discussion of the enzymes and hormones involved in digestion. The chapter then presented the pharmacokinetics, pharmacodynamics, pharmacotherapeutics, adverse drug reactions, and nursing implications of adsorbents, antiflatulents, and digestants. Here are the highlights of the chapter:

• Enzymes and hormones secreted by the liver, pancreas, stomach, and duodenum work together to digest food in the body.

• Major disturbances of digestion in the GI tract include gastric bloating with or without flatulence, and inadequate or incomplete digestion.

• An adsorbent is an agent that attracts molecules of a liquid, gas, or dissolved substance to its surface. Adsorbents are used to prevent the absorption of toxins in the GI tract in acute poisonings.

• The adsorbent activated charcoal is a chemically inert powder that is neither absorbed nor metabolized by the body. Activated charcoal is excreted unchanged in the feces. If given within 30 minutes of acute poisoning, activated charcoal will bind the toxin and thus inhibit its absorption.

• Antiflatulents are mixtures of liquid dimethylpolysiloxanes and silica gel that disperse and prevent the formation of mucus-enclosed gas pockets in the GI tract.

• The antiflatulent simethicone is a physiologically inactive substance that is clinically safe when used to treat conditions in which excess gas is a problem.

• Specific digestants include hydrochloric acid, glutamic acid hydrochloride, bile acids, bile salts, and pancreatic enzymes.

• Digestants aid the patient who lacks one or more of the specific digestive substances produced by the body.

• Patients receiving digestants need specific instructions concerning both the purpose of these drugs and the precautions to take during administration.

BIBLIOGRAPHY

Brimioulle, S., et al. "Hydrochloric Acid Infusion for Treatment of Metabolic Alkalosis: Effects on Acid-Base Balance and Oxygenation," *Critical Care Medicine.* 13:738, September 1985.

Clavert, R., et al. "Dietary Fiber and Intestinal Adaption: Effects on Intestinal and Pancreatic Digestive Enzyme Activities," *American Journal of Clinical Nutrition.* 41:1249, June 1985.

Kulig, K., et al. "Management of Acutely Poisoned Patients Without Gastric Emptying," *Annals of Emergency Medicine.* 14:562, June 1985.

Olkkola, K.T., et al. "Do Gastric Contents Modify Antidotal Efficacy of Oral Activated Charcoal?" *British Journal of Clinical Pharmacology.* 18:663, November 1984.

Sato, T., et al. "Gastric Acid Secretion and Gut Hormone Release in Patients Undergoing Pancreaticoduodenectomy," *Surgery.* 99:728, June 1986.

Van Ness, M.M., et al. "Flatulence: Pathophysiology and Treatment," *American Family Physician.* 31:198, April 1985.

CHAPTER 48

ANTIDIARRHEAL AND LAXATIVE AGENTS

OBJECTIVES

After reading and studying this chapter, you should be be able to:

1. Identify the various antidiarrheal agents indicated for acute, nonspecific diarrhea and chronic diarrhea.

2. Explain the mechanism of action of opium tincture in alleviating diarrhea.

3. Identify the potential adverse effects of opium tincture and paregoric, and describe the related nursing implications.

4. Explain how loperamide and diphenoxylate decrease gastrointestinal (GI) motility.

5. Describe the effectiveness of kaolin and pectin in treating the different kinds of diarrhea.

6. Identify the contraindications and precautions the nurse should be aware of when administering antidiarrheals.

7. Describe the general mechanism of action of laxatives.

8. Identify the clinical indications for hyperosmolar, bulk-forming, emollient, stimulant, and lubricant laxatives.

9. Identify the range of adverse reactions associated with hyperosmolar laxatives.

INTRODUCTION

Diarrhea and constipation represent the two major symptoms related to disturbances of the large intestine. Diarrhea refers to the increased frequency or weight and liquidity of stools produced by the rapid movement of fecal material through the large intestine. Constipation refers to the decreased movement of fecal matter through the large intestine.

Significant disorders involving diarrhea include ulcerative colitis, enteritis, and psychogenic diarrhea. Ulcerative colitis, a nonspecific inflammatory disease of the large intestine, is characterized by multiple ulcerations throughout the mucosal and submucosal linings of the intestine as well as repeated diarrheal stools. Though the cause of ulcerative colitis remains unclear, emotional

factors as well as specific infectious bacteria may contribute to it. Enteritis is an infection of the large intestine caused by either a virus or bacteria. Enteritis is typically an acute problem resulting in diarrhea, whereas ulcerative colitis is more often chronic in nature, marked by acute exacerbations and remissions. Psychogenic diarrhea is marked by excessive activation of the parasympathetic branch of the autonomic nervous system resulting in enhanced motility and secretion in the large intestine. This acute condition triggers a brief episode of self-limiting diarrhea.

Over time, the decreased peristaltic movements that characterize constipation may cause the production and accumulation of hard feces in the lower bowel, producing a decreased frequency, weight, and volume of stool passed. Most cases of constipation arise from poor bowel habits established in childhood and maintained through adulthood. This voluntary inhibition of normal defecation reflexes can weaken normal intestinal action. Long-term laxative abuse also impairs normal intestinal tone and peristaltic response, leading to an atonic bowel. Bowel retraining programs emphasize the gastrocolic and duodenocolic reflexes that are activated after a meal high in both content and fluids. Poor dietary habits are also a major cause of constipation, and constipation occasionally occurs from spasm of the sigmoid colon wall. The health care professional may detect chronic constipation in patients who complain of repeated patterns of constipation and mucoid diarrhea. Both diarrhea and constipation are common effects of many drugs, such as antacids.

Both diarrhea and constipation involve debilitating physiologic sequelae that may interfere with an individual's ability to perform the activities of daily living. Diarrhea may precipitate abdominal discomfort, malaise, and lethargy from dehydration. Constipation may be harmful in patients who should not strain, such as those with recent myocardial infarction. Drugs designed to control the symptoms of diarrhea and constipation are invaluable for patients with these problems.

Discussions in this chapter center on the following classes of drugs: (1) antidiarrheals, including opium tincture, paregoric, loperamide, diphenoxylate, and kaolin and pectin mixtures and (2) stool softeners and laxatives, including lactulose, glycerin, and saline compounds (hyperosmolar laxatives), dietary fiber and other bulk-forming laxatives, emollient laxatives, and stimulant laxatives. The discussion includes natural, synthetic, and semisynthetic drugs.

For a summary of representative drugs, see *Selected major drugs: Antidiarrheal and laxative agents* on page 761.

ANTIDIARRHEAL AGENTS

Antidiarrheals reduce the fluidity of the stool and the frequency of defecation. Antidiarrheals act either systemically or locally. Opium tincture, paregoric, loperamide, and diphenoxylate—all opiates—are systemic agents. The combination of kaolin and pectin is a local agent.

LAXATIVES

Laxatives and cathartics include various drugs that stimulate defecation. Laxatives exert their effects by increasing the water content of the feces and increasing the movement of the intestinal materials from the colon and rectum. The term *cathartic* implies a fluid evacuation in contrast to the term *laxative*, which implies the elimination of a soft, formed stool.

The major classes of laxatives include the hyperosmolar agents, dietary fiber and related bulk-forming substances, emollients, stimulants, and lubricants. The U.S. Food and Drug Administration Advisory Review Panel has approved various laxative-cathartic drugs as over-the-counter (OTC), nonprescription drugs. Laxatives are at times abused, and frequent use can result in physical dependence for maintenance of bowel pattern.

ANTIDIARRHEALS: OPIUM PREPARATIONS

Opium tincture and camphorated opium tincture, also called paregoric, are effective in treating acute, nonspecific diarrhea; however, these drugs should not be used for diarrhea from toxic chemicals or organisms. The drugs, which are well absorbed, produce some of the systemic effects of morphine in high doses.

History and source

Opium is obtained from the juice of the poppy, *Papaver somniferum*. The Greek Theophrastus first noted the psychological effects of opium in the 3rd century B.C. By the middle of the 19th century, researchers were aware that opium contained at least 20 separate alkaloids. The use of opium to relieve diarrhea preceded its use as an analgesic, perhaps by many centuries. The term opioid is a generic word referring to all drugs with morphinelike actions, whether natural or synthetic.

PHARMACOKINETICS

Opium tincture and camphorated opium tincture have similar pharmacokinetic properties. Both are absorbed systemically, metabolized by the liver, and excreted by the kidneys. The onset of action occurs within 1 hour of administration.

Absorption, distribution, metabolism, excretion

When administered orally, opium tincture and camphorated opium tincture are quickly absorbed from the GI tract. After absorption, the drugs are distributed to various parenchymatous tissues, specifically the kidneys, lungs, liver, and spleen. Metabolism and detoxification via conjugation with glucuronic acid occur in the liver. Approximately 90% of the opioid metabolites are excreted by the kidneys, while the remainder is excreted as bile products in the feces.

Onset, peak, duration

When given orally, opium tincture and camphorated opium tincture have an onset of action that occurs within the first hour and concentration levels that peak within 2 to 3 hours. The duration of action is approximately 4 hours.

PHARMACODYNAMICS

The morphine in opium tincture and camphorated opium tincture decreases GI motility and peristaltic movements.

Mechanism of action

The binding or receptor sites for opium tincture and camphorated opium tincture are found in the nerve plexuses and exocrine glands of the stomach and large and small intestines. The morphine decreases hydrochloric acid secretion and stomach motility while it increases antral tone. It also decreases propulsive contractions in the small intestine.

Opium tincture and camphorated opium tincture exert an antidiarrheal effect by: (1) slowing the effects of the mesenteric plexus of the intestine, (2) inhibiting intestinal peristalsis by direct central action on the brain, (3) decreasing propulsive contractions, (4) enhancing anal sphincter tone, and (5) enhancing ileocecal valve tone.

PHARMACOTHERAPEUTICS

Physicians use opium tincture and camphorated opium tincture to treat acute, nonspecific diarrhea. These opium preparations are frequently used in combination with kaolin, pectin, and bismuth salts for their adsorbent and protective effects. In large doses, opium tincture may affect the central nervous system (CNS).

opium tincture. A Schedule II drug, opium tincture is used to treat acute, nonspecific diarrhea.
USUAL ADULT DOSAGE: 0.6 ml (range 0.3 to 1 ml) P.O. q.i.d. The maximum dose is 6 ml/day.

paregoric or camphorated opium tincture. A Schedule III drug, paregoric is used to treat diarrhea. This drug is more dilute than opium tincture and is easier to measure.
USUAL ADULT DOSAGE: 5 to 10 ml P.O. daily to q.i.d., until acute diarrhea subsides.
USUAL PEDIATRIC DOSAGE: 0.25 to 0.5 ml/kg/day daily to q.i.d., until diarrhea subsides.

Drug interactions

Opium tincture and paregoric can enhance the depressant effects of alcohol, barbiturates, tranquilizers, and other CNS depressants. The drugs have an additive effect of constipation when used with anticholinergic drugs.

ADVERSE DRUG REACTIONS

Some adverse effects result from opium tincture and paregoric, however these effects are mostly mild with usual doses.

Predictable reactions

The predictable reactions to opium tincture and paregoric include nausea, vomiting, dizziness, dysphoria, constipation, and increased biliary tract pressure.

Unpredictable reactions

Unpredictable reactions include allergic reactions, such as urticaria and contact dermatitis. Anaphylactoid reactions are rare. Patients over age 60 experience more frequent allergic reactions and decreased sensitivity to pain.

NURSING IMPLICATIONS

Opium tincture and paregoric effectively treat diarrhea. However, the nurse should use caution when administering these drugs.
• Opium tincture and paregoric are contraindicated in acute diarrhea from organisms that may penetrate the intestinal mucosa.
• These drugs should not be used in patients with diarrhea caused by poisoning until toxic substances are eliminated by gastric lavage or cathartics.
• Administer these drugs cautiously with other analgesics, sedatives, and narcotics.
• Administer opium tinctures cautiously to a patient with a decreased respiratory rate (less than 12 breaths/minute).
• Administer these drugs cautiously to patients with asthma, benign prostatic hypertrophy, narcotic dependence, and liver dysfunction.
• Closely monitor the long-term use of opium preparations because of possible physical dependence.
• Observe proper procedures for storing and handling Schedule II and III drugs.
• Monitor the patient's GI response to the drug; record the frequency and amount of bowel movements per day; replace fluid as necessary.
• Consult with the physician if the patient's diarrhea lasts longer than 48 hours or if fever and abdominal pain develop during treatment with opium preparations.
• Be aware that the opium content of opium tincture is 25 times greater than that of camphorated opium tincture, and that the two drugs should never be used interchangeably.
• Be aware that a milky fluid normally forms when camphorated opium tincture is added to water.
• Inform the patient to take the drug as prescribed to avoid dependence.

ANTIDIARRHEALS: LOPERAMIDE AND DIPHENOXYLATE

Loperamide and diphenoxylate are synthetic drugs related to meperidine. Both drugs decrease peristalsis in the intestines. Loperamide produces less severe CNS effects than does diphenoxylate, which is combined with atropine to prevent abuse.

History and source

Meperidine, a synthetic analgesic, was introduced in 1939 by Eisleb and Schaumann. Physicians use meperidine predominantly for its analgesic effect; they use loperamide and diphenoxylate only for their constipating effects.

PHARMACOKINETICS

Diphenoxylate has better absorption, a faster onset of action, and a shorter duration of action than loperamide.

Absorption, distribution, metabolism, excretion

Loperamide, which is not well absorbed after oral administration, does not penetrate well into the brain. Diphenoxylate, however, is readily absorbed into the gastrointestinal tract and, at high doses (40 to 60 mg), penetrates well into the brain. After oral administration, loperamide and diphenoxylate enter the GI tract to bind with receptor sites in the mucosal layers of the large and small intestines. Both drugs are distributed in the serum. Metabolism occurs with the detoxification process in the liver. Diphenoxylate is metabolized to diphenoxylic acid, its biologically active, major metabolite. Both drugs are excreted primarily in the feces.

Onset, peak, duration

Concentration levels of loperamide peak in 4 to 5 hours after oral administration. The duration of action of loperamide is 7 to 10 hours, with a half-life of 7 to 14 hours. The peak concentration level of diphenoxylate is probably within 2 to 3 hours after administration. Diphenoxylate has a shorter duration of action and half-life than loperamide. Diphenoxylate has a half-life of about 2½ hours, while its active metabolite has a half-life of 3 to 12 hours. Diphenoxylate's duration of action is 3 to 4 hours.

PHARMACODYNAMICS

Both loperamide and diphenoxylate decrease peristalsis in the large and small intestine.

Mechanism of action

Loperamide and diphenoxylate decrease GI motility by depressing the circular and longitudinal muscle action in the large and small intestines. Both drugs also decrease propulsive contractions throughout the entire colon. Diphenoxylate may provide an antisecretory effect as well, but has little analgesic effect.

Diphenoxylate is administered in combination with atropine. Atropine, an anticholinergic agent, is added to discourage the potential abuse of diphenoxylate. Its addition is effective because the toxic effects of atropine occur before the narcotic effects of diphenoxylate. The symptoms of atropine toxicity (dry mouth, urinary retention, tachycardia, and hyperthermia) tend to discourage diphenoxylate abuse. Loperamide produces little CNS effect in usual doses.

PHARMACOTHERAPEUTICS

Physicians use loperamide and diphenoxylate to treat acute, nonspecific diarrhea. Loperamide is also used for chronic diarrhea. Large doses of diphenoxylate may affect the CNS, especially the brain, whereas loperamide does not readily enter the CNS.

loperamide (Imodium). This drug is used to treat acute, nonspecific diarrhea and chronic diarrhea.
USUAL ADULT DOSAGE: for acute, nonspecific diarrhea, 4 mg P.O. initially, then 2 mg after each unformed stool to a maximum dose of 16 mg/day; for chronic diarrhea, 4 mg P.O. initially, then 2 mg after each unformed stool until diarrhea subsides. Then the dosage is adjusted to the patient's response.
USUAL PEDIATRIC DOSAGE: for acute diarrhea, initially 1 mg P.O. t.i.d. for children age 2 to 5, liquid form only; 2 mg P.O. b.i.d. for children age 5 to 8; 2 mg P.O. t.i.d. for children age 8 to 12; after the first dose, 1 mg/kg is administered after a loose stool only.

diphenoxylate hydrochloride (Lomotil). A Schedule V drug, diphenoxylate is given with atropine for acute, nonspecific diarrhea.
USUAL ADULT DOSAGE: for acute, nonspecific diarrhea, 5 mg P.O. q.i.d. initially; thereafter, the dose is adjusted to the patient's response.
USUAL PEDIATRIC DOSAGE: 0.3 to 0.4 mg/kg q.i.d. for children above age 2, in liquid form only; dosage may be reduced to as low as one-fourth the initial dose as soon as initial symptoms have been controlled.

Drug interactions

Loperamide and diphenoxylate may enhance the depressant effects of barbiturates, alcohol, narcotics, tranquilizers, and sedatives.

ADVERSE DRUG REACTIONS

The predictable reactions to loperamide and diphenoxylate include nausea, vomiting, abdominal discomfort or distention, drowsiness and fatigue, CNS depression, tachycardia, paralytic ileus, and possible physical dependence with long-term use. Adverse reactions to atropine include flushing, diminished secretions, hyperthermia, tachycardia, urinary retention, miosis, nystagmus, and blurred vision. Allergic responses, such as rash and urticaria, may occur as unpredictable responses to both loperamide and diphenoxylate.

NURSING IMPLICATIONS

Physicians frequently prescribe loperamide and diphenoxylate for inpatients with acute diarrhea. The nurse must monitor the clinical response and general condition of the patient during therapy and be aware of the following implications:

- When administering loperamide or diphenoxylate for acute nonspecific diarrhea, withhold the drug and consult the physician if the patient shows no improvement in 48 hours; in chronic diarrhea, withhold the drug and consult the physician if no improvement occurs after 16 mg/day for at least 10 days.
- Monitor the patient's fluid and electrolyte status as well as the frequency and amount of bowel movements to ensure adequate fluid volume.
- Withhold the drug and consult the physician if the patient exhibits symptoms of abdominal distention, which may indicate toxic megacolon, especially in ulcerative colitis.
- Loperamide and diphenoxylate are contraindicated in patients with acute diarrhea caused by organisms that penetrate the intestinal mucosa and in patients with pseudomembranous colitis caused by broad-spectrum antibiotics.

- Do not administer these drugs for diarrhea caused by poisonings until the toxic substance has been removed by gastric lavage or cathartics.
- Administer loperamide and diphenoxylate cautiously to patients with liver dysfunction, glaucoma, severe prostatic hypertrophy, narcotic dependence, ulcerative colitis, or to pregnant patients. Neither drug is recommended for children under age 2.
- When administering diphenoxylate, observe for signs of atropine overdose (dry mouth, blurred vision, flushing, tachycardia, and urinary retention), and reduce dosage as prescribed by the physician.
- Observe for signs of hypoperistalsis, and consult a physician if it occurs. (See *Signs of hypoperistalsis* for more details regarding this condition.)
- If respiratory depression occurs, administer naloxone.
- Advise the patient not to use alcohol or any other CNS depressant while taking loperamide or diphenoxylate as an outpatient.

Signs of hypoperistalsis

Watch for the following signs and symptoms of hypoperistalsis while administering loperamide or diphenoxylate. If hypoperistalsis occurs, withhold the next dose of the drug and notify the physician.
- Anorexia and nausea in early stage
- Abdominal distention
- Auscultation of rushes or high-pitched sounds over the abdomen
- Eventually a "silent abdomen"—absent bowel sounds
- Possible percussion of air or fluid over abdomen
- Absence of flatus
- Absence of bowel movements
- Possible vomiting with resultant fluid and electrolyte imbalance

ANTIDIARRHEALS: KAOLIN AND PECTIN

Kaolin and pectin, which are locally acting antidiarrheals, act as adsorbents. Physicians use these drugs to treat acute diarrhea from various causes. Although the effectiveness of kaolin and pectin has not been firmly established through clinical studies, these preparations are sold over the counter and are widely used.

Kaolin is a hydrated aluminum silicate. Pectin is a purified carbohydrate product obtained from the acid extraction of citrus fruit rinds or from apple pomace.

PHARMACOKINETICS

Because kaolin and pectin are locally acting antidiarrheals, they are not absorbed and, therefore, not distributed throughout the body tissues. Up to 90% of a dose is metabolized in the GI tract. The drugs and their metabolites are excreted in the feces.

The onset of action of kaolin and pectin occurs within 30 minutes of oral administration. Duration of action is 4 to 6 hours.

PHARMACODYNAMICS

Kaolin and pectin produce their antidiarrheal effects by acting as adsorbents and protectants on the intestinal mucosa.

Mechanism of action

Kaolin and pectin act as adsorbents, binding with bacteria, toxins, and other irritants on the intestinal mucosa. Pectin decreases the pH in the intestinal lumen and provides a soothing demulcent effect on the irritated mucosa. Both drugs protect the intestinal mucosa.

PHARMACOTHERAPEUTICS

Kaolin and pectin are used to relieve mild to moderate acute diarrhea. They also may be used to temporarily relieve chronic diarrhea until the cause has been determined and definitive treatment instituted. These agents are used safely in diarrhea of unknown cause, even if toxins or bacteria are suspected as the etiology. In the home, they are most frequently used to treat simple gastroenteritis. Kaolin and pectin preparations have been established as minimally effective for mild to moderate acute diarrhea, but they are of little value in severe diarrhea. These drugs are generally mild; however, kaolin and pectin may impair the absorption of other medications, such as digoxin and lincomycin.

kaolin and pectin mixtures (Kaopectate, Pecto Kay). Available over the counter, kaolin and pectin mixtures are used for mild to moderate nonspecific diarrhea. Both drugs prove generally effective for 48 hours.
USUAL ADULT DOSAGE: for regular-strength suspension, 60 to 120 ml; for concentrated suspension, 45 to 90 ml. Administer regular or concentrated suspension after each loose bowel movement, usually up to eight doses per day.

Drug interactions

Kaolin and pectin mixtures interfere with lincomycin absorption if administered within 2 hours before or 3 to 4 hours after lincomycin. The antidiarrheals also can interfere with absorption of digoxin or other drugs from the intestinal mucosa if administered concurrently.

ADVERSE DRUG REACTIONS

Kaolin and pectin mixtures cause few adverse reactions. Constipation may occur, especially in elderly and debilitated patients, or with overdose and prolonged use, but the constipation is usually mild and transient. Rarely, fecal impaction occurs in infants and debilitated patients.

NURSING IMPLICATIONS

The nurse may administer kaolin and pectin mixtures to inpatients or provide information about the drugs for outpatients. Though both kaolin and pectin are relatively safe, the nurse should be aware of the following implications:
● Kaolin and pectin mixtures are contraindicated in patients with suspected bowel obstruction.
● Administer with caution to children under age 3 and adults over age 60, as well as in debilitated patients.
● Do not administer kaolin and pectin concurrently with other medications.
● Monitor the patient's fluid and electrolyte status as well as bowel pattern while administering kaolin and pectin.
● Administer these drugs as adjuncts to rest, increased fluid intake, and appropriate diet.
● Advise the patient to avoid self-medication for longer than 48 hours. Instruct the patient to consult a physician if diarrhea persists.

HYPEROSMOLAR LAXATIVES

Hyperosmolar laxatives include lactulose, saline compounds (magnesium salts, sodium biphosphate, and sodium phosphate), and glycerin. The hyperosmolar laxatives produce an osmotic effect in the intestinal lumen that causes fluid accumulation, intestinal distention, and eventual peristalsis. (See Chapter 54, Cation-Exchange, Resin and Ammonia-Detoxicating Agents, for more about lactulose as an ammonia-detoxicating agent.)

PHARMACOKINETICS

These agents are poorly absorbed. They act within 30 minutes to 2 days.

Absorption, distribution, metabolism, excretion

Lactulose enters the GI tract and is absorbed only to a minor degree; thus, the drug is distributed only in the intestine. Its site of action is the colon. Because lactulose is not hydrolyzed in the small intestine, it is not absorbed, and water and electrolytes are retained in the intestinal lumen because of the osmotic effect of the lactulose. In the distal ileum and colon, the unabsorbed lactulose is metabolized by the intestinal microflora into lactate and other organic acids, thereby significantly reducing the fecal pH. Blood ammonia concentration levels are reduced 25% to 50% via the movement of the fluid and electrolytes into the intestinal lumen. This effect is also useful in the treatment of systemic portal encephalopathy in patients with chronic liver disease. Lactulose is excreted in the feces.

The saline compounds are natural substances used primarily in clinical situations requiring prompt bowel evacuation. Because saline compounds are hypernatremic solutions, they produce hypertonicity within the intestine. Once they are introduced into the GI tract, some absorption of the component ions occurs.

Approximately 20% of the magnesium in magnesium salts is absorbed systemically and excreted in the urine. The patient's renal function must be adequate or toxicity may occur.

Approximately 10% of the sodium in sodium phosphate and sodium biphosphate enemas may be absorbed and excreted in the urine.

Glycerin acts by osmotic fluid pressure shifts. Once inside the intestinal lumen, glycerin pulls water from the extraluminal spaces into the feces and stimulates reflex evacuation. Glycerin is introduced into the large intestine and is not absorbed systemically.

Onset, peak, duration

Bowel evacuation should occur 1 to 2 days after administration of lactulose. Saline cathartics produce a watery stool evacuation within 1 to 3 hours after administration. Acting in the distal colon, glycerin usually causes bowel evacuation 15 to 30 minutes after administration.

PHARMACODYNAMICS

The hyperosmolar laxatives produce bowel evacuation by drawing water into the intestine. Distention of the bowel from fluid accumulation promotes peristalsis and bowel movement.

Mechanism of action

Lactulose usually produces a laxative effect by drawing water into the intestinal lumen. Lactulose promotes water and electrolyte retention in the intestine, and unabsorbed the drug is metabolized into lactate and other organic acids that decrease the fecal pH.

The laxative effect of saline cathartics, including magnesium salts and sodium phosphate, has two results: (1) hypernatremia leading to hypertonicity within the lumen, which produces an osmotic effect on water; as a result, water rapidly enters the intestine, producing hypervolemia; and (2) stimulation of cholecystokinin secretion, which produces a spasm of Oddi's sphincter, the passage of bile into the duodenum, stimulation of intestinal motility, and inhibition of fluid and electrolyte absorption from the jejunum and ileum.

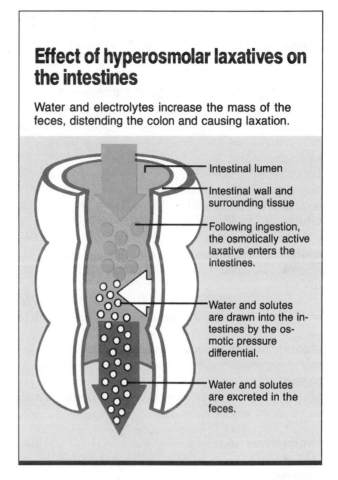

Effect of hyperosmolar laxatives on the intestines

Water and electrolytes increase the mass of the feces, distending the colon and causing laxation.

- Intestinal lumen
- Intestinal wall and surrounding tissue
- Following ingestion, the osmotically active laxative enters the intestines.
- Water and solutes are drawn into the intestines by the osmotic pressure differential.
- Water and solutes are excreted in the feces.

Glycerin, like the other hyperosmolar laxatives, draws water into the intestinal lumen, producing bowel hypervolemia and a watery stool evacuation. (See *Effects of hyperosmolar laxatives on the intestines* for a depiction of this mechanism of action.)

PHARMACOTHERAPEUTICS

Lactulose is used to treat chronic constipation and reduce ammonia production and absorption from the intestines in liver disease. Saline compounds are used when prompt and complete bowel evacuation is required. Glycerin is helpful in bowel retraining. (See *Bowel retraining program* on page 756 for points to teach when instituting such a program.)

lactulose (Cephulac, Chronulac). Primarily used to reduce ammonia levels in liver dysfunction when the patient has systemic portal encephalopathy, lactulose is also used clinically to manage chronic constipation. The nurse should use caution when giving lactulose to patients with diabetes mellitus and those requiring low-galactose diets.

USUAL ADULT DOSAGE: for constipation, 10 to 20 grams (15 to 30 ml) P.O. daily; for systemic portal encephalopathy, 20 to 30 grams (30 to 45 ml) P.O. t.i.d. or q.i.d., until two to three soft stools are produced daily.

magnesium salts [magnesium citrate, magnesium hydroxide, magnesium sulfate] (Milk of Magnesia). Administered to relieve chronic constipation, magnesium salts are also used for complete bowel evacuation and as a general laxative.

USUAL ADULT DOSAGE: for chronic constipation and bowel evacuation; 15 grams of the sulfate salt P.O. in a glass of water, or 240 ml of the citrate salt h.s.; as a laxative, 15 to 40 ml of the hydroxide salt P.O. h.s.

sodium phosphate or sodium biphosphate (Fleet Enema, PhosphoSoda). These drugs are used as a laxative.

USUAL ADULT DOSAGE: oral solution, 20 to 30 ml mixed with a glass of water; enema, 120 ml (4 ounces).

glycerin. Suppositories are administered primarily to re-establish proper bowel patterns in laxative-dependent patients.

USUAL ADULT DOSAGE: 3 grams by suppository; 5 to 15 ml as an enema.

Drug interactions

Hyperosmolar laxatives do not interact significantly with other drugs.

Contraindications of saline cathartics

Saline cathartics should not be ordered in the following patient groups. Milder, safer laxatives such as the emollients should be used.
- elderly patients
- patients with unstable chronic congestive heart failure
- patients with acute left ventricular failure
- patients with chronic or acute renal failure
- patients who have had intracranial surgery
- patients with decreased systemic arterial pressure
- patients with chronic emphysema accompanied by cor pulmonale
- patients with severe liver dysfunction

Adverse effects of saline cathartics

The following electrolyte imbalances may occur with excessive use of saline cathartics. Watch for the signs and symptoms of such imbalances.

Hypernatremia	• tachycardia • hypotension • dry mucous membranes • oliguria • thirst • dehydration • coma
Hypermagnesemia	• muscle weakness • nausea • vomiting • diminished reflexes • drowsiness • tachycardia • hypotension • flaccid paralysis • coma • respiratory distress
Hypocalcemia	• generalized neuromuscular irritability • facial spasming • grimace • laryngospasm • positive Chvostek's sign • tetany • convulsions • cardiac dysrhythmias • cardiac arrest
Hypovolemic shock	• hypotension • tachycardia • oliguria • decreased central venous pressure • decreased cardiac output • diminished vital organ perfusion

ADVERSE DRUG REACTIONS

The adverse reactions to hyperosmolar laxatives involve fluid and electrolyte imbalances. Although lactulose administration has little risk of toxicity, predictable adverse reactions include abdominal distention, flatulence, and abdominal cramps in approximately 20% of patients taking full doses. Other adverse reactions include nausea, vomiting, diarrhea, hypokalemia, hypovolemia, increased blood glucose level in patients with impaired glucose tolerance, and increased systemic portal encephalopathy in patients with severe liver dysfunction.

Preventing constipation

Review the following measures when teaching patients how to avoid constipation and therefore minimize the use of laxatives.
● Maintain a regular diet with adequate amounts of dietary fiber and fluids.
● Maintain regularity of dietary consumption; consume meals at approximately the same time each day.
● Allow time each day to use the toilet; do not ignore urge to defecate.
● Adhere to a regular daily exercise regimen.
● Avoid the habitual use of laxatives or cathartics.

Predictable adverse reactions to saline compounds include weakness and lethargy, dehydration from hypernatremia and resultant hypovolemia, hypermagnesemia, hyperphosphatemia, hypocalcemia, cardiac dysrhythmias from electrolyte imbalance, and hypovolemic shock. (See *Adverse effects of saline cathartics* for the signs and symptoms of these imbalances.)

Glycerin administration, which is quite safe, produces relatively few adverse reactions. The predictable ones may include weakness and fatigue. Severe diarrhea and hypovolemia may also occur, but rarely.

NURSING IMPLICATIONS

The hyperosmolar laxatives can be used safely in some patients, providing the nurse carefully monitors the patient's fluid status and the effect of the medication. In addition, the nurse should know the following implications:
● Lactulose is contraindicated in patients who need a low-galactose diet and should be administered cautiously to patients with diabetes mellitus.
● Hyperosmolar laxatives are contraindicated in patients with abdominal pain, nausea, vomiting, or other symptoms of appendicitis or acute surgical abdomen. The laxatives are also contraindicated in intestinal obstruction or perforation, edema, congestive heart failure, megacolon, impaired renal function, and in patients on a salt-restricted diet. (See *Contraindications of saline cathartics* for additional circumstances in which these laxatives should not be administered.)
● Do not administer lactulose to pregnant or lactating women because its safety has not been established.
● Store lactulose below 86° F. (30° C.); however, do not allow the drug to freeze.

● Dilute lactulose with water or juice prior to administration to dilute the sweetness and to prevent patient nausea.
● Monitor the patient's fluid and electrolyte status during administration, and replace fluids if diarrhea occurs.
● Monitor the patient's bowel patterns over the course of therapy.
● Encourage adequate fluid intake before administering sodium phosphate or magnesium salts.
● When administering magnesium salts, do not give other oral medications 1 to 2 hours before administration.
● Instruct the patient about the proper use of laxatives and about laxative dependence.

DIETARY FIBER AND RELATED BULK-FORMING LAXATIVES

Health care professionals consider a diet rich in fiber to be the most natural method of both preventing or treating constipation. Dietary fiber refers to the amount of plant food that is not digested in the small intestine. The bulk-forming laxatives, which resemble dietary fiber, contain natural and semisynthetic polysaccharides and cellulose. The bulk-forming laxatives include psyllium hydrophilic mucilloid and methylcellulose. Dietary fiber and bulk-forming laxatives increase fecal bulk and water content, thereby promoting peristalsis and elimination.

PHARMACOKINETICS

Dietary fiber and bulk-forming laxatives are not absorbed. The onset of action for both agents is slow.

Absorption, distribution, metabolism, excretion
Dietary fiber and related bulk-forming laxatives are ingested into the GI tract but are not absorbed systemically. Both act primarily in the small intestine and the colon. Polysaccharides in these agents are metabolized by intestinal bacterial flora into osmotically active metabolites. Both dietary fiber and bulk-forming laxatives are excreted in the feces.

Onset, peak, duration
Fecal softening occurs 1 to 3 days after the initiation of treatment. Continued administration of these agents re-

sults in a maximum effect in 3 to 4 days, and the duration of action depends on continued administration.

PHARMACODYNAMICS

Both dietary fiber and bulk-forming laxatives increase stool mass, which in turn increases peristalsis.

Mechanism of action

The laxative effect of dietary fiber and bulk-forming laxatives depends upon the hydrophilic bulk-forming properties of the polysaccharides in these agents. These bulk-forming properties increase the mass and water content of the stool; these form a viscous solution that promotes peristalsis and increases the elimination rate. The component polysaccharides are metabolized by the intestinal bacterial flora. Metabolism causes the accumulation of osmotically active metabolites, which increase water and solute transport into the intestinal lumen.

PHARMACOTHERAPEUTICS

Physicians prefer bulk-forming laxatives for most simple cases of constipation, especially for constipation from a low-fiber or low-fluid diet. These agents also are indicated for patients recovering from acute myocardial infarction or cerebral aneurysms who need to avoid Valsalva's maneuver and maintain soft feces. Physicians also use bulk-forming laxatives to manage patients with irritable bowel syndrome and diverticulosis.

dietary fiber. To prevent constipation, adults should consume 6 to 10 grams of dietary fiber daily. Dietary fiber is a major component of bran, whole grain cereals, fresh fruits and vegetables, and legumes.

psyllium hydrophilic mucilloid (Metamucil). Adults use this laxative to prevent constipation.
USUAL ADULT DOSAGE: 1 to 2 teaspoonfuls P.O. in a full glass of water b.i.d. or t.i.d. followed by a second glass of water; or 1 packet P.O. dissolved in water b.i.d. or t.i.d.

methylcellulose (Cologel). Adults should take these drugs in the morning or evening.
USUAL ADULT DOSAGE: 5 to 20 ml liquid P.O. t.i.d. with a full glass of water.

Drug interactions

No significant drug interactions occur with the use of dietary fiber or bulk-forming laxatives.

Bowel retraining program

Follow these points when instituting a bowel retraining program in patients with chronic constipation.

See that the patient's meals are high in fluid content and adequate in solid bulk (especially breakfast).

Have the patient eat breakfast at approximately the same time each day.

Place the patient on toilet or commode 15 to 30 minutes after the meal.

If reflex defecation does not occur, insert a lubricated glycerin suppository as prescribed.

If defecation does not follow the suppository insertion, administer a Fleet Enema as prescribed.

Eventually, the patient will defecate on a regular schedule on the basis of the meal plus the suppository.

The ultimate goal is reflex defecation based on the meal's content and the time of day, without the use of suppositories.

ADVERSE DRUG REACTIONS

Administration of dietary fiber or bulk-forming laxatives in the recommended amounts involves a minimal toxicity risk. Predictable reactions include flatulence, a subjective sense of abdominal fullness, intestinal obstruction, impaction, esophageal obstruction (if sufficient liquid has not been administered with the agent), and severe diarrhea. Allergic reactions rarely occur.

NURSING IMPLICATIONS

The nurse can administer dietary fiber and bulk-forming laxatives safely to patients if bowel obstruction is not suspected and sufficient fluid intake accompanies administration. Nonetheless, the nurse should be aware of the following implications:
- Dietary fiber and bulk-forming laxatives are contraindicated in patients with partial bowel obstruction, dysphagia, or intestinal ulceration.
- Evaluate the effectiveness of daily dietary fiber or bulk-forming laxatives on bowel evacuation pattern.
- For bowel retraining, administer glycerin suppositories daily as prescribed until defecation occurs naturally. (See *Bowel retraining program* for further details.)
- Monitor the patient for either laxative dependence or diarrhea.
- Advise patients with restricted sugar and salt intake against the frequent use of these agents because these laxatives contain varying amounts of sugar and salt.
- Teach the patient to take each dose with one glass of water and to increase fluid intake during the day to prevent impaction.
- Inform patients with chronic constipation about how diet, exercise, and fluid intake can help treat constipation. (See *Preventing constipation* on page 755.)

EMOLLIENT LAXATIVES

Emollients are also known as stool softeners. Usually safe, emollients are used to prevent constipation in patients who should avoid straining during defecation. Emollients reduce the surface tension of interfacing liquid bowel contents, thereby promoting fluid accumulation in the bowel and softening the stool. Emollients include the calcium, potassium, and sodium salts of docusate and poloxamer 188.

History and source

The pharmaceutical industry has used emollients for many years as wetting agents in topical drugs. Emollients have been used as laxatives since 1955.

PHARMACOKINETICS

Administered orally or rectally, emollients are absorbed and excreted through bile in the feces. Stool softening occurs within several days after administration.

Absorption, distribution, metabolism, excretion

Emollients are usually surface-acting agents. The degree of absorption after oral or rectal administration remains unknown, but some absorption through the duodenum and jejunum occurs after oral administration. Emollients concentrate in the liver, and excretion occurs through bile in the feces.

Onset, peak, duration

After oral administration, the onset of action is within 12 to 72 hours for docusate salts and within 3 to 5 days for poloxamer 188.

PHARMACODYNAMICS

Emollients soften the stool and ease defecation by emulsifying the fat and water components of feces in the small and large intestines. This detergent action allows water and lipids to penetrate the fecal material, thereby producing net fluid accumulation. Emollients also stimulate electrolyte and fluid secretion from intestinal mucosal cells.

PHARMACOTHERAPEUTICS

Emollients are the drugs of choice for softening stool in patients who should avoid straining during defecation. Such patients include those who have had recent myocardial infarction or surgery and those with a disease of the anus or rectum, increased intracranial pressure, or hernias. Children with hard dry stools can be administered emollients safely. Emollients also may be given before rectal cathartics to treat fecal impaction.

docusate calcium (Surfak). Docusate calcium is used to soften the stool of patients who should not strain during defecation.
USUAL ADULT DOSAGE: 240 mg P.O. daily until bowel movements are normal.

docusate potassium (Kasof, Dialose). Docusate potassium is a stool softener that can be administered orally or rectally.

USUAL ADULT DOSAGE: as stool softener, 100 to 300 mg P.O. daily until bowel movements are normal.

docusate sodium (Colace, Doxinate, Regutol). A stool softener, docusate sodium is frequently prescribed for hospitalized and nonhospitalized patients.

USUAL ADULT DOSAGE: 50 to 300 mg P.O. daily until bowel movements are normal.

USUAL PEDIATRIC DOSAGE: 1.25 mg/kg P.O. up to q.i.d.

poloxamer 188 (Alaxin). Poloxamer 188 is also a stool softener.

USUAL ADULT DOSAGE: 240 mg P.O. daily to t.i.d. until bowel movements are normal.

Drug interactions

Administration of emollients with aspirin may increase the mucosal damage caused by aspirin. The nurse should not administer oral emollients with oral mineral oil because they enhance the systemic absorption of the mineral oil and may result in tissue deposition. Because emollients may enhance the absorption of many oral drugs, the nurse should not administer them concurrently with oral drugs having low therapeutic indexes.

ADVERSE DRUG REACTIONS

Adverse drug reactions with emollients rarely occur. However, mild, transient abdominal cramping; a bitter taste; diarrhea; and irritation to the throat may occur.

NURSING IMPLICATIONS

Emollients are safe and simple to use. The nurse should administer these agents cautiously to patients with cardiac and renal disease. The nurse also should be aware of the following nursing implications:

• Potassium salts of docusate are contraindicated in renal dysfunction.

• Administer sodium salts of docusate cautiously to patients on sodium-restricted diets and to patients with edema, congestive heart failure, or renal dysfunction.

• Store emollients at 59° to 86° F. (15° to 30° C.). Protect liquid preparations from light.

• Give liquid emollients in milk or fruit juice to mask the bitter taste.

• Advise the patient to increase dietary bulk, fluid intake, and exercise to enhance the emollient's effect.

STIMULANT LAXATIVES

Stimulant laxatives, also known as irritant cathartics, may either directly irritate the intestinal mucosa or activate the intramural nerve plexus of the intestinal smooth muscle, thus increasing intestinal motility. Stimulant laxatives also alter electrolyte and fluid absorption, and some cause active ion secretion by intestinal mucosal cells, leading to net fluid accumulation in the intestines. The stimulant laxatives include bisacodyl, phenolphthalein, cascara sagrada, senna, and castor oil. These laxatives are used in constipation produced by medications, by neurologic disorders, and by irritable bowel syndrome. These laxatives are also used to empty the bowel before surgery, radiologic procedures, and endoscopy.

History and source

Most of the stimulant laxatives derive from natural plant sources. For example, phenolphthalein was first used in making adulterated wine in Hungary in 1902. Cascara sagrada was introduced by Bundy in 1877. Some of these laxatives, such as castor oil, have been used since the time of the early Egyptians. Others were developed as late as the 1950s.

PHARMACOKINETICS

Stimulant laxatives are slightly absorbed and are metabolized in the liver. The metabolites are excreted either in the urine or the feces.

Absorption, distribution, metabolism, excretion

Bisacodyl and phenolphthalein represent the diphenylmethane group of stimulant laxatives. Both laxatives are minimally absorbed, distributed to breast milk, metabolized by the liver, and excreted in the feces or urine.

Cascara sagrada and senna are of the anthraquinone group of stimulant laxatives. Both laxatives are only slightly absorbed from the small intestine. Unabsorbed drug is hydrolyzed by colonic flora, thus becoming pharmacologically active. Cascara sagrada and senna are metabolized by the liver and distributed into some body tissues, including breast milk. They are excreted through bile in the feces and in the urine.

Researchers do not know whether castor oil is significantly absorbed from the small intestine. In the small intestine, castor oil is hydrolyzed to ricinoleic acid, its active ingredient.

Onset, peak, duration

The diphenylmethane stimulants produce evacuation within 6 to 8 hours of oral administration and within 15 minutes to 1 hour after rectal administration. The duration of a single dose of phenolphthalein may be several days.

Cascara sagrada and senna produce an onset of action within 6 to 12 hours of oral administration and within ½ to 2 hours of rectal administration. Castor oil acts more quickly, with loose bowel movements occurring 2 to 3 hours after oral administration.

PHARMACODYNAMICS

Stimulant laxatives have several mechanisms of action to produce effective laxation.

Mechanisms of action

Stimulant laxatives stimulate peristalsis and induce defecation by either irritating the intestinal mucosa or stimulating nerve endings of the intestinal smooth muscle. These drugs also alter fluid and electrolyte absorption. Some stimulant laxatives produce active ion secretion by first inducing colonic mucosal cells to produce a net fluid accumulation in the bowel and laxation. All stimulant laxatives act on the colon, and castor oil and phenolphthalein increase the peristaltic activity of the small intestine as well.

PHARMACOTHERAPEUTICS

Physicians regard stimulant laxatives as the preferred laxatives to empty the bowel before general surgery, sigmoidoscopic or proctoscopic procedures, and radiologic procedures such as barium studies of the GI tract. Stimulant laxatives are also used for constipation from prolonged bed rest, neurologic dysfunction of the colon, and constipating drugs such as narcotics. Physicians may use these drugs for constipation associated with pregnancy or delivery, but usually prescribe other, milder laxatives because these agents may stimulate uterine contractions. Stimulant laxatives are never used in lactating women.

bisacodyl (Dulcolax). Administered for chronic constipation, bisacodyl is also used before delivery, surgery, or rectal or bowel examination.

USUAL ADULT DOSAGE: 10 to 15 mg P.O. in the evening or before breakfast up to 30 mg for thorough evacuation; 10 mg as a rectal suppository or 1.25-ounce (37.5 ml) enema.
USUAL PEDIATRIC DOSAGE: 5 to 10 mg P.O. in the evening or before breakfast; 10 mg rectally as a suppository for children age 2 and over, 5 mg for those under age 2.

cascara sagrada (Cas-Evac). Administer cascara sagrada for acute constipation or before bowel or rectal examination.
USUAL ADULT DOSAGE: one 325-mg tablet P.O. h.s.; 1 ml fluid extract P.O. daily; 5 ml aromatic fluid extract P.O. daily.

castor oil (Neoloid). Administer castor oil before rectal or bowel examination or surgery, or for acute constipation.
USUAL ADULT DOSAGE: 15 to 60 ml P.O. as liquid.

phenolphthalein (Alophen, Ex-Lax). Administer phenolphthalein for acute constipation.
USUAL ADULT DOSAGE: 60 to 194 mg P.O. h.s.

senna (Senokot, X-Prep). Administer senna for acute constipation or before bowel or rectal examination.
USUAL ADULT DOSAGE: 2 to 4 tablets P.O.; ½ to 4 teaspoons of granules added to liquid; 1 to 2 teaspoonfuls syrup; 1 to 2 suppositories h.s.

Drug interactions

No significant drug interactions occur with the stimulant laxatives.

ADVERSE DRUG REACTIONS

Stimulant laxatives provide relatively safe treatment of short-term or acute constipation. Because these drugs produce increased intestinal motility, they reduce the absorption of concomitantly administered oral drugs.

Predictable reactions

Predictable adverse reactions to stimulant laxatives include weakness, nausea, abdominal cramps, and mild proctitis. Rectal administration of bisacodyl can produce a burning sensation. Phenolphthalein can cause a reddish discoloration in alkaline urine. Cascara sagrada and senna cause a reddish-pink or brown to black discoloration of urine. Castor oil may cause pelvic congestion in menstruating women. With long-term use or overdose, stimulant laxatives may cause electrolyte disturbances, including hypokalemia, hypocalcemia, metabolic alkalosis, or acidosis. Malabsorption and weight loss may also occur. Habitual use may lead to cathartic colon with atony and dilation.

Unpredictable reactions
Stimulant laxatives can cause allergic reactions such as rash and pruritus. Phenolphthalein allergy may result in renal, cardiac, and respiratory dysfunction.

NURSING IMPLICATIONS
The nurse frequently administers stimulant laxatives preoperatively or before procedures requiring bowel evacuation. The nurse incorporates administration into the preoperative routine. Before using stimulant laxatives, the nurse should be aware of the following implications:
• Stimulant laxatives are contraindicated in patients with abdominal pain, nausea, vomiting, or other symptoms of appendicitis or acute surgical abdomen. The drugs are also contraindicated in patients with intestinal obstruction or perforation, fecal impaction, and anal or rectal fissures.
• Castor oil is contraindicated in pregnant or menstruating women.
• Administer stimulant laxatives cautiously in patients with rectal bleeding.
• Administer castor oil on an empty stomach for best results.
• Mix castor oil with juice or carbonated beverage to mask the preparation's oily taste. Tell the patient to hold ice in the mouth before taking castor oil to help decrease the taste.
• Store castor oil below 40° F. (4.4° C.), but do not freeze; shake the emulsion well.
• Monitor the patient's fluid and electrolyte status as well as the bowel evacuation pattern.
• Explain to the patient that increasing dietary bulk, fluid intake, and exercise can enhance the laxative's effectiveness.
• Alert the patient that phenolphthalein may discolor the urine pink to red and that cascara sagrada and senna may discolor alkaline urine to pink-red and acidic urine to brown.
• Advise the patient using phenolphthalein to avoid the sun and to discontinue the drug if a rash occurs.

LUBRICANT LAXATIVE

Mineral oil, a lubricant laxative, increases water retention in the stool by creating a barrier between the colon wall and feces. This barrier prevents colonic reabsorption of fecal water. Mineral oil is used to treat constipation in patients who must avoid straining, including patients with recent myocardial infarction, increased intracranial pressure, or fecal impaction. Mineral oil carries some risk for children and elderly or debilitated patients, who may aspirate the mineral oil and develop lipid pneumonia. Long-term use of mineral oil may impair the absorption of lipid-soluble vitamins.

History and source
Mineral oil is a complex mixture of saturated hydrocarbons derived from crude petroleum and refined for human use.

PHARMACOKINETICS
In its nonemulsified form, mineral oil is minimally absorbed; in the emulsified form, about half is absorbed. Defecation occurs 6 to 8 hours after oral administration and within 2 hours of rectal administration.

Absorption, distribution, metabolism, excretion
Absorption of nonemulsified mineral oil is minimal following oral and rectal administration. Following oral administration, 30% to 60% of emulsified mineral oil is absorbed. Absorbed mineral oil is distributed to the mesenteric lymph nodes as well as to the intestinal mucosa, liver, and spleen. Mineral oil is metabolized by the liver and excreted in the feces.

Onset, peak, duration
The onset of action occurs in 6 to 8 hours after the oral administration of mineral oil and in ½ to 2 hours after rectal administration. The duration of action depends on continuing administration of the agent.

PHARMACODYNAMICS
Mineral oil acts as a lubricant in the colon to produce-laxation.

Mechanism of action
Mineral oil lubricates the feces and the intestinal mucosa by preventing water reabsorption from the lumen of the

Antidiarrheal and laxative agents

The following chart summarizes the use of selected antidiarrheals and laxatives discussed in this chapter.

DRUG	MAJOR INDICATIONS	USUAL ADULT DOSAGES	NURSING IMPLICATIONS
Antidiarrheals			
opium tincture	Acute, nonspecific diarrhea	0.6 ml (range 0.3 to 1 ml) P.O. b.i.d.; maximum dose, 6 ml daily	• Use cautiously in conjunction with other analgesics, sedatives, and narcotics. • Administer cautiously to patients with asthma, benign prostatic hypertrophy, narcotic dependence, or liver dysfunction. • Long-term use may cause physical dependence. • Monitor GI response to therapy.
camphorated opium tincture	Acute, nonspecific diarrhea	5 to 10 ml P.O. daily to q.i.d. until acute diarrhea subsides	
loperamide	Acute, nonspecific diarrhea; chronic diarrhea	4 mg P.O., then 2 mg after each unformed stool; maximum dose, 16 mg/day	• Discontinue use if no improvement occurs in 48 hours (when used for acute diarrhea). • Discontinue use if no improvement occurs after giving 16 mg/day for at least 10 days (when used for chronic diarrhea). • Monitor fluid and electrolyte status as well as bowel pattern. • Withhold drug if symptoms of abdominal distention occur. • Administer cautiously to patients with benign prostatic hypertrophy, liver dysfunction, or narcotic dependence. • Monitor the patient's response to drug therapy.
diphenoxylate (with atropine)	Acute, nonspecific diarrhea; chronic diarrhea	5 mg P.O. q.i.d.; thereafter, the dose is adjusted to individual response	• Monitor fluid and electrolyte status to ensure adequate fluid volume before treatment. • Withhold drug if symptoms of abdominal distention occur. • Administer cautiously to patients with liver dysfunction, narcotic dependence, or benign prostatic hypertrophy.
Laxatives			
lactulose	Chronic constipation; reduction of ammonia level in patients with systemic portal encephalopathy	Chronic constipation: 10 to 20 grams P.O. daily Systemic portal encephalopathy: 20 to 30 grams (30 to 45 ml) P.O. t.i.d. or q.i.d. until two to three soft stools are produced daily	• Monitor fluid and electrolyte status during administration. • Monitor bowel response pattern over the course of therapy. • Note any complications, such as dehydration, acid-base abnormalities, electrolyte imbalance, or hypovolemia (especially in patients susceptible to laxative dependence. • Store lactulose below 86° F. (30° C.); do not freeze.
saline compounds	Prompt and complete bowel evacuation	15 grams magnesium sulfate P.O. in a glass of water; 10 to 20 ml of concentrated Milk of Magnesia; 240 ml of magnesium citrate at bedtime. Oral solution of sodium phosphates given 20 to 30 ml with a glass of water, or enema 120 ml (4 oz).	• Monitor fluid and electrolyte status during administration. • Monitor bowel response pattern over the course of therapy. • Note any complications, such as dehydration, acid-base abnormalities, electrolyte imbalance, or hypovolemia (especially in patients susceptible to laxative dependence.)

continued

SELECTED MAJOR DRUGS			
Antidiarrheal and laxative agents continued			
DRUG	**MAJOR INDICATIONS**	**USUAL ADULT DOSAGES**	**NURSING IMPLICATIONS**
Laxatives			
glycerin	Establishment of proper bowel patterns in laxative-dependent adults	3-gram suppository; 5 to 15 ml as an enema	• Monitor fluid and electrolyte status during administration. • Monitor bowel response pattern over the course of therapy. • Note any complications, such as dehydration, acid-base abnormalities, electrolyte imbalance, or hypovolemia (especially in patients susceptible to laxative dependence).
psyllium hydrophilic mucilloid	Prevention of constipation	1 to 2 teaspoonfuls P.O. in a glass of water b.i.d. or t.i.d. followed by a second glass of water; 1 packet dissolved in water b.i.d. or t.i.d..	• Advise patients with dietary restrictions of salt or sugar to read labels carefully. • Monitor bowel response to these agents. • Monitor for development of laxative dependence or diarrhea. • Caution the patient to consume liquids with these agents. • Teach the patient how to prevent and treat the constipation.
methylcellulose	Prevention of constipation	5 to 20 ml liquid P.O. t.i.d. with a full glass of water	
docusate sodium	To produce softer stools for patients at risk for chronic constipation	100 to 300 mg P.O. daily as a single or divided doses	• Before use for chronic constipation, assess daily dietary pattern, fluid intake, and exercise pattern; educate the patient as needed. • Time administration so that bowel evacuation will not interfere with sleep pattern. • Monitor serum electrolyte levels with prolonged use.

bowel. The increased fluid content of the feces increases peristalsis. Emulsified mineral oil provides slightly more effective action than the nonemulsified form. Rectal administration via an enema also produces laxation by physical distention.

PHARMACOTHERAPEUTICS

Physicians use mineral oil to treat constipation and maintain soft stools when straining is contraindicated (after recent myocardial infarction to avoid Valsalva's maneuver, after eye surgery to prevent increased intraocular pressure, and after cerebral aneurysm repair to avoid increased intracranial pressure). Mineral oil is also used to treat patients with fecal impaction and is administered either orally or by enema. Bulk-forming laxatives and emollients are usually considered to provide milder action than mineral oil.

mineral oil (Agoral Plain, Fleet Mineral Oil Enema). Used to treat constipation, mineral oil is also used to

maintain soft stools when straining during defecation is contraindicated.

USUAL ADULT DOSAGE: 15 to 30 ml P.O., usually h.s.; or 4-ounce (120 ml) enema.

Drug interactions

Mineral oil may impair the absorption of many oral medications, including fat-soluble vitamins, oral contraceptives, and anticoagulants. Mineral oil may also interfere with the antibacterial activity of nonabsorbable sulfonamides.

ADVERSE DRUG REACTIONS

Adverse reactions involving mineral oil include rectal irritation, aspiration, interference with nutrient absorption, and systemic absorption of the mineral oil.

Predictable reactions

Mineral oil may produce nausea, vomiting, diarrhea, and abdominal cramping. Seepage from the rectum after rectal administration may result in anal irritation, pruritus ani, infection, and impaired healing. Chronic oral use of nonemulsified mineral oil may impair absorption of fat-soluble vitamins (A,D,E, and K), causing vitamin deficiency. Lipid pneumonitis may result from the aspiration of orally administered mineral oil, especially in young children and elderly and debilitated patients.

Unpredictable reactions

The systemic absorption of mineral oil can lead to granulomatous reactions in mesenteric lymph nodes, the liver, and the spleen.

NURSING IMPLICATIONS

The nurse should use caution when administering mineral oil to some patients. Furthermore, the drug should not be given with meals or other medications. The nurse should be aware of the following implications before administering mineral oil:

• Mineral oil is contraindicated in patients with abdominal pain, nausea, vomiting, or other symptoms of appendicitis or acute surgical abdomen. The drug is also contraindicated in patients with intestinal obstruction or perforation; in children younger than age 6; in bedridden, elderly, debilitated, or pregnant patients; and in patients with esophageal or gastric retention, dysphagia, or hiatal hernia.

• Do not give mineral oil with or directly after meals or medications.

• Mix mineral oil with fruit juices or carbonated beverages to disguise its taste.

• Monitor the patient's fluid status and the effect of the laxative.

• Instruct the patient to avoid using mineral oil for more than 1 week to prevent dependence and nutrient malabsorption.

• Explain to the patient that increased dietary bulk, fluid intake, and exercise enhance mineral oil's effect.

CHAPTER SUMMARY

Chapter 48 contained information about the pharmacokinetics, pharmacodynamics, pharmacotherapeutics, adverse drug reactions, and nursing implications of antidiarrheal and laxative agents. Here are the highlights of the chapter:

• Diarrhea refers to the increased frequency or weight and liquidity of stools produced by the rapid movement of feces through the large intestine. Constipation refers to the decreased movement of fecal matter through the large intestine.

• Significant antidiarrheals include opium tincture, paregoric, diphenoxylate, loperamide, and kaolin and pectin mixtures. Antidiarrheals are indicated for the treatment of acute, nonspecific diarrhea or chronic diarrhea.

• Opium tincture and paregoric: (1) slow the effects of the mesenteric plexus of the intestine, (2) inhibit intestinal peristalsis by direct central action on the brain, (3) decrease propulsive contractions, (4) enhance anal sphincter tone, and (5) enhance the tone of the ileocecal valve.

• Loperamide and diphenoxylate decrease GI motility by depressing the action of the circular and longitudinal muscles of the large and small intestine.

• Kaolin and pectin act as adsorbents, binding with irritants on the intestinal mucosa. These antidiarrheals prove most effective for mild diarrhea.

• The long-term administration of certain antidiarrheals, especially opium tincture and paregoric, may precipitate some degree of physical dependence. Antidiarrheals can also cause nausea, vomiting, dizziness, dysphoria, and constipation.

• Use antidiarrheals cautiously in patients with asthma, benign prostatic hypertrophy, narcotic dependence, or liver dysfunction.

• The nurse must closely monitor the patient's GI response to these drugs, documenting the frequency and consistency of bowel movements per day. Fluids and electrolytes should be replaced as needed.

• Laxatives exert their effect by increasing fecal water content and increasing fecal movement from the colon and rectum.

• Hyperosmolar laxatives include lactulose, saline compounds, and glycerin. Lactulose is used to reduce ammonia levels in patients with liver dysfunction and to treat chronic constipation. Saline compounds are used for complete bowel evacuation and for chronic constipation. Physicians prescribe glycerin to reestablish proper bowel patterns.

• Hyperosmolar laxatives can produce adverse reactions ranging from abdominal distention, flatulence, and abdominal cramps to weakness and lethargy.

• The intake of dietary fiber is the most natural way to treat or prevent constipation.

• Emollients, administered orally or rectally, are used to soften stools in patients who should avoid straining during defecation. These drugs are safe; however, they have a bitter taste.

• Stimulant laxatives are used for constipation produced by drugs, neurologic disorders, and irritable bowel syndrome. They also are used to empty the bowel before surgery.

• The excessive use of laxatives, especially in susceptible patients, may result in severe problems, such as habitual dependence, fluid and electrolyte imbalances, acid-base abnormalities, dehydration, and cardiac dysrhythmias. For habitual users of laxatives, the nurse should teach bowel retraining regimens and interventions to prevent chronic constipation.

BIBLIOGRAPHY

American Hospital Formulary Service. *Drug Information '87.* McEvoy, G.K., ed. Bethesda, Md.: American Society of Hospital Pharmacists, 1987.

Behm, R.M. "A Special Recipe to Banish Constipation," *Geriatric Nursing* 6:216, July/August 1985.

Cummings, J.H. "Constipation, Dietary Fibre and the Control of Large Bowel Function," *Postgraduate Medicine Journal* 60:811, November 1984.

DuPont, H.L. "Nonfluid Therapy and Selected Chemoprophylaxis of Acute Diarrhea," *American Journal of Medicine* 78:81, June 1985.

Forbes, D.A., et al. "Laxative Abuse and Secondary Diarrhea," *Archives of Diseases of Children* 60:58, January 1985.

Goodman, A.G., et al, eds. *Goodman and Gilman's The Pharmacological Basis of Therapeutics,* 7th ed. New York: Macmillan Publishing Co, 1985.

Goth, A. *Medical Pharmacology.* St. Louis: C.V. Mosby Co., 1978.

Hope, A.K., et al. "Dietary Fibre and Fluid in the Control of Constipation in a Nursing Home Population," *Medical Journal of Australia* 144:306, March 17, 1986.

Lewis, B. "Streamlining the Process of Elimination," *American Journal of Nursing* 85:774, July 1985.

Marks, J. "Opium, the Religion of the People," *Lancet* 22:1439, June 1985.

Mumford, S. "Nutrition. 4: High Fibre Diets," *Nursing Mirror* 160:36, March 6, 1985.

Resnick, B. "Constipation: Common but Preventable," *Geriatric Nursing* 6:213, July/August 1985.

Tedisco, F.J., et al. "Laxative Use in Constipation, American College of Gastroenterology's Committee on FDA-Related Matters," *American Journal of Gastroenterology* 80:303, April 1985.

CHAPTER 49

EMETIC AND ANTIEMETIC AGENTS

OBJECTIVES

After reading and studying this chapter, you should be able to:

1. Explain the physiology of nausea and vomiting.

2. Describe physiologically how motion sickness, labyrinthitis, chemotherapy, and narcotics produce nausea and vomiting.

3. Explain at least five of the ways that nausea and vomiting can adversely affect the patient.

4. Delineate the pharmacokinetic, pharmacodynamic, and pharmacotherapeutic properties of the emetic agents apomorphine hydrochloride and ipecac syrup.

5. Identify the drug interactions, adverse reactions, and nursing implications for the emetic agents apomorphine and ipecac syrup.

6. List the components of patient teaching that should be included with the use of ipecac syrup in the home.

7. Differentiate among the pharmacokinetic, pharmacodynamic, and pharmacotherapeutic properties of the antihistamine and phenothiazine antiemetics, as well as those of other antiemetics, including benzquinamide hydrochloride, scopolamine, metoclopramide hydrochloride, diphenidol, dronabinol, and nabilone.

8. Identify the drug interactions, adverse reactions, and nursing implications for the antihistamine and phenothiazine antiemetics, as well as the other antiemetic agents, including benzquinamide, scopolamine, metoclopramide, diphenidol, dronabinol, and nabilone.

9. Discuss the technique for properly administering transdermal scopolamine.

INTRODUCTION

The emetics and antiemetics represent two groups of drugs with opposing actions. The emetic drugs, which are derived from plants, produce vomiting upon administration. The antiemetic drugs decrease nausea and hence, the urge to vomit. Physicians prescribe emetics primarily to induce vomiting in the emergency treatment of acute poisonings. The induced vomiting empties the stomach and prevents absorption of the ingested toxin. Generally, emetics should be administered immediately after a poisoning is discovered; however, they may prove effective even upon delayed administration if the ingested toxin is one that slowly empties from the stomach.

Emetics, although usually safe, should not be used indiscriminately. Vomiting should not be induced in poisonings involving caustic substances, such as lye, or petroleum distillates, such as gasoline, because the vomiting may cause further injury. Also, emetics should not be used by those with anorexia nervosa or bulimia.

The emergency use of emetics combined with other measures can be lifesaving in the treatment of acute poisonings. Indeed, the American Academy of Pediatrics recommends to parents of young children that emetics be kept on hand in case of accidental poisoning.

Antiemetics relieve nausea and vomiting from various causes. While the physiology of vomiting is relatively well understood, the complex physiology of nausea is not. The vomiting, or emetic, center, located in the reticular formation of the medulla, integrates the nausea response and coordinates the resulting vomiting reflex. The nausea response can be initiated when the upper gastrointestinal (GI) tract sends nerve impulses to the vomiting center along the vagus and the sympathetic nerves. Several conditions stimulate these nerve impulses. Irritation of mucosal receptors in the GI tract may provide input to the vomiting center. The emetic ipecac, which directly irritates the gastric mucosa; radiation therapy injury to the GI mucosa; and malignant disease of the GI tract all may stimulate nausea and vomiting via the vomiting center pathway.

Nausea and vomiting may also be induced via a second, more complex pathway. Another nucleus of cells, called the chemoreceptor trigger zone (CTZ), is also located in the medulla, close to the vomiting center. By itself, the CTZ cannot mediate the act of vomiting; however, activation of the CTZ can stimulate the vomiting center, which in turn initiates emesis. The CTZ contains dopamine receptors that can be activated by many stimuli, including narcotics, cancer chemotherapeutic drugs, vestibular motion or inflammation, ketoacidosis, and uremia.

Nausea and vomiting are common symptoms almost universally listed as adverse effects for many drugs. Both nausea and vomiting also frequently occur after surgery from the anesthetic and surgical manipulation. Whether or not the nausea and vomiting originate inside or outside the gastrointestinal tract, the physician should identify and directly treat the underlying cause. For example, parasitic intestinal disease, acute appendicitis, migraine headache, and diabetes cause nausea. Each of these conditions can be identified and treated medically. Nonetheless, the physician cannot always treat the underlying cause of nausea, making symptomatic treatment necessary. For example, the nausea from a viral illness may require treatment for the duration of the disease.

Motion sickness results from stimulation of the vestibular apparatus of the ear. During motion sickness, stimulation of the CTZ activates the vomiting center. People who know that they may experience motion sickness under certain circumstances can use an antiemetic prophylactically to avoid the nausea and vomiting.

Another form of nausea from stimulation of the vestibular apparatus of the ear is labyrinthitis. With labyrinthitis, inflammation of the vestibular apparatus causes nausea, vomiting, dizziness, and hearing loss. Meniere's disease, which involves a dilation of the endolymphatic channels in the cochlea, also produces nausea as well as dizziness, tinnitus, and hearing loss. The symptoms of Meniere's disease may last from several days to months and may recur without warning. During exacerbations of the disease, an antiemetic drug is indicated.

Cancer chemotherapy can directly or indirectly (through the CTZ) stimulate the vomiting center, causing severe nausea and vomiting. As with motion sickness, the administration of antiemetic drugs before the chemotherapy may prevent or decrease the severity of these symptoms.

Narcotics, such as morphine and meperidine, stimulate two pathways to produce nausea and vomiting. The drugs not only directly stimulate the CTZ, which in turn activates the vomiting center, but they also sensitize the vestibular apparatus of the ear. As a result, nausea occurs more often in ambulatory patients taking narcotics than among bedridden patients. Narcotic-induced nausea may be mild, occurring only with the first dose

of the narcotic, or it may be more severe, resulting in vomiting that require antiemetic medication. In anticipation that they will cause severe narcotic-induced nausea, some narcotics are premixed with an antiemetic. Mepergan, for example, is a combination of the narcotic meperidine and the antiemetic promethazine.

Many women experience nausea and vomiting during early pregnancy (morning sickness), a condition that poses treatment problems. The dilemma arises from the belief that any drug used during the first trimester of pregnancy may act teratogenically. Physicians usually prescribe supportive measures as the initial therapy, reserving drug use for the point at which the potential benefits of antiemetic therapy outweigh the risk to both mother and fetus. This point usually occurs when the nausea and vomiting so incapacitate the patient that a nutritional deficiency is possible.

Nausea and vomiting may lead to many other deleterious effects. Vomiting, for example, may lead to esophageal injury or, postoperatively, to disrupted sutures. Prolonged vomiting may lead to dehydration and the loss of gastric secretions, which in turn causes electrolyte, acid-base, nutritional, and fluid abnormalities. While vomiting, a person may also aspirate gastric contents into the lungs, resulting in an aspiration pneumonitis. Finally, nausea and vomiting can interrupt the absorption of some drugs, thus preventing the benefits of certain drug therapies.

For a summary of representative drugs, see *Selected Major Drugs: Emetic and antiemetic agents* on pages 779 and 780.

EMETICS

Emetics are used to induce vomiting after the ingestion of toxic substances. While many substances were used in the past to induce vomiting, only two drugs, apomorphine and ipecac syrup, are now available for use as emetics. Most physicians consider ipecac syrup the emetic of choice to treat toxic ingestions because the drug is the most effective and is less likely to cause problems than other emetics or mechanical stimulation. Household emetics, such as sodium chloride (salt) solutions, can cause fatalities from electrolyte imbalances (hypernatremia). Researchers have not determined the safety and efficacy of soaps and detergents as emetics. Studies of mechanically stimulated vomiting, such as placing a finger or spoon in the throat to cause a gag reflex, have shown this method to be much less effective than the administration of ipecac syrup.

History and source

Ipecac is an extract of alkaloids from the roots and rhizomes of the plants *Cephaelis ipecacuanha* and *Cephaelis acuminata*, which are indigenous to Brazil and Central America, respectively. Apparently, Central and South American Indians first used ipecac. Records indicate that Aztec physicians used ipecac as a standard medicinal. A Jesuit friar first described the drug in 1601, and in 1672 Le Gras introduced ipecac to Europe. By 1690, ipecac was well known in Europe as a medicinal. Today in the United States, many people with young children recognize the benefits of keeping ipecac syrup on hand.

Opium, the forerunner to apomorphine and other opiate alkaloids, has been used since antiquity. In 1803, Sertürner, a German pharmacist, discovered morphine, the first alkaloid of opium. When scientists treated morphine with hydrochloric acid in an attempt to increase the drug's analgesic potency, they obtained apomorphine, a chemical with decreased analgesic but stronger emetic properties than morphine. Apomorphine also retained the respiratory depressant properties of the narcotics.

PHARMACOKINETICS

Very little information exists concerning the absorption, distribution, and excretion of ipecac syrup. Apomorphine, which is absorbed well from the injection site, provides a quicker onset of action than ipecac.

Absorption, distribution, metabolism, excretion

Researchers have noted some absorption of ipecac. In one study, the alkaloids of ipecac administered to patients were later found in the serum of those patients; however, the amount of the drug present in the serum varied considerably among patients.

Apomorphine administered by either intramuscular or subcutaneous injection produces an emetic action that is more predictable than that produced by oral administration. The drug is well absorbed from the injection site and metabolized by the liver. Metabolites of the drug are excreted by the kidneys. Both ipecac syrup and apomorphine distribute to breast milk.

Onset, peak, duration

After administration of ipecac syrup, a delay of approximately 10 minutes usually occurs before the onset of vomiting. About 50% of the patients receiving ipecac will begin vomiting in less than 15 to 20 minutes, and about 90% will vomit within 30 minutes.

The onset of action of apomorphine is very fast, with emesis usually induced within 5 minutes after subcutaneous administration and with approximately 90% of patients vomiting within 15 minutes. The onset of action of apomorphine may occur more rapidly than that of ipecac syrup because apomorphine reaches its site of action more quickly. The narcotic sedative effect of apomorphine occurs within several minutes and lasts for about 2 hours after a dose.

PHARMACODYNAMICS

Both ipecac syrup and apomorphine induce vomiting by stimulating the vomiting center located in the medulla of the brain.

Mechanism of action

Ipecac syrup induces vomiting by producing both a local effect on the gastric mucosa and a central effect on the CTZ. After the administration of ipecac syrup, the initial episode of vomiting is probably from the local effect of the ipecac on the stomach, although subsequent episodes of vomiting may be from CTZ stimulation. Ipecac produces a regurgitation of the contents of the stomach and upper duodenum, but not of any contents further along the gastrointestinal tract. Most patients will vomit two or three times during the first hour after administration and will be able to resume normal eating in several hours.

Apomorphine produces its emetic effect by directly stimulating the dopamine receptors located in the CTZ. Like ipecac, apomorphine induces a regurgitation of the contents of the stomach and upper duodenum, but not of any contents in the lower gastrointestinal tract. Excitation of vestibular centers may also be involved in producing apomorphine-induced vomiting, since movement intensifies the emetic effect of the drug.

Apomorphine produces some of the same pharmacologic effects as other narcotics. It may cause central nervous system (CNS) stimulation or depression. The drug also produces respiratory depression, hypotension, and sedation similar to those same effects produced by the other narcotics.

PHARMACOTHERAPEUTICS

Since most poisonings and overdoses involve ingestion of a toxin, the primary objective in treatment is to prevent the ingested substance from being absorbed into the body. To attain this goal, treatment involves one of three mechanisms: gastric emptying, binding of the substance in the stomach, and to a lesser extent, the stimulation of gastrointestinal motility, which decreases the time the toxin travels through the GI tract. Gastric emptying involves physical removal of the toxic substance from the stomach, using either an emetic or gastric lavage. Administered activated charcoal binds with the toxic substance and prevents its absorption. Cathartics stimulate gastrointestinal motility and help the system quickly eliminate any unabsorbed poison in the feces.

Ipecac syrup is considered the therapy of choice for emptying the stomach because of its effectiveness and low incidence of adverse effects. It can be purchased without a prescription and stored in the home for emergencies.

Although the parenteral route of administration for apomorphine limits its use in the home, the drug is used occasionally in the emergency department. Apomorphine is as effective as ipecac syrup in removing toxic substances from the stomach, and has a slightly more rapid onset of action. However, the more rapid action may be outweighed by the longer time required for the patient to reach the emergency department to receive the drug.

ipecac syrup. This drug is available for use without a prescription in 1-ounce (30-ml) containers. Ipecac fluid extract, which is 14 times more potent than ipecac syrup, is no longer marketed; however, it may still be in use. If administered, ipecac fluid extract may contribute to significant toxicity or death from improper doses.
USUAL ADULT DOSAGE: 15 to 30 ml P.O. followed by 200 to 300 ml of water.
USUAL PEDIATRIC DOSAGE: for children over age 1, 15 ml P.O. followed by 200 ml of water or milk; for children under 1 year old, 5 to 10 ml P.O. followed by 100 ml of water or milk.

If vomiting does not occur within 30 minutes, repeat the initial dose. If the second dose does not produce emesis, initiate other measures, such as gastric lavage and activated charcoal, to minimize absorption and prevent toxicity from both the ipecac syrup and the poison.

apomorphine hydrochloride. A Schedule II drug, apomorphine is used to induce vomiting in poisoning. If emesis does not follow the initial dose of apomorphine, *do not* administer a subsequent dose because it is not likely to be any more effective.
USUAL ADULT DOSAGE: 5 to 6 mg S.C. or I.M. preceded by 200 to 300 ml of water or milk.
USUAL PEDIATRIC DOSAGE: 0.07 to 0.1 mg/kg S.C. or I.M. preceded by 100 to 200 ml of water or milk. The I.V. dose, which is rarely used, is 0.01 mg/kg for both children and adults.

Drug interactions

Because ipecac syrup and apomorphine are used only in acute situations, drug interactions rarely occur. If poisoning is from ingestion of a phenothiazine, the phenothiazine's antiemetic effect on the CTZ may decrease the emetic effect of both ipecac syrup and apomorphine. The administration of activated charcoal should be delayed until emesis has occurred because activated charcoal must remain in the gastrointestinal tract to be effective. If activated charcoal and ipecac syrup are administered together, the activated charcoal may be vomited or become bound with the ipecac syrup, inactivating it.

ADVERSE DRUG REACTIONS

Apomorphine produces many of the same adverse effects as other narcotics; ipecac syrup causes very few adverse effects.

Predictable reactions

Like other narcotics, apomorphine directly affects the central nervous system (CNS). The drug may cause euphoria, restlessness, tachypnea, tremors, and profound CNS depression ranging from stupor to coma. Apomorphine also may produce acute circulatory depression, usually manifested by orthostatic hypotension. Acute circulatory depression occurs especially in elderly and debilitated patients using apomorphine. Respiratory depression occurs when large or repeated doses of apomorphine are administered. Administering the narcotic antagonist naloxone may relieve the CNS and respiratory depressant effects as well as the protracted emesis produced by apomorphine.

Ipecac syrup rarely produces adverse effects when used in the recommended doses. Almost all reports of problems from ipecac involved massive overdose, chronic use, a congenital abnormality, complications in elderly patients, or poisoning with phenothiazine ingestion. As for adverse effects involving children, prolonged vomiting for more than 1 hour or repeated vomiting involving more than six episodes in 1 hour occurred in about 9% of the children given ipecac syrup. Also, about 3% of all the children had subsequent lethargy, and about 1.5% had diarrhea. Ipecac contains a specific cardiotoxin that, in high doses, may cause cardiac dysrhythmias or fatal myocarditis, especially in elderly patients. Heart failure is usually the cause of death after ipecac overdose.

Because the effects of using either ipecac syrup or apomorphine during pregnancy remain unknown, the drugs should be administered only when clearly indicated. Both drugs distribute to breast milk, so exercise caution when administering either one to lactating women.

Unpredictable reactions

People with eating disorders (for example, anorexia nervosa and bulimia) who abuse ipecac syrup can have serious, potentially fatal adverse reactions. These adverse reactions usually include generalized myopathy or cardiomyopathy. Other unpredictable adverse reactions include fixed eruptions and toxic epidermal necrolysis as well as tears in the esophagus (Mallory-Weiss syndrome) from protracted, severe vomiting.

NURSING IMPLICATIONS

Ipecac syrup and apomorphine are both contraindicated in those poisonings for which emesis should be avoided. Optimum results depend upon the proper administration of both drugs.

- Both ipecac syrup and apomorphine are contraindicated in semicomatose or unconscious patients and in patients with severe inebriation, convulsions, shock, or loss of gag reflex.
- These drugs are contraindicated in poisonings involving petroleum distillates (for example, gasoline, kerosene, lighter fluids, or paint and lacquer thinners) or volatile oils; vomiting may cause the victim to aspirate gastric contents into the lungs, causing an aspiration pneumonitis.
- These drugs are also contraindicated in poisonings involving caustic substances, such as ammonia, battery acid, lye, drain cleaners, and oven or toilet bowl cleaners because additional injuries to the esophagus and mediastinum may occur.
- Administer apomorphine cautiously to patients with impaired cardiac function and sclerotic changes of blood vessels because severe vomiting may cause hemorrhage and infarction in these patients.
- Apomorphine is contraindicated in patients with a known hypersensitivity to narcotic analgesics.
- Do not confuse ipecac syrup with fluid extract of ipecac. Check to be sure that the word *syrup* appears on the bottle.
- When administering apomorphine, have available the narcotic antagonist naloxone to reverse respiratory or CNS adverse reactions or prolonged vomiting.

Home use of ipecac syrup

Include poison prevention counseling for parents as part of either the 6-month or 1-year well-child examination for all children. Advise parents to purchase a 1-ounce (30-ml) bottle of ipecac syrup for poisoning emergencies, and teach them how to use the drug. Include the following points in the teaching:
- Keep ipecac syrup and all other medications out of the child's reach.
- Before using ipecac syrup to induce vomiting after poisoning, contact your physician, a poison control center, or emergency department. (Provide the parent with the appropriate telephone numbers.)
- Do not give ipecac syrup to unconscious or very drowsy children because vomited material may enter the lungs and cause pneumonia.
- Have the poisoned child drink a glass of water (approximately 6 to 8 ounces) immediately after taking ipecac syrup to help induce vomiting.
- Do not give the child milk unless otherwise instructed because milk will bind with the ipecac and prevent its vomiting effect.
- If the child does not vomit within 30 minutes, repeat the dose, and take the child to an emergency department. If the child does vomit, seek the physician's advice about follow-up medical care.

- Administer activated charcoal following emesis, unless otherwise contraindicated.
- For the usual subcutaneous administration of apomorphine, dissolve a 6-mg soluble tablet in 1 to 2 ml of 0.9% saline solution or sterile water for injection. Then purify the solution by passing it through a 0.22-micron filter before administration.
- After administering either ipecac syrup or apomorphine, you can induce early effects by moving the patient or gently bouncing a child.
- Teach parents that they should not administer ipecac syrup to a child unless advised by a poison control center or other qualified health care personnel. (See *Home use of ipecac syrup* for specific information to include in teaching.)

ANTIHISTAMINE ANTIEMETICS

The antihistamine antiemetics consist of drugs that are closely related in chemical structure, all of which block the histamine (H_1) receptors and decrease nausea, vomiting, and vertigo. A number of antihistamine derivatives exist; however, those groups with the greatest antiemetic activity are the ethanolamine derivatives, including dimenhydrinate and diphenhydramine hydrochloride, and the piperazine derivatives, including buclizine hydrochloride, cyclizine hydrochloride, meclizine hydrochloride, hydroxyzine pamoate, and hydroxyzine hydrochloride. Trimethobenzamide is structurally related to the ethanolamine antihistamines.

History and source
Bovet and Staub in 1937 discovered drugs with histamine-blocking activity, but these drugs were too toxic for human use. Then in the mid-1940s in France, a derivative that was not too toxic was found. Early work on the antihistamines focused on finding a drug that would prevent an allergic reaction by blocking the effects of histamine. While developing this histamine-blocking quality, researchers discovered the antiemetic effect of these drugs.

PHARMACOKINETICS

Antihistamines are well absorbed from the gastrointestinal tract and are metabolized primarily by the liver. Their inactive metabolites are excreted in the urine.

Absorption, distribution, metabolism, excretion
Though most antihistamines are generally well absorbed from the GI tract, the slower absorption of some accounts for their slower onset of action and longer duration of action. Little is known about the distribution, metabolism, and excretion of most antihistamines, but information about the few drugs studied may apply to all of the antihistamine antiemetics. Diphenhydramine, which has been widely studied, is well distributed to the central nervous system and throughout the body. Researchers believe that most of the antihistamine antiemetics are also distributed to breast milk. The antihistamine antiemetics are metabolized almost completely to inactive metabolites by the liver. The inactive metabolites are excreted by the kidneys within 24 hours.

Onset, peak, duration
The antihistamine antiemetics usually produce an onset of action 30 minutes after oral administration. The drug effects peak within 1 to 2 hours and last up to 6 hours. Some of the antihistamine antiemetics provide longer durations of action. For example, both hydroxyzine and meclizine may provide a duration of action up to 24 hours.

With trimethobenzamide, the onset of antiemetic action is 10 to 40 minutes, and drug action lasts up to

4 hours after oral administration. The onset and duration from rectal administration should be similar to that of oral administration. After intramuscular injection of trimethobenzamide, the onset of antiemetic action is 15 to 35 minutes, and the duration is from 2 to 3 hours.

PHARMACODYNAMICS

The antihistamine antiemetics exert several biochemical and physiologic effects. All bind with the H_1 receptors to prevent histamine action during allergic reactions, and as antiemetics, these drugs penetrate the central nervous system, where they exert antiemetic and some adverse effects. Most of the antihistamine antiemetics also inhibit the response to acetylcholine at the muscarinic receptors and, therefore, produce an anticholinergic effect characterized by dry mouth, blurred vision, urinary retention, or constipation.

Mechanism of action
The mechanism of action that produces the antiemetic effect of the antihistamines remains unclear. The drugs have been shown to inhibit vestibular stimulation of the ear, one of the primary causes of motion sickness. Also, the anticholinergic effects of antihistamines in the central nervous system may play an important role. Cholinergic stimulation in the vestibular and reticular systems may cause the nausea and vomiting of motion sickness. The antihistamines, through their anticholinergic action, block this stimulation and produce an antiemetic effect that helps treat motion sickness.

Finally, all of the antihistamine antiemetics produce a generalized CNS depressant effect, which probably accounts for some of their antiemetic effect.

Of the major antihistamine antiemetics, only trimethobenzamide can inhibit the emetic effects of apomorphine: that is, direct stimulation of the CTZ. Therefore, researchers believe that trimethobenzamide produces its antiemetic effect differently from the other antihistamines by inhibiting stimuli to the CTZ. Because of its direct inhibitory ability, trimethobenzamide produces a less specific antiemetic effect on the vestibular system of the ear. As a result, trimethobenzamide provides a general antiemetic effect regardless of the underlying cause. (See *Mechanism of action of antihistamine antiemetics* for a diagramatic representation of the mechanisms of action of this drug group and of trimethobenzamide in particular.)

PHARMACOTHERAPEUTICS

With the exception of trimethobenzamide, the antihistamines are fairly specific antiemetics for the nausea and vomiting from inner ear stimulation. As a consequence,

Mechanism of action of antihistamine antiemetics

The antihistamine antiemetics prevent nausea and vomiting by inhibiting impulses from the inner ear to the vestibular nuclei, as well as by inhibiting cholinergic stimulation of the chemoreceptor target zone (CTZ) and vomiting center from the vestibular nuclei. The vestibular pathway produces the nausea and vomiting of motion sickness and other labyrinth disorders. Trimethobenzamide directly inhibits dopaminergic stimulation of the CTZ, thus providing a general antiemetic effect.

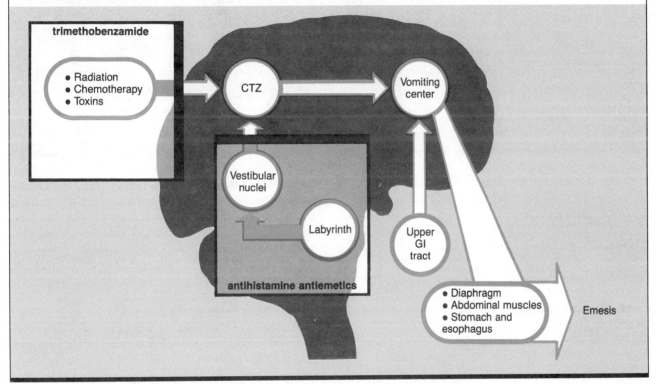

these drugs prevent and treat motion sickness. They usually prove effective when given prophylactically before activities that produce motion sickness; the drugs are much less effective when nausea or vomiting has begun. If administered after nausea or vomiting has begun, they probably will not alleviate further episodes.

Although scopolamine, which is not an antihistamine antiemetic, may be the most effective drug for motion sickness, its use may be limited by its anticholinergic adverse effects. Therefore, many physicians prefer the antihistamine antiemetics to treat motion sickness. Furthermore, antihistamine antiemetics provide a longer duration of action than does oral scopolamine (though not its transdermal form). (See page 777 for more information about scopolamine.)

The antihistamine antiemetics are used extensively to treat diseases that produce vertigo by affecting the vestibular system. Such diseases include labyrinthitis and Meniere's disease. Although studies have not proven conclusively that antihistamine antiemetics benefit patients with these diseases, they relieve some of the symptoms and are therefore useful for preventing or treating an acute attack.

Trimethobenzamide, used to control nausea and vomiting, is not as effective as the phenothiazine antiemetics but may be less toxic. Trimethobenzamide may be preferable to the phenothiazine antiemetics for long-term therapy because the risk of extrapyramidal reactions in the patient is lower.

buclizine hydrochloride (Bucladin-S Softab). This drug is supplied as a chewable tablet, which the patient can swallow whole, dissolve in the mouth and swallow, or chew before swallowing.
USUAL ADULT DOSAGE: for control of vertigo, 50 mg P.O. one to three times daily; for motion sickness, 50 mg P.O. every 4 to 6 hours.

DRUG INTERACTIONS

Antihistamine antiemetics

The following chart presents the important drug interactions for the major antihistamine antiemetics discussed in this chapter.

DRUG	INTERACTING DRUGS	POSSIBLE EFFECTS	NURSING IMPLICATIONS
buclizine, cyclizine, dimenhydrinate, diphenhydramine, hydroxyzine, meclizine, trimethobenzamide	CNS depressants, including barbiturates, tranquilizers, alcohol, and opiates	Produce additive CNS depression	• Use caution when administering concurrently to avoid excessive CNS depression or sedation. • Inform ambulatory patients of the possible additive effect.
	anticholinergic drugs, including tricyclic antidepressants, phenothiazines, and anti-parkinsonian drugs	Produce additive anticholinergic effects	• Assess for signs of increased anticholinergic activity (constipation, dry mouth, visual disturbances, and urinary retention).

cyclizine hydrochloride (Marezine). Cyclizine hydrochloride is for oral use; cyclizine lactate is the form for intramuscular injection.
USUAL ADULT DOSAGE: 50 mg P.O. or I.M. every 4 to 6 hours.

dimenhydrinate (Dramamine). Given orally, dimenhydrinate is probably the most frequently used drug for motion sickness because of its relatively low incidence of adverse effects.
USUAL ADULT DOSAGE: 50 to 100 mg P.O. q 4 to 6 hours.

diphenhydramine hydrochloride (Benadryl). Although this drug produces an antiemetic effect, its use is limited by the sedation it usually produces.
USUAL ADULT DOSAGE: 25 to 50 mg P.O. or I.M. q 4 to 6 hours.

hydroxyzine pamoate (Vistaril), **hydroxyzine hydrochloride** (Atarax). Also limited by its sedative effects, hydroxyzine produces a synergistic analgesic effect with narcotic analgesics and also decreases the nausea associated with narcotic administration.
USUAL ADULT DOSAGE: for antiemetic effects, 25 to 100 mg P.O. or I.M. t.i.d. to q.i.d.

meclizine hydrochloride (Antivert, Bonine). This drug provides a slower onset of action and longer duration of action than the other antihistamine antiemetics.
USUAL ADULT DOSAGE: for motion sickness, 25 to 50 mg P.O. daily at least one hour before travel; for vertigo, 25 to 100 mg P.O. daily in divided doses.

trimethobenzamide hydrochloride (Tigan). This drug is administered orally, rectally, or intramuscularly to treat nausea and vomiting. Administer rectally or by intramuscular injection for prevention of postoperative nausea and vomiting.
USUAL ADULT DOSAGE: 250 mg P.O. or 200 mg rectally or I.M., t.i.d. to q.i.d.

Drug interactions
Antihistamine antiemetics can produce an additive pharmacologic effect when they interact with other drugs that also produce an anticholinergic effect. The same is true for the sedative effect produced by antihistamines. (See *Drug interactions: Antihistamine antiemetics* for the common interactions and their nursing implications.)

ADVERSE DRUG REACTIONS

Most adverse reactions involving the antihistamine antiemetics are predictable, mild, and usually easy to control.

Predictable reactions
All antihistamine antiemetics produce some dose-related drowsiness. Reducing the dose may decrease the drowsiness without compromising the antiemetic effect. Paradoxical CNS stimulation has occurred, more often in children than adults. Symptoms of paradoxical CNS stimulation may range from restlessness, insomnia, and euphoria to tremors and even seizures. Other CNS adverse reactions include dizziness, headache, and lassitude.

The antihistamine antiemetics themselves may cause mild nausea or epigastric distress. Administering the drug with food or milk may decrease these symptoms. Anorexia may also occur and last for several weeks from long term administration of an antihistamine antiemetic.

The anticholinergic effect of the antihistamines may cause constipation. Other anticholinergic effects include dry mouth and throat, dysuria, urinary retention, and impotence. The anticholinergic action of antihistamines may also produce visual and auditory disturbances, such as blurred vision or tinnitus.

Besides the previously mentioned reactions, trimethobenzamide may produce extrapyramidal symptoms, such as acute dystonia and dyskinesis, that require discontinuation of the drug.

Unpredictable reactions

Hypersensitivity reactions, as manifested by rashes and photosensitivity, may occur. Blood dyscrasias have occurred, but rarely. These include agranulocytosis, hemolytic anemia, leukopenia, thrombocytopenia, and pancytopenia. (See *Adverse drug reactions to antiemetics* on page 776 for a list of reactions associated with the antihistamine antiemetics.)

NURSING IMPLICATIONS

Individual response to the drug and dosage may vary with these agents.
• Because of the anticholinergic effects of these drugs, administer them with caution, if at all, to patients with narrow-angle glaucoma, urinary retention, peptic ulcer disease, gastric obstruction, prostatic hypertrophy, or asthma.
• To prevent motion sickness, advise the patient to ingest the drug 30 to 60 minutes before the activity that might produce nausea and vomiting. Patients usually develop tolerance to motion sickness; therefore, only short-term therapy is usually needed.
• When one antihistamine antiemetic fails to produce the desired effects, a change in dose or derivative may produce results.
• If the patient vomits before drug administration, consider giving a rectal suppository or intramuscular injection.
• Alert the patient to the sedative effects, and advise the patient not to drive or participate in other activities that require mental alertness. Alert the patient not to drink alcohol or take other CNS depressants because doing so can result in the additive sedative effect of antihistamines.

PHENOTHIAZINE ANTIEMETICS

The phenothiazines primarily are used to treat psychotic disorders. Yet, some of the phenothiazines are used to prevent and treat severe nausea and vomiting from various causes. Phenothiazine antiemetics are not as effective as the antihistamine antiemetics for nausea from motion sickness or vestibular dysfunction. The phenothiazines most frequently used for their antiemetic effect include chlorpromazine hydrochloride, promethazine, prochlorperazine maleate, thiethylperazine, perphenazine, triflupromazine hydrochloride, and trimeprazine tartrate.

History and source

In 1945, promethazine was marketed as an antihistamine, which was not surprising because the chemical structures of the antihistamines and the phenothiazines closely resemble one another. The phenothiazines became the first specific class of general antiemetics. Since the 1950s, they have served as the mainstay of antiemetic therapy. The phenothiazines were not used as antipsychotic drugs until 1951. Since the early 1970s, additional interest in the antiemetic effects of the phenothiazines has been generated because of their effectiveness in preventing and treating nausea and vomiting from cancer chemotherapy and radiotherapy.

PHARMACOKINETICS

The phenothiazine antiemetics are well absorbed, extensively metabolized by the liver, and excreted in the urine and feces.

Absorption, distribution, metabolism, excretion

Phenothiazines are usually well absorbed from the gastrointestinal tract from both the oral and rectal routes of administration. The drugs are also well absorbed from injection sites.

Phenothiazines are distributed to most body tissues and fluids, including breast milk. These drugs cross into the central nervous system with fairly high concentration levels and become highly protein bound in the plasma.

Phenothiazines are metabolized by the liver to a number of metabolites, a few of which are pharmacologically active. After undergoing enterohepatic circulation, these metabolites are excreted in both the feces and urine.

Onset, peak, duration

The onset of action of chlorpromazine occurs shortly after oral, rectal, and parenteral administration. Concentration levels peak in about 1 to 2 hours, and duration of action is usually 4 to 5 hours. For other phenothiazine products, onset of action and peak concentration levels may not occur as quickly, though duration of action may be slightly longer.

PHARMACODYNAMICS

The biochemical and physiologic effects of the phenothiazines as antipsychotic drugs are well researched. Many of the effects of these drugs result from their antidopaminergic properties in the central nervous system. (See Chapter 33, Antipsychotic Agents, for a more in-depth discussion of the action of the phenothiazines.)

Mechanism of action

Phenothiazines produce their antiemetic effect by blocking the dopaminergic receptors in the CTZ. The phenothiazines may also directly depress the vomiting center.

PHARMACOTHERAPEUTICS

Phenothiazine antiemetics control severe nausea and vomiting from various causes. When vomiting becomes severe and potentially hazardous, the phenothiazines are the drugs of choice, providing effective treatment for postoperative nausea and vomiting and for the nausea and vomiting from viral illnesses. Physicians prescribe phenothiazines extensively to control the nausea and vomiting of cancer chemotherapy and radiotherapy. Phenothiazines, however, are not as effective as the antihistamine antiemetics in controlling the nausea and vomiting from vertigo, motion sickness, or direct irritation of the stomach. Although not all the phenothiazines with antiemetic effects have been compared in controlled trials, those drugs that have been studied and compared displayed little difference in their antiemetic effects.

The phenothiazines are the most effective general antiemetics; however, their use is limited to short-term therapy because the potential for serious adverse reactions is higher with these drugs than with the antihistamine antiemetics. The phenothiazine antiemetics are effective in treating morning sickness during pregnancy; however, their safety during pregnancy has not been established. As a result, phenothiazines should be used only when the potential benefits outweigh the potential risks.

The phenothiazines include several major drugs that share the same antiemetic use. The phenothiazine antiemetics are equally efficient in treating the nausea and vomiting from infection, uremia, cancer chemotherapy,

radiation, anesthesia, or drug toxicity. The choice of a phenothiazine antiemetic, therefore, depends upon the drug's potential for adverse effects.

Physicians reserve the parenteral route of administration for the phenothiazines for patients under direct observation, although they use the rectal route more often in an outpatient setting, where parenteral administration proves less practical or when vomiting reduces the effectiveness of the oral preparations.

chlorpromazine hydrochloride (Thorazine). This drug is more often used as an antipsychotic than as an antiemetic.
USUAL ADULT DOSAGE: 10 to 25 mg P.O. or 25 mg I.M. every 4 to 6 hours; 100 mg rectally every 6 to 8 hours.

promethazine (Phenergan). This drug is often used preoperatively and postoperatively or as an adjunct to narcotic analgesics for sedation and nausea control.
USUAL ADULT DOSAGE: 12.5 to 25 mg P.O., I.M., or rectally every 4 to 6 hours.

prochlorperazine maleate (Compazine). This drug is primarily used to control nausea and vomiting.
USUAL ADULT DOSAGE: 5 to 10 mg P.O. or I.M. t.i.d. to q.i.d.; rectally, 25 mg b.i.d.

Prochlorperazine is also available as a sustained-release capsule, administered twice daily. However, sustained-release antiemetics offer no advantages and are more expensive than other forms.

thiethylperazine (Torecan). Thiethylperazine is another major phenothiazine antiemetic.
USUAL ADULT DOSAGE: 10 mg one to three times daily, with oral, rectal, or intramuscular administration.

perphenazine (Trilafon). This antipsychotic agent is also used to treat severe nausea and vomiting.
USUAL ADULT DOSAGE: 8 to 16 mg P.O. daily, divided in two to four doses; 5 mg I.M.

triflupromazine hydrochloride (Vesprin). This drug is sometimes used to manage nausea and vomiting.
USUAL ADULT DOSAGE: 20 to 30 mg P.O. daily; 1 mg I.V. for a maximum of 3 mg daily; or 5 to 15 mg I.M. every 4 to 6 hours, up to a maximum of 60 mg daily.

trimeprazine tartrate (Temaril). This agent is used more frequently as an antipruritic than as an antiemetic.
USUAL ADULT DOSAGE: 2.5 mg P.O. q.i.d.

DRUG INTERACTIONS

Phenothiazine antiemetics

The following chart lists the major phenothiazine antiemetics discussed in this chapter and summarizes the drug interactions associated with this class. The additive CNS depressant and anticholinergic effects, as well as decreased antiemetic efficacy, require patient monitoring and teaching.

DRUG	INTERACTING DRUGS	POSSIBLE EFFECTS	NURSING IMPLICATIONS
chlorpromazine, promethazine, prochlorperazine, thiethylperazine	CNS depressants, including barbiturates, tranquilizers, alcohol, and opiates	Produce additive CNS depression	• Use caution when administering concurrently to avoid excessive CNS depression or sedation. • Inform ambulatory patients of the possible additive effect.
	anticholinergic drugs, including tricyclic antidepressants, phenothiazines, and anti-parkinsonian drugs	Produce additive anticholinergic effects	• Assess for signs of increased anticholinergic activity (constipation, dry mouth, visual disturbances, and urinary retention).
	antacids	Decrease phenothiazine absorption	• Administer doses with at least 2 hours intervening.
	barbiturates	Decrease phenothiazine effect	• Monitor the patient for decreased antiemetic effect.
	anticonvulsants	Lower seizure threshold	• Anticonvulsant drug doses may need to be increased.

Drug interactions

The drug interactions of the phenothiazine antiemetics resemble those of the antihistamine antiemetics. Phenothiazine antiemetics may produce an additive effect with the CNS depressant action of other depressants, such as narcotics, sedatives, or alcohol; they may also have an additive anticholinergic effect when used with other drugs with anticholinergic action. (See *Drug interactions: Phenothiazine antiemetics* for details.)

ADVERSE DRUG REACTIONS

Phenothiazines used in larger dosages as antipsychotics can produce numerous adverse reactions. When used as antiemetics, however, the drugs primarily produce sedation, hypotension, and extrapyramidal effects.

Predictable reactions

Central nervous system adverse reactions number among the major problems associated with the use of phenothiazine antiemetics. Mild to moderate sedation occurs in 50% to 80% of the patients who receive these drugs, with chlorpromazine producing the greatest incidence. Tolerance to the sedative effect usually develops over several days of therapy. Other CNS adverse reactions associated with phenothiazine antiemetics include anxiety, euphoria, agitation, depression, headache, insomnia, restlessness, and weakness. Use of these drugs can also lower the threshold for seizures. Therefore, use caution when administering these drugs to patients who are predisposed to seizures. Typical adverse anticholinergic reactions include dry mouth, blurred vision, constipation, and urinary retention.

Hypotension and postural hypotension with tachycardia, syncope, and dizziness frequently occur as adverse reactions to the phenothiazine antiemetics. Chlorpromazine, again, produces the highest incidence of hypotensive effects, with the lowest incidence occurring with prochlorperazine and thiethylperazine. Tolerance to the hypotensive effects usually develops.

Extrapyramidal reactions may occur with phenothiazine antiemetics. Such reactions are usually dose related and, therefore, relatively rare at antiemetic doses.

Unpredictable reactions

Phenothiazines used as antipsychotics can produce many unpredictable reactions, but these reactions rarely occur when the drugs are used as antiemetics. Agranulocytosis, although rare, is the most frequently reported adverse hematologic effect. Agranulocytosis usually occurs after prolonged phenothiazine therapy not associated with nausea and vomiting.

Adverse drug reactions to antiemetics

The following table indicates the incidence of adverse drug reactions from the different kinds of antiemetics. The number and frequency of these reactions may vary according to the specific class of drug and may affect drug selection by the physician.

	NAUSEA AND VOMITING	ANTICHOLINERGIC REACTIONS	SEDATION	EXTRAPYRAMIDAL REACTIONS	DIZZINESS AND OTHER C.N.S. REACTIONS	DERMATOLOGIC REACTIONS
antihistamine antiemetics	+	+ +	+ + +	0	+ +	+
phenothiazine antiemetics	0	+ +	+ +	+ +	+	+ +
scopolamine	0	+ + +	+ + +	0	+ +	0

Key:
    0 = none
    + = low incidence
  + + = moderate incidence
+ + + = high incidence

The phenothiazines also produce many dermatologic effects; again, these are more common with long-term therapy. Photosensitivity also may occur with short-term therapy.

Hypersensitivity reactions manifested as cholestatic jaundice, blood dyscrasias, dermatologic reactions, and photosensitivity have occurred, usually within the first few months of phenothiazine therapy. (See *Adverse drug reactions to antiemetics* for the major adverse reactions to the phenothiazine antiemetics.)

NURSING IMPLICATIONS

Phenothiazine antiemetics are contraindicated in patients with many CNS disorders, cardiovascular disease, and hepatic disease. Alert patients that these drugs may cause sedation, hypotension, and photosensitivity.

• Phenothiazine antiemetics are contraindicated in phenothiazine hypersensitivity, coma from any cause, CNS depression, bone marrow depression, and subcortical brain damage. The drugs are also contraindicated in pediatric surgery.

• Administer these drugs with caution to patients with encephalitis, Reye's syndrome, encephalopathy, meningitis, or tetanus because the adverse reactions from phenothiazine therapy are similar to the signs and symptoms of these conditions, increasing the risk of misdiagnosis.

• Administer these drugs with caution to patients with hepatic disease, cardiovascular disease (may cause sudden drop in blood pressure), exposure to extreme heat or cold (including antipyretic therapy), respiratory disorders, hypocalcemia, convulsive disorders or severe reactions to insulin or electroshock therapy, suspected brain tumor, intestinal obstruction, glaucoma, prostatic hypertrophy, or to elderly or debilitated patients.

• Administer cautiously to children with acute illnesses, such as chicken pox, measles, gastroenteritis, CNS infection, or dehydration, because of the increased incidence of extrapyramidal reactions.

• Alert the patient that these drugs are not effective for motion sickness.

• When preparing or administering these drugs, avoid skin contact with oral solutions and injections, which can cause contact dermatitis.

• Alert the patient that use of phenothiazine antiemetics may impair the ability to perform activities requiring mental alertness or physical coordination, such as driving or operating machinery. Also inform the patient that alcohol or other sedatives will potentiate the sedative effect of the phenothiazines.

• Inform the patient about the possibility of hypotension, and instruct the patient to remain recumbent for 30 to 60 minutes after receiving the drug. Inform the patient that urine may become pink or red-brown.

• Alert the patient to avoid prolonged exposure to sunlight or to wear protective clothing and sunscreen because phenothiazines may produce photosensitivity.

OTHER ANTIEMETICS

Other drugs, unrelated to either the antihistamines or phenothiazines, also act effectively to prevent and treat nausea and vomiting.

benzquinamide hydrochloride (Emete-con). This drug is a benzquinoline derivative available as an antiemetic in parenteral form. Though not related chemically to either the antihistamines or phenothiazines, benzquinamide does produce antiemetic, antihistamine, anticholinergic, vasopressor, and sedative effects. Benzquinamide probably produces its antiemetic effect by a direct depressant action on the CTZ.

Benzquinamide is indicated for the prevention and treatment of nausea and vomiting associated with anesthesia and surgery. This drug may be preferred in some circumstances because it does not produce CNS or respiratory depression. Furthermore, benzquinamide does not produce the extrapyramidal effects or hypotension associated with the phenothiazines.

Benzquinamide is rapidly absorbed after intramuscular administration. After I.M. injection, onset of action is within 15 minutes, and duration of action is from 3 to 4 hours. The drug is metabolized by the liver, and its metabolites are excreted in both the urine and feces. Adverse reactions to benzquinamide usually involve the central nervous system, with drowsiness the most common. Anticholinergic adverse reactions frequently occur. USUAL ADULT DOSAGE: 50 mg I.M., repeated in 1 hour if necessary. Subsequent doses may be given every 3 to 4 hours.

scopolamine (Triptone, Transderm-Scop). This drug has long been used to prevent motion sickness; however, physicians limit the drug's use because of its sedative and anticholinergic effects. One scopolamine transdermal preparation (Transderm-Scop) provides highly effective action without producing scopolamine's usual adverse reactions. (See *Facts about scopolamine patches* on page 778 for an illustration and explanation of transdermal scopolamine.) Drowsiness and dry mouth from the anticholinergic action of scopolamine are the most frequent adverse reactions. Patients usually tolerate these reactions well because the reactions are not pronounced. The nurse should observe the common anticholinergic precautions, such as administering scopolamine cautiously to patients with glaucoma or with gastrointestinal or urinary obstruction.

USUAL ADULT DOSAGE: 0.4 to 0.8 mg P.O. t.i.d. or q.i.d.; 0.25 mg P.O. 1 hour before travel and repeated in 4 hours; 1 transdermal patch applied to postauricular skin 4 hours before travel.

metoclopramide hydrochloride (Reglan). This drug is used to manage gastrointestinal motility disorders. The drug's effectiveness is partially attributed to its antagonistic effect on dopamine in the central nervous system. Apparently, metoclopramide is also antagonistic to dopamine in the CTZ, thereby suppressing the impulse to vomit. Metoclopramide may also decrease direct impulses from the gastrointestinal tract to the vomiting center.

Metoclopramide, used for many years in Europe to prevent motion sickness, is currently being used in the United States prophylactically to prevent cancer chemotherapy–induced nausea and vomiting. USUAL ADULT DOSAGE: to treat cancer chemotherapy–induced emesis, 2 mg/kg, a relatively high dose, by I.V. infusion 30 minutes before the administration of a highly nauseating drug. The dose is repeated twice at 2-hour intervals after the initial dose. Lower doses, sometimes administered orally, are effective for less nauseating drugs.

diphenidol (Vontrol). Structurally unrelated to either the antihistamine or phenothiazine antiemetics, diphenidol appears to provide a dual effect, inhibiting impulse conduction from the vestibular area of the ear to the vomiting center and directly suppressing the CTZ. Thus, the drug not only effectively prevents vertigo, but it also prevents and treats generalized nausea and vomiting. Diphenidol, which has a relatively long half-life of 4 hours, is well absorbed from the gastrointestinal tract and is metabolized by the liver. Its metabolites are excreted by the kidneys. The drug produces typical anticholinergic adverse reactions. Its use is limited because of the auditory and visual hallucinations, confusion, and disorientation that occur in 0.5% of patients. These adverse reactions occur within the first 3 days of therapy and usually disappear within 3 days after the therapy is discontinued. USUAL ADULT DOSAGE: 25 to 50 mg P.O. q 4 hours.

dronabinol (Marinol). A Schedule II drug, dronabinol is the synthetic equivalent of the isomer of delta-9-tetrahydrocannabinol (THC), the principal psychoactive component in marijuana. Dronabinol is indicated for the nausea and vomiting from cancer chemotherapy in patients who do not adequately respond to conventional antiemetics. Although its use is controversial, dronabinol appears to be an effective antiemetic in cancer chemotherapy. After oral administration, dronabinol is extensively metabolized on its first pass through the liver.

Facts about scopolamine patches

Apply the transdermal scopolamine patch behind the ear. For optimal effect, apply the patch at least 4 hours before the need for its antiemetic action. Remove the patch after it is no longer needed or after 72 hours.

Why the transdermal route for motion sickness?
• The nerve fibers in the inner ear's vestibular apparatus help people maintain balance. But for some, motion increases the activity of these fibers, causing dizziness, nausea, and vomiting. The transdermal scopolamine patch helps reduce the activity of these inner ear fibers.
• The patch releases minute amounts of scopolamine that permeate the intact skin at a programmed rate, minimizing adverse reactions. Scopolamine is directly absorbed into the bloodstream, quickly achieving and maintaining an optimal dose for up to 72 hours. That prevents the nausea and vomiting of motion sickness.

• The patch is a flexible, adhesive disk of four layers, as shown in the illustration.
• The priming dose of scopolamine rapidly achieves the required steady-state blood level. Over the 3-day lifetime of the patch, the drug is delivered at a nearly constant rate.
• The drug passes by diffusion through the membrane from the higher concentration inside the patch's reservoir to the lower concentration outside the reservoir.
• The amount of drug delivered through diffusion is regulated by the membrane thickness, surface area and composition of the patch, and the drug concentration on each side of the membrane.

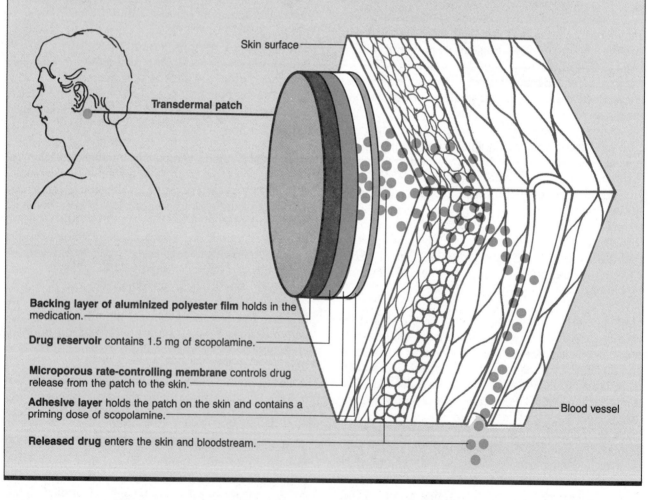

Skin surface

Transdermal patch

Backing layer of aluminized polyester film holds in the medication.

Drug reservoir contains 1.5 mg of scopolamine.

Microporous rate-controlling membrane controls drug release from the patch to the skin.

Adhesive layer holds the patch on the skin and contains a priming dose of scopolamine.

Released drug enters the skin and bloodstream.

Blood vessel

Some of the metabolites are also psychoactive. Serum concentration levels peak within 3 hours after the oral dose, and excretion occurs primarily through the feces. USUAL ADULT DOSAGE: 5 to 7 mg/m² P.O. q 3 to 4 hours beginning 4 hours before chemotherapy and con-

tinuing for 8 to 24 hours after chemotherapy. Dronabinol can accumulate in the body, and the patient can develop tolerance or physical and psychological dependence. The most prominent potential adverse reactions occur in the CNS and include mood changes (euphoria, panic, and paranoia), loss of memory, sleep disturbances, hallucinations, alterations of time perception, and poor impulse control. The nurse should advise patients not to drive or participate in any activity requiring mental alertness. Furthermore, a responsible adult should monitor the patient taking the drug.

nabilone (Cesamet). A Schedule II drug, nabilone is another synthetic derivative of THC and is used to treat nausea and vomiting from cancer chemotherapy when conventional antiemetics are ineffective.

USUAL ADULT DOSAGE: 1 to 2 mg P.O. every 6 to 12 hours. Maximum daily dose is 6 mg t.i.d. The nurse should administer the first dose 1 to 3 hours before chemotherapy.

Psychological changes (euphoria, anxiety, inability to concentrate, hallucinations, disorientation, and depression) may occur during treatment and for 48 to 72

SELECTED MAJOR DRUGS
Emetic and antiemetic agents

The following chart summarizes the major emetic and antiemetic drugs discussed in this chapter. Physicians currently use all of these drugs in the clinical setting; however, the differences in the indications, dosages, and nursing implications may affect drug selection by the physician.

DRUG	MAJOR INDICATIONS	USUAL ADULT DOSAGES	NURSING IMPLICATIONS
Emetic			
ipecac syrup	Emesis of ingested poisons	15 to 30 ml P.O. followed by 200 to 300 ml of water; dose may be repeated in 30 minutes if vomiting is not induced	• Drug is contraindicated in semicomatose or unconscious patients, or those with severe inebriation, convulsions, shock, or loss of gag reflex. • Drug is contraindicated in poisonings with petroleum distillates and caustic substances. • Administer only ipecac syrup, not fluid extract.
Antihistamine antiemetics			
dimenhydrinate	To prevent motion sickness and to prevent and treat nausea from vestibular disturbances	50 to 100 mg P.O. q 4 to 6 hr for motion sickness	• Administer with caution to patients with seizure disorders, narrow-angle glaucoma, or prostatic hypertrophy. • Undiluted injectable solution is irritating and may cause sclerosis; dilute in 10 ml of normal saline solution and infuse over 10 minutes for I.V. administration. • Inform the patient of the sedative effects; advise the patient not to drive or participate in activities that require mental alertness. • Parenteral preparation is incompatible when mixed with many solutions.
meclizine	To prevent motion sickness	25 to 50 mg P.O. daily at least 1 hour before travel	• Inform the patient of the sedative effects; advise the patient not to drive or participate in activities that require mental alertness.
trimethobenzamide	To prevent and treat mild to moderate nausea and vomiting	250 mg P.O. t.i.d. to q.i.d. or 200 mg I.M. or rectally t.i.d. to q.i.d.	• Administer cautiously in the treatment of vomiting in children; the use of centrally acting antiemetics in children with viral illnesses has been associated with an increased risk for developing Reye's syndrome. • Inform the patient of the sedative effects; advise the patient not to drive or participate in activities that require mental alertness.

continued

Emetic and antiemetic agents continued

DRUG	MAJOR INDICATIONS	USUAL ADULT DOSAGES	NURSING IMPLICATIONS
Phenothiazine antiemetics			
prochlorperazine	To prevent and treat severe nausea and vomiting of various etiologies	5 to 10 mg P.O. or I.M. t.i.d. or q.i.d.; or 25 mg rectally b.i.d.	• Elderly patients may be more susceptible to hypotension and neuromuscular reactions; observe closely and administer lower doses as prescribed. • Children may be more prone to extrapyramidal reactions; administer lowest possible dose. • Drug is contraindicated in patients with phenothiazine hypersensitivity, coma from any cause, CNS depression, bone marrow depression, brain damage, or in pediatric surgery. • Administer with caution to patients with hepatic disease, cardiovascular disease, exposure to extreme heat or cold, respiratory disorders, hypocalcemia, convulsive disorders, severe reactions to insulin or electroshock therapy, suspected brain tumors, intestinal obstruction, glaucoma, or prostatic hypertrophy, and to elderly or debilitated patients. • Avoid skin contact with oral solutions and injections because dermatitis can occur in rare instances. • Dilute oral concentrate before administration. • Inform the patient about sedative effects and precautions to take to avoid photosensitivity. • Do not administer subcutaneously or interarterially.
promethazine	To prevent and treat severe nausea and vomiting	12.5 to 25 mg P.O., I.M., or rectally every 4 to 6 hours	• Same implications listed for prochloroperazine.

hours afterward. Other adverse reactions include drowsiness, vertigo, ataxia, headache, visual disturbances, parasthesias, orthostatic hypotension, tachycardia, dry mouth, and increased appetite. The nurse should not administer nabilone with any other CNS depressant and should administer the drug cautiously to elderly patients and those with cardiovascular disease. The nurse should supervise all patients on nabilone therapy and advise them not to drive or engage in any activity that requires sound judgment and unimpaired coordination.

CHAPTER SUMMARY

Chapter 49 discussed the pharmacokinetics, pharmacodynamics, and pharmacotherapeutics of emetics and antiemetics, as well as their adverse reactions and the nursing implications associated with these drugs. Here are the highlights of the chapter:
• The emetics form the basis for the treatment of poisoning by ingestion. Drug-induced emesis removes the toxic substance from the stomach, thus preventing its absorption.
• Ipecac syrup has become the emetic of choice because of its effectiveness in evacuating the stomach and its relatively low incidence of adverse reactions. The American Academy of Pediatrics recommends that all homes with small children keep ipecac syrup on hand for the

emergency treatment of poisonings. When ipecac syrup is obtained, the nurse should teach safe home use of the drug and tell the parent to contact a physician before any use of the drug.

• The three basic groups of antiemetics include the antihistamines, the phenothiazines, and others, such as scopolamine. Some antiemetics control the nausea and vomiting from disturbances of the inner ear; others control generalized nausea and vomiting that arise from other causes.

• The antihistamine antiemetics and scopolamine are frequently used to prevent motion sickness; however, these drugs are not usually effective after the nausea has begun.

• Antihistamine antiemetics and scopolamine are also used to treat the vertigo from disturbances of vestibular function. The symptomatic relief provided by these drugs for the vertigo of labyrinthitis or Meniere's disease varies among patients.

• The most pronounced adverse reactions from antihistamine antiemetics and scopolamine include drowsiness and anticholinergic effects.

• Physicians usually treat generalized nausea and vomiting with phenothiazine antiemetics. Generalized nausea and vomiting, usually mediated through the CTZ of the medulla, may have various causes, including cancer chemotherapy and radiotherapy, infections, anesthesia and surgery, and drugs such as narcotics. Some beneficial therapies may be refused by the patient if nausea and vomiting are not prevented. Also, further complications can result if the vomiting is not treated.

• The adverse reactions associated with phenothiazines resemble those of the antihistamines and include sedation and anticholinergic effects. Phenothiazine antiemetics also produce hypotension that may be additive to that of the anesthetics.

• Benzquinamide does not produce hypotensive effects, which sometimes makes its use preferable in postoperative conditions.

• Metoclopramide effectively prevents or treats motion sickness and cancer chemotherapy–induced nausea and vomiting. Dronabinol and nabilone, both THC derivatives, represent nontraditional approaches to treating nausea caused by cancer chemotherapy.

BIBLIOGRAPHY

Albibi, R., and McCallum, R.W. "Metoclopramide: Pharmacology and Clinical Application," *Annals of Internal Medicine* 98:86, January 1983.

American Hospital Formulary Service. *Drug Information '86.* Edited by McEvoy, G.K., et al. Bethesda, Md.: American Society of Hospital Pharmacists, 1986.

Baldessarini, R.J. "Drugs and the Treatment of Psychiatric Disorders," in *Goodman and Gilman's The Pharmacological Basis of Therapeutics,* 7th ed. New York: Macmillan Publishing Co., 1985.

Carey, M.P., et al. "Delta-9-tetrahydrocannabinol in Cancer Therapy: Research Problems and Issues," *Annals of Internal Medicine* 99:106, July 1983.

Chaffee-Bahamon, C., et al. "Risk Assessments of Ipecac in the Home," *Pediatrics* 75:1105, June 1985.

Dipalma, J.R. "Drugs for Nausea and Vomiting of Pregnancy," *American Family Practice* 28:272, October 1983.

Douglas, W.W. "Histamine and 5-Hydroxytryptamine (Serotonin) and Their Antagonists," in *Goodman and Gilman's The Pharmacological Basis of Therapeutics,* 7th ed. New York: Macmillan Publishing Co., 1985.

Fortner, C.I., et al. "Combination Antiemetic Therapy in the Control of Chemotherapy-Induced Emesis," *Drug Intelligence and Clinical Pharmacy* 19:21, January 1985.

Gralla, R.J. "Metoclopramide: A Review of Antiemetic Trials," *Drugs* 25:63, February 1983.

Isselbacher, K.J. "Anorexia, Nausea and Vomiting," in *Harrison's Principles of Internal Medicine,* 10th ed. New York: McGraw-Hill Book Co., 1983.

Johnson, P.E. "Nausea and Vomiting," in *Applied Therapeutics: The Clinical Use of Drugs,* 3rd ed. San Francisco: Applied Therapeutics, Inc., 1983.

Laszlo, J. *Antiemetics and Cancer Chemotherapy.* Baltimore: Williams & Wilkins Co., 1983.

Laszlo, J. "Selecting an Antiemetic for the Individual Patient," *Drugs* 25:81, February 1983.

Lipscomb, J.W., et al. "Response in Children to 15-ml or 30-ml Doses of Ipecac Syrup," *Clinical Pharmacy* 5:234, March 1986.

Mofensan, H.C., and Carauccio, T.R. "Benefits/Risks of Syrup of Ipecac," *Pediatrics* 77:551, April 1986.

Stoudemire, A., et al. "Recent Advances in the Pharmacologic and Behavioral Management of Chemotherapy-Induced Emesis," *Archives of Internal Medicine* 144:1029, May 1984.

Toriozzi, P., and Laszlo, J. "Nausea & Vomiting," in *Conn's Current Therapy.* Edited by Rakel, R.E. Philadelphia: W.B. Saunders Co., 1986.

CHAPTER 50

PEPTIC ULCER AGENTS

OBJECTIVES

After reading and studying this chapter, you should be able to:

1. Explain the physiologic processes of peptic ulcer formation, concentrating on the role played by acetylcholine, gastrin, and histamine.

2. Differentiate among the ways in which antacids, histamine$_2$ (H$_2$)-receptor antagonists, and sucralfate decrease peptic ulcer formation.

3. Describe the mechanism of action of antacids.

4. Explain why patients are often not compliant when taking antacids.

5. Describe the mechanism of action of H$_2$-receptor antagonists.

6. Discuss why the H$_2$-receptor antagonists are the treatment of choice for both duodenal and gastric ulcers.

7. Identify the major clinical indications for both oral and parenteral H$_2$-receptor antagonists.

8. Explain the mechanism of action of sucralfate in promoting the healing of duodenal ulcers.

INTRODUCTION

A peptic ulcer is an open lesion of the epithelial, mucosal membranes of the lower esophagus, stomach, or duodenum. Between 5% and 10% of the U.S. population can expect to experience peptic ulcers; 3 to 4 million cases of active peptic ulcers occur each year. Several factors may contribute to the development of peptic ulcer disease, including smoking and the use of aspirin, nonsteroidal anti-inflammatory drugs (NSAIDs), or corticosteroids. Although stress and the consumption of coffee and alcohol are associated with peptic ulcer disease, health care professionals continue to debate the effect of these factors on peptic ulcer development.

Most experts believe that an imbalance between the damaging effects of acid and pepsin and the normal or decreased gastrointestinal (GI) tract defense mechanisms is the underlying cause of peptic ulcers. This imbalance damages the mucosal membranes and protective mechanisms. Some ulcers develop when in-

creased acid secretions overcome the protective mechanisms of the GI tract, while other ulcers develop from an impairment of these protective mechanisms. The combination of these two etiologies accounts for the development of peptic ulcers.

The rate of pepsin secretion is usually directly proportional to the rate of acid secretion, and many patients with duodenal ulcers display a hypersecretion of both acid and pepsin. Several factors contribute to the hypersecretion of acid and pepsin. An increased cell mass of the parietal and chief cells, which are the secretory cells of the stomach, leads to higher-than-normal acid and pepsin output. Cholinergic stimulation via the vagus nerve and gastrin release in the postprandial state enhance gastric acid response. The hormones gastrin, histamine, and acetylcholine stimulate acid secretion from the parietal cells and pepsin secretion from the chief cells. Furthermore, acid secretion from food stimulation increases, partially in response to an impaired feedback mechanism that permits gastrin release and partially in response to an increased sensitivity of the parietal cells to gastrin and possibly histamine.

The timing of acid hypersecretion is also important. Researchers have found nocturnal acid secretion to be higher in some individuals. Because the nocturnal acid may be unopposed by food in the stomach, an ulcer can result. Nocturnal acid secretion can also inhibit ulcer therapy.

Nonetheless, not all patients with duodenal ulcers have hypersecretion of acid and pepsin. Some duodenal ulcers and most gastric ulcers are caused by a breakdown in the mucosal resistance to the effects of acid, pepsin, and other stomach contents. The gastric mucosal barrier is a complex defense system that allows hydrochloric acid to diffuse into the lumen of the stomach but prevents the return of such acid, thereby protecting the gastric mucosa from digesting itself. (See *Mucosal defense*

Mucosal defense mechanisms

Acetylcholine, gastrin, and histamine stimulate the release of hydrochloric acid from the parietal cells.

Acetylcholine is released after cholinergic stimulation from vagal fibers or from local neurons after distention of the stomach resulting from the ingestion of food. The released acetylcholine increases gastric acid directly by stimulating acid secretion and indirectly by sensitizing the parietal cells to the effects of gastrin and histamine and stimulating the release of gastrin. These effects can be decreased by blocking the cholinergic receptor with an anticholinergic such as atropine.

Gastrin is the most potent stimulant of gastric acid secretion. It is stored in the G cells, which are interspersed among the other epithelial cells of the stom-

ach. Gastrin also stimulates pepsin secretion and GI motility, promotes closure of the esophageal sphincter, and stimulates hepatic bile flow and pancreatic secretions. Some researchers think that blocking the action of gastrin may serve as the goal for developing future antiulcer drugs.

Histamine in body tissues mediates many reactions, including allergic ones. Histamine is secreted by the gastric mucosa to stimulate the release of acid. However, the histamine receptors in the GI tract are not blocked by the typical antihistamine drugs. The GI tract receptors, the histamine$_2$ (H$_2$) receptors, are blocked only by the H$_2$-receptor antagonists, drugs that represent a major advance in treating peptic ulcer disease.

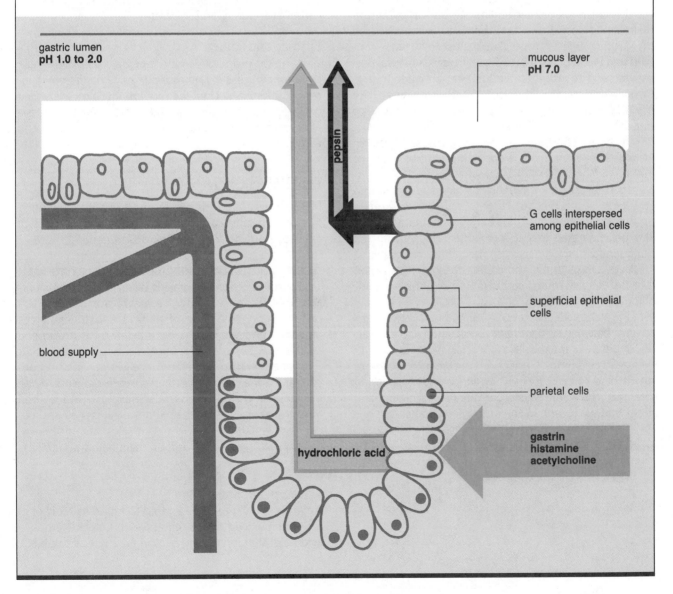

gastric lumen
pH 1.0 to 2.0

mucous layer
pH 7.0

pepsin

G cells interspersed among epithelial cells

superficial epithelial cells

blood supply

parietal cells

hydrochloric acid

**gastrin
histamine
acetylcholine**

mechanisms on page 783 for the details of this protective system.) This protective response is referred to as cytoprotection. Cytoprotective drugs prevent mucosal damage and enhance the protective effect. Factors important to mucosal protection include mucous secretion, bicarbonate secretion, mucosal perfusion, and cellular repair.

In opposition to the parietal cells and chief cells, which secrete acid and pepsin, other epithelial cells in the stomach secrete mucus and bicarbonate. Brunner's glands and surface epithelial cells in the duodenum also secrete mucus and bicarbonate. The mucous secretion provides a protective layer along the walls of the stomach and duodenum. The bicarbonate secretion maintains the pH of the mucous layer at about 7.0, which protects the stomach from the acidic pH of 1.0 to 2.0 found in the gastric lumen. The mucous barrier also protects against pepsin and other injurious agents.

Endogenous prostaglandins are also important in maintaining normal mucosal defenses. Synthesized by the gastric mucosa, prostaglandins act to increase mucous and bicarbonate secretion, to increase mucosal perfusion, and to enhance cellular repair after injury. Prostaglandins are, therefore, cytoprotective. The NSAIDs and aspirin may cause damage to the gastric mucosa because they inhibit prostaglandin synthesis.

If the mucosal defense system is impaired, peptic ulcer disease may occur. Pepsin, mechanical forces of the stomach, or other substances may increasingly damage the mucous layer. Hypersecretory states may thin and damage the mucous layer. Mucus or bicarbonate production may decline, thus thinning the mucous layer and presenting an inadequate buffer. The quality but not quantity of mucus may become abnormal, resulting in ulcers. Drugs that could correct these defects in the mucosal defense mechanisms would be important additions to peptic ulcer treatment.

Physicians direct peptic ulcer therapy at the imbalance between acid and pepsin secretion and the mucosal defense mechanisms. Peptic ulcer drugs (1) neutralize acid in the GI tract, (2) reduce acid secretion, or (3) bind to the ulcer, protecting it and neutralizing local acid. Researchers are currently investigating new drugs that act by enhancing mucosal resistance to acid.

For a summary of representative drugs, see *Selected Major Drugs: Peptic ulcer agents* on page 793.

ANTACIDS

The antacids, which are over-the-counter (OTC) medications, are used extensively both alone and in combination with other drugs to treat peptic ulcer disease. The subject of extensive advertising, antacids are sometimes used indiscriminately by the public for a wide variety of conditions.

Antacids are compounds that consist of a metallic cation (positively charged molecule) and a basic anion (negatively charged molecule). Frequently occuring cations are aluminum, magnesium, and calcium. The basic anion neutralizes acid, thereby producing the therapeutic effect of the antacid. Hydroxide is the most frequently employed anion; other anions include carbonate, bicarbonate, citrate, and trisilicate.

History and source

The antacid properties of the inorganic salts carbonate, bicarbonate, citrate, and trisilicate have been known for over 2,000 years. Until the modern era, however, their use was mainly empirical and subjective. Today, the effect and proper use of the antacids is well-known and respected.

PHARMACOKINETICS

Most modern antacids are formulated with aluminum, magnesium, and calcium cations. The effectiveness of antacids does not require their absorption.

Absorption, distribution, metabolism, excretion

The onset of action of antacids takes place in the stomach. Absorption is neither necessary nor desired. Depending upon the type of antacid and the patient's physical condition, problems may result if absorption takes place. For example, hypermagnesemia can occur if a patient with renal failure receives an antacid containing magnesium. Hypermagnesemia develops when the kidneys do not excrete the magnesium absorbed from the antacid. Acid-base abnormalities may also occur with antacid absorption. Antacids are distributed throughout the GI tract and are eliminated primarily in the feces.

Onset, peak, duration

Antacids usually provide a rapid to immediate onset of action. However, the speed at which antacids produce acid neutralization depends upon their rate of solubility.

Selected antacids

The nurse administering antacids should be familiar with the ingredients of some frequently used antacids, their sodium content, and their acid-neutralizing effect.

PRODUCT	INGREDIENTS	SODIUM CONTENT mg/5 ml	ACID NEUTRALIZING CAPACITY (mEq/5 ml)
ALternaGel	aluminum hydroxide	2.5	16
Gaviscon	magnesium carbonate; sodium alginate	13	1
Gelusil	magnesium and aluminum hydroxides, simethicone	0.7	12
Gelusil—II	magnesium and aluminum hydroxides, simethicone	1.3	24
Maalox	magnesium and aluminum hydroxides	1.4	13.3
Maalox Plus	magnesium and aluminum hydroxides, simethicone	1.2	13.3
Mylanta	magnesium and aluminum hydroxides, simethicone	0.68	12.7
Mylanta—II	magnesium and aluminum hydroxides, simethicone	1.141	25.4
Riopan	magaldrate (aluminum-magnesium complex)	0.1	15
Riopan Plus	magaldrate (magnesium-aluminum complex)	0.1	15
Titralac	calcium carbonate	11	19

Sodium bicarbonate is the most rapidly solubilized antacid, but is no longer recommended because of its high sodium content. Magnesium hydroxide is the second most rapidly solubilized antacid, followed by magnesium carbonate, calcium carbonate, and aluminum hydroxide. Because magnesium trisilicate is the least-soluble antacid, health care professionals question its usefulness.

The duration of action for antacids taken on an empty stomach is about 1 hour. Duration increases to 3 hours for antacids taken after a meal because food delays the gastric emptying time, which allows the antacid more time in the stomach to neutralize acid. Because of the short duration of action, frequent dosings of antacids are needed.

PHARMACODYNAMICS

The acid-neutralizing action of antacids reduces the total acid load in the GI tract, which allows peptic ulcers to heal. Because pepsin acts more effectively in an acid medium, antacids also reduce its activity. Antacids do not coat the lining of peptic ulcers or the GI tract.

Mechanism of action

The anions of an antacid combine with the acidic hydrogen cations secreted by the stomach to form water, thereby increasing the pH of the stomach contents. Antacids do not neutralize all the stomach acid and generally do not increase the pH above 4.0 or 5.0. By increasing gastric pH from the normal 1.3 to 2.3, an antacid neutralizes about 90% of the gastric acid. By increasing the pH further to 3.3, the antacid neutralizes 99% of the gastric acid. This change in pH also affects the activity of pepsin. Pepsin activity is greatest at a pH of 1.5 to 2.5. By increasing the pH, the antacid decreases proteolytic activity, which becomes minimal at a pH above 4.0.

Increasing the pH and decreasing the pepsin activity provide symptomatic relief from peptic ulcer disease and, if adequately maintained, facilitate healing. Neither the amount nor the duration of neutralization for the optimal healing of peptic ulcer disease is known; however, most clinicians recommend that the pH be maintained at 3.0 to 3.5 throughout each 24-hour period. For this reason, regular, rather than p.r.n., doses of the antacid are needed in the treatment of peptic ulcer disease.

DRUG INTERACTIONS
Antacids

The nurse should be aware of the following drug interactions involving antacids, the possible effects of the interactions, and the administration implications.

DRUG	INTERACTING DRUGS	POSSIBLE EFFECTS	NURSING IMPLICATIONS
antacids	digoxin, indomethacin, iron salts, tetracyclines	Decrease rate or extent of absorption by GI binding	• Do not administer the drugs within 1 hour of each other. • Monitor the patient for decreased therapeutic effects of the medication. • Monitor the patient's serum drug levels of digoxin.
	amphetamines, quinidine	Increase urine pH; decrease excretion of weakly basic drugs	• Do not administer the drugs within 1 hour of each other. • Monitor the patient for increased therapeutic effects of the medications. • Monitor the patient's serum quinidine levels.
	salicylates	Increase urine pH; increase excretion of weakly acidic drugs	• Do not administer the drugs within 1 hour of each other. • Monitor the patient for decreased salicylate effects or decreased serum salicylate levels.

PHARMACOTHERAPEUTICS

Physicians use antacids, either alone or combined with other drugs, primarily to relieve pain and promote healing in peptic ulcer disease. Antacids are also used for the relief of esophageal reflux, acid indigestion, heartburn, and dyspepsia. Antacids are used prophylactically during times of severe physical stress in critically ill patients to prevent stress ulcers and GI bleeding. Physicians prescribe aluminum hydroxide antacids to control hyperphosphatemia in renal failure because the aluminum cation binds with phosphate in the GI tract, thus preventing phosphate absorption.

Antacids appear to effectively treat both gastric and duodenal ulcers. When used alone in large doses over 4 weeks of treatment, they are as effective as any other therapy for peptic ulcer disease. They may also be used with histamine$_2$-receptor antagonists to help control or prevent pain.

Antacids are often used in combination with simethicone, a drug with antiflatuent properties; however, physicians do not usually use this combination to treat peptic ulcer disease unless concurrent symptoms require both effects. The combination of aluminum hydroxide and magnesium hydroxide is often used because one drug tends to offset the adverse effect of the other; that is, the aluminum hydroxide is constipating and the magnesium hydroxide has a laxative effect.

Antacids cause frequent and sometimes serious adverse effects. Patient acceptance and compliance may be lower than with other peptic ulcer medications because the patient must take the antacid frequently and use the liquid form. Palatability of the antacid also adversely affects compliance. For these reasons, antacids are no longer the first choice to treat peptic ulcer disease.

Not all antacids neutralize a given amount of gastric acid to the same extent. The physician must take into consideration the known *in vivo* neutralizing capacity for each antacid when calculating the dose of a specific antacid. Calcium carbonate antacids provide the most acid-neutralizing capacity, followed by those containing magnesium salts and aluminum salts.

In most cases, the adult doses of an antacid should neutralize more than 1,000 mEq of acid daily. The large amount needed to accomplish this goal is administered in divided doses. A dose is given 1 hour after each meal, and again 3 hours after each meal, and at bedtime. The regimen requires seven doses. For example, using Mylanta-II, a dose of 30 ml would be given for each of these seven doses. The 30-ml dose is the usual dose for the concentrated forms of antacids, and a 60-ml dose is usual for the unconcentrated forms. The treatments continue from 4 to 6 weeks for duodenal ulcers and until healing is complete for gastric ulcers.

magnesium hydroxide and aluminum hydroxide with simethicone (Maalox TC, Mylanta-II, Gelusil-II). These drugs represent concentrated antacids.
USUAL ADULT DOSAGE: 10 to 30 ml P.O. 1 hour and 3 hours after each meal and h.s.

magaldrate or aluminum-magnesium complex (Riopan, Riopan Plus). This antacid comes as a suspension, tablet, and chewable tablet.
USUAL ADULT DOSAGE: 540 to 1080 mg (5 to 10 ml) of the suspension P.O. with water between meals and h.s., or 480 to 960 mg or 1 to 2 tablets P.O. with water between meals and h.s., or 480 to 960 mg or 1 to 2 chewable tablets chewed before swallowing between meals and h.s.

calcium carbonate (Alka-Mints, Calcilac, Dicarbosil, Tums). This antacid is available as a suspension or chewable tablet.
USUAL ADULT DOSAGE: 1-gram tablet 4 to 6 times daily, chewed well and taken with water, or 1-gram suspension (5 ml of most products) 1 hour after meals and h.s. (See *Selected antacids* on page 786 for information on some other frequently used antacids.)

Drug interactions
All antacids can interfere with the absorption of concomitantly administered oral drugs by either binding with them or changing the GI transit time. Antacids also increase urine pH, which in turn increases the excretion of weakly acidic drugs and decreases the excretion of weakly basic drugs. However, aluminum and magnesium antacids do not affect urine pH. (See *Drug Interactions: Antacids* for a list of interacting drugs and possible effects.)

ADVERSE DRUG REACTIONS
The most common adverse reactions involving antacids occur in the GI tract.

Predictable reactions
Diarrhea and constipation frequently result from long-term antacid use. Aluminum hydroxide is particularly constipating. Constipation can be severe, and, if accompanied by dehydration or fluid restriction, may lead to intestinal obstruction. Hemorrhoids, rectal fissures, and fecal impaction may occur from hard stools. Conversely, magnesium-containing antacids provide a laxative effect and with frequent use can produce diarrhea and electrolyte abnormalities. Physicians most often prescribe aluminum hydroxide and magnesium-containing antacids in combination, which usually produces a mild laxative effect.

Most antacid products have been recently reformulated to decrease their sodium content. Furthermore, all antacids that contain more than 0.2 mEq of sodium per dose must be labeled with the amount. Patients on a sodium restriction because of hypertension, congestive heart failure, renal failure, or other conditions should pay particular attention to the sodium content of antacids. Some antacids may also possess a high potassium load, so patients on a potassium restriction should note the product label.

When used in patients with renal failure, aluminum-containing antacids may produce a hyperaluminemia state, in which aluminum accumulates in bones, lungs, and nerve tissue. Osteomalacia and dementia may occur. Hypophosphatemia, with anorexia, malaise, and muscle weakness, may also occur from prolonged administration of aluminum-containing antacids.

Hypermagnesemia characterized by hypotension, nausea, vomiting, electrocardiogram (EKG) changes, respiratory or mental depression, and coma has occurred in patients with renal failure taking magnesium-containing antacids.

Most physicians do not recommend calcium-containing antacids to treat peptic ulcer disease, but do recommend such antacids for short-term therapy for other GI conditions. When calcium carbonate is used, a hypersecretion of gastric acid and an acid rebound occur. Calcium carbonate may also cause the milk-alkali syndrome characterized by hypercalcemia, metabolic alkalosis, and renal impairment.

Unpredictable reactions
All adverse reactions involving antacids are dose related and predictable. No unpredictable reactions occur.

NURSING IMPLICATIONS
The antacids are nonprescription medications frequently used by the public. In ascertaining their use by a patient, the nurse must obtain a comprehensive drug history. The nurse should also be aware of the following implications:
• Magnesium-containing antacids are contraindicated in patients with severe renal disease; hypermagnesemia can result.
• Calcium-containing antacids are contraindicated in severe renal disease; hypercalcemia can result with prolonged therapy.
• Do not administer calcium carbonate for long-term therapy of peptic ulcer disease because gastric hypersecretion and acid rebound may occur.
• Use caution when giving magnesium-containing antacids to elderly patients and to patients with mild renal

impairment; hypermagnesemia and fluid and electrolyte imbalances may occur.
- Administer calcium- and aluminum-containing antacids cautiously to elderly patients, especially those with decreased bowel motility (those receiving antidiarrheals, antispasmodics, or anticholinergics), dehydration, fluid restriction, chronic renal disease, and suspected intestinal obstruction because severe constipation and fecal impaction can result.
- Shake suspensions well and give with a small amount of water.
- Have the patient thoroughly chew antacid tablets before swallowing, then have the patient drink 6 to 8 ounces of water.
- Because antacids impair the absorption of many other drugs, do not give other oral medications within 1 to 2 hours of antacid administration.
- Because antacids may cause enteric-coated drugs to be released prematurely in the stomach, separate the administration of antacids and enteric-coated drugs by 1 hour.
- Consider having the patient sample various antacids to determine individual taste preferences.
- Explain to the patient that antacid therapy may make stools appear speckled or whitish in color.

HISTAMINE$_2$-RECEPTOR ANTAGONISTS

The histamine$_2$ (H$_2$)-receptor antagonists, used to treat both duodenal and gastric ulcers, are the most frequently prescribed antiulcer drugs in the United States. The H$_2$-receptor antagonists act by blocking the histamine-receptor sites on the parietal cells of the stomach. These drugs inhibit not only histamine-stimulated acid secretion, but also basal-, postprandial-, and gastrin-stimulated acid secretion. The H$_2$-receptor antagonists available in the United States include cimetidine, ranitidine, and famotidine.

History and source
The concept of histamine-stimulated acid secretion in the parietal cells was first described by Ash and Schild in 1966. In 1972, Black and his colleagues described the first H$_2$-receptor antagonist. These investigations led to the development of cimetidine in 1975 and ranitidine several years later. Famotidine was discovered in Japan and introduced into the United States in late 1986.

PHARMACOKINETICS
Cimetidine, ranitidine, and famotidine share a somewhat similar pharmacokinetic profile.

Absorption, distribution, metabolism, excretion
Both cimetidine and ranitidine are rapidly and completely absorbed from the GI tract, while famotidine is incompletely absorbed. Food and antacids may impair the absorption of H$_2$-receptor antagonists. All three H$_2$-receptor antagonists undergo hepatic first-pass metabolism, with cimetidine displaying a bioavailability of 65% to 80%, ranitidine 40% to 90%, and famotidine 40%. These drugs are widely distributed throughout the body, though ranitidine is minimally distributed into the central nervous system (CNS). The extent to which famotidine is distributed into the CNS is unknown. All three H$_2$-receptor antagonists are only mildly protein bound (approximately 20%).

Cimetidine and ranitidine are metabolized by the liver, but over 50% of each drug is excreted unchanged in the urine. Famotidine is also metabolized by the liver, with over 70% of the dose being excreted unchanged in the urine. The bioavailability is increased and the half-life for cimetidine and ranitidine is slightly prolonged in patients with liver disease. The effects of liver dysfunction on famotidine half-life are unknown. A decrease in renal function will also prolong the half-lives of the H$_2$-receptor antagonists.

Onset, peak, duration
Cimetidine and ranitidine reach peak concentration levels in about 1 to 2 hours, while famotidine attains a peak concentration level in 1 to 3½ hours. The half-life of cimetidine is about 2 hours, while that of ranitidine is 2 to 3 hours and famotidine is 2½ to 4 hours. Ranitidine and famotidine, which are more potent than cimetidine and are administered at lower doses, remain effective longer.

PHARMACODYNAMICS
The H$_2$-receptor antagonists block the stimulant action of histamine on the acid-secreting parietal cells of the stomach. Ranitidine is 4 to 10 times more potent in suppressing histamine-induced acid secretion than cimetidine, and famotidine is 20 times more potent than cimetidine.

Mechanism of action
Because the chemical structure of cimetidine resembles that of histamine, the drug readily binds with H$_2$ receptors on the parietal cells as well as with other histamine receptor sites throughout the body, including those lo-

DRUG INTERACTIONS

H₂-receptor antagonists

The following chart contains information about drug interactions involving H₂-receptor antagonists, the possible effects from the interactions, and important nursing implications.

DRUG	INTERACTING DRUGS	POSSIBLE EFFECTS	NURSING IMPLICATIONS
cimetidine, ranitidine	antacids	Inhibit cimetidine and ranitidine absorption	• Do not administer within 1 hour of one another. • Monitor the patient for decreased therapeutic effects.
cimetidine	coumarin anticoagulants, propranolol, labetalol, possibly other beta-blockers, benzodiazepines, tricyclic antidepressants, theophylline, procainamide, quinidine, lidocaine, phenytoin	Inhibit hepatic enzyme metabolism of these drugs, thereby increasing their levels and effects	• Avoid concurrent administration if possible. • Monitor the patient for increased sedation from the benzodiazepines. Oxazepam, lorazepam, and temazepam are eliminated differently and are not affected by cimetidine. • Monitor the patient for drug toxicity. • Monitor the patient's serum levels of procainamide, phenytoin, quinidine, and lidocaine.
	carmustine (BCNU)	Increases bone marrow toxicity	• Monitor the patient's blood cell counts carefully if concurrent use is necessary.
	ethyl alcohol	Increases alcohol absorption and decreases metabolism	• Caution the patient about the risk of increased alcohol effects.

cated in androgen receptors, the hepatic oxidase system, and peripheral lymphocytes. The chemical structures of famotidine and ranitidine differ from the structure of histamine, but both famotidine and ranitidine bind competitively to the H₂ receptors. Unlike cimetidine, famotidine and ranitidine are specific and do not bind to other receptor sites. The specific binding may explain why ranitidine does not produce some of the serious adverse reactions of cimetidine.

Acid secretion by the stomach depends on the binding of gastrin, acetylcholine, and histamine to their respective receptors on the parietal cells. If the binding of any one of these hormones becomes blocked, a reduction in acid secretion occurs. Thus, by binding with H₂ receptors, the H₂-receptor antagonists reduce acid secretion. A cimetidine dose of 300 mg reduces basal acid output by 90% and reduces meal-stimulated acid secretion by 66%. The usual 150-mg dose of ranitidine twice daily reduces gastric acid by 70%. Cimetidine, ranitidine, and famotidine suppress nocturnal acid secretion by approximately 90%.

PHARMACOTHERAPEUTICS

As the drugs of choice to treat peptic ulcers, the H₂-receptor antagonists promote the healing of both duodenal and gastric ulcers. These drugs are also used for long-term treatment of pathologic GI hypersecretory conditions, such as Zollinger-Ellison syndrome or hyperhistaminemia. Physicians prescribe the H₂-receptor antagonists to reduce the output of gastric acid and prevent stress ulcers in severely ill patients and in those with reflux esophagitis or upper GI bleeding. Antacids may be used with the H₂-receptor antagonists to control pain, but their addition does not appear to increase the ulcer healing.

While cimetidine, ranitidine, and famotidine appear to be equally effective in healing peptic ulcers, famotidine and ranitidine provide several advantages over cimetidine. The effects of famotidine and ranitidine last longer than those of cimetidine, and famotidine and ranitidine cause fewer adverse reactions and drug interactions.

The final daily dose of the H₂-receptor antagonists should be given at bedtime. While oral administration is usually as effective as parenteral administration, the parenteral route may be preferred for hospitalized patients with pathologic hypersecretory conditions, intract-

Monitoring for adverse reactions of H$_2$-receptor antagonists

The following should help the nurse assess and intervene while caring for a patient receiving H$_2$-receptor antagonists.

ADVERSE REACTIONS	SIGNS AND SYMPTOMS	INTERVENTIONS
Headache	General headache, at times severe	Administer mild analgesics as prescribed.
Blood dyscrasias	Easy bruising, more frequent infections, granulocytopenia, leukopenia, or thrombocytopenia	Consult the physician to discontinue the medication.
Mental status changes	Confusion, agitation, depression, hallucinations. Usually occurs in severely ill or elderly patients or patients with renal failure.	Consult the physician to substitute ranitidine for patients on cimetidine or to discontinue drug use; discontinue drug use with patients on ranitidine.
Anti-androgen effects	Gynecomastia, impotence	Consult the physician to discontinue the drug or bedtime dose. Ranitidine may not cause this effect.
Changes in blood chemistry	Small increases in serum creatinine without increases in blood urea nitrogen	Continue to monitor the patient's renal function.
	Increases in hepatic enzymes	Monitor the patient for hepatic toxicity, especially in high-dose I.V. therapy.

able ulcers, or an inability to take oral medication. To treat active gastric bleeding, an I.V. loading dose of the H$_2$-receptor antagonist followed by an I.V. infusion has been shown in experimental trials to be more effective than bolus injections.

cimetidine (Tagamet). This H$_2$-receptor antagonist is the least potent of the agents used to treat peptic ulcer disease.
USUAL ADULT DOSAGE: for active peptic ulcer disease, 800 mg P.O. daily h.s.; 300 mg I.V. every 6 to 8 hours. The parenteral dose may be increased to a maximum of 2.4 grams in 24 hours.

ranitidine (Zantac). Ranitidine is used primarily to treat peptic ulcer disease.
USUAL ADULT DOSAGE: for active peptic ulcer disease, 150 mg P.O. b.i.d., with the second dose h.s., or 300 mg P.O. daily h.s., or 50 mg I.V. or I.M. every 6 to 8 hours; dosage may be increased to 400 mg in 24 hours.

famotidine (Pepcid). This drug is the newest H$_2$-receptor antagonist on the market.
USUAL ADULT DOSAGE: for active peptic ulcer disease, 20 mg P.O. b.i.d. with the second dose h.s., or 40 mg P.O. daily h.s.; I.V., 20 mg every 12 hours; maintenance dose, 20 mg P.O. daily h.s.

Drug interactions

The concomitant administration of antacids and H$_2$-receptor antagonists may decrease the absorption of the H$_2$-receptor antagonists. To prevent any potential problems, the nurse should not administer the drugs within 1 hour of each other. Cimetidine partially inhibits the hepatic cytochrome P450 enzyme system and consequently decreases the clearance or prolongs the half-lives of drugs that are metabolized by this system. Famotidine and ranitidine do not produce this effect. (See *Drug Interactions: H$_2$-receptor antagonists* on page 789 for details about other interactions.)

ADVERSE DRUG REACTIONS

The histamine$_2$-receptor antagonists produce few adverse reactions, most of which are relatively minor.

Predictable reactions

Both cimetidine and ranitidine may produce headache, dizziness, malaise, myalgia, nausea, diarrhea or constipation, skin rashes, pruritus, loss of libido, and impotence. Cimetidine, however, is more likely to produce these adverse reactions. Cimetidine probably produces sexual dysfunction and gynecomastia through its binding to the androgen receptor. Substituting ranitidine or famotidine decreases these adverse reactions. Famotidine produces very few adverse reactions, with headache being the most frequent (about 2% of patients), followed by constipation or diarrhea and skin rash.

Reversible mental confusion, agitation, depression, and hallucinations can result. However, these reactions occur much more frequently in patients receiving cimetidine, especially in severely ill or elderly patients. The reactions, which are usually associated with a decrease in renal function, may also occur with overdose.

When given by rapid I.V. injection, H_2-receptor antagonists can produce profound bradycardia and other cardiotoxic effects. Pain at the injection site occasionally occurs.

Unpredictable reactions

The H_2-receptor antagonists rarely cause hypersensitivity reactions. Some patients develop increased hepatic enzyme levels, but this reaction is also rare. Cimetidine has been associated with hematologic adverse reactions, such as thrombocytopenia and granulocytopenia, and seizures if drug accumulation occurs. (See *Monitoring for adverse reactions of H_2-receptor antagonists* for additional information about the reactions involving these drugs.)

NURSING IMPLICATIONS

Before administering the H_2-receptor antagonists, the nurse must be familiar with the following implications:
• Intravenous H_2-receptor antagonists are often administered prophylactically to critically ill patients to prevent GI bleeding.
• Use caution when giving cimetidine, ranitidine, and famotidine to patients with impaired renal or hepatic function.
• Reduced doses are usually administered to elderly patients because of their decreased acid and pepsin secretion. Be aware that cimetidine especially can induce confusion.
• Histamine-receptor antagonists may be administered without regard to meals.
• Dilute cimetidine, ranitidine, and famotidine before I.V. administration. Dilute cimetidine and ranitidine in 20 ml of 0.9% sodium chloride solution or another compatible I.V. solution.
• I.V. solutions compatible with cimetidine, ranitidine, and famotidine include 0.9% sodium chloride, 5% or 10% dextrose (and combinations of these), lactated Ringer's, and 5% sodium bicarbonate. Do not use sterile water for injection as a diluent.
• Discourage patients from smoking, which impairs the effectiveness of H_2-receptor antagonists.

SUCRALFATE

Physicians prescribe sucralfate for the short-term treatment of duodenal ulcers. Sucralfate acts through a different mechanism of action than do the antacids and H_2-receptor antagonists, apparently binding to the ulcer site and producing a protective barrier. Sucralfate, however, is not used as extensively as the antacids or H_2-receptor antagonists for peptic ulcer disease.

History and source
In 1932, Babkin and Kimarov described chondroitin sulfate, a sulfated polysaccharide, as a possibly active agent in the gastric mucosa. Since then, researchers have worked to develop synthetic sulfated polysaccharides for the treatment of peptic ulcer disease. In the early 1970s, the Chugai Pharmaceutical Company of Japan began investigating one of these compounds, sucralfate. In 1981, sucralfate was introduced into the United States.

PHARMACOKINETICS

Because sucralfate is only minimally absorbed after oral administration, researchers have not conducted extensive pharmacokinetic evaluations.

Absorption, distribution, metabolism, excretion
The minimal absorption of sucralfate from the GI tract is appropriate because sucralfate exerts its effects locally, rapidly reacting with hydrochloric acid in the GI tract to form a highly condensed, viscous, adhesive, pastelike substance that adheres to the gastric mucosa and especially to ulcer sites. The drug is minimally distributed to other areas of the body and is excreted in the feces.

Onset, peak, duration
The onset of action of sucralfate is rapid once the drug reaches the GI tract. The duration of action for sucralfate depends upon how long the drug remains in contact with its action site. The drug's viscosity, adhesiveness, and affinity for damaged mucosa prolong this contact. Usually, the duration of action is up to 6 hours after administration.

PHARMACODYNAMICS

By binding to the ulcer site, sucralfate protects the ulcer from the damaging effects of acid and pepsin and permits healing.

Mechanism of action

In an acid environment, sucralfate becomes a pastelike material that is negatively charged, highly viscous, and adhesive. This material binds to the positively charged proteins, such as albumin, fibrinogen, damaged mucosal cells, and dead leukocytes, found at the base of an ulcer. By forming a barrier at the ulcer site, sucralfate protects the ulcer against the ulcerogenic effects of gastric acid, pepsin, and bile. Thus, the ulcer is allowed to heal. The action of sucralfate in actively inhibiting pepsin and in absorbing bile acids may also play a role in its mechanism of action.

PHARMACOTHERAPEUTICS

Sucralfate is used for short-term treatment (up to 8 weeks) of duodenal ulcers. For this condition, sucralfate acts as effectively as H_2-receptor antagonists and antacids. Sucralfate has also been used successfully for the short-term treatment of gastric ulcers. Physicians also prescribe sucralfate for preventing recurrent ulcers, NSAID-induced ulcers, and stress ulcers.

Antacids may be used with sucralfate to relieve pain, but the antacids do not increase the ulcer healing. When combined with sucralfate, H_2-receptor antagonists increase the cost of therapy but do not offer any advantages. Therefore, the combination is not recommended.

Though sucralfate effectively treats ulcers, it is the least popular antiulcer agent. Compared to the H_2-receptor antagonists, sucralfate requires a cumbersome dosing schedule and produces a number of minor adverse reactions that lead to decreased patient compliance.

sucralfate (Carafate). The timing of sucralfate administration is important because the drug is more active in the lower pH of an empty stomach than in the higher pH of a stomach buffered by food.
USUAL ADULT DOSAGE: 1 gram P.O. q.i.d. taken on an empty stomach 1 hour before meals and h.s. Treatment should be continued 4 to 8 weeks unless radiographic or endoscopic examination indicates healing.

Drug interactions

When given orally with sucralfate, some drugs are bound in the GI tract, decreasing their absorption. Antacids, like food, increase the pH of the GI tract. If administered with sucralfate, antacids decrease its activity. Because sucralfate decreases the bioavailability of cimetidine, the nurse should give sucralfate 2 hours before or after the cimetidine dose.

ADVERSE DRUG REACTIONS

Usually, sucralfate is well tolerated. Though usually minor, adverse reactions may become bothersome for the patient. Constipation is the most frequent predictable adverse reaction, with an occurrence rate of about 2%. Nausea and a metallic taste may also accompany the use of sucralfate. Less frequently, sucralfate also may produce diarrhea, indigestion, dry mouth, back pain, dizziness, sleepiness, and vertigo. Sucralfate may unpredictably produce a rash and pruritus, but these reactions are rare.

NURSING IMPLICATIONS

When administering sucralfate, the nurse should be aware of the following implications:
• Sucralfate has no known contraindications.
• Administer sucralfate to the patient at least 1 hour before meals and at bedtime for the best results.
• If constipation becomes a problem, increase the patient's fluid and bulk intake or use laxatives as prescribed.

OTHER PEPTIC ULCER AGENTS

Most of the agents discussed in the following section are currently being investigated for their usefulness to treat peptic ulcer disease.

anticholinergic agents. The parasympathetic blockade produced by anticholinergic agents reduces gastric acid secretion. However, effective doses also produce severe systemic adverse reactions, such as urinary retention, constipation, dry mouth, and visual disturbances.

colloidal bismuth. Colloidal bismuth chelates with the base of the ulcer and protects the ulcer against the actions of acid, bile, and pepsin. This promotes the healing of duodenal ulcers with an effectiveness similar to cimetidine and is also effective against gastric ulcers. Colloidal bismuth has been used extensively in Europe.

proton-pump inhibitors. A new class of drugs, the proton-pump inhibitors block the transport of acid across the cell membrane of the parietal cells. This action produces a profound, almost total suppression of acid secretion.

Peptic ulcer agents

The following chart is a handy reference tool for indications, dosages, and nursing implications for selected peptic ulcer agents.

DRUG	MAJOR INDICATIONS	USUAL ADULT DOSAGES	NURSING IMPLICATIONS
Antacids			
magnesium hydroxide, aluminum hydroxide with simethicone, magaldrate or aluminum-magnesium complex	Symptomatic and therapeutic treatment of peptic ulcer disease	10 to 30 ml P.O. 1 and 3 hours after each meal and h.s. for magnesium hydroxide and aluminum hydroxide with simethicone; 480 to 960 mg P.O. with water between meals and h.s. for magaldrate or aluminum magnesium complex	• Patient on sodium-restricted or low-sodium diet should receive an antacid low in sodium. • Sodium bicarbonate is absorbed and may lead to metabolic alkalosis if used regularly. • Magnesium-containing products may produce a laxative effect; aluminum-containing products may cause constipation. • Magnesium-containing antacids are contraindicated in patients with renal failure; hypermagnesemia may result. • Calcium carbonate and sodium bicarbonate may cause rebound hyperacidity and milk-alkali syndrome. Administer only occasionally as prescribed. • Antacids impair the absorption of many medications. Do not administer other oral drugs within 1 to 2 hours of an antacid. • Administer liquid preparations in the treatment of peptic ulcer disease unless extenuating circumstances exist. • Encourage the patient to chew tablets thoroughly before swallowing; follow with 6 to 8 ounces of water.
Histamine$_2$-receptor antagonists			
cimetidine	Treatment and prophylaxis of peptic ulcer disease	800 mg P.O. daily h.s.; 300 mg I.V. q 6 to 8 hours	• Drug causes a greater incidence of adverse reactions and drug interactions than other H$_2$-receptor antagonists. • Administer with caution to patients with impaired renal function; reduce doses in these and elderly patients as prescribed. • Dilute cimetidine before direct I.V. administration in 20 ml of 0.9% sodium chloride solution or other compatible solution. • Compatible I.V. solutions are 0.9% sodium chloride, 5% or 10% dextrose (and combinations of these), lactated Ringer's, and 5% sodium bicarbonate. Do not use sterile water for injection.
ranitidine	Treatment and prophylaxis of peptic ulcer disease	150 mg P.O. b.i.d., 300 mg P.O. h.s. or 50 mg I.V. or I.M. q 6 to 8 hours	• Dilute ranitidine before direct I.V. administration in 20 ml of 0.9% sodium chloride solution or other compatible solution. • Compatible I.V. solutions are 0.9% sodium chloride, 5% or 10% dextrose (and combinations of these), lactated Ringer's, and 5% sodium bicarbonate. Do not use sterile water for injection.

continued

SELECTED MAJOR DRUGS

Peptic ulcer agents continued

DRUG	MAJOR INDICATIONS	USUAL ADULT DOSAGES	NURSING IMPLICATIONS
famotidine	Treatment and prophylaxis of peptic ulcer disease	20 mg P.O. b.i.d., 40 mg P.O. h.s., or 20 mg I.V. q 12 hours; for maintenance, 20 mg P.O. h.s.	• Before direct I.V. administration, dilute 2 ml of famotidine solution (10 mg/ml) with 0.9% sodium chloride or other compatible solution to a total volume of either 5 or 10 ml and injected over a period of not less than 2 minutes. • Famotidine may be administered as an I.V. infusion of 2 ml/100 ml of 5% dextrose or other compatible solution and administered over 15 to 30 minutes.
Sucralfate			
sucralfate	Treatment of active peptic ulcer disease	1 gram P.O. q.i.d. for 4 to 8 weeks	• Administer sucralfate to the patient 1 hour before each meal and at bedtime. • Instruct the patient to keep taking the medication unless otherwise directed by the physician, even if the ulcer pain has subsided. • Inform the patient that constipation may become a problem and can be treated with minor laxatives. • Sucralfate is as effective as antacids or H_2-receptor antagonists in healing duodenal ulcers.

prostaglandins. Researchers are investigating synthetic analogues of naturally occurring prostaglandins for the treatment of peptic ulcer disease. Administered orally or intravenously, these drugs inhibit gastric acid secretion, stimulate gastric bicarbonate secretion, and may produce a cytoprotective effect by increasing mucous secretion and mucosal perfusion.

tricyclic antidepressants. Two tricyclic antidepressants, doxepin hydrochloride and trimipramine maleate, are being investigated for their use in treating peptic ulcer disease. The tricyclic antidepressants produce an H_2-receptor antagonist effect and an anticholinergic effect that may be beneficial in ulcer treatment.

CHAPTER SUMMARY

Chapter 50 discussed peptic ulcer drugs. Peptic ulcer therapy attempts to correct the imbalanced gastric acid and pepsin secretion and to repair inadequate mucosal defenses of the GI lining. Here are the highlights of the chapter:

• Peptic ulcer drugs: (1) neutralize acid in the GI tract, (2) reduce acid secretion, or (3) bind to the ulcer, protecting it and neutralizing local acid.

• The antacids act in the stomach to neutralize acid, thereby reducing the acid load in the GI tract and permitting ulcers to heal.

• Antacids treat peptic ulcer disease safely and effectively. However, the unpleasant taste and the frequent doses required make their use as the sole treatment of peptic ulcer disease less attractive than the H_2-receptor antagonists. Nonetheless, the antacids serve as excellent alternatives when patients cannot tolerate the H_2-receptor antagonists.

• Histamine$_2$-receptor antagonists used for 4 to 6 weeks with adjunctive antacid therapy for pain have become the treatment of choice for both duodenal and gastric ulcers.

• Histamine$_2$-receptor antagonists block histamine-receptor sites, thereby inhibiting histamine-stimulated acid secretion. The H_2-receptor antagonists include cimetidine, ranitidine, and famotidine. These drugs promote the healing of both duodenal and gastric ulcers.

- The H_2-receptor antagonists (especially cimetidine) can produce headache, dizziness, malaise, nausea, diarrhea or constipation, skin rashes, loss of libido, and impotence.
- The sulfated polysaccharide sucralfate binds to the ulcer site and produces a protective barrier.
- Sucralfate is used for short-term treatment of duodenal and gastric ulcers; however, the drug requires an inconvenient dosing schedule and produces numerous minor adverse reactions, including constipation, diarrhea, dry mouth, dizziness, and sleepiness.
- Researchers are currently investigating other peptic ulcer agents, including anticholinergic drugs, colloidal bismuth, proton-pump inhibitors, prostaglandins, and tricyclic antidepressants.

BIBLIOGRAPHY

American Hospital Formulary Service. *Drug Information 86.* McEvoy, G.K., ed. Bethesda, Md.: American Society of Hospital Pharmacists, 1986.

Berman, P.M. "Peptic Ulcer," *in Conn's Current Therapy.* Rakel, R.E., ed. Philadelphia: W.B. Saunders Co., 1986.

Bertaccini, G., and Corruzzi, G. "Pharmacology of the Treatment of Peptic Ulcer Disease," *Digestive Diseases and Sciences* 30:43, November 1985.

Blum, A.L. "Therapeutic Approach to Ulcer Healing," *American Journal of Medicine* 79:8, August 30, 1985.

Debas, H.T., and Mulholland, M.W. "New Horizons in the Pharmacologic Management of Peptic Ulceration," *American Journal of Surgery* 151:422, March 1986.

Douglas, W.W. "Histamine and 5-Hydroxy-tryptamine (Serotonin) and Their Antagonists," in *Goodman and Gilman's The Pharmacological Basis of Therapeutics,* 7th edition. Gilman, A.G., et al., eds. New York: Macmillan Publishing Co., 1985.

Feldman, M. "Inhibition of Gastric Acid Secretion by Selective and Nonselective Anticholinergics," *Gastroenterology* 86(2):361, February 1984.

Halter, F. "The Other Option in Peptic Ulcer Therapy," *South African Medical Journal* 65:996, June 23, 1984.

Harvey, S.C. "Gastric Antacids, Miscellaneous Drugs for the Treatment of Peptic Ulcers, Digestants, and Bile Acids," in *Goodman and Gilman's The Pharmacological Basis of Therapeutics,* 7th edition. Gilman, A.G., et al., eds. New York: Macmillan Publishing Co., 1985.

Legerton, C.W. "Duodenal and Gastric Ulcer Healing Rates: A Review," *American Journal of Medicine* 77:2, November 19, 1984.

McGuigan, J.E. "Peptic Ulcer," in *Harrison's Principles of Internal Medicine,* 10th edition. Petersdorf, R.G., et al., eds. New York: McGraw-Hill Book Co., 1983.

Moran, D.M., et al. "Gastrointestinal Diseases," in *Applied Therapeutics: The Clinical Use of Drugs,* 3rd edition. Katcher, B.S., et al., eds. San Francisco: Applied Therapeutics, Inc., 1983.

Piper, D.W. "Drugs for the Prevention of Peptic Ulcer Recurrence," *Drugs* 26(5):439, November 1983.

Richardson, C.T. "Pathogenetic Factors in Peptic Ulcer Disease," *American Journal of Medicine* 79:1, August 30, 1985.

Siepler, J.K., et al. "Current Concepts in Clinical Therapeutics: Peptic Ulcer Disease," *Clinical Pharmacology* 5:128, February 1986.

Somerville, K.W., and Langman, M.J.S. "Newer Antisecretory Agents for Peptic Ulcer," *Drugs* 25(3):315, March 1983.

Zeldis, J.B., et al. "A New H_2-Receptor Antagonist," *New England Journal of Medicine* 309(22):1368, December 1983.

Zimmerman, T.W. "Problems Associated with Medical Treatment of Peptic Ulcer Disease," *American Journal of Medicine* 77:51, November 19, 1984.

DRUGS FOR FLUID, ELECTROLYTE, AND NUTRITIONAL BALANCE

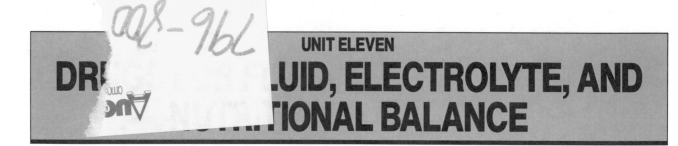

Illness can easily disturb the homeostatic mechanisms that help maintain the normal fluid, electrolyte, and nutritional balance. Such occurrences as loss of appetite, medication administration, vomiting, and diagnostic tests also can alter this delicate balance. Fortunately, physicians can use numerous drugs to correct fluid, electrolyte, acid-base, or nutritional imbalances. Unit Eleven provides a full range of information about these drugs.

Fluid and electrolyte balance

About 60% of an adult's body is made up of water: 60% of this body water is intracellular; 40% is extracellular. The ingestion of food and fluids and the metabolism of nutrients add water to the body—1,500 to 3,000 ml/day for an average adult. Ordinarily, the fluid intake equals the fluid output, but an illness can upset this delicate balance.

Intracellular and extracellular fluid compartments have specific chemical compositions of electrolytes. This unit will address the major electrolytes: sodium, potassium, chloride, calcium, phosphorus, magnesium, and bicarbonate. (See *Normal electrolyte concentration levels in intracellular and extracellular fluid* for detailed information about concentration levels.)

Many disorders and diseases can alter electrolyte concentration levels in the fluid compartments, profoundly affecting the body's water distribution, cell function, neuromuscular activity, and acid-base balance. When such imbalances occur, the agents discussed in this unit are used to reestablish homeostasis.

Nutritional balance

Unit Eleven also includes agents used to maintain nutritional balance or to correct a nutritional imbalance. Maintaining nutrition is important because the body relies on exogenous sources of carbohydrate, fat, and protein to sustain life. Malnutrition must be corrected because it can decrease the ability of organ systems to function, complicating a patient's treatment.

Nutritional assessment

Assessing the type and degree of malnutrition will help determine necessary nutritional support and the goals

Normal electrolyte concentration levels in intracellular and extracellular fluid

Blood contains both intracellular fluid (blood in red blood cells) and extracellular fluid (plasma fluid). Because their cells allow different substances to permeate, intracellular and extracellular fluids contain different electrolyte concentration levels. For example, intracellular fluid contains about 30 times more potassium than extracellular fluid, and extracellular fluid contains about 14 times more sodium than intracellular fluid.

Alterations in electrolyte balance will affect a patient's total physiologic functioning. Some drugs will alter that balance. Various electrolytes are ordered to treat electrolyte imbalance.

In the clinical setting, the nurse will see values reflecting the components of extracellular fluid only.

Be aware that standards for these values vary among institutions.

ELECTROLYTE	INTRACELLULAR CONCENTRATION	EXTRACELLULAR CONCENTRATION
Sodium	10 mEq/liter	136 to 146 mEq/liter
Potassium	140 mEq/liter	3.5 to 5.0 mEq/liter
Calcium	10 mEq/liter	4.5 to 5.8 mEq/liter
Magnesium	40 mEq/liter	1.6 to 2.2 mEq/liter
Chloride	4 mEq/liter	96 to 106 mEq/liter
Bicarbonate	10 mEq/liter	24 to 28 mEq/liter
Phosphate	100 mEq/liter	1 to 1.5 mEq/liter

of therapy. To assess malnutrition, the nurse can use laboratory tests and daily clinical evaluations, including the patient's daily weight and other anthropometric measurements to help determine the status of protein and fat reserves. A triceps skin-fold measurement estimates the body's fat reserve. Midarm muscle circumference indicates the protein deficit. The creatinine-height index helps evaluate muscle status. When assessing a patient, the nurse should compare the value of each measurement to the standard value to estimate the degree of depletion.

Certain laboratory tests can help assess visceral protein depletion. For example, a low serum albumin, serum transferrin, and total lymphocyte count may indicate this type of nutritional deficiency.

Nutritional supplements

A complete nutritional supplement will supply carbohydrates, protein, lipid electrolytes, vitamins, and trace elements. Patients need adequate nonprotein calories to allow optimal protein use, and carbohydrate calories should be given in amounts approximating the basal

---

Glossary

Abetalipoproteinemia: condition characterized by a lack of beta-lipoproteins in the blood.

Alkaline phosphatase: enzyme involved in bone mineralization that originates in the bone, liver, placenta, and other tissues.

Anion: negatively charged ion.

Beriberi: polyneuritis caused by a thiamine deficiency and characterized by spasmodic rigidity of the lower limbs, muscular atrophy, paralysis, anemia, and neuralgia.

Bilirubin: reddish bile pigment formed from the breakdown of hemoglobin in erythrocytes.

Buffer: any substance in a solution that decreases the change in pH when an acid or base is added.

Carbonic anhydrase: enzyme that catalyzes the breakdown of carbonic acid to carbon dioxide and water, or the formation of carbon dioxide and water to carbonic acid.

Carpopedal spasm: sudden, violent, involuntary muscle contraction in the hands or feet, accompanied by pain, distortion, and dysfunction in response to a decreased serum calcium level.

Cation: positively charged ion.

Chelation: process of binding a metallic ion with an organic compound to form a compound that sequesters the metallic ion from other interactions.

Electrolyte: ion that, when dissolved in solution, can conduct electricity.

Encephalopathy: any degenerative brain disease.

Extracellular fluid: fluid outside the cells that accounts for about 40% of the total body water and includes functional plasma and interstitial fluid. Some of the components of extracellular fluid are protein, magnesium, potassium, chloride, calcium, and certain sulfates.

Hyperbilirubinemia: excess bilirubin in the blood.

Hypercalcemia: excess calcium in the blood.

Hypercalciuria: excess calcium in the urine.

Hyperglycemia: excess glucose in the blood.

Hyperkalemia: excess potassium in the blood.

Hyperlipidemia: excess lipids in the blood.

Hypernatremia: excess sodium in the blood.

Hyperosmolality: excess solutes per unit of solvent in a solution.

Hyperphosphatemia: excess phosphate in the blood.

Hypervitaminosis: condition resulting from excessive intake of one or more vitamins.

Hypocalcemia: deficient calcium in the blood.

Hypoglycemia: deficient glucose in the blood.

Hypokalemia: deficient potassium in the blood.

Hypomagnesemia: deficient magnesium in the blood.

Hyponatremia: deficient sodium in the blood.

Hypophosphatemia: deficient phosphate in the blood.

Hypoprothrombinemia: deficient prothrombin in the blood.

Hypovolemia: abnormally decreased volume of circulatory body fluid.

Intracellular fluid: fluid inside the cells that accounts for 60% of the total body water, and includes intracellular and red blood cell fluid.

Lactic acidosis: decreased serum pH caused by the anaerobic metabolism of pyruvic acid to lactic acid.

Malabsorption: impaired absorption of nutrients.

Metabolic acidosis: decreased serum pH caused by an excess of hydrogen ions in the extracellular fluid.

Metabolic alkalosis: increased serum pH caused by excess bicarbonate in the extracellular fluid.

Mineral: naturally occurring inorganic substance with a distinctive chemical composition.

Nephrotoxic: property of being poisonous or destructive to kidney cells.

Neuritis: nerve inflammation, usually accompanied by pain, tenderness, anesthesia, paresthesia, paralysis, muscle wasting, and areflexia.

Nyctalopia: poor vision at night or in dim light, usually associated with vitamin A deficiency; also called night blindness.

continued

Glossary continued

Osmolality: solute concentration per unit of solvent in a solution.

Osteodystrophy: defective bone formation.

Osteomalacia: condition characterized by bone softening, pain, muscle weakness, anorexia, and weight loss; usually associated with vitamin D, calcium, or phosphorus deficiencies.

Osteoporosis: decrease in bone density caused by the failure of osteoblasts to form bone matrix.

Ototoxicity: property of being poisonous or destructive to the eighth cranial nerve or the organs of hearing and balance.

Paresthesia: abnormal burning or prickling sensation.

Pellagra: condition caused by a niacin deficiency and characterized by abnormalities in the integumentary, gastrointestinal, and nervous systems.

pH: abbreviation for the relative hydrogen ion concentration (acidity or alkalinity) of a solution; a pH of 7.0 is neutral; below 7 is acid; above 7 is alkaline.

Polycythemia: excess in the number of red blood cells.

Rickets: ossification disorder caused by a vitamin D deficiency, usually during childhood, characterized by abnormal bone formation.

Scurvy: condition caused by a vitamin C deficiency and characterized by weakness, anemia, spongy gums, mucocutaneous hemorrhages, and indurations of the leg muscles.

Systemic acidifier: agent that decreases serum pH level.

Systemic alkalinizer: agent that increases serum pH level.

Urinary acidifier: agent that decreases urine pH level.

Urinary alkalinizer: agent that increases urine pH level.

Vitamin: organic substance in food that is necessary for normal metabolism. Vitamins are classified as fat-soluble or water-soluble.

---

energy expenditure. Of the daily calorie requirements, 4% to 10% should include essential fatty acids. Daily protein requirements depend on the stress level because stress increases protein use. Maintenance therapy usually requires 0.5 to 1 gram of protein/kg/day; high-stress states or moderate protein repletion, 1.5 to 2 grams of protein/kg/day; extensive repletion, 2 to 4 grams of protein/kg/day. Physicians prescribe two types of nutritional supplements: enteral agents, administered through the alimentary canal, and parenteral agents, administered through other routes.

Enteral nutrition

Many physicians prefer enteral nutrition to parenteral nutrition for patients with functional gastrointestinal tracts because it uses the normal metabolic pathways and processes. It allows the body to use nutrients more efficiently and tends to cause fewer metabolic problems. Enteral nutrition is also much less expensive, averaging approximately 1/10 the cost of parenteral nutrition.

The nurse can administer enteral nutrition by the bolus, gravity drip, or continuous drip method. The bolus method delivers 240 to 400 ml of feeding solution by gravity over several minutes and is repeated every 4 to 6 hours. Because this method is poorly tolerated by most patients, its use is limited. The gravity drip method infuses 240 to 400 ml of feeding solution over 30 to 60 minutes and is repeated every 4 to 6 hours. This method is usually better tolerated than the bolus method. The continuous drip method delivers the feeding solution continuously over 24 hours, usually at a rate of 50 to 125 ml/hour. Ideally, an infusion pump is used to control the infusion rate. Studies show that this method is the most reliable and best tolerated of the three enteral nutrition methods.

Parenteral nutrition

Patients who cannot tolerate oral feeding or enteral nutrition may need parenteral nutrition. Total parenteral nutrition (TPN) provides carbohydrates, proteins, lipids, electrolytes, vitamins, and trace elements intravenously. It supplies carbohydrate as a dextrose solution, which provides 3.4 kcal/gram. Concentrations of dextrose 5% to 10% may be given via a peripheral vein, but hypertonic solutions greater than 12.5% must be given via a central catheter. Parenteral nutrition supplies protein in amino acid solutions that provide 4 kcal/gram, and lipids in 10% or 20% fat emulsions that provide 1.1 kcal/ml or 2 kcal/ml, respectively.

The nurse should initiate central TPN solutions slowly at about 40 to 50 ml/hour, increasing the rate over 24 to 48 hours to the maximum desired rate to avoid severe hyperglycemia. When discontinuing central TPN, the nurse must gradually taper the rate over 24 hours to avoid hypoglycemia.

Because some people are allergic to the egg protein in fat emulsions, therapy should begin with a test dose

Comparing types of parenteral nutrition

This chart summarizes the uses and special considerations of the various forms of parenteral nutrition, which may be used for a patient who needs nutritional supplementation.

SOLUTION COMPONENTS/LITER	USES	SPECIAL CONSIDERATIONS
Total parenteral nutrition (TPN) (via central venous line)		
• Dextrose 15% to 35% (1 liter dextrose 25% = 850 nonprotein calories) • Crystalline amino acids 2.5% to 5% • Electrolytes, vitamins, trace elements, insulin, and heparin as ordered • Fat emulsion 10% to 20% (usually infused as a separate solution; can be given peripherally or centrally)	• 1 week or more (long term) • For patients with large caloric and nutrient needs • Provides needed calories, essential vitamins, electrolytes, minerals, and trace elements; restores nitrogen balance • Promotes tissue synthesis, wound healing, and normal metabolic function • Allows bowel rest and healing; reduces activity in the gallbladder, pancreas, and small intestine	**Basic solution** • Is nutritionally complete • Requires minor surgical procedure for central line insertion • Delivers hypertonic solutions • May cause metabolic complications (glucose intolerance, electrolyte imbalances, essential fatty acid deficiency) **I.V. fat emulsion** • May not be used effectively in severely stressed patients (especially burn patients) • May interfere with immune mechanisms • Irritates peripheral vein in long-term use
Peripheral parenteral nutrition		
• Dextrose 5% to 10% • Crystalline amino acids 2.75% to 4.25% • Electrolytes, trace elements, and vitamins as ordered • Fat emulsion 10% or 20% (1 liter dextrose 10% and amino acids 3.5% infused at same time with 1 liter fat emulsion = 1,440 nonprotein calories: 340 from dextrose and 1,100 from fat emulsion) • Heparin or hydrocortisone as ordered	• 1 week or less • Maintains nutritional state in patients who can tolerate relatively high fluid volume, those who usually resume bowel function and oral feedings in a few days, and those who are susceptible to catheter-related infections of central venous TPN	**Basic solution** • Short-term use only; cannot be used in nutritionally depleted patients • Cannot be used in volume-restricted patients because higher volumes of solution are needed than with central venous TPN • Avoids insertion and maintenance of central catheter, but patient must have good veins; I.V. site should be changed every 48 hours • Does not require surgery for peripheral line insertion • Delivers less hypertonic solutions than central venous TPN • May cause phlebitis **I.V. fat emulsion** • Is as effective as dextrose for caloric source • Irritates vein in long-term use • Diminishes phlebitis if infused at same time as basic nutrient solution
Protein-sparing therapy		
• Crystalline amino acids in same amounts as TPN • Electrolytes, vitamins, and minerals as ordered	• 2 weeks or less • May preserve body protein in a stable patient • Augments oral or tube feedings	• Is nutritionally incomplete; may be initiated or stopped at any point in a patient's hospital stay • Allows administration of other I.V. fluids, medications, and blood by-products through same I.V. line • Is not as likely to cause phlebitis as peripheral parenteral nutrition
Standard I.V. therapy		
• Dextrose, water, electrolytes, and vitamins in varying amounts *Examples of frequently used parenteral fluids:* D_5W = 170 calories/liter $D_{10}W$ = 340 calories/liter 0.9% NaCl (normal saline solution) = 0 calories	• Less than 1 week as nutrition source • Maintains hydration (main function) • Facilitates and maintains normal metabolic function	• Is nutritionally incomplete; does not administer sufficient calories to maintain adequate nutritional status

of 1 ml/minute for 30 minutes. If no adverse reactions occur, the rate may be advanced to the desired rate. The nurse may give fat emulsions through a central or peripheral catheter, but should not use an in-line filter, because the fat particles are too large to pass through the pores. (See *Comparing types of parenteral nutrition* on page 799 for a summary of these nutritional supplements.)

Chapter 51
Vitamin and Mineral Agents

Chapter 51 focuses on the vitamin and mineral preparations used as nutritional supplements. It discusses the physiologic actions and clinical uses of the fat-soluble vitamins (A, D, E, and K), the water-soluble vitamins (B complex and C), and the minerals (iodine, fluoride, zinc, manganese, copper, selenium, cobalt, molybdenum, and chromium). It also emphasizes the patient education associated with these agents.

Chapter 52
Electrolyte Replacement Agents

Chapter 52 presents the agents used to replace electrolytes when an imbalance occurs: sodium, potassium, chloride, calcium, phosphorus, and magnesium. It also examines the signs and symptoms of electrolyte imbalances and the nursing implications associated with administering replacement agents.

Chapter 53
Alkalinizing and Acidifying Agents

Chapter 53 explores the systemic and urinary alkalinizing and acidifying agents. It discusses the use of systemic agents, such as sodium bicarbonate and ammonium chloride, to treat metabolic acidosis and alkalosis and the use of urinary alkalinizers, such as sodium bicarbonate and acetazolamide, to promote the excretion of certain weak acids and toxic drugs. The chapter also describes the use of ascorbic acid and ammonium chloride as urinary acidifiers to treat urinary tract infections. It concludes with a discussion of the adverse reactions to these agents and the associated nursing implications.

Chapter 54
Cation-Exchange Resin and Ammonia-Detoxicating Agents

Chapter 54 examines two types of agents used to treat toxic imbalances: a cation-exchange resin and ammonia-detoxicating agents. It discusses the cation-exchange resin, sodium polystyrene sulfonate, as a treatment for hyperkalemia. It then investigates the use of lactulose and neomycin, two ammonia-detoxicating agents, in re-ducing serum ammonia levels in patients with hepatic encephalopathy. The chapter details the adverse reactions and therapeutic responses to these agents and the nursing interventions associated with them.

Nursing diagnoses

Several nursing diagnoses may apply to a patient who requires pharmacologic agents to maintain normal fluid, electrolyte, and nutritional balance.
- Activity intolerance related to the specific imbalance
- Alteration in cardiac output: decreased, related to the specific imbalance
- Alteration in nutrition: less than body requirements, related to the specific imbalance or drug therapy
- Alteration in oral mucous membranes related to the specific imbalance or the drug therapy
- Alteration in thought processes related to the specific imbalance
- Altered growth and development related to the specific imbalance
- Anxiety related to the specific imbalance and the therapeutic outcome
- Fear related to the specific imbalance and the therapeutic outcome
- Fluid volume deficit/excess related to the specific imbalance or the drug therapy
- Impaired gas exchange related to the specific imbalance
- Impaired physical mobility related to the specific imbalance
- Knowledge deficit related to the specific imbalance or drug therapy
- Noncompliance related to the drug therapy
- Potential impairment of skin integrity related to the specific imbalance
- Self-care deficit related to the specific imbalance
- Sensory-perceptual alterations related to the specific imbalance.

CHAPTER 51

VITAMIN AND MINERAL AGENTS

OBJECTIVES

After reading and studying this chapter, you should be able to:

1. Explain the pharmacokinetics of the four fat-soluble vitamins (A, D, E, and K), including their routes of absorption, distribution, metabolism, and excretion.

2. Identify the signs of vitamin A and D toxicity.

3. Explain why vitamin K should not be administered undiluted by I.V. push.

4. Discuss the pharmacokinetics of the water-soluble vitamins (B and C) and explain why these preparations are less toxic than the fat-soluble vitamins.

5. Identify patient-teaching points concerning vitamins and food, storage, toxicity, and drug interactions.

6. Identify patient-teaching points concerning trace minerals and parenteral administration, gastric irritation, food, and drug interactions.

INTRODUCTION

Since the early 20th century, researchers have uncovered a wealth of information about the nutritional agents called vitamins and minerals. Evidence of the existence of vitamins and minerals was suggested by early research into the major nutritional-deficiency states, such as scurvy, night blindness, beriberi, and rickets. Despite years of study, experts possess incomplete knowledge about vitamins and minerals; indeed, only recently have experts understood the roles of these chemicals in the maintenance of normal growth, development, and metabolic function. Knowledge of vitamins and minerals will grow as research related to these substances continues.

Vitamins are organic chemicals that do not fit into the categories of protein, fat, or carbohydrate. Although the human body requires only small amounts of these chemicals, they are essential for the normal operation of various metabolic functions. With two exceptions, the source of vitamins is from outside the body, either from ingested foods or through an oral or parenteral supple-

ment. The two exceptions are vitamin D, which can be formed within the body through the action of ultraviolet radiation in sunlight on 7-dehydrocholesterol in the skin, and one form of vitamin K, which is synthesized by bacteria in the gastrointestinal (GI) tract.

Vitamins and minerals are naturally occurring substances; however, many vitamins can be synthesized, and natural and synthetic forms are commercially available. Both forms function identically, and claims for the increased nutritional value of natural vitamins are unfounded.

Vitamins are divided into two categories based on their solubility: fat-soluble and water-soluble.

Food sources of fat-soluble vitamins

The nurse should teach the patient about dietary sources of vitamins A, D, E, and K to prevent the development of chronic deficiencies.

VITAMIN	FOOD SOURCES
vitamin A	Dairy products, liver, egg yolks, fish, and yellow or green fruits and vegetables
vitamin D	Fortified milk and margarine
vitamin E	Vegetable oils, margarine, milk, eggs, meats, green leafy vegetables, whole grains, and animal fats
vitamin K	Liver, cheese, eggs, green leafy vegetables, tomatoes, meats, milk, and vegetable oils

FAT-SOLUBLE VITAMINS

The fat-soluble vitamins A, D, E, and K require the presence of bile salts, pancreatic lipase, and dietary fat for absorption into the body. Although their mechanisms of absorption and storage potential within the body are similar, each performs different functions. Adequate amounts of vitamin A are necessary for vision in dim light, skin and mucous membrane development, normal growth, and reproduction. Vitamin D—actually two related substances, cholecalciferol (D_3) and ergocalciferol (D_2)—plays a role in regulating calcium and phosphorus balance. Vitamin E acts as an antioxidant and enzyme cofactor. Vitamin K stimulates the synthesis of clotting factors by the liver. (See *Food sources of fat-soluble vitamins* on page 801 for a summary of the dietary sources of these vitamins.)

WATER-SOLUBLE VITAMINS

Water-soluble vitamins include B-complex vitamins (thiamine, riboflavin, nicotinic acid, pyridoxine, para-aminobenzoic acid, pantothenic acid, biotin, choline, inositol, folic acid, and cyanocobalamin), and vitamin C (ascorbic acid). Although different in structure and function, the B-complex vitamins are grouped together because they were originally derived from all liver and yeast foods that contained antiberiberi properties. This chapter will discuss thiamine (B_1), riboflavin (B_2), nicotinic acid or niacin (B_3), pyridoxine (B_6), and vitamin C in detail. (See Chapter 41, Hematinic Agents, for information about folic acid and cyanocobalamin [vitamin B_{12}] and their roles in hematopoiesis.) Although para-aminobenzoic acid (PABA) is not considered a true vitamin, it is a precursor to folic acid and therefore it will be discussed briefly in this chapter along with pantothenic acid, biotin, choline, and inositol.

The water-soluble vitamins are readily absorbed via the watery medium of the small intestine. They all function as coenzymes in various cellular enzymatic reactions, except vitamin C. Researchers believe that vitamin C participates in oxidation and reduction reactions used in cellular respiration. (See *Food sources of water-soluble vitamins* for a summary of the dietary sources of these vitamins.)

Food sources of water-soluble vitamins

The nuse should teach the patient about dietary sources of vitamins B and C to prevent the development of chronic deficiencies.

VITAMIN	FOOD SOURCES
thiamine (B_1)	Yeast, whole grain and enriched cereals and breads, legumes, nuts, pork, and organ meats
riboflavin (B_2)	Milk, cheese, organ meats, eggs, whole grain and enriched cereals and breads, and green leafy vegetables
nicotinic acid (B_3)	Meats, liver, poultry, fish, eggs, yeast, whole grain and enriched cereals and breads, nuts, and legumes
pyridoxine (B_6)	Meats, eggs, liver, whole grain cereals and breads, soybeans, and vegetables
ascorbic acid (C)	Citrus fruits, tomatoes, strawberries, cabbage greens, and potatoes

MINERALS (TRACE ELEMENTS)

Minerals are inorganic chemicals that are components of all living tissues. Like vitamins, they play a role in various metabolic functions. Because the body cannot manufacture any of the minerals, they must be obtained from some exogenous source, usually food. This chapter discusses the trace minerals (or trace elements) iodine, fluoride, zinc, manganese, copper, selenium, cobalt, molybdenum, and chromium.

Other minerals required by the body, such as calcium, sodium, and potassium, are discussed in Chapter 52, Electrolyte Replacement Agents. Iron is discussed in Chapter 41, Hematinic Agents. Other minerals, especially the heavy metals lead, mercury, and arsenic, are nontherapeutic elements that are toxic even in trace amounts. A brief discussion of heavy metals and heavy metal antagonists appears in Appendix 3.

RECOMMENDED DAILY ALLOWANCE (R.D.A.)

In the United States, the Food and Nutrition Board of the National Academy of Sciences establishes recommended daily allowances (RDAs) of nutrients. These RDAs are periodically updated and serve as goals for good nutrition. Other countries have similar boards or committees that assess their populations' requirements.

RDAs are noted in the following discussion of each vitamin. The Food and Drug Administration requires that labels of all vitamin products indicate the amount of the vitamin and the proportion of the RDA each vitamin product provides.

For a summary of representative drugs, see *Selected major drugs: Vitamin and mineral agents* on pages 823 to 825.

VITAMIN A

Vitamin A, a fat-soluble vitamin, is used to prevent and treat vitamin A deficiency. The RDA of vitamin A is 5,000 International Units (IU) for males, 4,000 IU for females, 5,000 IU for pregnant women, and 6,000 IU for lactating women.

History and source
Night blindness was described in Egypt as early as 1500 B.C. Not until the 1800s, however, was this disorder linked to a nutritional deficiency. By 1913, researchers had discovered that some factor contained in egg yolks, butter, and cod-liver oil could be used to treat drying and thickening of the conjunctiva of the eye, a condition known as xerophthalmia. In 1919, Steenbock observed that the vitamin A content of vegetables varied with their degree of pigmentation. This led Euler and associates to discover that the plant pigment carotene was an excellent source of vitamin A. Adults receive about half of their vitamin A from foods containing carotene. In 1931, Karrer and associates determined the structural formula of retinol, the form in which vitamin A exists in animals.

Vitamin A is present in dairy products, liver, egg yolks, fish, and yellow or green fruits and vegetables.

PHARMACOKINETICS

Vitamin A exists as beta carotene, provitamin A, in plants and as the retinyl ester in animals. Both are converted to forms of retinol in the intestines, where they are absorbed.

Absorption, distribution, metabolism, excretion
Physiologic doses of oral vitamin A preparations are readily and completely absorbed from the small intestine in the presence of bile salts, pancreatic lipase, protein, and dietary fat. Absorption is incomplete after the administration of large doses or in persons with fat malabsorption, low protein intake, intestinal infections, and hepatic or pancreatic disease. Absorption of vitamin A occurs via active transport and passive diffusion. Water-miscible preparations of vitamin A are absorbed more rapidly from the GI tract than oil solutions. Retinol is esterified in the intestines primarily to the retinyl pal-

mitate form, which is then carried by lymph to the liver and blood.

Vitamin A, existing as retinyl palmitate, retinol, and retinal, is distributed to and stored primarily in Kupffer's cells in the liver. Lesser amounts are stored in the kidneys, lungs, adrenal glands, retinas, and intraperitoneal fat. Beta carotene is widely distributed in the body and is deposited in skin and body fat. Normal body stores of vitamin A are sufficient to supply body needs for up to 2 years. Vitamin A appears in breast milk, but it does not readily cross the placenta.

Retinal is released from the liver in response to physiologic needs and is transported in the blood bound to retinol-binding protein (RBP). Retinol is metabolized in the liver to a beta glucuronide, which undergoes enterohepatic circulation and oxidation to retinal and retinoic acid. Retinal, retinoic acid, and other water-soluble metabolites are excreted in the urine and feces via bile.

Onset, peak, duration
The onset of action of vitamin A depends on body requirements. In a patient with vitamin A deficiency, administration of vitamin A results in increased concentrations, first in the retinas, then in the liver. Retinal correction does not begin for 2 weeks to 2 months.

Peak plasma concentration levels of retinol esters occur 4 to 5 hours after oral administration of retinol in oil solution; 3 to 4 hours after using water-miscible preparations.

PHARMACODYNAMICS

Vitamin A plays a role in the prevention of night blindness and is essential for growth and development of epithelial tissues, bone growth, human reproduction, and embryonic development. Vitamin A also plays a role in many biochemical reactions, including steroid metabolism and cholesterol synthesis.

Mechanism of action
Vitamin A deficiency interferes with vision in dim light. This condition is known as night blindness, or nyctalopia. Adaptation to dark is a function of chemical reactions occurring within the rods and cones of the retina. During the chemical reactions, photosensitive pigments in the retina initiate a receptor potential, allowing vision to occur. Primary adaptation occurs via the cones and takes place within several minutes. Secondary adaptation is a function of the rods and may take 30 minutes or longer.

A chemical reaction, the adaptation process results in formation of photosensitive pigments in the retina. The rod's photosensitive pigment, called rhodopsin, forms when the protein opsin combines with the vitamin A derivative 11-*cis* retinal. The cone's photosensitive pigment forms when retinal combines with a protein similar to opsin. When these pigments are exposed to light, they undergo a chemical reaction that initiates a receptor potential in the retina, resulting in vision.

Vitamin A is essential for the growth and development of basal epithelial cells, which it stimulates to produce mucus-secreting or keratinizing tissues. Excessive retinol may inhibit keratinization by decreasing the number of mucus-producing goblet cells, leading to epithelial atrophy. The basal epithelial cells will continue to grow even without goblet cells, but the resulting keratinized epithelium is easily irritated and infected.

PHARMACOTHERAPEUTICS

Vitamin A is used primarily to treat vitamin A deficiency, which rarely occurs in well-nourished individuals. Conditions that may lead to this deficiency include biliary tract or pancreatic disease, extreme dietary inadequacy, or malabsorption syndromes. The first step in the treatment of vitamin A deficiency is correction of poor dietary habits. Because vitamin A deficiencies may be accompanied by other vitamin deficiencies, multivitamin preparations are usually administered. The use of water-miscible preparations of vitamin A may be beneficial in patients with GI disorders in which vitamin A absorption may be decreased.

beta carotene (Solatene). This preparation is used to reduce the severity of photosensitivity reactions in patients with erythropoietic protoporphyria, an inherited disorder characterized by production of large amounts of porphyrins (iron- or magnesium-free pyrrole derivatives) in the blood-forming tissue of the bone marrow. Dosage is adjusted according to the severity of symptoms and patient response.
USUAL ADULT DOSAGE: 30 to 300 mg P.O. daily, which may be administered as a single dose or in divided doses, preferably with meals.
USUAL PEDIATRIC DOSAGE: 30 to 150 mg P.O. daily.

isotretinoin (Accutane). A retinoid preparation, isotretinoin is used to treat severe recalcitrant cystic acne by reducing sebum secretions. The dosage should be individualized according to clinical response, adverse reactions, and body weight.
USUAL ADULT DOSAGE: 0.5 to 2 mg/kg/day P.O. in two divided doses for 15 to 20 weeks.

vitamin A (as retinol, retinyl palmitate, or retinyl acetate) (Aquasol A). These preparations are used to prevent and treat symptoms of vitamin A deficiency.

USUAL ADULT DOSAGE: for treatment of severe deficiency with corneal changes, 500,000 IU P.O. for 3 days, followed by 50,000 IU P.O. daily for 2 weeks, then maintenance doses of 10,000 to 20,000 IU P.O. daily for 2 months. For treatment of vitamin A deficiency without corneal changes, 100,000 IU P.O. or I.M. daily for 3 days, then 50,000 IU P.O. or I.M. daily for 14 days, then maintenance doses of 10,000 to 20,000 IU P.O. daily for 2 months. For malabsorption syndromes, parenteral therapy is desired. 50,000 to 100,000 IU may be given I.M. daily for 3 days, followed by 50,000 IU I.M. daily for 2 weeks.
USUAL PEDIATRIC DOSAGE: for children ages 1 to 8, 17,500 to 35,000 IU I.M. daily for 10 days; for children under age 1, 7,500 to 15,000 IU I.M. daily for 10 days; for children over age 8, use adult dosage.

Drug interactions

Vitamin A interacts with mineral oil, resulting in decreased absorption of vitamin A.

ADVERSE DRUG REACTIONS

Because the primary functions of vitamin A relate to vision, development of epithelial tissues, and bone growth, adverse reactions to this drug tend to alter these functions. Changes in liver metabolism are also possible, because the liver is the primary site of vitamin A storage.

Predictable reactions

Most adverse reactions to vitamin A appear to be dose-related. Toxicity, known as hypervitaminosis A, may be acute or chronic; signs of acute toxicity have occurred after administration of very large vitamin A doses over a short time or with a single dose. In adults, this results from doses in the range of 25,000 IU per kilogram.

In adults, chronic toxicity usually results from doses of 4,000 IU per kilogram for 6 to 15 months. Possible manifestations of toxicity include fatigue, malaise, lethargy, abdominal discomfort, anorexia, nausea, and vomiting. Changes in epithelial tissues, including dry itchy skin, dry nose and mouth, inflammation of oral mucous membranes, or hair loss, may appear. Skeletal changes, including thickening of long bones, slowed growth, and migratory bone pain, have also been reported. Signs of increased intracranial pressure, such as headache and irritability, papilledema, and exophthalmos, may occur. Other signs are hypoplastic anemia, a broad category of anemias characterized by decreased red blood cells, and leukopenia, an abnormal decrease in white blood cells. Also, because large amounts of vitamin A accumulate in the liver, an overdose may result in jaundice, hepatomegaly, and a rise in liver enzymes.

Adverse reactions to isotretinoin, a metabolite of vitamin A used to treat acne, are similar to those described on the opposite page. Also, eye irritation, conjunctivitis, and cheilosis (scaly, cracked lips) tend to be prominent. Elevated serum triglyceride levels and photosensitivity may also result from use of this drug. Isotretinoin may also cause fetal abnormalities and should not be used during pregnancy.

Unpredictable reactions

Anaphylactic reactions and shock have occurred after intravenous administration of vitamin A. Parenteral vitamin A should be administered intramuscularly.

NURSING IMPLICATIONS

In addition to knowing the signs and symptoms of vitamin A toxicity, the nurse must be aware of the importance of patient teaching and the following considerations:

• Oral administration of vitamin A is contraindicated in patients with malabsorption syndrome; if malabsorption is the result of inadequate bile secretion, the oral route may be used with concurrent administration of bile salts (dehydrocholic acid). Vitamin A is also contraindicated in patients with hypervitaminosis A.

• Intravenous administration of vitamin A is contraindicated except for special water-miscible forms intended for infusion with large parenteral volumes. Vitamin A should not be administered by I.V. push because anaphylaxis or anaphylactoid reactions and death can result when the drug is administered by this route.

• Monitor the patient's vitamin A intake from fortified foods, dietary supplements, self-administered drugs, and prescription drugs to avoid possible toxicity.

• Instruct the patient to take vitamin A with food, which helps stimulate bile secretion, thereby aiding absorption and reducing nausea.

• Instruct the patient to avoid using mineral oil during vitamin A and other fat-soluble vitamin therapy because it decreases absorption.

• Teach the patient to recognize the signs and symptoms of vitamin A toxicity and to notify the physician if any of these symptoms appear.

• Caution the patient receiving isotretinoin as treatment for a skin disorder to avoid prolonged exposure to sunlight or to use a sunscreen to avoid photosensitivity reactions.

• Caution the pregnant patient not to take doses larger than the RDA (5,000 IU) of vitamin A.

• Stress that the patient should not share prescribed vitamins with family members or friends.

• Instruct the patient to protect vitamin A preparations from light and heat to prevent their deterioration.

• Caution the patient to avoid self-administration of non-prescribed megadoses of vitamin A.

• Teach the patient the food sources of vitamin A. Also teach proper storage procedures to avoid loss of vitamin A; 5% to 10% of vitamin A activity is lost when frozen foods are stored for 12 months at $-23°$ C.

VITAMIN D

Vitamin D is a fat-soluble vitamin with a biologically active form that is also considered a hormone. The main role of vitamin D is aiding in the absorption of ingested calcium from the GI tract. Vitamin D is the name applied to two related substances, cholecalciferol (D_3) and ergocalciferol (D_2). (See Chapter 57, Parathyroid Agents, for a detailed discussion of the vitamin D analogues calcifediol, calcitriol, and dihydrotachysterol as calcium regulators.

Severe nutritional deficiency of vitamin D produces rickets in infants and children. Disturbances in metabolism of vitamin D result in metabolic rickets in children and osteomalacia in adults. Hypophosphatemic vitamin D–resistant rickets is an X-linked inherited disorder of calcium and phosphate metabolism and is not a result of a disturbance in vitamin D metabolism. Vitamin D–dependent rickets is an inherited, autosomal recessive disorder, probably an inborn error of vitamin D metabolism whereby vitamin D is not converted to its active form. Renal osteodystrophy, also called renal rickets, results from chronic renal failure and the inability of the kidneys to convert vitamin D to its active form. The RDA of vitamin D is 200 IU for adults age 23 and older; 400 IU for children and pregnant and lactating women; and 500 IU if pregnant and lactating women are ages 19 to 22.

History and source

The discovery of vitamin D was stimulated by the observation that a significant number of children living in cities, particularly in the temperate zones, developed rickets. By 1920, researchers knew that lack of sunshine and fresh air and a dietary deficiency played a part in the development of this vitamin D deficiency. In 1952, Carlson demonstrated that physiologic doses of vitamin D promote mobilization of calcium from bone. In the mid-1970s, Kodicek, DeLuca, and Schnoes described the vitamin's physiologic metabolism.

DRUG INTERACTIONS
Vitamin D

Drug interactions with vitamin D can lead to decreased vitamin D absorption and, in serious interactions with digitalis glycosides, to cardiac dysrhythmias.

DRUG	INTERACTING DRUGS	POSSIBLE EFFECTS	NURSING IMPLICATIONS
vitamin D	mineral oil	Decreases absorption of vitamin D	• Larger doses of vitamin D may be required in patients who chronically use mineral oil.
	cholestyramine	Decreases absorption of vitamin D by decreasing bile acids	• Separate administration times as far as possible for both agents.
	digitalis glycosides	Produce possible cardiac dysrhythmias related to increased plasma calcium levels	• Monitor the patient's pulse rate and EKG.

Vitamin D is synthesized in the skin by sunlight and is also present in fortified milk and margarine.

PHARMACOKINETICS

Vitamin D taken orally is readily absorbed from the GI tract in the presence of bile. Traveling in the blood bound to protein, vitamin D is stored mostly in fat and muscle, metabolized in the liver and kidney, and excreted via bile in feces. A small amount is excreted in urine.

Absorption, distribution, metabolism, excretion

Oral vitamin D is readily absorbed from the small intestine in the presence of bile. Vitamin D_3 may be absorbed more rapidly and completely than vitamin D_2. GI absorption is reduced in the presence of hepatic or biliary disease and malabsorption syndromes.

Absorbed vitamin D circulates in the blood with vitamin D–binding protein. This protein is an alphaglobulin, specific for vitamin D. Vitamin D is stored primarily in fat and muscle. Although the plasma half-life is only 9 to 25 hours, vitamin D is stored in fat for prolonged periods of time.

Vitamin D is metabolized in the liver and kidneys. Ultraviolet light from the sun converts plant and animal steroidlike substances (sterols) to provitamin D. Vitamin D is converted into active metabolites in the liver and further metabolized in the kidneys to even more active metabolites.

Excretion of vitamin D occurs primarily in the feces via bile; a small amount is excreted in urine.

Onset, peak, duration

After oral or I.M. administration of natural vitamin D, the onset of action is 10 to 24 hours. Peak concentration levels occur about 4 weeks after daily administration of a fixed dose, and the duration of action of the drug can be 2 months or longer.

PHARMACODYNAMICS

Active forms of vitamin D maintain calcium and phosphorus homeostasis in humans primarily by facilitating their absorption, enhancing their mobilization from bone, and decreasing their renal excretion. (See also Chapter 57, Parathyroid Agents, for actions of vitamin D in calcium regulation.)

Mechanism of action

Low serum calcium or phosphorus levels lead to the release of parathyroid hormone from the parathyroid gland. This hormone, as well as estrogen and prolactin, may increase the activity of enzymes in the kidneys that facilitate conversion of vitamin D to its active forms, 1,25-dihydroxyergocalciferol and calcitriol. Active vitamin D increases the gastrointestinal absorption of calcium and phosphorus from the jejunum and enhances the mobilization of calcium and phosphorus from bone. Active vitamin D also increases urinary retention of calcium and phosphorus by enhancing proximal tubular reabsorption of these substances. Thus, calcium and phosphorus are maintained at plasma concentration levels necessary for normal neuromuscular activity, bone mineralization, and other calcium-dependent functions.

PHARMACOTHERAPEUTICS

Vitamin D is most frequently used as a dietary supplement. Nutritional rickets results from a lack of exposure to sunlight or a vitamin D–deficient diet. Because ergocalciferol is added to milk in the United States, rickets rarely occurs. Therefore, vitamin D is required as a supplement only in certain circumstances, as in persons with malabsorption syndrome, in breast-fed and premature infants, and in individuals receiving fewer than 10 mcg daily from food.

Patients with vitamin D–dependent rickets usually respond best to calcitriol (one of the vitamin D analogues).

Ergocalciferol and dihydrotachysterol have been used with oral calcium therapy to treat osteoporosis. However, further studies are needed to determine the efficacy of vitamin D therapy in osteoporosis.

cholecalciferol, or vitamin D₃. This vitamin is used as a dietary supplement and for treatment or prophylaxis of vitamin D deficiency.
USUAL ADULT DOSAGE: 400 to 1,000 IU P.O. daily or every other day. Dosage can be increased as needed every 4 weeks.

ergocalciferol, or vitamin D₂ (Calciferol). This vitamin is used to treat patients with familial hypophosphatemia (vitamin D–resistant rickets).
USUAL ADULT DOSAGE: for familial hypophosphatemia, 50,000 to 500,000 IU P.O. or I.M. daily; for hypoparathyroidism, 50,000 to 200,000 IU P.O. or I.M. daily; for renal osteodystrophy, 20,000 IU P.O. or I.M. daily. Calcitriol and calcifediol (vitamin D analogues) have also been used, because they function to a degree without being renally metabolized. If renal dysfunction becomes severe, dihydrotachysterol may be the drug of choice because it does not require renal conversion to the active form. For osteomalacia and rickets caused by dietary deficiency of vitamin D, 1,000 to 5,000 IU P.O. or I.M. daily.
USUAL PEDIATRIC DOSAGE: for vitamin D deficiency, 1,000 to 4,000 IU P.O. daily; for hypoparathyroidism, 50,000 to 200,000 IU P.O. daily.

Patients receiving long-term phenobarbital or phenytoin anticonvulsant therapy may develop low plasma concentrations of vitamin D and calcium. Rickets or osteomalacia rarely develop in these patients. If either occurs, treatment with ergocalciferol helps reverse the disorder. Some physicians use ergocalciferol prophylaxis for patients on long-term anticonvulsant therapy.

Drug interactions
Drugs that interact with vitamin D frequently do so by decreasing the absorption of vitamin D or by interacting with an altered state of homeostasis which may result from large doses of Vitamin D. (See *Drug Interactions: Vitamin D* for a discussion of these interactions.)

ADVERSE DRUG REACTIONS

As with other fat-soluble vitamins, vitamin D is stored in the body, and excessive ingestion over time can produce toxicity. The range between therapeutic and toxic levels is narrow. Hypercalcemia, hypercalciuria, and hyperphosphatemia can result from vitamin D overdose and are responsible for many of the adverse reactions reported. Similar toxicity occurs if vitamin D is administered with high doses of calcium and phosphorus. Maintenance of normal serum calcium and phosphorus levels, however, does not ensure the absence of adverse effects.

Predictable reactions
High doses of vitamin D stimulate increased absorption of calcium and phosphorus from the GI tract and increase mobilization of calcium and phosphorus from bone. If serum levels of calcium and phosphorus rise to a particularly critical level in relation to each other, calcium phosphate precipitates and calcification of soft tissues results. The kidneys, heart, muscles, blood vessels, eyes, and lungs may be affected. This can result in renal insufficiency with polyuria, hypertension, dysrhythmias, muscle pain, renal calculi, and conjunctivitis. Demineralization of bone can result in bone pain and osteoporosis in adults and growth retardation in children.

Other reactions associated with vitamin D toxicity include nausea, vomiting, anorexia, headache, weakness, and diarrhea or constipation. Elevations of serum glutamic-oxaloacetic transaminase (SGOT) and serum glutamic-pyruvic transaminase (SGPT) levels may also occur. Increased SGOT levels may indicate general cellular damage; increased SGPT levels, liver damage.

Unpredictable reactions
Some vitamin D preparations contain tartrazine. Individuals susceptible to this ingested chemical may develop an allergic response.

NURSING IMPLICATIONS

High doses of vitamin D should be administered only under the direction and supervision of a physician, and the nurse must be aware of the following implications, especially the importance of patient teaching.

• Vitamin D is contraindicated in patients with vitamin D toxicity, hypercalcemia, and renal osteodystrophy with hyperphosphatemia.

• Administer vitamin D cautiously to patients receiving digitalis preparations because hypercalcemia may precipitate cardiac dysrhythmias.

• During therapy, frequently monitor serum and urine calcium levels and serum levels of phosphorus, magnesium, blood urea nitrogen (BUN) and alkaline phosphatase. The product of serum calcium and serum phosphorus levels (serum calcium level multiplied by serum phosphorus level) should remain below 70 to avoid calcification of soft tissue. A decrease in the serum level of alkaline phosphatase usually precedes hypercalcemia.

• Before administering vitamin D containing tartrazine, inquire about tartrazine or aspirin hypersensitivity. Patients who are aspirin-sensitive frequently have a sensitivity to tartrazine as well. The sensitive patient should receive a test dose or another product. Monitor the patient closely for signs and symptoms of an allergic reaction.

• Monitor the patient's eating and bowel habits; dry mouth, nausea, vomiting, metallic taste, and diarrhea or constipation can be early signs of toxicity.

• Before vitamin D therapy begins, evaluate the patient's usual patterns of diet and exposure to sunlight to avoid overadministration: foods, such as milk and cereals, are fortified with vitamin D; sunlight is also a source of vitamin D. Monitor the diet to ensure that the patient obtains sufficient amounts of calcium to enhance the effectiveness of vitamin D.

• Caution the patient to take vitamin D with food whenever possible to prevent gastrointestinal adverse reactions and to promote better absorption.

• If the I.V. route is necessary, use only water-miscible solutions intended for dilution in large-volume parenteral fluids.

• Teach the patient the signs and symptoms of hypercalcemia and the importance of reporting them to the physician.

• Caution women age 23 and older not to exceed the RDA (400 IU) during pregnancy or lactation. Higher doses in children have not been demonstrated to be safe.

• Advise the patient that these vitamins are potent drugs that can be toxic to anyone for whom they were not prescribed.

VITAMIN E

Vitamin E is a fat-soluble vitamin whose exact functions, mechanisms of action, and nutritional significance remain unclear. Chemically, vitamin E is alpha-tocopherol, one of three tocopherols present in wheat germ oil, egg yolk, cereals, and beef liver.

Studies have shown that vitamin E deficiency in animals has various effects on the reproductive, nervous, muscular, cardiovascular, and hematopoietic systems. However, little evidence indicates that deficiency produces these same effects in humans. Therefore, no absolute daily requirement of vitamin E has been established; however, the RDAs are 15 IU for adult males, 12 IU for adult females, 4 to 6 IU for infants up to 1 year, 7 to 10 IU for children over 1 year, 15 IU for pregnant females, and 16 IU for lactating females.

History and source

The first evidence of the existence of vitamin E resulted from studies by Evans and Bishop in 1922. Their work suggested that female rats fed a deficient diet were unable to carry a pregnancy to term. The responsible agent remained a mystery until work by Evans led to the isolation of the vitamin in 1936.

Vitamin E is present in vegetable oils, margarine, milk, eggs, meat, green leafy vegetables, whole grains, and animal fats.

PHARMACOKINETICS

Vitamin E, a fat-soluble vitamin that exhibits poor absorption and wide distribution, is metabolized in the liver and excreted via the bile.

Absorption, distribution, metabolism, excretion

The absorption of vitamin E from the GI tract depends on the presence of bile. Only 20% to 60% of the vitamin obtained from dietary sources is absorbed. As the dosage of vitamin E increases, the fraction of vitamin E absorbed decreases. Water-miscible preparations are better absorbed than oil solutions.

After absorption, vitamin E is incorporated into lymphatic chylomicrons, which are then transported to the systemic circulation. Vitamin E circulates attached to beta-lipoproteins. It is widely distributed to all tissues and is stored in adipose tissue. Total body stores of vitamin E are estimated at 3 to 8 grams, which will meet the body's requirements for 4 years or more even if the diet is deficient in vitamin E. Placental transfer of vitamin

E is incomplete, and neonates have low plasma tocopherol levels.

Vitamin E is metabolized in the liver. Excretion occurs via bile in feces, and small amounts of the metabolite are excreted in urine as glucuronides.

Information on onset of action, peak concentration levels, and duration of action is not available.

PHARMACODYNAMICS

Vitamin E exists in foods as alpha-, beta-, delta-, and gamma-tocopherols and tocotrienols. The most biologically active form is d-alpha-tocopherol.

Mechanism of action
The exact biological function of vitamin E in humans is unknown. Vitamin E may act as an antioxidant, protecting fatty acids and other oxygen-sensitive substances, such as vitamin A and ascorbic acid, from oxidation. (The oxidation process uses oxygen to chemically alter a substance by freeing electrons, which results in energy production and an increased positive charge on the substance.) Vitamin E may also play a role in decreasing platelet aggregation.

PHARMACOTHERAPEUTICS

Because vitamin E is abundant in normal diets, deficiency of this vitamin does not normally occur. Deficiencies may occur in persons with abetalipoproteinemia, abnormal fat absorption, or malabsorption syndromes. The only established use for vitamin E is for the treatment or prevention of vitamin E deficiency.

vitamin E (Aquasol E, Solucap E). Usually administered orally, the drug may be given I.M. when oral administration is not possible or malabsorption is suspected. Vitamin E should not be given intravenously. Water-miscible oral vitamin E preparations are preferred in patients with malabsorption syndromes.

Because the potencies of the several forms of vitamin E vary, dosages are standardized into International Units, based on activity. For example, 1 mg of *dl*-alpha-tocopheryl acetate equals 1 IU, whereas 1 mg of *d*-alpha-tocopherol is 1.49 IU.

Free tocopherols may be oxidized and destroyed when exposed to air and light. The ester and the acetate and succinate forms are stable in light and air.
USUAL ADULT DOSAGE: to treat vitamin E deficiency, 60 to 75 IU P.O. or I.M. daily; to prevent vitamin E deficiency, 30 IU P.O. daily with other vitamins.
USUAL PEDIATRIC DOSAGE: 5 IU P.O. daily to prevent vitamin E deficiency in premature, low-birth weight neonates.

Drug interactions
Drugs that interact with vitamin E generally do so by decreasing the absorption of the vitamin. Mineral oil and cholestyramine, for example, may decrease vitamin E absorption. Large doses of vitamin E may increase the anticoagulant effects of warfarin by interfering with the synthesis of vitamin K–dependent clotting factors.

ADVERSE DRUG REACTIONS

Vitamin E tends to be a relatively nontoxic drug when administered within established dosing guidelines. As with the other fat-soluble vitamins, large doses can result in toxicity.

Predictable reactions
Doses of vitamin E above 300 IU per day have resulted in various adverse reactions. Gastrointestinal symptoms, such as nausea, diarrhea, and abdominal cramping, tend to predominate. Fatigue, weakness, headache, blurred vision, and rash have also been reported after vitamin E administration.

Vitamin E has been linked to increases in serum cholesterol and triglyceride levels and to decreases in serum thyroxine and triiodothyronine levels. Increases in urinary estrogen and androgen levels have also been noted.

Unpredictable reactions
At least two non-dose-related adverse reactions have been linked to vitamin E. Sterile abscesses have been documented after intramuscular injection of vitamin E; for this reason, the oral route is preferred. Hair regrowth that is white has been reported after oral administration of vitamin E for skin disorders with associated alopecia.

NURSING IMPLICATIONS

Vitamin E is readily available in the foods in normal diets, so deficiency of this vitamin is unusual. Numerous claims have been made of the benefits of vitamin E therapy for reversing some of the effects of aging; however, no conclusive evidence indicates that this vitamin is beneficial in any human disorder except vitamin E deficiency. Therefore, patient teaching is critical, especially since this drug can be purchased without a prescription.
● Caution the patient about the potential adverse effects of self-medication with high doses of vitamin E.
● Instruct the patient to store vitamin E in a cool, dark place.

VITAMIN K

Vitamin K, a fat-soluble vitamin, is essential for the normal biosynthesis of several factors required for blood clotting.

Vitamin K deficiency can result from inadequate intake, lack of absorption or utilization of the vitamin by the body, or from the actions of a vitamin K antagonist, such as warfarin. The RDAs have not been officially established.

History and source

Initial work leading to the discovery of vitamin K is attributed to Dam. In 1929, his studies of chickens fed a deficient diet described a state characterized by low prothrombin levels and bleeding. Further research by Dam and associates in 1935 and 1936 demonstrated that this condition could be rapidly corrected by the administration of an unidentified fat-soluble substance, which Dam called vitamin K. At about the same time, other researchers were observing prothrombin deficiencies and bleeding in patients with biliary tract disease. This led to the discovery in 1938 that the administration of vitamin K along with bile salts could effectively treat coagulation problems in individuals with jaundice.

Vitamin K as phytonadione (vitamin K_1) is present in liver, cheese, eggs, green leafy vegetables, tomatoes, meat, milk, and vegetable oils.

PHARMACOKINETICS

Vitamin K is absorbed from the GI tract and concentrates in the liver immediately after absorption. Metabolism occurs in the liver, and metabolites are excreted in bile and urine.

Absorption, distribution, metabolism, excretion

Phytonadione (vitamin K_1) and menaquinone (vitamin K_2) are absorbed from the GI tract only in the presence of bile. Absorption is an energy-requiring process occurring in the proximal small intestine. Menadione (vitamin K_3), a synthetic product, is no longer commercially available. However, menadiol sodium diphosphate, a synthetic water-soluble derivative of menadione, is available. It is absorbed in the absence of bile, by diffusion in the distal portions of the small intestine and colon. After I.M. injection, phytonadione is readily absorbed.

After absorption, phytonadione is concentrated in the liver, where it is metabolized to water-soluble metabolites. Only small amounts of phytonadione are stored in body tissues. Vitamin K crosses the placenta to a limited extent but is secreted in breast milk.

Excretion of phytonadione occurs via bile and urine. A high fecal concentration level of vitamin K results from intestinal bacterial synthesis of the vitamin.

Onset, peak, duration

Blood coagulation factors may increase in 6 to 12 hours after oral administration of phytonadione and in 1 to 2 hours after parenteral administration. Bleeding may be controlled in 3 to 8 hours, and a normal prothrombin time may be obtained 12 to 14 hours after parenteral administration. The onset of action of parenteral menadiol sodium diphosphate may require 8 to 24 hours.

PHARMACODYNAMICS

Synthesis of vitamin K occurs by bacteria in the intestinal tract. The body uses vitamin K to synthesize clotting factors and maintain hemostasis.

Mechanism of action

Vitamin K_1, or phytonadione, is the only natural vitamin K available for therapeutic use. Vitamin K_2, or menaquinone, is the vitamin K produced by gram-positive bacteria in the intestines; menadiol sodium diphosphate, is a synthetic form of vitamin K.

In normal individuals, phytonadione has no pharmacodynamic activity. In persons deficient in vitamin K, exogenous administration of phytonadione will promote the hepatic synthesis of vitamin K-dependent clotting factors. These include prothrombin (Factor II), proconvertin (Factor VII), plasma thromboplastin component (PTC, Christmas factor, or Factor IX), and the Stuart factor (Factor X).

Vitamin K–dependent clotting factors remain as inactive precursors in the liver in the absence of vitamin K or in the presence of coumarin-type anticoagulants. Vitamin K is an essential cofactor in activating these precursors. This is done by conversion of multiple peptide-bound residues of glutamic acid to gamma-carboxyglutamic acid in the completed precursor protein. This protein can then bind calcium, a necessary event for clot formation.

PHARMACOTHERAPEUTICS

Vitamin K is used to prevent and treat hypoprothrombinemia secondary to vitamin K deficiency. Although vitamin K is the drug of choice for impending or actual hemorrhage, its long onset of action may necessitate the use of fresh frozen plasma or whole blood in an acute situation.

Vitamin K is also used to treat anticoagulant-induced hypoprothrombinemia. Phytonadione is the drug of choice for treating a moderate to severe hemorrhage caused by excessive doses of coumarin or indanedione anticoagulants. Menadiol sodium diphosphate is less effective in treating anticoagulant-induced hypoprothrombinemia. Vitamin K derivatives do not antagonize the effects of heparin. Excessive dosages of phytonadione leading to normal prothrombin times may restore the condition that originally required administration of oral anticoagulant therapy. (See Chapter 42, Anticoagulant Agents, for more details about anticoagulants.)

Phytonadione is the drug of choice for treating and preventing hemorrhagic disease in newborns. For several days after birth, newborns may be hypoprothrombinemic secondary to vitamin K deficiency. Menadiol sodium diphosphate can produce anemia, hyperbilirubinemia, kernicterus, and death in newborns and should not be used. Phytonadione is also effective in preventing neonatal hemorrhage resulting from anticonvulsants used during pregnancy.

Other causes of hypoprothrombinemia, such as malabsorption syndromes and drug therapy with salicylates, sulfonamides, quinine, quinidine, or broad-spectrum antibiotics, are also treated with phytonadione, which is more effective than synthetic vitamin K. Patients with hepatocellular damage may not be able to produce vitamin K-dependent clotting factors even in the presence of excessive vitamin K.

menadiol sodium diphosphate (Synkayvite). This drug is a synthetic, water-soluble form of vitamin K_3 that may be administered orally or by subcutaneous, I.M., or I.V. routes. I.M. or S.C. administration may be contraindicated in patients with hypoprothrombinemia because hemorrhage or hematoma may develop.
USUAL ADULT DOSAGE: for hypoprothrombinemia secondary to obstructive jaundice and biliary fistulas, 5 mg P.O. daily; for bleeding secondary to drug therapy, 5 to 10 mg P.O. daily. If the parenteral route is required, 5 to 15 mg may be given one or two times daily.

phytonadione (AquaMEPHYTON, Konakion, Mephyton). This drug is a derivative identical to the naturally occurring vitamin K_1. Although both forms may be given orally or intramuscularly, only AquaMEPHYTON may also be given subcutaneously or intravenously. I.M. or S.C. administration may be contraindicated in patients with hypoprothrombinemia because hemorrhage or hematoma may develop.

AquaMEPHYTON administered I.V. should be given at a rate not to exceed 1 mg/minute, and slower rates may be safer. The drug should always be diluted in D_5W, 0.9% saline solution, or dextrose 5% in normal saline solution. Never give AquaMEPHYTON undiluted by I.V. push. The I.V. route should be restricted for use with those patients for whom other routes are not feasible and the serious risk is justified.
USUAL ADULT DOSAGE: for anticoagulant-induced hypoprothrombinemia, 2.5 to 10 mg P.O., I.M., S.C., or I.V. Use the lowest dose possible so refractoriness to further anticoagulant treatment is minimized. If the initial response is not satisfactory, the dose may be repeated in 12 to 48 hours after an oral dose, or 6 to 8 hours after a parenteral dose. For hypoprothrombinemia secondary to other causes, 2 to 25 mg P.O., I.M., or S.C. Doses larger than 25 mg are rarely required, and 10 mg will usually suffice. For prevention of hypoprothrombinemia associated with vitamin K deficiency in patients on prolonged total parenteral nutrition (TPN), 5 to 10 mg I.M. weekly.
USUAL PEDIATRIC DOSAGE: for hemorrhagic disease of the newborn, 0.5 to 1 mg I.M. or S.C. Higher doses may be needed if mother was taking anticoagulants or anticonvulsants during pregnancy.

Drug interactions

Vitamin K antagonizes the effect of coumarin and indanedione anticoagulants by increasing the synthesis of vitamin K–dependent clotting factors.

ADVERSE DRUG REACTIONS

In most cases, vitamin K is relatively nontoxic when administered in the usual adult dosages. Most adverse reactions occur after parenteral administration. Severe hypersensitivity-like reactions have occurred after oral and parenteral administration.

Predictable reactions

The adverse reactions to vitamin K administration primarily depend on the route of administration. Nausea, vomiting, and headache may occur with oral administration. Rapid parenteral administration may lead to transient flushing and, occasionally, dizziness, rapid and weak pulse, transient hypotension, dyspnea, cyanosis, or chest pain. Slow I.V. administration should help prevent these reactions.

Infants may develop hyperbilirubinemia and jaundice with parenteral administration of phytonadione. This is particularly a problem in premature infants.

Unpredictable reactions

Allergic responses may occur after vitamin K administration. These reactions can range from skin rashes and urticaria to severe and sometimes fatal anaphylactic reactions. Shock and cardiac or respiratory arrest have occurred with parenteral administration despite adequate dilution and slow administration.

NURSING IMPLICATIONS

Although vitamin K is relatively nontoxic when administered in therapeutic doses, this drug has important nursing implications.

• Menadiol sodium diphosphate is contraindicated in patients with hereditary hypoprothrombinemia, because vitamin K can paradoxically worsen it; hepatocellular disease, unless it is caused by biliary obstruction; and heparin-induced bleeding.

• Phytonadione is contraindicated in patients with hereditary hypoprothrombinemia because vitamin K can paradoxically worsen the hypoprothrombinemia; bleeding secondary to heparin therapy or overdose; and hepatocellular disease, unless it is caused by biliary obstruction. Oral administration is contraindicated if bile secretion is inadequate, unless supplemented with bile salts.

• Administer phytonadione cautiously, if at all, to patients with glucose-6-phosphate dehydrogenase deficiency to avoid hemolysis. Also administer large doses cautiously to those with severe hepatic disease.

• Safe usage during pregnancy has not been established. Small amounts of vitamin K cross the placenta. These drugs are particularly contraindicated during the last weeks of pregnancy. Phytonadione is preferred over menadiol sodium diphosphate in premature infants because of the risk of hemolytic anemia and hyperbilirubinemia.

• Be aware that severe adverse reactions may result from I.V. administration of AquaMEPHYTON, particularly if it is given rapidly. This route is reserved for situations in which rapid correction of hypoprothrombinemia is necessary. If this drug must be given intravenously, be careful to dilute it according to the manufacturer's guidelines and to administer it very slowly, never faster than 1 mg/minute. Observe the patient closely for signs of allergic reactions, and notify the physician immediately if they appear. Be prepared to intervene should hypotension, bronchospasm, or cardiac or respiratory arrest occur.

• Be aware that improvement in prothrombin time takes at least 1 to 2 hours after parenteral administration and 6 to 12 hours after oral administration of phytonadione, and 8 to 24 hours after parenteral administration of menadiol sodium diphosphate. Normal prothrombin levels usually occur in 12 to 14 hours after parenteral adminsitration of phytonadione. Monitor the patient for continued bleeding, as indicated by hematuria, oozing around I.V. catheters, petechiae, and bruising or bleeding from mucous membranes, until prothrombin times

return to normal. Apply pressure to control bleeding after I.M. administration.

• Monitor bilirubin levels in neonates receiving vitamin K.

• Caution the patient to take oral vitamin K with food to promote absorption and decrease nausea.

• Instruct patients receiving oral vitamin K for vitamin K deficiency to increase their dietary intake of vitamin K to decrease the risk of developing an ongoing deficiency.

• Store parenteral products in light-resistant containers.

THIAMINE (VITAMIN B₁)

Deficiency of thiamine, a B-complex vitamin, produces a form of polyneuritis known as beriberi. The RDA of this water-soluble vitamin is 1.4 mg for adult males and 1 mg for adult females. Pregnant women require 1.4 mg and lactating women require 1.5 mg.

History and source

In the 19th century, rice mills that removed the vitamin-containing husks to produce polished rice were introduced. As a result, beriberi increased in cultures that depended on rice as the mainstay of their diet.

Admiral Takaki of the Japanese navy is credited with demonstrating the relationship between beriberi and a dietary deficiency. In 1880, he changed the standard Japanese navy diet of rice to one that contained fish, meat, grains, and vegetables. This led to a reduction of the incidence of the disease in sailors. The first scientific evidence of the relationship between beriberi and nutritional deficiencies came in 1897, when Eijkman, a Dutch physician, produced a syndrome similar to beriberi in fowl by feeding them a diet of polished rice. He reversed this disorder by returning the rice husks to their diet. In 1911, Funk isolated the active factor and placed it in a new class of dietary substances, which he called "vitamines." The chemical structure of thiamine, the first identified B-complex vitamin, was later reidentified by Williams in 1936.

Thiamine is present in yeast, legumes, nuts, pork, organ meats, and whole grain and enriched cereals and breads.

PHARMACOKINETICS

Readily absorbed orally, thiamine is widely distributed into body tissues, metabolized in the liver, and excreted in the urine.

Absorption, distribution, metabolism, excretion

After administration of small oral doses, thiamine is readily absorbed. Absorption occurs through sodium-dependent active transport and is usually limited to 8 to 15 mg per day. At high concentrations, passive diffusion also occurs. Absorption may be improved by giving divided doses with food. Rapid and complete absorption occurs with I.M. administration.

Thiamine is widely distributed into body tissues. Body stores equal about 30 mg, and about 1 mg is lost each day from this supply. The body stores equal about 3 weeks' supply of the body's thiamine requirements.

Thiamine undergoes extensive metabolism in the liver.

With physiologic doses, little or no thiamine is excreted unchanged in the urine. With large doses, unchanged thiamine and its metabolites are excreted in the urine after tissue stores are saturated.

Onset, peak, duration

Exact information about thiamine's onset of action, peak concentration levels, and duration of action is not available. However, thiamine replacement usually produces rapid improvement in patients with thiamine deficiency.

PHARMACODYNAMICS

Thiamine plays an important part in carbohydrate metabolism by acting as a coenzyme. However, it shows no pharmacodynamic activity when given in therapeutic doses to normal individuals.

Mechanism of action

Thiamine combines with adenosine triphosphate (ATP) to form thiamine pyrophosphate, the active form of vitamin B_1. Thiamine pyrophosphate acts as a coenzyme in carbohydrate metabolism.

Related to metabolic rate, thiamine requirements increase as carbohydrate use increases. This may be important in patients maintained on TPN, who receive most of their calories as dextrose.

Thiamine may also modulate neuromuscular transmission.

PHARMACOTHERAPEUTICS

Thiamine is used primarily to prevent and treat thiamine deficiency syndromes, such as beriberi, Wernicke's en-

cephalopathy, and peripheral neuritis associated with pellagra. Alcoholics deficient in thiamine may exhibit Wernicke's encephalopathy and Korsakoff's psychosis. Beriberi can lead to cardiac failure. Wernicke's encephalopathy and cardiac failure are medical emergencies.

Malabsorption of thiamine may occur in patients with alcoholism, cirrhosis, or GI disease, necessitating supplementation. Increased thiamine requirements may be associated with pregnancy, increased physical activity, hyperthyroidism, infection, and hepatic disease. Because normal carbohydrate metabolism increases thiamine metabolism, administration of glucose may precipitate symptoms of thiamine deficiency. However, because of increased intake of dietary thiamine or thiamine supplements, thiamine deficiency is rarely noted in these cases.

thiamine, or vitamin B_1 (Betaline S, Thia). This vitamin may be given orally, intramuscularly, or intravenously. USUAL ADULT DOSAGE: 5 to 30 mg P.O. daily as a dietary supplement. Beriberi with cardiac failure (wet beriberi) is an emergency and should be treated with 30 mg I.V. t.i.d. Beriberi alone may be treated with 10 to 20 mg I.M. t.i.d. for 2 weeks. Oral multivitamin preparations with 5 to 10 mg of thiamine should be given daily for 1 month. For Wernicke's encephalopathy, 100 mg I.V. daily may be given.

Drug interactions

Thiamine has been reported to enhance the effect of neuromuscular blocking agents. The clinical significance of this interaction is unknown.

ADVERSE DRUG REACTIONS

In most cases, thiamine administration does not result in adverse reactions or toxicity. Because excess amounts are excreted in the urine, overdose cannot occur. Those adverse reactions which have been reported occur rarely and seem to be non-dose-related.

Unpredictable reactions

Various nonspecific reactions have been reported with thiamine administration, including nausea, anxiety, sweating, and sensations of warmth. Allergic reactions have also occurred with parenteral administration, ranging from itching and urticaria to cardiovascular failure and death.

NURSING IMPLICATIONS

Thiamine is relatively nontoxic, but the nurse should be aware of the following implications:

• Thiamine is contraindicated in patients with hypersensitivity to thiamine products. Administration by I.V. push is contraindicated, except when treating life-threatening cardiac failure in wet beriberi. Give I.V. doses slowly. Patients with a history of hypersensitivity should receive a skin test before therapy. Have epinephrine on hand to treat anaphylaxis should it occur after administration of a large parenteral dose.

• Do not administer thiamine with alkaline solutions (carbonates, citrates) because it is unstable.

• Teach the patient that thiamine is readily available and well absorbed from many grains, fresh vegetables, nuts, pork, beef and liver. Encourage patients with thiamine deficiency to increase their dietary intake of these foods.

• Teach patients requiring doses of thiamine above 15 mg per day to take the vitamin in divided doses with food.

• Teach pregnant patients and those who have hyperthyroidism, an infection, or hepatic disease or who increase physical activity or carbohydrate intake to be alert to the need for increased amounts of thiamine.

• As with all water-soluble vitamins, thiamine should be stored in a cool, dark place. Because potency tends to diminish rapidly, teach the patient to check expiration dates and to avoid purchasing more than a 3-month supply.

RIBOFLAVIN (VITAMIN B₂)

Ariboflavinosis, vitamin B_2 deficiency, rarely occurs in the United States. The RDA for water-soluble riboflavin is 1.6 mg for adult males, 1.2 mg for adult females, 1.5 mg for pregnant females and 1.7 mg for lactating females.

History and source
The history of riboflavin dates to 1879, when the name "flavin" was assigned to a family of yellow-pigmented substances. Its existence became clearer when research with "vitamin B" demonstrated two separate substances: a heat-labile factor, which was effective against beriberi, and a heat-stable factor, which was growth-promoting. Later research determined that this factor had a yellow color when concentrated. In 1932, Warburg and Christian identified an enzyme in yeast with a yellow color. In 1933, the yellow pigment of the enzyme was identified as riboflavin.

Riboflavin is present in milk, cheese, organ meats, eggs, green leafy vegetables, and whole grain and enriched cereals and breads.

PHARMACOKINETICS
Riboflavin is readily absorbed from the upper GI tract after oral administration. It is widely distributed throughout the body and is metabolized in GI mucosal cells, red blood cells, and the liver. Elimination is via the urine and feces.

Absorption, distribution, metabolism, excretion
GI absorption increases when riboflavin is taken with food and decreases in patients with hepatitis, cirrhosis, or biliary obstruction.

Riboflavin, as flavin-adenine dinucleotide (FAD) and flavin mononucleotide (FMN), is widely distributed to body tissues. Riboflavin is stored in limited amounts in the liver, spleen, kidneys, and heart, mostly as FAD. It crosses the placenta and appears in breast milk.

Riboflavin is metabolized to FMN in GI mucosal cells, red blood cells, and the liver. FMN is metabolized to FAD in the liver.

About 9% of a physiologic dose of riboflavin will appear in the urine. The fate of the remainder of the vitamin dose is unknown. Doses above the minimum requirement result in larger amounts excreted unchanged in the urine. Riboflavin also appears in the feces, probably as a result of synthesis by intestinal bacteria.

Onset, peak, duration
The half-life of riboflavin is 66 to 84 minutes after oral or I.M. administration of a single dose.

PHARMACODYNAMICS
Riboflavin, a water-soluble B-complex vitamin, plays an important role in tissue respiration.

Mechanism of action
Humans require an exogenous source of riboflavin. Some riboflavin is produced by intestinal bacteria, but this is not absorbed systemically.

FMN and FAD are the active forms of riboflavin. Functioning as coenzymes, they work with respiratory flavoproteins, which are involved in the metabolism of organic substrates used in tissue respiration. Riboflavin also helps maintain erythrocyte integrity.

PHARMACOTHERAPEUTICS

Riboflavin is used to prevent and treat riboflavin deficiency, which is rarely severe in humans but frequently mild. Such deficiency is characterized by digestive disturbances, burning sensations of the skin and eyes, inflammation and cracking at the corners of the mouth (cheilosis), inflammation of the tongue (glossitis), headache, scaly dermatitis around the nose, mental depression, and forgetfulness.

riboflavin, or vitamin B₂. This drug is used to prevent or treat riboflavin deficiency.
USUAL ADULT DOSAGE: as a dietary supplement, 1 to 4 mg P.O. daily; in deficiency states, 5 to 30 mg P.O. daily. Ocular and dermatologic manifestations may improve within several days.
USUAL PEDIATRIC DOSAGE: in deficiency states, 3 to 10 mg P.O., S.C., I.M., or I.V. daily.

Drug interactions

Propantheline and other anticholinergic drugs may increase the amount of riboflavin absorbed when taken concomitantly.

ADVERSE DRUG REACTIONS

Riboflavin is considered nontoxic. Despite the administration of large quantities of the vitamin, no adverse reactions have been reported. This may be related to its short half-life in the body and the rapid excretion of excess amounts in the urine.

NURSING IMPLICATIONS

Although riboflavin is nontoxic, the nurse must be aware of some important implications.
• Inform the patient that riboflavin colors the urine bright yellow. This may interfere with urinalysis based on spectrometry methods or color reactions.
• Teach the patient with riboflavin deficiency to increase the dietary intake of riboflavin-rich foods, such as milk, meats, eggs, nuts, and green vegetables. To preserve this water-soluble vitamin, foods that require cooking in water should be steamed or prepared in the smallest amount of water possible and covered during cooking.
• Instruct the patient to take oral riboflavin with food to improve absorption.
• Be alert to the potential need for increased amounts of riboflavin in patients with liver disease, such as hepatitis, cirrhosis, or biliary tract obstruction.
• Advise the patient to store the drug in a light-resistant container.

NICOTINIC ACID, NIACIN (VITAMIN B₃)

Nicotinic acid, also called niacin or vitamin B₃, is a water-soluble vitamin. *Niacin* was introduced as a term for this vitamin to avoid confusing the vitamin with nicotine, an alkaloid. Deficiency of this vitamin results in pellagra. The RDA of nicotinic acid is 18 mg for adult males, 13 mg for adult females, 15 mg for pregnant females, and 18 mg for lactating females.

History and source

The identification of nicotinic acid began in 1914, when Funk suggested that the disease pellagra might be related to a nutritional deficiency, which was later confirmed by the studies of Goldberger and associates. They produced a syndrome similar to pellagra in dogs fed a deficient diet and then reversed it by correcting those deficiencies. In 1935, Warburg and associates isolated nicotinic acid amide (nicotinamide) from a coenzyme in equine red blood cells. In 1937, Elvehjem and associates identified nicotinamide as the factor responsible for the effectiveness of liver extract in reversing pellagra.

Nicotinic acid is present in meats, fish, eggs, liver, poultry, nuts, legumes, yeast, and whole grain and enriched cereals and breads.

PHARMACOKINETICS

Nicotinic acid is well absorbed after oral, I.M., and S.C. administration and is widely distributed to all tissues. Nicotinic acid is metabolized in the liver, and the metabolites are excreted in the urine.

Absorption, distribution, metabolism, excretion

Nicotinic acid and nicotinamide are readily absorbed from all portions of the GI tract after oral administration. These drugs are also well absorbed from I.M. and S.C. injection sites.

Nicotinic acid is widely distributed to all tissues in the body and is secreted in breast milk.

Nicotinic acid is converted to nicotinamide in the body, then metabolized in the liver.

The metabolites of nicotinic acid are excreted in the urine. Normally, very little nicotinic acid is excreted unchanged, although greater amounts are excreted unchanged as the dose increases.

Onset, peak, duration

After oral administration, nicotinic acid–induced vasodilation may occur within 20 minutes and may persist for 20 to 60 minutes. Peak serum concentration levels occur within 45 minutes, and the plasma half-life is 45 minutes.

PHARMACODYNAMICS

Nicotinic acid and nicotinamide are water-soluble B-complex vitamins. Nicotinic acid is required for lipid metabolism, tissue respiration, and glycogenolysis (splitting of glycogen in the body, yielding glucose the primary carbohydrate in the body).

Mechanism of action

The body converts nicotinic acid to nicotinamide. Nicotinamide is subsequently incorporated in nicotinamide-adenine dinucleotide (NAD) and nicotinamide-adenine dinucleotide phosphate (NADP). NAD and NADP function as coenzymes that carry hydrogen in tissue respiration, glycogenolysis, and lipid metabolism.

Large doses of nicotinic acid produce vasodilation. The cutaneous blood vessels of the face, neck, and chest are most affected. Tolerance to this effect may occur within 2 weeks. Nicotinamide does not cause this reaction.

Doses of nicotinic acid greater than 1 gram per day decrease serum low-density lipoproteins (LDL) and very low-density lipoproteins (VLDL).

PHARMACOTHERAPEUTICS

Nicotinic acid and nicotinamide are used to prevent and treat nicotinic acid deficiency and pellagra. Pellagra may result from dietary deficiency, isoniazid therapy, or certain neoplasms. Nicotinamide is preferred by some users because it does not produce the vasodilating effects of nicotinic acid.

Nicotinic acid is also used as an adjunct to dietary therapy in the treatment of hyperlipidemia.

nicotinic acid, niacin, or vitamin B$_3$ (Nicobid, Nico-Span). This drug may be given orally, intramuscularly, subcutaneously, or very slowly intravenously. For I.V. administration, dilute the drug to 10 mg/ml and infuse it at a rate not to exceed 2 mg/minute. Begin oral administration with small doses to avoid vasodilation reactions.
USUAL ADULT DOSAGE: for nicotinic acid deficiency, 10 to 20 mg P.O. daily; for pellagra, 300 to 500 mg P.O. daily, given in divided doses. If the I.V. route is required, give 25 to 100 mg of niacin two or more times daily. For intramuscular injections, give 50 to 100 mg five or more times daily. For hyperlipidemia, 1 to 2 grams P.O. t.i.d., not to exceed 6 grams per day.
USUAL PEDIATRIC DOSAGE: up to 300 mg P.O. or 100 mg I.V. daily, depending on severity of the disease.

nicotinamide, or niacinamide. Used by the body as a source of nicotinic acid, nicotinamide does not possess the vasodilating or hypolipidemic effects of niacin. It is used to prevent and treat pellagra.
USUAL ADULT DOSAGE: 50 mg P.O. 3 to 10 times per day.

Drug interactions

Nicotinic acid may potentiate the hypotensive effects of ganglionic blocking and antihypertensive drugs. This drug has also been reported to produce a false-positive reaction to the cupric sulfate (Benedict's reagent) urine glucose test.

ADVERSE DRUG REACTIONS

Although nicotinic acid and nicotinamide may be used interchangeably to correct niacin deficiency, nicotinamide produces fewer adverse reactions. The vasodilating properties of nicotinic acid may be troublesome to some patients, but these effects usually diminish with continued administration.

Predictable reactions

The most common adverse reaction to nicotinic acid is vasodilation. Sensations of flushing and warmth, itching, tingling, and hypotension have been reported with oral and parenteral administration. Gastrointestinal reactions may also occur, including nausea, vomiting, diarrhea, and abdominal pain.

Hyperglycemia and hyperuricemia may occur with nicotinic acid therapy. Abnormalities of liver function tests, including increased serum bilirubin, have been documented.

Unpredictable reactions

Some nicotinic acid products contain tartrazine, which may cause allergic-type responses in sensitive individuals.

NURSING IMPLICATIONS

Most of the nursing implications, especially those concerning precautions, are related to nicotinic acid because nicotinamide has fewer adverse effects.
• Nicotinic acid is contraindicated in patients with hepatic dysfunction, active peptic ulcer disease, severe hypotension, or arterial hemorrhage. Administer the drug cautiously to patients with gallbladder disease, diabetes

mellitus, or gout. During therapy, check liver function tests, blood glucose levels, and serum uric acid levels frequently.

• Before administering nicotinic acid products with tartrazine, inquire about tartrazine or aspirin hypersensitivity. Patients who are aspirin-sensitive frequently have sensitivity to tartrazine as well. The sensitive patient should receive a test dose or another product. Monitor the patient closely for signs and symptoms of an allergic response.

• Be aware that a false-positive reaction may occur with the cupric sulfate (Benedict's reagent) urine glucose test.

• Give nicotinic acid with meals to minimize gastrointestinal reactions.

• Administer I.V infusions slowly. Explain the harmlessness of the vasodilation to the patient.

• Teach the patient that the vitamin is a drug. Explain the importance of adhering to the therapeutic regimen.

• Teach patients with nicotinic acid deficiency which foods they may eat to increase the niacin content of their diet.

• Women who are pregnant or lactating should not exceed the RDA of nicotinic acid except under the guidance of a physician. The safety of large doses during pregnancy has not been established.

• The safety of large doses for young children also has not been established.

PYRIDOXINE (VITAMIN B$_6$)

Vitamin B$_6$ occurs in nature as pyridoxine, pyridoxal, and pyridoxamine. Symptoms of pyridoxine deficiency relate to changes in the skin, the nervous system, and erythropoiesis. The RDA for water-soluble pyridoxine is 2.2 mg for adult males, 2 mg for adult females, 2.6 mg for pregnant females and 2.5 mg for lactating females.

History and source
The discovery of pyridoxine stemmed from the study of riboflavin. In 1926, rats fed a diet deficient in riboflavin developed dermatitis. In 1936, György found that the dermatitis resulted from a deficiency of another related substance, which he named vitamin B$_6$. Its structure was identified in 1939.

Pyridoxine is present in meats, eggs, liver, whole-grain cereals and breads, soybeans, and vegetables.

PHARMACOKINETICS

Pyridoxine is well absorbed after oral administration and is stored primarily in the liver. Pyridoxine metabolism occurs in red blood cells and in the liver, and metabolites are excreted in the urine.

Absorption, distribution, metabolism, excretion
Pyridoxine is well absorbed from the GI tract after oral administration. Absorption may be decreased in patients with malabsorption syndromes or gastric resection.

Pyridoxine is stored mainly in the liver, with smaller amounts in the muscle and brain. The physiologically active forms of vitamin B$_6$ are found in the blood as pyridoxal phosphate and pyridoxamine phosphate, which are highly protein-bound. Pyridoxine readily crosses the placenta and appears in breast milk.

Pyridoxine is converted to pyridoxal phosphate in red blood cells and in the liver. Pyridoxamine phosphate is metabolized in the liver. Pyridoxine's metabolites are excreted in the urine.

Onset, peak, duration
The half-life of pyridoxine is 15 to 20 days.

PHARMACODYNAMICS

All forms of vitamin B$_6$ are water-soluble. Pyridoxine is used in the metabolism of proteins, carbohydrates, and fats and acts as a coenzyme in many other metabolic reactions.

Mechanism of action
All three forms of vitamin B$_6$ are converted to pyridoxal phosphate, the active form of vitamin B$_6$.

Humans require exogenous pyridoxine for amino acid metabolism. Pyridoxine is also involved in carbohydrate and lipid metabolism. The active form of vitamin B$_6$ acts as a coenzyme in many metabolic reactions and serves as a cofactor in the production of several neurotransmitters and proteins.

PHARMACOTHERAPEUTICS

Although vitamin B$_6$ exists as pyridoxine, pyridoxal, and pyridoxamine, the therapeutic preparation is called pyridoxine. Pyridoxine is used to prevent and treat vitamin B$_6$ deficiency. Deficiencies may occur in patients with uremia, alcoholism, cirrhosis, or malabsorption syndromes and in those receiving isoniazid (INH), cycloserine, hydralazine, ethionamide, penicillamine, or oral contraceptives. Clinical signs of deficiency are rare.

DRUG INTERACTIONS

Pyridoxine

Drug interactions with pyridoxine occur with some frequently administered drugs. The nurse must be aware of the following interactions and nursing implications.

DRUG	INTERACTING DRUGS	POSSIBLE EFFECTS	NURSING IMPLICATIONS
pyridoxine	levodopa	Accelerates metabolism of levodopa, decreases control of parkinsonism	• Consult the physician about administering carbidopa to prevent this reaction. • Monitor the patient for increased signs and symptoms of Parkinsonism.
	isoniazid (INH), penicillamine	Increase urinary excretion of pyridoxine	• Observe the patient for signs of pyridoxine deficiency.
	phenobarbital, phenytoin	Decrease serum concentrations of anticonvulsants	• Monitor the patient for decreased serum levels and seizure control.

Infants exposed to high amounts of pyridoxine in utero may become pyridoxine-dependent after birth. Pyridoxine is used to treat seizures unresponsive to standard therapy in these infants.

Pyridoxine is used as an adjunct therapy with other measures to treat toxicity from INH, cycloserine, or hydralazine overdose. INH-induced seizures may also be treated with pyridoxine and other anticonvulsants.

pyridoxine, or vitamin B₆ (Bee Six, Hexa-Betalin). Requirements are higher in those receiving INH or oral contraceptives. Pyridoxine may be given orally or by the I.M., I.V., or S.C. route.

USUAL ADULT DOSAGE: to treat dietary deficiency, 10 to 20 mg P.O. daily for 3 weeks, with recommended follow-up treatment with multivitamins containing 2 to 5 mg of pyridoxine; to prevent pyridoxine deficiency in patients receiving INH or penicillamine, 6 to 25 mg P.O. daily; to prevent seizures in patients receiving cycloserine, 100 to 300 mg P.O. daily in divided doses; to treat seizures induced by acute INH intoxication, give pyridoxine in doses approximating the amount of INH ingested, along with other anticonvulsant therapy. Administer 1 to 4 grams of pyridoxine I.V., followed by 1 gram I.M. every 30 minutes until the entire dose is given.

USUAL PEDIATRIC DOSAGE: for pyridoxine-dependent infants, 10 to 100 mg I.M. or I.V. for seizure activity. If the response to pyridoxine is positive, these infants may require oral doses of 2 to 100 mg of pyridoxine daily for life.

Drug interactions

Pyridoxine interacts with levodopa, INH, penicillamine, phenobarbital, and phenytoin. (See *Drug Interactions: Pyridoxine* for a discussion of these interactions.)

ADVERSE DRUG REACTIONS

In therapeutic doses, pyridoxine results in few, if any, adverse reactions. Very large doses, roughly 1,000 times the RDA, have resulted in nervous system damage.

Patients have reportedly developed difficulty with balance and a sensory neuropathy after ingestion of 2 to 6 grams of pyridoxine. Other nervous system effects, such as drowsiness and paresthesias, have occurred with smaller doses of this vitamin.

NURSING IMPLICATIONS

Patient teaching is the most important nursing implication with this drug.

• Teach patients with pyridoxine deficiency to increase their dietary intake of foods containing this vitamin.

• Assess for pyridoxine deficiency infants of women who have received large doses of pyridoxine. They may become pyridoxine–dependent after exposure to large amounts in utero.

• Advise a lactating patient that large doses of pyridoxine may suppress lactation through its inhibitory effect on prolactin.

• Instruct the patient to store the drug in a light-resistant container.

OTHER B-COMPLEX VITAMINS

Other water-soluble B-complex vitamins include para-aminobenzoic acid, pantothenic acid, biotin, choline, and inositol.

Para-aminobenzoic acid (PABA) is not a true vitamin, but is part of the B-complex group because it is a precursor of folic acid. Present in small amounts in cereal, eggs, milk, and meats, PABA has no known nutrient value; however it is used topically as a sunscreen agent.

Pantothenic acid is abundant in beef, egg yolks, and organ meats; therefore, deficiency in humans is rare. Although no clearly defined uses for this vitamin exist, it is frequently included in multivitamin preparations.

Biotin appears in yeast, grains, nuts, vegetables, fruits, organ meats, egg yolks, poultry, and seafood and is synthesized in the GI tract. It may play a role in fat and carbohydrate metabolism.

Choline, present in vegetable and animal fat and in egg yolks, is not considered an essential vitamin. It plays a role in fat metabolism and is a precursor of the neurotransmitter acetylcholine.

Inositol is present in plants, fruits, and whole-grain cereals and is synthesized in the GI tract. Inositol is not an essential vitamin; however, it plays some role in fat metabolism.

VITAMIN C (ASCORBIC ACID)

Vitamin C, a water-soluble vitamin, is responsible for a number of biochemical reactions in the body, mostly involving oxidation. Vitamin C deficiency can lead to scurvy, a disease characterized by degenerative changes in capillaries, bone, and connective tissue. Mild vitamin C deficiency is usually manifested by impairment in bone and tooth development, bleeding gums, loose teeth, fever, and infections. The RDA for adults is 60 mg, 80 mg for pregnant women, and 100 mg for lactating women.

History and source

Scurvy has been recognized since the time of the Crusades, particularly in northern Europe, where fresh fruits and vegetables were unavailable during the winter. The introduction of the potato reduced the incidence of scurvy somewhat, but the disease continued to plague sailors on long voyages. In the 1500s, the Canadian Indians taught European sailors how to cure the disease by ingesting spruce leaves. Lind, a British Royal Navy physician, demonstrated in 1747 that the disease could be rapidly reversed by the administration of lemon juice and citrus fruit. In 1928, Szent-Györgyi discovered a reducing agent in cabbage and the adrenal glands that was identified in 1932 by Waugh and King as the same factor in lemon juice that prevented scurvy.

Vitamin C is present in citrus fruits, tomatoes, strawberries, cabbage greens, and potatoes.

PHARMACOKINETICS

Well absorbed after oral administration, vitamin C is widely distributed throughout the body and excreted in the urine.

Absorption, distribution, metabolism, excretion

Vitamin C is readily absorbed after oral administration. The absorption of dietary ascorbic acid is 80% to 90% complete.

Vitamin C is widely distributed into body tissues and is found in large concentrations in the liver, leukocytes, platelets, glandular tissues, and the lens of the eye. Ascorbic acid crosses the placenta and appears in breast milk.

Vitamin C is reversibly oxidized to dehydroascorbic acid and inactive compounds, which are eliminated in the urine as an oxalate. If high doses of absorbic acid are administered, tissue stores become saturated and excess ascorbic acid is excreted unchanged in the urine.

Onset, peak, duration

Vitamin C administration begins to reverse the skeletal changes and hemorrhagic disorders reported in scurvy patients within 2 days to 3 weeks.

PHARMACODYNAMICS

Vitamin C possesses few pharmacologic actions. However, it functions in many important biochemical reactions in the body.

Mechanism of action

Vitamin C functions in many oxidative biochemical reactions. It is involved in steroid synthesis, the conversion of folic acid to folinic acid, and microsomal drug metabolism.

Vitamin C plays a role in tyrosine metabolism and as an intracellular cement in the synthesis of many intracellular substances, such as collagen, tooth and bone matrix, and capillary endothelium.

PHARMACOTHERAPEUTICS

Vitamin C is used primarily as a dietary supplement to prevent or treat vitamin C deficiency. It is also used to treat scurvy, the result of severe vitamin C deficiency. Vitamin C can also be used as a urinary acidifier.

vitamin C, or ascorbic acid (Cecon, Ce-Vi-Sol). This drug may be administered orally, intramuscularly, intravenously, or subcutaneously.
USUAL ADULT DOSAGE: for prophylaxis against scurvy, 75 to 150 mg P.O. daily; to treat scurvy, 300 mg to 1 gram P.O. should be given in divided doses daily for 2 to 3 weeks; to acidify the urine, 4 to 12 grams daily in divided doses.

Drug interactions

No clinically significant interactions occur with vitamin C. However, vitamin C may increase iron absorption and decrease warfarin effects. The excretion of acidic and basic drugs is affected by concomitant administration of vitamin C.

ADVERSE DRUG REACTIONS

As with other water-soluble vitamins, few adverse reactions are associated with ascorbic acid administration. However, because many people use large doses of vitamin C to treat such conditions as the common cold, the nurse should be aware of the adverse reactions.

Predictable reactions

Adverse reactions to ascorbic acid are related to the dose size or the administration route. Dose-related reactions include diarrhea and the precipitation of oxalate or urate renal calculi. The development of renal calculi results from urine acidification.

Adverse reactions to almost every administration route of ascorbic acid have been described. Dental erosion has occurred with the long-term use of chewable vitamin C. Patients may complain of tenderness at the injection site after I.M. administration. Rapid I.V. administration may cause brief dizziness.

Unpredictable reactions

Some ascorbic acid products contain tartrazine, which may cause allergic responses in sensitive individuals.

NURSING IMPLICATIONS

When administering vitamin C, the nurse must be aware of some important implications.
• Administer vitamin C cautiously to patients with G-6-PD deficiency.
• When administering ascorbic acid products with tartrazine, inquire about tartrazine or aspirin hypersensitivity. Patients who are aspirin–sensitive frequently have sensitivity to tartrazine as well. The sensitive patient should receive a test dose or another product. Monitor the patient closely for signs and symptoms of an allergic response.
• Be aware that large doses of vitamin C can cause false-negative urine glucose determinations when using the glucose oxidase methods or false-positive results when using cupric sulfate (Benedict's reaction). Large doses may also cause false-positive reaction to a fecal occult blood test.
• Teach patients with diabetes mellitus or a history of renal calculi and those who are receiving oral antico-

---

Food sources of trace minerals

Patients may know generally what foods contain which vitamins but probably will not be aware of the food sources of trace minerals. This list can serve as a useful tool for teaching patients about such foods. The nurse must remember, however, that the mineral content of foods depends on the mineral content of the soil, water and grazing land.

MINERAL	FOOD SOURCE
iodine	Iodized salt, seafood
fluoride	Fluoridated water, seafood
zinc	Whole grains, meats, dairy products, seafood
manganese	Green leafy vegetables, whole grains, legumes
copper	Meats, seafood, legumes, whole grain cereals, liver
selenium	Meats, seafood, dairy products, whole grains, vegetables
cobalt	Meats, dairy products, liver
molybdenum	Liver, milk, vegetables, legumes, cereal grains
chromium	Yeast, cereal grains, meats

agulants to avoid large doses of ascorbic acid. Ascorbic acid can interfere with urine testing for glucose or cause precipitation of renal calculi and may interfere with the action of oral anticoagulants.

● Instruct the patient to store vitamin C tablets in a closed container in a cool, dark place because ascorbic acid is rapidly destroyed by exposure to air and heat.

MINERALS (TRACE ELEMENTS)

INTRODUCTION

This section discusses minerals that are used as nutritional supplements, including iodine, fluoride, zinc, manganese, copper, selenium, cobalt, molybdenum, and chromium. (See Chapter 41, Hematinic Agents, for a discussion of iron, another mineral).

These minerals are inorganic chemicals found in all living tissues. Because most are required in very small quantities in the diet, they are known as *trace elements*. Usually, minerals are widely available in foods in the normal diet. Deficiencies are unusual unless some factor inhibits absorption or a patient requires long-term TPN and is not adequately supplemented. Research into the effects of trace mineral deficiencies has been difficult because of the small amounts of the minerals needed to maintain health and their widespread availability in the diet. For these reasons, RDAs for many minerals have not been established.

Minerals perform a wide variety of functions in the body. Many function as components of enzyme systems, regulating or enhancing enzyme reactions. Some act as building materials for cells, bones, and teeth. Others play a role in such essential body processes as nerve transmission, cellular respiration, glucose metabolism, or hormone functions. In some of these functions, the involved mineral is recognized as an essential component for normal functioning; for others, the evidence is not as clear. Additional research is needed to expand knowledge about these elements.

No significant drug interactions occur with the use of minerals, so this topic is not discussed in this section.

History and source

All trace elements enter the food chain when taken up by plants from the soil, eventually becoming part of the tissues of animals. The study of iron, copper, and iodine began more than a century ago, but most of what is known about the role of trace elements in human nutrition has been learned within the past 30 to 50 years. (See *Food sources of trace minerals* for a discussion of dietary sources of these substances.)

PHARMACOKINETICS

The pharmacokinetics of the trace minerals iodine, fluoride, zinc, manganese, copper, selenium, cobalt, molybdenum, and chromium are discussed below.

Absorption, distribution, metabolism, excretion

Iodine is rapidly and completely absorbed from the GI tract as iodide. The highest concentration of iodine is in the thyroid gland. Iodine is not metabolized, but is incorporated into the tyrosine residues of thyroglobulin to produce thyroid hormones. When broken down, these hormones release iodine, which is reabsorbed by the thyroid. Unabsorbed iodine is 40% to 80% excreted in the urine.

Fluoride, as sodium fluoride, is completely absorbed from the GI tract after oral administration, but calcium fluoride and bone meal are slowly and variably absorbed. Fluoride is distributed mostly to bone and developing teeth. Fluoride is not metabolized and is excreted mainly in the urine.

Many factors influence zinc absorption. Amino acids and vitamin C increase zinc absorption; calcium and phosphate decrease zinc absorption. Zinc is distributed to bone and hepatic, pancreatic, retinal, and gonadal tissues. It is not metabolized and is excreted in urine, feces, and perspiration.

Manganese is poorly absorbed from the GI tract. It is widely distributed to bone, the pituitary gland, liver, pineal gland, and lactating mammary glands. High concentrations are found in mitochondria and cell nuclei. Manganese is not metabolized and is excreted mainly in the feces via bile.

Copper is absorbed after oral administration and is distributed mostly to the liver. It is excreted in the feces via bile.

Selenium is well absorbed after oral administration and is distributed to the kidneys, liver, muscle, and skin. Selenium is incorporated into glutathione peroxidase but otherwise is not metabolized. It is excreted primarily in the urine, although significant losses occur in the feces.

Cobalt is also well absorbed after oral administration and undergoes increased absorption in iron deficiency states. It is excreted in the urine.

Molybdenum is well absorbed after oral administration and is distributed mostly to the liver, kidneys, spleen, lungs, brain, and muscle. Molybdenum is not known to undergo metabolism other than its incorporation into enzymes. It is excreted primarily in the urine, with small amounts lost in the feces via bile.

Chromium, poorly absorbed after oral administration, is widely distributed to many tissues. It is excreted in the urine.

PHARMACODYNAMICS

The pharmacodynamics of the trace elements iodine, fluoride, zinc, manganese, copper, selenium, cobalt, molybdenum, and chromium are discussed below.

Mechanism of action

Iodine is essential in manufacturing thyroid hormones. By itself, it has no known metabolic function.

Fluoride is incorporated into teeth and bone. Deposited in tooth enamel, it makes teeth resistant to acid dissolution and to formation of dental caries. Oral fluoride works best in developing teeth. After tooth calcification is complete, fluoride strengthens surface enamel. Fluoride also increases skeletal mass and density.

Zinc acts as a component of many zinc metalloenzymes and metalloproteins, such as alcohol dehydrogenase and carbonic anhydrase. It is involved in ribonucleic acid and protein metabolism, acts as a stabilizer of cell membranes, and interacts with insulin. Physiologic functions of zinc include cell growth and proliferation, sexual maturation and reproduction, taste, wound healing, and immune defenses.

Manganese is involved in activating many metalloenzymes, such as pyruvate carboxylase and superoxide dismutase. Manganese and other metals activate enzymes involved in the metabolism of carbohydrates, proteins, and lipids.

Copper functions as a component of enzymes involved in red blood cell formation, white blood cell formation, cellular energy production, elastin and collagen synthesis, and glucose and catecholamine metabolism.

Selenium functions as an antioxidant. By incorporation into glutathione peroxidase, it helps protect cell membranes and structures from destruction by oxidation.

Cobalt functions as a component of vitamin B_{12}.

Molybdenum functions as a component of xanthine oxidase, sulfite oxidase, and aldehyde oxidase, all enzymes integral to a number of metabolic reactions.

Chromium potentiates the action of insulin and is involved in the regulation of lipoprotein metabolism.

PHARMACOTHERAPEUTICS

The pharmacotherapeutics of the trace elements iodine, fluoride, zinc, manganese, copper, selenium, cobalt, molybdenum, and chromium are discussed below.

iodine (SSKI Solution). Used to treat goiter and hypothyroidism secondary to iodine deficiency, iodine may suppress mild forms of hyperthyroidism and thyroid crisis. It is used to prepare hyperthyroid patients for thyroidectomy and may be used as an expectorant. The RDA for iodine is 150 mcg for adults, 175 mcg for pregnant females, and 200 mcg for lactating females. USUAL ADULT DOSAGE: for patients on TPN, 1 to 2 mcg/kg/day; for thyroid crisis, 250 to 500 mg I.V. daily of sodium iodide or 50 to 100 mg P.O. daily of potassium iodide solution in water or juice; to prepare hyperthyroid patients for thyroidectomy, 2 to 6 drops of strong iodine solution t.i.d. for 10 days before surgery.

fluoride (Luride, Pediaflor Drops). Used to prevent dental caries, to desensitize dentin, and to treat bone diseases such as osteoporosis, fluoride may be administered orally as sodium fluoride or topically onto teeth as stannous fluoride or sodium fluoride. Oral fluorides should be used if public water fluoride concentration levels are 0.7 parts per million or less. No guidelines for adult dosages exist. Topical fluorides, except those present in toothpaste or rinsing solutions, are applied by dental personnel only.

zinc (Orazinc, Zinctrace). This mineral is used to treat zinc deficiencies. The RDA is 15 mg for adults, 20 mg for pregnant females, and 25 mg for lactating females. USUAL ADULT DOSAGE: in zinc deficiency states, 200 to 220 mg P.O. t.i.d. (equal to 135 to 150 mg of elemental zinc daily, nine times the adult RDA). This amount may be increased in patients with diarrhea. Zinc may be added to solutions for patients receiving TPN, usually 2.5 to 6 mg I.V. daily.

manganese (Manganese Gluconate, Mangatrace). This mineral is used as a dietary supplement only. The need for manganese in human nutrition has been established; however, no RDA has been determined. USUAL ADULT DOSAGE: as a dietary supplement, 5 to 50 mg P.O. daily. Those receiving TPN should receive 0.15 to 0.8 mg/day added to the solution.

copper (Coppertrace). Used primarily as a supplement in TPN, copper also is used in patients on vegetarian diets and in those with disease states that affect the absorption or excretion of copper, such as sprue, nephrosis, cancer, or burns. Copper deficiency may also result in patients receiving molybdenum. The daily dose of copper varies with age and health status. USUAL ADULT DOSAGE: 0.5 to 1.5 mg I.V. daily or 2 to 3 mg P.O. daily.

Vitamin and mineral agents

The following chart summarizes the major indications, dosages, and nursing implications of the fat-soluble and water-soluble vitamins and of trace minerals.

DRUG	MAJOR INDICATIONS	USUAL ADULT DOSAGES	NURSING IMPLICATIONS
Fat-soluble vitamins			
vitamin A	Severe vitamin A deficiency with corneal changes	500,000 IU P.O. for 3 days, followed by 50,000 IU P.O. daily for 2 weeks, then maintenance doses of 10,000 to 20,000 IU P.O. daily for 2 months	• Vitamin A is contraindicated in patients with hypervitaminosis A; oral administration is contraindicated in the presence of malabsorption syndrome; I.V. administration is contraindicated except for special water-miscible forms, and these preparations should not be given by I.V. push. • Administer with food for better absorption. • Avoid concurrent administration of mineral oil. • Teach the patient the signs and symptoms of toxicity, primarily changes in skin and mucous membranes. • Caution patients on isotretinoin to use a sunscreen.
cholecalciferol (vitamin D_3)	Cholecalciferol deficiency	400 to 1,000 IU P.O. daily	• Contraindicated in patients with vitamin D toxicity, hypercalcemia, and renal osteodystrophy with hyperphosphatemia.
ergocalciferol (vitamin D_2)	Familial hypophosphatemia	50,000 to 500,000 IU P.O. or I.M. daily	• Administer vitamin D cautiously to patients receiving digitalis preparations; hypercalcemia may precipitate cardiac dysrhythmias. • Monitor the patient's serum calcium, phosphorus, magnesium, blood urea nitrogen, and alkaline phosphatase levels during therapy. • Administer vitamin D with food to increase absorption and decrease adverse effects.
menadiol sodium diphosphate (vitamin K)	Hypoprothrombinemia secondary to obstructive jaundice and biliary fistulas	5 mg P.O. daily	• Give oral vitamin K with food to improve tolerance and increase absorption.
phytonadione (vitamin K)	Anticoagulant-induced hypoprothrombinemia	2.5 to 10 mg P.O., I.M., S.C. or I.V.	• Phytonadione is contraindicated in patients with hereditary hypoprothrombinemia, bleeding secondary to heparin therapy, and hepatocellular disease, unless caused by biliary obstruction. • Oral administration of phytonadione is contraindicated if bile secretion is inadequate, unless supplemented with bile salts. • Administer phytonadione cautiously, if at all, to patients with G-6-PD deficiency. • If administering phytonadione I.V., follow the manufacturer's directions for dilution and rate of administration to avoid possible severe adverse reactions.

continued

SELECTED MAJOR DRUGS

Vitamin and mineral agents continued

DRUG	MAJOR INDICATIONS	USUAL ADULT DOSAGES	NURSING IMPLICATIONS
Water-soluble vitamins			
thiamine (B$_1$)	Thiamine deficiency	5 to 30 mg P.O. daily	• Thiamine is contraindicated in patients with hypersensitivity. • Administration of thiamine by I.V. push is contraindicated except when treating life-threatening myocardial failure in wet beriberi. • Follow the manufacturer's directions when administering I.V. • Have epinephrine available to treat possible anaphylaxis after a large parenteral dose. • Administer oral thiamine with food.
riboflavin (B$_2$)	Riboflavin deficiency	5 to 30 mg P.O., daily	• Administer with food to improve absorption. • Drug may turn urine bright yellow.
nicotinic acid (niacin, vitamin B$_3$)	Nicotinic acid deficiency	10 to 20 mg P.O. daily	• Nicotinic acid is contraindicated in patients with hepatic dysfunction, active peptic ulcer disease, severe hypotension, or arterial hemorrhage. • Administer nicotinic acid cautiously to patients with gallbladder disease, diabetes mellitus, or gout. • Monitor the patient's liver function tests and blood glucose and serum uric acid levels frequently. • Nicotinic acid products may contain tartrazine; observe the patient for signs of allergic response. • Administer nicotinic acid with food to minimize GI adverse effects.
pyridoxine (vitamin B$_6$)	Pyridoxine deficiency	10 to 20 mg P.O. daily for 3 weeks, ollowed by 2 to 5 mg P.O. daily	• Large doses of pyridoxine in pregnant women may produce dependency in the neonate and suppress lactation after delivery.
ascorbic acid (vitamin C)	Ascorbic acid deficiency Scurvy	70 to 150 mg P.O. daily 300 mg to 1 gram P.O. in divided doses for 2 to 3 weeks	• Administer ascorbic acid cautiously to patients with G-6-PD deficiency. • Ascorbic acid products contain tartrazine; observe the patient for signs of allergic response. • Teach the patient who has a history of renal calculi or who is taking oral anticoagulants to avoid large doses of vitamin C. • Tell the patient to store tablets or powder in a cool, dark place.
Trace minerals			
iodine	Thyroid storm Additive to TPN solution	30 drops of super-saturated potassium iodide solution 1 to 2 mcg/kg/day	• Dilute liquid preparations well and administer with food to improve absorption and tolerance. • Document any patient allergy to iodine or shellfish before administration.

continued

SELECTED MAJOR DRUGS

Vitamin and mineral agents continued

DRUG	MAJOR INDICATIONS	USUAL ADULT DOSAGES	NURSING IMPLICATIONS
fluoride	Prevention of dental caries, treatment of specific bone diseases	Dose dependent upon amount obtained from water source	• Do not administer oral preparations with dairy products because absorption will be decreased. • Rinses and gels should be used after brushing the teeth and before going to bed.
zinc	Zinc deficiency Additive to TPN solution	200 to 220 mg P.O. t.i.d. 2.5 to 6 mg I.V. daily	• Do not administer oral preparations with dairy products or foods with a high fiber content because absorption will be decreased. • Parenteral zinc should be well diluted and administered via a central vein.

selenium (Selenitrace). Used primarily as a supplement in TPN, selenium is also used in patients with neoplasms.
USUAL ADULT DOSAGE: 40 to 100 mcg I.V. daily, or 50 to 200 mcg P.O. daily.

cobalt. Deficiency states of this mineral are not known to exist in humans other than in vitamin B_{12} deficiency. Excess cobalt leads to polycythemia.

molybdenum (Molybdenum Solution, Molypen). This mineral is indicated primarily in patients receiving long-term TPN.
USUAL ADULT DOSAGE: 20 to 120 mcg I.V. daily. This may be increased to 163 mcg I.V. daily in deficiency states.

chromium (Chrometrace, Chromic Chloride). This mineral is indicated primarily in patients receiving long-term TPN.
USUAL ADULT DOSAGE: 10 to 20 mcg I.V. daily or 50 to 200 mcg P.O. daily.

ADVERSE DRUG REACTIONS

With many minerals, the margin of safety between therapeutic and toxic levels is fairly narrow because of the body's limited ability to eliminate excess amounts. Most adverse reactions are related to administration of large doses of minerals. Concentrated amounts of minerals also tend to irritate tissues they contact. GI symptoms may occur with oral administration. Phlebitis may develop if minerals are inadequately diluted before parenteral administration.

Predictable reactions

Overdose is the most common cause of adverse reactions to minerals. The patient should be monitored for toxicity any time a mineral is administered in amounts above the recommended dose.

Iodine therapy may produce metallic taste, skin lesions, tenderness of mouth, gums, and salivary glands, eyelid swelling, increased saliva production, iodide goiter (thyroid gland enlargement that results from high ingestion of high concentrations of iodide), bloody diarrhea, fever, or depression.

The patient on fluoride therapy may develop nausea, vomiting, diarrhea, abdominal pain, nervous system hyperirritability, tetany and paresthesias related to hypocalcemia, hypoglycemia, or cardiac and respiratory failure.

Zinc therapy can result in stomach irritation, gastric ulceration, diarrhea, vomiting, elevated serum amylase levels, hypothermia, or hypotension accompanied by signs and symptoms of shock.

Manganese therapy may cause anorexia, diarrhea, headache, or Parkinson-like symptoms such as altered gait and speech impairment.

Copper therapy may produce diarrhea, lethargy, altered behavior, diminished reflexes, photophobia, or liver and kidney damage.

Adverse reactions to selenium therapy may include alopecia, skin lesions, GI irritation, depression, or garlic odor of breath and sweat. Acute poisoning has led to multiple organ failure and death.

With cobalt therapy, polycythemia can occur; with molybdenum therapy, goutlike symptoms.

Chromium therapy may produce nausea, vomiting, gastric ulceration, rash, joint swelling, bronchospasm, convulsions, coma, or kidney and liver damage.

Unpredictable reactions

Hypersensitivity reactions have occurred following iodine administration. The use of stannous fluoride solutions has led to tooth discoloration. Allergy to fluoride has resulted in rash. Some products contain tartrazine, which may cause allergic-type reactions in sensitive individuals.

NURSING IMPLICATIONS

Most of the nursing implications involving trace elements are related to patient teaching.

• When administering parenteral mineral solutions, be certain they are well diluted and administered via a central vein to decrease vessel irritation. Solutions containing minerals should be discarded within 24 hours after mixing.

• To help prevent mineral toxicity, evaluate the mineral content of the patient's diet, and consider this in addition to the mineral supplements being taken. Watch for signs of toxicity, particularly if the patient has renal failure or hepatic disease. Monitor the patient for signs of adequate therapy so that doses of minerals can be decreased or discontinued.

• Before administering medication containing tartrazine, inquire about tartrazine or aspirin hypersensitivity. Patients who are aspirin-sensitive are also frequently tartrazine-sensitive. Sensitive patients should receive another product or should be monitored.

• Document any patient history of allergy to iodine or shellfish before administering preparations containing iodine. Be prepared to intervene if an allergic response occurs.

• Dilute liquid preparations well before administration to improve taste and decrease gastric irritation.

• Do not administer mineral preparations with other medications because many combinations are incompatible.

• Teach the patient that the best way to prevent mineral deficiencies is to eat a well-balanced diet of fresh foods, especially whole grain products, fruits, and vegetables. Deficiencies may develop if the patient usually eats large amounts of highly processed foods.

• Teach the patient to preserve minerals by cooking foods in the smallest amount of water possible.

• Teach the patient to avoid GI irritation by taking minerals with or immediately after meals, except for fluoride and zinc. These minerals should not be taken with dairy products, and zinc should not be taken with high-fiber foods, such as bran, which interfere with its absorption.

• Teach the patient with small children to buy mineral preparations in containers with child-proof caps and to store them in a safe place, out of children's reach.

• Teach the patient that fluoride rinses or gels used for dental prophylaxis are most effective if used immediately after brushing teeth and before bedtime. Instruct the patient to avoid eating or drinking for ½ hour after rinsing with fluoride.

CHAPTER SUMMARY

Chapter 51 presented the vitamin and mineral preparations that are used as nutritional supplements. The three categories of drugs highlighted are fat-soluble vitamins, water-soluble vitamins, and minerals (trace elements). Here are the highlights of the chapter:

• Fat-soluble vitamins are organic chemical substances required in small amounts in the diet.

• Vitamin A is necessary for vision in dim light, healthy skin and mucous membranes, and normal growth and reproduction. Vitamin D plays a role in regulating calcium and phosphorus. Vitamin E acts as an antioxidant and enzyme cofactor. Vitamin K stimulates the synthesis of clotting factors by the liver.

• The fat-soluble vitamins are absorbed with dietary fats in the small intestine, so they require bile salts and pancreatic lipase for absorption.

• All of the fat-soluble vitamins are stored, but the amount stored varies with each vitamin.

• The primary clinical indication for fat-soluble vitamins is dietary supplementation to compensate for low levels of the vitamin, which may result from inadequate intake, decreased absorption, or increased excretion. Vitamin D is also used to treat calcium and phosphorus imbalances; vitamin K has been used to treat acquired hypoprothrombinemia.

• Adverse reactions caused by fat-soluble vitamins vary; however, nausea and vomiting occur frequently with all of them. Vitamin A may produce changes in the skin and mucous membranes and congenital anomalies. Vitamin D may result in hypercalcemia. Severe hypersensitivity-like reactions and death have been noted after I.V. administration of vitamin K.

• Because these drugs can accumulate in the body, the nurse must monitor patients for signs of toxicity and educate them about the potential hazards.

• Water-soluble vitamins are organic chemical substances required in small quantities in the diet.

• The water-soluble vitamins, except vitamin C, all function as coenzymes in various metabolic functions. Vitamin C functions in many oxidative biochemical reactions in the body and is involved in the synthesis of intracellular substances.

• The water-soluble vitamins are readily absorbed from the small intestine.

• Because the water-soluble vitamins are not stored to a great extent, body supplies must be replenished frequently to avoid deficiency.

• Clinical indications for these drugs include inadequate intake, impaired absorption, increased demand, or increased excretion.

• Although generally considered nontoxic, water-soluble vitamins can cause adverse reactions, including nausea, vomiting, flushing, rashes, diarrhea, neuropathy, polycythemia, renal calculi, and cardiovascular collapse.

• Water-soluble vitamins can be destroyed by heat and light and should be stored in a cool, dark place. Also, because of the rapidity with which they lose their potency, they should not be stored for long periods of time.

• Water-soluble vitamins should be taken with food to decrease GI adverse effects and to improve absorption.

• Trace minerals are inorganic chemical substances that are components of all living tissues.

• Trace minerals cannot be manufactured by the body and therefore must be obtained from exogenous sources, usually food. All are stored by the body and, in many cases, are difficult for the body to eliminate. Mineral levels may therefore become toxic.

• Trace minerals function primarily as components of other substances, such as enzymes, hormones, bones, and teeth.

• The primary clinical indication for trace minerals is to treat deficiency states and as a nutritional supplement, particularly in patients receiving TPN.

• The most common adverse reaction to trace minerals is GI irritation, which can usually be prevented by administering them with food.

• Nurses should be aware of the symptoms indicating toxic levels of trace minerals. Toxicity can usually be prevented by limiting the patient's intake of minerals to levels within the RDAs, unless otherwise prescribed.

• When administering trace minerals parenterally, the nurse must ensure that they are well diluted and administered via a central vein.

BIBLIOGRAPHY

Baumgartner, T.G., ed. *Clinical Guide to Parenteral Micronutrition.* Melrose Park, Ill.: Educational Publications Ltd., 1984.

Brewer, G.J., et al. Interactions of Trace Elements: Clinical Significance. *Journal of the American College of Nutrition* 4:33, 1985.

Drug Information for the Health Care Provider, vol. 1, 7th ed., Rockville, Md.: The United States Pharmacopeial Convention, Inc., 1987.

Gilman, A.G., et al., eds. *Goodman and Gilman's The Pharmacological Basis of Therapeutics,* 7th ed. New York: Macmillan Publishing Co., 1985.

Kastrup, E.K., ed. *Facts and Comparisons.* St. Louis: Facts and Comparisons Division, J.B. Lippincott Co., 1986.

Katcher, B.S., et al., eds. *Applied Therapeutics: The Clinical Use of Drugs.* San Francisco: Applied Therapeutics, 1983.

Levine, M. "New Concepts in the Biology and Biochemistry of Ascorbic Acid," *New England Journal of Medicine* 314:892, April 3, 1986.

McEvoy, G.K., ed. *American Hospital Formulary Service—Drug Information 1986.* Bethesda, Md.: American Society of Hospital Pharmacists, 1986.

Ovesen, L. "Vitamin Therapy in the Absence of Obvious Deficiency: What is the Evidence?" *Drugs* 27:148, February 1984.

Rombeau, J.L., and Caldwell, M.D., eds. *Parenteral Nutrition.* Philadelphia: W.B. Saunders Co., 1986.

Williams, S.R. *Nutrition and Diet Therapy.* St. Louis: Times Mirror/Mosby College Publishing, 1985.

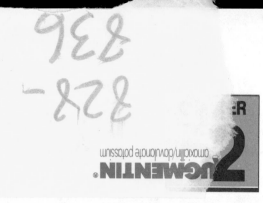

ELECTROLYTE REPLACEMENT AGENTS

OBJECTIVES

After reading and studying this chapter, you should be able to:

1. Explain the physiology of fluid and electrolyte balance.

2. Identify the roles of the major electrolytes in maintaining homeostasis.

3. Describe the pharmacokinetics, pharmacodynamics, and pharmacotherapeutics of potassium, as well as its adverse effects.

4. Describe the pharmacokinetics, pharmacodynamics, and pharmacotherapeutics of calcium, as well as its adverse effects.

5. Discuss the specific nursing actions associated with administration of the major electrolyte replacement agents.

6. Explain the normal functions of magnesium and sodium, their causes of insufficiency, and replacement therapy.

INTRODUCTION

Electrolyte replacement agents are mineral salts that increase depleted or deficient electrolyte levels, thus helping to maintain homeostasis, or stability in body fluid composition and volume. Chapter 52 discusses the primary intracellular fluid (ICF) electrolyte, potassium; a major extracellular fluid (ECF) electrolyte, calcium; and two other electrolytes essential for homeostasis: magnesium (in ICF) and sodium (in ECF).

Physiology of fluid and electrolyte balance

Homeostasis depends on a complex interrelationship among water, electrolyte, and acid-base metabolisms. Because they are so closely related, an alteration in any one of these factors can affect the others profoundly. (Acid-base balance is discussed more fully in Chapter 53, Alkalinizing and Acidifying Agents.)

Water makes up 45% to 75% of body weight. This water is present either within the cells (ICF) or outside the cells (ECF). It must be present in sufficient volume for metabolic processes to take place.

ICF and ECF contain electrolytes, substances that separate into ions when in solution and conduct a weak electrical current—hence their name. For an environment conducive to proper cell functioning, fluid volume must be adequate, and ICF and ECF must be balanced electrically—that is, the number of negatively charged ions (anions) must equal the number of positively charged ions (cations). ICF and ECF differ in electrolyte composition: ICF primarily contains the cations potassium and magnesium and the anion phosphate; ECF primarily contains the cations sodium and calcium and the anions chloride and bicarbonate.

These electrolytes profoundly affect water distribution, osmolality, acid-base balance, and neuromuscular irritability. Normally, the body maintains fluid volume and electrolyte concentrations within narrow limits despite a varied diet and often-changing metabolic activity. When this balance is disturbed, it causes a profound change in cells' ability to function and in muscles' ability to respond to nerve transmission.

The four major electrolytes are potassium, sodium, calcium, and magnesium. Potassium is the electrolyte most often replaced, because it is not stored in the body, and the kidneys excrete almost all that is taken in daily. Replacement therapy for sodium depletion depends on the amount of water in the body. For example, in water intoxication, the amount of water taken in exceeds the amount excreted, thereby diluting the sodium in ECF. This can occur in patients with congestive heart failure or renal failure, or during I.V. fluid replacement. In these cases, the treatment is to restrict water intake rather than replace sodium. When sodium is lost through burns, diarrhea, vomiting, diuretics, salt-losing renal disorders, or adrenal insufficiency, its replacement is essential to electrolyte balance.

Calcium and magnesium are stored in bone and can be mobilized if needed. Even so, losses of these electrolytes can exceed the body's ability to mobilize them.

For a summary of representative drugs, see *Selected major drugs: Electrolyte replacement agents* on page 834.

POTASSIUM

Potassium is the major positively charged ion (cation) in ICF. It has an important role in maintaining the electrical excitability of nerve and muscle cells, thus enhancing nerve impulse transmission and muscle contraction. Potassium also helps maintain acid-base balance, cellular function, and enzyme action necessary to change carbohydrates into energy and to reassemble amino acids into protein.

Because the body cannot store potassium, adequate amounts must be ingested daily. If this is not possible, potassium replacement can be accomplished either orally or intravenously with potassium salts.

PHARMACOKINETICS

Oral potassium is readily absorbed from the GI tract. Extended-release preparations embedded in a wax matrix are absorbed slowly as they move through the intestine, helping minimize small bowel ulcerations associated with potassium salts. I.V. potassium is effective immediately. After absorption into ECF, 98% of the potassium passes into ICF.

Normal serum levels of potassium are maintained by the kidneys, which excrete almost 90% of excessive potassium intake. The rest is excreted in feces (9%) and sweat (1%).

The onset of action of oral potassium (liquid or powder) is usually within 30 minutes. Extended-release forms have a slower onset of action, usually 1 to 2 hours.

PHARMACODYNAMICS

Potassium moves quickly into ICF to restore depleted potassium levels and reestablish homeostasis. Potassium is an essential element in determining cell membrane potentials and excitability. It is, therefore, necessary for proper functioning of all nerve and muscle cells and for nerve impulse transmission. Potassium also is essential for tissue growth and repair and maintenance of acid-base balance.

PHARMACOTHERAPEUTICS

Hypokalemia is a common occurrence in conditions that increase potassium excretion. These include malabsorption, excessive vomiting or diarrhea, polyuria, diabetes, some kidney diseases, cystic fibrosis, burns, an excess of antidiuretic hormone (ADH), or therapy with potassium-depleting diuretics. Other causes of potassium depletion include alkalosis and insufficient potassium intake from starvation or I.V. solutions that contain insufficient potassium.

Apart from its role in preventing or reversing hypokalemia, potassium also is used to decrease the toxic effects of digitalis. Because potassium inhibits the excitability of the heart, insufficient potassium enhances digitalis action, which may result in toxicity.

Potassium is available in several salts. These can be administered alone or with other potassium salts or electrolytes. (For information on commercially available combination products, see *Combination potassium replacement agents* on page 830.)

potassium bicarbonate (K-Lyte). Available as effervescent tablets for oral solution, potassium bicarbonate is used to treat symptomatic hypokalemia.
USUAL ADULT DOSAGE: 25 to 50 mEq P.O. dissolved in ½ to 1 glass of cold water once daily or b.i.d.

potassium chloride (Kaochlor; Slow-K). Chloride depletion frequently occurs simultaneously with potassium depletion. Oral potassium chloride is most commonly used by patients taking potassium-depleting diuretics.
USUAL ADULT DOSAGE: to prevent hypokalemia, 20 mEq P.O. daily in two to three divided doses; to treat symptomatic hypokalemia, 40 to 96 mEq extended-release capsules P.O. daily in two to three divided doses, or 20 mEq P.O. diluted in ½ glass of cold water or juice once daily to q.i.d., or, when oral replacement is not feasible or hypokalemia is life-threatening, 10 mEq I.V. hourly in concentration of 40 mEq/liter or less, to a maximum of 200 mEq daily based on the patient's serum potassium levels.

potassium gluconate (Kaon). This potassium salt is used to replace and maintain potassium levels.
USUAL ADULT DOSAGE: to treat hypokalemia, 5 to 20 mEq P.O. b.i.d. to q.i.d. Further doses are based on serum potassium determinations.

Combination potassium replacement agents

Several potassium salts are available as combination products to be given orally as electrolyte replenishers.

PRODUCT	DOSAGE	NURSING IMPLICATIONS
potassium bicarbonate and potassium chloride (Klorvess, K-lyte/Cl, Potassium-Sandoz)	20 mEq daily or b.i.d.	• Completely dissolve effervescent tablets or powder in 120 to 240 ml of cold water or juice.
potassium chloride, potassium bicarbonate, and potassium citrate (Kaochlor-Eff)	20 mEq daily to q.i.d.	• Completely dissolve effervescent tablets in 120 to 240 ml of cold water or juice.
potassium bicarbonate and potassium citrate (K-Lyte DS)	50 mEq daily or b.i.d.	• Be careful not to confuse these double-strength tablets with regular-strength medications. • Completely dissolve effervescent tablets in 120 to 240 ml of cold water or juice.
potassium gluconate and potassium chloride (Kolyum)	20 mEq b.i.d. to q.i.d. (children, 20 to 40 mEq/m^2 or 2 to 3 mEq/kg/day in divided doses)	• Dissolve liquid or powder in 30 ml of cold water or juice.
potassium gluconate and potassium citrate (Bi-K, Twin-K)	20 mEq b.i.d. to q.i.d. (children, 20 to 40 mEq/m^2 or 2 to 3 mEq/kg/day in divided doses)	• Dilute in 120 ml of cold water or juice.
potassium gluconate, potassium citrate, and ammonium chloride (Twin-K-Cl)	15 mEq b.i.d. to q.i.d.	• Dilute in 120 to 240 ml of cold water or juice.
potassium acetate, potassium bicarbonate, and potassium citrate (Potassium Triplex, Tri-K)	15 mEq t.i.d. to q.i.d. (children, 15 to 30 mEq/m^2 or 2 to 3 mEq/kg/day in divided doses)	• Dilute in 120 ml of cold water or juice.
potassium and sodium phosphate tablets (Uro-KP-Neutral)	2 tablets t.i.d.	• Dissolve in 240 ml of water or juice. • Primarily prescribed to replace phosphorus.
potassium and sodium phosphate capsules for oral solution (Neutra-Phos)	1 capsule q.i.d.	• Dissolve contents of capsule in 75 ml of water or juice; patient must not swallow filled capsule. • Primarily prescribed to replace phosphorus.
potassium and sodium phosphate powder for oral solution (Neutra-Phos)	75 ml of reconstituted solution q.i.d. (children age 4 and over, same as adult; under age 4, 60 ml q.i.d.)	• Do not dilute solution. • Primarily prescribed to replace phosphorus.

potassium phosphate. (Neutra-Phos-K). Recommended as an oral supplement for phosphorus deficiency, potassium phosphate also is used to treat hypokalemia.

USUAL ADULT DOSAGE: 1 capsule P.O. emptied and mixed into 75 ml of cold water q.i.d. (provides 14.25 mEq of potassium and phosphate and 250 mg of phosphorus) or, when oral replacement is not feasible or hypokalemia is life-threatening, 3.3 ml/day diluted in I.V. solution (supplies 14.5 mEq of potassium and 935 mg of phosphate).

Drug interactions

Potassium should be used cautiously in patients receiving potassium-sparing diuretics, such as amiloride, spironolactone, or triamterene, to avoid hyperkalemia. Potassium causes no significant drug interactions.

ADVERSE DRUG REACTIONS

Many of the adverse reactions caused by potassium can be prevented by careful monitoring of serum potassium levels during therapy.

Administration of potassium preparations may produce hyperkalemia if the patient's serum potassium levels are not closely monitored. Hyperkalemia causes paresthesia of the extremities, listlessness, mental confusion, weakness and heaviness of limbs, and flaccid paralysis. Cardiovascular signs may include EKG changes (prolonged PR interval; wide QRS complex; depressed ST segment; and tall, tented T waves), peripheral vascular collapse with a fall in blood pressure, cardiac dysrhythmias, heart block, and possible cardiac arrest.

Oral potassium sometimes causes nausea, vomiting, abdominal pain, and diarrhea. Enteric-coated tablets may cause small-bowel ulceration, stenosis, hemorrhage, and obstruction. Because wax-matrix tablets have largely replaced enteric-coated tablets, however, this adverse reaction is no longer common.

I.V. infusion of potassium preparations can cause pain at the site and phlebitis. Infusion of potassium in patients with decreased urine production increases the risk of hyperkalemia.

NURSING IMPLICATIONS

Both oral and I.V. potassium supplements are commonly administered; the nurse must be aware of the following implications:

• Tell the patient to take oral potassium with or after meals to minimize GI symptoms.
• Direct the patient to dissolve all powders and tablets in at least 120 ml of water or fruit juice, as directed, and to sip the solution slowly over 5 to 10 minutes.
• Make sure the patient knows to take capsules with plenty of liquid.
• Remind the patient not to crush or chew extended-release tablets, which will defeat the purpose of the special coating but will not affect bioavailability of the potassium.
• Be aware that tablets in wax matrix sometimes lodge in the esophagus and cause ulceration in a cardiac patient who has esophageal compression from an enlarged left atrium; with such a patient, and in one with esophageal stasis or obstruction, use liquid potassium.
• Remind the patient that although remnants of the wax matrix may appear in feces, the drug will be absorbed.
• Always dilute I.V. potassium preparations before infusion; never give as a bolus or I.M.

• Never mix I.V. potassium phosphate in a solution that contains calcium or magnesium because precipitates will occur.
• Give diluted potassium slowly I.V.; potentially fatal hyperkalemia may result from too-rapid infusion.
• Monitor serum potassium levels closely in all patients taking potassium; make sure outpatients understand the need to have frequent blood tests.
• If hyperkalemia occurs, review the patient's diet to see if the patient eats large amounts of high-potassium foods.
• Instruct outpatients to report symptoms of hyperkalemia or GI upset to the physician.

CALCIUM

Calcium is a major positively charged ion (cation) in ECF. Almost all the calcium in the body—99%—is stored in bone, where it can be mobilized if necessary. It is the small amount of extracellular ionized calcium that plays an essential role in normal nerve and muscle excitability. Calcium also is integral to normal functioning of the heart, kidneys, and lungs, and it affects the blood coagulation rate and cell membrane and capillary permeability. Calcium also is a factor in neurotransmitter and hormone activity, amino acid metabolism, vitamin B_{12} absorption, and gastrin secretion. It plays a major role in normal bone and teeth formation.

When dietary intake is insufficient to meet metabolic needs, calcium stores in bone are reduced. Chronic insufficient calcium intake can result in bone demineralization. Calcium is replaced either orally or intravenously with calcium salts.

PHARMACOKINETICS

Oral calcium is absorbed readily from the duodenum and proximal jejunum. A pH of 5.0 to 7.0, parathyroid hormone, and vitamin D all aid calcium absorption. Absorption also depends on dietary factors, such as calcium binding to fiber, phytates, and oxalates and to fatty acids, with which calcium salts form insoluble soaps. Calcium is distributed primarily in bone. About 80% of calcium salt is eliminated in feces; the rest is excreted in urine. I.V. calcium infusion raises blood levels immediately; levels return to normal in 30 minutes to 2 hours.

Calcium replacement agents

Although the drug interactions involving calcium are few, they are potentially lethal and the nurse must be aware of them.

DRUG	INTERACTING DRUGS	POSSIBLE EFFECTS	NURSING IMPLICATIONS
calcium replacement agents	digitalis glycosides (digoxin, digitoxin)	Precipitate cardiac dysrhythmias	• To administer calcium and digitalis glycosides simultaneously, give small amounts slowly, as prescribed.
	calcium channel blockers (verapamil, nifedipine)	Reduce response to the calcium channel blockers	• Monitor the patient's therapeutic response to the calcium channel blockers, and expect dosage adjustments, as needed.

PHARMACODYNAMICS

Calcium moves quickly into ECF to restore calcium levels and reestablish homeostasis. Its action is particularly crucial in the heart, nervous system, and bone.

PHARMACOTHERAPEUTICS

The major clinical indication for I.V. calcium is to treat acute hypocalcemia, in which a rapid increase in serum calcium levels is needed. Conditions that create this need are tetany, vitamin D deficiency, and alkalosis. I.V. calcium also is used to prevent a hypocalcemic reaction during exchange transfusions. Calcium is helpful in treating magnesium intoxication and in strengthening myocardial tissue after defibrillation or after a poor response to epinephrine.

Oral calcium commonly is used to supplement a calcium-deficient diet or to prevent osteoporosis. Pregnancy and lactation create a need for calcium replacement, as do periods of bone growth during childhood and adolescence. Chronic hypocalcemia from such conditions as chronic hypoparathyroidism, osteomalacia, rickets, and vitamin D deficiency also is treated with oral calcium.

Calcium is available in several salts, which can be administered alone or with other calcium salts.

calcium carbonate (Cal-Bid, Os-Cal). Available as regular and chewable tablets, calcium carbonate is the most efficient form of calcium. It contains 40% calcium by weight and is also used as an antacid and as a treatment for hyperphosphatemia.
USUAL ADULT DOSAGE: as a dietary supplement, 500 mg P.O. b.i.d. to q.i.d. 1 to 2 hours after meals.

calcium chloride. Available in injectable form, calcium chloride is used in acute situations that demand immediate increases in serum calcium levels. These include tetany and cardiac arrest.
USUAL ADULT DOSAGE: for hypocalcemia, 500 mg to 1 gram I.V. solution (1 gram equals 13.6 mEq of calcium) at a rate no faster than 1 ml/minute (repeated in 1 to 3 days as determined by serum calcium levels); for cardiac arrest, 500 mg to 1 gram I.V. or 200 to 400 mg injected directly into ventricle as a single dose.

calcium citrate (Calcigard, Citracal). Available in tablet form, calcium citrate is better absorbed from the GI tract than is calcium carbonate.
USUAL ADULT DOSAGE: as a dietary supplement, 950 mg to 1.9 grams P.O. t.i.d. or q.i.d. 1 to 2 hours after meals.

calcium glubionate (Neo-Calglucon Syrup). Calcium glubionate is used as a dietary supplement and as a replacement for calcium deficiency. In children, it is used as a dietary supplement during periods of bone growth.
USUAL ADULT DOSAGE: as a dietary supplement, 5.4 grams t.i.d. or q.i.d. before meals.
USUAL PEDIATRIC DOSAGE: as a dietary supplement in children up to age 1, 1.8 grams five times a day before meals; in children ages 1 to 4, 3.6 grams t.i.d. before meals; in children over age 4, same as adult dosage.

calcium gluconate (Calcet, Kalcinate). Available in oral and I.V. forms, calcium gluconate has the same clinical indications as calcium glubionate and is used for magnesium toxicity as well.
USUAL ADULT DOSAGE: as a dietary supplement, 11 grams P.O. daily in divided doses after meals; for hy-

pocalcemic tetany, 4.5 to 10 mEq I.V. slowly at a rate not exceeding 5 ml/minute; for magnesium toxicity, 4.5 to 10 mEq I.V. slowly at a rate no faster than 5 ml/minute.
USUAL PEDIATRIC DOSAGE: as a dietary supplement, 500 to 720 mg/kg of body weight P.O. daily in divided doses after meals.

calcium lactate. Calcium lactate is used primarily as a dietary supplement.
USUAL ADULT DOSAGE: 7.7 grams P.O. daily in divided doses after meals.
USUAL PEDIATRIC DOSAGE: 345 to 500 mg/kg of body weight P.O. daily in divided doses after meals.

Drug interactions
Calcium preparations interact with digitalis glycosides and calcium channel blockers. (See *Drug interactions: Calcium replacement agents* for more information, including nursing implications.)

ADVERSE DRUG REACTIONS
Calcium preparations may produce hypercalcemia if blood levels are not closely monitored. Early signs of hypercalcemia include drowsiness, lethargy, muscle weakness, headache, constipation, and a metallic taste in the mouth. EKG changes include a shortened Q-T interval and heart block. Severe hypercalcemia can cause cardiac dysrhythmias and, eventually, coma. Because calcium is excreted by the kidneys, high levels sometimes predispose patients to renal calculi.

I.V. administration of calcium may cause venous irritation; I.M. injection may cause severe local reactions, such as burning, necrosis, and tissue sloughing.

NURSING IMPLICATIONS
Because calcium is commonly prescribed, the nurse must be aware of the following implications:
• Keep in mind that calcium absorption is decreased in the elderly, so oral doses of calcium may need adjustment.
• Advise the patient to avoid eating large amounts of spinach, rhubarb, bran, whole grain cereals and bread, and fresh fruits and vegetables when taking calcium because these foods interfere with calcium absorption. Or, unless ordered otherwise, the patient can take calcium tablets 1 to 2 hours after eating these foods.
• Suggest that the patient eat foods containing vitamin D, which enhances calcium absorption.
• Administer I.V. calcium cautiously in children—their small veins are extremely sensitive to irritation.

• Warm an I.V. infusion to body temperature before administering it.
• Administer an I.V. infusion slowly to prevent high concentrations from reaching the heart and causing cardiac dysrhythmias and arrest.
• After injecting calcium, keep the patient recumbent for 15 minutes.
• If extravasation occurs, discontinue the I.V. infusion; infiltrate the area with 1% procaine and hyaluronidase to reduce vasospasm and dilute calcium; and apply warm, moist compresses to the area, as prescribed.
• Use the I.M. route in an emergency, only when the I.V. route is impossible to use; if the I.M. route is necessary, give the injection in the gluteal muscle in adults and in the lateral thigh in infants and small children.

OTHER ELECTROLYTES

Besides potassium and calcium, several other electrolytes are needed in proper amounts to maintain the body's acid-base balance and to ensure proper organ functioning. Magnesium and sodium are the most important of the other electrolytes.

Magnesium is the second most common positively charged ion (cation), after potassium, in ICF. It is essential in transmitting nerve impulses to muscle and in activating enzymes necessary for carbohydrate and protein metabolism. It also stimulates parathyroid hormone secretion, thus regulating ICF calcium levels, and aids in cell metabolism and in the movement of sodium and potassium across cell membranes.

Approximately 66% of the body's magnesium is stored in bone, 1% is in plasma and interstitial fluid, and the rest is in cells.

Magnesium stores may be depleted by malabsorption, chronic diarrhea, prolonged treatment with diuretics, nasogastric suctioning, prolonged therapy with parenteral fluids not containing magnesium, hyperaldosteronism, hypoparathyroidism, hyperparathyroidism, and excessive release of adrenocortical hormones.

Magnesium sulfate is the drug of choice for replacement therapy in magnesium deficiency. Severe cases can be treated using an I.V. infusion. The usual adult dosage is 5 grams in 1 liter of dextrose 5% in water (D_5W) or normal saline solution administered over 4 hours.

SELECTED MAJOR DRUGS

Electrolyte replacement agents

This chart summarizes the major electrolyte replacement agents currently in clinical use.

DRUG	MAJOR INDICATIONS	USUAL ADULT DOSAGES	NURSING IMPLICATIONS
potassium bicarbonate	Replacement electrolyte for symptomatic hypokalemia	25 to 50 mEq P.O. dissolved in ½ to 1 glass of cold water daily or b.i.d.	• Contraindicated in patients with severe renal impairment, acute dehydration, or hyperkalemia. • Dissolve effervescent tablets in ½ to 1 glass of water and give with meals to avoid gastric upset.
potassium chloride	Prevention of hypokalemia Replacement electrolyte for symptomatic hypokalemia	20 mEq P.O. daily in two to three divided doses 40 to 96 mEq extended-release capsules P.O. daily in two to three divided doses, or 20 mEq P.O. diluted in ½ glass of cold water or juice daily to q.i.d., or 10 mEq I.V. hourly in concentration of 40 mEq/liter or less, to a maximum of 200 mEq daily based on patient's serum potassium levels	• Contraindicated in patients with severe renal impairment, acute dehydration, or hyperkalemia. • Tell the patient to swallow capsule whole without chewing. • If giving oral solution, dilute well and give with meals to avoid gastric upset. • Potassium chloride I.V. usually is prescribed only when oral replacement is not feasible or hypokalemia is life-threatening. • If giving potassium chloride I.V., monitor the patient closely for EKG changes; measure urinary output; and monitor serum electrolyte levels frequently. • Give I.V. infusion slowly; rapid infusion causes pain or burning at the infusion site and may cause cardiac dysrhythmias.
calcium carbonate	Replacement electrolyte for hypocalcemia	500 mg P.O. b.i.d. to q.i.d 1 to 2 hours after meals	• Contraindicated in patients with hypercalcemia. • Administer cautiously to patients on digitalis therapy: calcium enhances digitalis effect and may cause dysrhythmias. • Give after meals to enhance absorption.
calcium chloride	Replacement electrolyte for hypocalcemia in acute conditions, such as tetany and cardiac arrest	500 mg to 1 gram I.V. solution at a rate no faster than 1 ml/min; or 500 mg to 1 gram I.V. or 200 to 400 mg injected directly into ventricle as a single dose	• Contraindicated in patients with hypercalcemia. • Administer cautiously to patients on digitalis therapy: calcium enhances digitalis effect and may cause dysrhythmias. • Never mix I.V. calcium chloride in a solution containing carbonates, bicarbonates, phosphates, sulfates, or tartrates.
calcium glubionate	Replacement electrolyte for hypocalcemia	5.4 grams t.i.d. or q.i.d. before meals	• Contraindicated in patients with hypercalcemia. • Administer cautiously to patients on digitalis therapy: calcium enhances digitalis effect and may cause dysrhythmias. • Give before meals to avoid patient gastric upset.
calcium gluconate	Dietary supplement Replacement electrolyte for severe hypocalcemic tetany	11 grams P.O. daily in divided doses after meals 4.5 to 10 mEq I.V. at a rate no faster than 5 ml/min	• Contraindicated in patients with hypercalcemia. • Administer cautiously to patients on digitalis therapy: calcium enhances digitalis effect and may cause dysrhythmias. • Give after meals to enhance absorption. • Tell the patient to chew tablets before swallowing.

I.M. injection also may be used. For severe deficiency, the dosage is 250 mg/kg I.M. within 4 hours. For mild deficiency, the dosage is 1 gram as a 50% solution administered I.M. every 6 hours for a maximum of four doses per 24 hours.

Magnesium sulfate also is used to treat convulsions, severe toxemia, and acute nephritis in children. (For more information on magnesium sulfate as an anticonvulsant, see Chapter 24, Anticonvulsant Agents.)

Sodium is the major positively charged ion (cation) in ECF. It maintains the osmotic pressure and concentration of ECF, acid-base balance, and water balance; contributes to nerve conduction and neuromuscular function; and plays a role in glandular secretion. Sodium is readily absorbed by the small intestine, and 90% of absorbed sodium can be found in ECF. It is excreted through the skin and by the kidneys.

Sodium replacement is necessary in conditions that rapidly deplete it, such as excessive loss of GI fluids or excessive perspiration. Diuretics and tap water enemas also can deplete sodium, particularly when fluids are replaced by plain water. Sodium can be lost in trauma or wound drainage, adrenal gland insufficiency, cirrhosis of the liver with ascites, inappropriate ADH secretion, and prolonged I.V. infusion of dextrose in water without other solutes.

Severe symptomatic sodium deficiency may be treated by I.V. infusion of 3% or 5% saline solution. Other I.V. solutions containing saline include D_5W and saline 0.9%; D_5W and saline 0.45%; dextrose 2.5% and saline 0.45%; and saline 0.9%. These solutions are used to prevent sodium depletion in those conditions that predispose the patient to sodium loss, such as severe vomiting, excessive perspiration, or fever.

Injectable sodium salts (sodium bicarbonate injection and sodium lactate injection) also are used to treat metabolic acidosis.

I.V. solutions containing multiple electrolyte salts for treating dehydration with accompanying acidosis are available from various manufacturers.

CHAPTER SUMMARY

Chapter 52 presented the role of electrolyte replacement agents in maintaining homeostasis, or stability in body fluid composition and volume. Chapter highlights include:

• Fluid and electrolyte balance is essential for proper cell functioning. Water in ICF and ECF must be present in sufficient volume for metabolic processes to take place.

• Electrolytes are substances that separate into ions when in solution and conduct a weak electrical current. Those with a negative charge are anions; those with a positive charge are cations. To maintain homeostasis, the number of anions must equal the number of cations.

• Potassium, magnesium, and phosphate ions are found mainly in ICF; sodium, chloride, calcium, and bicarbonate are found mainly in ECF.

• Electrolytes profoundly affect water distribution, osmolality, acid-base balance, and neuromuscular irritability.

• Potassium is the main cation in ICF; sodium the main cation in ECF.

• Magnesium is the second most common cation in ICF; calcium is a major cation in ECF.

• Electrolytes are primarily absorbed through the GI tract and excreted by the kidneys. With the exception of calcium and magnesium, which are stored in bone, electrolytes are excreted by the kidneys within 24 hours. Any conditions that increase excretion or decrease absorption of electrolytes can lead to a deficiency state that disturbs homeostasis.

• Electrolytes can be replaced orally or parenterally. Calcium chloride can be injected directly into the ventricle in emergency situations to increase ventricular muscle tone.

• When administering replacement electrolytes, the nurse must monitor for elevated blood levels of the electrolyte. An excess of electrolytes can cause as serious an alteration in homeostasis as a deficit can.

BIBLIOGRAPHY

American Hospital Formulary Service. *Drug Information 87.* McEvoy, G. K., et al., eds. Bethesda, Md.: American Society of Hospital Pharmacists, 1987.

Anthony, C., and Thibodeau, G. *Textbook of Anatomy and Physiology.* St. Louis: C.V. Mosby Co., 1983.

Dickerson, R., and Brown, R. "Hypo-Magnesemia in Hospitalized Patients Receiving Nutritional Support," *Heart and Lung* 14(6):561-68, 1985.

Drug Information for the Health Care Provider, 7th ed. Rockville, Md.: United States Pharmacopeial Convention, Inc., 1987.

Dudek, S. *Nutrition Handbook for Nursing Practice.* Philadelphia: J.B. Lippincott Co., 1987.

Elbaum, N. "With Cancer Patients, Be Alert for Hypercalcemia," *Nursing84* 14(8):58-59, 1984.

Folk-Lightly, M. "Solving the Puzzles of Patient Fluid Imbalances," *Nursing84* 14(2):34, 1984.

Gilman, A.G., et al., eds. *Goodman and Gilman's The Pharmacological Basis of Therapeutics,* 7th ed. New York: Macmillan Publishing Co., 1985.

Goth, A. *Medical Pharmacology: Principles and Concepts,* 11th ed. St. Louis: C.V. Mosby Co., 1984.

Hansten, P. *Drug Interactions,* 5th ed. Philadelphia: Lea & Febiger, 1985.

Keyes, J. *Fluid, Electrolyte and Acid-Base Regulation.* Belmont, Calif.: Wadsworth Inc., 1985.

Knapil, J. "The Buffering and Excretion of Acids...Biochemical Features," *Nursing Mirror* 156(18):41-43, 1983.

Knapil, J. "Water Balance," *Nursing Mirror* 157(5):28, 1983.

Maziak, M., et al. *Fluids and Electrolytes Through the Life Cycle.* East Norwalk, Conn.: Appleton-Century-Crofts, 1985.

McCormack, A. "RN Master Care Plan—Preventing Electrolyte Imbalances," *RN* 47(11):32-33, 1984.

McFadden, E., et al. "Hypocalcemia," *American Journal of Nursing* 83(2):227-30, 1983.

Metheney, N., and Snively, W. *Nurses' Handbook of Fluid Balance.* Philadelphia: J.B. Lippincott Co., 1983.

Monrow-Black, J. "The ABC's of Total Parenteral Nutrition," *Nursing84* 14(2):50, 1984.

Stroot, V., et al. *Fluids and Electrolytes—A Practical Approach.* Philadelphia: F.A. Davis, 1984.

CHAPTER
53

ALKALINIZING AND ACIDIFYING AGENTS

OBJECTIVES

After reading and studying this chapter, you should be able to:

1. Describe the homeostatic buffer systems and the compensatory mechanisms that maintain the acid-base balance in the blood.

2. Explain why sodium bicarbonate is used in cardiac arrest.

3. Explain how ammonium chloride, arginine chloride, and hydrochloric acid are used to treat metabolic alkalosis.

4. Explain the way acetazolamide acidfies the blood and aklalinizes the urine.

5. Discuss the action of urine-alkalinizing agents when they are used to treat drug overdose.

6. Explain why ascorbic acid is used to treat urinary tract infections.

7. Compare cranberry juice and ascorbic acid as treatments for urinary tract infections.

8. Explain why the sodium content of certain alkalinizing agents must be carefully monitored in some patients.

9. Discuss the adverse reactions associated with each alkalinizing and acidifying agent.

INTRODUCTION

Alkalinizing and acidifying agents act to correct acid-base imbalances in the blood: they are commonly used to treat metabolic acidosis and alkalosis. An alkalinizing agent will increase the pH (hydrogen ion concentration) of the blood; an acidifying agent will decrease the pH. Some of these agents also alter urine pH, making them useful in treating some urinary tract infections and overdoses of certain drugs.

Acid-base balance and imbalance

The basis for all acid-base relationships is the hydrogen ion concentration, or pH. To maintain normal blood pH (between 7.35 and 7.45) and normal acid-base balance, the body must constantly engage in a delicate homeostatic process, balancing anions (negatively charged ions, such as bicarbonate [HCO_3-]) with cations (positively charged ions, such as hydrogen [H^+]). The body of a person consuming the typical American diet produces 40 to 80 mEq of hydrogen ions every day from protein metabolism, and this excess is easily offset as part of the homeostatic process. However, disorders such as chronic obstructive pulmonary disease (COPD) and normal events such as exercise can disrupt this process, altering blood pH and causing acid-base imbalance.

When an acid-base imbalance occurs, the body activates homeostatic buffer systems and compensatory mechanisms to counteract the problem. Blood buffer systems neutralize excess acids and alkalies by reducing high levels of hydrogen ions or by generating hydrogen ions when levels are too low. Blood buffer systems include the bicarbonate, phosphate, and sulfate systems; of these, perhaps the most important is the bicarbonate system. This system regulates shifting of bicarbonate and carbonic acid levels in the blood to offset shifts in the hydrogen ion concentration, or pH.

Besides the buffer systems, the respiratory and renal systems act as compensatory mechanisms to counteract acid-base imbalances. The lungs alter the carbon dioxide levels in the blood by increasing or decreasing the rate and depth of respirations, thus increasing or decreasing carbon dioxide elimination. The kidneys offset hydrogen ion levels by increasing or decreasing the reabsorption of bicarbonate ions. The two organ systems work closely together: If an acid-base imbalance occurs in one, the other will try to compensate for it. For example, if a disease such as COPD causes respiratory acidosis, the kidneys will try to compensate by retaining bicarbonate. (See *Compensatory mechanisms* on page 838.)

Despite the day-to-day reliability of the body's pH-regulating processes, which can function adequately even under the stress of a disorder such as COPD, alkalinizing or acidifying agents are sometimes needed to correct the acid-base disorders: respiratory or metabolic acidosis or alkalosis. They may even be given concomitantly to a severely ill patient who has a mixed acid-

Compensatory mechanisms

The lungs and kidneys work closely together to compensate for acid-base imbalances. When an imbalance is respiratory, the kidneys try to compensate by altering the formation or excretion of bicarbonate ions. When the imbalance is metabolic, the lungs try to compensate by altering the carbon dioxide concentration. The chart below shows these organ systems' compensatory responses to the effects of various acid-base imbalances.

DISORDER	EFFECTS		COMPENSATORY RESPONSE
Metabolic acidosis caused by diabetic ketoacidosis	↓ HCO_3^-	↓ blood pH	Lungs ↓ pCO_2
Respiratory acidosis caused by COPD	↑ pCO_2	↓ blood pH	Kidneys ↑ HCO_3^-
Metabolic alkalosis caused by excessive diuretic administration	↑ HCO_3^-	↑ blood pH	Lungs ↑ pCO_2
Respiratory alkalosis caused by hyperventilation syndrome	↓ pCO_2	↑ blood pH	Kidneys ↓ HCO_3^-

base disorder; for example, when a patient has respiratory acidosis from COPD complicated by metabolic alkalosis from excessive diuretic administration.

These agents may also be used to acidify or alkalinize the urine, which they do by affecting the kidneys' buffer systems or hydrogen ion excretion.

This chapter will cover the alkalinizing and acidifying agents as they are used to treat certain acid-base disorders.

For a summary of representative drugs, see *Selected major drugs: Alkalinizing and acidifying agents* on page 845.

ALKALINIZING AGENTS

Four alkalinizing agents are used to increase blood pH: sodium bicarbonate, sodium citrate, sodium lactate, and tromethamine. Sodium bicarbonate is also used to increase urine pH, as is the carbonic anhydrase inhibitor acetazolamide (which, paradoxically, lowers the blood pH).

PHARMACOKINETICS

All of the alkalinizing agents are well absorbed when given orally. Sodium lactate and sodium citrate are metabolized to the active ingredient, bicarbonate. Sodium

bicarbonate is not metabolized. Tromethamine and acetazolamide undergo little or no metabolism and are excreted unchanged in the urine.

Absorption, distribution, metabolism, excretion

After oral administration, sodium bicarbonate is absorbed rapidly and completely. It is the active moiety (the molecule with the characteristic pharmaceutical property), so it acts without needing to be metabolized. It is excreted as carbon dioxide from the lungs and as bicarbonate in the urine.

After oral administration of sodium citrate in Shohl's solution (a mixture of sodium citrate and citric acid) or in modified Shohl's solution (a mixture of sodium and potassium citrate with citric acid), the drug is metabolized by oxidation to form bicarbonate. Less than 5% of sodium citrate is excreted unchanged in the urine.

Sodium lactate is slowly metabolized in the liver to form bicarbonate (the alkalinizing metabolite) and glycogen. Conversion to bicarbonate usually occurs 1 to 2 hours after intravenous (I.V.) administration.

After I.V. administration, tromethamine combines with hydrogen ions and associated acid anions to form salts that are excreted by the kidneys.

When given orally, acetazolamide is well absorbed from the gastrointestinal (GI) tract, widely distributed in body tissues, and excreted unchanged by the kidneys.

Onset, peak, duration

Onset of the alkalinizing agents is rapid after oral administration and immediate after I.V. administration. These drugs' duration of action varies widely, however, depending on use and underlying disorders.

PHARMACODYNAMICS

All of the alkalinizing agents act by decreasing the hydrogen ion concentration and increasing pH. Sodium bicarbonate and tromethamine do this directly, but sodium lactate and citrate must first undergo conversion to bicarbonate.

Mechanism of action

Sodium bicarbonate dissociates in the blood to provide bicarbonate ions that are used in the bicarbonate blood buffer system to decrease the hydrogen ion concentration and raise the blood pH. As the bicarbonate ions are excreted in the urine, urine pH rises. Sodium citrate and lactate, after conversion to bicarbonate, alkalinize the blood and urine in the same way.

Tromethamine acts by combining with hydrogen ions to alkalinize the blood; the resulting tromethamine-hydrogen ion complex is excreted in the urine.

Acetazolamide promotes renal excretion of sodium, potassium, bicarbonate, and water; the bicarbonate ion excretion alkalinizes the urine and, by reducing blood bicarbonate levels, also acidifies the blood.

PHARMACOTHERAPEUTICS

Physicians most commonly use these agents to treat metabolic acidosis. Other uses for these agents include raising the urine pH to help remove certain substances, as in a phenobarbital overdose.

sodium bicarbonate. Administered I.V. or orally, this alkalinizing agent is used to treat metabolic acidosis related to cardiac arrest as well as metabolic acidosis from chronic renal failure and other disorders. The drug is used to alkalinize the urine and thus increase the excretion of weak acids, such as cystine or uric acid, that may accumulate as a result of gout or chemotherapy for soft-tissue cancer. Alkalinizing the urine is also done to facilitate excretion of excess barbiturates, salicylates, and other toxic agents.

Sodium bicarbonate is not usually administered during cardiac arrest unless the patient's blood pH falls below 7.1 or the plasma bicarbonate level falls below 8 mEq/liter. When used to treat cardiac arrest, bicarbonate administration offsets the excess hydrogen ions (acidosis) generated by lactic acid produced during the arrest. It also helps prevent ventricular fibrillation, which tends to occur in patients with severe metabolic acidosis caused by cardiac arrest.

Mild metabolic acidosis may not require treatment, but oral or I.V. sodium bicarbonate can be used to treat severe acidosis. No matter which route is used, the dosage must be determined separately for each patient. The base-deficit formula provides the ideal method for dosage calculation. First, determine the patient's base deficit by subtracting the serum bicarbonate level from the desired one. Then use that figure in the following formula:

$$\text{sodium bicarbonate dosage (in mEq)} = 0.4 \times \text{body weight (kg)} \times \text{base deficit}$$

For example, if the patient's actual serum bicarbonate level is 8 mEq/liter and the desired level is 22 mEq/liter, then the patient's base deficit is 14. If this patient weighs 70 kg, then the calculation is:

$$\text{sodium bicarbonate dosage (in mEq)} = 0.4 \times 70 \times 14$$

Thus, the dosage would be 392 mEq of sodium bicarbonate.

USUAL ADULT DOSAGE: for severe metabolic acidosis in cardiac arrest, initially, half of the dosage calculated using the base-deficit formula, with subsequent dosages recalculated based on regularly monitored serum bicarbonate levels; or 1 mEq/kg I.V. initially, followed by 0.5 mEq/kg every 10 minutes; for less severe forms of metabolic acidosis, 2 to 5 mEq/kg I.V. infused over 4 to 8 hours; for acidosis related to chronic renal failure, 20 to 36 mEq P.O. daily in divided doses to achieve serum bicarbonate level of 18 to 20 mEq/liter; for urine alkalinization, 20 to 36 mEq P.O. daily in divided doses.

USUAL PEDIATRIC DOSAGE: for metabolic acidosis in cardiac arrest in a pediatric patient, 1 to 2 mEq/kg every 10 minutes; in a neonate, 2 mEq/kg by slow I.V. infusion at a rate of less than 2 mEq/kg/minute.

sodium citrate [Shohl's solution]. Usually administered orally as Shohl's solution for correction of metabolic acidosis, sodium citrate must be diluted with 60 to 90 ml of water. Refrigeration may help to make the drug more palatable.

USUAL ADULT DOSAGE: for correction of metabolic acidosis, 10 to 30 ml of Shohl's solution P.O. after meals and at bedtime.

USUAL PEDIATRIC DOSAGE: for correction of metabolic acidosis, 5 to 15 ml of Shohl's solution P.O. after meals and at bedtime.

sodium lactate. This alkalinizing agent is administered I.V. to treat patients with moderate metabolic acidosis who cannot tolerate oral products. It cannot be used in its alkalinizing metabolite—occurs in the liver. As with

DRUG INTERACTIONS

Alkalinizing agents

Drug interactions involving alkalinizing agents may be severe and may increase or decrease another drug's pharmacologic action.

DRUG	INTERACTING DRUGS	POSSIBLE EFFECTS	NURSING IMPLICATIONS
sodium bicarbonate, sodium citrate, sodium lactate	amphetamines	Decrease amphetamine excretion, resulting in increased stimulant effects	• Monitor the patient closely for indications of increased amphetamine effects, such as rapid heart rate, increased blood pressure, and restlessness.
	chlorpropamide	Increase chlorpropamide clearance and decrease chlorpropamide's serum half-life	• Assess the patient for signs of decreased chlorpropamide effectiveness, such as elevated blood glucose level.
	flecainide	Decrease flecainide excretion	• Monitor the patient for signs of flecainide toxicity, such as reduced heart rate and hypotension.
	ketoconazole	Decrease ketoconazole absorption	• Avoid concomitant use with oral alkalinizing agents.
	lithium	Increase lithium excretion	• Monitor the patient for signs of decreased lithium effectiveness, such as increased manic-depressive behavior. • Monitor the patient's lithium blood levels regularly.
	methenamine	Decrease conversion of methenamine to formaldehyde, resulting in decreased antibacterial action	• Avoid concomitant use with alkalinizing agents.
	quinidine	Decrease quinidine excretion, resulting in increased blood levels of quinidine	• Monitor the patient for signs of quinidine toxicity, such as tinnitus and a widened Q-T interval on electrocardiograph (EKG) tracings.
	salicylates	Increase salicylate excretion if salicylate dosage exceeds 50 mg/kg/day	• Monitor the patient for signs of decreased salicylate effectiveness, such as increased pain and inflammation, at sites where relief had previously been obtained.

sodium bicarbonate, the dosage of sodium lactate is based on the patient's base deficit:

sodium lactate dosage (in ml of ⅙ molar solution) =
0.8 × body weight (lb) × base deficit

USUAL ADULT DOSAGE: for correction of moderate metabolic acidosis, an individually calculated dosage based on the base deficit I.V. as a ⅙ molar solution at a rate no greater than 300 ml/hr; for alkalinizing the urine, 30 ml/kg of body weight of a ⅙ molar solution; P.O. in divided doses over 24 hours.

tromethamine (Tham). Tromethamine is administered I.V. to treat metabolic acidosis associated with cardiac bypass surgery, cardiac arrest, or cardiac disease. The drug is used to avoid the high sodium load that can occur with sodium bicarbonate, citrate, or lactate. (A high sodium load can cause water retention and expansion of the extracellular fluid compartment, worsening cardiac function in these conditions.) This alkalinizing agent may also be used to treat metabolic acidosis in a patient with impaired ability to excrete sodium or carbon dioxide—for example, a patient with COPD.

Whether this drug is administered by slow I.V. infusion or with an infusion pump (during cardiac bypass surgery), the dosage must be individualized using the base deficit in the following calculation:

$$\text{tromethamine dosage (in ml of 0.3 molar solution)} =$$
$$\text{body weight (kg)} \times \text{base deficit (mEq/liter)}.$$

USUAL ADULT DOSAGE: to correct metabolic acidosis associated with cardiac bypass surgery, cardiac arrest, or cardiac disease, an individually calculated dosage based on the base deficit and infused over 1 hour or more. The dosage may range from 3.5 to 6 ml/kg of the 0.3 molar solution in cardiac arrest. Additional therapy is based on serial determination of bicarbonate levels.

acetazolamide (Diamox). Acetazolamide may be used to alkalinize urine in treating phenobarbital, lithium, or salicylate overdose. Acetazolamide is not recommended to treat salicylate overdose, however, because both drugs can cause metabolic acidosis. (See Chapter 38, Diuretic Agents, for information about other uses of acetazolamide.)

USUAL ADULT DOSAGE: for urinary alkalinization in drug overdose, individualized oral or I.V. dosage based on the overdosed drug and pertinent laboratory results.

Drug interactions

Alkalinizing agents can interact with a wide range of drugs to increase or decrease their pharmacologic effects. (See *Drug interactions: Alkalinizing agents* for further information.)

ADVERSE DRUG REACTIONS

These agents may cause severe adverse reactions, which are usually predictable and related to overdose. Unpredictable reactions occur only with acetazolamide.

Predictable reactions

Oral sodium bicarbonate may produce gastric distention and flatulence as it combines with hydrochloric acid in the stomach to release carbon dioxide. Shohl's solution, which produces less gastric upset than sodium bicarbonate, is usually preferred for this reason. I.V. administration of sodium bicarbonate can cause extravasation that may result in tissue sloughing, ulceration, and necrosis. The most severe adverse reaction (causing hyperirritability, tetany, or both) is metabolic alkalosis related to sodium bicarbonate overdose. In a patient with diabetic ketoacidosis, rapid administration of sodium bicarbonate that corrects acidosis too quickly may cause cerebral dysfunction, tissue hypoxia, and lactic acidosis. The high sodium content (12 mEq or 276 mg/

gram) in this drug may cause water retention and edema in some patients, especially those with renal disease, congestive heart failure (CHF), or other disorders that can cause fluid imbalance.

Sodium citrate normally produces few adverse reactions, but an overdose may cause metabolic alkalosis or tetany or may aggravate existing cardiac disease by decreasing serum calcium levels. Oral sodium citrate can have a laxative effect.

Sodium lactate also causes few adverse reactions except for metabolic alkalosis (from an overdose) and extravasation. Because the sodium content is high (8 to 9 mEq or 204 mg/gram), this alkalinizing agent may cause water retention and edema in a patient whose ability to excrete sodium is impaired, particularly by a renal disease or CHF.

Adverse reactions to tromethamine may be mild, such as phlebitis or irritation at the injection site, or severe, such as hypoglycemia, respiratory depression (especially in a patient who already has depressed respirations or is receiving drugs that depress respirations), extravasation, and hyperkalemia. In a patient with impaired renal function, this renally excreted drug may accumulate to toxic levels. In a severely ill neonate, hypertonic tromethamine given through the umbilical vein can cause hepatic necrosis. Because of these adverse reactions, tromethamine administration should not exceed 1 day for most patients.

A wide range of predictable adverse reactions can occur with acetazolamide. GI tract signs and symptoms include nausea, vomiting, diarrhea, anorexia, and weight loss. Central nervous system (CNS) reactions may include sedation, headache, confusion, and paresthesias. This drug can also elevate blood glucose levels in a diabetic patient; decrease uric acid excretion, leading to gout; cause metabolic acidosis; and precipitate hepatic coma in a patient with severe liver disease.

Unpredictable reactions

Unpredictable adverse reactions to acetazolamide include hypersensitivity reactions, such as cholestatic jaundice, fever, rash, skin eruptions, and bone marrow depression (which may lead to aplastic anemia).

NURSING IMPLICATIONS

Whenever treatment with an alkalinizing agent is required, the nurse should monitor the patient for metabolic alkalosis and extravasation (with I.V. administration) and be aware of the following considerations:

• Treat extravasation by elevating the affected extremity, applying warm compresses, and administering lidocaine, hyaluronidase, or both, as prescribed.

• Advise the patient receiving prolonged therapy with sodium bicarbonate tablets that GI distress and flatulence may occur and should be reported to the physician. GI distress can lead to noncompliance and subsequent acute acidosis, so expect an order for an alternate alkalinizing agent if the patient reports GI distress.

• Dilute Shohl's solution with water before administering it, refrigerate it to improve the taste, and administer it after meals to prevent its laxative effects.

• Teach the patient to recognize the signs and symptoms of sodium and water retention (for example, swelling of ankles and tightening of rings). Emphasize the importance of reporting these signs and symptoms immediately to the physician.

• Monitor the patient's urine pH frequently when sodium bicarbonate or acetazolamide is used to alkalinize the urine.

ACIDIFYING AGENTS

Certain disorders cause alkalosis, or excess base in the blood. To correct this type of acid-base imbalance, the blood pH can be lowered by administering drugs that provide hydrogen ions or drugs that interfere with bicarbonate metabolism and decrease blood bicarbonate levels.

Three acidifying agents—ammonium chloride, arginine hydrochloride, and hydrochloric acid—are used to correct metabolic alkalosis. Ammonium chloride and ascorbic acid may serve as urine-acidifying agents. Because they acidify the urine, all these agents may be used to increase the effectiveness of certain urinary antibacterial agents and to enhance drug excretion in patients with overdoses of certain drugs.

One additional substance, cranberry juice, has commonly been used as a urine-acidifying agent, even though it is probably ineffective and is certainly less effective than ascorbic acid or ammonium chloride. (For additional information, see *The cranberry juice controversy* on page 844.)

History and source
Ammonium chloride is prepared from an inorganic salt and hydrochloric acid from a chemical reagent. Arginine hydrochloride is a synthetic form of the essential amino acid L-arginine.

PHARMACOKINETICS

Acidifying agents are usually administered I.V. (Ammonium chloride and ascorbic acid may be administered orally.) Ammonium chloride and arginine hydrochloride are metabolized and release hydrochloric acid, the acidifying agent.

Absorption, distribution, metabolism, excretion
When ammonium chloride is administered orally, it is completely absorbed in 3 to 6 hours. It is metabolized in the liver to form urea, which is excreted by the kidneys, and hydrochloric acid, the acidifying agent.

When used to treat metabolic alkalosis, arginine hydrochloride is administered I.V. The drug is metabolized in the liver to ornithine and urea, which are excreted by the kidneys, and to hydrochloric acid.

When administered I.V., hydrochloric acid is used directly as hydrogen ions.

After oral administration, ascorbic acid is usually well absorbed. However, absorption of a large dose may be limited, because the body's stores fill and level off at the renal threshold, and the excess is excreted. When this occurs, no additional ascorbic acid will be absorbed, even if more is administered. Ascorbic acid is widely distributed in body tissues and metabolized in the liver. Metabolites are excreted in the urine along with excess ascorbic acid, which is excreted unchanged because it remains unabsorbed.

PHARMACODYNAMICS

When alkalosis occurs, therapy must increase the hydrogen ion concentration to correct the acid-base imbalance. Acidifying agents can increase the concentration directly—by providing hydrogen ions from metabolic release of hydrochloric acid—or indirectly—by interfering with bicarbonate metabolism.

Mechanism of action
Ammonium chloride lowers the blood pH after being metabolized to urea and to hydrochloric acid, which provides hydrogen ions to acidify the blood or urine. Arginine hydrochloride also provides hydrogen ions via metabolism to hydrochloric acid. Hydrochloric acid lowers blood pH directly by acidifying the blood with hydrogen ions.

Ascorbic acid directly acidifies the urine, providing hydrogen ions and lowering the urine pH.

PHARMACOTHERAPEUTICS

A patient with metabolic alkalosis requires therapy with an acidifying agent that provides hydrogen ions; such a patient may need chloride ion therapy as well. Although the patient can receive both in a hydrochloric acid infusion, this infusion is difficult to prepare, and an overdose can produce severe adverse reactions. That is why most patients receive both types of ions in oral or parenteral doses of ammonium chloride, a safer drug that is easy to prepare.

A patient with a urinary tract infection or a drug overdose may benefit from receiving a urine-acidifying agent.

ammonium chloride. This acidifying agent is used to treat metabolic alkalosis related to chloride loss, which may result from vomiting, gastric suctioning, fistula drainage, pyloric stenosis, or the use of a chloride-wasting diuretic, such as hydrochlorothiazide or furosemide. It is effective for 3 to 4 days, until the kidneys' compensatory responses take effect and they begin to excrete the same amount of acid as the patient receives. Discontinuation of ammonium chloride for several days lets the compensatory mechanisms return to normal, when ammonium chloride therapy, reinitiated, will again be effective for several days.

This agent may also be used to acidify the urine of a patient with a urinary tract infection. This use is discouraged, however, because it can produce metabolic acidosis. Ammonium chloride may be administered by the oral or I.V. route.

USUAL ADULT DOSAGE: for metabolic alkalosis, 0.9 to 1.3 ml/minute I.V. of a 2.14% solution, or 20 ml of a 26.75% solution in 500 ml of normal saline solution I.V. at a rate of 5 ml/minute or less; as a urine acidifying agent, 4 to 12 grams P.O. daily in divided doses every 4 to 6 hours.

USUAL PEDIATRIC DOSAGE: as an acidifying agent, 75 mg/kg/day in four divided doses.

DRUG INTERACTIONS

Acidifying agents

Drug interactions involving acidifying agents can be severe and may increase or decrease another drug's pharmacologic action.

DRUG	INTERACTING DRUGS	POSSIBLE EFFECTS	NURSING IMPLICATIONS
ammonium chloride	chlorpropamide	Decreases chlorpropamide excretion	• Monitor the patient for signs of hypoglycemia, such as diaphoresis, tachycardia, and tremors. • Monitor the patient's blood glucose levels.
	flecainide	Increases flecainide excretion and decreases flecainide serum half-life	• Assess the patient for recurring dysrhythmias.
	methadone	Increases renal clearance of methadone	• Monitor the patient for decreased methadone effect, indicated by signs of withdrawal, such as stomach cramps, diaphoresis, and a runny nose.
	mexiletine	Increases mexiletine excretion	• Assess the patient for recurring dysrhythmias.
	spironolactone	Impairs excretion of hydrogen ions, resulting in metabolic acidosis	• Monitor the patient for signs of metabolic acidosis, such as headache, lethargy, decreasing level of consciousness, and abnormal respirations.

arginine hydrochloride. Like ammonium chloride, arginine hydrochloride is used to treat metabolic alkalosis related to chloride loss. (See Chapter 58, Pituitary Agents, for information about other uses of arginine.) It is available as a 100 mg/ml I.V. solution. The following formula can be used to calculate the correct dosage:

$$\text{arginine dosage (in grams)} = \frac{\text{base deficit} \times \text{body weight (kg)}}{9.6}$$

USUAL ADULT DOSAGE: for metabolic alkalosis, dosage calculated using the patient's base deficit.

hydrochloric acid. In a dilute solution, hydrochloric acid can be used to treat metabolic alkalosis, but it must be given I.V. after preparation in the pharmacy under carefully controlled aseptic conditions. (See Chapter 47, Adsorbent, Antiflatulent, and Digestive Agents, for information about other uses of hydrochloric acid.)
USUAL ADULT DOSAGE: for metabolic alkalosis, 0.1 or 0.2 molar solution administered I.V. at a rate of 0.2 mEq/kg/hour or less through a central venous line. Subsequent doses must be based on arterial blood gas measurements taken every 4 hours during the infusion.

The cranberry juice controversy

Cranberry juice has been used to acidify the urine for many years. More than 100 years ago, researchers discovered that eating cranberries increased hippuric acid excretion. Then, in the 1920s, a study demonstrated that eating cranberries acidified the urine of one patient. Repeated publication of this study's results led to widespread use of cranberries and cranberry juice as urine-acidifying agents.

Although the exact mechanism of action of cranberry juice remains unknown, some researchers theorize that acidic substances, such as benzoic acid, are metabolized from the quinic acid in cranberries and that these substances acidify the urine. But up to the present, few studies support these theories, and most people do not consume enough cranberries or cranberry juice to produce the desired effect.

The cranberry juice drink sold in most grocery stores actually contains only 10% cranberry juice, so the amount of it needed to acidify the urine would be too large to consume. Although no studies have proved that cranberry juice can acidify the urine, one recent study found that consumption of 3 to 10 ounces of cranberries produced mild acidosis in the blood. However, routine cranberry consumption—about 1 ounce—is not nearly enough to produce this effect.

ascorbic acid [vitamin C] (Ascorbicap, Ascorbineed). Administered orally, this drug is used to maintain the urine acidity needed for effective action of urinary antibacterial agents, such as methenamine mandelate (Mandelamine), which can only be converted to its active ingredient in an acidic environment. In addition, the acidic environment itself helps decrease bacterial growth in the urine. Some physicians, however, question ascorbic acid's effectiveness. (See Chapter 51, Vitamin and Mineral Agents, for information about the other uses of ascorbic acid.)
USUAL ADULT DOSAGE: as a urine acidifier, 4 to 12 grams daily P.O. in divided doses.

Drug interactions
These acidifying agents can interact with various drugs, primarily by their action of altering the acid-base environment, which in turn modifies the other drugs' action or excretion. (See *Drug interactions: Acidifying agents* on page 843 for detailed information.)

ADVERSE DRUG REACTIONS
Adverse reactions to acidifying agents are usually mild—for example, GI distress. However, overdose can occur, especially with parenteral administration, and may lead to acidosis.

Predictable reactions
Oral administration of ammonium chloride may cause nausea, vomiting, anorexia, and thirst. Large doses may cause metabolic acidosis and loss of electrolytes, especially potassium. Rapid I.V. administration may cause pain and irritation at the infusion site. Ammonium toxicity may also occur, producing twitching and hyperreflexia.

Adverse reactions to arginine hydrochloride typically result from too-rapid I.V. administration and include flushing, nausea, vomiting, headache, numbness, and irritation at the infusion site.

With hydrochloric acid administration, metabolic acidosis may occur with an overdose.

In high doses, ascorbic acid can produce GI distress, such as nausea, vomiting, diarrhea, and abdominal cramps, and flushing, headache, and insomnia. In a patient with glucose-6-phosphate dehydrogenase (G6PD) deficiency, hemolytic anemia may develop after administration of a high dose of ascorbic acid.

Unpredictable reactions
In some patients, arginine hydrochloride causes a hypersensitivity reaction consisting of a macular rash with redness and edema of the hands and face; these disappear when the drug is discontinued. This agent may also cause other hypersensitivity reactions.

SELECTED MAJOR DRUGS

Alkalinizing and acidifying agents

This chart summarizes the major alkalinizing and acidifying agents currently in clinical use.

DRUG	MAJOR INDICATIONS	USUAL ADULT DOSAGES	NURSING IMPLICATIONS
Alkalinizing agents			
sodium bicarbonate	Severe metabolic acidosis in cardiac arrest	1 mEq/kg I.V. initially, followed by 0.5 mEq/kg every 10 minutes; or an individualized dosage	• Monitor the patient's serum sodium level to detect any increase. • Assess the patient for gastric distention and flatulence.
	Less severe metabolic acidosis	2 to 5 mEq/kg I.V. infused over 4 to 8 hours	
	Systemic or urine alkalinization	20 to 36 mEq/kg P.O. daily in divided doses	
sodium citrate	Metabolic acidosis	10 to 30 ml of Shohl's solution P.O. after meals and at bedtime	• Monitor the patient's serum sodium level to detect any increase. • Refrigerate the drug to make it more palatable. • Dilute the drug before administration. • Administer after meals to minimize the laxative effect.
Acidifying agent			
ammonium chloride	Metabolic alkalosis related to chloride loss	0.9 to 1.3 ml/minute I.V. of a 2.14% solution	• Monitor the I.V. infusion continuously to prevent overdose and acidosis. • Monitor the patient's blood pH.
	Urine acidification	4 to 12 grams P.O. daily in divided doses every 4 to 6 hours	

NURSING IMPLICATIONS

Because acidifying agents can cause severe adverse reactions, the nurse must monitor the patient carefully and be aware of the following considerations:

• Monitor the patient for signs of metabolic acidosis, such as CNS depression, abnormal respirations, and abnormal laboratory values of arterial blood pH, serum bicarbonate, serum chloride, or serum potassium.

• Prepare acidifying agents for I.V. administration under aseptic conditions, preferably in a laminar airflow hood. Expect the pharmacy to prepare a hydrochloric acid infusion, because the acid is extremely caustic.

• Inform the patient receiving ascorbic acid to take it exactly as directed, to report severe GI adverse reactions, and to monitor the urine pH regularly.

CHAPTER SUMMARY

Chapter 53 covered alkalinizing and acidifying agents as they are used to treat certain acid-base disorders and to regulate blood and urine pH. Here are the highlights of the chapter:

• Homeostatic buffer systems and compensatory mechanisms help keep blood pH within a narrow normal range—between 7.35 and 7.45. Certain disorders can upset this delicate acid-base balance, which may be corrected by the administration of alkalinizing or acidifying agents.

• Alkalinizing agents, such as tromethamine and sodium bicarbonate, citrate, and lactate, are used to treat metabolic acidosis by alkalinizing the blood. They do this by decreasing the hydrogen ion concentration. Sodium bicarbonate is also used when treating cardiac arrest to correct acidosis and prevent dysrhythmias.

• Some alkalinizing agents, such as sodium bicarbonate and acetazolamide, can also alkalinize the urine. They are useful for promoting the excretion of certain weak acids, such as uric acid, or toxic drugs, such as phenobarbital.

• Acidifying agents, such as ammonium chloride, arginine hydrochloride, and hydrochloric acid, are used to correct metabolic alkalosis by acidifying the blood. They do this by increasing the hydrogen ion concentration.

• Ammonium chloride and large doses of ascorbic acid may be used to acidify the urine in patients with urinary tract infections. Although cranberry juice is widely used as a urine acidifying agent, it is largely ineffective.

• Alkalinizing and acidifying agents can cause some adverse reactions. Most result from overdose of the agents. Sodium bicarbonate, citrate, and lactate may cause water retention and edema in patients with impaired ability to excrete sodium from disorders such as CHF or renal dysfunction.

• Alkalinizing and acidifying agents can interact with a wide variety of drugs, increasing or decreasing their pharmacologic action.

BIBLIOGRAPHY

American Hospital Formulary Service. *Drug Information 87.* McEvoy, G.K., ed. Bethesda, Md.: American Society of Hospital Pharmacists, 1987.

Der Marderosian, A.H. "Cranberry Juice," *Drug Therapy* 7:151, 157, 160, November 1977.

Hansten, P.D. *Drug Interactions,* 5th ed. Philadelphia: Lea & Febiger, 1985.

Kaehny, W.D. "Respiratory Acid-Base Disorders," *Medical Clinics of North America* 67:915, July 1983.

Mangini, R.J., ed. *Drug Interaction Facts.* St. Louis: Facts and Comparisons Division, J.B. Lippincott Co., 1984.

Masoro, E.J. "An Overview of Hydrogen Ion Regulation," *Archives of Internal Medicine* 142:1019, May 1982.

Windus, D.W. "Fluids and Electrolytes," in *Manual of Medical Therapeutics,* 25th ed. Boston: Little, Brown & Co., 1986.

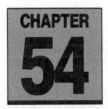

CHAPTER 54

CATION-EXCHANGE RESIN AND AMMONIA-DETOXICATING AGENTS

OBJECTIVES

After reading and studying this chapter, you should be able to:

1. Describe how the cation-exchange resin sodium polystyrene sulfonate acts to remove endogenous substances from the body.

2. Explain the significance of monitoring electrolytes such as calcium, magnesium, and sodium during sodium polystyrene sulfonate therapy.

3. Explain why sorbitol is administered with sodium polystyrene sulfonate.

4. Describe how the acidification of the colon contents after lactulose therapy reduces the absorption of ammonia.

5. Explain the significance of closely monitoring diabetic patients who are receiving lactulose.

6. Identify the signs and symptoms and nursing interventions for nephrotoxicity and ototoxicity from neomycin therapy.

INTRODUCTION

Chapter 54 describes drugs that decrease toxic levels of endogenous substances via the gastrointestinal (GI) tract. The body naturally contains both potassium and ammonia. When the serum concentration levels of these substances are within normal range, potassium and ammonia participate in the normal metabolic function of the internal environment. When the serum concentration levels increase, both of these substances can lead to harmful and potentially fatal effects.

A cation-exchange resin, also called a potassium-removing resin, is an insoluble compound of high molecular weight, capable of exchanging sodium ions for potassium ions in surrounding solution. Sodium polystyrene sulfonate is a synthetic cation-exchange resin used to remove potassium from the body of a patient with hyperkalemia. Sodium polystyrene sulfonate may be used alone, if potassium concentration levels are only slightly elevated, or in combination with other drugs to treat higher serum potassium concentration levels.

Ammonia is formed in the body in several ways: (1) by the liver during deamination of amino acids, (2) by epithelial cells of the proximal and distal tubules and collecting duct of the nephron, as part of regulation of hydrogen ion, and (3) by bacteria in the gastrointestinal tract acting on urea or dietary protein. A normally functioning liver then converts the absorbed ammonia to urea, a less toxic substance. Urea is excreted by the kidneys in the urine.

Liver damage or the shunting of blood flow around the liver can inhibit the conversion of ammonia to urea. The resulting elevated blood ammonia concentration levels can lead to a disorder known as hepatic encephalopathy, which may cause a decreased level of consciousness, an altered mental state, impaired neuromuscular functioning, or death.

Neomycin and lactulose help reduce blood ammonia levels. The antibiotic neomycin is formed naturally by a particular bacterial strain. When administered orally, neomycin will also eliminate the normal bacterial flora of the GI tract and may lead to superinfection. (See Chapter 66, Antibacterial Agents, for additional information regarding the antimicrobial uses of neomycin.) Lactulose is a synthetic derivative of lactose. Lactulose is also used to treat constipation. (See Chapter 48, Antidiarrheal and Laxative Agents, for additional information about the use of lactulose as a laxative.)

For a summary of representative drugs, see *Selected major drugs: Cation-exchange resin and ammonia-detoxicating agents* on page 855.

CATION-EXCHANGE RESIN

Sodium polystyrene sulfonate is the only commercially available drug that is effective as a cation-exchange resin. The drug exchanges sodium ions for potassium ions in the gastrointestinal tract. This action of sodium polystyrene sulfonate makes the resin useful for treating hyperkalemia.

PHARMACOKINETICS

Because sodium polystyrene sulfonate is insoluble, the resin remains available for binding potassium, which exists in high concentration in the large intestine.

Absorption, distribution, metabolism, excretion

Sodium polystyrene sulfonate is not absorbed from the gastrointestinal tract. Theoretically, each gram of the resin may bind with up to 3.1 mEq of potassium; however, because other cations, such as calcium and magnesium, also bind to sodium polystyrene sulfonate, an actual exchange capacity greater than 1 mEq of potassium per gram of resin is unlikely.

Each gram of sodium polystyrene sulfonate powder contains about 4.1 mEq of sodium. While only 33% of the resin's sodium content is distributed systemically, a daily administration of 15 to 60 grams of the drug may also result in the administration of 30 to 80 mEq of sodium.

Distribution of the resin is limited to the gastrointestinal tract. Sodium polystyrene sulfonate is not metabolized to any extent, and nearly 100% of a dose is excreted from the intestinal tract in the feces, primarily as potassium polystyrene sulfonate.

Onset, peak, duration

The potassium-lowering effects of sodium polystyrene sulfonate are slow and unpredictable. Onset of action may not occur for 2 to 24 hours after oral administration. The onset of action after rectal administration is somewhat shorter. The duration of action for sodium polystyrene sulfonate is about 4 to 6 hours.

PHARMACODYNAMICS

Sodium polystyrene sulfonate is a cation-exchange resin used to reduce elevated body potassium levels.

Mechanism of action

After oral administration of sodium polystyrene sulfonate, sodium ions are exchanged with hydrogen ions found in the stomach's acidic environment. As the resin passes through the gastrointestinal tract, hydrogen ions are released in exchange for other cations present in higher concentrations. Because of the high concentration of potassium in the large intestine, potassium readily exchanges with hydrogen ions. The modified resin, which includes small amounts of other cations besides potassium, is then eliminated in the feces. After rectal administration of sodium polystyrene sulfonate, sodium ions are released directly in exchange for potassium ions.

PHARMACOTHERAPEUTICS

Oral or rectal sodium polystyrene sulfonate is used to lower serum potassium concentration levels in the treatment of hyperkalemia when urgent reduction of potassium levels is not necessary. Since effective lowering of the serum potassium concentration level with sodium polystyrene sulfonate may take hours to days, physicians first treat life-threatening hyperkalemia with prompt-acting, shorter-duration measures to reduce the serum potassium level. Therapies that rapidly lower serum potassium levels include I.V. sodium bicarbonate or glucose and insulin. These therapies produce a transient intracellular shift of potassium, thus lowering plasma concentration levels. I.V. calcium decreases myocardial irritability caused by hyperkalemia, but does not correct hyperkalemia. Hemodialysis also rapidly and effectively reduces serum potassium levels and does so much longer than other therapies.

sodium polystyrene sulfonate (Kayexalate, SPS). During treatment, the dose and duration of sodium polystyrene sulfonate therapy must be individualized and depend on the daily assessment of total body potassium. USUAL ADULT DOSAGE: orally, 15 grams one to four times daily. Give each dose as a suspension in 20 to 100 ml of water or syrup. Using 70% sorbitol as a vehicle for administering this agent may prevent constipation because of sorbitol's laxative effect. As a retention enema, 30 to 50 grams rectally every 1 to 2 hours initially, then every 6 hours, or as needed. The agent should be retained at least 20 to 30 minutes to be effective.
USUAL PEDIATRIC DOSAGE: 1 gram for each mEq of potassium to be removed.

Drug interactions

Drugs that contain certain cations (such as calcium, magnesium, aluminum) have a propensity to interfere with sodium polystyrene sulfonate's effectiveness by competing for binding sites. Foods or liquids that contain potassium may also reduce sodium polystyrene sulfonate's effectiveness. (See Drug interactions: Cation-ex-

DRUG INTERACTIONS

Cation-exchange resin

Although drug interactions involving the cation-exchange resin rarely occur, the nurse should take precautions during the simultaneous administration of electrolyte solutions and some antacids.

DRUG	INTERACTING DRUGS	POSSIBLE EFFECTS	NURSING IMPLICATIONS
sodium polystyrene sulfonate	electrolyte-containing solutions	Reduce effectiveness of sodium polystyrene sulfonate	• Monitor serum electrolytes, especially sodium and potassium.
	calcium or magnesium antacids, such as calcium carbonate or magnesium hydroxide	Cause possible metabolic alkalosis occurring as the antacids neutralize gastric hydrochloric acid, forming magnesium or calcium chloride; in the small intestine, these antacids normally interact with bicarbonate to form magnesium or calcium carbonate; sodium polystyrene sulfonate prevents this reaction by binding calcium and magnesium; hydrogen ion is then lost without a concomitant loss of bicarbonate	• If used concurrently, watch for signs of alkalosis: pH above 7.45, confusion, and irritability.
		Cause cations to bind sodium polystyrene sulfonate, reducing its ability to bind potassium	• Monitor for continued hyperkalemia.
	aluminum-containing antacids	Cause additive constipation effect, possible fecal impaction	• If these drugs must be administered concurrently, watch for signs of constipation.

change resin for a list of the interacting drugs and their possible effects.)

ADVERSE DRUG REACTIONS

Sodium polystyrene sulfonate administration can cause numerous adverse drug reactions and, therefore, requires close patient monitoring. The most common adverse reactions involve altered GI function, primarily GI upset, and altered elimination patterns. Alterations of electrolyte balance, particularly of sodium, potassium, calcium, and magnesium, may also occur.

Predictable reactions

Sodium polystyrene sulfonate's potential to produce electrolyte imbalances can cause the drug's most serious adverse effect. Because the mechanism of action of sodium polystyrene sulfonate involves an exchange of sodium ions for potassium ions, use of the drug will alter

levels of these electrolytes. The patient will retain sodium ions and lose potassium ions.

Serious hypokalemia may develop from sodium polystyrene sulfonate therapy. Hypokalemia may cause disturbances of muscle function, cardiac rhythm, acid-base balance, and deep tendon reflexes, as well as potential digitalis toxicity. Sodium polystyrene sulfonate administration is usually discontinued when serum potassium concentration levels begin to approach the normal range.

Though sodium polystyrene sulfonate primarily affects sodium and potassium balance, the drug may also affect other electrolytes. Deficiencies of calcium and magnesium have been noted during therapy with cation-exchange resin.

Patients may complain of GI tract disturbances, such as nausea, vomiting, or anorexia, during sodium polystyrene sulfonate therapy. These symptoms may be from the drug's taste, the patient's feelings of fullness, or slowing of GI motility. Constipation is a serious problem because it may cause fecal impaction. To help the patient avoid constipation, the nurse can mix the sodium polystyrene sulfonate with 70% sorbitol, which draws water into the GI tract, thereby helping to keep stools soft and promoting elimination. However, patients may develop diarrhea from taking the sorbitol.

Unpredictable reactions
Some patients receiving sodium polystyrene sulfonate and aluminum hydroxide gel antacids concurrently have experienced intestinal obstruction when these drugs combine to form a hard mass in the intestinal tract. Correcting the problem may require surgical intervention.

NURSING IMPLICATIONS

During treatment with the cation-exchange resin, the nurse must monitor the patient closely for signs of hypokalemia as well as normokalemia, which indicates the effectiveness in treating hyperkalemia. Other important nursing implications include proper administration of the cation-exchange resin and patient teaching.
• Administer sodium polystyrene sulfonate cautiously to patients unable to tolerate a sodium load. Carefully monitor patients with hypertension, congestive heart failure, or edema for signs of sodium and fluid overload. Also monitor their serum sodium concentration levels.
• Sodium polystyrene sulfonate is administered to lower the serum potassium concentration level; therefore, treatment may cause potassium deficiency. Monitor the serum potassium level at least once daily, and observe for signs of hypokalemia, including irritability, confusion, cardiac dysrhythmias, and muscle weakness.
• Always closely monitor electrocardiograms and the patient's clinical condition because serum potassium concentration levels may not reflect intracellular potassium deficiency. Furthermore, identify and eliminate if possible any exogenous sources of potassium the patient may be receiving (in diet, medications, and blood products).
• Administer sodium polystyrene sulfonate either orally or by retention enema. The enema route seems to work more rapidly but is less reliable because patients often expel part or all of the suspension.
• When administering sodium polystyrene sulfonate by enema, be certain to place it at least 20 cm (8 inches) into the colon. The patient should retain the enema for 20 to 30 minutes or as prescribed. If the patient experiences difficulty retaining the enema, elevate the patient's hips on pillows, have the patient assume a knee-chest position, or instill the enema through a catheter with an inflatable balloon.

• Mix sodium polystyrene sulfonate with fruit juice, water, syrup, or soft drinks to increase its palatability for oral administration. However, avoid fluids with high potassium content, including citrus juices, prune juice, milk, and apricot nectar. Sodium polystyrene sulfonate should be given in suspension. Do not administer the drug as a paste since its effectiveness greatly diminishes in that form.
• Monitor bowel function frequently to be certain that the patient is eliminating the resin. For patient constipation, add 70% sorbitol in volumes sufficient to produce one or two soft stools daily.
• If the patient is receiving aluminum hydroxide gel antacids concurrently, consult the physician about withholding this drug until the sodium polystyrene sulfonate therapy has ended.
• Teach patients taking sodium polystyrene sulfonate mixed with sorbitol at home to take the preparation early in the day. Taking the drug early should prevent problems with diarrhea at night.
• Be aware that the premixed preparations may be more desirable for the patient to use at home.

AMMONIA-DETOXICATING AGENTS

The ammonia-detoxicating drugs lactulose and neomycin commonly are used to lower blood ammonia concentration levels in patients with hepatic encephalopathy. The two drugs, however, lower blood ammonia concentration levels by different mechanisms. Lactulose produces acidification of the colon contents, thereby trapping ammonia in the GI tract. Neomycin, an aminoglycoside, acts by eliminating colonic bacteria that form ammonia.

History and source
In 1930, researchers at the Bureau of Standards of the United States Department of Commerce first synthesized lactulose. It was first used as a drug in 1959 when Mayerhofer and Petuely described its effect in treating chronic constipation in adults. Ingelfinger first suggested using lactulose to treat chronic hepatic coma, and clinical trials for this application began in 1965.

The aminoglycoside family of antibiotics, to which neomycin belongs, resulted from an intensive scientific search for drugs that would effectively act against gram-negative bacteria. In 1944, Waksman and co-workers announced the discovery of the first drug in this class, streptomycin. In 1949, Waksman and Lechevalier isolated neomycin from substances produced by the soil organism *Streptomyces fradiae.*

PHARMACOKINETICS

Lactulose remains in the gastrointestinal tract, where it acts to reduce ammonium ion absorption. Neomycin also remains in the gastrointestinal tract, where it acts to sterilize the bowel.

Absorption, distribution, metabolism, excretion

After oral administration, lactulose is absorbed from the GI tract, but only to a minor degree. Distribution of lactulose then occurs throughout the gastrointestinal tract.

The unabsorbed lactulose is metabolized by colonic bacteria to lactic, acetic, and formic acids. The small quantity of lactulose absorbed is not metabolized and is excreted unchanged in the urine, bile, and feces. Excretion of lactulose is complete within 24 hours.

About 1% to 3% of a neomycin dose is absorbed from the GI tract after oral or rectal administration; however, more may be absorbed in certain circumstances, such as impaired gastrointestinal motility.

Because most of an oral or rectal dose of neomycin remains in the gut, drug distribution is limited to the GI tract. The small amount of neomycin that is absorbed systemically is distributed mostly into the extracellular fluid. Neomycin is not metabolized, and 97% to 99% of a dose remains unchanged in the gut. This unabsorbed neomycin is excreted in the feces, whereas the small percentage of absorbed neomycin is eliminated in the urine.

Onset, peak, duration

The onset of action for lactulose varies depending on the route of administration and on the patient's clinical condition. With rectal administration, the lactulose may produce beneficial effects in 2 to 12 hours, while orally administered lactulose may not produce beneficial effects for 24 to 48 hours. The duration of effect for a single dose may be from 6 to 8 hours.

The onset of action for neomycin to reduce blood ammonia concentration levels also varies. Theoretically, neomycin should begin to decrease the number of ammonia-producing bacteria when the drug reaches the large intestine. Reaching this destination, however, may take up to several hours, depending on the activity in the patient's gut.

Peak plasma concentration levels from the absorbed portion of neomycin may occur 1 to 4 hours after oral or rectal administration.

The duration of action for neomycin to treat hepatic encephalopathy is about 4 to 6 hours. Administering the neomycin dose every 6 hours should maintain adequate concentration levels of the drug in the bowel.

PHARMACODYNAMICS

Lactulose is a disaccharide sugar. When metabolized, the drug acts to decrease blood ammonia concentration levels, thereby reducing the degree of hepatic encephalopathy. Neomycin is an aminoglycoside antibiotic used to sterilize the bowel.

Mechanism of action

The disaccharide sugar lactulose consists of galactose and fructose. The metabolism of lactulose by colonic bacteria produces lactic, acetic, and formic acids. These organic acids acidify the colon from its normal pH of 7.0 to a pH of 5.0. Acidification of the colon contents converts nonionized ammonia to ionized ammonia, preventing its absorption.

Nonionized ammonia can diffuse from the blood into the colon. In the colon, the nonionized ammonia is converted to relatively nonabsorbable ammonium ions. These ammonium ions remain trapped in the gut. The following represents the progress from nonionized ammonia to the nonabsorbable ammonium ion:

$$\text{Blood} \quad \text{Intestine}$$
$$NH_3 \rightarrow NH_3 + H^+ \rightarrow NH_4{}^+$$

The acidification of the colon maintains the ammonium ion in its ionized state. The charged ions cannot readily be absorbed through the lipid layer of the intestine. Furthermore, colon acidification encourages the growth of weak ammonia-producing bacteria, such as *Lactobacillus acidophilus,* over ammonia producers such as *Escherichia coli.* Lactulose may also produce an osmotic diarrhea that decreases the intestinal transit time available for ammonia production and absorption.

The mechanism by which neomycin lowers blood ammonia concentration levels relates to its ability to decrease the number of ammonia-producing bacteria such as *E. coli* in the gut. As with other aminoglycosides, neomycin exerts its antibacterial activity directly on the ribosomes of susceptible organisms, among them *E. coli,* by inhibiting protein synthesis via direct action on ribosomal subunits. When these bacteria are present, they convert urea to ammonia. Neomycin is bactericidal in high concentrations and bacteriostatic in low concentrations.

DRUG INTERACTIONS

Ammonia-detoxicating agents

The following chart summarizes the drug interactions of lactulose and neomycin. Each interaction necessitates additional patient monitoring.

DRUG	INTERACTING DRUGS	POSSIBLE EFFECTS	NURSING IMPLICATIONS
lactulose	laxatives	Cause possible misinterpretation of loose stools as achievement of adequate lactulose dose	• Do not administer with lactulose if the dose is being titrated according to the presence of loose stools.
	neomycin and other anti-infective agents	Eliminate, in theory, bacteria responsible for conversion of lactulose into organic acids, preventing colonic acidification; however, evidence indicates that lactulose remains active when used with neomycin in patients with hepatic encephalopathy	• None.
neomycin	dietary carbohydrate, protein, lipid	Decrease absorption because to malabsorption	• Patient may require increased amounts of nutrients.
	digoxin, penicillin, vitamin K, methotrexate	Decrease absorption because to malabsorption	• Monitor patient for effectiveness of therapy.
	oral anticoagulants	Increase effect of oral anticoagulants	• Monitor patient for bleeding gums, oozing from I.V. sites, blood in urine, or epistaxis. • Monitor prothrombin time and bleeding time.
	aminoglycosides	Produce additive nephrotoxicity	• Monitor renal function.
	furosemide (Lasix)	Produces additive ototoxicity	• Monitor patient for hearing loss; inform patient to report signs and symptoms of ototoxicity: hearing loss, tinnitus, dizziness, headache, nausea, and vomiting.
	neuromuscular blockers	Cause possible potentiation of neuromuscular blockade	• Observe for respiratory depression.

PHARMACOTHERAPEUTICS

Lactulose serves as an adjunct to protein restriction and supportive therapy to prevent or treat hepatic encephalopathy. Lactulose can also be used to prevent or treat hepatic encephalopathy from surgical portocaval shunts and chronic hepatic diseases, such as cirrhosis. The drug may reduce ammonia levels by 25% to 50%, usually accompanied by an improved mental status. Clinical responses occur in 75% to 85% of the patients undergoing lactulose therapy. Patients unresponsive to neomycin and protein restriction therapy also may respond to lactulose; however, studies have shown that lactulose and neomycin are about equally effective.

Because neomycin destroys bacteria, whereas lactulose requires bacterial metabolism, some researchers have theorized that the concomitant use of these drugs may be counterproductive. In actual practice, however, lactulose seems to remain active even in the presence of neomycin. In fact, some evidence seems to indicate that concomitant use of lactulose and neomycin may be more beneficial than using either drug alone. Neomycin serves as an adjunct to protein restriction and lactulose therapy in the treatment of hepatic encephalopathy. Health care professionals use neomycin as a preoperative intestinal antiseptic and for the treatment of diarrhea caused by enteropathogenic *E. coli*.

Though clinical trials have shown neomycin to be as effective as lactulose to reduce elevated blood ammonia concentration levels, toxicities occurring from the systemic absorption of neomycin may be significant, especially with prolonged therapy. Therefore, lactulose may be more suitable for patients who need more than 2 to 3 days of therapy or for those with compromised renal function. Lactulose is also used to treat constipation because it produces an osmotic diarrhea.

lactulose (Cephulac, Chronulac). Doses of lactulose can be given orally or rectally.
USUAL ADULT DOSAGE: orally, 20 to 30 grams (30 to 45 ml) t.i.d. or q.i.d. Adjust the dosage every 1 to 2 days as needed to produce two to three soft stools daily. The dose may also be adjusted by measuring the stool pH, that is, the acidity of the colon contents, until the pH approximates 5.0. For most patients, typical dosages range from 60 to 100 grams (90 to 150 ml) daily. Hourly doses of 30 to 45 ml may induce rapid defecation in acute situations.

For rectal administration, dilute 200 grams (300 ml) in 700 ml of tap water or normal saline solution. Repeat the dose every 4 to 6 hours. If the patient does not retain the enema for 30 minutes, repeat the dose immediately.

neomycin (Mycifradin Sulfate, Neobiotic). Neomycin therapy usually accompanies other mechanisms of reducing blood ammonia concentration levels. These mechanisms might include using a low-protein diet and cleansing the GI tract of old blood.
USUAL ADULT DOSAGE: Orally as adjunctive treatment of hepatic encephalopathy, 4 to 12 grams/day in four divided doses. Therapy should continue for 5 to 6 days. Chronic hepatic insufficiency may require 4 grams/day for an indefinite time.

Rectally, administer a 1% solution as a retention enema for 20 to 60 minutes q.i.d.

Drug interactions

Anti-infective agents such as neomycin may eliminate colonic bacteria responsible for converting lactulose into organic acids. Existing data are contradictory regarding the importance of this interaction between neomycin and lactulose.

Loose stools help assure the adequacy of lactulose therapy. Concomitant laxative therapy also produces loose stools. As a result, the nurse may misinterpret the laxative-induced stool as evidence of adequate lactulose therapy. Oral neomycin may produce a reversible malabsorption syndrome that can affect the absorption of many foods and drugs. Vitamin K absorption may also decrease, increasing the oral anticoagulant effects.

During chronic treatment in renal dysfunction, the patient may systemically absorb a substantial quantity of neomycin. The concomitant use of other nephrotoxic or ototoxic drugs may increase nephrotoxicity or ototoxicity. (See *Drug interactions: Ammonia-detoxicating agents* for a list of interacting drugs and the nursing implications for the different effects.)

ADVERSE DRUG REACTIONS

Lactulose is administered via the GI tract, and little of the drug is absorbed systemically. As a result, most adverse reactions to lactulose involve the gastrointestinal tract. Because lactulose is a disaccharide, the small amount that is absorbed may increase the blood glucose concentration level in patients with impaired glucose tolerance. The aminoglycoside antibiotics are powerful antimicrobial drugs noted for their potential to produce ototoxicity and nephrotoxicity. Despite the limited absorption of oral neomycin, long-term therapy with high doses of the drug administered concurrently with other aminoglycoside antibiotics can lead to serious adverse effects.

A number of factors tend to increase the likelihood of the patient developing adverse reactions to neomycin. Patients with decreased GI motility or mucosal ulceration tend to absorb larger amounts of neomycin, thereby increasing their serum concentration levels of the drug. Most of the toxic effects relate directly to the concentration level and duration of action of high blood concentration levels of neomycin. Serum concentration levels of neomycin are also likely to be higher in patients who are elderly, dehydrated, experiencing renal failure, or taking potent diuretic drugs.

Predictable reactions

GI symptoms represent the most frequent adverse reactions to lactulose administration. As intestinal bacteria metabolize lactulose to lactic, acetic, and formic acid, hydrogen gas is released. As a result, patients may experience gaseous abdominal distention, abdominal pain, belching, or flatulence. Some patients have reported nausea and vomiting after lactulose ingestion. These symptoms may represent the patient's reaction to the extremely sweet taste of the drug.

Diarrhea, sometimes accompanied by abdominal cramping, may result from too much lactulose because some metabolites of lactulose produce a laxative action. Lactulose also exerts an osmotic effect, drawing water into the large intestine. This effect, increased with large doses, may produce frequent, loose stools. If the patient exhibits severe hepatic encephalopathy with high blood ammonia concentration levels, diarrhea may be considered an acceptable adverse reaction.

Identifying and preventing neomycin toxicity

Because neomycin therapy produces nephrotoxicity and ototoxicity, the nurse must know the signs and symptoms of these adverse effects as well as how to prevent them.

SIGNS AND SYMPTOMS	PREVENTION
Nephrotoxicity	
• Impaired urine concentrating ability evidenced by decreased specific gravity and urine osmolality • The appearance of protein or granular or hyaline casts in the urine • Increasing serum creatinine	• Do not administer neomycin to patients with decreased gastric motility or GI ulceration because these conditions cause increased neomycin absorption; do not administer to patients with dehydration or renal failure, or in combination with potent diuretics. • Avoid concurrent use with other drugs that can produce nephrotoxicity. • Monitor serum neomycin concentration levels. • Monitor urine specific gravity, urinalysis, and serum creatinine levels before, during, and after neomycin therapy. • Monitor intake, output, and weights daily, remembering that renal failure from neomycin is frequently non-oliguric.
Ototoxicity	
• The onset of a high-pitched tinnitus may be the initial symptom • Hearing loss later in therapy; loss of high-frequency sounds • Vestibular damage may result in an initial headache, later followed by dizziness, nausea, vomiting, and difficulty with coordination	• Do not administer neomycin to patients with decreased gastric motility or GI ulceration because these conditions lead to increased neomycin absorption; do not administer to patients with preexisting hearing loss. • Avoid concurrent administration of other drugs that might cause ototoxicity. • Inform the patient to report any ringing in the ears or headache. • Consider audiometric evaluation before, during, and after neomycin therapy.

As previously mentioned, small amounts of orally administered lactulose are converted to galactose and fructose, which may be absorbed from the small intestine. After large doses of lactulose, these sugars may be absorbed in amounts sufficient to produce hyperglycemia in patients with diabetes mellitus.

Because nephrotoxicity can result from neomycin, the nurse should closely monitor the patient for signs of impaired renal function. Furthermore, the signs of nephrotoxicity may not appear until after neomycin therapy has been discontinued. The nephrotoxic changes from neomycin are usually reversible over time.

Ototoxicity from damage to the vestibular and auditory branches of the eighth cranial nerve may also result from neomycin therapy. Auditory changes are more frequent than vestibular changes, but vestibular effects tend to be more reversible. (See *Identifying and preventing neomycin toxicity* for preventive measures for nephrotoxicity and ototoxicity.)

Nausea, vomiting, and diarrhea probably represent the most frequent adverse reactions to neomycin. Diarrhea may result from malabsorption of fat, xylose, glucose, or other substances. It may also be from superinfection with bacteria after normal bowel flora destruction by neomycin. *Clostridium difficile* infection leading to pseudomembranous colitis can be a particularly devastating result.

The potential for neuromuscular blockade also exists after neomycin administration. This reaction occurs less frequently with oral administration, but the nurse should never discount the problem. Neuromuscular blockade probably results when the release of acetylcholine at the nerve synapse becomes inhibited. Most cases of neuromuscular blockade have occurred when high doses of neomycin were administered concurrently with neuromuscular blocking drugs (such as tubocurarine and succinylcholine) or with general anesthesia. Hypocalcemia or myasthenia gravis also seems to increase the risk of neuromuscular blockade. The effects of neuromuscular blockade usually include a decreased rate and depth of respiration and acute muscle paralysis. The administration of calcium gluconate and perhaps neostigmine usually reverses these effects.

Unpredictable reactions

Though unpredictable reactions to ammonia-detoxicating agents do not frequently occur, some reactions have resulted from neomycin. These unpredictable reactions include skin rashes, fever, angioedema, stomatitis, and anaphylactic shock.

Cation-exchange resin and ammonia-detoxicating agents

The following chart summarizes the major cation-exchange resin and ammonia-detoxicating agents discussed in this chapter.

DRUG	MAJOR INDICATIONS	USUAL ADULT DOSAGES	NURSING IMPLICATIONS
Cation-exchange resin			
sodium polystyrene sulfonate	Hyperkalemia	15 grams P.O. one to four times daily or 30 to 50 grams every 1 to 6 hours rectally	• Administer cautiously to patients who cannot tolerate sodium loads, such as those with congestive heart failure. • Administer in a suspension. • Usually mix with 70% sorbitol to promote excretion. • Check that the patient retains the rectally administered drug for 20 to 30 minutes. • Monitor fluid, electrolyte, and acid-base balance carefully during therapy. • Assess bowel function to be certain the drug is eliminated. • Do not give concurrently with aluminum hydroxide gel antacids.
Ammonia-detoxicating agents			
lactulose	Hepatic encephalopathy Constipation	Initial dose: for hepatic encephalopathy, 20 to 30 grams (30 to 45 ml) P.O. t.i.d. to q.i.d. Acute toxicity: 30 to 45 ml every hour Rectally: 200 grams (300 ml) in 700 ml water or normal saline solution	• Agent is contraindicated in patients who need a low-galactose diet; it should be administered cautiously in patients with diabetes mellitus. • Use a catheter with a large inflatable balloon to improve lactulose retention during enema administration. • Monitor the number and consistency of stools; fluid, electrolyte, and acid-base balance; blood ammonia concentration levels; and the patient's level of consciousness. • A stool pH of 5.0 indicates adequate acidification of colon contents. • Avoid using other laxative agents or enemas during lactulose therapy. • Check to be sure the patient retains rectally administered drug for 30 to 60 minutes.
neomycin	Hepatic encephalopathy Preoperative bowel sterilization Diarrhea resulting from enteropathogenic *E. coli*	Orally: 4 to 12 grams in four divided doses for 5 to 6 days Rectally: 1% solution retained for 20 to 60 minutes, q.i.d.	• Agent is contraindicated in pregnant patients, in those with known hypersensitivity or intestinal obstruction, and possibly in those with GI ulceration. • Administer cautiously in the presence of neuromuscular blocking agents, general anesthesia, myasthenia gravis, renal failure, advanced age, dehydration, hearing impairment, hypocalcemia, and with other nephrotoxic and ototoxic drugs. • Monitor renal, auditory, and vestibular function carefully before, during, and after therapy. • Monitor the patient's level of consciousness and muscle coordination as indicators of clinical improvement. • Notify the physician if diarrhea occurs. • Monitor the adequacy of respiration and motor function in the presence of neuromuscular blocking agents.

NURSING IMPLICATIONS

The nurse must be aware of some important implications when using ammonia-detoxicating drugs, especially neomycin.

• Be aware that lactulose is contraindicated in patients who need a low-galactose diet. Administer lactulose cautiously to patients with diabetes mellitus.

• Also be aware that lactulose is contraindicated in patients with inflammatory bowel disease and chronic constipation. Consult the physician before administration if the patient displays symptoms of bowel obstruction, GI bleeding, or acute abdominal pain. Research has not established the safe use of lactulose during pregnancy and lactation.

• Know that neomycin is contraindicated in pregnant patients as well as in patients with known hypersensitivity and intestinal obstruction. Neomycin may also be contraindicated in patients with GI ulceration. Administer neomycin cautiously in the presence of neuromuscular blocking agents, general anesthesia, myasthenia gravis, renal failure, advanced age, dehydration, hearing impairment, hypocalcemia, and with other nephrotoxic or ototoxic drugs.

• During lactulose therapy, monitor the number and consistency of the patient's stools. Normally, consider the dose to be adequate if the patient has two to three soft stools per day. In acute situations, the large amounts of prescribed lactulose may cause diarrhea. If diarrhea occurs, monitor the patient for fluid, electrolyte, and acid-base disturbances, particularly dehydration, hypokalemia, and acidosis. Institute measures to protect the patient's perianal skin from the irritation caused by frequent stools.

• During treatment with either lactulose or neomycin, monitor the patient for signs of effective therapy. Evaluation should include assessments of the patient's level of consciousness, asterixis, muscle coordination, and blood ammonia concentration levels. All of these factors should improve as blood ammonia concentration levels decrease.

• To test for muscle coordination, have the patient provide a signature or draw a five-pointed star each day. As the hepatic encephalopathy improves, muscle coordination should improve, and the patient's signature and drawings will become clearer. The patient's level of consciousness should also improve.

• Check the pH of the stool periodically. A pH of 5.0 or less indicates that the colon contents are acidic enough to trap ammonia ions, thereby reducing ammonia absorption.

• Monitor blood glucose levels in diabetic patients, and carefully evaluate all patients' renal function before, during, and after neomycin therapy. Always document information about the patient's auditory and vestibular function before the onset of neomycin therapy, and ask the patient to report any changes.

• Closely monitor the rate and depth of respiration and motor function in patients who risk developing a neuromuscular blockade. Have calcium gluconate and neostigmine readily available if administering neomycin to these patients.

• Note that lactulose may be mixed in a beverage such as juice, a soft drink, milk, or water to improve its palatability and decrease nausea and vomiting.

• When giving rectal lactulose, use a catheter with a large balloon for inflation. Administer the drug deep into the rectum, at least 20 cm. After administration, the patient should retain the drug for 30 to 60 minutes. Inflating the rectal catheter balloon improves retention. Do not use cleansing enemas containing soapsuds or alkaline agents with rectally administered lactulose because the soapsuds and alkalines interfere with the drug's effectiveness.

CHAPTER SUMMARY

Chapter 54 covered the cation-exchange resin and ammonia-detoxicating agents. Both kinds of drugs decrease toxic levels of endogenous substances by increasing the elimination or decreasing the production of these substances in the gastrointestinal tract. Here are the highlights of the chapter:

• Sodium polystyrene sulfonate is a nonabsorbable resin that releases sodium and absorbs potassium in the GI tract. Physicians use sodium polystyrene sulfonate to treat hyperkalemia.

• The onset of action of sodium polystyrene sulfonate is quite slow, and changes in the serum potassium concentration level may not occur for 2 to 24 hours. Do not use this cation-exchange resin alone in the presence of life-threatening serum potassium concentration levels because it may not remove the excess potassium quickly enough.

• Sodium polystyrene sulfonate may be administered orally or via retention enema.

• Sodium polystyrene sulfonate may absorb electrolytes other than potassium, primarily calcium and magnesium. The resin also may release sodium in quantities sufficient to cause problems for patients who cannot tolerate a sodium load. The nurse should closely monitor the signs and symptoms of fluid and electrolyte concentration balance as well as the serum electrolyte concentration levels.

• Sodium polystyrene sulfonate tends to solidify in the GI tract, and fecal impaction may result. To prevent fecal impaction, the nurse can administer the drug with 70% sorbitol, which forms softer stools and helps excrete the resin.

• Lactulose and neomycin reduce blood ammonia concentration levels in patients with hepatic encephalopathy. Lactulose, a synthetic derivative of lactose, is a disaccharide sugar composed of galactose and fructose. Neomycin is an aminoglycoside antibiotic that is minimally absorbed from the GI tract.

• Lactulose is metabolized by colonic bacteria to lactic, acetic, and formic acid, thereby acidifying the colon contents. As the colon contents become more acidic, ammonia within the bowel and from the serum is trapped in the stool and excreted from the body.

• Effective lactulose therapy generally results in two to three soft stools per day. Diarrhea may result if large doses are used to treat acute toxicity.

• Neomycin lowers blood ammonia concentration levels by acting in the gut to eliminate bacteria that form ammonia from urea.

• As with all aminoglycoside antibiotics, neomycin can produce serious toxicity. Nephrotoxicity, ototoxicity, and neuromuscular blockade may result from the prolonged administration of neomycin.

BIBLIOGRAPHY

American Hospital Formulary Service. *Drug Information 1986*. McEvoy, G.K., et al., eds. Bethesda, Md.: American Society of Hospital Pharmacists, 1986.

Crossley, I.R., and Williams, R. "Progress in the Treatment of Chronic Portasystemic Encephalopathy," *Gut* 25:85, January 1984.

Fraser, C.L., and Arieff, A.I. "Hepatic Encephalopathy," *The New England Journal of Medicine* 313:865, October 3, 1985.

Gilman, A.G., et al., eds. *Goodman and Gilman's The Pharmacological Basis of Therapeutics*, 7th ed. New York: Macmillan Publishing Co., 1985.

Guyton, A.C. *Textbook of Medical Physiology*. Philadelphia: W.B. Saunders Co., 1986.

Kastrup, E.K., ed. *Drug Facts and Comparisons*. Philadelphia: J.B. Lippincott Co., 1985.

Katcher, B.S., et al., eds. *Applied Therapeutics: The Clinical Use of Drugs*. San Francisco: Applied Therapeutics, Inc., 1983.

Nelson, D.C., et al. "Hypernatremia and Lactulose Therapy," *Journal of the American Medical Association* 249:1295, March 11, 1983.

Schablik, J.K. "Hepatic Failure: Etiologies, Manifestations, and Management," *Critical Care Nurse* 5:60, January/February 1985.

DRUGS TO TREAT ENDOCRINE SYSTEM DISORDERS

Endocrine pharmacology encompasses a wide range of agents, including natural hormones and their synthetic analogues, hormonelike substances, and drugs that stimulate or suppress hormone secretion. To understand endocrine pharmacology, the nurse needs to know about the endocrine system and its hormones. (See *Endocrine hormones* on page 861 for an illustration of endocrine glands and the substances they secrete.)

Pancreatic hormones
The pancreas secretes two hormones, insulin and glucagon, from special cells in the islets of Langerhans. The beta cells produce insulin; the alpha cells secrete glucagon.

Insulin promotes the uptake, storage, and use of glucose; glucagon increases glycogenolysis and gluconeogenesis. Insulin also inhibits lipolysis and promotes cellular uptake of amino acids and protein synthesis. Blood glucose levels primarily control insulin and glucagon secretion. At a normal fasting blood glucose level, (70 to 110 mg/dl), little insulin is secreted. When the blood glucose level rises above 110 mg/dl, insulin secretion rapidly increases. When it falls below 70 mg/dl, glucagon secretion increases, rapidly increasing hepatic glucose production. Thus, glucagon prevents hypoglycemia and insulin prevents hyperglycemia.

Thyroid hormones
The thyroid gland secretes triiodothyronine (T_3) and thyroxine (T_4), which influence the body's metabolic rate, and calcitonin, which helps regulate calcium metabolism. Secretion of these thyroid hormones is controlled primarily by thyroid-stimulating hormone, which is secreted by the anterior pituitary gland.

The thyroid gland secretes more T_4 than T_3. Although the hormones function the same physiologically, they differ in onset and intensity of action: T_3 is about four times as potent as T_4 and produces effects much more rapidly. Yet both hormones increase protein synthesis, stimulate cellular enzyme activity, promote growth, and enhance carbohydrate and fat metabolism. They also increase cardiac output and heart rate, respiratory rate and depth, and gastrointestinal (GI) motility.

Calcitonin is secreted primarily by the thyroid gland. When the serum calcium level is high, calcitonin secretion increases. Calcitonin reduces the serum calcium level by inhibiting bone resorption, reducing osteoclast activity, and increasing renal excretion of calcium.

Parathyroid hormone
The parathyroid glands' secretion of parathyroid hormone is regulated primarily by the concentration of plasma calcium. Any physiologic or pathologic alteration that increases the serum calcium level will suppress parathyroid gland secretion. Any decrease in serum calcium level will increase parathyroid gland secretion.

Parathyroid hormone stimulates the resorption of calcium and phosphate from bone. It also increases GI absorption, and decreases renal excretion of calcium.

Anterior pituitary hormones
The anterior pituitary gland secretes six hormones that help control metabolic processes throughout the body: growth hormone (GH), adrenocorticotropic hormone (ACTH), thyroid-stimulating hormone (TSH), prolactin, follicle-stimulating hormone (FSH), and luteinizing hormone (LH).

GH, also called somatotropic hormone or somatotropin, promotes growth by increasing protein synthesis, decreasing carbohydrate use, and increasing the mobilization and use of fats for energy.

ACTH, also called adrenocorticotropin or corticotropin, controls cortisol secretion and enhances androgen production by the adrenal gland. It also influences aldosterone secretion.

TSH, or thyrotropin, stimulates the thyroid gland to increase T_3 and T_4 production and secretion. Normally, thyroid hormone levels remain fairly constant because of an effective feedback mechanism. Increased levels of thyroid hormone inhibit TSH secretion from the pituitary gland; decreased levels stimulate TSH secretion. A hypothalamic hormone, thyrotropin-releasing hormone, regulates the increase in TSH secretion.

Prolactin promotes mammary gland development and milk production. Prolactin secretion is predominantly under the negative control of the hypothalamus, which synthesizes a hormone that suppresses its secre-

Glossary

Adrenocorticotropin: anterior pituitary hormone that stimulates the adrenal cortex.

Anabolism: constructive process by which living cells convert simple substances into more complex compounds.

Androgenic: producing masculine characteristics.

Atrophic vaginitis: postmenopausal inflammation of the vagina characterized by vaginal burning, vaginal and vulvar itching, dyspareunia, and possibly blood-flecked discharge.

Calcitonin: thyroid hormone that decreases serum calcium levels.

Chvostek's sign: facial muscle spasm elicited by tapping the muscles or facial nerve in hypocalcemic individuals.

Cretinism: chronic condition caused by congenital hypothyroidism, characterized by arrested physical and mental development, osteodystrophy, and a decreased basal metabolic rate.

Cryptorchidism: developmental defect in which the testes fail to descend into the scrotum.

Desquamation: shedding of skin and other epithelial elements.

Diabetes insipidus: metabolic disorder characterized by extreme polyuria and polydipsia from deficient secretion of antidiuretic hormone or the inability of kidney tubules to respond to ADH.

Diabetes mellitus: metabolic disorder in which the ability to metabolize carbohydrates is lost because of decreased insulin secretions, characterized by hyperglycemia, glycosuria, polyuria, polydipsia, polyphagia, emaciation, and weakness.

Diabetic ketoacidosis: acute life-threatening complication of uncontrolled diabetes mellitus. The patient appears flushed; has hot, dry skin; is restless, uncomfortable, agitated, and diaphoretic; and has a fruity breath odor.

Dwarfism: abnormal underdevelopment of the body.

Eclampsia: severe toxemia of pregnancy characterized by convulsions, coma, hypertension, edema, and proteinuria.

Endometrium: mucous lining of the uterus, which varies in thickness and structure during the menstrual cycle.

Epiphysis: end of a long bone, usually wider than the shaft, that is either entirely cartilaginous or separated from the shaft by a cartilaginous disk.

Euthyroid: with a normal thyroid gland.

Galatorrhea: excessive or spontaneous milk flow not associated with childbirth or nursing.

Gluconeogenesis: carbohydrate formation from protein molecules.

Glycogenolysis: breakdown of the polysaccharide glycogen in body tissues.

Gonadotropin: hormonal substance that stimulates the ovaries or testes.

Gynecomastia: excessive development of male mammary glands.

Hyperglycemia: abnormally high blood glucose level.

Hyperglycemic hyperosmolar nonketotic coma: loss of consciousness caused by hyperglycemia and characterized by extreme hypovolemia.

Hypoglycemia: abnormally low blood glucose level.

Hypogonadism: condition resulting from abnormally decreased functioning of the ovaries or testes, characterized by retarded growth and sexual development.

Iodism: toxicity from excessive ingestion of iodine, characterized by glandular atrophy, coryza, frontal headache, emaciation, weakness, and skin eruptions.

Kraurosis vulvae: postmenopausal disorder characterized by dryness, atrophy, pain, redness, and itching of the external genitalia.

Lipoatrophy: wasting of the body's fatty tissues.

Lipodystrophy: disturbance of fat metabolism involving regional loss of subcutaneous fat.

Lipohypertrophy: excessive enlargement of fatty tissues.

Lipolysis: breakdown of fat.

Lymphadenopathy: lymph node disease.

Myometrium: smooth muscle layer of the uterus.

Myxedema: condition resulting from hypothyroidism and characterized by dry, waxy, nonpitting edema; abnormal mucin deposits in the skin; swollen lips; and a thickened nose.

Nephrocalcinosis: condition characterized by calcium phosphate precipitation in the renal tubules, often accompanied by renal insufficiency.

Nephrolithiasis: condition characterized by renal calculi.

Oligospermia: deficiency in the number of spermatozoa in semen.

Osteodystrophy: defective bone formation.

Osteolysis: bone dissolution, particularly the loss of calcium from bone.

Osteomalacia: condition characterized by loss of calcification of the bone matrix, resulting in bone softening, accompanied by pain, tenderness, weakness, anorexia, and weight loss. This condition is caused by a deficiency of phosphorus, calcium, or vitamin D or a lack of sunlight exposure.

Osteoporosis: abnormal decrease in bone density caused by failure of the osteoblasts to lay down bone matrix.

Paget's disease: progressive metabolic bone disease characterized by enlargement, bowing, destruction or deformity of the bones, tenderness, and dull, aching pain.

Panhypopituitarism: pituitary insufficiency.

Polydipsia: excessive, persistent thirst.

continued

Glossary continued

Polyphagia: excessive or voracious eating.

Polyuria: excretion of a large amount of urine.

Preeclampsia: toxemia of late pregnancy characterized by hypertension, proteinuria, and edema.

Priapism: persistent abnormal erection of the penis, usually without sexual desire.

Rickets: disturbance of normal ossification caused by vitamin D deficiency and characterized by soft, pliable bones causing bowlegs and knock-knees, nodular enlargements on the ends and sides of bones and other bone deformities; usually seen in childhood.

Somogyi phenomenon: hypoglycemia followed by a compensatory period of rebound hyperglycemia, usually during sleep.

Tetany: manifestation of abnormal calcium metabolism by sharp flexion of the wrist and ankle joints (carpopedal spasms), muscle twitching, muscle cramps, convulsions, and stridor.

Thyroglobulin: iodine-containing protein in the colloid of thyroid gland follicles, which stores thyroid hormones.

Thyroiditis: thyroid gland inflammation.

Thyrotoxicosis: disorder caused by overactivity of the thyroid gland; hyperthyroidism.

Thyrotropin: anterior pituitary hormone that stimulates the thyroid gland.

Tocolytic agent: drug that inhibits uterine contractions, labor, or childbirth.

Trousseau's sign: carpopedal spasm elicited by putting pressure on large nerves in patients with hypocalcemia.

---

tion from the pituitary gland. During lactation, however, formation of this prolactin inhibitory hormone is suppressed, and suckling or breast manipulation stimulates prolactin secretion.

FSH and LH are gonadotropic hormones secreted in response to a hypothalamic releasing hormone and regulated by plasma estrogen and progesterone levels. During each female reproductive cycle, FSH and LH plasma levels increase and decrease. During the first phase of the cycle, increased secretion of the hormones stimulates new follicle growth in the ovaries. Eventually, one follicle becomes more highly developed than the others and begins to secrete large amounts of estrogen, which triggers a feedback mechanism that inhibits FSH secretion by the anterior pituitary. This makes the other follicles stop growing and involute. The one large follicle continues to grow through the self-stimulating effect of the secreted estrogen. Shortly before ovulation, LH and FSH secretion by the anterior pituitary increases markedly, producing rapid swelling of the follicle that culminates in ovulation.

Posterior pituitary hormones

The posterior pituitary gland secretes antidiuretic hormone (ADH) and oxytocin. Nerve impulses originating in the hypothalamus regulate the secretion of these hormones.

ADH, or vasopressin, increases water reabsorption in the collecting ducts of the nephrons. Its production is regulated by osmotic receptors and volume receptors. Concentration of body fluids stimulates the osmotic receptors in the hypothalamus, increasing the impulses transmitted to the posterior pituitary to stimulate ADH secretion, which increases the collecting ducts' permeability to water.

Blood loss stimulates the volume receptors: atrial stretch receptors and baroreceptors in the carotid, aortic, and pulmonary arteries, precipitating a marked increase in ADH secretion. ADH also exerts a potent pressor effect to maintain arterial blood pressure.

Oxytocin produces uterine contractions and the release of breast milk from the breast alveoli into the milk ducts. At the end of pregnancy, stretching or irritation of the uterine cervix transmits a neurogenic reflex to the posterior pituitary, which stimulates increased oxytocin secretion and, subsequently, uterine contraction.

Gonadal hormones

The testes secrete testosterone, the major male gonadal hormone, and other male sex hormones, or androgens. These hormones produce androgenic (masculinizing) effects but also exert some anabolic effects. The adrenal gland also secretes androgens, but they are much less potent and do not produce significant androgenic effects.

The ovaries secrete estrogens and progesterone in response to FSH and LH. Estrogens stimulate the cellular proliferation and growth of sexual organs and related reproductive tissues. They also affect skeletal growth, fat deposition, skin vascularity, and various intracellular functions. Progesterone promotes secretory changes in the endometrium to prepare the uterus for implantation of the fertilized ovum. It also evokes secretory changes in the fallopian tubes and breasts.

Estrogen or progesterone can inhibit ovulation by a negative feedback effect on the hypothalamus and subsequent suppression of FSH and LH release.

Endocrine hormones

In the endocrine system, various glands secrete different endocrine hormones, as indicated below. These hormones stimulate or inhibit the activity of target glands or cells to maintain homeostasis.

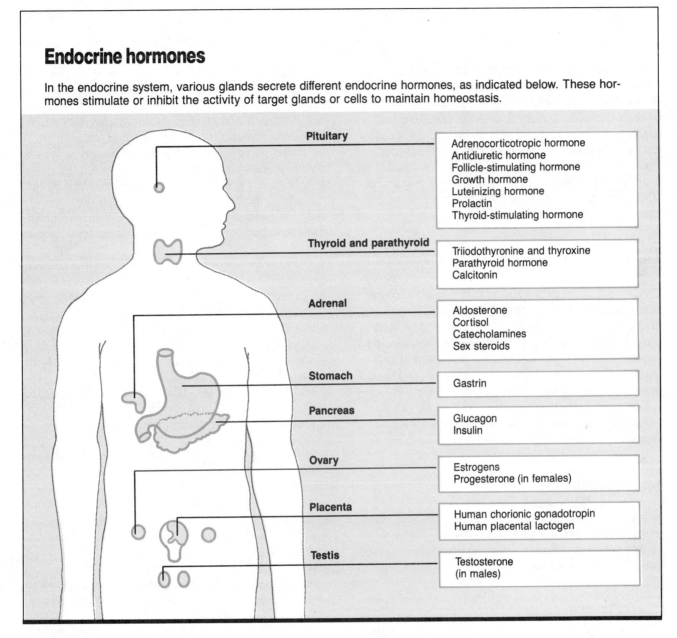

Pituitary

Adrenocorticotropic hormone
Antidiuretic hormone
Follicle-stimulating hormone
Growth hormone
Luteinizing hormone
Prolactin
Thyroid-stimulating hormone

Thyroid and parathyroid

Triiodothyronine and thyroxine
Parathyroid hormone
Calcitonin

Adrenal

Aldosterone
Cortisol
Catecholamines
Sex steroids

Stomach

Gastrin

Pancreas

Glucagon
Insulin

Ovary

Estrogens
Progesterone (in females)

Placenta

Human chorionic gonadotropin
Human placental lactogen

Testis

Testosterone
(in males)

Chapter 55
Hypoglycemic Agents and Glucagon

Chapter 55 begins by differentiating between Type I and Type II diabetes mellitus. Then it presents the role of insulin and the sulfonylureas, or oral hypoglycemic agents, in treating hyperglycemic states. It concludes with a discussion of glucagon, a hyperglycemic agent used to treat hypoglycemic states.

Chapter 56
Thyroid and Antithyroid Agents

Chapter 56 discusses the normal anatomy and physiology of the thyroid gland and the biosynthesis and physiologic effects of T_3 and T_4. Then it investigates the pharmacotherapeutic uses of thyroid and antithyroid agents.

Chapter 57
Parathyroid Agents

Chapter 57 presents the agents that regulate serum calcium levels: parathyroid hormone, calcitonin, etidronate disodium, and the vitamin D analogues. It compares their actions and adverse effects.

Chapter 58
Pituitary Agents

Chapter 58 first explores the normal functions of anterior and posterior pituitary hormones and then details the pharmacologic preparations of corticotropin, vasopressin, and oxytocin.

Chapter 59
Androgenic and Anabolic Steroid Agents

Chapter 59 differentiates between agents used primarily as androgenic agents and those used mainly as anabolic ones. It discusses the pharmacologic properties of the predominantly androgenic agents, including the testosterones, danazol, fluoxymesterone, and methyltestosterone; the predominantly anabolic agents, including oxandrolone, testolactone, and oxymetholone; and related agents, emphasizing their pharmacotherapeutic uses and adverse effects.

Chapter 60
Estrogens, Progestins, and Oral Contraceptive Agents

Chapter 60 presents the agents that mimic the physiologic effects of female gonadal hormones. After a review of the normal physiology of the female reproductive cycle, it discusses estrogen and progestin pharmacologic agents. Then it explores specific administration procedures, including their therapeutic rationales, and details patient education information. The chapter also discusses oral contraceptives, which are usually estrogen-progestin combinations, delineating their other therapeutic uses and adverse effects.

Chapter 61
Fertility Agents

Chapter 61 discusses the drugs used to treat infertility, including gonadotropins, clomiphene, bromocriptine, progesterone, and danazol. It outlines the process of conception, then explores the pharmacotherapeutic uses, for the various agents.

Chapter 62
Uterine Motility Agents

Chapter 62 addresses the uterine-stimulating agents (oxytocin, the prostaglandins, and the ergot alkaloids) and the uterine-inhibiting, or tocolytic agents (ritodrine, terbutaline, magnesium sulfate, and ethanol). It examines their physiologic actions, therapeutic uses, and adverse effects.

Nursing diagnoses

For patients who receive drugs to treat endocrine system disorders, the following nursing diagnoses may apply:
• Alteration in bowel elimination: constipation or diarrhea, related to an endocrine system disorder or thyroid, parathyroid, pituitary, or uterine motility drug therapy
• Alteration in cardiac output: decreased, related to an endocrine system disorder or drug therapy

• Alteration in comfort: pain, related to uterine stimulant therapy
• Alteration in fluid volume: excess or deficit, related to an endocrine system disorder or drug therapy
• Alteration in nutrition: more or less than body requirement, related to an endocrine system disorder or drug therapy
• Alteration in urinary elimination patterns related to an endocrine system disorder or drug therapy
• Altered growth and development related to an endocrine system disorder
• Anticipatory grieving related to an endocrine system disorder, infertility, or altered uterine motility
• Anxiety related to drug therapy or a disorder, such as diabetes, hypothyroidism, infertility, or abnormal uterine motility
• Disturbance in self-concept related to an endocrine system disorder or drug therapy
• Fear related to an endocrine system disorder, drug therapy, or life-style changes
• Hopelessness related to an endocrine system disorder or infertility
• Impaired physical mobility related to an endocrine system disorder or drug therapy
• Impaired social interaction related to an endocrine system disorder or drug therapy
• Impairment of skin integrity: actual, related to an endocrine system disorder or drug therapy
• Ineffective family coping: compromised, related to an endocrine system disorder, drug therapy, or life-style changes
• Ineffective individual coping related to an endocrine system disorder, drug therapy, or life-style changes
• Knowledge deficit related to all aspects of an endocrine system disorder or drug therapy
• Noncompliance related to drug therapy
• Potential alteration in body temperature related to an endocrine system disorder or thyroid, pituitary, estrogen, or progestin drug therapy
• Potential for infection related to an endocrine system disorder or drug therapy
• Sexual dysfunction related to an endocrine system disorder or drug therapy
• Sleep pattern disturbance related to an endocrine system disorder.

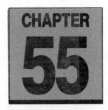
HYPOGLYCEMIC AGENTS AND GLUCAGON

OBJECTIVES

After reading and studying this chapter, you should be able to:

1. Differentiate between Type I and Type II diabetes mellitus, and describe the patient's needs in each.

2. Identify the different sources of insulins and describe how they are classified.

3. Describe the mechanisms of action by which insulin decreases blood glucose level.

4. Explain the important points the nurse should teach a diabetic patient about taking insulin.

5. Explain why different insulin regimens exist.

6. Describe the clinical uses of sulfonylureas, and explain the pancreatic and extrapancreatic actions of these drugs.

7. Describe important nursing implications related to oral hypoglycemic agents.

8. Explain how glucagon increases blood glucose level.

9. Explain the nursing implications for glucagon administration.

INTRODUCTION

Scattered throughout the pancreas are cell clusters known as islets of Langerhans. Beta cells in the islets of Langerhans produce insulin; alpha cells in the islets of Langerhans produce glucagon. Insulin decreases the blood glucose level, while glucagon increases the level.

During normal carbohydrate metabolism, insulin facilitates the cellular uptake of glucose, as well as its storage (in the form of glycogen and fat) and metabolism. Insulin also plays an important role in the metabolism of protein and fat. During protein metabolism, insulin increases protein synthesis and inhibits protein breakdown. In fat metabolism, insulin stimulates triglyceride synthesis and inhibits fat breakdown. Without insulin, the body cannot metabolize glucose, and must, as an alternative, break down protein and fat for fuel.

Glucagon opposes the actions of insulin. It stimulates the conversion of glycogen to glucose, a process known as glycogenolysis. It also stimulates the production of glucose from plasma amino acids resulting from

protein breakdown (gluconeogenesis). Furthermore, glucagon increases the breakdown of fats (lipolysis) and inhibits the storage of triglycerides.

An absolute or relative insulin deficiency causes diabetes mellitus. This disorder is characterized by hyperglycemia. Diabetes mellitus is categorized into the following types:

• *Type I diabetes mellitus.* The etiology of Type I diabetes mellitus, also called insulin-dependent diabetes mellitus or IDDM, remains unknown. However, genetic factors, viral infections, and an autoimmune disease probably play a role. In Type I diabetes mellitus, the pancreas cannot produce sufficient insulin. A patient with this disorder depends upon exogenous sources of insulin for survival. Diet and exercise are other essential components of the therapy for patients with Type I diabetes mellitus.

• *Type II diabetes mellitus.* Also called noninsulin-dependent diabetes mellitus or NIDDM, Type II diabetes mellitus is characterized by a relative deficiency of insulin and insulin resistance. Relative deficiency describes a condition in which a patient produces normal to excessive amounts of insulin, but cannot maintain normal blood glucose levels. The inability to maintain glucose levels is a result of aberrant glucose metabolism. Patients with Type II diabetes mellitus need not depend upon exogenous insulin for survival although they may at times require exogenous insulin to maintain blood glucose control within acceptable limits.

Diet and exercise are essential for achieving blood glucose control in Type II diabetes mellitus. Therapy may also include oral hypoglycemic agents if diet alone cannot maintain blood glucose within acceptable limits. The etiology of Type II diabetes mellitus is unknown, although obesity seems to play a role in genetically predisposed persons. (See *Type I and Type II diabetes mellitus* on page 864 for a comparison of characteristics.)

• *Other types of diabetes mellitus.* Other types of diabetes mellitus may occur secondary to drug therapy or to another disease or condition. Such cases of diabetes may be temporary conditions.

Type I and Type II diabetes mellitus

The information in this table is for comparative purposes, but all patients do not fit the age and weight patterns.

CHARACTERISTIC	TYPE I	TYPE II
Age	Usually diagnosed before age 20	Usually diagnosed after age 40
Weight	Usually underweight or thin	Usually overweight or obese
Endogenous insulin production	Decreased or absent	Slightly decreased, normal, or increased
Exogenous insulin requirement	Present	None, except during periods of stress
Risk of ketoacidosis	Present	None

Patients with blood glucose levels that are above normal but not diagnostic for diabetes mellitus are considered as having an impaired glucose tolerance.

Insulin and oral hypoglycemic preparations are classified as antidiabetic or hypoglycemic agents. Glucagon is classified as a hyperglycemic agent.

For a summary of representative drugs, *see Selected major drugs: Hypoglycemic agents and glucagon* on page 879.

INSULIN

Patients with Type I diabetes mellitus require exogenous insulin to control blood glucose. Insulin may also be given to patients with Type II and other types of diabetes mellitus. Insulin decreases blood glucose levels by facilitating glucose cellular uptake and metabolism during normal carbohydrate metabolism.

History and source
Banting and Best, working in 1921 at the University of Toronto with Macleod, isolated insulin. Testing of insulin in humans began in 1922; the commercial production followed in 1923. That same year, Banting and Macleod won the Nobel prize in physiology and medicine. With the availability of insulin to prevent ketoacidosis, deaths among patients with diabetes mellitus declined dramatically.

Since the first insulin became available to the public, the product has undergone modifications of source, duration of action, purity, and concentration. Today, four sources of insulin are available:
- beef insulin, from the bovine pancreas
- pork insulin, from the porcine pancreas
- "human" insulin, from a recombinant DNA process in which the insulin is synthesized in *Escherichia coli* bacteria that have been genetically altered by adding a human gene
- "human" insulin, from an enzymatic conversion of pork insulin through which the pork insulin molecule becomes identical to that produced by the human pancreas.

Three concentrations of insulin are available: U-40, or 40 units of insulin per millilter; U-100, or 100 units of insulin per milliliter; and U-500, or 500 units of insulin per milliliter.

PHARMACOKINETICS

The absorption, distribution, metabolism, and excretion of different insulins are quite similar. However, their onset, peak, and duration of action vary considerably.

Absorption, distribution, metabolism, excretion
Insulin is *not* effective when taken orally because the digestive tract breaks down the protein molecule before it reaches the bloodstream. All insulins, however, may be given by subcutaneous injection. Absorption of subcutaneously injected insulin varies according to the injection site, the degree of tissue hypertrophy at the injection site, and the vascular supply at the injection site. (See *Subcutaneous insulin injection* for further details.)

Subcutaneous insulin injection

Subcutaneous insulin is absorbed most rapidly at abdominal injection sites, more slowly at sites on the arms, and slowest at sites on the anterior thigh. Absorption of insulin into the subscapular areas and the upper-outer quadrant of the buttocks is less predictable.

The greater the degree of tissue hypertrophy at the injection site, the greater the time required for the tissue to absorb the insulin.

If the vascular supply to the injection site increases, the time required for the tissue to absorb the insulin decreases. The vascular supply can be altered by temperature, massage, and exercise. Injection of the insulin deeper into the tissue also increases the rate of absorption.

Also, regular (unmodified) insulin may be given intravenously or intramuscularly, as well as in dialysate fluid infused into the peritoneal cavity for patients on peritoneal dialysis therapy.

After absorption into the bloodstream, insulin is distributed throughout the body. Insulin-responsive tissues are located in the liver, adipose tissue, and muscle.

Insulin is metabolized primarily in the liver, to a lesser extent in the kidneys, and in the muscle tissue. Enzymes degrade the insulin protein into two amino acid chains, with a resulting loss of activity. Insulin is excreted in the feces and urine.

Onset, peak, duration

Insulins are categorized as rapid-acting, intermediate-acting, and long-acting. In general, following subcutaneous administration, rapid-acting insulins act in ½ to 1 hour, reach peak levels in 2 to 10 hours, and have a duration of action of 5 to 16 hours. Intermediate-acting insulins act in 1 to 2 hours and reach peak levels in 4 to 15 hours. Duration of intermediate-acting insulins is from 22 to 28 hours. Long-acting insulins act in 4 to 8 hours, and reach peak levels in 10 to 30 hours. Duration of action can be 36 or more hours. Without insulin-binding antibodies, insulin circulating in the bloodstream has a half-life of 5 to 10 minutes.

The exact times for onset of action, peak concentration levels, and duration of action, however, are not absolute. They vary not only from patient to patient, but also from injection to injection in the same patient. If insulin absorption is altered, insulin onset, peak, and duration of action are also altered. If insulin absorption occurs more rapidly, the onset and peak times occur

more rapidly. Conversely, if insulin absorption is prolonged, insulin onset and peak are delayed and duration is prolonged.

PHARMACODYNAMICS

Insulin is an anabolic, or building, hormone. It promotes the storage of glucose as glycogen, increases protein and fat synthesis, and inhibits the breakdown of glycogen, protein, and fat. Although it has no antidiuretic effect, insulin can correct the polyuria and polydipsia associated with the osmotic diuresis of hyperglycemia. Insulin also facilitates the movement of potassium from the extracellular fluid into the cell.

Mechanism of action

Insulin decreases blood glucose by facilitating the uptake and metabolism of glucose by insulin-dependent target cells located in both striated muscle and adipose tissue. (See *Mechanism of action for insulin* on page 866 for an illustration of how insulin works with target cells.) Insulin also inhibits hepatic glucose production and the breakdown of glycogen, protein, and fat while it promotes the storage of energy in the form of glycogen, protein, and triglycerides. When insulin and glucose levels are sufficient in the postprandial period, the body will use glucose for fuel rather than break down protein and fat. In a fasting state, however, fats are the primary energy source for the body. In muscle, insulin increases the active transport of amino acids, thereby increasing protein synthesis. In adipose tissue, insulin facilitates the uptake of glucose and its transformation to fat.

PHARMACOTHERAPEUTICS

Insulin is indicated for Type I diabetes mellitus. It is also administered to patients with Type II and other types of diabetes mellitus when other methods of maintaining normal blood glucose level are ineffective or contraindicated. Patients with Type II diabetes mellitus may find the usual methods of maintaining normal blood glucose level ineffective during periods of emotional or physical stress (infection, surgery) or contraindicated because of pregnancy or an allergy. These patients may need insulin administration to control blood glucose more stringently. Insulin is also indicated for two of the comas that are complications of diabetes: diabetic ketoacidosis (DKA), more common with Type I diabetes mellitus, and hyperglycemic hyperosmolar nonketotic coma (HHN), more common with Type II.

Physicians sometimes prescribe insulin for patients who do not have diabetes mellitus. Because insulin stimulates the cellular uptake of potassium, it may be administered with hypertonic glucose to patients with

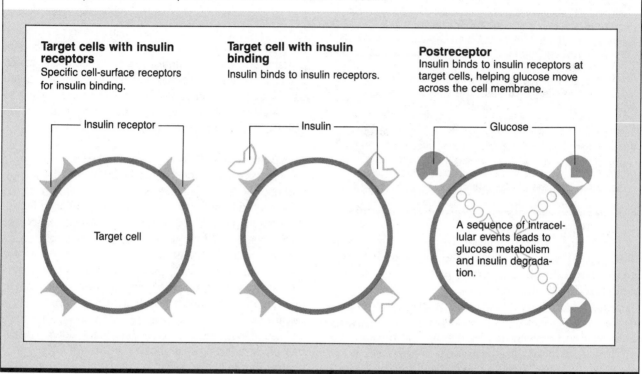

Mechanism of action for insulin

This three-part illustration depicts the mechanism of action of insulin.

Target cells with insulin receptors
Specific cell-surface receptors for insulin binding.

Insulin receptor

Target cell

Target cell with insulin binding
Insulin binds to insulin receptors.

Insulin

Postreceptor
Insulin binds to insulin receptors at target cells, helping glucose move across the cell membrane.

Glucose

A sequence of intracellular events leads to glucose metabolism and insulin degradation.

severe hyperkalemia. This insulin and glucose mixture produces a shift of serum potassium into cells, and lowers serum potassium levels. Health care professionals may also administer insulin to patients receiving hyperalimentation if the patients cannot maintain a normal or near-normal blood glucose level.

All insulins have the same effect within the body. The advantages or disadvantages of a particular kind of insulin reflect the differences in onset of action, peak concentration levels, and duration of action, as well as in concentration, source, and purity. Thirty-three different insulin preparations are available on the U.S. market. Several of these are available in more than one concentration. (See *Available insulins* for the manufacturer and species of the various preparations.)

In most cases, the physician selects for the patient an insulin that will provide a normal or near-normal blood glucose level throughout the day with minimal risk and disruption to the patient's life. To achieve this goal, the physician chooses a particular insulin category (rapid-, intermediate-, or long-acting) or a combination of categories. For example, a patient with fairly predictable episodes of hyperglycemia and hypoglycemia might be put on a regimen involving multiple injections of rapid-acting insulin throughout the day and night. The patient, however, may prefer a different regimen that causes less disruption in life-style. For such a patient, the physician might recommend intermediate- or long-acting insulin, or a combination of rapid-, intermediate-, and long-acting insulins. (See *Selected insulin regimens* on page 868 for some frequently used regimens.)

Insulin concentration is measured in units of insulin per milliliter (ml). Insulin is available as U-40 (40 units/ml), U-100 (100 units/ml), and U-500 (500 units/ml). Although U-100 is by far the most frequently used, U-40 and U-500 may be used for patients who take either very small or very large amounts of insulin in one injection. For example, a patient might need 4 units of insulin for an injection. This amount would require 0.04 ml of U-100 or 0.10 ml of U-40. Because 0.04 ml could be difficult for the patient to withdraw accurately from the insulin vial, U-40, with its 0.10-ml dose, would be the preferable insulin. Another patient who needs 250 units of insulin for injection would require 2.5 ml of U-100 or 0.5 ml of U-500. Because a 2.5-ml dose is too large for one subcutaneous injection, the patient would use U-500.

Available insulins

The insulins currently available are divided into rapid-acting, intermediate-acting, and long-acting categories, with an additional division for standard and purified preparations.

Standard			Purified		
TRADE NAME	**MANUFACTURER**	**SPECIES**	**TRADE NAME**	**MANUFACTURER**	**SPECIES**
Rapid-Acting					
Regular Iletin I	Lilly	beef and pork	Regular Iletin II	Lilly	pork
Regular	Squibb-Novo	pork	Regular Purified Pork Insulin Injection (formerly Actrapid)	Squibb-Novo	pork
Semilente Iletin I	Lilly	beef and pork	Velosulin R	Nordisk	pork
Semilente Insulin	Squibb-Novo	beef	Semilente Purified Pork Prompt Insulin Zinc Suspension (formerly Semitard)	Squibb-Novo	pork
			Humulin R	Lilly	human*
			Novolin R (formerly Actrapid Human)	Squibb-Novo	human†
Intermediate-Acting					
NPH Iletin I	Lilly	beef and pork	NPH Iletin II	Lilly	beef
Lente Iletin I	Lilly	beef and pork	NPH Iletin II	Lilly	pork
NPH Isophane	Squibb-Novo	beef	Lente Iletin II	Lilly	beef
Lente	Squibb-Novo	beef	Lente Iletin II	Lilly	pork
			NPH Purified (formerly Protaphane)	Squibb-Novo	pork
			Lente Purified (formerly Monotard)	Squibb-Novo	pork
			Insulatard NPH	Nordisk	pork
			Mixtard‡	Nordisk	pork
			Humulin L	Lilly	human*
			Humulin N	Lilly	human*
			Novolin L	Squibb-Novo	human†
			Novolin N	Squibb-Novo	human†
Long-Acting					
Ultralente Iletin I	Lilly	beef and pork	Protamine Zinc & Iletin II	Lilly	beef
Protamine Zinc & Iletin I	Lilly	beef and pork	Protamine Zinc & Iletin II	Lilly	pork
Ultralente	Squibb-Novo	beef	Ultralente Purified	Squibb-Novo	beef

*Recombinant DNA alteration of *E. coli*
†Enzymatic conversion of porcine insulin
‡30% Velosulin R, 70% Insulatard NPH

Some insulins are made from a single animal species; others from a combination. Mixtures of beef and pork insulins may have slight batch-to-batch variations of beef and pork percentages. A small percentage of individuals may develop an allergy to animal insulins, with beef insulin considered more antigenic than pork insulin. Human insulin is the least antigenic. Beef insulin differs from human insulin by three amino acids, while pork insulin differs from human insulin by one amino acid.

Animal insulins are obtained by cleaving the insulin protein from a larger polypeptide called proinsulin. Standard insulins contain no more than 25 parts per million (ppm) of proinsulin and related contaminants that result from an incomplete conversion of proinsulin. Purified insulins contain less than 10 ppm of proinsulin and related contaminants. These contaminants may cause adverse effects, including allergy, the formation of antibodies, and lipodystrophy. Such adverse effects, however, occur in only a few patients. Purified insulins, which cost more than standard forms, are indicated for patients with insulin allergy, severe insulin resistance from insulin antibodies, lipoatrophy, an onset of diabetes during pregnancy, or an acute problem that requires short-term or intermittent insulin therapy.

Adult dosages of insulin, which vary widely, represent the amount needed to keep the blood glucose at normal or near-normal levels. The dose varies from person to person as well as at different times for the same person. Insulin requirements are increased by growth, pregnancy, increased food intake, stress, surgery, infection, illness, increased insulin antibodies, and some medications. Insulin requirements are decreased by hypothyroidism, decreased food intake, exercise, and some medications.

The diagnosis of Type I or Type II diabetes mellitus gives no clue to dosage requirements. Although the individual with Type II diabetes mellitus does not depend upon exogenous insulin for survival, that patient may receive a dose exceeding 200 units/day if insulin resistance is present.

Drug interactions

Some drugs interact with insulin to alter its ability to decrease the blood glucose level; other drugs directly alter the patient's blood glucose level. If a medication that produces hypoglycemia is added to the patient's drug regimen, the insulin dose may need to be decreased. If a medication that produces hyperglycemia is added, the insulin dose may need to be increased.

Alcohol consumption is particularly risky for individuals with diabetes mellitus. Alcohol itself can contribute to hypoglycemia. Alcohol's adverse effects may also mask the symptoms of hypoglycemia. Patients with dia-

Selected insulin regimens

A patient on insulin therapy might experience various regimens. The four most frequently encountered ones are detailed here.

REGIMEN	TYPES OF INSULIN	ADMINISTRATION TIMES
Single-dose	Intermediate-acting	Before breakfast. Little insulin activity during morning and night.
Mixed-dose	Rapid-acting and intermediate-acting	30 minutes before breakfast. Little insulin activity during the night.
	Rapid-acting, intermediate-acting, and long-acting	30 minutes before breakfast.
Split-mixed dose	Rapid-acting and intermediate acting	In two injections: 30 minutes before breakfast and 30 minutes before dinner.
Multiple dose	Rapid-acting and intermediate-acting	In four injections: rapid-acting taken 30 minutes before each meal; intermediate-acting taken at bedtime.
	Rapid-acting and long-acting	In three injections: long-acting and rapid-acting taken 30 minutes before breakfast; rapid-acting taken 30 minutes before lunch and dinner.
	Rapid-acting	In multiple injections, perhaps via an insulin pump.

DRUG INTERACTIONS
Insulin

Insulin interactions with other drugs can either increase or decrease the effect of insulin, resulting in inappropriately altered blood glucose levels for the patient. The nurse must be aware of these interactions.

DRUG	INTERACTING DRUGS	POSSIBLE EFFECTS	NURSING IMPLICATIONS
insulin	alcohol	Causes hypoglycemia	• Discourage the patient's consumption of alcohol. • Monitor the patient for hypoglycemia. Symptoms include hunger, diaphoresis, weakness, tremors, dizziness, and tachycardia. • Decrease the insulin dose as prescribed.
	anabolic steroids, clofibrate, fenfluramine, guanethidine, salicylates, sulfonamides, tetracycline	Cause hypoglycemia	• Monitor the patient for hypoglycemia. Symptoms include hunger, diaphoresis, weakness, tremor, dizziness, and tachycardia. • Decrease the insulin dose as prescribed.
	corticosteroids, glucagon, isoniazid, oral contraceptives, phenothiazines, sympathomimetic agents, thiazide diuretics, thyroid hormone preparations	Cause hyperglycemia	• Monitor the patient for hyperglycemia. Symptoms include thirst, polyuria, rapid weak pulse, and stupor. • Increase the insulin dose as prescribed.
	beta-blockers	Modify symptoms of hypoglycemia; delay recovery from hypoglycemia	• Teach the patient the atypical symptoms of hypoglycemia, including the typical tachycardia and tremors, but without diaphoresis. • Monitor the patient for prolonged hypoglycemia.

betes mellitus should not drink alcohol, but if they do, they must take care to eat adequately and to include these beverages in their dietary exchanges. Patients drinking alcohol may be tempted not to eat to limit calorie consumption, however, not eating further increases the chance of hypoglycemia. (See *Drug interactions: Insulin* for a list of drugs that lead to hypoglycemia and hyperglycemia.)

ADVERSE DRUG REACTIONS

The patient may experience dose-related complications or idiosyncratic complications from contaminants within the insulin.

Predictable reactions

Hypoglycemia, below-normal levels of blood glucose, is a relatively frequent adverse reaction to insulin. Hypoglycemia usually results from too much insulin, too little food, too much exercise, or some combination of these. While no absolute correlation exists between hypoglycemic symptoms and blood glucose levels, symptoms typically appear when the blood glucose level falls below 50 mg/dl.

Specific symptoms may vary and include nervousness or shakiness, sweating, weakness, light-headedness, confusion, paresthesias, irritability, headache, hunger, tachycardia, and changes in speech, hearing, or vision. If untreated, symptoms may progress to unconsciousness, convulsions, coma, and death. The symptoms of hypoglycemia result from an adrenergic reaction as well as from cellular malnutrition, primarily at the neurologic level.

The Somogyi phenomenon, another potential complication of insulin therapy, occurs when a patient experiences hypoglycemia followed by a compensatory period of rebound hyperglycemia as the body increases glucose production to correct the problem. The Somogyi phenomenon typically occurs during the late night or early morning when the patient is asleep. During this time, insulin continues to be absorbed from the subcutaneous (S.C.) injection site, although insufficient glucose may be present for it to act on. As a result, the blood glucose level drops rapidly. In response, the body secretes glucagon, norepinephrine, and corticosteroids to correct the hypoglycemia. An overshot phenomenon occurs, resulting in hyperglycemia. Though the patient awakens with symptoms of hyperglycemia, hypoglycemia is the condition that must be corrected.

Unpredictable reactions

A patient can develop a local or systemic allergy to any type of insulin, but such reactions to purified and human insulin are unlikely. Local reactions are characterized by redness, itching, or burning at the injection site. Local allergies generally disappear after 1 or 2 months of continued insulin use. If the patient is currently using a standard insulin, he can be switched to a purified insulin. If the patient is uncomfortable, the physician may prescribe an antihistamine.

A systemic allergic reaction to insulin is characterized by generalized urticaria (hives), angioedema (swelling of submucosa), dyspnea, tachycardia, and possibly anaphylactic shock. Systemic allergic reactions rarely occur. Treatment involves discontinuing the offending insulin and introducing insulin from another source; desensitization therapy may also be required.

Two kinds of lipodystrophy, or disturbance in fat metabolism, can occur with insulin injections. Lipoatrophy, a loss of fat tissue at the injection site, can be improved when purified insulins are injected into the area; lipohypertrophy, thickening of subcutaneous fat tissue, is not influenced by the purity of the insulin. Rotation of insulin injection sites is essential to prevent lipoatrophy and lipohypertrophy. Injecting room-temperature, not cold, insulin also helps prevent the two kinds of lipodystrophy.

Patients can develop a resistance to insulin. While anti-insulin antibodies may play a role, insulin resistance is usually produced by a decreased number of insulin receptors, a variety of postreceptor defects in insulin action, or an excess of hormones antagonistic to insulin. A characteristic of Type II diabetes mellitus, insulin resistance can also occur in poorly controlled Type I diabetes mellitus, but improves with insulin therapy. Insulin resistance associated with Type II diabetes mellitus may be at least partially reversed with treatments such as a weight-reducing diet or insulin therapy. Insulin antibodies seem more likely to develop during episodic insulin therapy with Type II diabetes mellitus. As a consequence, physicians prefer human insulin for episodic insulin therapy because no antibodies are formed against human insulin.

NURSING IMPLICATIONS

The nurse should be aware of the following implications, particularly those for patients with Type I diabetes mellitus who are on long-term insulin therapy.

• Teach the patient about the numerous insulins available so that the patient monitors for the correct dose of the proper insulin.

• To avoid dosage errors, measure U-100 insulin in U-100 insulin syringes and U-40 insulin in U-40 insulin syringes.

• Because no U-500 insulin syringe exists, prepare the dose with extreme caution. A small, inadvertent overdose of U-500 insulin could cause death.

• Observe for signs and symptoms of hypoglycemia and hyperglycemia. Be sure the patient knows the signs and symptoms of both disorders. The peak action for each category of insulin represents the most likely time for a hypoglycemic episode. Hyperglycemia typically occurs when fewer calories are burned and used for energy or the patient has an excessive intake of calories.

• Ensure that the patient realizes the importance of eating sufficient calories each day in the prescribed number of meals. A readily available source of glucose or glucagon followed by a complex carbohydrate snack is the treatment of choice for hypoglycemia.

• Include the calories in I.V. solutions in the patient's daily caloric intake.

• Untreated hyperglycemia can lead to DKA or HHNK. Patients with DKA or HHNK present with dehydration and an intracellular potassium deficit, although serum potassium levels may be normal or high. Ketosis is present with DKA and absent or nearly absent with HHNK; dehydration is usually more severe with HHNK. Therefore, be prepared to administer I.V. fluids, insulin, and potassium as prescribed.

• Instruct the patient on insulin therapy to carry or wear medical identification and to have ready access to glucose, such as hard candy. (See *Individual identification* for an example of a wallet card.)

• Instruct the patient not to change the manufacturer, type, purity, species, or dosage of insulin unless instructed to do so by the physician.

• Instruct the patient that a change in diet or amount of exercise, the presence of an infection, and possibly starting or stopping cigarette smoking may require alterations in insulin dosage.

• Be aware that all insulins may be administered subcutaneously. Regular insulin may be given I.V. and I.M.; it may also be mixed with dialysate and infused into the peritoneal cavity for patients on insulin therapy who require peritoneal dialysis.

• Teach the patient how to monitor blood glucose levels. Monitoring blood glucose is especially important for patients requiring rigid control of their blood glucose level and for those on sliding-scale insulin coverage (dose varies according to the body's need). Patients should also be instructed to monitor blood glucose levels during times of stress or when infection is present. Some patients may monitor urine glucose levels rather than blood glucose levels, although this indirect method for estimating the blood glucose level typically provides less accurate and less reliable information.

• Teach the patient how to monitor urine acetone levels. This procedure is especially important during illness, when oral intake of food and fluids may decrease.

• Instruct the patient using an insulin pump how to care for the device.

• Be sure the patient knows how to withdraw insulin from the vial into the proper syringe. The patient must use a U-40 insulin syringe with U-40 insulin and a U-100 syringe with U-100 insulin.

• Inform the patient with decreased vision of the numerous aids available to help withdraw the correct amount of insulin into a syringe.

• Instruct patients who mix insulins always to follow the same order when drawing the insulins into the syringe (typically the rapid-acting insulin is drawn first). (See *Mixing insulins* on page 872 for the sequence for withdrawing two insulins into one syringe.)

• Instruct the patient using mixtures to either withdraw and administer the mixture within 5 minutes or store the mixture in the refrigerator and administer after the binding period (15 minutes for regular insulin with NPH insulins; 24 hours for regular insulin with lente insulins).

• Instruct the patient about proper procedures for administering insulin; explain that handwashing and skin preparation are essential components of aseptic technique.

• Teach the patient that proper rotation of subcutaneous injection sites helps prevent the complications of lipodystrophy.

• Instruct the patient to store insulin at a temperature less than 80° F. (27° C.) and greater than 36° F. (2° C.). Insulin can be refrigerated (store unopened vials in the refrigerator) but should never be frozen or left in direct sunlight.

• Instruct the patient to allow insulin to reach room temperature before injection because cold insulin can cause lipodystrophy.

• Instruct the patient to rotate vials of intermediate- and long-acting insulin gently before withdrawing the dose; doing so ensures proper dispersion of the suspension.

• Never shake insulin because the resulting froth prevents withdrawal of an accurate dose and may damage protein molecules.

Individual identification

This is a sample identification card that a diabetic patient should carry.

I HAVE DIABETES

I am not intoxicated. If I am unconscious or my behavior is peculiar, I may be having a reaction associated with diabetes or its treatment.

EMERGENCY TREATMENT
If I can swallow, give me sugar in some form—candy, syrup, cola or similar beverage. Call a doctor or the emergency squad. If I cannot swallow, call a doctor or emergency squad immediately.

ORAL HYPOGLYCEMIC AGENTS

Oral hypoglycemic agents are given to patients with Type II diabetes mellitus when those patients cannot maintain normal or near-normal blood glucose levels with exercise and a controlled diet. All oral hypoglycemic agents approved for use in the United States are sulfonylureas. These drugs act to stimulate pancreatic beta-cell production of insulin and increase tissue sensitivity to insulin.

History and source

In Germany in the 1920s, Frank, Nothmann, and Wagner attempted to synthesize an oral hypoglycemic agent; however, the drug was abandoned because of its severe adverse effects. During World War II, the French researcher Janbon used sulfonamides for their antibiotic properties but noticed that many patients developed hypoglycemia. Another French investigator, Loubatieres, performed extensive laboratory investigations on the sulfonamides. Continuing research resulted in the introduction of the sulfonylureas, which are chemical derivatives of the sulfonamides. The sulfonylureas do not, however, have antibacterial activity. Since the mid-

Mixing insulins

The patient may withdraw two different types of insulin into the same syringe. In this series of diagrams, a rapid-acting insulin (R vial) is combined with an intermediate-acting insulin (I vial).

1 After cleansing the rubber stopper on both vials with an alcohol wipe, inject the amount of air equal to the dose of the intermediate-acting insulin into the I vial.

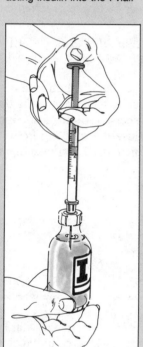

2 Inject the amount of air equal to the dose of the rapid-acting insulin into the R vial.

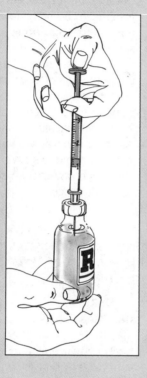

3 Withdraw the correct amount of rapid-acting insulin.

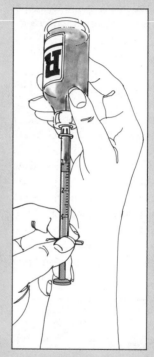

4 Withdraw the correct amount of intermediate-acting insulin. (Note: Pull the plunger down to the unit mark that equals the dose of rapid-acting insulin *plus* the dose of intermediate-acting insulin. The insulins will mix immediately in the syringe. If too large an amount of intermediate-acting insulin is withdrawn, the entire contents of the syringe must be discarded.)

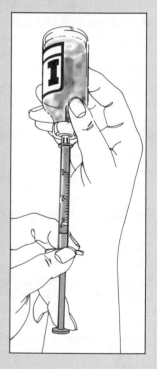

1950s, health care professionals have used sulfonylureas in the treatment of Type II diabetes mellitus.

The initially developed drugs, known as first-generation sulfonylureas, include acetohexamide, chlorpropamide, tolazamide, and tolbutamide. The second-generation sulfonylureas were developed more recently. Glipizide and glyburide are the only second-generation sulfonylureas currently approved for use in the United States. Both drugs were approved in 1984.

PHARMACOKINETICS

The absorption and distribution of oral hypoglycemic agents are similar. These drugs, however, vary in metabolism, excretion, and onset of action, peak concentration levels, and duration of action as well as in the hypoglycemic activity of their metabolites.

Absorption, distribution, metabolism, excretion

Available only in oral forms, sulfonylureas are well absorbed after administration. Absorption varies, depending on whether the patient takes the drug while fasting or with food. Absorption occurs more rapidly when a patient is fasting.

Sulfonylureas are absorbed from the gastrointestinal tract and distributed via the bloodstream throughout the body. Both first- and second-generation sulfonylureas rapidly bind to plasma proteins. Only a small portion of a sulfonylurea dose is left free to produce an effect.

The oral hypoglycemic agents are metabolized primarily in the liver, and the activity of their metabolites varies significantly. Of the first-generation sulfonylureas, only tolbutamide metabolites are inactive; tolazamide and chlorpropamide metabolites are weak, but the metabolites of acetohexamide are quite active. The acetohexamide metabolites provide a hypoglycemic effect 2½ times as potent as acetohexamide itself. Metabolites of the second-generation agents are inactive.

The sulfonylureas are excreted primarily in the urine, with some biliary excretion. Glyburide is excreted equally in the urine and feces. Patients with renal dysfunction taking these drugs require careful monitoring for signs of hypoglycemia and metabolite accumulation.

Onset, peak, duration

Oral hypoglycemic agents reach peak concentration levels within 2 to 6 hours of administration. The half-life and duration of action of these drugs vary considerably. (See *Pharmacokinetics of sulfonylureas* for specific peak, half-life, and duration times.)

PHARMACODYNAMICS

Both first- and second-generation sulfonylureas stimulate insulin release and appear to work by the same mechanism of action, which is not completely understood.

Mechanism of action

Generally accepted theory suggests that oral hypoglycemic agents provide both pancreatic and extrapancreatic actions to regulate blood glucose. These drugs probably stimulate pancreatic beta cells to release insulin. While the mechanism of stimulation remains unknown, the pancreas must already be functioning at a minimal level. Within a few weeks to a few months of the initial response to the sulfonylureas, pancreatic insulin secretion drops to pretreatment levels, however, blood glucose levels remain normal or near-normal. Extrapancreatic actions of oral hypoglycemic agents prob-

Pharmacokinetics of sulfonylureas

The pharmacokinetic information on the oral hypoglycemic agents indicates that the action of second-generation sulfonylureas more closely resemble one another than do the first-generation drugs.

	PEAK SERUM CONCENTRATION (HOURS)	HALF-LIFE (HOURS)	DURATION (HOURS)
First-generation sulfonylureas			
acetohexamide	2	5 to 8	10 to 24
chlorpropamide	4	32 to 40	36 to 72
tolazamide	6	6 to 8	12 to 24
tolbutamide	2	4 to 6	6 to 12
Second-generation sulfonylureas			
glipizide	2	2 to 4	18 to 24
glyburide	4	10	24

ably maintain this continued control of blood glucose.

The oral hypoglycemic agents may provide several extrapancreatic actions to decrease and control blood glucose. The drugs probably decrease glucose production by the liver. They may also increase the number of cellular insulin receptors. With more available receptors, the cells can bind insulin sufficiently to initiate the process of glucose metabolism. Oral hypoglycemic agents may also partially reverse the postreceptor deficit in insulin action, enabling the completion of intracellular glucose metabolism. The ability to restore tissue sensitivity to insulin at the receptor and postreceptor level is not restricted to sulfonylureas; weight reduction and exercise probably provide similar effects.

PHARMACOTHERAPEUTICS

Oral hypoglycemic agents are indicated for patients with Type II diabetes mellitus if diet and exercise do not maintain blood glucose at normal or near-normal levels. These agents are not indicated for patients with Type I diabetes mellitus because pancreatic beta cells are not functioning at a sufficient level.

Combining oral hypoglycemic agents and insulin may be indicated for a small number of patients who do not respond to either therapy alone. Combination therapy, which has not been tested extensively, is infrequently used. Sulfonylureas are contraindicated for pregnant women, patients undergoing surgery, and patients experiencing severe stress such as accompanies infection or trauma.

Compared to insulin, the oral hypoglycemic agents provide one major advantage, oral administration, and several disadvantages:
• The patient must have endogenous insulin; the beta cells must be functioning.
• Oral hypoglycemic agents cannot be used if the patient has been ordered not to take anything by mouth.
• Oral hypoglycemic agents may not sufficiently control blood glucose during periods of acute injury, stress, or infection.
• Oral hypoglycemic agents are contraindicated during pregnancy and lactation because their effects on the fetus and breast-feeding infant remain unknown.

acetohexamide (Dymelor). A first-generation sulfonylurea, acetohexamide produces a diuretic effect and increases the urinary excretion of uric acid.
USUAL ADULT DOSAGE: 250 to 1,500 mg P.O. daily or divided into two doses during the day.

chlorpropamide (Diabinese, Glucamide). A first-generation sulfonylurea, chlorpropamide produces a potent antidiuretic effect and can cause water retention and hyponatremia. Because chlorpropamide potentiates the action of antidiuretic hormone, it may be used in the treatment of mild diabetes insipidus.
USUAL ADULT DOSAGE: 100 to 750 mg P.O. daily.

tolazamide (Tolinase). A first-generation sulfonylurea, tolazamide produces a diuretic effect.
USUAL ADULT DOSAGE: 100 to 1,000 mg P.O. daily or divided into two doses during the day.

tolbutamide (Orinase). Tolbutamide is a first-generation sulfonylurea.
USUAL ADULT DOSAGE: 250 to 3,000 mg P.O. divided into two or three doses during the day.

glipizide (Glucotrol). A second-generation sulfonylurea, glipizide has a mild diuretic effect.
USUAL ADULT DOSAGE: 2.5 to 40 mg P.O. daily or divided into two doses during the day.

glyburide (DiaBeta, Micronase). A second-generation sulfonylurea, glyburide produces a mild diuretic effect.
USUAL ADULT DOSAGE: 1.25 to 20 mg P.O. daily or divided into two doses during the day.

Drug interactions

Some drugs interact with the oral hypoglycemic agents and alter their ability to decrease the blood glucose level, but other drugs directly alter the patient's blood glucose level. If a drug that produces hypoglycemia is added to the patient's medication regimen, the sulfonylurea dose may need to be decreased. If a drug that produces hyperglycemia is added to the patient's medication regimen, the sulfonylurea dose may need to be increased. Although not all drug interactions involving oral hypoglycemic agents are serious, the nurse should use caution when giving a sulfonylurea in combination with any of the interacting drugs. (See *Drug interactions: Oral hypoglycemic agents,* for further details.)

Alcohol consumption proves particularly risky for the patient on an oral hypoglycemic agent. Alcohol itself produces a hypoglycemic effect, but some alcoholic beverages may increase the blood glucose level because of their carbohydrate content. Alcohol and oral hypoglycemic agents also can interact to cause a disulfiram (Antabuse)-like reaction. During such a reaction, the patient

DRUG INTERACTIONS
Oral hypoglycemic agents

Numerous drugs can interact with the sulfonylureas to produce hypoglycemia or hyperglycemia.

DRUG	INTERACTING DRUGS	POSSIBLE EFFECTS	NURSING IMPLICATIONS
acetohexamide, chlorpropamide, tolazamide, tolbutamide, glipizide, glyburide	alcohol	Causes hypoglycemia or hyperglycemia	• Monitor the patient for both hyperglycemia (thirst, polyuria, rapid weak pulse, and stupor) and hypoglycemia (hunger, diaphoresis, weakness, tremors, dizziness, and tachycardia). • Discourage the consumption of alcohol. • Teach the patient about the possibility of a disulfiram-like reaction.
	diazoxide	Causes hypoglycemia or hyperglycemia	• Monitor the patient for both hypoglycemia (hunger, diaphoresis, weakness, tremors, dizziness, and tachycardia), and hyperglycemia (thirst, polyuria, rapid weak pulse, and stupor).
	dicumarol	Causes hypoglycemia, increases anticoagulant effect	• Monitor the patient for signs of hypoglycemia. • Monitor the patient for increased anticoagulant effect. • The patient may need to be changed to another medication for anticoagulant therapy.
	allopurinol, chloramphenical, clofibrate, fenfluramine, guanethidine, methyldopa, monoamine oxidase inhibitors, oxyphenbutazone, phenylbutazone, probenecid, salicylates, sulfonamides, tetracycline	Cause hypoglycemia	• Monitor the patient for hypoglycemia. • Decrease the oral hypoglycemic agent as prescribed.
	beta-blockers, calcium channel blockers, corticosteroids, estrogen, indomethacin, isoniazid, nicotinic acid, oral contraceptives, phenothiazines, phenytoin, rifampin, sympathomimetic agents, thiazide diuretics, thyroid hormone preparations	Cause hyperglycemia	• Beta-blockers will block the epinephrine-induced symptoms of hypoglycemia but not alter the hypoglycemia itself. • Increase the oral hypoglycemic agent as prescribed.
	beta-blockers, clonidine	Produce modified symptoms of hypoglycemia	• Monitor the patient for hypoglycemia. • Teach the patient the atypical symptoms of hypoglycemia, including the typical tachycardia and tremors, but without diaphoresis.

may experience various symptoms, including flushing, nausea and vomiting, headache, syncope, dyspnea, and tachycardia. Although the disulfiram-like reaction occurs most frequently with chlorpropamide, it can occur with any of the first-generation sulfonylureas, and, though rarely, with second-generation sulfonylureas.

ADVERSE DRUG REACTIONS

Patients may develop adverse reactions to sulfonylureas, but other than hypoglycemia and drug failure, these occur infrequently.

Predictable reactions

Hypoglycemia, the major adverse reaction to oral hypoglycemic agents, typically results from too little food or too much medication. Some patients, especially the elderly, may decide to skip a meal because they are not hungry. Hypoglycemia can also occur after an incorrect dose or, more likely, from drug or metabolite accumulation in the body. Patients with decreased liver or kidney function and those taking chlorpropamide must be especially careful to note signs of hypoglycemia.

Other relatively infrequent reactions involving oral hypoglycemic agents include gastrointestinal effects (nausea, vomiting, cholestasis), skin reactions (rashes, pruritis, photosensitivity), a diffuse pulmonary reaction, hematologic reactions (leukopenia, thrombocytopenia, hemolytic anemia), hepatic effects (abnormal liver function tests), and renal effects (severe diuretic or antidiuretic effect).

In 1970, the University Group Diabetes Project reported an increase in the incidence of cardiovascular mortality among patients using oral hypoglycemic agents. Since that time, the finding has been widely disputed. Today, health care professionals generally consider the cardiovascular mortality reported by the Diabetes Project to have been caused by other individual risk factors related to cardiovascular disease.

Unpredictable reactions

Oral hypoglycemic agents are contraindicated for patients allergic to sulfonylureas.

When a patient does not initially respond to sulfonylurea therapy, the patient is said to exhibit primary failure. Primary failure occurs in approximately 20% of the patients on oral hypoglycemic agents; the mechanism of drug failure is unknown. In secondary failure, the sulfonylurea maintains a normal or near-normal blood glucose level for a time, but then, for unknown reasons, can no longer do so. Each year, secondary failure occurs in 5% to 10% of the patients taking oral hypoglycemic agents.

NURSING IMPLICATIONS

The nurse caring for patients receiving oral hypoglycemic agents must be aware of numerous implications.
• Observe the patient for signs of both hypoglycemia and hyperglycemia.
• Encourage the patient to eat meals on a regular schedule; skipping a meal increases the risk of hypoglycemia.
• Patients with decreased hepatic or renal function and patients on chlorpropamide are at particular risk for hypoglycemia. When patients on oral hypoglycemic agents with long half-lives experience hypoglycemia, they re-

quire careful observation for 3 to 5 days and may need hospitalization.
• Hyperglycemia is typically related to fewer calories being burned and used for energy, to an excessive intake of calories, or to drug failure.
• Instruct the patient receiving a sulfonylurea to have glucose readily available to treat hypoglycemia and to carry or wear identification.
• Advise the patient to adjust the dose of sulfonylurea *only* under medical supervision. A change in body weight, diet, or the amount of exercise may require a change in the drug dosage. Severe stress may also require a change in dosage or the addition of insulin to the regimen.
• Because the rate of drug absorption from the gut varies from fasting to nonfasting states, give oral hypoglycemic agents 30 minutes before breakfast; if the drug dose is divided, give the second dose 30 minutes before dinner. The patient taking tolbutamide three times during the day should take a dose before each meal. Oral hypoglycemic agents should be taken on a regular schedule to minimize wide fluctuations in blood glucose levels.
• Teach the patient how to monitor blood glucose levels. Blood glucose determinations better indicate diabetic management than urine glucose measurements because of individual variations in the renal threshold for glucose.
• Teach the patient how to monitor urine acetone. Ketoacidosis becomes a potential complication of Type II diabetes mellitus during episodes of severe stress such as during an illness or infection.
• Instruct the patient about insulin administration. Because the oral hypoglycemic agent may not provide adequate management of blood glucose, the patient may require temporary insulin therapy (especially during a period of severe stress) to supplement or replace oral hypoglycemic therapy.

GLUCAGON

Whereas insulin and oral hypoglycemic agents decrease the blood glucose level, glucagon, a hyperglycemic agent, increases the blood glucose level. Glucagon is a hormone normally produced by the alpha cells of the islets of Langerhans in the pancreas.

History and source

Lane discovered the pancreatic alpha cells in 1907, and Murlin and co-workers discovered glucagon in 1923.

Glucagon was of little interest, however; it was not purified until the 1950s. In 1962, immunofluorescence staining techniques helped researchers identify the alpha cells as the source of glucagon. Another source of glucagon exists somewhere in the body, but researchers have not yet identified its location. Many investigators believe that the extrapancreatic glucagon is produced in the gastrointestinal tract. Purified and crystallized in the laboratory, glucagon is used to treat hypoglycemia.

PHARMACOKINETICS

Glucagon acts to increase blood glucose through both glycogenolysis and gluconeogenesis. When the body is in a resting or near-resting state, the liver must replace approximately 10 grams of glucose each hour. The brain requires approximately 6 of these 10 grams of glucose per hour, and other tissues consume the remaining 4 grams. Hepatic glucose production must equal the glucose demands of the brain and other tissues. Except during meals and extended fasting, glucagon is responsible for hepatic glucose production. Glucagon also increases the breakdown of protein and fat, which provides additional fuel for cellular metabolism.

Absorption, distribution, metabolism, excretion

Following subcutaneous, intramuscular, or intravenous injection, glucagon is rapidly absorbed. Glucagon cannot be taken orally because it is a protein, and it would be destroyed in the gastrointestinal tract. Glucagon is distributed throughout the body, although its effect occurs primarily in the liver, where it increases glycogenolysis and gluconeogenesis. The exact metabolic fate of glucagon is not known, although it is extensively degraded in the liver. Glucagon is removed from the body by the liver and kidneys.

Onset, peak, duration

The blood glucose level begins to increase within 5 to 20 minutes of glucagon administration. The half-life of glucagon in plasma is approximately 3 to 6 minutes. The ability of glucagon to increase hepatic glucose production begins to decline after 1 to 2 hours, and glucose production returns to the original level. This decrease in hepatic glucose production is in part secondary to the inhibitory effect of the hyperglycemia produced by the glucagon.

PHARMACODYNAMICS

Glucagon regulates the rate of glucose production through both glycogenolysis, gluconeogenesis, and lipolysis. A glucagon deficiency results in hypoglycemia.

Although glucagon stimulates insulin secretion, insulin antagonizes glucagon's actions through a negative feedback system.

PHARMACOTHERAPEUTICS

Glucagon is indicated for the emergency treatment of severe hypoglycemia. Health care professionals also use glucagon during radiologic examination of the gastrointestinal tract to produce a hypokinetic state.

glucagon. Used for emergency treatment of severe hypoglycemia, glucagon also serves as a diagnostic aid. USUAL ADULT DOSAGE: for hypoglycemia, 0.5 to 1 mg S.C., I.M. or I.V. If the patient does not awaken from the hypoglycemic coma within 5 to 20 minutes of the first injection, the dose should be repeated once or twice. As a diagnostic aid, the dose ranges from 0.25 to 2 mg I.M. or I.V.

Drug interactions

As a normal body protein, glucagon interacts adversely with very few drugs. Also, no evidence of glucagon toxicity exists. Some drugs, however, decrease the ability of glucagon to stimulate glucose production in the liver. (See *Drug interactions: Glucagon* on page 878.)

Although glucagon does not interact adversely with any food, it is ineffective in poorly nourished or starving patients. If the patient has no glycogen stored in the liver, glycogenolysis cannot occur even with glucagon.

ADVERSE DRUG REACTIONS

Adverse reactions to glucagon are rare. Nausea and vomiting may occur occasionally. Although the nausea and vomiting may be related to glucagon's inhibitory effect on gastrointestinal motility, these adverse reactions may also be from hypoglycemia. Because of the short half-life of glucagon, overdose is unlikely. With large doses or prolonged treatment with glucagon, hypokalemia can result.

Because glucagon is a protein, a patient can develop an allergy to it, but this reaction is rare. Patients can also develop antibodies to glucagon, although the effect of such antibodies remains unknown.

NURSING IMPLICATIONS

The nurse must be aware of the following implications when caring for a patient with diabetes mellitus who requires glucagon to correct hypoglycemia.
• Give the patient with Type I diabetes mellitus a complex carbohydrate snack as soon as possible to restore the liver glycogen and prevent secondary hypoglycemia.

DRUG INTERACTIONS
Glucagon

This chart contains drug interactions and nursing implications for glucagon.

DRUG	INTERACTING DRUGS	POSSIBLE EFFECTS	NURSING IMPLICATIONS
glucagon	alcohol	Causes limited or no hyperglycemic response	• Monitor blood glucose level.
	beta-blockers	Decrease beta blockade	• Monitor the patient's vital signs closely.
	sulfonylureas, insulin	Decrease the hypoglycemic effect of hypoglycemic agents	• Monitor the patient for signs of hyperglycemia (thirst, polyuria, rapid weak pulse, and stupor).
	oral anticoagulants	Increase anticoagulant effect	• Monitor the patient for signs of bleeding.

Patients with Type I diabetes mellitus typically have limited amounts of glycogen stored in the liver, and glycogen must be available before glucagon can act effectively.

• Contact a physician immediately to begin I.V. glucose if the patient does not respond to glucagon as prescribed because of the potential harmful effects of cerebral hypoglycemia.

• Administer intravenous glucose with glucagon as prescribed if the patient is in a deep coma or does not awaken from the coma after glucagon administration.

• Instruct family members or others likely to be with the patient how to prepare and administer glucagon should an emergency arise. Glucagon is supplied as a white powder with an accompanying vial of solution. The diluent provided should be used only for the preparation of glucagon. Do not mix the glucagon solution with solutions containing calcium, potassium, or sodium chlorides because precipitation may occur. Glucagon does not precipitate in dextrose solution.

• Monitor the patient's blood glucose levels frequently, and observe for symptoms of hypoglycemia. However, if a severe episode of hypoglycemia does occur, notify the physician; the dose of oral hypoglycemic agents may need to be altered.

• Instruct the family members about the emergency treatment of hypoglycemia.

• If the patient receives insulin via an infusion pump, the patient should have a readily available supply of glucagon. Furthermore, family members should know how to administer glucagon. Ideally the insulin pump eliminates the sudden drop in blood glucose level; however, a sudden drop in blood glucose level can occur from mechanical malfunction or patient manipulation of the insulin pump. In such circumstances, the patient requires glucagon.

CHAPTER SUMMARY

Chapter 55 included discussions of insulin, the sulfonylureas, and glucagon. Because these drugs are used to treat diabetes mellitus, this disease was also discussed briefly. Here are chapter highlights:

• The patient with Type I diabetes mellitus cannot produce enough insulin to maintain normal blood glucose levels. This patient depends upon exogenous insulin for survival. The patient with Type II diabetes mellitus displays a relative insulin deficiency and insulin resistance. The patient does not require exogenous insulin, though the patient may need it at times, especially during periods of stress.

• Insulin is a normal body protein produced by the pancreas. With variations in manufacturer, source, purity, and concentration, over 33 insulins are currently marketed in the United States.

• Insulins may vary in onset of action, peak concentration levels, and duration of action but are similar in absorption, distribution, metabolism, and excretion. All insulins treat hyperglycemia by facilitating the uptake and metabolism of glucose.

Hypoglycemic agents and glucagon

This chart contains important information for the nurse on selected antidiabetic agents.

DRUG	MAJOR INDICATIONS	USUAL ADULT DOSAGES	NURSING IMPLICATIONS
First-generation sulfonylureas			
acetohexamide	Hyperglycemia	250 to 1,500 mg P.O. daily	• Administer with caution to patients with impaired renal or hepatic function. • Monitor the patient for dehydration. • Monitor the patient for a decrease in uric acid; drug may be preferred for patients with gout.
chlorpropamide	Hyperglycemia	100 to 750 mg P.O. daily	• Administer with caution to patients with impaired renal or hepatic function. • Monitor the patient for fluid retention. • Monitor the patient for hyponatremia. • Caution the patient against the use of alcohol. • Monitor the patient for hypoglycemia. • Should hypoglycemia occur, continue to monitor the patient for 3 to 5 days.
tolazamide	Hyperglycemia	100 to 1,000 mg P.O. daily	• Administer with caution to patients with impaired renal or hepatic function. • Monitor the patient for dehydration.
tolbutamide	Hyperglycemia	250 to 3,000 mg P.O. daily	• Administer with caution to patients with impaired hepatic function.
Second-generation sulfonylureas			
glipizide	Hyperglycemia	2.5 to 40 mg P.O. daily	• Administer with caution to patients with impaired hepatic function. • Adverse drug interactions are less likely with second-generation sulfonylureas.
glyburide	Hyperglycemia	1.25 to 20 mg P.O. daily	• Administer with caution to patients with impaired hepatic function. • Adverse drug interactions are less likely with second-generation sulfonylureas.

• Hypoglycemia is the most frequent adverse reaction to insulin therapy.

• The nurse can help the patient on insulin therapy balance diet, exercise, and insulin requirements. The nurse also plays a major role in teaching the patient how to prevent complications of both diabetes mellitus and insulin therapy.

• All oral hypoglycemic agents currently on the market in the United States are sulfonylureas. If the patient displays sufficient pancreatic beta-cell function, the sulfonylureas may act effectively to regulate blood glucose at normal or near-normal levels.

• The sulfonylureas vary considerably in metabolism, excretion, and onset of action, peak concentration levels, and duration of action. The hypoglycemic activity of sulfonylurea metabolites also varies.

• Sulfonylureas are used to treat hyperglycemia; hypoglycemia is a potential adverse reaction.

• The nurse plays a significant role in helping the patient receiving sulfonylureas to understand the importance of diet and exercise. The nurse should also teach the patient how to prevent complications.

● Glucagon is a normal body protein produced by the pancreas and used for the emergency treatment of severe hypoglycemia.

● Glucagon acts to produce glucose through glycogenolysis, gluconeogenesis, and lipolysis. Glucagon produces few adverse reactions.

● The nurse should instruct the patient and the patient's family how and when to administer glucagon.

BIBLIOGRAPHY

American Diabetes Association. *Glucagon: For Emergency Treatment of Insulin Shock.* Indianapolis: Eli Lilly and Company, 1986.

Baba, S., et al. *Diabetes Mellitus: Recent Knowledge on Aetiology, Complications, and Treatment.* Sydney, Australia: Academic Press, 1984.

Bliss, M. *The Discovery of Insulin.* Chicago: University of Chicago Press, 1982.

Donohue-Porter, P. "Insulin-Dependent Diabetes Mellitus," *Nursing Clinics of North America.* 20:191, March 1985.

Dukes, M.N.G., and Elis, J., eds. *Side Effects of Drugs Annual 8.* New York: Elsevier Science Publishers, 1984.

Ellenberg, M., and Rifkin, H., eds. *Diabetes Mellitus: Theory and Practice,* 3rd edition. New Hyde Park, N.Y.: Medical Examination Pub. Co., 1983.

Essig, M. "Update Your Knowledge of Oral Antidiabetic Agents," *Nursing83.* 13:58, October 1983.

Hussar, D.A. "New Drugs," *Nursing85.* 15:33, June 1985.

Klosiewski, M. "Hypoglycemia—What Does the Diabetic Experience?" *Diabetes Educator.* 10:18, Fall 1984.

Leske, J.S. "Hyperglycemic Hyperosmolar Nonketotic Coma: A Nursing Care Plan," *Critical Care Nurse.* 5:49, September/October 1985.

McCarthy, J.A. "The Continuum of Diabetic Coma," *American Journal of Nursing.* 85:878, August 1985.

Miller, V.G. "Diabetes: Let's Stop Testing Urine," *American Journal of Nursing.* 86:54, January 1986.

Morrisett, W.R. "The Role of Sulfonylureas in Managing Type II Diabetes," *Physician Assistant.* 8:33, August 1984.

Moss, J.M., and Delawter, D.E. "The New Oral Antidiabetic Drugs," *American Family Physician.* 30:119, November 1984.

Pepper, G.A. "What's News in Insulin?" *The Nurse Practitioner.* 11:62, January 1986.

Poole, D. "Type II Diabetes Mellitus Update: Diagnosis and Management," *Nurse Practitioner.* 11:26, August 1986.

Price, M.J. "Insulin and Oral Hypoglycemic Agents." *Nursing Clinics of North America.* 18:687, December 1983.

Rifkin, H., ed. *The Physician's Guide to Type II Diabetes (NIDDM): Diagnosis and Treatment.* New York: American Diabetes Association, 1984.

Robertson, C. "When an Insulin-Dependent Diabetic Must be NPO," *Nursing86.* 16:30, June 1986.

Shinn, A.F., et al., eds. *Evaluations of Drug Interactions.* St. Louis: C.V. Mosby Co., 1985.

Thatcher, G. "Insulin Injections: The Case Against Random Rotation," *American Journal of Nursing.* 85:690, June 1985.

Uranic, M., et al., eds. *Comparison of Type I and Type II Diabetes.* New York: Plenum Press, 1985.

Volk, W., and Arquilla, E.R., eds. *The Diabetic Pancreas,* 2nd edition. New York: Plenum Publishing Co., 1985.

CHAPTER 56

THYROID AND ANTITHYROID AGENTS

OBJECTIVES

After reading and studying this chapter, you should be able to:

1. Describe the normal anatomy and physiology of the thyroid gland, and explain how thyroid hormones function.
2. Describe how synthetic thyroid agents act as hormones.
3. Recognize the physiologic effects of insufficient hormone levels, and identify pharmacologic interventions.
4. Describe the pharmacokinetics, pharmacodynamics, and pharmacotherapeutics of thyroid USP (dessicated), levothyroxine sodium, liothyronine sodium, liotrix, and thyroglobulin.
5. Recognize the physiologic effects of excess hormone levels, and identify pharmacologic interventions.
6. Explain how antithyroid agents interfere with hormone secretion.
7. Describe the pharmacokinetics, pharmacodynamics, and pharmacotherapeutics of methimazole, propylthiouracil, iodine, and radioactive iodine.
8. Identify the major drug interactions, adverse reactions, and nursing implications for the major classes of thyroid and antithyroid agents.

INTRODUCTION

Thyroid and antithyroid agents are drugs that function to correct the thyroid hormone imbalances hypothyroidism and hyperthyroidism. This chapter discusses the use of thyroid agents as replacement therapy in patients with hypothyroidism. It also describes antithyroid agents and their ability to interfere with thyroid hormone synthesis in patients with hyperthyroidism.

Anatomy of the thyroid

The thyroid gland secretes two significant hormones, triiodothyronine (T_3) and thyroxine (T_4). Located just below the larynx and anterior to the trachea, the thyroid gland has two lateral lobes, one on each side of the trachea, that give it a butterfly shape. A narrow band of tissue, called the isthmus, connects the lobes. The parathyroid glands are usually located on the posterior surface of the lobes. Recurrent laryngeal nerves run medial to the lobes in the cleft between the trachea and the esophagus. Four major arteries supply blood to the thyroid gland, making it highly vascular.

On a cellular level, the gland is composed of many nodules, actually groups of closed follicles. Epithelial cells line the follicles and secrete a substance called colloid into them. Colloid contains a large glycoprotein, thyroglobulin, which contains thyroid hormones in its molecule. The release of colloid initiates thyroid hormone secretion.

Thyroid hormone production and function

Thyroid hormone secretion is controlled primarily by thyrotropin, the thyroid-stimulating hormone (TSH) secreted by the anterior pituitary gland. TSH is in turn stimulated by thyrotropin-releasing hormone (TRH) from the hypothalamus. Iodine and circulating thyroid levels are key factors in the storage and secretion of thyroid hormones. Iodine is essential for thyroid hormone formation, and circulating levels of thyroid hormone act as a feedback mechanism, telling the body to increase or decrease the hormone secretion rate.

Besides the two major thyroid hormones, the thyroid also secretes calcitonin to help regulate calcium. The thyroid's follicles include the parafollicular, or C, cells, which secrete calcitonin (thyrocalcitonin). Calcitonin and parathyroid hormone produce opposite effects on blood calcium levels. Calcitonin rapidly decreases blood calcium levels, but its effects last only a few days at most. Parathyroid hormone, however, increases blood calcium levels for a long time.

Calcitonin's primary target site is bone. But T_3 and T_4 have as their primary target site almost all body tissue. Their primary function is to increase the metabolic processes throughout the body.

Thyroid hormone storage and release

Thyroid cells store a hormone precursor, colloidal iodinated thyroglobulin, which contains iodine and thyroglobulin. When stimulated by TSH, a follicular cell takes up some of the stored thyroglobulin. The cell membrane extends fingerlike projections into the colloid, then pulls portions of it back into the cell. Lysosomes in the cell fuse with the colloid, which is then degraded by proteolysis into T_3 and T_4, which are released into the circulation and the lymphatic system by exocytosis.

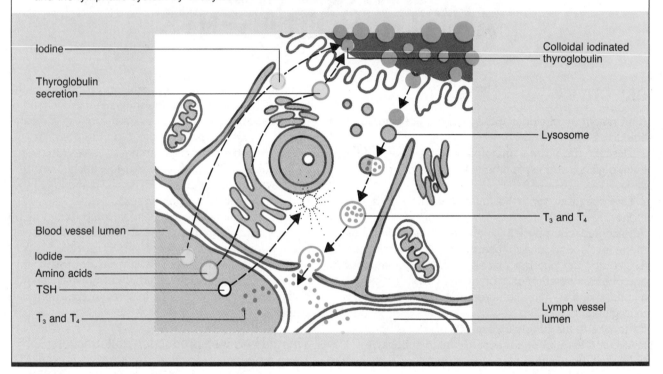

Iodine

Thyroglobulin secretion

Blood vessel lumen

Iodide

Amino acids

TSH

T_3 and T_4

Colloidal iodinated thyroglobulin

Lysosome

T_3 and T_4

Lymph vessel lumen

Iodine, a major component of T_3 and T_4, must be present in the body for thyroid hormone synthesis to occur. The optimum daily iodine requirement for adults is 150 to 300 mcg. In the United States, the average intake is 200 to 500 mcg daily from water, food, and medicine. Iodized table salt, iodine-rich foods such as shellfish, and foods such as milk that use iodophors (sterilizing agents with iodine) add iodine to the diet. After ingestion, iodine is broken down into iodide.

The process of thyroid hormone synthesis and release involves six steps: (1) entrapment of iodide, (2) oxidation of iodide, (3) combination of iodide with tyrosine to form monoiodotyrosine (MIT) and diiodotyrosine (DIT), (4) coupling of MIT and DIT to form T_3 and T_4, (5) storage of T_3 and T_4, and (6) hormone release.

After the synthesis process is complete, the thyroid hormone can be stored or released. Thyroglobulin molecules can store T_3 and T_4 for up to several months. This long-term storage explains why the effects of hormone deficiency may not appear for several months, even when hormone synthesis has ceased.

When the body needs thyroid hormones, TSH stimulates the release of T_3 and T_4. They diffuse through the base of the thyroid cell into the blood of the surrounding capillaries. The thyroid cell also releases MIT and DIT, which are deiodinated (iodine is cleaved from them by deiodinase enzyme) so that the iodine can be reused.

In the blood, most of the hormones combine with plasma proteins, mainly thyroxine-binding globulin (TBG), thyroxine-binding prealbumin (TBPA), and thyroxine-binding albumin (TBA). Very little of the hormone circulates freely in the blood. A bound hormone has a long half-life in circulation because it is protected from metabolism and excretion.

TBG, which is synthesized by the liver, transports about 75% of the T_3 and T_4 in the serum. T_4 is deiodinated in the liver and kidneys to produce about 80% of the T_3, which is 3 to 4 times more potent than T_4. Breakdown of T_4 also produces metabolically inert reverse T_3 (rT_3). In the liver, T_3 and T_4 are conjugated (joined) with acids and excreted by the biliary tract. Then they are hydrolyzed in the intestines, and most of them reenter the blood by the hepatic portal vessel. About 20% of these thyroid hormones is excreted unchanged in the feces. T_4 has a half-life of 6 to 7 days, whereas T_3 has a half-life of 2 days or less because of its lower affinity for protein binding.

Thyroid hormones affect the body in various ways. For example, they regulate growth and development through their influence on the central nervous system and somatotropin (growth hormone); produce heat by increasing the metabolic rate of body tissues; stimulate the cardiovascular system; and increase protein, lipid, and carbohydrate metabolism.

For a summary of representative drugs, see *Selected major drugs: Thyroid and antithyroid agents,* on page 893.

THYROID AGENTS

Thyroid agents can be natural or synthetic and may contain T_3, T_4, or both. Natural thyroid agents, which are derived from animal thyroid, include thyroid USP (dessicated) and thyroglobulin. Both contain T_3 and T_4. Synthetic thyroid agents are actually the sodium salts of the L-isomers of the hormones. These synthetic hormones include levothyroxine sodium, which contains T_4, liothyronine sodium, which contains T_3, and liotrix, which contains T_3 and T_4. All of these agents are used for exogenous replacement of thyroid hormone.

History and source
In 1874, Gull wrote about thyroid gland atrophy, describing the symptoms of hypothyroidism for the first time. Seventeen years later, Murray treated a patient with hypothyroidism by injecting an extract of sheep thyroid gland. In the same year, Fenwick wrote a treatise on the diuretic effect of thyroid juices. Around the same time, Howitz, Mackenzie, and Fox investigated the effectiveness of thyroid tissue given orally. In 1895, Magnus-Levy discovered that thyroid administration to a hypothyroid or euthyroid (normal) individual increased oxygen consumption.

Kendall first isolated T_4 crystals from a thyroid hydrolysate in 1915. In 1926, Harington derived the structural formula of T_4. The next year, he synthesized the hormone with his partner, Barger.

In the early 1950s, researchers detected, isolated, and synthesized T_3. Later studies revealed that T_3 was much more potent than T_4.

PHARMACOKINETICS
Thyroid hormones are variably absorbed from the gastrointestinal (GI) tract and distributed in plasma bound to serum proteins. They are metabolized through deiodination, primarily in the liver, and excreted unchanged in the feces.

Absorption, distribution, metabolism, excretion
The body absorbs natural and synthetic thyroid hormones in a similar way. About 50% to 80% of orally administered levothyroxine is absorbed from the GI tract, primarily in the ileum and colon. Absorption increases with fasting and decreases with malabsorption states. Two other factors may influence the absorption of different brands of levothyroxine sodium tablets: particle size and solubility. About 95% of orally administered liothyronine is absorbed from the GI tract.

I.M. administration of levothyroxine and liothyronine is not preferable, because absorption may be variable, even poor. When synthetic hormones must be given parenterally, I.V. administration of levothyroxine is preferred over liothyronine.

All of the thyroid agents are distributed in the plasma. They are reversibly bound to protein, mainly TBG.

The primary method of metabolism of the T_4 in these drugs is deiodination, which produces T_3 and physiologically inactive rT_3. Then T_3 and rT_3 are deiodinated to form an inactive metabolite in plasma. The thyroid gland uses the liberated iodine for hormone synthesis, or the body excretes the liberated iodine in feces, bile, or urine.

After conjugation in the liver, T_4 is distributed by the biliary system to the intestines. Although some of the T_4 is hydrolyzed and reabsorbed, 20% to 40% of it is excreted unchanged in the feces.

Onset, peak, duration
The fastest-acting thyroid agent is liothyronine. Maximum effects occur 24 to 72 hours after oral therapy is begun, and the drug continues to work for up to 72 hours after discontinuation. Its half-life is short—1 to 2 days.

Levothyroxine and thyroglobulin have a much slower onset of action and longer duration of action. Their full effects occur 1 to 3 weeks after therapy has begun. However, an initial I.V. dose of levothyroxine administered to a patient in hypothyroid coma will demonstrate effectiveness in 6 to 8 hours and will reach peak concentration levels within 24 hours.

Levothyroxine, which has a great affinity for protein binding, is eliminated much more slowly from the body than liothyronine. Levothyroxine's average half-life is 6 to 7 days, although the plasma half-life of any thyroid

Therapeutic effectiveness of thyroid agents

In hypothyroidism, drug therapy includes triiodothyronine (T_3), thyroxine (T_4), or combinations of these hormones. Although most T_4 is converted to T_3, the prolonged action and long half-life of T_4 make it the treatment of choice. T_3, a short-acting drug, and combinations of T_3 and T_4 have varying durations of action, depending on their relative concentrations.

DRUG	EQUIVALENT DOSE	CONTENTS	RELATIVE DURATION
levothyroxine	100 mcg	T_4	Long (Effects occur in 1 to 3 weeks.)
liothyronine	25 mcg	T_3	Short (Effects occur in 24 to 72 hours.)
liotrix	62.5 to 75 mcg	T_4 and T_3 in 4:1 ratio	Intermediate*
thyroglobulin	65 mg	T_4 and T_3 in 2.5:1 ratio	Intermediate*
thyroid USP	65 mg	T_4 and T_3 in variable ratios	Intermediate*

*Those with higher T_4 concentrations are longer acting; those with lower T_4 concentrations are shorter acting.

agent is decreased in patients with hyperthyroidism and increased in patients with hypothyroidism.

Liotrix is an intermediate-acting agent. (See *Therapeutic effectiveness of thyroid agents* for a comparison of these agents' effects.)

PHARMACODYNAMICS

Natural and synthetic thyroid agents act as essential hormones, affecting many physiologic processes.

Mechanism of action

Research continues to determine how thyroid agents work in the body. Some researchers believe that the mechanism of action is related to nucleoproteins that have an extremely high affinity for thyroid hormones.

In the adult, thyroid hormones act on tissues through various mechanisms, including intracellular transport of amino acids and electrolytes, synthesis of specific intracellular enzymes, and enhancement of intracellular processes that lead to changes in cell size and number.

The principal pharmacologic effect of exogenous thyroid hormones is an increased metabolic rate in body tissues. These hormones affect protein and carbohydrate metabolism and stimulate protein synthesis. They promote gluconeogenesis (carbohydrate formation from noncarbohydrate molecules) and increase the use of glycogen stores. By decreasing hepatic and serum cholesterol concentrations, thyroid hormones affect lipid metabolism. They stimulate the heart and increase cardiac output. They may even increase the heart's sensitivity to catecholamines and increase the number of myocardial beta-adrenergic receptors. Thyroid hor-

mones may increase renal blood flow and the glomerular filtration rate in hypothyroid patients, producing diuresis within 24 hours after administration.

PHARMACOTHERAPEUTICS

Thyroid agents act as replacement or substitute hormones when the body's hormone level cannot meet its needs. For this reason, they are used to treat the many forms of hypothyroidism (thyroid hormone deficiency). Primary hypothyroidism results from thyroid gland malfunction, which can be related to reduced functional thyroid tissue mass or to impaired synthesis or release of hormones. This malfunction can be congenital, as in cretinism, or acquired. The congenital malfunction may result from the thyroid gland's absence or underdevelopment, resulting in cretinism if left untreated. Treatment with thyroid hormone replacement has the best results when begun in patients under age 3 months. Children metabolize thyroid hormone more quickly than adults, so pediatric doses are usually higher. The acquired malfunction may result from neoplasms, thyroidectomy, radiation therapy, iodine deficiency, or excess consumption of antithyroid agents. Secondary hypothyroidism results from pituitary dysfunctions such as neoplasms, postpartum pituitary necrosis, or pituitary insufficiency that results in insufficient TSH secretion. Tertiary hypothyroidism results from hypothalamic dysfunction. Myxedema is a severe form of hypothyroidism.

Physicians may also use thyroid agents in combination with antithyroid agents to prevent goitrogenesis (goiter formation) and hypothyroidism. In diagnostic tests, these agents help differentiate between primary and secondary hypothyroidism. Treating papillary or follicular thyroid carcinoma may also require their use.

Although thyroid USP (dessicated) is the oldest thyroid agent, it presents the problem of variable absorption. Its potency also may vary from batch to batch. Most physicians consider levothyroxine the drug of choice for thyroid hormone replacement and TSH suppression therapy. It is available in I.V. form and has a relatively long half-life, so that administration once a day is acceptable. Liothyronine has a faster onset of action. But because it has a short half-life and causes problems with laboratory monitoring, it is recommended for short-term suppression of TSH. The combination drug liotrix is expensive and may result in excess serum concentration levels of T_3.

thyroid USP (dessicated) (S-P-T, Thyrar, Thyro-Teric). Used for thyroid hormone replacement in hypothyroidism, thyroid USP (dessicated) is cleaned, dried, and powdered thyroid gland obtained from domesticated animals, such as pigs, sheep, and cattle. It is also used to suppress thyrotropin secretion in patients with simple goiter or chronic lymphocytic thyroiditis, to reduce goiter size, and to treat cretinism.

USUAL ADULT DOSAGE: for mild hypothyroidism, initially 60 mg P.O. daily, increased in 60-mg increments at 30-day intervals until the desired response is achieved;

for severe hypothyroidism, initially 15 mg P.O. daily, increased to 30 mg/day after 2 weeks and to 60 mg/day after 4 weeks, then if laboratory results do not improve, increase to 120 mg/day, and finally to 180 mg/day; for maintenance, 60 to 180 mg P.O. daily; for adult myxedema, 16 mg P.O. daily, may double dose every 2 weeks to a maximum of 120 mg daily.

USUAL PEDIATRIC DOSAGE: for cretinism and juvenile hypothyroidism, children 1 year and older may approach adult dose (60 to 180 mg P.O. daily), depending on response; children 4 to 12 months, 30 to 60 mg P.O. daily; children 1 to 4 months, initially, 15 to 30 mg P.O. daily, increased at 2-week intervals; for maintenance, 30 to 45 mg P.O. daily.

levothyroxine sodium [T_4 or L-thyroxine sodium] (Levothroid, Noroxine, Synthroid). Levothyroxine is the preferred agent for thyroid hormone replacement in primary hypothyroidism and cretinism. It is also used in secondary hypothyroidism. Its standard hormone content makes its effects predictable. Although usually administered orally, it can be given I.M. or I.V.

USUAL ADULT DOSAGE: for mild hypothyroidism, initially 50 mcg P.O. daily, increased every 2 to 4 weeks by 25 to 50 mcg until the desired effect is achieved; for an otherwise healthy adult with recent onset of hypothyroidism, initially 100 to 200 mcg P.O. daily; for severe

DRUG INTERACTIONS

Thyroid agents

Thyroid agents interact with several common drugs, including oral anticoagulants, insulin, oral hypoglycemic agents, cholestyramine, and phenytoin. The nurse should monitor any patient who is receiving these drugs and taking thyroid agents.

DRUG	INTERACTING DRUGS	POSSIBLE EFFECTS	NURSING IMPLICATIONS
levothyroxine, liothyronine, liotrix, thyroglobulin, thyroid USP	oral anticoagulants	Increase anticoagulant effect	• Monitor the patient for signs of bleeding. • Monitor the patient's prothrombin time (PT) and partial thromboplastin time. • Reduce the anticoagulant dosage, as prescribed, when thyroid therapy begins and readjust it according to the PT results.
	insulin and oral hypoglycemic agents	Decrease the insulin or oral hypoglycemic agent effect	• Monitor the patient's blood glucose levels. • Observe the patient for signs and symptoms of hyperglycemia.
	cholestyramine	Binds T_3 and T_4 in the GI tract, preventing absorption and recirculation of hormones	• Administer these medications at least 4 hours apart.
	phenytoin	Increases serum T_4 levels	• Monitor the patient's serum thyroid levels. • Adjust thyroid dosage, as prescribed.

hypothyroidism, initially 12.5 to 25 mcg P.O. daily, increased every 2 to 4 weeks by 25 to 50 mcg; for an elderly hypothyroid patient, initially 12.5 to 50 mcg daily, increased every 3 to 8 weeks until the desired effect is achieved; for maintenance, 100 to 400 mcg P.O. daily or 80 to 300 mcg P.O. daily for an elderly patient; for parenteral administration, about half of the oral adult dose; for myxedema coma, initially 400 mcg I.V. in a concentration of 100 mcg/ml, increased by 100 to 300 mcg or more on the second day if improvement has not occurred; for parenteral maintenance, 50 to 200 mcg I.V. daily until the patient is stabilized and can take oral medication.

liothyronine sodium [T_3] (Cytomel). Liothyronine has a rapid onset of action and short duration of action. Because of these qualities, some physicians prefer to use it for a rapid effect. Used primarily in the T_3 suppression test, liothyronine can differentiate hyperthyroidism from euthyroidism in patients with borderline to high values on the ^{131}I thyroid uptake test. It is usually administered orally, but researchers are investigating a parenteral preparation.
USUAL ADULT DOSAGE: for mild hypothyroidism, initially 25 mcg P.O. daily, increased by 12.5 to 25 mcg every 1 to 2 weeks; for maintenance, 25 to 75 mcg P.O. daily; for severe hypothyroidism, initially 5 mcg P.O. daily, increased every 1 to 2 weeks by 5 to 10 mcg; for maintenance, 50 to 100 mcg daily; for an elderly patient, initially 5 mcg P.O. daily, increased every 1 to 2 weeks by 5 mcg; for myxedema coma, 200 mcg I.V. initially, followed by 10 to 25 mcg I.V. every 8 to 12 hours until the patient stabilizes; for use in the T_3 suppression test, 75 to 100 mcg P.O. daily for 7 days. (A ^{131}I uptake test is performed at the beginning and end of this medication regimen.)

liotrix (Euthroid, Thyrolar). Liotrix is a synthetic combination of T_4 and T_3 in a 4:1 ratio by weight and a 1:1 ratio in terms of physiologic activity. However, the total amount of hormone varies between drugs from different manufacturers. For example, Euthroid-1 contains 60 mcg of T_4 and 15 mcg of T_3; Thyrolar-1 contains 50 mcg of T_4 and 12.5 mcg of T_3. Liotrix may be used as a replacement agent in hypothyroidism, but its use remains controversial because it may result in excessive T_3 concentrations with normal T_4 concentrations.
USUAL ADULT DOSAGE: for hypothyroidism, Euthroid-½ (30 mcg T_4 and 7.5 mcg T_3) or Thyrolar-¼ (12.5 mcg T_4 and 3.1 mcg T_3) or Thyrolar-½ (25 mcg T_4 and 6.25 mcg T_3) P.O. daily initially, before breakfast, increased every 1 to 2 weeks, as needed. Dosages are individualized to approximate the deficit in the patient's thyroid secretion.

thyroglobulin (Proloid). Obtained from hog thyroid glands, this agent's T_4 and T_3 content is standardized. Each 65 mg of thyroglobulin equals approximately 60 to 65 mg of thyroid USP, 100 mcg of levothyroxine, or 25 mcg of liothyronine. Although thyroglobulin is used as a replacement agent in hypothyroidism, it has no clinical advantage over thyroid USP.
USUAL ADULT DOSAGE: for hypothyroidism, initially 32 mg P.O. daily, increased gradually by 32 mg every 1 to 2 weeks; for maintenance, 65 to 200 mg P.O. daily.

Drug interactions
Thyroid agents interact with several common medications. For instance, they may decrease the effectiveness of insulin and oral hypoglycemic agents or increase an anticoagulant's effect. (See *Drug interactions: Thyroid agents* on page 885 for further information.)

ADVERSE DRUG REACTIONS
Most adverse reactions to thyroid agents occur because of overdose. Discontinuation of the drugs will reverse the signs and symptoms.

Predictable reactions
Common GI effects of a thyroid medication overdose include diarrhea, abdominal cramps, weight loss, and increased appetite. Cardiovascular signs and symptoms may also occur, including palpitations, sweating, tachycardia, increased blood pressure, angina pectoris, and dysrhythmias. Other signs and symptoms of overdose may include headache, tremors, insomnia, nervousness, fever, heat intolerance, and menstrual irregularities. These effects usually subside when the drug is temporarily discontinued. Thyroid USP, thyroglobulin, and levothyroxine should be discontinued for 2 to 7 days; liothyronine, for 2 to 3 days. When the patient starts to take the medication again, the dose must be decreased.

Elderly patients beginning thyroid therapy require close monitoring, because if coronary artery disease is present, the thyroid agent's cardiostimulatory effect may produce angina pectoris or a myocardial infarction.

A patient with adrenal insufficiency should receive corticosteroids to correct the insufficiency before thyroid therapy begins. Because thyroid agents increase tissue demand for adrenal hormones, thyroid therapy could precipitate an acute adrenal crisis in a patient with adrenal insufficiency.

Unpredictable reactions
Euthroid and Synthroid tablets contain tartrazine yellow dye, which may produce bronchial asthma and other allergic reactions in a susceptible individual. Although

Myxedema coma

Chronic untreated hypothyroidism or abrupt withdrawal of thyroid medication may lead to myxedema coma. Because its mortality is 50% to 80%, myxedema coma is a medical emergency. Listed below are the causes, the signs and symptoms, treatment, and nursing implications of myxedema coma.

In a patient with a thyroid disorder, other causes of myxedema coma may include thyroidectomy; infection; decreased pituitary stimulation of the thyroid; sedatives, narcotics, or anesthesia; hypothermia; stress; respiratory acidosis and carbon dioxide narcosis from hypoventilation; and hypoglycemia.

Signs and symptoms
- lethargy, stupor, or a decreased level of consciousness
- dry skin and hair
- delayed deep-tendon reflexes
- progressive respiratory center depression
- decreased cardiac output, bradycardia, and hypotension
- weight gain
- progressive cerebral hypoxia
- decreased serum levels of free T_4, dilutional hyponatremia (low sodium levels caused by excessive water in the bloodstream), serum hypoosmolarity, and highly concentrated urine
- hypothermia
- hypoglycemia.

Treatment
- Establish and maintain a patent airway.
- Assist with ventilation if respiratory failure occurs.

- Establish an I.V. line to administer fluids and medications and to maintain fluid volume as prescribed.
- Establish a normal thyroid hormone level by administering T_3 or T_4 I.V. or through a nasogastric tube as prescribed. (The usual dose of liothyronine sodium is 200 mcg I.V. initially, and 10 to 25 mcg I.V. every 8 to 12 hours until the patient is stable. The usual dose of levothyroxine sodium is 400 mcg I.V. initially, 100 to 300 mcg I.V. on the 2nd day, and thereafter 50 to 200 mcg I.V. daily until the patient can take oral medication.)
- Possibly administer glucocorticoids as prescribed after adrenal function laboratory work is complete.

Nursing implications
- Be aware that hypothermia can be present without shivering and that the use of a hypothermia blanket is not recommended because active warming may cause peripheral vasoconstriction and shock in a patient with intense peripheral vasoconstriction.
- Be aware that aggressive replacement of thyroid hormones may cause serious cardiac dysrhythmias and precipitate a myocardial infarction.
- Be aware that dosage adjustment is necessary when adminsitering narcotics or sedatives to the severely hypothyroid patient to avoid further compromise of the patient's respiratory status.

rare, these reactions are more likely to occur in a patient who is sensitive to aspirin. A lactose-sensitive patient may need to avoid Levothroid, because it contains lactose. A patient who is sensitive to pork may experience GI symptoms when taking thyroid USP or thyroglobulin.

NURSING IMPLICATIONS

Adult hypothyroidism and myxedema cause characteristic changes: tiredness, apathy, inattention, and a feeling of being overwhelmed by simple activities. Patient teaching is extremely important, because the patient must continue to take the medication even after the physical symptoms disappear and the sense of well-being returns. If the patient discontinues the medication, the signs and symptoms of hypothyroidism will recur. The nurse must stress the importance of a lifetime medication regimen and regular follow-up.

- Do not administer thyroid agents to a patient with myocardial infarction, hyperthyroidism, or uncorrected adrenal insufficiency.
- Administer thyroid agents with extreme caution to a patient with angina pectoris, hypertension, other cardiovascular disorders, or renal insufficiency or ischemia.
- Administer thyroid agents carefully to a patient with myxedema, because thyroid hormone sensitivity is likely. Abrupt withdrawal of a thyroid agent in such a patient may precipitate myxedema coma. (See *Myxedema coma* for a summary of the causes and treatments of this disorder.)
- Assess for any history of pork sensitivity before administering thyroid USP or thyroglobulin, lactose sensitivity before administering Levothroid, and aspirin sensitivity before administering Euthroid or Synthroid. If a history of sensitivity exists, consult the physician about use of a different thyroid preparation.
- Evaluate the patient's response to therapy regularly. Appropriate treatment should restore normal serum lev-

els of T_3 and T_4. With thyroid USP or levothyroxine, expect to see a change in the patient's physical appearance and well-being in 1 to 3 weeks. With liothyronine, expect a change in 1 to 3 days.

• Monitor for cardiac problems if your patient is elderly or has a history of cardiac disease, because T_4 may aggravate angina and lead to myocardial infarction.

• Reassure a child on thyroid agents (and the parents) that partial hair loss during the first months of therapy is normal and temporary.

• Be aware that thyroid agents may alter thyroid function test results.

• Monitor the patient's prothrombin time and partial thromboplastin time, and adjust anticoagulant dosages, as ordered. Alert the patient to report any unusual bleeding or bruising.

• Reconstitute levothyroxine for injection immediately before administration. Do not add it to other I.V. fluids. Discard any unused portions.

• Teach the patient to recognize and report the signs and symptoms of hyperthyroidism, such as fatigue, breathlessness, and heat intolerance. Also instruct the patient to report any headaches, palpitations, or nervousness—symptoms of thyroid hormone overdose.

• Discuss the prescribed medication regimen with the patient. A prescription for T_3 may require the patient to take it two to three times per day because of its rapid plasma half-life, whereas a T_4 prescription usually specifies that it be taken once a day. Remind the patient to take levothyroxine on an empty stomach to promote regular absorption and to take it in the morning to help prevent insomnia and to mimic normal hormone release.

• Remind the patient to store thyroid medication in a tightly capped, light-resistant container at 59° to 86° F. (15° to 30° C.) to prevent deterioration.

• Teach the patient that different brands of thyroid agents may vary slightly in concentration. Instruct the patient to check that the physician orders the drug by brand name and that the pharmacist does not substitute a different brand.

OTHER THYROID AGENTS

Several thyroid agents are used in diagnostic tests. The most common ones—thyrotropin and protirelin—help differentiate between the various forms of hypothyroidism.

thyrotropin [thyroid-stimulating hormone or TSH] (Thytropar). Made from bovine pituitary glands, thyrotropin aids in the differential diagnosis of primary and secondary hypothyroidism. Parenteral administration of 10 IU of thyrotropin for 1 to 3 days precedes serum T_3 and T_4 measurements.

protirelin [thyrotropin-releasing hormone or TRH] (Relefact-TRH, Thypinone). A synthetic version of the natural hypothalamic tripeptide hormone, protirelin assists in the differential diagnosis of secondary and tertiary hypothyroidism. After a baseline TSH level is drawn, the patient receives 400 to 500 mcg of protirelin I.V. A second TSH level is drawn 30 minutes after administration and a third is drawn 30 minutes later. The patient requires careful monitoring for 1 hour after injection because complications can occur, including transient hypotension or hypertension.

ANTITHYROID AGENTS

A number of agents act as antithyroid agents, or thyroid antagonists. These agents function by interfering with hormone synthesis, modifying tissue response to hormones, or destroying the thyroid gland. Used for patients with hyperthyroidism (thyrotoxicosis), these agents include the thionamides (propylthiouracil and methimazole) and the iodides (stable iodine and radioactive iodine).

History and source
A decrease in circulating thyroid hormone can increase thyrotropin secretion and result in thyroid hypertrophy, or goiter. Researchers discovered this fact when test rabbits on a cabbage diet developed goiter because thiocyanate ion precursors in the cabbage blocked iodine uptake. In 1923, Plummer reported on the successful use of stable iodine in preparing patients with Graves' disease (a severe form of hyperthyroidism) for surgery. Mackenzies and McCollum in 1941 and Richter and Clisby in 1942 discovered two substances that produced goiters in animals—sulfaguanidine and phenylthiourea. Further research by Astwood in 1945 indicated that the substances inhibited thyroid hormone formation and that the goiter was a compensatory change resulting from this induced hypothyroidism. Related substances are the major antithyroid agents in clinical use today. Also in the 1940s, two forms of radioactive iodine were introduced: [130]I in 1941 and ^{131}I in 1946. These break-

throughs in the treatment of hyperthyroidism led to the birth of nuclear medicine. Then in 1976, the discovery that iopanoic acid decreased serum T_3 levels and increased rT_3 levels in normal patients opened a new area of research regarding antithyroid agents.

PHARMACOKINETICS

The thionamides and the iodides are absorbed through the GI tract, concentrated in the thyroid, metabolized by conjugation, and excreted in the urine.

Absorption, distribution, metabolism, excretion

Propylthiouracil is rapidly absorbed, but its bioavailability ranges from 50% to 80%. In contrast, methimazole is absorbed at variable rates, but its bioavailability approaches 100%. Both are distributed by the blood, concentrated in the thyroid, metabolized in the liver, and excreted by the kidneys. The kidneys excrete most of a propylthiouracil dose in 24 hours and 60% to 75% of a methimazole dose in 48 hours.

Stable iodine is reduced to iodide in the GI tract, absorbed in the small intestine, concentrated in the thyroid and epithelial cells, and excreted by the kidneys. Radioactive iodine is rapidly absorbed after oral administration, concentrated by the thyroid, and incorporated into storage follicles in the thyroid gland. It is excreted in the urine.

Onset, peak, duration

The thionamides inhibit the synthesis, rather than the release, of hormones. Therefore, their onset of action may take 3 to 4 weeks. A patient whose thyroid gland contains a relatively high concentration level of iodine (from ingestion or from administration during a radiologic diagnostic test) may respond slowly to an antithyroid agent. The thionamides reach peak plasma concentration levels about 1 hour after administration. The plasma half-life of propylthiouracil is 1½ to 2 hours; that of methimazole is 6 to 13 hours. Because the follicular cells of the thyroid accumulate these agents, their effective half-life is much longer than the serum half-life. Their duration of action varies: for example, 100 mg of propylthiouracil can inhibit hormone synthesis for 7 hours, and 10 mg of methimazole can inhibit most of it for 8 hours.

Because iodides inhibit hormone release, their onset of action is faster than that of the thionamides. Improvement in symptoms can appear with the iodides in 2 to 7 days; peak concentration levels occur in 10 to 15 days. The serum half-life of plasma iodide is approximately 8 hours.

PHARMACODYNAMICS

The thionamides prevent thyroid hormone synthesis by blocking the combination of iodide and tyrosine. Stable iodine also inhibits hormone synthesis, but it does so through the Wolff-Chaikoff effect, in which above-critical concentrations of intracellular iodide seem to deter hormone synthesis. Radioactive iodine limits hormone secretion by destroying thyroid tissue.

Mechanism of action

The thionamides have distinct mechanisms of action in treating Graves' disease and other forms of hyperthyroidism. They inhibit hormone production by reducing the combination of iodide and tyrosine and the coupling of MIT and DIT. One thionamide, propylthiouracil, limits T_3 production. All of the thionamides act as immunosuppressants, which may help decrease the concentration levels of thyroid-stimulating antibody (TSAb) acting on thyroid cells.

Pharmacologic doses of stable iodine rapidly produce a critical level of iodide in the thyroid. This results in the Wolff-Chaikoff effect, significantly decreasing the rate of thyroid hormone synthesis. However, this effect is temporary. In a few days, the thyroid begins to synthesize hormones again in spite of the high iodine intake. This phenomenon occurs because the body adapts to the high iodine levels by decreasing iodide transport and lowering the intracellular iodide concentration level. Iodine can also limit the release of thyroid hormones by inhibiting thyroglobulin endocytosis, which results in colloid accumulation in the follicles.

Radioactive iodine works in two ways: by inducing acute radiation thyroiditis and chronic gradual thyroid atrophy. These mechanisms destroy thyroid tissue. Acute radiation thyroiditis usually occurs 3 to 10 days after administering radioactive iodine. Chronic thyroid atrophy may take several years to appear.

PHARMACOTHERAPEUTICS

Antithyroid agents are frequently used to treat hyperthyroidism, especially in the form of Graves' disease, which accounts for 85% of all hyperthyroidism. (Other causes of hyperthyroidism that require therapy include toxic multinodular goiter, thyroiditis, excessive intake of thyroid hormones, and neoplasms.) Graves' disease is an autoimmune disorder that affects only the thyroid gland and may be caused by an inherited defect in the manufacture of TSAb. The goal of treatment is to produce a temporary euthyroid state that will allow the autoimmune response to recede either spontaneously or from the medication's immunosuppressive properties. Propylthiouracil, which lowers serum T_3 levels faster than methimazole, is usually used for rapid improvement of severe hyperthyroidism. It is also the thionamide of choice in pregnancy because its rapid action lessens placental transfer and it doesn't cause aplasia cutis (a severe dermatologic disorder) in the fetus. Because methimazole blocks thyroid hormone formation for a longer time, it is better suited for administration once a day to patients with mild to moderate hyperthyroidism. Therapy may continue for 12 to 24 months before remission.

To help treat hyperthyroidism, the thyroid gland may be removed by surgery or destroyed by radiation. Preoperatively, stable iodine is used to prepare the gland for surgical removal by firming it and decreasing its vascularity. Stable iodine is also used after radioactive iodine therapy to control symptoms of hyperthyroidism while the radiation takes effect.

methimazole [thiamazole] (Tapazole). Used to treat hyperthyroidism, methimazole can also serve as an adjunct before thyroid surgery and with radioactive iodine therapy. It is approximately 10 times as potent as propylthiouracil.
USUAL ADULT DOSAGE: initially, for hyperthyrodism, 5 to 20 mg P.O. t.i.d.; for maintenance, 5 to 20 mg/day. Dosages for preoperative preparation are the same.

propylthiouracil [PTU]. Because propylthiouracil takes effect faster than methimazole, it is used to treat severe hyperthyroidism. It is also used to treat thyroid crisis (thyroid or thyrotoxic storm) because it inhibits the conversion of T_4 to T_3. It can also be used to prepare the thyroid before surgery or radioactive iodine therapy. Finally, it is the agent of choice in pregnancy because it is safer for the fetus.
USUAL ADULT DOSAGE: 100 to 200 mg P.O. t.i.d.; for thyroid crisis, dosage may be increased up to 1,200 mg/day; for maintenance, 50 to 200 mg/day.

iodine (Potassium Iodide Solution, USP; Sodium Iodide, USP; Strong Iodine Solution, USP). Used for the rapid treatment of hyperthyroidism, iodine produces visible effects in 3 days. More often, it is used to prepare the thyroid gland for surgery, because it firms the gland and reduces its vascularity. Iodine is usually administered orally as strong iodine solution or Lugol's solution (5 grams iodine and 10 grams potassium iodide per 100 ml of solution, yielding 6 mg iodine per drop) or as saturated solution of potassium iodide or SSKI (100 grams potassium iodide per 100 ml of solution, yielding 50 mg iodide per drop).
USUAL ADULT DOSAGE: for hyperthyroidism, 3 to 5 drops of Lugol's solution t.i.d. or 1 drop of SSKI t.i.d.; as a preoperative agent, 3 to 5 drops of Lugol's solution t.i.d. or 1 to 5 drops of SSKI t.i.d. for 10 to 14 days

before surgery; for thyroid crisis, 1 gram I.V. of sodium iodide or 10 drops of SSKI every 8 hours or 30 drops of Lugol's solution P.O. or by nasogastric tube daily.

radioactive iodine [^{131}I, sodium iodine-131]. Administering radioactive iodine is often the preferred treatment for hyperthyroidism. It exposes only the thyroid tissue to altering radiation, eliminates the problems of surgery, and allows the patient to be treated as an outpatient. However, the use of radioactive iodine can create problems for young adults because it may cause neoplastic changes in the gland later in life, may induce delayed hypothyroidism, and may require months to take effect. Therefore, it is usually used with older patients and those with cardiac disease rather than as surgical intervention. It is the treatment of choice when hyperthyroidism persists after a thyroidectomy or when drug therapy has not produced remission. Administered orally, it can be given as a capsule or dissolved in a half glass of water. After a tracer dose is administered, a patient's optimal dosage can be calculated based on the iodine accumulated by the gland, the rate of iodine loss, and the estimated weight of the gland.
USUAL ADULT DOSAGE: for hyperthyroidism, 4 to 10 mCi P.O.; for thyroid cancer, 50 to 150 mCi P.O. Radioactive iodine is contraindicated in pregnant women because of the potential adverse effects to the fetus. It is also contraindicated in lactating women because it is secreted in breast milk and can affect the infant. Its use in children is still under investigation.

Drug interactions
Iodide preparations may react synergistically with lithium, causing hypothyroidism. Other interactions have not proven clinically significant.

ADVERSE DRUG REACTIONS
Thionamides can produce toxic reactions, such as hypersensitivity reactions and granulocytopenia. The iodides can produce iodism, or chronic iodine poisoning.

Predictable reactions
The most serious adverse reaction to thionamide therapy is potentially fatal granulocytopenia. It typically appears after 4 to 8 weeks of treatment and usually produces a precipitous drop in white blood cell count. The patient may develop a sore throat or fever, which should be reported immediately to the physician so that throat culture and blood count with differential can be done. If the laboratory results reveal fewer than 1,500 granulocytes/mm^3, the drug will be discontinued and the patient will begin taking antibiotics.

Thyroid crisis

A medical emergency, thyroid crisis occurs when a hyperthyroid patient becomes critically thyrotoxic. Its mortality ranges from 20% to 40%. Sometimes called thyroid storm, thyroid crisis has a rapid onset and may be triggered by excess intake of thyroid hormones; abrupt withdrawal of antithyroid agents; radioactive iodine therapy; thyroidectomy, if antithyroid agents were not given preoperatively; infection; trauma; and severe stress. Listed below are the signs and symptoms, treatment, and nursing implications of thyroid crisis.

Signs and symptoms
• fever
• hot, flushed skin
• tachycardia and tachydysrhythmia
• agitation and restlessness
• confusion and psychosis
• GI disturbances, such as diarrhea and abdominal pain
• apathy, severe myopathy, congestive heart failure, profound weight loss, and atrial fibrillation in elderly patients
• elevated serum levels of free T_4
• elevated T_3 levels
• elevated serum levels of total and free calcium
• abnormal liver function test, especially in elderly patients
• a progression from stupor to coma, hypotension, and vascular collapse.

Treatment
• Begin treatment quickly, or patient could die within 48 hours.
• Initiate I.V. fluid replacement as prescribed.

• Block thyroid hormone release with sodium iodide as prescribed. (The usual dosage is initially 1 to 2 g I.V. repeated every 12 to 24 hours, or 1 g every 8 hours by continuous infusion.)
• Block thyroid hormone synthesis with propylthiouracil as prescribed. (The usual dosage is initially 600 to 1,000 mg P.O., then 300 mg P.O. every 6 hours.)
• Block the peripheral effects of thyroid hormones with propranolol as prescribed.
• Replace glucocorticoids with hydrocortisone as prescribed.
• Treat fever with a hypothermia blanket and nonsalicylate antipyretics as prescribed.

Nursing implications
• Be aware that aspirin may interfere with the binding of T_3 and T_4 to circulating protein.
• Be aware that excess thyroid hormones may increase glycogenolysis (carbohydrate breakdown), causing hyperglycemia.
• Be aware that excess thyroid hormones increase metabolic rate.

Iodism, chronic toxicity related to iodine therapy, is dose-dependent. It can produce an unpleasant brassy taste and burning sensation in the mouth and increased salivation and swelling of the parotid and submaxillary glands. Other signs and symptoms may include headache, rhinitis, conjunctivitis, gastric irritation, bloody diarrhea, anorexia, and depression. These reactions should disappear a few days after iodine therapy is discontinued. Radioactive iodine can produce a feeling of fullness in the neck and a metallic taste and can increase the risk of birth defects and leukemia.

Unpredictable reactions

Hypersensitivity reactions to the thionamides frequently produce pruritus, rash, or fever in the first 3 weeks of treatment.

Rarely, I.V. iodine administration can cause an acute hypersensitivity reaction with angioedema, hemorrhagic skin lesions, and serum sickness. Radioactive iodine can also cause a rare—but acute—reaction 3 to 14 days after administration. During this time, thyroglobulin pours out of damaged follicles and can lead to acute

exacerbation of hyperthyroidism and thyroid crisis. (See *Thyroid crisis* for further information about this disorder.) Thyroid crisis may also occur after propylthiouracil withdrawal or after administering iodine or iodinated contrast dye.

NURSING IMPLICATIONS

Because of the antithyroid agents' potential for adverse effects, the nurse must make patient teaching a priority. The patient must understand the importance of follow-up care and of continuing to take the medication even if the feeling of well-being returns. If the thyroid gland is destroyed radioactively or removed surgically, the patient also must understand the importance of taking replacement hormones to prevent hypothyroidism. The nurse must be aware of the following considerations:
• Do not administer iodides to patients who are pregnant or lactating. Thionamides may be administered cautiously in pregnancy but are contraindicated during lactation.

• Do not administer potassium iodide to patients with tuberculosis, iodide hypersensitivity, hyperkalemia, laryngeal edema, and swelling of the salivary glands.

• Evaluate the patient's response to treatment. With propylthiouracil, expect the serum T_4 level to return to normal 14 to 60 days after the therapy begins. The average time to reach a euthyroid state is 42 to 49 days, but this can vary with drug dosage. Signs and symptoms of increased sympathetic activity, such as tachycardia, palpitations, and tremors, usually reverse rapidly. Signs and symptoms of increased catabolic activity, such as weight loss and myopathy, will take longer to improve.

• Monitor the patient for signs of overdose, such as thyroid gland enlargement. Also monitor for signs and symptoms of hypothyroidism, such as mental depression, cold intolerance, and nonpitting edema.

• Monitor the patient's complete blood count periodically to detect impending granulocytopenia, leukopenia, and thrombocytopenia.

• Institute full radiation precautions for 24 hours after a patient receives a dose of radioactive iodine for hyperthyroidism, because the patient will have slightly radioactive urine and saliva for 24 hours, and highly radioactive vomitus for 6 to 8 hours. Teach the patient to use appropriate disposal methods for soiled tissues after coughing and expectorating.

• Isolate a patient who receives a dose of radioactive iodine for thyroid cancer, because the patient will have radioactive urine, saliva, and perspiration for 3 days. Observe the following precautions: ensure that pregnant personnel do not take care of the patient, use disposable eating utensils and linens, and instruct the patient to save all urine in a lead container for 24 to 48 hours so that the laboratory can measure the amount of radioactive material excreted. Advise the patient to drink as much fluid as possible for 48 hours after drug administration to facilitate excretion. Limit contact with the patient to 30 minutes per person per shift on the first day and 1 hour on the second day.

• Advise the patient who is discharged in fewer than 7 days after receiving radioactive iodine for thyroid cancer to avoid close prolonged contact with small children. Also instruct the patient not to sleep in the same room with anyone else for 7 days after treatment because of the risk of thyroid cancer to people exposed to radioactive iodine. Inform the patient that using the same bathroom as the rest of the family is safe.

• Instruct the patient to call the physician immediately if a sore throat and fever develop. Explain that the physician may need to order blood tests and a throat culture if these symptoms appear. Inform the patient that these symptoms are most likely to occur 4 to 8 weeks after drug therapy begins.

• Teach the patient to recognize the signs and symptoms of a hypersensitivity reaction, such as pruritus and a rash. Explain that these symptoms may occur during the first 3 weeks of therapy, and if they do, the physician may prescribe a different medication or treat the reaction with an antihistamine.

• Document any patient history of iodine allergies, and describe the signs and symptoms of iodism if the patient is receiving iodine. Tell the patient that these symptoms will disappear a few days after the drug is discontinued.

• Teach the patient to recognize the signs and symptoms of hypothyroidism that may occur after radioactive iodine therapy.

• Advise a pregnant patient that she should not receive radiation therapy. Also recommend that she wait several months after therapy before becoming pregnant. Advise a male patient not to father a child for several months after therapy.

• Teach the patient to keep antithyroid agents in light-resistant containers.

• Advise the patient to take antithyroid agents with meals to prevent GI adverse reactions. Radioactive iodine, however, requires overnight fasting before administration. Instruct the patient to dilute potassium iodide with water, milk, or fruit juice to mask the salty taste, and to drink it through a straw to avoid tooth discoloration.

• Advise the patient to consult the physician before eating iodized salt and iodine-rich foods such as shellfish during treatment with antithyroid agents. The patient should also consult the physician before using any over-the-counter cough medicines, because they may contain iodine.

OTHER ANTITHYROID AGENTS

Other agents may be used as thyroid antagonists, although they are not currently used as first-line drug therapy for hyperthyroidism. These agents include ionic inhibitors, primarily perchlorate; adrenergic blocking agents, primarily propranolol; and ipodate, a cholecystographic agent used experimentally to decrease serum T_3 levels.

Ionic inhibitors interfere with the thyroid gland's ability to concentrate iodide ions. One of the ionic inhibitors, perchlorate, is concentrated in the thyroid gland

SELECTED MAJOR DRUGS

Thyroid and antithyroid agents

This chart summarizes the drugs most commonly used in treating hypothyroidism and hyperthyroidism.

DRUG	MAJOR INDICATIONS	USUAL ADULT DOSAGES	NURSING IMPLICATIONS
Thyroid agents			
thyroid USP	Mild hypothyroidism	60 mg P.O. daily initially, increased until desired response is achieved	• Assess patient for history of pork sensitivity before administering drug. • Monitor serum thyroid levels periodically to determine therapeutic effectiveness. Expect to see a change in the patient's physical appearance and well-being in 1 to 3 weeks. • Assess patient for history of lactose sensitivity before administering Levothroid, and aspirin sensitivity before administering Synthroid. • Reconstitute levothyroxine for injection immediately before administration. Do not add it to other I.V. fluids. Discard any unused portions. • Remind the patient to take levothyroxine on an empty stomach, and to take it in the morning.
	Adult myxedema	16 mg P.O. daily; may double dose every 2 weeks to a maximum 120 mg daily	
levothyroxine	Mild hypothyroidism	50 mcg P.O. daily initially, increased by 25 to 50 mcg every 2 to 4 weeks; 100 to 400 mcg P.O. daily for maintenance	
	Myxedema coma	400 mcg I.V. initially in a concentration of 100 mcg/ml, increased by 100 to 300 mcg or more, if needed	
Antithyroid agents			
propylthiouracil	Hyperthyroidism, adjunct preparation before thyroid surgery or radioactive iodine therapy, thyroid crisis	100 to 200 mg P.O. t.i.d., increased up to 1,200 mg/day for thyroid crisis if needed; 50 to 200 mg P.O. daily for maintenance	• Evaluate the patient's response to treatment. Expect the serum T_4 level to return to normal 14 to 60 days after therapy begins. • Do not administer to a lactating patient.
iodine	Adjunct preparation before thyroid surgery	3 to 5 drops t.i.d. of Lugol's solution or 1 to 5 drips t.i.d. of SSKI for 10 to 14 days before surgery	• Document patient history of iodine allergies and teach the patient the signs and symptoms of iodism. • Instruct the patient to dilute potassium iodide with water, milk, or fruit juice to mask its salty taste, and to drink it through a straw to avoid tooth discoloration.
	Thyroid crisis	1 g I.V. of sodium iodide or 10 drops of SSKI every 8 hours, or 30 drops of Lugol's solution P.O. or by nasogastric tube daily	
	Hyperthyroidism	3 to 5 drops t.i.d. of Lugol's solution or 1 drop of SSKI t.i.d.	

and excreted unchanged by the kidneys. However, the occasional incidence of granulocytopenia has limited its use.

Researchers have recently recognized lithium as a cation-exchange agent that induces hypothyroidism. But they have not yet established indications for lithium therapy in hyperthyroidism.

Adrenergic blocking agents deplete catecholamines or prevent their release. These agents, which include propranolol, guanethidine, and reserpine, have been used to reduce the signs and symptoms of hyperthyroidism, such as nervousness, tremors, palpitations, tachycardia, and diaphoresis. Currently, propranolol is used as a short-term adjunct treatment in hyperthyroidism when tachycardia is a problem. The dosage ranges from 10 to 30 mg P.O. three to four times daily. Although propranolol reduces conversion of T_4 to T_3, it is not effective when used alone. And because it tends to weaken myocardial contractions, propranolol is contra-indicated in patients with heart failure.

Ipodate (Oragraffin) is an oral cholecystographic agent that has decreased serum T_3 levels in experiments. When given to a hyperthyroid patient, it can reduce serum T_3 levels by almost 70% in 48 hours. Researchers have discovered no toxic effects in the experimental group receiving ipodate therapy. The dosage is 3 grams P.O. once every 3 days for five doses, or 1 gram every day P.O. for 21 days. Ipodate shows promise for use in the short-term management of hyperthyroidism, as an adjunct therapy after radioactive iodine administration, for more rapid control of hyperthyroidism when given with thionamides, and in preparation for thyroid surgery.

CHAPTER SUMMARY

This chapter presented the normal anatomy of the thyroid gland as well as the physiology of the thyroid hormones. It then discussed the thyroid agents used to treat hypothyroidism and antithyroid agents used to treat hyperthyroidism. Here are the highlights of the chapter:
• The body synthesizes thyroid hormones after ingestion of iodine, which is a natural part of the diet. The thyroid gland can store hormones for several months.
• The two major thyroid hormones are triiodothyronine (T_3) and thyroxine (T_4).
• Thyroid-stimulating hormone (TSH), or thyrotropin, primarily controls the release of thyroid hormones. TSH is secreted by the anterior pituitary, which is stimulated by thyrotropin-releasing hormone (TRH) from the hypothalamus.
• Thyroid agents are natural or synthetic preparations that contain T_3 and T_4. Although the onset of effect varies widely among thyroid agents, their principal pharmacologic effect is the same: an increase in the metabolic rate of body tissues.
• Thyroid agents are used as replacements when the body's thyroid hormone level cannot meet its needs.
• Levothyroxine sodium is usually the drug of choice for thyroid hormone replacement and TSH suppression therapy. Liothyronine sodium is used for short-term or rapid-acting therapy.
• Some thyroid agents are also used in diagnostic tests to differentiate among primary, secondary, and tertiary hypothyroidism.
• Antithyroid agents are used to treat hyperthyroidism. Major drugs in this class include the thionamides (pro-pylthiouracil and methimazole) and the iodides (stable iodine and radioactive iodine).
• Antithyroid agents function by interfering with hormone synthesis, modifying the tissue response to hormones, or destroying the thyroid gland.
• A patient receiving thyroid therapy must learn the signs and symptoms of hypothyroidism and hyperthyroidism, the importance of compliance with the medication regimen, the need for follow-up care, and the signs and symptoms of adverse drug reactions.

BIBLIOGRAPHY

American Hospital Formulary Service. *Drug Information 87.* McEvoy, G., ed. Bethesda, Md.: American Society of Hospital Pharmacists, 1987.

DeGroot, L., et al. *The Thyroid and Its Diseases,* 5th ed. New York: John Wiley and Sons, 1984.

Endocrine Disorders. Nurse's Clinical Library. Springhouse, Pa.: Springhouse Corp., 1984.

Evangelisti, J., and Thorpe, C. "Thyroid Storm—A Nursing Crisis," *Heart & Lung* 12:184, March 1983.

Geffner, E., ed. *Compendium of Drug Therapy.* New York: Biomedical Information Corp., 1985.

Gilman, A.G., et al. *Goodman and Gilman's The Pharmacological Basis of Therapeutics,* 7th ed. New York: Macmillan Publishing Co., 1985.

Goth, A. *Medical Pharmacology Principles and Concepts.* St. Louis: C.V. Mosby Co., 1984.

Hollister, L.H., ed. *1986—The Year Book of Drug Therapy.* Chicago: Year Book Medical Pubns., 1986.

Ingbar, S., and Braverman, L., eds. *Werner's The Thyroid: A Fundamental and Clinical Text,* 5th ed. Philadelphia: J.B. Lippincott Co., 1986.

Kastrup, E., et al., eds. *Facts and Comparisons.* St. Louis: Facts and Comparisons Division, J.B. Lippincott Co., 1986.

Katzung, B., ed. *Basic and Clinical Pharmacology,* 3rd ed. Los Altos, Calif.: Lange Medical Pubns., 1987.

Krieger, D., and Badin, C., eds. *Current Therapy in Endocrinology, 1983-1984.* Philadelphia: B.C. Decker Inc., 1983.

Krupp, M., and Chatton, M., eds. *Current Medical Diagnosis and Treatment, 1984.* Los Altos, Calif.: Lange Medical Pubns., 1984.

Wyngaarden, J.B., and Smith, L.H., eds. *Cecil Textbook of Medicine,* 17th ed. Philadelphia: W.B. Saunders Co., 1985.

CHAPTER 57

PARATHYROID AGENTS

OBJECTIVES

After reading and studying this chapter, you should be able to:

1. Describe how parathyroid hormone (PTH) functions physiologically to increase the serum calcium concentration.

2. Describe the absorption, distribution, metabolism, and excretion of calcitonin, etidronate disodium, and vitamin D analogues.

3. Describe the mechanism of action of calcitonin, etidronate disodium, and vitamin D analogues.

4. Identify the diagnostic and therapeutic uses of the calcium-regulating drugs.

5. Identify interactions among the calcium regulators, foods, and other drugs.

6. Explain why calcium-regulating drugs can cause hypercalcemia or hypocalcemia.

7. Identify adverse reactions associated with the calcium-regulating drugs.

8. Identify at least four major nursing implications associated with the use of calcitonin, etidronate disodium, and vitamin D analogues.

9. Describe the procedures for checking Chvostek's and Trousseau's signs to help assess for hypocalcemia.

INTRODUCTION

The parathyroid glands secrete parathyroid hormone (PTH), which is the principal hormone regulating calcium metabolism.

Hormones are mammalian metabolites, either steroidal or derived from peptides of amino acids. The parathyroid hormone consists primarily of various sizes of peptides in simple chains. Each parathyroid gland is a red-brown oval structure approximately 0.5 cm in length and is composed of two cell types: chief cells and oxyphil cells. While the function of the oxyphil cells remains unknown, the chief cells secrete PTH and are rich in

ribonucleic acid (RNA). Any decrease in extracellular calcium levels stimulates the chief cells to secrete PTH, thus increasing the amount of circulating calcium.

Understanding the importance of calcium metabolism requires knowing the vital role that calcium plays in the body's physiologic processes. Calcium, an important constituent of biological membranes, affects the permeability and electrical properties of those membranes. For example, calcium ions are instrumental in regulating heart rhythm. Calcium also acts to stabilize neuromuscular activity. An increase or decrease in the serum calcium concentration alters neuron permeability and nerve tissue excitability, resulting in altered muscle function. Calcium is also involved in the release of preformed hormones (hormones that are stored in glands in active form and do not require metabolism or cleavage to exert their effects) by endocrine cells and in the secretion of transmitter substances at synaptic junctions. Calcium also serves as an important component in the adhesive that binds cells, in enzyme activity, and in blood coagulation.

PTH primarily increases the serum calcium concentration by mobilizing calcium from bone. The action of the hormone depends upon activation of cyclic AMP (adenosine 3':5'-monophosphate) and, possibly, upon the increased entry of magnesium ions into the cells. An abundant blood supply is needed for PTH to effectively regulate calcium. PTH action also stimulates osteoclastic activity (breakdown and resorption of bone tissue).

While PTH acts on the kidneys to inhibit reabsorption of phosphate in the proximal tubules, it acts to increase renal tubular reabsorption of calcium, which, in turn, increases the serum calcium concentration levels. PTH also increases calcium absorption in the gut by promoting the renal synthesis of 1,25-dihydroxycholecalciferol, the active form of vitamin D. By maintaining an inverse relationship between serum calcium and phosphate concentration levels, PTH facilitates the normal excitability of nerves and muscles. Finally, PTH inhibits magnesium excretion.

This chapter includes discussions of the following calcium-regulating drugs: parathyroid hormone, calcitonin, etidronate disodium, and vitamin D analogues (calcifediol, calcitriol, and dihydrotachysterol). (See Chapter 51, Vitamin and Mineral Agents, for a discussion of vitamin D [cholecalciferol, vitamin D$_2$; and ergocalciferol, vitamin D$_3$].)

Although no therapeutic use of exogenous PTH currently exists, the drug was formerly used to elevate serum calcium concentration levels. Today, PTH remains available for diagnostic and research purposes only. The effects of vitamin D analogues on serum calcium concentration levels resemble the effect of endogenous and exogenous PTH; however, other drugs discussed in this chapter—calcitonin, etidronate disodium—produce effects opposite to those of the parathyroid hormone.

For a summary of representative drugs, see *Selected major drugs: Parathyroid hormone agents* on page 905.

CALCIUM REGULATORS

Calcitonin, a polypeptide hormone, is produced in mammals by the parafollicular C cells, primarily of the thyroid gland, but also of the parathyroid and thymus glands. Calcitonin is a single-chain polypeptide composed of 32 amino acids. When required for therapeutic purposes, calcitonin is isolated from salmon and pigs (porcine calcitonin). In salmon and other submammalian vertebrates, calcitonin is secreted from the ultimobrachial glands that are adjacent to the thyroid glands. (In mammals, these glands are incorporated into the thyroid gland.) Salmon calcitonin is more potent and lasts longer than calcitonin derived from pigs. Calcitonin acts to inhibit bone resorption, increase the renal excretion of calcium, and decrease the gastrointestinal absorption of calcium. The regulating actions of calcitonin decrease the extracellular serum calcium concentration. The actions of calcitonin are usually antagonistic to the actions of PTH.

Etidronate disodium, a synthetic compound, inhibits bone metabolism. The compound functions as a calcium regulator primarily by preventing PTH-induced bone resorption, slowing bone metabolism, and decreasing bone formation and bone turnover.

Vitamin D analogues (calcifediol, calcitriol, and dihydrotachysterol) are synthetic parathyroid drugs that act like hormones to stimulate calcium transport from bone to serum.

History and source

The parathyroid glands were discovered in 1880 by Sandström, but the importance of the glands in terms of calcium regulation was not documented until 1909 by MacCallum and Voegtlin. This documentation led to many unsuccessful attempts to isolate parathyroid secretions. Finally, in 1924 through 1925, Berman, Collip, and Hanson obtained active extracts of the glands for use in clinical trials, successfully establishing the therapeutic benefits of the parathyroid extract and heralding the beginning of laboratory studies to synthesize it.

The development of synthetic analogues was a major step in endocrine therapy. Synthetically produced analogues resemble the natural hormones somewhat and are compatible with receptor sites, but differ enough to prevent their destruction by enzyme activity; therefore, they have the added advantage of being more useful therapeutically than the natural substances.

Another important discovery, by Sutherland and Rall, involved adenylate cyclase, a protein enzyme essential for the cellular activity of protein hormones. Adenylate cyclase catalyzes the conversion of adenosine triphosphate (ATP) to cyclic AMP. The hormone-receptor complex on the cell membrane can either enhance or inhibit the activation of adenylate cyclase, thereby altering the rate of synthesis of cyclic AMP from ATP. Cyclic AMP regulates many internal activities of the cell, including hormonal action. (See *The cyclic AMP mechanism of action of parathyroid hormone.*)

In 1959, Berson, Yallow, and Edmans developed radioimmunoassay, a technology for identifying amino acid sequences. This simplified the chemical synthesis of calcium-regulating drugs. In the 1960s, the Merrifield solid-phase synthesis of peptides represented another major development. This process, now automated and commercially feasible, has been extended to include peptides containing 24 to 32 amino acids. Calcitonin, discovered and named by Copp in 1962, is a polypeptide hormone that can be synthesized by the Merrifield solid-phase process. Etidronate disodium is a more recently developed synthetic compound.

By 1920, the work of Mellanby and Huldschinsky indicated the benefit of vitamin D to prevent or cure rickets (deficiency of vitamin D and calcium). Then, in 1952, Carlsson demonstrated that physiologic doses of vitamin D mobilized calcium from bone and increased serum calcium concentration levels.

The cyclic AMP mechanism of action of parathyroid hormone

The parathyroid hormone uses the cyclic AMP mechanism to stimulate target tissues. The parathyroid hormone binds with receptor cells on the cell membrane of the target cells. The binding of the hormone and the receptor activates the protein enzyme adenylate cyclase, which enters the cytoplasm and facilitates the conversion of ATP to cyclic AMP. Cyclic AMP stimulates or activates a cascade of enzymes and protein synthesis to implement the hormonal action of regulating calcium.

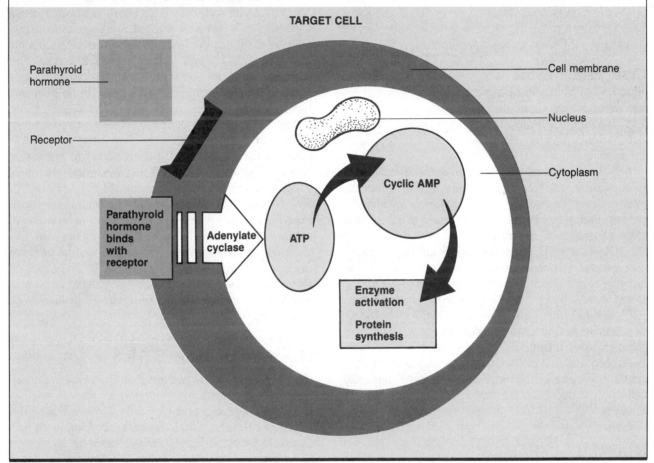

PHARMACOKINETICS

Most of the synthetic calcium regulators provide the advantages of oral administration and longer duration of action. As a result, the synthetic calcium regulators provide better long-term therapeutic effects than PTH—no longer used therapeutically.

Absorption, distribution, metabolism, excretion

The onset of action of parenterally administered calcitonin is within 15 minutes. The hormone is rapidly metabolized by conversion to smaller inactive fragments, primarily in the kidneys, but also in the blood and peripheral tissues. A small amount of unchanged hormone and its inactive metabolites are excreted in the urine.

Calcitonin will not cross the placental barrier, and its passage to cerebrospinal fluid and breast milk is uncertain. Salmon calcitonin is considerably more potent than either the porcine or human variety; it is also cleared more slowly from the system.

Etidronate disodium absorption is dose-dependent and progressive. For example, on the average, about 1% of an oral dose of 5 mg/kg of body weight daily would be absorbed; however, as the dose increases, so does the percent absorbed. At 20 mg/kg daily, approximately 6% would be absorbed. Food in the gastrointestinal tract reduces absorption. Etidronate disodium is mainly distributed into bone and is not metabolized. Unabsorbed drug is slowly eliminated intact in the feces.

Within 24 hours, half of the absorbed drug is excreted unchanged in urine. Etidronate disodium does not cross the placental barrier; however, its distribution into breast milk is uncertain.

Administered orally, the vitamin D analogues (calcifediol, calcitriol, and dihydrotachysterol) are well absorbed from the small intestine, though bile is essential for adequate intestinal absorption. The drugs are distributed throughout the body and are stored in fat deposits for long periods. Metabolism occurs in the liver. Excretion is primarily through bile in feces, with a small percentage of the drugs appearing in urine.

Onset, peak, duration

After I.M. or S.C. administration, calcitonin onset of action occurs within 15 minutes, with a peak concentration level reached in 4 hours. The duration of action is from 8 to 24 hours. The half-life of calcitonin is approximately 10 minutes.

Etidronate disodium's onset of action is slow, with therapeutic effects occurring as long as 1 to 3 months after initiation of therapy. Remissions (decreased bone pain and other symptoms) may last for 3 to 12 months after the drug is discontinued.

The vitamin D analogues calcifediol and calcitriol both produce an onset of action in about 2 hours. The hypercalcemic effect of these drugs peaks in 10 hours. Duration of action is about 3 to 5 days. Dihydrotachysterol, another vitamin D analogue, produces an onset of action several hours after administration. The drug's hypercalcemic effect peaks within 1 to 2 weeks. With the discontinuation of therapy, the serum calcium concentration levels of dihydrotachysterol drop markedly within 4 to 5 days, and the drug's effect disappears after 2 weeks.

PHARMACODYNAMICS

Calcium-regulating calcitonin, etidronate disodium, and the vitamin D analogues produce their effects by inhibiting or promoting bone resorption, by increasing or decreasing bone formation and mineral deposition, and by regulating serum calcium concentrations. (See *Serum calcium regulation by parathyroid hormone* for a diagram of that metabolic activity.)

Mechanism of action

A rise in the blood concentration level of calcium stimulates secretion of naturally occurring calcitonin, which is thought to increase cyclic AMP in bone cells not activated by PTH. Calcitonin decreases osteoclastic activity as well as the rate at which mesenchymal stem cells convert to osteoclasts. By binding to specific receptor sites on the osteoclast cell membrane and decreasing

the transmission of calcium and phosphorus, calcitonin acts antagonistically to PTH and its action. Initially, the use of exogenous calcitonin enhances the activity of the osteoblasts, but this effect decreases with prolonged use. Calcitonin increases the renal excretion of calcium, phosphorus, sodium, and water. It may also inhibit the intestinal absorption of calcium. The hypocalcemic effect of calcitonin is rapid but transitory; however, its effects on bone metabolism are more long-term.

Etidronate disodium decreases the number of osteoclasts, inhibits bone resorption and regeneration, and appears to reduce the rate of bone turnover. Etidronate disodium is used to treat Paget's disease, a disease characterized by increased skeletal remodeling (increased bone resorption and bone formation), bone pain and deformity, neurologic disorders, and elevated cardiac output. Etidronate disodium lowers serum alkaline phosphatase and urinary hydroxyproline levels and reduces elevated cardiac output by decreasing the bone vascularity. The drug also enhances hyperphosphatemia, which is reversible upon discontinuation of therapy.

Vitamin D analogues stimulate calcium absorption from the gastrointestinal tract and promote secretion of calcium from bone to blood, thereby raising serum calcium concentration levels. (See *Effects of parathyroid hormone on target tissues* on page 900 for an illustration of how increased naturally occurring parathyroid hormone secretion increases the serum concentration levels of calcium.)

PHARMACOTHERAPEUTICS

Calcitonin and etidronate disodium decrease serum alkaline phosphatase concentration levels, urinary hydroxyproline levels, and blood flow in the bone. The action of calcitonin and etidronate disodium leads to a decline in the rate of bone turnover and to the restoration of normal bone structure. These effects make calcitonin and etidronate disodium the drugs of choice in the treatment of Paget's disease. One major disadvantage of calcitonin is that patients frequently develop resistance to the hormone. Calcitonin is contraindicated in patients sensitive to fish or to the gelatin diluent used to prepare the drug, in patients with a history of allergy, and during pregnancy. Safe use of calcitonin for children has not been established. Vitamin D analogues are the drugs of choice for increasing serum calcium concentration levels.

calcitonin-salmon (Calcimar). Calcitonin is used to treat hypercalcemia of infancy, vitamin D intoxication, postmenopausal osteoporosis, osteolytic bone metastases, and occasionally hyperphosphatemia. Calcitonin is also

Serum calcium regulation by parathyroid hormone

Homeostatic serum calcium concentration levels are maintained by an elaborate feedback system that begins with the stimulation or inhibition of PTH secretion. The increase or decrease of PTH level elicits concurrent responses in the renal, gastrointestinal, and skeletal systems. These responses return the serum calcium concentration level to a normal level.

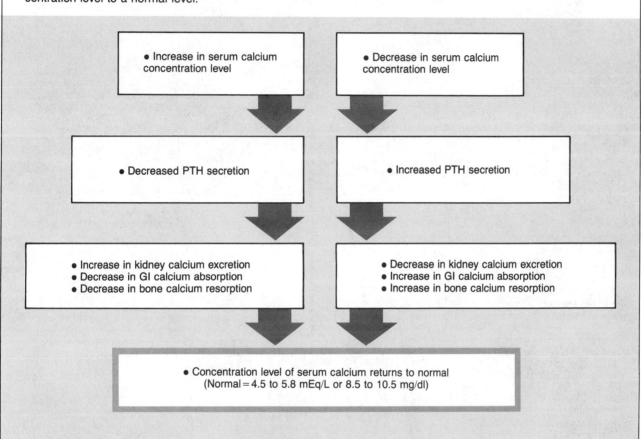

- Increase in serum calcium concentration level

- Decrease in serum calcium concentration level

- Decreased PTH secretion

- Increased PTH secretion

- Increase in kidney calcium excretion
- Decrease in GI calcium absorption
- Decrease in bone calcium resorption

- Decrease in kidney calcium excretion
- Increase in GI calcium absorption
- Increase in bone calcium resorption

- Concentration level of serum calcium returns to normal
(Normal = 4.5 to 5.8 mEq/L or 8.5 to 10.5 mg/dl)

an important therapeutic agent in treating Paget's disease (osteitis deformans). This bone disease, of unknown etiology, is marked by increased bone resorption and disordered bone formation. Calcitonin therapy can relieve bone pain and alleviate the neurologic and biochemical complications that may accompany Paget's disease. Calcitonin is also used with plicamycin to control Paget's disease and to treat the severe hypercalcemia associated with cancer.

USUAL ADULT DOSAGE: for hypercalcemia, 4 International Units (IU)/kg S.C. or I.M. every 12 hours; if no response, dosage may be increased to 8 IU/kg every 12 hours; for Paget's disease, an initial dose of 100 IU S.C. or I.M. daily for first few months, then followed by 50 to 100 IU daily or every other day; for postmenopausal osteoporosis, 100 IU S.C. or I.M. daily.

etidronate disodium (Didronel). A drug of choice for Paget's disease, etidronate disodium slows the accelerated bone turnover of the disease. Reduced bone pain usually accompanies the reduced bone turnover. Etidronate disodium is also used to prevent and treat heterotopic ossification, a nonmalignant overgrowth of bone, which may occur for unknown reasons or may follow total hip replacement or spinal cord injury.

USUAL ADULT DOSAGE: for Paget's disease, 5 to 10 mg/kg P.O. daily for no more than 6 months, or 11 to 20 mg/kg P.O. daily for no more than 3 months. Doses above 10 mg/kg P.O. daily for no more than 3 months are reserved for the prompt reduction of increased cardiac output or bone turnover suppression (retreatment may be instituted after a drug-free interval of 3 months). In the treatment of heterotopic ossification *with total hip*

Effects of parathyroid hormone on target tissues

Increased naturally occurring PTH hormone secretion acts on bone, the kidneys, and the intestines to increase the concentration level of calcium in the extracellular fluid.

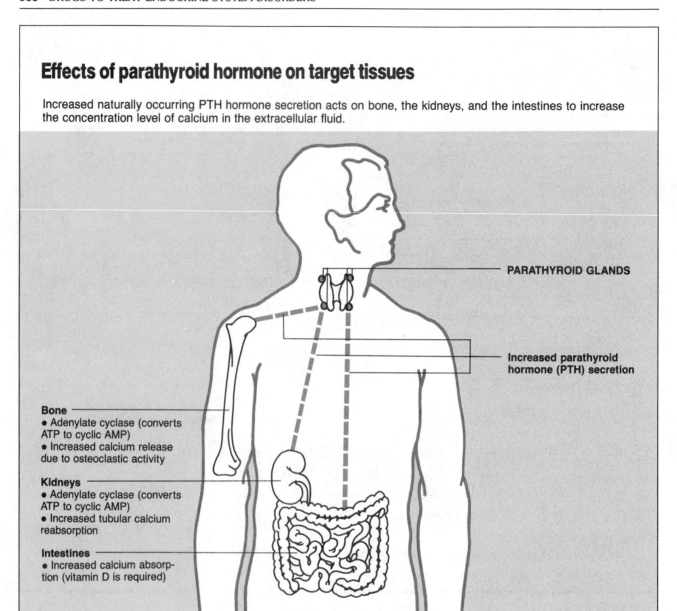

PARATHYROID GLANDS

Increased parathyroid hormone (PTH) secretion

Bone
• Adenylate cyclase (converts ATP to cyclic AMP)
• Increased calcium release due to osteoclastic activity

Kidneys
• Adenylate cyclase (converts ATP to cyclic AMP)
• Increased tubular calcium reabsorption

Intestines
• Increased calcium absorption (vitamin D is required)

replacement, the suggested dosage is 20 mg/kg P.O. daily for 1 month preoperatively, then 20 mg/kg P.O. daily for 3 months postoperatively. In heterotopic ossification *with spinal cord injury,* an initial dose of 20 mg/kg P.O. daily for 2 weeks, followed by 10 mg/kg/day P.O. for 10 weeks.

calcifediol (Calderol). This vitamin D analogue is used primarily in the management of metabolic bone disease associated with renal failure.
USUAL ADULT DOSAGE: 50 to 100 mcg P.O. daily.

calcitriol [1,25-dihydroxycholecalciferol] (Rocaltrol). A vitamin D analogue, 1,25-dihydroxycholecalciferol is used primarily to treat hypocalcemia in patients under-

going chronic dialysis and in patients with hypoparathyroidism and pseudohypoparathyroidism.
USUAL ADULT DOSAGE: to treat hypocalcemia in patients undergoing chronic dialysis, 0.25 mcg P.O. daily, possibly increased by 0.25 mcg P.O. daily at 2- to 4-week intervals, with maintenance dosages of 0.25 mcg P.O. every other day, up to 0.5 to 1.25 mcg P.O. daily. For management of adults and children age 1 and older with hypoparathyroidism and pseudohypoparathyroidism, 0.25 mcg P.O. daily, with dosages possibly increased at 2- to 4-week intervals. Maintenance dosages are 0.25 to 2 mcg P.O. daily.

dihydrotachysterol (DHT Intensol, DHT Oral Solution, Hytakerol). Major uses of this vitamin D analogue in-

clude the treatment of hypocalcemia associated with hypoparathyroidism and pseudohypoparathyroidism, and treatment of renal osteodystrophy in chronic uremia.
USUAL ADULT DOSAGE: for hypocalcemia due to hypoparathyroidism or pseudohypoparathyroidism, 0.8 to 2.4 mg P.O. daily for several days, with maintenance doses of 0.2 to 1 mg P.O. daily as required to maintain normal serum calcium concentration levels. For renal osteodystrophy in chronic uremia, 0.1 to 0.6 mg P.O. daily.
USUAL PEDIATRIC DOSAGE: for hypocalcemia caused by hypoparathyroidism or pseudohypoparathyroidism, 1 to 5 mg P.O. for several days; pediatric maintenance doses, for children age 6 and older, 0.5 mg to 2 mg, for children ages 1 to 5, 0.25 to 0.75 mcg daily as required to maintain normal serum calcium levels.

Drug interactions
Several types of drugs and some foods can interact with the calcium regulators to alter their therapeutic effects. (See *Drug interactions: Calcium regulators* on page 902.)

ADVERSE DRUG REACTIONS

The use of these agents to regulate calcium and bone metabolism may produce hypercalcemia; however, because some of these drugs work in opposition to each other, hypocalcemia may also result. With the use of vitamin D analogues, vitamin D intoxication associated with hypercalcemia may occur. (See *Adverse drug reactions: Calcium regulators* on page 903.)

Predictable reactions
Clinical use of calcitonin can cause flushing, nausea, vomiting, and urticaria. Because calcitonin is also protein in nature, a severe systemic reaction may occur. Long-term calcitonin therapy often produces swelling and tenderness of the hands. Diarrhea and neurologic symptoms, such as headache, may also occur.

Adverse reactions to etidronate disodium are dose-related and infrequent. Most commonly affecting the gastrointestinal tract, adverse reactions include nausea, vomiting, cramps, and diarrhea. Also, increased serum phosphate concentrations may occur.

Normal dosages of vitamin D analogues produce no significant predictable adverse reactions.

Unpredictable reactions
Calcitonin antibody formation may result from the activation of the body's antigen-antibody complex. A local inflammatory reaction at the injection site has been documented following long-term use. In rare instances, hypocalcemic tetany has been observed.

Etidronate disodium use may cause hypocalcemic crisis in which the threshold potential of the neuron is lowered, enabling the neurons to fire more easily. This enhanced motor nerve activity is accompanied by sensory symptoms, including numbness, tingling, muscle twitches, and cramps. Finally, suppressed bone mineralization in the uninvolved skeleton increases the risk of bone fractures in patients with Paget's disease. These patients also experience increased bone pain at the pagetic sites as well as at previously uninvolved sites.

Adverse reactions associated with excessive dosages of vitamin D analogues and an increased responsiveness to normal amounts of vitamin D represent a clinical syndrome that probably results from deranged calcium metabolism. The syndrome involves vitamin D intoxication associated with hypercalcemia. Initial signs and symptoms include weakness, fatigue, lassitude, headache, nausea, vomiting, and diarrhea. Symptoms caused by the impairment of renal function from hypercalcemia include polyuria, polydipsia, nocturia, decreased urinary concentrating ability, and proteinuria. During chronic hypercalcemia, calcium deposits occur in soft tissue, especially the kidneys, which can lead to nephrolithiasis (kidney stones) and nephrocalcinosis (calcium deposits in the kidneys leading to infection, hematuria, renal colic, and decreased renal function). Osteoporosis may occur during vitamin D intoxication from the mobilization of calcium from bone. Some infants may exhibit hyperactivity even when small dosages of vitamin D are administered.

NURSING IMPLICATIONS

The control of serum calcium in the body sometimes requires the use of exogenous calcium regulators. Because most of the products are protein in nature, the nurse must be especially aware of allergies as well as the signs and symptoms of hypocalcemia and hypercalcemia. The nurse must also understand the factors regarding the administration of these agents.
● Calcitonin is contraindicated in patients with hypersensitivity to fish or with a history of allergy to calcitonin or to the gelatin composition of its diluent. Calcitonin is also contraindicated in breast-feeding and pregnant women and in children.
● Use calcitonin cautiously with patients experiencing renal dysfunction, pernicious anemia, osteoporosis, and Zollinger-Ellison syndrome (a condition characterized by severe peptic ulceration and other gastric disorders).
● Use caution when administering etidronate disodium to patients with enterocolitis or renal dysfunction, to pregnant or breast-feeding patients, or to patients with restricted calcium and vitamin D intake.

DRUG INTERACTIONS
Calcium regulators

Drug interactions involving calcium regulators can increase or decrease bone resorption, kidney reabsorption, and gut absorption of calcium. These interactions can produce hypercalcemia or hypocalcemia.

DRUG	INTERACTING DRUGS	POSSIBLE EFFECTS	NURSING IMPLICATIONS
calcitonin	theophylline, isoproterenol	Increase bone resorption, gut absorption, and kidney reabsorption of calcium	• Monitor the patient's calcium and phosphate levels. • Observe for signs and symptoms of calcium imbalance.
etidronate disodium	Foods and drugs containing calcium, iron, magnesium, or aluminum	Decrease absorption of etidronate disodium	• Administer the drug between meals. • See that the patient does not ingest interacting substances within 2 hours after administration of this drug. • Monitor for signs and symptoms of calcium imbalance.
vitamin D analogue (calcifediol)	cholestyramine	Decreases absorption of calcifediol	• Observe the patient closely for desired therapeutic effect of calcifediol if given with cholestyramine.

• Vitamin D analogues are contraindicated in patients with hypercalcemia and vitamin D intoxication. Use caution when administering calcifediol and calcitriol to patients receiving digitalis preparations because hypercalcemia may precipitate cardiac dysrhythmias. Calcitriol and dihydrotachysterol are not recommended for use in breast-feeding women.

• Calcitonin and PTH produce many of the same adverse reactions. A systemic allergic reaction may result from use of either drug. The patient usually receives a skin test before the administration of either drug. The appearance of more than mild erythema 15 minutes after injection constitutes a positive test, indicating that the drug should not be administered.

• During calcitonin treatment, have available for emergency care oxygen, epinephrine, and steroids should a systemic allergic reaction occur. Calcium should also be available for the emergency treatment of hypocalcemic tetany, which may also result from use of calcitonin.

• Hypocalcemic tetany may be demonstrated by a positive Chvostek's sign or Trousseau's sign and by serum calcium concentration levels of 7 to 8 mg/dl (latent tetany) or below 7 mg/dl (manifest tetany). (See *Assessing hypocalcemic tetany* on page 904.) Both Chvostek's and Trousseau's signs can sometimes be elicited in patients with normal calcium concentration levels; however, the strength of the muscle contraction will be much less severe in those patients than in hypocalcemic patients.

Trousseau's sign is definitely the more reliable of the two diagnostic tests.

• The use of etidronate disodium results in relatively few adverse reactions; however, hypocalcemia can occur.

• To prevent vitamin D intoxication, administer the drug in dosages and at dosage intervals as prescribed, and monitor serum calcium concentration levels. Serum calcium level multiplied by serum phosphate level should not exceed 70. The patient must also receive adequate daily intake of calcium.

• When administering any calcium regulator, perform the following: closely monitor serum calcium concentration levels, monitor for signs of hypocalcemic tetany, report the earliest signs of tetany, and ascertain drug compliance if a relapse occurs.

• Until calcium levels are effectively restored in hypocalcemic patients, provide seizure precautions, such as padded side rails, the bed in a low position, a suction setup, and a padded tongue depressor. In addition, reduce sound and light stimuli by placing the hypocalcemic patient in a quiet room with dim lights.

• Calcitonin is commercially prepared in 200 MRC units per ml, packaged in gelatin. Refrigerate the reconstituted drug to maintain its potency.

• Food, especially milk and antacids high in metals (calcium, iron, magnesium, or aluminum), reduces etidronate disodium absorption. Instruct the patient to avoid such foods within 2 hours of drug ingestion. Administer etidronate disodium (oral tablet form) with a full glass of water or juice to reduce gastric irritation.

● To prevent loss of potency, protect calcitriol and dihydrotachysterol from heat and light. Do not refrigerate dihydrotachysterol.

● When teaching the patient to self-administer calcitonin, demonstrate the preferred subcutaneous route. For doses of calcitonin exceeding 2 ml, instruct the patient to use the intramuscular route and to rotate the sites.

● Teach the patient to use aseptic method when reconstituting calcitonin and when administering the injection, and to recognize and seek advice about local inflammation at injection sites.

● The patient receiving calcitonin therapy must know the signs and symptoms of hypocalcemia. Explain to the patient that the initial nausea and vomiting tend to disappear with continued therapy. Inform the patient that facial flushing and warmth occur in some patients within minutes of a calcitonin injection, and assure the patient that these effects usually last no longer than 1 hour. Stress the importance of having periodic urine tests to assess renal function.

● Advise the patient taking calcitonin to consult a physician before using over-the-counter (OTC) preparations during treatment because some combination vitamins, hematinics, and antacids contain calcium. The patient using calcitonin may have to reduce dietary calcium intake. High-calcium foods include green, leafy vegetables and milk and other dairy products.

● With etidronate disodium therapy, teach the patient and family to maintain a well-balanced diet with an adequate intake of calcium and vitamin D. Advise the patient to include milk and other dairy products, as well as green, leafy vegetables, in the diet; however, advise the patient not to eat such foods within 2 hours of taking the drug.

● Because the risk of adverse reactions increases with high doses of etidronate disodium, instruct the patient to report promptly the sudden onset of unexplained bone pain. Urge the patient to keep follow-up appointments for periodic evaluation of clinical tests.

● The patient receiving vitamin D analogues should maintain the prescribed diet and calcium supplementation and avoid OTC drugs. Teach the patient to report signs and symptoms of hypercalcemia and to store the drugs properly. Also, explain to the patient that although these drugs are vitamins, they are potent and must not be taken by anyone for whom they were not prescribed because serious toxicities may result.

Calcium regulators: Summary of adverse reactions

The primary adverse reactions involving parathyroid hormone agents (calcium regulators) include hypersensitivity, hypercalcemia, and hypocalcemia, any of which can produce serious consequences. The nurse must observe for the early signs and symptoms of such reactions.

DRUG	REACTION
calcitonin	Hypersensitivity to salmon, hypocalcemic tetany, facial flushing and urticaria, local inflammation at injection site, nausea
etidronate disodium	Increased bone pain, nausea and diarrhea
vitamin D analogues	Vitamin D intoxication associated with hypercalcemia (weakness, fatigue, lassitude, headache, nausea, vomiting, and diarrhea), altered renal function from hypercalcemia (possible polyuria, polydipsia, nocturia, decreased urinary concentrating ability, and proteinuria)

CHAPTER SUMMARY

Chapter 57 presented the physiology of the parathyroid glands, the hormone they secrete (parathyroid hormone) and the mechanism of action of this hormone on various target organs and tissues. The chapter also described the pharmacokinetics, pharmacodynamics, and pharmacotherapeutics of the major parathyroid agents (calcium regulators). Finally, the predictable and unpredictable adverse drug reactions and interactions were explored and nursing implications described. Here are the highlights of the chapter:

● The parathyroid glands contain chief cells that secrete PTH into the blood. PTH acts as a calcium regulator, responding to blood calcium concentration levels. Any lowering of these levels stimulates the release of PTH to increase the circulating calcium. This hormonal action is dependent on the activation of cyclic AMP.

● Endogenous PTH regulates serum calcium by acting

on the bone, the kidneys, and the gastrointestinal system. The role of PTH in the regulation of calcium is a vital one for the body because calcium ions play an important part in the functioning of the cardiac and neuromuscular systems, in cell binding, in enzyme activity, and in blood coagulation.

• The major calcium regulators include calcitonin, etidronate disodium, and vitamin D analogues. Vitamin D analogues increase the serum calcium levels, while calcitonin and etidronate disodium decrease these levels.

• Protein hormones are easily degraded in the gastrointestinal tract and are best given parenterally. Natural hormones are metabolized rapidly in the body and provide a short duration of action. Most synthetic analogues provide more effective therapeutic results because the body metabolizes them more slowly and they provide a longer duration of action. Calcitonin is metabolized by the kidneys and is excreted in the urine. Etidronate disodium is excreted as unchanged drug, primarily in the urine. Vitamin D analogues are metabolized in the liver and eliminated through the bile in feces.

• Most adverse reactions involving calcium regulators are dose-dependent. Since some calcium regulators increase serum calcium concentration levels while others decrease these levels, toxicity can result as either hypercalcemia or hypocalcemia. A systemic allergic reaction may occur with calcitonin administration.

• Nursing interventions include monitoring for allergic reactions, for signs and symptoms of hypercalcemia or hypocalcemia, and for kidney function. Besides teaching the patient about the specific drug and its administration, the nurse should instruct the patient in following a prescribed diet and avoiding over-the-counter products, especially those containing calcium.

Assessing hypocalcemic tetany

Severe hypocalcemia may cause tetany and spasms of the skeletal muscles. The effects of severe hypocalcemia can ultimately progress to cardiac arrest. Chvostek's sign and Trousseau's sign are two methods of assessing hypocalcemic tetany.

Elicit Chvostek's sign by tapping or stroking the area over the facial nerve in front of the ear. Then observe the lips and cheek for twitching, a positive sign.

Evoke Trousseau's sign by applying a blood pressure cuff to the arm, inflating the cuff between diastolic and systolic blood pressure levels, and maintaining the inflation for 3 minutes. Then observe for carpal spasm as evidenced by palmar flexion, a positive sign.

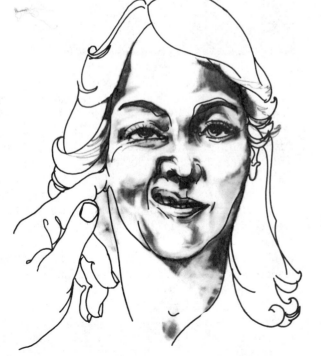

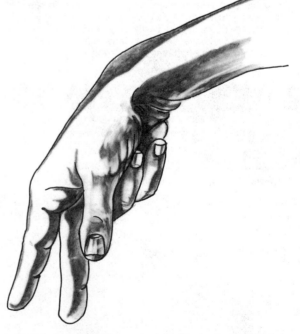

SELECTED MAJOR DRUGS

Parathyroid hormones (Calcium regulators)

The drugs discussed in this chapter and selected for this chart are representative of the class as a whole.

DRUG	MAJOR INDICATIONS	USUAL ADULT DOSAGES	NURSING IMPLICATIONS
calcitonin-salmon	Paget's disease	100 International Units/day S.C., I.M. for first few months then 50 to 100 IU daily or every other day	• Drug is contraindicated in patients with hypersensitivity to fish or to the gelatin composition of the diluent; also contraindicated in breast-feeding or pregnant women and in children. • Use caution when administering to patients with renal impairment, pernicious anemia, osteoporosis, and Zollinger-Ellison syndrome. • Assess for hypocalcemic tetany during administration.
etidronate disodium	Paget's disease	5 to 10 mg/kg/day P.O. for 6 months or less or 11 to 20 mg/kg P.O. daily for 3 months or less	• Use caution when administering to patients with enterocolitis or patients with renal dysfunction and in pregnant or breast-feeding patients who have restricted calcium and vitamin D intake. • Monitor urinary hydroxyproline and serum alkaline phosphatase levels. • Teach the patient to include adequate calcium and vitamin D in diet. • Instruct the patient to take drug between meals.
calcitriol	Hypoparathyroidism and pseudohypoparathyroidism	0.25 mcg P.O. daily with dosages possibly increased at 2- to 4-week intervals	• Drug is contraindicated in hypercalcemia and vitamin D toxicity. • Use caution when administering to patients receiving digitalis. • Monitor serum calcium levels: serum calcium level times serum phosphate level should not exceed 70. • Teach the patient to include adequate daily intake of calcium in diet. • Warn the patient that although calcitriol is a vitamin, it is a potent drug that must not be taken by anyone for whom it was not prescribed; it can cause serious toxicities.

BIBLIOGRAPHY

AMA Division of Drugs. *AMA Drug Evaluations,* 6th edition. New York: John Wiley & Sons, 1986.

American Hospital Formulary Service. *Drug Information 85.* McEvoy, G.K., et al. (eds.). Bethesda, Md.: American Society of Hospital Pharmacists, 1985.

Covington, T.R., and Walker, J.I. *Current Geriatric Therapy.* Philadelphia: W.B. Saunders Co., 1984.

Dukes, M.N.G. *Myler's Side Effects of Drugs: An Encyclopedia of Reaction and Interactions,* 10th edition. New York: Elsevier Science Publishing Co., 1984.

Esselstyn, C., Jr., et al. "Hyperparathyroidism after Radioactive Iodine Therapy for Graves' Disease," *Surgery* 92(5):811, November 1982.

Fischbach, F.T. *A Manual of Laboratory Diagnostic Tests,* 2nd edition. Philadelphia: J.B. Lippincott Co., 1984.

Gilman, A.G., et al., eds. *Goodman and Gilman's The Pharmacological Basis of Therapeutics,* 7th edition. New York: Macmillan Publishing Co., 1985.

Tyler, V.E., et al. *Pharmacognosy,* 6th edition. Philadelphia: Lea & Febiger, 1981.

United States Pharmacopeial Convention, Inc. *Drug Information for the Health Care Provider, 1984, Vol. 1.* Oradell, N.J.: Medical Economics Books, 1984.

CHAPTER 58

PITUITARY AGENTS

OBJECTIVES

After reading and studying this chapter, you should be able to:

1. Describe the roles of anterior pituitary hormones in controlling the structure and function of the body.

2. Compare the absorption, distribution, metabolism, and excretion of the anterior pituitary hormones.

3. Describe several diagnostic and therapeutic uses of the anterior pituitary hormone drugs corticotropin, cosyntropin, and somatrem.

4. Explain why you must carefully monitor the patient for unpredictable adverse reactions during adrenocorticotropic hormone therapy.

5. Identify the uses of the posterior pituitary hormone drugs.

6. Differentiate between the dosage form and route of administration for vasopressin and vasopressin tannate.

7. Describe the advantages and disadvantages of the nasal route for administering posterior pituitary hormone drugs.

8. Identify the nursing implications for administration of vasopressin, desmopressin, lypressin, and oxytocin.

INTRODUCTION

The pituitary gland, approximately 1.25 cm (½ inch) in diameter, lies buried in the sella turcica, a pouchlike sac at the base of the brain. The gland consists of an anterior lobe (adenohypophysis) and a posterior lobe (neurohypophysis). Between these two lobes is a small avascular area called the pars intermedia. The pars intermedia, almost absent in humans, remains functional in lower animals.

Often called the master gland, the anterior lobe of the pituitary secretes six major hormones, four of which regulate the functions of other endocrine glands. The major hormones include growth hormone (GH), adrenocorticotropic hormone (ACTH), thyroid-stimulating hormone (TSH), follicle-stimulating hormone (FSH), luteinizing hormone (LH), and prolactin. The secretion of the hormones of the anterior lobe is controlled by neurohormonal-stimulating and neurohormonal-inhibiting release factors secreted from the hypothalamus into the pituitary portal system.

The hormones of the anterior pituitary are secreted in minuscule amounts that produce important effects on the function and structure of the human body. These hormones also regulate the synthesis and secretion of other hormones in target organs and tissues.

The posterior pituitary gland secretes two hormones: antidiuretic hormone (ADH, vasopressin) and oxytocin. The secretion of ADH regulates fluid balance in the body and occurs in response to hypovolemia and increased serum osmolality. An increased secretion of oxytocin (in response to estrogen levels and nipple stimulation) stimulates the smooth muscle contraction of the pregnant uterus and milk ejection during lactation.

Pituitary hormones are mammalian metabolites produced by the endocrine glands. When released into the bloodstream, these hormones elicit a biological effect on specific organs and tissues. The pituitary hormones are derived from amino acid chains, the building blocks of protein. Because the natural pituitary hormones extracted from animals contain proteins that can precipitate hypersensitivity reactions, synthetically prepared pituitary substances are preferable. In some instances, however, the naturally occurring hormones provide therapeutic effects superior to those of the synthetically prepared analogues. That is particularly true for a synthetic extract that does not exactly mirror the natural hormone it is replacing.

For a summary of representative drugs, *see Selected major drugs: Pituitary agents* on pages 919 and 920.

ANTERIOR PITUITARY HORMONES

The protein hormones produced in the anterior pituitary regulate growth, development, and sexual characteristics by stimulating the actions of other endocrine glands. The anterior pituitary hormone drugs may be used either diagnostically or therapeutically. Anterior pituitary hormone drugs include the adrenocorticotropics (corticotropin, cosyntropin), growth hormone (somatrem), the gonadotropics (chorionic gonadotropin, menotropins), and the thyrotropics (TSH, or thyrotropin, and protirelin). (See Chapter 61, Fertility Agents, for a detailed discussion of the gonadotropics, and Chapter 56, Thyroid and Antithyroid Agents, for a discussion of the thyrotropics.)

History and source

As with other endocrine products, the therapeutic use of pituitary hormones is an outgrowth of organotherapy, a practice dating to the 13th century and Magnus's use of powdered hog testis to treat male impotence. The word pituitary derives from the Latin *pituita,* which means "phlegm," and early scientists believed that the pituitary contained secretions that moistened the nasal membranes. In 1887, Minkowski made the connection between acromegaly and a tumor of the pituitary gland. In 1900, Hutchinson concluded that the pituitary served as the growth control center for the body. In 1921, Evans and Long produced growth in rats using pituitary extract injections. Further research into the correlation between pituitary secretions and growth was conducted by Aschner (1909) and Smith (1930). Aron, Loeb, and Bassett identified TSH in 1929. In 1933, an important milestone in endocrine research, Collip prepared an adrenotropic substance, Riddle named prolactin, and Fevold identified FSH and LH.

Though the origin and early development of endocrine therapy was empiric, most current knowledge comes from continuous study over the past 30 years. The development in the 1960s of the Merrifield solid-phase synthesis of peptides made endocrine therapy commercially feasible. The discovery of recombinant DNA techniques in the late 1970s also began an entirely new chapter in the therapeutic use of endocrine hormones. For example, somatrem is a purified polypeptide hormone of recombinant DNA origin and displays an amino acid chain identical to that of the pituitary-derived natural growth hormone. Productive research with recombinant DNA continues.

Problems remain, however, with both natural and synthetic hormone extracts. For example, most animal hormones differ in amino acid structure from human hormones. As a result, animal hormones may precipitate antigen-antibody reactions. Furthermore, natural mammalian hormone extracts produce multiple effects on the system from considerable interaction among the basic units of the hormones. This interaction makes obtaining extracts with only one hormonal action very difficult. The short biological half-life of these hormones also has presented technical barriers to their synthetic production. The aim of current research is to purify hormone synthesis, thereby eliminating patient hypersensitivity reactions, and to produce single-action hormones.

PHARMACOKINETICS

The anterior pituitary hormones have peptide links, which enable peptidases in the digestive tract to destroy the hormones. Therefore, oral administration proves ineffective. Some of these hormones can be administered topically, but most require injection. Though the precise pharmacokinetic fate of some anterior pituitary hormones remains unknown, these drugs produce rapid therapeutic results. Usually, natural hormones are absorbed, distributed, and metabolized rapidly. Some analogues, however, are absorbed and metabolized more slowly, providing a prolonged duration of therapeutic activity. Anterior pituitary hormones are metabolized at the receptor site and also by the liver and kidneys. The hormones are excreted primarily in urine.

Absorption, distribution, metabolism, excretion

Corticotropin (ACTH) is rapidly absorbed when administered parenterally. The drug is usually administered I.M., but is also given I.V. or subcutaneously. Repository corticotropin contains ACTH in gelatin, designed to delay absorption and extend the period of therapeutic effectiveness. Repository corticotropin is usually given I.M. or subcutaneously. Corticotropin zinc hydroxide, a combination of ACTH and zinc, also is absorbed slowly. This drug, like repository corticotropin, provides extended effectiveness; it is administered I.M. The distribution information regarding these three drugs is imprecise, but all three are metabolized at the receptor site and by the liver and kidneys, and all are excreted in the urine.

Cosyntropin is rapidly absorbed following I.M. administration. The specific rate of cosyntropin metabolism remains unknown; however, the drug is rapidly removed from the plasma by the tissues and is excreted in the urine.

The control and effects of the anterior pituitary hormones

The hypothalamus (by the hypothalamic neurohormonal releasing factors) and stress stimulate the anterior pituitary to secrete hormones that act on various target organs in the endocrine system. The following illustration summarizes the specific action of each hormone and the target organs involved.

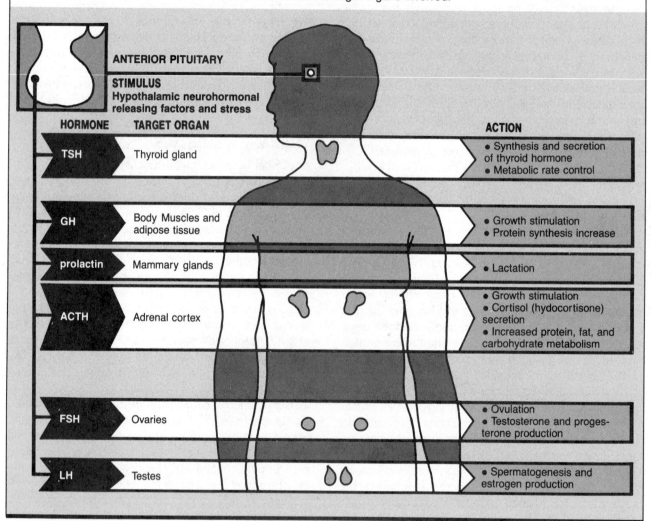

ANTERIOR PITUITARY

STIMULUS
Hypothalamic neurohormonal releasing factors and stress

HORMONE	TARGET ORGAN	ACTION
TSH	Thyroid gland	• Synthesis and secretion of thyroid hormone • Metabolic rate control
GH	Body Muscles and adipose tissue	• Growth stimulation • Protein synthesis increase
prolactin	Mammary glands	• Lactation
ACTH	Adrenal cortex	• Growth stimulation • Cortisol (hydocortisone) secretion • Increased protein, fat, and carbohydrate metabolism
FSH	Ovaries	• Ovulation • Testosterone and progesterone production
LH	Testes	• Spermatogenesis and estrogen production

Clinical tests have shown somatrem to be the pharmacokinetic equivalent of the natural pituitary growth hormone. When administered parenterally, somatrem is well absorbed, distributed, metabolized in the liver, and excreted in the urine.

Onset, peak, duration

When administered parenterally, corticotropin acts within 5 minutes, with a duration of 2 to 4 hours. The plasma level half-life is less than 20 minutes. For repository and zinc hydroxide preparations, onset of action is 6 hours, with a duration of 18 to 72 hours.

Cosyntropin acts in 5 minutes and peaks in 1 hour after I.V. administration. The duration of effect is 2 to 4 hours. The action of cosyntropin can be monitored by plasma cortisol levels.

The effects of somatrem begin immediately and last several days. The plasma level half-life is 15 to 50 minutes.

PHARMACODYNAMICS

The anterior pituitary hormones exert a profound effect on the body's growth and development. Under the control of neurohormonal-stimulating and neurohormonal-inhibiting release factors from the hypothalamus, these hormones alter the functions of their target tissues. The concentration of hormones in the circulating blood helps determine hormone production rate. Increasing hormone levels inhibit hormone production, while too little circulating hormone causes an increase in production and secretion. The relationship between hormone concentration and hormone production critically affects the regulation of hormone levels.(See *The control and effects of the anterior pituitary hormones* for a summary of the target organs and actions of these hormones.)

Mechanism of action

Anterior pituitary hormones interact with specific plasma membrane receptors to produce enzymatic actions. The hormone-receptor interaction induces direct changes in membrane permeability or stimulates adenosine 3',5'-monophosphate (cyclic AMP) production, which transmits the hormone signal within the cell. Both effects of the hormone-receptor interaction affect the metabolic rate of target organs.

PHARMACOTHERAPEUTICS

The clinical indications for anterior pituitary hormone drugs are both diagnostic and therapeutic. Because of their protein structure, pituitary tropic drugs (drugs that act on one of the target organs) prove ineffective when administered orally; as a result, they are not routinely used for hormone replacement in deficiency states. Instead, oral preparations of hormones normally produced by the target glands (corticosteroids, thyrotropic and gonadotropic hormones) are prescribed to maintain normal body function. Somatrem is an exception and is used to treat pituitary dwarfism. Gonadotropics may also prove effective in treating infertility from pituitary hypofunction. Some anterior pituitary hormone drugs are used diagnostically to differentiate between primary and secondary failure of the thyroid gland and adrenal cortex. Finally, ACTH is used to treat certain progressive diseases.

corticotropin [ACTH] (Acthar), **corticotropin repository** (ACTH Gel, Cortigel, Cortrophin Gel, H.P. Acthar Gel), **and corticotropin zinc hydroxide** (Cortrophin-Zinc). Used for the diagnostic testing of adrenocortical function, these drugs are also used to treat adrenal insufficiency from long-term use of corticosteroids. The drugs are also used like glucocorticoids, as anti-inflammatory and immunosuppressant agents, as well as for their effect on the hematopoietic and lymphatic systems. These characteristics make the corticotropins useful for treating dermatologic, allergic, ophthalmic, respiratory, edematous, hematologic, and gastrointestinal diseases. Corticotro-

pin, generally referred to as ACTH, is also used to treat the symptoms of acute episodes of multiple sclerosis and to increase muscle strength in patients with myasthenia gravis. It may also be used in treating collagen diseases, rheumatoid arthritis, and acute rheumatic fever. Miscellaneous uses include treating tubercular meningitis with subarachnoid block and hypercalcemia associated with cancer.

USUAL ADULT DOSAGE: for adrenal function tests, possibly as much as 80 units in a single injection. An I.V. infusion of 10 to 25 units (aqueous form) in 500 ml D_5W is administered over 8 hours. Deficiency states require a corticotropin injection, either I.M. or S.C., of 20 units q.i.d.; repository preparations, 40 to 80 units I.M. or S.C. every 24 to 72 hours; or zinc hydroxide preparations, 40 units I.M. every 12 to 24 hours. Multiple sclerosis episodes respond to the I.M. administration of 80 to 120 units per day for 2 to 3 weeks.

cosyntropin (Cortrosyn, Synacthen Depot). Physicians use cosyntropin strictly as a diagnostic drug to differentiate primary (adrenal) from secondary (pituitary) adrenal insufficiency.

USUAL ADULT DOSAGE: for the rapid screening test, 0.25 to 0.75 mg I.M. over 2 minutes, or 0.25 mg I.V. over 4 to 8 hours at a rate of 40 mcg/hour over 6 hours.

somatrem (Protropin). Used to treat linear growth failure from hormonal deficiency, the drug may also be used as replacement therapy before epiphyseal closure in patients with GH deficiency. Somatrem produces an increase in the size and number of muscle cells, thereby affecting organ growth, as well as protein, carbohydrate, lipid, mineral, and connective tissue metabolism.

USUAL PEDIATRIC DOSAGE: up to 0.1 mg (0.2 IU) per kg of body weight I.M. three times weekly; to avoid adverse effects, do not exceed this dosage.

arginine HCl (R-Gene 10). An amino acid used diagnostically to test pituitary function, the drug is not intended for therapeutic use. With intact pituitary function, arginine HCl results in elevated plasma levels of human GH. Arginine HCl can also be used as a diagnostic aid in such conditions as panhypopituitarism, pituitary dwarfism, acromegaly, and linear growth problems.

USUAL ADULT DOSAGE: 30 grams of a 10% solution administered I.V. over 30 minutes.

Drug interactions

When administered with aspirin, corticotropin (ACTH) decreases the blood levels of the salicylate. Because of the hyperglycemic activity of ACTH, diabetic patients

DRUG INTERACTIONS

Anterior pituitary agents

Anterior pituitary hormone drug interactions produce adverse physiologic and therapeutic effects, sometimes reducing the effectiveness of therapy and, in some instances, creating additional pathologies.

DRUG	INTERACTING DRUGS	POSSIBLE EFFECTS	NURSING IMPLICATIONS
corticotropin	immunosuppressants	Cause neurologic complications	• Assess the neurologic system.
	aspirin	Decreases salicylate levels	• Assess for decreased therapeutic effects of aspirin.
	diuretics	Cause electrolyte losses	• Monitor electrolytes, particularly potassium.
cosyntropin	amphetamines, estrogens, lithium	Produce altered test results	• Obtain a complete current drug history. • Consult with the physician to reschedule the test.
somatrem	thyroid hormone and androgens (concurrently)	Cause epiphyseal closure precipitated	• Assess the patient annually for bone age.
	corticosteroids	Cause diminished growth response; decreased hyperglycemia and sensitivity to insulin	• Carefully document pretreatment growth rate for 6 to 12 months. • Instruct parent to record child's accurate height measurements at intervals. • Continuously monitor for glycosuria or increased blood glucose levels.

may need increased insulin or oral antidiabetic agents. Corticotropin with diuretics may cause increased electrolyte losses.

Amphetamines, estrogens, and lithium alter cortisol levels and, when taken with cosyntropin, may alter diagnostic test results. Radioactive scans should not be scheduled within 1 week of a cosyntropin test because cosyntropin may alter the results of the scan.

Concomitant glucocorticoid therapy may diminish the growth-stimulating potential of somatrem and act synergistically with it to increase blood glucose levels by producing insulin resistance. Thyroid hormone and androgens given simultaneously may precipitate epiphyseal closure, reducing the effectiveness of somatrem. (See *Drug interactions: Anterior pituitary agents* for a summary of the drug interactions that affect these hormones.)

ADVERSE DRUG REACTIONS

Because of the polypeptide nature of all of the pituitary hormones, the major adverse drug reactions are allergic reactions. Short-term, intensive hormone therapy with animal preparations increases the possibility of an allergic reaction; however, allergic reactions occur less frequently when the therapy involves synthetic hormone drugs. The incidence of allergic reactions has decreased from advancements in bioassay, immunoassay, and radioimmunoassay techniques, which have improved the quality, quantity, and refinement of both natural protein hormones and synthetic analogue extracts. Other possible adverse reactions can lead to electrolyte and mineral imbalances.

Because the physiologic need for hormones fluctuates greatly with the patient's age, state of health, stress level, and other variables, dosages must vary. Continuous assessment of the patient's response to therapy also helps determine the hormone drug regimen. Since dosage must vary, the number and types of adverse reactions vary also. (See *Anterior pituitary agents: Summary of adverse reactions* for a list of possible reactions.)

Predictable reactions

The most frequently documented dose-related reactions from corticotropin include sodium and water retention, impaired wound healing, dizziness, convulsions, and euphoria. Other, less frequent dose-related reactions include potassium loss, hypertension, ketosis, immunosuppression, skin hyperpigmentation, and mood elevation. Long-term use of corticotropin can cause iatrogenic Cushing's syndrome indistinguishable from the naturally occurring condition. Cosyntropin administration can cause pruritus and flushing.

Somatrem may cause glucose intolerance and hypothyroidism. A large percentage of patients treated with somatrem develop antibodies to the hormone; however, the antibodies do not seem to interfere with the therapy's effectiveness. Arginine HCl can produce nausea, vomiting, headache, flushing, numbness, and local infusion site irritation in a few patients.

Unpredictable reactions

Hypersensitivity reactions occur frequently during therapy with anterior pituitary hormone drugs. Allergic reactions to cosyntropin rarely occur, probably because it

Anterior pituitary agents: Summary of adverse reactions

The dose-related adverse reactions from anterior pituitary hormone drugs vary greatly. Many of the reactions have long-term physiologic ramifications for the patient.

DRUG	REACTION
corticotropin	Hypersensitivity, iatrogenic Cushing's syndrome (with long-term therapy), electrolyte imbalances, hyperpigmentation, immunosuppression, impaired wound healing, mood elevation, hypertension
cosyntropin	Hypersensitivity, pruritus, facial flushing
somatrem	Pain at injection site, glucose intolerance, transient hypothyroidism during treatment, development of antibodies that interfere with treatment (rare)
arginine HCl	Nausea and vomiting, headache, flushing, irritation at infusion site

is produced synthetically and used only diagnostically. Hypersensitivity with arginine HCl also rarely occurs.

NURSING IMPLICATIONS

Because anterior pituitary hormone drugs are protein in nature (except for the synthetic products), the nurse must carefully monitor the patient for allergic reactions. Other important nursing implications follow:

• Corticotropin is contraindicated to treat conditions involving adrenocortical hyperfunction and in primary adrenal insufficiency. Intravenous administration of corticotropin is contraindicated except in patients with idiopathic thrombocytopenic purpura and in diagnostic tests for determining adrenocortical function.

• Do not administer corticotropin to patients who have had recent surgery or to patients with ocular herpes simplex, congestive heart failure, scleroderma, osteoporosis, fungal infections, hypertension, or hypersensitivity to porcine proteins.

• The administration of corticotropin during pregnancy and lactation necessitates careful consideration of the risk-benefit ratio of the therapy. Prolonged corticotropin therapy in children will inhibit linear growth.

• Live vaccines are contraindicated during corticotropin therapy; in fact, any immunization procedure should be performed with caution. The drug should be used cautiously in patients with latent tuberculosis, hypothyroiditis, impaired hepatic function, diabetes, abscesses, pyogenic infections, or diverticulitis.

• Cosyntropin exhibits some immunosuppressive activity and contains no foreign animal protein. Cosyntropin is safer to use than corticotropin.

• Do not administer cosyntropin to patients with known hypersensitivity to the drug or with a known allergic reaction to corticotropin. Also, do not administer cosyntropin with hydrocortisone on the day of testing.

• Somatrem is contraindicated in patients with closed epiphyses, evidence of underlying intracranial lesion, or known sensitivity to benzyl alcohol. As a precaution when using somatrem, frequently assess patients with growth deficiency secondary to an intracranial lesion to determine the stability of the underlying problem.

• Continued assessment for glucose intolerance is necessary during somatrem therapy. Periodic thyroid function tests are suggested because hypothyroidism interferes with the therapeutic effects of somatrem.

• Arginine HCl is contraindicated in patients with allergic tendencies. The drug should be used cautiously in high doses in patients with renal insufficiency or electrolyte imbalances.

• Before administering any anterior pituitary hormone, always perform a hypersensitivity skin test. After the test, document the result; if it is negative, therapy can begin.

• Before administering the drug, check to be sure that epinephrine 1:1,000 is readily available for the emergency treatment of an allergic reaction.

• A patient's adverse reactions to the anterior pituitary hormone drugs may be prevented or minimized by implementing the following actions: check the urinary and plasma corticosteroid values to measure the adrenal response before administering corticotropin; restrict dietary supplementation; restrict sodium and encourage potassium intake to reduce the edema and hypokalemia from overstimulation of the adrenal cortex during corticotropin therapy; and monitor glucose intolerance and thyroid function when using somatrem.

• During corticotropin therapy, perform the following important nursing interventions: observe the patient closely for hypersensitivity reactions during the first 15 minutes of I.V. administration or immediately after I.M. or S.C. injection; monitor the patient for the unpredictable signs and symptoms of adverse reactions, such as skin reactions, dizziness, nausea, vomiting, mild fever, wheezing, and circulatory failure, and be aware that respiratory or cardiac arrests can occur; assess the patient for infection or a peptic ulcer, for a history of tuberculosis, and for diabetes mellitus; assess before and after I.V. infusions for hypercortisolism by checking plasma cortisol levels and 24-hour urinary 17-ketosteroid and 17-hydroxycorticosteroid levels; and monitor and record weight changes, intake and output data, and resting blood pressures until an effective drug dose is attained. After the cosyntropin test (rapid ACTH test), observe the patient for signs of hypersensitivity including urticaria, tachycardia, and pruritus.

• When administering somatrem, monitor the blood glucose level, blood urea nitrogen, electrolytes, and thyroid function.

• I.V. infusions of corticotropin require aqueous solutions, while I.M. and S.C. injections require suspension and gelatin solutions. Use caution when matching the type of preparation to the method of administration.

• Corticotropin repository is viscid at room temperature. Corticotropin zinc and corticotropin repository are not suitable for I.V. use and should be shaken before injecting into the gluteal muscle.

• Taper high dosage levels of corticotropin rather than suddenly withdrawing the drug because withdrawal usually causes a 2- to 5-day period of hypofunction.

• Protect corticotropin solutions from heat, freezing, and agitation to avoid denaturing the protein molecules in the drug.

• Cosyntropin, a synthetic peptide powder, requires reconstitution. Add 1 ml of normal saline solution to a 0.25-mg vial to provide 0.25 mg/ml. Reconstituted solutions have a pH of 5.5 to 7.5 and remain stable for 12 hours at room temperature, or 21 days if refrigerated.

• Each 5-mg vial of somatrem should be reconstituted with 1 to 5 ml of bacteriostatic water for injection. For the bacteriostatic water, use benzyl alcohol, preserved only. To prepare the solution, inject the bacteriostatic water into the 5-mg vial, aiming the stream against the glass wall. Then, rotate the vial gently without shaking it. The contents of the vial should be clear after reconstitution. Discard any drug that appears cloudy or contains particulate material. Use small syringes to validate the accuracy of the dose and a needle of adequate length (1 inch [2.5 cm] or greater) to ensure muscle insertion.

• Refrigerate the drug for storage but avoid freezing. Use the contents of reconstituted vials within 1 week.

• Invert and inspect each bottle of arginine HCl to be sure that the contents are clear. Discard any bottle that has cloudy contents or lacks a vacuum.

• A patient receiving corticotropin therapy should be taught stress-management techniques and the importance of reporting symptoms of infection, peptic ulcer disease, glucose imbalance, or hypercortisolism. Inform the patient that immunization is contraindicated during treatment. Encourage a low-sodium, high-protein diet during the therapy. Finally, warn the patient that corticotropin injections are painful.

• Before cosyntropin test (rapid ACTH test), explain the test's purpose. Advise the patient to fast for 12 hours, rest for 30 minutes before the test, and not take any ACTH or steroids before the test.

• Impart similar information to a patient before the pituitary (growth hormone) function test with arginine HCl. The patient must observe the dietary, activity, and medication restrictions prescribed to obtain accurate test results.

POSTERIOR PITUITARY HORMONES

Protein hormones synthesized by the nerve bodies of the hypothalamus and stored in the posterior pituitary have a pressor effect from arteriole and capillary vasoconstriction; an antidiuretic action from increased reabsorption of water in the renal tubular and collecting duct; and a stimulation effect on smooth muscles in the body. These hormones are secreted into the blood by the pituitary gland. Posterior pituitary hormone drugs include all forms of the antidiuretic hormone (ADH), such as lypressin, desmopressin, vasopressin, and vasopressin tannate; and oxytocin.

History and source

As with the hormones of the anterior pituitary, the medicinal use of natural and synthetic posterior pituitary hormones is a 20th-century innovation. Over the past 30 years, advances in technology have led to the identification of the structure and function of many hormones in the body. Both ADH and oxytocin are nonapeptides (a peptide containing nine amino acids) with similar structures, differing only in one or two amino acids. Thus, no clear-cut separation of the physiologic properties or pharmacologic actions of these two hormones can be made until the hormones are compared quantitatively rather than qualitatively. For example, in tests with rats, oxytocin is about 100 times less potent than ADH in antidiuretic and pressor effects, but ADH is about 20 times less potent than oxytocin at stimulating the rat uterus. In stimulating the contractile activity of the nonpregnant human uterus, ADH proves more potent than oxytocin; however, late in pregnancy oxytocin becomes steadily more potent until, at term, it is much more effective than ADH.

In 1954, duVigneaud and his associates identified the structures of ADH and oxytocin, and that year, duVigneaud was awarded the Nobel prize in chemistry. The development of the Merrifield solid-phase synthesis of peptides made the synthesis of ADH analogues possible. In 1967, Zaoral synthesized desmopressin, which resists degradation by the action of peptidases, making desmopressin a much more effective antidiuretic than the natural hormone. Since 1982, scientists have developed and tested a series of analogues known as synthetic ADH antagonists. Scientists see a potential clinical benefit of the synthetic ADH antagonists, which act to reverse the water intoxication resulting from the action of ADH.

PHARMACOKINETICS

Because enzymes in the digestive tract can destroy all protein hormones, oral administration of the hormones proves ineffective. Preparations of posterior pituitary hormones may be given by injection or topical intranasal spray. Blood peptidases destroy some of the administered hormone; some binds to receptors on the myo-

metrium; and one third to one half of any given dose reaches the receptors of the renal tubules, where it stimulates water reabsorption. Target tissues degrade much of the hormone, with less than 20% being excreted unchanged in the urine.

Absorption, distribution, metabolism, excretion

The antidiuretic hormone vasopressin tannate is absorbed more slowly than the aqueous solution vasopressin. Both vasopressin (aqueous) and vasopressin tannate are distributed throughout the extracellular fluid, metabolized in the liver and kidneys, and excreted in the urine. Following an S.C. dose of vasopressin (aqueous), 5% is excreted unchanged in the urine after approximately 4 hours; after I.V. administration, 5% to 15% of the dose appears in the urine.

Both desmopressin and lypressin are effectively absorbed following intranasal administration. Though the quantitative absorption data for lypressin are currently unavailable, 10% to 20% of the desmopressin dose is absorbed via this route. Desmopressin and lypressin are distributed throughout the extracellular fluid, metabolized by the liver and kidneys, and excreted in the urine.

The precise pharmacokinetics of the oxytocic drugs remains unclear. Like other natural hormones, however, oxytocic drugs are usually absorbed, distributed, and metabolized rapidly. Parenterally administered oxytocin is absorbed rapidly, but when administered intranasally, the absorption is erratic. Oxytocin is distributed throughout the extracellular fluid, rapidly metabolized by the liver and kidneys, and excreted in the urine. Oxytocinase, an enzyme produced in the placenta, helps to degrade oxytocin, thereby controlling the concentration of oxytocin in the uterus.

Onset, peak, duration

Administered subcutaneously, vasopressin (aqueous) onset is within 1 hour and lasts 2 to 8 hours. With I.M. injection, the onset varies, and duration is 6 to 12 hours. Following I.V. administration, vasopressin onset is within 1 minute and half-life is 1 to 20 minutes. After an I.M. injection, vasopressin tannate becomes effective within 1 hour, with a duration from 24 to 96 hours.

Desmopressin and lypressin act within 1 hour. Concentration levels of desmopressin peak in 1 to 4 hours and last 8 to 20 hours; lypressin concentration levels peak in ½ to 2 hours and last 3 to 8 hours.

Uterine response to oxytocin occurs 3 to 7 minutes after I.M. administration and lasts 30 to 60 minutes. After I.V. administration, oxytocin's onset of action is 1 minute, with a shorter duration. Response occurs in 5 to 10 minutes following nasal spray. The plasma half-life of oxytocin is 1 to 6 minutes.

The control and effects of the posterior pituitary hormones

The hypothalamus (by direct hypothalamic neurocontrol) stimulates the posterior pituitary to secrete hormones that act on specific target organs. This illustration summarizes the specific action of each hormone and the target organs involved.

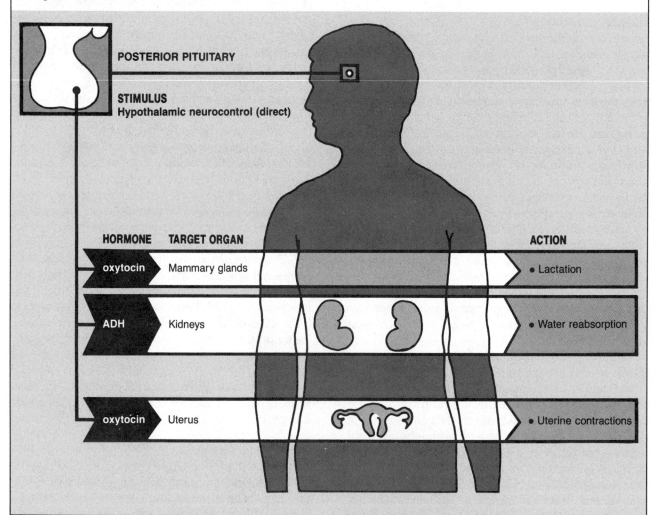

HORMONE	TARGET ORGAN	ACTION
oxytocin	Mammary glands	• Lactation
ADH	Kidneys	• Water reabsorption
oxytocin	Uterus	• Uterine contractions

POSTERIOR PITUITARY

STIMULUS
Hypothalamic neurocontrol (direct)

PHARMOCODYNAMICS

The posterior pituitary hormones, under neural control, affect smooth muscle contraction in the uterus, bladder, and gastrointestinal tract; fluid balance via renal reabsorption of water; and blood pressure via stimulation of the arterial wall muscles. (See *The control and effects of the posterior pituitary hormones* for a summary of the target organs and actions of these hormones.)

Mechanism of action

As with other protein hormones, an increase in cyclic AMP in the target cells mediates the effects of ADH. In the kidneys, ADH is bound by receptors on the surfaces of collecting duct cells, thereby regulating the threshold for water reabsorption by the distal tubules, collecting tubules, and collecting ducts. High doses of ADH stimulate vasculature contraction, producing pressor effects and increasing blood pressure. Oxytocin may stimulate uterine contractions by increasing the permeability of uterine cell membranes to sodium ions.

PHARMACOTHERAPEUTICS

Physicians prescribe ADH for hormone replacement therapy in patients affected by neurogenic diabetes insipidus. ADH, however, does not effectively treat nephrogenic diabetes insipidus. ADH treatment is short-term for patients with transient diabetes insipidus after head injury or surgery, but may be lifelong for patients with idiopathic hormone deficiencies. The drugs of choice for chronic deficiency, the synthetic extracts desmopressin and lypressin are administered intranasally two to four times a day based on the degree of polyuria. Desmopressin and lypressin prove particularly useful for patients allergic or refractory to vasopressin of animal origin. If desmopressin and lypressin prove ineffective, vasopressin tannate is administered every 2 to 3 days. The dosage of vasopressin tannate depends upon the amount of urine output. Vasopressin treatment also elevates the blood pressure in patients experiencing hypotension from lack of vascular tone and relieves postoperative intestinal gaseous distention.

The oxytocics are used to induce labor and promote incomplete abortions. The short biological half-lives of oxytocin and vasopressin can offer advantages or disadvantages, depending upon the therapeutic objectives. The short duration of oxytocin is an advantage in the therapeutic roles of this drug. However, when vasopressin is employed as replacement therapy to manage diabetes insipidus, an increased duration of action is needed. As a result, physicians usually prescribe vasopressin tannate.

posterior pituitary injection (Pituitrin, Pituitrin-S Ampoules). This natural extract with oxytocic, vasopressor, and antidiuretic properties has a rapid pressor effect that makes its use hazardous; most physicians now use more refined drugs with specific oxytocic or antidiuretic properties. Posterior pituitary injection can be used to treat postoperative ileus; stimulate gas expulsion; achieve homeostasis in esophageal varices; treat diabetes insipidus; and stimulate the uterus after incomplete expulsion of the placenta. Posterior pituitary injection can also serve to help treat shock. The use of this hormone to treat enuresis accompanying diabetes insipidus is not curative. USUAL ADULT DOSAGE: 5 to 20 units, preferably I.M. or S.C.

posterior pituitary intranasal (Posterior Pituitary). A natural hormone with antidiuretic properties, posterior pituitary intranasal can control the polyuria, polydipsia, and dehydration associated with diabetes insipidus from an ADH deficiency.

USUAL ADULT DOSAGE: not specified; instead, individualized doses are determined and administered three to four times daily.

vasopressin (Pitressin) **and vasopressin tannate** (Pitressin Tannate). These natural antidiuretic hormones are used to treat diabetes insipidus; to relieve postoperative intestinal gaseous distention; to dispel gas shadows appearing before abdominal roentgenography (X-rays); and to treat transient polyuria from an ADH deficiency following trauma.

USUAL ADULT DOSAGE: for abdominal distention, an initial dose of 5 units vasopressin, given I.M., followed by 10 units every 3 to 4 hours; for diabetes insipidus, 5 to 10 units, S.C. or I.M., b.i.d. to t.i.d.; for abdominal roentgenography, two injections of 10 units each, the first administered 2 hours and the second ½ hour before the films are exposed; and for polyuria due to ADH deficiency, 5 to 10 units intranasally, S.C., or I.M., every 8 to 12 hours.

Vasopressin tannate, used primarily to treat diabetes insipidus, is administered in dosages of 0.3 to 1 ml I.M. and then repeated as ordered.

desmopressin acetate (DDAVP). This synthetic antidiuretic hormone is used to treat diabetes insipidus, hemophilia A, von Willebrand's disease, and temporary polyuria and polydipsia associated with pituitary trauma or surgery.

USUAL ADULT DOSAGE: for diabetes insipidus and polyuria with pituitary trauma, 0.1 to 0.4 ml/day, intranasal, either in single or divided doses (most patients require 0.2 ml/day in two doses adjusted according to the pattern of response); for hemophilia A and von Willebrand's disease, 0.3 mcg/kg of body weight diluted in 50 ml of sterile saline solution, infused I.V. slowly over 15 to 30 minutes.

lypressin (Diapid Nasal Spray). A synthetic ADH analogue that produces minimal vasopressor or oxytocic effect, lypressin is primarily used to treat diabetes insipidus of neurogenic origin and is very useful in patients allergic or refractory to vasopressin of animal origin.

USUAL ADULT DOSAGE: from 1 to 10 sprays into each nostril every 3 to 4 hours; however, 4 sprays in each nostril is the maximum that can be absorbed at any one time. One spray provides 2 Posterior Pituitary (Pressor) Units. The usual dose is 1 or 2 sprays into each nostril q.i.d. The frequency of administration is governed by increased urination or severe thirst.

oxytocin (Pitocin, Syntocinon) **and oxytocin citrate** (Pitocin Citrate). Synthetic compounds identical to the natural hormone, oxytocin and oxytocin citrate treat uterine inertia and induce labor in cases of erythroblastosis fetalis. These drugs are also used to treat preeclampsia, eclampsia, and the premature rupture of membranes. Physicians also prescribe oxytocin to control postpartum hemorrhage and uterine atony, hasten uterine involution, and complete inevitable abortions after the 20th week of pregnancy.

USUAL ADULT DOSAGE: for inducing labor, preeclampsia, eclampsia, and premature rupture of membranes, via I.V. infusion (drip) method, initial dose should not exceed 1 to 2 mU/minute (0.001 to 0.002 units/minute). The dose can be gradually increased by 1 to 2 mU/minute at 15- to 30-minute intervals until a normal contraction pattern is established. The maximum dose should not exceed 20 mU/minute. For reducing postpartum bleeding, 10 to 40 units are added to 1,000 ml of physiologic electrolyte solution and infused at a rate necessary to control uterine atony. Also, 10 units may be administered I.M. after the delivery of the placenta. In treating an incomplete abortion, an I.V. infusion of 10 units in 500 ml of solution is administered at a rate of 10 to 20 mU/ml (20 to 40 drops) per minute. For stimulating lactation, the nasal spray (40 units/ml), sprayed once into one or both nostrils 2 to 3 minutes before nursing proves effective.

Drug interactions

Drug interactions with posterior pituitary hormones include decreased antidiuretic properties when combined with alcohol, phenytoin, demeclocycline, epinephrine, heparin, and lithium; and increased antidiuretic activity when combined with acetaminophen (Tylenol), cyclophosphamide, indomethacin, chlorpropamide, clofibrate, and carbamazepine. Also, either barbiturate sedation or cyclopropane anesthesia may produce synergistic and additive effects with vasopressin. The resulting potentiation of the antidiuretic effect may lead to coronary insufficiency and cardiac dysrhythmias. Ephedrine, methoxamine, and other vasopressors can potentiate the effect of oxytocin, possibly resulting in severe hypertension and the rupture of cerebral blood vessels postpartum. (See *Drug interactions: Posterior pituitary agents.*)

ADVERSE DRUG REACTIONS

The major adverse drug reaction to natural posterior pituitary hormone extracts is hypersensitivity. Administering synthetic hormone drugs markedly reduces the probability of hypersensitivity. Large doses of antidiuretic hormones can cause gastrointestinal upsets and cardiovascular pathologies. Vasopressin tannate administration may result in sterile abscesses at the injection site and sufficient peripheral vasoconstriction to produce gangrene. (See *Posterior pituitary agents: Adverse reactions* on page 918.)

Predictable reactions

Frequently observed and documented dose-related reactions with natural antidiuretic hormone therapy include circumoral and facial pallor, increased gastrointestinal motility, and abdominal and uterine cramps. Other adverse reactions can include tinnitus, anxiety, hyponatremia, albuminuria, eclamptic attacks, mydriasis, and transient edema. Nasal preparations can induce irritation, rhinorrhea, and nasal passage ulceration. Accidental deep inhalation of the powder preparation into the bronchial passages may cause substernal tightness, coughing, and transient dyspnea. Large doses may increase blood pressure. Anaphylaxis has occurred after injection.

Adverse reactions from synthetic drugs are rare, although high doses can cause transient headaches, nausea, nasal congestion, rhinitis, flushing, mild abdominal cramps, and vulval pain. Decreasing the dose usually reduces such reactions.

Synthetic extracts have entirely replaced natural oxytocics. Synthetic oxytocin, however, can cause uterine problems for the pregnant woman and hypertensive disorders for both her and the fetus. The adverse reactions involving uterine problems and hypertensive disorders include fetal bradycardia, neonatal jaundice, postpartum hemorrhage, and cardiac dysrhythmias. Other adverse reactions with synthetic oxytocin include gastrointestinal disturbances, diaphoresis, headache, dizziness, and tinnitus. Excessive dosages as well as sensitivity to the drug may result in uterine hypertonicity, tetany, or uterine rupture. Severe water intoxication has been associated with slow oxytocin infusion over 24 hours.

Unpredictable reactions

Hypersensitivity reactions are the most common unpredictable reactions associated with the administration of both antidiuretic hormone drugs and oxytocics. These reactions occur more frequently with natural hormone extracts than with synthetic drug preparations.

DRUG INTERACTIONS

Posterior pituitary agents

Posterior pituitary hormone drug interactions can be antagonistic, synergistic, or potentiating. Patients receiving hormone therapy need to be monitored continually for drug interactions that can alter the desired therapeutic effect.

DRUG	INTERACTING DRUGS	POSSIBLE EFFECTS	NURSING IMPLICATIONS
vasopressin and its derivatives	alcohol, phenytoin, demeclocycline, epinephrine, heparin, lithium	Decrease ADH activity	● Monitor for dehydration (acute weight loss, increased pulse, dry skin and mucous membranes, decreased postural systolic blood pressure, decreased skin turgor, thirst, oliguria, and fatigue). ● Monitor urine output and specific gravity and serum osmolality. ● Monitor vital signs and weight. ● Monitor laboratory values (hematocrit, hemoglobin, red blood cell count, and blood urea nitrogen).
	chlorpropamide, clofibrate, carbamazepine, acetaminophen, cyclophosphamide, indomethacin	Increase ADH activity	● Monitor for water intoxication (drowsiness, increased blood pressure, dyspnea, headache, confusion, and weight gain). ● Monitor urine output and specific gravity and serum osmolality. ● Monitor vital signs and weight. ● Monitor laboratory values (hematocrit, hemoglobin, and red blood cell counts).
	barbiturate or cyclopropane anesthesias	Produce synergistic effects leading to coronary insufficiencies, cardiac dysrhythmias	● Monitor vital signs.
oxytocin	cyclophosphamide	Increases oxytocic effects	● Monitor uterine contractions. ● Monitor for signs of water intoxication.
	vasoconstrictors (anesthetics, ephedrine, methoxamine)	Increase possibility of severe hypertension	● Monitor vital signs.

NURSING IMPLICATIONS

The posterior pituitary hormones can produce potent effects. The nurse must be aware of contraindications and precautions when administering dosages, as well as proper administration methods. The nurse should also realize the importance of patient teaching.

● Before using antidiuretic hormone drugs, assess patient sensitivity to the drug or to products of animal origin. Antidiuretic hormone drugs may be contraindicated and should be used cautiously in patients who have severe symptomatic cardiovascular disease, are elderly, are pregnant, or are in any state in which rapid increased extracellular water may result in further damage to the body (epilepsy, migraine headaches, asthma).

● Oxytocin is contraindicated in unfavorable fetal positions requiring surgical intervention, cephalopelvic disproportion, fetal distress where delivery is not imminent, cord prolapse, placenta previa, and prematurity. Oxytocin is also contraindicated in a previous cesarean section, uterine overdistention, grand multiparity, a history of uterine sepsis, traumatic delivery, and invasive cervical carcinoma.

● Exercise caution when using oxytocics concomitantly with cyclopropane anesthesia or vasoconstrictive drugs.

● With antidiuretic hormone drugs and oxytocic drugs, assess for allergic reactions and be prepared to deliver emergency treatment should such reactions occur.

● No known specific antidote for water intoxication caused by antidiuretic hormone drugs exists; however, use of a loop diuretic such as furosemide can induce diuresis.

● Have available magnesium sulfate during the I.M. administration of oxytocin to produce relaxation of the endometrium.

Posterior pituitary agents: Summary of adverse reactions

The major adverse drug reactions with posterior pituitary hormone drugs include hypersensitivity, gastrointestinal disorders, and cardiovascular pathologies. Other significant adverse reactions can occur.

DRUG	REACTION
posterior pituitary injection	Tremors, diaphoresis, vertigo, circumoral and facial pallor, increased gastrointestinal motility, abdominal and uterine cramps, tinnitus, anxiety, albuminuria, eclamptic attacks, mydriasis, urticaria, and angioneurotic edema and anaphylaxis
vasopressin	Facial pallor, gastrointestinal disturbances, water intoxication and hyponatremia, hypertension, hypersensitivity (high doses)
desmopressin acetate	Transient headaches, nausea, nasal congestion, rhinitis, flushing, abdominal cramps (rare and dose-dependent)
lypressin	Same as vasopressin, nasal congestion, pruritus, rhinorrhea, heartburn
oxytocin	Uterine contractions and ruptured uterus, cardiac dysrhythmias, neurologic disorders, water intoxication and hyponatremia, gastrointestinal disturbances, and anaphylactic reactions, postpartum hemorrhage, fetal bradycardia, neonatal jaundice

• With antidiuretic hormone therapy, monitor the patient's blood pressure closely for 30 minutes after administration and assess for early signs of water intoxication (drowsiness, headache, vomiting). Monitor fluid intake and output to estimate the patient's response to the antidiuretic hormone drug. Also check the patient's skin turgor and the condition of the mucous membranes. Finally, assess the patient for bowel sounds, the passage of flatus, and the resumption of bowel movements during antidiuretic hormone therapy used to improve peristalsis in the gastrointestinal tract.

• Because vasopressin tannate is in an oil suspension, never use I.V. administration. Before withdrawing the dose for I.M. injection, warm the vial to body temperature and shake. Giving the patient one or two glasses of water with vasopressin tannate administration may reduce some adverse reactions and improve therapeutic results.

• When administering desmopressin, check the expiration date on the label because nasal solutions expire 1 year after the date of manufacture. Store parenteral and nasal desmopressin in a refrigerator at 39° F. (4°C.). Discard any cloudy or discolored solution.

• A physician must always be present when the nurse administers oxytocin.

• Nursing responsibilities during oxytocin administration include assessment of the fetal heart rate and uterine contractions. Intravenous oxytocin is stopped immediately and oxygen is administered if the following occur: contractions more frequent than every 2 minutes and lasting longer than 60 seconds without uterine relaxation; contractions excessively strong or exceeding 50 mm Hg as measured on a monitor; or fetal heart rate indicating bradycardia, tachycardia, or irregular rhythm as measured by a monitor.

• During oxytocin therapy, frequently assess the fundus of the obstetric patient and the lochia of the postpartum patient. Carefully monitor fluid intake and output and be alert for alterations in the level of consciousness and orientation, which might indicate water intoxication.

• When local or regional anesthesia is given to a patient receiving oxytocin, monitor the patient closely for signs or symptoms of a hypertensive crisis.

• When administering nasal oxytocin, keep the plastic nasal tube for administration clean and dry. The dosage measurement of nasal oxytocin must be exact because the drug is potent.

• During I.V. administration of oxytocin, gently rotate the solution container to distribute the drug throughout the solution. Use a Y connection to the infusion tubing; the Y connection provides an alternate route for another solution that may be required to maintain the patency of the vein if the oxytocin needs to be discontinued. Oxytocin administration should always be controlled by an infusion pump and should never be administered via more than one route at a time.

• Oxytocin is incompatible with infusions of fibrinolysin, norepinephrine, prochlorperazine, protein hydrolysate, and warfarin, but it is compatible with dextrose-Ringer's combinations, dextrose-lactated Ringer's combinations, dextrose in water, and dextrose–saline solution mixtures.

• To reconstitute oxytocin, add 1 ml (10 units) to 1,000 ml of normal saline or other I.V. fluid to provide a solution containing 10 mU/ml (0.01 units/ml).

• Patient teaching is critical with antidiuretic hormone therapy because these drugs exert potent systemic effects. During patient or family teaching, address the following major issues: administration techniques; the signs and symptoms of adverse reactions, such as drowsiness, lethargy, headache, dyspnea, heartburn, nausea, abdominal cramps, vulval pain, or nasal congestion; and methods for monitoring fluid intake and output, including the recommended amounts of fluid.

• Instruct the patient never to increase the number of intranasal vasopressin sprays without checking with a physician.

• Since intravenous oxytocin is always administered under the supervision of a physician, explain the procedure to the patient and describe the expected outcome. Instruct the patient to clear the nasal passages before administering nasal oxytocin, to hold the squeeze bottle upright, and to spray into the nostril while sitting with the head vertical. Nasal oxytocin is contraindicated if administered while patient is lying down or with the head tilted back.

SELECTED MAJOR DRUGS

Pituitary agents

The drugs discussed in this chapter and selected for this chart are those most frequently used for diagnostic and clinical purposes.

DRUG	MAJOR INDICATIONS	USUAL ADULT DOSAGES	NURSING IMPLICATIONS
Anterior pituitary hormones			
corticotropin	Diagnosis of adrenal function	80 units in a single injection; 10 to 25 units/500 ml D₅W over 8 hrs I.V. Repository: 40 to 80 units q 24 to 72 hrs I.M., S.C. Zinc hydroxide preparation: 40 units I.M. q 12 to 24 hrs.	• Drug is contraindicated in patients with adrenocortical hyperfunction and primary adrenal insufficiency. • Intravenous administration is contraindicated except in patients with idiopathic thrombocytopenic purpura and for diagnostic tests for determining adrenocortical function. • Do not give corticotropin to patients with ocular herpes simplex, recent surgery, congestive heart failure, scleroderma, osteoporosis, fungal infections, hypertension, or hypersensitivity to porcine proteins. • Use cautiously in pregnant or breast-feeding women and in women of childbearing age; in patients being immunized; and in patients with latent tuberculosis, hypothyroiditis, impaired hepatic function, diabetes, abscesses, pyogenic infections, or diverticulitis. • Provide potassium intake during treatment. • Assess for euphoria, nervousness, insomnia, or depression.
cosyntropin	Diagnostic testing of adrenocortical function	0.25 to 0.75 mg I.M. over 2 min or 0.25 mg I.V. over 4 to 8 hrs	• Cosyntropin is contraindicated in patients with known hypersensitivity to the drug or a known allergic reaction to corticotropin.
somatrem	Promote linear and skeletal growth due to deficiency of GH secretion	0.1 mg (0.2 IU)/kg I.M. three times/week at 48-hr intervals	• Somatrem is contraindicated in individuals with closed epiphyses, evidence of underlying intracranial lesion, or known sensitivity to benzyl alcohol. • Examine patients frequently for progression or recurrence of the underlying disease when the GH deficiency results from an intracranial lesion. • Measure the patient's height monthly. • Check for glycosuria. • Assess for acidosis and hyperglycemia.

continued

SELECTED MAJOR DRUGS

Pituitary agents continued

DRUG	MAJOR INDICATIONS	USUAL ADULT DOSAGES	NURSING IMPLICATIONS
Posterior pituitary hormones			
posterior pituitary injection	Postoperative ileus	5 to 20 units I.M. or 10 units S.C.	• The drug is contraindicated in toxemia of pregnancy, cardiac disease, hypertension, epilepsy, and advanced arteriosclerosis. • Assess for allergic reaction. • Monitor blood pressure closely.
vasopressin	Diabetes insipidus	5 to 10 units two to three times/day, S.C., I.M. Tannate: 0.3 to 1 unit I.M.	• Vasopressin is contraindicated in chronic nephritis with nitrogen retention. • Use cautiously in children, elderly patients, pregnant women, and patients with epilepsy, migraine headaches, asthma, cardiovascular disease, or fluid overload. • Assess fluid intake and output. • Do not administer vasopressin tannate in oil I.V. • Monitor for dehydration. • Monitor blood pressure at least twice a day.
oxytocin	Induce labor	1 to 2 mU/min I.V.; the dose can be gradually increased not to exceed 20 mU/min.	• Oxytocin is contraindicated in the following conditions: significant cephalopelvic disproportion, unfavorable fetal position, fetal distress where delivery is not imminent, cord prolapse, placenta previa, prematurity of the fetus, a previous cesarean section, uterine overdistention, grand multiparity, a history of uterine sepsis, traumatic delivery, or invasive cervical carcinoma. • Make sure physician is available during oxytocin administration. • Assess uterine tone and fetal heart rate. • Assess for water intoxication. • Monitor vital signs at least once each hour.

CHAPTER SUMMARY

Chapter 58 presented discussions of the physiology of the pituitary gland, its hormones, and the effects of those hormones on body structure and function. The chapter identified and described the anterior pituitary hormones and the posterior pituitary hormones, elaborating on their pharmacokinetics, pharmacodynamics, and pharmacotherapeutics. The drug reactions, interactions, adverse effects, and nursing implications associated with pituitary hormone drugs were also explored. Here are the highlights of the chapter:

• The pituitary gland is divided into the anterior lobe and the posterior lobe. Each lobe of the pituitary secretes different hormones that produce widespread physiologic effects on body structure and function. Hypothalamic release factors stimulate or inhibit secretion of pituitary hormones as necessary.

• The hormones of the anterior pituitary act on other endocrine glands, such as the thyroid, adrenals, and ovaries, to control their structure and function. Anterior pituitary hormones also play a direct role in sexual maturity, reproduction, and linear growth. The three major anterior pituitary hormone drugs are corticotropin, cosyntropin, and somatrem.

• The hormones of the posterior pituitary regulate fluid volume and stimulate smooth muscle contraction. Posterior pituitary hormones include antidiuretic hormone and oxytocics. The major posterior pituitary hormone drugs include posterior pituitary injection, vasopressin, desmopressin, lypressin, and oxytocin.

• Endocrine therapy has benefited greatly from innovations in technology, physiology, and biochemistry during the past 30 years. Present research in the areas of recombinant DNA and ADH antagonist development is providing new therapeutic possibilities.

• Pituitary hormones are mammalian metabolites with protein structures. Pituitary hormone drugs occur as natural hormones and synthetically produced analogues.

• Because protein hormones are easily destroyed in the gastrointestinal tract by peptidases, oral administration of pituitary hormone drugs is not effective. Pituitary hormones can be administered parenterally or, for some drugs, intranasally. Natural pituitary hormone drugs are absorbed rapidly, metabolized by the kidneys and liver, and excreted in the urine. Natural hormone drugs have a short duration of action. Synthetic analogues are metabolized more slowly, providing a longer therapeutic duration, which makes them more clinically useful.

• The most significant adverse reaction associated with protein hormones results from a sensitivity to natural hormone extracts. Administering synthetic hormone analogues markedly decreases the incidence of sensitivity reactions.

• Interactions between pituitary hormones and other drugs can produce vasoconstriction and vasopressor activities that can cause cardiovascular crisis and water intoxication.

• The nursing interventions associated with pituitary hormone therapy include: assessing for allergic reactions and providing emergency treatment; assessing for signs of water intoxication; monitoring the cardiovascular system for signs of impending distress; and patient teaching.

• Patient teaching should explain hormone therapy, teach accurate dosages and correct administration, and emphasize compliance with prescribed drug regimens.

BIBLIOGRAPHY

Billups, N.F., and Billups, S.M., *American Drug Index 1984*, 28th ed. Philadelphia: J.B. Lippincott Co., 1984.

Dukes, M.N.G. *Myler's Side Effects of Drugs: An Encyclopedia of Reaction and Interactions*, 10th ed. New York: Elsevier Publishing Co., 1984.

Franklin, D. "Growing up Short," *Science News* 125(6):92, February 6, 1984.

Gever, L.N. "Synthetic is Better," *Nursing83* 13:6, December 1983.

Greenblatt, D.J., and Shader, R.I. *Pharmacokinetics in Clinical Practice.* Philadelphia: W.B. Saunders Co., 1985.

Hansten, D. *Drug Interactions,* 5th ed. Philadelphia: Lea & Febiger, 1985.

Hauser, S.I., et al. "Intensive Immunosuppression in Progressive Multiple Sclerosis. A Randomized, Three-Arm Study of High Dose Cyclophosphamide, Plasma Exchange and ACTH," *The New England Journal of Medicine* 308(4):173, January 27, 1983.

McEvoy, G.K., ed. *Drug Information 84.* Bethesda, Md.: American Society of Hospital Pharmacists, 1984.

Tyler, V.E., et al. *Pharmacognosy,* 8th ed. Philadelphia: Lea & Febiger, 1981.

Uhrig, J., and Hurley, R. "Chlorpropamide in Pregnancy and Transient Neonatal Diabetes Insipidus," *Canadian Medical Association Journal* 128(4):368, February 15, 1983.

ANDROGENIC AND ANABOLIC STEROID AGENTS

OBJECTIVES

After reading and studying this chapter, you should be able to:

1. Differentiate between the effects of the androgenic and anabolic steroid agents.

2. Identify the androgenic and anabolic steroid agents that are associated with hepatic disorders.

3. Explain why these agents are used to treat hypogonadism and related disorders; breast engorgement, breast cancer, and related disorders; and osteoporosis, anemias, and tissue-development problems.

4. Describe the mechanisms of action of these agents.

5. Describe the major drug interactions that occur with androgenic and anabolic steroid agents.

6. Describe the common adverse reactions to these agents and explain how to manage them.

INTRODUCTION

Androgenic steroids stimulate the growth of male accessory sex organs and produce masculinizing effects, such as facial hair growth and voice deepening. Anabolic steroids promote a positive nitrogen balance in the body, which stimulates tissue building and reverses tissue depletion.

In reality, these sharp distinctions are blurred; no purely androgenic or anabolic steroids exist. All androgenic steroids provide some anabolic effects, and all anabolic steroids provide some androgenic effects. Yet the distinctions remain useful because one effect always predominates. Predominantly androgenic steroid agents include danazol, fluoxymesterone, methyltestosterone, and all forms of testosterone. Predominantly anabolic steroid agents include ethylestrenol, nandrolone decanoate and phenpropionate, oxandrolone, oxymetholone, stanozolol, and testolactone.

Researchers derived many of the androgenic and anabolic steroid agents from testosterone, the male hormone secreted by the testes and, in smaller amounts,

by the ovaries and adrenal cortex. They modified testosterone's base molecule to try to minimize the androgenic effects and maximize the anabolic effects. Today, the search continues for an anabolic agent that can promote tissue building without producing masculinizing effects.

For a summary of representative drugs, see *Selected major drugs: Androgenic and anabolic steroid agents* on pages 926 and 927.

ANDROGENIC AND ANABOLIC STEROIDS

These steroid agents have many clinical uses. In androgen-deficient males, predominantly androgenic agents can correct hypogonadism and related disorders. In females, they can prevent postpartum breast engorgement and may be used to treat certain types of breast cancer and related disorders. Predominantly anabolic agents can promote weight gain in underweight patients affected by a catabolic disorder or drug. They also may be used to treat certain types of osteoporosis and anemias.

History and source

Just before World War II, scientists discovered the tissue-building effects of male sex hormones when they injected testosterone into castrated laboratory animals and observed a marked reduction in protein breakdown. A few years later, others applied this discovery by administering male sex hormones to promote muscle weight gain in German concentration camp survivors who were recovering from disease or starvation. Since the 1950s, physicians have treated many disorders with androgenic and anabolic steroid agents.

PHARMACOKINETICS

Anabolic and androgenic steroid agents are rapidly absorbed and highly bound to plasma proteins. These lipid-soluble agents are widely distributed throughout the body, metabolized in the liver, and excreted mainly by the kidneys.

Absorption, distribution, metabolism, excretion

Although oral and parenteral forms of testosterone are readily absorbed, they undergo such rapid hepatic metabolism that they produce little response. To overcome this problem, researchers modified the testosterone molecule or placed it in a special vehicle. Today, alkylated steroids allow rapid absorption but retard hepatic metabolism, making oral administration possible. Testosterone cypionate and enanthate use an oil base to prolong absorption and allow effective parenteral administration. After absorption, all androgenic and anabolic steroid agents are widely distributed throughout the body and highly bound to plasma proteins.

Testosterone and all other androgenic and anabolic steroid agents are excreted in the urine or feces as metabolites or unchanged drug.

Onset, peak, duration

The onset of action, peak concentration levels, and duration of action vary with the testosterone molecule modification. After oral administration, for example, the 17-alpha-alkylated steroids (oxymetholone, oxandrolone, ethylestrenol, and stanozolol) provide a short duration of action. After parenteral administration, the 17-beta esters (nandrolone decanoate and phenpropionate) offer a longer duration of action. Parenteral administration of testosterone cypionate and enanthate also provides an extended duration of action.

PHARMACODYNAMICS

Steroid agents produce either predominantly androgenic or anabolic effects, depending on the agent used. A predominantly androgenic agent will act as an exogenous replacement, stimulating normal development in androgen-deficient males. A predominantly anabolic agent will stimulate cellular protein synthesis, promoting a positive nitrogen balance and tissue development.

Mechanism of action

Agents such as testosterone produce androgenic and anabolic effects by binding to androgen receptors in target organs, such as skeletal muscle, the prostate gland,

and bone marrow. Receptor binding not only stimulates development in these organs, but also increases protein synthesis. These actions produce dramatic effects in androgen-deficient patients, such as castrated men, men with pituitary hormone deficiencies, and normal women.

Steroid agents may promote anabolic effects by blocking cortisol uptake in muscle and liver cells. Cortisol, secreted by the adrenal gland, normally acts as a catabolic agent, increasing muscle breakdown and body stress mechanisms. By blocking cortisol uptake in muscle cells, steroid agents reduce muscle breakdown and increase muscle mass; by blocking cortisol uptake in liver cells, they maximize its effect on body stress reactions. Steroid agents also decrease plasma protein synthesis in the liver, which enhances their effects by increasing the amount of free, or unbound, drug in the plasma.

The anabolic steroid agents reduce urinary excretion of nitrogen and electrolytes, causing water retention and weight gain.

PHARMACOTHERAPEUTICS

Although each agent produces androgenic and anabolic effects, one effect always predominates and helps determine the agent's clinical indications.

Androgenic agents such as testosterone cypionate and enanthate best serve as androgen replacements for castrated and hypogonadal males. They produce pronounced effects in prepubertal males. Some predominantly anabolic agents, such as oxymetholone, can stimulate erythropoiesis (red blood cell production) in the bone marrow, which makes them effective against aplastic and other anemias in 25% of patients. Danazol and other agents can be used to treat hereditary angioedema (an immune disorder that causes transient attacks of subcutaneous, submucosal, or visceral edema) because they can stabilize the immune defect by increasing or restoring components in the complement system. Testosterone propionate and related agents can provide palliative treatment for some hormone-sensitive breast cancers. (See Chapter 76, Hormonal Antineoplastic Agents, for additional information on the use of androgens for treating breast cancer.) Predominantly anabolic steroid agents such as oxandrolone sometimes are used to treat malnourished patients. For some, they can promote a positive nitrogen balance, enhance the appetite, and increase the sense of well-being.

In recent years, healthy people have taken predominantly anabolic steroids to increase their muscle mass and enhance their athletic performance. However, medical studies have not proved that these agents can enhance athletic performance, so these dubious claims of enhancement should be weighed against these agents' adverse reactions.

danazol (Danocrine). Administered primarily for its androgenic effects, danazol may be used to treat endometriosis and fibrocystic breast disease in women. It can also be used to prevent hereditary angioedema.

USUAL ADULT DOSAGE: for endometriosis, 200 to 400 mg P.O. b.i.d. uninterrupted for 3 to 6 months (may continue for 9 months); for fibrocystic breast disease, 100 to 400 mg P.O. daily in two divided doses for 2 to 6 months; for hereditary angioedema, 200 mg P.O. b.i.d. or t.i.d. until the desired response is achieved, then decreased by half every 1 to 3 months to determine lowest effective dose.

fluoxymesterone (Halotestin). Because of its predominantly androgenic activity, fluoxymesterone is used to treat hypogonadism and impotence caused by a testicular deficiency. It can also reduce postpartum breast engorgement and act as a palliative treatment for breast cancer in women.

USUAL ADULT DOSAGE: for hypogonadism and impotence, 5 to 20 mg P.O. daily; for postpartum breast engorgement, 2.5 mg P.O. when active labor begins, followed by 5 to 10 mg daily for 5 days; for breast cancer, 10 to 30 mg P.O. daily in divided doses, adjusted to the individual's needs and reduced to a minimum when desired effects are noted.

methyltestosterone (Metandren). A predominantly androgenic agent, methyltestosterone can be used to treat eunuchoidism (deficient testicular secretion), eunuchism (underdeveloped sex organs), male climacteric symptoms (reduced sexual activity), and postpubertal cryptorchidism (failure of one or both testes to descend normally). It also is used to treat breast cancer 1 to 5 years after menopause and postpartum breast engorgement in women.

USUAL ADULT DOSAGE: for eunuchoidism, eunuchism, and male climacteric symptoms, 10 to 40 mg P.O. daily or 5 to 20 mg buccally daily; for postpubertal cryptorchidism, 30 mg P.O. daily or 15 mg buccally daily; for breast cancer, 200 mg P.O. daily or 100 mg buccally daily; for postpartum breast engorgement, 80 mg P.O. daily or 40 mg buccally daily.

testosterone (Histerone, Testoject). Used primarily for its androgenic effects, testosterone is indicated for eunuchoidism, eunuchism, and male climacteric symptoms. It also can be used to treat breast cancer in postmenopausal women and postpartum breast engorgement.

USUAL ADULT DOSAGE: for eunuchoidism and related disorders, 10 to 25 mg I.M. two to three times weekly; for breast cancer, 100 mg I.M. three times weekly as long as improvement is maintained; for postpartum breast engorgement, 25 to 50 mg I.M. daily for 3 to 4 days starting at delivery.

testosterone cypionate (Andro-Cyp, Depo-Testosterone). Also used primarily as an androgen, this form of testosterone can help treat eunuchism, male hormone deficiency after castration, and male climacteric symptoms. It also may be used to treat metastatic breast cancer in women.

USUAL ADULT DOSAGE: for eunuchism and related disorders, 50 to 400 mg I.M. every 2 to 4 weeks; for breast cancer, 200 to 400 mg I.M. every 2 to 4 weeks.

testosterone enanthate (Android-TLA, Andryl). Another agent used chiefly for its androgenic effects, this form of testosterone is indicated for eunuchism, eunuchoidism, male hormone deficiency after castration, and male climacteric symptoms. It also may be used to treat metastatic breast cancer in women and oligospermia (insufficient sperm in the semen).

USUAL ADULT DOSAGE: for eunuchism and related disorders, 50 to 400 mg I.M. every 4 weeks; for breast cancer, 200 to 400 mg I.M. every 2 to 4 weeks; for oligospermia, 100 to 200 mg I.M. every 4 to 6 weeks.

testosterone propionate (Androlan, Testex). This form of testosterone is used chiefly for its androgenic effects in treating eunuchism, eunuchoidism, male climacteric symptoms, and impotence. It also may be used to treat metastatic breast cancer in women.

USUAL ADULT DOSAGE: for eunuchism and related disorders, 10 to 25 mg I.M. two to four times weekly; for breast cancer, 50 to 100 mg I.M. three times weekly.

ethylestrenol (Maxibolin). Used primarily for its anabolic effects, ethylestrenol can promote weight gain and combat tissue depletion from refractory anemias, corticosteroid therapy, osteoporosis, prolonged immobilization, and various debilitated states. For an adult or child, therapy should not exceed 6 weeks. However, after a 4-week interval, treatment may be repeated.

USUAL ADULT DOSAGE: for weight gain, tissue depletion, and debilitation, 4 to 8 mg P.O. daily, decreased to the lowest effective maintenance dose as soon as the desired response is achieved.

USUAL PEDIATRIC DOSAGE: for weight gain, tissue depletion, and debilitation, 1 to 3 mg P.O. daily, individualized to the patient's needs.

nandrolone decanoate (Deca-Durabolin). Predominantly used as an anabolic agent, nandrolone decanoate is indicated to treat refractory anemia and to build tissue.

USUAL ADULT DOSAGE: for refractory anemia, 50 to 200 mg deep I.M. weekly, preferably in the gluteal muscle; for tissue building, 50 to 100 mg deep I.M. every 3 to 4 weeks.

nandrolone phenpropionate (Durabolin). Also used primarily as an anabolic agent, nandrolone phenpropionate is indicated for control of metastatic breast cancer.
USUAL ADULT DOSAGE: 50 to 100 mg deep I.M. weekly, preferably in the gluteal muscle.

oxandrolone (Anavar). Used primarily for its anabolic effects, oxandrolone is indicated as an adjunct treatment to promote weight gain after extensive surgery, chronic infection, trauma, or other medically related weight loss. It also may be used to relieve bone pain in osteoporosis or to offset catabolism from long-term corticosteroid use.
USUAL ADULT DOSAGE: for weight gain, osteoporosis, or catabolism, 5 to 10 mg P.O. daily, increased, if needed, to 20 mg daily for 2 to 4 weeks.
USUAL PEDIATRIC DOSAGE: for weight gain, osteoporosis, or catabolism, 0.1 to 0.25 mg/kg P.O. daily for 2 to 4 weeks. Continuous therapy should not exceed 3 months.

oxymetholone (Anadrol-50). A predominantly anabolic agent, oxymetholone is used to treat anemias caused by deficient red blood cell production, myelofibrosis, and myelotoxic drugs as well as acquired and congenital aplastic anemias.
USUAL ADULT DOSAGE: 1 to 5 mg/kg P.O. daily.

stanozolol (Winstrol). Primarily used for its anabolic activity, stanozolol can be used to treat hereditary angioedema.
USUAL ADULT DOSAGE: for hereditary angioedema, initially, 2 mg P.O. t.i.d.; maintenance dose, 2 mg daily.

testolactone (Teslac). This predominantly anabolic agent is indicated as an adjunct in treating advanced or disseminated postmenopausal breast cancer.
USUAL ADULT DOSAGE: 250 mg P.O. q.i.d.

Drug interactions
Although testosterone and its salts produce no significant drug interactions, other androgenic and anabolic steroid agents can cause a few. The oral anabolic agents may increase oral anticoagulants' effects, and all anabolic agents may increase the effects of insulin and hypoglycemic agents. These agents also may interact with high-sodium foods, causing sodium and fluid retention.

ADVERSE DRUG REACTIONS

Androgenic and anabolic steroid agents can cause many adverse reactions, ranging from changes in sexual characteristics to life-threatening liver failure.

Predictable reactions
In women, long-term or high-dose use may cause masculinizing reactions, including hoarseness or deepening of the voice, male-pattern hair distribution, menstrual irregularities, acne, increased libido, and clitoral enlargement. Discontinuation of the drug may reverse many of these reactions.

In men, adverse reactions result from the conversion of steroids to female sex hormone metabolites in the body. This commonly causes gynecomastia—especially in adolescent males—and may also produce testicular atrophy, decreased levels of pituitary reproductive hormones, and prostatic hypertrophy. Other adverse reactions may include priapism (persistent erection), increased libido, and oligospermia.

In children, androgenic and anabolic steroid agents may cause premature epiphyseal closure (closure of the growth plate in the body's long bones), thus retarding growth. Prepubertal boys may develop secondary sex characteristics prematurely.

These agents can produce serious toxic effects. In many patients, they elevate liver enzyme levels, causing jaundice. In some patients, peliosis hepatis (blood-filled liver cysts) may occur, leading to liver failure. In others, long-term oral steroid use may cause liver cancer.

Androgenic and anabolic steroids can affect metabolism in several ways. They commonly increase serum cholesterol levels and decrease high-density lipoprotein levels, predisposing the patient to atherosclerotic heart disease. These agents may increase serum calcium to dangerous levels in a patient with metastatic bone disease or parathyroid hormone oversecretion. They may also cause sodium and water retention, leading to edema.

Unpredictable reactions
Androgenic and anabolic steroid agents do not appear to precipitate allergic or other unpredictable reactions.

NURSING IMPLICATIONS

To promote the therapeutic effects and reduce the adverse effects of these agents, the nurse must implement a well-defined teaching plan and understand the following considerations:
• Be aware that androgenic and anabolic steroid agents are contraindicated in pregnant patients, children, in-

(Text continues on page 928.)

Androgenic and anabolic steroid agents

The following chart summarizes the major androgenic and anabolic steroids currently in clinical use.

DRUG	MAJOR INDICATIONS	USUAL ADULT DOSAGES	NURSING IMPLICATIONS
fluoxymesterone	Hypogonadism and impotence caused by testicular deficiency	5 to 20 mg P.O. daily	• Be aware that cholestatic hepatitis and jaundice may occur with relatively low doses of fluoxymesterone.
	Breast cancer in women	10 to 30 mg P.O. daily in divided doses, adjusted to individual's needs and reduced to minimum when effects are noted	• Advise the patient to report androgenic effects, such as voice changes, male-pattern hair distribution, hirsutism, acne, clitoral enlargement, and menstrual irregularities, in women; testicular atrophy and gynecomastia in men; phallic enlargement and facial hair growth in prepubertal boys; and premature epiphyseal closure in children.
	Postpartum breast engorgement	2.5 mg P.O. when active labor begins, followed by 5 to 10 mg P.O. daily for 5 days	• Assess the patient for signs of peliosis hepatis, such as right upper quadrant pain. • Assess the patient for and report any change in serum cholesterol levels. • Observe the geriatric male patient closely for signs of prostatic hypertrophy. • Advise the patient to report anabolic effects, such as weight gain and edema. • Assess the patient's sclera and skin for jaundice. • Monitor the patient's laboratory studies for hepatic function, CBC, fasting blood sugar, and serum electrolytes before and periodically during therapy. • Monitor urine glucose and ketones for a diabetic patient.
testosterone cypionate	Eunuchism, male hormone deficiency after castration, and male climacteric symptoms	50 to 400 mg I.M. every 2 to 4 weeks	• Advise the patient to report androgenic effects, such as voice changes, male-pattern hair distribution, hirsutism, acne, clitoral enlargement, and menstrual irregularities, in women; testicular atrophy and gynecomastia in men; phallic enlargement and facial hair growth in prepubertal boys; and premature epiphyseal closure in children.
	Metastatic breast cancer in women	200 to 400 mg I.M. every 2 to 4 weeks	• Assess the patient for signs of peliosis hepatitis, such as right upper quadrant pain. • Assess the patient for and report any change in serum cholesterol levels. • Observe the geriatric male patient closely for signs of prostatic hypertrophy. • Advise the patient to report anabolic effects, such as weight gain and edema. • Assess the patient's sclera and skin for jaundice. • Monitor the patient's laboratory studies for hepatic function, CBC, fasting blood sugar, and serum electrolytes before and periodically during therapy. • Monitor the patient's urine glucose and ketones for a diabetic patient. • Administer testosterone cypionate in oil only. Avoid giving it with a wet needle or syringe, which could turn the solution cloudy. Be sure to warm or shake the vial to dissolve any crystals.

SELECTED MAJOR DRUGS

Androgenic and anabolic steroid agents continued

DRUG	MAJOR INDICATIONS	USUAL ADULT DOSAGES	NURSING IMPLICATIONS
nandrolone deca-noate	Management of refractory anemia Tissue building	50 to 200 mg deep I.M. weekly 50 to 100 mg deep I.M. every 3 to 4 weeks	• Inject nandrolone decanoate deeply into the gluteal muscle. • Teach the patient to follow a diet to promote weight gain. • Assess the patient for peripheral edema. • Observe for development of masculinizing effects, such as voice changes, male-pattern hair distribution, hirsutism, acne, clitoral enlargement, and menstrual irregularities, in women; phallic enlargement and facial hair growth in prepubertal boys; and premature epiphyseal closure in children. • Advise the patient to report anabolic effects, such as weight gain and edema. • Assess the patient's sclera and skin for jaundice. • Monitor the patient's laboratory studies for hepatic function, CBC, fasting blood sugar, and serum electrolytes before and periodically during therapy. • Monitor the patient's urine glucose and ketones for a diabetic patient.
oxandrolone	Weight gain after medically related weight loss, bone pain in osteoporosis, catabolism from long-term corticosteroid therapy	5 to 10 mg P.O. daily, increased, if needed, to 20 mg daily for 2 to 4 weeks	• Assess the patient's sclera and skin for jaundice. • Observe for development of masculinizing effects, such as voice changes, male-pattern hair distribution, hirsutism, acne, clitoral enlargement, and menstrual irregularities, in women; phallic enlargement and facial hair growth in prepubertal boys; and premature epiphyseal closure in children. • Monitor the patient's laboratory studies for hepatic function, CBC, fasting blood sugar, and serum electrolytes before and periodically during therapy. • Monitor the patient's urine glucose and ketones for a diabetic patient.
stanozolol	Hereditary angioedema	2 mg P.O. t.i.d. initially, decreased to a maintenance dose of 2 mg daily	• Monitor the patient for edema. • Advise the patient to check and record body weight daily. • Assess the patient's sclera and skin for jaundice. • Observe for development of masculinizing effects, such as voice changes, male-pattern hair distribution, hirsutism, acne, clitoral enlargement, and menstrual irregularities, in women; phallic enlargement and facial hair growth in prepubertal boys; and premature epiphyseal closure in children. • Monitor the patient's laboratory studies for hepatic function, CBC, fasting blood sugar, and serum electrolytes before and periodically during therapy. • Monitor the patient's urine glucose and ketones for a diabetic patient.

fants, and men with hormone-dependent cancers such as prostatic or breast cancer. When used in pregnancy, these agents can masculinize the female fetus and cause labial fusion. In infants and children, they may cause premature epiphyseal closure and cessation of long-bone growth. In men with prostatic cancer, they can cause further prostatic hypertrophy.

• Administer androgenic or anabolic steroid agents with caution in a patient with a cardiac, renal, or hepatic disorder. Drug-induced sodium and fluid retention can cause edema, which can worsen these disorders.

• Perform a complete assessment of the patient's physical and nutritional status before therapy. This information will serve as a baseline for determining the drug's therapeutic or adverse effects. Include the patient's blood pressure, pulse rate, and respirations in the physical assessment. Monitor serum protein determinations, which indicate nitrogen and protein balance, as part of the nutritional assessment. Also monitor baseline values for the patient's complete blood count, serum cholesterol and serum calcium levels, and hepatic and cardiac function.

• Prepare the patient for changes in appearance, and encourage expression of concerns or fears about these changes.

• Monitor the patient's fluid intake and output and weigh the patient regularly during dosage determination. Instruct the patient to report to the physician any weight gain of more than 2 lb/week or any signs of edema, such as swelling in the feet or ankles. Expect to administer a diuretic and a low-sodium diet, as prescribed, to alleviate any water retention.

• Advise the female patient to report to her physician any masculinizing effects, such as hoarseness or voice changes, facial hair growth, clitoral enlargement, acne, libido increase, and menstrual irregularities. She should be alert particularly for a libido increase, which may be an early indication of toxicity.

• Reassure the female patient that such effects as facial hair growth and acne should disappear with drug discontinuation. Other effects, such as voice changes caused by structural alterations in the larynx, may be irreversible.

• Advise the male patient to report to his physician any libido increase, priapism, or urinary hesitancy. These reactions may require a dosage reduction or drug discontinuation.

• Advise the prepubertal boy and his family that steroid therapy may cause premature development of secondary sex characteristics, such as facial hair and phallic enlargement. The patient or family should report any of these changes to the physician.

• Assess the patient's sclera and skin for jaundice in natural—not fluorescent or incandescent—light. If jaundice exists, notify the physician.

• Assess the patient for and report other signs of hepatotoxicity, such as nausea, vomiting, an increased prothrombin time, and increased bilirubin, serum glutamic oxaloacetic transaminase, and alkaline phosphatase levels.

• Assess the patient for signs of hypercalcemia, such as muscle weakness, dysrhythmias, and bone pain in a patient with metastatic bone cancer. Monitor the patient's serum calcium levels and administer fluids to decrease the risk of renal calculi, which may develop with hypercalcemia and cause flank pain, fever, and hematuria.

• Help the patient cope with body changes by providing emotional support and a positive attitude. Encourage the patient's family and friends to do the same.

• Teach the patient to take the drug *exactly* as prescribed for the specified duration. Advise the patient not to eliminate any doses or discontinue the drug without consulting the physician.

• Advise the patient receiving parenteral steroid agents to report any irritation at the injection site.

• Tell the patient to store oral steroid agents in a dry, light-resistant, tightly closed container.

• Instruct the patient to carry a Medic Alert card or other drug information source.

• Advise the patient to return as directed for follow-up laboratory tests and physician consultations.

• Help the patient maximize tissue building by establishing a diet that includes calcium, protein, vitamins, adequate calories, and ample fluids.

• Warn the patient not to take androgenic or anabolic steroid agents for bodybuilding or aphrodisiac effects. The risks outweigh the benefits.

CHAPTER SUMMARY

A steroid agent produces a predominantly androgenic, or masculinizing, effect or a predominantly anabolic, or protein-sparing, effect. These agents can be used in males to treat hypogonadism and related disorders, in females to treat breast cancer and related disorders, and in both sexes to stimulate weight gain and tissue and bone development.

Here are the chapter highlights:

• Androgenic and anabolic steroid agents include testosterone—a hormone produced in the testes, ovaries, and adrenal glands—and its chemical derivatives.

• Oral and parenteral steroid agents are well absorbed and distributed throughout the body.

• The duration of action of an androgenic or anabolic steroid depends on its chemical structure.

• Oral steroid agents can cause various hepatic disorders, including jaundice, hepatic carcinoma, and peliosis hepatis.

• The nurse must monitor closely a patient receiving an androgenic or anabolic steroid agent because of adverse reactions ranging from changes in sexual characteristics to liver failure.

BIBLIOGRAPHY

Haupt, H.A., and Rovere, G.D. "Anabolic Steroids: A Review of the Literature," *American Journal of Sports Medicine* 12(6):469-84, 1984.

Lamb, D.R. "Anabolic Steroids in Athletics—How Well Do They Work and How Dangerous Are They?" *American Journal of Sports Medicine* 12(1):31-38, 1984.

Mellion, M.B., "Anabolic Steroids in Athletics," *American Family Physician* 30(1):113-19, 1984.

Murad, F., and Haynes, R.C., Jr. "Anabolic Steroids," in *Goodman and Gilman's The Pharmacological Basis of Therapeutics*, 7th ed. Edited by Gilman, A.G., et al. New York: Macmillan Publishing Co., 1985.

Perlmutter, G., and Lowenthal, D.T. "Use of Anabolic Steroids by Athletes," *American Family Physician* 32(4):208-10, 1985.

CHAPTER 60

ESTROGENS, PROGESTINS, AND ORAL CONTRACEPTIVE AGENTS

OBJECTIVES

After reading and studying this chapter, you should be able to:

1. Describe the major physiologic actions of estrogen and progesterone.

2. Explain the relationship of first-pass metabolism to estrogen and progestin dosages.

3. Describe the therapeutic uses of estrogens and progestins.

4. Identify the major adverse reactions to estrogens, progestins, and oral contraceptives.

5. Describe how oral contraceptives prevent pregnancy.

6. Explain the similarities and differences among the monophasic, biphasic, and triphasic oral contraceptives.

7. Discuss the nursing implications—especially those involving patient education—for the estrogens, progestins, and oral contraceptives.

INTRODUCTION

Estrogens, progestins, and oral contraceptives mimic the physiologic effects of the naturally occurring female sex hormones, the estrogens and progesterone. The naturally occurring estrogens and progesterone serve a vital function in the development of the female reproductive tract and secondary sex characteristics. Also, estrogens and progesterone are responsible for the maturation of the ovum and its development after fertilization. Therapy with estrogens and progestins includes their use as contraceptives and as replacement therapy after menopause.

Hormonal control of the menstrual cycle

A woman's reproductive years are characterized by monthly rhythmic changes in the secretion of estrogens and progesterone. The hypothalamus and pituitary gland control the changing concentrations of these hormones. The gonadotropic hormones—follicle-stimulating hormone (FSH) and luteinizing hormone (LH)—secreted by the anterior pituitary gland stimulate the ovaries to secrete estrogen and progesterone. Elevated concentration levels of estrogen and progesterone produce negative feedback on the hypothalamus and pituitary gland. This leads to reduced concentration levels of FSH and LH, ultimately reducing the ovarian secretion of estrogens and progesterone. (See *The female sex cycle* for an illustration of how the various hormones interrelate.)

Physiology of the menstrual cycle

Menstrual bleeding is caused by desquamation of the endometrium. The first day of menstrual bleeding represents the beginning of the female sex cycle. During the next few days, the concentration levels of FSH and LH rise, stimulating the growth of 6 to 12 follicles within the ovaries. One follicle becomes predominant and begins to secrete large amounts of estrogen, which causes reduction in FSH and LH concentration levels via a negative feedback mechanism. The diminished levels of FSH and LH result in degeneration of the remaining follicles and stimulation of growth of a new endometrial lining. This process, known as the *proliferation phase,* occurs during the 2 weeks after menstruation.

After the proliferation phase and about 2 weeks after onset of menstruation, LH secretion rises sharply, signaling that ovulation is about to occur. At this time, the endometrial glands secrete a thin, stringy mucus, deposited mainly in the region of the cervix, that helps channel sperm into the uterus.

Once ovulation has occurred, the remaining cells of the estrogen-secreting follicle become the *corpus luteum,* which produces large quantities of estrogen, progesterone, and inhibin in the days after ovulation. Under the influence of these hormones, the endometrium undergoes a second developmental process. This is known as the *secretory phase,* when progesterone causes swelling and accumulation of secretory substances in the endometrial lining. These changes allow accumulation of large stores of nutrients and provide appropriate conditions for the implantation of a fertilized ovum.

The female sex cycle

This figure illustrates the interrelationships among hormones involved in the female sex cycle. The first panel shows the changes in follicle-stimulating hormone (FSH) and luteinizing hormone (LH) concentration levels. The second panel displays the cyclic nature of estrogen and progesterone concentration levels. The third panel illustrates the changes in the ovaries and endometrial tissue produced by FSH, LH, estrogens, and progesterone.

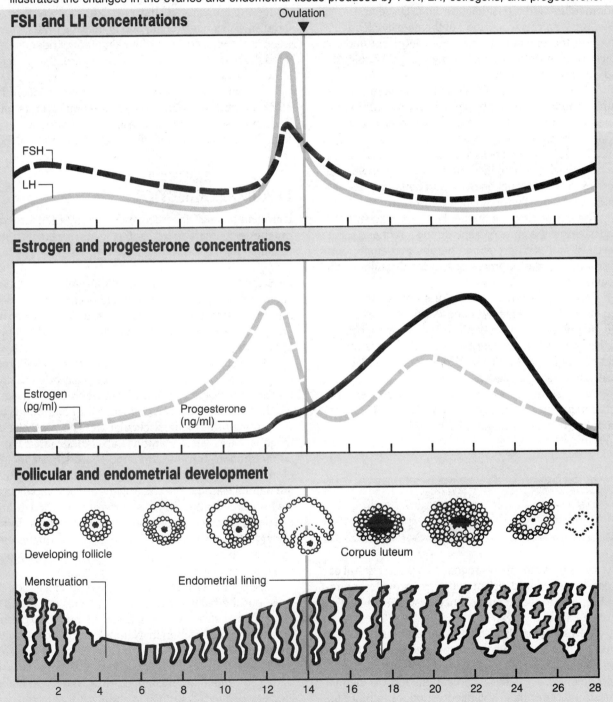

FSH and LH concentrations

Ovulation

FSH

LH

Estrogen and progesterone concentrations

Estrogen
(pg/ml)

Progesterone
(ng/ml)

Follicular and endometrial development

Developing follicle

Corpus luteum

Menstruation

Endometrial lining

2   4   6   8   10   12   14   16   18   20   22   24   26   28

DAYS OF FEMALE SEX CYCLE

The postovulation surge in estrogen and progesterone production causes FSH and LH concentration levels to decline sharply because of the negative feedback effect. The corpus luteum can no longer survive unless implantation of the fertilized ovum occurs. Degeneration of the corpus luteum results in sharply decreased estrogen and progesterone concentration levels, causing desquamation of the superficial layers of the endometrium and menstrual bleeding. These hormonal decreases also cause cessation of the negative feedback effect on the pituitary, thereby allowing FSH and LH levels to increase and initiate a new cycle of follicular and endometrial growth.

If implantation occurs, the fertilized ovum secretes human chorionic gonadotropin, which prevents the degeneration of the corpus luteum and thus promotes the continued secretion of estrogens and progesterone. The corpus luteum continues its secretory action until about the 12th week of pregnancy. At that point, the placenta secretes sufficient quantities of estrogens and progesterone to sustain the pregnancy on its own.

The elevated concentration levels of estrogens and progesterone that are present during pregnancy suppress LH and FSH secretion, thereby preventing ovulation and the development of follicles throughout the pregnancy.

This chapter covers the natural and synthetic estrogens, used to correct estrogen-deficient states and to prevent pregnancy; the natural and synthetic progestins, used to restore or regulate the menstrual cycle and to treat premenstrual syndrome (PMS); and the oral contraceptives, used to prevent pregnancy.

For a summary of representative drugs, see *Selected major drugs: Estrogens, progestins, and oral contraceptive agents* on pages 947 and 948.

ESTROGENS

Physicians prescribe the estrogens to replace natural estrogen in estrogen-deficient states, to provide contraception, and to treat certain cancers, such as breast or prostate cancer.

The estrogens discussed in this section include the natural products (estradiol, estrone, and conjugated estrogenic substances) as well as the synthetic estrogens (chlorotrianisene, dienestrol, diethylstilbestrol, diethylstilbestrol diphosphate, esterified estrogens, ethinyl estradiol, estradiol cypionate and valerate, and quinestrol).

History and source

In 1900, Knauer and Halban described hormonal control of the female reproductive system and demonstrated that the ovaries are vital to normal female sexual development and function. In 1926, Loewe and Lange isolated a female sex hormone from the urine of menstruating women and showed that its concentration varied with the phase of the menstrual cycle. Also in 1926, Zondek demonstrated that pregnant women excreted large amounts of estrogen, and in the late 1920s, chemists Butenandt and Doisy (working independently) isolated the active hormone. Soon afterward, the chemical structure of estrogen was determined.

Commercially prepared estrogen first appeared in 1935. Since then, pharmaceutical manufacturers have developed several synthetic estrogen compounds in efforts to improve the effectiveness of the natural hormone.

PHARMACOKINETICS

Estrogens are well absorbed and are distributed throughout the body. Metabolized in the liver, they are excreted primarily by the kidneys.

Absorption, distribution, metabolism, excretion

After oral administration, naturally occurring estrogens and their derivatives are rapidly and well absorbed, but first-pass metabolism limits their potency by shortening their duration of action.

After absorption from the gastrointestinal (GI) tract, naturally occurring estrogens that are orally administered travel via the portal vein to the liver, where large amounts are then rapidly metabolized to inactive compounds before entering the general circulation. The synthetic estrogens are also rapidly absorbed after oral administration, but they undergo less first-pass metabolism. As a result, they provide greater oral potency than the natural estrogens do. Estrogens are also rapidly and well absorbed after administration via the skin (transdermally) or mucous membranes; because they do not undergo first-pass metabolism, estrogens administered by these routes reach higher levels in the body than orally administered preparations do.

Estrogens are distributed throughout most body tissues, but the highest concentration levels are found in fat deposits. Estrogens are 50% to 80% bound to plasma proteins, primarily albumin. Naturally occuring estrogens are primarily metabolized in the liver. Most of an orally administered dose is inactivated via first-pass metabolism. The remaining unchanged drug and the metabolites are converted further in the liver to more water-soluble compounds.

Researchers have not fully determined the metabolic fate of the synthetic estrogens, but it appears to resemble that of the naturally occurring estrogens.

Estrogens and their metabolites are excreted primarily in urine, with small amounts excreted in feces.

Onset, peak, duration

Estrogens exert their pharmacologic effects via protein synthesis at the cellular level. The time required for this process varies greatly among the preparations available.

Although estrogens reach peak plasma concentration levels within hours of administration, their onset of action may not occur for days, weeks, or even months after initiation of therapy. Their duration of action is also unrelated to their plasma concentration levels: their plasma half-life is much shorter than their biological half-life.

PHARMACODYNAMICS

The estrogens primarily promote the growth and development of the female reproductive system. At puberty, estrogen secretion by the ovaries increases about twentyfold, precipitating several major physiologic events—the female sex organs increase in size and become functional, the endometrium undergoes proliferation and becomes glandular in nature, and the vaginal epithelium becomes secretory. Furthermore, estrogen-induced metabolic changes result in the development of secondary female sex characteristics and cause increased fat deposition in the subcutaneous tissues. Estrogen also increases skeletal osteoblastic activity, causing a growth spurt as the woman reaches her reproductive years. After a few years, however, estrogen-stimulated fusion of the epiphysis and the shafts of the long bones halts further growth. For this reason, women rarely reach the height of men.

As discussed in the introduction to this chapter, estrogen is responsible for the reepithelialization and proliferation of the endometrium before the ovulation phase of each female sex cycle. The highly secretory endometrium contains large amounts of nutrients to support growth of a fertilized ovum. At the end of the female sex cycle, estrogen and progesterone secretion declines, resulting in the abrupt breakdown of endometrial tissue and menstrual bleeding.

Mechanism of action

The exact mechanism of action of estrogen is not well understood but is believed to involve cytoplasmic receptor proteins found in estrogen-responsive tissues in the female breast and genitourinary tract. After estrogen binds to these cytoplasmic receptors, the resulting estrogen-receptor complex is transported into the nu-

Mechanism of action of estrogens and progestins

This figure illustrates how estrogens and progestins exert their pharmacologic effects. The hormone (H) passes through the cell membrane and into the cell cytoplasm, where it binds with a cytoplasmic receptor (R). The resulting hormone-receptor (H-R) complex is transported through the cytoplasm and into the cell nucleus, where it stimulates DNA to produce messenger RNA (mRNA). The mRNA contains the genetic coding for the production of specific proteins responsible for structural and functional changes in the cell; these changes produce the physiologic effects of the hormone.

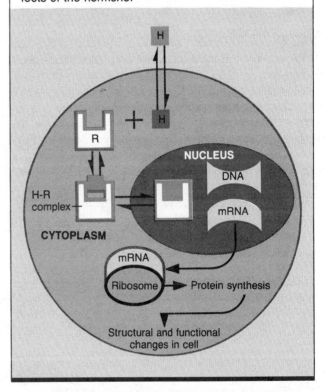

cleus. This action stimulates the synthesis of messenger ribonucleic acid (mRNA) and deoxyribonucleic acid (DNA), which in turn promotes the synthesis of specific proteins responsible for the actions of the estrogens. (See *Mechanism of action of estrogens and progestins* for a schematic representation.)

PHARMACOTHERAPEUTICS

Physicians prescribe estrogens primarily for hormonal replacement therapy in postmenopausal women for the relief of symptoms caused by loss of ovarian function.

Specific postmenopausal indications include the relief of vasomotor symptoms (so-called hot flashes) and urogenital atrophy as well as the prevention of osteoporosis. Estrogens are also used, less frequently, for hormonal replacement therapy in patients with primary ovarian failure or female hypogonadism and in patients who have undergone surgical castration. Estrogens are also used to prevent postpartum breast engorgement in women who are not breast-feeding and palliatively to treat advanced, inoperable breast cancer in postmenopausal women and prostate cancer in men. (See Chapter 76, Hormonal Antineoplastic Agents, for additional information about the use of estrogens in cancer patients.)

Estrogen therapy has been linked with increased risk of endometrial cancer, thromboembolism, hypertension, and other, less serious, adverse reactions. Adding progestin to estrogen therapy may reduce the risk of some of these reactions, particularly endometrial cancer. Because some data suggest an association between estrogen therapy and breast cancer, estrogenic agents are not recommended for women at high risk for breast cancer.

Estrogens are administered most commonly in a cyclic manner during 3 out of 4 weeks of a calendar month; however, this method can cause confusion because therapy may start or end on a different day each month. As an alternative method, the patient may take the drug for the first 25 days of the month, not take the drug for the remaining 5 to 6 days, then resume the therapy. This regimen may prove easier to follow because it starts on the first day of the calendar month and always ends on the 25th day. If a progestin is added, it is administered during the last 10 days of each 25-day cycle. (See *Estrogen regimens* for illustrations.)

Because orally administered estrogens undergo first-pass metabolism, they are more frequently associated with adverse reactions involving the liver, such as alterations in hepatic lipid metabolism thought to be responsible for thromboembolic diseases. To avoid first-pass metabolism, a transdermal delivery system for estradiol (Estraderm) has been developed.

chlorotrianisene (TACE). A synthetic estrogen, chlorotrianisene is administered orally or I.M. to relieve vasomotor symptoms of menopause and to treat atrophic vaginitis, female hypogonadism, and postpartum breast engorgement.
USUAL ADULT DOSAGE: for menopausal symptoms, 12 to 25 mg P.O. daily in 21-day cycles; for atrophic vaginitis, 12 to 25 mg P.O. daily for 30 to 60 days; for female hypogonadism, 12 to 25 mg P.O. for 21 days, followed by one dose of 100 mg I.M. progesterone or 5 to 10 mg/day medroxyprogesterone during the last 5 days of therapy; for postpartum breast engorgement, 72

Estrogen regimens

The first panel illustrates the traditional estrogen regimen: 3 weeks of therapy followed by 1 drug-free week. In the example, the second cycle starts on the 29th and ends on the 18th of the next month. The second panel illustrates an alternative 25-day regimen. Because this regimen starts on the first day and ends on the 25th day of each month, it is easier for the patient to follow month by month. In either regimen, progestin can be co-administered during the last 10 days of the cycle as a precaution against endometrial cancer.

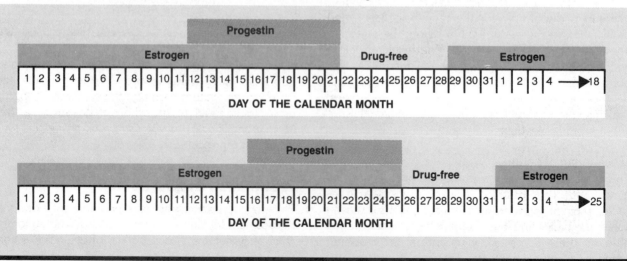

DRUG INTERACTIONS

Estrogens

Clinically significant drug interactions involving the estrogens are relatively minor; most result in decreased therapeutic activity of the estrogen.

DRUG	INTERACTING DRUGS	POSSIBLE EFFECTS	NURSING IMPLICATIONS
chlorotrianisene, conjugated estrogenic substances, dienestrol, diethylstilbestrol, esterified estrogens, estradiol, estrone, ethinyl estradiol, quinestrol	rifampin, barbiturates, carbamazepine, phenytoin, primidone	Decrease estrogen activity by increasing hepatic metabolism of estrogen	• Adjust the estrogen dosage as prescribed. • Monitor the patient for loss of therapeutic effect and possible return of symptoms.
	bishydroxycoumarin	Decrease anticoagulant effect	• Increase the anticoagulant dosage as prescribed. • Monitor the patient for signs of clotting, such as calf pain, edema, and tenderness. • Monitor the patient's prothrombin time.

mg P.O. b.i.d. for 2 days, 50 mg every 6 hours for six doses, or 12 mg q.i.d. for 7 days, starting within 8 hours after delivery.

dienestrol (DV Cream, Ortho Dienestrol). A synthetic estrogen cream, dienestrol is administered vaginally to treat atrophic vaginitis and kraurosis vulvae (atrophy of the female external genitalia).
USUAL ADULT DOSAGE: for atrophic vaginitis or kraurosis vulvae, 1 to 2 applications daily for 2 weeks, then half-doses for 2 weeks.

diethylstilbestrol [DES] and **diethylstilbestrol diphosphate** (Stilphostrol). Administered orally or by vaginal suppository, these synthetic estrogens are used to relieve vasomotor symptoms of menopause and to treat atrophic vaginitis, kraurosis vulvae, female hypogonadism, surgical castration, primary ovarian failure, and postpartum breast engorgement. They are also used as a postcoital contraceptive.
USUAL ADULT DOSAGE: for atrophic vaginitis or kraurosis vulvae, 0.1 to 1 mg by vaginal suppository daily for 10 to 14 days, or up to 5 mg/week by vaginal suppository; for female hypogonadism, surgical castration, or primary ovarian failure, 0.2 to 0.5 mg P.O. daily; for menopausal symptoms, 0.1 to 2 mg P.O. daily in 21-day cycles; for postcoital contraception ("morning-after" pill), 25 mg P.O. b.i.d. for 5 days, starting within 72 hours after coitus; for postpartum breast engorgement, 5 mg P.O. daily or t.i.d., up to 30 mg.

esterified estrogens (Estratab, Estratest, Menest). These naturally occurring estrogen esters, administered orally, are used to relieve postmenopausal symptoms and to treat female hypogonadism, surgical castration, and primary ovarian failure.
USUAL ADULT DOSAGE: for female hypogonadism, surgical castration, or primary ovarian failure, 2.5 mg P.O. daily to t.i.d. in 21-day cycles; for menopausal symptoms, 0.3 to 1.25 mg P.O. in 21-day cycles.

estradiol (Estrace, Estrace Vaginal Cream), **estradiol transdermal system** (Estraderm), **estradiol cypionate** (Depo-Estradiol Cypionate, Dura-Estrin, Estroject-LA), and **estradiol valerate** (Delestrogen, Duragen, Estradiol L.A., Valergen). Administered orally, I.M., or transdermally, these natural (estradiol) and synthetic estrogens are used to relieve vasomotor symptoms of menopause and to treat atrophic vaginitis, kraurosis vulvae, female hypogonadism, surgical castration, primary ovarian failure, and postpartum breast engorgement.
USUAL ADULT DOSAGE: for atrophic vaginitis or kraurosis vulvae, 2 to 4 grams estradiol vaginal cream daily for 1 to 2 weeks with a maintenance dose of 1 gram one to three times weekly, or 1 to 2 mg estradiol P.O. daily in 21-day cycles; for female hypogonadism, surgical castration, primary ovarian failure, or menopausal symptoms, 1 to 2 mg estradiol P.O. daily in 21-day cycles, 1 to 5 mg estradiol cypionate I.M. monthly, 5 to 20 mg estradiol valerate I.M. every 4 weeks, or 0.05 to 0.1 mg/day estradiol transdermal patch twice weekly in 21-day cycles; for postpartum breast engorgement, 10 to 25 mg estradiol valerate I.M. at the end of the first stage of labor.

estrogenic substances, conjugated (Estrocon, Premarin). Administered orally, I.M., or I.V., these naturally occurring estrogenic substances are used to relieve vasomotor symptoms of menopause and to treat atrophic vaginitis, kraurosis vulvae, female hypogonadism, surgical castration, primary ovarian failure, postpartum breast engorgement, osteoporosis, and abnormal uterine bleeding from hormonal imbalance.

USUAL ADULT DOSAGE: for atrophic vaginitis or kraurosis vulvae, 0.3 to 1.25 mg P.O. daily or 2 to 4 grams vaginal cream daily in 21-day cycles; for female hypogonadism, 2.5 mg P.O. b.i.d. or t.i.d. for 20 consecutive days each month; for surgical castration or primary ovarian failure, 1.25 mg P.O. daily in 21-day cycles; for menopausal symptoms, 0.3 to 1.25 mg P.O. daily in 21-day cycles; for postpartum breast engorgement, 3.75 mg P.O. every 4 hours for five doses or 1.25 mg P.O. every 4 hours for 5 days; for osteoporosis, 0.625 mg P.O. daily in 21-day cycles; for abnormal uterine bleeding caused by hormonal imbalance, 25 mg I.V. or I.M., repeated in 6 to 12 hours, as ordered.

estrone (Bestrone, Kestrone-5, Theelin). A naturally occurring estrogen, estrone is administered I.M. to relieve menopausal symptoms and to treat atrophic vaginitis, kraurosis vulvae, female hypogonadism, and primary ovarian failure.

USUAL ADULT DOSAGE: for menopausal symptoms, atrophic vaginitis, and kraurosis vulvae, 0.1 to 0.5 mg I.M. two or three times weekly; for female hypogonadism and primary ovarian failure, 0.1 to 2 mg I.M. weekly.

ethinyl estradiol (Estinyl, Feminone). A synthetic estrogen administered orally, ethinyl estradiol is used to relieve menopausal symptoms and to treat female hypogonadism.

USUAL ADULT DOSAGE: for menopausal symptoms, 0.02 to 0.05 mg P.O. daily in 21-day cycles; for female hypogonadism, 0.05 mg P.O. daily to t.i.d. for 2 weeks per month, followed by 2 weeks of progesterone therapy, continued for 3 to 6 monthly cycles, followed by 2 months off therapy.

quinestrol (Estrovis). A long-acting synthetic estrogen, quinestrol is used to relieve menopausal symptoms and to treat female hypogonadism, primary ovarian failure, atrophic vaginitis, and kraurosis vulvae.

USUAL ADULT DOSAGE: for all indications, 100 mcg/day for 7 days, then no drug for 7 days, after which a maintenance dose of 100 mcg/week is begun; the dosage may be increased to 200 mcg/week.

Drug interactions

Relatively few interactions occur involving the estrogens and other drugs; those that do occur generally result in decreased estrogenic activity and are not significant. (See *Drug interactions: Estrogens* on page 935 for the significant interactions between estrogens and other drugs.) No significant interactions occur between the estrogens and food.

ADVERSE DRUG REACTIONS

Most of the adverse reactions associated with estrogen replacement therapy are mild and do not have serious long-term consequences. However, endometrial cancer and possibly breast cancer may be more likely to occur in women taking estrogens. Most of the risk appears to be dose-related, so that taking higher doses over longer periods of time increases the risk.

Predictable reactions

The risk of endometrial cancer increases fourfold to eightfold in women taking estrogens. However, mortality in this group does not seem to increase, probably because of the closer monitoring of patients on estrogen therapy and the less aggressive nature of these estrogen-induced cancers. An increased risk of breast cancer associated with low-dose estrogen replacement therapy has not been definitely determined. Evidence exists that progestin therapy (medroxyprogesterone 5 to 10 mg/day) added to the last 5 to 10 days of an estrogen therapy cycle reduces the risk of developing endometrial cancer, and may reduce the risk of developing breast cancer.

The increased risk of thromboembolic disorders associated with oral contraceptive use has not been clearly linked to estrogen replacement therapy in postmenopausal women. However, the nurse should closely monitor such patients for thromboembolic disorders, which may occur.

The incidence of gallbladder disease increases with the use of estrogens. Increased blood pressure may also occur; although such increases are usually minor and reversible, some women may develop hypertension.

Metabolic adverse reactions may include decreased glucose tolerance, altered thyroid function test results, increased serum lipoprotein levels, fluid retention, decreased dietary folic acid absorption, cholestatic jaundice, and alterations in liver function test results.

Genitourinary adverse reactions may include breakthrough bleeding, spotting, altered menstrual flow, dysmenorrhea, amenorrhea, and increased risk of vaginal candidiasis. Central nervous system (CNS) adverse reactions may include mental depression, migraine headaches, dizziness, and altered libido. Changed corneal curvature may cause contact lens intolerance. Adverse reactions involving the skin include melasma and acne. Breast tenderness, enlargement, and secretions can also occur.

Estrogen patient-teaching tips

The nurse should advise the patient to read the patient package insert before starting estrogen therapy. This insert provides information about the adverse reactions of estrogens and explains what precautions the patient should take while on estrogen therapy. The patient should know the drug name, dosage, and schedule. The following material will help answer the patient's questions.

Why is this estrogen being prescribed?
● Estrogens are hormones produced by the body. When these naturally occurring hormones are deficient, synthetic estrogens are used in women to relieve unpleasant menopausal symptoms and medical problems (hot flashes, sweating, and brittle bones). Estrogens are also prescribed to treat some forms of cancer, including breast cancer and, in men, prostate cancer.

How should the estrogen be used?
● Estrogens are available in tablets, which should be swallowed whole.
● Estrogens also are available as vaginal creams or as suppositories to be inserted into the vagina. The physician, nurse, or pharmacist should explain to the patient exactly how to insert these products. The patient may want to use a sanitary napkin to avoid soiling clothing.
● Estrogens also are available as patches to be stuck on the skin like adhesive tape.
● Some estrogens are injected into muscle.

What special instructions should the patient receive about using an estrogen?
● The patient should report suspected or confirmed pregnancy to the physician immediately.
● The patient should keep all appointments for checkups so that the physician can check for any

problems that may occur while the patient is taking estrogen.
● The patient should inform the physician of the estrogen therapy before any type of laboratory test is performed.

How should estrogen be stored?
● The drug should be stored in its original container.
● The patient should keep this and all other medications out of the reach of children.

What should the patient do if she forgets to take a dose?
● The patient should take the dose as soon as she discovers the oversight, but should not take two doses at the same time to make up for a missed dose.

What can the patient do about adverse reactions?
● The patient can eat a light snack to help relieve nausea, which should disappear after the estrogen has been taken for a while. However, the patient should inform her physician if nausea continues.
● The patient should not worry about breast tenderness or fullness, which is harmless.
● The patient should inform the physician about ankle puffiness or swelling and any weight gain, leg cramps, vaginal bleeding or discharge, or pain or tenderness in the groin or calf.

Unpredictable reactions

Urticaria, skin rash, and very rare hypersensitivity reactions may occur.

NURSING IMPLICATIONS

The estrogens are associated with a number of contraindications, precautions, and adverse reactions. To ensure the safe use of these drugs, the nurse should be aware of the following considerations and pay particular attention to patient education. (See *Estrogen patient-teaching tips* for additional important nursing implications.)
● Do not administer estrogens to patients with known or suspected pregnancy or to patients with thrombophlebitis or other thromboembolic disorders, undiagnosed abnormal genital bleeding, or estrogen-

dependent cancer of the breast or reproductive organs, except when the drugs are being used as palliative therapy for advanced, inoperable cancer in men or postmenopausal women.
● Administer estrogens cautiously in patients with conditions that may be aggravated by fluid retention—such as asthma, hypertension, congestive heart failure, migraine, and renal or hepatic insufficiency—and in patients with mental depression, metabolic bone disease, blood dyscrasias, gallbladder disease, seizure disorders, diabetes mellitus, amenorrhea, or a family history (involving mother, grandmother, or sister) of breast or genital cancer.
● Take a complete pretreatment medical history and perform a physical examination before the start of estrogen therapy and every 6 to 12 months thereafter.

Pay special attention to examinations or tests involving the patient's blood pressure, breasts, abdomen, pelvic organs, and hepatic function as well as to Papanicolaou (Pap) tests.

• Be aware that estrogens may interfere with the following diagnostic or laboratory tests: metapyrone test, norepinephrine-induced platelet aggregation, sulfobromophthalein, some thyroid function tests, prothrombin time (PT), serum folate levels, serum triglyceride levels, phospholipid levels, and liver function tests. When any relevant specimen is submitted, inform the pathologist that the patient is receiving estrogen.

• Because some I.M. products are dispersed in natural oils (sesame, peanut, or castor oil), ask the patient about related hypersensitivities before administration.

• Roll the vial between the palms to mix the contents completely.

• Administer I.M. injections deeply into large muscles.

• Instruct the patient to report any abdominal pain or mass, severe headache, slurred speech, vomiting, dizziness or faintness, weakness or numbness, calf pain, heaviness in the chest, shortness of breath, blurred vision or blind spots, vaginal bleeding or discharge, breast lumps, swelling of hands or feet, yellow skin and sclera, dark urine, or light-colored stools.

• Inform sexually active women of childbearing age to use effective means of contraception because estrogens (especially diethylstilbestrol) are associated with congenital fetal malformations.

• Inform the patient that estrogens are secreted into breast milk and, therefore, should not be used by lactating women.

• Inform the male patient that long-term estrogen therapy can lead to gynecomastia or impotence but that these conditions will resolve when therapy is discontinued.

• Be aware that diabetic patients may require adjustment of their antidiabetic (hypoglycemic) medication.

• Inform the patient that problems with fitting hard or rigid gas-permeable contact lenses may occur because of corneal curvature changes.

• Explain to the patient on cyclic therapy for postmenopausal symptoms that withdrawal bleeding may occur but does not indicate that fertility has been restored.

• Teach female patients breast self-examination.

• Advise the patient to read the patient package insert. Also, provide verbal explanation and reinforcement of the information.

PROGESTINS

Progestins have pharmacologic properties similar to those of the natural female sex hormone progesterone, which acts primarily to prepare the endometrium for pregnancy and the breasts for lactation. Progestins are used to regulate or restore the menstrual cycle and to treat endometrial or renal cancer, endometriosis, and PMS. In combination with estrogens, progestins are also used as oral contraceptives.

Progesterone is the major naturally occurring hormone in this drug category, but it has limited potency (a short duration of action) when administered orally because it undergoes rapid and extensive first-pass metabolism in the liver. To overcome this disadvantage, researchers have developed several synthetic progestins that remain active when administered orally. Of these, medroxyprogesterone acetate, norethindrone, and norethindrone acetate are most frequently used. Hydroxyprogesterone caproate is a synthetic agent that is administered I.M.

History and source

In the 1920s, Corner and Allen first isolated progesterone from the corpora lutea of sows. However, further research into the functions of progesterone was hampered by the small amounts available and by its short duration of action. By the 1950s, however, longer-acting synthetic hormones were being produced in quantities sufficient to allow their use in clinical settings.

PHARMACOKINETICS

Progestins are well absorbed and distributed throughout the body. After metabolism in the liver, they are excreted primarily by the kidneys.

Absorption, distribution, metabolism, excretion

Naturally occurring and synthetic progestins are rapidly and well absorbed when administered orally; however, they have limited potency because first-pass metabolism shortens their duration of action. Naturally occurring progestins are, therefore, most active when administered parenterally. Like naturally occurring progesterone, orally administered synthetic progestins also undergo first-pass metabolism, but not as extensively as the naturally occurring agents do. Progestins are rapidly and well absorbed through the skin and mucous membranes.

Progestins are 80% to 95% bound to the plasma proteins albumin and sex hormone–binding globulin; small amounts are stored in body fat.

Progestins are primarily metabolized in the liver. Most of an orally administered dose is inactivated via first-pass metabolism. The remaining unchanged drug and the metabolites are converted further in the liver to more water-soluble compounds.

Progestins and their metabolites are excreted primarily in urine, with small amounts excreted in feces.

Onset, peak, duration

Like estrogens, progestins exert their pharmacologic effects via protein synthesis at the cellular level. Although these drugs reach peak plasma concentration levels within hours of administration, their onset of action may not occur for days or weeks after initiation of therapy. Their duration of action is also unrelated to their plasma concentration levels. Their plasma half-life is much shorter than their biological half-life.

PHARMACODYNAMICS

Progesterone is often termed the *pregnancy hormone* because it functions primarily to prepare the uterus to receive and nourish the fertilized ovum. Under the influence of progesterone, the endometrium swells and becomes highly secretory. Progesterone also decreases the frequency of uterine muscle contractions, thereby preventing expulsion of the implanted ovum, and stimulates the secretory cells of the breast (the alveoli). Finally, the cyclic withdrawal of progesterone toward the end of the menstrual cycle leads to breakdown of the endometrium, beginning menstruation.

Mechanism of action

At the cellular level, progestins act on receptor proteins in cellular cytoplasm. The resulting progesterone-receptor complex is transported into the cell nucleus, where the synthesis of mRNA is stimulated. Under the direction of mRNA, the cell produces various proteins that are responsible for the pharmacologic effects of the progestins.

PHARMACOTHERAPEUTICS

Natural progesterone and its synthetic derivatives are used to treat ovarian disorders. The primary clinical indications for progestin therapy are amenorrhea and abnormal uterine bleeding caused by hormonal imbalance. These conditions are characterized by an absent or abnormal menstrual flow, so the goal of therapy is to restore a regular menstrual cycle. This goal is accomplished by administering both estrogens and progestins in a cyclic pattern that resembles the natural secretion pattern of estrogen and progesterone.

Continuous progestin therapy is used to treat endometriosis by preventing menstruation for several months, thereby relieving the symptoms and promoting the regression of the ectopic endometrial growths.

Singly and in combination with estrogens, progestins also are frequently used as oral contraceptives. (See the section "Oral Contraceptives" later in this chapter for a complete discussion of this use.) They also are used, less frequently, to treat PMS and to provide palliative therapy for advanced metastatic endometrial and renal cancer. (See Chapter 76, Hormonal Antineoplastic Agents, for information about the use of progestins in cancer patients.)

Despite their therapeutic value, progestins have some disadvantages. For example, when they are used for prolonged periods, such as for endometriosis, ovulation may not resume for several months after discontinuation of therapy. Also, use of progestins should be avoided during pregnancy because the drugs can lead to congenital fetal defects.

hydroxyprogesterone caproate (Delalutin, Duralutin). A synthetic progestin administered I.M., hydroxyprogesterone is used to treat amenorrhea and abnormal uterine bleeding caused by hormonal imbalance. Hydroxyprogesterone has a long duration of action (7 to 14 days).
USUAL ADULT DOSAGE: for amenorrhea or abnormal uterine bleeding, 375 mg I.M. every 4 weeks if needed, not to extend beyond four cycles.

medroxyprogesterone acetate (Amen, Curretab, Depo-Provera, Provera). A synthetic preparation administered orally or I.M., medroxyprogesterone is used to treat amenorrhea and abnormal uterine bleeding caused by hormonal imbalance. The injectable form, Depo-Provera, has a long duration of action and is recommended only for cancer treatment.
USUAL ADULT DOSAGE: for amenorrhea or abnormal uterine bleeding, 5 to 10 mg P.O. daily for 5 to 10 days beginning on the 16th day of the menstrual cycle; if the patient has received estrogen previously, 10 mg P.O. daily for 10 days beginning on the 16th day of the menstrual cycle.

norethindrone (Norlutin). An orally active synthetic agent, norethindrone is used to treat amenorrhea, abnormal uterine bleeding caused by hormonal imbalance, and endometriosis.
USUAL ADULT DOSAGE: for amenorrhea or abnormal uterine bleeding, 5 to 20 mg P.O. daily from the 5th through the 25th day of the menstrual cycle; for en-

dometriosis, initially, 10 mg P.O. daily for 14 days, then increased by 5 mg/day at 14-day intervals up to a total of 30 mg/day.

norethindrone acetate (Aygestin, Norlutate). Twice as potent as norethindrone, this oral synthetic agent is used to treat amenorrhea, abnormal uterine bleeding caused by hormonal imbalance, and endometriosis.
USUAL ADULT DOSAGE: for amenorrhea or abnormal uterine bleeding, 2.5 to 10 mg P.O. daily from the 5th through the 25th day of the menstrual cycle; for endometriosis, initially, 5 mg P.O. daily for 14 days, then increased by 2.5 mg/day at 14-day intervals up to a total of 15 mg/day.

progesterone (Femotrone, Profac-O, Progelan, Progest-50, Progestaject-50). This natural progestin preparation, administered I.M. or by vaginal or rectal suppository, is used to treat amenorrhea, abnormal uterine bleeding from hormonal imbalance, and PMS.
USUAL ADULT DOSAGE: for amenorrhea, 5 to 10 mg I.M. daily for 6 to 8 days starting 8 to 10 days before the anticipated start of menstruation; for abnormal uterine bleeding, 5 to 10 mg I.M. daily for 6 days, or as a single 50- to 100-mg I.M. dose; for PMS, 200- to 400-mg suppository once or twice a day, administered vaginally or rectally.

Drug interactions
No clinically significant interactions between progestins and other drugs or food have been reported.

ADVERSE DRUG REACTIONS

The progestins produce several minor predictable adverse reactions, such as changes in vaginal bleeding patterns; breast tenderness; and edema. Unpredictable hypersensitivity reactions are rare but may occur.

Predictable reactions
Breakthrough bleeding, spotting, changes in menstrual flow, and amenorrhea are the most common adverse reactions to the progestins. Cervical erosions or abnormal secretions, uterine fibromas, vaginal candidiasis, edema, weight gain or loss, mental depression, cholestatic jaundice, and melasma may also occur. Occasional adverse CNS reactions include migraine headaches, dizziness, nervousness, insomnia, and fatigue. Rare reactions include breast tenderness and galactorrhea.

Progestins and estrogens used in combination as oral contraceptives have been associated with an increased risk of thrombophlebitis, pulmonary embolism, and cerebral embolism. Because these disorders also may occur in patients receiving progestins alone, the nurse should monitor all patients receiving these agents for signs and symptoms of these disorders.

Unpredictable reactions
Hypersensitivity reactions, including urticaria, pruritus, angioedema, and generalized skin rash (with or without pruritus) have occurred. Anaphylaxis is rare.

NURSING IMPLICATIONS

A number of contraindications, precautions, and patient-teaching requirements are associated with use of the progestins. To ensure safe and proper use of progestins, the nurse should be aware of the following considerations. (See *Progestin patient-teaching tips* for additional implications.)
• Be aware that the use of progestins is contraindicated in patients with the following conditions: thrombophlebitis, thromboembolism, pregnancy or suspected pregnancy, breast cancer or cancer of the female reproductive organs (except in a patient selected for palliative therapy), hepatic disease or dysfunction, undiagnosed abnormal vaginal bleeding, or missed abortion. Use of progestins is also contraindicated as a pregnancy test.
• Administer progestins cautiously to patients with conditions that may be aggravated by fluid retention (for example, asthma, cardiac or renal insufficiency, seizure disorders, or migraine headaches) and to patients with mental depression or diabetes mellitus.
• Be aware that progestins may interfere with the following diagnostic or laboratory tests: urine pregnanediol determination, serum alkaline phosphatase levels, plasma amino acid levels, and urinary nitrogen levels. When relevant specimens are submitted, inform the pathologist that the patient is receiving progestins.
• Expect to adjust the dosage of antidiabetic medication for a patient who is also receiving a progestin.
• Because I.M. solutions are dispersed in natural oils (sesame, castor, or peanut oil), ask the patient about related hypersensitivities before administration.
• Roll the vial between the palms to mix its contents.
• Administer an I.M. injection deeply in a large muscle.
• Teach the patient to report any signs of thromboembolic disorders, including pain in the chest, groin, or calf; headache or changes in vision; shortness of breath; or slurred speech.
• Advise sexually active women of childbearing age to use effective contraception because progestins may cause congenital fetal defects.
• Advise lactating women not to use progestins because the drugs are secreted in breast milk.

Progestin patient-teaching tips

The nurse should see that the patient receives and reads the patient package insert, which provides information about the adverse reactions of progestins and explains what precautions to take while on progestin therapy. The patient should know the drug name, dosage, and schedule. The following material will help answer the patient's questions.

Why is this progestin being prescribed?
• Progestins are hormones produced by the body. They are used in women to regulate the menstrual cycle and to treat endometriosis and selected cases of breast and kidney cancer.

How should the progestins be used?
• Some progestins are taken in tablet form; others are injected into muscle.

What special instructions should the patient receive while using a progestin?
• The patient should stop taking the drug and inform the physician immediately if pregnancy is suspected or confirmed.
• The patient should keep all appointments for checkups so that the physician can check for any problems that may occur during progestin therapy.
• The patient should inform the physician of the progestin therapy before any type of laboratory test is performed.

How should progestin be stored?
• The drug should be stored in its original container.
• The patient should keep this and all other medications out of the reach of children.

What should the patient do if she forgets to take a dose?
• The patient should take the dose as soon as she discovers the oversight, but should not take two doses at the same time to make up for a missed dose.

What can the patient do about adverse reactions?
• The patient can eat a light snack to help relieve nausea.
• The patient should expect breast tenderness or fullness, which is harmless.
• The patient should inform the physician about ankle puffiness or swelling and any weight gain, leg cramps, vaginal bleeding or discharge, or pain or tenderness in the groin or calf.

• Explain to the patient that routine follow-up examinations should be performed every 6 to 12 months with special attention given to breast and pelvic organs, the Pap test, and liver function tests.
• Teach female patients breast self-examination.
• Advise the patient to read the patient package insert. Also, provide verbal explanation and reinforcement of the information.

ORAL CONTRACEPTIVES

The oral contraceptives were the first drugs developed for use in healthy individuals. They are used not to cure disease, but to prevent a condition that arises from normal physiologic events. Most contraceptive agents are combinations of estrogens and progestins, but a few contain only progestin.

History and source
Rock, Pincus, and Garcia, in the 1950s, were the first to study the effects of progestin on ovulation. Their studies demonstrated that ovulation could be suppressed for as long as desired by the cyclic ingestion of daily doses of progestins.

Oral contraceptives first became commercially available in the United States in the early 1960s. These early oral contraceptives were combination products containing 50 to 150 mcg of estrogen and 1 to 10 mg of progestin in each tablet. Other contraceptive agents soon became available that required two types of tablets to be taken in sequence. They were removed from the market in 1976 because of their low efficacy and suspected association with endometrial cancer.

The currently available contraceptive agents are combination products containing 50 mcg or less of estrogen and 1 mg or less of progestin. The few progestin-only preparations are known as *minipills*.

PHARMACOKINETICS

The pharmacokinetic profiles of the oral contraceptives are the same as those described in the sections on estrogens and progestins in this chapter.

Absorption, distribution, metabolism, excretion
Oral contraceptives are well absorbed and are distributed throughout the body. Metabolized in the liver, they are excreted primarily by the kidneys.

Only two estrogens, ethinyl estradiol and mestranol, are used currently in oral contraceptives. Ethinyl estradiol, regarded as the more potent of the two agents, is used in nearly all of the low-dose preparations. Mestranol, found primarily in the high-dose products, is metabolized to ethinyl estradiol in the liver. Among the progestins used in the various oral contraceptives, norethynodrel, ethynodiol diacetate, and norethindrone acetate are metabolized to norethindrone by the liver.

Onset, peak, duration

The onset of action of the oral contraceptives is somewhat delayed because of their mechanisms of action. Full contraceptive benefits are not experienced until the contraceptive agents have been taken for at least 10 days. As a result, women starting contraceptive therapy should use back-up means of contraception, such as condoms, a diaphragm, or spermicidal foam, during the first month.

Oral contraceptives remain effective throughout the 21-day cycle. When the woman has taken all of the tablets properly, the contraceptive efficacy extends through the 7-day contraceptive-free period each month. If doses are missed immediately before or after the contraceptive-free period, however, the likelihood of breakthrough ovulation and contraceptive failure is great; this is especially true for low-dose products containing estrogen and progestin.

Ovulation usually resumes within three to six menstrual cycles after discontinuation of oral contraceptives. Women are advised to wait to become pregnant until three menstrual cycles have passed after the discontinuation of oral contraceptives, because the endometrium may require as long as 3 months to regain its normal physiology.

PHARMACODYNAMICS

Estrogens and progesterone are endogenous substances that are responsible for ovulation and the nurturing of the fertilized ovum after implantation. Exogenously administered estrogens and progestins can promote changes in the female reproductive organs that help prevent fertilization and implantation even if ovulation occurs.

Mechanism of action

Estrogens act as contraceptives by suppressing ovulation and inhibiting implantation of the fertilized ovum. Oral contraceptives create negative feedback upon the hypothalamus and pituitary gland, reducing FSH and LH concentration levels. The diminished FSH concentration level prevents follicle development, and the absence of the midcycle surge of LH prevents ovulation. Although estrogens are 95% to 98% effective in inhibiting ovulation, the chance of ovulation increases when doses are missed and when low doses of estrogen are used.

Estrogens can interfere with implantation of the fertilized ovum by altering ovum transport and by inhibiting the normal secretory development of the endometrium. Alteration of ovum transport can cause the fertilized ovum to be delivered to the uterus at a time improper for implantation; inhibited secretory development of the endometrium can result in unfavorable conditions for implantation. Interference with ovum implantation is the main mechanism of action of the estrogen only postcoital contraceptives.

Progestins also inhibit ovulation via the negative feedback mechanism, making combinations of estrogen and progestin nearly 100% effective. However, noncompliance and low doses of progestin reduce the efficacy of these products.

Besides inhibiting ovulation, pharmacologically increased concentrations of progestin occurring during the first half of the female sex cycle promote changes in the endometrium that make it unsuitable for ovum implantation. Progestins also thicken cervical mucus, blocking sperm migration toward the ovum. Finally, progestins can slow ovum transport through the fallopian tubes; this may be why women taking the minipill have a higher incidence of tubal and ectopic pregnancies.

PHARMACOTHERAPEUTICS

Oral contraceptives are used primarily to prevent pregnancy and are the most effective form of reversible contraception available. With proper administration, the theoretical failure rate is less than one pregnancy per 100 women per year. Higher failure rates occur with irregular use, missed doses, and estrogen doses less than 20 mcg.

Oral contraceptives containing high doses of estrogen and progestin may be used to treat hypermenorrhea and endometriosis and to promote cyclic withdrawal bleeding. Progestin-dominant oral contraceptives (those providing mainly progestin effects) are sometimes used to treat dysmenorrhea. Because most of the severe adverse reactions associated with oral contraceptives are dose-related, the trend is toward use of lower-dose contraceptives.

Several types of combination oral contraceptives are available; most are monophasic, providing fixed doses of estrogen and progestin throughout the 21-day

DRUG INTERACTIONS

Oral contraceptives

This table summarizes the major interactions that can occur between the oral contraceptives and other drugs.

DRUG	INTERACTING DRUGS	POSSIBLE EFFECTS	NURSING IMPLICATIONS
all combination oral contraceptives, especially the low-dose monophasic and the biphasic and triphasic products	barbiturates, carbamazepine, phenylbutazone, phenytoin, primidone, rifampin	May cause rapid metabolism of oral contraceptives, leading to breakthrough bleeding and decreased contraceptive efficacy	• Advise the patient to use an alternative method of contraception if therapy with known enzyme-inducers is necessary.
	ampicillin, chloramphenicol, neomycin, penicillin V, nitrofurantoin, sulfonamides, tetracycline	May alter GI bacterial flora, leading to decreased contraceptive efficacy and breakthrough bleeding	• Advise the patient to use an alternative means of contraception for the duration of anti-infective therapy and for 1 week after discontinuation of the anti-infective agent.
	benzodiazepines	Decrease oxidative metabolism of some benzodiazepines (chlordiazepoxide, diazepam) and increase glucuronide conjugation of others (lorazepam, oxazepam)	• Monitor the patient for enhanced therapeutic effects of oxidatively metabolized benzodiazepines (alprazolam, chlordiazepoxide, clorazepate, diazepam, flurazepam, halazepam, and prazepam). • If the patient requires higher doses of a benzodiazepine eliminated via glucuronide conjugation (lorazepam, oxazepam, and temazepam), administer as ordered.
	beta-adrenergic blocking agents	May decrease metabolism of the beta-adrenergic blocking agent	• Monitor the patient for signs of increased effects of the beta-adrenergic blocking agent.
	corticosteroids	Enhance anti-inflammatory actions of corticosteroids	• Observe the patient for signs of excessive corticosteroid effects. • Alterations in corticosteroid dosage may be necessary when oral contraceptives are started or discontinued; alter the dosage as ordered.

cycle. One biphasic product delivers a constant amount of estrogen throughout the 21-day cycle but an increased amount of progestin for the last 11 days. The newest oral contraceptives are triphasic formulations. Two of these provide fixed doses of estrogen throughout the 21-day cycle, with progestin doses varying every 7 days, and the others are tablets that vary both the estrogen and progestin doses every 7 days throughout the 21-day cycle.

ethinyl estradiol/ethynodiol diacetate (Demulen 1/35-21, Demulen 1/50-21, Demulen 1/50-28). This monophasic oral contraceptive provides relatively well-balanced estrogen and progestin effects.
USUAL ADULT DOSAGE: for contraception with the 21-day products, one tablet P.O. daily, followed by 7 days without a dose before beginning the next cycle of tablets; for contraception with the 28-day product, one tablet P.O. daily.

ethinyl estradiol/levonorgestrel (Levlen, Nordette, Tri-Levlen, Triphasil). Levlen and Nordette are monophasic oral contraceptives with slightly progestin-dominant formulations. Tri-Levlen and Triphasil are triphasic products that provide relatively well-balanced estrogen and progestin activity throughout the 21-day cycle.
USUAL ADULT DOSAGE: for contraception with the 21-day products, one tablet P.O. daily, followed by 7 days without a dose before beginning the next cycle of tablets; for contraception with the 28-day products, one tablet P.O. daily.

ethinyl estradiol/norethindrone (Brevicon, Genora 1/35, Modicon, Norinyl 1+35, Ortho-Novum 1/35, Ortho-Novum 7/7/7, Ortho-Novum 10/11, Ovcon-35, Ovcon-50, Tri-Norinyl). Ovcon, Brevicon, and Modicon are slightly estrogen-dominant monophasic oral contraceptives. Genora, Norinyl, and Ortho-Novum 1/35 are also monophasic preparations, but they provide relatively well-balanced estrogen and progestin effects. A biphasic formulation, Ortho-Novum 10/11, provides estrogen-dominant effects during days 1 to 10, then relatively well-balanced estrogen and progestin effects during days 11 to 21 of the 21-day cycle. Ortho-Novum 7/7/7 and Tri-Norinyl are triphasic oral contraceptives that provide relatively well-balanced estrogen and progestin effects during the 21-day cycle; both products are slightly estrogen-dominant during days 1 to 7 and slightly progestin-dominant during days 15 to 21.

USUAL ADULT DOSAGE: for contraception with the 21-day products, one tablet P.O. daily, followed by 7 days without a dose before beginning the next cycle of tablets; for contraception with the 28-day products, one tablet P.O. daily.

ethinyl estradiol/norethindrone acetate (Loestrin 1/20, Loestrin 1.5/30, Loestrin Fe 1/20, Loestrin Fe 21 1.5/30, Norlestrin 1/50, Norlestrin 2.5/50, Norlestrin Fe 1/50, Norlestrin Fe 2.5/50). These oral contraceptives are monophasic formulations. Loestrin products are progestin-dominant; Norlestrin products provide relatively well-balanced estrogen and progestin effects.

USUAL ADULT DOSAGE: for contraception with the 21-day products, one tablet P.O. daily, followed by 7 days without a dose before beginning the next cycle of tablets; for contraception with the 28-day products, 1 tablet P.O. daily.

ethinyl estradiol/norgestrel (Lo/Ovral, Ovral). These monophasic oral contraceptives include Ovral, a progestin-dominant formulation, which is also used for postcoital contraception. Lo/Ovral provides relatively well-balanced estrogen and progestin effects.

USUAL ADULT DOSAGE: for contraception with the 21-day products, one tablet P.O. daily, followed by 7 days without a dose before beginning the next cycle of tablets; for contraception with the 28-day products, one tablet P.O. daily; for postcoital contraception, two tablets P.O. within 24 to 72 hours of unprotected intercourse and two more tablets 12 hours later.

mestranol/ethynodiol diacetate (Ovulen). A high-dose monophasic oral contraceptive, Ovulen provides relatively well-balanced estrogen and progestin effects.

USUAL ADULT DOSAGE: for contraception with the 21-day product, one tablet P.O. daily, followed by 7 days without a dose before beginning the next cycle of tablets; for contraception with the 28-day product, one tablet P.O. daily.

mestranol/norethindrone (Genora 1/50, Norinyl 1+50, Norinyl 1+80, Norinyl 2 mg, Ortho-Novum 1/50, Ortho-Novum 1/80, Ortho-Novum 2 mg). Norinyl 2 mg and Ortho-Novum 2 mg are monophasic progestin-dominant oral contraceptives also used to treat hypermenorrhea. Genora 1/50, Norinyl 1+50, and Ortho-Novum 1/50 provide relatively well-balanced estrogen and progestin effects. Norinyl 1+80 and Ortho-Novum 1/80 are estrogen-dominant products.

USUAL ADULT DOSAGE: for contraception with the 21-day products, one tablet P.O. daily, followed by 7 days without a dose before beginning the next cycle of tablets; for contraception with the 28-day products, 1 tablet P.O. daily; for hypermenorrhea, a 3-month course of therapy with Norinyl 2 mg, one tablet P.O. daily for 20 days, followed by 8 days without a dose before beginning the next cycle of tablets; or a 3-month course of therapy with Ortho-Novum 2 mg, one tablet P.O. daily for 21 days, followed by 7 days without a dose before beginning the next cycle of tablets.

mestranol/norethynodrel (Enovid, Enovid-E). These products are estrogen-dominant monophasic formulations. Enovid-E is used as a contraceptive, and Enovid is used to treat endometriosis and hypermenorrhea.

USUAL ADULT DOSAGE: for contraception with Enovid-E, one tablet P.O. daily, followed by 7 days without a dose before beginning the next cycle of tablets; for severe hypermenorrhea, 20 to 30 mg of Enovid P.O. daily until bleeding is controlled, then 10 mg P.O. daily through day 24 of the cycle; for endometriosis, 5 or 10 mg of Enovid P.O. daily for 14 days, increased by 5 or 10 mg every 14 days until a total daily dose of 20 mg is achieved, then 20 mg/day continuously for 6 to 9 months.

norethindrone (Micronor, Nor-Q.D.). This is a noncyclic, progestin-only oral contraceptive.

USUAL ADULT DOSAGE: one tablet P.O. every day on a continuous basis.

norgestrel (Ovrette). This is a noncyclic, progestin-only oral contraceptive.

USUAL ADULT DOSAGE: one tablet P.O. every day on a continuous basis.

Drug interactions

Relatively few interactions occur between oral contraceptives and other drugs; however, those few interactions are clinically significant. No interactions between oral contraceptives and food have been documented. (See *Drug interactions: Oral contraceptives* on page 943 for details.)

Oral contraceptives: Summary of adverse reactions

This table summarizes the adverse reactions of oral contraceptives that are related to excessive or deficient amounts of estrogen and progestin.

Estrogen excess

General effects
- Nausea and vomiting
- Dizziness
- Cyclic headaches
- Irritability and bloating
- Edema and fluid retention
- Cyclic weight gain
- Altered fit of contact lenses

Reproductive effects
- Breast tenderness and cystic changes
- Uterine enlargement
- Leukorrhea
- Hypermenorrhea
- Suppression of lactation

Estrogen deficiency

General effects
- Spotting and breakthrough bleeding on days 1 through 7
- Amenorrhea or decreased menstrual flow

Menopause-like effects
- Irritability
- Nervousness
- Mental depression
- Decreased libido
- Hot flashes and other vasomotor symptoms
- Atrophic vaginitis
- Dyspareunia

Progestin excess

General effects
- Noncyclic weight gain and increased appetite
- Fatigue and weakness
- Decreased menstrual flow
- Monilial vaginitis

Androgenic effects
- Oily skin and scalp
- Acne
- Hirsutism
- Mental depression

Pill-free day effects
- Nausea and vomiting
- Dizziness
- Cyclic headaches
- Edema and bloating
- Cyclic weight gain
- Breast tenderness

Progestin deficiency

General effects
- Breakthrough bleeding on days 8 through 21
- Heavy menstrual flow and clotting
- Delayed withdrawal bleeding
- Weight loss

ADVERSE DRUG REACTIONS

The oral contraceptives can produce various adverse reactions: some can be severe; others may be only annoying.

Predictable reactions
Many of the common adverse reactions are related to the estrogen content of oral contraceptives. The reactions tend to be most pronounced during the first cycle of oral contraceptive therapy and usually abate after three or four cycles.

The most common adverse reaction is nausea. Other GI reactions can include vomiting, abdominal cramping, diarrhea, and constipation.

Melasma is the most common dermatologic adverse reaction: facial hyperpigmentation may develop 1 month to 2 years after the initiation of oral contraceptive therapy, fades very slowly, and may be permanent. Paradoxically, acne may improve or develop: estrogen-dominant products tend to improve it; progestin-dominant products tend to cause or worsen it.

Serious cardiovascular reactions can accompany oral contraceptive use. The incidence of hypertension in women using oral contraceptives is about two to three times that of nonusers; researchers have not determined whether estrogen or progestin is primarily responsible. Women taking oral contraceptives also are at greater risk for developing myocardial infarction (MI)—a risk that increases with age; duration of oral contraceptive use; and, especially, cigarette smoking.

Oral contraceptives are also associated with an increased risk of thromboembolic disorders because of their estrogen and progestin content. (The lower-dose formulations used today, however, are less likely to cause thromboembolic disorders than the original formulations.) The risk of developing cerebrovascular accidents and subarachnoid hemorrhage, also increased in patients taking oral contraceptives, is further increased if the patient smokes or has hypertension.

Endocrine and metabolic adverse reactions can occur. Decreased glucose tolerance appears to be related primarily to estrogen, but progestin may also be in-

---

Oral contraceptive patient-teaching tips

The nurse should see that the patient receives and reads the patient package insert before starting oral contraceptive therapy. This insert provides information about adverse reactions of oral contraceptives and explains what precautions to take while using them. The patient should know the drug name, dosage, and schedule. The following information will help answer the patient's questions.

Why is this oral contraceptive being prescribed?
• Oral contraceptives (birth control pills) contain two female sex hormones that prevent the release of an egg from the ovaries each month, thus preventing pregnancy. Oral contraceptives, the most effective method of birth control, can almost completely prevent unplanned pregnancy if taken correctly.

How should the oral contraceptive be used?
• Oral contraceptives are pills that should be swallowed whole.
• The patient should use an alternative method of contraception (condom, spermicides, or diaphragm) for the first cycle (3 weeks) to ensure full protection.
• Oral contraceptives come in packs containing either 21 or 28 pills. In the 28-pill pack, the last seven pills are colored differently and are inactive. The patient should expect her period to begin while taking these last seven pills. If the patient is using the 21-pill pack, her period should begin a few days after taking the last pill in the pack.
• The physician will tell the patient how to start the first cycle. One way is to start taking the pills on the 5th day of menstrual bleeding. The other way is to take the first pill on the first Sunday after the patient's period begins. If her period begins on Sunday, she should take the first pill on that day.
• The pills must be taken exactly on schedule to ensure effectiveness. The patient should take the pill at the same time each day— for example, at bedtime or with breakfast.

What special instructions should the patient follow when using an oral contraceptive?
• The patient should stop taking the pills and contact the physician if pregnancy is suspected or confirmed.
• The patient should keep all appointments for checkups so that the physician can check for any problems that may occur.

What can the patient do about adverse reactions?
• Although spotting or bleeding may occur during the first two cycles of birth control pills, the patient should report to the physician any spotting or bleeding that persists after the second cycle. Mild reactions, including nausea, weight gain, breast tenderness, and skin blotching, are not unusual. They should not cause alarm.
• Severe adverse reactions, such as blood clots, rarely occur but can produce pain in the chest, arms, or legs; numbness; dizziness; headaches; or vision changes. If any of these symptoms appear, the patient should contact the physician immediately.

How should oral contraceptives be stored?
• The oral contraceptives should be stored in their original container.
• The patient should keep this and all other medications out of the reach of children.

What should the patient do if she forgets to take a dose?
• If the patient misses one pill, she should take it as soon as she remembers. (If she does not remember it until the next day, the patient should take two pills— the one she forgot and the one scheduled for that day.)
• If the patient misses two pills in a row, she should take two pills daily for the next 2 days and use an alternative method of contraception during the rest of the cycle.
• If the patient misses three or more pills in a row, she should not take any more pills from that cycle and should discard the pack. She should use an alternative method of contraception until her period begins, then start a new pack on the regular schedule.

SELECTED MAJOR DRUGS

Estrogens, progestins, and oral contraceptive agents

This chart summarizes the major estrogens, progestins, and oral contraceptives currently in clinical use.

DRUG	MAJOR INDICATIONS	USUAL ADULT DOSAGES	NURSING IMPLICATIONS
Estrogens			
conjugated estrogenic substances	Atrophic vaginitis or kraurosis vulvae	0.3 to 1.25 mg P.O. daily or 2 to 4 grams vaginal cream daily in 21-day cycles	• Conjugated estrogenic substances are contraindicated in patients with known or suspected pregnancy, thrombophlebitis or thromboembolic disorders, estrogen-dependent cancer of the breast or reproductive organs (except when used as palliative therapy for inoperable cancer in postmenopausal women), and undiagnosed abnormal uterine bleeding.
	Female hypogonadism	2.5 mg P.O. b.i.d. or t.i.d. for 20 consecutive days each month	
	Surgical castration or primary ovarian failure	1.25 mg P.O. daily in 21-day cycles	• Administer these agents cautiously to patients with conditions that may be aggravated by fluid retention or to patients with mental depression, metabolic bone disease, blood dyscrasias, gallbladder disease, seizure disorders, diabetes mellitus, amenorrhea, or a family history of breast or genital cancer.
	Menopausal symptoms	0.3 to 1.25 mg P.O. daily in 21-day cycles	
	Postpartum breast engorgement	3.75 mg P.O. every 4 hours for five doses or 1.25 mg P.O. every 4 hours for 5 days	• Monitor the patient for any signs of blood clotting and for vaginal bleeding or discharge, breast lumps, edema of hands or feet, yellow skin or sclera, dark urine, or light-colored stools.
	Osteoporosis	0.625 mg P.O. daily in 21-day cycles	• I.M. or I.V. administration is preferred for rapid treatment of abnormal uterine bleeding or reduction in surgical bleeding.
	Abnormal uterine bleeding caused by hormonal imbalance	25 mg I.V. or I.M., repeated in 6 to 12 hours as ordered	
Progestin			
medroxyprogesterone acetate	Amenorrhea or abnormal uterine bleeding from hormonal imbalance	5 to 10 mg P.O. daily for 5 to 10 days beginning on 16th day of menstrual cycle; if the patient has received estrogen, 10 mg P.O. daily for 10 days beginning on 16th day of cycle	• This drug is contraindicated in patients with thromboembolic disorders, thrombophlebitis, known or suspected pregnancy, cancer of the breast or reproductive organs (except in selected patients for palliative therapy), hepatic disease or dysfunction, undiagnosed abnormal uterine bleeding, and missed abortion. The drug is also contraindicated as a test for pregnancy.
			• Monitor the patient for signs of blood clotting and for changes in vaginal bleeding pattern, mental depression, yellow sclera, jaundice, or dark-colored stools.
Oral contraceptives			
estrogen-progestin combination products	Contraception	*21-tablet therapy:* one tablet P.O. at the same time each day for 21 days beginning on the 5th day of the menstrual cycle; after 7 days, the patient should begin a new pill pack	• These combination products are contraindicated in patients with known or suspected pregnancy, thrombophlebitis or thromboembolic disorders, estrogen-dependent cancer of the breast or reproductive organs (except when used as palliative therapy in postmenopausal women), and undiagnosed abnormal uterine bleeding.
		28-tablet therapy: one active tablet P.O. at the same time each day for	• Administer these products cautiously to patients with conditions that may be aggravated by fluid retention or to patients with mental de-

continued

Estrogens, progestins, and oral contraceptive agents continued

DRUG	MAJOR INDICATIONS	USUAL ADULT DOSAGES	NURSING IMPLICATIONS
estrogen-progestin combination products (continued)		21 days beginning on the 5th day of the menstrual cycle, then one inactive tablet P.O. daily for 7 days; when all 28 tablets have been taken, the patient should start a new pill pack *28-tablet therapy:* Sunday-start products, one active tablet P.O. daily for 21 days beginning on the first Sunday of the menstrual cycle, then one inactive tablet P.O. daily for 7 days; when all 28 tablets have been taken, the patient should start a new pill pack	pression, metabolic bone disease, blood dyscrasias, gallbladder disease, seizure disorders, diabetes mellitus, amenorrhea, or a family history of breast or genital cancer. • Monitor the patient for signs of blood clotting and for uterine bleeding or discharge, breast lumps, edema of hands or feet, yellow skin and sclera, dark urine, or light-colored stools. • Be aware that these products should be discontinued at least 1 week before surgery. • Advise the patient of the increased risks associated with smoking while on oral contraceptive therapy. • Advise the patient to use an alternative means of contraception during the first cycle of oral contraceptive therapy. • Stress the importance of semiannual Pap tests and blood pressure checks and annual gynecologic examinations to the patient taking oral contraceptives.

volved. Estrogens can increase the concentration levels of high-density lipoprotein cholesterol; progestins can decrease it. Thus, the overall effect of an oral contraceptive on cholesterol levels depends on whether it is estrogen- or progestin-dominant. Oral contraceptive use also may lead to folate deficiency.

Oral contraceptives can affect several serum proteins produced by the liver, elevate thyroxine-binding globulin concentration levels, and variously affect albumin and immunoglobulin concentration levels. Users of oral contraceptives also have an increased incidence of liver tumors, primarily benign hepatic adenomas, and gallbladder disease.

Recent epidemiologic studies indicate that oral contraceptives may not be as carcinogenic as was once believed. For example, none of the currently available oral contraceptives increases the risk of endometrial cancer; however, these formulations may increase the risk of cervical cancer. Recent studies have found no association between oral contraceptive use and breast cancer.

Various genitourinary adverse reactions may occur, depending on the estrogen or progestin dominance of oral contraceptives. (See *Oral contraceptives: Summary of adverse reactions* on page 945 for a summary of hormone-related effects.)

Dizziness, headache, mental depression, lethargy, decreased libido, fluid retention, and edema also are associated with oral contraceptive use. Oral contraceptives also may worsen myopia and astigmatism and may alter the fit of rigid contact lenses.

Unpredictable reactions

Some users of oral contraceptives have experienced hypersensitivity reactions including skin rashes, urticaria, and pruritus.

NURSING IMPLICATIONS

Use of oral contraceptives is associated with numerous contraindications and precautions. Also, patient teaching plays an important role in ensuring patient compliance and product effectiveness. The nurse should be aware of the following considerations. (See *Oral contraceptive patient-teaching tips* on page 946 for additional implications.)

• Oral contraceptives are contraindicated in lactating patients and in those with thromboembolic disorders, cerebrovascular or coronary artery disease, MI, known or suspected cancer of the breast or reproductive organs, benign or cancerous liver tumors, undiagnosed or abnormal vaginal bleeding, and known or suspected pregnancy. Oral contraceptives also are contraindicated in adolescents with incomplete epiphyseal closure, in women age 35 or older who smoke more than 15 cigarettes per day, and in all women over age 40.

- Oral contraceptives should be used cautiously in patients with systemic lupus erythematosus, hypertension, mental depression, migraine, epilepsy, asthma, diabetes mellitus, renal disease, gallbladder disease, amenorrhea, scanty or irregular periods, fibrocystic breast disease, or a family history (involving mother, grandmother, or sister) of breast disease or genital cancer. Instruct the patient to report any worsening of the medical conditions listed to her physician.
- Inform the patient of the importance of semiannual Pap tests and blood pressure checks and annual gynecologic examinations.
- Teach female patients breast self-examination.
- Advise patients who smoke to stop; explain the increased risks of smoking while using oral contraceptives.
- Instruct the patient to weigh herself at least twice a week and to report any sudden weight gain or swelling to her physician.
- Advise the patient of alternate methods of contraception before surgery to decrease the risk of thromboembolism.
- Advise the patient to avoid exposure to ultraviolet light and prolonged exposure to sunlight.
- Instruct the patient to report the following symptoms to the physician immediately: abdominal pain, chest pain, headache, eye problems, or severe leg pain. Also instruct the patient to report any undiagnosed vaginal bleeding or discharge, two consecutive missed menstrual periods, lumps in the breast, and swelling of the hands or feet.
- Advise the patient to take the oral contraceptive pills at the same time every day. A regular schedule is especially important for the low-dose products. Explain that if headache or nausea occurs, taking the dose at bedtime may reduce its severity.
- Explain to the patient that oral contraceptives must be taken on a daily basis to be effective. Check that the patient understands the sequence to follow in taking the pills.
- Instruct the patient beginning oral contraceptive therapy to use an additional form of birth control for the first oral contraceptive cycle.
- Explain to the patient that if she misses one dose, she should either take the missed dose as soon as she remembers it or take two pills the next day. She should then resume her usual daily dosage. Also explain that if she misses two doses, she should take two pills for the next 2 days, then resume her usual daily dosage and use a backup means of contraception for the rest of the cycle. Finally, explain that if the patient misses three doses, she should discard the pill pack, wait 4 days, then start a new pack. Be sure the patient understands that missing doses immediately before or immediately after the 7-day pill-free period greatly increases the risk of pregnancy.
- Explain to the patient that if she misses one menstrual period after having taken all the pills on time, she should start her next cycle of pills at the regularly scheduled time. However, if she misses one menstrual period and has not taken all the pills on time, or if she misses two consecutive menstrual periods even though she has taken all the pills on time, she should stop taking the pills and have a pregnancy test. Explain to the patient that progestins and estrogens can cause birth defects if taken early in pregnancy.
- Explain to the patient that nausea, headache, dizziness, breast tenderness, spotting, and breakthrough bleeding are common adverse reactions that usually resolve after three to six oral contraceptive cycles. If breakthrough bleeding does not resolve, a dosage adjustment may be necessary.
- Explain to the patient that achieving pregnancy may be difficult for a short time after oral contraceptives are discontinued. Advise her to wait 3 months before trying to become pregnant, using an alternative means of contraception in the interim, because the endometrium may take up to 3 months to return to normal.

CHAPTER SUMMARY

Chapter 60 covered the estrogens, progestins, and oral contraceptives as they are used to regulate the function of the female reproductive tract, relieve menopausal and postmenopausal symptoms, treat diseases of female reproductive organs, and prevent pregnancy. Here are the highlights of the chapter:

- Estrogens and progesterone are hormones that play a vital role in the development of the female reproductive tract and secondary sex characteristics. These hormones also are responsible for the maturation of the ovum and its development after fertilization. Both estrogen and progesterone are necessary for development of the endometrial lining during the female sex cycle and for the maintenance of pregnancy.
- Many orally administered estrogens and progestins undergo first-pass metabolism. After absorption from the GI tract, these agents are transported via the portal vein to the liver, where large amounts of both agents are

rapidly metabolized to inactive compounds before entering the general circulation. To achieve therapeutic effects, oral doses of these estrogens and progestins must be much higher than parenterally administered doses, which do not undergo first-pass metabolism.

• Physicians prescribe estrogens primarily for hormonal replacement therapy in postmenopausal women. These agents are also used as contraceptives, either alone or in combination with progestins.

• Progestins are used to treat abnormal menstrual flow, endometriosis, PMS, and advanced metastatic endometrial or renal cancer. They also are used as contraceptives, either alone or in combination with estrogens.

• Therapy with estrogens, progestins, and oral contraceptives is associated with a number of adverse reactions. The most severe involve the cardiovascular system and include hypertension, stroke, thromboembolism, and MI. Women who smoke while on oral contraceptive therapy have a greatly increased risk of developing cardiovascular adverse reactions. Research has shown that the risk of cervical cancer also increases with oral contraceptive use.

• Oral contraceptives act primarily by inhibiting ovulation. Large doses of estrogenic oral contraceptives (the so-called morning-after pills) interfere with implantation of the fertilized ovum. Progestins act by preventing sperm migration toward the ovum and creating a hostile environment within the uterus that is unsuitable for ovum implantation even if fertilization occurs.

• Oral contraceptives also are used to treat hypermenorrhea, endometriosis, and dysmenorrhea and to promote cyclic withdrawal bleeding.

• Most currently available oral contraceptives contain estrogen and progestin. The monophasic preparations provide fixed doses of both hormones throughout the 21-day cycle. The biphasic preparations deliver a constant amount of estrogen throughout the 21-day cycle but an increased amount of progestin during the last 11 days. The progestin dose in triphasic preparations varies every 7 days; the estrogen dose may remain fixed throughout the 21-day cycle or may also vary every 7 days.

BIBLIOGRAPHY

American Hospital Formulary Service. *Drug Information 87.* McEvoy, G.K., et al., eds. Bethesda, Md.: American Society of Hospital Pharmacists, 1987.

American Society of Hospital Pharmacists. *Medication Teaching Manual: A Guide for Patient Counseling,* 3rd ed. Bethesda, Md.: American Society of Hospital Pharmacists, 1983.

Gilman, A.G., et al., eds. *Goodman and Gilman's The Pharmacological Basis of Therapeutics,* 7th ed. New York: Macmillan Publishing Co., 1985.

Guyton, A.G. *Textbook of Medical Physiology,* 7th ed. Philadelphia: W.B. Saunders Co., 1986.

Hansten, P.D. *Drug Interactions: Clinical Significance of Drug-Drug Interactions,* 5th ed. Philadelphia: Lea & Febiger, 1985.

Huppert, L.C. "Hormonal Replacement Therapy: Benefits, Risks, Doses," *Medical Clinics of North America* 71:23, 1987.

Judd, H.L., et al. "Estrogen Replacement Therapy: Indications and Complications," *Annals of Internal Medicine* 98:195, 1983.

Kastrup, E.K., et al., eds. *Facts and Comparisons.* St. Louis: Facts and Comparisons Division, J.B. Lippincott Co., 1987.

Katcher, B.S., et al. *Applied Therapeutics: The Clinical Use of Drugs,* 3rd ed. Spokane, Wash.: Applied Therapeutics Inc., 1983.

Miller, L.G. "Update on the New Triphasic Oral Contraceptives," *Clinical Pharmacy* 4:24, September/October 1985.

Nursing88 Drug Handbook. Springhouse, Pa.: Springhouse Corp., 1988.

Petersdorf, R.G., et al, eds. *Harrison's Principles of Internal Medicine,* 10th ed. New York: McGraw-Hill Book Co., 1983.

Smith, M.A., and Youngkin, E.Q. "Current Perspectives on Combination Oral Contraceptives," *Clinical Pharmacy* 3:485, January/February 1984.

United States Pharmacopeial Convention (USPDI). *Drug Information for the Health Care Provider,* vol. 1, 7th ed. Rockville, Md.: United States Pharmacopeial Convention Inc., 1987.

FERTILITY AGENTS

OBJECTIVES

After reading and studying this chapter, you should be able to:

1. Discuss the causes of infertility.

2. Describe the hormonal physiology of ovulation and spermatogenesis.

3. Discuss the clinical indications for the various fertility agents.

4. Identify the target organs of the various fertility agents.

5. Discuss the contraindications and adverse reactions associated with fertility agents.

6. Discuss the nursing implications for fertility agents, especially those involving patient education.

INTRODUCTION

For a couple to be fertile, the male and female must produce several different hormones in the proper sequence, in the right amounts, and at the appropriate time. The combined actions of the central nervous system; the hypothalamus, pituitary, thyroid, and adrenal glands; and the ovaries and testes enable conception to occur and the fetus to grow and develop properly. (See *Hormonal physiology of ovulation* on page 952 and *Hormonal physiology of spermatogenesis* on page 953 for details and illustrations.)

For pregnancy to occur, the female must be capable of ovulation; her fallopian tubes must be free of obstruction; her uterine lining must accept the fertilized ovum; and the quantity and quality of her cervical mucus must be adequate for sperm motility. The male must produce sufficient numbers of normal sperm, and the sperm must possess sufficient progressive motility and ability to penetrate and fertilize the egg.

Fertility agents are used to help the female ovulate or to treat diseases, such as endometriosis, which may cause infertility. Because the etiology of male infertility is much less understood, treatment for the male is limited; however, some fertility agents are used in males to aid spermatogenesis. The fertility agents discussed in this chapter include human chorionic gonadotropin (HCG);

human menopausal gonadotropin (HMG), or menotropins; gonadotropin-releasing hormone (Gn-RH); clomiphene citrate; bromocriptine mesylate; progesterone; and danazol.

For a list of representative drugs, *see Selected major drugs: Fertility agents* on page 958.

GONADOTROPINS

The gonadotropin agents mimic or replace the physiologic action of the naturally occurring gonadotropins, which help control male and female sexual function. Follicle–stimulating hormone (FSH) and luteinizing hormone (LH) are two major hormones secreted by the anterior pituitary gland. Chorionic gonadotropin (CG) is secreted by the placenta. The following section presents information on several gonadotropin agents used to treat male and female infertility, including HCG, HMG, and Gn-RH.

History and source

HCG is a placental hormone agent extracted from the urine of pregnant women. HMG is a purified preparation of FSH and LH extracted from the urine of postmenopausal women.

Gn-RH, a drug available since the 1970s, was not widely used until the early 1980s, when new information about pulsatile Gn-RH became available. Once researchers understood that Gn-RH is released in pulsations throughout the day, they developed a pump that would mimic normal Gn-RH release. (For additional information, see *Pulsatile Gn-RH* on page 954.)

Hormonal physiology of ovulation

The central nervous system (CNS) stimulates the hypothalamus to emit gonadotropin-releasing hormone (Gn-RH), which in turn excites the anterior pituitary gland to secrete follicle-stimulating hormone (FSH) and luteinizing hormone (LH). FSH stimulates the ovary to produce and mature a follicle. The developing follicle secretes estrogen, which causes the hypothalamus and pituitary gland to suppress FSH secretion and increase LH secretion. Estrogen also stimulates the endometrium to become prolific and influences the quantity and quality of cervical mucus, which facilitates sperm migration.

The LH surge triggers ovulation, after which the LH level drops. Under the influence of progesterone, the endometrium becomes secretory. The ovary feedback to the CNS influences the hypothalamus and pituitary to suppress gonadotropin secretion. Without gonadotropin, the corpus luteum begins to deteriorate and progesterone and estrogen levels drop. Without progesterone, the endometrial lining of the uterus cannot continue to accumulate, and menses occurs. Without estrogen and progesterone inhibition, the CNS stimulates the hypothalamus, and the cycle repeats itself.

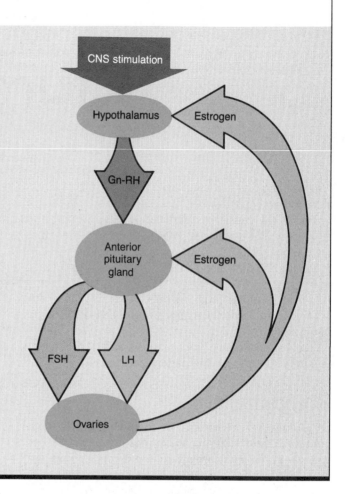

PHARMACOKINETICS

Because the gonadotropin agents are destroyed by the gastrointestinal (GI) tract, they are administered parenterally. These drugs are specific to receptors in the ovaries and testes. Following I.M. administration, HCG is distributed mainly to the ovaries and the testes; smaller amounts are distributed to the proximal tubules of the kidneys. HMG also is administered I.M. The metabolism of HMG is unknown, but about 8% of a dose is excreted unchanged in the urine. Gn-RH is administered S.C. or I.V; it is metabolized in the liver and excreted in the urine.

HCG reaches peak concentration levels in 5 to 6 hours; it has a half-life of 12 hours. The half-life of HMG is several hours. The half-life of Gn-RH is short, and regular pulsatile support is needed.

PHARMACODYNAMICS

HCG initiates ovulation in the female and spermatogenesis in the male; its target organs are the ovaries and the testes. HMG is used as replacement therapy in patients with FSH and LH deficiencies; its target organs are also the ovaries and testes. Gn-RH stimulates the secretion of gonadotropic hormones from its target organ, the anterior pituitary gland.

Mechanism of action

In the female, HCG mimics the action of LH and allows ovarian follicle rupture. HCG also stimulates the corpus luteum to produce progesterone, which is needed to sustain the fertilized ovum. In the male, HCG stimulates Leydig's cells in the testes to secrete testosterone, which is needed for spermatogenesis.

HMG produces the physiologic effects of FSH by stimulating development and maturation of the ovarian follicle. HMG also mimics LH, causing ovulation and

Hormonal physiology of spermatogenesis

The central nervous system (CNS) stimulates the hypothalamus to emit gonadotropin-releasing hormone (Gn-RH), which excites the anterior pituitary to secrete follicle-stimulating hormone (FSH) and luteinizing hormone (LH). FSH stimulates the Sertoli's cells in the seminiferous tubules of the testes to produce sperm. The Sertoli's cells also secrete the hormone inhibin, which feeds back to the hypothalamus and pituitary, thereby suppressing FSH but increasing LH. LH stimulates the Leydig's cells in the seminiferous tubules to produce testosterone, the most important male sex hormone. Testosterone works on the accessory male organs to ensure the production of adequate secretions and the normal maturation of sperm.

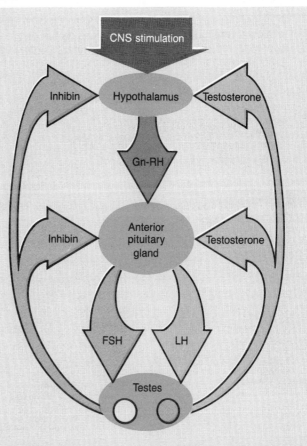

stimulating development of the corpus luteum in females; HMG stimulates spermatogenesis in males.

Gn-RH, which is synthesized in the hypothalamus, stimulates the synthesis and secretion of FSH and LH by the anterior pituitary, thereby allowing follicular growth and maturation.

PHARMACOTHERAPEUTICS

HMG and HCG are indicated to treat anovulation due to absent or inadequate FSH or LH and to treat luteal phase defect. These gonadotropic agents also are used to stimulate ovulation for in vitro fertilization programs. Patients must be pretreated with HMG for HCG to be effective. These agents should not be used in patients with primary ovarian failure.

Hypogonadotropic males may respond to HCG alone, or in combination with HMG, with increased sperm counts. Prepubertal cryptorchidism (undescended testes) also may respond to HCG.

Gn-RH has been used investigationally to stimulate ovulation in patients with hypothalamic dysfunction who do not respond to HMG and HCG. This drug offers advantages over other treatments—lower overall expense and fewer adverse effects. A disadvantage: it must be given S.C. or I.V. in a pulsatile manner every 90 to 120 minutes.

human chorionic gonadotropin [HCG] (Follutein, Pregnyl). HCG facilitates ovulation after follicular stimulation. In males it is used to stimulate spermatogenesis. Dosages vary, depending on indication, the patient's age and weight, and the physician's preference.
USUAL ADULT DOSAGE: for the female, 5,000 to 10,000 IU I.M. at the time of ovulation or on the day after discontinuing HMG; for the male, 4,000 IU I.M. three times/week for 3 weeks, or 5,000 IU I.M. every other day for 4 doses, or 500 to 1,000 IU I.M. for 15 doses

Pulsatile Gn-RH

Doses of gonadotropin-releasing hormone (Gn-RH) can be delivered in an interval or pulsatile fashion that closely mimics normal physiology. Such devices as the pulsatile pump and the button infuser and pen pump will allow women to receive Gn-RH at home in close-to-normal levels. For the woman who is trying to conceive, this new method (adapted from the insulin pump that has allowed diabetics to maintain a normal life-style while maintaining normal insulin levels) provides possibilities not available just a few years ago.

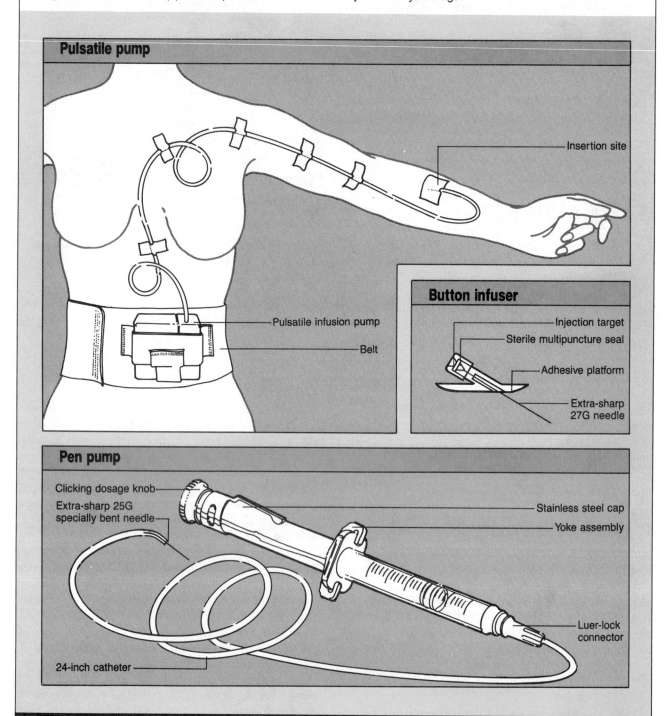

Pulsatile pump

- Insertion site
- Pulsatile infusion pump
- Belt

Button infuser

- Injection target
- Sterile multipuncture seal
- Adhesive platform
- Extra-sharp 27G needle

Pen pump

- Clicking dosage knob
- Extra-sharp 25G specially bent needle
- Stainless steel cap
- Yoke assembly
- Luer-lock connector
- 24-inch catheter

over 6 weeks, or 500 IU I.M. three times/week for 6 to 9 months. If the male patient's testosterone level (needed for production and maturation of sperm) does not rise significantly, dosage may be changed to 2,000 IU I.M. twice weekly in conjunction with HMG for 6 to 12 weeks.

human menopausal gonadotropin [HMG] (Pergonal). In females, HMG is used primarily to initiate ovulation, and HMG also is used to stimulate ovulation for several special procedures. In males, HMG is used to treat hypogonadotropic hypogonadism and prepubertal cryptochiaism.

USUAL ADULT DOSAGE: for the female, dosage depends on whether the drug is used to initiate ovulation or to stimulate ovulation for special procedures, such as an in vitro fertilization attempt, Gamete Intra-fallopian Transfer (GIFT), or egg donation. However, the usual initial dosage is 1 ampule (containing 75 IU of FSH and 75 IU of LH) I.M. once a day for 9 to 12 days followed the day after the last dose with 5,000 to 10,000 IU I.M. of HCG. For the male, pretreatment consists of HCG 5,000 IU three times/week until normal testosterone levels are achieved. Then 1 ampule (containing 75 IU of FSH and 75 IU of LH) I.M. three times/week along with 2,000 IU I.M. of HCG twice a week for 4 months.

gonadotropin-releasing hormone [Gn-RH] (Factrel). Used primarily to diagnose the cause of hypogonadism in males and females; as an investigational treatment it is used to stimulate ovulation in patients with hypothalmic dysfunction. Gn-RH causes fewer multiple births than HMG and is less expensive. Promising results have been obtained, especially when the drug is used on a pulse-dosing schedule.

Drug interactions
No significant drug interactions occur with HCG or HMG. However, significant interactions can occur between Gn-RH and other drugs. To avoid interactions, Gn-RH should not be mixed with other drugs (estrogens, progesterones, androgens, or glucocorticoids) that affect pituitary secretion of gonadotropins.

ADVERSE DRUG REACTIONS

Adverse drug reactions associated with HCG are predictable and dose-related. They include headache, irritability, fatigue, depression, weight gain associated with fluid retention, and gynecomastia. HCG also can produce ovarian hyperstimulation and multiple births. The patient may experience pain at the injection site.

The most common adverse reaction to HMG is ovarian enlargement. Mild to moderate uncomplicated ovarian enlargement may be accompanied by lower abdominal pain and distention. Ovarian hyperstimulation syndrome (OHSS), which occurs much less frequently but may be life-threatening, does not occur unless HCG has also been administered. In severe cases, OHSS may include ovarian enlargement, ascites, and pleural effusion. Electrolyte imbalance, increased capillary permeability, and hypercoagulability also may accompany the syndrome.

Other adverse reactions to HMG include hemoperitoneum from ruptured ovarian cysts, and arterial thromboembolism.

The predictable adverse reactions from Gn-RH include headache, nausea, light-headedness, abdominal discomfort, and swelling and pain at the injection site. Hypersensitivity reactions, though rare, include tachycardia, flushing, and urticaria.

NURSING IMPLICATIONS

The nurse should be aware of the following implications when working with patients receiving HCG, HMG, or Gn-RH:
• Administer HCG cautiously to patients with asthma, seizure disorders, migraine headaches, or cardiac or renal disease; androgen secretion may cause fluid retention.
• Inform the patient when and how to administer HCG, and about the timing of intercourse in relation to HCG administration (usually 24 to 36 hours after the injection).
• Instruct the female patient to continue recording her basal body temperature and to test for pregnancy if no menses occurs within 16 days of the injection.
• HMG is contraindicated in patients with thyroid or adrenal dysfunction, pituitary tumor, abnormal uterine bleeding, ovarian cysts, testicular enlargement, or a history of thrombophlebitis. HMG is also contraindicated during pregnancy and in patients on anticoagulant therapy.
• Explain to the patient that HMG therapy is expensive, warrants close monitoring by an infertility specialist, and often involves traveling to a facility offering the treatment. Also explain that HCG injections are required to initiate ovulation.

OTHER FERTILITY AGENTS

Other fertility agents to be discussed in this section include clomiphene, bromocriptine, progesterone, and danazol. (See Chapter 60, Estrogens, Progestins, and Oral Contraceptive Agents, for more information about progesterone.)

History and source

For more than 20 years after its discovery, clomiphene is still the most commonly used drug to initiate ovulation in women. Clomiphene also is used to treat menstrual abnormalities, gynecomastia, and, in rare cases, fibrocystic breast disease, persistent lactation, and hyperplasia. More recently, clomiphene has been used to treat oligospermia in males, but this use is not approved. Bromocriptine is a semisynthetic ergot alkaloid that has been used to suppress lactation and more recently has been approved for treating anovulation (absence of ovulation) from hyperprolactinemia. Danazol is an androgenic synthetic compound used to treat infertility associated with endometriosis.

PHARMACOKINETICS

After oral administration, clomiphene is readily absorbed, metabolized in the liver, and excreted in the feces. Its half-life is 5 days, but the drug can be found in the feces up to 6 weeks after administration.

After oral administration, 28% of bromocriptine is absorbed from the GI tract, but only 6% reaches the systemic circulation because of the first-pass effect through the liver. It is excreted in the urine and feces. Its half-life allows for once daily dosing. Danazol is well absorbed by the oral route and is metabolized in the liver. Its peak effect usually occurs after 6 to 8 weeks of therapy. Danazol has a half-life of approximately 4.5 hours.

PHARMACODYNAMICS

Clomiphene stimulates increased gonadotropin secretion from the anterior pituitary. Bromocriptine inhibits prolactin release from the anterior pituitary but does not interfere with the production of other pituitary hormones. Suppression of prolactin allows restoration of ovulation. Danazol's target organ is the pituitary gland.

Mechanism of action

Clomiphene is an antiestrogenic agent that occupies estrogen receptor sites in the hypothalamus, preventing estrogen from binding to these sites. In turn, the hypothalamus stimulates the pituitary to release greater amounts of FSH and LH, which then initiate and enhance the growth of an ovarian follicle in the female and spermatogenesis in the male.

Bromocriptine reduces serum prolactin levels by inhibiting prolactin release from the anterior pituitary or by stimulating postsynaptic dopamine receptors in the hypothalamus to release prolactin inhibiting factor. These effects allow FSH and LH production to return to normal.

Research in animals and humans has shown that danazol reduces ovarian estrogen production by depressing the pre-ovulatory surge in output of FSH and LH, thus mimicking menopause and causing atrophy of the endometrium. The suppression of the ovarian function creates a hypoestrogenic state manifested by amenorrhea and anovulation. Ovulation and menses resume 60 to 90 days after discontinuation of the drug.

PHARMACOTHERAPEUTICS

In the female, clomiphene is indicated for anovulation, cycle regulation where ovulatory cycles are shorter than 23 days or longer than 37 days, oligo-ovulation, polycystic ovary disease, and luteal phase defect (LPD). Clomiphene also is used to treat menstrual abnormalities, gynecomastia, fibrocystic breast disease, persistent lactation, and hyperplasia.

Bromocriptine is indicated for hyperprolactinemia, which leads to irregular menses, amenorrhea with or without galactorrhea, and hypogonadism. Bromocriptine also is used to induce ovulation and to treat prolactin-secreting adenomas of the pituitary, LPD, acromegaly, postpartum lactation, and parkinsonian syndrome.

Physicians prescribe danazol to treat endometriosis, benign breast disease, and precocious puberty.

clomiphene citrate (Clomid, Serophene). Easily administered, clomiphene does not require extensive monitoring.
USUAL ADULT DOSAGE: 50 mg P.O. daily from the 5th to the 9th day of the cycle; if the patient has had no recent uterine bleeding, the medication may be started at any time after a negative pregnancy test. If ovulation does not occur, the dosage may be increased by 50 mg increments each cycle until ovulation occurs or a daily dose of 200 mg is reached. Adjuvants to clomiphene include estrogens, glucocorticoids, HCG, HMG, and progesterone.

bromocriptine mesylate (Parlodel). Bromocriptine is used for patients with hypergonadism or amenorrhea associated with galactorrhea; it should be discontinued immediately upon diagnosis of pregnancy.

USUAL ADULT DOSAGE: for the female, 1.25 to 2.5 mg P.O. at bedtime, increasing dosage every 2 to 3 days by 2.5 mg until ovulation occurs or the maximum daily dose of 7.5 mg is reached; for the male, 2.5 mg P.O. daily.

danazol (Danocrine). Danazol exerts weak androgenic properties but no estrogenic or progestogenic activity. It is used in the treatment of endometriosis which may result in infertility and fibrocystic breast disease.
USUAL ADULT DOSAGE: for endometriosis, 100 to 400 mg P.O. b.i.d., depending on the degree of disease and the patient's response; for fibrocystic breast disease, 50 to 200 mg P.O. b.i.d.

Drug interactions

No significant drug interactions occur with clomiphene, progesterone, or danazol. The effectiveness of bromocriptine may be decreased with concurrent use of phenothiazines. Larger doses of bromocriptine may be required to lower prolactin levels if given concurrently with phenothiazines.

ADVERSE DRUG REACTIONS

Clomiphene, bromocriptine, and danazol share many of the same predictable adverse reactions, such as light-headedness, dizziness, depression, and fatigue. Their unpredictable adverse reactions vary.

Predictable reactions

The predictable adverse reactions specific to clomiphene include insomnia; hypertension; blurred vision; nausea and vomiting; bloating; photophobia; urinary frequency and polyuria; and ovarian enlargement and cyst formation, both of which regress spontaneously when the drug is discontinued. Occasionally, hyperglycemia occurs. Other predictable reactions to clomiphene include hot flashes, reversible alopecia, breast discomfort, and multiple births.

The predictable adverse reactions specific to bromocriptine may be reduced by beginning with a lowered dosage and administering the medication at bedtime. Reactions include mania, delusions, nasal congestion, hypotension, syncope, tinnitus, blurred vision, nausea and vomiting, abdominal cramps, and urinary retention. Pulmonary infiltration, pleural effusion, and coolness and pallor of the fingers and toes also have been reported.

Besides light-headedness, dizziness, depression, and fatigue, danazol produces androgenic effects, including edema, acne, mild hirsutism, decreased breast size, weight gain, and deepening of the voice. Flushing and sweating may occur. These androgenic effects may not be reversible even when drug is discontinued.

Unpredictable reactions

Clomiphene can produce urticaria, rash, and dermatitis. Other unpredictable reactions include female masculinization, early spontaneous abortion, and subfertility from the antiestrogenic effect on cervical mucus. Endometriosis may recur when danazol is discontinued.

NURSING IMPLICATIONS

The nurse should be aware of the following implications, which apply to clomiphene, bromocriptine, and danazol:
• Do not administer clomiphene to pregnant patients or patients with liver disease, abnormal uterine bleeding, or cancer of the breast or reproductive organs.
• Caution the patient taking clomiphene to avoid hazardous tasks requiring mental alertness or physical coordination, because the drug can produce visual disturbances, dizziness, or light-headedness.
• Teach the female patient how and when to take basal body temperatures and how to calculate the menstrual cycle length (1st day of flow is 1st day of new cycle).
• Inform the patient that maximum fertility time is usually 10 to 12 days after the last clomiphene tablet is taken.
• Encourage the patient to have intercourse every 36 to 40 hours during the maximum fertility time.
• Stress the importance of having a pregnancy test if no menses occurs after 16 days from the last clomiphene tablet.
• Instruct the patient about the proper timing of and injection method for administering HCG if it is combined with clomiphene.
• Instruct the patient to stop the drug and call the physician immediately if abdominal pain occurs; this could indicate ovarian enlargement or ovarian cyst.
• Do not administer bromocriptine to patients who display a hypersensitivity to ergot derivatives and in patients with renal or liver disease.
• Check to be sure the patient has been examined for pituitary tumor before beginning bromocriptine therapy.
• Administer progesterone cautiously to patients with a history of asthma, seizure disorders, migraines, cardiac or renal disease, depression, or thrombophlebitis.
• Do not administer danazol to patients with undiagnosed abnormal uterine bleeding or with liver, renal, or cardiac problems. Danazol is also contraindicated during pregnancy and lactation.

SELECTED MAJOR DRUGS

Fertility agents

This chart summarizes the major fertility agents currently in clinical use.

DRUG	MAJOR INDICATIONS	USUAL ADULT DOSAGES	NURSING IMPLICATIONS
human chorionic gonadotropin (HCG)	Ovulation induction, spermatogenesis	For females, 5,000 to 10,000 IU I.M. at ovulation time or on the day after discontinuing HMG; for males, 4,000 IU I.M. three times a week for 3 weeks; or 5,000 IU I.M. every other day for 4 doses; or 500 to 1,000 IU I.M. for 15 doses over 6 weeks; or 500 IU I.M. three times/week for 6 to 9 months	• Advise the patient about the proper timing of drug injection and subsequent intercourse. • Instruct the female patient how to record basal body temperature. • Advise the patient to obtain a pregnancy test if menses does not occur within 18 days of the start of therapy.
human menopausal gonadotropin (HMG)	Ovulation stimulation, hypogonadotropic hypogonadism	For females, 75 IU I.M. once daily for 9 to 12 days followed the day after the last dose by 5,000 to 10,000 IU I.M. of HCG; for males, 75 IU three times a week plus 2,000 IU I.M. of HCG twice a week for 4 months	• Explain to the patient that HCG is necessary to complete ovulation. • Inform the patient that hyperstimulation syndrome may occur. • Stress the importance of keeping follow-up appointments.
clomiphene	Anovulation, oligo-ovulation, short or long ovulation cycle	50 mg/day P.O. from the 5th through the 9th day of the ovulation cycle until desired effects are achieved or increase dose each cycle by 50 mg until a maximum dose of 200 mg/day is reached	• Ensure that the patient has received pretreatment screening (female: basal body temperature, cervical mucus, endometrial biopsy; male: semen analysis, testosterone, follicle-stimulating hormone). • Advise the patient to match the time of the administration of the fertility agent and intercourse. • Advise the patient to obtain a pregnancy test if menses does not occur within 16 days after therapy begins.
bromocriptine	Hyperprolactinemia, amenorrhea with or without galactorrhea, prolactin-secreting adenomas, hypogonadism	For females, 1.25 to 2.5 mg/day P.O. at bedtime; for males, 2.5 mg P.O. daily	• Advise the patient to take the drug at bedtime to help prevent nausea. • Stress the importance of follow-up prolactin therapy, as prescribed. • Instruct the female patient how to record basal body temperature.

• Inform the patient of the adverse reactions to danazol's androgenic effect. These include edema, acne, mild hirsutism, decreased breast size, weight gain, deepening of the voice, and emotional lability (rare). The patient may also experience hot flashes and sweating.

• Instruct the patient to begin danazol therapy during menses or after a negative pregnancy test.

• Advise the patient taking any of these agents to continue with follow-up visits.

CHAPTER SUMMARY

Chapter 61 presented discussions of fertility agents. Therapy with fertility agents is directed primarily toward stimulating or enhancing ovulation and facilitating sperm transportation in the female, and stimulating spermatogenesis in the male. Here are chapter highlights:

• For a couple to be fertile, both male and female must produce FSH and LH.

• Clomiphene and Gn-RH stimulate FSH and LH secretion. HMG, HCG, and progesterone provide replacement therapy. Bromocriptine is used to treat hyperprolactinemia and to induce ovulation. Danazol is used to treat endometriosis.

• Because gonadotropic agents are destroyed in the GI tract, they are administered parenterally.

• No significant drug interactions are associated with the fertility agents.

• The nurse should stress to the patient the importance of timing the fertility agent's administration and of having intercourse during the maximum fertility time.

• The nurse must also be familiar with the various fertility agents available and their indications, usual dosage ranges, monitoring techniques, contraindications, and adverse reactions.

BIBLIOGRAPHY

American Hospital Formulary Service. *Drug Information 87*. Maryland: American Society of Hospital Pharmacists, 1987.

American Medical Association Division of Drugs. *AMA Drug Evaluation*, 5th ed. Philadelphia: W.B. Saunders Co., 1985.

Charney, C.W. "Testosterone Rebound Therapy," in *Current Therapy of Infertility*. Garcia, C.R., ed. St. Louis: C.V. Mosby Co., 1984.

Flamigni, C., et al. "Use of Human Urinary Follicle Stimulating Hormone in Infertile Women with Polycystic Ovaries," *Journal of Reproductive Medicine* 30:184, 1985.

Hammond, C.B. "Bromocriptine Mesylate in Hyperprolactinemia Infertility: A Review" *Advances in Therapy* 1:285, 1985.

Hammond, M.G. "Monitoring Techniques for Improved Pregnancy Rates During Clomiphene Ovulation Induction," *Fertility and Sterility* 42:499, 1984.

McArdle, C., et al. "The Diagnosis of Ovarian Hyperstimulation (OHS): The Impact of Ultrasound," *Fertility and Sterility* 39:464, 1983.

Marcovitz, S., and Hardy, J. "Combined Medical and Surgical Treatment of Prolactin-Producing Pituitary Tumors," *Reproductive Endocrine* 2:73, 1984.

Maxsom, W.S., and Hammond, C.B. "When and How to Treat Patients with Prolactin Disorders," *Contemporary OB/GYN* 19:67, 1983.

Maxsom, W.S., et al. "Antiestrogenic Effect of Clomiphene Citrate: Correlation with Serum Estradiol Concentrations," *Fertility and Sterility* 42:536, 1984.

Pepperell, B.J. "A Rational Approach to Ovulation Induction," *Fertility and Sterility* 40:1, 1983.

CHAPTER 62

UTERINE MOTILITY AGENTS

OBJECTIVES

After reading and studying this chapter, you should be able to:
1. Differentiate among the uterine-stimulating agents: oxytocin, the prostaglandins, and the ergot alkaloids.
2. Distinguish between uterine-stimulating agents and uterine-inhibiting (tocolytic) agents.
3. Discuss the pharmacokinetics of each class of drug that affects uterine motility.
4. Identify the major drug interactions, adverse reactions, and nursing implications associated with the four classes of uterine motility agents.

INTRODUCTION

Uterine motility agents are drugs that either stimulate or inhibit uterine contractions. Those that stimulate contractions are used primarily to induce or augment labor, to abort pregnancy, or to control postpartum hemorrhage; those that inhibit contractions are used to prevent or stop preterm labor. Chapter 62 discusses the three classes of uterine-stimulating agents—oxytocin, the prostaglandins, and the ergot alkaloids—and the single class of uterine-inhibiting agents, also known as tocolytic agents.

Physiology of labor and delivery

Although both hormonal and mechanical factors are involved in producing uterine contractions during labor, the ratio of estrogen to progesterone appears to be crucial. Progesterone inhibits uterine contractions, and estrogen stimulates them. Until the 7th month of pregnancy, both hormones are secreted in progressively greater quantities. From that point on, however, estrogen secretion continues to increase, while progesterone secretion decreases slightly. This increasing estrogen-progesterone ratio promotes onset of uterine contractions.

Oxytocin and the prostaglandins are other hormones that stimulate uterine contractions. Produced by the hypothalamus and stored in the pituitary gland, oxy-tocin is secreted in increasing amounts by both mother and fetus in late pregnancy. The fetal membranes release high concentrations of prostaglandins during labor.

The mechanical factors that stimulate uterine contractions include muscle stretch and cervical irritation. The smooth muscles of the uterus are stretched continuously as the fetus grows and intermittently as it moves. Apparently this stretching helps stimulate contraction of the uterus when labor begins.

How cervical irritation stimulates uterine contractions is unknown. One theory suggests that irritation of neuronal cells in the cervix sets up reflex contractions in the uterus.

Uterine motility agents are used to prevent or treat problems that occur during labor and delivery. Uterine-stimulating agents are used to induce labor when early vaginal delivery is desired, such as when the mother has Rh incompatibility, diabetes, preeclampsia near or at term, or premature rupture of the membranes. They also stimulate or reinforce contractions and help control severe bleeding in the third stage of labor and postpartum hemorrhage.

Uterine-inhibiting (tocolytic) agents are used to prevent or treat preterm labor.

For a summary of representative drugs, see *Selected major drugs: Uterine motility agents* on page 968.

OXYTOCIN

Oxytocin is a hormone secreted by the pituitary gland that stimulates uterine contractions. It is the drug of choice for inducing or stimulating labor during term pregnancy. It is also used to prevent or treat postpartum hemorrhage and to stimulate milk ejection.

History and source

Oxytocin was first identified in 1954 by duVigneaud and co-workers. Their synthesis of antidiuretic hormone (ADH) and oxytocin led to a Nobel prize for duVigneaud. Commercial preparations of oxytocin are now made synthetically. The purified oxytocin preparations cause fewer vasopressor and antidiuretic actions than the naturally occurring hormone.

PHARMACOKINETICS

The pharmacokinetics of oxytocin are not completely understood, but parenteral doses are absorbed and distributed better than oral doses. Oxytocin is metabolized in the liver, kidneys, and mammary glands and excreted by the kidneys.

Absorption, distribution, metabolism, excretion

After oral administration, oxytocin is rapidly destroyed by the intestinal enzyme chymotrypsin, so only 0.1% of a dose reaches the systemic circulation. After I.M. administration, oxytocin is rapidly and completely absorbed, but its effects are erratic and difficult to regulate. Oxytocin has the best bioavailability when it is administered I.V. Oxytocin is distributed throughout the maternal extracellular fluid, but only small amounts are detectable in the fetal circulation. It is rapidly metabolized in the liver and kidneys and inactive metabolites are excreted in urine.

Onset, peak, duration

I.V. administration of oxytocin produces an immediate onset of action; its duration of action is short. Uterine activity decreases to pretreatment levels within 20 minutes after the infusion stops. The intranasal route also produces a rapid onset of action, with a duration of action of 20 minutes. Oxytocin's half-life is 1 to 6 minutes.

PHARMACODYNAMICS

Oxytocin's principal actions are stimulation of uterine smooth muscle contraction and facilitation of milk ejection.

Mechanism of action

Oxytocin indirectly stimulates uterine contraction by increasing myofibril cell-membrane permeability to sodium. Circulating prostaglandin levels increase significantly after oxytocin administration; this may enhance the drug's effects on smooth muscle. The response of the uterus to oxytocin increases throughout pregnancy and peaks in the last 9 weeks.

Mammary gland myoepithelium (a smooth muscle network) is also highly responsive when exposed to oxytocin. Myoepithelial cells contract, forcing milk into the large ducts where milk ejection will occur. Oxytocin may also stimulate ADH-like activity and transiently relax vascular smooth muscle.

PHARMACOTHERAPEUTICS

Oxytocin is used primarily to induce or augment labor at term, and it is the drug of choice to induce labor in pregnancies associated with preeclampsia, eclampsia, maternal diabetes, or erythroblastosis fetalis or other fetal distress syndromes. It is also indicated in postterm pregnancies (gestational age 42 weeks or more). I.V. infusion of oxytocin immediately after delivery hastens placental expulsion and helps control uterine bleeding. Occasionally, however, oxytocin has the opposite effect, inhibiting expulsion of the placenta and increasing the risk of hemorrhage and infection.

Other indications for oxytocin include adjunctive treatment of incomplete or inevitable abortion, promotion of milk ejection, and reduction of postpartum breast engorgement. Oxytocin is also used in the oxytocin challenge test to assess fetal respiratory capability in high-risk pregnancy, although this use is not included in United States product labeling.

oxytocin (Oxytocin, Pitocin, Syntocinon). Oxytocin is available as a parenteral injection (10 units/ml) and as a nasal solution or spray (40 units/ml).
USUAL ADULT DOSAGE: for induction or augmentation of labor, initially, 1 ml (10 units) in 1,000 ml of dextrose 5% in water (D_5W) or normal saline solution (0.9% sodium chloride solution) I.V., infused at 0.1 to 0.2 ml (1 to 2 milliunits)/minute, rate increased at 15- to 30-minute intervals to a maximum of 2 ml (20 milliunits)/minute, rate decreased when labor is firmly established; for reduction of postpartum bleeding after expulsion of placenta, 1 to 4 ml (10 to 40 units) in 1,000 ml D_5W or normal saline solution I.V., infused at a rate necessary to control bleeding, usually 20 to 40 milliunits/minute, or 10 units I.M. after delivery of the placenta; for incomplete or inevitable abortion, 1 ml (10 units) in 500 ml dextrose 5% in normal saline solution I.V., infused at a rate of 20 to 40 milliunits/minute; for promoting milk ejection, one spray or three drops of nasal solution in one or both nostrils 2 to 3 minutes before breast-feeding or pumping breasts; for the oxytocin challenge test, initially, 1 ml (10 units) in 1,000 ml D_5W or normal saline solution I.V., infused at 0.05 ml (0.5 milliunits)/minute and doubled every 20 minutes as necessary to reach an effective dose, usually 0.5 to 0.6 ml (5 to 6

milliunits)/minute, and discontinued when three moderate contractions of 40 to 60 seconds occur within a 9- to 10-minute interval.

Drug interactions

Drug interactions are uncommon with oxytocin, but co-administration with other uterine-stimulating agents will cause additive effects. (For a list of representative substances that interact with oxytocin, see *Drug interactions: Posterior pituitary agents* in Chapter 58, Pituitary Agents.)

ADVERSE DRUG REACTIONS

Most adverse reactions to oxytocin are extensions of the drug's actions.

Predictable reactions

Adverse reactions to oxytocin may be uterine, extra-uterine, or fetal. Uterine reactions include rupture, impaired blood flow, increased postpartum bleeding, and amniotic fluid embolism. Extrauterine reactions include hypertension, tachycardia, and dysrhythmias—most serious in patients who have valve disease or who are receiving an epidural or a spinal anesthetic. Water intoxication manifested by seizures has been associated with infusing oxytocin for periods exceeding 24 hours. Fetal adverse reactions are related to impaired uterine blood flow and the resulting fetal hypoxia, which may lead to intracranial hemorrhage, bradycardia, or tachycardia.

Unpredictable reactions

Hypersensitivity reactions, the major unpredictable reactions to oxytocin, include urticaria, pruritus, and hypotension. Commercially available synthetic preparations cause fewer hypersensitivity reactions than the naturally occurring hormone does.

NURSING IMPLICATIONS

To administer oxytocin safely, the nurse must understand the contraindications and precautions associated with its use. These are summarized in the following nursing considerations:

• Be aware that oxytocin is contraindicated in patients with severe toxemia, hypertonic uterine contractions, uterine scarring (which can lead to uterine rupture), cephalopelvic disproportion, uterine infection, umbilical cord prolapse, placenta previa, unfavorable fetal position requiring surgical intervention, traumatic delivery, grand multiparity, or hypersensitivity to the drug and in patients for whom vaginal delivery is contraindicated. It is also contraindicated in fetal distress when delivery is not imminent. Oxytocin nasal spray is contraindicated during pregnancy.

• Oxytocin is administered by I.V. infusion, not by bolus injection, with an infusion pump or a drip regulator to ensure accurate delivery.

• Never give oxytocin by more than one route simultaneously.

• Monitor and record the following for the mother and fetus at least every 15 minutes: uterine contractions, maternal and fetal heart rate, blood pressure, and blood loss; discontinue the drug at the first sign of uterine hyperactivity or fetal distress.

• Dosage is adjusted individually based on maternal and fetal response; reduce the dosage in patients with cardiovascular, hypertensive, or renal disease.

PROSTAGLANDINS

Prostaglandins (PGs) are derivatives of fatty acids (lipid acids) found in virtually every tissue and fluid in the body. As uterine-stimulating agents, they are used clinically mainly to abort pregnancy.

The three endogenous prostaglandins available for use as abortifacients (agents that induce expulsion of the fetus) are carboprost tromethamine, dinoprostone, and dinoprost tromethamine.

History and source

Prostaglandins were first observed in the 1930s by von Euler and by Kurzrok and Lieb, who noticed that strips of human uterine tissue contracted when exposed to human semen. Von Euler coined the term *prostaglandin,* believing the chemical substance was produced by prostate gland tissue. In the early 1960s, Bergström and Sjovall isolated pure prostaglandin and were able to identify its chemical structure. Since then, six primary prostaglandins have been identified: PGA, PGB, PGC, PGD, PGE, and PGF.

PHARMACOKINETICS

The pharmacokinetics of the prostaglandins remain incompletely understood, even though they have been used clinically for more than 15 years.

Absorption, distribution, metabolism, excretion

Carboprost is absorbed slowly after I.M. administration. After vaginal insertion of a dinoprostone suppository, the drug slowly diffuses across the vaginal wall into the maternal blood and is widely distributed. Dinoprost, administered I.V. or intraamniotically, is widely distributed in both mother and fetus and appears to concentrate in the fetal liver.

Little is understood about the metabolism and excretion of these agents, but dinoprostone and dinoprost appear to be rapidly metabolized to inactive metabolites in the maternal lungs and liver. After metabolism, both parent compounds and metabolites are excreted primarily in urine, but small amounts have been detected in feces.

Onset, peak, duration

Carboprost's onset of action occurs approximately 16 hours after I.M. injection, but is shorter with increased gravidity (number of pregnancies) or parity (number of live births) and longer with increased gestational age. Onset of action with dinoprostone suppositories usually occurs within 10 minutes of administration. Dinoprost's onset of action occurs within 30 minutes.

The half-life of dinoprostone and dinoprost usually ranges from less than 1 minute to 10 minutes. After intraamniotic injection, dinoprost has an extended half-life of 3 to 6 hours, probably from delayed transport to the maternal circulation.

PHARMACODYNAMICS

Although their mechanism of action has not been completely established, the abortifacient prostaglandins carboprost, dinoprostone, and dinoprost appear to act directly on the myometrium of the uterus. They stimulate uterine contractions similar to those that occur during labor, inducing fetal expulsion. They also facilitate cervical dilation and softening.

PHARMACOTHERAPEUTICS

Prostaglandins used primarily to terminate pregnancy include carboprost, dinoprostone, and dinoprost.

carboprost tromethamine (Prostin/15M). The primary clinical indication for this drug is termination of pregnancy between the 13th and the 20th weeks of gestation. I.M. administration makes it the drug of choice for patients with profuse vaginal bleeding or ruptured placental membranes. It also is used to treat postpartum hemorrhage from uterine atony. Carboprost is available in 1–ml ampules containing 250 mcg/ml.

USUAL ADULT DOSAGE: for abortion, 250 mcg deep I.M.—if necessary, repeated doses of 250 to 500 mcg I.M. every 1½ to 3½ hours—with total dose not to exceed 12 mg, nor should the drug be administered repeatedly for more than 48 hours; for postpartum hemorrhage, 250 mcg deep I.M.—if necessary, repeated doses every 15 to 90 minutes—with total dose not to exceed 2 mg.

dinoprostone (Prostin E_2). The primary indication for dinoprostone is termination of pregnancy from the 12th to the 20th week of gestation. Available as 20-mg intravaginal suppositories, dinoprostone stimulates uterine contractions similar to those of labor. It also is used to soften the cervix before induction of labor. Continuous I.V. infusion of dilute oxytocin may be administered with dinoprostone to hasten the onset of uterine contractions, thus shortening the time required for uterine evacuation. USUAL ADULT DOSAGE: one 20-mg suppository inserted high into the vagina; after insertion, the patient should remain supine for at least 10 minutes to allow adequate absorption; additional suppositories may be administered every 3 to 5 hours as necessary until abortion occurs or symptoms of intolerance develop.

dinoprost tromethamine (Prostin F_2 Alpha). The primary indication for dinoprost is termination of pregnancy between the 16th and the 20th weeks of gestation. Slowly injected into the amniotic sac, the drug stimulates the uterus to contract in a manner similar to labor contractions. The average time for expulsion of the fetus is approximately 22 hours but ranges from 4 to 54 hours. The drug also is used to ripen the cervix before induction of labor. Dinoprost is available in 4-ml and 8-ml ampules in a concentration of 5 mg/ml. USUAL ADULT DOSAGE: after transabdominal tapping of the amniotic sac and withdrawal of 1 ml of amniotic fluid, 40 mg is injected slowly into the amniotic sac through an intraamniotic catheter, with the first 5 mg administered at a rate no faster than 1 mg/minute; if no adverse reactions (vomiting, hypertension, bronchospasm) occur, the remaining drug is infused over 5 minutes; if the patient fails to respond within 24 hours, a second intraamniotic dose of 10 to 40 mg may be administered; with continued unresponsiveness, a third dose of 25 mg may be administered 24 hours later, provided the fetal membranes remain intact.

Drug interactions

The major interactions between the prostaglandins and other drugs involve oxytocin and alcohol. Alcohol antagonizes the action of dinoprostone. Oxytocin enhances the effect of carboprost and dinoprostone. Use extreme caution when administering these drugs together. Frequent monitoring of uterine contractions and cervical dilation is essential.

ADVERSE DRUG REACTIONS

Adverse reactions to the endogenous prostaglandins are diverse, mimicking the effects observed with naturally occurring prostaglandins.

Prostaglandins cause gastrointestinal (GI), vascular, bronchial, and uterine adverse reactions. GI stimulation causes the most common adverse reactions. Nausea and vomiting occur in 60%, and diarrhea in 20%, of patients receiving prostaglandins. Other predictable adverse reactions include coughing, pain, and fever, which occur in more than half the patients receiving the drugs.

Unpredictable adverse reactions to prostaglandins are potentially life-threatening and include bronchospasm, seizures, hypotension, and cardiac arrest. The most severe reactions usually occur in patients with underlying cardiovascular disease, asthma, or seizure disorders.

NURSING IMPLICATIONS

To ensure patient safety during prostaglandin administration, the nurse must be aware of the following considerations:
• Prostaglandins are contraindicated in a patient who is hypersensitive to them or who has a history of pelvic inflammatory disease.
• Administer cautiously to a patient who has cervical lacerations or uterine rupture because severe bleeding or placental retention may occur. Also administer cautiously to a patient with a history of seizures or pelvic surgery or with uterine fibroids, cervical stenosis, glaucoma, hypertension, cardiovascular disease, anemia, or diabetes mellitus.
• Closely monitor a patient who has a history of seizures.
• Remember that temperature increases occur in more than half the patients taking prostaglandins; this drug fever may be misinterpreted for infection or may mask concomitant infection. It does not respond to antipyretics such as aspirin, but sponge baths with water or alcohol may be effective.
• Monitor the patient for signs of infection.
• Premedicate the patient with antiemetics such as prochlorperazine and antidiarrheal agents such as a diphenoxylate, as ordered, to decrease the risk of GI adverse reactions.

• Store dinoprost and carboprost in a refrigerator at 35.6° to 39.2° F. (2° to 4° C.); store dinoprostone suppositories in a freezer at temperatures below −4° F. (20° C.), but bring them to room temperature before use.
• Before administering dinoprost, instruct the patient to empty her bladder.
• After administering dinoprost, monitor the patient's vital signs and uterine contractions.
• Observe and record the character and amount of the patient's vaginal bleeding that occurs with dinoprost administration.
• After termination of pregnancy, observe the patient for postabortion hemorrhage by frequently monitoring blood pressure, pulse rate, and vaginal discharge.

ERGOT ALKALOIDS

Ergot alkaloids are naturally occurring substances that markedly increase the motor activity of uterine smooth muscle. They are used to clinically control postpartum or postabortion hemorrhaging from uterine atony or subinvolution. Ergonovine maleate and its semisynthetic derivative, methylergonovine maleate, are the ergot alkaloids used as uterine motility agents.

History and source

Ergot is a product of *Claviceps purpurea*, a fungus that grows on rye and other grains and that can cause death if contaminated grains are eaten. (This effect was recognized for centuries.) The effect of ergot alkaloids during pregnancy was first recognized in 1582 by Lonicer; however, it was not until 1931 that Barger isolated the major ergot alkaloids. After isolation and chemical identification, detailed study of the alkaloids' biological activities began.

PHARMACOKINETICS

Ergot alkaloids are rapidly absorbed and distributed and appear to be metabolized in the liver and excreted in feces.

Absorption, distribution, metabolism, excretion

Ergonovine and methylergonovine are rapidly absorbed after oral and I.M. administration. Bioavailability of oral methylergonovine is approximately 60%. Although their distribution is not entirely understood, both ergot alkaloids are rapidly distributed to plasma and extracellular fluid. Methylergonovine has been detected in breast milk; however, concentrations are too low to affect a breast-feeding infant. Besides their probable metabolism in the liver and excretion in feces, only limited information exists concerning the metabolism and excretion of ergonovine and methylergonovine.

Onset, peak, duration

After oral administration, the onset of action for both drugs usually occurs within 5 to 15 minutes, with the time of peak concentration varying from 30 minutes to 3 hours and the duration of action lasting 3 hours or longer. Also with both drugs, I.M. administration produces an onset of action in 2 to 5 minutes, with a duration of action of at least 3 hours; I.V. administration causes immediate uterine contractions that last for 45 minutes.

PHARMACODYNAMICS

Ergonovine and methylergonovine are pharmacologically similar, directly stimulating uterine and vascular smooth muscle contractions. Both drugs increase the amplitude and frequency of uterine contractions, thus impeding uterine blood flow by vasoconstriction. Cervical smooth muscle contractions are also increased by both agents.

PHARMACOTHERAPEUTICS

The ergot alkaloids are used to prevent and treat postpartum and postabortion hemorrhage from uterine atony or subinvolution. They should *not* be used to induce or augment labor. Ergonovine also has been used to diagnose coronary artery spasm in patients with variant (Prinzmetal's) angina.

ergonovine maleate (Ergotrate Maleate). To treat postpartum and postabortion hemorrhage, ergonovine is available in both oral and parenteral forms.
USUAL ADULT DOSAGE: for postpartum and postabortion hemorrhage, 0.2 mg I.M. every 2 to 4 hours, to a maximum of five doses; for severe vaginal bleeding, 0.2 mg I.V. over 1 minute while blood pressure and uterine contractions are monitored, diluting the I.V. dose to a volume of 5 ml with normal saline solution; after initial I.M. or I.V. dose, 0.2 to 0.4 mg P.O. every 6 to 12 hours for 2 to 7 days, decreasing dose if severe uterine cramping occurs.

methylergonovine maleate (Methergine). To treat postpartum and postabortion hemorrhage, methylergonovine is available in both oral and parenteral forms.
USUAL ADULT DOSAGE: for postpartum and postabortion hemorrhage, 0.2 mg I.M. every 2 to 4 hours to a maximum of five doses; for severe vaginal bleeding, 0.2 mg I.V. over 1 minute while blood pressure and uterine contractions are monitored, diluting the I.V. dose to a volume of 5 ml with normal saline solution; after initial I.M. or I.V. dose, 0.2 to 0.4 mg P.O. every 6 to 12 hours for 2 to 7 days, decreasing dose if severe uterine cramping occurs.

Drug interactions

Few—but potentially harmful—drug interactions occur with the ergot alkaloids. The combined use of dopamine or other vasoconstrictors with ergot alkaloids may cause increased peripheral vasoconstriction, resulting in cyanosis and tissue necrosis.

ADVERSE DRUG REACTIONS

Most adverse reactions to the ergot alkaloids occur when the drugs are administered incorrectly—either in undiluted form or too rapidly.

The most common adverse reactions are nausea and vomiting. These may be minimized by administering prochlorperazine or another phenothiazine antiemetic before administering the ergot alkaloid, as prescribed.

Other adverse reactions include dizziness, headache, tinnitus, diaphoresis, palpitations, temporary chest pain, and dyspnea. Hypertension may also occur, most commonly with ergonovine; its incidence increases if the ergot alkaloid is administered undiluted, too rapidly, or concomitantly with vasoconstrictors or a regional anesthetic. Patients with a history of eclampsia or hypertension are at greater risk. With severe overdosage, ergot poisoning, characterized by seizures and gangrene, may occur. Other manifestations include numbness and coldness of the extremities, hypercoagulability, and confusion. Hypersensitivity reactions, including shock, have also been reported.

NURSING IMPLICATIONS

When administering ergot alkaloids, the following considerations are important for ensuring patient safety and drug effectiveness:
• Ergot alkaloids are contraindicated in patients with hypertension, eclampsia, or a hypersensitivity to these drugs.

● Administer cautiously to a patient with sepsis, obliterative vascular disease, hepatic or renal impairment, or cardiac disease.

● Avoid concomitant administration with vasoconstrictors, vasopressors, or a regional anesthetic.

● Monitor the patient for hypotension and bronchospasm because prolonged use may produce ergot poisoning.

● Dilute I.V. preparations to a volume of 5 ml with normal saline solution, and administer over at least 1 minute.

● Store ergot alkaloids in tightly closed, light-resistant containers; discard discolored solution.

● Monitor the patient's blood pressure, pulse, uterine contractions, and vaginal bleeding; report sudden changes in vital signs, frequent periods of uterine relaxation, and any change in the character and amount of vaginal bleeding.

TOCOLYTIC AGENTS

Uterine-inhibiting (tocolytic) agents, most commonly magnesium sulfate and the beta-receptor agonists ritodrine hydrochloride and terbutaline sulfate, are used to inhibit uterine contractions in preterm labor. Ethyl alcohol also relaxes uterine smooth muscle, but it is rarely used in clinical practice.

History and source

In 1925, Rucker first observed that small doses of epinephrine inhibited uterine contractions. In 1948, Ahlquist hypothesized that this effect was caused by beta-receptor stimulation of the uterine smooth muscle. Since then, several beta-receptor agonists have been noted to have uterine-inhibiting properties. Ritodrine was developed principally for obstetric use and is the only agent approved by the Food and Drug Administration (FDA) for use in the United States to treat preterm labor; however, terbutaline also is commonly used.

PHARMACOKINETICS

The tocolytic agents readily cross the placenta and appear in breast milk. When administered I.V., they have a rapid onset of action.

Absorption, distribution, metabolism, excretion

After oral administration, terbutaline and ritodrine are absorbed from the GI tract, with a bioavailability of 30% to 50%, and 30%, respectively. Both agents cross the placenta and appear in breast milk. Magnesium sulfate is administered I.V. and distributed widely. The beta-

---

DRUG INTERACTIONS

Tocolytic agents

The drug interactions involving the tocolytic agents are summarized in this chart.

DRUG	INTERACTING DRUGS	POSSIBLE EFFECTS	NURSING IMPLICATIONS
ritodrine, terbutaline	corticosteroids	Cause pulmonary edema	● If concomitant administration is unavoidable, monitor the patient's breath sounds.
	beta-adrenergic blocking agents	Antagonize uterine-inhibiting action	● Avoid concomitant administration. ● Monitor the patient's uterine contractions frequently.
	sympathomimetics	Increase the sympathomimetic effect	● Administer concomitantly with caution. ● Monitor the patient's vital signs.
	Monamine oxidase inhibitors	Cause hypertensive crisis	● Avoid concomitant administration. ● Monitor the patient's blood pressure.
magnesium sulfate	neuromuscular blocking agents	Enhance neuromuscular blockade	● Avoid concomitant administration. ● Monitor the patient's vital signs.
	barbiturates, narcotic agents, benzodiazepines	Increase respiratory depression	● Avoid concomitant administration. ● Monitor the patient's respiratory rate.

receptor agonists are metabolized in the liver. All the tocolytic agents and their metabolites are excreted in urine; 90% to 98% of a magnesium sulfate dose is excreted in urine, and the remainder in feces.

Onset, peak, duration

Administered I.V., tocolytic agents have a rapid onset of action; ritodrine reaches peak concentration levels after 50 minutes. Terbutaline I.V. reaches peak concentration levels in 30 to 60 minutes and has a duration of action of 1½ to 4 hours. Magnesium sulfate's duration of action is 30 minutes. Oral ritodrine has an onset of action of 30 to 60 minutes and reaches peak concentration levels in 30 to 60 minutes. Oral terbutaline has an onset of action of 30 minutes and reaches peak concentration levels in 2 hours. Ritodrine's half-life is 15 to 17 hours after I.V. administration and 12 to 20 hours after oral administration.

Therapeutic blood level for magnesium sulfate is 6 mEq/liter; when this level falls, uterine contractions may recur.

PHARMACODYNAMICS

The mechanisms of action for the tocolytic agents vary. However, all three agents directly affect uterine muscle.

Mechanism of action

Ritodrine and terbutaline, the beta-receptor agonists, interact with beta receptors in the uterus. That stimulates release of adenylate cyclase, thus increasing the production of cyclic adenosine monophosphate (AMP). The increased production of cyclic AMP causes an increased uptake and sequestration of intracellular calcium. The final result is inhibition of uterine smooth muscle contractions with decreased intensity and frequency of contractions.

Magnesium sulfate's mechanism of action as a tocolytic agent is not known. The present theory is that magnesium sulfate successfully competes with calcium in uterine smooth muscle, preventing calcium from triggering uterine contractions.

PHARMACOTHERAPEUTICS

The tocolytic agents initially are administered I.V. for rapid inhibition of uterine contractions. Then, once contractions are under control, oral beta-receptor agonists are used to maintain the initial effect.

magnesium sulfate. Administered I.V., magnesium sulfate is used to treat hypomagnesemia, to prevent or control seizures in preeclampsia or eclampsia, and to control preterm labor.

USUAL ADULT DOSAGE: for prevention or control of seizures in preeclampsia or eclampsia, initially, 4 grams I.V. in 250 ml D₅W and 4 grams deep I.M. into each buttock, then 4 grams deep I.M. into alternate buttock every 4 hours as necessary or, alternatively, 4 grams I.V. as a loading dose followed by 1 to 2 grams hourly as an I.V. infusion; for control of preterm labor, initially, 6 grams I.V. of a 10% solution as a loading dose, given slowly at a rate of 150 mg/minute until contractions stop or adverse reactions occur; maintenance dose, 2 grams/hour I.V. infusion, keeping magnesium levels between 4 and 6 mEq/liter.

ritodrine hydrochloride (Yutopar). This is the beta-receptor agonist approved by the FDA for the inhibition of preterm uterine contractions.

USUAL ADULT DOSAGE: initially, 50 to 100 mcg/minute I.V., increasing every 10 minutes by 50 mcg/minute to a maximum of 350 mcg/minute until contractions stop or adverse reactions occur; maintenance dose, 10 mg P.O. 30 minutes before stopping the I.V. infusion, repeated every 2 hours for the first 24 hours, then 10 to 20 mg P.O. every 4 to 6 hours, not to exceed 120 mg/day.

Physiologic effects of magnesium levels

Maternal reactions to magnesium sulfate administration depend on the serum magnesium level. The list below indicates the serum magnesium levels and their corresponding physiologic effects.

MAGNESIUM LEVEL (mEq/liter)	PHYSIOLOGIC EFFECTS
1.5 to 3	Normal serum levels; no adverse physiologic effects
4 to 7	Therapeutic level for preventing or controlling seizures associated with preeclampsia or eclampsia and for controlling preterm labor contractions
8 to 10	Loss of deep tendon reflexes; hypotension; central nervous system depression
12 to 15	Respiratory paralysis
>15	Cardiac conduction dysrhythmias
>25	Cardiac arrest

Uterine motility agents

This chart summarizes the major uterine motility agents currently in clinical use.

DRUG	MAJOR INDICATIONS	USUAL ADULT DOSAGES	NURSING IMPLICATIONS
oxytocin	Induction or augmentation of labor	1 ml (10 units) in 1,000 ml D_5W or normal saline solution I.V., infused at 0.1 to 0.2 ml (1 to 2 milliunits)/minute; increase rate at 15- to 30-minute intervals to a maximum rate of 2 ml until desired contraction pattern is established	• Administer I.V. by infusion, not by bolus injection. Always use an infusion pump or a drip regulator to ensure accurate delivery. • Monitor maternal and fetal heart rate, CNS status, blood pressure, and maternal uterine contractions and blood loss every 15 minutes.
	Postpartum bleeding after expulsion of the placenta	1 to 4 ml (10 to 40 units) in 1,000 ml D_5W or normal saline solution I.V., infused at a rate to control bleeding, usually 20 to 40 milliunits/minute; or 10 units I.M. after delivery of the placenta	
carboprost	Termination of pregnancy between the 13th and 20th weeks of gestation	250 mcg deep I.M.; repeated doses of 250 to 500 mcg at 1½- to 3½-hour intervals; total dose should not exceed 12 mg	• Administer cautiously to a patient who has cervical lacerations or uterine rupture. • Store drug in a refrigerator at 35.6° to 39.2° F. (2° to 4° C.).
ergonovine	Postpartum and postabortion hemorrhage from uterine atony or subinvolution	0.2 mg I.M. every 2 to 4 hours to a maximum of five doses	• Monitor the patient's blood pressure, pulse rate, uterine contractions, and vaginal bleeding; report sudden changes in vital signs, frequent periods of uterine relaxation, and any change in the character or amount of vaginal bleeding. • Dilute I.V. preparations to a volume of 5 ml with normal saline solution and administer over at least 1 minute.
	Severe vaginal bleeding	0.2 mg I.V. diluted in normal saline solution; after initial I.M. or I.V. dose, 0.2 to 0.4 mg P.O. every 6 to 12 hours for 2 to 7 days	
ritodrine	Inhibition of preterm uterine contractions	50 to 100 mcg/minute I.V. initially, increased by 50 mcg/minute every 10 minutes to a maximum of 350 mcg/minute until contractions stop or adverse reactions occur; maintenance dose, 10 mg P.O. 30 minutes before stopping infusion, followed by 10 mg every 2 hours for 24 hours, then 10 to 20 mg P.O. every 4 to 6 hours not to exceed 120mg/day	• Monitor the patient's blood glucose, urine glucose, and potassium levels, especially in diabetic patients. • Monitor the patient's uterine activity and fetal heart rate continuously during therapy. • Monitor the patient for chest tightness and pain, palpitations, and dyspnea.

terbutaline sulfate (Brethine, Bricanyl). Although it is not approved for use as a tocolytic agent, terbutaline is commonly used to treat preterm labor.

USUAL ADULT DOSAGE: initially, 2.5 mcg/minute I.V., increasing every 20 minutes by 2.5 mcg/minute to a maximum of 17.5 mcg/minute until contractions stop or adverse reactions occur; once contractions cease, continue I.V. infusion for 60 minutes to determine the lowest effective dose; continue lowest effective dose for at least 12 hours, then begin 15 mg P.O./day maintenance therapy.

Drug interactions

The drug interactions associated with the tocolytic agents are typical of the other agents in their respective classes. (For additional information on the interacting drugs, their possible effects, and related nursing implications, see *Drug interactions: Tocolytic agents* on page 966.)

ADVERSE DRUG REACTIONS

Tocolytic agents cause many minor adverse reactions and a few that can be severe, including cardiovascular reactions, electrolyte imbalances, and seizures.

Predictable reactions

Most adverse reactions to the beta-receptor agonists ritodrine and terbutaline are extensions of their actions. Common maternal adverse reactions to these agents include an increase in heart rate by 20 to 40 beats/minute, increased cardiac output, hypotension, hyperglycemia, increased insulin secretion, increased free fatty acid release, hypokalemia, anxiety, headache, nausea, vomiting, nervousness, and tremors. Because these agents cross the placenta, the neonate may also experience adverse reactions, including increased heart rate, hypotension, and hypocalcemia.

Adverse reactions to magnesium sulfate generally depend on the drug dose, the rapidity of administration, and the serum magnesium level. (For a correlation between various blood levels of magnesium and the adverse reactions associated with them, see *Physiologic effects of magnesium levels* on page 967.)

Unpredictable reactions

The beta-receptor agonists ritodrine and terbutaline can cause unpredictable maternal adverse reactions, including pulmonary edema, chest tightness or pain, dysrhythmias, palpitations, acute congestive heart failure, and hypertensive crisis. Unpredictable neonatal adverse reactions include respiratory depression, paralytic ileus, and pulmonary edema (rare).

NURSING IMPLICATIONS

Tocolytic agents require careful administration and close patient monitoring. To administer these agents safely and correctly, the nurse must understand the following considerations:

• Be aware that the beta-receptor agonists ritodrine and terbutaline are contraindicated in patients who have a history of hypersensitivity to these agents or who have hypervolemia, cardiac disease, hyperthyroidism, uncontrolled hypertension, uncontrolled diabetes, or severe vaginal bleeding.

• Carefully assess maternal vital signs and a 20- to 30-minute fetal monitor strip before initiating beta-receptor agonist therapy; assess maternal heart rate and blood pressure before increasing the infusion rate.

• Monitor uterine activity and fetal heart rate continuously during beta-receptor agonist therapy.

• Carefully monitor the hydration status of patients receiving beta-receptor agonists to be sure they are not hypovolemic or hypervolemic; the I.V. infusion rate should not exceed 150 ml/hour.

• Be prepared to administer repeated I.V. doses of beta-receptor agonists, because standard dosages do not always induce therapeutic effects and uterine contractions may recur.

• With a diabetic patient receiving beta-receptor agonists, monitor blood glucose, urine glucose, and potassium levels. Also assess the patient's fluid intake and output.

• With the nondiabetic patient receiving beta-receptor agonists, monitor blood glucose levels before and periodically during therapy.

• Monitor the patient receiving beta-receptor agonists for chest tightness and pain, palpitations, and dyspnea.

• Magnesium sulfate is contraindicated in the patient with heart block or myocardial damage.

• When administering magnesium sulfate, monitor the patient's vital signs, knee jerk reflex, and fluid intake and output.

• Monitor the patient's magnesium levels every 4 to 6 hours until they stabilize.

• Administer a bolus dose of magnesium sulfate slowly, at a rate of 150 mg/minute, to prevent nausea, vomiting, headache, palpitations, and flushing.

• Administer magnesium sulfate cautiously to the patient with impaired renal function.

• Remember that administration of magnesium sulfate with other central nervous system (CNS) depressants may have an additive depressant effect.

• Remember that magnesium sulfate enhances the effects of neuromuscular blocking agents.

• Monitor infants born to patients receiving magnesium sulfate for hypermagnesemia, hypotonia, CNS depression, and respiratory depression.

CHAPTER SUMMARY

Uterine motility agents as they are used to induce or augment labor, to terminate pregnancy, to control postpartum hemorrhage, and to stop preterm labor were discussed in Chapter 62. Here are the highlights of the chapter:

• Uterine motility agents include uterine-stimulating agents and uterine-inhibiting (tocolytic) agents.

• Uterine-stimulating agents include oxytocin, the prostaglandins, and the ergot alkaloids.

• Uterine-inhibiting agents include magnesium sulfate and the beta-receptor agonists ritodrine and terbutaline.

• Oxytocin is the drug of choice for inducing labor at term, for evacuating uterine contents after delivery, and for preventing or stopping postpartum hemorrhage. It is preferred because it is associated with few adverse reactions and minimal drug interactions.

• Two ergot alkaloids are commercially available: ergonovine and its semisynthetic derivative, methylergonovine. Both are used—less commonly than oxytocin, however—to prevent and treat postpartum hemorrhage.

• The three endogenous prostaglandins used as abortifacients (agents that induce the expulsion of the fetus) are carboprost, dinoprostone, and dinoprost.

• The beta-receptor agonists ritodrine and terbutaline are considered the drugs of choice to stop uterine contractions in preterm labor, although the use of magnesium sulfate is increasing. Used correctly, these agents are safe and cause few major adverse reactions.

BIBLIOGRAPHY

American Hospital Formulary Service. *Drug Information 87.* McEvoy, G.K., et al., eds. Bethesda, Md.: American Society of Hospital Pharmacists, 1987.

American Medical Association. *Drug Evaluations,* 6th ed. Philadelphia: W.B. Saunders Co., 1986.

Anderson, K.E., et al. "Pharmacology of Labor," *Clinical Obstetrics and Gynecology* 26:56, 1983.

Cano, A., et al. "Metabolic Disturbances During Intravenous Use of Ritodrine: Increased Insulin Levels and Hypokalemia," *Obstetrics and Gynecology* 65:356, March 1985.

Caritis, S.N. "Treatment of Preterm Labour: A Review of the Therapeutic Options," *Drugs* 26:243, September 1983.

Eggleston, K.M. "Management of Preterm Labor and Delivery," *Clinical Obstetrics and Gynecology* 29:230, June 1986.

Elliott, J.P., and Colnel, L. "Magnesium Sulfate as a Tocolytic Agent," *American Journal of Obstetrics and Gynecology* 147:277, October 1983.

Finley, J., et al. "Cardiovascular Consequences of Beta-Agonist Tocolysis: An Echocardiographic Study," *Obstetrics and Gynecology* 64:787, December 1984.

Frederiksen, M.C. "Tocolytic Therapy with Beta-Adrenergic Agonist," *Rational Drug Therapy* 17:1, June 1983.

Fuchs, A., et al. "Oxytocin and the Initiation of Human Parturition (Part 2)," *American Journal of Obstetrics and Gynecology* 141:694, November 15, 1981.

Gonik, B., and Greasy, R.K. "Preterm Labor: Its Diagnosis and Management," *American Journal of Obstetrics and Gynecology* 154:3, January 1986.

Hansten, P.D. *Drug Interactions,* 5th ed. Philadelphia: Lea & Febiger, 1986.

Husslein, P., et al. "Oxytocin and the Initiation of Human Parturition (Part 1)," *American Journal of Obstetrics and Gynecology* 141:688, November 15, 1981.

Konturek, S.J., and Pawlik, W. "Physiology and Pharmacology of Prostaglandins," *Digestive Diseases and Sciences* 3:6s, February 1986.

Moncada, S., et al. "Prostaglandins, Prostacyclin, Thromboxane A_2, and Leukotriene," in *Goodman and Gilman's The Pharmacological Basis of Therapeutics,* 7th ed. Gilman, A.G., et al., eds. New York: Macmillan Publishing Co., 1985.

Pitt, B., et al. "Prostaglandins and Prostaglandin Inhibitors in Ischemic Heart Disease," *Annals of Internal Medicine* 99:83, July 1983.

Slater, R.M., et al. "Anaphylactoid Reaction to Oxytocin in Pregnancy," *Anesthesia* 40:566, July 1985.

Toaff, M.E., et al. "Induction of Labour by Pharmacological and Physiological Doses of Intravenous Oxytocin," *British Journal of Obstetrics and Gynaecology* 85:101, February 1978.

DRUGS TO CONTROL INFLAMMATION, ALLERGY, AND ORGAN REJECTION

The chapters in this unit focus on drugs used to control inflammation, allergy, and organ rejection. Some drugs are used for more than one purpose. The glucocorticoids, for example, exert anti-inflammatory and immunosuppressant effects, and the antiallergy drugs block inflammation caused by antigen-antibody reactions. Immunosuppressant drugs, however, are used specifically to prevent organ rejection. To understand the mechanisms of action of these drugs, the nurse needs an overview of the immune and inflammatory responses.

Immune and inflammatory responses

Immune and inflammatory responses protect the body from foreign substances and insults. These responses usually help maintain homeostasis but sometimes are inappropriate, as in a patient undergoing organ transplantation or experiencing autoimmune disease. In such instances, drugs are used to suppress these responses.

The immune system's complex network of specialized cells degrades and removes damaged or dead cells and prevents the growth and development of abnormal cells. The immune system generates two types of response: cell-mediated and humoral.

The cell-mediated response depends on the T lymphocyte (T cell) system. Stem cells in the bone marrow give rise to T cell precursors, which are later released from the thymus as mature T cells. (The name T cell comes from thymus.) T cells may be helper or suppressor cells. Helper T cells enhance the body's immune response; suppressor T cells inhibit it. Helper T cells usually outnumber suppressor T cells by two to one. In a disease such as acquired immune deficiency syndrome (AIDS), however, the number of helper T cells drops to almost zero.

In an autoimmune disease, such as systemic lupus erythematosus or rheumatoid arthritis, the cell-mediated response is activated by the individual's cells, which the immune system treats as foreign substances.

The humoral response depends on B lymphocyte (B cell) activity. B cells (lymphocytes that originate as stem cell precursors in the bone marrow) respond to an

Glossary

Allergen: substance capable of producing a hypersensitivity reaction.

Allergy: hypersensitivity reaction acquired through exposure to an allergy that results in an increased reaction to reexposure.

Allograft, allogenic graft, or **homograft:** tissue transplanted between genetically different individuals of the same species.

Antibody: immunoglobulin synthesized by lymphoid tissue in response to an antigenic stimulus.

Antigen: high-molecular-weight foreign protein or protein-polysaccharide complex that can stimulate the synthesis of a specific antibody.

Autoimmunity: abnormal reactivity of the body to its own tissue.

Basophil: granulocytic leukocyte characterized by a lobulated nucleus and coarse, large, round, irregular bluish cytoplasmic granules. In an allergic reaction, basophils release histamine, bradykinin, heparin, and serotonin.

B cell: bursal lymphocyte responsible for humoral immunity.

Chemotaxis: movement of an organism in response to a chemical stimulus.

Complement: serum substance that combines with an antibody-antigen complex, producing antigen lysis.

Conjunctivitis: inflammation of the mucous membrane lining the eyelids and covering the exposed surface of the eyeball.

continued

Glossary continued

Creatinine clearance: volume of plasma cleared of creatinine per unit of time; the normal average value is 120 ml/minute.

Dermatitis: skin inflammation.

Dermatosis: any skin disorder.

Diuretic: agent that promotes urine excretion.

Dyskinesia: impairment of the ability to execute voluntary movements.

Ecchymosis: skin discoloration caused by extravasation of blood into subcutaneous tissue; bruise.

Exocrine gland: gland that secretes externally through a duct to the skin.

Fibroblast: connective tissue cell.

Globulin: class of proteins characterized by solubility in saline solutions but not in water.

Glucocorticoid: adrenocortical hormone that increases gluconeogenesis, raising the concentration of liver glycogen and blood glucose, and inhibits the inflammatory response.

Gout: condition caused by abnormal purine metabolism, characterized by increased serum uric acid levels, acute arthritic episodes, and formation of chalky urate deposits in the joints.

Hepatotoxic: destructive or poisonous to liver cells.

Histamine: powerful tissue substance, released during allergic reactions, that dilates capillaries, contracts most smooth muscles, increases heart rate, and stimulates gastric secretions.

Hypercalcemia: excess calcium in the blood.

Hyperglycemia: excess glucose in the blood.

Hypernatremia: excess sodium in the blood.

Hypersensitivity: exaggerated immune system reaction, with characteristic symptoms, to contact with certain substances (allergens) that are innocuous to nonsensitized individuals.

Hyperuricemia: excess uric acid in the blood.

Hypocalcemia: calcium deficiency in the blood.

Hypokalemia: potassium deficiency in the blood.

Immunology: study of the immune system and its reactions to antigens.

Immunosuppression: inhibition of the body's immune response to foreign substances.

Inflammation: tissue response to injury characterized by pain, heat, redness, edema, and sometimes loss of function.

Labyrinthitis: inner ear inflammation.

Lymphocyte: white blood cell with a single nucleus and nongranular protoplasm that arises from the reticular tissue of the lymph gland.

Lymphokine: soluble substance released by a lymphocyte when stimulated by an antigen.

Lysosome: minute cellular body containing hydrolytic enzymes that are released upon injury to the cell.

Macrophage: large mononuclear cell that ingests microorganisms, other cells, or foreign particles.

Mast cell: large connective tissue cell that secretes heparin, histamine, bradykinin, and serotonin in response to an allergic or inflammatory stimulus.

Mineralocorticoid: adrenocortical hormone that increases sodium retention and potassium excretion.

Myelosuppression: inhibition of the bone marrow's production of blood cells.

Myopathy: skeletal muscle disorder.

Nephritis: kidney inflammation.

Nephrotoxic: destructive or poisonous to kidney cells.

Paresthesia: abnormal burning, prickling, or tingling sensations.

Percutaneous: performed through the skin, as the instillation of fluid in a cavity using a needle.

Phagocytosis: engulfment of microorganisms, cells, or foreign particles by reticuloendothelial cells, polymorphonuclear leukocytes, monocytes, or macrophages.

Polymorphonuclear leukocyte: white blood cell with a lobed nucleus that responds to allergic and inflammatory stimuli.

Proteolysis: enzymatic hydrolysis of proteins into proteose, peptone, and other by-products.

Pruritus: itching.

Rheumatoid arthritis: disease characterized by connective tissue inflammation, especially in the muscles and joints.

Rhinitis: inflammation of nasal mucous membranes.

Rhinorrhea: discharge of thin nasal mucus.

Seborrhea: sebaceous gland dysfunction characterized by excessive secretion of sebum that forms white or yellowish greasy scales or cheesy plugs.

Striae: streaks or lines, especially on the skin.

Telangiectasia: condition characterized by capillary and minute artery dilation, which serves as the basis for various angiomas.

T helper cell: cell released by T lymphocytes in response to an antigen that activates other T cells, B cells, and macrophages.

Tophi: chalky urate deposits in the tissue around joints in individuals with gout.

T suppressor cell: cell released by T lymphocytes in response to an antigen that prevents other T cells from producing an excessive immune response that might severely damage the body.

Tussive: pertaining to a cough.

Uricosuric: agent that promotes uric acid excretion.

Urticaria: skin reaction characterized by transient wheals that are paler or redder than the surrounding skin and are often accompanied by severe itching.

antigen by differentiating into plasma cells that secrete antigen-specific antibodies. This antigen-antibody reaction activates the complement system, which causes lysis of antigenic cells. (See *Immune responses* on page 974 for a summary of cell-mediated and humoral responses.)

Immune responses commonly result in inflammation, the local reaction of vascularized tissue to injury. When injury occurs, chemical reactions involving bradykinin, prostaglandins, and histamines ensue. These reactions cause vasodilation at the injury site, which increases blood flow, redness, and warmth. Capillary permeability also increases, causing edema (swelling). Pain results from the edema and the effects of histamine and bradykinin on nerve endings. Leukocyte migration to the area to remove cellular debris contributes to the edema and pain.

An exaggerated immune response, hypersensitivity reaction, can occur in a sensitized individual. Reexposure to an allergen can cause such symptoms as rhinitis, wheezing, and red, tearing eyes.

Chapter 63
Antihistaminic Agents

Chapter 63 investigates the antihistaminic agents: the ethanolamines, ethylenediamines, alkylamines, phenothiazines, and piperazines. First, it describes the events that occur in a Type I hypersensitivity reaction and discusses the histamine (H_1)-receptor antagonists. Then it explores the mechanisms of action and clinical uses of the antihistaminic agents. It concludes with a discussion of related nursing implications, including patient education.

Chapter 64
Corticosteroids and Other Immunosuppressant Agents

Chapter 64 focuses on anti-inflammatory and immunosuppressant agents, including the glucocorticoids, mineralocorticoids, cyclosporine, azathioprine, cyclophosphamide, antilymphocyte globulin, antithymocyte globulin, and muromonab CD3. It introduces adrenal anatomy and physiology and presents the pharmacologic properties of the drug classes, emphasizing the clinical uses for the agents and their long-term adverse effects. The chapter also discusses nursing implications and patient education, including ways to help patients prevent secondary infections and cope with adverse reactions.

Chapter 65
Uricosurics, Other Antigout Agents, and Gold Salts

Chapter 65 presents the antigout agents and gold salts. After discussing the causes and signs and symptoms of gout and rheumatoid arthritis, the chapter details the pharmacologic properties of the agents used to treat these disorders. It provides detailed nursing implications and patient education that stresses detection, prevention, and response to adverse reactions.

Nursing diagnoses

One or more of the following nursing diagnoses may be appropriate for the nurse caring for a patient receiving antihistaminic, systemic or topical corticosteroid, immunosuppressant, uricosuric, antigout, or gold salt agents:

• Alteration in bowel elimination: constipation or diarrhea, related to illness or drug therapy

• Alteration in family process related to illness, medical or surgical interventions, drug therapy, or life-style changes

• Alteration in fluid volume: excess, related to illness or drug therapy

• Alteration in health maintenance related to illness or drug therapy

• Alteration in nutrition: more or less than body requirements, related to illness or drug therapy

• Alteration in oral mucous membrane related to illness or drug therapy

• Alteration in thought processes related to illness or drug therapy

• Alteration in urinary elimination patterns related to illness or drug therapy

• Altered growth and development related to illness or drug therapy

• Anticipatory grieving related to illness, medical or surgical interventions, drug therapy, or life-style changes

• Anxiety related to illness, medical or surgical interventions, drug therapy, or life-style changes

• Disturbance in self-concept related to illness, medical or surgical interventions, drug therapy, or life-style changes

• Fear related to illness, medical or surgical interventions, drug therapy, or life-style changes

• Hopelessness related to illness, medical or surgical interventions, drug therapy, or life-style changes

• Hyperthermia related to drug therapy

• Impaired home maintenance management related to illness, medical or surgical interventions, drug therapy, or life-style changes

Immune responses

When an antigen stimulates the bone marrow stem cells, the immune system produces cell-mediated and humoral responses in different ways.

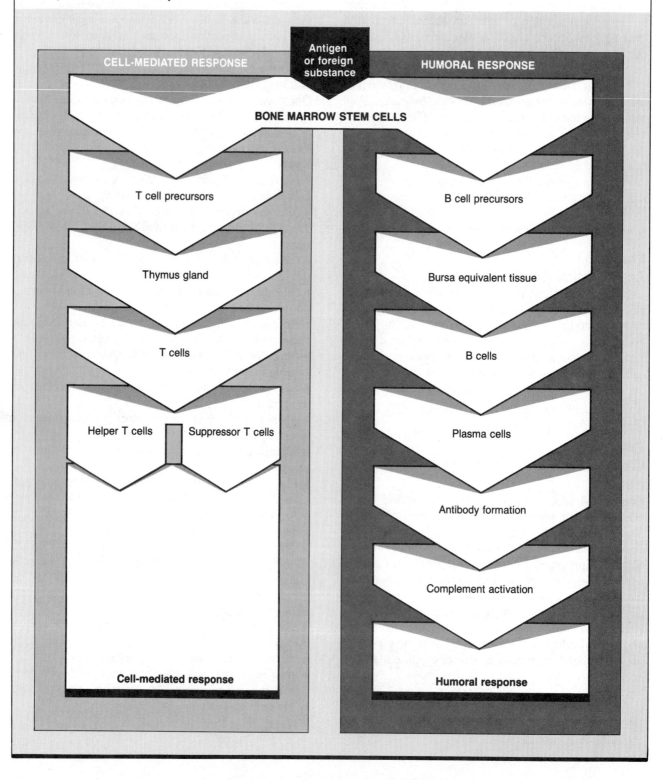

- Impaired physical mobility related to illness or drug therapy
- Impaired social interaction related to illness or drug therapy
- Impairment of skin integrity: actual, related to illness, medical or surgical interventions, or drug therapy
- Ineffective family coping: compromised, related to illness, medical or surgical interventions, drug therapy, or life-style changes
- Ineffective individual coping related to illness, medical or surgical interventions, drug therapy, or life-style changes
- Knowledge deficit related to illness, medical or surgical interventions, or drug therapy
- Noncompliance related to medical interventions or drug therapy
- Potential alteration in body temperature related to illness or drug therapy.
- Potential for infection related to illness, medical or surgical interventions, or drug therapy
- Potential for injury related to drug therapy
- Powerlessness related to illness, medical or surgical interventions, or drug therapy
- Self-care deficit related to illness, medical or surgical interventions, or drug therapy
- Sensory-perceptual alteration related to illness or drug therapy
- Sexual dysfunction related to illness or drug therapy
- Sleep pattern disturbance related to illness or drug therapy
- Social isolation related to illness or drug therapy.

CHAPTER 63

ANTIHISTAMINIC AGENTS

OBJECTIVES

After reading and studying this chapter, you should be able to:
1. Describe the sequence of physiologic events in a type I hypersensitivity reaction.
2. Discuss the mechanism of action of H_1-receptor antagonists and explain how they relieve allergy symptoms.
3. Identify the major adverse reactions to the H_1-receptor antagonists.
4. Discuss the interactions between H_1-receptor antagonists and other drugs.
5. Discuss the nursing implications for antihistaminic agents.

INTRODUCTION

Antihistamines primarily act to block histamine effects that occur in a type I, or immediate, hypersensitivity reaction, commonly called an allergic reaction. A review of the immunologic sequence and the antigen-antibody reaction will help explain the antihistamines' mechanism of action.

The human immune system reacts to agents that it recognizes as foreign to the host. These foreign substances, or antigens, stimulate the production of antibodies that help defend the body against bacterial, viral, or other invasion. An allergy occurs when an individual has an antigen response to an ordinary substance in the environment. Most people with allergies have inherited an immune system deficiency that makes them more vulnerable than others to foreign substances.

Type I hypersensitivity develops after the first exposure to a protein or other substance that the host recognizes as foreign. This antigen, or allergen, stimulates production of unusual amounts of immunoglobulin E (IgE) antibodies, which normally are present in very small quantities. These antibodies sensitize mast cells (connective tissue cells that contain histamine) and basophils (a type of leukocyte) by attaching to their surfaces. Later, when the sensitized cells are reexposed to the antigen, a reaction occurs between the antigen and

the IgE antibodies. This antigen-antibody reaction stimulates the sensitized cells to release chemical mediators, including histamine, bradykinin, prostaglandins, chemotactic factors (substances that produce cell movement), and slow-reacting substance of anaphylaxis (SRS-A). The body responds to these mediators by dilating the veins and arteries, increasing capillary permeability, constricting smooth muscles (except arterioles), and increasing the secretions of exocrine glands, such as parietal cells and lacrimal glands.

Histamine is the major chemical mediator in this reaction and is responsible for producing most of the allergy symptoms. When histamine binds to H_1 receptors on effector tissues (tissues that contract or secrete in response to nerve impulses), it produces profound peripheral vasodilation and capillary permeability. This in turn leads to edema and constriction of bronchial smooth muscles. (See *The allergic response* for a summary of this process.)

Antihistamine therapy works to block histamine's binding to H_1 receptors. By doing this, antihistamines diminish most histamine effects and relieve the symptoms of a type I hypersensitivity reaction. They are available alone or in combination products, by prescription or over the counter.

For a summary of representative drugs, see *Selected major drugs: Antihistaminic agents* on pages 985 and 986.

H_1-RECEPTOR ANTAGONISTS

The term antihistamine refers to drugs that act as H_1-receptor antagonists. Drugs that antagonize H_2 receptors are not considered antihistamines and are discussed separately. (See Chapter 50, Peptic Ulcer Agents, for a

The allergic response

This illustration traces the cellular and systemic events that occur in an allergic response, or type I hypersensitivity reaction.

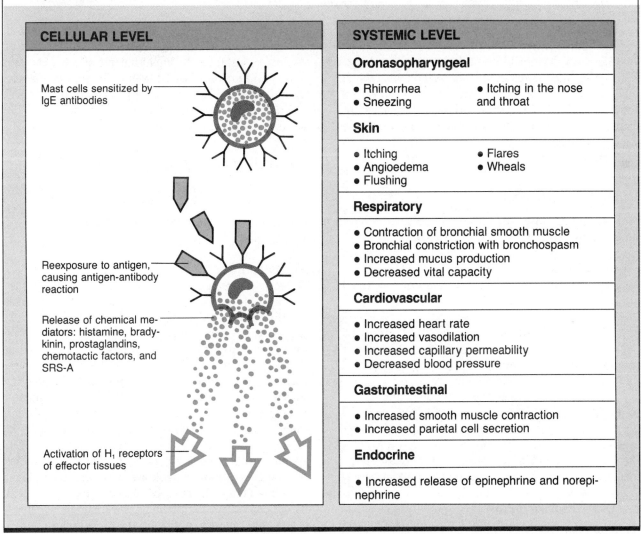

CELLULAR LEVEL

Mast cells sensitized by IgE antibodies

Reexposure to antigen, causing antigen-antibody reaction

Release of chemical mediators: histamine, bradykinin, prostaglandins, chemotactic factors, and SRS-A

Activation of H_1 receptors of effector tissues

SYSTEMIC LEVEL

Oronasopharyngeal

- Rhinorrhea
- Sneezing
- Itching in the nose and throat

Skin

- Itching
- Angioedema
- Flushing
- Flares
- Wheals

Respiratory

- Contraction of bronchial smooth muscle
- Bronchial constriction with bronchospasm
- Increased mucus production
- Decreased vital capacity

Cardiovascular

- Increased heart rate
- Increased vasodilation
- Increased capillary permeability
- Decreased blood pressure

Gastrointestinal

- Increased smooth muscle contraction
- Increased parietal cell secretion

Endocrine

- Increased release of epinephrine and norepinephrine

discussion of these drugs.) Based on chemical structure, antihistamines are categorized into six major classes: ethanolamines, ethylenediamines, alkylamines, phenothiazines, piperazines, and miscellaneous agents.

The ethanolamines include carbinoxamine maleate, clemastine fumarate, dimenhydrinate, diphenhydramine hydrochloride, doxylamine succinate, phenyltoloxamine, and phenyltoloxamine citrate. The ethylenediamines are pyrilamine maleate and tripelennamine. The alkylamines include brompheniramine, chlorpheniramine maleate, dexchlorpheniramine maleate, and triprolidine hydrochloride. The phenothiazines include methdilazine hydrochloride, promethazine

hydrochloride, and trimeprazine tartrate. The piperazine class consists of chlorcyclizine hydrochloride, cyclizine lactate, hydroxyzine hydrochloride, hydroxyzine pamoate, and meclizine hydrochloride. Azatadine maleate, cyproheptadine hydrochloride, phenindamine tartrate, and terfenadine are miscellaneous antihistamines.

All classes of antihistamines competitively block the binding of histamine to H_1-receptor sites on effector tissues. This blocking action can halt the progression of a type I hypersensitivity reaction but cannot reverse effects that are already present. Certain H_1-receptor antagonists can also counteract motion sickness, vertigo, nausea, and vomiting.

History and source

Bovet and Staub discovered histamine-blocking activity in 1937 during laboratory experiments with guinea pigs. Subsequent testing of amine and phenolic ether synthesis helped to produce pyrilamine maleate in 1944. By the 1950s, many histamine-blocking compounds, including diphenhydramine and tripelennamine, were available.

But histamine-receptor activity remained undiscovered until 1966, when Ash and Schild tried to learn why antihistamines did not block all histamine effects. Explaining that antihistamines worked only on one type of histamine receptor, Ash and Schild termed this an H_1 receptor. In the 1970s, Black and his colleagues identified H_2-receptor antagonists, drugs that selectively blocked histamine effects on gastric parietal cells, which are unresponsive to H_1-receptor antagonists.

PHARMACOKINETICS

Studies of three compounds—brompheniramine, chlorpheniramine, and diphenhydramine—have provided most of the information about the fate of antihistamines in the body. These studies show that antihistamines are metabolized by the liver, with most metabolites excreted in the urine in 24 hours.

Absorption, distribution, metabolism, excretion

H_1-receptor antagonists are well absorbed after oral or parenteral administration. Onset of action, toxicity, and duration of action vary among the drugs.

Antihistamines are widely distributed throughout the body and central nervous system (CNS), with the highest concentration in the lungs and lower concentrations in the kidneys, brain, spleen, muscles, and skin. The only exception is terfenadine, a new "nonsedating" antihistamine, which penetrates the blood-brain barrier so poorly that very little of it is distributed in the CNS.

These drugs are metabolized by hepatic enzymes and excreted in the urine, almost entirely as degradation products of metabolism. Terfenadine is excreted in the feces. The drugs are almost entirely excreted 24 hours after administration. Small amounts are excreted in breast milk.

Onset, peak, duration

After oral administration of the H_1-receptor antagonists, symptom relief begins in about 30 minutes. Onset of action is from 15 to 60 minutes. After parenteral administration, onset of action occurs in 20 to 30 minutes. Effects of rectal suppositories develop 30 to 40 minutes after administration. Terfenadine's onset of action is somewhat delayed; effects begin in 1 to 2 hours.

Peak concentration levels vary with the drug used but usually occur 1 to 2 hours after administration. Studies indicate that diphenhydramine reaches a peak blood concentration level after about 2 hours, remaining there for another 2 hours before the level begins to fall. Terfenadine also achieves a peak blood concentration level in about 2 hours but does not reach peak effects for 3 to 4 hours.

Usually, the duration of action varies from 4 to 8 hours, although some drugs have a longer duration of action. For instance, the antihistaminic effects of terfenadine and azatadine last 12 hours. The plasma half-life for most antihistamines is about 4 hours, but longer-acting drugs have longer half-lives. Terfenadine's half-life, for example, is 20 hours.

PHARMACODYNAMICS

Most H_1-receptor antagonists are used to block the effects of histamine in allergic reactions. Their histamine-blocking action, however, also makes them useful in treating other disorders.

Mechanism of action

H_1-receptor antagonists competitively antagonize histamine at H_1-receptor sites on effector cells in the small blood vessels, smooth muscles, peripheral nerves, adrenal medulla, exocrine glands, and brain. Through this antagonism, histamine binding on these target tissues is blocked, but the overall release of histamine continues. This action prevents further responses to histamine but does not reverse histamine's present effects. That means that continued exposure to the allergen will cause continued release of histamine. If the amount of histamine increases rapidly, antihistamines may not be able to block the numerous histamine molecules from the receptors. When that happens, epinephrine or another physiologic histamine antagonist must be administered to produce the opposite effects of histamine: constricting small blood vessels and relaxing bronchial smooth muscles.

H_1-receptor antagonists effectively block histamine's action on the small blood vessels. They can decrease small arteriole dilation and engorgement of related tissues. They significantly reduce capillary permeability, decreasing interstitial leakage of plasma proteins and fluids and lessening edema.

H_1-receptor antagonists inhibit most smooth muscle responses to histamine. In particular, they block the constriction of bronchial, gastrointestinal (GI), and vascular smooth muscle. They are less effective on histamine-induced vasodilation; however, administration of an H_2-receptor antagonist may correct this problem.

Antihistamine effects

The effects of antihistamines vary among the classes of drugs and among the specific drugs in each class. The following chart summarizes the general effects for each pharmacologic class.

ANTIHISTAMINE CLASS	SEDATIVE EFFECTS	ANTICHOLINERGIC EFFECTS	ANTIEMETIC EFFECTS
ethanolamines	Moderate to high	High	Moderate to high
ethylenediamines	Low to moderate	Low	Low
alkylamines	Low	Moderate	Low
phenothiazines	Low to high	High	Very high
piperazines	Low to moderate	Moderate	Low
others (azatadine, cyproheptadine, phenindamine, terfenadine)	Moderate (azatadine) Low (others)	Low (terfenadine) Moderate (others)	Low

---

H_1-receptor antagonists also relieve symptoms by acting on the skin's terminal nerve endings. Nerve endings stimulated by histamine produce a flare (redness around an urticarial lesion) and itching. H_1-receptor antagonists suppress both symptoms, possibly by blocking histamine receptors that occupy nerve endings.

The drugs also selectively suppress adrenal medulla stimulation, autonomic ganglia stimulation, and exocrine gland secretion, such as lacrimal and salivary secretion. Although these anticholinergic properties may contribute to the drugs' adverse effects, they allow them to be used as antimuscarinics, which inhibit responses to acetylcholine. The drugs, however, do not affect parietal cell secretion, which is more effectively suppressed by H_2-receptor antagonists.

Several antihistaminic agents have a high affinity for H_1 receptors in the brain and are used for their CNS effects. The CNS effects of diphenhydramine make it useful as a sedative-hypnotic. Dimenhydrinate, diphenhydramine, promethazine, and various piperazine derivatives serve as effective antiemetic and antivertigo agents, although their exact mechanisms of action are unknown. Diphenhydramine can act as an antidyskinetic (a drug that corrects impaired involuntary movements) because of its ability to inhibit the responses to acetylcholine. Diphenhydramine also suppresses the cough center in the medulla, making it an effective antitussive agent. (See *Antihistamine effects* for a summary of the effects of each class of antihistamine.)

PHARMACOTHERAPEUTICS

The ability of these drugs to block H_1 receptors throughout the body helps to explain their broad spectrum of activity and multiple indications for use. Antihistaminic agents are used to treat the symptoms of type I hypersensitivity reactions, such as allergic rhinitis, vasomotor rhinitis, allergic conjunctivitis, urticaria (hives), and angioedema (submucosal swelling in the hands, face, and feet). They are also used as adjunctive therapy to treat anaphylactic reactions after acute manifestations are controlled. Additional clinical indications include nausea, vomiting, motion sickness, vertigo, and preoperative sedation. In fact, some of these drugs are primarily used as antiemetics. (See Chapter 49, Emetic and Antiemetic Agents, for more information on this use.) Diphenhydramine can help treat Parkinson's disease (parkinsonism) and drug-induced extrapyramidal reactions. Because of its antiserotonin qualities, cyproheptadine may be used to treat Cushing's disease, serotonin-associated diarrhea, vascular cluster headaches, and anorexia nervosa.

Most antihistamines lack specificity for selective H_1 receptors. Although nonspecificity promotes multiple use, it causes a major disadvantage: sedation. Most antihistamines readily cross the blood-brain barrier and bind to H_1 receptors in the brain. That leads to CNS depression, which can be an undesired effect, depending on the treatment goal. Ethanolamines, in particular, can produce extreme CNS depression and sedation.

carbinoxamine maleate (Cardec, Clistin, Rondec). An ethanolamine derivative, carbinoxamine is available by itself or in combination with other drugs, such as pseudoephedrine, dextromethorphan, acetaminophen, and phenylephrine. Although this drug produces fewer CNS effects than the other ethanolamines, it should not be used with neonates.

USUAL ADULT DOSAGE: 4 to 8 mg P.O. t.i.d. or q.i.d. by itself; 4 mg P.O. q.i.d. when taken in a fixed combination with pseudoephedrine.

clemastine fumarate (Tavist). An ethanolamine derivative, clemastine is used to relieve the symptoms of histamine-induced allergic reactions. Its most common adverse reaction is drowsiness.

USUAL ADULT DOSAGE: 1.34 mg P.O. b.i.d. or 2.68 mg P.O. one to three times a day, depending on the patient's age and condition. The lower dose is usually indicated for an elderly patient or a patient with rhinitis and other allergy symptoms; the higher dose, for a younger patient or a dermatologic condition. Dosage should not exceed 8.04 mg/day.

dimenhydrinate (Dimentabs, Dramamine, Dymenate, Marmine). An ethanolamine derivative, dimenhydrinate is also an anticholinergic that acts principally through CNS depression. Through its depressant action on hyperstimulated labyrinthine function, it can prevent and treat the nausea, vomiting, and vertigo associated with motion sickness. It can also relieve the symptoms of labyrinthitis, Ménière's disease, and other diseases affecting the vestibular system. Most oral forms of the drug are available over the counter, but parenteral forms require a prescription.

USUAL ADULT DOSAGE: 50 mg to 100 mg P.O. every 4 to 6 hours p.r.n.; 50 to 100 mg every 4 hours I.M. p.r.n.; 50 mg I.V. in 10 ml of saline solution injected over at least 2 minutes, every 4 hours p.r.n. Dosage should not exceed 400 mg/day.

diphenhydramine hydrochloride (Allerdryl, Benadryl, Benahist, Bendylate, Caladryl, Compoz, Nordryl, Nytol, Sominex Formula 2, Valdrene). An ethanolamine derivative, diphenhydramine is probably the broadest-spectrum antihistamine. It has strong central and peripheral actions. Its central action makes diphenhydramine useful for preventing or treating motion sickness and nausea and vomiting associated with amphotericin administration and cancer chemotherapy. It is effective as a preoperative sedative and as a nighttime sleep aid, appearing in many over-the-counter (OTC) products, such as Compoz, Nytol, and Sominex. In syrup form, it is used to treat coughs related to colds or allergy. The drug's central action may inhibit the action of acetyl-

choline mediated by muscarinic receptors. As a result, it is useful as an antidyskinetic and antimuscarinic, especially in some elderly patients with Parkinson's disease or drug-induced dyskinesias who should not take stronger drugs.

Because of diphenhydramine's peripheral action, this drug can be used to relieve allergy symptoms and prevent transfusion reactions in sensitized patients who are receiving platelet transfusions.

Although oral administration is preferred, the drug may be given by deep I.M. or I.V. injection. The parenteral form is available in 10 and 50 mg per ml. Diphenhydramine is also available in topical 1% and 2% creams and lotions (Caladryl). In these forms, it temporarily relieves itching associated with skin conditions.

USUAL ADULT DOSAGE: for allergy symptoms or motion sickness, 25 to 50 mg P.O. t.i.d. or q.i.d.; 10 to 50 mg deep I.M. or I.V. For prophylaxis before transfusions, cancer chemotherapy, or amphotericin administration, 25 to 50 mg P.O. For dyskinesias, 50 to 150 mg P.O. daily or 10 to 50 mg deep I.M. or I.V. For hypnotic effects, 50 to 100 mg P.O. at bedtime. For coughs, 25 mg of syrup P.O. every 4 hours. For itching, topical application t.i.d. or q.i.d.

doxylamine succinate (Decapryn, Unisom). An ethanolamine derivative, this drug is used primarily for sedation and for symptomatic relief of coughs, colds, and histamine-induced allergic reactions. Doxylamine is available over the counter.

USUAL ADULT DOSAGE: as a sleep aid, 25 mg P.O. 30 minutes before bedtime; for antihistaminic effects, 7.5 to 12.5 mg P.O. every 4 to 6 hours, not to exceed 75 mg/day. The physician may increase this dosage to 25 mg P.O. every 4 to 6 hours, or a maximum of 150 mg/day. Because the effects of doxylamine on the fetus have not yet been fully determined, pregnant patients should avoid taking this drug. Lactating patients should also avoid its use.

phenyltoloxamine (Tussionex) and **phenyltoloxamine citrate** (Naldecon). An ethanolamine derivative, phenyltoloxamine is combined with other compounds to increase their effectiveness. In Tussionex, phenyltoloxamine boosts the antitussive effects of hydrocodone, a systemic opioid analgesic. In Naldecon, phenyltoloxamine citrate works with chlorpheniramine maleate and two sympathomimetic amines, phenylpropanolamine hydrochloride and phenylephrine hydrochloride, to relieve congestion and the symptoms of hay fever and other allergies.

USUAL ADULT DOSAGE: for cough, one capsule, tablet, or 5-ml suspension of Tussionex P.O. every 6 to 8 hours p.r.n. (a patient susceptible to respiratory depression may require a smaller dose). To relieve allergy symptoms, 5 ml of Naldecon syrup P.O. every 3 to 4 hours, not to exceed four doses in 24 hours; or one sustained-release tablet of Naldecon P.O. every 8 hours p.r.n. Tablets must be swallowed whole to be effective.

pyrilamine maleate (Dormarex, Quiet World). An ethylenediamine derivative, pyrilamine is available by itself or in combination products and provides symptomatic relief for allergic reactions. In combination products, this drug also acts as a nighttime sleep aid.
USUAL ADULT DOSAGE: for allergies, 25 to 50 mg P.O. t.i.d.; as a sleep aid, 50 mg P.O. at bedtime.

tripelennamine (PBZ, PBZ-SR, Pyribenzamine, Ro-Hist). An ethylenediamine, this drug comes in two forms: tripelennamine citrate and tripelennamine hydochloride. Both forms can be given orally, but the hydrochloride salt can also be administered topically as a cream. Tripelennamine relieves allergy symptoms.
USUAL ADULT DOSAGE: 37.5 to 75 mg of tripelennamine citrate P.O. every 4 to 6 hours, not to exceed 900 mg per day; 25 to 50 mg of tripelennamine hydrochloride P.O. every 4 to 6 hours, not to exceed 600 mg per day; or 100 mg of sustained-release tripelennamine hydrochloride P.O. b.i.d. or t.i.d.

brompheniramine (Bromphen, Dimetane, Dimetane Extentabs, Veltane). An alkylamine, brompheniramine is available as an elixir, in regular and sustained-release tablets, and in injectable form and is used to treat allergy symptoms. In combination with other drugs, brompheniramine is used to treat seasonal and perennial allergic rhinitis and upper respiratory symptoms in the common cold.
USUAL ADULT DOSAGE: 4 mg P.O. every 4 to 6 hours, not to exceed 24 mg/day; 8 to 12 mg P.O. every 8 to 12 hours of the sustained-release form; or 10 mg I.V., I.M., or S.C. every 6 to 12 hours p.r.n., not to exceed 40 mg/day.

chlorpheniramine maleate and **dexchlorpheniramine maleate** (Chlor-Trimeton, Chlor-Trimeton Repetabs, Dexchlor, Polaramine, Teldrin). An alkylamine used to treat rhinitis and allergy symptoms, chlorpheniramine maleate is available in various forms: capsules; solutions; regular, chewable, and sustained-release tablets; parenteral injections; and in combination products. The parenteral form is also indicated to relieve symptoms of anaphylaxis and allergic reactions to blood or plasma.

Dexchlorpheniramine is available in tablets, repeat-action tablets, and syrups.
USUAL ADULT DOSAGE: chlorpheniramine maleate, 4 mg P.O. every 4 to 6 hours, not to exceed 4 mg/day. For sustained-release tablets, 8 to 12 mg P.O. b.i.d., not to exceed 24 mg per day. For anaphylaxis or severe allergic reactions, 10 to 20 mg I.V. or I.M. For uncomplicated allergic reactions or when oral administration is contraindicated, 5 to 20 mg I.V. or I.M. The maximum parenteral dose is 40 mg/day; dexchlorpheniramine, 2 mg P.O. every 4 to 6 hours, or 4 to 6 mg P.O. every 8 to 10 hours for repeat-action tablets.

triprolidine hydrochloride (Actidil). An alkylamine derivative, triprolidine is used to relieve symptoms of colds and allergies. It is available in solutions, tablets, and with pseudoephedrine hydrochloride in combination products, such as Actifed.
USUAL ADULT DOSAGE: 2.5 mg P.O. every 4 to 6 hours, not to exceed 10 mg/day.

methdilazine hydrochloride (Tacaryl). A phenothiazine derivative, this drug comes in tablets, chewable tablets, and solutions. It is used primarily to relieve symptoms of pruritus associated with urticaria.
USUAL ADULT DOSAGE: 8 mg P.O. b.i.d. to q.i.d.

promethazine hydrochloride (Pentazine, Phenergan). A phenothiazine derivative, promethazine is a potent antihistamine that is primarily used for its CNS effects. Dosage forms include tablets, syrups, rectal suppositories, and I.V. and I.M. injections. The preferred route of administration is oral. Promethazine commonly produces sedation, which limits its usefulness in allergy relief for an ambulatory patient. This action, however, makes promethazine useful as a preoperative and postoperative sedative, an adjunct to analgesics for controlling postoperative pain, an antianxiety agent, and a hypnotic. Although not fully understood, its actions on the CNS also make this drug useful in treating nausea, vomiting, and motion sickness. Promethazine can also be used to control minor allergic transfusion reactions.
USUAL ADULT DOSAGE: for motion sickness, initially, 25 mg P.O. 30 to 60 minutes before traveling; then 8 to 12 hours later p.r.n., and b.i.d. thereafter, taken immediately upon arising in the morning and before the evening meal. For nausea and vomiting, initially, 25 mg P.O., I.M., or rectally, followed by 12.5 to 25 mg every 4 to 6 hours p.r.n. For preoperative and postoperative prevention of nausea and vomiting, initially, 25 mg P.O. or I.M., followed by 25 mg every 4 to 6 hours. For

DRUG INTERACTIONS

Antihistaminic agents

Antihistamines can increase the anticholinergic effects of anticholinergic drugs and the sedative effects of CNS depressants, such as tricyclic antidepressants, tranquilizers, reserpine, barbiturates, and alcohol. The combination of these drugs with antihistamines can cause life-threatening consequences.

DRUG	INTERACTING DRUGS	POSSIBLE EFFECTS	NURSING IMPLICATIONS
carbinoxamine, clemastine, dimenhydrinate, diphenhydramine, doxylamine, phenyltoloxamine, pyrilamine, tripelennamine, brompheniramine, chlorpheniramine, dexchlorpheniramine, triprolidine, chlorcyclizine, cyclizine, hydroxyzine, meclizine, methdilazine, promethazine, trimeprazine	CNS depressant drugs (barbiturates, tranquilizers, alcohol, tricyclic antidepressants, depressant analgesics, antianxiety agents, sedatives, and antimuscarinics)	Produce profound CNS depression	• Administer a reduced dosage of the interacting drug as ordered. • Monitor the patient for changes in level of consciousness.
	MAO inhibitors and other drugs with anticholinergic effects	Prolong and intensify anticholinergic effects	• Monitor the patient's therapeutic response.
	ototoxic medications (aminoglycosides, salicylates, cisplatin)	Mask signs and symptoms of ototoxicity	• Monitor the patient for signs of hearing loss and conduct an audiometric test weekly or biweekly.
	procarbazine	Increases CNS depression	• Monitor the patient for changes in level of consciousness.
	epinephrine	Reverses epinephrine's vasopressor effect, causing vasodilation, increased heart rate, and further decreased blood pressure	• Monitor the patient's heart rate and blood pressure.

sedation or for postoperative sedation with analgesics, 25 to 50 mg P.O. For preoperative sedation, 50 mg P.O. the night before surgery. For allergy, 12.5 mg P.O. before meals and at bedtime p.r.n., or 25 mg P.O. at bedtime. For minor transfusion reactions, 25 mg I.M. or I.V., repeated in 2 hours, if necessary.

trimeprazine tartrate (Temaril). A phenothiazine derivative, trimeprazine is a stronger histamine antagonist than promethazine but produces fewer anticholinergic and CNS depressant effects. It can alleviate histamine-induced urticaria and pruritus and is available in tablets, sustained-release capsules, and syrups.
USUAL ADULT DOSAGE: 2.5 mg P.O. q.i.d. p.r.n. for tablets or syrups; 5 mg P.O. every 12 hours p.r.n. for sustained-release capsules.

chlorcyclizine hydrochloride (Fedrazil). A piperazine, chlorcyclizine is the oldest H_1-receptor antagonist in this group. Available over the counter in combination with pseudoephedrine hydrochloride, it has a prolonged action and relatively low incidence of drowsiness.
USUAL ADULT DOSAGE: 50 mg P.O. b.i.d.

cyclizine lactate (Marezine). A piperazine, cyclizine is used as an antiemetic to prevent or treat motion sickness. The drug probably acts indirectly on the medullary chemoreceptor trigger zone, diminishes vestibular stimulation, and depresses labyrinthine function. It is available in tablet and injection form.
USUAL ADULT DOSAGE: 50 mg P.O. or I.M. 30 minutes before traveling, repeated every 4 to 6 hours p.r.n.

hydroxyzine hydrochloride (Atarax) and **hydroxyzine pamoate** (Vistaril). A piperazine, hydroxyzine acts on the subcortical areas of the CNS to produce sedation and relieve anxiety. The sedative effects may explain how it helps manage histamine-induced pruritus.
USUAL ADULT DOSAGE: for pruritus, 25 to 100 mg P.O. t.i.d. or q.i.d.; for preoperative and postoperative sedation, 25 to 100 mg I.M.

meclizine hydrochloride (Antivert, Bonine). A piperazine, meclizine is used to prevent and treat motion sickness and relieve vertigo associated with vestibular disturbances, such as Meniere's disease.

USUAL ADULT DOSAGE: for motion sickness, 25 to 50 mg P.O. 1 hour before traveling, repeated every 24 hours p.r.n. For vertigo, 25 to 100 mg P.O. daily in divided doses.

azatadine maleate (Optimine). A miscellaneous antihistaminic agent, azatadine relieves the symptoms of allergic rhinitis and chronic urticaria. In a fixed combination product with pseudoephedrine hydrochloride, azatadine can treat the symptoms of upper respiratory tract congestion associated with allergic rhinitis.
USUAL ADULT DOSAGE: 1 to 2 mg P.O. b.i.d., determined by patient response.

cyproheptadine hydrochloride (Periactin). A miscellaneous antihistaminic agent, cyproheptadine is used primarily to relieve pruritus and cold urticaria (edema and wheals caused by exposure to cold). Research on its antiserotonin properties may lead to Food and Drug Administration (FDA) approval of its use in producing clinical remissions in Cushing's disease caused by pituitary disorders and in managing the symptoms of anorexia nervosa, carcinoid syndrome, vascular cluster headaches, galactorrhea-amenorrhea syndrome, and other antiserotonin-responsive disorders.
USUAL ADULT DOSAGE: for allergy symptoms, 4 mg P.O. t.i.d. or q.i.d., not to exceed 0.5 mg/kg/day.

phenindamine tartrate (Nolahist, Nolamine). A miscellaneous antihistaminic agent, phenindamine is used to treat allergic reactions. It is available in tablet form over the counter.
USUAL ADULT DOSAGE: 25 mg P.O. every 4 to 6 hours, not to exceed 150 mg/day.

terfenadine (Seldane). A miscellaneous antihistaminic agent, terfenadine is a new "nonsedating" antihistamine. It slowly binds to H$_1$ receptors to form a stable complex from which it slowly dissociates. It does not readily cross the blood-brain barrier and, in normal doses, does not appear to affect H$_1$ receptors in the CNS. As a result, terfenadine produces fewer CNS effects, such as sedation, than the other antihistamines. Also, it does not increase the sedative effects of CNS depressants, such as diazepam and alcohol, when given concurrently. Available in tablets, terfenadine effectively relieves rhinorrhea, sneezing, oronasopharyngeal irritation or itching, lacrimation, and red, irritated, or itching eyes associated with seasonal allergic rhinitis. It is less effective in relieving nasal congestion.
USUAL ADULT DOSAGE: 60 mg P.O. b.i.d.

Drug interactions

When given with other drugs, antihistamines may cause one of three different interactions. The first type of interaction may occur when a patient simultaneously receives two or more drugs that have similar effects. The patient will display additive or cumulative drug effects characteristic of drug overdose. Drugs that are likely to cause this interaction with antihistamines include CNS depressants, antimuscarinics, tricyclic antidepressants, and monoamine oxidase (MAO) inhibitors.

The second type of interaction may occur when an antihistamine blocks or reverses the effects of another drug. For instance, if epinephrine is administered to a patient receiving one of the phenothiazines, the antihistamine may block, or even reverse, the intended vasopressor effect. If a vasopressor is required for a patient receiving phenothiazines, norepinephrine or phenylephrine should be used. Similarly, antihistamines may block H$_1$ receptors in the skin, suppressing the flare reaction to antigen skin testing. That is why antihistamines should be discontinued for 4 days before skin testing, whenever possible.

The third type of interaction occurs when antihistamine use masks the toxic signs and symptoms of another drug. For example, an antihistamine used to depress vestibular stimulation and labyrinthine function in motion sickness and vertigo can mask the signs of ototoxicity associated with aminoglycosides or large doses of salicylates. If antihistamines must be given with aminoglycosides, the physician or nurse must monitor the patient closely for signs of ototoxicity. (See *Drug interactions: Antihistaminic agents* for further details.)

ADVERSE DRUG REACTIONS

Used as antiallergy agents, antihistamines produce many predictable adverse reactions, especially CNS depression. However, this adverse reaction and others have been exploited widely and now provide the pharmacologic basis for many other antihistamine uses. Because a predictable adverse reaction may be a desired therapeutic response or a dose-related drug reaction, the nurse must consider the goal of antihistaminic treatment before determining that a predictable adverse reaction is undesirable. Not all adverse reactions are predictable, however; unpredictable reactions to antihistamines include hematologic and hypersensitivity reactions.

Predictable reactions

The incidence and severity of adverse reactions vary among the antihistamines, but severe toxicity rarely occurs, and a dosage reduction or the use of a different antihistamine will usually relieve a mild reaction. Susceptibility to adverse reactions varies among patients. For instance, an elderly patient is more likely than a younger adult to develop dizziness, sedation, and hypotension.

The most common adverse reaction is CNS depression, which can produce sedation and other symptoms. Occurring with usual doses, sedation can range from mild drowsiness to deep sleep. Occasionally, other reactions may include dizziness, lassitude, disturbed coordination, and muscular weakness. After 2 to 3 days of antihistamine therapy, these adverse reactions may spontaneously disappear. Less common reactions include CNS excitation, restlessness, insomnia, palpitations, and seizures. Because of this, antihistamines should be administered cautiously to a patient with a seizure disorder.

The next most common adverse reactions are GI symptoms, including epigastric distress, loss of appetite, nausea, vomiting, constipation, and diarrhea. Giving the drug with meals or with milk may reduce these symptoms.

The third most common reactions are the anticholinergic effects, which occur especially with the ethanolamines. Dryness of the mouth, nose, and throat and thickening of bronchial secretions commonly occur and may be desired. But in a patient with asthma or chronic obstructive pulmonary disease, they may lead to airway obstruction. Such a patient should use antihistamines with caution and only under a physician's direction. Other anticholinergic effects include urinary retention and dysuria; vertigo, tinnitus, and labyrinthitis; vision disturbances, such as diplopia and blurred vision; and cardiovascular effects, such as hypotension, hypertension, tachycardia, and extrasystoles. The anticholinergic effects of antihistamines can exacerbate some underlying conditions. Therefore, antihistamines—especially the ethanolamines—should be administered with extreme caution to a patient with narrow-angle glaucoma, peptic ulcer disease, cardiovascular disease, hyperthyroidism, prostatic hypertrophy, or bladder neck obstruction.

Unpredictable reactions

Unpredictable adverse reactions of antihistamines occur much less frequently but may include hypersensitivity, drug fever, hematologic complications, and teratogenic effects (effects that interfere with fetal development). Hypersensitivity manifested by urticaria, drug rash, and photosensitivity may occur with oral drug administration, but usually results from topical application. Once local hypersensitivity has occurred, topical or systemic reuse of the drug or any drug in the same chemical class will produce a similar reaction.

Although rare, hematologic complications include leukopenia, granulocytopenia, hemolytic anemia, thrombocytopenia, and pancytopenia.

Antihistamines have been used extensively to control nausea and vomiting during pregnancy; however, evidence regarding their teratogenic effects is limited. Meclizine and dimenhydrinate offer the lowest risk of teratogenicity. The teratogenic effects of the other antihistamines are not fully known. Therefore, a pregnant patient should take antihistamines only under the direction of her physician. Because some antihistamines appear in breast milk, a breast-feeding patient should avoid using them.

Drug fever is a sign of a toxic reaction or overdose. Because of the wide use and ready availability of OTC antihistamines, acute poisoning frequently occurs, especially in children. The drugs' CNS effects pose the greatest threat and account for most of the signs and symptoms of poisoning: hallucinations, excitement, ataxia, athetosis, involuntary movements, and convulsions. Fever is more common in children than in adults. Fixed, dilated pupils accompany other anticholinergic effects and may be followed by coma and death. Because no specific therapy exists for H_1-receptor antagonist poisoning, treatment aims at relieving these symptoms and providing systems support.

NURSING IMPLICATIONS

The nurse must pay particular attention to patient education about the proper use of antihistamines, the identification of predictable adverse reactions, and the measures to take if adverse reactions occur. The nurse must also be aware of the following implications:
• When administering sustained-release capsules or long-acting tablets, encourage the patient to take the medication in its whole form. Remind the patient not to break, cut, crush, or chew the medication.
• Monitor a child on antihistamines for excitation or reduced mental alertness. Report these adverse reactions to the physician.
• Consult the physician to discontinue antihistamines for 4 days before the patient receives an allergy skin test to avoid masking positive results.
• Review CNS, anticholinergic, and GI adverse reactions with the patient.
• Explain to the patient that antihistamines can produce drowsiness and reduce alertness. Taking the drug at bedtime can minimize these symptoms but may cause continued drowsiness in the morning. These effects may lessen after 2 to 3 days of use. Advise the patient not

SELECTED MAJOR DRUGS

Antihistaminic agents

This chart summarizes the major antihistamines currently in clinical use.

DRUG	MAJOR INDICATIONS	USUAL ADULT DOSAGES	NURSING IMPLICATIONS
Ethanolamines			
dimenhydrinate	Nausea, vomiting, and vertigo associated with motion sickness; vestibular system diseases	50 to 100 mg P.O. every 4 to 6 hours, p.r.n.; 50 to 100 mg I.M. every 4 hours p.r.n.; or 50 mg I.V. in 10 ml of saline solution injected over 2 minutes every 4 hours, p.r.n., not to exceed 400 mg/day	• Administer the drug with caution to elderly patients and children; they may be more sensitive to the medication. • Administer the drug with caution to patients with prostatic hypertrophy, bladder neck obstruction, narrow-angle glaucoma, bronchial asthma, or cardiac dysrhythmias and whenever anticholinergic drug effects can aggravate other conditions. • Advise a lactating patient to avoid using the drug because small amounts of it may appear in breast milk and harm the infant.
diphenhydramine	Motion sickness; rhinitis and other allergy symptoms Dyskinesias and Parkinson's disease Hypnotic effects	25 to 50 mg P.O. t.i.d. or q.i.d., or 10 to 50 mg deep I.M. or I.V. 50 to 150 mg P.O. daily or 10 to 50 mg deep I.M. or I.V. 50 to 100 mg P.O. at bedtime	• Administer the drug with caution to a patient receiving an aminoglycoside, and monitor the patient closely. • Advise the patient to take dimenhydrinate or diphenhydramine at least 30 minutes, and preferably 1 to 2 hours, before traveling. • Advise the patient that drowsiness may occur and to avoid operating machinery or taking other sedating drugs or alcohol.
Ethylenediamines			
tripelennamine	Allergy symptoms	37.5 to 75 mg P.O. in elixir form every 4 to 6 hours not to exceed 900 mg/day; 25 to 50 mg P.O. in regular tablets every 4 to 6 hours, not to exceed 600 mg/day; 100 mg P.O. b.i.d. or t.i.d. in sustained-release tablets	• Do not administer 100-mg sustained-release tablets of tripelennamine to children. • Administer the drug with caution to elderly patients, because they are susceptible to dizziness, hypotension, and sedation. • Tripelennamine is usually contraindicated in patients with prostatic hypertrophy, bladder neck obstruction, narrow-angle glaucoma, and bronchial asthma. • Avoid administering the drug to a pregnant or lactating patient. • Administer the drug with caution to infants and children. Do not administer the drug to neonates.
Alkylamines			
brompheniramine	Allergy symptoms; seasonal and perennial allergic rhinitis	4 mg P.O. in regular tablets every 4 to 6 hours, not to exceed 24 mg/day; 8 to 12 mg P.O. in sustained-release tablets every 8 to 12 hours; 10 mg I.V., I.M., or S.C. every 6 to 12 hours, not to exceed 40 mg/day	• Do not administer sustained-release tablets to children under age 6, and administer the drug to children aged 6 to 12 as ordered. • Administer the drug with caution to elderly patients, because they are susceptible to dizziness, hypotension, and sedation. • Alkylamines are usually contraindicated in patients with prostatic hypertrophy, bladder neck obstruction, narrow-angle glaucoma, and bronchial asthma.

continued

SELECTED MAJOR DRUGS

Antihistaminic agents continued

DRUG	MAJOR INDICATIONS	USUAL ADULT DOSAGES	NURSING IMPLICATIONS
chlorpheniramine	Allergy symptoms; transfusion and drug reactions	4 mg P.O. in regular tablets every 4 to 6 hours, not to exceed 24 mg/day; 8 to 12 mg P.O. b.i.d. of sustained-release tablets; 5 to 20 mg I.V.	• Administer as ordered to children under age 6. Do not administer to neonates. • When administering intravenously, ensure that the patient is lying down. Sweating, fainting, and hypotension may occur with I.V. use. Use only preservative-free solutions for I.V. administration.
	Anaphylactic reactions	10 to 20 mg I.V. or I.M.	
Miscellaneous antihistaminic agents			
terfenadine	Allergic rhinitis	60 mg P.O. b.i.d.	• Avoid administering terfenadine to a pregnant or lactating patient. • Avoid administering terfenadine to children because its safety and effectiveness in children has not been established. • Advise the patient that drowsiness may occur and to avoid driving and other activities that require mental concentration until the patient's response to the drug is known. • Administer the drug cautiously to patients with prostatic hypertrophy, bladder neck obstruction, narrow-angle glaucoma, bronchial asthma, cardiac dysrhythmias, epilepsy, or seizure disorders and whenever anticholinergic drug effects can aggravate other conditions, such as hypertensive crisis.

to drive or engage in activities that require mental alertness until the patient's reactions to the drug are known.
• Know that combining antihistamines with alcohol or other CNS depressants adds to the drugs' sedative effects. Advise the patient taking antihistamines to consult the physician before taking any CNS depressants, such as narcotics, sedatives, barbiturates, OTC sleep aids, tranquilizers, tricyclic antidepressants, muscle relaxants, anesthetics, and alcohol.
• Suggest that the patient take the medication with food, milk, or water to avoid GI adverse reactions.
• If an antihistamine is prescribed for motion sickness, instruct the patient to take it at least 30 minutes—but preferably 1 to 2 hours—before traveling.
• Remind the patient to keep this and other drugs out of the reach of children. Instruct the patient to be alert for signs of an overdose, such as clumsiness, unsteadiness, convulsions, severe drowsiness, and hallucinations. Advise the patient to get help immediately if an overdose is suspected.
• Advise a patient with a severe allergy to carry identification or wear an identification band that lists the type of allergy, the usual treatment, and the physician's name.

• Instruct the patient to report adverse reactions to the physician because a change in dosage may be indicated.
• Instruct the patient to drink fluids, chew sugarless gum, or suck on sugarless candy if the medication produces a dry mouth.
• Review all contraindications with the patient. Advise against using antihistamines during pregnancy, while breast-feeding, or if the patient has a history of asthma, enlarged prostate, cardiovascular disease, hypertension, intestinal blockage, kidney disease, overactive thyroid, stomach ulcer, or urinary tract blockage. Caution the patient against taking antihistamines concurrently with antimuscarinics (muscle relaxants and antispasmodics), MAO inhibitors, or drugs that can produce ringing in the ears or balance problems, such as aspirin, other salicylates, cisplatin, paramomycin, and aminoglycosides.
• When administering an antihistamine parenterally, administer deep I.M. using the Z-track method to prevent subcutaneous irritation.

CHAPTER SUMMARY

Chapter 63 included discussions of the antihistaminic agents, specifically H_1-receptor antagonists. Here are the highlights of the chapter:

• Antihistamines antagonize H_1 receptors, blocking the effects of histamine on target tissues. Most useful in exudative allergies, such as seasonal rhinitis and conjunctivitis, the drugs relieve symptoms without altering the antigen-antibody reaction. Additional uses exploit the drugs' sedative and antimuscarinic effects.

• The classes of antihistamines include ethanolamines, ethylenediamines, alkylamines, phenothiazines, piperazines, and miscellaneous agents.

• Ethanolamines are potent and effective H_1-receptor antagonists that produce significant antimuscarinic and anticholinergic effects. Sedation, the major adverse reaction, occurs in about half of all patients taking these drugs and ranges from drowsiness to deep sleep. GI adverse reactions, however, occur less frequently in this class than in the others. The ethanolamines are carbinoxamine, clemastine, dimenhydrinate, diphenhydramine, doxylamine, and phenyltoloxamine.

• The ethylenediamine class contains the oldest, the best known, and the most specific of the H_1-receptor antagonists. Ethylenediamines include pyrilamine and tripelennamine. In most cases, these drugs produce weak central effects, although sedation does occur. Stomach upset or discomfort are more common.

• Because alkylamines are the most potent H_1-receptor antagonists, they produce the same effects as other antihistamines when given in smaller doses. Their low production of CNS effects makes them suitable for daytime use. Although drowsiness may occur, CNS stimulation is more commonly associated with these drugs. Alkylamines include brompheniramine, chlorpheniramine, and triprolidine.

• Phenothiazines have significant anticholinergic and antimuscarinic activity. Primarily used for their antiemetic effects, phenothiazines also depress the CNS, which makes them useful for preoperative and postoperative sedation and for postoperative pain management with analgesics. The phenothiazines are methdilazine, promethazine, and trimeprazine.

• The piperazines, a class of long-acting H_1-receptor antagonists, significantly depress the CNS. In fact, this depressant action may contribute to their usefulness in managing allergic pruritus. The piperazines can also help prevent and treat motion sickness. This class consists of chlorcyclizine, cyclizine, hydroxyzine, and meclizine.

• Miscellaneous antihistaminic agents include azatadine, cyproheptadine, phenindamine, and terfenadine. Each of these drugs relieves some allergy symptoms and has unique considerations.

BIBLIOGRAPHY

American Hospital Formulary Service. *Drug Information 87.* McEvoy, G.K., et al., eds. Bethesda, Md.: American Society of Hospital Pharmacists, 1986.

Douglas, W.W. "Histamine and 5-Hydroxytryptamine (Serotonin) and Their Antagonists," in *Goodman and Gilman's The Pharmacological Basis of Therapeutics,* 7th ed. Gilman, A.G., et al., eds. New York: Macmillan Publishing Co., 1985.

Fastner, Z. "Antihistamines," in *Meyler's Side Effects of Drugs,* 10th ed. Dukes, M.N.G., ed. New York: Elsevier Publishing Co.,1984.

Hansten, P.D. *Drug Interactions,* 5th ed. Philadelphia: Lea & Febiger, 1985.

"Histamines and Antihistamines," in *Drug Evaluations,* 5th ed. American Medical Association. Philadelphia: W.B. Saunders Co., 1983.

Kastrup, E.K., et al., eds. *Facts and Comparisons.* St. Louis: Facts and Comparisons Division, J.B. Lippincott Co., 1985.

Labson, L.H. "Doctor, I Can't Stand This Itching," *Patient Care* 18:89, October 15, 1984.

Leatham, A.M. "Safety and Efficacy of Antiemetics Used to Treat Nausea and Vomiting in Pregnancy," *Clinical Pharmacy* 5:660, August 1986.

USPDI, vol. 1. *Drug Information for the Health Care Provider,* 6th ed. Rockville, Md.: United States Pharmacopeial Convention, 1986.

USPDI, vol. 2. *Advice for the Patient,* 6th ed. Rockville, Md.: United States Pharmacopeial Convention, 1986.

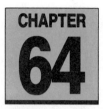

CHAPTER 64

CORTICOSTEROID AND OTHER IMMUNOSUPPRESSANT AGENTS

OBJECTIVES

After reading and studying this chapter, you should be able to:
1. Discuss the mechanisms of action of the systemic and topical corticosteroids (glucocorticoids and mineralocorticoids).
2. Identify the common clinical uses of the systemic and topical corticosteroids.
3. List the most common adverse reactions to the systemic and topical corticosteroids.
4. Discuss nursing implications appropriate to administration of the systemic and topical corticosteroids.
5. Discuss the mechanisms of action of the immunosuppressants.
6. Identify the common clinical uses of the immunosuppressants.
7. List the most common adverse reactions to the immunosuppressants.
8. Discuss nursing implications appropriate to administration of the immunosuppressants.

INTRODUCTION

Corticosteroid drugs, which are available as natural or synthetic steroids, are used to suppress the body's immune responses and to reduce inflammation. Natural corticosteroids are hormones produced by the adrenal cortex; most corticosteroid drugs are synthetic forms of these hormones. These drugs are classified according to their biological activities. The glucocorticoids, such as cortisone and dexamethasone, affect carbohydrate and protein metabolism; the mineralocorticoids, such as aldosterone and desoxycorticosterone acetate, regulate electrolyte and water balance.

Besides their primary uses as anti-inflammatory and immunosuppressant agents, glucocorticoids and mineralocorticoids are used for replacement therapy in patients with adrenocortical insufficiency (decreased secretion of endogenous corticosteroids) and for suppression of adrenocortical hyperfunction in patients with adrenogenital syndrome.

The noncorticosteroid immunosuppressant agents include antithymocyte globulin (ATG), azathioprine, cyclophosphamide, cyclosporine, and muromonab-CD3. Except for cyclophosphamide, they are used to prevent rejection of transplanted organs and experimentally to treat various autoimmune disorders. These drugs and the glucocorticoids and mineralocorticoids are the subjects of this chapter. Cyclophosphamide is used primarily to treat cancer. (See Chapter 73, Alkylating Agents, for details.)

Physiology of the adrenal glands

The adrenal glands, which lie at the superior poles of the kidneys, consist of an inner medulla and an outer cortex. (See *Anatomy of the adrenal glands* for information about their composition and function.) The medulla secretes the hormones epinephrine and norepinephrine. The three cortical layers secrete three classes of adrenocortical hormones: glucocorticoids, mineralocorticoids, and androgens.

The glucocorticoids, of which the most prominent is hydrocortisone (cortisol), are synthesized in the zona fasciculata, the middle layer of the adrenal cortex. (Their synthesis is controlled by another hormone, adrenocorticotropic hormone [ACTH], secreted by the pituitary gland.) In a 24-hour period, the adrenal cortex produces about 30 mg of glucocorticoids. Acute stress, such as from infection, trauma, or surgery, may increase glucocorticoid production tenfold. This increase occurs because stress stimulates secretion of the hormone corticotropin-releasing factor by the hypothalamus, which in turn activates pituitary secretion of ACTH, thereby increasing glucocorticoid secretion.

Acute stress also causes a sharp rise in levels of mineralocorticoids, which are synthesized in the zona glomerulosa—the outermost layer of the adrenal cortex. Production of these hormones is controlled by the level of potassium in the blood and by the renin-angiotensin

Anatomy of the adrenal glands

The adrenal glands are paired structures located retroperitoneally, one atop each kidney. Each gland consists of cortex, composed of three layers, and medulla, as shown in the cross section on the right. The outer layer of the cortex, the zona glomerulosa, produces mineralocorticoids; the middle layer, the zona fasciculata, produces glucocorticoids; and the innermost layer, the zona reticularis, produces androgen. The medulla stores catecholamines (epinephrine and norepinephrine).

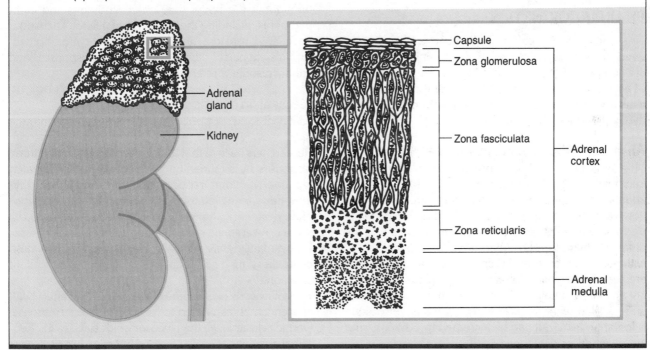

system. Aldosterone, the major mineralocorticoid, is secreted in response to sodium depletion rather than to ACTH secretion. Aldosterone causes retention of sodium at the distal convoluted tubule of the kidney, thus maintaining extracellular fluid volume and adequate circulation. The mineralocorticoids and the glucocorticoids share many functions in maintaining the cardiovascular tone essential for homeostasis.

The amount of androgens synthesized in the zona reticularis, the innermost layer of the adrenal cortex, is far less than the amount secreted by the gonads. Although androgens are secreted by the adrenal gland, they are not considered corticosteroids. Androgens are used to treat endocrine system disorders. (See Chapter 59, Androgenic and Anabolic Steroid Agents, for detailed information about these agents.)

For a summary of representative drugs, see *Selected major drugs: Corticosteroids and other immunosuppressant agents* on pages 1006 to 1009.

SYSTEMIC GLUCOCORTICOIDS

Most of the glucocorticoid drugs are synthetic analogues of hormones secreted by the zona fasciculata of the adrenal cortex. They exert anti-inflammatory, metabolic, and immunosuppressant effects. Drugs in this class include beclomethasone dipropionate, betamethasone, cortisone acetate, dexamethasone, hydrocortisone, methylprednisolone, paramethasone, prednisolone, prednisone, and triamcinolone and their derivatives.

History and source
Research conducted between 1855 and 1856 by Addison and Brown-Séquard established that the adrenal glands were essential to life. In the 1930s, the neuro-

surgeon Cushing described the complex of symptoms now known as Cushing's syndrome. In the 1940s, two types of adrenocortical hormones were identified, and five active glucocorticoids were isolated. Since that time, 70 different corticosteroids have been isolated from the adrenal gland. Drugs in this class are also synthesized through microbiological conversion of other corticosteroids to adrenocortical hormones.

PHARMACOKINETICS

The glucocorticoids are well absorbed when administered orally or topically. After I.M. administration, they are completely absorbed, but their onset and duration of action may vary. Glucocorticoids are bound to proteins and distributed via the blood with metabolism in the liver and excretion by the kidneys.

Absorption, distribution, metabolism, excretion

Most of the systemic glucocorticoids are absorbed well and quickly from the gastrointestinal (GI) tract after oral administration. Absorption after parenteral administration (except I.V.) varies. Glucocorticoids combined with freely soluble salts, such as sodium phosphate and sodium succinate, are absorbed rapidly; those combined with poorly soluble esters, such as acetate and acetonide, are absorbed slowly but completely. The glucocorticoids are absorbed equally well from the mucous membranes and the skin when applied topically. Rectal absorption is less than 20% but can be increased to 50% if tissues are inflamed or damaged.

All glucocorticoids are distributed to the tissues by the blood bound to corticosteroid-binding globulin and corticosteroid-binding albumin. They cross the placenta and are distributed into breast milk. Metabolism to the active drug prednisolone occurs in the liver, with the kidneys excreting the inactive metabolites.

Onset, peak, duration

The systemic glucocorticoids have a rapid onset of action and reach peak concentration levels within 1 hour of oral administration. The onset of action for parenteral and topical forms varies with the drug combination and the administration route. The peak concentration levels for forms combined with sodium phosphate or sodium succinate are attained in 1 hour when given I.M. For forms combined with acetate, the peak concentration level is attained in 24 to 48 hours when given I.M. or intraarticularly. The glucocorticoids' duration of action depends on the dosage form, administration route, and individual patient factors. No positive correlation exists between these drugs' half-life and their biological effects: glucocorticoid preparations may be short-acting (half-life of 8 to 12 hours), intermediate-acting (half-life of 18

to 36 hours), or long-acting (half-life of 36 to 54 hours), but their pharmacologic effects can last days, weeks, or longer. In fact, after prolonged therapy with large doses of these drugs, adrenal suppression of the ACTH response may persist for up to 12 months.

PHARMACODYNAMICS

Because of the systemic glucocorticoids' distribution throughout the body, they enter all tissues and compartments, including the cerebrospinal fluid. They influence lipid, protein, and carbohydrate metabolism, suppress hypersensitivity and immune responses, and enhance sodium retention.

Mechanism of action

Glucocorticoids suppress hypersensitivity and immune responses through a process not entirely understood. Researchers believe that the glucocorticoids inhibit these responses by suppressing or preventing cell-mediated immune reactions; reducing the concentration of thymus-dependent leukocytes, monocytes, and eosinophils; decreasing the binding of immunoglobulins to cell surface receptors; and inhibiting interleukin synthesis. Unfortunately, this clinically useful process may also mask the signs and symptoms of serious concomitant infections.

Glucocorticoids suppress the redness, edema, heat, and tenderness associated with the inflammatory response. On the cellular level, the glucocorticoids stabilize the lysosomal membranes so that they do not release their store of hydrolytic enzymes into the cells. The drugs also prevent plasma exudation, suppress the migration of polymorphonuclear leukocytes, inhibit phagocytosis, decrease antibody formation in injured or infected tissues, and disrupt histamine synthesis, fibroblast development, collagen deposition, microvasculature dilatation, and capillary permeability.

PHARMACOTHERAPEUTICS

Besides their use in replacement therapy for patients with adrenocortical insufficiency, the glucocorticoids are prescribed for their anti-inflammatory and immunosuppressant properties and their effects on the blood and lymphatic systems. Specific indications include suppression of adrenocortical hyperfunction in patients with adrenogenital syndrome and treatment of hypercalcemia in patients with cancer with bone metastases, such as breast cancer (glucocorticoids increase calcium excretion); multiple myeloma; and vitamin D intoxication. In patients with rheumatoid arthritis, osteoarthritis, rheumatic fever, nephrotic syndrome, inflammatory bowel disease, or collagen diseases, glucocorticoids are used for their anti-inflammatory effects: they may cause a rapid and marked reduction in symptoms but do not affect the progression of the disease. The glucocorticoids also are used to relieve hypersensitivity reactions by suppressing the inflammatory response in patients with asthma, food and drug hypersensitivities, bee stings, hay fever, contact or exfoliative dermatitis, ulcerative colitis, or vasculitis. These drugs also contribute antilymphocytic effects in treating leukemias, lymphomas, and myelomas; reduce or prevent the cerebral edema associated with neoplasms, neurosurgery, and trauma; are used in chronic obstructive pulmonary disease; and are combined with other immunosuppressants to prevent or treat transplant rejection. Finally, glucocorticoids are commonly used to decrease ocular inflammatory processes.

Patient factors, such as response to therapy and occurrence and types of adverse reactions, must be taken into account in selecting glucocorticoids and dosages for individual patients.

beclomethasone dipropionate (Beclovent, Vanceril). A synthetic drug, beclomethasone is used primarily as an inhalant to treat bronchial asthma that has not responded to conventional therapy or as an alternative to oral systemic corticosteroids for patients who need reduced dosages to decrease the risk or severity of adverse reactions. It is a potent anti-inflammatory agent and is contraindicated in acute asthmatic episodes.
USUAL ADULT DOSAGE: 2 to 4 inhalations of 42 mcg each, t.i.d. or q.i.d., up to 20 sprays daily.

betamethasone (Celestone). A synthetic drug, betamethasone has potent anti-inflammatory and immunosuppressant properties. Because of its minimal mineralocorticoid effects, it cannot be used alone to manage adrenocortical insufficiency. It is used for its anti-inflammatory properties in local injections into affected joints. The administration route and the dosage depend on the condition being treated and the patient's response.
USUAL ADULT DOSAGE: as an anti-inflammatory, initially, 0.6 to 7.2 mg P.O. daily or 0.5 to 9 mg I.M. daily, followed by individualized dosages for further therapy; for joint inflammation, 0.25 to 2 ml injected into the affected joint or bursa.

cortisone acetate (Cortone). Cortisone is usually the drug of choice for replacement therapy in patients with adrenocortical insufficiency. It has both glucocorticoid and mineralocorticoid properties. Dosage varies greatly,

depending on the nature and severity of the disease. It is not given I.V.
USUAL ADULT DOSAGE: initially, 25 to 300 mg P.O. or 20 to 300 mg I.M. daily; further therapy must be individualized for each patient.

dexamethasone (Decadron, Hexadrol). A potent anti-inflammatory agent, dexamethasone is used to treat acute self-limiting allergic disorders or exacerbation of chronic allergies. It also is used as a diagnostic aid to test for Cushing's syndrome and depression.
USUAL ADULT DOSAGE: 0.75 to 9 mg P.O. daily, usually in two to four divided doses.

dexamethasone acetate (Decadron-LA). A delayed-onset, long-acting salt of dexamethasone, dexamethasone acetate is not given when an immediate, short-term effect is needed. It is used to treat inflammatory conditions and cancer.
USUAL ADULT DOSAGE: for inflammatory conditions, 8 to 16 mg I.M. or 4 to 16 mg I.M. injected into the joint or soft tissue every 1 to 3 weeks; for cancer, 0.8 to 1.6 mg injected into the lesions every 1 to 3 weeks.

dexamethasone sodium phosphate (Decadron Phosphate, Hexadrol Phosphate). Another salt of dexamethasone, dexamethasone sodium phosphate is used in emergencies, such as cerebral edema or unresponsive shock, or when oral therapy is not possible. It is available in oral, inhalant, and parenteral forms.
USUAL ADULT DOSAGE: for bronchospasm or asthma, initially 0.5 to 9 mg I.M. or I.V. daily, or three inhalations (300 mcg) b.i.d. or q.i.d., up to 1,200 mcg daily; for inflammatory conditions, 2 to 4 mg I.M. into large joints, 0.8 to 1 mg I.M. into small joints; for cerebral edema, initially 10 mg I.V., then 4 to 6 mg I.M. every 6 hours for 2 to 4 days, then tapered over 5 to 7 days.

hydrocortisone (Cortef, Hydrocortone). The prototype systemic glucocorticoid, hydrocortisone is used to treat adrenocortical insufficiency and severe inflammation. Dosage varies greatly, depending on the nature and severity of the disease.
USUAL ADULT DOSAGE: 10 to 320 mg P.O. daily in three or four divided doses.

hydrocortisone acetate (Hydrocortone Acetate). A salt of hydrocortisone, hydrocortisone acetate is used to treat adrenocortical insufficiency and severe inflammation. The dosage depends on where the drug is administered: into soft tissue lesions, bursae, joints, or ganglia. It is not given I.V.

DRUG INTERACTIONS

Systemic corticosteroids

The corticosteroids interact with many other drugs. The nurse must be aware that these interactions affect electrolyes as well as medication dosages.

DRUG	INTERACTING DRUGS	POSSIBLE EFFECTS	NURSING IMPLICATIONS
systemic glucocorticoids, mineralocorticoids	barbiturates, phenytoin, rifampin	Decrease corticosteroid effect by speeding hepatic metabolism	• The corticosteroid dosage may need to be increased.
	furosemide	Increases incidence or severity of hypokalemia	• Monitor the patient's serum potassium levels; watch for signs and symptoms of hypokalemia. • Administer potassium supplements, as ordered. • Recommend foods high in potassium (for example, bananas, grapes).
	erythromycin, troleandomycin	Decrease corticosteroid metabolism	• The corticosteroid dosage may need to be decreased. • Observe for signs and symptoms of increased corticosteroid effects.
	salicylates	Increase risk of GI ulceration; decrease salicylate effect	• Watch for signs and symptoms of GI irritation (heartburn) and ulceration (melena). • As ordered, increase the dosage of a salicylate administered concomitantly with a corticosteroid. • During weaning, observe the patient for indications of salicylate intoxication (for example, tinnitus or hyperventilation) when the corticosteroid dosage is decreased.
	nonsteroidal anti-inflammatory agents	Increase risk of peptic ulcer	• Watch for signs and symptoms of GI irritation.
	vaccines, toxoids	Decrease the patient's response to vaccines and toxoids; may increase replication of attenuated viruses	• Administer with extreme caution and only as ordered. • After administration, observe for signs and symptoms of specific viral infection.
	warfarin	Decreases effect of anticoagulant because of corticosteroid-induced hypercoagulability	• The anticoagulant dosage may need to be increased. • Monitor the patient's prothrombin time.
	estrogen	Enhances corticosteroid effect	• Observe for signs and symptoms of increased corticosteroid effects. • The corticosteroid dosage may need to be reduced.

USUAL ADULT DOSAGE: 25 to 75 mg into soft tissue; 5 to 12.5 mg into tendon sheath; 25 to 50 mg into bursae and large joints; 10 to 25 mg into ganglia and small joints. Injections may be repeated.

hydrocortisone sodium phosphate (Hydrocortone Phosphate). A salt of hydrocortisone, hydrocortisone sodium phosphate is a parenteral drug used to treat adrenocortical insufficiency and severe inflammation. Dosage varies greatly, depending on the nature and severity of the disease.

USUAL ADULT DOSAGE: initially, 15 to 240 mg I.M., I.V., or S.C. daily; further therapy must be individualized for each patient.

hydrocortisone sodium succinate (A-HydroCort, Solu-Cortef). A salt of hydrocortisone, hydrocortisone sodium succinate is a parenteral drug used to treat adrenocortical insufficiency and severe inflammation. Dosage varies greatly, depending on the nature and severity of the disease.
USUAL ADULT DOSAGE: initially, 100 to 500 mg I.M. or I.V., then every 2 to 10 hours as needed; further therapy must be individualized for each patient.

methylprednisolone (Medrol). Methylprednisolone is used primarily as an anti-inflammatory or immunosuppressant agent; because it has minimal mineralocorticoid effects, it cannot be used alone to manage adrenocortical insufficiency.
USUAL ADULT DOSAGE: initially, 2 to 60 mg P.O. daily; further therapy must be individualized for each patient.

methylprednisolone acetate (Depo-Medrol, Medrol Acetate). The acetate salt of methylprednisolone is used for its anti-inflammatory properties.
USUAL ADULT DOSAGE: 10 to 80 mg I.M. or 4 to 80 mg injected into joints or soft-tissue lesions.

methylprednisolone sodium succinate (Solu-Medrol). Used with prednisone and prednisolone, this drug has been used in "pulse therapy" for patients with severe lupus nephritis or incapacitating rheumatoid arthritis. Successful "pulse therapy" induces a temporary remission.
USUAL ADULT DOSAGE: 10 to 250 mg I.M. or I.V. every 4 to 6 hours.

paramethasone acetate (Haldrone). Paramethasone is used primarily as an anti-inflammatory or immunosuppressant agent; because it has minimal mineralocorticoid effects, it cannot be used alone to manage adrenocortical insufficiency.
USUAL ADULT DOSAGE: initially, 2 to 24 mg P.O. daily in three or four divided doses; further therapy must be individualized for each patient.

prednisolone (Cortalone, Delta-Cortef, Fernisolone-P). Prednisolone is used primarily as an anti-inflammatory or immunosuppressant agent.
USUAL ADULT DOSAGE: initially, 5 to 60 mg P.O. daily in two to four divided doses; further therapy must be individualized for each patient.

prednisolone acetate (Key-Pred 25, Predcor-25). The acetate salt of prednisolone is used primarily as an anti-inflammatory or immunosuppressant agent. It is not given I.V.
USUAL ADULT DOSAGE: initially, 4 to 60 mg I.M. daily; further therapy must be individualized for each patient.

prednisolone sodium phosphate (Hydeltrasol). This drug is used primarily as an anti-inflammatory or immunosuppressant agent.
USUAL ADULT DOSAGE: 2 to 30 mg injected into joints, repeated every 3 days to 3 weeks, or 4 to 60 mg I.M. or I.V. daily initially; maintenance dose, 10 to 400 mg I.M. or I.V. daily.

prednisolone tebutate (Hydeltra-TBA). Used for its anti-inflammatory effects, prednisolone tebutate is injected into joints, soft-tissue, or lesions. It is not given I.V.
USUAL ADULT DOSAGE: 4 to 40 mg injected into joints, soft-tissue, or lesions every 2 to 3 weeks.

prednisone (Deltasone, Orasone). Prednisone is the oral glucocorticoid of choice for anti-inflammatory or immunosuppressant effects.
USUAL ADULT DOSAGE: initially, 5 to 60 mg P.O. daily; further therapy must be individualized for each patient.

triamcinolone (Aristocort, Kenacort). Triamcinolone is used primarily as an anti-inflammatory or immunosuppressant agent; because it has minimal mineralocorticoid effects, it cannot be used alone to manage adrenocortical insufficiency.
USUAL ADULT DOSAGE: 4 to 48 mg P.O daily in one to four divided doses.

triamcinolone acetonide (Azmacort, Kenalog). A slowly absorbed derivative of triamcinolone, triamcinolone acetonide is available as an inhalant for long-term therapy for bronchial asthma; it is also used I.M. for its anti-inflammatory and immunosuppressant properties.
USUAL ADULT DOSAGE: for bronchial asthma, 600 to 800 mcg (100 mcg/spray) by oral inhalation daily divided into three or four doses, or 4 to 48 mg P.O. daily divided into two to four doses; for anti-inflammatory or immunosuppressant action, 60 mg I.M. or 2.5 to 40 mg injected into the affected joint, bursa, or tendon sheath.

triamcinolone diacetate (Amcort, Aristocort Forte Parenteral). Triamcinolone diacetate is used for its anti-inflammatory and immunosuppressant properties.
USUAL ADULT DOSAGE: 4 to 48 mg P.O. daily divided into one to four doses, 40 mg I.M. weekly, or 2 to 40 mg injected into the joint, soft-tissue, or lesion.

Drug interactions
Many drugs interact with the systemic glucocorticoids. (For additional information on the interacting drugs and their possible effects, see *Drug interactions: Systemic corticosteroids.*)

ADVERSE DRUG REACTIONS

Because glucocorticoids affect nearly every body system, they can cause widespread adverse reactions. Such reactions are unlikely to occur with short-term administration, even of large doses. But when glucocorticoids are given for more than a brief period, devastating reactions can occur. If long-term therapy with these drugs is necessary, alternate-day therapy may decrease the severity of adverse reactions.

Predictable reactions

Long-term therapy with glucocorticoids may cause some degree of adrenocortical insufficiency, depending on the dosage frequency and, especially, on the duration of glucocorticoid therapy. For example, rapid withdrawal

---

Predictable adverse reactions to systemic corticosteroids

Systemic corticosteroids—the glucocorticoids and mineralocorticoids—affect almost all body systems, so they can cause widespread adverse reactions. Here, the most common of these reactions are listed by body system.

Central nervous system

- Behavioral changes ranging from mood alterations to psychoses and suicidal behavior
- Insomnia
- Increased intracranial pressure
- Seizures
- Cerebral edema
- Blunting of sensorium

Endocrine system

- Diabetes mellitus
- Hyperlipidemia
- Adrenal atrophy
- Hypothalamic-pituitary axis suppression
- Truncal obesity
- Dysmenorrhea

Fluid and electrolytes

- Increased retention of sodium and water
- Increased excretion of potassium

Immune system

- Suppressed immune response
- Suppressed inflammation
- Increased susceptibility to infection
- Suppressed signs and symptoms of infection

Musculoskeletal system

- Osteoporosis
- Aseptic necrosis of bone
- Increased susceptibility to fractures
- Muscle wasting
- Myopathy
- Arthralgia
- Muscle weakness

Gastrointestinal system

- Intestinal perforation
- Peptic ulcer
- Pancreatitis

Cardiovascular system

- Hypertension
- Edema
- Hypercoagulability
- Thrombophlebitis
- Embolism
- Atherosclerosis
- Polycythemia

Integumentary system

- Impaired wound healing
- Hirsutism
- Ecchymoses
- Acne
- Striae
- Thin, fragile skin

Metabolic system

- Alterations in protein, fat, and carbohydrate metabolism and protein catabolism
- Cushingoid symptoms
- Increased serum cholesterol levels
- Inhibited protein synthesis

Ophthalmic system

- Glaucoma
- Posterior subcapsular cataracts

of glucocorticoids after long-term therapy will cause acute adrenocortical insufficiency. The withdrawal syndrome is characterized by arthralgia, myalgia, anorexia, lethargy, weakness, depression, hypotension, and hypoglycemia. To prevent this syndrome requires gradual drug withdrawal. Although the adrenal glands almost always return to normal after a period of glucocorticoid-induced adrenocortical insufficiency, the patient may need replacement therapy during stressful situations—such as surgery, severe infection, or trauma—for up to a year. (See *Predictable adverse reactions to systemic corticosteroids* for a summary.)

Weakness of the proximal muscles of the extremities, shoulders, and pelvic muscles occurs occasionally in patients receiving large doses of glucocorticoids; this severe complication may force cessation of therapy. Even then, recovery is often slow and incomplete.

Prolonged therapy with systemic glucocorticoids causes abnormal fat distribution, depleting it in the extremities and increasing its deposition in the face and abdomen and between the shoulder blades. (See *Assessing cushingoid symptoms* for more information.) Glucocorticoids also can lead to catabolism (protein destruction) and inhibited protein synthesis, which results in muscle wasting, weakness, osteoporosis, poor wound healing, and immunosuppression.

These drugs alter carbohydrate metabolism by promoting glyconeogenesis and glycogenolysis and by antagonizing the action of insulin. This can result in diabetes mellitus in susceptible people; it may also cause hyperglycemia, glycosuria, and an increase in the severity of existing diabetes mellitus.

The immunosuppressant and anti-inflammatory effects of the glucocorticoids often delay detection of major infections and profoundly compromise patient resistance. The most common adverse reaction to oral inhalation therapy, for example, is fungal *(Candida albicans)* infection of the mouth and pharynx. Although usually of little clinical significance, such infections require antifungal therapy.

GI tract adverse reactions to glucocorticoids include abdominal distention, pancreatitis, ulcerative esophagitis, gastric irritation, and weight gain caused by increased appetite. Occasionally, these drugs play a role in peptic ulcer formation, reactivation, perforation, hemorrhage, or delayed healing.

Posterior subcapsular cataracts, particularly in children, may occur with prolonged use of glucocorticoids. So may exophthalmos or increased intraocular pressure, occasionally causing glaucoma and damaging the optic nerve. Glucocorticoids also may induce secondary fungal or viral eye infections.

Assessing cushingoid symptoms

Prolonged corticosteroid therapy may result in the signs and symptoms associated with Cushing's syndrome, in which fat is distributed in the face, in pads between the shoulders, and around the waist.

Assessment:
● Observe the patient for the cushingoid signs and symptoms illustrated here and for muscle weakness, atrophy, hyperglycemia, renal disorders, mental changes ranging from euphoria to depression, and lowered resistance to infection.
● Be aware of and record the patient's dietary and fluid intake and output.
● Monitor the patient's emotional state and record those situations that the patient finds disturbing.
● Observe female patients for hirsutism and masculinizing tendencies that the patient may find distressing.

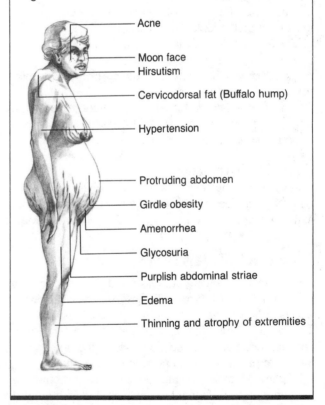

- Acne
- Moon face
- Hirsutism
- Cervicodorsal fat (Buffalo hump)
- Hypertension
- Protruding abdomen
- Girdle obesity
- Amenorrhea
- Glycosuria
- Purplish abdominal striae
- Edema
- Thinning and atrophy of extremities

Various dermatologic effects are associated with glucocorticoid therapy. These include skin atrophy and thinning, acne, striae formation, excessive diaphoresis, hirsutism, facial erythema, petechiae, ecchymoses, and easy bruising. Parenteral therapy sometimes results in scarring, induration, and sterile abscesses.

Glucocorticoids may cause adverse neurologic reactions as well, including insomnia, vertigo, headache, increased motor activity, restlessness, and seizures. Alterations in behavior can range from mood swings, anxiety, depression, and euphoria to frank psychoses. Patients sometimes become suicidal.

Fluid and electrolyte disturbances such as sodium retention may result in edema, weight gain, hypertension, and potassium loss, leading to hypokalemic alkalosis. Glucocorticoids also promote calcium excretion, which may cause hypocalcemia.

Because glucocorticoids inhibit ACTH secretion by the pituitary glands, the adrenal glands are not stimulated and may eventually atrophy. The resulting decrease in adrenal function means the patient must receive increased amounts of glucocorticoids (and mineralocorticoids) during periods of stress such as surgery.

Glucocorticoids also can increase red blood cell and hemoglobulin concentrations, leading to polycythemia; enhance coagulability, resulting in increased incidence of emboli and thrombi; decrease gastric absorption and increase renal excretion of calcium, resulting in decreased serum calcium levels; retard normal growth in children by its effect on the epiphyseal cartilage; and cause alterations in behavior ranging from mood elevation and anxiety to psychosis.

In children, even small doses of glucocorticoids can inhibit or even arrest growth by interfering with deoxyribonucleic acid (DNA) synthesis and cell division.

Unpredictable reactions

Reported anaphylactic reactions in patients receiving parenteral glucocorticoids may be from hypersensitivity to the preservative used in some parenteral formulations.

NURSING IMPLICATIONS

Every patient receiving glucocorticoid therapy requires close monitoring because of these drugs' widespread effects and potential to cause severe adverse reactions. This is particularly important for patients receiving long-term glucocorticoid therapy. Therefore, the nurse must be aware of the following nursing considerations:
• In general, avoid administering glucocorticoids to women who are pregnant or lactating; to children; and to patients with Cushing's syndrome, a known hypersensitivity to corticosteroids, active or untreated tuberculosis, severe infections, or acute psychoses.
• Administer prednisone cautiously in patients with severe hepatic dysfunction because it must be metabolized in the liver to prednisolone, the active drug.
• Keep in mind that oral inhalation therapy with beclomethasone is contraindicated in the treatment of acute asthmatic episodes because of its delayed onset of action.
• Administer glucocorticoids cautiously to patients with any of the following conditions: diabetes mellitus, hypothyroidism, congestive heart failure (CHF), cardiac disease, hypertension, fungal infections, herpes simplex, emotional instability or a history of psychoses, glaucoma, liver disease, diverticulitis, gastritis, peptic ulcer disease, metastatic cancer, osteoporosis, kidney disorders, sensitivity to tartrazine, myasthenia gravis, thromboembolic disorders, and latent tuberculosis or positive Mantoux tests.
• Obtain baseline data before a patient begins long-term glucocorticoid therapy. Such data may include an EKG, chest and spinal X-rays, a glucose tolerance test, a Mantoux test for tuberculosis, and measurements of blood pressure, body weight, and hypothalamic-pituitary-adrenal axis function.
• During systemic glucocorticoid therapy, monitor the patient's serum glucose levels, body weight, blood pressure, complete blood count (CBC), blood chemistries (particularly electrolytes), and ocular pressure, and regularly obtain chest and spine X-rays, as prescribed.
• Monitor the patient for signs of Cushing's syndrome. (See *Assessing cushingoid symptoms* on page 995 for details.)
• Monitor the patient's fluid and electrolyte balance, observing for signs and symptoms of hypernatremia, hypokalemia, and hypocalcemia.
• To prevent severe GI complications, assess the patient for epigastric pain 1 to 3 hours after meals and for nausea, vomiting, bloody stools, hematemesis, "coffee-ground" vomitus, decreases in hematocrit and hemoglobin levels, and a positive guaiac stool test.
• Because the patient taking glucocorticoids is more susceptible to infections than usual, monitor closely for signs of delayed wound healing, fever, and a decreased white blood cell (WBC) count, and be meticulous when handling or dressing all wounds, sites, tubes, and catheters.
• Observe for and report any emotional changes; suicide precautions may be needed for severely depressed patients.
• Monitor immobilized and elderly patients and postmenopausal women for signs and symptoms of osteoporosis.
• Monitor the patient for myopathy by assessing the patient's muscle strength and reported weakness.
• Patients with diabetes mellitus need special care. Measurement of fasting blood glucose levels and testing of urine are essential. Also, assess for the signs and symptoms of hyperglycemia, such as polyuria, polydipsia, polyphagia, and decreased or blurred vision.

• Periodically monitor all patients receiving glucocorticoids for signs and symptoms of hyperglycemia.

• Monitor the patient for signs of adrenocortical insufficiency—including hypotension, dehydration, fatigue, hyponatremia, diarrhea, and anorexia—during and after glucocorticoid therapy.

• Assess the patient for potential stressors (such as surgery, trauma, and infections) and adjust the dosage accordingly, as prescribed.

• For patients requiring short-term oral therapy (2 weeks or less), administer the daily dosage in four equally divided doses or in one single dose in the early morning. (Early-morning administration simulates the natural circadian rhythm of corticosteroid secretion—higher in the morning, lower in the evening.)

• Be aware that alternate-day therapy (a single dose administered every other morning) minimizes the risk or severity of adverse reactions when long-term therapy (longer than a month) is necessary.

• Administer oral glucocorticoids to a patient with food or milk to decrease the risk of gastric irritation.

• Because I.M. glucocorticoid preparations may produce atrophy at injection sites, inject them deeply into gluteal muscle, and avoid using the same site for repeated injections. Subcutaneous injection is usually contraindicated.

• When oral inhalation therapy with beclomethasone is indicated, teach the patient the correct way to use the inhaler: shake the inhaler well immediately before use; invert the inhaler; exhale completely; place the mouthpiece of the inhaler in the mouth and close the lips around it; while pressing the metal canister down with a finger, inhale slowly and deeply through the mouth; after holding the breath as long as possible, remove the mouthpiece and exhale as slowly as possible. Wait 1 minute (breathing normally) before inhaling again.

• Make sure the patient and the patient's family have a clear understanding of why the glucocorticoid drug has been prescribed and what risks are associated with taking it. Advise the patient who is taking the drug for more than 1 week not to stop taking it abruptly. Explain that the dosage must be decreased gradually before the drug can be discontinued.

• Instruct the patient about the name of the drug; its dosage, storage requirements, and rate of administration; adverse reactions it may cause; and the importance of taking it as prescribed. (See *Answers to patients' questions about prednisone therapy* for more information.)

• Review guidelines for missed doses with the patient. In general, a missed daily dose should be taken as soon as the patient remembers it (but not the next day— doses should never be doubled). The patient who misses one portion of a divided daily dose should take the next

---

Answers to patients' questions about prednisone therapy

Teach the patient why taking prednisone is necessary, why taking it as directed is important, and which adverse reactions it may cause.

Q. My doctor has prescribed prednisone. Why?

A. Prednisone is similar to a substance called cortisone that is made by your body. The drug helps decrease the pain, heat, or swelling that accompany arthritis, so-called allergic reactions, and other inflammatory conditions.

Q. How should I take it?

A. Your physician will give you instructions on how to take the medication. Follow the directions on the prescription's label. If you do not understand the directions, be sure to ask the pharmacist or your physician to clarify them for you. Take the drug regularly with food or milk, as prescribed.

Q. Is there anything special I need to know about taking prednisone?

A. Yes. Follow these guidelines:
• Weigh yourself daily. Report any unusual weight gain to your physician.
• Report to your physician any sore throat, cold, or infection that lasts an unusually long time.
• Report to your physician any changes in your appearance, moods, behavior, or (if female) menstrual periods.
• Report any occurrence of muscle weakness, frequent heartburn, or black, tarry stools.
• Tell your dentist or any other physician you consult that you are taking prednisone.
• Limit your salt intake and intake of sodium from other products, such as diet soda.
• Do not take aspirin or over-the-counter products containing aspirin.
• Wear or carry some form of medical alert identification that indicates you are taking prednisone.

Q. Is it okay to stop taking the drug when I feel better?

A. No. Do not stop taking your prednisone. When you no longer need the medication, your physician will gradually taper your dosage before discontinuing it completely.

---

dose on schedule. A patient on alternate-day therapy should not take a missed dose, even if it is remembered that same morning. Instead, the patient should take the missed dose the next morning, skip a day, then resume alternate-day therapy on the following day.

• Advise the patient to avoid the use of alcohol, cigarettes, caffeine, aspirin, or aspirin-containing compounds without consulting the physician.

• Teach the patient to recognize the signs and symptoms of GI disorders and to notify the physician immediately if they appear.

• Advise the patient to take extra medication along when traveling in case the trip lasts longer than expected. Another travel tip: Advise the patient not to pack the medication in a suitcase, but to carry it at all times.

• Instruct the patient to wear a medical identification tag or to carry a wallet card at all times; these are available at pharmacies. The patient also should notify any health care provider (dentists or oral surgeons, for example) about the glucocorticoid therapy before undergoing any other kind of treatment.

• To reduce the risk of infection, teach the patient self-care practices to prevent skin injury as well as techniques to take care of minor injuries.

• Instruct the patient to call the physician if signs or symptoms of infection, such as fever, develop.

• Advise the patient to avoid people with infections, especially respiratory infections.

• Stress to the patient the importance of periodic blood tests to monitor WBC function.

• For a patient on oral inhalation therapy, stress the importance of scrupulous oral hygiene, especially immediately after treatment.

• Inform the patient receiving long-term glucocorticoid therapy about the possibility of changes in appearance, such as fat deposits in the face, acne, hirsutism, and truncal obesity. Reassure the patient that these changes are therapy-related.

• Inform the patient that the glucocorticoids may cause emotional changes that should be reported to the physician.

• Instruct the patient about therapy-related dietary precautions, including adequate intake of proteins, vitamins, and calcium. Foods high in potassium and low in sodium also may be prescribed. Have the patient keep a weekly weight record and report any gain over 5 lb.

• Explain the need for the patient to keep active to prevent osteoporosis. (Periodic X-rays also may be required to monitor bone status.)

TOPICAL GLUCOCORTICOIDS

Topical glucocorticoids—available as creams, ointments, gels, aerosols, lotions, solutions, and drug-impregnated tape—are used to treat a number of skin diseases, principally for their anti-inflammatory and antiproliferative effects. The numerous preparations available have similar uses and actions and can cause similar adverse reactions.

The history and source of the topical glucocorticoids are covered in the "History and source" section of the systemic glucocorticoids on page 989.

PHARMACOKINETICS

The topical glucocorticoids are absorbed through the skin in varying degrees and enter the circulation. They then are metabolized in the liver and excreted by the kidneys.

Absorption, distribution, metabolism, excretion

Topical glucocorticoids are applied for their local effects on the epidermis or dermis. The skin is usually an effective barrier against percutaneous absorption; however, some absorption does occur. The most important factors determining the amount of percutaneous absorption are the vehicle used in the formulation and the degree of skin moisture. For example, occlusive dressings that prevent air circulation keep the skin moist and promote drug penetration. Other factors affecting absorption include drug concentration (the mechanism for absorption is passive diffusion), any break in the skin, the length of time the drug stays on the skin, the amount of drug applied, and the site of application (the face has the thinnest layer of skin, and the soles and palms have the thickest). Once the topical glucocorticoid enters the circulation, most of it is metabolized in the liver and excreted by the kidneys.

PHARMACODYNAMICS

The major actions of the topical glucocorticoids are anti-inflammatory and antiproliferative.

Mechanism of action

The anti-inflammatory effects of the topical glucocorticoids result partly from vasoconstriction, but the exact sequence of events is unknown. The vasoconstriction may be a direct or indirect effect exerted by the reduction of catecholamine, prostaglandin, or histamine levels at target cell sites. The drugs' anti-inflammatory effects may also result from interference with the migration of polymorphonuclear leukocytes through the capillary walls and from decreased adherence of WBCs to the capillary endothelium.

The glucocorticoids also exert anti-inflammatory effects by interfering with the function of lymphocytes and macrophages and by decreasing the action of lymphokines. (Lymphokines are released in the presence of an antigen and play a role in macrophage activation, lymphocyte transformation, and cell-mediated immunity.) The glucocorticoids also decrease the permeability of the cell membrane, impair the release of toxins or lysosomal enzymes, and inhibit the release or action of other chemical mediators during the inflammatory process.

Topical glucocorticoids that are more potent than hydrocortisone produce an antiproliferative effect on epidermal cells and dermal fibroblasts. In the epidermis, the drugs reduce ribonucleic acid (RNA) transcription, with a resultant decrease in DNA synthesis. When used to treat psoriasis, the topical glucocorticoids may interfere with the re-formation of the granular layer.

PHARMACOTHERAPEUTICS

All topical glucocorticoids are used to treat acute and chronic inflammatory dermatoses, psoriasis, atopic eczema, pruritus ani, neurodermatitis, contact dermatitis, seborrheic dermatitis, and exfoliative dermatitis. Because they evaporate, glucocorticoid creams are used on acute, wet lesions. Glucocorticoid ointments moisturize and are used on chronic, dry, scaly lesions. Any specific indications are noted in the listing that follows.

amcinonide (Cyclocort).
USUAL ADULT DOSAGE: 0.1% cream or ointment applied b.i.d. or t.i.d.

betamethasone dipropionate (Diprosone, Lotrisone).
USUAL ADULT DOSAGE: 0.05% cream, ointment, or lotion applied daily to q.i.d.; or 0.1% aerosol, one 3-second spray t.i.d. or q.i.d.

betamethasone valerate (Betatrex, Valisone).
USUAL ADULT DOSAGE: 0.1% cream, ointment, or lotion, applied b.i.d. or t.i.d.

clobetasol propionate (Temovate). To avoid percutaneous absorption, do not cover clobetasol with an occlusive dressing.
USUAL ADULT DOSAGE: 0.05% cream or ointment applied b.i.d. to a maximum of 50 grams/week and a total treatment time of 14 days.

clocortolone pivalate (Cloderm). Besides the usual indications, clocortolone is indicated for corticosteroid-responsive dermatoses.
USUAL ADULT DOSAGE: 0.1% cream applied daily to q.i.d.

desonide (DesOwen, Tridesilon). Desonide is indicated for acne rosacea as well as seborrheic dermatitis.
USUAL ADULT DOSAGE: 0.05% cream or ointment applied b.i.d. to q.i.d.

desoximetasone (Topicort).
USUAL ADULT DOSAGE: 0.05% or 0.25% cream applied b.i.d., or 0.05% gel applied b.i.d., or 0.25% ointment applied b.i.d.

dexamethasone (Aeroseb-Dex, Decaderm, Decaspray).
USUAL ADULT DOSAGE: 0.1% gel applied t.i.d. or q.i.d., or 0.01% or 0.04% aerosol b.i.d. to q.i.d. sprayed from 6 inches above the surface for 1 to 2 seconds.

diflorasone diacetate (Florone, Maxiflor).
USUAL ADULT DOSAGE: 0.05% cream or ointment applied b.i.d. to q.i.d.

fluocinolone acetonide (Fluonid, Synalar, Synemol).
USUAL ADULT DOSAGE: 0.01% to 0.2% cream, ointment, or solution applied b.i.d. to q.i.d.

fluocinonide (Lidex).
USUAL ADULT DOSAGE: 0.05% cream, ointment, solution, or gel applied t.i.d. or q.i.d.

flurandrenolide (Cordran).
USUAL ADULT DOSAGE: 0.05% or 0.025% cream or ointment applied b.i.d. or t.i.d., or 0.05% lotion applied b.i.d. or t.i.d., or 4 mcg/cm^2 drug-impregnated tape applied daily or b.i.d.

halcinonide (Halog).
USUAL ADULT DOSAGE: 0.1% or 0.025% cream applied b.i.d. to t.i.d., or 0.1% ointment or solution applied b.i.d. or t.i.d.

hydrocortisone (Aeroseb-HC, Cort-Dome, Dermacort).
USUAL ADULT DOSAGE: 0.25% or 2.5% cream or lotion, 0.5% to 2.5% ointment, 1% gel, or 0.5% aerosol sprayed daily to q.i.d.

methylprednisolone acetate (Medrol Acetate).
USUAL ADULT DOSAGE: 0.25% or 1% ointment applied daily to q.i.d.

triamcinolone acetonide (Aristocort, Kenalog).
USUAL ADULT DOSAGE: 0.025% or 0.5% cream, ointment, or lotion applied b.i.d. to q.i.d.

Drug interactions

No significant interactions occur between other drugs and the topical glucocorticoids themselves; however, chemicals used in formulating the various preparations do interact with certain drugs. Ethylenediamine, a stabilizer in certain preparations, interacts with systemic aminophylline, antazoline, antazoline hydrochloride ophthalmic solution, and edetate disodium, a preservative common in ophthalmic solutions. The interaction may cause allergic contact dermatitis, urticaria, and systemic eczematous contact-type dermatitis. Parabens are commonly added as preservatives to topical glucocorticoid preparations, especially creams. These parabens interact with such other paraben-containing formulations as toothpaste, cosmetics, and soaps, resulting in allergic contact dermatitis and urticaria.

ADVERSE DRUG REACTIONS

Many adverse reactions can occur with use of topical glucocorticoids. These effects are more pronounced with fluorinated preparations and when glucocorticoids are used with occlusive dressings.

Predictable reactions

Long-term use of the more potent topical glucocorticoids can cause atrophic changes in the epidermis and dermis, including striae, telangiectasia, subcutaneous fat wasting or muscle wasting, ecchymoses, and increased skin fragility. These changes may result from decreased synthesis of fibrous tissue by fibroblasts and increased breakdown of collagen. Facial skin eruptions usually result from improper use of fluorinated topical glucocorticoids. Steroid rosacea eruptions range from skin reddening to papulopustular lesions. Perioral dermatitis appears as a reddened papular eruption.

The anti-inflammatory action of topical glucocorticoids can mask the characteristic signs of certain conditions, such as tinea and scabies. Inappropriate use of these preparations may lead to superinfections or impetigo. Indiscriminate use of topical glucocorticoids in or around the eye may result in periorbital swelling, glaucoma, or cataracts.

Unpredictable reactions

Absorption of the topical glucocorticoids through the skin can cause the same adverse reactions as those occurring with systemic glucocorticoids. Allergic contact dermatitis is usually caused by chemicals added to the preparations.

NURSING IMPLICATIONS

The major consideration for nurses administering topical glucocorticoids is correct application: inappropriate administration may lead to severe adverse reactions.

- When applying topical glucocorticoids, use the smallest amount and the lowest concentration possible.
- Wash the patient's skin before applying the medication.
- Use caution when applying topical glucocorticoids in areas of thin or broken skin around the patient's eyes.
- Do not use fluorinated glucocorticoid preparations on the patient's face except as ordered.
- Do not apply high-potency glucocorticoid preparations on the patient's face, axilla, or groin except as prescribed.
- Report any infection, rash, pruritus, atrophic change, or purpura to the physician.
- Report any vision changes or unusual appearance of the patient's eyes.
- If the patient's body temperature rises after an occlusive dressing is used, remove the dressing and notify the physician.
- Do not use solutions on dry lesions (except as ordered) because they will cause further drying and itching; solutions also are contraindicated for use in the perineal area, where they can cause burning.
- Use gels and lotions for glucocorticoid application to the scalp or other hairy areas, as prescribed.
- To prevent skin damage, apply creams, lotions, ointments, solutions, or gels gently, leaving a thin coat; to apply medication to the scalp or other hairy areas, part the patient's hair and apply the medication directly to the lesion.
- When using an aerosol preparation, spray at least 6 inches above the site for 1 to 2 seconds; also, protect the patient's and your nose and mouth to prevent inhalation.
- When an occlusive dressing is necessary, apply medication as indicated; cover the area with a light gauze dressing followed by a layer of impermeable plastic (such as plastic wrap); seal the edges with hypoallergenic or paper tape; secure the dressing with a stockinette or an elastic bandage; and leave it in place for as long as prescribed. This technique is not usually used if infection is present or if the lesion is wet or exudative.
- Teach the patient that topical glucocorticoid preparations are for external use only and that overuse may cause adverse reactions.
- Teach the patient the proper technique for applying the prescribed glucocorticoid medication and any dressing needed.

• Emphasize that these preparations should not be used for purposes other than those prescribed, nor should they be shared with other family members. For other patient-teaching information, see the "Nursing implications" of the systemic glucocorticoids on page 996.

MINERALOCORTICOIDS

The mineralocorticoid drugs—administered orally, I.M., or as implanted pellets—are synthetic analogues of hormones secreted by the zona glomerulosa layer of the adrenal cortex. In general, these drugs affect electrolyte and water balance and are used for replacement therapy in patients with adrenocortical insufficiency. Drugs in this class include desoxycorticosterone acetate, desoxycorticosterone pivalate, and fludrocortisone acetate. Aldosterone, a natural mineralocorticoid, is the prototype drug in this class, but its use has been limited by its high cost, limited availability, and requirement of parenteral administration.

History and source
The principal endogenous mineralocorticoid, aldosterone was identified in the late 1950s, 25 years after the mineralocorticoid desoxycorticosterone acetate was isolated from the adrenal cortex by Reichstein.

PHARMACOKINETICS
The mineralocorticoids are well absorbed and distributed to all parts of the body. Some of the drug is metabolized to inactive forms by the body tissues, but the liver is the major metabolic site. The mineralocorticoids are excreted by the kidneys, primarily as inactive metabolites.

Onset, peak, duration
The onset of action, peak concentration levels, and duration of action of the mineralocorticoids vary widely—from minutes to months—depending on the preparation used, the dosage, and the administration route. The plasma half-life of desoxycorticosterone acetate injection is 70 minutes. The duration of action for the pellet form of this drug is 8 to 12 months; for the I.M. form, 1 to 2 days. The desoxycorticosterone pivalate repository injection has a duration of action of 4 weeks. After oral administration, fludrocortisone has an onset of action of 30 minutes and a duration of action of 1 to 2 days.

PHARMACODYNAMICS
The mineralocorticoids affect fluid and electrolyte balance by acting on the distal renal tubule to enhance the reabsorption of sodium and the secretion of potassium and hydrogen. The glomerular filtration rate is increased, favoring sodium excretion; however, the mineralocorticoids' net effect is usually sodium retention.

PHARMACOTHERAPEUTICS
The mineralocorticoids are used as part of replacement therapy for patients with adrenocortical insufficiency. They also are used to treat salt-losing congenital adrenogenital syndrome after the patient's electrolyte balance has been restored.

desoxycorticosterone acetate (Doca Acetate, Percorten Acetate). The most potent mineralocorticoid, desoxycorticosterone acetate is used to treat salt-losing adrenogenital syndrome and, with glucocorticoids, adrenocortical insufficiency.
USUAL ADULT DOSAGE: 1 to 5 mg I.M. daily, may range up to 10 mg. Once a maintenance dose has been established and administered for 2 to 3 months, a pellet may be implanted subcutaneously; one pellet is equal to 0.5 mg. Pellet implantation is repeated every 8 to 12 months.

desoxycorticosterone pivalate (Percorten Pivalate). This mineralocorticoid is used only for maintenance therapy for patients with salt-losing adrenogenital syndrome. With glucocorticoids, it also is used to treat adrenocortical insufficiency.
USUAL ADULT DOSAGE: 25 to 100 mg I.M. every 4 weeks.

fludrocortisone acetate (Florinef Acetate). Almost always given with cortisone or hydrocortisone, fludrocortisone is used to treat salt-losing adrenogenital syndrome and adrenocortical insufficiency.
USUAL ADULT DOSAGE: 0.1 to 0.2 mg P.O. daily with 10 to 37.5 mg cortisone P.O. daily or with 10 to 30 mg hydrocortisone P.O. daily in three or four divided doses.

Drug interactions
The drug interactions associated with the mineralocorticoids are similar to those associated with the systemic glucocorticoids. (See *Drug interactions: Systemic corticosteroids* on page 992 for additional information on interacting drugs and their possible effects.)

ADVERSE DRUG REACTIONS

Desoxycorticosterone has virtually no glucocorticoid effects, so the adverse reactions associated with it are limited to fluid and electrolyte imbalances and the signs and symptoms they cause. These include edema, hypertension, CHF, hypernatremia, hypokalemia, and hypocalcemia.

Although it is a very potent mineralocorticoid, fludrocortisone exhibits adverse reactions associated with both the glucocorticoids and the mineralocorticoids. (See *Predictable adverse reactions to systemic corticosteroids* on page 994 for more details.) The mineralocorticoids do not themselves cause hypersensitivity reactions, but chemicals used in their preparation may do so.

NURSING IMPLICATIONS

Because the mineralocorticoids are usually used for replacement therapy for patients with adrenocortical insufficiency, their use may be long-term; therefore, patient teaching and proper administration are very important. Besides the nursing considerations below, the nurse should be aware that the "Nursing implications" for systemic glucocorticoids (covered on pages 996 to 998) also apply to mineralocorticoid administration.
• Administer these drugs cautiously to pregnant patients and patients with CHF, diabetes mellitus, or hypertension.
• Monitor the patient closely for blood pressure elevation, edema, excessive weight gain, muscle weakness, dysrhythmias, or paresthesias.
• Inject I.M. desoxycorticosterone acetate only in the upper outer quadrant of the buttock; rotate injection sites, but never use the patient's arms to administer the drug.
• Inject desoxycorticosterone pivalate in the upper outer quadrant of the buttock with a 20-gauge needle.
• Teach the patient the importance of periodic evaluations of serum electrolyte levels and blood pressure.
• Advise the patient to control salt intake and to keep track of daily weight; teach the patient the signs of edema, such as swollen ankles and feet.

IMMUNOSUPPRESSANTS

Several drugs used for their immunosuppressant effects in patients undergoing allograft transplantation (for example, patients receiving kidney, bone marrow, heart, or skin allografts) are also used experimentally to treat autoimmune diseases. Drugs in this immunosuppressant class include azathioprine, cyclosporine, muromonab-CD₃, lymphocyte immune globulin, antithymocyte globulin (equine) (ATG). Cyclophosphamide, classified as an alkylating agent, is also used as an immunosuppressant, but it is primarily used to treat cancer. (See Chapter 73, Alkylating Agents, for information about this agent.)

History and source

The idea of using antilymphocyte compounds such as ATG to suppress the body's immune response was first expressed by Metchnikoff in 1899, but the first clinical use occurred only recently, in 1966. ATG is prepared from the plasma or serum of healthy horses hyperimmunized with human thymus lymphocytes. The monoclonal antibody muromonab-CD3 was developed by Kung and associates in 1979 and introduced clinically by Cosimi and associates in 1981. Stable hybridomas now provide a limitless supply of muromonab-CD3 antibodies.

PHARMACOKINETICS

The drugs in this category vary greatly in structure, and their pharmacokinetics are equally varied.

Absorption, distribution, metabolism, excretion

Azathioprine and cyclosporine are administered orally whenever possible, but they may also be administered I.V. Azathioprine is readily absorbed from the G.I. tract, whereas absorption of cyclosporine is varied and incomplete. ATG and muromonab-CD3 are administered I.V.

The distribution of azathioprine is not fully understood, but it is partially bound to serum protein; the unbound drug rapidly clears from the blood. Cyclosporine and muromonab-CD3 are widely distributed throughout the body, and about 90% of cyclosporine is protein-bound mainly to lipoproteins. Both azathioprine and cyclosporine cross the placenta. The distribution of ATG is not clearly defined, but it may be distributed in breast milk.

Azathioprine is metabolized in the liver, primarily to mercaptopurine. The metabolic pathway is unknown. Cyclosporine is metabolized in the liver. Muromonab-CD3 is consumed by T cells circulating in the blood; it does not react with other cells or tissues in the body.

Azathioprine and ATG are excreted in the urine, whereas cyclosporine is principally excreted in the bile.

DRUG INTERACTIONS

Immunosuppressants

Interactions involving the immunosuppressants and other drugs can greatly increase the patient's risk of infection. The nurse should assess the patient carefully and continuously for fever, malaise, and other signs and symptoms of infection.

DRUG	INTERACTING DRUGS	POSSIBLE EFFECTS	NURSING IMPLICATIONS
ATG	other immunosuppressant agents (except corticosteroids)	Increase risk of infection and lymphoma	• Monitor the patient for signs of infection.
azathioprine	allopurinol	Increases blood levels of azathioprine by slowing its metabolism	• An azathioprine dosage decrease is mandatory when these drugs are administered concomitantly.
cyclosporine	acyclovir, aminoglycosides, amphotericin B	Increase potential for nephrotoxicity	• Monitor the patient's blood urea nitrogen (BUN) and serum creatinine levels. • Monitor intake and output. • The dosage of nephrotoxic drugs may need to be decreased.
	other immunosuppressant agents (except corticosteroids)	Increase risk of infection and lymphoma	• Monitor the patient for signs of infection.
	ketoconazole	Increases serum cyclosporine levels	• Monitor the patient for excessive cyclosporine effect (neurotoxicity). • Monitor BUN and serum creatinine levels. • Monitor intake and output. • The dosage of cyclosporine may need to be decreased.
	rifampin, phenytoin, sulfamethazine, trimethoprim	Decrease plasma cyclosporine levels	• The dosage of cyclosporine may need to be increased.
	cimetidine	Increases plasma cyclosporine levels	• The dosage of cyclosporine may need to be decreased.
muromonab-CD3	other immunosuppressants agents	Increase immunosuppressant effectiveness	• Monitor the patient for signs and symptoms of infection.

Onset, peak, duration

Azathioprine reaches peak concentration levels 2 hours, cyclosporine 3½ hours, after oral administration. Peak serum levels of ATG depend on the patient's ability to catabolize foreign immunoglobulin G (IgG).

Muromonab-CD3's onset of action begins within minutes of I.V. administration. During treatment with 5 mg/day for 14 days, the patient's serum levels of muromonab-CD3 rise over the first 3 days, leveling off to 0.9 mcg/ml on days 3 through 14.

The estimated half-life of azathioprine is 5 hours, with 50% excreted in the urine within 24 hours. The clinical effects of immunosuppression, however, may persist for long periods after the drug is eliminated. The half-life of cyclosporine ranges from 10 to 27 hours. The plasma half-life of ATG is about 6 days but may range from 1½ to 12 days.

PHARMACODYNAMICS

Because of the varied structure of these drugs, they have a wide range of actions.

Mechanism of action

The action of azathioprine has not been precisely determined. It is an antagonist to metabolism of the amino acid purine and may therefore inhibit RNA and DNA synthesis. The drug also may alter RNA and DNA in some way, resulting in chromosome breaks, malfunctioning of the nucleic acids, or manufacture of fraudulent proteins. It also may inhibit coenzyme formation and function, thus interfering with cellular metabolism, and may act to prevent mitosis. In patients receiving kidney allografts, the drug suppresses cell-mediated hypersensitivities and produces various alterations in antibody production.

Cyclosporine's precise mechanism of action is also unknown, but experimental data suggest that the drug inhibits the helper T cells and the suppressor T cells. Its effectiveness in suppressing B cells is controversial. Cyclosporine does not affect the nonspecific immune system (the macrophages), nor does it cause significant leukopenia and lymphopenia. Unlike azathioprine, cyclosporine lacks myelosuppressive action.

Muromonab-CD3 is a monoclonal antibody that preferentially reacts with the T_3 complex and thus blocks the function of T cells. ATG has an unknown mechanism of action, but it may eliminate antigen-reactive T cells in peripheral blood and/or alter T-cell function.

PHARMACOTHERAPEUTICS

The immunosuppressant drugs are used mainly to prevent organ transplant rejection in patients who undergo organ transplantation.

lymphocyte immune globulin, antithymocyte globulin (equine) (Atgam). ATG is used as adjunctive therapy to prevent and/or treat rejection of kidney allografts. However, recent controlled studies have shown that it effectively treats acute rejections as well. ATG also has been used to treat aplastic anemia, with good results. It has been used with some success to treat acute graft-versus-host disease in patients with bone marrow allografts, but corticosteroids are still the therapy of choice. Finally, ATG has been effective in preventing rejection of skin allografts and has had some success as part of immunosuppressive protocols for the prevention and/or treatment of heart allograft rejection.

USUAL ADULT DOSAGE: for prevention of kidney allograft rejection, 15 mg/kg I.V. daily for 14 days, starting within 24 hours before or after surgery, followed by alternate-day therapy with the same dose for an additional 14 days; for the management of acute rejection, 10 to 15 mg/kg I.V. daily for 14 days, followed by alternate-day therapy with the same dose for up to another 14 days if necessary; for aplastic anemia, 10 to 15 mg/kg I.V. daily for 10 to 14 days, followed by alternate-day therapy with the same dose for 14 additional days; for prevention of graft-versus-host disease in patients with bone marrow allografts, 7 to 10 mg/kg I.V. every other day for a total of six doses; for the management of acute graft-versus-host disease, 7 mg/kg I.V. every other day for a total of six doses; for prevention of skin allograft rejection, 10 mg/kg I.V. 24 hours before the first allograft, followed by a maintenance dose of 10 to 15 mg/kg every other day.

azathioprine (Imuran). Used with corticosteroids, local radiation, and other cytotoxic agents, azathioprine helps prevent rejection of kidney allografts. It also is used to treat severe rheumatoid arthritis unresponsive to conventional therapies.

USUAL ADULT DOSAGE: for prevention of kidney allograft rejection, 3 to 5 mg/kg P.O. daily starting on the day of transplantation or 1 to 3 days before; after transplantation, the same dosage I.V. until the patient can tolerate oral dosing (usually in 1 to 4 days); for rheumatoid arthritis, 1 mg/kg P.O. daily; if necessary, after 6 to 8 weeks of therapy, the dosage may be increased by 0.5 mg/kg/day P.O. up to a maximum of 2.5 mg/kg/day; if the patient exhibits no therapeutic response in 12 weeks, therapy should be discontinued.

cyclosporine (Sandimmune). Used to prevent organ allograft rejection, cyclosporine is always given with corticosteroids. The drug also is used to treat chronic rejection in patients previously treated with other immunosuppressant agents to prolong graft survival of allogenic transplants and prophylactically to ameliorate or prevent graft-versus-host disease after bone marrow transplantation.

USUAL ADULT DOSAGE: 15 mg/kg P.O. 4 to 12 hours before transplantation; postoperatively, the same daily dose for 1 to 2 weeks, followed by doses decreased 5% per week to a maintenance level of 5 to 10 mg/kg/day; when cyclosporine cannot be administered orally, it may be given I.V. at one-third the oral dose (5 mg/kg I.V. daily), but the patient should be switched to oral administration as soon as possible.

muromonab-CD3 (Orthoclone OKT3). Muromonab-CD3 is used as first-line therapy or to "rescue" allograft rejection that has not responded to other therapies. It is also effective in preventing allograft rejection.

USUAL ADULT DOSAGE: 5 mg I.V. daily for 10 to 14 days.

Drug interactions

Most drug interactions with this class of drugs involve other immunosuppressant and anti-inflammatory agents and various antibiotic and antimicrobial drugs. (For additional information, see *Drug interactions: Immunosuppressants* on page 1003.)

ADVERSE DRUG REACTIONS

The immunosuppressant drugs can have multisystemic toxic effects and should be administered only under close medical supervision.

Predictable reactions

The primary adverse reaction to azathioprine is bone marrow depression, evidenced by leukopenia, macrocytic anemia, pancytopenia, and thrombocytopenia; this may alter clotting mechanisms and cause hemorrhaging. Nausea, vomiting, anorexia, and diarrhea can occur with large doses; mouth ulcerations, esophagitis, and steatorrhea are other complications. In a small number of patients, hepatic dysfunction has been reported. Other adverse reactions to azathioprine include alopecia, arthralgia, retinopathy, Raynaud's disease, and pulmonary edema.

The most severe adverse reaction to cyclosporine is nephrotoxicity, usually characterized by increased blood urea nitrogen (BUN) and serum creatinine levels. Thus, differentiating between allograft rejection and an adverse reaction to cyclosporine can be difficult. More common adverse reactions include hyperkalemia, hyperuricemia, decreased serum bicarbonate levels, hypertension, tremors, gingival hyperplasia, hirsutism, diarrhea, nausea, vomiting, generalized abdominal discomfort, and infection. Less common are gastritis, hiccups, and peptic ulcer. Occasional complaints include central nervous system effects (flushing, paresthesias, headache) and hepatotoxicity (usually occurring during the first month of therapy and with higher doses). Leukopenia, thrombocytopenia, and anemia are uncommon, and hematuria and psychiatric disorders are rare. In 3% of patients undergoing cyclosporine therapy, sinusitis and gynecomastia have been reported; conjunctivitis, hearing loss, tinnitus, hyperglycemia, edema, fever, and muscle pain have been reported in 2% or fewer.

With ATG therapy, the most common adverse reaction is fever accompanied by chills. Up to 20% of patients receiving kidney allografts experience leukopenia and/or thrombocytopenia while receiving these drugs. Early myelosuppression also may occur and force discontinuation of ATG. The immunosuppressant effects of ATG may cause local and systemic infections. Nausea, vomiting, diarrhea, stomatitis, hiccups, epigastric pain, and abdominal distention also may occur. Rash, pruritus, urticaria, and erythema have been reported in 10% to 15% of patients. Cardiovascular adverse reactions to ATG, such as hypotension, hypertension, tachycardia, edema, pulmonary edema, iliac vein obstruction, and renal artery stenosis, are uncommon.

Most adverse reactions to muromonab-CD3 occur during the first 2 days of therapy, the most common being fever and chills. Others include dyspnea, chest pain, vomiting, wheezing, nausea, diarrhea, and tremors. Severe (potentially fatal) pulmonary edema is reported in 2% or fewer of patients receiving this drug. The incidence of infection associated with muromonab-CD3 therapy is comparable to that associated with high doses of corticosteroids; the most common infections occurring during the first 45 days of therapy involve cytomegalovirus and herpes simplex.

Unpredictable reactions

All the drugs in this class can cause hypersensitivity reactions, which range from rash and serum sickness to anaphylaxis. A hypersensitivity pancreatitis may occur with azathioprine.

NURSING IMPLICATIONS

Suppressing the body's natural responses to foreign-body invasion requires drugs so highly potent that their use can also lead to life-threatening adverse reactions. Therefore, when administering immunosuppressant drugs, the nurse must exercise caution and monitor the patient closely. The nurse should also be aware of the following nursing considerations:

• Remember that the immunosuppressant drugs are contraindicated in pregnant patients.

• Monitor the patient for signs and symptoms of infection throughout the immunosuppressant therapy, keeping in mind that classic signs of infection may be suppressed.

• Monitor the patient's CBC (including platelets) and liver function tests frequently during azathioprine therapy.

• Evaluate the patient's liver enzymes and BUN, serum creatinine, and bilirubin levels frequently during cyclosporine therapy.

• Monitor cyclosporine blood levels periodically for patients receiving oral cyclosporine.

• Perform an intradermal skin test before administering the first dose of ATG, to assess the patient's risk of severe systemic adverse reactions.

• Document that the patient starting muromonab-CD3 therapy has had a chest X-ray 24 hours before receiving the first dose; the chest must be clear of fluid.

• Monitor the patient's WBC and differential counts and T cell assays at intervals during muromonab-CD3 therapy.

• Administer azathioprine in divided doses and/or after meals, as ordered, to reduce the risk or severity of adverse GI reactions.

(Text continues on page 1009.)

Corticosteroid and other immunosuppressant agents

This chart summarizes a sampling of these agents in clinical use today.

DRUG	MAJOR INDICATIONS	USUAL ADULT DOSAGES	NURSING IMPLICATIONS
Systemic glucocorticoids			
cortisone	Replacement therapy for adrenocortical insufficiency; anti-inflammatory conditions	25 to 300 mg P.O. daily or 20 to 300 mg I.M. daily	• The drug is contraindicated in systemic fungal infections. • Use cautiously in patients with GI ulceration, renal disease, hypertension, osteoporosis, varicella, vaccinia, exanthema, diabetes mellitus, hypothyroidism, thromboembolic disorders, seizures, myasthenia gravis, congestive heart failure (CHF), tuberculosis, ocular herpes simplex, hypoalbuminemia, emotional instability, or psychoses.
dexamethasone sodium phosphate	Cerebral edema	Initially, 10 mg I.V., then 4 to 6 mg I.M. every 6 hours for 2 to 4 days, then taper over 5 to 7 days	
prednisone	Inflammatory conditions and those requiring immunosuppression	Initially, 5 to 60 mg P.O. daily; further therapy must be individualized	• Gradually reduce dosage after long-term therapy; tell the patient not to discontinue the drug abruptly or without the physician's consent. • The patient may need a potassium supplement and a salt-restricted diet. • Report sudden weight gain or edema to the physician. • Observe the patient for signs of infection, especially after withdrawal from the drug. • Monitor serum electrolyte and blood glucose levels. • Inform a patient on long-term therapy about cushingoid symptoms. • Administer with milk or food to reduce the risk or severity of gastric irritation. • Instruct the patient to carry a card indicating the need for supplemental glucocorticoids during stressful periods. • Do not administer cortisone or prednisone I.V. • Observe for additional potassium depletion when administering the drug with diuretics or amphotericin B. • Immunizations may yield a decreased antibody response. • Teach the patient the signs and symptoms of early adrenocortical insufficiency: fatigue, muscle weakness, joint pain, fever, anorexia, nausea, dyspnea, dizziness, fainting.
methylprednisolone	Inflammatory conditions and those requiring immunosuppression	Initially, 2 to 60 mg P.O. daily; further therapy must be individualized	• Follow nursing implications for cortisone, dexamethasone, and prednisone above. • Watch for depression or psychotic episodes, especially in patients receiving high-dose therapy. • Inspect the patient's skin for petechiae; warn the patient about easy bruising. • A diabetic patient may need increased insulin.
Topical glucocorticoids			
betamethasone valerate	Inflammatory conditions such as corticosteroid-responsive dermatoses	0.1% cream, ointment, or lotion applied b.i.d. or t.i.d.	• Topical glucocorticoids are contraindicated in patients with viral skin diseases, such as varicella, vaccinia, and herpes simplex; fungal

SELECTED MAJOR DRUGS

Corticosteroid and other immunosuppressant agents continued

DRUG	MAJOR INDICATIONS	USUAL ADULT DOSAGES	NURSING IMPLICATIONS
betamethazone valerate (continued)			infections and skin tuberculosis; and impaired circulation. • Avoid application in or near the eyes. • Beware of systemic absorption with occlusive dressings, prolonged treatment, or extensive body-surface application. • Stop the drug and notify the physician if the patient develops signs of systemic absorption, skin irritation or ulceration, hypersensitivity, or infection. • Before applying the medication, gently wash the patient's skin; to prevent skin damage, rub the medication in gently, leaving a thin coat; to apply to hairy sites, part the hair and apply the medication directly to lesions. • For a patient with eczematous dermatitis who may develop irritation from adhesive material, hold the dressing in place with gauze, elastic bandages, or stockings. • Tell the physician and remove any occlusive dressing if the patient's body temperature rises. • Change the dressing as ordered, inspecting the patient's skin for infection, striae, and atrophy; discontinue the drug and notify the physician if any of these occurs. • Instruct the patient to report signs or symptoms of a hypersensitivity reaction to the drug.
fluocinolone	Inflammatory conditions such as corticosteroid-responsive dermatoses	0.01% to 0.2% cream, ointment, or solution applied t.i.d. or q.i.d	
flurandrenolide	Inflammatory conditions such as corticosteroid-responsive dermatoses	0.05% or 0.025% cream or ointment applied t.i.d. or q.i.d., or 4 mcg/cm² drug-impregnated tape applied daily or b.i.d.	
triamcinolone acetonide	Inflammatory conditions such as corticosteroid-responsive dermatoses	0.025% or 0.5% cream, ointment, or lotion applied b.i.d. to q.i.d.	
Mineralocorticoids			
desoxycorticosterone acetate, desoxycorticosterone pivalate	Adrenocortical insufficiency, salt-losing adrenogenital syndrome	1 to 5 mg (acetate) I.M. daily, or 1 pellet (125 mg) implanted subcutaneously for each 0.5 mg of the daily maintenance dose; 25 to 100 mg (pivalate) I.M. every 4 weeks	• The drug is contraindicated in patients with hypertension, CHF, or cardiac disease. • Use cautiously in patients with Addison's disease, who may have exaggerated adverse reactions. • Report significant weight gain and any evidence of edema, hypertension, or cardiac symptoms to the physician. • Monitor sodium and potassium levels and fluid intake; the patient may need a salt-restricted diet and a potassium supplement. • Watch for additional potassium depletion from diuretics and amphotericin B.
fludrocortisone	Adrenocortical insufficiency, salt-losing adrenogenital syndrome	0.1 to 0.2 mg P.O. daily with 10 to 37.5 mg cortisone P.O. daily or with 10 to 30 mg hydrocortisone P.O. daily in three or four divided doses	• The drug is contraindicated in patients with systemic fungal infections. • Use cautiously in patients with GI ulceration, renal disease, hypertension, osteoporosis, varicella, vaccinia, exanthema, diabetes mellitus, cushingoid symptoms, thromboembolic disorders, myasthenia gravis, metastatic cancer, CHF, tuberculosis, ocular herpes simplex, hypoalbuminemia, emotional instability, or psychoses. • Reduce the dosage gradually, as ordered, after long-term therapy; tell the patient not to discontinue the drug abruptly or without consulting the physician. • Monitor the patient's blood pressure and serum electrolyte levels.

continued

Corticosteroid and other immunosuppressant agents continued

DRUG	MAJOR INDICATIONS	USUAL ADULT DOSAGES	NURSING IMPLICATIONS
fludrocortisone (continued)			• Weigh the patient daily, and report a sudden weight gain to the physician. • Stress (for example, fever, trauma, surgery, or emotional problems) may increase adrenocortical insufficiency, so the drug dosage may have to be increased. • Instruct the patient to carry a card indicating the need for supplemental mineralocorticoids during periods of stress. • Teach the patient with adrenocortical insufficiency to watch for and report any occurrence of fatigue, muscle weakness, joint pain, fever, anorexia, nausea, dyspnea, dizziness, or fainting. • Inform the patient that mild peripheral edema is common and may occur. • Monitor for depression or psychotic episodes, especially in patients receiving high-dose therapy. • Inspect the patient's skin for petechiae; warn the patient about easy bruising. • Unless contraindicated, provide a salt-restricted diet rich in potassium and protein; a potassium supplement may be needed. • Give P.O. doses with food when possible. • Watch for additional potassium depletion from diuretics or amphotericin B.
Immunosuppressants			
azathioprine	Prevention of kidney allograft rejection	3 to 5 mg/kg P.O. daily, starting on the day of transplant or 1 to 3 days before; after transplant, the same dose I.V. until the patient can tolerate oral dosing	• Use cautiously or avoid in patients with hepatic or renal dysfunction. • Watch for clay-colored stools, dark urine, pruritus, and yellow skin and sclera and for increased alkaline phosphatase, bilirubin, SGOT, and SGPT levels. • For a patient undergoing kidney allograft transplantation, start the drug 1 to 5 days before surgery and continue it 24 to 96 hours after surgery, as ordered. • Check the patient's hemoglobin, WBC, and platelet counts at least once a week, and more often at the beginning of treatment; stop the drug immediately, as ordered, when the patient's WBC count is less than 3,000/mm³, to prevent irreversible bone marrow depression. • Warn the patient to report even mild symptoms of infection, such as coryza, fever, sore throat, or malaise. • To reduce the risk or severity of nausea, administer an antiemetic before administering the drug. • Strongly urge a female patient to avoid conception during therapy and for up to 4 months after stopping it. • Warn the patient that alopecia may occur. • Avoid I.M. injections in patients with severely depressed platelet counts (thrombocytopenia), to prevent hemorrhage.

Corticosteroid and other immunosuppressant agents continued

DRUG	MAJOR INDICATIONS	USUAL ADULT DOSAGES	NURSING IMPLICATIONS
ATG	Prevention or delay of allograft rejection	15 mg/kg I.V. daily for 14 days, followed by alternate-day therapy with the same dose for an additional 14 days	• Fever with chills is the most common adverse reaction. Premedicate the patient with an common adverse reaction. Premedicate the patient with an antipyretic and/or antipyretic and/or an antihistamine. • Strongly urge a female patient to avoid conception during therapy and for up to 4 months after stopping it. • Monitor the patient for leukopenia and thrombocytopenia. • Perform an intradermal skin test before the first dose; monitor the test site for at least 1 hour after injection. • Emphasize the patient's need for scrupulous personal hygiene. • Tell the patient to avoid crowds and persons with infections. • Teach the patient the signs and symptoms of infection and instruct him to notify the physician if they occur.
	Prevention of graft-versus-host disease after bone marrow allograft transplantation	7 to 10 mg/kg I.V. every other day for six doses	
	Management of acute allograft rejection	10 to 15 mg/kg I.V. daily for 14 days, followed by alternate-day therapy with the same dose for up to another 14 days	
	Treatment of graft-versus-host disease after bone marrow allograft transplantation	7 mg/kg I.V. every other day for six doses	
muromonab-CD3	Treatment or "rescue" of allograft rejection unresponsive to other therapies; prevention of allograft rejection	5 mg I.V. daily for 10 to 14 days	• Monitor the patient closely for 48 hours after the first dose. • To decrease the risk or severity of adverse reactions associated with the first dose, administer methylprednisolone sodium succinate 1 mg/kg I.V. before the first dose; 30 minutes after the first dose, administer hydrocortisone sodium succinate 100 mg I.V. • Give acetaminophen and antihistamines concomitantly to decrease the risk and severity of early adverse reactions. • Monitor the patient's temperature, which should not exceed 100° F. (37.8° C.) at the time of the first dose. • A chest X-ray performed 24 hours before the therapy begins must be clear of fluid; the patient's weight must be less than or equal to 3% above minimum weight in the week before treatment begins. • Monitor the patient's WBC count, differential count, and T cell assays. • Strongly urge a female patient to avoid conception during therapy and for up to 4 months after it. • Inform the patient that reactions to the first dose will reduce in severity with subsequent doses.

• Administer azathioprine I.V., as ordered, if the patient cannot tolerate it orally, but resume oral therapy as soon as possible.

• Give I.V. azathioprine as a bolus or diluted in normal saline solution or dextrose 5% in water (D_5W) and infuse over a period of 30 to 60 minutes.

• Mix oral cyclosporine with milk or orange juice at room temperature to increase its palatability, stir well, and administer the drink immediately; then put a little more milk or orange juice in the container and have the patient drink it, thus receiving the entire dose.

• If I.V. infusion of cyclosporine is ordered, dilute each milliliter in 20 to 100 ml of normal saline solution or D_5W immediately before administration and infuse over a period of 2 to 6 hours; ensure that the solution is free of particulate matter and discoloration. If it isn't, discard it and start over.

• Always give I.V. ATG as an infusion, diluted in 250 to 1,000 ml of normal or 0.45% saline solution over a period of 4 to 8 hours.

• Refrigerate ATG solution if it will not be given immediately; if refrigeration time plus infusion time exceeds 12 hours, do not use the solution.

• Administer ATG solution into high-flow veins to decrease the risk of phlebitis and thrombosis, and always use an in-line filter; make sure the solution is free of particulate matter and discoloration.

• Before administering muromonab-CD3 I.V. therapy, give the patient 1 mg/kg methylprednisolone sodium succinate I.V., as prescribed, to reduce the risk of a first-dose reaction.

• Thirty minutes after muromonab-CD3 I.V. administration, administer 100 mg of hydrocortisone sodium succinate I.V., as prescribed, to reduce the risk of a first-dose reaction.

• Be prepared to use acetaminophen and antihistamines to treat or reduce the severity of a first-dose reaction.

• Inspect the muromonab-CD3 solution for particulate matter; use a filtered needle to draw it up; and use a new needle for I.V. bolus administration.

• Administer muromonab-CD3 I.V. bolus in less than 1 minute; do not administer it as an infusion or with other solutions.

• Give the patient a complete explanation of the immunosuppressant's therapeutic purpose and its action in the body.

• Make the patient aware that infection, which can be life-threatening, is the most common hazard associated with immunosuppressant therapy.

• Emphasize that preventing infection requires scrupulous oral and personal hygiene while the patient is receiving immunosuppressant therapy.

• Advise the patient to avoid crowds and people who have infections while taking immunosuppressants.

• Urge the patient to postpone immunizations until after cessation of immunosuppressant therapy.

• Strongly urge a female patient to avoid conception during immunosuppressant therapy and for up to 4 months afterward.

• Emphasize that prescribed laboratory tests and periodic monitoring by the physician are essential.

CHAPTER SUMMARY

Chapter 64 discussed the systemic and topical corticosteroid and other immunosuppressant agents as they are used to suppress the inflammatory response and the allograft rejection response and to treat adrenocortical insufficiency. Here are the highlights of the chapter:

• Systemic and topical corticosteroids affect nearly every body system and have the potential to cause severe adverse reactions.

• Systemic glucocorticoids are synthetic analogues of natural corticosteroids secreted by the adrenal cortex. They are mainly used as replacement therapy for patients with adrenocortical insufficiency.

• Because the systemic glucocorticoids are distributed throughout the body, they can cause widespread adverse reactions that can be life-threatening. The best known is Cushing's syndrome.

• Nursing implications for the systemic glucocorticoids include the requirement for close monitoring of patients because of these drugs' widespread effects and potential to cause severe adverse reactions. Also emphasized is the importance of teaching patients correct timing and self-administration of doses and the signs and symptoms of expected and unexpected adverse reactions.

• Topical glucocorticoids' anti-inflammatory and antiproliferative effects make them useful in treating various skin disorders.

• Adverse reactions to the topical glucocorticoids are usually reversible.

• Nursing implications for the topical glucocorticoids include applying them correctly, understanding which formulations to use for which types of lesions, and teaching patients proper application techniques.

• Mineralocorticoids are also synthetic analogues of corticosteroids excreted by the adrenal cortex. They exert their principal effect on fluid and electrolyte balance and extracellular fluid volume. They are used principally for replacement therapy in patients with adrenocortical insufficiency.

• Nursing implications for the mineralocorticoids include preparing patients for long-term use of the drugs.

• The major immunosuppressant drugs, used to prevent or treat allograft rejection, are highly potent and can cause severe—even life-threatening—adverse reactions.

• Nursing implications for the immunosuppressant drugs include taking all possible measures to prevent infection, teaching the patient the importance of preventing infection, and explaining the need for the patient to report any change in health status because it may signal infection.

BIBLIOGRAPHY

American Hospital Formulary Service. *Drug Information 87*. McEvoy, G.K., et al., eds. Bethesda, Md.: American Society of Hospital Pharmacists, 1987.

Ballou, S., et al. "Intravenous Pulse Methylprednisolone Followed by Alternate-Day Corticosteroid Therapy in Lupus Erythematosus: A Prospective Evaluation," *Journal of Rheumatology* 12(5):944-48, October 1985.

Gilman, A.G., et al., eds. *Goodman and Gilman's The Pharmacological Basis of Therapeutics*, 7th ed. New York: Macmillan Publishing Co., 1985.

Goldstein, G., ed. "Monoclonal Antibody Therapy with Orthoclone OKT_3 in Renal Transplantation," *Transplantation Proceedings* 17(4):925-56, 1986.

Griffin, P., et al. "Antilymphocyte Globulin for the Treatment of Steroid Non-Responsive Acute Renal Allograft Rejection," *Clinical Nephrology* 21(2):115-17, February 1984.

Hahn, A., et al. *Pharmacology in Nursing*, 16th ed. St. Louis: C.V. Mosby Co., 1986.

Hansten, P. *Drug Interactions*, 5th ed. Philadelphia: Lea & Febiger, 1985.

Jamieson, T. "Corticosteroids for Rheumatic Disease. 1. Physiology, Pharmacology, and Therapeutic Strategies," *Postgraduate Medicine* 79(5):239-44, April 1986.

Matas, A., et al. "ALG Treatment of Steroid-Resistant Rejection in Patients Receiving Cyclosporine," *Transplantation* 41(5):579-83, May 1986.

Ortho Multicenter Transplant Study Group. "A Randomized Clinical Trial of OKT_3 Monoclonal Antibody for Acute Rejection of Cadaveric Renal Transplants," *New England Journal of Medicine* 313(6):337-42, August 8, 1985.

Weiner, M., and Pepper, G. *Clinical Pharmacology and Therapeutics in Nursing*, 2nd ed. New York: McGraw-Hill Book Co., 1985.

CHAPTER 65

URICOSURICS, OTHER ANTIGOUT AGENTS, AND GOLD SALTS

OBJECTIVES

After reading and studying this chapter, you should be able to:

1. Briefly describe the etiology and clinical signs and symptoms of gout and rheumatoid arthritis.

2. Identify the specific clinical indications for the following drugs: probenecid, sulfinpyrazone, colchicine, allopurinol, auranofin, aurothioglucose, and gold sodium thiomalate.

3. Describe the mechanism of action of the uricosurics probenecid and sulfinpyrazone and the antigout agents colchicine and allopurinol.

4. Identify the pharmacotherapeutic advantages and disadvantages of the uricosurics, other antigout drugs, and gold salts.

5. Describe the adverse drug reactions to the major drugs used to treat acute gouty attacks and rheumatoid arthritis.

6. Differentiate between the pharmacokinetic parameters of parenteral and oral gold salt preparations.

7. Identify the nursing implications for gold salt therapy.

INTRODUCTION

Physicians can select from many drugs to treat joint inflammation, depending upon the etiology. For example, gout and rheumatoid arthritis produce joint inflammation that responds to quite different drug interventions. Gout, a hereditary disease involving an error in an individual's metabolism, leads to hyperuricemia and the formation of monosodium urate crystals. Deposition of the monosodium urate crystals in and about a joint causes the inflammation and resultant pain.

Gout is best treated with uricosuric drugs, such as probenecid and sulfinpyrazone, or other antigout medications, such as colchicine and allopurinol. Indomethacin, naproxen, and phenylbutazone are also used to treat gout; these drugs are discussed in other chapters in this text.

In rheumatoid arthritis, inflammation and destruction occur primarily in the peripheral joints, producing pain. Treatment of rheumatoid arthritis, however, differs markedly from that of gout. The drugs of choice include auranofin, an oral gold salt, or aurothioglucose and gold sodium thiomalate, two parenteral forms of gold salt therapy. These drugs are used only after other drugs, such as nonsteroidal anti-inflammatory agents, have failed to work effectively.

For a summary of representative drugs, see *Selected major drugs: Uricosurics, other antigout agents, and gold salts* on page 1024.

URICOSURICS

The two major uricosurics are probenecid and sulfinpyrazone, which act by increasing excretion of uric acid in the urine. The primary goal in using the uricosurics is to prevent or control the frequency of gouty arthritis attacks.

History and source

In the 1940s, penicillin, just introduced, was in extremely short supply. The rapid renal excretion of penicillin also required that the drug be given frequently. Consequently, Beyer began a study to find an organic acid that would depress the tubular secretion of penicillin, which led to the discovery of probenecid in 1951.

Investigators discovered sulfinpyrazone while looking for drugs that would provide the anti-inflammatory effects of phenylbutazone without its adverse effects.

PHARMACOKINETICS

Uricosurics are absorbed from the gastrointestinal (GI) tract and metabolized in the liver.

Absorption, distribution, metabolism, excretion

Probenecid and sulfinpyrazone are rapidly and completely absorbed from the GI tract after oral administration. Distribution of the two drugs is also similar, with 75% to 95% of probenecid and 98% of sulfinpyrazone being protein bound. Metabolism of the drugs occurs in the liver; probenecid is metabolized slowly. Excretion takes place within the renal system, where small amounts of both drugs are filtered by the glomeruli. However, both probenecid and sulfinpyrazone are primarily secreted at the proximal tubule. Only small amounts of these two drugs are excreted in the feces. Sulfinpyrazone is excreted primarily unchanged.

Onset, peak, duration

The onset of action for probenecid and sulfinpyrazone usually occurs rapidly, within 30 minutes of oral administration. Maximal renal clearance of uric acid also occurs within 30 minutes of administering probenecid. Peak plasma concentration levels of probenecid are reached in 2 to 4 hours, while the peak concentration level for sulfinpyrazone is reached within 1 to 2 hours. The duration of action for both drugs usually ranges from 4 to 6 hours but may last as long as 10 hours. Half-life varies: probenecid's half-life is from 4 to 17 hours; that of sulfinpyrazone is much shorter, only 3 hours. (See *Pharmacokinetics of the uricosurics* for a depiction of the onset, peak, and duration.)

PHARMACODYNAMICS

Both probenecid and sulfinpyrazone competitively inhibit the active reabsorption of uric acid at the proximal convoluted tubules. As a result, urinary excretion of uric acid and a subsequent reduction of serum urate concentration are achieved.

Probenecid and sulfinpyrazone produce minimal, if any, analgesic or anti-inflammatory effect. Instead, by promoting a decrease in serum urate concentration, they reduce chronic joint destruction and tophi (sodium urate deposits around a joint) formation. The goal of using the uricosuric drugs is to reduce the frequency of gouty arthritis attacks.

PHARMACOTHERAPEUTICS

Probenecid and sulfinpyrazone, which lower serum urate concentrations, are indicated for patients with chronic gouty arthritis and tophaceous gout. An elevated serum urate concentration without symptoms of gouty arthritis is usually not considered an indication for uricosuric therapy. However, when the serum urate level exceeds 9 mg/dl, therapy is sometimes started to prevent joint changes and renal impairment, which can occur above that level.

Uricosuric drugs are also used in patients with visible tophi, with a serum urate concentration above 8.5 to 9 mg/dl, and with a family history of tophi or decreased uric acid excretion. Probenecid and sulfinpyrazone are contraindicated during an acute gouty attack; if taken at that time, the drugs only prolong inflammation.

Probenecid and sulfinpyrazone are also used to promote uric acid excretion in patients experiencing hyperuricemia secondary to thiazide and other related diuretics. Neither drug is indicated, however, for hyperuricemia secondary to cancer chemotherapy because of the risk of increasing uric acid nephropathy.

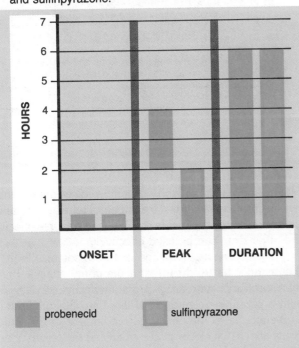

Pharmacokinetics of the uricosurics

This graph illustrates the onset of action, peak concentration levels, and duration of action of probenecid and sulfinpyrazone.

probenecid   sulfinpyrazone

DRUG INTERACTIONS

Uricosurics

All drug interactions involving the uricosurics represent potentially serious complications for the patient.

DRUG	INTERACTING DRUGS	POSSIBLE EFFECTS	NURSING IMPLICATIONS
probenecid, sulfin-pyrazone	weak organic acids (penicillin, cephalosporins)	Increase plasma concentration of the antibiotics	• Monitor serum antibiotic concentration levels frequently.
	anticoagulants	Enhance oral anticoagulant activity by increasing blood levels of anticoagulants	• Monitor closely when adding or discontinuing either drug. • Teach the patient the signs and symptoms of bleeding (bleeding gums, nosebleeds, easy bruising). • Monitor for changes in red blood cell count, hemoglobin, and hematocrit. • Monitor the patient for blood in urine, feces, or vomitus.
	thiazide diuretics	Enhance diuretic effect, inhibiting the action of uricosurics, which may precipitate an acute gouty attack	• Use caution when giving these drugs together. • Monitor serum uric acid levels.
	salicylates	May cause serious prolongation of bleeding time; may antagonize the action of probenecid and sulfinpyrazone	• Explain to the patient that prolonged use of salicylates is contraindicated. • Administer acetaminophen if an analgesic or antipyretic is needed. • Monitor for signs and symptoms of bleeding (bleeding gums, nosebleeds, easy bruising). • Monitor the platelet count.
	sulfonamides	Increase the activity and toxicity of sulfonamides because of a decrease in renal excretion	• Use caution when giving these drugs together. • Monitor fluid intake and output. • Urge the patient to consume enough fluids to produce a urine output of 1,500 ml daily.
	oral hypoglycemic agents	Enhance hypoglycemic action	• Use caution when giving these drugs together. • Teach the patient the signs and symptoms of hypoglycemia (hunger, nausea, lethargy, sweating, tachycardia). • Monitor blood for glucose levels.
	antineoplastic drugs	May increase serum urate concentrations	• Do not administer these drugs together.

Both probenecid and sulfinpyrazone work effectively when given in combination with allopurinol. Even though they promote the excretion of allopurinol's active metabolite, the uricosurics produce an additive effect and are of therapeutic value. Nonetheless, when one of the uricosurics is administered concomitantly with allopurinol, smaller doses of each drug are advised.

Probenecid, which is often considered the preferred drug of the two uricosurics, produces less severe GI and hematologic adverse effects than sulfinpyrazone. On the other hand, sulfinpyrazone produces fewer rashes and hypersensitivity reactions. If a patient is refractory to one uricosuric drug or is unable to tolerate its adverse effects, the other drug can be used effectively.

The major disadvantage of the uricosurics is that they cannot be used to treat acute gouty attacks. Furthermore, uricosuric drugs prove ineffective in patients with a creatinine clearance of less than 30 ml/minute. Probenecid also may increase the chance of an acute gouty attack, which can occur whenever the serum urate doses during the first 3 to 6 months of probenecid therapy.

probenecid (Benemid, SK-Probenecid). Used to treat chronic gouty arthritis and tophaceous gout, probenecid is also used to treat hyperuricemia secondary to diuretic use.

USUAL ADULT DOSAGE: 250 mg P.O. b.i.d. during the first week of therapy; after the first week, dosage is increased to 500 mg b.i.d. If symptoms are not controlled, the dosage can be increased by 500 mg every 4 weeks, up to 2 to 3 grams daily. If after 6 months of therapy no gouty attacks occur and the serum uric acid level falls within normal limits, the daily dosage may be decreased by 500 mg every 6 months.

sulfinpyrazone (Anturane). Used to treat chronic gouty arthritis, sulfinpyrazone is also used to treat tophaceous gout and hyperuricemia secondary to diuretic therapy.

USUAL ADULT DOSAGE: 100 to 200 mg P.O. b.i.d. during the first week of therapy; after the first week, the dosage is gradually increased until the full maintenance dosage of 200 to 400 mg b.i.d. is reached. The maximum dosage is 800 mg/day in divided doses.

Drug interactions

Numerous drugs interact with uricosurics. Although some of these interactions can be potentially harmful, others can prove beneficial. For example, probenecid elevates and prolongs the plasma concentration levels of penicillin. This dual therapy, while not often used, is primarily indicated to treat patients with sexually transmitted diseases requiring high plasma and tissue concentration levels of the antibiotic. The nurse should monitor for adverse reactions in patients taking uricosurics in combination with other drugs. (See *Drug interactions: Uricosurics* for a summary of the common drug interactions.)

Interactions between uricosurics and food do not seem to present problems. In fact, the patient should take uricosurics with meals, milk, or antacids to prevent adverse GI reactions.

ADVERSE DRUG REACTIONS

Though the uricosurics are usually well tolerated, some predictable and unpredictable adverse reactions can occur.

Predictable reactions

When given in therapeutic doses, probenecid is usually well tolerated by patients. Its most frequent adverse reactions are headache and GI distress, including anorexia, nausea, and vomiting. Other adverse reactions include flushing, dizziness, frequent urination, sore gums, and anemia.

When given in theurapeutic doses, sulfinpyrazone is usually well tolerated. Nausea, dyspepsia, GI pain, and blood loss are the most frequently reported adverse reactions to sulfinpyrazone. Reactivation or aggravation of peptic ulcer disease can also occur. Other adverse reactions include dizziness, rash, vertigo, tinnitus, and edema. Blood dyscrasias such as anemia, leukopenia, agranulocytosis, and thrombocytopenia are reported, but rarely.

Some patients taking either probenecid or sulfinpyrazone may form uric acid calculi. This usually occurs upon initiation of therapy. Acute gouty attacks also can occur in some patients during the first 6 to 12 months of therapy.

Unpredictable reactions

Hypersensitivity reactions can occur in some patients taking probenecid. Signs and symptoms of such reactions may include dermatitis, pruritus, fever, sweating, or hypotension. On rare occasions, a patient may experience an anaphylactic reaction, nephrotic syndrome, hepatic necrosis, or aplastic anemia. Unpredictable reactions to sulfinpyrazone may include skin rash, blood dyscrasias (anemia, leukopenia, agranulocytosis, thromboctyopenia, or aplastic anemia), and bronchoconstriction. Some patients have experienced reversible renal dysfunction following sulfinpyrazone therapy.

NURSING IMPLICATIONS

When administering the uricosurics, the nurse should:
• Initiate therapy cautiously in patients with a history of peptic ulcer disease, because uricosuric therapy is contraindicated in patients with active peptic ulcer disease.
• Be aware that probenecid is contraindicated in patients with known blood dyscrasias or with a history of uric acid calculus formation.
• Know that sulfinpyrazone is contraindicated in patients with a known hypersensitivity to the drug or in patients who are allergic to other pyrazole derivatives, such as phenylbutazone.
• Recommend that the patient take the drug with food, milk, or an antacid to prevent discomfort from GI distress, the most common adverse reaction to the uricosurics.
• Be aware that administering colchicine concurrently with the uricosurics may help to prevent the acute attack of gouty arthritis that occasionally occurs at the start of therapy.
• Assess the appropriate laboratory values, including a complete blood count (CBC), urinalysis, and serum uric acid levels.

- Monitor renal function tests and blood urea nitrogen regularly.
- Encourage the patient to drink between ten and twelve 8-ounce (240-ml) glasses of water daily. Maintaining a high fluid intake minimizes the probability of calculus formation.
- Encourage the patient to ingest a high-vegetable diet to alkalinize the urine. Maintaining an alkaline urine decreases the formation of uric acid calculi.
- Instruct the patient to take the drug as ordered and not to stop the drug without consulting the physician because gout symptoms may reappear.
- Instruct the patient to notify the physician if persistent GI distress or other symptoms occur.
- Alert the patient not to take aspirin during uricosuric therapy. If an analgesic or antipyretic is needed, the patient should take acetaminophen.
- Advise the patient to avoid drinking alcohol and eating foods high in purine, such as organ meats, while taking uricosuric agents.
- Be certain that the patient understands that uricosurics should not be taken during an acute attack of gout. Explain that using the drugs at that time will only prolong the symptoms of the gouty attack. Uricosurics are usually not started until 2 to 3 weeks after an acute attack.
- Alert diabetic patients who test their urine with Clinitest of the possibility of false-positive test results. Recommend, therefore, that the patient use Clinistix or some other urine glucose testing product.

OTHER ANTIGOUT AGENTS

Physicians frequently prescribe two other drugs, colchicine and allopurinol, to treat gout. Colchicine, the use of which is relatively specific, is indicated to treat acute gouty attacks. Allopurinol is not indicated for an acute attack but is used instead to inhibit uric acid synthesis, thereby reducing the metabolic pool of uric acid in the body and preventing gouty attacks.

History and source
Colchicine, a derivative of the crocus plant, the oldest drug available for treating gouty inflammation, has been used since the 6th century A.D.

Hitchings, Elion, and associates originally introduced allopurinol as a candidate antineoplastic agent. Allopurinol, however, lacked the antimetabolite activity necessary for an antineoplastic. During further investi-

gation, researchers found allopurinol to be a substrate for and inhibitor of xanthine oxidase. Furthermore, plasma concentration levels and renal excretion of uric acid were reduced in its presence. Rundles and co-workers then introduced allopurinol in clinical trials for treating gout. As a result of these successful trials, allopurinol was introduced as an antigout medication.

PHARMACOKINETICS
The pharmacokinetic properties of colchicine and allopurinol vary greatly. The variations in these drugs are discussed in the following paragraphs.

Absorption, distribution, metabolism, excretion
After oral administration, colchicine is absorbed from the GI tract and then partially metabolized in the liver. The drug and its metabolites then reenter the intestinal tract via biliary secretions. After reabsorption from the intestines, colchicine is distributed to various tissues throughout the body, including the kidneys, liver, spleen, and intestinal tract. The highest concentration level of colchicine, however, can be found in leukocytes. The drug is excreted primarily in the feces and to a lesser degree in the urine.

Allopurinol is rapidly absorbed from the GI tract after oral administration and is metabolized in the liver. The drug and its inactive metabolite alloxanthine are distributed throughout the tissue fluid, with the exception of the brain, where its concentration is about one third of that found in other tissues. Allopurinol is rapidly cleared from plasma, with small amounts excreted unchanged in the urine within 6 hours of ingestion. Small amounts are also excreted unabsorbed in the feces. Most of the drug, however, is slowly excreted in the urine as the metabolite alloxanthine.

Onset, peak, duration
Colchicine rapidly achieves peak concentration levels in the plasma within ½ to 2 hours. The pain that accompanies an acute gouty attack is alleviated within 12 to 48 hours after oral administration and 4 to 12 hours after I.V. therapy. The duration of action for colchicine varies, as plasma concentration levels decline 1 to 2 hours after ingestion and then rise as the drug recycles. After I.V. administration, the half-life of colchicine is 20 minutes. In leukocytes, however, where the highest concentration level of colchicine exists, the half-life is 60 hours.

Allopurinol appears in plasma within 30 to 60 minutes after oral administration. Its metabolite, alloxanthine, reaches peak concentration levels in 2 to 6 hours,

Sites of allopurinol action

This diagram depicts allopurinol's mechanism of action. Alloxanthine, the primary metabolite, inhibits the enzyme xanthine oxidase, which converts hypoxanthine to xanthine and then acts on xanthine to form uric acid. By blocking xanthine oxidase, alloxanthine inhibits uric acid production.

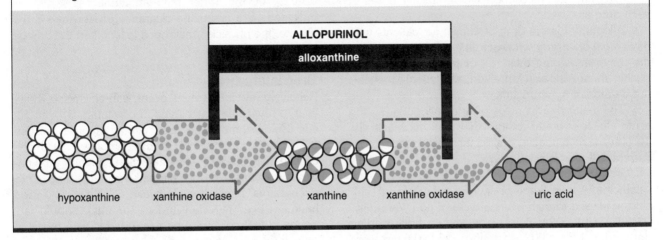

with a duration of action of 2 to 3 days. At that time, serum and urinary uric acid levels begin to fall. The half-life of allopurinol is 2 to 3 hours, during which time the drug is converted to alloxanthine. Alloxanthine, however, has a plasma half-life of 18 to 30 hours. The long half-life of alloxanthine contributes significantly to xanthine oxidase inhibition.

PHARMACODYNAMICS

The mechanism of action of allopurinol is much better understood than that of colchicine, even though colchicine has been in use for a longer period. Colchicine, however, appears to reduce the body's inflammatory response to monosodium urate crystals deposited in joint tissues. Colchicine may produce its effects by interfering with the polymorphonuclear leukocyte activity that results when metabolism, mobility, chemotaxis, or other leukocyte functions become inhibited.

Allopurinol lowers serum and urinary uric acid levels in the treatment of primary gout. Allopurinol and its primary metabolite alloxanthine inhibit xanthine oxidase, the enzyme responsible for converting hypoxanthine to xanthine as well as xanthine to uric acid. The inhibition of xanthine oxidase contributes to the pharmacologic effectiveness of allopurinol. (See *Sites of allopurinol action* for a more complete description of allopurinol's mechanism of action.)

PHARMACOTHERAPEUTICS

Colchicine is used to relieve acute attacks of gouty arthritis. When initiated early enough and in adequate amounts, the drug proves especially effective in relieving the pain. Colchicine is also recommended to treat recurrent gouty arthritis prophylactically. Also, colchicine administered during the first several months of allopurinol, probenecid, or sulfinpyrazone therapy may prevent the acute gouty attacks that sometimes accompany the use of these drugs.

Colchicine can be especially valuable in the diagnosis of gouty arthritis. When a small joint is involved, synovial fluid is unavailable for examination. If the condition is from gouty arthritis, therapeutic response occurs within 48 hours of the oral administration of colchicine and within 12 hours of I.V. injection. This consistent response to colchicine occurs only with gouty arthritis.

The use of colchicine has its advantages and disadvantages. The use of the drug in diagnosing gouty arthritis is of primary value. Colchicine is also effective in treating crystalline-induced arthropathies. Unfortunately, the drug produces several adverse effects, with those affecting the GI tract being the most severe. Colchicine is ineffective against non-gouty arthritis and does not affect uric acid metabolism.

Allopurinol is used to treat primary gout and gout associated with blood dyscrasias and related therapy. Allopurinol is recommended for primary or secondary uric acid nephropathy, with or without the accompanying symptoms of gout, and for patients with recurrent uric acid calculus formation. Allopurinol also proves effective in patients who respond poorly to maximal doses of uricosuric agents or who have allergic reactions or intolerance to uricosuric drugs. Allopurinol is useful in the prophylactic treatment of hyperuricemia in patients who are receiving cancer chemotherapy for myeloproliferative disorders. It is also effective when given in combination with the uricosurics, where smaller doses of each drug are used.

Allopurinol is the drug of choice for patients who have renal disease or who excrete excessive uric acid in the urine, increasing their risk of renal calculi. By reducing urinary uric acid formation, allopurinol eliminates the hazards of hyperuricuria.

The major disadvantage of using allopurinol is the acute attack of gouty arthritis that may occur initially. To prevent such attacks, physicians may prescribe concurrent use of colchicine.

colchicine. Administered orally and intravenously, colchicine is used to treat acute attacks of gouty arthritis. USUAL ADULT DOSAGE: for acute gouty arthritis, starting dose of 1 to 1.2 mg P.O.; thereafter, 0.5 to 0.6 mg every hour, or 1 to 1.2 mg every 2 hours until pain ceases or until nausea, vomiting, or diarrhea ensues. The total oral dose in a course of therapy for acute gouty arthritis may range from 4 to 8 mg. Given intravenously, the initial dose is 2 mg, followed by 0.5 mg every 6 hours until a satisfactory response is achieved. The total daily dose of I.V. colchicine should not exceed 4 mg.

As prophylactic or maintenance therapy for acute attacks of gout, the amount prescribed depends upon the number of attacks a patient has. For patients with less than one attack per year, the usual oral dose is 0.5 to 0.6 mg one to four times a week; in patients who have more than one attack per year, 0.5 to 0.6 mg/day. Some patients, however, may need up to 1.5 to 1.8 mg/day to achieve the benefit of prophylactic therapy. For I.V. prophylactic treatment, 0.5 to 1 mg is given once or twice daily. However, oral administration is preferred.

To prevent an attack of gout in patients with gouty arthritis who are undergoing surgery, use a dose of 0.5 to 0.6 mg P.O. t.i.d. for 3 days before and after surgery.

allopurinol (Zyloprim). Administered orally, allopurinol is available in 100-mg and 300-mg tablets. USUAL ADULT DOSAGE: to treat gout and hyperuricemia, an initial dosage of 100 mg P.O. daily; increased at weekly intervals by 100 mg to a maximum of 800 mg or until a serum uric acid level of 6 mg/dl or less is attained. Never exceed maximum dosage in an attempt to reach a normal serum uric acid level. Divide daily doses that exceed 300 mg.

Patients with renal failure require dosage adjustments. To estimate these dosage adjustments, the health care professional must first obtain a serum creatinine level and a 12- or 24-hour urine creatinine level to calculate a creatinine clearance. With a creatinine clearance of 10 to 20 ml/minute, the daily dose is 200 mg. When the creatinine clearance is less than 10 ml/minute, the dose is 100 mg. When renal impairment is severe, as indicated by a creatinine clearance of less than 3 ml/minute, the physician may need to lengthen the dosage schedule.

Drug interactions

Relatively few interactions occur with colchicine, however, a reversible malabsorption of vitamin B_{12} can occur. Sympathomimetics and central nervous system (CNS) depressants, when given in combination with colchicine, may interact, with interaction enhancing the patient's response to the sympathomimetics and CNS depressants. Interactions between colchicine and food have not been reported. In fact, the nurse should recommend that colchicine be administered with meals to reduce GI adverse reactions.

In combination with other drugs, allopurinol can create interactions that can seriously affect the patient. Anticoagulants, diuretics, iron salts, oral hypoglycemics, and certain cancer chemotherapeutic drugs can interact with allopurinol.

No known interactions between allopurinol and food occur. The drug should be given after meals to prevent GI upset. For reasons distinct from those in allopurinol therapy, gout patients should avoid the consumption of alcohol and foods high in purine content (kidney, liver, sardines, and anchovies). Avoiding such foods will minimize the number of acute gouty attacks. (See *Drug interactions: Other antigout agents* for a more detailed presentation of the drug interactions related to colchicine and allopurinol.)

ADVERSE DRUG REACTIONS

Both colchicine and allopurinol can affect the GI and integumentary systems. The adverse reactions to both drugs are discussed in the following section.

Predictable reactions

The most frequent adverse reactions to orally administered colchicine include nausea, vomiting, abdominal discomfort, and diarrhea. These reactions usually occur with doses used to achieve a therapeutic level of colchicine. But these reactions also indicate drug toxicity, and the physician should discontinue the colchicine. Therapy can be resumed after the symptoms have disappeared, usually within 24 to 48 hours. Gastrointestinal

DRUG INTERACTIONS

Other antigout agents

When given in combination with other drugs, colchicine and allopurinol can potentially cause interactions that affect the patient adversely. The nurse must exercise caution and monitor the patient closely.

DRUG	INTERACTING DRUGS	POSSIBLE EFFECTS	NURSING IMPLICATIONS
colchicine	vitamin B_{12}	Interferes with vitamin B_{12} absorption from the GI tract, apparently by altering the function of the ileal mucosa	• Avoid the use of oral vitamin B_{12} preparations. If necessary, give vitamin B_{12} intramuscularly or subcutaneously. • Monitor for signs and symptoms of vitamin B_{12} deficiency. • Inform the patient that the malabsorption is reversible.
	sympathomimetic and CNS depressants	Enhance response to CNS depressants	• Use caution when giving these drugs in combination. • Assess level of consciousness frequently.
allopurinol	oral anticoagulants	May inhibit the metabolism of the anticoagulants, leading to a prolonged anticoagulant half-life	• Monitor prothrombin time. • Teach the patient the signs and symptoms of bleeding. • Monitor the patient for blood in urine, feces, and emesis.
	diuretics	Enhance allopurinol toxicity	• Use caution when giving these drugs in combination.
	oral hypoglycemic agents	May reduce renal excretion, thereby enhancing hypoglycemic activity	• Use caution when giving these drugs together. • Teach the patient the signs and symptoms of hypoglycemia. • Monitor blood glucose levels.
	mercaptopurine or azathioprine	Increases antimetabolite effect of these drugs	• Consult the physician for appropriate dosage adjustments.

symptoms can also occur when colchicine is administered intravenously, but these adverse reactions usually occur only when the recommended dosage is exceeded.

Other predictable adverse reactions involving colchicine primarily affect the skin, vascular system, and CNS. The most frequent skin problems include dermatitis, urticaria, and alopecia. Hematologic problems from bone marrow depression that follows prolonged administration may include aplastic anemia, agranulocytosis, leukopenia, and thrombocytopenia. The only adverse reaction affecting the CNS is peripheral neuritis. Other known but rarely occurring adverse reactions include renal damage, muscular weakness, reversible azospermia, and increased serum concentration levels of alkaline phosphatase.

The most frequent predictable reaction to allopurinol is a skin rash, which is usually maculopapular. Gastrointestinal reactions include nausea, vomiting, diarrhea, and intermittent abdominal pain. Less frequent reactions include those that cause hematopoietic changes, such as agranulocytosis, anemia, aplastic anemia, and bone marrow depression. However, these adverse reactions usually result from the combined use of allopurinol and any drug known to cause such reactions. Peripheral neuritis and drowsiness can also occur.

Unpredictable reactions
Though colchicine produces few unpredictable reactions, some have been reported. These unpredictable reactions include bladder spasms, paralytic ileus, stomatitis, hypothyroidism, and nonthrombocytopenic purpura. Fever, chills, leukopenia, eosinophilia, arthralgias, skin rash, and pruritus may also be present. Rare instances of alopecia and altered liver function test results have occurred during allopurinol therapy.

NURSING IMPLICATIONS

The nurse must be aware of the following implications, which relate to the use, administration, specific interventions, and patient teaching regarding colchicine and allopurinol:

• Use caution when giving colchicine to elderly and debilitated patients because of possible drug accumulation.

• Be aware that colchicine is contraindicated in patients with serious GI distress, including nausea, vomiting, abdominal discomfort, and diarrhea. To avoid or ease less extreme adverse reactions, administer colchicine orally with food or milk. (Paregoric has been suggested as a remedy for diarrhea; however, prophylactic use of paregoric is not recommended because it may mask colchicine toxicity.)

• Prevent extravasation of colchicine into surrounding tissues during I.V. administration. To ensure correct I.V. administration, properly position the needle in the vein and check for good blood return before injecting the drug. Should extravasation occur, apply heat or cold to relieve the discomfort. Analgesics may also be given.

• Do not give more than 12 tablets of oral colchicine for any single acute attack in a 24-hour period. Oral colchicine is available in 0.5- and 0.6-mg tablets.

• When administering parenteral colchicine, do not give more than 4 mg/ml I.V. during a 24-hour period. Parenteral colchicine is available in a strength of 0.5 mg/ml given I.V. by diluting the drug with normal saline solution.

• Instruct the patient to discontinue the drug if nausea, vomiting, or diarrhea occurs.

• Tell the patient to keep colchicine readily available so that it can be taken as soon as symptoms of an acute gouty attack occur. Explain to the patient that a delay in taking the drug can impair its effectiveness.

• Instruct the patient to store colchicine in a tightly closed, light-resistant container.

• Do not give allopurinol to breast-feeding or pregnant women, or women who might be pregnant.

• Be aware that allopurinol is contraindicated in patients who report a severe reaction to the drug during prior use.

• To prevent an acute patient attack of gouty arthritis during allopurinol therapy, colchicine is often given prophylactically. GI distress can also accompany treatment; encourage the patient to take allopurinol after meals to decrease these GI reactions.

• Before therapy and periodically throughout treatment with colchicine or allopurinol, obtain and monitor CBC, urinalysis, serum uric acid level, and liver and kidney function test results.

• Instruct the patient to discontinue allopurinol and to notify the physician at the first sign of skin rash because this reaction may precede a severe hypersensitivity reaction.

• Inform the patient that drowsiness occasionally accompanies the use of allopurinol.

• Instruct the patient taking allopurinol to exercise caution when engaging in activities that require alertness.

• Instruct the patient taking colchicine or allopurinol to maintain a fluid intake of approximately 2,000 ml of water per day.

• Instruct the patient to store the drug in an airtight container.

GOLD SALTS

Gold salts are administered orally and parenterally, primarily to treat rheumatoid arthritis. The oral gold salt is auranofin, and the parenteral forms are gold sodium thiomalate and aurothioglucose.

History and source

In the 1960s, parenteral gold salts were introduced to treat rheumatoid arthritis because researchers thought that chronic arthritis might have a tubercular origin. In 1890, Koch had demonstrated in the laboratory that gold inhibited *Mycobacterium tuberculosis*. Subsequent to the introduction of parenteral gold salts, rheumatoid arthritis and tuberculosis were determined to be separate diseases. Nonetheless, the use of parenteral gold salts had been beneficial for rheumatoid arthritis patients; as a result, the drug was maintained as treatment for that condition. Introduced as an alternative to injectable gold therapy, oral gold salts came onto the market in late 1985.

PHARMACOKINETICS

The pharmacokinetics of gold salts vary depending upon their route of administration.

Absorption, distribution, metabolism, excretion

Absorption of auranofin, or the oral form of gold salts, takes place in the GI tract. Approximately 20% to 25% of auranofin is absorbed after an oral dose. Distribution of auranofin is primarily related to its binding with erythrocytes. Within an erythrocyte, 90% of auranofin is distributed intracellularly, while the remaining 10% is membrane bound. The metabolic fate of auranofin is not completely understood. Approximately 60% of the absorbed auranofin is excreted in the urine, with the remainder excreted in the feces. The unabsorbed auranofin is excreted primarily in the feces.

The parenteral forms of the gold salts, gold sodium thiomalate and aurothioglucose, differ in their ability to be absorbed. Gold sodium thiomalate is rapidly absorbed after I.M. administration; aurothioglucose is more slowly and irregularly absorbed. The parenteral gold salts are distributed throughout the body, with concentrations occurring in the kidneys, liver, spleen, bone marrow, and the reticuloendothelial cells of the lymph nodes. The metabolic fate of the parenteral gold salts remains obscure. Gold sodium thiomalate and aurothioglucose are both slowly excreted from the body, with approximately 70% excreted in the urine and the remaining 30% excreted in the feces.

Onset, peak, duration

Gold salts exhibit a slow onset of action. Benefits occur approximately 8 to 12 weeks after the initiation of therapy, and in some patients therapeutic benefits may not occur for 6 months or longer. Peak serum concentration levels, however, are found within a couple of hours of administration.

The duration of action of gold salts increases with each dose. The half-life changes dramatically depending on the administration mode. After 6 months of daily oral therapy, auranofin has a half-life ranging from 26 to 81 days. Parenterally administered gold salts have a half-life of 14 to 40 days after only 3 weeks of weekly injections. After the eleventh weekly dose of a parenteral gold salt, the half-life increases to 168 days.

PHARMACODYNAMICS

The complexity of the disease and the pharmacologic effects of gold salts makes understanding the mechanism of action of these drugs difficult. These drugs may act by decreasing liposomal enzyme release and altering the immune response.

Like the uricosurics, gold salts do not provide a direct analgesic action. Pain relief occurs from the anti-inflammatory and antiarthritic effects these drugs provide.

PHARMACOTHERAPEUTICS

Gold salts are one of a group of drugs referred to by rheumatologists as "remittive agents," which may block the inflammatory disease process rather than just provide anti-inflammatory action and pain relief.

Physicians prescribe gold salts only for patients who have an established diagnosis of rheumatoid arthritis and display an insufficient therapeutic response to an adequate trial of one or more nonsteroidal anti-inflammatory drugs (NSAIDs). NSAIDs are used primarily to decrease the number of painful, tender, swollen joints, to shorten the duration of morning stiffness, and to improve grip strength. Nondrug therapies, such as physical therapy, always accompany the use of gold salts in the management plan.

Using gold salts to treat rheumatoid arthritis has both advantages and disadvantages. When effective, these drugs can have dramatic effects. By slowing the progress of joint destruction, gold salts can effectively decrease the signs and symptoms that accompany rheumatoid arthritis. On the other hand, gold salts can be toxic—the primary reason why they are prescribed only after other treatments have failed.

A major benefit of auranofin is its oral administration. Auranofin also produces fewer toxic effects than parenterally administered gold, with mucocutaneous reactions and diarrhea being the most frequent adverse reactions. As a result, substantially fewer patients withdraw from therapy because of adverse reactions. Unfortunately, auranofin therapy usually proves slightly less effective than parenteral gold therapy, and the drug is likely to be discontinued because of the patient's poor or inadequate response.

Parenteral gold therapy is slightly more effective than auranofin, and fewer patients discontinue treatment because of poor therapeutic response. Parenteral gold also produces its therapeutic effects sooner and with more pronounced results than does oral gold. As a result, physicians prefer parenteral gold therapy to treat rheumatoid arthritis. Parenteral gold therapy is also preferred in patients with severe or rapidly progressing arthritis and in patients for whom compliance with the daily dosing regimen presents problems. The numerous, severe adverse effects of parenteral gold represent this therapy's major disadvantage. The patient also must make frequent office visits, which can be costly, to receive the parenteral administration of the drug. Because of the slow therapeutic response to gold salts, physicians usually prescribe the concurrent use of an NSAID or salicylate until the patient begins to experience symptomatic relief. If cartilage and bone destruction have also occurred, gold salts cannot reverse the structural damage to the joints.

auranofin (Ridaura). Available in a 3-mg capsule, auranofin is used to treat active synovitis associated with classical or definite rheumatoid arthritis. Auranofin is usually given concurrently with an NSAID.

DRUG INTERACTIONS
Gold salts

Gold salts are toxic drugs. The nurse should exercise caution when administering them with other drugs.

DRUG	INTERACTING DRUGS	POSSIBLE EFFECTS	NURSING IMPLICATIONS
auranofin, auro-thioglucose, gold sodium thiomalate	phenytoin	May increase blood phenytoin concentration levels	• Administer together cautiously. • Monitor serum phenytoin levels.
	parenteral gold, penicillamine, immunosuppressive agents, corticosteroids	Safety of concomitant administration has not been established	• Do not administer together.
	antimalarials, immunosuppressive agents, penicillamine, phenylbutazone	May produce blood dyscrasias and other potentially severe adverse reactions	• Administer together cautiously.

USUAL ADULT DOSAGE: 6 mg P.O. daily as a single dose or in two divided doses. Should adverse GI reactions occur, the dose will be reduced to 3 mg daily. Also the dosage will be reduced if the patient does not tolerate a 6-mg dose. If the patient's response is inadequate, dosage will be increased to 9 mg/day P.O. (3 mg t.i.d.). If patient response continues to be inadequate after 3 months of 9 mg/day P.O., therapy will be discontinued.

aurothioglucose (Solganal). The oil-based form of injectable gold, aurothioglucose is available in a suspension of 50 mg/ml. Parenteral gold salts are initially administered at weekly intervals. During the first week, an initial test dose of 10 mg is given.
USUAL ADULT DOSAGE: initial test dose of 10 mg I.M. followed in the second and third weeks by a dose of 25 mg; thereafter, weekly injections of 50 mg until 0.8 to 1 gram has been administered. Therapy must be reevaluated when the patient has received 1 gram of parenteral gold salt. If the patient shows signs of improvement without any toxic effects with 25- to 50-mg injections every third to fourth week, therapy will be continued indefinitely. Discontinue therapy in patients who receive the initial 1-gram dosage and show no clinical improvement.

gold sodium thiomalate (Myochrysine). The water-based form of injectable gold, gold sodium thiomalate is available in doses of 10, 25, and 50 mg/ml. The drug is initially administered at weekly intervals. During the first week, an initial test dose of 10 mg I.M. is given.
USUAL ADULT DOSAGE: initial dose of 10 mg followed in the second and third weeks by a dose of 25 mg I.M.; thereafter, weekly injections of 50 mg until 1 gram has been administered. The therapy will be reevaluated when the patient has received 1 gram I.M. of parenteral gold salt. If the patient experiences a favorable response, continued maintenance therapy at 25 to 50 mg I.M. every 2 weeks for 2 to 20 weeks will be given. Thereafter, if the clinical course of the patient remains stable, expect to give injections of 25 to 50 mg I.M. every third to fourth week indefinitely. Therapy will be discontinued in patients who receive the initial 1-gram dosage and have no clinical improvement.

Drug interactions
Though few drug interactions occur with gold salts, some occur that can produce blood dyscrasias. The safety of using auranofin concomitantly with injectable gold, penicillamine, immunosuppressive agents, or high doses of corticosteroids has not been established. No known interactions between gold salts and food occur. (See *Drug interactions: Gold salts* for a list of possible effects and nursing implications.)

ADVERSE DRUG REACTIONS
The numerous adverse reactions from gold salts explain why physicians do not use these drugs as the first line in treating rheumatoid arthritis.

Predictable reactions
Most adverse drug reactions involving the gold salts occur during the first 6 months of therapy. However, reactions can occur at any time, and the nurse must continually observe the patient on maintenance therapy for such reactions.

The most frequent adverse reactions to auranofin therapy involve the GI system. More than 50% of patients taking auranofin experience diarrhea. Nausea, vomiting, anorexia, abdominal cramps, and flatulence also occur but less frequently. Ulcerative enterocolitis is rare but serious.

Patients on oral gold therapy also experience mucocutaneous reactions. A rash, often preceded by pruritus, occurs in about 25% of patients taking auranofin. Other mucocutaneous reactions include conjunctivitis, glossitis, and stomatitis. Stomatitis occurs in approximately 13% of patients and produces shallow ulcers on the buccal membranes, palate, pharynx, and borders of the tongue. Alopecia, a dermatologic reaction, can also occur with gold salt therapy.

Other less frequent adverse reactions to auranofin involve the renal and hematologic systems. Renal effects include nephrotic syndrome and glomerulonephritis with proteinuria and hematuria. Blood dyscrasias, including leukopenia, thrombocytopenia, and anemia, have occurred.

Most adverse reactions to parenteral gold therapy occur during the second or third month of treatment after a total of 250 to 500 mg of the drug has been given. An estimated 25% to 30% of patients receiving parenteral gold discontinue therapy because of adverse reactions.

The most frequent adverse reactions involve mucocutaneous conditions, including stomatitis, gingivitis, glossitis, pharyngitis, tracheitis, and vaginitis. Parenteral gold salts can also produce severe blood dyscrasias, as well as renal and hepatic damage, which warrant immediate attention. Adverse gastrointestinal reactions rarely develop.

Unpredictable reactions

Most unpredictable reactions seem to occur with the parenteral gold salts. Up to 5% of patients receiving gold sodium thiomalate experience a vasomotor reaction, often referred to as the nitritoid reaction. This reaction is characterized by flushing, dizziness, nausea, weakness, tachycardia, and syncope. Having the patient lie down can alleviate the nitritoid reaction; then the patient should be switched to aurothioglucose.

Rare incidents of anaphylactic shock, syncope, bradycardia, difficulty swallowing, and angioedema have occurred with injectable gold. These reactions usually occur immediately or within 10 minutes of injection.

NURSING IMPLICATIONS

Because the gold salts are effective but potentially toxic drugs, the nurse should administer them cautiously and observe the following:

- Note that gold salt therapy is contraindicated in any patient who has experienced an adverse reaction to previous gold salt therapy or to other heavy metals.
- Be aware that gold salt therapy is also contraindicated in patients with urticaria, eczema, colitis, hemorrhagic conditions, and systemic lupus erythematosus. Patients who have recently received radiation therapy or who are severely debilitated should not receive gold therapy.
- Know that parenteral gold salt therapy is contraindicated in patients with Sjögren's syndrome.
- Instruct the patient to report diarrhea that persists longer than 3 to 4 days or that interferes with normal daily activities.
- Minimize or prevent diarrhea, the most common adverse reaction to auranofin therapy, by having the patient use antidiarrheal medications. Concomitant administration of an oral iron preparation may also prove effective. Also encourage the patient to increase the amount of dietary fiber.
- Advise the patient to avoid exposure to sunlight to prevent the aggravation of gold-induced dermatitis.
- Treat a patient's localized skin eruptions with topical corticosteroids as prescribed; more severe or generalized rashes may require oral antihistamines. Consider any skin eruption a reaction to the gold salts until proven otherwise.
- Explain to the patient that rinsing the mouth with 1 teaspoon salt in 8 ounces (240 ml) of water can help treat the symptomatic mild mouth ulcers.
- Remind the patient not to swallow any of the salt solution. Assess appropriate laboratory values before treatment and at monthly intervals. A urinalysis, CBC, and platelet count provide the baseline information to which subsequent monthly laboratory values will be compared in assessing the patient's response to therapy.
- Monitor the toxicity of the gold salts by questioning the patient at each visit about any signs and symptoms that indicate an adverse reaction.
- Administer auranofin orally; give aurothioglucose and gold sodium thiomalate intramuscularly, preferably intragluteally.
- Because aurothioglucose is an oil-based suspension, take special care to withdraw a uniform suspension from the vial. To do so, immerse the vial in warm water and then remove the medication with a dry needle and syringe.
- Instruct the patient to lie down during administration and to remain lying down for 10 minutes. Continue to observe the patient for adverse reactions for another 15 minutes.
- Explain to the patient that the therapeutic effects of the gold salts may not be experienced for 3 to 4 months.

Uricosurics, other antigout agents, and gold salts

Listed below are the drugs used most often to treat gout and rheumatoid arthritis.

DRUG	MAJOR INDICATIONS	USUAL ADULT DOSAGES	NURSING IMPLICATIONS
Uricosuric			
probenecid	Chronic gouty arthritis and tophaceous gout	250 mg P.O. b.i.d. during first week, then 500 mg b.i.d. Can be increased by 500 mg every 4 weeks until a daily maximum of 2 to 3 grams is achieved.	• Do not administer to a patient with active peptic ulcer disease or known blood dyscrasias. • Instruct the patient to take the drug with food to minimize GI distress. • Drug may be given concomitantly with colchicine. • Assess CBC, urinalysis, and serum uric acid level prior to beginning therapy. • Instruct the patient to maintain a high fluid intake while receiving this drug.
Other antigout agents			
colchicine	Relief of acute gouty arthritis	Oral: starting dose of 1 to 1.2 mg, then 0.5 to 0.6 mg every hour, or 1 to 1.2 mg every 2 hours. I.V.: 2 mg followed by 0.5 mg every 6 hours until satisfactory response occurs.	• Administer cautiously to debilitated or elderly patients. • When using an oral preparation, give with food or milk. • Consult with the physician to discontinue drug if nausea, vomiting, or diarrhea occurs.
allopurinol	Primary gout and gout arising secondary to hyperuricemia	100 mg P.O. daily; increased at weekly intervals by 100 mg to maximum of 800 mg or until uric acid level reaches 6 mg/dl or less	• Instruct the patient to take with meals to decrease GI symptoms. • Assess CBC, urinalysis, and serum uric acid level before therapy. • Frequently monitor appropriate laboratory values. • Consult with the physician to discontinue the drug at first sign of patient skin rash.
Gold salts			
auranofin	Rheumatoid arthritis	6 mg P.O. daily in single or divided doses	• This is a potentially toxic drug; administer with caution. • Instruct the patient to minimize the possibility of skin rash by avoiding exposure to sunlight. • Assess CBC, urinalysis, and platelet count at start of treatment and at monthly intervals. • Caution the patient that therapeutic effects may not be seen for 3 to 4 months.
aurothioglucose	Rheumatoid arthritis	10 mg I.M. during first week, 25 mg I.M. during second and third week, then 50 mg I.M. weekly until 0.8 to 1 gram I.M. is administered. Maintenance: 25 to 50 mg I.M. every 3 to 4 weeks.	• Caution the patient to return to the physician for regularly scheduled appointments. • Teach the patient the signs and symptoms of decreased platelet count. • Caution the patient to report any skin changes, diarrhea, or metallic taste to the physician.

• Instruct the patient to keep regularly scheduled appointments with the physician.

• Explain that monthly platelet counts are needed, and teach the patient the signs and symptoms of decreased platelet count (purpura, ecchymoses, petechiae, bleeding gums). Should the platelet count drop below 100,000/cu mm, the drug may be discontinued.

• Inform the patient that a metallic taste often precedes a sore mouth and other oral adverse reactions.

• Instruct the patient to store oral gold in a tight, light-resistant container and to use capsules before their expiration date, 4 years after the date of manufacturing.

CHAPTER SUMMARY

Chapter 65 presented the uricosurics, other antigout agents, and gold salts. Here are its highlights:

• Uricosurics and other antigout preparations are used to treat gout. The gold salts are used to treat rheumatoid arthritis. The drugs indicated for the treatment of gout cannot be used to treat rheumatoid arthritis, nor can gold salts be used to treat gout.

• The drug administered to treat gout depends upon the acuity of the disease. During an acute patient attack of gout, physicians prescribe colchicine or allopurinol. The uricosurics, including probenecid, are used only when a patient has chronic gouty arthritis or hyperuricemia, which places the patient at risk for an acute attack of gout.

• The use of gold salts can help a patient with rheumatoid arthritis achieve a remission. The effects of gold salts can be dramatic, but the drugs can be toxic.

• The uricosurics, antigout agents, and gold salts exert their effects through their anti-inflammatory actions; they are not analgesics.

• Administering these drugs is not without risk. The nurse should educate the patient about the risks and benefits of specific treatments. The nurse should also closely monitor the patient for adverse drug reactions. Monitoring involves comparing periodic laboratory test results and discussing with the patient the response to drug therapy.

BIBLIOGRAPHY

Abruzzo, J.L. "Auranofin: A New Drug for Rheumatoid Arthritis," *Annals of Internal Medicine* 105:274, August 1986.

Adramowicz, M. "Auranofin," *Medical Letter* 27:89, October 25, 1985.

American Hospital Formulary Service. *Drug Information 86.* Edited by McEvoy, G.K., et al. Bethesda, Md.: American Society of Hospital Pharmacists, 1986.

Gilman, A.G., et al., eds. *Goodman and Gilman's The Pharmacological Basis of Therapeutics,* 7th ed. New York: Macmillan Publishing Co., 1985.

Johnson, G. *Blue Book of Pharmacologic Therapeutics.* Philadelphia: W.B. Saunders Co., 1985.

Lo, B. "Hyperuricemia and Gout," *Topics in Primary Care Medicine* 142:20, January 1985.

Rodman, G., and Schumacher, R. *Primer on the Rheumatic Diseases.* Atlanta: Arthritis Foundation, 1983.

DRUGS TO PREVENT OR TREAT INFECTIONS

Attempts to treat systemic microbial infections with chemicals date back to the 16th century when mercury was used to treat syphilis. Organometallic compounds, such as mercury, arsenic, and bismuth, were introduced during the 1920s to treat syphilis, malaria, and other parasitic diseases. Compounds containing arsenic, an antimony, still are used to treat protozoa and other parasites. With the introduction of sulfanilamide in 1936, a new era began in treating infectious diseases. In 1941, penicillin was introduced as the first antimicrobial that could be mass-produced, making it available to treat a wide patient population. Since then, numerous other antimicrobials have been introduced.

The antimicrobial spectrum

The currently available antimicrobial drugs vary in their degree of effectiveness against different microorganisms. A drug's *spectrum of activity* refers to the number and type of organisms vulnerable to its action. Broad-spectrum antimicrobials affect a wide variety of pathogens, and narrow-spectrum drugs affect a few. Antimicrobials tend to affect pathogens with similar biochemical characteristics. The most common method used to distinguish among various microorganisms is the Gram stain, which uses laboratory dyes to stain organisms; the reactions reveal chemical differences in the cell wall. Organisms that are stained by the Gram stain are called gram-positive; those that are not are called gram-negative. For some bacteria, Gram staining is not a useful diagnostic tool. Some of these organisms, such as mycobacteria, can be stained with carbolfuchsin, then decolorized with ethyl alcohol and hydrochloric acid. They are classified as acid-fast if they retain the stain. Spirochetes can be visualized only by special techniques such as dark-field examination. Other important stains used to identify bacteria include Giminez stain for *Rickettsia*, Giemsa and Wright's stain for parasites and intracellular microorganisms, and fluorescent antibody for various organisms. Organisms with similar staining properties tend to be susceptible to the same antimicrobial agents. Therefore, a drug's antimicrobial spectrum may be de-scribed by its activity against gram-negative, gram-positive, or acid-fast bacilli. (See *Gram-negative and gram-positive bacteria* on page 1029 for examples of these organisms.)

Organisms also are classified as aerobes—those that can live and grow in the presence of oxygen—or as anaerobes—those that can live or grow without oxygen.

Microbial resistance

One factor limits the usefulness of antimicrobial agents: Pathogens may develop resistance to a drug's action. *Resistance* is the ability of a microorganism to live and grow in the presence of an antibacterial agent that is usually bactericidal or bacteriostatic. Resistance usually results from genetic events that develop mutant strains of the microorganism; these mutant strains resist a drug's activity by enhancing the action of specific enzymes that break down the chemical structure of the drug, restricting uptake of the drug or altering critical cellular target sites.

Drug selection

Selecting an appropriate antimicrobial agent to treat a specific infection involves several important factors. First, the microorganism must be isolated and identified. Then, its susceptibility to various drugs must be determined. The lowest antimicrobial concentration that prevents visible growth after an 18- to 24-hour incubation is known as the minimal inhibitory concentration (MIC). The minimal bactericidal concentration (MBC) is defined as the lowest antimicrobial concentration that totally suppresses growth after overnight incubation. Because culture and sensitivity results take 48 hours, treatment usually is initiated on clinical assessment and then re-evaluated when test results are complete.

Another important factor in choosing an antimicrobial is the infection site. For antimicrobial therapy to be effective, an adequate concentration of the drug must be delivered to the infection site. That means the local antimicrobial concentration should equal at least the MIC for the infecting organism. Other factors in selecting an antimicrobial are the relative cost of the drug, its potential adverse effects, and patient allergies.

Glossary

Acetylation: metabolic process that introduces an acetyl group into the molecule of an organic compound.

Acid fast: organism that retains carbolfuchsin stain after being decolorized with 95% ethyl alcohol and 3% hydrochloric acid—a unique characteristic of mycobacteria.

Aerobe: microorganism that can live and grow only in the presence of molecular oxygen.

Amoebicidal: pertaining to an agent that destroys amoebas, one-celled protozoa.

Anaerobe: microorganism that can live and grow only in the complete, or almost complete, absence of molecular oxygen.

Anaphylaxis: life-threatening reaction of a person to a foreign protein or other substance.

Antibacterial: substance, derived from cultures or semi-synthetically produced, that inhibits bacterial growth or kills bacteria.

Antibiotic: substance, derived from cultures or semi-synthetically produced, that inhibits growth of or kills other organisms, such as parasites.

Antimicrobial: substance, either antibiotic or chemotherapeutic, used to treat infection with pathogenic microorganisms.

Arthralgia: joint pain.

Ataxia: lack of muscular coordination or irregularity of muscle action.

Bacillus: any rod-shaped, gram-positive, spore-forming microorganism.

Bacteremia: presence of bacteria in the blood.

Bacteria: a group of single-cell organisms, usually possessing a rigid cell wall, dividing by binary fission, and exhibiting either round, rodlike, or spiral form.

Bactericidal: pertaining to an agent that destroys bacteria.

Bacteriostatic: pertaining to an agent that inhibits growth or multiplication of bacteria.

Bacteriuria: presence of bacteria in the urine.

Cestode: any tapeworm or platyhelminth that has a head, or scolex, and segmented joints, or proglottids.

Coccus: a spherical bacterial cell, usually slightly less than 1 micron in diameter.

Conjugation: chemical combination of a toxic product with a substance in the body to form a detoxified product that is then excreted.

Creatinine clearance: amount of plasma cleared of creatinine, a by-product of muscle metabolism, per unit of time; the normal average value is 120 ml/minute.

Dermatophytosis: fungal skin infection (in many cases, of the feet).

Encephalitis: inflammation of the brain.

Enterohepatic circulation: portal system transport of substances from the bowel directly to the liver.

Flaccid paralysis: loss or impairment of motor and sensory function, partially caused by a lesion in the neural or muscular mechanisms, accompanied by loss of muscle tone and absence of reflexes.

Fungicidal: pertaining to an agent that destroys fungi.

Fungistatic: pertaining to an agent that inhibits fungal growth.

Gram stain: laboratory dye used to differentiate organisms. An organism that retains the dye is classified as gram-positive; otherwise, the organism is gram-negative.

Hansen's disease: chronic communicable disease caused by *Mycobacterium leprae,* characterized by granulomatous lesions in the skin, mucous membranes, and peripheral nervous system; also called leprosy.

Helminth: worm or wormlike parasite.

Hemodialysis: extracorporeal removal of certain elements from the blood by differential diffusion through a semipermeable membrane.

Hepatotoxicity: quality or property of exerting a destructive or poisonous effect upon liver cells.

Hydrolysis: splitting of a compound into fragments by adding water, with the hydroxyl group incorporated in one fragment and the hydrogen atom in the other.

Induction: stimulation of the hepatic microsomal enzyme system by one drug, which increases metabolism of another drug.

Infection: reactions of tissues to invading pathogenic microorganisms and the toxins they generate.

Iatrogenic: caused by a treatment or diagnostic procedure.

Malaria: infectious febrile disease caused by protozoa transmitted by the bites of infected mosquitoes; characterized by periodic attacks of chills, fever, and diaphoresis.

Meningitis: inflammation of the membranes that envelop the brain and spinal cord.

Microbial: pertaining to minute living organisms capable of producing diseases, including bacteria, protozoa, and fungi.

Microorganism: any microscopic organism, including bacteria, spiral organisms, *Rickettsiae,* viruses, molds, yeasts, and protozoa.

Morphologic: pertaining to the science of the physical forms and structures of an organism.

Mycobacteria: slender, gram-positive, acid-fast, rod-shaped microorganisms.

Mycoses: diseases caused by fungi.

Nematode: multicellular parasite, such as roundworm or threadworm.

Nephrotoxicity: quality or property of exerting a destructive or poisonous effect upon kidney cells.

continued

Glossary continued

Neuritis: inflammation of a nerve, characterized by pain, tenderness, anesthesia, paresthesia, paralysis, wasting, and absent reflexes.

Nosocomial: pertaining to a hospital.

Ototoxicity: quality or property of exerting a destructive or poisonous effect upon the eighth cranial nerve or the organs of hearing and balance.

Parasite: plant or animal that lives upon or within another living organism, at whose expense it obtains some advantage without return compensation.

Paresthesia: abnormal burning or prickling sensation.

Pathogen: any disease-producing microorganism or material.

Peritoneal dialysis: removal of certain elements from the blood by differential diffusion through the peritoneal membrane.

Phlebitis: inflammation of a vein, characterized by thrombus formation, edema, stiffness, pain, and redness.

Phosphorylation: chemical process of introducing the trivalent phosphoryl group into an organic molecule.

Prophylaxis: disease prevention.

Protozoa: unicellular organisms constituting the lowest division of the animal kingdom.

Resistance: an organism's natural ability to ward off deleterious effects of noxious agents, such as toxins, poisons, irritants, or pathogenic microorganisms.

Ribosome: one of the minute granules composed of nucleic acid, attached to the membranes of the endoplasmic reticulum of a cell where cellular protein synthesis occurs.

Schistosome: blood fluke that is a type of trematode parasite.

Sepsis: poisoning from pathogenic organisms or their toxins.

Serum sickness: type of immune complex hypersensitivity occurring 6 to 14 days after injection with foreign serum; characterized by edema, fever, inflammation of the blood vessels and joints, and urticaria.

Spastic paralysis: loss or impairment of motor and sensory function, partially caused by a lesion in the neural or muscular mechanisms; accompanied by muscle rigidity and heightened deep tendon reflexes.

Spectrum: range of bacteria affected by an antibacterial agent.

Sterol: monohydroxyl alcohol of high molecular weight, frequently classified as a lipid.

Superinfection: condition produced by the sudden overgrowth of resistant bacteria or fungi, which can occur in a patient on antibiotic therapy.

Thrush: fungal infection characterized by whitish spots and shallow ulcers in the oral cavity, fever, and gastrointestinal irritation; usually from superinfection.

Toxicity: quality of being poisonous.

Trematode: parasite resulting from ingestion of fluke-contaminated uncooked fish, crustaceans, or vegetation.

Trough levels: the lowest serum therapeutic concentration of a drug.

Tuberculosis: infectious disease caused by a species of *Mycobacterium*, characterized by small rounded nodules in the tissues, as well as fever, emaciation, and night sweats.

Virulence: degree of pathogenicity of a microorganism as indicated by case fatality rates or its ability to invade host tissues.

Virus: group of minute infectious agents characterized by a lack of independent metabolism and by ability to replicate within living host cells only.

Xanthine: white amorphous base formed by the oxidation of hypoxanthine and oxidized to uric acid.

Dosage and route of administration

The patient's clinical condition determines when antimicrobial therapy is started and how it is administered. If the patient is stable, therapy may be delayed until culture and sensitivity test results are available. Unstable patients usually are treated immediately with broad-spectrum agents. Patients with serious infections usually need higher and more predictable blood concentration levels, necessitating intravenous (I.V.) therapy. In less severe infections, intramuscular (I.M.) or oral therapy can be used.

Mixed infections

Mixed infections are caused by two or more organisms, such as gram-positive, gram-negative, and anaerobic organisms, each of which may be sensitive to different drugs. Examples are peritoneal or pelvic infections caused by mixed bowel flora and diabetic foot infections. They respond best to treatment with a selected combination of antimicrobial drugs.

Prevention of resistance

Antimicrobial drugs should not be used indiscriminately, because unnecessary exposure of organisms to these agents encourages resistant strains. The drugs should be

Gram-negative and gram-positive bacteria

The bacteria listed below are grouped as gram-negative or gram-positive, which means that an antibacterial agent that is effective against any gram-negative or gram-positive bacteria may be effective against all others in that group. Knowing which organisms are classified gram-negative or gram-positive helps the nurse understand the clinical use of antibacterial agents.

Gram-negative bacteria

Acinetobacter calcoaceticus	Legionella pneumophila
Bacteroides fragilis	Morganella morganii
Bartonella bacilliformis	Neisseria gonorrhoeae
Bordetella pertussis	Neisseria meningitidis
Brucella abortus	Pasteurella multocida
Brucella canis	Proteus mirabilis
Brucella melitensis	Proteus morgani
Brucella suis	Proteus vulgaris
Campylobacter faecalis	Providencia stuartii
Campylobacter fetus	Providencia rettgeri
Citrobacter diversus	Pseudomonas aeruginosa
Citrobacter freundii	Salmonella choleraesuis
Enterobacter cloacae	Salmonella enteritidis
Escherichia coli	Salmonella typhosa
Francisella tularensis	Serratia marcescens
Fusobacterium nucleatum	Shigella dysenteriae
Hemophilus ducreyi	Shigella flexneri
Hemophilus influenzae	Spirillum minus
Hemophilus parahemolyticus	Streptobacillus moniliformis
Hemophilus parainfluenzae	Veillonella
Klebsiella pneumoniae	Vibrio cholerae
Legionella micdadei	Vibrio parahaemolyticus
	Yersinia enterocolitica

Gram-positive bacteria

Actinomyces israelii	Listeria monocytogenes
Arachnia propionica	Nocardia asteroides
Bacillus anthracis	Peptococcus
Bacillus cereus	Peptostreptococcus
Clostridium botulinum	Propionibacterium acnes
Clostridium butyricum	Staphylococcus aureus
Clostridium difficile	Staphylococcus epidermidis
Clostridium perfringens	Streptococcus bovis
Clostridium septicum	Streptococcus faecalis
Clostridium sordellii	Streptococcus pneumoniae
Clostridium tetani	Streptococcus pyogenes
Corynebacterium diphtheriae	Streptococcus sanguis
Erysipelothrix insidiosa	Streptococcus viridans
Eubacterium alactolyticum	

reserved for patients with infections caused by susceptible organisms and should be used in high enough doses and for appropriate duration to eradicate even the most resistant mutants. Administration of subtherapeutic doses may allow resistant mutant strains to proliferate. New antimicrobial agents should be reserved for severely ill patients with serious infections that do not respond to conventional drugs.

Adverse reactions to antimicrobial agents

All antimicrobials can produce beneficial and adverse reactions in a patient. The adverse reactions can be classified as direct toxic effects upon such organs as the gastrointestinal tract, kidneys, and liver or the auditory, optic, and peripheral nerves; allergic reactions and other kinds of hypersensitivity reactions affecting the skin and other organs and structures, including the bone marrow and blood; and superinfections resulting from drug-induced overgrowths of resistant bacterial strains or fungal organisms.

Chapter 66
Antibacterial Agents

Chapter 66 discusses agents used to treat systemic bacterial infections. It emphasizes the mechanisms of action and clinical indications for the aminoglycosides, penicillins, cephalosporins, tetracyclines, sulfonamides, chloramphenicol, erythromycin, clindamycin, lincomycin, vancomycin, and imipenem/cilastatin. Also provided are the spectrum of activity, nursing implications, and patient teaching for each drug class. Tables detail specific clinically significant information, such as a drug's effects on laboratory tests.

Chapter 67
Antitubercular and Antileprotic Agents

The anti-infective agents used to treat diseases caused by organisms of the genus *Mycobacterium* are the focus of Chapter 67. The two major diseases addressed are tuberculosis and Hansen's disease, or leprosy. The mechanisms of action of these drugs are delineated as well as their adverse effects. The nursing implications focus on patient education because of the necessary prolonged use of these drugs.

Chapter 68
Antiviral Agents

Discussion in Chapter 68 begins with an overview of the difficulties inherent in developing antiviral agents that are not toxic to host cells. Then the current major drugs—including acyclovir, vidarabine, amantadine, ribavirin, and zidovudine—are explored. The adverse reactions to these agents are emphasized as are their nursing implications.

Chapter 69
Antimycotic (Antifungal) Agents

Chapter 69 discusses the various classes of antifungal agents used to treat diseases ranging from athlete's foot to exotic systemic infections. The mechanisms of actions of the four major drug classes—polyene antibiotics, imidazoles, antimetabolites, and superficial agents—are delineated. The clinical uses for these agents are described as is associated patient teaching. Nursing interventions and associated rationales are detailed.

Chapter 70
Anthelmintic Agents

Chapter 70 discusses those agents used to treat helminthic infections. The chapter begins with an overview of the various types of helminths, including their site of entry into the host and infection site. Then the specific drugs, their mechanisms of action, clinical uses, and associated nursing implications are presented.

Chapter 71
Antimalarial and Other Antiprotozoal Agents

Chapter 71 focuses on agents used to treat human protozoal diseases. The mechanisms of action of these agents in treating and providing prophylaxis for persons with malaria are detailed. Also discussed are agents used to manage other protozoal infections, such as amebiasis, *Pneumocystis carinii* pneumonia, and giardiasis. Associated nursing implications are delineated, and reasons for the increased number of protozoal diseases in the United States are suggested.

Chapter 72
Urinary Antiseptic Agents

Agents used to treat bacterial infections in the urine usually are not effective in treating systemic infections. Chapter 72 begins by reviewing those individuals at greatest risk for developing urinary tract infections. Then the specific agents are presented, with an emphasis on the spectrum of antibacterial activity. Associated nursing implications and patient education are highlighted.

Nursing diagnoses

The nursing diagnoses most applicable in caring for patients receiving drugs to prevent or treat infections are:
● Activity intolerance related to the effects of pathogenic organisms
● Alteration in bowel elimination: diarrhea, related to the effects of pathogenic organisms or drug therapy
● Alteration in cardiac output: decreased, related to the effect of pathogenic organisms
● Alteration in comfort: pain, related to the effects of pathogenic organisms or drug therapy

- Alteration in family processes related to the effects of pathogenic organisms or drug therapy
- Alteration in fluid volume: potential excess or deficit, related to the effects of pathogenic organisms or drug therapy
- Alteration in health maintenance related to the effects of pathogenic organisms or drug therapy
- Alteration in nutrition: less than body requirements, related to the effects of pathogenic organisms or drug therapy
- Alteration in oral mucous membranes related to the effects of pathogenic organisms or drug therapy
- Alteration in thought processes related to the effects of pathogenic organisms and drug therapy
- Alteration in urinary elimination patterns related to the effects of pathogenic organisms or drug therapy
- Altered sexuality patterns related to the effects of pathogenic organisms or drug therapy
- Anxiety related to the effects of pathogenic organisms or drug therapy
- Disturbance in self-concept related to the effects of pathogenic organisms or drug therapy
- Diversional activity deficit related to the effects of pathogenic organisms or drug therapy
- Fear related to the effects of pathogenic organisms or drug therapy
- Hopelessness related to the effects of pathogenic organisms
- Impaired gas exchange related to the effects of pathogenic organisms
- Impaired home maintenance related to the effects of pathogenic organisms or drug therapy
- Impaired skin integrity related to the effects of pathogenic organisms or drug therapy
- Impaired social interactions related to the effects of pathogenic organisms or drug therapy
- Impaired tissue integrity related to the effects of pathogenic organisms or drug therapy
- Ineffective airway clearance related to the effects of pathogenic organisms
- Ineffective breathing patterns related to the effects of pathogenic organisms
- Ineffective family coping: compromised, related to the effects of pathogenic organisms or drug therapy on the patient
- Ineffective individual coping related to the effects of pathogenic organisms or drug therapy
- Knowledge deficit related to the effects of pathogenic organisms and drug therapy
- Noncompliance related to drug therapy

- Potential alteration in body temperature related to the effects of pathogenic organisms or drug therapy
- Potential for infection related to the effects of pathogenic organisms or drug therapy
- Self-care deficit related to the effects of pathogenic organisms or drug therapy
- Sensory-perceptual alterations related to the effects of pathogenic organisms or drug therapy
- Sleep pattern disturbances related to the effects of pathogenic organisms or drug therapy.

CHAPTER 66

ANTIBACTERIAL AGENTS

OBJECTIVES

After reading and studying this chapter, you should be able to:
1. Identify the predictable adverse reactions associated with the aminoglycosides.
2. Discuss the reasons for ordering serum aminoglycoside peak and trough serum concentration levels.
3. Compare the antibacterial activity of the penicillinase-resistant penicillins to that of the extended-spectrum penicillins.
4. Describe the signs and symptoms of penicillin allergy, and explain the importance in antibacterial therapy of assessing penicillin allergy.
5. Describe the differences among the first-, second-, and third-generation cephalosporins.
6. Identify the predictable adverse reactions to tetracyclines.
7. Discuss why chloramphenicol still is used, even though it may cause aplastic anemia.
8. Explain how clindamycin can produce pseudomembranous colitis.
9. Discuss why erythromycin has been improved since its introduction.
10. Describe the common adverse reactions to the sulfonamides.
11. Describe the hypotension reaction associated with vancomycin administration.
12. Discuss why imipenem and cilastatin have been combined to make a new antibacterial drug.

INTRODUCTION

The discovery of drugs that prevent and treat infection from pathogenic microorganisms was one of the most important pharmacologic developments in modern medicine. The era of antimicrobial therapy began with the discovery and clinical use of the sulfonamides in 1936, followed by the discovery of the therapeutic value of penicillin and streptomycin in the 1940s. Since the 1950s, a new antimicrobial agent has been introduced almost every year.

Some of the newly developed drugs act against antibiotic-resistant bacteria; others are more effective against a specific organism or are less toxic than older drugs. However, every antimicrobial agent that selectively kills pathogens can also inflict damage on the patient. Therefore, before prescribing and instituting antimicrobial drug therapy, the physician must identify the infecting organism and consider the appropriate drug's pharmacologic and toxicologic characteristics. The physician also must consider the selected drug's pharmacokinetic characteristics and its ability to diffuse into the infection site. (For information on topical antibacterial agents, see Chapter 78, Integumentary System Agents.)

This chapter describes drugs used mainly to treat systemic bacterial infections. The antibacterial classes discussed include aminoglycosides, penicillins, cephalosporins, tetracyclines, chloramphenicol, clindamycin and lincomycin, erythromycin, sulfonamides, vancomycin, and imipenem/cilastatin.

Because polymyxin B sulfate and spectinomycin dihydrochloride have been replaced largely by more effective and less toxic antibiotics, they will not be covered in detail in this chapter. Polymyxin B is indicated only for treating urinary tract and meningeal infections caused by organisms that are resistant to other antibiotics. Spectinomycin is used to treat penicillinase-producing strains of *Neisseria gonorrheae*. It is also used to treat patients who are allergic to penicillin, cephalosporins, probenecid, and tetracycline and those who would not comply with multiple-dose tetracycline therapy.

For a summary of representative drugs, see *Selected major drugs: Antibacterial agents* on pages 1071 to 1077.

AMINOGLYCOSIDES

The aminoglycosides are primarily used to treat gram-negative bacterial infections. They also are used with beta-lactam agents such as penicillin and cephalosporins to treat the critically ill patient who has peritonitis or pneumonia. The aminoglycosides provide effective bactericidal activity against aerobic gram-negative bacilli, some aerobic gram-positive bacteria, mycobacteria, and some protozoa. They all contain aminosugars in glycosidic linkage, and all display a similar antimicrobial spectrum of activity, a similar pharmacokinetic profile, and similar toxicities.

Although streptomycin sulfate was at first clinically useful, bacterial resistance to it developed rapidly. Subsequently, neomycin sulfate and kanamycin sulfate were introduced, but their usefulness was limited by their potential toxicity and by bacterial resistance to them. Currently, gentamicin sulfate, tobramycin sulfate, netilmicin sulfate, and amikacin sulfate are the most frequently prescribed aminoglycosides for serious gram-negative bacillary infections.

History and source
The inability of penicillin G to treat gram-negative infections prompted investigators to search for new antimicrobial agents. Waksman and associates isolated the first aminoglycoside, streptomycin, in 1944. Unfortunately, susceptible bacteria rapidly developed resistance to streptomycin; today, it is used primarily to treat tuberculosis.

In 1949, neomycin was isolated; however, it proved too toxic for systemic administration. Paromomycin sulfate, with an antimicrobial spectrum of activity identical to neomycin, was isolated next. In 1957, Japanese investigators isolated kanamycin, which subsequently was replaced by agents that were active against *Pseudomonas aeruginosa*. In 1963, Weinstein and associates isolated gentamicin, still one of the most frequently prescribed aminoglycosides.

The antibacterial compound tobramycin was produced in the early 1970s. Tobramycin is more effective than gentamicin in treating serious *P. aeruginosa* infections. The two newest aminoglycosides, netilmicin and amikacin, are semisynthetic products.

PHARMACOKINETICS

The various aminoglycosides have similar pharmacokinetic properties. All contain highly polarized molecules,
are absorbed poorly after oral administration, and are excreted almost entirely unchanged in the urine by glomerular filtration.

Absorption, distribution, metabolism, excretion
After oral administration, aminoglycosides are poorly absorbed from the gastrointestinal (GI) tract. However, after intravenous (I.V.) and intramuscular (I.M.) administration, aminoglycoside absorption is complete and rapid if impaired tissue perfusion does not exist. In patients with serious infections, I.V. administration is used to ensure optimal reliable serum concentration levels.

The aminoglycosides are distributed widely in the extracellular fluid. Small amounts are distributed to bile, sweat, tears, saliva, sputum, and breast milk. Concentration levels in the renal cortex and the perilymph of the inner ear far exceed plasma levels; however, concentration levels in bronchial secretions attain only about 20% of plasma levels. When administered in therapeutic doses, aminoglycosides readily cross the placenta. They do not cross the blood-brain barrier even in patients with inflamed meninges. As a result, intraventricular administration is proposed for gram-negative bacillary meningitis in adults. Drug concentration levels in prostatic fluid and bile are significantly lower than plasma levels. In the urine, aminoglycoside concentration levels exceed plasma levels by 25 to 100 times. Aminoglycosides are not metabolized.

Aminoglycosides are excreted primarily via the kidneys. From 40% to 97% of a single dose is excreted within 24 hours of administration. Complete urine recovery can be seen 20 to 30 days after administration of the last dose. Because aminoglycosides are excreted by the kidneys, decreased renal function can increase the serum half-life from the normal 2 to 3 hours and between 50 to 60 hours in uremic patients. In patients with diminished renal glomerular function, the total daily dose must be reduced. Less than 1% of a given dose appears in the feces.

Onset, peak, duration
After I.M. administration, peak concentration levels usually are achieved in 1 hour. With I.V. administration, peak concentration levels occur 30 to 45 minutes after the infusion ends. The recommended length of infusion to achieve peak concentration levels is 30 minutes. In adults with normal renal function, gentamicin, tobramycin, and netilmicin are administered every 8 hours; amikacin and kanamycin usually are administered every 12 hours. In the patient with impaired renal function, the dosage interval may be increased to 24 hours or longer.

PHARMACODYNAMICS

The aminoglycosides act as bactericidal agents against susceptible organisms by binding irreversibly to their ribosomal subunits, thus inhibiting protein synthesis.

Mechanism of action

Aminoglycosides are transported across cell membranes to bind within the pathogen to ribosomes, which process genetically coded information. As a result, protein synthesis required for maintaining the bacterial cell's structure and metabolic activity is inhibited.

Bacterial resistance to an aminoglycoside may be related to the drug's failure to cross the cell membrane, an altered binding to ribosomes, or destruction of the drug by bacterial enzymes. Some gram-positive cocci (enterococci) resist aminoglycoside transport across the cell membrane. When penicillin is used with aminoglycoside therapy, the cell wall is altered, enabling the aminoglycoside to penetrate the bacterial cell.

PHARMACOTHERAPEUTICS

Aminoglycosides are most useful in treating infections caused by aerobic gram-negative bacilli. They also are valuable in treating serious nosocomial infections in critically ill patients, such as gram-negative bacteremia, peritonitis, and pneumonia. Urinary tract infections caused by enteric bacilli that are resistant to less toxic antibiotics, such as penicillins and cephalosporins, frequently respond to aminoglycosides. Infections of the central nervous system and the eye require local instillation. Streptomycin is active against many strains of mycobacteria, including *Mycobacterium tuberculosis,* and against gram-positive bacteria *Nocardia* and *Erysipelothrix.* Gentamicin, tobramycin, netilmicin, and amikacin are active against *Acinetobacter, Citrobacter, Enterobacter, Klebsiella, Proteus* (indole-positive and indole-negative), *Providencia, Serratia, Escherichia coli,* and *Pseudomonas aeruginosa.* Because susceptibility of these organisms to the particular aminoglycoside varies with time and clinical setting, a culture and sensitivity test should be performed during therapy.

Against gram-positive organisms, aminoglycosides are used as synergistic combinations with penicillins to treat staphylococcal or enterococcal infections. Aminoglycosides are inactive against anaerobic bacteria.

Potentially serious toxicity limits the usefulness of the aminoglycosides; all display the same spectrum of toxicity, which can damage auditory, vestibular, and renal functions.

To assess the effectiveness of aminoglycoside therapy and to monitor for toxicity, the nurse should monitor aminoglycoside levels. (See *Serum aminoglycoside levels* for details.)

streptomycin sulfate. Used to treat plague, tularemia, and tuberculosis, streptomycin is also used with penicillin to treat bacterial endocarditis. The route of administration usually is intramuscular.
USUAL ADULT DOSAGE: 250 to 1,000 mg I.M. every 12 hours; smaller daily doses should be used for elderly patients and those with renal impairment.
USUAL PEDIATRIC DOSAGE: with normal renal function, 20 to 40 mg/kg I.M. daily in divided doses.

neomycin sulfate (Mycifradin, Neobiotic). Used as an adjunct to treat hepatic coma and as a bowel antiseptic before intestinal surgery, neomycin is administered orally.
USUAL ADULT DOSAGE: for hepatic encephalopathy, 4 to 12 grams P.O. daily in divided doses; for preoperative intestinal antisepsis, 1 gram of neomycin and 1 gram of erythromycin base administered at 1 p.m., 2 p.m., and 11 p.m. the day before a scheduled 8 a.m. surgery.

paromomycin sulfate (Humatin). Paromomycin has been used as adjunctive therapy to treat hepatic coma, but is not commonly used today. Because paromomycin

---

Serum aminoglycoside levels

Periodic assessment of aminoglycoside serum peak and trough concentration levels is needed to assess therapeutic efficacy and toxicity. That is especially important in patients with changing renal function and in those on concomitant therapy with an extended-spectrum penicillin. The goal is to obtain a peak serum concentration level between 4 and 8 mcg/ml for gentamicin and tobramycin, 4 and 10 mcg/ml for netilmicin, and 15 and 30 mcg/ml for kanamycin and amikacin. These therapeutic peak concentration levels will vary depending on the pathogen and the site of infection. Serum trough concentration levels for gentamicin, tobramycin, and netilmicin are generally lower than 2 mcg/ml; for amikacin and kanamycin, lower than 5 mcg/ml. High trough levels correlate with nephrotoxicity; high peak levels with ototoxicity and nephrotoxicity.

Blood for serum aminoglycoside trough levels should be obtained within ½ hour before the next dose. Blood for peak concentration levels should be obtained 1 hour after the administration of an I.M. dose and ½ hour after the end of a 30-minute infusion. Each specimen must be dated and timed.

DRUG INTERACTIONS

Aminoglycosides

The following chart summarizes significant interactions between aminoglycosides and other drugs. The nurse must be familiar with these interactions to provide efficient care.

DRUG	INTERACTING DRUGS	POSSIBLE EFFECTS	NURSING IMPLICATIONS
all aminoglycosides	dimenhydrinate	Masks ototoxicity	● Monitor the patient for hearing loss.
	ethacrynic acid	Increases ototoxicity	● Monitor the patient for hearing loss.
	methoxyflurane	Produces additive nephro-toxicity	● Do not administer together.
kanamycin, tobra-mycin, gentamicin, neomycin, strepto-mycin	neuromuscular blocking agents	Increase neuromuscular blockade	● Administer calcium and anticholinergic agents as prescribed.
gentamicin, tobra-mycin	carbenicillin, ticarcillin, azlocillin, mezlocillin, pi-peracillin	Inactivate the aminoglyco-sides	● Never mix these two types of antibacterials; if the patient is on combined therapy administer the doses at least 1 hour apart.
neomycin	digitalis glycosides	Inhibits GI absorption of digitalis glycosides	● Monitor the patient's serum digoxin levels, and adjust dosage as prescribed.
	penicillin V	Decreases absorption of penicillin V	● Monitor the patient frequently for reduced therapeutic effects.
gentamicin	amphotericin B, cephalosporins	Produce nephrotoxicity	● Monitor renal function tests frequently for the patient on combination therapy.

is amebicidal, it sometimes is used to treat intestinal amebiasis and other parasitic infections.

USUAL ADULT DOSAGE: for intestinal amebiasis, 25 to 35 mg/kg P.O. daily in three divided doses.

USUAL PEDIATRIC DOSAGE: 7.5 mg/kg I.M. or I.V. every 12 hours.

kanamycin sulfate (Kantrex). Kanamycin is effective against infections caused by *E. coli, Proteus* species, *Enterobacter aerogines, Serratia marcescens, Klebsiella pneumoniae,* and *Acinetobacter* species. It is ineffective against *P. aeruginosa.*

USUAL ADULT DOSAGE: 7.5 mg/kg I.M. or I.V. every 12 hours, not to exceed 1.5 grams/day; for inhalation therapy, 250 mg diluted in 3 ml of normal saline solution and nebulized b.i.d. to q.i.d.; for intraperitoneal therapy, 500 mg in 20 ml of sterile water instilled into the peritoneal cavity.

USUAL PEDIATRIC DOSAGE: 7.5 mg/kg I.M. or I.V. every 12 hours, not to exceed 30 mg/kg/day.

gentamicin sulfate (Garamycin). The most widely used aminoglycoside, gentamicin has been limited by the increasing numbers of gentamicin-resistant gram-negative bacilli. It is the drug of choice for suspected infection from *P. aeruginosa, E. coli, Staphylococcus, Serratia, Citrobacter,* indole-positive and indole-negative *Proteus, Providencia, Klebsiella, Enterobacter,* and other gram-negative aerobic bacteria.

USUAL ADULT DOSAGE: 1 to 1.75 mg/kg I.V. or I.M. every 8 hours; dosage adjustment is required for patients with renal impairment.

USUAL PEDIATRIC DOSAGE: 2 to 2.5 mg/kg I.V. or I.M. every 8 hours.

tobramycin sulfate (Nebcin). The antimicrobial spectrum of tobramycin resembles that of gentamicin, with greater activity against *P. aeruginosa* demonstrated in vitro.

USUAL ADULT DOSAGE: 1 to 1.75 mg/kg I.V. or I.M. every 8 hours; dosage adjustment is required for patients with renal impairment.
USUAL PEDIATRIC DOSAGE: 1.5 to 1.9 mg/kg I.M. or I.V. every 8 hours.

netilmicin sulfate (Netromycin). Made available in 1983, netilmicin resembles gentamicin and tobramycin, but may be less likely to produce ototoxicity and nephrotoxicity.
USUAL ADULT DOSAGE: 1.5 to 2 mg/kg I.V. or I.M. every 8 to 12 hours; dosage adjustment is required for patients with renal insufficiency.

amikacin sulfate (Amikin). Amikacin is active against many aminoglycoside-resistant gram-negative bacilli. With restricted use, bacterial resistance may be prevented.
USUAL ADULT DOSAGE: 7 to 7.5 mg/kg I.V. or I.M. every 12 hours; dosage adjustment is required for patients with renal impairment.

Drug interactions

The use of various aminoglycosides with extended-spectrum penicillins (carbenicillin, ticarcillin, mezlocillin, piperacillin, and azlocillin) can inactivate the aminoglycosides when the drugs are mixed together or administered simultaneously. This interaction is clinically important for patients with impaired renal function or those on high doses of extended-spectrum penicillins. Serum aminoglycoside levels should be monitored to ensure adequate therapy. (See *Drug interactions: Aminoglycosides* on page 1035 for additional information.)

ADVERSE DRUG REACTIONS

Serious adverse reactions limit the use of aminoglycosides, all of which display the same spectrum of toxicity. Careful patient monitoring using appropriate laboratory tests can help reduce the incidence of toxicity. The total dosage and duration of therapy contribute to toxicity.

Predictable reactions

The most notable adverse reactions to aminoglycosides are ototoxicity and nephrotoxicity. These occur most often in elderly patients, dehydrated patients, those with renal impairment, and those receiving concurrent ototoxic or nephrotoxic drugs.

Aminoglycosides can produce irreversible eighth cranial nerve damage. High-frequency tone loss usually occurs before clinical hearing loss. Audiometric testing can help prevent permanent hearing loss. These drugs can induce vestibular symptoms, such as dizziness, nystagmus, vertigo, and ataxia.

Aminoglycosides can produce renal tubular necrosis, resulting in elevated serum creatinine and blood urea nitrogen (BUN) levels. Nephrotoxicity is related to high drug concentration levels that accumulate in the renal cortex. Renal tubular damage usually is reversible after discontinuation of the drug. Monitoring the patient's renal function and serum aminoglycoside levels and making appropriate dosage adjustments may decrease the severity of nephrotoxicity and renal tubular damage.

Aminoglycosides can produce neuromuscular reactions ranging from peripheral nerve toxicity to neuromuscular blockade. Reactions frequently occur after local, peritoneal, pleural, or wound instillation. Neuromuscular reactions also can occur when aminoglycosides are administered to patients immediately after surgery. Neomycin and netilmicin produce the most potent neuromuscular reactions.

The most common adverse reactions to orally administered aminoglycosides are nausea, vomiting, and diarrhea.

Unpredictable reactions

Allergic reactions to aminoglycosides are rare. Rash, urticaria, stomatitis, pruritus, generalized burning, fever, and eosinophilia occasionally occur.

NURSING IMPLICATIONS

Because the aminoglycosides can cause serious toxicity, the nurse should be aware of the following implications:
• Assess the patient's renal function using BUN and serum creatinine levels; assess the patient's hearing using audiometric testing before instituting aminoglycoside therapy.
• Collect appropriate specimens (blood, urine, sputum, wound) for culture and sensitivity tests before beginning aminoglycoside therapy.
• Ensure that the patient is well hydrated before therapy unless otherwise contraindicated.
• Refrigerate prepared aminoglycoside solution until use; infuse the drug over a 30-minute interval.
• Monitor serum creatinine levels to help detect changes in renal function. Serum creatinine levels should be monitored every other day in the patient with unstable renal function and at least once weekly in the patient with normal renal function.

• Be aware that routine urinalysis that indicates casts or protein in the urine may indicate renal damage caused by the aminoglycoside.

• Do not mix aminoglycosides in the same solution with extended-spectrum penicillins; the aminoglycosides may be inactivated.

• Administer aminoglycosides and extended-spectrum penicillins at least 2 hours apart to the patient with normal renal function; for the patient with renal impairment, give amikacin with the extended-spectrum penicillin as prescribed.

• Monitor the respiratory rate and heart rhythm of the patient receiving aminoglycosides after surgery or receiving two or more aminoglycosides simultaneously, to detect neuromuscular blockade.

PENICILLINS

The era of chemotherapy began with the development of penicillin during World War II. Penicillin remains one of the most important and useful antibacterials despite the availability of numerous others. In the years since penicillin's discovery, researchers have developed natural and semisynthetic congeners. The penicillins can be divided into four groups: natural penicillins, penicillinase-resistant penicillins, aminopenicillins, and extended-spectrum penicillins. (See *Penicillins and their pharmacotherapeutic uses* on page 1040 for how these penicillins are classified according to their antimicrobial spectrum of activity.)

History and source

In 1929, Fleming isolated penicillin from a blue-green bread mold. The work of Florey, Chain, and associates made possible the commercial production of penicillin G in 1941. This group determined that penicillin was active against staphylococci and streptococci and was not toxic in experimentally infected animals. The need for a reliably safe and effective antimicrobial to treat wounded soldiers during World War II intensified efforts to produce penicillin in large quantities. By the summer of 1943, penicillin was used throughout the U.S. armed forces medical services.

In 1959, Batchelor and associates isolated the penicillanic acid nucleus; newer penicillins were developed by adding semisynthetic side chains to the nucleus. Methicillin sodium, the first semisynthetic penicillin, was active against beta-lactamase–producing *Staphylococcus aureus*. Methicillin was followed by ampicillin, which was active against selected gram-negative bacilli, then by carbenicillin disodium, active against *Pseudomonas aeruginosa*.

PHARMACOKINETICS

Clinical use of penicillin G, the first penicillin introduced, has been limited because it is readily hydrolyzed by penicillinase and because many organisms have developed a resistance to it. Over the years, new forms superior to penicillin G have been developed.

Absorption

After oral administration, the penicillins are absorbed mainly in the duodenum and the upper jejunum. Extent of absorption of oral dosage forms varies and depends on such factors as the particular penicillin, the patient's gastric and intestinal pH, and the presence of food. Penicillin G is inactivated rapidly within the stomach's acidic environment, and only 15% to 30% of an orally administered dose is absorbed in healthy, fasting adults. The presence of food in the GI tract also contributes to penicillin G destruction. Because penicillin V, a phenoxymethyl derivative, resists acid hydrolysis, it is better absorbed after oral administration. From 60% to 70% of a dose of oral penicillin V is absorbed in an adult; food intake has minimal effect.

Methicillin, which is acid-labile, is inactivated by gastric contents after oral administration; it must be administered parenterally. Oxacillin sodium, cloxacillin sodium, nafcillin sodium, and dicloxacillin sodium are acid-stable but are incompletely and erratically absorbed after oral administration. In healthy, fasting adults, 30% to 35% of an oxacillin dose, 37% to 60% of a cloxacillin dose, and 35% to 76% of a dicloxacillin dose are absorbed after oral administration. The percentage of nafcillin absorbed varies considerably among individuals.

Ampicillin is 35% to 66% absorbed; amoxicillin and cyclacillin are stable in the presence of acidic gastric secretions and are well absorbed after oral administration. Bacampicillin hydrochloride is a prodrug of ampicillin; it is absorbed rapidly and becomes effective when hydrolyzed to ampicillin after oral administration. Food decreases the rate and extent of absorption of ampicillin. Food lowers and delays the peak concentration levels of amoxicillin trihydrate; however, it does not affect the

Peak concentration levels and durations of action for penicillins

The following chart provides pharmacokinetic information about the different penicillins and their administration in fasting adults.

DRUG	ADMINISTRATION ROUTES	PEAK CONCENTRATION LEVELS	DURATIONS OF ACTION
penicillin G, penicillin V	Oral	½ to 1 hour	6 hours
penicillin G potassium, penicillin G sodium	I.M.	15 to 30 minutes	3 to 6 hours
penicillin G procaine	I.M.	1 to 3 hours	1 to 2 days
penicillin G benzathine	I.M.	13 to 24 hours	1 to 4 weeks
cloxacillin, dicloxacillin, nafcillin, oxacillin	Oral	½ to 2 hours	4 to 6 hours
methicillin, nafcillin, oxacillin	I.M.	½ to 1 hour	4 to 6 hours
methicillin, nafcillin, oxacillin (1 gram)	I.V.	Immediately after infusion	2 to 3 hours
amoxicillin, ampicillin	Oral	1 to 2 hours	6 to 8 hours
ampicillin	I.M.	1 hour	6 to 8 hours
ampicillin	I.V. (30 minutes)	Immediately after infusion	6 hours
bacampicillin	Oral	½ to 1½ hours	6 to 8 hours
cyclacillin	Oral	½ to 1 hour	4 hours
carbenicillin, mezlocillin, piperacillin, ticarcillin	I.M.	½ to 2 hours	6 to 8 hours
azlocillin, carbenicillin, mezlocillin, piperacillin, ticarcillin	I.V.	Immediately after infusion	6 to 8 hours

total amount of drug absorbed. Food does not alter the absorption of bacampicillin or cyclacillin.

Azlocillin sodium, carbenicillin, mezlocillin sodium, piperacillin sodium, and ticarcillin disodium are not absorbed well from the GI tract and must be given parenterally. Only carbenicillin is available orally in ester form, which is acid-stable, allowing carbenicillin to be absorbed partially from the small intestine. After absorption, the ester is hydrolyzed, and free carbenicillin appears in the systemic circulation.

Intramuscular administration is indicated primarily when compliance with an oral regimen is inconvenient or questionable. Because long-acting preparations of penicillin G (penicillin G benzathine and penicillin G procaine) are relatively insoluble, they must be administered by the I.M. route. Penicillin G benzathine is slowly absorbed after I.M. administration and is detectable even

after 28 days. Penicillin G procaine usually is preferred for I.M. administration because it provides more consistent steady-state levels for up to 24 hours. Also, penicillin G procaine provides the local anesthetic properties of procaine, thereby reducing pain at the injection site.

Distribution

Penicillins are distributed widely to most areas of the body, including the lungs, liver, kidneys, muscle, bone, and placenta. The highest concentration levels occur in the plasma, where much of a dose is reversibly bound to plasma albumin. Because of their lipid insolubility, penicillins do not penetrate cell membranes well. Distribution of the penicillins to the eyes, cerebrospinal fluid, and prostate is poor in the absence of inflammation;

inflammation alters normal barriers and enhances penicillin distribution. High concentration levels appear in the urine even with moderately reduced renal function, making penicillins useful in treating urinary tract infections.

Metabolism

Penicillins are metabolized to a limited extent in the liver to inactive metabolites.

Excretion

Penicillins are excreted 60% unchanged by the kidneys, largely by glomerular filtration and active tubular secretion. Because excretion into the urine is rapid, penicillins have a short half-life, ranging from less than 30 minutes for penicillin G to 72 minutes for carbenicillin. Biliary excretion is important for nafcillin only. Reduced renal function (creatinine clearance less than 30 to 40 ml/minute) may necessitate reduced doses of certain penicillins, such as penicillin G, carbenicillin, ticarcillin, azlocillin, mezlocillin, and piperacillin.

Onset, peak, duration

Peak concentration levels and durations of action for the penicillins vary, depending on the specific drug and the route of administration. (See *Peak concentration levels and durations of action for penicillins* for specific data.)

PHARMACODYNAMICS

Penicillins usually are bactericidal in action. Traditionally, penicillins have been thought to inhibit the last step of mucopeptide synthesis in the bacterial cell wall. Recent studies suggest a more complicated mechanism of action.

Mechanism of action

Although the exact mechanism of action of penicillins is not understood, research has shown that penicillins bind reversibly to several enzymes outside the bacterial cytoplasmic membrane. These enzymes, known as penicillin-binding proteins (PBPs), are involved in cell-wall synthesis and cell division. Interference with these processes increases internal osmotic pressure and ruptures the cell.

The antibacterial activity of penicillins depends partly on their ability to bind to the target enzymes. The cell walls of gram-positive bacteria are relatively permeable to most penicillins, especially natural penicillins. However, gram-negative bacteria possess an outer membrane around the cell wall that decreases accessibility to the PBPs. The production of penicillinases (enzymes that convert penicillin to inactive penicilloic acid)

by the bacteria also contributes to bacterial resistance. Aminopenicillins and extended-spectrum penicillins penetrate the outer membranes of gram-negative bacteria more readily than either the natural penicillins, such as penicillin G, or penicillinase-resistant penicillins, such as cloxacillin, dicloxacillin, methicillin, nafcillin, and oxacillin. The greater ability of the penicillin derivatives to gain access to the PBPs may relate to their increased antibacterial activity against these gram-negative organisms.

PHARMACOTHERAPEUTICS

No other class of antibacterials provides as wide a spectrum of antimicrobial activity as the penicillins.

Natural penicillins and their derivatives are used to treat many common infections. Therapeutic indications include streptococcal pharyngitis, streptococcal endocarditis, staphylococcal infections, pneumococcal pneumonia, meningococcal meningitis, gonorrhea, syphilis, GI infections caused by *Shigella* and *Salmonella*, upper respiratory tract infections, otitis media, sinusitis caused by *Hemophilus influenzae*, and various gram-negative bacillary infections. (See *Penicillins and their pharmacotherapeutic uses* on page 1040 for more details.)

Concurrent administration of probenecid increases the serum concentration levels of penicillins by 50% to 100%, because probenecid blocks tubular secretion of penicillin. Combined probenecid-penicillin therapy is used to treat bacterial endocarditis and acute gonorrhea.

penicillin G aqueous. A natural penicillin and the prototype for all penicillins, penicillin G is available for I.M. or I.V. administration in two salts, penicillin G potassium and penicillin G sodium. Aqueous penicillin G is used intravenously when a rapid effect or high serum concentration levels are desired, as in meningitis, septicemia, pericarditis, endocarditis, severe pneumonia, and other serious infections.
USUAL ADULT DOSAGE: 600,000 to 5 million units I.V. or I.M. every 4 to 6 hours.
USUAL PEDIATRIC DOSAGE: 100,000 to 250,000 units/kg I.V. or I.M. daily in divided doses every 4 hours.

penicillin G procaine (Wycillin). Used when a long-acting preparation is preferred and high blood concentration levels are not required, this suspension is administered I.M. only.
USUAL ADULT AND PEDIATRIC DOSAGE: for moderately severe penicillin G–sensitive systemic infection, 600,000 to 1.2 million units I.M. daily.

Penicillins and their pharmacotherapeutic uses

Natural or semisynthetic derivatives of the *Penicillium* fungus, penicillins are prepared by chemically modifying a natural penicillin. The resulting drugs are classified according to their antimicrobial spectrum of activity.

DRUG	ANTIMICROBIAL SPECTRUM
Natural penicillins	

penicillin G benzathine
penicillin G potassium
penicillin G procaine
penicillin G sodium
penicillin V potassium
	Gram-positive organisms:
	  Actinomyces israelii
	  Staphylococcus aureus (non-penicillinase-producing strains)
	  Streptococci (groups A,B,C, and D)
	Streptococcus viridans
	  Streptococcus faecalis
	  Beta-hemolytic streptococci
	  Streptococcus bovis
	  Streptococcus (Diplococcus) pneumoniae
	  Eubacterium species
	  Bacillus anthracis
	  Peptostreptococcus species
	  Clostridium tetani
	  Clostridium perfringens
	  Listeria monocytogenes
	Gram-negative organisms:
	  Bacteroides (all species except for many strains of *B. fragilis*)
	  Neisseria gonorrhoeae
	  Neisseria meningitidis
	  Pasteurella multocida
	  Spirillum minor
	  Streptobacillus moniliformis
	  Salmonella species
	  Shigella species
	  Enterobacter species
	Anaerobic oganisms:
	  Treponema pallidum
	  Treponema pertenue
	  Borrelia recurrentis
	  Leptospira icterohaemorrhagiae

DRUG	ANTIMICROBIAL SPECTRUM
Penicillinase-resistant penicillins	
cloxacillin dicloxacillin methicillin nafcillin oxacillin	*Staphylococcus aureus* *Staphylococcus epidermidis* streptococci (some species)
Aminopenicillins	

amoxicillin
ampicillin
bacampicillin
cyclacillin
	Gram-positive organisms:
	  staphylococci (non-penicillinase–producing
	  streptococci (some species)
	Gram-negative organisms:
	  Escherichia coli
	  Hemophilus influenzae
	  Neisseria gonorrhoeae
	  Proteus mirabilis
	  Salmonella species
	  Shigella species

Extended-spectrum penicillins	

azlocillin
carbenicillin
mezlocillin
piperacillin
ticarcillin
	Gram-positive and gram-negative organisms that natural penicillins and aminopenicillins are active against, plus:
	  Pseudomonas aeruginosa
	  Proteus species (indolepositive)
	  Providencia species
	  Enterobacter species
	  Citrobacter species
	  Serratia species
	  Acinetobacter species
	  Veillonella species

penicillin G potassium (Pentids). This oral form of penicillin G is used to treat mild to moderate bacterial infections.

USUAL ADULT DOSAGE: for mild streptococcal upper respiratory tract infection (URI), 200,000 to 250,000 units P.O. every 6 to 8 hours for 10 days; for moderately severe URI, 400,000 to 500,000 units P.O. every 8 hours for 10 days or 800,000 units every 12 hours P.O.; for mild to moderate pneumococcal respiratory tract infection, 400,000 to 500,000 units P.O. every 6 hours for at least 2 days; for staphylococcal infection, 200,000 to 500,000 units P.O. every 6 to 8 hours until therapy is effective.

USUAL PEDIATRIC DOSAGE: for the same indications as adults, 25,000 to 90,000 units/kg P.O. daily in three to six divided doses.

penicillin G benzathine (Bicillin, Bicillin L-A). Penicillin G benzathine is used in the definitive management of streptococcal upper respiratory infections and syphilis, and in the prophylaxis of rheumatic fever. It should not be used to treat gonorrhea because peak concentration levels are too low for satisfactory results. The suspension form can be given I.M. only.

USUAL ADULT DOSAGE: for group A streptococcal upper respiratory infections, 1.2 million units I.M. in a single injection or 400,000 to 600,000 units P.O. every 4 to 6 hours for 10 days; for prophylaxis of poststreptococcal rheumatic fever, 1.2 million units I.M. once a month, 600,000 units I.M. twice a month, or 200,000 units P.O. b.i.d.; for syphilis of less than 1 year's duration, 2.4 million units I.M. in a single dose; for syphilis of more than 1 year's duration, 2.4 million units I.M. weekly for 3 successive weeks.

USUAL PEDIATRIC DOSAGE: for congenital syphilis in children age 2 and under, 50,000 units/kg I.M. as a single dose; for group A streptococcal upper respiratory infections, 25,000 to 90,000 units/kg P.O. daily in three to six divided doses, or 900,000 units I.M. in a single injection for children over 27 kg, or 300,000 to 600,000 units I.M. in a single injection for children under 27 kg; for prophylaxis of poststreptococcal rheumatic fever, 1.2 million units I.M. once a month, 600,000 units I.M. twice a month, or 200,000 units P.O. b.i.d.

penicillin V or **penicillin V potassium [phenoxymethyl penicillin]** (Pen-Vee K, V-Cillin K). This drug is acid-stable; when given orally, it provides higher peak serum concentration levels than a similar dose of penicillin G does. Penicillin V is not a substitute for parenterally administered penicillin G. Penicillin V is used to treat mild infections of the throat, respiratory tract, or soft tissues.

USUAL ADULT DOSAGE: 125 to 500 mg P.O. every 6 hours.

USUAL PEDIATRIC DOSAGE: 25 to 50 mg/kg P.O. daily every 6 to 8 hours.

methicillin sodium (Staphcillin). First of the semisynthetic penicillinase-resistant penicillins, methicillin is effective against S. aureus. Because it is inactivated by gastric acid, methicillin must be administered parenterally. Methicillin seems to be associated with interstitial nephritis and is currently used less frequently than oxacillin or nafcillin.

USUAL ADULT DOSAGE: 1 to 3 grams I.M. or I.V. every 4 to 6 hours.

USUAL PEDIATRIC DOSAGE: 100 to 300 mg/kg I.M. or I.V. daily in divided doses every 4 to 6 hours.

oxacillin sodium (Prostaphlin). A penicillinase-resistant penicillin, oxacillin is as effective as methicillin against staphylococcal infections and causes less interstitial nephritis. Orally administered oxacillin does not produce as predictable serum concentration levels as dicloxacillin does.

USUAL ADULT DOSAGE: 2 to 4 grams P.O. daily in divided doses every 6 hours, or 2 to 12 grams I.M. or I.V. daily in divided doses every 4 to 6 hours.

USUAL PEDIATRIC DOSAGE: for children under 40 kg, 30 to 40 mg/kg P.O. daily in divided doses every 6

hours, or 50 to 200 mg/kg I.M. or I.V. daily in divided doses every 4 to 6 hours; for children over 40 kg, same as adult.

nafcillin sodium (Unipen). Similar to oxacillin in its activity against S. aureus, nafcillin is a penicillinase-resistant penicillin. Nafcillin is excreted in bile; therefore, dosage adjustment in renal impairment is unnecessary.

USUAL ADULT DOSAGE: 2 to 4 grams P.O. daily in divided doses every 6 hours, or 2 to 12 grams I.M. or I.V. daily in divided doses every 4 to 6 hours.

USUAL PEDIATRIC DOSAGE: 50 to 100 mg/kg P.O. daily in divided doses every 4 to 6 hours or 100 to 200 mg/kg I.M. or I.V. daily in divided doses every 4 to 6 hours.

dicloxacillin sodium (Dynapen). This penicillinase-resistant penicillin is the oral drug of choice against staphylococci because of its superior absorption and lower minimum inhibitory concentration levels.

USUAL ADULT DOSAGE: 125 to 250 mg P.O. every 6 hours.

USUAL PEDIATRIC DOSAGE: 25 to 50 mg/kg P.O. daily divided into four doses.

cloxacillin sodium (Tegopen). Used to treat infections caused by penicillinase-producing staphylococci, this penicillinase-resistant penicillin is less well absorbed than dicloxacillin is after oral administration.

USUAL ADULT DOSAGE: 250 to 500 mg P.O. every 6 hours.

USUAL PEDIATRIC DOSAGE: 50 to 100 mg/kg P.O. daily in divided doses every 6 hours.

ampicillin (Omnipen). An aminopenicillin, ampicillin is acid-stable and penicillinase-sensitive. When ampicillin was first introduced, most Escherichia coli, H. influenzae, Neisseria gonorrhoeae, and Proteus mirabilis strains were sensitive. Today, ampicillin-resistant strains have emerged.

USUAL ADULT DOSAGE: for systemic infections, 250 to 500 mg P.O. every 6 hours, or 1 to 3 grams I.M. or I.V. every 6 hours; for uncomplicated gonorrhea, 3.5 grams P.O. with 1 gram of probenecid as a single dose along with 500 mg of tetracycline P.O. q.i.d. for 7 days.

USUAL PEDIATRIC DOSAGE: for acute and chronic urinary tract or respiratory infections caused by gram-positive or gram-negative organisms, 50 to 100 mg/kg P.O. daily in divided doses every 6 hours, or 100 to 200 mg/kg I.M. or I.V. daily in divided doses every 6 hours; for meningitis, up to 300 mg/kg I.V. daily in divided doses every 4 hours.

DRUG INTERACTIONS
Penicillins

The interactions between penicillins and other drugs produce various effects that the nurse needs to know about before administering penicillins.

DRUG	INTERACTING DRUGS	POSSIBLE EFFECTS	NURSING IMPLICATIONS
penicillins	methotrexate	Interferes with renal tubular secretion of methotrexate	• Monitor the patient for enhanced action and possible methotrexate toxicity.
	tetracyclines	Interfere with bactericidal action of penicillin	• Separate the doses of these drugs by several hours if they are used together.
oxacillin	sulfonamides	Inhibit GI absorption of oxacillin	• Avoid concurrent therapy if possible.
extended-spectrum penicillins: azlocillin, carbenicillin, mezlocillin, piperacillin, ticarcillin	aminoglycosides	Inactivate aminoglycosides	• Do not mix these drugs; separate doses by at least 1 hour.

amoxicillin trihydrate (Amoxil). An analogue of ampicillin similar in spectrum of activity and pharmacology, amoxicillin is an aminopenicillin. Amoxicillin is absorbed better than ampicillin and is less likely to cause diarrhea; however, it is less effective against shigellosis.
USUAL ADULT DOSAGE: for systemic infections including acute and chronic urinary tract infections caused by susceptible strains of gram-positive and gram-negative organisms, 750 mg to 1.5 grams P.O. daily in divided doses every 8 hours; for uncomplicated gonorrhea, 3 grams P.O. with 1 gram of probenecid as a single dose along with 500 mg of tetracycline P.O. q.i.d. for 7 days.
USUAL PEDIATRIC DOSAGE: 20 to 40 mg/kg P.O. daily in divided doses every 8 hours.

cyclacillin (Cyclapen-W). Although closely related to ampicillin, this aminopenicillin is less likely to cause diarrhea than ampicillin or amoxicillin are.
USUAL ADULT DOSAGE: for systemic and urinary tract infections caused by gram-negative and gram-positive organisms, 250 to 500 mg P.O. every 6 hours.
USUAL PEDIATRIC DOSAGE: 50 to 100 mg/kg P.O. daily in four divided doses.

bacampicillin hydrochloride (Spectrobid). This aminopenicillin is an ester of ampicillin and is hydrolyzed to ampicillin during absorption from the GI tract; however, bacampicillin is more completely absorbed than ampicillin.

USUAL ADULT DOSAGE: 400 to 800 mg P.O. every 12 hours; for gonorrhea, 1.6 grams P.O. with 1 gram of probenecid as a single dose.
USUAL PEDIATRIC DOSAGE: in children under 25 kg, 12.5 to 25 mg/kg P.O. every 12 hours; for children 25 kg and over, same as adult.

carbenicillin disodium (Geopen). An extended-spectrum penicillin, carbenicillin has an antibacterial spectrum of activity similar to ampicillin's with important added activity against *P. aeruginosa,* the indole-positive *Proteus,* and *Enterobacter.* Large parenteral doses are necessary to treat serious *Pseudomonas* infections outside the urinary tract. With large doses of carbenicillin, the patient receives significant amounts of sodium, which can be problematic for patients with hypertension or congestive heart failure.
USUAL ADULT DOSAGE: for systemic infections caused by susceptible strains of gram-positive and especially gram-negative organisms (*Proteus, P. aeruginosa*), 30 to 40 grams I.V. infusion daily in divided doses every 4 to 6 hours or given by continuous I.V. infusion; for urinary tract infections, 200 mg/kg I.M. or I.V. infusion daily in divided doses every 4 to 6 hours or given by continuous I.V. infusion.
USUAL PEDIATRIC DOSAGE: for systemic infections caused by susceptible strains of gram-positive and gram-negative organisms, 250 to 500 mg/kg I.V. infusion daily in divided doses every 4 to 6 hours or given by contin-

uous I.V. infusion; for urinary tract infections, 50 to 200 mg/kg I.M. or I.V. infusion daily in divided doses every 4 to 6 hours.

carbenicillin indanyl sodium (Geocillin). As an extended-spectrum penicillin and oral form of carbenicillin, this drug is used only to treat certain urinary tract infections and prostatitis. Carbenicillin indanyl sodium should not be used to treat systemic infections because blood concentration levels remain too low. The drug is not recommended for pediatric use.
USUAL ADULT DOSAGE: for urinary tract infections and prostatitis caused by susceptible strains of gram-negative organisms, 382 to 764 mg P.O. q.i.d.

ticarcillin disodium (Ticar). An extended-spectrum penicillin, ticarcillin is similar to carbenicillin but is more active against *P. aeruginosa*. Like carbenicillin, ticarcillin is synergistic with aminoglycosides against *P. aeruginosa*. Ticarcillin and carbenicillin have a similar sodium content; however, ticarcillin delivers less sodium because the total daily dosage is smaller. No oral form is available.
USUAL ADULT DOSAGE: for uncomplicated urinary tract infections, 1 gram I.V. or I.M. every 4 to 6 hours; for complicated urinary tract infections, 3 grams I.V. every 4 to 6 hours; for septicemia, 3 grams I.V. every 3 to 6 hours.
USUAL PEDIATRIC DOSAGE: for neonates up to 2 kg, 100 mg/kg I.M. initially, then 75 mg/kg every 8 hours; for neonates 2 kg and over, 100 mg/kg I.M. initially, then 75 mg/kg every 4 to 6 hours; for children up to 40 kg, 25 to 75 mg/kg every 4 to 8 hours; for children over 40 kg, same as adult.

mezlocillin sodium (Mezlin). An extended-spectrum penicillin, mezlocillin's activity against *P. aeruginosa* is similar to ticarcillin's. Mezlocillin has some activity against *Klebsiella pneumoniae;* however, it is used primarily in combination with an aminoglycoside. Of all extended-spectrum penicillins, mezlocillin contains the least amount of sodium.
USUAL ADULT DOSAGE: 100 to 300 mg/kg I.V. or I.M. daily in divided doses every 4 to 6 hours.
USUAL PEDIATRIC DOSAGE: 50 mg/kg I.V. every 4 hours.

piperacillin sodium (Pipracil). The most active of the extended-spectrum penicillins against *P. aeruginosa*, piperacillin provides increased activity against *K. pneumoniae* in vitro. Clinical trials have not shown that piperacillin is more effective than carbenicillin or ticarcillin when used with aminoglycosides. Piperacillin should be reserved for clinical situations in which a deleterious platelet dysfunction or salt loading may occur

with carbenicillin or ticarcillin, or for situations in which the infecting organism is sensitive to piperacillin only. This drug can also be used with amikacin as empiric therapy for the febrile neutropenic patient.
USUAL ADULT DOSAGE: 12 to 24 grams I.V. daily, or 100 to 300 mg/kg I.M. or I.V. every 4 to 12 hours; for prophylaxis against surgical infections, 2 grams I.V. 30 to 60 minutes before surgery; may be repeated during and after surgery.
USUAL PEDIATRIC DOSAGE: for age 12 and older, same as adult; for under age 12, dosage not established.

azlocillin sodium (Azlin). An extended-spectrum penicillin, azlocillin is as active as piperacillin against *P. aeruginosa* but is less active against most Enterobacteriaceae and anaerobes. Azlocillin is used primarily with an aminoglycoside to treat *Pseudomonas* infections in patients with extensive burns or cystic fibrosis.
USUAL ADULT DOSAGE: 100 to 300 mg/kg I.V. daily in four to six divided doses.
USUAL PEDIATRIC DOSAGE: for acute exacerbation of cystic fibrosis, 75 mg/kg I.V. every 4 hours or 100 to 200 mg/kg I.V. every 8 hours; maximum daily dose, 24 grams.

amoxicillin/clavulanate potassium (Augmentin). The clavulanic acid inhibits beta-lactamases that usually inactivate amoxicillin. This combination provides an antibacterial spectrum of activity similar to that of amoxicillin, with added coverage for *S. aureus* and *Klebsiella*. It is used to treat skin infections caused by beta-lactamase–producing staphylococci, otitis caused by *H. influenzae,* and urinary tract infections caused by beta-lactamase–producing *E. coli* and *Klebsiella*.
USUAL ADULT DOSAGE: 250 mg of amoxicillin/125 mg of clavulanic acid P.O. every 8 hours; 250- and 500-mg tablets both contain 125 mg of clavulanic acid.
USUAL PEDIATRIC DOSAGE: 20 to 40 mg/kg P.O. daily in divided doses every 8 hours.

ticarcillin disodium/clavulanate potassium (Timentin). This combination contains 3 grams of ticarcillin and 100 mg of clavulanic acid. Its antibacterial spectrum resembles that of ticarcillin, with added coverage for *S. aureus* and *Klebsiella*.
USUAL ADULT DOSAGE: 3.1 grams I.V. every 4 to 6 hours.
USUAL PEDIATRIC DOSAGE: for age 12 and older, same as adult; for under age 12, dosage not established.

amdinocillin (Coactin). Formerly called mecillinam, amdinocillin is ineffective against gram-positive organisms but is *effective against ampicillin-resistant E. coli, Shi-*

gella, Salmonella, Klebsiella, Enterobacter, and *Citrobacter* species. Amdinocillin acts synergistically with other penicillins and cephalosporins but not with aminoglycosides.

USUAL ADULT DOSAGE: 10 mg/kg I.V. or I.M. *every 4 to 6 hours.*

USUAL PEDIATRIC DOSAGE: for age 12 and older, same as adult; for under age 12, dosage not established.

Drug interactions

High doses of penicillin G and extended-spectrum penicillins (azlocillin, carbenicillin, mezlocillin, piperacillin, and ticarcillin) inactivate aminoglycosides. This interaction is clinically relevant in patients with poor renal function, because elevated blood concentration levels of both agents may exist simultaneously. Penicillins should not be mixed in the same I.V. fluid with aminoglycosides.

Inactivation of aminoglycosides by penicillins depends on the penicillin concentration level, the temperature of the blood sample, and the duration of contact between the two drugs. When serum aminoglycoside levels are measured, the sample should be kept on ice while being transported to the laboratory and should be stored in the laboratory until the assay can be made. The presence of penicillins in the serum samples may result in falsely decreased aminoglycoside concentration levels. (See *Drug interactions: Penicillins* on page 1042 for additional interactions.)

ADVERSE DRUG REACTIONS

The low incidence of serious toxicity and the relatively low cost make penicillins the drugs of choice for treating susceptible organisms in nonallergic patients. Toxic effects include hypersensitivity reactions, neurotoxicity, nephrotoxicity, electrolyte imbalances, and hematologic reactions.

Predictable reactions

Certain extended-spectrum penicillins (carbenicillin and ticarcillin) are administered as disodium salts. The increased intake of sodium or potassium with these drugs may pose a therapeutic problem for patients with cardiac disease or decreased renal function. The nurse should be aware that the patient may have sodium overload and hyperkalemia or hypokalemia and should monitor the patient for these imbalances.

Penicillins can produce hematologic reactions. A positive Coombs' test for hemolytic anemia (evidenced by a fall in hemoglobin concentration levels) can occur in patients receiving high doses of I.V. penicillin G (in excess of 10 million units a day in uremic patients, or 40 million units a day in patients with normal renal function). Withdrawing the penicillin usually returns the hemoglobin to the baseline normal value. Penicillins (especially carbenicillin and ticarcillin) may induce platelet dysfunction, causing prolonged bleeding time. This is significant in patients with uremia or hepatic disease. Platelet function returns to normal when the drug is discontinued.

Hepatotoxicity has occasionally developed during oxacillin therapy. GI adverse reactions are usually associated with oral use. GI symptoms (glossitis, nausea, vomiting, and diarrhea) occur most frequently with ampicillin. The aminopenicillins and the extended-spectrum penicillins can produce pseudomembranous colitis.

Convulsions or coma secondary to direct central nervous system (CNS) irritation can occur with penicillin G doses greater than 20 million units daily in patients with decreased renal function.

Unpredictable reactions

Allergic reactions are the major adverse reactions to penicillins. Penicillin allergy occurs in 3% to 5% of the population and in up to 10% of those who have received penicillin previously. Large doses or prolonged therapy may lead to allergic reactions. Allergic reactions occur less frequently when the drugs are administered orally and more frequently when given parenterally. Penicillin hypersensitivity may occur as anaphylactic reactions, serum sickness, drug fever, or various skin rashes.

Anaphylactic shock is a syndrome characterized by rapidly developing dyspnea and hypotension. Immediate treatment includes epinephrine, corticosteroids, antihistamines, and other resuscitative measures. Serum sickness usually occurs 7 to 10 days after penicillin treatment is initiated, but is uncommon today. Signs and symptoms may include fever, urticaria (hives), joint pains, or angioneurotic edema. Patients with infectious mononucleosis will develop a macular or maculopapular erythematous skin rash when given ampicillin.

Renal failure and interstitial nephritis may occur in patients receiving large parenteral doses of penicillin G or methicillin. Usually, the reaction begins within 5 to 10 days after therapy begins. Signs and symptoms may include fever, eosinophilia, hematuria, proteinuria, or pyuria. Renal biopsy has revealed tubular damage and interstitial mononuclear cells and eosinophils, considered to be components of a hypersensitivity reaction. This reaction usually subsides when the penicillin is discontinued. In some cases, corticosteroids may be administered to improve renal function.

Some patients may experience an allergic reaction to tartrazine, a dye contained in certain penicillin preparations.

NURSING IMPLICATIONS

Whenever penicillin therapy is considered, the nurse must obtain a thorough patient history to assess the risk of allergic reaction. The nurse should ask the patient about previous penicillin use (name of drug, route of administration, type of adverse reaction, and date of occurrence). If a patient is allergic to penicillin and its derivatives, alternative therapy should be considered. The nurse should also consider the following implications:

• Monitor all patients on penicillins for allergic reactions; patients may become sensitized to penicillin through exposure. Have epinephrine readily available to treat anaphylaxis.
• Monitor the patient for GI symptoms, changes in liver function tests, coagulation tests, and urinalysis results.
• Monitor the patient's electrolyte levels if the patient is receiving penicillins high in sodium.
• Do not mix aminoglycosides with extended-spectrum penicillins.
• Administer oral forms of penicillins 1 hour before or 2 hours after meals to ensure optimal serum concentration levels.
• Advise the patient to complete the course of penicillin therapy.
• Advise the patient who is allergic to penicillins to wear a Medic Alert necklace or bracelet stating this information.

CEPHALOSPORINS

Most of the antibacterial agents introduced for clinical use in recent years have been cephalosporins, and they account for a large percentage of the nationwide escalating health care budget. Because penicillins and cephalosporin molecules have a beta-lactam structure, some cross-sensitivity occurs. The pharmacokinetic properties and mechanisms of action of the cephalosporins resemble those of the penicillins. Cephalosporins are categorized into groups called generations, based on their antibacterial spectra of activity. (See *Antibacterial activity of cephalosporins* on page 1046 for the specific drugs in each generation.)

History and source

The discovery of cephalosporins dates to 1945, when Brotzu began searching for antibiotic-producing micro-organisms. Brotzu isolated the fungus *Cephalosporium acremonium* from seawater near a sewer outlet off the coast of Sardinia. The fungus was active against numerous gram-positive and gram-negative bacteria. In 1948, at Oxford, Abraham and colleagues isolated the active antibacterial factors from a culture of *Cephalosporium acremonium* sent from Brotzu and called them cephalosporin C, cephalosporin N, and cephalosporin P. Cephalosporin C, the major product, formed the basis for the new drugs. Since cephalothin sodium was introduced for clinical use in 1962, basic structural modification has produced more effective drugs with differing bacterial spectra, pharmacokinetics, and pharmacodynamics.

PHARMACOKINETICS

A few cephalosporins are administered orally. Because most are not absorbed from the GI tract, they must be administered parenterally; I.M. injections may be painful. The degree of protein binding and renal excretion varies.

Absorption, distribution, metabolism, excretion

Despite the large number of cephalosporins, only cephradine, cephalexin monohydrate, cefadroxil monohydrate, and cefaclor are absorbed from the GI tract and administered orally. Food usually delays the absorption of the oral cephalosporins, resulting in lower peak serum concentration levels. However, peak concentration levels of cefadroxil are not affected by food. Many cephalosporins are administered intramuscularly, although peak concentration levels are higher when the drugs are administered intravenously.

After absorption, the cephalosporins are distributed widely, although they are not distributed into the CNS. Most are poorly distributed into cerebrospinal fluid (CSF), even when meninges are inflamed, but several (cefuroxime sodium, cefotaxime sodium, moxalactam disodium, cefoperazone sodium, ceftizoxime sodium, ceftriaxone sodium, and ceftazidime) penetrate CSF sufficiently to be useful for treating meningitis.

The cephalosporins are distributed widely to tissues and fluids, including pleural, pericardial, and synovial fluids, bone, and the placenta. Biliary levels are usually high, especially after cefoperazone administration. (See *Distribution of cephalosporins* on page 1047 for an illustration of distribution sites.)

Cephalothin sodium, cephapirin sodium, and cefotaxime are metabolized to the desacetyl forms and provide less antibacterial activity than the parent compounds do. Ceftriaxone is metabolized to a small extent in the intestines to inactive metabolites, which are excreted via the biliary system.

Antibacterial activity of cephalosporins

This chart shows the generations of cephalosporins and the basis for those generations—their antibacterial spectrum of activity.

CEPHALOSPORINS	ANTIBACTERIAL SPECTRUM OF ACTIVITY
First-generation cephalosporins	
cefadroxil	Gram-positive organisms:
cefazolin	Most staphylococci
cephalexin	Groups A and B hemo-
cephalothin	lytic streptococci
cephapirin	Most streptococci
cephradine	Gram-negative organisms:
	Escherichia coli
	Klebsiella species
	Proteus mirabilis
	Hemophilus influenzae
Second-generation cephalosporins	
cefaclor	All of the above
cefamandole	Gram-negative organisms:
cefonicid	*Neisseria gonorroheae*
ceforanide	*Neisseria meningitidis*
cefoxitin	Indole-positive *Proteus*
cefuroxime	species
	Providencia species
	Enterobacter species
	Citrobacter species
	Anaerobic organisms:
	Clostridium species
	Peptococcus species
	Peptostreptococcus species
	Fusobacterium species
	Bacteroides species
Third-generation cephalosporins	
cefoperazone	All of the above
cefotaxime	Gram-negative organisms:
cefotetan	*Pseudomonas aerugi-*
ceftazidime	*nosa*
ceftizoxime	*Serratia* species
ceftriaxone	*Acinetobacter* species
moxalactam	

All cephalosporins are excreted primarily unchanged by the kidneys with the exception of cefoperazone and ceftriaxone, which are excreted in the feces via bile. Renal elimination occurs via glomerular filtration and tubular secretion. Dosage adjustments are necessary in patients with renal insufficiency, because serum concentration levels will increase. Dosages need not be altered for cefoperazone or ceftriaxone in patients

with impaired renal function unless hepatic impairment exists also. As with the penicillins, oral probenecid slows excretion of cephalosporins, especially those eliminated by renal tubular secretion.

Onset, peak, duration

After a 30-minute I.V. infusion, onset of action is rapid. Peak concentration levels are usually achieved within 1 hour. After I.V. administration of 1 gram, peak concentration levels are 50 to 100 mcg/ml for most cephalosporins. The higher concentration levels of cefazolin sodium given intravenously or intramuscularly is a considerable advantage over other first-generation cephalosporins. After I.M. administration, the onset of action usually is delayed. The peak concentration levels achieved are approximately 50% of those achieved after I.V. administration.

The serum half-life of cephalosporins in adults with normal renal function ranges from 0.4 to 10.9 hours. Among first-generation cephalosporins, cefazolin has the longest half-life, 2.2 hours, which allows an every-8-hour dosage schedule. Cefonicid sodium is the longest-acting second-generation cephalosporin, with a serum half-life of nearly 6 hours and 90% to 98% of the drug bound to serum proteins. The drug is normally given once daily. In patients with renal impairment, dosages and frequency of cefonicid administration depend on creatinine clearance. Among the third-generation cephalosporins, ceftriaxone displays the highest degree of plasma protein binding (85% to 95%) and the longest serum half-life (up to 10.9 hours). Ceftriaxone usually is administered once daily. Dosage adjustments of ceftriaxone usually are unnecessary in patients with impaired renal or hepatic function. The remaining cephalosporins have a serum half-life of 0.5 to 2 hours. They usually are administered at every-4-to-6-hour intervals in patients with normal renal function.

PHARMACODYNAMICS

The mechanism of action of the beta-lactam antibacterials is related to interference with cell-wall synthesis similar to penicillins. Rapidly growing organisms are more susceptible to these antibacterials.

Mechanism of action

Cephalosporins inhibit cell-wall synthesis by binding to bacterial enzymes (PBPs) located on the cell membrane. These enzymes are important for the biosynthesis of bacterial cell-wall components. The antibacterial action of cephalosporins depends on their ability to penetrate the bacterial cell wall and bind with proteins in the cy-

Distribution of cephalosporins

Therapeutic levels of cephalosporins are achieved in most tissues, but some cephalosporins are more effective than others in treating infections in certain areas. This illustration shows which cephalosporins are distributed most effectively to specific body parts or systems.

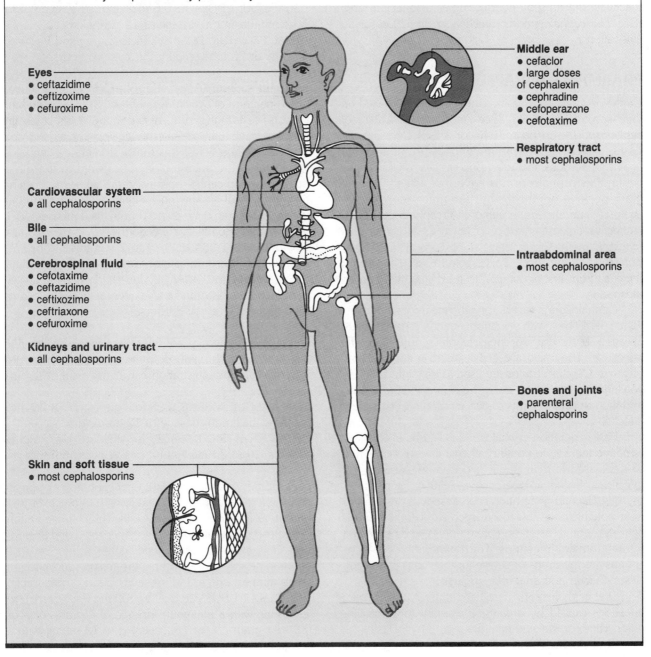

Eyes
- ceftazidime
- ceftizoxime
- cefuroxime

Cardiovascular system
- all cephalosporins

Bile
- all cephalosporins

Cerebrospinal fluid
- cefotaxime
- ceftazidime
- ceftixozime
- ceftriaxone
- cefuroxime

Kidneys and urinary tract
- all cephalosporins

Skin and soft tissue
- most cephalosporins

Middle ear
- cefaclor
- large doses of cephalexin
- cephradine
- cefoperazone
- cefotaxime

Respiratory tract
- most cephalosporins

Intraabdominal area
- most cephalosporins

Bones and joints
- parenteral cephalosporins

toplasmic membrane. Once the drug damages the cell wall by binding with the PBPs, the body's natural defense mechanisms destroy the bacteria. To produce a bactericidal effect on the cell, the cephalosporins must reach the PBPs in sufficient concentrations to inhibit cell-wall synthesis and must resist the destructive action of the beta-lactamases produced by some bacteria, which inactivate the drug by hydrolyzing its beta-lactam ring. (See *The cephalosporins' mechanism of action* for an illustration.)

PHARMACOTHERAPEUTICS

Cephalosporins are classified into generations based on their spectra of activity. (See *Antibacterial activity of cephalosporins* on page 1046 for a list.) Cefoxitin sodium, a second-generation cephalosporin, is active against anaerobes, including *Bacteroides fragilis*. Third-generation cephalosporins have less activity against gram-positive organisms but are much more active against *Pseudomonas aeruginosa*. All cephalosporins are ineffective against enterococci (such as *Streptococcus faecalis)*, methicillin-resistant staphylococci, and beta-hemolytic streptococci. Toxicity and cost of the drugs increase from first-generation to third-generation cephalosporins.

Cephalosporins are among the most prescribed antibacterials. They, with or without aminoglycosides, have always been the drugs of choice to treat serious *Klebsiella* infections. They also are widely used in surgical prophylaxis. Cephalosporins are used to treat infections involving the respiratory tract, the skin and soft tissues, and the bones and joints as well as certain urinary tract infections.

First-generation cephalosporins can be used as alternative therapy in patients allergic to penicillin. They also are used to treat staphylococcal and streptococcal infections, including pneumonia, cellulitis, and osteomyelitis. Second-generation cephalosporins are used to treat polymicrobial infections, such as diabetic foot ulcers, nosocomial aspiration pneumonias, and pelvic and intraabdominal infections. Third-generation cephalosporins are the drugs of choice for infections caused by *Acinetobacter* and anaerobic organisms.

Oral cephalosporins are used to treat urinary tract infections caused by organisms resistant to ampicillin, tetracycline, or the sulfonamides.

Cephalosporins are effective and well tolerated. Their major disadvantages are their cost and the emergence of gram-negative resistance.

cephalothin sodium (Keflin). The earliest available cephalosporin and the most stable against staphylococcal beta-lactamase, cephalothin is used to treat severe staph-

ylococcal infections. Incidence of nephrotoxicity increases with concurrent use of cephalothin and gentamicin. This first-generation cephalosporin is not well absorbed after oral administration and is administered parenterally only. Cephalothin usually is administered intravenously because it causes pain at the I.M. injection site.
USUAL ADULT DOSAGE: 0.5 to 2 grams I.V. every 4 to 6 hours; maximum dosage of 12 grams/day.
USUAL PEDIATRIC DOSAGE: 14 to 27 mg/kg I.V. every 4 hours or 20 to 40 mg/kg I.V. every 6 hours.

cefazolin sodium (Ancef, Kefzol). Cefazolin's antibacterial spectrum of activity resembles that of cephalothin. Because of its high serum concentration levels, cefazolin is more active than cephalothin against *Escherichia coli* and *Klebsiella* species. It is the best-tolerated cephalosporin for I.M. administration. Compared to the other first-generation cephalosporins, cefazolin has a substantially longer half-life and much higher peak concentration levels. A 500-mg dose every 8 hours is equivalent to 1 gram of cephalothin every 6 hours.
USUAL ADULT DOSAGE: 0.25 to 1.5 grams I.V. or I.M. every 6 to 8 hours; maximum dosage of 12 grams/day.
USUAL PEDIATRIC DOSAGE: for children over age 1 month, 6.25 to 25 mg/kg I.V. every 6 hours or 8.3 to 33.3 mg/kg I.V. every 8 hours.

cephapirin sodium (Cefadyl). Pharmacologically, this first-generation cephalosporin resembles cephalothin. Intramuscular administration can cause pain at the injection site.
USUAL ADULT DOSAGE: 0.25 to 2 grams I.V. every 4 to 6 hours; maximum dosage of 12 grams/day.
USUAL PEDIATRIC DOSAGE: for children over age 3 months, 10 to 20 mg/kg I.M. or I.V. every 6 hours.

cephradine (Anspor, Velosef). Oral cephradine appears to be chemically interchangeable with cephalexin; the parenteral form resembles cefazolin. This first-generation cephalosporin is unmetabolized; after rapid oral absorption, it is excreted unchanged in the urine. Because cephradine is so well absorbed, the serum concentration levels after an oral or I.M. dose are nearly comparable.
USUAL ADULT DOSAGE: 250 to 500 mg P.O. every 6 to 12 hours, with a maximum dosage of 4 grams/day; or 0.5 to 1 gram I.V. or I.M. every 6 to 12 hours, with a maximum dosage of 8 grams/day.
USUAL PEDIATRIC DOSAGE: 6.25 to 25 mg/kg P.O. every 6 hours.

cephalexin monohydrate (Keflex). Acid-stable and well absorbed from the GI tract, this first-generation cephalosporin is excreted unchanged in the urine. It is used

The cephalosporins' mechanism of action

An understanding of the cephalosporins' mechanism of action requires an understanding of the structure of a bacterial cell. Outside the *cytoplasmic membrane* lies a chemically complex, rigid cell wall that protects the cell against osmotic pressure and the outside environment. This cell wall contains a *mucocomplex layer,* which forms a sac around the bacterium. Acting as a filter, this layer prevents large molecules from passing through it. Gram-positive bacteria have a thick mucocomplex layer extending from the cytoplasmic membrane to the *teichoic acid layer* that coats the cell's exterior. In contrast, the mucocomplex layer in gram-negative cells is thin and supported by a complex outer cell wall composed of polysaccharides, lipids, and proteins. The gram-negative cell also contains *periplasmic space,* which lies between the cytoplasmic membrane and the cell wall.

Both gram-positive and gram-negative bacterial cell walls contain chemically similar *peptidoglycans,* the basic building blocks of the mucocomplex layer, which are necessary for cell-wall strength and rigidity. Cephalosporins inhibit the synthesis of these cell walls apparently by interfering with enzymatic action and preventing cross-linkage of these peptidoglycan chains.

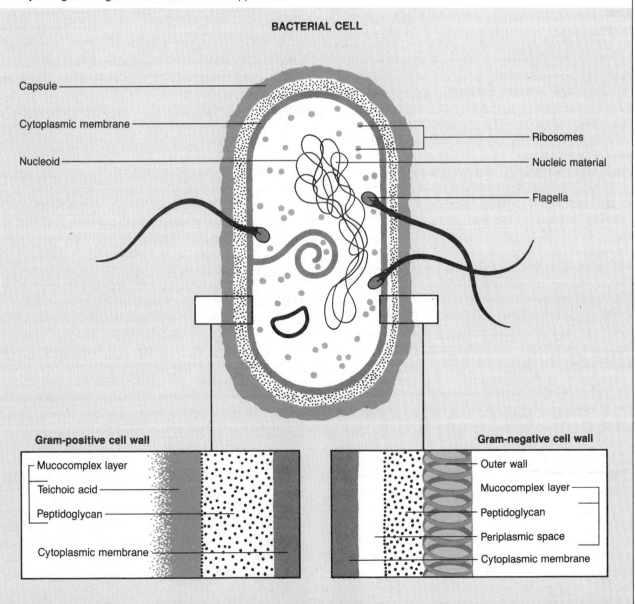

BACTERIAL CELL

Capsule
Cytoplasmic membrane
Nucleoid

Ribosomes
Nucleic material
Flagella

Gram-positive cell wall

Mucocomplex layer
Teichoic acid
Peptidoglycan
Cytoplasmic membrane

Gram-negative cell wall

Outer wall
Mucocomplex layer
Peptidoglycan
Periplasmic space
Cytoplasmic membrane

to treat urinary tract infections. Cephalexin is interchangeable with oral cephradine.

USUAL ADULT DOSAGE: 250 mg to 1 gram P.O. every 6 hours; maximum dosage of 4 grams/day.

USUAL PEDIATRIC DOSAGE: 6 to 12 mg/kg P.O. every 6 hours; maximum dosage of 25 mg/kg/day.

cefadroxil monohydrate (Duricef, Ultracef). Acid-stable, this first-generation cephalosporin is absorbed completely from the GI tract and has a long half-life. Unlike other oral cephalosporins, cefadroxil's absorption is not affected by food.

USUAL ADULT DOSAGE: 500 mg to 2 grams P.O. every 12 to 24 hours; maximum dosage of 2 grams/day.

USUAL PEDIATRIC DOSAGE: 30 mg/kg/day P.O. in two divided doses.

cefaclor (Ceclor). Acid-stable and well absorbed from the GI tract, cefaclor is used to treat respiratory tract infections and otitis media. The serum concentration levels after an oral dose are about 50% of those achieved after equivalent oral doses of cephalexin. However, this second-generation cephalosporin is more active against *Hemophilus influenzae, E.coli,* and *Proteus mirabilis* when compared to the first-generation oral cephalosporins.

USUAL ADULT DOSAGE: 250 to 500 mg P.O. every 8 hours; maximum dosage of 4 grams/day.

USUAL PEDIATRIC DOSAGE: 20 mg/kg P.O. daily in divided doses every 8 hours; maximum dosage of 1 gram/day.

cefamandole nafate (Mandol). A second-generation cephalosporin, cefamandole is more active than first-generation cephalosporins against gram-negative organisms such as *H. influenzae, Enterobacter,* and indole-positive *Proteus;* it also is used for gram-positive cocci. Because cefamandole is not absorbed orally, it must be administered parenterally.

USUAL ADULT DOSAGE: 500 mg to 2 grams I.V. or I.M. every 4 to 8 hours; maximum dosage of 12 grams/day.

USUAL PEDIATRIC DOSAGE: 50 to 100 mg/kg/day I.V. or I.M. in divided doses every 4 to 8 hours.

cefoxitin sodium (Mefoxin). A derivative of cephamycin C, produced by *Streptomyces lactamdurans,* cefoxitin is highly beta-lactamase resistant and provides excellent activity against anaerobes, especially *B. fragilis.* This second-generation cephalosporin is somewhat less active than cefamandole and the first-generation cephalosporins against gram-positive organisms but is more active against gram-negative bacteria, such as indole-positive *Proteus,* penicillinase-producing *Neisseria gonorrhoeae,* and some strains of *Serratia marcescens.* Cefoxitin's

special role is to treat certain mixed anaerobic-aerobic infections, such as diabetic foot ulcers, pelvic inflammatory disease, lung abscess, and aspiration pneumonia. Because cefoxitin causes pain at the I.M. injection site, it usually is administered intravenously.

USUAL ADULT DOSAGE: 1 to 2 grams I.V. or I.M. every 6 to 8 hours; maximum dosage of 12 grams/day.

USUAL PEDIATRIC DOSAGE: 80 to 160 mg/kg/day I.V. or I.M. in divided doses every 4 to 6 hours.

cefuroxime sodium (Zinacef). Cefuroxime's antibacterial spectrum of activity resembles that of cefamandole, but cefuroxime also can penetrate inflamed meninges. It is the only second-generation cephalosporin approved to treat bacterial meningitis *H. influenzae, Neisseria meningitidis,* and *Streptococcus pneumoniae.* Cefuroxime has a serum half-life of 1.5 hours as compared with 0.5 hour for cefamandole. Cefuroxime can be administered every 8 hours.

USUAL ADULT DOSAGE: 750 mg to 1.5 grams I.V. or I.M. every 8 hours, usually for 5 to 10 days; maximum dosage of 9 grams/day.

USUAL PEDIATRIC DOSAGE: 50 to 100 mg/kg/day I.M. or I.V. in divided doses every 6 to 8 hours; not for infants under age 3 months.

cefonicid sodium (Monocid). A second-generation cephalosporin, cefonicid's spectrum of activity resembles cefamandole's. The serum half-life of cefonicid is 4.5 hours, and only one daily dose is necessary. Cefonicid is used in single-dose surgical prophylaxis and for patients in nursing home and home care programs who require antibiotic therapy.

USUAL ADULT DOSAGE: 1 gram I.V. or I.M. daily; maximum dosage of 2 grams/day.

USUAL PEDIATRIC DOSAGE: not established.

ceforanide (Precef). A second-generation cephalosporin, ceforanide's structure and antibacterial spectrum of activity resemble those of cefamandole; however, ceforanide can be administered twice daily because its serum half-life is about 3 hours. It is used to treat pneumonia and soft-tissue and urinary tract infections.

USUAL ADULT DOSAGE: 0.5 to 1 gram I.V. or I.M. every 12 hours.

USUAL PEDIATRIC DOSAGE: 20 to 40 mg/kg/day in divided doses every 12 hours.

cefotetan disodium (Cefotan). A semisynthetic parenteral cephamycin derivative, cefotetan has a spectrum of activity somewhere between the second- and third-generation cephalosporins; however, it is usually considered a third-generation cephalosporin. The in vitro activity against gram-negative bacilli resembles that of cefotaxime; however, cefotetan is less active against *Enterobacter* and *Serratia* species and has no useful activity against *P. aeruginosa*. Compared with cefoxitin, cefotetan is less active against *B. fragilis*. Cefotetan can be given every 12 hours.

USUAL ADULT DOSAGE: 1 to 2 grams I.V. or I.M. every 12 hours; maximum dosage of 6 grams/day.
USUAL PEDIATRIC DOSAGE: not established.

cefotaxime sodium (Claforan). The first of the third-generation cephalosporins available in the United States, cefotaxime has an enhanced spectrum of activity against gram-negative aerobic organisms except *P. aeruginosa*. Used to treat gram-negative meningitis, cefotaxime provides effective activity against gram-positive organisms except enterococci and exhibits poor activity against anaerobes, such as *B. fragilis*. Cefotaxime is metabolized to desacetyl cefotaxime, which is less active than the parent compound.

USUAL ADULT DOSAGE: 1 to 2 grams I.V. or I.M. every 4 to 8 hours; maximum dosage of 12 grams/day.
USUAL PEDIATRIC DOSAGE: for neonates up to age 1 week, 50 mg/kg I.V. every 12 hours; for neonates over age 1 week, 50 mg/kg I.V. every 8 hours; for children up to 50 kg, 8.3 to 30 mg/kg I.M. or I.V. every 4 hours or 12.5 to 45 mg/kg I.M. or I.V. every 6 hours; for children over 50 kg, same as adult.

moxalactam disodium (Moxam). A semisynthetic 1-oxa-beta-lactam, moxalactam differs structurally from the other third-generation cephalosporins. This difference greatly enhances its antibacterial activity, particularly against gram-negative bacteria. Compared to cefotaxime, moxalactam is less active against staphylococci and enterococci but is equally effective against most of the Enterobacteriaceae. Numerous reports of bleeding and enterococcal superinfections caused by moxalactam do not occur with other cephalosporins.

USUAL ADULT DOSAGE: 1 to 4 grams I.V. or I.M. every 8 to 12 hours for up to 14 days; maximum dosage of 12 grams/day.
USUAL PEDIATRIC DOSAGE: for children, 50 mg/kg I.M. or I.V. every 6 to 8 hours; for neonates, 50 mg/kg I.M. or I.V. every 8 to 12 hours.

cefoperazone sodium (Cefobid). Less active than cefotaxime against the Enterobacteriaceae, this third-generation cephalosporin has greater activity against *P. aeruginosa*. The dose need not be adjusted in renal impairment. Although it achieves adequate CNS levels, cefoperazone is not indicated to treat meningitis.

USUAL ADULT DOSAGE: 1 to 2 grams I.V. or I.M. every 12 hours; maximum dosage of 12 grams/day.
USUAL PEDIATRIC DOSAGE: not established.

ceftizoxime sodium (Cefizox). A third-generation cephalosporin, ceftizoxime's spectrum of activity resembles that of cefotaxime; however, ceftizoxime has a longer serum half-life and can be administered every 8 to 12 hours instead of every 4 to 8 hours. Dosage adjustment is necessary in patients with renal insufficiency.

USUAL ADULT DOSAGE: 1 to 2 grams I.V. or I.M. every 8 to 12 hours; maximum dosage of 12 grams/day.
USUAL PEDIATRIC DOSAGE: for children over age 6 months, 50 mg/kg I.V. every 6 to 8 hours.

ceftriaxone sodium (Rocephin). Ceftriaxone's antibacterial spectrum of activity is similar to that of ceftizoxime and cefotaxime. Ceftriaxone has the longest half-life of all the third-generation cephalosporins (about 9 hours), which allows for once-daily dosage. Ceftriaxone is used to treat meningitis caused by susceptible organisms and penicillinase-producing *N. gonorrhoeae*. Dosage adjustment is not necessary in patients with renal insufficiency.

USUAL ADULT DOSAGE: 1 to 2 grams I.V. or I.M. every 12 to 24 hours (maximum dosage of 4 grams/day); for meningitis, 100 mg/kg I.V. or I.M. in divided doses every 12 hours; may administer 75 mg/kg as a loading dose.
USUAL PEDIATRIC DOSAGE: 25 to 37.5 mg/kg I.V. or I.M. every 12 hours.

ceftazidime (Fortaz, Tazicef, Tazidime). Ceftazidime's spectrum of activity is excellent against *P. aeruginosa* and good against the Enterobacteriaceae (resembling that of cefotaxime), but ceftazidime exhibits the poorest activity among all third-generation cephalosporins against gram-positive organisms and *B. fragilis*. Ceftazidime is used to treat *P. aeruginosa* meningitis and CNS infections caused by *H. influenzae* and *N. meningitidis*. Dosage adjustment is necessary in patients with renal impairment.

USUAL ADULT DOSAGE: 1 gram I.V. or I.M. every 8 to 12 hours; maximum dosage of 6 grams/day.
USUAL PEDIATRIC DOSAGE: for neonates up to age 1 month, 30 mg/kg I.V. every 12 hours; for children over age 1 month to 12 years, 30 to 50 mg/kg I.V. every 8 hours; maximum dosage of 6 grams/day.

Drug interactions

Patients receiving cefamandole, cefoperazone, or moxalactam who drink alcoholic beverages concurrently or up to 72 hours after drug administration may experience acute alcohol intolerance with symptoms similar to disulfiram (Antabuse) reaction. Patients may experience headache, flushing, dizziness, nausea, vomiting, or abdominal cramps within 30 minutes of alcohol ingestion.

Concomitant use of cephalosporins and imipenem/cilastatin can antagonize the antibacterial activity of the beta-lactam cephalosporins.

Uricosurics, such as probenecid and sulfinpyrazone, can block the renal tubular secretion of some cephalosporins. Probenecid is used therapeutically to increase and prolong cephalosporin plasma concentration levels.

ADVERSE DRUG REACTIONS

Cephalosporins are relatively safe, but with the development of newer and more potent second- and third-generation cephalosporins, adverse reactions have increased.

Predictable reactions

Intramuscular administration of cephalothin and cefoxitin frequently produces pain, induration, and tenderness at the injection site. Thrombophlebitis is associated most commonly with I.V. cephalothin. Frequent changes of I.V. sites may be necessary.

High doses of cephalosporins administered to patients with impaired renal function may produce confusion and convulsions. Seizures associated with high doses of cefazolin also can occur.

Serious bleeding related to hypoprothrombinemia, thrombocytopenia, or platelet dysfunction can occur in patients receiving moxalactam or cefoperazone. This coagulation disorder is a problem in elderly and poorly nourished patients and in those with renal failure.

Orally administered cephalosporins frequently produce nausea, vomiting, and diarrhea. These adverse reactions, which are usually mild and transient, may be alleviated by administering the drug with food. Antibiotic-associated pseudomembranous colitis caused by *Clostridium difficile* may occur during or after cephalosporin therapy, especially with the third-generation cephalosporins.

Cephalosporins may produce nephrotoxicity. High doses of cephalothin can lead to acute tubular necrosis, and usual doses of 8 to 12 grams/day can be nephrotoxic in patients with renal disease. Cephalothin administered with an aminoglycoside, such as gentamicin, can be nephrotoxic.

Unpredictable reactions

Hypersensitivity reactions are the most common systemic adverse reactions to cephalosporins. Allergic reactions range in severity from mild to life-threatening.

Usual allergic reactions appear as urticaria, pruritus or morbilliform eruptions, and serum sickness reactions. Anaphylaxis is rare.

Because of the similarities between penicillins and cephalosporins, a 5% to 10% cross-reactivity may occur. No cephalosporin skin test can predict whether a patient will have an allergic reaction. Patients with a history of mild penicillin reactions are at low risk for developing an allergic reaction to cephalosporins; however, patients who have had severe immediate reactions to penicillin are at high risk and should be monitored carefully when they are administered cephalosporin.

NURSING IMPLICATIONS

Because cephalosporins are among the most frequently prescribed antibacterials, the nurse will encounter them frequently and should be aware of these implications:
• Avoid administering cephalosporins to a patient who recently has experienced a severe, immediate reaction to penicillins or cephalosporins. Obtain a thorough drug history, and screen patients for possible allergy and cross-reactions with cephalosporins.
• Infuse all I.V. cephalosporins over 30 minutes to prevent pain and irritation.
• Decrease pain at the injection site during I.M. administration of cefoxitin and ceftriaxone by reconstituting drugs with a 0.5% to 1% lidocaine injection.
• Monitor the patient closely for signs and symptoms of superinfection, such as diarrhea, sore mouth (oral thrush), and vaginal itching. To prevent intestinal superinfection, advise the patient to ingest yogurt or buttermilk, which replenishes normal gut flora.
• Advise the patient taking moxalactam, cefoperazone, cefamandole, or cefotetan to avoid food or other medications containing alcohol (elixirs).
• Advise the diabetic patient taking cephalosporins to test urine glucose levels with Tes-Tape or Clinistix (not Clinitest).

TETRACYCLINES

Although among the most commonly prescribed antibacterials in the world, tetracyclines rarely are considered drugs of choice for most common bacterial infections. Overuse of tetracyclines has led to the emergence of tetracycline-resistant bacteria.

History and source

Development of the tetracyclines resulted from a systematic screening of antibacterial-producing microorganisms in soil collected from many parts of the world. In 1948, Duggar discovered the first compound, chlortetracycline hydrochloride. In 1950, oxytetracycline hydrochloride was derived. The third member of this group, tetracycline hydrochloride, was produced in 1952 by chemically modifying chlortetracycline. The most recently introduced semisynthetic second-generation tetracyclines were doxycycline hyclate (1966) and minocycline hydrochloride (1967).

PHARMACOKINETICS

The tetracycline analogues are classified as (1) short-acting compounds (chlortetracycline, oxytetracycline, and tetracycline), (2) intermediate-acting compounds (demeclocycline hydrochloride and methacycline hydrochloride), and (3) long-acting compounds (doxycycline and minocycline). Both doxycycline and minocycline provide an improved antibacterial spectrum of activity; because of their lipid solubility, they also have improved tissue penetration and a longer half-life.

Absorption, distribution, metabolism, excretion

After oral administration, tetracyclines are absorbed rapidly from the duodenum. Absorption is impaired by intake of dairy products; it is drastically reduced by iron preparations or the concomitant administration of antacids containing calcium, magnesium, or aluminum salts. Food interferes little with doxycycline and minocycline absorption; both drugs usually are taken with food to minimize possible GI irritation. However, food does affect the absorption of other tetracyclines, which should be taken on an empty stomach 1 hour before or 2 hours after meals. Absorption of various tetracyclines differs: doxycycline and minocycline are well absorbed (90% to 100%); oxytetracycline and tetracycline are poorly absorbed. Tetracyclines are poorly and erratically absorbed after I.M. administration.

The tetracyclines are distributed widely into body tissues and fluids, including pleural fluid, synovial fluid, bronchial secretions, sputum, and prostatic fluid. Intravenous administration of a tetracycline results in a CSF concentration of approximately 25% of serum concentration levels. Oral or I.M. administration results in an even lower CSF concentration level. Meningeal inflammation is not required for tetracycline penetration into the CSF. Because doxycycline and, to a greater extent, minocycline are more lipid-soluble than other tetracyclines, they penetrate most body tissues and fluids well. Relatively high concentration levels of minocycline are found in tears and saliva, and minocycline is used as an alternative to rifampin to eradicate *Neisseria meningitidis* from asymptomatic carriers. All tetracyclines are distributed into bile; the tetracyclines cross the placenta, and relatively high concentration levels appear in breast milk.

The tetracyclines concentrate in bile. Biliary concentration levels average 5 to 10 times higher than corresponding serum concentration levels. Obstruction of the hepatobiliary tract decreases the biliary concentration levels of tetracyclines. Minocycline is partially metabolized in the liver to at least six metabolites. Doxycycline is partially inactivated in the intestine. Demeclocycline, methacycline, oxytetracycline, and tetracycline are not metabolized in the liver.

With the exception of doxycycline and minocycline, tetracyclines are primarily excreted by the kidneys. Oxytetracycline and tetracycline are excreted almost entirely unchanged in urine. About 60% of the active drug is recovered in the urine; 40%, in the feces. Demeclocycline and methacycline also are excreted primarily by the kidneys; about 60% of methacycline and 40% of demeclocycline are excreted unchanged. Doxycycline is excreted independent of renal and hepatic function. Researchers believe that doxycycline is inactivated by chelate formation in the intestine and is excreted in the feces. Minocycline undergoes enterohepatic recirculation; only about 10% of the active drug is excreted in the urine. Other tetracyclines should not be used in patients with impaired renal function because azotemia, metabolic acidosis, and hepatotoxicity can result.

Onset, peak, duration

Oral administration of the tetracyclines results in detectable serum concentration levels in 30 minutes; peak concentration levels are reached in 1 to 4 hours. After oral administration of 500 mg of tetracycline or 100 mg of doxycycline or minocycline, peak serum concentration levels are reached in 2 hours. Peak serum concentration levels are reached 1 hour after I.V. administration of 500 mg of tetracycline or 100 mg of doxycycline or minocycline. Because of a prolonged serum half-life of about 20 hours, doxycycline and minocycline can maintain adequate serum concentration levels with administration every 12 to 24 hours. The serum half-life of tetracycline is about 8.5 hours; the patient should receive a dose every 6 hours. After I.M. administration of oxytetracycline or tetracycline, peak serum concentration levels are reached in 30 minutes to 1 hour. With usual dosages, the serum concentration levels achieved after I.M. administration are lower than those after oral administration.

PHARMACODYNAMICS

All tetracyclines are primarily bacteriostatic. Like the aminoglycosides, they interfere with protein synthesis.

Mechanism of action

The tetracyclines penetrate the interior of the bacterial cell by an energy-dependent process. Once within the cell, the tetracyclines reversibly bind primarily to a subunit of the ribosome, thereby inhibiting access of transfer RNA–amino acid complexes to the messenger RNA–ribosome complex. This action prevents the addition of new amino acids to the peptide chain.

PHARMACOTHERAPEUTICS

The tetracyclines provide a broad spectrum of activity against gram-positive, gram-negative, aerobic, and anaerobic bacteria, and spirochetes, mycoplasmas, rickettsiae, chlamydiae, and some protozoa. In general, doxycycline and minocycline provide more action against various organisms than the other tetracyclines do. Tetracyclines are used to treat Rocky Mountain spotted fever, Q fever, Lyme disease, brucellosis, and tularemia. They are the drugs of choice for treating nongonococcal urethritis caused by *Chlamydia* and *Ureaplasma urealyticum.*

Tetracycline or erythromycin is the drug of choice for treating *Mycoplasma pneumoniae* infections. Combination therapy with a tetracycline and streptomycin is the most effective treatment for brucellosis. Tetracyclines also can be used to treat syphilis and gonorrhea in patients allergic to penicillin. The tetracyclines effectively treat acne because they can decrease the fatty acid content of sebum: low-dose tetracycline (250 mg b.i.d.) is used for this condition. Although the tetracyclines are active against many aerobic gram-positive cocci, they are not used to treat staphylococcal, group A beta-hemolytic streptococcal, or pneumococcal infections because of the tetracycline resistance displayed by these bacteria.

chlortetracycline hydrocholoride (Aureomycin). Available as a 3% ointment for topical use, chlortetracycline is indicated for infection prophylaxis in minor skin abrasions and for treating superficial skin infections. The preparation may stain clothing. Chlortetracycline is also available as a 1% ophthalmic ointment, which is used to treat bacterial conjunctivitis.
USUAL ADULT DOSAGE: for skin infections, applied to the affected area b.i.d. or t.i.d.; for conjunctivitis, approximately 1 cm of ointment applied to the conjunctival sac every 2 to 4 hours.

demeclocycline hydrochloride (Declomycin). Demeclocycline is used to successfully treat susceptible gram-negative and gram-positive infections. Photosensitivity reactions to demeclocycline occur more frequently and more severely than with other tetracyclines.
USUAL ADULT DOSAGE: for infections caused by susceptible gram-negative and gram-positive organisms, *Chlamydia trachomatis,* and rickettsiae, 150 to 300 mg P.O. every 6 hours or 300 mg P.O. every 12 hours; for gonorrhea, 600 mg P.O. initially, then 300 mg P.O. every 12 hours for 4 days.
USUAL PEDIATRIC DOSAGE: for children over 8 years old, 6 to 12 mg/kg P.O. daily in divided doses every 6 to 12 hours.

doxycycline hyclate (Vibramycin). Doxycycline does not accumulate in patients with renal or hepatic dysfunction. It is effective as a prophylactic treatment for traveler's diarrhea caused by toxigenic strains of *Escherichia coli* and frequently is used to treat pelvic inflammatory disease and cervicitis caused by *C. trachomatis.* Doxycycline and rifampin have been used as an alternative to erythromycin to treat pneumonia caused by *Legionella pneumophila.*
USUAL ADULT DOSAGE: for infections caused by sensitive gram-negative and gram-positive organisms, *C. trachomatis,* and rickettsiae, 100 mg P.O. every 12 hours on first day followed by 100 mg P.O. daily, or 200 mg I.V. on the first day in one or two infusions followed by 100 to 200 mg I.V. daily; administer the I.V. infusion slowly (minimum of 1 hour); complete the infusion within 12 hours (within 6 hours in lactated Ringer's solution or dextrose 5% in lactated Ringer's solution); for gonorrhea in patients allergic to penicillin, 200 mg P.O. initially, followed by 100 mg P.O. at bedtime and 100 mg P.O. b.i.d. for 3 days, or 300 mg P.O. initially with the dose repeated in 1 hour; for primary or secondary syphilis in patients allergic to penicillin, 300 mg P.O. daily in divided doses for 10 days; for uncomplicated urethral, endocervical, or rectal infections caused by *C. trachomatis* or *U. urealyticum,* 100 mg P.O. b.i.d. for at least 7 days; to prevent traveler's diarrhea caused by enterotoxigenic *E. coli,* 100 mg P.O. daily.
USUAL PEDIATRIC DOSAGE: for children 45 kg and under, 2.2 to 4.4 mg/kg P.O. or I.V. once daily or 1.1 to 2.2 mg/kg P.O. or I.V. every 12 hours; for children over 45 kg, same as adult.

methacycline hydrochloride (Rondomycin). Although methacycline is indicated to treat *M. pneumoniae,* uncomplicated gonorrhea, and syphilis, it is used rarely. Tetracycline and doxycycline have replaced methacycline because they are recommended by the Centers for Disease Control (CDC).

USUAL ADULT DOSAGE: 150 to 300 mg P.O. every 6 to 12 hours.

USUAL PEDIATRIC DOSAGE: for children age 8 and over, 1.65 to 3.3 mg/kg P.O. every 6 hours or 3.3 to 6.6 mg/kg P.O. every 12 hours; not recommended for children under age 8.

minocycline hydrochloride (Minocin). Because it enters salivary secretions, minocycline is effective in treating asymptomatic carriers of *Neisseria meningitidis*. Minocycline also is used to treat severe acne because of its high lipophilicity. However, minocycline should not be administered to patients with renal insufficiency.

USUAL ADULT DOSAGE: for infections caused by sensitive gram-negative and gram-positive organisms, *C. trachomatis,* or amebiasis, 200 mg P.O. or I.V. initially, followed by 100 mg every 12 hours or 50 mg P.O. every 6 hours; for gonorrhea in patients sensitive to penicillin, 200 mg P.O. initially followed by 100 mg every 12 hours for 4 days; for syphilis in patients sensitive to penicillin, 200 mg P.O. initially followed by 100 mg P.O. every 12 hours for 10 to 15 days; for meningococcal carrier state, 100 to 200 mg P.O. every 12 hours for 5 days; for uncomplicated urethral, endocervical, or rectal infection caused by *C. trachomatis* or *U. urealyticum,* 100 mg P.O. b.i.d. for at least 7 days; for uncomplicated gonococcal urethritis in males, 100 mg P.O. b.i.d. for 5 days.

USUAL PEDIATRIC DOSAGE: for infections caused by sensitive gram-negative and gram-positive organisms, *C. trachomatis,* or amebiasis, for children over 8 years old, 4 mg/kg P.O. or I.V. initially, followed by 4 mg/kg P.O. daily in divided doses every 12 hours; administer I.V. in 500 to 1,000 ml of solution without calcium over 6 hours. Not recommended for use in children under age 8.

oxytetracycline hydrochloride (Terramycin). Oral administration of oxytetracycline is preferred; I.M. administration produces pain and lower serum concentration levels. Intravenous therapy may lead to thrombophlebitis. Because oxytetracycline is excreted in urine to a great degree, it is ideal for treating urinary tract infections.

USUAL ADULT DOSAGE: for infections caused by sensitive gram-negative and gram-positive organisms, *C. trachomatis,* or rickettsiae, 250 mg P.O. every 6 hours, or 100 mg I.M. every 8 to 12 hours, 250 mg I.M. every 12 hours, or 250 to 500 mg I.V. every 6 to 12 hours; for brucellosis, 500 mg P.O. q.i.d. for 3 weeks, given with 1 gram of streptomycin sulfate I.M. every 12 hours the 1st week and once daily the 2nd week; for syphilis in patients sensitive to penicillin, 30 to 50 grams in a total dose P.O. divided equally over 10 to 15 days; for gonorrhea in patients sensitive to penicillin, 1.5 grams

P.O. initially, followed by 0.5 gram q.i.d. for a total of 9 grams.

USUAL PEDIATRIC DOSAGE: for infections caused by sensitive gram-negative and gram-positive organisms, *C. trachomatis,* and rickettsiae in children over 8 years old, 25 to 50 mg/kg P.O. daily in divided doses every 6 hours, or 15 to 25 mg/kg I.M. daily in divided doses every 8 to 12 hours, or 10 to 20 mg/kg I.V. daily in divided doses every 12 hours.

tetracycline hydrochloride (Achromycin, Sumycin). This drug is used frequently to treat acute exacerbations of chronic bronchitis, infections caused by *Mycoplasma pneumoniae,* urinary tract infections, gonorrhea, and syphilis in penicillin-allergic patients. Phlebitis and pain at the infusion site limit I.V. use to those situations in which oral administration is not feasible. Intramuscular injection is not recommended because of pain on injection.

USUAL ADULT DOSAGE: for infections caused by sensitive gram-negative and gram-positive organisms, rickettsiae, and *Mycoplasma,* 250 to 500 mg P.O. every 6 hours, 250 mg I.M. daily, 150 mg I.M. every 12 hours, or 250 to 500 mg I.V. every 8 to 12 hours (for I.M. and I.V., hydrochloride salt only); for uncomplicated urethral, endocervical, or rectal infection caused by *C. trachomatis,* 500 mg P.O. q.i.d. for at least 7 days; for brucellosis, 500 mg P.O. every 6 hours for 3 weeks with 1 gram of streptomycin I.M. every 12 hours the 1st week and daily the 2nd week; for gonorrhea in patients sensitive to penicillin, 1.5 grams P.O. initially, followed by 500 mg every 6 hours for a total of 9 grams; for syphilis in patients sensitive to penicillin, 30 to 50 grams total in equally divided doses over 10 to 15 days; for acne in adults and adolescents, 250 mg P.O. every 6 hours initially, followed by 125 to 500 mg P.O. daily or every other day; for shigellosis, 2.5 grams P.O. in one dose.

USUAL PEDIATRIC DOSAGE: for children over 8 years old, 25 to 50 mg/kg P.O. daily in divided doses every 6 hours, 15 to 25 mg/kg/day (maximum dosage of 250 mg) I.M. as a single dose or in divided doses every 8 to 12 hours, or 10 to 20 mg/kg I.V. daily in divided doses every 12 hours.

Drug interactions

The nurse should be aware of the numerous significant interactions between tetracyclines and other drugs. (See *Drug interactions: Tetracyclines* on page 1056 for a summary.)

ADVERSE DRUG REACTIONS

Tetracyclines produce many of the same adverse reactions that the other antibacterials do, such as super-

DRUG INTERACTIONS
Tetracyclines

This chart summarizes the interactions between the tetracyclines and other drugs that the nurse should know.

DRUG	INTERACTING DRUGS	POSSIBLE EFFECTS	NURSING IMPLICATIONS
chlortetracycline, demeclocycline, doxycycline, methacycline, minocycline, oxytetracycline, tetracyline	antacids with divalent or trivalent cations, such as aluminum and magnesium	Inhibit oral absorption of tetracyclines	• Separate doses by 1 to 2 hours.
	diuretics	Elevate BUN levels	• Do not administer tetracyclines to patients taking diuretics.
	methoxyflurane	Produces nephrotoxicity	• Avoid tetracycline use in patients who are to receive anesthesia with methoxyflurane.
tetracycline, oxytetracycline, methacycline, doxycycline	ferrous sulfate	Impairs GI absorption of tetracyclines	• Administer ferrous sulfate 3 hours before or 2 hours after tetracyclines.
doxycycline	alcohol	Enhances doxycycline metabolism	• Avoid concurrent use; if necessary, assess the patient for reduced antibacterial effect.
	barbiturates	Enhance doxycycline metabolism	• Avoid concurrent use.
	carbamazepine	Enhances doxycycline metabolism	• Avoid concurrent use.

infection (overgrowth of tetracycline-resistant organisms) and GI disturbances. Because these drugs can significantly affect tooth enamel development, they are not recommended for children under age 8 or for pregnant patients.

Predictable reactions
GI adverse reactions resulting from oral administration include nausea, vomiting, abdominal distress and distention, and diarrhea. Diarrhea frequently is related to alterations in the enteric flora. Doxycycline affects gut flora less than tetracycline. The diarrhea usually subsides when the drug is stopped; prolonged symptoms from pseudomembranous colitis have occurred.

Photosensitivity reactions (red rash on areas exposed to sunlight) occur most frequently in patients receiving demeclocycline and doxycycline. However, photosensitivity reactions can occur with any tetracycline.

The tetracyclines cause permanent gray-brown to yellow discoloration of the teeth when administered during tooth formation. Darkening of permanent teeth may be related to the total dosage of tetracycline. Bone deposition from a tetracycline temporarily halts bone growth. The tetracyclines should not be administered to pregnant patients or to children under age 8, the period when tooth enamel is forming.

Hepatotoxic reactions to tetracyclines include fatty infiltration of the liver associated primarily with I.V. tetracyclines. This reaction is most significant in pregnant patients given doses greater than 2 grams/day and in patients with an excessive serum concentration level caused by renal failure.

Nephrotoxicity develops in patients with renal failure; the antianabolic effects of tetracyclines may increase BUN and serum creatinine levels. Outdated or degraded tetracycline can produce a reversible Fanconi-like syndrome with renal tubular acidosis. However, because tetracycline preparations that have produced this syndrome have been reformulated, this complication is unlikely to recur.

CNS toxicity, including vestibular disturbances, occurs primarily with minocycline. Light-headedness, loss of balance, dizziness, and tinnitus usually begin on the 2nd or 3rd day of therapy and occur more frequently in women than men. Symptoms are reversible within several days after discontinuing the drug.

As with the use of any antibiotic, superinfection frequently develops during tetracycline therapy. Overgrowth of yeast frequently occurs, and oral or vaginal moniliasis requires specific therapy. Staphylococcal enterocolitis caused by tetracycline-resistant staphylococci can lead to severe diarrhea, dehydration, and possible circulatory collapse.

Unpredictable reactions

Hypersensitivity reactions to tetracyclines include anaphylaxis, urticaria, periorbital edema, fixed drug eruptions, and morbilliform rashes. These unpredictable reactions occur infrequently.

NURSING IMPLICATIONS

Because tetracyclines are prescribed frequently, the nurse should be aware of these implications:
• Avoid administration in children under age 8 and in older children exhibiting delayed or arrested growth and development.
• Assess patients for hypersensitivity, renal impairment, pregnancy, and lactation before initiating tetracycline therapy.
• Administer oral preparations with 8 fluid ounces (240 ml) of water to prevent esophageal irritation and possible ulcer formation.
• Monitor the patient for signs and symptoms of hepatotoxicity or nephrotoxicity.
• Dilute I.V. preparations in large volumes of fluids and administer them by continuous slow drip.
• Check orders for I.M. injections because I.M. administration is usually not recommended. If I.M. injections must be administered, inject the drug deep into a large muscle.
• Know that the tetracyclines alter laboratory results. (See *How tetracyclines affect laboratory tests* for details.)
• Advise the patient not to ingest milk, milk products, or drugs containing calcium, magnesium, aluminum, or iron at the same time as tetracycline, because these products bind with tetracycline and prevent absorption. (This does not occur with minocycline or doxycycline.)
• Advise the patient to take tetracyclines on an empty stomach if possible.
• Advise the patient to avoid direct sunlight, cover exposed skin, or use a sunscreen with an SPF of 15 or higher.
• Be aware that some tetracyclines contain tartrazine, a dye which can cause an allergic reaction in a sensitive patient.

CHLORAMPHENICOL

Chloramphenicol was released for clinical use in 1949. Soon afterward, drug-induced aplastic anemia limited its clinical usefulness; today, chloramphenicol is reserved for treating serious infections. In recent years, however,

How tetracyclines affect laboratory tests

Tetracyclines can alter the results of blood, urine, and liver function tests. Specific tests in each category are listed on this chart.

Blood tests	Altered results
Serum amylase level	Increased
Indirect Coombs' test	False positive
Lupus erythematosus cell preparation	False positive
Hemoglobin value	Decreased
Platelet count	Decreased
Serum glucose level	Variable, depending on testing method
Urine tests	
Serum creatinine level	Increased
Urine protein level	Increased
Urea nitrogen level	Increased
Urine glucose level	Variable, depending on testing method
Urine catecholamine level	Increased
Liver function tests	
Blood ammonia level	Decreased
Bilirubin level	Increased
Alkaline phosphatase level	Increased
Serum glutamic-oxaloacetic transaminase (SGOT), or aspartate aminotransferase (AST), level	Increased
Serum glutamic-pyruvic transaminase (SGPT), or alanine aminotransferase (ALT), level	Increased
Lactic dehydrogenase (LDH) level	Increased

an increased awareness of the pathogenicity of anaerobic organisms and the development of ampicillin-resistant *Hemophilus influenzae* have revived the clinical interest in chloramphenicol.

History and source

Chloramphenicol was originally produced by *Streptomyces venezuelae,* discovered in soil samples from Venezuela in 1947 by Burkholder and in compost by workers at the University of Illinois. The drug was synthesized in 1948 and marketed for general use in 1949. The importance of this broad-spectrum antibacterial was quickly recognized; however, incidences of serious blood dyscrasias caused it to fall into disfavor as early as 1950. The drug is now produced synthetically.

PHARMACOKINETICS

Chloramphenicol is available in capsules for oral treatment and in ointment for topical treatment of ophthalmic or otic infections. It also is available as chloramphenicol palmitate in oral suspensions, and as chloramphenicol succinate for I.V. administration. Chloramphenicol salts must be hydrolyzed to free chloramphenicol before pharmacologic action can occur.

Absorption, distribution, metabolism, excretion

Chloramphenicol is absorbed rapidly and completely from the GI tract and is not impaired by the concomitant administration of food or antacids. Chloramphenicol salts are hydrolyzed slowly to free drug by pancreatic lipases in the duodenum; as a result, peak serum concentration levels are somewhat lower and delayed compared with those of chloramphenicol. Intravenous preparations must also be hydrolyzed before they can provide antibacterial activity. When chloramphenicol is administered orally, hydrolysis occurs in the GI tract; hydrolysis occurs in the plasma after I.V. administration.

After absorption, chloramphenicol is widely distributed to body fluids and tissue. The drug's lipid solubility permits penetration across lipid barriers. Peak concentration levels are high in the CNS even without inflammation. Levels in the CSF, with or without meningitis, are usually one third to three fourths of the peak serum concentration levels. Chloramphenicol crosses the blood-ocular barrier. Lipid solubility also accounts for increased uptake by alveolar macrophages. Chloramphenicol crosses the placenta to the fetal circulation but appears in negligible amounts in the amniotic fluid. Chloramphenicol is excreted in breast milk.

In patients with normal hepatic function, free chloramphenicol is metabolized primarily in the liver by glucuronide conjugation. The nontoxic glucuronide metabolite is excreted in inactive form by the kidneys. Glucuronyl transferase, the enzyme that metabolizes chloramphenicol, is not very active in newborns or in adults with serious hepatic dysfunction; administering usual doses of chloramphenicol to such patients can lead to increased serum concentration levels of biologically active drug.

Only 5% to 10% of an administered dose is recovered in urine as biologically active chloramphenicol. The rest is metabolized by the liver. If the patient has no renal disease, concentration levels of 150 to 200 mcg/ml of active drug are achieved, sufficient to treat urinary tract infections. However, urine concentration levels are decreased greatly in patients with renal failure.

Onset, peak, duration

Peak serum concentration levels occur 2 to 3 hours after oral administration. Peak concentration levels occur 1 to 2 hours after I.V. infusion. Chloramphenicol is 50% to 60% bound to serum albumin. Plasma half-life in adults with normal liver function is 1.5 to 3.5 hours. The half-life is prolonged greatly in patients with immature or inadequate liver function, lasting 24 hours or longer in neonates.

Therapeutic peak concentration levels are 10 to 25 mcg/ml. Levels exceeding 25 mcg/ml may lead to reversible bone marrow suppression; levels greater than 40 mcg/ml have been associated with gray syndrome in neonates and encephalitis in adults.

PHARMACODYNAMICS

Chloramphenicol usually is bacteriostatic and may be bactericidal against some organisms.

Mechanism of action

Chloramphenicol, which inhibits protein synthesis of susceptible organisms, also inhibits protein synthesis in cells that proliferate rapidly, such as bone marrow cells. The inhibition can lead to bone marrow suppression. The major mechanism of resistance in gram-negative bacilli other than *Pseudomonas aeruginosa* is enzymatic acetylation, which is plasmid-mediated. *P. aeruginosa* and some strains of *Proteus* and *Klebsiella* resist via nonenzymatic mechanisms, including an induced block that prevents chloramphenicol from entering the bacterial cell.

PHARMACOTHERAPEUTICS

Chloramphenicol is active against various organisms, including bacteria, spirochetes, rickettsiae, chlamydiae, and mycoplasmas. Easily reached serum concentration levels of chloramphenicol inhibit most gram-positive and gram-negative aerobic bacteria, but more active and less toxic agents are available. Chloramphenicol is extremely active against anaerobic bacteria, including *Bacteroides fragilis*. It is the drug of choice for treating ampicillin-resistant typhoid fever and other systemic *Salmonella* infections. It also is effective for brain abscesses and certain types of bacterial meningitis. Because of the increasing resistance of *Hemophilus influenzae* to ampicillin, ampicillin given with chloramphenicol is the currently recommended regimen for initial treatment of *H. influenzae* meningitis. Topical chloramphenicol is used to treat eye and external ear infections.

chloramphenicol (Chloromycetin). The oral formulation has greater bioavailability than chloramphenicol sodium succinate, the I.V. form. Whenever possible, oral administration is preferable because it costs less. Because of potential toxicity, chloramphenicol should be reserved for serious infections in which the infection site and pathogen susceptibility indicate limited treatment alternatives. Careful monitoring of serum concentration levels is essential.
USUAL ADULT DOSAGE: 50 to 100 mg/kg/day P.O. in divided doses every 6 hours.
USUAL PEDIATRIC DOSAGE: for neonates up to 2 weeks old, 6.25 mg/kg P.O. every 6 hours; for children over 2 weeks old, 12.5 mg/kg P.O. every 6 hours or 25 mg/kg P.O. every 12 hours.

chloramphenicol palmitate (Chloromycetin Palmitate). Oral suspension is available as 150 mg per 5 ml; it should be administered to patients who cannot swallow capsules.
USUAL ADULT DOSAGE: 50 to 100 mg/kg/day P.O. in divided doses every 6 hours.
USUAL PEDIATRIC DOSAGE: for neonates up to 2 weeks, 6.25 mg/kg P.O. every 6 hours; for children over 2 weeks, 12.5 mg/kg P.O. every 6 hours or 25 mg/kg P.O. every 12 hours.

chloramphenicol sodium succinate (Chloromycetin Sodium Succinate). This preparation is used for I.V. administration. Because the ester must be hydrolyzed to its active form, a time lag follows infusion before adequate serum concentration levels are reached.
USUAL ADULT DOSAGE: 50 to 100 mg/kg/day I.V. in four divided doses every 6 hours.
USUAL PEDIATRIC DOSAGE: for neonates up to 2 weeks, 6.25 mg/kg I.V. every 6 hours; for children over 2 weeks, 12.5 mg/kg I.V. every 6 hours or 25 mg/kg I.V. every 12 hours.

Drug interactions
Chloramphenicol may inhibit the metabolism of oral hypoglycemic agents such as chlorpropamide and tolbutamide, anticonvulsants such as phenytoin, and oral anticoagulants such as dicumarol. This inhibited metabolism can lead to hypoglycemia, phenytoin toxicity, or hemorrhage. The dosages of oral hypoglycemics, anticonvulsants, and anticoagulants may need to be decreased.

ADVERSE DRUG REACTIONS
The clinical use of chloramphenicol is limited by its potential toxicities. When the drug is used, the nurse must recognize the patient's adverse reactions.

Predictable reactions
GI adverse reactions to oral chloramphenicol may include nausea, vomiting, glossitis, unpleasant taste, stomatitis, diarrhea, and perineal irritation.
Gray syndrome, a potentially fatal adverse reaction associated with excessive chloramphenicol serum concentration levels, occurs most frequently in neonates. Initial manifestations include abdominal distention, vomiting, anorexia, tachypnea, cyanosis, green stools, lethargy, and an ashen color. These symptoms are followed by circulatory collapse and death. Gray syndrome results from the neonate's decreased ability to conjugate chloramphenicol and to excrete the active form in urine, especially when the drug is given within the first 48 hours of life. Gray syndrome also may occur in older children or adults receiving excessive chloramphenicol doses resulting in serum concentration levels greater than 40 to 200 mcg/ml.
Bone marrow suppression is the most toxic reaction to chloramphenicol. Reversible bone marrow suppression results from inhibiting mitochondrial protein synthesis. Signs and symptoms of bone marrow suppression include granulocytopenia, reticulocytopenia, anemia, leukopenia, and thrombocytopenia. These symptoms correlate with daily doses greater than 4 grams/day, duration of treatment, and serum concentration levels exceeding 25 mcg/ml. Bone marrow suppression is reversible when chloramphenicol is discontinued.

Unpredictable reactions
Aplastic anemia, which is usually irreversible, may occur after chloramphenicol is discontinued. The peripheral blood shows pancytopenia. Aplastic anemia is produced by a different mechanism than the direct bone marrow suppression; it may be an allergic reaction. Aplastic anemia occurs in about 1 in 40,000 or more patients taking chloramphenicol. Mortality is greater than 50%.

Hypersensitivity reactions, including fever, macular and vesicular rashes, angioedema, urticaria, and anaphylaxis, have been reported.

NURSING IMPLICATIONS

Because chloramphenicol can produce serious adverse reactions, the nurse must be aware of the following implications when administering this agent:
• Screen patients for history of chloramphenicol hypersensitivity before starting therapy.
• Screen patients for liver function impairment and recent or concurrent use of drugs that inhibit liver microsomal enzymes.
• Monitor the patient for signs and symptoms of bone marrow suppression throughout treatment. Monitor that the patients complete blood counts are performed at regular intervals.
• Advise the patient to notify the physician if fever, sore throat, fatigue, unusual bleeding, or bruising occurs.

CLINDAMYCIN AND LINCOMYCIN

Clindamycin and lincomycin hydrochloride are lincosamide antibacterials with similar spectra of activity. Clindamycin usually is more effective than lincomycin, which remains particularly important in treating certain anaerobic infections. With its limited indications and greater incidence of adverse effects, lincomycin is mainly of historic interest.

History and source

Lincomycin was isolated in 1962 from *Streptomyces lincolnensis* obtained from soil samples near Lincoln, Nebraska. Chemical modification of lincomycin resulted in clindamycin, which provides increased antibacterial potency, better oral absorption, and fewer adverse reactions. Clindamycin was approved by the FDA for oral use in 1970 and for I.M. and I.V. administration in 1972. Although both lincomycin and clindamycin are available, most physicians prefer clindamycin.

PHARMACOKINETICS

Clindamycin and lincomycin can be administered orally, intramuscularly, or intravenously. After oral administration, clindamycin is well absorbed and widely distributed in the body. Lincomycin is more poorly absorbed. Clindamycin and lincomycin are eliminated primarily via hepatic metabolism and renal and biliary excretion.

Absorption, distribution, metabolism, excretion

Clindamycin hydrochloride is rapidly and almost completely (about 90%) absorbed from the GI tract. The presence of food slightly delays but does not decrease the drug's absorption. Lincomycin is only 20% to 30% absorbed in the fasting state and the presence of food greatly decreases its absorption.

Clindamycin and lincomycin are well distributed to most body tissues with the exception of the CSF. Even when the meninges are inflamed, only small concentration levels of clindamycin are found in the CSF. Clindamycin's concentration levels in bone is 60% to 80% that of serum concentration levels. Clindamycin readily crosses the placenta and enters fetal blood and tissues.

Most of a clindamycin dose is metabolized in the liver to N-demethyl-clindamycin (more active than the parent compound) and clindamycin sulfoxide (less active than the parent compound). Both of these metabolites may appear in bile and urine but not in serum.

About 10% of active clindamycin is excreted unchanged in urine, and only small quantities are excreted in feces. However, excretion in feces is increased in patients with impaired renal function. About 40% of oral lincomycin is excreted unchanged in the feces. About 30% of I.V. or I.M. lincomycin is excreted in the urine. The normal half-life of clindamycin is 2.4 hours; lincomycin's half-life is 4.5 hours. In patients with severe renal failure, the half-life of clindamycin increases to about 6 hours and lincomycin increases to 9 hours. Appreciable dosage adjustments should be made when a patient has severe renal and hepatic disease concomitantly.

Onset, peak, duration

After oral administration of clindamycin, peak serum concentration levels are reached earlier and are at least twice as high as those of lincomycin. Mean peak serum concentration levels in adults after a single oral dose are reached in 1 hour. After I.M. administration, which causes little pain, mean peak serum concentration levels are reached in 3 hours. With I.V. infusion, peak concentration levels are reached when the infusion is complete.

PHARMACODYNAMICS

Clindamycin and lincomycin have the same mechanism of action as chloramphenicol and erythromycin. Clindamycin and lincomycin may compete for the same binding sites on the ribosomes.

Mechanism of action

Clindamycin and lincomycin inhibit bacterial protein synthesis; they may inhibit the binding of bacterial ribosomes. At therapeutically attainable concentration levels, clindamycin and lincomycin are primarily bacteriostatic against most organisms.

PHARMACOTHERAPEUTICS

Because of its greater activity, enhanced absorption properties, and smaller potential for toxicity, clindamycin is preferred over lincomycin; however, because of its potential for serious toxicity and pseudomembranous colitis, clindamycin is limited to a few clinical indications where safer alternative antibacterials are not available.

Clindamycin is more potent than lincomycin against most aerobic gram-positive organisms, including staphylococci, streptococci (except *Streptococcus faecalis*), and pneumococci. Clindamycin is effective against most of the clinically important anaerobes, particularly *B. fragilis;* however, resistance to clindamycin has been found in 5% to 15% of *B. fragilis* strains. Clindamycin and lincomycin are inactive against aerobic gram-negative bacilli.

Clindamycin is used primarily to treat anaerobic intraabdominal or pleuropulmonary infections caused by *B. fragilis*. Clindamycin is used as an alternative to penicillin in treating *Clostridium perfringens* infections. It also may be used as an alternative to penicillin in treating staphylococcal infections; however, clindamycin is an unreliable bactericidal. It should not be used for deep-seated staphylococcal infections, particularly endocarditis.

clindamycin hydrochloride (Cleocin). Available as 75- and 150-mg capsules, clindamycin hydrochloride is used to treat soft-tissue and respiratory tract infections.
USUAL ADULT DOSAGE: 150 to 450 mg P.O. every 6 hours.
USUAL PEDIATRIC DOSAGE: for children over age 1 month, 2 to 6.3 mg/kg P.O. every 6 hours or 2.7 to 8.3 mg/kg P.O. every 8 hours.

clindamycin palmitate hydrochloride (Cleocin Pediatric). This suspension preparation of flavored granules, at 75 mg of clindamycin per milliliter, is convenient for children and elderly patients who are unable to swallow capsules. The water-soluble clindamycin compound is hydrolyzed in vivo to the active drug.
USUAL ADULT DOSAGE: 150 mg P.O. every 6 to 8 hours.
USUAL PEDIATRIC DOSAGE: for children over age 1 month, 2 to 6.3 mg/kg P.O. every 6 hours or 2.7 to 8.3 mg/kg P.O. every 8 hours.

clindamycin phosphate (Cleocin Phosphate). This preparation is supplied for I.M. or I.V. use as a solution of 150 mg/ml in 2-, 4-, and 6-ml vials. For treating serious infections caused by aerobic gram-positive cocci and anaerobes, this parenteral form of clindamycin should be administered initially.
USUAL ADULT DOSAGE: 300 to 600 mg I.V. or I.M. every 6 hours.
USUAL PEDIATRIC DOSAGE: for children over age 1 month, 3.75 to 10 mg I.M. or I.V. every 6 hours or 5 to 13.3 mg/kg I.M. or I.V. every 8 hours.

lincomycin hydrochloride (Lincocin). Largely replaced by clindamycin, lincomycin is less active and more toxic.
USUAL ADULT DOSAGE: 500 mg P.O. every 6 to 8 hours, 600 mg to 1 gram I.V. every 12 hours, or 600 mg I.M. every 12 to 24 hours.
USUAL PEDIATRIC DOSAGE: for children over age 1 month, 7.5 to 15 mg/kg P.O. every 6 hours or 10 to 20 mg/kg P.O. every 8 hours; 10 mg/kg I.M. every 12 to 24 hours, 3.3 to 6.7 mg/kg I.V. every 8 hours or 5 to 10 mg/kg I.V. every 12 hours.

Drug interactions

Because erythromycin acts as an antagonist that may block access of clindamycin to its action site, erythromycin and clindamycin should not be used together. Clindamycin may block neuromuscular transmission and may enhance the action of neuromuscular blocking agents. Clindamycin phosphate in solution is incompatible with ampicillin, aminophylline, calcium gluconate, and magnesium sulfate.

ADVERSE DRUG REACTIONS

Clindamycin and lincomycin can produce severe and even fatal toxicities. As a result, these drugs are reserved for serious infections for which less toxic antibacterial agents are unavailable.

Predictable reactions

During clindamycin therapy, diarrhea occurs in about 80% of patients, most frequently with oral administration. Diarrhea, which can be severe, may begin a few days after initiation of therapy or days to weeks after the drug is discontinued.

Pseudomembranous colitis, characterized by severe diarrhea, abdominal pain, fever, and mucus and blood in stools, has occurred. This syndrome, which can be fatal, is caused by a toxin secreted by *Clostridium difficile* that overgrows in the presence of clindamycin or lincomycin. Pseudomembranous colitis occurs in 0.01%

to 10% of clindamycin-treated patients. Prompt discontinuation of the antibacterial is essential. Use of antiperistaltic drugs, which may aggravate the condition, should be avoided. Oral vancomycin in doses of 125 to 500 mg every 6 hours for 5 to 10 days is the treatment of choice for pseudomembranous colitis. Oral administration of clindamycin can also produce stomatitis, nausea, and vomiting.

Clindamycin is an irritating substance. When administered intravenously, it can damage tissue. Intramuscular administration can produce pain, induration, and sterile abscess.

Unpredictable reactions

Hypersensitivity reactions in the form of skin rashes occur in approximately 10% of patients treated with clindamycin. The skin rashes resemble those seen in patients receiving ampicillin.

Stevens–Johnson–like syndrome has occurred infrequently with this drug, and a few instances of anaphylactic reactions have occurred.

NURSING IMPLICATIONS

Clindamycin is used frequently to treat serious nosocomial infections. The nurse should be aware of the following implications:
- Screen patients for a history of intestinal disease, particularly colitis. If persistent diarrhea occurs during clindamycin therapy, consult the physician.
- Monitor the patient's liver function tests during prolonged clindamycin therapy.
- Do not refrigerate reconstituted oral clindamycin palmitate hydrochloride solution because it thickens and becomes difficult to measure accurately. The solution remains stable for 2 weeks at room temperature.
- Explain to the patient that I.M. injections of clindamycin may be painful. Rotate injection sites and inject the drug deep into the muscle.
- Be aware that clindamycin capsules contain tartrazine, which can cause an allergic reaction in a sensitive individual.

ERYTHROMYCIN

A macrolide antibacterial, erythromycin contains a large macrocyclic lactone ring. Erythromycin is used to treat a number of commonly encountered infections. Because this highly effective drug is considered one of the safest antibiotics, clinical indications for erythromycin continue to increase.

History and source

Erythromycin was derived in 1952 by McGuire and associates from a strain of *Streptomyces erythraeus* obtained from Philippine soil. Since its introduction into clinical medicine, erythromycin has proved to be safe and effective for many common infections.

PHARMACOKINETICS

Erythromycin, the unmodified drug, is a bitter, crystalline compound that dissolves poorly in water. It is rapidly inactivated by gastric acid. Investigators have modified the drug and its preparations to improve absorption and increase serum concentration levels.

Absorption, distribution, metabolism, excretion

Because gastric acid destroys erythromycin, preparations are made with an acid-resistant film coating that delays drug dissolution until it reaches the small intestine. Erythromycin esters and ester salts, which are more acid-stable and tasteless, form a stable suspension in water. Because of their characteristics, the esters and ester salts are used in liquid suspension for children.

Erythromycin is absorbed intact. The type of tablet and the patient's food intake affect absorption.

Erythromycin is distributed well to most tissues and body fluids except for the CSF. Limited data on CSF concentration levels in patients with meningitis suggest that large parenteral doses may be effective against only highly susceptible organisms, such as the pneumococci. Protein binding varies from 70% to 90%. The drug persists longer in tissues than in serum.

Erythromycin has poor penetration into the synovial fluid. Concentrations achieved in the middle ear in otitis media and in the sputum and sinus secretions are adequate to treat infections caused by pneumococci and group A streptococci but are not adequate to eradicate *Hemophilus influenzae* consistently. Erythromycin is transported across the placenta and is excreted in breast milk.

Erythromycin is metabolized by the liver and excreted in bile in high concentrations. After oral administration, large concentration levels of erythromycin, representing both unabsorbed drug and some excreted by the biliary tract, appear in the stool.

Small amounts of erythromycin, ranging from about 2% of an oral dose to about 15% of a parenteral dose, are excreted in urine. Active transport and net tubular reabsorption of erythromycin may occur. The normal serum half-life of erythromycin is about 1.2 to 2.6 hours. In anuric patients, the serum half-life is increased to about 6 hours.

Onset, peak, duration

Peak serum concentration levels obtained after administration of various erythromycin preparations depend on several factors, including the chemical structure, coating, and number of doses of the drug, and whether the patient is fasting. Enteric-coated erythromycin provides excellent bioavailability. Mean peak serum concentration levels occur 2 to 4 hours after a single 250-mg dose in the fasting patient.

PHARMACODYNAMICS

Erythromycin is a bacteriostatic antibacterial that inhibits protein synthesis similarly to chloramphenicol, clindamycin, and lincomycin. Acting on the ribosomal subunit, erythromycin inhibits RNA-dependent protein synthesis by blocking translocation of peptides. The antibacterial spectrum of activity of chloramphenicol, clindamycin, and lincomycin may be affected by erythromycin because of competition for common binding sites.

PHARMACOTHERAPEUTICS

Erythromycin provides a broad spectrum of antimicrobial activity against gram-positive and gram-negative bacteria, including actinomycetes and mycobacteria, treponemas, mycoplasmas, rickettsiae, and chlamydiae. Erythromycin also is effective against pneumococci and group A streptococci. Most clinical isolates of *Staphylococcus aureus* are sensitive to erythromycin; however, resistant strains may emerge during therapy. Erythromycin is the drug of choice for treating *Mycoplasma pneumoniae* infections. It also is the preferred drug for treating pneumonia caused by *Legionella pneumophila*. In patients who are allergic to penicillin, erythromycin is effective for infections produced by group A beta-hemolytic streptococci or *Streptococcus pneumoniae*. It also may be used to treat gonorrhea and syphilis in patients who cannot tolerate penicillin G or the tetracyclines. Erythromycin also may be used to treat minor cutaneous staphylococcal infections, although the semisynthetic penicillins, cephalosporins, and vancomycin are used to treat serious staphylococcal infections.

erythromycin (E-Mycin, Ery-Tab, Ilotycin). No one oral preparation provides any clinical advantages over another. Erythromycin appears to be the best absorbed. It is available as enteric-coated and film-coated tablets.

USUAL ADULT DOSAGE: 250 mg P.O. every 6 hours.
USUAL PEDIATRIC DOSAGE: 7.5 to 25 mg/kg P.O. every 6 hours or 15 to 50 mg/kg P.O. every 12 hours.

erythromycin estolate (Ilosone). Erythromycin estolate is available in tablet, capsule, and liquid forms. There is a higher incidence of hepatotoxicity associated with erythromycin estolate than with other forms. The liquid form is well absorbed and used mostly for pediatric patients.
USUAL ADULT DOSAGE: 250 mg P.O. every 6 hours.
USUALY PEDIATRIC DOSAGE: 7.5 to 25 mg/kg P.O. every 6 hours or 15 to 50 mg/kg P.O. every 12 hours.

erythromycin ethylsuccinate (E.S.S., Pediamycin). This preparation is not affected by food. A 400-mg erythromycin ethylsuccinate dose produces the same free erythromycin serum concentration levels as 250 mg of erythromycin stearate or estolate.
USUAL ADULT DOSAGE: 400 mg every 6 hours.
USUAL PEDIATRIC DOSAGE: 7.5 to 25 mg/kg P.O. every 6 hours or 15 to 50 mg/kg P.O. every 12 hours.

erythromycin stearate (Erythrocin). An acid-stable preparation available as film-coated tablets, erythromycin stearate should not be administered with food. After dissociation in the duodenum, it is absorbed as free erythromycin.
USUAL ADULT DOSAGE: 250 mg P.O. every 6 hours.
USUAL PEDIATRIC DOSAGE: 7.5 to 25 mg/kg P.O. every 6 hours or 15 to 50 mg/kg P.O. every 12 hours.

erythromycin glucceptate (Ilotycin). The nurse should dilute this preparation in 100 to 200 ml of solution and infuse it intravenously over 30 to 60 minutes. The serum concentration levels achieved are much higher than those with any oral preparations.
USUAL ADULT DOSAGE: 250 to 500 mg I.V. every 6 hours.
USUAL PEDIATRIC DOSAGE: 3.75 to 5 mg/kg I.V. every 6 hours.

erythromycin lactobionate (Erythrocin Lactobionate). This preparation is the most common salt form used for I.V. administration.
USUAL ADULT DOSAGE: 250 to 500 mg I.V. every 6 hours.
USUAL PEDIATRIC DOSAGE: 3.75 to 5 mg/kg I.V. every 6 hours.

Drug interactions

Concurrent use of erythromycin in patients receiving high doses of theophylline can decrease theophylline clearance and increase theophylline concentration levels. The theophylline dose may have to be decreased to avoid toxicity.

ADVERSE DRUG REACTIONS

Few adverse reactions are associated with erythromycin. Significant toxicity has been reported with use of erythromycin estolate only.

Predictable reactions
Dose-related GI reactions (epigastric distress, nausea, vomiting, and diarrhea) occur most frequently, especially with large doses. Stomatitis, heartburn, anorexia, and melena have occurred.

Although rare, reversible sensorineural hearing loss can occur with I.V. erythromycin lactobionate. This adverse reaction is most likely to occur in patients with renal failure who are receiving high doses of erythromycin. Venous irritation and thrombophlebitis have occurred after I.V. administration of erythromycin gluceptate or erythromycin lactobionate.

Unpredictable reactions
Allergic reactions, including rashes, fever, eosinophilia, and anaphylaxis, have occurred.

The most serious toxicity is a characteristic syndrome of cholestatic hepatitis most commonly associated with erythromycin estolate and erythromycin ethylsuccinate. The syndrome consists of nausea, vomiting, and abdominal pain followed by jaundice, fever, and abnormal liver function test results that are consistent with cholestatic hepatitis. These symptoms sometimes are accompanied by rash, leukocytosis, and eosinophilia. The syndrome may represent a hypersensitivity reaction to the specific structure of the estolate compound. The cholestatic jaundice and hepatocellular necrosis may resolve within days to a few weeks after discontinuing the drug.

NURSING IMPLICATIONS

Although erythromycin is one of the safest antibacterials in clinical use, the nurse should be aware of the following implications:
- Assess the patient for previous allergic reaction to erythromycin. Sensitivity to tartrazine (frequently reported in patients with aspirin allergy) can produce an allergic response to erythromycin.
- Assess the patient for hepatic dysfunction. Patients on long-term therapy should receive frequent liver function tests and physical assessment for signs of liver failure.
- Monitor the patient on I.V. erythromycin lactobionate therapy for changes in hearing, especially elderly patients and those with renal insufficiency.

- Do not administer erythromycin by I.M. injection; the injection is painful and may cause abscess or local tissue necrosis.
- Do not mix I.V. erythromycin with vitamins B complex and C, cephalothin, tetracycline, heparin, or chloramphenicol because they are incompatible. Reconstitute erythromycin solutions in normal saline solution or dextrose 5% in water (D_5W) and administer the solutions within 4 hours after preparation.

SULFONAMIDES

The sulfonamides were the first effective systemic antibacterials. Today, they are less useful because resistant strains of bacteria have emerged. By modifying the sulfonamides, researchers have developed other useful drugs, including para-aminosalicylic acid (for treating tuberculosis), carbonic anhydrase inhibitor diuretics, sulfonylurea hypoglycemics, and thiouracil antithyroids.

History and source
In 1908, German chemists synthesized a series of dyes containing a chemical group called sulfonamide. However, the therapeutic value of these dyes was not studied for almost 25 years. In 1932, the modern era of antibacterial chemotherapy began when Domagk reported the protective activity of Prontosil, a bright red dye, against experimental streptococcal infection in mice. Prontosil (sulfamidochrysoidine) exerted its antibacterial activity via the release of para-aminobenzenesulfonamide, or sulfanilamide. During the late 1930s, the basic sulfanilamide compound was modified to expand its spectrum of activity and decrease its adverse effects.

PHARMACOKINETICS

Most sulfonamides are absorbed well and distributed widely in the body. They are metabolized in the liver to inactive metabolites.

Absorption, distribution, metabolism, excretion
The sulfonamides differ markedly in their absorption. With the exception of sulfapyridine and sulfasalazine, which are poorly absorbed, sulfonamides are well absorbed after oral administration. From 70% to 90% of an oral dose is absorbed from the GI tract. Food can delay but cannot reduce absorption.

Sulfonamides enter the cerebrospinal, synovial, pleural, and peritoneal fluids with concentration levels of 80% of serum concentration levels. Sulfonamides readily cross the placenta; fetal plasma concentration levels may exceed 50% of maternal plasma concentration levels. Sulfonamides also are distributed into breast milk.

Most sulfonamides are metabolized in the liver by acetylation and glucuronidation. The metabolites lack antibacterial activity and usually are acetyl metabolites, which are less water-soluble than the parent sulfonamide.

Sulfonamides and their metabolites are excreted primarily by the kidneys via glomerular filtration. Partial reabsorption and active tubular secretion also are involved. The rates of excretion and solubility characteristics of the drugs vary widely with urine pH. Alkalinizing the urine increases renal excretion and decreases sulfonamide blood concentration levels.

Onset, peak, duration

Sulfonamides are classified as short-acting, intermediate-acting, and long-acting, depending on their absorption and excretion rates. Sulfisoxazole, sulfacytine, and sulfasalazine are considered short-acting, with plasma half-lives of about 4 to 8 hours. Sulfadiazine, sulfamethoxazole, and sulfapyridine are intermediate-acting, with plasma half-life of about 7 to 17 hours. Sulfadoxine (in combination with pyrimethamine as Fansidar) is the only long-acting sulfonamide available in the United States. Sulfadoxine has a half-life of 100 to 250 hours and is used as treatment and prophylaxis of malaria caused by chloroquine-resistant *Plasmodium falciparum*. See Chapter 71, Antimalarial and Other Antiprotozoal Agents, for further information on this drug.

Peak plasma concentration levels usually are reached within 2 to 4 hours after oral administration of short-acting sulfonamides. Intermediate-acting sulfonamides are absorbed more slowly, with peak concentration levels occurring within 3 to 17 hours, depending on the specific drug used.

Widely varying blood concentration levels occur among patients receiving identical doses of the same sulfonamide. Blood concentration levels are based on total sulfonamide concentration, even though only free (unmetabolized and unbound) sulfonamides are microbiologically active. Optimal blood concentration levels of 60 to 150 mcg/ml have been reported. Those greater than 200 mcg/ml increase the incidence of toxicity.

PHARMACODYNAMICS

Sulfonamides are bacteriostatic agents that prevent the growth of microorganisms by inhibiting the production of folic acid.

Mechanism of action

Sulfonamides competitively inhibit the incorporation of para-aminobenzoic acid (PABA) into dihydropteroic acid and subsequently into dihydrofolic acid, thereby inhibiting folic acid synthesis. The decreased folic acid synthesis decreases bacterial nucleotides and inhibits bacterial growth.

PHARMACOTHERAPEUTICS

Sulfonamides are used primarily to treat acute urinary tract infections. With recurrent or chronic urinary tract infections, the infecting organism may or may not be susceptible to sulfonamides. The choice of therapy should be based on bacteria susceptibility tests. Sulfonamides also are used to treat infections caused by *Nocardia asteroides*, *Toxoplasma gondii*, and *Chlamydia trachomatis* and to treat chronic ulcerative colitis. Sulfonamides exhibit a wide spectrum of activity against gram-positive and gram-negative bacteria; however, the increasing resistance of formerly susceptible bacteria has decreased the clinical usefulness of these drugs. Sulfonamides effectively prevent recurrent attacks of rheumatic fever caused by group A beta-hemolytic streptococcal infections, but are ineffective against established streptococcal pharyngitis. Sulfonamide prophylaxis against *Neisseria meningitidis* is variably effective.

sulfadiazine (Microsulfon). An intermediate-acting sulfonamide, sulfadiazine is absorbed and excreted rapidly after oral administration. It may be used as prophylaxis against sulfonamide-sensitive meningococcus and is the drug of choice for nocardiasis.
USUAL ADULT DOSAGE: for urinary tract infections, initially, 2 to 4 grams P.O., then 500 mg to 1 gram P.O. every 6 hours; for adjunctive treatment in toxoplasmosis, 2 to 8 grams P.O. in divided doses every 6 hours for 3 to 4 weeks, discontinued for 1 week, the administered with 25 mg of pyrimethamine P.O. daily for 3 to 4 weeks; for nocardiasis, 4 to 8 grams P.O. daily in divided doses for 6 weeks.
USUAL PEDIATRIC DOSAGE: for urinary tract infections, initially, 75 mg/kg P.O., then 150 mg/kg P.O. in four to six divided doses daily to a maximum daily dosage of 6 grams; for rheumatic fever prophylaxis (as an alternative to penicillin), for children over 30 kg, 1 gram P.O. daily, and for children under 30 kg, 500 mg P.O. daily;

DRUG INTERACTIONS
Sulfonamides

The following chart summarizes the significant interactions between sulfonamides and other drugs.

DRUG	INTERACTING DRUGS	POSSIBLE EFFECTS	NURSING IMPLICATIONS
sulfadiazine, sulfamethoxazole, sulfapyridine, sulfisoxazole, sulfacytine, sulfasalazine	local anesthetics (benzocaine, procaine, tetracaine, butacaine)	Decrease the antibacterial activity	• Use alternative local anesthetics, such as dibucaine or lidocaine.
	para-aminobenzoic acid	Decreases the antibacterial activity	• Avoid concurrent use.
sulfisoxazole	thiopental	Prevents plasma protein binding of thiopental	• If used together, thiopental dosage may need to be reduced.
	methotrexate	Prevents plasma protein binding of methotrexate	• Avoid concurrent use.
sulfasalazine	phenobarbital	Increases biliary excretion of sulfasalazine	• Therapeutic effect is not altered.
	digoxin	Reduces bioavailability of digitalis	• Monitor the patient's serum digoxin levels, and adjust the dosage, as ordered.

for adjunctive treatment of toxoplasmosis, 100 to 200 mg/kg P.O. in divided doses every 6 hours for 3 to 4 weeks, then administered with 2 mg/kg pyrimethamine daily for 3 days, then 1 mg/kg daily for 3 to 4 weeks.

sulfamethoxazole (Gantanol). An intermediate-acting sulfonamide, sulfamethoxazole is absorbed and excreted more slowly than sulfisoxazole. It is also less water-soluble. Sulfamethoxazole is often used with trimethoprim to prevent acute and recurrent urinary tract infections and otitis media.

USUAL ADULT DOSAGE: for urinary tract and systemic infections, initially, 2 grams P.O., then 1 gram P.O. b.i.d. to t.i.d. for severe infections; for lymphogranuloma venereum (genital, inguinal, or anorectal infections), 1 gram/day in two divided doses for at least 2 weeks.

USUAL PEDIATRIC DOSAGE: for urinary tract and systemic infections in children over age 2 months, initially, 50 to 60 mg/kg P.O. every 12 hours, then 25 to 30 mg/kg P.O. every 12 hours; maximum dosage of 75 mg/kg/day.

sulfapyridine. An intermediate-acting sulfonamide, sulfapyridine is absorbed slowly and incompletely from the GI tract. It is not used as an antibacterial agent because of its toxicity; however, sulfapyridine may be used to treat dermatitis herpetiformis when sulfones are not tolerated or are contraindicated.

USUAL ADULT DOSAGE: for dermatitis herpetiformis, 500 mg P.O. q.i.d. until improvement is noted, then the dosage is decreased by 500 mg every 3 days until a minimum effective maintenance dose is achieved.

sulfisoxazole (Gantrisin). A short-acting sulfonamide, sulfisoxazole is absorbed readily from the GI tract and excreted rapidly. Because of its low cost and high water-solubility, sulfisoxazole is considered the sulfonamide of choice. It frequently is used to treat urinary tract infections.

USUAL ADULT DOSAGE: for urinary tract and systemic infections, initially, 2 to 4 grams P.O., then 1 to 2 grams P.O. q.i.d.; or 4 to 5 grams P.O. of sustained-release suspension every 12 hours.

USUAL PEDIATRIC DOSAGE: for urinary tract and systemic infections in children over age 2 months, initially, 75 mg/kg P.O. daily in divided doses every 6 hours, then 150 mg/kg P.O. daily in divided doses every 6 hours; for sustained-release suspension, 60 to 75 mg/kg P.O. every 12 hours, then 120 to 150 mg/kg P.O. daily in divided doses.

sulfacytine (Renoquid). A short-acting sulfonamide, sulfacytine is absorbed rapidly and almost completely from the GI tract and is excreted rapidly by the kidneys. Sulfacytine is indicated to treat acute urinary tract infections.
USUAL ADULT DOSAGE: 500 mg P.O. initially, followed by 250 mg P.O. q.i.d. for 10 days.
USUAL PEDIATRIC DOSAGE: for children age 14 and older, same as adult. Not recommended for children under age 14.

sulfasalazine (Azulfidine). Poorly absorbed from the GI tract, this short-acting sulfonamide is administered for local effect in the gut and is used to treat ulcerative colitis.
USUAL ADULT DOSAGE: for mild to moderate ulcerative colitis and as adjunctive therapy in severe ulcerative colitis, initially, 3 to 4 grams P.O daily in evenly divided doses; usual maintenance dose, 1.5 to 2 grams P.O. daily in divided doses every 6 hours; may need to start with 1 to 2 grams, gradually increasing the dose to minimize adverse reactions.
USUAL PEDIATRIC DOSAGE: for children over age 2, initially, 40 to 60 mg/kg P.O. daily in three to six divided doses, then 30 mg/kg daily in four doses; may need to start at a lower dose if GI intolerance occurs.

Drug interactions
PABA and local anesthestics that contain PABA may directly decrease the antibacterial activity of the sulfonamides. Sulfisoxazole prevents plasma protein binding of thiopental when given concurrently, increasing serum concentration levels of free thiopental. This decreases the amount of thiopental needed for anesthesia and shortens wake-up time. Sulfisoxazole also prevents plasma protein binding of methotrexate, possibly inhibiting renal tubular excretion and increasing the serum concentration levels of free methotrexate. These drugs should not be administered concurrently.

Because sulfasalazine reduces digoxin bioavailability, serum digoxin levels should be monitored and dosages should be adjusted as needed if these drugs are administered concurrently. (See *Drug interactions: Sulfonamides* for a summary.)

ADVERSE DRUG REACTIONS
The sulfonamides produce numerous predictable and unpredictable adverse reactions.

Predictable reactions
Excessively high doses of less water-soluble sulfonamides can produce crystalluria and tubular deposits of sulfonamide crystals. These complications can be minimized by maintaining high urine flow rates and alkalinized urine. These complications usually do not occur with newer water-soluble sulfonamides. Nausea, vomiting, and diarrhea are common.

Unpredictable reactions
Agranulocytosis, the most common unpredictable reaction, is reversible upon drug discontinuation. Extremely rare reactions, such as aplastic anemia and hemolytic anemia, have been reported.

The incidence of hypersensitivity reactions appears to increase as the dosage increases. Various dermatologic reactions, including rash, pruritus, erythema nodosum, erythema multiforme of the Stevens-Johnson type, and exfoliative dermatitis, can occur. Sulfonamide also can produce photosensitivity; the patient should be cautioned against exposure to ultraviolet light or prolonged exposure to sunlight.

Fever may develop 7 to 10 days after the initial sulfonamide dose. Serum sickness–like reactions, including fever, joint pain, urticarial eruptions, bronchospasm, and leukopenia, can occur.

NURSING IMPLICATIONS
Although the sulfonamides are less frequently used today, the nurse should still be aware of the following implications:
• Obtain a careful patient history before initiating sulfonamide therapy. Ask the patient about skin rashes, reduced urine output, and kidney dysfunction.
• Rule out pregnancy, lactation, and the recent use of PABA (a sulfonamide antagonist) before initiating therapy.
• Administer oral preparations of sulfonamides with ample fluids.
• Advise the patient to avoid direct sunlight to help prevent a photosensitivity reaction.
• Advise the patient to call the physician if signs of hematologic reactions, such as sore throat, pallor, purpura, jaundice, or weakness, occur.

VANCOMYCIN

Vancomycin hydrochloride is used increasingly to treat methicillin-resistant *Staphylococcus aureus*, which has become a major concern in the United States and other parts of the world.

History and source

Vancomycin, introduced in 1956, was obtained from *Streptomyces orientalis,* a microorganism isolated from soil samples in Indonesia and India. Clinical use of vancomycin declined rapidly because of impurities in early preparations that resulted in hypersensitivity and other adverse reactions. The advent of semisynthetic penicillins (methicillin in 1959) and cephalosporins (cephalothin in 1962) contributed to vancomycin's further decline in popularity. In recent years, however, vancomycin has been used more frequently because of an increase in methicillin-resistant *S. aureus* and because of the recognition of *Clostridium difficile* as the cause of pseudomembranous colitis.

PHARMACOKINETICS

Vancomycin is absorbed poorly when administered orally. For systemic infections, vancomycin is administered intravenously. Intramuscular administration is not recommended because of injection pain and tissue necrosis. Peak serum concentration levels of vancomycin occur 1 to 2 hours after I.V. administration.

Absorption, distribution, metabolism, excretion

Vancomycin is absorbed poorly from the GI tract and is used orally only to treat *C. difficile*–induced pseudomembranous colitis and staphylococcal enterocolitis. To treat systemic infections, vancomycin is administered by intermittent I.V. infusion over 30 to 60 minutes. Rapid or bolus administration is dangerous and can cause flushing and anaphylactic reactions.

Vancomycin diffuses well into pleural, pericardial, synovial, and ascitic fluids. Only small amounts are found in bile. Vancomycin is not found in normal CSF, but bactericidal levels have been found in patients with inflamed meninges.

Vancomycin is eliminated from the body almost exclusively by glomerular filtration. Approximately 85% of the dose is excreted unchanged in urine within 24 hours. A small amount may be eliminated via the liver and biliary tract. The half-life of vancomycin is 4 to 6 hours in patients with normal renal function. In patients with anuria, half-life may be up to 10 days. In such patients, as little as 1 gram of vancomycin may be administered every 7 to 10 days. Because high and potentially toxic serum concentration levels of vancomycin can occur in patients with renal insufficiency, dosage adjustments must be made. Vancomycin is not removed by hemodialysis or peritoneal dialysis.

PHARMACODYNAMICS

Vancomycin has a narrow spectrum of antibacterial activity.

Mechanism of action

Vancomycin is a complex soluble glycopolypeptide that is not chemically related to any other antibacterial agent. It inhibits biosynthesis of peptidoglycan, the major structural component of the bacterial cell wall. When the bacterial cell wall is damaged, the body's natural defenses can attack the organism.

PHARMACOTHERAPEUTICS

Vancomycin is active against gram-positive organisms such as *S. aureus, Staphylococcus epidermidis, Streptococcus pyogenes,* and *Streptococcus pneumoniae.* Gram-negative organisms, fungi, and yeasts are resistant to vancomycin. Intravenous vancomycin is the therapy of choice in patients with serious staphylococcal infections; methicillin-, oxacillin-, nafcillin-, or cephalosporin-resistant organisms; or intolerance to those drugs.

Vancomycin, when used in combination with an aminoglycoside, is also the treatment of choice for *Streptococcus faecalis* (enterococcal) endocarditis in patients who are allergic to penicillin. (Vancomycin alone is not a dependable bactericide against all the indicated streptococci.) Orally administered vancomycin is the drug of choice for treating seriously ill patients with antibiotic-associated *C. difficile* colitis. This organism is highly susceptible to vancomycin. Intravenous vancomycin is not as reliable for treating this disorder, but may be used concomitantly.

vancomycin hydrochloride (Vancocin). Available in 500-mg or 1-gram vials, vancomycin is administered intravenously to treat serious systemic infections.
USUAL ADULT DOSAGE: 500 mg I.V. every 6 hours or 1 gram I.V. every 12 hours; maximum dosage, 2 gram/day.
USUAL PEDIATRIC DOSAGE: 44 mg/kg I.V. daily in divided doses; for neonates, 10 mg/kg I.V. daily every 6 to 12 hours.

vancomycin hydrochloride pulvules (Vancocin). Administered orally, this vancomycin preparation is used to treat staphylococcal enterocolitis or antibiotic-associated pseudomembranous colitis caused by *C. difficile.* It is available as 125- or 250-mg capsules as well as 1- or 10-gram powder for oral solutions.
USUAL ADULT DOSAGE: 125 to 500 mg P.O. every 6 hours for 7 to 10 days.

USUAL PEDIATRIC DOSAGE: 44 mg/kg P.O. daily in divided doses every 6 hours.

Drug interactions

Vancomycin may enhance the possibility of additive toxicities when administered concurrently with other nephrotoxic drugs, such as aminoglycosides, amphotericin B, and cisplatin.

ADVERSE DRUG REACTIONS

With purified vancomycin preparations now available and with clinicians more aware of the drug's potential toxicity, adverse reactions occur less frequently.

Predictable reactions

Ototoxicity is the most serious adverse reaction to parenteral vancomycin. It is most likely to occur in patients with renal impairment and those receiving long-term high-dose I.V. vancomycin. Vancomycin may damage the auditory branch of the eighth cranial nerve. Permanent deafness has occurred. Tinnitus may precede deafness and necessitates drug discontinuation. Hearing loss occasionally improves when the drug is discontinued, but in many cases, deteriorates further.

Transient or reversible nephrotoxicity was a relatively common adverse reaction with early impure vancomycin preparations, especially when high doses were given. Occasional mild hematuria, proteinuria, casts in the urine, and azotemia may occur. High doses of parenteral vancomycin should be avoided. The nurse should monitor serum concentration levels when other nephrotoxic drugs are administered concurrently. A higher incidence of nephrotoxicity occurs when vancomycin is administered concurrently with an aminoglycoside.

Parenteral vancomycin must be administered intravenously only, and care must be taken to avoid extravasation. Pain and thrombophlebitis may occur after I.V. administration.

Hypotensive reaction associated with rapid I.V. administration of vancomycin is characterized by a sudden blood pressure decrease, which can be severe and may be accompanied by a maculopapular or erythematous rash on the face, neck, chest, and arms. The reaction usually begins a few minutes after the infusion is started and resolves spontaneously several hours after the infusion is discontinued.

Unpredictable reactions

Hypersensitivity reactions occur in 5% to 10% of patients receiving vancomycin. Anaphylactic reactions, eosinophilia, and drug fever have occurred. Neutropenia, which is rapidly reversible after discontinuation, can occur.

NURSING IMPLICATIONS

Because of the changing nature of infectious diseases in recent years, vancomycin is being prescribed with increasing frequency. The nurse should be aware of the following implications:

• Do not administer vancomycin by I.M. injection, because it is painful and can produce tissue necrosis.

• Know that because oral vancomycin is absorbed poorly, it does not reach serum concentration levels adequate to treat systemic infections.

• Do not administer vancomycin by rapid I.V. route. It should be infused slowly over 30 to 60 minutes in a large volume of fluid to avoid hypotensive reaction.

• Monitor the patient for phlebitis at the infusion site.

• Assess the patient's renal status before initiating vancomycin therapy. Monitor vancomycin serum concentration levels (peak and trough levels) and serum creatinine levels if the patient is concurrently receiving other ototoxic or nephrotoxic drugs.

• If possible, perform a baseline audiogram before initiating vancomycin therapy. Assess the patient's hearing (complaints of tinnitus) while the patient is on vancomycin. Instruct the patient to report fullness or ringing in the ears to the physician.

• Do not mix vancomycin with other drugs in the same I.V. solution.

IMIPENEM/CILASTATIN

A fixed combination, imipenem/cilastatin sodium is the first of a new class of beta-lactam antibacterials called carbapenems. Imipenem/cilastatin's antibacterial spectrum of activity is broader than that of any other antibacterial studied to date and includes gram-positive, gram-negative, and anaerobic organisms. Imipenem/cilastatin has been used to treat many clinically important infections, especially those acquired nosocomially.

History and source

Imipenem is a semisynthetic carbapenem antibiotic and a derivative of thienamycin. Carbapenems are beta-lactam antibiotics that contain a fused beta-lactam ring and a five-member ring system similar to that contained in penicillins. Thienamycin was derived from *Streptomyces cattleya,* which was discovered in soil samples from New Jersey by American and Spanish scientists in the early 1970s.

Cilastatin is a specific and reversible inhibitor of dehydropeptidase-I, an enzyme present on the brush border of proximal renal tubular cells that inactivates imipenem by hydrolyzing the beta-lactam ring.

PHARMACOKINETICS

To be effective, imipenem must be given with cilastatin, otherwise, imipenem would be hydrolyzed rapidly in the brush border of the renal tubules, rendering it ineffective. After parenteral administration, imipenem/cilastatin is absorbed well and distributed widely. It is metabolized by several mechanisms and excreted primarily in the urine.

Absorption, distribution, metabolism, excretion

Imipenem/cilastatin is not absorbed after oral ingestion because of the molecule's instability in gastric acid. It must be administered parenterally. Imipenem is incompletely absorbed after I.M. administration. The bioavailabilities of imipenem and cilastatin are 60% and 100%, respectively, after I.M. administration in healthy adults. I.V. infusion studies have shown high serum levels.

After I.V. administration, imipenem is not destroyed in the circulation and is distributed widely to various body compartments, including sputum, bone, aqueous humor, and pleural and peritoneal fluids. In the absence of meningeal inflammation, only minor amounts of imipenem enter the CSF. With meningeal inflammation, CSF concentration levels usually are 1% to 10% of concurrent serum concentration levels. Imipenem is distributed into breast milk.

Imipenem is metabolized to some extent by a nonrenal mechanism unrelated to dehydropeptidase-I. Approximately 25% of an imipenem dose is inactivated by nonspecific hydrolysis of the beta-lactam ring. Cilastatin is metabolized partially in the kidneys to N-acetyl cilastatin, which is also an effective inhibitor of dehydropeptidase-I. Less than 1% of an imipenem dose and less than 2% of a cilastatin dose are excreted in feces after I.V. administration.

Imipenem is excreted primarily by glomerular filtration. Tubular secretion also assists in drug elimination. Imipenem is metabolized by dehydropeptidase-I at the brush border of the renal tubular cells. Cilastatin, a dehydropeptidase-I inhibitor, blocks this peptidase in the renal tubular cells, increasing excretion of active imipenem into the luminal tubular urine. Cilastatin has no

antibacterial activity, nor does it alter the antibacterial activity of imipenem. Approximately 70% of an imipenem dose is recovered in urine when imipenem is administered with cilastatin.

Both imipenem and cilastatin have a half-life of about 1 hour. In patients with decreased renal function, the serum half-life of the imipenem/cilastatin combination increases to 4 hours. Therefore, the imipenem/cilastatin dose should be reduced by at least 50% when the patient's creatinine clearance is below 30 ml/minute. Fortunately, the drug combination is hemodialyzable, and 40% to 82% of the imipenem is removed in a dialysis session, depending on the technique used.

Onset, peak, duration

After 20 to 30 minutes of infusion of 250 mg of imipenem/cilastatin, mean peak serum concentration levels of imipenem are 14 to 24 mcg/ml. With 500 mg of each, mean peak serum concentration levels are 21 to 58 mcg/ml. From 4 to 6 hours after administration, serum concentration levels decline to 1.5 mcg/ml or less. In adults who receive 500 mg of imipenem/cilastatin by I.V. infusion over 30 minutes every 6 hours, peak serum imipenem concentration levels are 19.3 to 38.3 mcg/ml, and trough concentration levels average 1 mcg/ml.

PHARMACODYNAMICS

Imipenem is usually bactericidal. Imipenem exerts its antibacterial activity by inhibiting mucopeptide synthesis in the bacterial cell wall. Because of its spatial configuration, imipenem is particularly resistant to beta-lactamase.

Mechanism of action

Imipenem binds to all of the PBPs, but most avidly and most importantly to penicillin-binding protein 2. Imipenem's binding to penicillin-binding protein 2 in the cell wall causes the bacterium to develop into a round, osmotically unstable form, which then lyses.

PHARMACOTHERAPEUTICS

Imipenem has a broader spectrum of activity than that of other currently available beta-lactam antibiotics. It displays excellent in vitro activity against aerobic gram-positive species such as the streptococci, *Staphylococcus aureus,* and *Staphylococcus epidermidis.* The majority of Enterobacteriaceae are inhibited by imipenem concentration levels less than or equal to 1 mcg/ml. *Pseudomonas aeruginosa,* including strains resistant to piperacillin and ceftazidime, is inhibited by imipenem.

(Text continues on page 1077.)

SELECTED MAJOR DRUGS

Antibacterial agents

This chart summarizes representative drugs from each class of antibacterials.

DRUG	MAJOR INDICATIONS	USUAL ADULT DOSAGES	NURSING IMPLICATIONS
Aminoglycosides			
gentamicin	Infections caused by sensitive *Pseudomonas aeruginosa, Escherichia coli, Proteus, Providencia, Klebsiella, Serratia, Enterobacter, Citrobacter, Staphylococcus*	1 to 1.75 mg/kg I.V. or I.M. every 8 hours; may be administered every 6 hours; dosage adjustment required for patients with renal impairment	• Administer cautiously to patients with impaired renal function and in neonates, infants, and elderly patients. • Obtain specimens for culture and sensitivity tests before first dose. • Weigh the patient and obtain baseline renal function studies before therapy begins. • Monitor renal function (output, urinalysis, BUN and creatinine levels, and creatinine clearance). Notify the physician of signs of decreasing renal function. • Maintain adequate patient hydration during therapy to minimize chemical irritation of the renal tubules. • After completing I.V. infusion, flush the line with normal saline solution or D_5W. • Evaluate the patient's hearing before and during therapy. Notify the physician if the patient complains of tinnitus, vertigo, or hearing loss. • Monitor the patient for bacterial or fungal superinfection caused by overgrowth of resistant organisms. • Usual duration of therapy is 7 to 10 days. If no response occurs in 3 to 5 days, therapy should be stopped, as ordered, and new specimens obtained for culture and sensitivity tests. • Monitor the patient's peak concentration levels. Peak serum concentration levels above 10 mcg/ml and trough concentration levels above 2 mcg/ml are associated with a higher incidence of toxicity. • Draw blood for gentamicin peak concentration level 1 hour after I.M. injection and 30 minutes after I.V. infusion ends; for trough concentration levels, draw blood just before next dose.
Penicillins			
penicillin G aqueous	Moderate to severe systemic infections	600,000 to 5 million units I.V. or I.M. every 4 to 6 hours	• Administer cautiously to patients with other drug allergies, especially to cephalosporins. • Obtain specimens for culture and sensitivity tests before first dose. • Before giving penicillin, obtain a history to determine if the patient has had allergic reactions to this drug. However, a negative history of penicillin allergy is no guarantee against a future allergic reaction. • Instruct the patient to take the medication exactly as prescribed. The entire quantity prescribed should be taken.

continued

SELECTED MAJOR DRUGS

Antibacterial agents continued

DRUG	MAJOR INDICATIONS	USUAL ADULT DOSAGES	NURSING IMPLICATIONS
penicillin G aqueous (continued)			• Advise the patient to call the physician if rash, fever, or chills develop. • Food may interfere with absorption, so give the drug 1 to 2 hours before or 2 to 3 hours after meals. • I.M. administration is extremely painful. Inject deep into large muscle. • When giving I.V., mix with D_5W or saline solution. • Give by intermittent I.V. to prevent vein irritation. Change the administration site every 48 hours. • Large doses may produce increased yeast growths. Report symptoms to the physician. • With prolonged therapy, bacterial or fungal superinfections may occur, especially in elderly patients, debilitated patients, or those with low resistance to infection from immunosuppressives or irradiation. Observe the patient closely for signs and symptoms of infection.
ampicillin	Systemic infections Uncomplicated gonorrhea	250 to 500 mg P.O. every 6 hours, or 1 to 3 grams I.M. or I.V. every 6 hours 3.5 grams P.O. with 1 gram of probenecid as a single dose along with 500 mg of tetracycline P.O. q.i.d. for 7 days	• Administer cautiously to patients with other drug allergies, especially to cephalosporins, and patients with mononucleosis—a high incidence of maculopapular rash occurs in those receiving ampicillin. • Obtain specimens for culture and sensitivity tests before the first dose. • Before giving ampicillin, obtain a history to determine if the patient has had allergic reactions to penicillin. However, a negative history of penicillin allergy is no guarantee against a future allergic reaction. • Instruct the patient to take the medication exactly as prescribed. The entire quantity prescribed should be taken. • Advise the patient to call the physician if rash, fever, or chills develop. A rash is the most common allergic reaction, especially if the patient is also taking allopurinol. • Food may interfere with absorption, so give the drug 1 to 2 hours before or 2 to 3 hours after meals. • Dosage should be altered in patients with impaired hepatic and renal function. • When giving I.V., mix with D_5W or saline solution. Do not mix with other drugs or solutions: they might be incompatible. • Administer by intermittent I.V. to prevent vein irritation. Change administration site every 48 hours. • Large doses may cause increased yeast growths. Report symptoms to the physician. • With prolonged therapy, bacterial or fungal superinfection may occur, especially in elderly patients, debilitated patients, or those with low resistance to infection from immunosuppressives or irradiation. Close observation is essential.

SELECTED MAJOR DRUGS

Antibacterial agents continued

DRUG	MAJOR INDICATIONS	USUAL ADULT DOSAGES	NURSING IMPLICATIONS
ticarcillin	Septicemia	3 grams I.V. every 3 to 6 hours	• Administer cautiously to patients with other drug allergies, especially to cephalosporins, and in patients with impaired renal function, hemorrhagic conditions, hypokalemia, or sodium restrictions (drug contains 5.2 mEq sodium per gram).
	Complicated urinary tract infections	3 grams I.V. every 4 to 6 hours	• Obtain specimens for culture and sensitivity tests before the first dose.
	Uncomplicated urinary tract infections	1 gram I.M. or I.V. every 4 to 6 hours	• Before giving ticarcillin, obtain a history to determine if the patient has had allergic reactions to penicillin. However, a negative history of penicillin allergy is no guarantee against a future allergic reaction.
			• Expect dosage alterations in patients with impaired hepatic and renal function.
			• Monitor the patient's complete blood count (CBC) frequently. Ticarcillin may cause thrombocytopenia.
			• When giving I.V., mix with D_5W or other suitable I.V. fluids.
			• Give by intermittent I.V. to prevent vein irritation. Change administration site every 48 hours.
			• Administer deep I.M. into large muscle.
			• With prolonged therapy, bacterial or fungal superinfections may occur, especially in elderly patients, debilitated patients, or those with low resistance to infection from immunosuppressives or irradiation. Close observation is essential.

Cephalosporins

DRUG	MAJOR INDICATIONS	USUAL ADULT DOSAGES	NURSING IMPLICATIONS
cefadroxil monohydrate	Urinary tract infections caused by *Escherichia coli, Proteus mirabilis,* or *Klebsiella* species; skin and soft-tissue infections; and streptococcal pharyngitis	500 mg to 2 grams P.O. every 12 to 24 hours, depending on the infection being treated; total daily dosage should not exceed 2 grams	• Cefadroxil is contraindicated in patients with hypersensitivity to other cephalosporins. Administer cautiously to patients with impaired renal status and in those with a history of sensitivity to penicillin.
			• Before administering first dose, obtain a history to determine if the patient has had reaction to previous cephalosporin or penicillin therapy.
			• Prolonged use may result in bacterial or fungal superinfection. Careful observation of the patient is essential.
			• Obtain specimens for culture and sensitivity tests before first dose, but therapy may begin pending test results.
			• If creatinine clearance is below 50 ml/minute, the dosage interval should be lengthened so that the drug does not accumulate.
			• Advise the patient to take the medication exactly as prescribed, even with condition improvement.
			• Instruct the patient to call the physician if skin rash develops.
			• Since absorption is not delayed by the presence of food, advise the patient to take the drug with food or milk to lessen GI discomfort.

continued

Antibacterial agents continued

DRUG	MAJOR INDICATIONS	USUAL ADULT DOSAGES	NURSING IMPLICATIONS
ceftizoxime	Serious infections of the lower respiratory and urinary tracts, gynecologic infections, bacteremia, septicemia, meningitis, intraabdominal infections, and skin infections	1 to 2 grams I.V. or I.M. every 8 to 12 hours; total daily dosage should not exceed 12 grams	• Ceftizoxime is contraindicated in patients with hypersensitivity to other cephalosporins. Administer cautiously to patients with impaired renal function and to those with a history of sensitivity to penicillin. • Before administering the first dose, obtain history to determine if the patient has had reaction to previous cephalosporin or penicillin therapy. • Prolonged use may result in bacterial or fungal superinfection. Observe the patient carefully. • Obtain specimens for culture and sensitivity tests before the first dose. • Dilute reconstituted solution in any of the following fluids: sodium chloride injection; 5% or 10% dextrose injection; 5% dextrose and 0.9%, 0.45%, or 0.2% sodium chloride injection; Ringer's injection; lactated Ringer's injection; invert sugar 10% in sterile water for injection; and 5% sodium bicarbonate in sterile water for injection.
Tetracyclines			
tetracycline	Infections caused by sensitive gram-negative and gram-positive organisms, rickettsiae, and *Mycoplasma*	250 to 500 mg P.O. every 6 hours; 250 mg I.M. daily or 150 mg I.M. every 12 hours; 250 to 500 mg I.V. every 8 to 12 hours (I.M. and I.V., hydrochloride salt only)	• Administer with extreme caution in patients with impaired renal or hepatic function. Use during last half of pregnancy and in children younger than age 8 may cause permanent tooth discoloration, enamel defects, and retarded bone growth. • Obtain specimens for culture and sensitivity before starting therapy. • Explain to the patient that effectiveness is reduced when the drug is taken with milk or other dairy products, food, antacids, or iron products. Instruct the patient to take each dose with a full glass of water on an empty stomach, at least 1 hour before or 2 hours after meals, and at least 1 hour before bedtime to prevent esophagitis. • The patient may develop thrombophlebitis with I.V. administration. Avoid extravasation. • Check drug expiration date. Outdated or deteriorated tetracycline may cause nephrotoxicity. • Discard I.M. solutions after 24 hours because they deteriorate. Discard Achromycin solution in 12 hours. • Do not expose these drugs to light or heat. • Inject I.M. dose deeply. Warn the patient that administration may be painful. Rotate sites. I.M. preparations in many cases contain a local anesthetic; ask the patient about hypersensitivity to local anesthetics. • Monitor the patient for superinfection. Assess the patient's tongue for signs of monilia infection. Stress good oral hygiene. If superin-
	Uncomplicated urethral, endocervical, or rectal infections caused by *Chlamydia trachomatis*	500 mg P.O. q.i.d. for at least 7 days	
	Brucellosis	500 mg P.O. every 6 hours for 3 weeks with 1 gram of streptomycin I.M. every 12 hours during 1st week and daily during 2nd week	
	Gonorrhea in patients sensitive to penicillin	1.5 grams P.O. initially, then 500 mg every 6 hours for a total of 9 grams	
	Syphilis in patients sensitive to penicillin	30 to 50 grams total in equally divided doses over 10 to 15 days	
	Acne	250 mg P.O. initially every 6 hours, then 125 to 500 mg P.O. daily or every other day	

SELECTED MAJOR DRUGS

Antibacterial agents continued

DRUG	MAJOR INDICATIONS	USUAL ADULT DOSAGES	NURSING IMPLICATIONS
tetracycline (continued)	Shigellosis	2.5 grams P.O. in one dose	fection occurs, the drug should be discontinued. • Advise the patient to avoid direct sunlight and ultraviolet light. A sunscreen may help prevent photosensitivity reactions. Photosensitivity persists for some time after drug discontinuation. • Advise the patient to take medication exactly as prescribed, even if the condition improves. • For I.V. use, reconstitute 100 mg and 250 mg powder for injection with 5 ml sterile water; reconstitute 500 mg for 10-ml injection. Further dilute in 100 to 1,000 ml of dextrose 5% in normal saline solution. Refrigerate diluted I.V. solution and use within 24 hours. Use Achromycin solution immediately. • Do not mix tetracycline solution with any other I.V. additive.
minocycline	Infections caused by sensitive gram-negative and gram-positive organisms, *Chlamydia trachomatis,* amebiasis	200 mg P.O. or I.V. initially; then 100 mg every 12 hours or 50 mg P.O. every 6 hours	• Administer with extreme caution to patients with impaired renal or hepatic function. Use during last half of pregnancy and in children younger than age 8 may cause permanent tooth discoloration, enamel defects, and retarded bone growth. • The patient may develop thrombophlebitis with I.V. administration of this drug. Avoid extravasation. • Obtain specimens for culture and sensitivity tests before starting therapy. • Do not expose this drug to light or heat. Keep cap tightly closed. • Monitor the patient for superinfection. Assess the patient's tongue for signs of monilia infection. Stress good oral hygiene. If superinfection occurs, drug should be discontinued. • Observe the patient for diarrhea, which may result from local irritation or superinfection. • Minocycline may be taken with food. Advise the patient to take the medication exactly as prescribed, even if the condition improves. • Reconstitute 100 mg powder with 5 ml sterile water for injection, with further dilution of 500 to 1,000 ml for I.V. infusion. Drug remains stable for 24 hours at room temperature.
	Gonorrhea in patients sensitive to penicillin	200 mg P.O. initially, then 100 mg every 12 hours for 4 days	
	Syphilis in patients sensitive to penicillin	200 mg P.O. initially, then 100 mg every 12 hours for 10 to 15 days	
	Meningococcal carrier state	100 to 200 mg P.O. every 12 hours for 5 days	
	Uncomplicated urethral, endocervical, or rectal infection caused by *Chlamydia trachomatis* or *Ureaplasma urealyticum*	100 mg P.O. b.i.d. for at least 7 days	
	Uncomplicated gonococcal urethritis in males	100 mg P.O. b.i.d. for 5 days	

Sulfonamides

sulfamethoxazole	Urinary tract and systemic infections	2 grams P.O. initially, then 1 gram P.O. b.i.d. to t.i.d for severe infections	• Contraindicated in patients with porphyria or in infants younger than age 2 months (except in congenital toxoplasmosis). Administer cautiously and in reduced dosages to patients with impaired hepatic or renal function and in those with severe allergy or bronchial asthma, glucose-6-phosphate dehydrogenase (G6PD) deficiency, or blood dyscrasias. • Advise the patient to drink a full glass of water with each dose and to drink plenty of water
	Lymphogranuloma venereum (genital, inguinal, or anorectal infections)	1 gram/day in two divided doses for at least 2 weeks	

continued

SELECTED MAJOR DRUGS

Antibacterial agents continued

DRUG	MAJOR INDICATIONS	USUAL ADULT DOSAGES	NURSING IMPLICATIONS
sulfamethoxazole (continued)			during the day to prevent crystalluria. Monitor fluid intake and urine output. • To help prevent crystalluria, sodium bicarbonate may be administered to alkalinize urine, as prescribed. Monitor urine pH daily. • Advise the patient to take medication for as long as prescribed, even if the condition improves. • Advise the patient to avoid direct sunlight and ultraviolet light to prevent a photosensitivity reaction. • Monitor urine culture, CBC, and urinalysis before and during therapy to assess efficacy of treatment.
Vancomycin			
vancomycin hydrochloride	Severe staphylococcal infections when other antibacterials are ineffective or contraindicated	500 mg I.V. every 6 hours, or 1 gram I.V. every 12 hours; total daily dosage should not exceed 2 grams	• Vancomycin is contraindicated in patients receiving other neurotoxic, nephrotoxic, or ototoxic drugs. Administer cautiously to patients with impaired hepatic or renal function; to those with hearing loss; to patients over age 60; and in patients with allergies to other antibiotics. • Advise the patient to take the medication exactly as directed, even if the condition improves. • Monitor the patient's auditory function tests before and during therapy. • Advise the patient to report adverse reactions at once, especially ringing in the ears. Stop the drug immediately if these occur. • Do not give drug I.M. • For I.V. infusion, dilute in 100 ml sodium chloride injection or 5% glucose solution and infuse over 30 minutes. Monitor the site daily for phlebitis and irritation. Report pain at infusion site. Avoid extravasation: severe irritation and necrosis can result. • The infusion rate should not exceed 500 mg in 30 minutes; more rapid infusion may cause an erythema multiforme–like rash involving the face, neck, upper trunk, and back. • Refrigerate I.V. solution after reconstitution and use within 96 hours. • Monitor renal function (BUN and serum creatinine levels, urinalysis, creatinine clearance, urine output) before and during therapy. • Monitor for signs of superinfection. • Refrigerated oral preparation remains stable for 2 weeks.
Chloramphenicol			
chloramphenicol	*Hemophilus influenzae* meningitis, *Salmonella* infection, rickettsiae, lymphogranuloma, psittacosis, *Bacteroides fragilis,* and other gramnegative organisms caus-	50 to 100 mg/kg/day P.O. or I.V. in divided doses every 6 hours	• Administer cautiously to patients with impaired hepatic or renal function, and with other drugs causing bone marrow suppression or blood disorders. • Obtain specimens for culture and sensitivity tests before first dose and as needed. • Monitor the patient's CBC, platelets, serum

SELECTED MAJOR DRUGS

Antibacterial agents continued

DRUG	MAJOR INDICATIONS	USUAL ADULT DOSAGES	NURSING IMPLICATIONS
chloramphenicol (continued)	ing meningitis, bacteremia, or other serious infections		iron, and reticulocyte count before and every 2 days during therapy. Stop drug immediately if anemia, reticulocytopenia, leukopenia, or thrombocytopenia develops. • Instruct the patient to report adverse reactions to the physician, especially nausea, vomiting, diarrhea, fever, confusion, sore throat, or mouth sores. • Advise the patient to take the medication for as long as prescribed, exactly as directed, even if the condition improves. • Reconstitute a 1-gram vial of powder for injection with 10 ml sterile water. Concentration will be 100 mg/ml and will remain stable for 30 days at room temperature, but refrigeration is recommended. Do not use cloudy solutions. • Monitor the patient for evidence of superinfection by nonsusceptible organisms.
Clindamycin			
clindamycin	Infections caused by certain staphylococci, streptococci, pneumococci, *Bacteroides fragilis, Clostridium perfringens,* and other aerobic and anaerobic organisms	150 to 450 mg P.O. every 6 hours; 300 to 600 mg I.M. or I.V. every 6 hours	• Clindamycin is contraindicated in patients with a known hypersensitivity to the antibiotic congener lincomycin and in patients with a history of GI disease, especially colitis. Administer cautiously to neonates and to patients with renal or hepatic disease, asthma, or significant allergies. • Monitor renal, hepatic, and hematopoietic function during prolonged therapy. • Obtain specimens for culture and sensitivity tests before starting treatment. • Don't refrigerate reconstituted oral solution, because it will thicken. Drug is stable for 2 weeks at room temperature. • Instruct the patient to report adverse reactions to the physician, especially diarrhea. • Advise a patient taking the capsule form to take it with a full glass of water to prevent dysphagia.

Imipenem inhibits most anaerobic species, including *Bacteroides fragilis.* The precise clinical role of imipenem/cilastatin is not clear. It may be used alone for mixed aerobic and anaerobic infections; as therapy for serious hospital-contracted infections or infections in immunocompromised hosts; and as treatment for those infections normally requiring combinations of antibiotics.

imipenem/cilastatin sodium (Primaxin). With its wide antibacterial spectrum of activity, imipenem/cilastatin is effective against gram-positive, gram-negative, and anaerobic organisms. It is especially useful against hospital-acquired (iatrogenic) infections. Before initiating imipenem/cilastatin therapy, verify that appropriate specimens have been obtained for culture and sensitivity testing. Because resistant strains of *P. aeruginosa* have developed during imipenem/cilastatin therapy, concomitant therapy with an aminoglycoside is recommended when treating infections caused by this organism.

USUAL ADULT DOSAGE: 250 mg imipenem/250 mg cilastatin or 500 mg imipenem/500 mg cilastatin for more serious infections, administered via intermittent I.V.

USUAL PEDIATRIC DOSAGE: for children age 12 and over, same as adult; not recommended for children under age 12.

Drug interactions

Only a few significant interactions occur between imipenem/cilastatin and other drugs. Concomitant administration of probenecid and imipenem/cilastatin produces higher and prolonged serum concentration levels of cilastatin but only slightly higher serum concentration levels of imipenem. Consequently, concomitant use of these drugs is not recommended.

The combination of imipenem/cilastatin and an aminoglycoside acts synergistically against *Streptococcus faecalis* but is not effective against most strains of *P. aeruginosa*. Chloramphenicol can decrease the bactericidal activity of imipenem against *Klebsiella pneumoniae*.

ADVERSE DRUG REACTIONS

The adverse reactions associated with the imipenem/cilastatin combination are neither common nor particularly serious.

Predictable reactions

Elderly patients and patients with a history of previous seizure activity, underlying CNS disease, or renal insufficiency may experience seizures. The most common adverse reactions are nausea, vomiting, and diarrhea. In some instances, nausea is related to rapid infusion and is reduced by increasing the administration time. Pseudomembranous colitis caused by *Clostridium difficile* has been reported.

Phlebitis, thrombophlebitis, and pain at the infusion site can occur. Transient elevations in liver function values (SGOT, SGPT, LDH) may occur.

Unpredictable reactions

Allergic reactions, such as rashes, have occurred in clinical trials. No anaphylactic reactions have been reported. Patients with a history of serious beta-lactam allergy should not receive imipenem/cilastatin.

NURSING IMPLICATIONS

Imipenem/cilastatin is a new antibacterial combination drug that may be used with increasing frequency. The nurse should be aware of the following implications:
• Know that prolonged use of imipenem/cilastatin may result in bacterial or fungal superinfection.
• Assess the patient for a history of hypersensitivity to beta-lactam antibacterials.
• Assess the patient for history of CNS disorders (brain lesions, seizures) and compromised renal function.

• Do not mix imipenem/cilastatin with, or add to, other antibiotics.
• Administer imipenem/cilastatin by intermittent I.V. infusion over a 30-minute interval.

CHAPTER SUMMARY

Chapter 66 described the clinically important antibacterial drugs used to treat systemic infections. Here are the highlights:
• Aminoglycosides are the mainstay in the treatment of serious nosocomial gram-negative bacterial infections. Currently, gentamicin, tobramycin, netilmicin, and amikacin are the most commonly prescribed.
• In patients with renal insufficiency, aminoglycoside dosage adjustments must be made to avoid serious toxicities and damage to the auditory, vestibular, and renal functions. Periodic assessment of aminoglycoside serum peak concentration and trough concentration levels is needed to assess therapeutic efficacy and toxicity.
• Penicillins remain one of the most important and useful antibacterial groups available for clinical use. No other class of antibacterial has as wide a spectrum of activity as the penicillins, which are used to treat gram-positive and gram-negative aerobic bacteria as well as anaerobic bacteria. Because penicillins have a low incidence of serious toxicity and are relatively inexpensive, they are the drugs of choice to treat susceptible organisms in nonallergic patients.
• Cephalosporins are frequently prescribed. Many new cephalosporins have been introduced for clinical use in recent years. The available cephalosporins are classified into three generations based on their spectra of activity.
• Patients taking penicillins and cephalosporins concurrently may develop cross-sensitivities.
• Tetracyclines rarely are considered the drug of choice to treat most common bacterial infections; however, they are among the most commonly prescribed antibacterials in the world. The tetracyclines are primarily bacteriostatic.
• Chloramphenicol-induced aplastic anemia has limited the use of the drug. This broad-spectrum antibacterial usually is reserved for treating serious infections.
• Clindamycin is more effective than lincomycin against susceptible bacteria. Clindamycin remains particularly

important in treating certain anaerobic infections. Diarrhea occurs in 20% or more of the patients receiving clindamycin (most frequently with oral administration).

• Erythromycin is used to treat a number of commonly encountered infections. A bacteriostatic antibacterial, erythromycin inhibits protein synthesis, as do chloramphenicol, clindamycin, and lincomycin. Erythromycin is the drug of choice to treat *Mycoplasma pneumoniae* infections as well as *Legionella* pneumonia. The drug's adverse effects are few.

• Sulfonamides were the first effective systemic agents to be used to treat bacterial infections. Today, the emergence of resistant strains of bacteria has reduced sulfonamide effectiveness. These drugs are used primarily to treat certain acute community-acquired urinary tract infections.

• Vancomycin is experiencing a resurgence in popularity because of increasing problems with methicillin-resistant *Staphylococcus aureus*, which has become a major concern in the United States and throughout the world.

• Imipenem/cilastatin is the first of a new class of beta-lactam antibacterials called carbapenems. Imipenem/cilastatin's antibacterial spectrum of activity is broader than that of any other antibacterial studied to date. Imipenem/cilastatin is used to treat many clinically important infections, especially those acquired nosocomially. Elderly patients with renal insufficiency or a history of seizures are prone to drug-induced seizures.

BIBLIOGRAPHY

American Hospital Formulary Service. *Drug Information 87.* McEvoy, G.K., et al., eds. Bethesda, Md.: American Society of Hospital Pharmacists, 1987.

Birnbaum, J., et al. "Carbapenems: A New Class of Beta-Lactam Antibiotics," *American Journal of Medicine* 78:3, June 1985.

Clissold, S.P., et al. "Imipenem/Cilastatin: A Review of Its Antibacterial Activity, Pharmacokinetic Properties and Therapeutic Efficacy," *Drugs* 33:183, March 1987.

Edson, R.S., and Keys, T.F. "The Aminoglycosides: Streptomycin, Kanamycin, Gentamicin, Tobramycin, Amikacin, Netilmicin, Sisomicin," *Mayo Clinic Proceedings* 58:99, February 1983.

Geraci, J.E., and Hermans, P.E. "Vancomycin," *Mayo Clinic Proceedings* 58:88, February 1983.

Lyon, J.A. "Imipenem/Cilastatin: The First Carbapenem Antibiotic," *Drug Intelligence and Clinical Pharmacy* 19:895, December 1985.

Mandell, G., et al., eds. *Principles and Practice of Infectious Diseases,* 2nd ed. New York: John Wiley & Sons, 1985.

Neu, H.C. "Carbapenems: Special Properties Contributing to Their Activity," *American Journal of Medicine* 78:33, June 1985.

Reed, M.D., et al. "Pharmacokinetics of Imipenem and Cilastatin in Patients with Cystic Fibrosis," *Antimicrobial Agents and Chemotherapy* 27:583, April 1985.

Thompson, R.L., and Wright, A.J. "Cephalosporin Antibiotics," *Mayo Clinic Proceedings* 58:79, February 1983.

Weintraub, M., and Evans, P. "Imipenem/Cilastatin: A Multipurpose Antibiotic from a New Chemical Class," *Hospital Formulary* 20:1138, 1985.

Wilson, W.R., and Cockerill, F.R., III. "Tetracyclines, Chloramphenicol, Erythromycin, and Clindamycin," *Mayo Clinic Proceedings* 58:92, February 1983.

Wright, A.J., and Wilkowske, C.J. "The Penicillins," *Mayo Clinic Proceedings* 58:21, January 1983.

CHAPTER 67

ANTITUBERCULAR AND ANTILEPROTIC AGENTS

OBJECTIVES

After reading and studying this chapter, you should be able to:

1. Identify the first-line agents employed in treating tuberculosis and Hansen's disease (leprosy).

2. Identify the major adverse drug reactions these agents produce and intervene appropriately.

3. Identify the genetic factors that can affect the actions of these agents.

4. Identify drug interactions associated with antitubercular and antileprotic agents.

5. Teach the patient with a mycobacterial infection about the disease and its drug therapy.

INTRODUCTION

Antitubercular and antileprotic agents are used to treat mycobacterial infections; tuberculosis, which is caused by *Mycobacterium tuberculosis;* and Hansen's disease (previously called *leprosy*), which is caused by *M. leprae.* These agents are also effective against less common mycobacterial infections caused by *M. kansasii, M. avium, M. fortuitum, M. intracellularis*, and related organisms. Not always curative, these agents can halt the progression of a mycobacterial infection.

Unlike most antibiotics, antitubercular and antileprotic agents may need to be administered over many months, or even years. This creates problems, such as patient noncompliance, the development of bacterial resistance, and drug toxicity. The nurse must be aware of these and other problems to assist the patient during the therapeutic process.

For a summary of representative drugs, see *Selected major drugs: Antitubercular and antileprotic agents* on page 1087.

ANTITUBERCULAR AGENTS

Isoniazid (INH), ethambutol hydrochloride, and rifampin are the mainstays of tuberculosis therapy. Streptomycin sulfate, the first effective antitubercular agent, is also used, but not as frequently. Other antitubercular agents are even less frequently used because they are less effective and more toxic. These include aminosalicylic acid, capreomycin sulfate, cycloserine, ethionamide, and pyrazinamide. Usually, these agents are used only when hypersensitivity, intolerance, or bacterial resistance to a first-line agent exists. (See the section "Other Antitubercular Agents" in this chapter for information about these secondary drugs.

History and source

In 1945, researchers discovered that nicotinamide was tuberculostatic—able to inhibit the growth of *M. tuberculosis*. Further examination of nicotinamide and related compounds, including INH, revealed that INH exhibited effective tuberculostatic action with a relatively low incidence of toxicity.

In 1959, researchers first isolated macrocyclic rifamycin antibiotics, derived from *Streptomyces mediterranei*. After extensive, prolonged research, they noted that one member of this group, rifampin, acted as a strong bactericide and also increased the activity of streptomycin and INH against *M. tuberculosis*. These discoveries helped make rifampin a major drug for tuberculosis therapy.

In 1961, Thomas and associates discovered the antitubercular activity of N,N¹-di-isopropyl-ethylenediamine in mice. Subsequent studies of its derivatives revealed that ethambutol had the strongest tuberculostatic effect among them.

PHARMACOKINETICS

These drugs are almost exclusively administered orally; only INH is commercially available parenterally. When administered orally, they are well absorbed from the gastrointestinal (GI) tract and widely distributed throughout the body. The drugs are primarily metabolized in the liver and excreted by the kidneys.

Absorption, distribution, metabolism, excretion

INH, readily absorbed from the GI tract and I.M. injection sites, is distributed into all body tissues and fluids, readily crossing the blood-brain barrier and the placenta. It is distributed into breast milk in concentration levels similar to those of the maternal plasma. INH is almost completely metabolized by enzymatic acetylation and hydrolysis in the liver. The rate of acetylation, however, is determined by race-linked genetic factors. (See *Isoniazid metabolism* for further information.) Although these genetic factors can produce significant variations in the rate of INH elimination, the drug is still effective when administered two or three times a week. Its effectiveness is reduced for some patients (fast acetylators), however, when administration is once weekly. From 75% to 95% of INH is excreted in the urine as metabolites and unchanged drug within 24 hours after administration. Small amounts are excreted in the saliva, sputum, and feces.

Rifampin is also well absorbed from the GI tract, although food in the stomach can reduce its rate and extent of absorption. The drug diffuses freely into most body tissues and fluids, including the cerebrospinal fluid (CSF), in concentration levels that are 10% to 20% of plasma concentration levels. It crosses the placenta and appears in breast milk. After metabolism in the liver, the drug is excreted primarily in the feces but also in urine and bile.

About 75% to 80% of an oral dose of ethambutol is rapidly absorbed from the GI tract. The drug is widely distributed into most body tissues and fluids, and about twice as much appears in erythrocytes as in plasma. (The erythrocytes may serve as a reservoir, slowly releasing the drug into the circulation.) Although it is not known if ethambutol crosses the placenta, it appears in breast milk in concentration levels roughly equal to those of blood plasma. The liver metabolizes up to 15% of ethambutol, and the kidneys excrete almost all of it, primarily unchanged.

Onset, peak, duration

After oral administration, INH reaches peak plasma concentration levels in 1 to 2 hours. The half-life of this drug ranges from 1 to 4 hours, but it may be longer for a patient with renal or hepatic impairment.

Rifampin reaches peak plasma concentration levels in 2 to 4 hours. Initially, its half-life ranges from 1½ to 5 hours and averages 3 hours, but because biliary excretion of rifampin increases during the first 2 weeks of therapy, the half-life gradually decreases to about 2 hours. Plasma concentration levels of rifampin are higher and more prolonged in a patient with hepatic dysfunction but unaffected in a patient with renal dysfunction.

After an oral dose of ethambutol, plasma concentration levels peak in 2 to 4 hours in proportion to the size of the dose. The drug's half-life in a patient with

Isoniazid metabolism

In the liver, the enzyme acetyltransferase metabolizes isoniazid (INH) to acetylisoniazid by a process called *acetylation*. Acetylisoniazid then is metabolized by hydrolysis to acetylhydrazine, a potentially hepatotoxic metabolite. This normal metabolic path of INH is illustrated below.

Race-linked genetic factors determine how fast acetylation occurs. About 50% of all whites and blacks are so-called slow acetylators. Because their supply of the enzyme acetyltransferase is below normal, they metabolize INH slowly and are more likely to experience adverse reactions such as peripheral neuritis. The remaining whites and blacks and about 90% of all Eskimos, Japanese, and Chinese are so-called fast acetylators. They have normal supplies of the enzyme, so they metabolize INH quickly. However, this makes fast acetylators more susceptible to the potentially hepatotoxic effects of the metabolite acetylhydrazine.

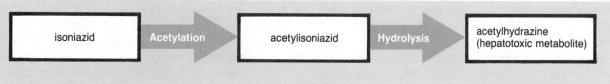

normal renal function is about 3 hours; in a patient with renal impairment, the drug will have a longer half-life, and a dosage adjustment may be necessary.

PHARMACODYNAMICS

Antitubercular agents are specific for mycobacteria. At usual doses, INH and ethambutol are tuberculostatic, inhibiting growth of *M. tuberculosis* bacteria. In contrast, rifampin is tuberculocidal, destroying the bacteria. Because bacterial resistance to INH and rifampin can develop rapidly, however, they are usually used in combination with other antitubercular agents.

Mechanism of action

Although INH's exact mechanism of action is not known, evidence suggests that the drug inhibits the synthesis of mycolic acids, important components of the mycobacterium cell wall. This inhibition alters the cell's acid-fastness and disrupts the cell wall. Because mycolic acid synthesis is unique to mycobacteria, this mechanism explains INH's high degree of specificity. Only INH-sensitive bacteria take up the drug, and only replicating, not resting, bacteria appear to be inhibited.

Rifampin inhibits ribonucleic acid (RNA) synthesis in susceptible organisms by acting on the beta subunit of the enzyme RNA polymerase. The drug is effective primarily in replicating bacteria but may have some effect on resting bacteria as well.

Ethambutol is most active against *M. tuberculosis* and *M. kansasii* but acts—to varying degrees—against all mycobacteria. Although mycobacteria rapidly take up ethambutol, the drug does not significantly inhibit their growth for approximately 24 hours. Its exact mechanism of action remains unclear but may be related to inhibition of cell metabolism. Ethambutol acts only against replicating bacteria.

PHARMACOTHERAPEUTICS

INH is usually used in combination with ethambutol, rifampin, or streptomycin. This is because combination therapy for tuberculosis and other mycobacterial infections can prevent or delay the development of bacterial resistance to the drug regimen.

isoniazid [INH] (Nydrazid, Teebaconin). Although INH is the most important drug for treating tuberculosis, bacterial resistance develops rapidly if it is used alone. However, resistance does not pose a problem when INH is used alone to prevent tuberculosis in individuals who have been exposed to the disease, and no evidence exists of cross-resistance between INH and other antitubercular agents. INH may be given I.M. or P.O., although I.M. administration offers no special advantages. Experiments with continuous and intermittent therapy may eventually lead to revision of current dosage and regimens.

USUAL ADULT DOSAGE: for treatment of tuberculosis, 5 to 10 mg/kg of body weight P.O. or I.M. daily as a single dose, up to a maximum of 300 mg daily for at least 1 year; for prevention of tuberculosis, 300 mg P.O. daily as a single dose for at least 1 year.

rifampin (Rifadin, Rimactane). A first-line agent for treating pulmonary tuberculosis, rifampin is particularly effective when combined with INH or another antitubercular agent. This drug combats many gram-positive and some gram-negative bacteria but is seldom used for nonmycobacterial infections because bacterial resistance develops rapidly. It is used to treat asymptomatic carriers of *Neisseria meningitidis* when the risk of meningitis is high, but it is not used to treat *N. meningitidis* infections because of the potential for bacterial resistance. Rifampin is usually used in combination with other drugs to treat Hansen's disease and is the drug of choice in treating dapsone-resistant Hansen's disease.

USUAL ADULT DOSAGE: for tuberculosis or Hansen's disease, 600 mg P.O. once daily 1 hour before or 2 hours after a meal; for asymptomatic carriers of *N. meningitidis,* 600 mg P.O. once daily 1 hour before or 2 hours after a meal for 4 days, or 600 mg b.i.d. for 2 days.

ethambutol hydrochloride (Myambutol). Ethambutol is used in combination with INH and rifampin to treat uncomplicated pulmonary tuberculosis in a patient who lives in a geographic area noted for a high incidence of bacterial resistance or who has been previously treated with antitubercular agents. The drug is also used to treat infections resulting from *M. bovis* and most strains of *M. kansasii.*

USUAL ADULT DOSAGE: for infections previously untreated with antitubercular agents, 15 mg/kg of body weight P.O. as a single daily dose. For previously treated infections, 25 mg/kg P.O. daily for 60 days, then the dose is decreased to 15 mg/kg P.O. daily as a single dose; for intermittent therapy, 50 mg/kg two to three times weekly. In a patient with renal impairment, the dose may be reduced or the interval between doses may be increased. For instance, if the creatinine clearance is 10 to 50 ml/minute, the interval may be increased to 24 to 36 hours; if the creatinine clearance is less than 10 ml/minute, the interval may be increased to 48 hours.

Drug interactions

Some evidence suggests that INH, cycloserine, and ethionamide may produce additive central nervous system (CNS) effects, such as drowsiness, dizziness, headache, lethargy, depression, tremor, anxiety, confusion, and tinnitus. Therefore, these drugs should be administered cautiously in combination. INH increases plasma concentration levels of phenytoin, increasing the likelihood of phenytoin toxicity in patients who are slow acetylators. Aluminum hydroxide, a common ingredient in antacids, significantly decreases INH absorption. INH administration with a corticosteroid decreases INH's effects and increases the corticosteroid's effects.

Rifampin can increase the rate of metabolism—and consequently decrease the plasma concentration level—of some drugs, including oral contraceptives, corticosteroids, methadone, oral hypoglycemics, warfarin, digitalis derivatives, and dapsone. The dosages of these agents may need to be increased during rifampin therapy. Aminosalicyclic acid may inhibit rifampin absorption.

Antacids that contain aluminum hydroxide or other aluminum salts may slightly decrease the GI absorption of ethambutol.

ADVERSE DRUG REACTIONS

The antitubercular agents' adverse reactions primarily affect the GI tract, the peripheral nervous system, and the hepatic system. Fortunately, these reactions are seldom severe enough to necessitate interruption of tuberculosis therapy.

Predictable reactions

Peripheral neuritis occurs in 20% of the patients receiving 6 mg/kg of INH daily, and higher doses increase the incidence of this reaction. Usually preceded by paresthesias of the feet and hands, peripheral neuritis is more likely to affect an alcoholic, diabetic, or other individual who is malnourished or predisposed to peripheral neuritis. It typically produces muscle twitching, dizziness, ataxia, stupor, and paresthesias. Daily administration of 10 to 50 mg of pyridoxine (vitamin B_6) may prevent this reaction. During the first 6 months of therapy, transient elevations occur in levels of the enzymes serum glutamic-pyruvic transaminase (SGPT), or alanine aminotransferase (ALT); and serum glutamic-oxaloacetic transaminase (SGOT), or aspartate aminotransferase (AST); and in bilirubin concentration levels in 10% to 20% of patients receiving INH. This drug may also produce hepatitis, especially in elderly patients and usually in the first 4 to 8 weeks of therapy.

The most common adverse reactions to rifampin include epigastric pain, nausea, vomiting, abdominal cramps, flatulence, anorexia, and diarrhea. Joint pain and muscle aches and cramps may also occur. All these reactions, which are most likely to occur during the first 2 weeks of therapy, may subside as biliary excretion of rifampin increases and its half-life decreases; interruption of therapy is seldom necessary. Rifampin can elevate ALT, AST, bilirubin, and alkaline phosphatase levels, possibly leading to eventual discontinuation of the drug. Transient asymptomatic jaundice and red-orange discoloration of sweat, tears, saliva, urine, and feces may also occur but do not necessitate discontinuation of drug therapy.

Optic neuritis is the only significant adverse reaction to ethambutol. Signs and symptoms include decreased visual acuity, loss of red-green color discrimination, visual field constriction, and central and peripheral scotomas (areas of depressed vision in the visual field). This adverse reaction occurs in only 0.8% of patients receiving 15 mg/kg, but its incidence increases in patients who receive higher doses or who have renal dysfunction. Discontinuing ethambutol usually reverses the optic neuritis—but if vision impairment is severe, recovery may be incomplete. Pruritus, joint pain, GI upset, malaise, headache, dizziness, and mental confusion have also been reported with ethambutol therapy.

Unpredictable reactions

Hypersensitivity reactions to INH occur rarely, producing fever, skin eruptions (morbilliform, maculopapular, purpuric, or exfoliative), lymphadenopathy, and vasculitis. These reactions usually appear 3 to 7 weeks after therapy begins. INH may precipitate seizures in a patient with a seizure disorder. It may also produce optic neuritis and atrophy; mental abnormalities, such as euphoria and memory impairment; and sedation or uncoordination.

Large (900- to 1,200-mg) intermittent doses of rifampin produce hypersensitivity reactions in about 1% of patients so treated. This reaction appears as a flulike syndrome characterized by dyspnea with or without wheezing; purpura associated with thrombocytopenia; leukopenia; and, rarely, anaphylaxis. A patient with this reaction will probably be able to tolerate a reduced rifampin dosage (only 3% of all patients require discontinuation of this drug).

The most commonly occurring unpredictable reactions to ethambutol are rash (in 10.5% of patients) and fever (in 0.3%). Hypersensitivity reactions occur rarely with ethambutol and tend to be mild. Leukopenia, anaphylaxis, and peripheral neuritis with paresthesias of the extremities have been reported. Occasionally, ethambutol therapy increases serum uric acid levels and precipitates an acute gout episode.

NURSING IMPLICATIONS

For antitubercular therapy to be successful, the nurse must teach the patient the consequences of noncompliance. The nurse must also monitor the patient for signs and symptoms of adverse reactions and intervene to minimize their effects.

• Administer INH when the patient's stomach is empty— 1 hour before meals or 2 hours after—and avoid concomitant administration of antacids.

• Instruct the patient to consult the physician if signs and symptoms of possible hepatic dysfunction appear, such as nausea, vomiting, fatigue, weakness, and anorexia.

• Conduct periodic eye examinations of the patient receiving INH, and monitor for visual disturbances.

• Advise the patient receiving INH to avoid consuming alcohol because of the risk of hepatotoxicity.

• Administer pyridoxine concurrently with INH, as prescribed, to prevent peripheral neuritis.

• Rifampin therapy is contraindicated in pregnant women because its safety in pregnancy has not been established. Counsel a lactating mother to consider alternatives to breast-feeding because rifampin is secreted in breast milk.

• Advise the patient taking rifampin that it may produce red-orange urine, tears, sputum, sweat, and feces that stain clothes, linen, and soft contact lenses.

• Advise a woman who is on rifampin therapy and taking oral contraceptives to use alternate forms of birth control.

• Monitor the patient's liver function tests for signs of rifampin toxicity.

• To help prevent rifampin hypersensitivity reactions, caution the patient against interrupting rifampin therapy.

• Reassure the patient who experiences adverse reactions early in rifampin therapy that most of them will subside with continued treatment.

• Monitor the patient's visual acuity before ethambutol therapy begins and monthly thereafter when doses exceed 15 mg/kg. Instruct the patient to report any visual changes immediately.

• Administer ethambutol as a single daily dose because divided doses may increase the incidence of visual disturbances.

• Monitor renal and hepatic function tests periodically for the patient receiving ethambutol.

• Ethambutol is contraindicated in pregnant women unless the benefits to the mother outweigh the risks to the fetus.

OTHER ANTITUBERCULAR AGENTS

Several other drugs are used as antitubercular agents, in combination with first-line agents. Because these drugs have a greater incidence of toxicity, they are primarily used when resistance or allergies to less toxic agents exist.

aminosalicylic acid (Para-Aminosalicytic Acid, P.A.S.). A tuberculostatic agent, aminosalicylic acid acts like a sulfonamide by decreasing bacterial synthesis of folic acid. The drug is readily absorbed, widely distributed, and rapidly metabolized by the liver and excreted by the kidneys. Its half-life is about 1 hour. The usual adult dosage is 8 to 12 grams P.O. daily given in three to four divided doses after meals. The potential for severe GI disturbances limits the use of aminosalicylic acid.

capreomycin sulfate (Capastat Sulfate). A polypeptide antibiotic, capreomycin inhibits the growth of mycobacteria. Its half-life is 4 to 6 hours, and it is primarily excreted unchanged in the urine. Administered I.M., the usual adult dosage is 15 mg/kg or 1 gram/day for 60 to 120 days, then 1 gram two to three times a week for 18 to 24 months.

cycloserine (Seromycin). An antibiotic derived from the *Streptomyces* genus, cycloserine acts against many strains of mycobacteria. After oral administration, cycloserine is well absorbed, widely distributed, and primarily excreted by the kidneys. It has a half-life of 10 hours. It is used in combination with other antitubercular agents, but its neurotoxicity and the rapid development of bacterial resistance limit its use. The usual adult dosage is 250 mg P.O. every 12 hours for 2 weeks, increased to a maximum of 1 gram/day.

ethionamide (Trecator-SC). A derivative of isonicotinic acid, ethionamide is used to treat tuberculosis and Hansen's disease. It is especially useful in treating Hansen's disease produced by dapsone-resistant *M. leprae*. Rapid absorption, wide distribution, hepatic metabolism, renal excretion, and a half-life of 3 hours characterize ethionamide. The usual adult dosage is 250 mg P.O. b.i.d., increased by 125 mg per day every 5 days up to 1 gram/ day with meals. GI disturbances are the most common adverse reactions to the drug.

pyrazinamide. A niacinamide derivative, pyrazinamide is highly specific for *M. tuberculosis*. Well absorbed and widely distributed, pyrazinamide is extensively metabolized by the liver and has a half-life of 9 to 10 hours. Because this drug commonly produces hepatotoxicity, a patient receiving it requires close monitoring. The usual adult dosage is 20 to 35 mg/kg P.O. daily in three to four divided doses. The maximum dose is 3 grams/day.

streptomycin sulfate. The first agent recognized as effective in treating tuberculosis, streptomycin is administered I.M. only. It appears to enhance the activity of oral antitubercular agents and is of greatest value in the early weeks to months of therapy. But I.M. administration limits its usefulness in long-term therapy. Rapidly absorbed from the I.M. injection site, streptomycin is primarily excreted by the kidneys as unchanged drug. The usual adult dosage is 0.5 to 1 gram I.M. every 12 hours. Most patients tolerate streptomycin well, but those receiving large doses may exhibit eighth cranial nerve toxicity. (See Chapter 66, Antibacterial Agents, for information about the other uses of streptomycin.)

ANTILEPROTIC AGENTS

The primary agent used to treat Hansen's disease (leprosy) is dapsone, a sulfone drug; however, rifampin and clofazimine are also used. Rifampin was discussed in the "Antitubercular Agents" section and clofazimine is included in the "Other Antileprotic Agents" section in this chapter. Ethionamide, an antitubercular agent, is used to treat dapsone-resistant Hansen's disease and is usually combined with rifampin, or clofazimine and rifampin.

History and source
Diaminodiphenysulfone—known as DDS or dapsone—was first synthesized in 1908, but its antibacterial activity was not reported until 1937. Four years later, a dapsone derivative, glucosulfone, was first used to treat Hansen's disease in humans. Dapsone itself was first used to treat Hansen's disease in 1946.

PHARMACOKINETICS

Dapsone is only administered orally. It is distributed into most body tissues and fluids, slowly metabolized in the liver, and excreted in the urine.

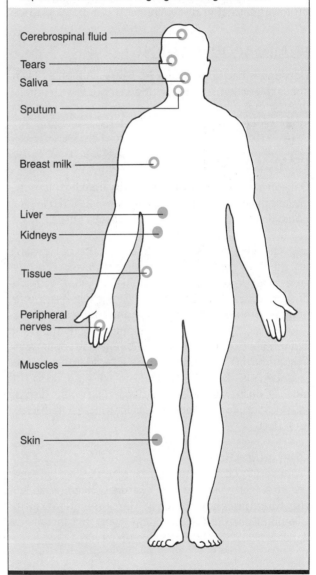

Dapsone distribution

The antileprotic agent dapsone is widely distributed in the body and retained in the liver, kidneys, skin, and muscles. The areas of greatest distribution are highlighted below as white dots, and the areas of dapsone retention are highlighted as green dots.

Cerebrospinal fluid
Tears
Saliva
Sputum
Breast milk
Liver
Kidneys
Tissue
Peripheral nerves
Muscles
Skin

Absorption, distribution, metabolism, excretion
After oral administration, dapsone is slowly—but completely—absorbed from the GI tract and is freely distributed throughout the body. It appears in most tissues and fluids but is retained in the skin, muscles, and especially in the liver and kidneys. (See *Dapsone distribution* for more information.) Dapsone is distributed into breast milk. Similar to INH, dapsone undergoes acety-

lation in the liver at a genetically determined rate. Approximately 20% of the drug is excreted unchanged in the urine, and the rest is excreted as metabolites.

Onset, peak, duration

Dapsone reaches peak serum concentration levels in 1 to 3 hours. The drug's half-life ranges from 10 to 50 hours, averaging 28 hours. Trace amounts may remain in the body 8 to 12 days after a single 200-mg dose or up to 35 days after discontinuation of repeated doses.

PHARMACODYNAMICS

Dapsone is bacteriostatic for *M. leprae.* Although its antibacterial action is not fully understood, it may parallel that of the sulfonamides. Like those drugs, dapsone inhibits folic acid synthesis by bacteria.

PHARMACOTHERAPEUTICS

Dapsone is the drug of choice for treating Hansen's disease because it is effective, inexpensive, and relatively nontoxic. It is also used to treat dermatitis herpetiformis.

dapsone. Dapsone is used to treat all forms of Hansen's disease, and bacterial resistance to it develops by degrees. The drug is used alone only after intensive multidrug treatment. Sulfone-sensitive infections usually require a combination of dapsone and rifampin; sulfone-resistant infections require combinations of rifampin and clofazimine or ethionamide. Treatment may continue for 6 months to life, depending on the severity of the disease. USUAL ADULT DOSAGE: for Hansen's disease, 50 to 100 mg P.O. daily as a single dose, depending on the disease classification; for dermatitis herpetiformis, 25 to 400 mg P.O. daily.

Drug interactions

Probenecid decreases urinary excretion of dapsone metabolites, increasing the drug's serum concentration levels. Rifampin may increase dapsone metabolism, lowering its serum concentration levels, but the clinical significance of this interaction is unknown.

ADVERSE DRUG REACTIONS

Dapsone produces relatively few adverse reactions, which seldom require interruption of therapy. The most serious are hematologic.

G6PD deficiency

Glucose-6-phosphate dehydrogenase (G6PD) deficiency affects many people, especially Blacks; Chinese; Thais; and Eastern Mediterranean peoples, such as Greeks, Sardinians, and Sephardic Jews. The more than 100 variants of this genetic chromosomal deficiency can produce varying degrees of erythrocyte hemolysis when affected individuals receive treatment with such drugs as dapsone, antimalarial agents, analgesics, sulfonamides, vitamin K, and probenecid. All these drugs should be administered cautiously to patients with G6PD deficiency. Complicating this risk, G6PD deficiency may also trigger erythrocyte hemolysis when an affected individual is subjected to the stress of metabolic acidosis, diabetic ketoacidosis, or a bacterial infection. Such stress shortens erythrocyte life span, decreasing the hemoglobin level (especially in older erythrocytes) and increasing the reticulocyte count. Thus, both an infection *and* the drug used to treat it pose special hazards for the person with G6PD deficiency.

Predictable reactions

Hemolytic anemia and methemoglobinemia are the most frequently occurring dose-related reactions to dapsone. Hemolysis can occur in varying degrees. It develops in almost every patient receiving 200 to 300 mg of dapsone daily but hardly ever affects those receiving 100 mg/day. Some degree of methemoglobinemia occurs in most patients receiving dapsone but usually does not necessitate discontinuation of therapy. Cyanosis may accompany mild methemoglobinemia. Although these adverse hematologic reactions pose no problems for most patients, dapsone may produce severe hemolysis and methemoglobinemia in a patient with glucose-6-phosphate dehydrogenase (G6PD) deficiency. (See *G6PD deficiency* for further information.)

Unpredictable reactions

Serious complications of dapsone therapy are uncommon, but may include granulocytosis and dapsone syndrome, which mimic infectious mononucleosis. Hypersensitivity to dapsone may produce adverse cutaneous reactions, such as exfoliative dermatitis, toxic erythema, erythema multiforme, urticaria, and erythema nodosum.

NURSING IMPLICATIONS

Long-term treatment is generally required with antileprotic agents. Because patient compliance tends to decrease over time, the nurse must stress the importance of compliance and be aware of the following considerations to ensure effective treatment:

• Dapsone is contraindicated in a patient with anemia.
• Dapsone is contraindicated in pregnant women unless the benefits to the mother outweigh the risks to the fetus.
• Monitor the patient's complete blood count weekly during the first 6 months of dapsone therapy and monthly thereafter.
• Administer dapsone cautiously in combination with nitrite, aniline, nitrofurantoin, primaquine, or other drugs that can induce hemolysis, particularly if the patient has G6PD deficiency.
• Instruct the patient to report sore throat, fever, purpura, or jaundice occurring during dapsone therapy.

OTHER ANTILEPROTIC AGENTS

The antitubercular agents rifampin and ethionamide are also important antileprotic agents. Their use and limitations in treating Hansen's disease mirror their role in tuberculosis treatment.

clofazimine (Lamprene). An investigational drug, clofazimine is available only through the Gillis W. Long Hansen's Disease Center at Carville, La. An effective antileprotic agent, the drug is used to treat the dapsone-

SELECTED MAJOR DRUGS

Antitubercular and antileprotic agents

This chart summarizes the first-line agents used to treat mycobacterial infections. Effective therapy usually combines these drugs with each other or with second-line agents.

DRUG	MAJOR INDICATIONS	USUAL ADULT DOSAGES	NURSING IMPLICATIONS
isoniazid (INH)	Tuberculosis	5 to 10 mg/kg P.O. or I.M. daily as a single dose, up to a maximum of 300 mg/day for at least 1 year	• Monitor the patient for signs and symptoms of hepatic disease. • Monitor the patient for vision disturbances. • Administer pyridoxine supplements concurrently, as prescribed, to reduce the risk of peripheral neuritis.
	Prevention of tuberculosis	300 mg P.O. daily as a single dose for at least 1 year	
rifampin	Tuberculosis and Hansen's disease	600 mg P.O. daily as a single dose 1 hour before or 2 hours after a meal	• Advise the patient that rifampin may produce orange-red tears, sweat, and urine that may stain clothes, linens, and soft contact lenses. • Monitor the patient's liver function tests for signs of toxicity. • Reassure the patient that any adverse reactions appearing early in therapy will subside without therapy discontinuation.
	Asymptomatic *Neisseria meningitidis* carriers	600 mg P.O. b.i.d. for 2 days or 600 mg P.O. once a day for 4 days	
ethambutol	Tuberculosis, *Mycobacterium bovis*, and *M. kansasii* infections	15 mg/kg P.O. in a single daily dose, if previously untreated; 25 mg/kg P.O. daily, for 60 days with dosage decreased to 15 mg/kg P.O. daily as a single dose	• Instruct the patient to immediately report any vision changes during ethambutol therapy. • Be aware that ethambutol is contraindicated for any patient whose visual acuity cannot be monitored. • Monitor the patient's renal and hepatic function tests periodically.
dapsone	Hansen's disease caused by *M. leprae*	50 to 100 mg P.O. daily as a single dose	• Monitor the patient's complete blood count weekly during the first 6 months of dapsone therapy and monthly thereafter. • Instruct the patient to report fever, purpura, jaundice, a sore throat, or signs of dapsone syndrome.
	Dermatitis herpetiformis	25 to 400 mg P.O. daily	

resistant lepromatous form of Hansen's disease. Perhaps the most serious form, lepromatous Hansen's disease causes invasion of virtually every organ system and of plaques and nodules in the skin. Clofazimine also acts an anti-inflammatory agent and is used to treat Hansen's disease reactions. These reactions include a delayed hypersensitivity reaction (to the bacterial load) and erythema nodosum leprosum, a reaction between circulating immune complexes and sensitized tissues. The primary adverse reaction to clofazimine is skin pigmentation.

CHAPTER SUMMARY

Chapter 67 covered the antitubercular and antileprotic agents as they are used to treat various mycobacterial infections. Here are the highlights of this chapter:

• Various chemically unrelated agents are used to treat mycobacterial infections. Although these agents show relatively high mycobacterial specificity and inhibition, M. tuberculosis and M. leprae infections remain difficult to eradicate and often require long-term treatment. In almost all compliant patients, however, combinations of antitubercular and antileprotic agents can successfully control these diseases.

• INH, rifampin, ethambutol, and sometimes streptomycin serve as the first-line agents for treating tuberculosis. Although they vary in terms of specific regimens and length of treatment required, these drugs produce similar therapeutic results.

• Antitubercular agents have a favorable benefit-to-risk ratio. Significant adverse reactions do occur, however, usually producing neurotoxic or hepatotoxic effects. Therapy may be continued, and these reactions usually subside with discontinuation of the drug.

• The development of bacterial resistance to these drugs is a constant threat. Fortunately, aggressive combination therapy can greatly minimize it.

• Dapsone, rifampin, ethionamide, and the investigational drug clofazimine currently dominate the treatment of Hansen's disease. Like most drugs used to treat mycobacterial infections, these antileprotic agents are used in combination to improve their effectiveness and reduce the likelihood of the development of bacterial resistance to them.

• Hematologic, immunologic, GI, and cutaneous disturbances can result from antileprotic therapy, but they seldom require interruption of therapy.

BIBLIOGRAPHY

American Hospital Formulary Service. *Drug Information 87.* McEvoy, G.K., et al., eds. Bethesda, Md.: American Society of Hospital Pharmacists, 1987.

Chemotherapy of Leprosy for Control Programmes. Technical Report Series No. 675. Geneva, Switzerland: World Health Organization, 1982.

Conn, H.F. *Current Therapy 1986.* Philadelphia: W.B. Saunders Co., 1986.

"Drugs for Tuberculosis," *Medical Letter on Drugs and Therapeutics* 28:6, January 17, 1986.

Grzybowski, S. "The Impact of Treatment Programmes on the Epidemiology of Tuberculosis," *Tubercle* 66:69, March 1985.

Hastings, R.C., ed. *Leprosy.* New York: Churchill Livingstone, 1985.

Jacobson, R.R. "Hansen's Disease Drugs in Use: Current Recommendations for Treatment," *The Star* 44:1, July/August 1985.

Lefrock, J.L., et al. "Tuberculosis Therapy," *American Family Physician* 127:261, March 1983.

Mitchison, D.A. "The Action of Antituberculosis Drugs in Short-Course Chemotherapy," *Tubercle* 66:219, September 1985.

Montaner, L.J., et al. "Adverse Effects of Antituberculosis Drugs Causing Changes in Treatment," *Tubercle* 63:291, December 1982.

Tanzania/British Medical Research Council. "Controlled Clinical Trial of Two 6-Month Regimens of Chemotherapy in the Treatment of Pulmonary Tuberculosis," *American Review of Respiratory Diseases* 131:727, May 1985.

"Treatment of Tuberculosis and Other Mycobacterial Diseases," *American Review of Respiratory Diseases* 127:790, June 1983.

CHAPTER 68

ANTIVIRAL AGENTS

OBJECTIVES

After reading and studying this chapter, you should be able to:

1. Discuss the indications, pharmacokinetics, and nursing implications for acyclovir.

2. Discuss the pharmacokinetics, pharmacotherapeutics, and nursing implications for vidarabine.

3. Discuss the pharmacotherapeutics and nursing implications for amantadine.

4. Discuss the pharmacokinetics, pharmacotherapeutics, and nursing implications for ribavirin.

5. Recognize the difficulties and dangers in administering parenteral antiviral agents.

6. Discuss the mechanism of action and adverse effects of zidovudine.

INTRODUCTION

Antiviral agents are drugs used to prevent or treat viral infections. They usually work by interfering with viral replication. The relatively few antiviral agents available for clinical use will kill a specific virus while leaving the host cell intact. Unlike other infecting organisms, viruses are intracellular parasites that survive and multiply through the metabolic processes of the invaded cell. Thus, any agent that kills the virus may also destroy the cells that harbor it. In fact, many experimental antiviral compounds are too toxic for human use. Although they inhibit viral deoxyribonucleic acid (DNA) or protein synthesis, they unfortunately inhibit these functions in host cells, too. Recently, significant progress has been made in producing antiviral agents with actions specific to viral function.

Chapter 68 discusses four major antiviral agents: acyclovir sodium, vidarabine monohydrate, amantadine hydrochloride, and ribavirin. For the most part, they are effective against herpes simplex virus (HSV) and influenza A and B viruses. Also discussed in this chapter is zidovudine, the first Food and Drug Administration

(FDA)–released antiviral drug for use against human immune virus (HIV) in the treatment of acquired immune deficiency syndrome (AIDS). The primary emphasis is on systemic therapy. Topical therapy, including dermatologic and ophthalmologic routes, is covered in more detail in Chapter 78, Integumentary System Agents, and Chapter 79, Ophthalmic Agents.

For a summary of representative drugs, *see Selected major drugs: Antiviral agents* on page 1098.

ACYCLOVIR

The anti-herpesvirus agent, acyclovir, produces marked antiviral activity and minimal cellular toxicity. It is 300 to 3,000 times more toxic to herpesviruses than it is to mammalian cells.

History and source

Acyclovir, formerly known as acylcoguanosine, was synthesized in 1974 during research on antineoplastic agents. Its effectiveness against herpesvirus infections was later discovered and has significantly advanced antiviral treatment.

PHARMACOKINETICS

Acyclovir is available in oral, intravenous (I.V.), and topical forms. The topical form of the drug is covered in Chapter 78, Integumentary System Agents.

Absorption, distribution, metabolism, excretion

Although gastrointestinal (GI) absorption of acyclovir is slow and only 15% to 30% complete, its resulting serum concentration levels are therapeutic. Acyclovir is distributed throughout the body and can be detected in the kidneys, brain, lungs, liver, intestines, spleen, uterus, muscles, vaginal mucosa and secretions, cerebrospinal fluid (CSF), and herpetic vesicular fluid. CSF concentration levels are approximately 50% of plasma concentrations. Acyclovir crosses the placenta. Data on breast milk distribution are lacking. The drug is 9% to 33% protein-bound.

Metabolism of acyclovir is complex. The drug has five metabolites: two produced from hepatic metabolism and three produced by cells infected by herpesviruses. Infected cells produce the inactive monophosphate and diphosphate metabolites and the active triphosphate metabolite, which is the antiviral form of the drug.

Acyclovir is excreted primarily in the urine via glomerular filtration and renal tubular secretion.

Onset, peak, duration
Acyclovir's onset of action, peak concentration level, and duration of action are related to the time the drug maintains a serum concentration level higher than the minimal inhibitory concentration level. Host defense mechanisms, such as white blood cell activity, also contribute to the drug's effectiveness and can extend its duration of action. Usually, average peak concentration levels of acyclovir are reached 1.5 to 2.5 hours after oral administration and immediately after I.V. administration.

Acyclovir's half-life in adults with normal renal function is between 2 and 3.5 hours. The half-life increases as renal function deteriorates, and anuria prolongs it to nearly 20 hours. Thus, the dosage needs to be adjusted in patients with renal impairment. (See *Dosage adjust-ments for acyclovir in patients with renal dysfunction* for more information.)

PHARMACODYNAMICS
To be effective, acyclovir must be metabolized to its active form in cells infected by the herpesvirus. Although metabolism to the active drug form also takes place in uninfected cells, it proceeds at a rate so slow and limited that it does not cause significant toxicity to uninfected cells.

Mechanism of action
Acyclovir enters virus-infected cells, where it is changed to an organic phosphate by a virus-specific enzyme called thymidine kinase. The resulting monophosphate metabolite of acyclovir is polarized and cannot readily diffuse out of the cell. This monophosphate form is then further converted by cellular enzymes to diphosphate and triphosphate forms. The latter—acyclovir triphosphate—is the effective antiviral compound that inhibits virus-specific DNA polymerase, an enzyme necessary for viral growth, and disrupts viral replication.

PHARMACOTHERAPEUTICS
The antiviral activity of acyclovir is limited to the herpesviruses, including HSV Types 1 and 2 and the varicella-zoster virus.

Oral acyclovir is used primarily to treat initial and recurrent genital HSV infections. Chronic suppressive oral acyclovir significantly decreases recurrence in patients with genital HSV infection, but all patients experience recurrent infection if acyclovir is discontinued.

Parenteral acyclovir has a number of clinical indications: to treat severe initial genital HSV infections in patients with normal immune systems; initial and recurrent mucocutaneous herpes simplex (HSV-1 and HSV-2) infections in immunocompromised patients; herpes zoster (shingles) infections caused by the varicella-zoster virus in immunocompromised patients; disseminated varicella-zoster virus in immunocompromised patients; and varicella (chicken pox) infections caused by varicella-zoster virus in immunocompromised patients. Although parenteral acyclovir therapy prevents new vesicle formation, it does not seem to reduce the frequency of recurrent genital herpes lesions.

Use of parenteral acyclovir in primary (self-limiting, acute) genital HSV infections reduces viral shedding, shortens healing time, and limits the duration of symptoms.

Dosage adjustments for acyclovir in patients with renal dysfunction

Adults and children age 12 or older with acute or chronic renal impairment require a reduction in acyclovir dosage, as summarized in this table.

CREATININE CLEARANCE (ml/min/1.73 m²)	DOSAGE INTERVALS (mg/kg)
50 or greater	5 mg/kg every 8 hours
25 to 50	5 mg/kg every 12 hours
10 to 25	5 mg/kg every 24 hours
0 to 10	2.5 mg/kg every 24 hours

DRUG INTERACTIONS
Acyclovir

Drug interactions with acyclovir therapy are infrequent, but potentially serious.

DRUG	INTERACTING DRUGS	POSSIBLE EFFECTS	NURSING IMPLICATIONS
acyclovir	probenecid	Increases plasma concentration and slows elimination of acyclovir	• Monitor the patient for signs of possible acyclovir toxicity, including hematologic reactions.
	nephrotoxic agents	Increase chance of renal dysfunction	• Monitor the patient's renal function. • Keep the patient well hydrated.
	interferon, intrathecal methotrexate	Cause neurotoxicity in patients who have experienced neurologic problems with interferon or methotrexate	• Observe the patient for sudden onset of neurologic problems. • Dosage of acyclovir may need to be decreased or discontinued.

acyclovir sodium (Zovirax). Available in both oral and parenteral forms, acyclovir is used to treat a variety of HSV-1, HSV-2, and varicella-zoster infections. Dosage must be reduced in patients with renal impairment (creatinine clearance < 50 ml/minute).

USUAL ADULT DOSAGE: for primary genital HSV infection, 200 mg P.O. every 4 hours while awake five times a day for 10 days, or with creatinine clearance greater than 50 ml/minute, 5 mg/kg of body weight I.V. every 8 hours for 5 to 7 days; for recurrent genital HSV infection, 200 mg P.O. five times a day for 5 days; for prophylaxis of recurrent genital HSV infections, 200 mg P.O. t.i.d. for 6 months; for varicella-zoster infections in patients with normal renal function, 5 to 10 mg/kg of body weight I.V. every 8 hours for 5 days; for varicella-zoster infections in immunocompromised patients, 500 mg/m² I.V. every 8 hours for 7 days; for herpes simplex encephalitis, 10 mg/kg of body weight I.V. every 8 hours for at least 10 days.

Drug interactions

Acyclovir has significant interactions with several other drugs, including probenecid, interferon, methotrexate, and nephrotoxic agents. (For additional information on the interacting drugs and their possible effects, see *Drug interactions: Acyclovir.*)

ADVERSE DRUG REACTIONS

Adverse reactions to oral and parenteral acyclovir are usually minimal—primarily because the drug is inactive until metabolized by the virus-infected cell. However, those that occur are significant.

Predictable reactions

Local reactions at the injection site, particularly with inadvertent extravasation, are the most frequent problems with parenteral acyclovir. These reactions include irritation, phlebitis, inflammation, and pain. Reversible renal impairment, demonstrated by transient rises in blood urea nitrogen (BUN) or serum creatinine levels and decreases in creatinine clearance, occurs in patients receiving parenteral acyclovir by rapid I.V. injection or infusion. Patients at greatest risk are dehydrated, have a low urine output, or have had a too-rapid infusion (less than 60 minutes).

Headache is very common with oral acyclovir, as are GI reactions such as nausea, vomiting, and diarrhea. Other reactions include vertigo and hematuria.

Patients receiving oral or parenteral acyclovir have reported infrequent diaphoresis, fatigue, insomnia, irritability, depression, and hypotension. Rarely, patients report muscle cramps and leg pain.

Unpredictable reactions

Unpredictable reactions include thrombocytosis, thrombocytopenia, transient lymphopenia, transient leukopenia, and bone marrow hypoplasia. Fever, rash, arthralgia, sore throat, lymphadenopathy, and inguinal adenopathy indicate hypersensitivity responses to acyclovir.

NURSING IMPLICATIONS

Acyclovir therapy has the potential for significant adverse reactions, especially with parenteral administration, and close monitoring is necessary during therapy. The nurse must:

• Be aware that acyclovir is contraindicated in patients who are hypersensitive to the drug.

• Be aware that dosage adjustment, especially with parenteral therapy, is needed in patients with decreased renal function.

• Monitor the patient's renal function, especially serum creatinine levels, closely during parenteral acyclovir therapy.

• Administer I.V. infusions of acyclovir slowly (over 60 minutes) to prevent drug crystals from precipitating in renal tubules.

• Keep the patient well hydrated during parenteral therapy to ensure good urine output.

• Administer acyclovir with caution in pregnant or lactating patients. Be aware that this drug is used only if the potential benefits outweigh the possible risks to the fetus or breast-feeding infant.

• Monitor the patient for signs and symptoms of neurotoxicity (especially with parenteral therapy), such as lethargy, tremors, obtundation, confusion, agitation, hallucinations, seizures, and coma.

• Remember that the serum concentration levels of acyclovir will increase when it is given concomitantly with probenecid.

• Monitor the patient's I.V. infusion sites closely, and rotate regularly to prevent irritation or phlebitis.

VIDARABINE

Vidarabine was the first important anti-herpesvirus drug clinically available for parenteral use. It is used to treat patients with herpes simplex encephalitis.

History and source
First introduced as an antineoplastic agent in 1960, vidarabine is also known as adenine arabinoside or Ara-A. Its antiviral activity was discovered in 1964, and it replaced the more toxic agent cytosine arabinoside (Ara-C). Vidarabine was the primary agent used to treat herpesvirus infections before the discovery of acyclovir.

PHARMACOKINETICS

Systemic vidarabine is administered by the I.V. route. The ophthalmic preparation is covered in more depth in Chapter 79, Ophthalmic Agents.

Absorption, distribution, metabolism, excretion
Vidarabine and its active metabolite Ara-Hx (arahypoxanthine) are widely distributed in body fluids and tissues. Drug and metabolite readily cross the blood-brain barrier and achieve adequate CSF concentration levels. Vidarabine crosses the placenta. Its presence in breast milk is unverified. The drug is 20% to 30% protein-bound.

Other than its change to Ara-Hx, vidarabine does not undergo significant metabolism. Both the unchanged drug and Ara-Hx are excreted primarily by the kidneys.

Onset, peak, duration
The half-life for vidarabine is 1 hour, and for Ara-Hx, 3.3 hours in adults with normal renal function.

Specific onset of action, peak concentration levels, and duration of action information on vidarabine is unavailable.

PHARMACODYNAMICS

Vidarabine was first produced as an antileukemic agent but was found to have antiviral activity.

The exact mechanism of action of vidarabine is unknown. It may be changed to an organic phosphate by cellular enzymes to its active form, vidarabine triphosphate, which blocks viral replication. Vidarabine and its metabolites appear to halt viral DNA synthesis by inhibiting viral DNA polymerase. Although Ara-Hx, vidarabine's primary metabolite, has 30 to 50 times less antiviral activity than vidarabine, it does appear to enhance vidarabine's action.

PHARMACOTHERAPEUTICS

Vidarabine is active against HSV-1 and HSV-2, varicella-zoster virus, cytomegalovirus, and vacinnia virus.

Intravenous vidarabine is primarily indicated to treat herpes simplex encephalitis and herpes zoster (shingles) caused by reactivated varicella-zoster infections in immunocompromised adults and children. Although vidarabine decreases mortality from herpes simplex encephalitis, it does not decrease the disease's neurologic aftereffects. Vidarabine is also used to treat varicella (chicken pox) in immunocompromised patients. Some physicians use vidarabine to treat disseminated herpesvirus infections in neonates. The major drawback to I.V. vidarabine therapy is its poor solubility, which necessitates diluting it in large volumes of I.V. fluids, which may cause heart failure and hyponatremia.

vidarabine monohydrate (Vira-A). Available only as a slow I.V. infusion, vidarabine is used to treat HSV-1 and HSV-2 and varicella-zoster viral infections. Dosages must be reduced in patients with renal impairment (creatinine clearance < 10 ml/minute). Specific guidelines have not been established, but the current recommendation is for a 25% reduction. Vidarabine is removed by hemodialysis, so a supplementary dose may be necessary after dialysis.

USUAL ADULT DOSAGE: for herpes simplex encephalitis, 15 mg/kg of body weight I.V. daily over 12 to 24 hours for 10 days; for varicella-zoster infections, 10 mg/kg of body weight I.V. daily over 12 to 24 hours for 5 days.

Drug interactions
Allopurinol inhibits formation of the metabolite xanthine arabinoside from Ara-Hx. This may increase the serum concentration level of Ara-Hx, causing tremors, anemia, nausea, pain, and pruritus.

ADVERSE DRUG REACTIONS

The primary adverse reactions of vidarabine involve the GI tract and central nervous system and are usually related to high serum concentrations of the drug.

Predictable reactions
Dose-related GI adverse reactions include nausea, vomiting, diarrhea, anorexia, and weight loss. These reactions are usually mild, occurring after 2 to 3 days of therapy and subsiding within 1 to 4 days while therapy continues. Central nervous system (CNS) problems include weakness, tremors, ataxia, hallucinations, malaise, and confusion. These subside once therapy is discontinued. Both GI and CNS reactions are more prevalent in patients receiving a vidarabine dose greater than 10 mg/kg/day and in patients with decreased renal function. Less frequently seen adverse reactions include local responses, such as pain and thrombophlebitis; transient elevations in liver function test results; and depressed leukocytes, platelets, and hemoglobin. Hyponatremia and the syndrome of inappropriate antidiuretic hormone (SIADH) occur rarely.

Unpredictable reactions
Hypersensitivity reactions, including rash and pruritus, may occur during vidarabine therapy.

NURSING IMPLICATIONS
Vidarabine carries the potential for significant adverse effects and presents major stability and solubility concerns. The nurse must:

● Be aware that the maximum amount of vidarabine in a liter of I.V. solution must not exceed 450 mg.
● Check to see that the solution is clear before infusion, and use an in-line 0.45-micron filter for the infusion.
● Administer vidarabine cautiously in women of child-bearing age to avoid any potential complications in future pregnancies. Because the drug may alter chromosomes, it should be used only if the potential benefits outweigh the risks.
● Monitor the patient's fluid balance closely, because patients can experience fluid overload.
● Monitor the patient's renal function, along with complete blood count and liver function.
● Know that vidarabine dosage must be adjusted in patients with depressed renal function.

AMANTADINE

Amantadine was the first oral antiviral drug available for clinical use. It is used to prevent or treat influenza A infections.

PHARMACOKINETICS

Amantadine is well absorbed in the GI tract after oral administration. Distribution is limited to saliva, CSF, nasal secretions, breast milk, and lung tissue. Amantadine is not metabolized and is primarily eliminated in the urine.

Amantadine reaches peak concentration levels in 1 to 4 hours. Its half-life in adults with normal renal function averages 15 hours, but is prolonged in patients with severe renal impairment. Unlike vidarabine, amantadine is only minimally removed by hemodialysis.

PHARMACODYNAMICS

The mechanism of action of amantadine appears to inhibit an early stage of viral replication, possibly the uncoating of the virus. In the presence of amantadine, the virus appears to attach normally to cells and is phagocytosed, but the virus then fails to uncoat and initiate the replication cycle.

PHARMACOTHERAPEUTICS

Amantadine has no activity against influenza B virus, but is active against most strains of influenza A. Its effectiveness depends on the concentration of both the virus and the drug and varies with the viral strain.

Amantadine, used to prevent and treat respiratory tract infections caused by influenza A virus strains, is a fairly effective prophylactic during influenza A epidemics. Amantadine is particularly useful because it can be administered to patients undergoing immunization and can protect them during the 2 weeks immunity takes to develop. It is also useful for those who cannot take the influenza vaccine because of hypersensitivity. When used to treat patients who have influenza A infections, amantadine reduces the severity and duration of fever and other symptoms.

Amantadine is also used to treat parkinsonian syndrome and drug-induced extrapyramidal reactions. These uses are described in Chapter 23, Antiparkinsonian Agents.

amantadine hydrochloride (Symmetrel). Amantadine is an oral drug effective in preventing and treating influenza A infections. Dosage must be reduced in patients with renal impairment. (See *Dosage adjustments for amantadine in patients with renal dysfunction* for additional information.) Dosage adjustments are also necessary for

patients with a history of seizure disorders. For these patients, the normal adult dosage of 200 mg/day must be reduced by half.

USUAL ADULT DOSAGE: 200 mg P.O. daily in a single dose or divided and given b.i.d.; to treat infection, the dose should be started 24 to 48 hours after the onset of symptoms and continue for at least 2 days after symptoms resolve; to prevent infection, therapy should begin immediately after an outbreak and continue until the risk of infection is eliminated.

Drug interactions

Significant reactions result when amantadine is given with large doses of anticholinergic drugs, triamterene, thiazide diuretics, and CNS stimulants. (For additional information on the interactions of these drugs and their possible effects, see *Drug interactions: Amantadine.*)

ADVERSE DRUG REACTIONS

Amantadine is usually well tolerated, with mild adverse reactions occurring in approximately 5% of patients. The most frequently reported adverse reactions are nausea, anorexia, nervousness, fatigue, mental depression, irritability, insomnia, psychosis, anxiety, confusion, forgetfulness, and hallucinations. Other CNS reactions include headache, dizziness, light-headedness, slurred speech, ataxia, tremors, and a sense of drunkenness. Patients with seizure disorders are more prone to seizures while using amantadine.

Other, less common, adverse reactions include congestive heart failure (CHF), orthostatic hypotension, edema, leukopenia, dermatitis, photosensitivity, dry mouth, rash, urinary retention, constipation, and vomiting. Neutropenia, visual disturbances, and oculogyric events are rare.

NURSING IMPLICATIONS

Amantadine has the potential for significant adverse effects, especially in patients with decreased renal function or a history of seizure disorders. Frequent monitoring is necessary during amantadine therapy. The nurse must:
• Avoid giving amantadine to pregnant or lactating patients, because safety during pregnancy has not been established; the drug is secreted in breast milk.
• Know that amantadine is contraindicated in patients who are hypersensitive to the drug.
• Administer amantadine cautiously in elderly patients and in those with a history of epilepsy, CHF, peripheral

---

Dosage adjustments for amantadine in patients with renal dysfunction

Adults with impaired renal function require an adjustment in the dosage of amantadine as summarized in this table.

CREATININE CLEARANCE (ml/min/1.73 m²)	DOSAGE INTERVALS
80 or greater	100 mg b.i.d.
60 to 79	200 mg once daily; 100 mg on alternate days
40 to 59	100 mg once daily
30 to 39	200 mg twice weekly
20 to 29	100 mg thrice weekly
10 to 19	200 mg; 100 mg alternating every 7 days

DRUG INTERACTIONS

Amantadine

Drug interactions with amantadine are serious because they usually involve either CNS toxicity or renal impairment.

DRUG	INTERACTING DRUGS	POSSIBLE EFFECTS	NURSING IMPLICATIONS
amantadine	anticholinergic agents	Enhance adverse reactions to anticholinergic agents	• Observe the patient for excessive anticholinergic effects, such as dry mouth, confusion, and urinary retention.
	triamterene, thiazide diuretics	Cause CNS intoxication by slowing renal elimination of amantadine	• Observe the patient for potential CNS toxicity.
	CNS stimulants	Enhance CNS irritability and may cause seizures	• Observe the patient for evidence of CNS hyperactivity and possible seizure activity.

edema, hepatic disease, mental illness, eczematoid rash, renal impairment, orthostatic hypotension, or cardiovascular disease.

• Have the patient take the drug after meals for best absorption.

• Instruct the patient to report adverse reactions, especially signs of CNS involvement (dizziness, depression, anxiety, and nausea) and any renal impairment.

• Have elderly patients take the drug in two daily doses rather than a single dose to avoid adverse neurologic reactions.

• Instruct the patient experiencing orthostatic hypotension to stand or change positions slowly.

• Tell the patient with insomnia to take the dose several hours before bedtime.

RIBAVIRIN

Ribavirin inhibits a number of ribonucleic acid (RNA) and DNA viruses, but is currently available only to treat respiratory syncytial virus (RSV) infections in children. It is administered by aerosol inhalation only.

History and source
Ribavirin, a recently approved antiviral agent, is now commercially available in the United States. It was synthesized in 1972 as part of a search for a compound with broad-spectrum antiviral activity but remained investigational for some time.

PHARMACOKINETICS

Ribavirin is administered via nasal or oral inhalation and is well absorbed by these routes. The drug has limited, specific distribution, with highest concentration levels found in the pulmonary tract and erythrocytes. Ribavirin is metabolized in the liver and by erythrocytes. The main route of excretion is via the kidneys, with some excretion in the feces. Onset of action and peak concentration levels of ribavirin are virtually simultaneous, occurring immediately after inhalation. The drug's half-life is $1\frac{1}{2}$ to $2\frac{1}{2}$ hours, and the plasma half-life is approximately 9 hours.

PHARMACODYNAMICS

The mechanism of action of ribavirin is not known, but the drug probably becomes effective after it is converted to an active metabolite.

Mechanism of action
Ribavirin is rapidly transported into virus-infected cells, where it is metabolized by cellular enzymes to monophosphate, diphosphate, and triphosphate derivatives. All three metabolites inhibit viral DNA and RNA synthesis, subsequently halting viral replication. Ribavirin does not seem to have the same affinity for host DNA and RNA synthesis.

PHARMACOTHERAPEUTICS

Ribavirin therapy is indicated in infants and young children who have severe lower respiratory tract infections caused by RSV. Ribavirin has also been used experimentally to treat respiratory infections involving influenza viruses A and B in elderly patients; however, no clinical guidelines are available for this application.

ribavirin (Virazole). Ribavirin sterile powder is reconstituted with sterile water and administered by aerosol inhalation using a Viratek Small-Particle Aerosol Generator (SPAG-2).
USUAL PEDIATRIC DOSAGE: 20 mg/ml solution administered via aerosol inhalant over 12 to 18 hours/day for 3 to 7 days; dosage depends on patient's lung pathology and ventilation.

Drug interactions

No significant drug interactions with ribavirin have been identified.

ADVERSE DRUG REACTIONS

Adverse reactions to ribavirin therapy have been infrequent and, in many cases, uncertain. Reactions include worsening of respiratory function, cardiac arrest, hypotension, and cardiac glycoside intoxication. Reticulosis has been reported along with an anemia, possibly from erythrocyte hemolysis. Other adverse reactions include rash, conjunctivitis, and erythema of the eyelids.

NURSING IMPLICATIONS

Ribavirin has the potential for complications during therapy, primarily from incorrect administration techniques. Thus, nursing considerations are primarily in the areas of drug administration and patient education. The nurse must:
• Remember that ribavirin is contraindicated for patients requiring mechanical ventilation; the drug can precipitate in the ventilatory apparatus, jeopardizing adequate ventilation.
• Be aware that ribavirin is contraindicated in women of childbearing age; the drug is teratogenic in all animal species tested.
• Prepare ribavirin solution by diluting 6 grams of ribavirin powder in 50 to 100 ml of sterile water; transfer the solution to an Erlenmeyer flask (which serves as the reservoir for the SPAG-2) and dilute further to a volume of 300 ml.

• Administer ribavirin with the SPAG-2; do not use any other aerosol-generating device.
• For reconstituting ribavirin powder that does not contain any antimicrobial agent, use sterile USP water for injection, not bacteriostatic water.
• Discard solutions placed in the SPAG-2 unit at least every 24 hours before adding newly reconstituted solutions.
• Store reconstituted solutions at room temperature for 24 hours.

ZIDOVUDINE

Zidovudine is the first drug to receive FDA approval for treating AIDS or AIDS-related complex (ARC). The drug, also known as azidothymidine or AZT, was initially studied as an antineoplastic agent.

PHARMACOKINETICS

Oral zidovudine is readily absorbed from the GI tract, and 34% to 38% of the drug is protein-bound. Zidovudine undergoes rapid hepatic metabolism to inactive metabolites. The drug is renally excreted. Zidovudine reaches peak concentration levels in 0.5 to 1.5 hours and has a duration of action of 4 hours. The half-life is approximately 1 hour.

PHARMACODYNAMICS

The mechanism of action of zidovudine is much like that of acyclovir. The drug is converted by cellular enzymes to an active form, zidovudine triphosphate. The metabolite inhibits RNA-dependent DNA polymerase produced by HIV, thus preventing viral DNA from replicating. The sensitivity of HIV to inhibition by zidovudine appears to depend on the duration of cell infection.

PHARMACOTHERAPEUTICS

Zidovudine has been used for patients with AIDS and ARC who have a history of *Pneumocystis carinii* pneumonia or a T lymphocyte count lower than 200 mm³. Clinical trials have demonstrated reduced mortality with the use of zidovudine. The drug also has reduced the incidence and severity of opportunistic infections.

DRUG INTERACTIONS

Zidovudine

The list of drugs that interact with zidovudine is incomplete because of the drug's newness. With zidovudine's continued use, other interactions may be discovered. The nurse must assess the patient for any drug interactions and adverse reactions.

DRUG	INTERACTING DRUGS	POSSIBLE EFFECTS	NURSING IMPLICATIONS
zidovudine	dapsone, pentamidine, flucytosine, vincristine, vinblastine, doxorubicin, interferon	Increase nephrotoxic and cytotoxic effects when administered together	• Avoid concurrent administration if possible; if not, monitor the patient's blood count and renal function frequently.
	probenecid, aspirin, acetaminophen, indomethacin	Inhibit metabolism of zidovudine; probable toxicity from either drug is increased	• Avoid concurrent use.

zidovudine (Retrovir). Zidovudine is used to treat AIDS and ARC and has been successful in reducing opportunistic infections in these patients.

USUAL ADULT DOSAGE: 200 mg P.O. every 4 hours around the clock. Doses are adjusted in relation to the anemia and granulocytopenia that usually occur.

Drug interactions

Many drug interactions occur with zidovudine. (For specific information, see *Drug interactions: Zidovudine.*)

ADVERSE DRUG REACTIONS

The most predictable reactions to zidovudine therapy are hematologic. Significant anemia occurs 4 to 6 weeks after therapy has begun, and agranulocytopenia appears within 6 to 8 weeks. When reductions in red and white blood cell counts occur, the dose is usually adjusted or stopped. Reducing or stopping therapy produces an immediate reversal of the abnormal blood cell counts. Research has yet to discover whether the drug is safe in pregnancy or lactation.

NURSING IMPLICATIONS

The nurse caring for a patient receiving zidovudine should remember the following considerations:
• Monitor the patient's blood counts, as prescribed.

• Instruct the patient to take the drug every 4 hours around the clock even though it means interrupting sleep.
• Instruct the patient that zidovudine does not reduce the risk of transmitting the virus to others through sexual contact or blood contamination.
• Caution the patient to avoid over-the-counter medications without first checking with the physician, pharmacist, or nurse.

CHAPTER SUMMARY

Chapter 68 presented the five antiviral agents available today: acyclovir, vidarabine, amantadine, ribavirin, and zidovudine (zidovudine has been approved by the FDA to treat AIDS). Here are the highlights of the chapter:
• Few antiviral agents are available because of the difficulty of developing drugs that selectively kill viruses and do not harm their host cells.
• Acyclovir is used to treat herpesvirus infections. It is available in oral, topical, and parenteral forms.
• Acyclovir is relatively safe, although it has the potential to be nephrotoxic. This danger can be reduced by infusing the drug slowly (over 60 minutes) and keeping the patient well hydrated.

SELECTED MAJOR DRUGS

Antiviral agents

This chart summarizes the major antiviral agents currently in clinical use.

DRUG	MAJOR INDICATIONS	USUAL ADULT DOSAGES	NURSING IMPLICATIONS
acyclovir	Primary genital HSV infection	5 mg/kg of body weight I.V. every 8 hours for 5 to 7 days in patients with creatinine clearance greater than 50 ml/minute; or 200 mg P.O. every 4 hours while awake, five times a day for 10 days	• Contraindicated in patients who are hypersensitive to the drug. • Monitor the patient's renal function and administer acyclovir cautiously to patients with decreased renal function; dosage adjustments are necessary. • Administer I.V. infusions over 60 minutes; too-rapid infusions will lead to acyclovir crystals precipitating in renal tubules. • Keep the patient well hydrated during parenteral therapy to ensure good urine output. • Administer cautiously to pregnant or lactating patients.
	Varicella-zoster infections	5 to 10 mg/kg of body weight I.V. every 8 hours for 5 days	
	Herpes simplex encephalitis	10 mg/kg of body weight I.V. every 8 hours	
	Recurrent genital HSV infection	200 mg P.O. five times a day for 5 days	
vidarabine	Herpes simplex encephalitis	15 mg/kg of body weight I.V. daily, infused over 12 to 24 hours for 10 days	• Contraindicated in patients who are hypersensitive to the drug. • Vidarabine requires large amounts of fluid for dissolution and administration. The maximum amount of vidarabine that can be added to 1 liter is 450 mg. • Use an in-line 0.45-micron filter for vidarabine infusions. • Do not administer by intramuscular or subcutaneous injections, because they are not well absorbed. • Administer cautiously to women of childbearing age. • Adjust dosage in patients with renal impairment as prescribed. • Monitor the patient's fluid balance during therapy. • Monitor the patient's renal, hematologic, and hepatic functions during therapy.
	Varicella-zoster infections	10 mg/kg of body weight I.V. daily, infused over 12 to 24 hours for 5 days	
amantadine	Respiratory tract infections from influenza virus A	200 mg P.O. daily	• Amantadine is contraindicated in patients who are hypersensitive to the drug. • Administer cautiously to pregnant or lactating patients. • Administer cautiously to elderly patients and those with a history of seizures, CHF, peripheral edema, hepatic disease, mental illness, eczematoid rash, renal impairment, or orthostatic hypotension. • Warn the patient about orthostatic hypotension; instruct the patient to go slowly from a lying or sitting to standing position. • Instruct the patient to report adverse reactions, such as dizziness, depression, anxiety, nausea, and urinary retention. • If insomnia develops, advise the patient to take the dose several hours before bedtime. • Warn the patient against discontinuing the drug abruptly when it is given for parkinsonism.

• Acyclovir has replaced vidarabine in treating severe types of viral infections, including herpes simplex encephalitis and herpes zoster infection.

• Vidarabine has long been used to treat herpes simplex encephalitis, but is being replaced by parenteral acyclovir. A major problem with parenteral vidarabine is its poor solubility, requiring large amounts of fluid for dissolution and administration. Patients can experience fluid overload or electrolyte abnormalities.

• Amantadine is an oral antiviral drug used to prevent or treat influenza A viral infections. The drug must be used with caution in patients with seizure disorders, and it can cause other CNS disturbances.

• Ribavirin, the only chemotherapeutic agent available to treat RSV in children, is available in aerosol form only. Development of other dosage forms of and indications for ribavirin is ongoing.

BIBLIOGRAPHY

American Hospital Formulary Service. *Drug Information 87.* McEvoy, G.K., et al., eds. Bethesda, Md.: American Society of Hospital Pharmacists, 1987.

Bean, B. "Acyclovir in the Treatment of Herpesvirus Infections," *Postgraduate Medicine* 73:297, March 1983.

Bryson, Y.J., et al. "Treatment of First Episodes of Genital Herpes Simplex Virus Infection with Oral Acyclovir: A Randomized Double-Blind Controlled Trial in Normal Subjects," *New England Journal of Medicine* 308:916, April 1983.

Centers for Disease Control. "Prevention and Control of Influenza," *Annals of Internal Medicine* 103(4):560, 1985.

Corey, L., and Holmes, K.K. "Genital Herpes Simplex Virus Infections: Current Concepts in Diagnosis, Therapy, and Prevention," *Annals of Internal Medicine* 98:973, June 1983.

Deeter, R., and Khanderia, U. "Recent Advances in Antiviral Therapy," *Clinical Pharmacy* 5(12):961, December 1986.

deMiranda, P., and Blum, M.R. "Pharmacokinetics of Acyclovir after Intravenous and Oral Administration," *Journal of Antimicrobial Chemotherapy* 12:29, 1983.

Douglas, R.G. "Antiviral Drugs 1983," *Medical Clinics of North America* 67(5):1163, 1983.

Fletcher, C., and Bean, B. "Evaluation of Oral Acyclovir Therapy," *Drug Intelligence and Clinical Pharmacy* 19:518, July/August 1985.

Gilman, A.G., et al., eds. *Goodman and Gilman's The Pharmacological Basis of Therapeutics,* 7th ed. New York: Macmillan Publishing Co., 1985.

Hall, C.B., et al. "Ribavirin Treatment of Respiratory Syncytial Viral Infection in Infants with Underlying Cardiopulmonary Disease," *Journal of the American Medical Association* 254:3047, December 6,1985.

Hermans, P.E., and Cockerill, F.R. "Antiviral Agents," *Mayo Clinic Proceedings* 58:217, April 1983.

Nahata, M.C. "Clinical Use of Antiviral Drugs," *Drug Intelligence and Clinical Pharmacy* 5:399, July/August 1987.

Nicholson, K.G. "Properties of Antiviral Agents," *Lancet* 2:503, September 1984.

Richards, D.M., et al. "Acyclovir: A Review of its Pharmacodynamic Properties and Therapeutic Efficacy," *Drugs* 26:378, November 1983.

True, B.L., and Carter, B.L. "Update on Acyclovir: Oral Therapy for Herpesvirus Infections," *Clinical Pharmacy* 3(6):607, November/December 1984.

USPDI: *Drug Information for the Health Care Provider,* Vol.1, 6th ed. Rockville, Md.: United States Pharmacopeial Convention, Inc., 1985.

CHAPTER 69

ANTIMYCOTIC (ANTIFUNGAL) AGENTS

OBJECTIVES

After reading and studying this chapter, you should be able to:

1. Describe the types of fungal infections that can affect humans.

2. Describe the antimycotic agents used to treat systemic fungal infections: amphotericin B, miconazole, ketoconazole, and flucytosine.

3. Describe the antimycotic agents used to treat topical fungal infections: nystatin, clotrimazole, griseofulvin, ketoconazole, and miconazole.

4. Explain the various antimycotic agents' actions on fungal cells.

5. Describe the pharmacokinetics of systemic and topical antimycotic agents.

6. Identify the adverse reactions caused by these agents, and describe ways to prevent or treat them.

7. Identify significant interactions between the antimycotic agents and other drugs.

8. Explain how certain antimycotic agents can be used together for synergistic effects.

INTRODUCTION

Antimycotic, or antifungal, agents include many drugs that are used to treat fungal infections. In humans, fungal infections can range from the common, such as tinea pedis (athlete's foot), to the rare and exotic, such as sporotrichosis (agranulomatous disease). Two general types of fungal infections exist: topical (superficial) infections, affecting the skin and mucous membranes, and systemic infections, affecting such areas as the lungs, central nervous system (CNS), and blood. Treating either type of infection requires a topical, oral, or parenteral agent chosen according to the infection's site and severity.

The patient's underlying condition usually determines the type of fungal infection the patient will acquire. For example, a severely immunocompromised patient is predisposed to develop a systemic infection, such as aspergillosis. In contrast, a patient who is receiving antibiotic therapy that eliminates the normal flora, has poor oral hygiene, or wears dentures is predisposed to develop a mucocutaneous infection, such as oral candidiasis (thrush). Thus, managing fungal infections not only calls for antimycotic drug therapy, but also requires modification or elimination of predisposing factors.

Of the two types, topical infections are more common and include candidiasis, tinea versicolor (pityriasis versicolor), and infections by dermatophytes (various skin fungi). Candidiasis affects certain mucosal sites such as the mouth, gastrointestinal (GI) tract, and vagina. It frequently follows antibiotic therapy that disrupts the natural flora, a physiologic change in the host, or immunosuppressive therapy. Therapy usually involves topical antimycotic agents. Tinea versicolor produces hypopigmented or hyperpigmented skin patches and usually requires topical treatment. Dermatophytes cause many common infections, such as tinea pedis (athlete's foot), tinea cruris (jock itch), tinea capitis (scalp ringworm), tinea corporis (body ringworm), and tinea unguium (onychomycosis, or nail infection). Most of these infections respond well to topical therapy; however, infected nail beds require long-term systemic treatment.

Systemic fungal infections can result from pathogenic fungi or from so-called opportunistic fungi, those that are normally nonpathogenic but that become pathogenic under certain circumstances, such as a decreased immune response. Opportunistic systemic fungal infections usually affect immunosuppressed or immunocompromised patients and may include systemic candidiasis and aspergillosis. Pathogenic systemic fungal infections can affect normal or immunocompromised patients and include histoplasmosis and coccidioidomycosis. Pathogenic fungi usually enter the host by the respiratory tract, but opportunistic fungi may invade the host through various other routes, including the GI tract and intravenous (I.V.) lines. Whether pathogenic or opportunistic, a systemic fungal infection almost always requires systemic antimycotic therapy.

Antimycotic agents are categorized in four basic groups: polyene antimycotics, which include amphotericin B and nystatin; imidazole agents, which include miconazole, ketoconazole, and clotrimazole; the antimetabolite antimycotic agent, flucytosine; and superficial antimycotic agents, which include griseofulvin and various topical drugs.

Because the pharmacotherapeutics and nursing implications of amphotericin B and nystatin are so different, this chapter discusses them separately. It covers the major systemic antimycotic agents and includes information on the topical antimycotic agents.

For a summary of representative drugs, see *Selected major drugs: Antimycotic agents* on page 1111.

AMPHOTERICIN B

This drug's potency has made it the most widely used antimycotic agent for severe systemic fungal infections. Unfortunately, it also causes a wide range of adverse reactions, especially when administered parenterally.

History and source
After nystatin, the first polyene antimycotic, proved to be extremely toxic when administered parenterally, researchers began to seek safer agents to treat fungal infections. Their search led to the discovery of amphotericin A and B.

Produced by the bacterium *Streptomyces nodosus,* amphotericin A and B were first isolated from Venezuelan soil samples in 1956. Today, because amphotericin B offers greater antimycotic activity, it is the only one of the two forms used clinically. The drug is named for its amphoteric property (the ability to act as both an acid and a base).

PHARMACOKINETICS
After I.V. administration, amphotericin B is distributed throughout the body and excreted by the kidneys. Its metabolic fate has not been conclusively demonstrated.

Absorption, distribution, metabolism, excretion
Because amphotericin B is poorly absorbed from the GI tract, it is usually administered by I.V. infusion to bypass the absorption process. The drug is essentially insoluble in water, so a colloidal suspension must be used. It may also be administered intrathecally.

After I.V. administration, the drug is quickly distributed to various body compartments and appears to cross the placenta. Its degree of binding to lipoproteins approaches 95%. Moderate concentration levels of amphotericin B appear in the aqueous humor and urine, and in pleural, peritoneal, and synovial fluids; high concentration levels occur in the kidneys, spleen, and lungs. With I.V. administration, amphotericin B concentration levels in the cerebrospinal fluid (CSF) are usually too low to inhibit fungal growth. With intrathecal administration, however, concentration levels in CSF are much higher.

Researchers have not yet discovered the metabolic fate of amphotericin B.

Although the major route of excretion of amphotericin B has not been clearly identified, the kidneys excrete less than 5% of the drug in the urine.

Onset, peak, duration
After I.V. administration, the onset of action of amphotericin B occurs almost immediately. In a patient with normal renal function, the drug's half-life is usually 24 hours. The half-life seems to lengthen as therapy continues, however; it may reach 15 days with long-term administration, possibly because of slow release of amphotericin B from tissue compartments. After therapy is discontinued, amphotericin B appears in the blood for up to 4 weeks and in the urine for 7 to 8 weeks.

PHARMACODYNAMICS
Amphotericin B acts primarily on sterols in fungal cells, binding with them to produce antimycotic effects.

Mechanism of action
The irreversible binding of amphotericin B to sterols in the membranes of amphotericin B–sensitive fungal cells seems to produce pores or channels that increase cell membrane permeability. The resulting permeability allows leakage of intracellular components, which prevents the fungal cell membrane from functioning normally as a barrier. Amphotericin B usually acts as a fungistatic agent, but can become fungicidal if it reaches high concentrations in the fungi.

DRUG INTERACTIONS

Amphotericin B

When given with the drugs listed below, amphotericin B may cause significant drug interactions. Some may be severe, such as nephrotoxicity and hypokalemia. Thus, a patient receiving concomitant therapy will need to be monitored closely.

DRUG	INTERACTING DRUGS	POSSIBLE EFFECTS	NURSING IMPLICATIONS
amphotericin B	aminoglycosides	Increase nephrotoxicity	• Monitor the patient's renal function by monitoring BUN and serum creatinine levels and intake and output patterns.
	cyclosporine	Increases nephrotoxicity	• Monitor the patient's renal function by monitoring BUN and serum creatinine levels and intake and output patterns.
	corticosteroids	Increase hypokalemia, possibly leading to cardiac dysfunction	• Monitor the patient's serum potassium levels. • Monitor the patient for signs and symptoms of cardiac dysfunction, such as palpitations, tachycardia, and hypotension.
	extended-spectrum penicillins	Increase hypokalemia	• Monitor the patient's serum potassium levels.
	digitalis glycosides	Increase hypokalemia, which may cause digitalis toxicity	• Monitor the patient's serum potassium levels. • Monitor the patient for signs and symptoms of hypokalemia, such as hypotension, muscle weakness, and confusion.
	nondepolarizing skeletal muscle relaxants (pancuronium bromide)	Increase muscle relaxant effects	• Monitor the patient's serum potassium levels. • Monitor the patient for muscle weakness and respiratory insufficiency. • Have emergency equipment available.
	miconazole	Decreases antimycotic effects	• Monitor the patient for signs of decreased therapeutic effect.
	electrolyte solutions	Precipitate and inactivate amphotericin B colloid	• Do not dilute amphotericin B in electrolyte solutions; use only D₅W or sterile water without bacteriostatic agents.
	flucytosine	Increases antimycotic effects	• Monitor the patient for signs of resistance to these drugs.

PHARMACOTHERAPEUTICS

Amphotericin B is usually administered to treat severe systemic fungal infections and meningitis caused by fungi sensitive to the drug. Because the drug is highly toxic, its use must be limited to patients who have been definitively diagnosed as having life-threatening infections and who are under close medical supervision.

amphotericin B (Fungizone). This potent antimycotic agent is effective against *Aspergillus fumigatus, Blastomyces dermatitidis, Candida* species, *Cryptococcus neoformans, Histoplasma capsulatum, Coccidioides im-* *mitis, Microsporum audouini, Paracoccidioides brasiliensis, Rhizopus* species, *Sporothrix schenckii, Torulopsis glabrata, Trichophyton* species, and *Rhodotorula* species. It can be used to treat aspergillosis; North American blastomycosis; pulmonary, disseminated, or meningeal coccidioidomycosis; disseminated candidiasis; pulmonary or disseminated cryptococcosis; and pulmonary or disseminated histoplasmosis. Amphotericin B is usually considered the drug of choice for severe infections caused by *Candida* species, *P. brasiliensis, B. dermatitidis, C. immitis, C. neoformans,* and *S. schenckii.* Because of the synergistic effects between flucytosine and amphotericin B, many physicians combine these two drugs in therapy for candidal or cryptococcal infections, especially for cryptococcal meningitis.

Amphotericin B therapy usually begins with a test dose that is increased daily until the desired dose is reached. The physician may increase the dose more rapidly to treat a life-threatening infection, such as fulminating cryptococcal meningitis. Duration of the therapy depends on the maturity and severity of the infection. Some patients may need months of therapy with total doses that range from 300 to 4,000 mg.

USUAL ADULT DOSAGE: as a test dose for infection, 1 mg in 250 ml of dextrose 5% in water (D$_5$W) infused over 2 to 4 hours initially, increased to 5 mg, 10 mg, 20 mg, and up each day; as a test dose for severe infections, 1 mg I.V. given over 30 to 60 minutes initially, increased to 0.25 mg/kg the same day. For systemic fungal infections and meningitis, 0.25 to 1.5 mg/kg/day I.V. is given—based on the organism present and the patient's drug tolerance—infused over 4 to 6 hours. For coccidioidal meningitis and cryptococcal meningitis, 0.025 to 1 mg is given intrathecally two to three times weekly. For coccidioidal arthritis or osteoarticular sporotrichosis, 5 to 15 mg is injected into the joint spaces. For candidal infections of the bladder, 50 mg in 1 liter of sterile water is continuously or intermittently instilled into the bladder. For topical application, 3% ointment, cream, or lotion is applied liberally and rubbed well into the affected area b.i.d. to q.i.d.

As an alternate method of I.V. administration, amphotericin B can be given every other day. To do this, the daily dose is doubled gradually and administered every 48 hours. Under no circumstances, however, should the daily dose exceed 1.5 mg/kg.

Drug interactions

Amphotericin B can produce significant interactions with many drugs. Some drug combinations may be unavoidable, however. In that situation, the patient will require close monitoring. When given with amphotericin B, several drugs can alter renal function and electrolyte balance. In addition, certain I.V. solutions can inactivate amphotericin B. (For detailed information, see *Drug interactions: Amphotericin B.*)

ADVERSE DRUG REACTIONS

Amphotericin B is probably the most toxic antibiotic in use today. Adverse reactions to I.V. amphotericin B therapy may include nephrotoxicity and hypokalemia. Adverse reactions to other forms of amphotericin therapy tend to be less severe.

Predictable reactions

Almost all patients receiving I.V. amphotericin B experience chills, fever, nausea, vomiting, anorexia, muscle and joint pain, headache, abdominal pain, weight loss, and dyspepsia, especially at the beginning of therapy with low doses. As therapy continues and the dose increases to the optimum level, these reactions usually subside. Most patients also develop normochromic normocytic anemia that significantly decrease the hematocrit level.

Up to 80% of patients receiving amphotericin B develop some degree of nephrotoxicity. With this adverse reaction, blood urea nitrogen (BUN) and serum creatinine levels rise, and the kidneys lose their concentrating ability. The latter promotes renal losses of potassium, bicarbonate, water, and phosphate. Nephrotoxicity usually disappears within 3 months after the drug is discontinued, but it sometimes leads to permanent renal impairment. A direct relationship may exist between the severity and permanency of the impairment and the total amphotericin B dosage. Permanent problems occur more frequently in patients who receive a total of 5 grams or more.

Up to 25% of patients receiving amphotericin B may develop hypokalemia, which can be severe and lead to extreme muscle weakness and electrocardiographic changes. Distal renal tubular acidosis commonly occurs, contributing to the development of hypokalemia.

Other predictable adverse reactions to I.V. amphotericin B therapy include phlebitis, thrombophlebitis, hypotension, flushing, paresthesias, and seizures.

Intrathecal administration may cause headache, leg and back pain, paresthesias, peripheral neuropathies, sensory loss, and urine retention. Topical application may result in pruritus, skin thickening and discoloration, dry skin, erythema, and contact dermatitis. Uncommon predictable reactions to amphotericin B include blurred or double vision, ventricular dysrhythmias, thrombocytopenia, leukopenia, agranulocytosis, tinnitus, and hearing loss.

Unpredictable reactions

Rarely, amphotericin B causes anaphylaxis or liver failure.

NURSING IMPLICATIONS

Because amphotericin B can cause serious drug interactions and adverse reactions, the nurse must monitor the patient carefully and understand the following considerations:

● Amphotericin B is usually contraindicated in a patient with known hypersensitivity to it. However, if a hyper-

sensitive patient has a life-threatening condition that can only be treated with amphotericin B, anticipate its use.
• Monitor the patient's BUN and serum creatinine levels before therapy begins, every other day during initiation of therapy, and once a week after the optimal dose is reached. Expect to administer a reduced dosage or to use alternate-day therapy if the serum creatinine level approaches 3 mg/dl.
• Monitor the patient's fluid intake and output, and observe for oliguria, hematuria, cloudy urine, or excessive urine output. These may be the first clinical signs of nephrotoxicity.
• Monitor the patient's serum electrolyte levels, particularly noting any changes in potassium, magnesium, calcium, and phosphorus levels. Potassium requires especially close monitoring in a patient who is receiving digitalis glycosides or potassium-wasting drugs, such as diuretics and extended-spectrum penicillins, or who is losing potassium because of severe vomiting or diarrhea. Watch for muscle weakness, cramping, and fatigue, which may be the first signs of hypokalemia. Expect to administer potassium supplements, as ordered.
• Instruct the patient to report tinnitus or any hearing loss.
• Monitor the patient for signs of an immediate hypersensitivity reaction, including dyspnea, wheezing, urticuria, pruritus, laryngeal edema, hypotension, and tachycardia..
• Monitor the patient's vital signs during I.V. infusion. Note that a fever may occur but will usually subside within 4 hours after the infusion is discontinued. To relieve the fever and chills associated with the infusion, expect to administer an antihistamine or antipyretic. Antiemetics are sometimes also used to relieve other symptoms, such as nausea and vomiting.
• Check the I.V. site for phlebitis. To reduce phlebitis, rotate the site routinely and add small doses of heparin or corticosteroids to the infusion, as ordered. Expect to use alternate-day therapy if phlebitis becomes severe. Some patients may receive amphotericin B via a central line, which permits greater drug dilution in the blood and decreases the severity of the phlebitis.
• Refrigerate amphotericin B until it is used.
• For infusion or injection, dilute amphotericin B in a D_5W solution with a pH greater than 4.2 or in sterile water. The drug is *not* compatible with any electrolyte solution.
• Before administration, shake the vial vigorously for at least 3 minutes to assure particle dispersion in the colloidal suspension.
• Infuse I.V. amphotericin B over 4 to 6 hours, or as ordered.

• For I.V. administration, use an in-line filter with a mean pore diameter of 1 micron or greater. Smaller filters will remove appreciable amounts of the drug from the solution.
• Infuse any other antibiotics separately; do not use the amphotericin B I.V. line.
• Do not administer the solution if it contains precipitate.
• Instruct the patient using topical amphotericin B to report dry skin, erythema, pruritus, or skin discoloration. Warn the patient that the drug may stain clothing.

NYSTATIN

Nystatin resembles amphotericin B in its chemical structure. Unlike amphotericin B, however, this drug is usually used only topically or orally to treat local infections, because it is extremely toxic when administered parenterally.

The first polyene antibiotic, nystatin was isolated from *Streptomyces noursei* in 1950. It was named after New York State, where the researchers who discovered it were working.

PHARMACOKINETICS

Oral nystatin undergoes little or no absorption, distribution, or metabolism. It is excreted as unchanged drug in the feces.

Topical nystatin is not absorbed through the skin or mucous membranes, and blood concentration levels are not measurable at therapeutic doses.

Because nystatin is not systemically absorbed, its onset of action, peak concentration levels, and duration of action are not significant.

PHARMACODYNAMICS

Like amphotericin B, nystatin acts by binding to sterols in fungal cells.

Mechanism of action

Nystatin binds to sterols in fungal cell membranes and alters the membranes' permeability, leading to loss of essential cell components. Nystatin can act as a fungicidal or fungistatic agent, depending on the organism present.

PHARMACOTHERAPEUTICS

Nystatin is primarily used to treat fungal skin infections. The drug is effective against *C. albicans, C. guilliermondi,* and other *Candida* species.

nystatin (Mycostatin, Nilstat). Different forms of nystatin are available for treating the different types of candidal infections. Topical nystatin is used to treat cutaneous or mucocutaneous *Candida* infections, such as thrush, diaper rash, vulvovaginitis, and intertriginous candidiasis. Oral nystatin is used to treat intestinal candidiasis and may be used as an adjunct to vaginal application in treating vulvovaginitis. Oral nystatin is also used to prevent fungal infection in a neutropenic patient receiving immunosuppressive therapy.

USUAL ADULT DOSAGE: for oral or esophageal candidiasis, 500,000 units of oral suspension, gargled and then swallowed, t.i.d. or q.i.d., or 500,000 units of oral tablets, dissolved in the mouth t.i.d. or q.i.d. for 10 days or until 48 hours after overt symptoms have subsided; for intestinal candidiasis, 500,000 to 1 million units of oral tablets t.i.d. or q.i.d.; for vaginal candidiasis, 100,000 units (one vaginal tablet) inserted vaginally once or twice daily for 14 days or longer; for cutaneous candidiasis, topical cream, ointment, lotion, or powder applied to the affected area b.i.d. or as directed for 14 days or longer.

Drug interactions

No significant drug interactions occur with nystatin use.

ADVERSE DRUG REACTIONS

Reactions to nystatin, which rarely occur, are usually mild. The patient may experience diarrhea, nausea, vomiting, and abdominal pain, especially with high doses; some patients also report a bitter taste. Topical nystatin may cause a skin irritation.

A hypersensitivity reaction may occur with oral or topical nystatin administration.

NURSING IMPLICATIONS

Although nystatin is usually safe when used to treat local fungal infections, the nurse should be aware of the following considerations:

• Instruct the patient taking nystatin in suspension form for oral candidiasis to divide the suspension for each dose in half, place one half in each side of the mouth, swish the suspension in the mouth for as long as possible, and then swallow it.

• Instruct the patient taking nystatin in tablet form for oral candidiasis to dissolve the tablet in the mouth. Emphasize that the patient must not chew it or swallow it whole.

• Advise the patient receiving topical nystatin to report any signs of a hypersensitivity reaction, such as redness or skin irritation.

• Teach the patient receiving topical nystatin the proper application techniques, and emphasize the importance of compliance and good hygiene.

• Instruct the patient receiving vaginal nystatin to insert the tablets high in the vagina. Also inform the patient that vaginal drainage from the tablets may stain clothing.

• Tell the patient using nystatin ointment or cream to avoid using occlusive dressings during nystatin therapy, because they provide a favorable environment for fungal growth.

• Advise the patient to apply a topical powder used for foot infections to both shoes and socks as a preventive measure.

• Expect to continue oral, topical, or vaginal nystatin therapy for 48 hours after the symptoms disappear.

• Advise the patient to take the drug for the full length of time prescribed—usually 14 days—even though symptomatic relief may occur in 14 to 72 hours.

ANTIMETABOLITE ANTIMYCOTIC AGENTS

Flucytosine is the only antimetabolite with antimycotic activity. It is primarily used with another antimycotic agent, such as amphotericin B, to treat systemic fungal infections.

Researchers initially synthesized flucytosine (also known as 5-fluorocytosine or 5-FC) for use as an antineoplastic agent but found it to be ineffective. Then they discovered its antimycotic effects—the drug's only therapeutic use today.

PHARMACOKINETICS

After oral administration, flucytosine is well absorbed and widely distributed. It usually undergoes little metabolism and is excreted primarily by the kidneys.

Absorption, distribution, metabolism, excretion

Flucytosine is rapidly and well absorbed from the GI tract. Although the presence of food in the stomach slows the rate of absorption, it does not affect its extent.

As a result of flucytosine's wide distribution throughout the body, it appears in the kidneys, liver, heart, spleen, aqueous humor, and bronchial secretions. It also reaches high concentration levels in the CSF. It is only 2% to 4% protein-bound.

Because flucytosine is not significantly metabolized, about 90% of it is excreted unchanged in the urine. Unchanged, unabsorbed flucytosine also appears in feces.

Onset, peak, duration

Therapeutic serum concentration levels of flucytosine range from 25 to 120 mcg/ml. The drug usually reaches peak concentration levels 2 to 4 hours after administration unless the patient's renal function is impaired; when the drug will reach peak concentration levels more slowly and maintain them longer. For a patient with normal renal function, flucytosine's half-life ranges from 2.5 to 8 hours. For a patient with renal impairment, the half-life can range from 1 to 10 days.

PHARMACODYNAMICS

Unlike the polyene antimycotic agents, flucytosine must be converted to its active metabolite within fungal cells.

Mechanism of action

Flucytosine penetrates fungal cells sensitive to it and there undergoes conversion to its active metabolite fluorouracil, a metabolic antagonist. Fluorouracil is then incorporated into the fungal cells' ribonucleic acid, altering the cells' protein synthesis to the point where cell death ensues. The drug displays selective toxicity against fungi. Most nonfungal cells do not take up and convert large quantities of flucytosine. Fungal resistance to flucytosine usually occurs when the drug is used alone to treat infections caused by *Cryptococcus*; resistance also occurs, to a lesser degree, when the drug is used alone to treat infections caused by *Candida, Torulopsis,* and *Cladosporium.*

PHARMACOTHERAPEUTICS

Some fungal species and strains are not susceptible to flucytosine. Therefore, susceptibility tests should be done before the drug is used. Also, because some fungi can develop a resistance to flucytosine when it is given alone, it is usually used with another antimycotic agent, such as amphotericin B. Flucytosine reaches high concentration levels in the CSF and urinary tract, so it is effective against fungal meningitis and urinary candidiasis.

flucytosine (Ancobon). Administered orally, flucytosine is used in combination therapy to treat systemic fungal infections caused by *Candida* and *Cryptococcus.* Although amphotericin B is considered the drug of choice for treating candidal and cryptococcal meningitis, endocarditis, pneumonia, septicemia, and urinary and ophthalmic infections, flucytosine is usually given with it to reduce the amphotericin B dose and toxicity. This combination therapy is the treatment of choice for cryptococcal meningitis. Flucytosine can be used alone to treat lower urinary tract *Candida* infections because it reaches high urinary concentration levels. It is also used effectively to treat infections caused by *T. glabrata, Phialophora* species, and *Aspergillus* species.

USUAL ADULT AND PEDIATRIC DOSAGE: for patients over 50 kg with normal renal function and fungal infections caused by *Candida* and *Cryptococcus,* 50 to 150 mg/kg P.O. daily, divided into four equal doses and administered every 6 hours; for a patient with impaired renal function, the dose and dosage interval should be altered as follows: 12.5 to 37.5 mg/kg every 12 hours for a patient with a creatinine clearance between 20 and 40 ml/minute; 12.5 to 37.5 mg/kg every 24 hours when the creatinine clearance ranges from 10 to 20 ml/minute; individualized doses based on the drug's serum concentration level when the creatinine clearance falls below 10 ml/minute; and 20 to 50 mg/kg after each dialysis treatment (every 48 to 72 hours) for a patient on hemodialysis therapy.

Drug interactions

Flucytosine can cause clinically significant interactions with several drugs, including amphotericin B (a complication of combination therapy), antacids, and bone marrow depressant drugs, such as antineoplastics. (See *Drug interactions: Flucytosine* for further information.) It may also interact with food, delaying drug absorption.

ADVERSE DRUG REACTIONS

Adverse reactions to flucytosine seem to involve rapidly proliferating cells in the bone marrow and the GI tract.

Predictable reactions

Typically associated with flucytosine serum concentration levels that exceed 100 mcg/ml, bone marrow depression may occur and lead to leukopenia, thrombocytopenia, anemia, pancytopenia, or agranulocytosis. It most frequently affects patients with renal failure who are undergoing combination therapy with amphotericin B or receiving large doses of flucytosine.

GI reactions may also occur with flucytosine therapy. They can be severe and may include nausea, vomiting, abdominal distention, diarrhea, and anorexia. Rarely, bowel perforation can occur, as can hepatotox-

DRUG INTERACTIONS

Flucytosine

Flucytosine can cause clinically significant interactions when administered with the drugs listed below.

DRUG	INTERACTING DRUGS	POSSIBLE EFFECTS	NURSING IMPLICATIONS
flucytosine	antacids	Delay rate of flucytosine absorption	• Administer these drugs several hours apart.
	amphotericin B	Decreases renal excretion of flucytosine, leading to elevated flucytosine blood levels and increased antimycotic activity	• Expect to administer smaller doses of amphotericin B, as ordered, to reduce its toxicity. • Anticipate giving flucytosine at longer dosage intervals as ordered.
	bone marrow depressants, such as antineoplastics, penicillamine, and gold compounds	Enhance bone marrow toxicity	• Monitor the patient's CBC frequently during therapy.

icity, manifested by elevated transaminase and alkaline phosphatase levels.

Unpredictable reactions

The drug may produce unpredictable adverse reactions, including confusion, headache, sedation, vertigo, hallucinations, and skin rashes.

NURSING IMPLICATIONS

Although flucytosine is a relatively safe antimycotic agent, the nurse must understand the following considerations:
• Be aware that flucytosine is contraindicated in a patient who is hypersensitive to it.
• Administer flucytosine cautiously to a patient with renal impairment or bone marrow depression, and especially with concomitant renal dysfunction.
• Monitor the patient's hematologic values and kidney and liver function tests during flucytosine therapy.
• Monitor flucytosine blood levels regularly during long-term therapy. Therapeutic serum concentrations range from 25 to 120 mcg/ml.
• Instruct the patient to report sore throat, fever, easy bruising or bleeding, unusual fatigue or weakness, severe nausea, vomiting, or skin rash.
• Emphasize the importance of the patient's compliance with therapy.
• Advise the patient taking flucytosine capsules to take them over 15 minutes to minimize nausea or vomiting.
• Instruct the patient to take a missed dose as soon as possible, but not to take a double dose. Explain that missing a dose is safer than overmedication with a double dose.

IMIDAZOLE ANTIMYCOTIC AGENTS

The imidazole group includes ketoconazole, miconazole, and clotrimazole. Ketoconazole and miconazole are used to treat systemic and topical fungal infections; clotrimazole, only topical ones. (See "Other Antimycotic Agents" on page 1110 for more information about clotrimazole.) Because ketoconazole provides effective antimycotic activity with oral administration, its use overshadows that of miconazole, which is available only in parenteral and topical preparations.

Although ketoconazole was introduced more than a decade ago, it did not become commercially available until 1981. Considered an important advance in fungal infection therapy, ketoconazole is the first effective oral antimycotic agent with a broad spectrum of activity.

PHARMACOKINETICS

After oral administration, ketoconazole is variably absorbed and widely distributed. It undergoes extensive metabolism and is excreted through the bile and feces.

After parenteral administration, miconazole is distributed throughout most of the body. It is metabolized in the liver and excreted in the feces and urine.

Absorption, distribution, metabolism, excretion

Ketoconazole usually is well absorbed from the GI tract. Its degree of absorption, however, depends on the pH of the GI tract. A normal acidic environment increases absorption; an alkaline environment, which may result from diseases, other drugs, or foods that reduce gastric acid, decreases absorption. The drug is absorbed best when the patient's stomach is empty.

Widely distributed throughout the body, ketoconazole appears in bile, saliva, serum, cerumen, and feces, and in the skin and soft tissues. It is poorly distributed in urine and CSF, however, where concentration levels usually are low. The drug crosses the placenta and appears in breast milk. Its protein binding—primarily to albumin—ranges from 84% to 99%.

After I.V. administration, miconazole achieves wide distribution, appearing in inflamed joints, the vitreous humor, and the peritoneum. It is poorly distributed in the CSF, saliva, and sputum. Intrathecal miconazole, however, can achieve therapeutic CSF concentration levels. About 90% is bound to plasma albumin.

Ketoconazole metabolism in the liver produces inactive metabolites; these metabolites and unchanged drug are excreted primarily in the feces.

In the liver, miconazole undergoes rapid metabolism to inactive metabolites. The kidneys excrete 14% to 22% of the drug in the urine, and the bowel excretes 50% in the feces.

Onset, peak, duration

When administered ½ to 1 hour after meals, ketoconazole reaches peak plasma concentration levels in 1 to 4 hours. The ensuing decline in plasma concentration levels appears to be biphasic. During the initial phase, the drug's half-life is about 2 hours; in the terminal phase, 8 hours.

After I.V. administration, miconazole begins to act immediately and reaches peak concentration levels in 15 minutes. Its half-life is about 24 hours.

PHARMACODYNAMICS

Like the polyene antimycotic agents, ketoconazole and miconazole act by affecting cell permeability. They usually produce fungistatic effects but can also produce fungicidal effects under certain conditions.

Mechanism of action

Within the fungal cells, ketoconazole interferes with sterol synthesis, damaging the cell membrane and increasing its permeability. That leads to a loss of essential intracellular elements and inhibition of cell growth.

At lower concentration levels, miconazole produces a fungistatic action; it alters the cell membrane by thickening it. At higher concentration levels, the drug has a fungicidal action; it impairs the endoplasmic reticulum, causing cell death.

PHARMACOTHERAPEUTICS

Ketoconazole is used to treat topical and systemic infections caused by susceptible fungi, which include dermatophytes and most other fungi. However, it should not be used to treat fungal meningitis, because it does not reach adequate concentration levels in the CSF. Ketoconazole is also active against some gram-positive bacteria, including *Staphylococcus epidermis, S. aureus, Nocardia* species, *Actinomadura* species, and enterococci.

Administered parenterally, miconazole is used to treat severe fungal infections and fungal meningitis; it is administered topically to treat topical fungal infections. Miconazole provides antimycotic action against *Candida albicans, C. parapsilosis,* and *C. tropicalis; Coccidioides immitis; Cryptococcus neoformans; Histoplasma capsulatum; Paracoccidioides brasiliensis; Aspergillus flavus; Microsporum canis;* and *Sporothrix schenckii.*

ketoconazole (Nizoral). Administered orally, this antimycotic agent can effectively treat topical and systemic fungal infections, including chronic mucocutaneous candidiasis. Mucosal infections respond in days; skin infections, in weeks; and nail infections, in months.

Other clinical indications for ketoconazole therapy include pulmonary and disseminated blastomycosis caused by *Blastomyces dermatitidis,* chromomycosis caused by *Phialophora* species, pulmonary and disseminated coccidioidomycosis caused by *Coccidioides immitis,* pulmonary and disseminated histoplasmosis caused by *Histoplasma capsulatum,* oral candidiasis caused by *Candida* species, and paracoccidioidomycosis caused by *Paracoccidioides brasiliensis.*
USUAL ADULT DOSAGE: 200 mg P.O. daily, increased to 400 mg/day if the infection is severe or does not respond. The duration of therapy varies with the organism and infection site as follows: 1 to 4 weeks for oral candidiasis; 1 to 2 months for most dermatophyte infections; 6 months for histoplasmosis; and 6 to 12 months for coccidioidomycosis, chromomycosis, chronic mucocutaneous candidiasis, and tinea unguium.

miconazole (Monistat) and **miconazole nitrate** (Mycatin). An imidazole derivative, miconazole may be used to treat systemic fungal infections—such as coccidioidomycosis, paracoccidioidomycosis, cryptococcosis, and candidiasis—and topical fungal infections such as chronic mucocutaneous candidiasis. The drug may be administered I.V. or intrathecally to treat fungal meningitis, or I.V. or in bladder irrigations to treat fungal bladder infections.

In general, miconazole is less effective than amphotericin B for treating systemic fungal infections. For this reason, it is usually reserved for patients who cannot tolerate amphotericin B.

USUAL ADULT DOSAGE: for severe systemic fungal infections, fungal meningitis, and chronic mucocutaneous candidiasis, 200 to 3,600 mg I.V. daily in normal saline or D_5W solution, given in three divided doses, each infused over 30 to 60 minutes; therapy may continue 1 to 20 weeks or longer, depending on the organism and infection site; for fungal meningitis, 20 mg intrathecally every 24 to 48 hours; for fungal bladder infections, 200 mg diluted in a normal saline solution and instilled into the bladder; for skin infections, cream or lotion applied b.i.d. to affected area for up to 2 weeks; for vaginal infections, one 100-mg suppository or one applicatorful of cream at bedtime inserted high in the vagina for 7 days, or one 200-mg suppository administered daily for 3 days.

Drug interactions

Use of ketoconazole with drugs that decrease gastric acidity, such as cimetidine, ranitidine, famotidine, antacids, and anticholinergics, may decrease its absorption and antimycotic effects. Concomitant administration with an oral anticoagulant can cause hemorrhage from the increased anticoagulant effect.

Miconazole may prolong the prothrombin time in a patient receiving oral anticoagulants. It may also antagonize the antimycotic effects of amphotericin B, contraindicating concomitant use of the two drugs.

ADVERSE DRUG REACTIONS

Although ketoconazole appears to be safer than amphotericin B and miconazole, it may produce adverse reactions primarily affecting the CNS, GI tract, and skin. I.V. miconazole can cause a wide range of adverse reactions because of its lipid vehicle, Cremaphor EL.

Predictable reactions

The most common predictable reactions to ketoconazole are nausea and vomiting; other reactions include pruritus, rash, dermatitis, urticaria, headache, insomnia, dizziness, vivid dreams, lethargy, paresthesias, diarrhea, flatulence, and abdominal pain. The patient may also experience endocrine effects, such as gynecomastia and

breast pain. Rarely occurring, hepatotoxicity is reversible with drug discontinuation.

The lipid vehicle in I.V. miconazole produces most of the drug's significant adverse reactions, including phlebitis, pruritus, nausea, fever, chills, rash, and hyperlipidemia. These adverse reactions, especially severe pruritus and hyperlipidemia, occur more frequently in patients receiving high doses. When phlebitis occurs, it can be severe, and effective administration may require replacement of the peripheral line with a central venous catheter.

Unpredictable reactions

Rarely, ketoconazole can cause anaphylaxis, arthralgia, chills, fever, tinnitus, impotence, and photophobia.

Unpredictable reactions to miconazole may include thrombocytopenia, anemia, hypersensitivity reactions, diarrhea, anorexia, and flushing. I.V. administration of miconazole may produce cardiac dysrhythmias, tachypnea, and cardiopulmonary arrest.

NURSING IMPLICATIONS

To ensure effective therapy with these broad-spectrum antimycotic agents, the nurse must understand the following considerations:

• Be aware that ketoconazole and miconazole are contraindicated in a patient with a known hypersensitivity to them.

• Do not administer ketoconazole with drugs that decrease gastric acidity, such as antacids and anticholinergics. Administer ketoconazole at least 2 hours before giving these other drugs, if they must be used.

• Ketoconazole requires gastric acidity for dissolution and absorption. A patient with achlorhydria may require small amounts of hydrochloric acid to enhance ketoconazole absorption. For this patient, dissolve ketoconazole in a dilute solution of normal hydrochloric acid. Give the patient a glass straw for drinking the solution, to avoid contact between the acid and the teeth.

• Give ketoconazole with food to minimize the risk of nausea and vomiting.

• Administer an I.V. infusion of miconazole over 30 to 60 minutes to reduce the risk of cardiac dysrhythmias, tachypnea, and cardiopulmonary arrest.

• Monitor the patient's liver function tests. Expect to discontinue the drug if test results show persistent elevations and the patient displays signs of hepatic injury, such as right upper abdominal quadrant pain, fatigue, or jaundice.

• Monitor the patient's serum electrolyte and lipid levels and complete blood count (CBC) before I.V. miconazole therapy begins and periodically during therapy.

• Check the miconazole I.V. site frequently, and rotate sites to prevent phlebitis.

• Expect to minimize nausea and vomiting associated with miconazole therapy by premedicating the patient with antiemetics, slowing the infusion rate, and reducing the dose, as ordered.

• Ketoconazole is not used to treat fungal meningitis.

• Administer ketoconazole cautiously to a pregnant or lactating patient.

• Administer miconazole cautiously to a pregnant patient or a child, because the effects of I.V. miconazole on these patients are unknown.

• Tell the patient to notify the physician if certain signs develop during ketoconazole therapy, such as dark or amber-colored urine, pale stools, abdominal pain, unusual fatigue, or yellowing of the eyes or skin, which could mean hepatic injury.

• Advise the patient to report occurrence of breast enlargement, breast pain, or a skin rash during ketoconazole therapy.

OTHER ANTIMYCOTIC AGENTS

Several other antimycotic agents offer alternate forms of treatment for topical fungal infections. These agents are effective against susceptible fungi and typically produce only mild, local adverse reactions.

Before ketoconazole was developed, griseofulvin was the only oral antimycotic agent available for effectively treating dermatophytic infections. In 1939, researchers isolated griseofulvin from *Penicillium griseofulvum*. Nearly 20 years later, physicians began to use the drug to treat fungal infections. Today, griseofulvin remains an important antimycotic agent for treating nonsystemic fungal infections. It is available in two oral forms—microsize and ultramicrosize—and is used to treat infections of the skin and nails.

Ciclopirox olamine, econazole nitrate, haloprogin, carbol-fushsin solution, tolnaftate, and undecylenic acid are only available as topical agents. (For information about these drugs, see Chapter 78, Integumentary System Agents.)

Clotrimazole comes in several forms for oral, vaginal, and topical use.

griseofulvin. Available in microsize form (Fulvicin-U/F, Grifulvin V, Grisactin) and in ultramicrosize form (Fulvicin P/G, Grisactin-Ultra, Gris-PEG), griseofulvin is used to treat fungal infections of the skin on the body in general (tinea corporis), feet (tinea pedis), groin (tinea cruris), and beard area (tinea barbae), and infections of the nails (tinea unguium) and scalp (tinea capitis). However, it is less effective against nail infections than skin infections.

To prevent a relapse, griseofulvin therapy must continue until the fungus is completely eradicated and the infected skin or nails are replaced. Because the infected areas grow at different rates, the duration of therapy varies with the site of infection.

For tinea corporis, the usual adult dosage is 500 mg P.O. of microsize griseofulvin daily or b.i.d. or 250 mg P.O. of ultramicrosize griseofulvin daily or b.i.d. with food for 2 to 4 weeks. The duration of therapy for other indications is 4 to 6 weeks for tinea capitis, 4 to 8 weeks for tinea pedis, 4 months or more for tinea unguium of the fingernails, and 6 months or more for tinea unguium of the toenails.

Most patients tolerate griseofulvin very well. When adverse reactions occur, they usually include nausea, vomiting, diarrhea, fatigue, mental confusion, and headaches. Headaches are common and can be severe, especially at the beginning of therapy, but they usually disappear as therapy continues. Other adverse reactions may include flatulence and excessive thirst.

Rarely, griseofulvin may cause such reactions as proteinuria, urticaria, rash, serum sickness (a hypersensitivity reaction), photosensitivity, hearing loss, paresthesias, dizziness, insomnia, and leukopenia. It may even cause oral candidiasis.

clotrimazole (Gyne-Lotrimin, Mycelex). An imidazole derivative, clotrimazole resembles miconazole and ketoconazole in chemical structure. It is used topically to treat dermatophyte and *Candida albicans* infections; orally to treat oral candidiasis; and vaginally to treat vaginal candidiasis. For topical treatment of tinea corporis, tinea pedis, tinea cruris, tinea versicolor, or candidiasis, the patient must apply clotrimazole cream, lotion, or solution b.i.d. for 2 to 4 weeks. For treatment of oral candidiasis, the patient must dissolve in the mouth—not chew—an oral troche five times a day for 14 days. For treatment of vaginal candidiasis, the patient must insert one 100-mg vaginal tablet or one applicatorful of cream into the vagina once a day for 7 days. As an alternate method, a nonpregnant patient may

SELECTED MAJOR DRUGS

Antimycotic agents

The following chart summarizes the major antimycotic agents currently in clinical use.

DRUG	MAJOR INDICATIONS	USUAL ADULT DOSAGES	NURSING IMPLICATIONS
amphotericin B	Life-threatening systemic fungal infections and meningitis	0.25 to 1.5 mg/kg/day I.V. infused over 4 to 6 hours	• Amphotericin B is contraindicated in a patient with known hypersensitivity to it. • Monitor the patient's BUN and serum creatinine levels before and during therapy. • Monitor the patient's urine output for signs of renal dysfunction. • Monitor the patient's serum electrolyte levels, especially the potassium, phosphorus, calcium, and magnesium levels. • Monitor the patient's vital signs closely during an infusion. Expect to premedicate the patient with an antipyretic and an antihistamine to prevent fever, chills, and tremors. • Monitor the patient closely for signs of phlebitis, such as redness, tenderness and heat. Expect to add small doses of heparin or corticosteroids to the infusion to prevent or relieve these reactions. • Assess the patient for signs of anemia, such as pallor and a decreased hematocrit level, which commonly occur with amphotericin B therapy. • Dilute amphotericin B with only D_5W or sterile water without bacteriostatic agents. All other solutions are incompatible. • Administer an I.V. infusion over 4 to 6 hours. • For I.V. administration, use an in-line filter with a mean pore diameter of 1 micron or greater. • Do not administer an I.V. solution that contains a precipitate. • Expect to use alternate-day infusions to reduce phlebitis, decrease the risk of nephrotoxicity, and give the patient greater mobility.
	Candidal infections of the bladder	50 mg in 1 liter sterile water injected or instilled into the bladder	
	Coccidioidal arthritis and osteoarticular sporotrichosis	5 to 15 mg injected into joint spaces	
	Coccidioidal meningitis and cryptococcal meningitis	0.025 to 1 mg given intrathecally two to three times weekly	
nystatin	Cutaneous candidiasis	Cream, lotion, ointment, or powder applied to the affected area b.i.d. or as directed	• Nystatin is contraindicated in a patient with known hypersensitivity to it. • Administer nystatin cautiously to a patient who is allergic to penicillin, because a cross-sensitivity may exist. • Instruct the patient using an oral suspension to place half of each dose in each side of the mouth and then swish the suspension around before swallowing. • Advise the patient receiving tablets for oral candidiasis to dissolve—not chew—them in the mouth. • Tell the patient using nystatin cream or ointment not to use an occlusive dressing on the affected area.
	Oral candidiasis	500,000 to 1 million units of oral suspension, gargled and then swallowed, t.i.d. or q.i.d., or 500,000 units of oral tablets, dissolved in the mouth, t.i.d. or q.i.d.	
	Vaginal candidiasis	100,000 units inserted vaginally one to two times per day	
	Intestinal candidiasis	500,000 to 1 million units of oral tablets t.i.d. or q.i.d.	
ketoconazole	Topical and systemic fungal infections, including chronic mucocutaneous	200 to 400 mg P.O. daily for 1 week to 12 months, depending on the organ-	• Ketoconazole is contraindicated in a patient with known hypersensitivity to it. • Administer this drug cautiously to the preg-

continued

SELECTED MAJOR DRUGS

Antimycotic agents continued

DRUG	MAJOR INDICATIONS	USUAL ADULT DOSAGES	NURSING IMPLICATIONS
ketoconazole (continued)	candidiasis, tinea infections, and pulmonary infections	ism and the infection site	nant or lactating patient. • Check the patient's records for drugs or diseases that could reduce gastric acidity and decrease ketoconazole absorption. • Administer ketoconazole with dilute hydrochloric acid as ordered to enhance drug absorption in a patient with achlorhydria. Have the patient drink the solution through a glass straw to avoid contact between the acid and the teeth. • Monitor the patient's liver function tests. • Tell the patient to report any occurrence of breast pain or gynecomastia.
flucytosine	Severe systemic fungal infections caused by *Candida* or *Cryptococcus;* frequently used in combination with amphotericin B	50 to 150 mg/kg P.O. daily divided in four equal doses and administered every 6 hours	• Flucytosine is contraindicated in a patient with known hypersensitivity to it. • Administer flucytosine cautiously to a patient with renal impairment or bone marrow depression. • Monitor the patient's renal function and hematologic studies frequently during therapy. • Emphasize to the patient the importance of compliance with medication therapy. • Expect to adjust the dose and dosage interval for a patient with renal impairment.

insert two vaginal tablets once a day for 3 days, although this method is somewhat less effective than the 7-day regimen.

Adverse reactions to the oral troches occur most frequently and may include elevated liver function test results, nausea, and vomiting. Adverse reactions to topical clotrimazole include localized blistering, stinging, pruritus, erythema, urticaria, and peeling.

CHAPTER SUMMARY

Chapter 69 covered antimycotic (antifungal) agents as they are used in the treatment of topical and systemic fungal infections. Here are the highlights of the chapter:
• The antimycotic agents used to treat systemic fungal infections include amphotericin B, miconazole, ketoconazole, and flucytosine. Nystatin, clotrimazole, and griseofulvin are used primarily to treat topical infections. Ketoconazole and miconazole may also be used for topical infections.
• Amphotericin B, a polyene antimycotic agent, is the most widely used antimycotic for severe systemic fungal infections. It is usually administered I.V. in D_5W or sterile water. Certain adverse reactions, however, limit its parenteral use. These include nephrotoxicity, phlebitis, hematologic effects, electrolyte imbalances, and immediate reactions, such as fever, chills, vomiting, and hypotension. Premedication with antipyretics, antiemetics, and antihistamines can reduce the immediate reactions' severity. With long-term amphotericin B therapy, phlebitis can be especially severe and may require placement of a central venous catheter. Because of these adverse reactions and certain drug interactions, parenteral amphotericin B therapy requires close monitoring. When given as a bladder irrigant, however, amphotericin B produces far fewer adverse reactions.
• Like amphotericin B, nystatin is a polyene antimycotic agent. Unlike amphotericin B, however, it cannot be given parenterally or used to treat systemic infections. Instead, it is administered as a tablet or suspension to treat oral, vaginal, and intestinal candidiasis. Its adverse reactions may affect the GI tract and the skin.
• For severe systemic fungal infections, miconazole offers one major advantage over amphotericin B. It doesn't cause nephrotoxicity. However, this imidazole agent's low effectiveness and high incidence of relapse limit its use in the treatment of systemic infections. Rapid infusion of I.V. miconazole can lead to severe toxicity.

- Ketoconazole, an oral imidazole antimycotic agent, can be used to treat topical and systemic fungal infections, including griseofulvin-resistant infections. Interactions between ketoconazole and other drugs may prevent ketoconazole absorption or alter the effectiveness of the other drug. A patient receiving ketoconazole as part of combination drug therapy requires close monitoring.

- Flucytosine, an oral antimycotic agent, is usually given with amphotericin B to treat severe systemic fungal infections. Because this antimetabolite antimycotic increases the effects of amphotericin B, the patient can receive lower amphotericin B doses, decreasing the risk of adverse drug reactions. When flucytosine is given alone, fungal resistance to the drug may develop. The most significant adverse reaction to flucytosine—bone marrow depression—can be severe enough to require drug discontinuation and usually occurs when the drug reaches high serum concentration levels. A patient with renal impairment will need dosage adjustments to prevent toxic serum concentration levels.

- Clotrimazole may be administered topically, orally, or vaginally to treat topical dermatophyte and candidal infections.

- Before the introduction of ketoconazole, griseofulvin was the only systemic antimycotic agent available for treating topical dermatophytic infections. Ketoconazole's popularity has decreased the use of griseofulvin. The older drug is now used primarily for treating dermatophytic infections that do not respond to topical therapy.

BIBLIOGRAPHY

American Hospital Formulary Service. *Drug Information 87.* McEvoy, G.K., et al., eds. Bethesda, Md.: American Society of Hospital Pharmacists, 1987.

Barton, C.H., et al. "Renal Magnesium Wasting Associated with Amphotericin B Therapy," *American Journal of Medicine* 77:471, September 1984.

Christiansen, K.I., et al. "Distribution and Activity of Amphotericin B in Humans," *Journal of Infectious Diseases* 152:1037, November 1985.

Dismukes, W.E., et al. "Treatment of Systemic Mycoses with Ketoconazole: Emphasis on Toxicity and Clinical Response in 52 Patients," *Annals of Internal Medicine* 98:13, January 1983.

Gilman, A.G., et al., eds. *Goodman and Gilman's The Pharmacological Basis of Therapeutics,* 7th ed. New York: Macmillan Publishing Co., 1985.

Gotz, V.P., et al. "Effect of Filtering Amphotericin B Infusions on the Incidence and Severity of Phlebitis and Selected Adverse Reactions," *Drug Intelligence and Clinical Pharmacology* 19:436, June 1985.

Hermans, P.E., and Keys, T.F. "Antifungal Agents Used for Deep-Seated Mycotic Infections," *Mayo Clinic Proceedings* 58:223, April 1983.

Smith, E.B., and Henry, J.C. "Ketoconazole: An Orally Effective Antifungal Agent: Mechanism of Action, Pharmacology, Clinical Efficacy, and Adverse Effects," *Pharmacotherapy* 4:199, July/August 1984.

USPDI: Drug Information for the Health Care Provider, Vol. 1, 6th ed. Rockville, Md.: United States Pharmacopeial Convention, Inc., 1985.

Van Tyle, J.H. "Ketoconazole: Mechanism of Action, Spectrum of Activity, Pharmacokinetics, Drug Interactions, Adverse Reactions, and Therapeutic Use," *Pharmacotherapy* 4:343, November/December 1984.

ANTHELMINTIC AGENTS

OBJECTIVES

After reading and studying this chapter, you should be able to:

1. Explain the physiology of helminth infections, distinguishing among nematodes, cestodes and trematodes.
2. Explain how the pharmacokinetics of the anthelmintic agents relates to their effectiveness.
3. Describe the mechanisms of action of the various anthelmintic agents.
4. Discuss the common adverse reactions to anthelmintic agents.
5. List the contraindications to the anthelmintic agents.
6. Instruct patients regarding proper administration, expected therapeutic effects, and possible adverse reactions to the anthelmintic agents.

INTRODUCTION

Anthelmintic agents destroy helminths—parasitic worms that infect humans. The three groups of helminths that infect humans include nematodes (roundworms), cestodes (tapeworms), and trematodes (flukes). Thus, the anthelmintic agents are classified as antinematode, anticestode, and antitrematode.

Although commonly believed to exist solely in tropic and subtropic areas, helminths are everywhere, and conservative estimates indicate that one fourth of the world's population is infected with them. The most commonly encountered helminth infection in North America is childhood enterobiasis, or pinworm infection. Hookworm, whipworm, tapeworm, and threadworm infections occur occasionally in adults and children living in the southern United States. Helminth infections are also found in recent immigrants and tourists from areas of the world where such infections are endemic.

Anthelmintic agents are a varied group: Their only common link is their effectiveness against helminth infection. Many were discovered by chance; others were first used in veterinary medicine, then adapted for human use. Some anthelmintics are highly toxic, so positive helminth identification is imperative before treatment

begins. Because of frequent patient reinfection and noncompliance, treatment must be repeated in many cases, usually with the same agent. (Secondary drugs are frequently less specific and more toxic than the drug of choice.)

Chapter 70 discusses anthelmintic agents currently used in North America, grouped according to the particular helminth group they combat most effectively. These agents include mebendazole, piperazine citrate, pyrantel pamoate, and thiabendazole (antinematode agents); mebendazole, niclosamide, paramomycin sulfate, and praziquantel (anticestode agents); and oxamniquine and praziquantel (antitrematode agents).

Physiology of helminth infection

Helminths are multicellular parasitic worms that vary in size from 4 inches to 7 yards and are different from other organisms that invade the body. For example, many require two hosts to complete their life cycles. One, *Taenia solium*, or pork tapeworm, develops partially in hog intestines and muscle, but cannot complete its life cycle unless the infected pork is ingested by a human, who becomes the new host.

Helminths usually infect humans by one of two routes: ingestion or intact-skin penetration. Inside the host, the helminth migrates to a predestined anatomic location, usually the lungs, liver, or intestines. There, the helminth progresses to its next developmental stage, whereupon it must leave the human host to complete its life cycle and reproduce. (With few exceptions, helminths cannot multiply within the primary host.)

Another difference between helminths and other invading organisms is that helminths, particularly those that migrate in human tissue, cause eosinophilia, an increase in white blood cells with special antiparasite functions.

In appearance, nematodes are cylindrical, unsegmented, elongated helminths that taper at each end; this shape has earned them the familiar designation *round-*

worms. Cestodes, better known as *tapeworms*, have bodies flattened front to back with distinct regular segments (proglottides) that carry the fertilized eggs out into the environment; tapeworms also have heads with suckers or sucking grooves. Trematodes have flattened, unsegmented bodies; many are leaflike in shape. They are called *blood, intestinal, lung,* or *liver flukes,* depending on their infection sites in human hosts.

Signs and symptoms of helminth infections are specific for each helminth and for each infection site and basically reflect disturbance in the affected organ or body system.

See *Selected major drugs: Anthelmintic agents* on page 1120 for a summary of representative drugs.

ANTINEMATODE AGENTS

The four drugs with specific antiparasitic action against nematodes, or roundworms, are mebendazole, piperazine, pyrantel pamoate, and thiabendazole.

History and source

The anthelmintic character of the colorless crystal compound piperazine, first observed by a French pharmacist, was first publicized by Fayard in 1949. (Piperazine previously had been used as an anticorrosive and an insecticide.) Thiabendazole and mebendazole, developed specifically for their anthelmintic activity, are among the most potent anthelmintic agents. Thiabendazole's activity against roundworms was described by Brown and co-workers in 1961, whereas mebendazole's action was described by Brugmans and co-workers in 1971. Pyrantel pamoate, a veterinary anthelmintic introduced in the mid-1960s, was first studied in humans by Bumbalo and others in 1969. Successful clinical trials have subsequently proven its effectiveness in treating nematode infections in humans.

PHARMACOKINETICS

Antinematode agents have individually distinctive pharmacokinetic properties.

Absorption, distribution, metabolism, excretion

Less than 10% of an oral mebendazole dose is absorbed from the gastrointestinal (GI) tract; the remainder is excreted unchanged in the feces. The absorbed drug is metabolized by the liver and excreted unchanged in the urine. It is well distributed and crosses the placenta. Like mebendazole, pyrantel pamoate is poorly absorbed from the GI tract. Less than 15% of a dose is excreted in the urine as unchanged drug or metabolites. Because these two drugs stay in the GI tract, they are particularly effective against roundworms that infect the intestines. Piperazine is readily absorbed after oral administration and widely distributed. A small portion is metabolized in the liver, but most of a piperazine dose is excreted unchanged in the urine. Thiabendazole is rapidly and almost completely absorbed from the GI tract. It is widely distributed in the body, rapidly metabolized by the liver, and excreted by the kidneys.

Onset, peak, duration

For anthelmintic agents, the onset of action varies and depends on when the agent comes in contact with the helminth. This, in turn, depends on the rate of drug uptake, which varies greatly between infected tissues, such as the lungs and liver.

The peak concentration level and duration of action have little effect on an agent's anthelmintic action. However, these pharmacokinetic processes affect the extent of systemic drug absorption, which determines whether or not toxic effects occur.

Peak plasma concentration levels of the antinematode agents have a wider than usual range, particularly with oral mebendazole, which reaches peak plasma concentration levels from 1½ to 7 hours after oral administration. Its half-life is 2.8 to 9 hours. Piperazine achieves peak plasma concentration levels in 2 to 4 hours. Its half-life varies considerably, but its metabolism is complete within 24 hours. Because more than 50% of pyrantel pamoate is eliminated unchanged in the feces, its elimination time depends on bowel transit time. Thiabendazole reaches peak plasma concentration levels within 1 to 2 hours after oral administration, and has a half-life of 1.2 to 1.7 hours. About 90% of an oral dose is eliminated from the body within 24 to 48 hours.

PHARMACODYNAMICS

The pharmacodynamic effects of the antinematode agents are diverse and include several mechanisms of action, most not fully understood. Antinematode agents immobilize or kill roundworms by impairing their ability to use energy from available sources or by interfering with their neurologic systems. The immobilized or dead roundworms are then eliminated from the GI tract by peristalsis.

Mechanism of action

Mebendazole interferes with the roundworm's micro-tubule system, thus preventing glucose uptake and distribution. As a result, the parasite depletes its energy stores and is immobilized or dies; actual expulsion from the GI tract can take several days. Piperazine paralyzes the roundworm by blocking the neurotransmitter acetylcholine at the myoneural junction, causing flaccid paralysis. The paralyzed roundworm, unable to counter peristalsis, is thus expelled from the GI tract. Pyrantel pamoate also acts by interfering with the roundworm's neuromuscular transmission, causing spastic paralysis by a process similar to that of the depolarizing neuromuscular blocking agents. Like mebendazole, thiabendazole acts on microtubules; it inhibits the action of fumarate reductase, an enzyme critical to the roundworm's anaerobic metabolism.

PHARMACOTHERAPEUTICS

The rule of thumb in treating nematode infection is to continue using the drug of choice for the particular invading organism until the organism is eradicated or the drug has clearly failed to eradicate it. Alternative choices are characteristically more toxic to the patient. Realistic cure rates range from 70% to 100%, depending on the drug and the type of roundworm. Repeat treatment is frequently necessary because of patient noncompliance or reinfection.

Mebendazole has broad anthelmintic activity and is the drug of choice against infection with *Trichuris trichiura* (whipworm), *Enterobius vermicularis* (pinworm), *Necator americanus* (hookworm), and *Ascaris lumbricoides* (giant intestinal roundworm). It is not effective against *Strongyloides stercoralis* (threadworm) infection. Mebendazole also has been tried with some success in patients with hydatid disease (systemic infection) from *Echinococcus granulosus*, a liver tapeworm. Mebendazole's advantages include low systemic toxicity because of its limited absorption.

Piperazine is no longer recommended as a first-line drug for treating roundworm infections, because other agents are more effective and less toxic. It is used primarily as an alternative drug to mebendazole in patients with large ascaris infections causing intestinal blockage. In these patients, piperazine relieves the blockage by promoting expulsion of volumes of paralyzed roundworms. Pyrantel pamoate is an alternative drug of choice for treating a number of nematode infections, including giant intestinal roundworm, hookworm, and pinworm infections. It has the advantage of one-time dosage.

Thiabendazole is the drug of choice to treat threadworm infection and also acts as an anti-inflammatory agent in trichinosis (caused by the nematode *Trichinella spiralis*).

mebendazole (Vermox). Available in 100-mg tablets, mebendazole may be administered either before or after meals; tablets should be chewed to enhance the drug's efficacy. Mebendazole is primarily used to treat roundworm infections.
USUAL ADULT AND PEDIATRIC DOSAGE: for *Ascaris* (giant intestinal roundworm), *Trichuris* (whipworm), and *Necator* (hookworm) infections, 100 mg P.O. b.i.d. for 3 days, may be repeated in 2 to 3 weeks; for *Enterobius* (pinworm) infection, one 100-mg tablet, repeated in 2 to 3 weeks. The dosage for children under age 2 has not been established.

piperazine citrate (Antepar). Piperazine is a secondary agent for all nematode infections, but principally for large *Ascaris* infections that cause intestinal blockage.
USUAL ADULT AND PEDIATRIC DOSAGE: for *Ascaris* infection, 75 mg/kg (to a maximum of 3.5 grams/day) P.O. as a single dose for 2 days; for enterobiasis, 65 mg/kg (to a maximum of 2.5 grams/day) P.O. for 7 days.

pyrantel pamoate (Antiminth). Available as an oral suspension, pyrantel pamoate is used as an alternate drug to treat nematode infections (hookworm, pinworm, and giant intestinal roundworm).
USUAL ADULT AND PEDIATRIC DOSAGE: 11 mg/kg (to a maximum 1 gram/day) P.O. as a one-time dose; may be repeated in 2 to 3 weeks if needed. The dosage for children under age 2 has not been established.

thiabendazole (Mintezol). Although effective against all nematodes, thiabendazole is highly toxic and therefore is the drug of choice for *Strongyloides* (threadworm) infections only; it is used to treat other nematode infections only when the drug of choice has clearly failed.
USUAL ADULT AND PEDIATRIC DOSAGE: for *Strongyloides* infections, 25 mg/kg (maximum of 3 grams/day) P.O. b.i.d. (or 50 mg/kg as a single dose) for 2 days, or 1.5 grams P.O. b.i.d for patients who weigh 155 lb (70 kg) or more; for trichinosis, 25 mg/kg (to a maximum of 3 grams/day) P.O. b.i.d. for 2 to 4 days.

Drug interactions

As a group, antinematode agents are associated with few drug interactions. In high concentration levels, piperazine may increase extrapyramidal effects and the potential for seizures in patients also receiving phenothiazines. The most important potential interaction, however, is between piperazine and pyrantel pamoate and relates to their mechanisms of action: because piperazine causes flaccid paralysis and pyrantel pamoate causes spastic paralysis, the possibility exists that they could cancel each other's effect if administered together. No special interactions between antinematode agents and food exist.

ADVERSE DRUG REACTIONS

Almost all the antinematode agents cause predictable GI adverse reactions ranging from abdominal pain to nausea, vomiting, and diarrhea. Other adverse reactions are less common. For example, mebendazole may rarely cause leukopenia, and piperazine occasionally causes headache, vertigo, and loss of coordination. Piperazine may also lower seizure thresholds, so it should not be used with phenothiazines or other drugs that have the same effect, particularly in patients with epilepsy. Pyrantel pamoate and thiabendazole sometimes cause headache, dizziness, drowsiness, and weakness; thiabendazole may also cause rash and hallucinations and rare occurrences of tinnitus and seizures.

NURSING IMPLICATIONS

To achieve the greatest patient benefit with the fewest adverse reactions, the nurse should be aware of the following considerations:
• Mebendazole, piperazine, pyrantel pamoate, and thiabendazole are contraindicated for patients who are hypersensitive to them.
• Avoid concomitant administration of piperazine and phenothiazines because of the increased risk of seizures.
• Do not administer piperazine to a patient with epilepsy because of the increased risk of seizures.
• Administer antinematode agents with caution to a patient with liver disease.
• Administer thiabendazole cautiously to a patient with renal dysfunction.
• To ensure correct dosage of agents available in suspension form (pyrantel pamoate and thiabendazole), shake the container well before administering either agent.
• Instruct the patient receiving thiabendazole or mebendazole tablets to chew them for greatest effectiveness.
• Keep in mind that reinfection is a major problem with nematode infection, especially with pinworms. Instruct patients to change and wash underclothes and bedding daily until the nematodes are eradicated; explain that washing the perineal area daily and the hands and fingernails after each bowel movement will also reduce the risk of reinfection.
• Remember that pinworm and other nematode infections may recur unless all family members are treated.
• Instruct the patient receiving thiabendazole to take doses immediately after meals to minimize GI distress.
• Inform the patient taking thiabendazole that urine may smell like asparagus but that the odor has no medical significance.
• Stress the importance of patient compliance with the antinematode agent dosage regimen to prevent treatment failure.

ANTICESTODE AGENTS

All cestode, or tapeworm, infections are acquired by ingestion and most are confined to the intestinal tract. The exception is *Echinococcus granulosus*, which causes hydatid disease with cystic lesions of the liver. If surgery, the treatment of choice, is not indicated, high-dose long-term mebendazole therapy may cure or suppress the infection. Although its use for this disorder is still experimental in the United States, recent reports seem to indicate that it is an effective treatment.

Two other agents, niclosamide and paromomycin sulfate, are used as anticestodes. Niclosamide acts specifically against tapeworm infection. Paromomycin, an aminoglycoside with antiamoebic action, also acts against tapeworms. A third agent, praziquantel, is currently used to treat trematode (fluke) infections, but is gaining wider use for treating tapeworms. The Food and Drug Administration (FDA), however, considers this use investigational.

History and source

Niclosamide, a derivative of the antifungal agent salicylanilide, was tested on *Taenia saginata* (beef tapeworm) in rats by Gönnert in 1960. Further trials showed it to be a highly effective, minimally toxic drug for treating tapeworm infection in humans. Praziquantel is a derivative of a class of compounds discovered in 1972. Its simplified dosage schedule accounts for its selection over paromomycin. Paromomycin is an aminoglycoside antibiotic with antiamoebic and anticestode action. It is now the third choice for treating tapeworm infection, after niclosamide and praziquantel.

PHARMACOKINETICS

Niclosamide and paromomycin are both negligibly absorbed from the GI tract. Therefore, their action against tapeworm infection remains confined to the intestinal tract. Because both drugs act locally in the GI tract, little systemic absorption occurs. Their onset of action, peak concentration levels, and duration of action vary greatly between individuals and indicate only the pharmacokinetics of the systemically absorbed drug. Neither drug is metabolized in the liver or elsewhere; both are excreted, unchanged, in the feces.

PHARMACODYNAMICS

Niclosamide and paromomycin have differing mechanisms of action. Niclosamide interferes with the tapeworm's ability to convert food into energy, either by inhibiting oxidative phosphorylation or by enhancing adenosine triphosphatase activity. Paromomycin is thought to inhibit the tapeworm's protein synthesis by causing misreading of messenger ribonucleic acid.

PHARMACOTHERAPEUTICS

Niclosamide and praziquantel, the emerging drugs of choice, are similarly effective against all varieties of tapeworm infection. The adverse reactions they cause are also similar, however, so neither offers a clear advantage. Paromomycin is an alternate choice if the patient cannot tolerate niclosamide or praziquantel. However, it has a more complex dosage schedule.

mebendazole (Vermox). Primarily an antinematode agent, mebendazole is also used to treat hydatid disease caused by *E. granulosus* (liver tapeworm).
USUAL ADULT AND PEDIATRIC DOSAGE: for liver tapeworm infection (hydatid disease), 13.3 to 16.7 mg/kg P.O. t.i.d. for 1 to 6 months. The dosage for children under age 2 has not been established.

niclosamide (Niclocide). Active against all intestinal tapeworm species, niclosamide tablets should be chewed thoroughly and taken with water after a light meal.
USUAL ADULT DOSAGE: for *Hymenolepsis nana* (dwarf tapeworm) infection, 2 grams P.O. once daily for 7 days or 2 grams P.O. for the first day and 1 gram P.O. for the next 6 days, repeated in 7 to 14 days, if needed; for *T. saginata* and *T. solium* infections, 2 grams P.O. as a single dose, repeated in 7 days if needed.
USUAL PEDIATRIC DOSAGE: for *H. nana*, 1 gram P.O. the first day and 500 mg P.O. the next 6 days for children who weigh from 11 to 34 kg, and 1.5 grams P.O. the first day and 1 gram P.O. the next 6 days (may be repeated in 7 to 14 days) for children who weigh more than 34 kg; for *T. saginata* or *T. solium* infections, 1 gram P.O. as a single dose for children who weigh from 11 to 34 kg, and 1.5 grams P.O. as a single dose (may be repeated in 7 days) for children who weigh more than 34 kg.

paromomycin sulfate (Humatin). Available as 250-mg capsules, paromomycin is considered by the FDA an investigational drug for treating tapeworm infections.
USUAL ADULT AND PEDIATRIC DOSAGE: for tapeworm infection, 25 to 35 mg/kg P.O. daily in three divided doses with meals for 5 to 10 days; for *H. nana* (dwarf tapeworm) infection, 45 mg/kg P.O. daily for 5 to 7 days.

praziquantel (Biltricide). Primarily an antitrematode agent, praziquantel is fast becoming a drug of choice for treating tapeworm infections.
USUAL ADULT AND PEDIATRIC DOSAGE: for *Taenia* infection, 10 to 25 mg/kg P.O. as a single dose; for *H. nana* infection, 25 mg/kg P.O. as a single dose that may be repeated in 1 to 2 weeks.

Drug interactions

No significant drug interactions involving niclosamide or paromomycin are known to occur.

ADVERSE DRUG REACTIONS

Adverse reactions to niclosamide are uncommon. They include nausea and abdominal pain; rarely, a hypersensitivity-like reaction may occur, producing headache, rash, or vertigo. Paromomycin's main adverse reactions affect the GI tract and include anorexia, nausea, vomiting, cramps, and diarrhea. Secondary infection of the intestinal tract may also occur. Theoretically, paromomycin could cause aminoglycoside-like nephrotoxicity or ototoxicity in patients with renal impairment; however, this has not been reported.

NURSING IMPLICATIONS

Tapeworm infections are the simplest of all helminth infections to treat, with few adverse reactions and contraindications. Nevertheless, the nurse must be aware of the following considerations:
• Remember that anticestode agents are contraindicated in patients with a history of hypersensitivity to them.
• Bear in mind that a hypersensitivity-like reaction may be a reaction to the antigens released from microfilaria (prelarval form of the worms) rather than to the drug

itself. This is an important factor in determining whether or not a patient is hypersensitive to the drug.

• Instruct the patient receiving niclosamide therapy to chew the tablets thoroughly and then drink water.

• Do not administer paromomycin to patients with renal insufficiency, because accumulated blood levels of the drug may cause ototoxicity or nephrotoxicity.

• Stress the importance of patient compliance with anticestode therapy, to prevent treatment failure.

• For patients on high-dose mebendazole therapy for systemic (hydatid) disease, monitor their complete blood count regularly to detect agranulocytosis, neutropenia, or leukopenia.

ANTITREMATODE AGENTS

Trematode, or fluke, infections are characterized according to their anatomic location: the blood, lungs, or liver. In endemic areas, fluke infections can be devastating, giving rise to many seemingly unrelated disorders such as hepatic cirrhosis, esophageal varices, pulmonary fibrosis, and cor pulmonale. The two drugs available to treat fluke infections are oxamniquine and praziquantel.

History and source

Oxamniquine is the most effective drug among a series of related compounds developed in the 1960s to treat schistosomiasis (blood fluke infection); however, it is no longer a drug of choice for treating fluke infections. Praziquantel is a derivative of a class of compounds that, in 1972, were found to have broad anthelmintic action; praziquantel is particularly effective against fluke infections that cause severe morbidity and mortality. Before the discovery of praziquantel, the drugs used had limited effectiveness against only one or two fluke strains.

PHARMACOKINETICS

Both oxamniquine and praziquantel, administered orally, are effective against systemic fluke infections.

Absorption, distribution, metabolism, excretion

Oxamniquine is well absorbed from the GI tract after oral administration, although the presence of food in the stomach interferes with both the rate and amount of absorption. Some of the drug is metabolized by the intestinal mucosa, but most is metabolized in the liver and excreted by the kidneys. Praziquantel is also readily absorbed (over 80%) after oral administration. It is distributed widely, crossing the blood-brain barrier. Praziquantel undergoes hepatic metabolism, and its metabolites are excreted in the urine.

Onset, peak, duration

Oxamniquine reaches peak plasma concentration levels within 3 hours after oral administration, whereas praziquantel reaches peak concentration levels within 1 to 2 hours. As with the other anthelmintic agents, the antitrematode agents act locally. Therefore, their onset of action, peak concentration levels, and duration of action, which relate to systemic absorption, do not indicate their therapeutic effect.

PHARMACODYNAMICS

Praziquantel has a known mechanism of action; oxamniquine's mechanism of action remains largely unknown.

Mechanism of action

Oxamniquine's known anticholinergic activity does not explain its antitrematode action. Oxamniquine is known, however, to induce schistosomes (blood fluke adults) to migrate from the mesenteric veins into the liver, where they eventually die. Praziquantel, like the antinematode agent pyrantel pamoate, causes spastic paralysis of the fluke's musculature; eventually, it disintegrates.

PHARMACOTHERAPEUTICS

Oxamniquine is no longer a drug of choice to treat fluke infections. It is effective against only one variety of blood fluke, *Schistosoma mansoni*, and its adverse reactions are significant, though rare. Praziquantel has swiftly become the drug of choice for all fluke infections because of its broad spectrum of action.

oxamniquine (Vansil). Available as a 250-mg capsule, oxamniquine is indicated for *S. mansoni*; it is ineffective against the other blood fluke species and fluke infections.
USUAL ADULT DOSAGE: for Western Hemisphere strains, 15 mg/kg P.O. as a one-time dose; for West African strains, 15 mg/kg P.O. b.i.d. for 2 days; for South American strains, 7.5 mg/kg I.M. as a single dose.
USUAL PEDIATRIC DOSAGE: for children who have Western Hemisphere strains and who weigh less than 30 kg, 10 mg/kg P.O. for two doses given 2 to 8 hours apart; the adult dosage applies for children who weigh more than 30 kg.

Anthelmintic agents

This chart summarizes the anthelmintic agents currently in clinical use.

DRUG	MAJOR INDICATIONS	USUAL ADULT DOSAGES	NURSING IMPLICATIONS
Antinematode agents			
mebendazole	*Ascaris* (roundworm), *Trichuris* (whipworm), and *Necator* (hookworm) infections	100 mg P.O. b.i.d. for 3 days	• Instruct the patient to chew the tablet to enhance mebendazole's effectiveness. • Stress attention to personal hygiene: hand washing and changing of underclothes and bedding daily.
	Enterobius (pinworm) infection	100 mg P.O. once; may be repeated in 2 to 3 weeks	
piperazine citrate	*Ascaris* (roundworm) infection	75 mg/kg (maximum of 3.5 grams/day) P.O. daily for 2 days	• Do not administer concomitantly with phenothiazines or other agents that lower seizure thresholds. • Piperazine is contraindicated in patients with epilepsy.
pyrantel pamoate	*Ascaris* (roundworm), *Necator* (hookworm), and *Enterobius* (pinworm) infections	11 mg/kg P.O. as a one-time dose to a maximum of 1 gram; may be repeated in 2 to 3 weeks	• Shake the suspension well to ensure the correct dosage. • Stress attention to personal hygiene.
thiabendazole	*Strongyloides stercoralis* (roundworm) infection	25 mg/kg (maximum of 3 grams/day) P.O. b.i.d. for 2 days	• Tell the patient to chew the tablets well or to shake suspension well before taking each dose. • Administer after meals to minimize immediate GI adverse reactions. • Prepare the patient for an asparagus-like urine odor while taking thiabendazole.
Anticestode agents			
praziquantel	*Taenia* infections	10 to 25 mg/kg P.O. as a single dose	• Halve or quarter the tablets to prepare an exact dose. • Instruct the patient to swallow the tablet whole; praziquantel is bitter and may cause gagging or vomiting if held in the mouth or chewed. • Caution the patient that the drug may cause drowsiness for 48 hours after beginning therapy.
	Hymenolepsis nana infection	25 mg/kg P.O. as a single dose; may be repeated in 1 to 2 weeks	
Antitrematode agents			
praziquantel	*Schistosoma* infections	20 mg/kg P.O. t.i.d. for 1 day	• Halve or quarter the tablets to prepare an exact dose. • Instruct the patient to swallow the tablets whole; praziquantel is bitter and may cause gagging or vomiting if held in the mouth or chewed. • Caution the patient that the drug may cause drowsiness for 48 hours after beginning therapy.
	Clonorchis infections	25 mg/kg P.O. t.i.d. for 1 to 3 days	
	Paragonimus infections	25 mg/kg P.O. t.i.d. for 1 to 2 days	

praziquantel (Biltricide). The first highly effective broad-spectrum antitrematode agent, praziquantel is the drug of choice for treating all fluke infections.

USUAL ADULT AND PEDIATRIC DOSAGE: for *Schistosoma* infections, 20 mg/kg P.O. t.i.d. for 1 day; for *Paragonimus* infections, 25 mg/kg P.O. t.i.d. for 1 to 2 days; for *Clonorchis* infections, 25 mg/kg P.O. t.i.d. for 1 to 3 days. The dosage for children under age 4 has not been established.

Drug interactions

The only significant drug interaction with this class of drugs involves interaction between the two antitrematode agents. One animal study indicated that concomitant administration of oxamniquine and praziquantel may enhance their effectiveness against *S. mansoni* (blood fluke). This is a preliminary finding, however; more studies are needed to determine its clinical relevance.

ADVERSE DRUG REACTIONS

Both oxamniquine and praziquantel have low human toxicity compared to their effects on target flukes. In about one third of patients, both agents cause transient drowsiness, dizziness, headache, nausea, and diarrhea. Praziquantel may also cause macular rash with pruritus. The most significant adverse reaction to oxamniquine is rare central nervous system (CNS) stimulation causing behavioral changes, seizures, or hallucinations. (The seizures usually occur in patients with a history of epilepsy.) Oxamniquine also causes orange-red urine that has no clinical significance but may alarm the patient and interfere with laboratory tests based on spectrometry or color reactions. Both drugs may be embryocidal or abortifacient, so they are contraindicated in pregnant patients. Some patients may experience a hypersensitivity reaction to the drugs.

NURSING IMPLICATIONS

When administering oxamniquine and praziquantel to patients with fluke infections, the nurse must keep the following considerations in mind:

• Remember that these agents, which may be embryocidal or abortifacient, are contraindicated in pregnant patients.

• Give oxamniquine as a single dose after meals to help prevent GI adverse reactions.

• Monitor for CNS adverse reactions in patients taking oxamniquine; seizures, although rare, occur most frequently in patients with a history of epilepsy.

• Inform the patient taking oxamniquine that the urine may turn orange or red.

• Caution the patient taking oxamniquine or praziquantel that drowsiness and dizziness may occur, necessitating curtailment of activities on the day of treatment and the day after.

• Remind patients taking praziquantel to take the tablet with meals to minimize adverse reactions; explain that the tablet is bitter and should be swallowed rapidly, or it may cause gagging or vomiting.

CHAPTER SUMMARY

Chapter 70 discussed the anthelmintic agents as they are used to treat nematode (roundworm), cestode (tapeworm), and trematode (fluke) infections. Here are the highlights of the chapter:

• Anthelmintic agents are categorized according to the helminth groups they combat most effectively. The three major classes of anthelmintic agents are antinematode (antiroundworm), anticestode (antitapeworm), and antitrematode (antifluke) agents.

• Two anthelmintic agents are used to treat more than one type of helminth infection: mebendazole is used to treat roundworm infections and a systemic tapeworm infection (hydatid disease) as well, and praziquantel is becoming the alternate drug of choice for all tapeworm infections besides its use as an antitrematode agent.

• The anthelmintic agents act primarily by disrupting the helminths' energy use or neurologic function.

• The anthelmintic agents' toxicities vary widely. Most of these agents cause GI signs and symptoms, and CNS, hepatic, and skin adverse reactions may also occur. Some of the toxicity attributed to the anticestode agents may actually represent reaction to the release of antigens when the tapeworms die.

• Helminth superinfection is not a major factor in treatment failure, as are patient noncompliance and reinfection.

BIBLIOGRAPHY

Abramowicz, M., ed. "Drugs for Parasitic Infections," *Medical Letter on Drugs and Therapeutics* 28:9, 1986.

American Hospital Formulary Service. *Drug Information 87.* McEvoy, G.K., ed. Bethesda, Md.: American Society of Hospital Pharmacists, 1987.

Davidson, R.A. "Issues in Clinical Parasitology: The Management of Hydatid Cyst," *American Journal of Gastroenterology* 79:397, May 1984.

Gilman, A.G., et al. *Goodman and Gilman's The Pharmacological Basis of Therapeutics*, 7th ed. New York: Macmillan Publishing Co., 1985.

Grove, D.I. "Treatment of Strongyloidiasis with Thiabendazole: An Analysis of Toxicity and Effectiveness," *Transactions of the Royal Society of Tropical Medicine and Hygiene* 76:114, 1982.

Hansten, P.D. *Drug Interactions*, 5th ed. Philadelphia: Lea & Febiger, 1985.

Kammerer, W.S., and Schantz, P.M. "Long-Term Follow-Up of Human Hydatid Disease (*Echinococcus granulosus*) Treated with a High-Dose Mebendazole Regimen," *American Journal of Tropical Medicine and Hygiene* 33:132, January 1984.

Katz, M. "Anthelmintics: Current Concepts in the Treatment of Helminthic Infections," *Drugs* 32:358, October 1986.

Katzung, B.G. *Basic and Clinical Pharmacology*, 3rd ed. East Norwalk, Conn.: Appleton & Lange, 1987.

Keystone, J.S., and Murdoch, J.K. "Mebendazole," *Annals of Internal Medicine* 91:582, October 1979.

Mandel, G.L., et al. *Principles and Practice of Infectious Diseases*, 2nd ed. New York: John Wiley & Sons, 1985.

Pearson, R.D., and Hewlett, E.L. "Niclosamide Therapy for Tapeworm Infections," *Annals of Internal Medicine* 102:550, April 1985.

Reynolds, J.E.F., ed. *Martindale: The Extra Pharmacopoeia*, 28th ed. London: The Pharmaceutical Press, 1982.

Seidel, J.S. "Treatment of Parasitic Infections," *Pediatric Clinics of North America* 32:1077, August 1985.

Warren, J.S., and Mahmoud, A.A.F., eds. *Tropical and Geographical Medicine*. New York: McGraw-Hill Book Co., 1984.

CHAPTER 71

ANTIMALARIAL AND OTHER ANTIPROTOZOAL AGENTS

OBJECTIVES

After reading and studying this chapter, you should be able to:

1. Discuss the major prophylactic and therapeutic indications for antimalarial agents and the major therapeutic indications for other antiprotozoal agents.

2. Discuss why some antiprotozoal agents require dosage adjustments for a patient with hepatic or renal disease.

3. Discuss the most frequent adverse effects of antimalarial and antiprotozoal agents, and explain how to minimize them during therapy.

4. Identify the contraindications for administering antiprotozoal agents.

5. Describe potential interactions between antimalarial or antiprotozoal agents and other drugs.

6. Explain how to monitor the patient receiving antiprotozoal therapy.

7. Identify alternate treatments if the antimalarial or antiprotozoal agent of choice is unavailable or contraindicated.

INTRODUCTION

Protozoal diseases, including malaria, have assumed critical importance in the United States for several reasons. An increase in the incidence and type of immune disorders that make the patient more susceptible to protozoal invasion, immigration from areas where protozoal diseases are endemic, and travel by Americans to those areas have all sharpened physicians' and nurses' focus on protozoal diseases and produced an increased need for effective antiprotozoal drugs. This chapter will discuss the most frequently used antimalarial and antiprotozoal drugs and their indications.

For a summary of representative drugs, see *Selected major drugs: Antimalarial and other antiprotozoal agents* on pages 1133 and 1134.

ANTIMALARIAL AGENTS

The major agents used to prevent and treat malaria are quinine sulfate, pyrimethamine, the 4-aminoquinolones (chloroquine phosphate, chloroquine hydrochloride, and hydroxychloroquine sulfate) and the 8-aminoquinolone primaquine phosphate. The sulfonamides, sulfones, and tetracyclines may also be used in combination with these agents. (See Chapter 66, Antibacterial Agents, for information about these ancillary antimalarial agents.)

Four parasites can transmit malaria to humans: *Plasmodium falciparum, P. malariae, P. ovale,* and *P. vivax.* Although their life cycles vary, all four species transmit malaria in the same way. (See *The malaria transmission cycle* on page 1124 for a description of this process.) Because drug therapy and drug resistance vary among species, the development of more powerful antimalarials continues.

History and source

Quinine is the major alkaloid of the South American Cinchona tree, also known as the fever tree. For more than two centuries, the tree's whole bark was used to treat malaria. Finally in 1820, researchers isolated the quinine and cinchonine alkaloids, which were the only antimalarials available until World War I. Chloroquine, hydroxychloroquine, and primaquine are synthetic compounds discovered during World War II in an attempt to find agents more effective and less toxic than quinine. Pyrimethamine, a synthetic drug originally developed as an antibacterial agent, was later found to possess antimalarial properties.

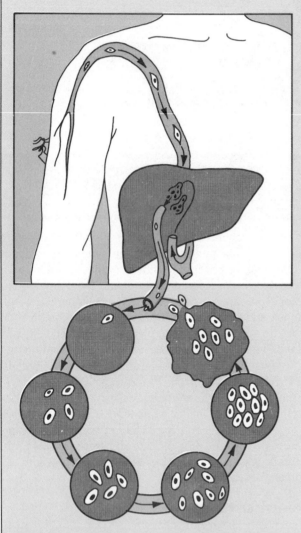

The malaria transmission cycle

When the carrier mosquito (genus *Anopheles*) draws blood from an infected person, it picks up malarial parasites. The mosquito bites the next victim **(A)** and infects that person with the parasites, which enter the bloodstream and travel to the liver.

Each parasite invades a separate liver cell, then multiplies, rupturing the host cell **(B)**.

Ten to fourteen days later, the parasites leave the liver and invade the red blood cells, where they feed on hemoglobin **(C)**.

They multiply again and rupture the cells **(D)**. At this stage, the victim experiences the symptoms of malaria: backache, chills, fever, and severe headache.

Free parasites enter other red blood cells to multiply again. Any mosquito that feeds on the victim may become infected, beginning a new transmission cycle.

PHARMACOKINETICS

After oral administration, the antimalarial agents are well absorbed and widely distributed throughout the body. The extent of metabolism among these agents varies, and excretion occurs primarily through the urine.

Absorption, distribution, metabolism, excretion

Quinine is almost completely absorbed from the gastro-intestinal (GI) tract. About 70% protein-bound, it is well distributed throughout the body. It readily crosses the placenta and appears in breast milk. Quinine and its alkaloids are extensively metabolized in the liver and excreted in the urine.

Chloroquine is also well absorbed from the GI tract, but only about 55% of it is serum protein-bound. Widely distributed, chloroquine appears in high concentrations in the liver, spleen, kidneys, lungs, heart, brain, melanin-containing tissues, and erythrocytes. It binds to platelets and granulocytes. Serum and tissue concentrations of chloroquine are higher than those in plasma. Low concentrations are found in the central nervous system (CNS) and in breast milk, and it appears to cross the placenta. Chloroquine is partially metabolized in the liver and slowly excreted in the urine: up to 70% of an oral dose may be excreted as unchanged drug. Hydroxy-chloroquine's pharmacokinetics are believed similar to chloroquine's except for metabolite formation.

After oral administration, primaquine is well absorbed from the GI tract. Little is known about its pharmacokinetics, but the drug is thought to be widely distributed with small concentrations appearing in the liver, lungs, heart, and skeletal muscles. Primaquine is rapidly metabolized in the liver and excreted in urine. Only about 1% of an oral dose is excreted unchanged.

Pyrimethamine is almost completely absorbed from the GI tract after oral administration. Approximately 80% protein-bound, this drug is widely distributed to the kidneys, lungs, liver, and spleen. Pyrimethamine also appears in breast milk. Although its metabolism and excretion are not well defined, pyrimethamine appears to be partially metabolized in the liver and excreted in urine.

Onset, peak, duration

Peak plasma concentrations of quinine usually occur 1 to 3 hours after oral administration. When therapy is discontinued, plasma concentrations decline to negligible levels within 24 hours. Both the drug's plasma concentrations and its half-life may be prolonged in a patient with impaired hepatic function accompanying active malaria. The half-life of quinine varies from 8 to 21 hours in patients with active malaria, and from 4 to 12 hours in healthy adults.

Because chloroquine is rapidly absorbed into the bloodstream, plasma concentrations occur 1 to 2 hours after oral administration. The half-life of chloroquine ranges from 72 to 120 hours in a healthy adult. Hydroxychloroquine is thought to act in a similar manner.

After oral administration, plasma concentrations of primaquine usually peak within 3 hours. The drug's plasma half-life varies greatly, ranging from 3.7 to 9.6 hours.

Peak plasma concentrations of pyrimethamine usually occur within 2 hours of oral administration. Its half-life is approximately 4 days.

PHARMACODYNAMICS

Although their exact mechanisms of action are not well understood, antimalarial agents seem to work in differing ways to kill malarial parasites or inhibit their reproduction. For instance, quinine, chloroquine, and hydroxychloroquine appear to work by interfering with protozoal deoxyribonucleic acid (DNA). Primaquine may disrupt cellular metabolism, and pyrimethamine appears to inhibit dihydrofolate reductase.

Mechanism of action

Quinine has diverse pharmacologic properties. Its antimalarial action may result from incorporation into the parasite's DNA, rendering it ineffective. Its action may also result from depression of the parasite's oxygen uptake and carbohydrate metabolism. In addition, quinine acts as a skeletal muscle relaxant, a local anesthetic, an antipyretic, and an analgesic, thus relieving malarial symptoms.

Chloroquine and hydroxychloroquine are thought to disrupt parasite protein synthesis. Also, the drugs may concentrate in the parasite's digestive vacuoles, increasing pH and and interfering with utilization of hemoglobin.

Primaquine appears to affect the parasite's mitochondria, eventually disrupting cellular metabolism.

Pyrimethamine selectively inhibits the enzyme dihydrofolate reductase, which impedes folic acid reduction and ultimately disrupts parasitic reproduction.

PHARMACOTHERAPEUTICS

The prevention and treatment of malaria is a continually changing process, primarily because of *P. falciparum's* increasing resistance to antimalarial drugs. Varying degrees of chloroquine resistance exist in parts of Africa, South America, Asia, India, and the South Pacific.

Yet chloroquine remains the drug of choice to prevent and treat all malaria strains, except chloroquine-resistant or multidrug-resistant strains of *P. falciparum*.

Hydroxychloroquine serves as an alternative when chloroquine is not available.

For acute attacks of chloroquine-resistant or multidrug-resistant strains of *P. falciparum*, quinine is the drug of choice and is given in combination with slower-acting antimalarial agents. Primaquine is the drug of choice to prevent *P. vivax* or *P. ovale* malaria relapse and during the last 2 weeks of several prophylactic regimens.

Pyrimethamine is used alone or with sulfadoxine (Fansidar) to prevent chloroquine-resistant malaria. However, the United States Centers for Disease Control (CDC) recommends that the pyrimethamine-sulfadoxine combination be used for prophylaxis only when the risk of chloroquine-resistant *P. falciparium* is high because of some fatalities that have occurred with use of this combination.

quinine sulfate (Quinamm, Strema) and **quinine dihydrochloride.** Available in tablets and capsules as quinine sulfate or in injection form as quinine dihydrochloride, quinine sulfate is the drug of choice for a patient with chloroquine-resistant *P. falciparum* malaria. If the patient cannot tolerate oral quinine sulfate, an I.V. preparation of quinine dihydrochloride may be obtained from the CDC. The I.V. form is also used for any patient with malaria who needs parenteral therapy. USUAL ADULT DOSAGE: 650 mg P.O. t.i.d. for 3 days given with pyrimethamine and sulfadiazine. Tetracycline may be substituted for pyrimethamine and sulfadiazine. The dihydrochloride salt dosage is 600 mg I.V. in 300 ml of normal saline solution given over 2 to 4 hours and repeated every 8 hours until oral therapy can begin; the maximum daily I.V. dose is 1,800 mg.

chloroquine hydrochloride/chloroquine phosphate (Aralen). Available in tablets as chloroquine phosphate or in injection form as chloroquine hydrochloride, chloroquine is the drug of choice to prevent and treat all types of malaria except for that caused by chloroquine-resistant *P. falciparum*. Chloroquine also serves as an adjunct in the management of hepatic abscess caused by *Entamoeba histolytica*.
USUAL ADULT DOSAGE: for preventing malaria in a person traveling to an area where chloroquine-resistant *P. falciparum* is not prevalent, 500 mg P.O. once a week for 1 week before departure and for 6 weeks after returning; for preventing malaria in a person traveling to an area where exposure to chloroquine-resistant *P. falciparum* is a moderate to high risk, 500 mg P.O. with 25 mg of pyrimethamine and 500 mg of sulfadoxine once a week for 1 week before departure and for 6 weeks after returning; for treating malaria caused by *P. malariae, P. ovale, P. vivax*, or susceptible strains of *P.*

DRUG INTERACTIONS

Antimalarial agents

Antimalarial agents can produce a variety of interactions. The most serious are additive, occurring with concomitant adminis-tration of drugs that produce similar adverse reactions.

DRUG	INTERACTING DRUGS	POSSIBLE EFFECTS	NURSING IMPLICATIONS
quinine	antacids that contain alu-minum	Delay or decrease quinine absorption	• Separate antacid doses as far as possible from quinine doses if these drugs must be used concomitantly.
	neuromuscular blocking agents (pancuronium, tub-ocurarine, succinylcholine)	Produce neuromuscular blockade, which may lead to respiratory arrest	• Monitor the patient's respirations. • Have emergency resuscitation equipment available. • Monitor the patient's arterial blood gases, as needed.
	oral anticoagulants (war-farin type)	Enhance hypoprothrom-binemia	• Monitor a patient receiving an oral anticoag-ulant for altered anticoagulant effect when qui-nine therapy begins or ends.
	cardiac glycosides (di-goxin, digitoxin)	Increase plasma levels of glycosides	• Monitor the patient's blood levels of cardiac glycosides, and adjust the dosages as or-dered.
chloroquine	oral antacids that contain magnesium trisilicate	Decrease chloroquine ab-sorption	• Separate antacid doses as far as possible from chloroquine doses if these drugs must be used concomitantly.
hydroxychloroquine	digoxin	Elevates digoxin levels	• Monitor a patient's serum digoxin level when hydroxychloroquine therapy begins or ends.
primaquine	quinacrine	Increases toxicity of pri-maquine	• Monitor the patient for adverse effects.
pyrimethamine	folic acid	Inhibits antimicrobial effect	• Monitor the patient for a decreased thera-peutic effect.

falciparum, 1 g P.O. initially, followed by 500 mg at 6, 24, and 48 hours (or 250 mg I.M. every 6 hours in a seriously ill patient). An infection caused by *P. vivax* or *P. ovale* will require concomitant or follow-up treatment with primaquine to prevent a relapse. For treating he-patic abscess caused by *E. histolytica,* after emetine hy-drochloride therapy, the dosage is 1 g P.O. daily for 2 days followed by 500 mg daily for 2 to 3 weeks with iodoquinol [diiodohydroxyquin].

hydroxychloroquine sulfate (Plaquenil Sulfate). When chloroquine is not available, this drug may be used to prevent and treat malaria caused by chloroquine-susceptible strains. A 400-mg dose of hydroxychloro-quine sulfate equals 500 mg of chloroquine sulfate.
USUAL ADULT DOSAGE: for preventing malaria in a per-son traveling to an endemic area, 400 mg P.O. once a week for 1 week before departure and for 6 weeks after

returning; for treating chloroquine-susceptible malaria, 800 mg P.O. initially, followed by 400 mg at 6, 24, and 48 hours.

primaquine phosphate. Available in tablets, primaquine is used to prevent *P. ovale* and *P. vivax* infection and relapse. It can also eliminate hepatic forms of the parasite not eradicated by chloroquine.
USUAL ADULT DOSAGE: to prevent infection, 26.3 mg P.O. daily for 14 days with last two weeks of chloroquine prophylaxis; or to prevent relapse, 79 mg P.O. once a week for 8 weeks or 26.3 mg P.O. daily for 14 days.

pyrimethamine (Daraprim). This drug is used to prevent and treat chloroquine-resistant malaria and to treat tox-oplasmosis. It is available alone in tablet form or in com-bination with sulfadoxine.
USUAL ADULT DOSAGE: for preventing chloroquine-resistant *P. falciparum* malaria in areas where the risk

Antimalarial agents: Summary of adverse reactions

This chart summarizes the adverse reactions to antimalarial agents, grouping them by frequency. Most of the adverse reactions result from high doses.

DRUG	COMMON	OCCASIONAL	RARE
quinine	Mild cinchonism	Moderate cinchonism, thrombocytopenic purpura, hypoprothrombinemia, hemolytic anemia, hearing disturbances, ventricular tachycardia, angina, fever, apprehension, hypothermia, restlessness, confusion, syncope, excitement, delirium	Severe cinchonism, granulocytopenia, optic atrophy, hepatitis, hypoglycemia, deafness, hypersensitivity reaction
chloroquine, hydroxychloroquine	Epigastric discomfort, anorexia, nausea, vomiting, abdominal cramps, diarrhea	Blurred vision, difficulty in focusing, corneal inclusions, corneal changes, skin rash, pruritus, changes in skin and mucosal pigment, hair bleaching, headache, fatigue, nervousness, anxiety, irritability, personality changes	Retinal changes, exfoliative dermatitis, psychotic episodes, seizures, hypotension, EKG changes, ototoxicity, tinnitus, neutropenia, granulocytopenia, aplastic anemia, thrombocytopenia, hemolytic anemia, neuropathy, neuromyopathy, hypersensitivity reaction
primaquine	Nausea, vomiting, epigastric distress, abdominal cramps	Headache, difficulty in focusing, pruritus, hemolytic anemia, methemoglobinemia, mild anemia, leukocytosis, leukopenia	Hypertension, dysrhythmias, granulocytopenia, extreme mental confusion, hypersensitivity reaction
pyrimethamine	Anorexia, vomiting, abdominal cramps	Megaloblastic anemia, leukopenia, thrombocytopenia, ataxia, tremors	Granulocytopenia, hemolytic anemia, seizures, respiratory failure, photosensitivity, malaise, fatigue, irritability, hypersensitivity reaction

of exposure is high, 25 mg P.O. of pyrimethamine and 500 mg P.O. of sulfadoxine once a week in addition to the standard prophylactic chloroquine regimen; for treating chloroquine-resistant *P. falciparum* malaria, 25 mg P.O. b.i.d. for 3 days with 500 mg of sulfadiazine q.i.d. for 5 days with quinine sulfate; for treating toxoplasmosis, 25 mg P.O. daily with 1 gram of sulfadiazine q.i.d. for 3 to 4 weeks.

Drug interactions

A variety of interactions can occur between antimalarial agents and other drugs. Many result from decreased absorption from the GI tract, from concomitant administration of other drugs that cause similar adverse effects, or protein binding displacement leading to elevated serum concentrations of the drug. (See *Drug interactions: Antimalarial agents* for further information.)

ADVERSE DRUG REACTIONS

In the low dosages used to prevent or treat malaria, these agents usually produce few serious adverse reactions. (See *Antimalarial agents: Summary of adverse reactions* for information about other adverse effects.)

Predictable reactions

GI complaints are the most common adverse reactions to the antimalarial agents. Adverse ocular effects have been reported for the 4-aminoquinolones, quinine, and primaquine. Cardiovascular reactions are most prominent with the administration of intravenous quinine. CNS reactions have been attributed to all these agents, and a unique toxic syndrome known as cinchonism can be seen with quinine.

Unpredictable reactions

Agranulocytosis can occur but is rare. Reported hypersensitivity reactions, which can range from mild to life-threatening, include severe bronchospasm, and skin reactions such as exfoliative dermatitis; Stevens-Johnson syndrome; and toxic epidermal necrolysis.

NURSING IMPLICATIONS

Because antimalarial therapy is complex, the nurse must carefully consider the contraindications for these agents and the guidelines for monitoring drug therapy.

• Quinine is contraindicated for a patient with a known hypersensitivity to the drug or a known or suspected history of glucose 6-phosphate dehydrogenase (G6PD) deficiency, thrombocytopenic purpura, Blackwater Fever (a complication of chronic *P. falciparum* malaria), tinnitus, or optic neuritis.

• Administer quinine cautiously to a patient with atrial fibrillation, and administer it by slow I.V. infusion to avoid adverse cardiovascular effects, such as severe hypotension, dysrhythmias, and acute circulatory failure.

• Chloroquine and hydroxychloroquine are contraindicated in a patient with a known hypersensitivity to them or with known retinal or visual field changes. Monitor routine eye examinations for a patient on long-term therapy, and advise the patient to report any vision or hearing disturbances.

• Administer chloroquine cautiously to a patient who has hepatic disease, alcoholism, or takes other hepatotoxic agents; because chloroquine is concentrated in the liver, it may cause further liver damage.

• Monitor a patient on long-term chloroquine therapy for signs of muscular weakness, and monitor the patient's complete blood count (CBC) regularly.

• Monitor a patient with a history of G6PD deficiency for signs of hemolysis.

• Avoid using chloroquine in a patient with psoriasis or porphyria, because it can exacerbate these disorders. Advise a patient who is receiving any other dermatitis-inducing medication that concomitant chloroquine use may provoke an adverse skin reaction.

• Primaquine is contraindicated in an acutely ill patient with a systemic disease that tends to produce granulocytopenia, such as active rheumatoid arthritis or systemic lupus erythematosus.

• Administer primaquine with extreme caution to a patient with a history of hypersensitivity to it or with a history of G6PD deficiency or nicotinamide-adenine dinucleotide (NAD) methemoglobin-reductase deficiency.

• Instruct the patient receiving primaquine to take the drug with food to minimize GI adverse reactions.

• Pyrimethamine is contraindicated in a patient with megaloblastic anemia from a folate deficiency.

• Monitor routine blood and platelet counts for a patient receiving pyrimethamine for toxoplasmosis, because the dosage may approach the toxic level.

• Initiate pyrimethamine therapy with caution for a patient with a history of a seizure disorder, to minimize CNS toxicity.

• Administer a pyrimethamine-sulfadoxine combination cautiously to a patient with impaired renal or hepatic function. Instruct the patient to maintain adequate fluid intake to avoid crystalluria and calculus formation. Also advise the patient to discontinue the medication and seek immediate medical attention if a sore throat, or pallor, fever, purpura, jaundice, erythema, rash, or glossitis appears.

• Instruct the patient to take quinine with meals to minimize GI adverse reactions. Describe the common adverse reactions and advise the patient to report any that become pronounced. Because quinine may produce blurred vision or dizziness, advise the patient not to drive or operate dangerous machinery.

• Explain to the patient that children are extremely sensitive to chloroquine and hydroxychloroquine and that accidental ingestion can cause death. Instruct the patient to keep these and all other medications out of the reach of children.

OTHER ANTIPROTOZOAL AGENTS

Physicians use many agents to treat protozoal infections, including some investigational new drugs (INDs) that can only be obtained from the CDC. These INDs include dehydroemetine, diloxanide furoate (Furamide), melarsoprol (Mel B, Arsobal), nifurtimox (Bayer 2502, Lampit), spiramycin (Rovamycin), stibogluconate sodium (Pentostam), suramin sodium (Germanin), and typarsamide.

Besides these INDs, paromomycin, co-trimoxazole, and amphotericin B are sometimes used as antiprotozoals. None of these drugs will be discussed in this chapter. (See Chapter 66, Antibacterial Agents, and Chapter 69, Antimycotic [Antifungal] Agents, for information about these drugs.) Instead, this chapter will focus on the readily obtainable antiprotozoal agents: pentamidine isethionate, metronidazole, iodoquinol, emetine, quinacrine hydrochloride, and furazolidone.

History and source
Pentamidine's antiprotozoal effects were discovered in the late 1930s. It was first used in the tropics to treat African trypanosomiasis and leishmaniasis in the 1940s.

Almost a decade later, pentamidine was introduced in Europe to treat *Pneumocystis carinii* pneumonia. In 1984, it became commercially available in the United States.

Cosar and Julou first reported the trichomonacidal and amebicidal properties of metronidazole (a synthetic nitroimidazole derivative) in 1959. In the following year, Durel and colleagues demonstrated its clinical use in patients with trichomoniasis. Since then, metronidazole has demonstrated an extremely broad range of antiprotozoal and antimicrobial activity.

Tenney and Craign investigated iodoquinol's effectiveness as a luminal amebicide in the 1930s and 1940s. Unfortunately, the indiscriminate use of iodoquinol to treat diarrhea led to a high incidence of adverse effects, and the drug's popularity waned.

Vedder first demonstrated emetine's ability to kill amoebas in 1912. Since then, emetine has been widely used to treat amoebic diseases.

Quinacrine was developed in Germany during World War I by Mauss and Mietzsch. During World War II, it became the drug of choice for treating malaria, but its popularity later declined because of its toxicity and ineffectiveness as a prophylactic agent. Historically, quinacrine has also been used to treat many parasitic infections, including tapeworm, giardiasis, amebiasis, and trichomoniasis. Today, quinacrine has been largely replaced by more effective, less toxic agents.

Furazolidone was studied extensively as an antibacterial by Dodd and Stillman in 1944. Later studies revealed its antiprotozoal activity and led to its current use in treating giardiasis.

PHARMACOKINETICS

The pharmacokinetic processes of the antiprotozoal agents vary widely and have not been completely defined.

Absorption, distribution, metabolism, excretion

Little is known about the pharmacokinetics of pentamidine after I.V. administration, although some evidence suggests that it is well absorbed after I.M. administration. Its distribution is not well understood, but research suggests that it is well distributed and/or highly protein-bound. It is probably not metabolized but excreted unchanged in the urine and feces.

After oral administration, 80% to 90% of a metronidazole dose is absorbed. It is widely distributed and reaches therapeutic concentrations in vaginal tissue, bone, saliva, and bile; in seminal, pleural, peritoneal, and cerebrospinal fluids; and in hepatic and cerebral abscesses. Less than 20% of metronidazole is protein-bound. It readily crosses the placenta and is well dis-

tributed in breast milk. Metronidazole is partially metabolized in the liver and excreted in the urine and, to a lesser degree, in the feces.

Although little information exists about iodoquinol's pharmacokinetics, researchers believe that only a small portion of an oral dose is absorbed from the GI tract and that most of it is excreted in the feces.

Emetine's pharmacokinetics are unclear, but some facts are known. After administration by deep S.C. or I.M. injection, high concentrations occur in the liver, kidneys, spleen, and lungs. Low concentrations occur in cardiac and striated muscle and in the intestinal lumen. It is eliminated primarily by the kidneys.

After oral administration, quinacrine is well absorbed from the GI tract and widely distributed. Highest concentrations appear in the pancreas, lungs, liver, bone marrow, spleen, erythrocytes, and skeletal muscles. The drug readily crosses the placenta, resulting in fetal tissue concentrations similar to those of the mother. Evidence suggests that quinacrine is slowly metabolized and eliminated primarily in the urine.

After oral administration, only a small fraction (about 5%) of a furazolidone dose is absorbed, producing high GI concentrations. The nonabsorbed portion is metabolized in the intestine and eliminated in the feces. The absorbed portion is excreted in the urine unchanged or as metabolites.

Onset, peak, duration

Very little is known about pentamidine's onset of action, peak concentrations, or duration of action. One study noted that peak plasma concentrations occurred about 1 hour after I.M. administration and did not vary much over 24 hours. The same study detected decreasing amounts of pentamidine in the urine up to 8 weeks after therapy was discontinued.

Peak plasma concentrations of metronidazole occur about 1 hour after I.V. administration and up to 2 hours after oral administration with food. The plasma half-life is about 6 to 8 hours for healthy adults but longer for patients with hepatic failure.

Little or no information exists about the onset of action, peak plasma concentrations, or duration of action of iodoquinol, emetine, quinacrine, and furazolidone. Some studies have detected small amounts of emetine in the urine 20 to 40 minutes after parenteral administration and for 40 to 60 days after discontinuation of therapy. Other research has determined that peak plasma concentrations of quinacrine occur about 8 hours after oral administration.

DRUG INTERACTIONS

Other antiprotozoal agents

Many interactions can occur between antiprotozoal agents and other drugs. Because most interactions are unpredictable, the nurse must monitor the patient closely.

DRUG	INTERACTING DRUGS	POSSIBLE EFFECTS	NURSING IMPLICATIONS
furazolidone	amphetamines, mono-amine oxidase (MAO) inhibitors, levodopa, tyramine	Increase pressor effect caused by inhibition of MAO metabolism	• Instruct the patient to avoid amphetamines, MAO inhibitors, levodopa, and tyramine-rich foods such as cheese, chocolate, and sausages. • Obtain an extensive patient drug history before administering furazolidone.
iodoquinol	preparations that contain iodine	Increase binding of iodine to protein, causing interference with thyroid function tests	• Explain to the patient that thyroid function tests may be abnormal for up to 6 months after iodoquinol therapy.
metronidazole	anticoagulants (warfarin type)	Enhance hypoprothrombinemia	• Monitor a patient receiving oral anticoagulants for altered anticoagulant effect when metronidazole therapy begins or ends.
	disulfiram	Produces acute psychotic reaction and confusion	• Monitor the patient's psychological status for changes.
pentamidine	aminoglycosides, cisplatin, amphotericin B	Increase nephrotoxic effects	• Reduce doses or adjust dose intervals, as ordered, when these nephrotoxic medications are used concomitantly. • Monitor the patient's renal function by measuring fluid intake and output and assessing the serum creatinine and blood urea nitrogen values.
quinacrine	primaquine	Increases toxicity of primaquine	• Monitor the patient for adverse reactions.

PHARMACODYNAMICS

The antiprotozoal agents act in very different ways, and many of their mechanisms of action are not well understood.

Mechanism of action

Pentamidine may work by several mechanisms that may vary with the protozoa involved. These mechanisms include inhibition of dihydrofolate reductase, interference with aerobic glycolysis, and inhibition of oxidative phosphorylation and nucleic acid synthesis.

Metronidazole's bactericidal, amebicidal, and trichomonacidal properties may result from disruption of protozoal DNA and inhibition of nucleic acid synthesis, eventually causing cellular death.

Iodoquinol is a contact or luminal amebicide that acts directly on protozoa in the GI tract.

Emetine acts directly on *E. histolytica* by inhibiting its polypeptide elongation. This action blocks protein synthesis in parasitic cells.

Quinacrine may act by coupling with DNA, which would make it unable to replicate or transcribe ribonucleic acid (RNA). This action would decrease protein synthesis and ultimately lead to ribosomal destruction.

Furazolidone may kill bacteria by interfering with their enzyme systems and by inhibiting monoamine oxidase.

PHARMACOTHERAPEUTICS

Antiprotozoal agents are used for a wide range of disorders, including *P. carinii* infections, amebiasis, giardiasis, trichomoniasis, toxoplasmosis, African trypanosomiasis, and leishmaniasis.

pentamidine isethionate (Pentam 300). Pentamidine is becoming more widely used to treat *P. carinii* pneumonia. A patient with renal impairment may require lower doses of this potentially nephrotoxic drug. Pentamidine can also be used to treat African trypanosomiasis and leishmaniasis.

USUAL ADULT DOSAGE: for *P. carinii* pneumonia, 4 mg/kg I.V. or I.M. once a day for 12 to 21 days; for African trypanosomiasis, 4 mg/kg I.M. or I.V. once a day for 10 days; for visceral leishmaniasis, 4 mg/kg I.M. or I.V. three times a week for 5 to 25 weeks.

metronidazole (Flagyl, Metryl, Satric). Metronidazole is the drug of choice in the treatment of amoebic hepatic abcess and mild, moderate, or severe intestinal amebiasis. It is also used to treat bacterial infections caused by anaerobic microorganisms and is the drug of choice for vaginal trichomoniasis; it is under investigation for use in treating giardiasis.

USUAL ADULT DOSAGE: for mild, moderate, and severe intestinal amebiasis or amoebic hepatic abscess, 750 mg P.O. t.i.d. for 10 days, given with iodoquinol; for bacterial infections, a loading dose of 15 mg/kg I.V. infused over 1 hour, decreased to 7.5 mg/kg I.V. or P.O. every 6 hours; for vaginal trichomoniasis, 2 g P.O. once or 250 mg P.O. t.i.d. for 7 days given to the patient and her sexual contacts.

iodoquinol [diiodohydroxyquin] (Moebiquin, Yodoxin). The drug of choice for treating asymptomatic amebiasis, iodoquinol can also be used in combination with metronidazole to treat mild, moderate, or severe intestinal amebiasis and hepatic abscess caused by *E. histolytica*.

USUAL ADULT DOSAGE: for asymptomatic amebiasis, 650 mg P.O. t.i.d. for 20 days; to treat mild, moderate, or severe intestinal amebiasis, or hepatic abscess due to *E. histolytica*, 650 mg P.O. t.i.d. for 20 days, with metronidazole.

emetine hydrochloride. Emetine is used to treat severe intestinal amebiasis and hepatic abscess, in combination with other antiparasitic drugs.

USUAL ADULT DOSAGE: to treat severe amoebic dysentery, 1 mg/kg/day up to 60 mg/day I.M. up to 5 days until symptoms of amebiasis are under control; for hepatic abscess, 1 mg/kg/day up to 60 mg/day I.M. for up to 5 days.

quinacrine hydrochloride (Atabrine). Quinacrine is the drug of choice for treating giardiasis caused by *Giardia lamblia*.

USUAL ADULT DOSAGE: 100 mg P.O. t.i.d. for 5 days.

furazolidone (Furoxone). Furazolidone serves as an alternate drug for treating of giardiasis.

USUAL ADULT DOSAGE: 100 mg P.O. q.i.d. for 7 to 10 days.

Drug interactions

Many interactions occur between antiprotozoal agents and other drugs. Some may result from interference of drug metabolism, concomitant adminstration of other drugs that cause similar adverse effects or protein binding displacement leading to elevated plasma levels. Because most of these interactions are unpredictable, the nurse must closely monitor the patient if other medications are given concurrently. (See *Drug interactions: Other antiprotozoal agents* for more information.)

ADVERSE DRUG REACTIONS

Several of the antiprotozoal agents can produce severe, even life-threatening, adverse reactions. The recommended doses and duration of therapy for these agents must not be exceeded. (See *Antiprotozoal agents: Summary of adverse reactions* on page 1132 for more details.)

Predictable reactions

GI adverse reactions have been reported with all of the antiprotozoal agents. Both emetine and pentamidine have adverse effects on the cardiovascular system, and nephrotoxicity is associated with pentamidine administration. The most serious adverse effect of iodoquinol is dose-related neurotoxicity. Both emetine and metronidazole can produce neuromuscular symptoms, and all of the antiprotozoal agents can produce blood dyscrasias.

Unpredictable reactions

Quinacrine and furazolidone can provoke intravascular hemolysis in patients with G6PD deficiency. Aplastic anemia has occurred after quinacrine administration, and iodoquinol has produced agranulocytosis. Pentamidine has been associated with Stevens-Johnson syndrome and toxic epidermal necrolysis, and quinacrine has been implicated in exfoliative dermatitis.

NURSING IMPLICATIONS

Because many antiprotozoal drugs can produce serious adverse reactions, the nurse must be particularly aware of the relative and absolute contraindications for these agents and be able to closely monitor the patient during therapy.

• Pentamidine should be administered cautiously to a patient with a history of hypotension, hypertension, hypoglycemia, hyperglycemia, hypocalcemia, leukopenia,

Antiprotozoal agents: Summary of adverse reactions

This chart summarizes the adverse reactions to other antiprotozoal agents by frequency.

DRUG	COMMON	OCCASIONAL	RARE
pentamidine	Nephrotoxicity, pain or induration at the injection site, elevated liver function tests, leukopenia, nausea, anorexia	Hypotension, phlebitis, pruritus, urticaria, hypoglycemia, hyperglycemia, thrombocytopenia, hypocalcemia, vomiting, sterile abscess	Stevens-Johnson syndrome, pancreatitis, anemia, neutropenia, thrombocytopenic purpura, toxic epidermal necrolysis
metronidazole	Nausea, headache, anorexia, dry mouth, metallic taste	Vomiting, diarrhea, epigastric distress, abdominal discomfort, constipation, dizziness, vertigo, uncoordination, ataxia, confusion, irritability, depression, weakness, insomnia, urethral burning, dysuria, vaginal dryness, dyspareunia, decreased libido	Pseudomembranous colitis, peripheral neuropathy, transient leukopenia, hypersensitivity reaction, furry tongue, glossitis, stomatitis, disulfiram-like reaction, flattening of T wave on EKG
iodoquinol	Anorexia, vomiting, diarrhea, abdominal cramps, constipation, pruritus ani	Neurotoxicity, optic neuritis, optic atrophy, peripheral neuropathy, iodism, subacute myelo-opticneuropathy (with muscle pain, weakness, optic atrophy, and ataxia), urticaria, pruritus, thyroid enlargement, fever, chills, headache, vertigo, malaise, discoloration of hair and nails	Agitation, amnesia, hair loss, granulocytopenia, hypersensitivity reaction
emetine	Diarrhea, abdominal cramps, nausea, vomiting, dizziness, headache; tenderness, aching, and muscle weakness at injection site	Cardiotoxicity, neuromuscular symptoms (weakness, aching, stiffness, tenderness, pain, tremors), generalized weakness; eczematous, urticarial, or purpuric lesions	Hypokalemia
quinacrine	Headache, dizziness, diarrhea, abdominal cramps, discolored urine	Nervousness, skin eruptions, vertigo, irritability, emotional changes, nightmares, psychosis, corneal deposits	Seizures, aplastic anemia, exfoliative dermatitis, retinopathy, hepatitis, hemolytic anemia
furazolidone	Nausea, vomiting	Abdominal pain, diarrhea, headache, malaise	Hypersensitivity reaction, hypoglycemia, granulocytopenia, hemolytic anemia, disulfiram-like reaction

thrombocytopenia, anemia, or hepatic or renal dysfunction.

• Pentamidine can precipitate severe hypotension and dysrhythmias. With the patient supine, monitor the blood pressure and electrocardiogram (EKG) before, during, and after administration, and infuse I.V. pentamidine over 1 hour to minimize these effects. Have emergency resuscitation equipment available.

• Monitor renal function closely for a patient receiving pentamidine by monitoring the blood urea nitrogen and serum creatinine concentrations before, during, and after therapy. Maintain adequate patient hydration to minimize the risk of nephrotoxicity.

• Monitor the blood glucose level for a patient receiving pentamidine during therapy and for several weeks afterward to detect hypoglycemia or hyperglycemia. Also monitor the patient's CBC, platelet count, liver function tests, and serum calcium level.

Antimalarial and other antiprotozoal agents

This chart summarizes the major antimalarial and other antiprotozoal agents currently in use.

DRUG	MAJOR INDICATIONS	USUAL ADULT DOSAGES	NURSING IMPLICATIONS
Antimalarial agents			
quinine sulfate	Treatment of chloroquine-resistant *Plasmodium falciparum* malaria	650 mg P.O. t.i.d. for 3 days with pyrimethamine and sulfadiazine	• Quinine is contraindicated in patients with known hypersensitivity, glucose 6-phosphate dehydrogenase (G6PD) deficiency, thrombocytopenic purpura, tinnitus, Blackwater Fever, or optic neuritis.
quinine dihydrochloride	Parenteral treatment of all malarial infections	600 mg I.V. in 300 ml of normal saline solution over 2 to 4 hours, repeated every 8 hours, up to a maximum of 1,800 mg/day, until oral therapy can begin	• Administer cautiously to a patient with atrial fibrillation. • Avoid rapid I.V. administration, to minimize cardiovascular effects. • Administer with food. • Advise the patient not to drive or to operate dangerous machinery, because quinine may cause blurred vision. • Advise the patient that quinine may produce diarrhea, nausea, stomach cramps or pain, vomiting, or ringing in the ears. Instruct the patient to notify the physician if symptoms become pronounced.
chloroquine hydrochloride, chloroquine phosphate	Malaria prevention in areas of low risk of exposure to chloroquine-resistant *P. falciparum* malaria	500 mg P.O. once a week beginning 1 week before exposure and continuing 6 weeks after exposure	• Chloroquine is contraindicated in patients with hypersensitivity or retinal or visual field changes. • Monitor routine eye examinations for a patient on long-term therapy. • Administer cautiously to a patient who has hepatic disease, G6PD deficiency, or a history of psoriasis or porphyria, or to a patient who is taking other hepatotoxic agents. • Administer with food. • Avoid concomitant administration of antacids. • Monitor the complete blood count (CBC) of a patient on long-term therapy. • Instruct the patient to take this drug exactly as prescribed and to contact the physician if visual disturbances or muscle weakness develops.
	Malaria prevention in the areas of moderate to high risk of exposure to chloroquine-resistant *P. falciparum* malaria	500 mg P.O. once a week beginning 1 week before exposure and continuing 6 weeks after exposure, plus pyrimethamine and sulfadoxine	
	Treatment of all malaria except chloroquine-resistant *P. falciparum*	1 g P.O. initially, then 500 mg at 6, 24, and 48 hours	
pyrimethamine	Malaria prevention only in areas of high risk of chloroquine resistance	25 mg of pyrimethamine and 500 mg of sulfadoxine P.O. once a week in combination with chloroquine prophylactic therapy	• Pyrimethamine is contraindicated in patients with known hypersensitivity or megaloblastic anemia caused by folate deficiency. • Administer cautiously to a patient with a history of seizures. • Monitor CBC and platelet counts in a patient on high-dose or long-term therapy. • Administer the pyrimethamine-sulfadoxine combination with caution to a patient with impaired renal or hepatic function, and encourage the patient to maintain an adequate hydration state.
	Treatment of chloroquine-resistant *P. falciparum* malaria	25 mg P.O. b.i.d. for 3 days in combination with sulfadiazine and quinine	

continued

SELECTED MAJOR DRUGS

Antimalarial and other antiprotozoal agents continued

DRUG	MAJOR INDICATIONS	USUAL ADULT DOSAGES	NURSING IMPLICATIONS
pyrimethamine (continued)			• Advise the patient to seek medical attention if sore throat, fever, yellowing of skin, inflammation of tongue, or rash develops.
Other antiprotozoal agents			
pentamidine isethionate	*Pneumocystis carinii* pneumonia	4 mg/kg I.M. or I.V. once a day for 12 to 21 days	• Administer cautiously to patients with hypotension, hypertension, hypoglycemia, hyperglycemia, hypocalcemia, leukopenia, thrombocytopenia, anemia, or hepatic or renal dysfunction.
	African trypanosomiasis	4 mg/kg I.M. or I.V. once a day for 10 days	• Encourage the patient to maintain a supine position during administration.
	Visceral leishmaniasis	4 mg/kg I.M. or I.V. three times a week for 5 to 25 weeks	• Monitor the patient's blood pressure; EKG; blood urea nitrogen, serum creatinine, blood glucose, and serum calcium levels; CBC; platelet counts; and liver function tests before, during, and after therapy.
			• Have emergency resuscitation equipment available.
			• Administer I.V. pentamidine over a period of 1 hour to minimize the risk of adverse reactions.
			• Be aware that the patient must remain well hydrated during therapy.
metronidazole	Mild, moderate, or severe intestinal amebiasis or amoebic hepatic abscess	750 mg P.O. t.i.d. for 10 days with iodoquinol	• Be aware that metronidazaole is contraindicated in patients with hypersensitivity to the drug or any nitroimidazole derivative.
	Vaginal trichomoniasis	2 g P.O. once or 250 mg P.O. t.i.d. for 7 days	• Administer cautiously to patients with a history of blood dyscrasias.
			• Advise the patient to take this drug with food to minimize the risk of adverse GI reactions.
			• Advise the patient that metronidazole may darken the urine and cause a metallic taste in the mouth.
quinacrine hydrochloride	Giardiasis	100 mg P.O. t.i.d. for 5 days	• Be aware that quinacrine is contraindicated in a patient receiving primaquine.
			• Administer cautiously to a patient with psoriasis, porphyria, or G6PD deficiency.
			• Administer cautiously to a patient with severe renal or cardiac disease, hepatic disease, or alcoholism, or in a patient with a history of psychosis or over age 60.
			• Monitor CBC in a patient on long-term therapy.
			• Advise the patient on long-term therapy to receive periodic eye examinations and to report any vision disturbance to the physician.

• Metronidazole is contraindicated in a patient with a history of hypersensitivity to this drug or to any other nitroimidazole derivative.

• Expect to decrease the metronidazole dosage in a patient with severe hepatic impairment, to avoid toxicity.

• Administer metronidazole with caution to a patient with a history of blood dyscrasias, and monitor the patient's total and differential leukocyte counts.

• Advise the patient that metronidazole may darken the urine and cause a lingering metallic taste in the mouth.

• Iodoquinol is contraindicated in a patient with optic neuropathy, hypersensitivity to iodine or 8-hydroxyquinolone compounds, hepatic disease, or renal disease. Administer this drug with caution to a patient with a thyroid disorder. Inform the patient that it can interfere with thyroid function tests. Discontinue iodoquinol immediately if a hypersensitivity reaction occurs.

• Emetine should only be given under direct medical supervision. Because it can be toxic, the patient should be hospitalized and confined to bed during therapy and for several days afterward. Closely monitor the patient's blood pressure, pulse rate, and EKG readings. Discontinue therapy as ordered if the patient experiences tachycardia, hypotension, neuromuscular symptoms, marked GI symptoms, or extreme weakness.

• Emetine should be administered with extreme caution to a debilitated or elderly patient. Do not administer it to a pregnant woman or a patient with organic heart disease or kidney disease. Emetine is also contraindicated in a patient who has received emetine less than 8 weeks previously or who has recently developed polyneuropathy or muscle weakness. Administer emetine only by deep I.M. injection.

• Do not administer quinacrine to a patient who is taking primaquine, and avoid concomitant use with other hepatotoxic drugs. Administer quinacrine cautiously to a patient with severe cardiac or renal disease, hepatic disease, alcoholism, or a history of psychosis, or in a patient over age 60.

• Monitor CBCs for a patient on prolonged quinacrine therapy. Advise a patient on long-term therapy to have periodic ophthalmologic examinations and to report any vision disturbances to the physician.

• Quinacrine should be administered to a patient with psoriasis, porphyria, or a history of G6PD deficiency *only* when the potential benefits outweigh the risks of therapy. Closely monitor this patient during therapy.

• Furazolidone should be administered with caution to a patient with a history of G6PD deficiency, to avoid hemolysis. Do not administer furazolidone to a patient hypersensitive to it.

• Advise the patient receiving metronidazole to take it with food to minimize the risk of adverse GI reactions. Also instruct the patient to avoid alcoholic beverages during therapy and for 48 hours after it is discontinued. During treatment for trichomoniasis, advise the patient to refrain from sexual intercourse or to have her partner use a condom to avoid reinfection. Recommend that the sexual partner(s) be evaluated for infection.

• Teach the patient about drug interactions that can occur with furazolidone. Tell the patient to avoid alcoholic beverages during therapy and for 4 days after it is discontinued. The patient should also avoid tyramine-rich foods, such as cheese, chocolate, and sausage meats; and over-the-counter medications containing sympathomimetics, such as cold capsules, allergy tablets, and anorexiants. Advise the diabetic patient that furazolidone may increase the effects of insulin and the sulfonylureas and may cause false-positive results in urine glucose tests.

CHAPTER SUMMARY

Chapter 71 discussed antimalarial and other antiprotozoal agents as they are used to prevent or treat malaria and other protozoal infections. Here are the highlights of the chapter:

• The major agents used to prevent and treat malaria include quinine, pyrimethamine, the 4-aminoquinolones (chloroquine and hydroxychloroquine), and the 8-aminoquinolone, primaquine.

• Different agents are used to manage amebiasis, giardiasis, leishmaniasis, *Pneumocystis carinii* infections, toxoplasmosis, trichomoniasis, and African trypanosomiasis. These agents include pentamidine, metronidazole, iodoquinol, emetine, quinacrine, and furazolidone.

• Four types of plasmodia cause malaria: *P. falciparum, P. malariae, P. ovale,* and *P. vivax.* In some areas of the world, strains of *P. falciparum* are chloroquine-resistant.

• Other organisms, such as *Pneumocystis carinii, G. lamblia,* and *E. histolytica,* produce disorders that are treated by the other antiprotozoal agents.

• Interactions occur when certain antimalarial drugs are used with antacids, neuromuscular blocking agents, oral anticoagulants, cardiac glycosides, digoxin, quinacrine, and folic acid.

• Certain other antiprotozoal agents will interact with other drugs, including amphetamines, monoamine oxidase inhibitors, levodopa, tyramine, iodine preparations, anticoagulants, disulfiram, aminoglycosides, cisplatin, amphotericin B, and primaquine. Interactions can be severe and unpredictable and may include nephrotoxicity, acute psychosis, and increased drug toxicity.

• Antimalarial drugs can produce a wide variety of adverse reactions. Quinine commonly produces cinchonism; the others typically produce adverse GI reactions. Less frequent adverse reactions range from blood disorders to deafness to psychotic episodes.

• The other antiprotozoal drugs also produce a range of adverse reactions, which include GI symptoms, CNS symptoms, and nephrotoxicity. More severe, but less common, adverse reactions affecting most body systems can occur.

● Because of the other antiprotozoal agents' potential toxicity and interactions with other drugs, a patient receiving an antiprotozoal agent will require close supervision during administration and regular monitoring for adverse reactions.

BIBLIOGRAPHY

Abramowicz, M., ed. "Drugs for Parasitic Infections," *Medical Letter on Drugs and Therapeutics* 28:9, January 31, 1986.

Abramowicz, M., ed. "Prevention of Malaria: Additional Notes," *Medical Letter on Drugs and Therapeutics* 28:44, April 11, 1986.

American Hospital Formulary Service. *Drug Information 86.* McEvoy, G.K., et al., eds. Bethesda, Md.: American Society of Hospital Pharmacists, 1986.

American Medical Association. *Drug Evaluations,* 5th ed. Bennett, D., et al., eds. Chicago: American Medical Association, 1983.

Andersen, R., et al. "Adverse Reactions Associated with Pentamidine Isethionate in AIDS Patients: Recommendations for Monitoring Therapy," *Drug Intelligence and Clinical Pharmacy* 20:862, November 1986.

Beaver, P.C., et al. *Clinical Parasitology,* 9th ed. Philadelphia: Lea & Febiger, 1984.

Bennett, W.M., et al. "Drug Prescribing in Renal Failure: Dosing Guidelines for Adults," *American Journal of Kidney Diseases* 3:155, November 1983.

Briggs, G.G., et al. *Drugs in Lactation and Pregnancy,* 2nd ed. Baltimore: Williams & Wilkins Co., 1986.

Brown, H.W., and Neva, F.A. *Basic Clinical Parasitology,* 5th ed. East Norwalk, Conn.: Appleton-Century-Crofts, 1983.

Campbell, W.C., and Rew, R.S., eds. *Chemotherapy of Parasitic Diseases.* New York: Plenum Press, 1986.

Centers for Disease Control. "Revised Recommendations for Preventing Malaria in Travelers to Areas with Chloroquine-Resistant *Plasmodium Falciparum,*" *Morbidity and Mortality Weekly Report* 34: 185, April 1985.

Centers for Disease Control. "STD Treatment Guidelines," *Morbidity and Mortality Weekly Report* 34:S75, October 18, 1985.

Drake, S., et al. "Pentamidine Isethionate in the Treatment of *Pneumocystis Carinii* Pneumonia, *Clinical Pharmacy* 4:507, September/October 1985.

Frisk-Holmberg, M., et al. "Chloroquine Serum Concentrations and Side Effects: Evidence for Dose-Dependent Kinetics," *Clinical Pharmacology and Therapeutics* 25:345, March 1979.

Furio, M.M., and Wordell, C.J. "Treatment of Infectious Complications of Acquired Immunodeficiency Syndrome," *Clinical Pharmacy* 4:539, September/October 1985.

Gilman, A.G., et al., eds. *Goodman and Gilman's The Pharmacological Basis of Therapeutics,* 7th ed. New York: Macmillan Publishing Co., 1985.

Goodman, L.S., and Gilman, A.G., eds. *The Pharmacological Basis of Therapeutics,* 4th ed. New York: Macmillan Publishing Co., 1970.

Hansten, P.D. *Drug Interactions,* 5th ed. Philadelphia: Lea & Febiger, 1985.

Kastrup, E.K., et al, eds. *Facts and Comparisons.* St Louis: Facts and Comparisons Division, J.B. Lippincott Co., 1986.

Levine, M.M. "Antimicrobial Therapy for Infectious Diarrhea," *Review of Infectious Diseases* 8:S207, June 1986.

Markell, E.K., et al. *Medical Parasitology,* 6th ed. Philadelphia: W.B. Saunders Co., 1986.

Parenti, D.M. "New Recommendations for Malaria Prophylaxis," *Drug Therapy* 16:107, April 1986.

Pearson, R.D., and Hewlett, E.L. "Pentamidine for the Treatment of *Pneumocystis Carinii* Pneumonia and Other Protozoal Diseases," *Annals of Internal Medicine* 103:782, 1985.

Reynolds, J., ed. *Martindale, The Extra Pharmacopoeia,* 28th ed. London: The Pharmaceutical Press, 1982.

Ruebush, T.K., et al. "Selective Primary Health Care: XXIV Malaria," *Review of Infectious Diseases* 8:454, May/June 1986.

Toumans, G.P., et al. *The Biologic and Clinical Basis of Infectious Diseases,* 3rd ed. Philadelphia: W.B. Saunders Co., 1985.

Warren, K.S., and Mahmoud, A.A.F., eds. *Tropical and Geographical Medicine.* New York: McGraw-Hill Book Co., 1984.

Williams, D.R., et al. "Common Intestinal Parasitic Infections," *Pharmacy Times* 52:120, November 1986.

Winstanley, P. "Malaria Prophylaxis," *Adverse Drug Reactions Bulletin* 4:436, 1986.

Zuger, A., et al. "Pentamidine-Associated Fatal Acute Pancreatitis," *Journal of the American Medical Association* 256:2383, November 7, 1986.

CHAPTER 72

URINARY ANTISEPTIC AGENTS

OBJECTIVES

After reading and studying this chapter, you should be able to:

1. Describe conditions that place patients at greater risk for developing urinary tract infections (UTIs).

2. Name the principal bacterial organism responsible for producing community-acquired UTIs.

3. Describe the mechanisms of action for the quinolones: nitrofurantoin, methenamine, and trimethoprim.

4. Describe drug interactions associated with methenamine and nitrofurantoin.

5. Explain how the nurse determines the efficacy of methenamine.

6. Describe adverse reactions, both unpredictable and predictable, associated with nitrofurantoin.

INTRODUCTION

Urinary tract infections frequently occur in community and hospital environments. Certain patients—including females, diabetics, paraplegics, pregnant patients, elderly males, and those with Cushing's syndrome—run the greatest risk of developing UTIs. Surgery and other medical procedures involving the urinary tract, including catheter placement, also increase the patient's risk.

Urinary antiseptic agents provide antibacterial effects that are limited to the urine. Physicians do not use urinary antiseptic agents to treat systemic infections because safe doses of the drugs do not reach effective concentration levels in the plasma. These drugs do, however, reach therapeutic concentration levels in the urine because they concentrate in the renal tubules during their excretion.

Before therapy with urinary antiseptic agents is initiated, a diagnosis based on the patient's symptoms and a urinalysis is made. Although the majority of community-acquired UTIs are caused by *Escherichia coli*, a urine culture and sensitivity test is necessary to confirm the infection, the specific organism, and appropriate antibiotics. More than 100,000 organisms per cubic milliliter cultured from a midstream urine specimen confirms the presence of a UTI. Treatment usually succeeds if an appropriate antimicrobial drug is administered at the proper dosage for an appropriate length of time and if the patient has no complications.

The most frequently used urinary antiseptics are the quinolones (nalidixic acid and its newer derivatives, cinoxacin and norfloxacin), methenamine, nitrofurantoin, and trimethoprim. These agents inhibit the growth of many species of bacteria in the urine and greatly diminish the symptoms of lower UTIs.

See *Selected major drugs: Urinary antiseptic agents* on pages 1143 and 1144 for a summary of these agents.

QUINOLONES

Nalidixic acid, cinoxacin, and norfloxacin are structurally similar synthetic chemotherapeutic agents. The nurse may administer any of these agents orally as prescribed to treat UTIs.

History and source

Introduced in 1964, nalidixic acid was the first quinolone derivative used for antibacterial therapy. Cinoxacin appeared on the market in 1981; norfloxacin, a synthetic fluoroquinolone, was released in 1986. Physicians prescribe norfloxacin as an alternative for patients who are allergic to penicillins, cephalosporins, and sulfonamides.

PHARMACOKINETICS

After oral administration, the quinolones are well absorbed, highly protein-bound, metabolized in the liver, and excreted primarily by the kidneys in the urine.

Absorption, distribution, metabolism, excretion

An entire dose of nalidixic acid is rapidly absorbed from the gastrointestinal (GI) tract after oral administration.

The drug is 93% to 97% protein-bound in plasma; it does not accumulate in the tissues, even during prolonged administration. Although nalidixic acid is not distributed to prostatic fluid, it does appear in seminal fluid and renal tissues. Nalidixic acid appears in breast milk and may harm the neonate. The drug is rapidly metabolized in the liver to active hydroxynalidixic acid and inactive monoglucoronide conjugates. Nalidixic acid and its metabolites, which attain concentration levels of 100 to 500 mcg/ml in the urine, are excreted rapidly. Nearly all of a dose is eliminated within 24 hours, 80% to 90% in conjugated inactive forms.

After oral administration, cinoxacin is absorbed rapidly and almost completely from the GI tract. Concomitant ingestion of food delays cinoxacin absorption and decreases plasma concentration levels by 30%. Approximately 70% of a cinoxacin dose is protein-bound in plasma. Peak concentration levels in the urine range from 88 to 925 mcg/ml within 4 to 6 hours after an oral dose; urine concentration levels may remain for up to 12 hours after the dose. Cinoxacin concentration levels in human prostatic tissue range from 0.6 to 6.3 mcg/g, whereas concentration levels in renal tissue exceed those in serum. Researchers do not know whether cinoxacin appears in breast milk. Approximately 40% of a cinoxacin dose is metabolized by the liver to at least four microbiologically inactive metabolites. About 60% of a dose is excreted unchanged in the urine.

Orally administered norfloxacin is readily absorbed from the GI tract. Food in the stomach may decrease drug absorption. From 10% to 15% of a norfloxacin dose is protein-bound in the plasma. Urine concentration levels of 200 mcg/ml are attained in 2 to 3 hours after an oral dose of 400 mg. Concentration levels in prostatic tissue range from 1 to 3 mcg/ml. Norfloxacin crosses the placenta, but researchers do not know if it appears in breast milk. About 30% of a dose is excreted in the urine as unmetabolized norfloxacin, with an additional 5% to 8% excreted as six active metabolites of lesser activity. Another 30% of the norfloxacin dose is excreted in the feces.

Onset, peak, duration

The onset of action of a nalidixic acid dose is approximately 30 minutes. Nalidixic acid's peak concentration levels of active drug average 20 to 50 mcg/ml 1 to 2 hours after a 1-gram dose. The plasma half-life of nalidixic acid ranges from about 2 hours in patients with normal renal function to 21 hours in anuric patients.

The onset of action of cinoxacin is about 30 minutes. Cinoxacin's peak concentration levels usually occur in 2 to 3 hours in the range of 15 to 28 mcg/ml after a 500-mg dose. Cinoxacin has a serum half-life of 1 hour,

which increases to more than 16 hours in patients with end-stage renal failure.

The onset of action for norfloxacin is about 30 minutes. Norfloxacin's peak concentration levels are 1.58 to 2.41 mcg/ml after 1 to 2 hours for doses of 400 mg and 800 mg. The plasma half-life of norfloxacin is 3 to 4 hours, increasing to 6.5 hours when creatinine clearances are below 30 ml/min/1.73 m².

PHARMACODYNAMICS

The quinolones' effectiveness in treating UTIs relates to an affinity for enzymes within the bacterial cell. The quinolones interrupt DNA synthesis during bacterial replication.

PHARMACOTHERAPEUTICS

The clinical use of nalidixic acid was restricted to UTIs because of its limited antibacterial spectrum and poor tissue penetration. The new quinolones, however, provide higher levels of antibacterial activity and penetrate body fluids and tissue more readily. Also, the new quinolones can be used to treat a wider variety of UTIs. All the quinolones require dosage reductions when they are used to treat patients with renal dysfunction.

nalidixic acid (NegGram). Used to treat acute and chronic UTIs, nalidixic acid has a limited antibacterial spectrum. Although the development of resistance may limit the usefulness of nalidixic acid against *E. coli., Proteus mirabilis,* other *Proteus* species, *Klebsiella,* and *Enterobacter,* nalidixic acid is bactericidal at easily achieved concentration levels the urine of 16 mcg/ml or less. *Pseudomonas* species are resistant.
USUAL ADULT DOSAGE: 1 g P.O. q.i.d. for 1 to 2 weeks, then 1 g P.O. b.i.d. if long-term treatment is needed.

cinoxacin (Cinobac). Indicated for acute and chronic uncomplicated UTIs, cinoxacin's antibacterial spectrum is somewhat greater than nalidixic acid's but less than norfloxacin's. Cinoxacin is effective against all *Proteus* species, *E. coli,* and most strains of *Klebsiella, Enterobacter, Citrobacter, Providencia,* and *Serratia* species. It is ineffective against *Pseudomonas, S. aureus,* and enterococci.
USUAL ADULT DOSAGE: for patients with normal renal function, 1 g P.O. daily in 2 or 4 divided doses for 7 to 14 days.

norfloxacin (Noroxin). Indicated for treating complicated and uncomplicated UTIs, norfloxacin is 100 times more active than nalidixic acid, with a similar spectrum. Norfloxacin also is effective against *Proteus aeruginosa, S. aureus,* and enterococci.

USUAL ADULT DOSAGE: for uncomplicated UTIs, 400 mg P.O. b.i.d. for 7 to 10 days; for complicated UTIs, 400 mg P.O. b.i.d. for 10 to 21 days. Dosages apply to patients with normal renal function.

Drug interactions

Few drug interactions are associated with the quinolones. Nalidixic acid may produce a false-positive reaction for glucose when the urine is tested with Benedict's solution (Clinitest), but not with glucose oxidase methods (Clinistix, Tes-Tape). Nalidixic acid may enhance the effects of oral anticoagulants, such as warfarin, by displacing significant amounts from serum albumin binding sites. Also, urinary excretion of cinoxacin and norfloxacin decreases with concomitant administration of probenecid.

ADVERSE DRUG REACTIONS

Well tolerated by patients, the quinolones produce few adverse reactions. Any adverse reactions that occur disappear with discontinuation of the drug. The most frequent predictable reactions affect the GI, central nervous, and integumentary systems and include nausea, vomiting, diarrhea, abdominal pain, headaches, drowsiness, seizures, visual disturbances, hallucinations, depression, agitation, and photosensitivity.

The quinolones can produce unpredictable hypersensitivity reactions that include urticaria, nonspecific rashes, pruritus, and edema. Rare reactions include hematologic problems, such as hemolytic anemia, that are associated with glucose-6-phosphate dehydrogenase (G6PD) deficiency.

NURSING IMPLICATIONS

Because the quinolones are used frequently, the nurse must be aware of these implications:
- Do not administer quinolones to a patient with a history of allergy to any one of the agents in this class. Also, do not administer nalidixic acid to a patient with a history of convulsive disorders.
- Do not administer cinoxacin or nalidixic acid to an anuric patient. Expect to adjust the dosage for a patient with impaired renal function, because the rate of elimination will decrease and the serum half-life will increase.
- Administer antacids at least 2 hours after administering norfloxacin.
- Advise the patient taking quinolones to use extreme caution when driving or operating machinery, because these drugs may cause dizziness.

- Instruct the patient to take protective measures against exposure to ultraviolet light or sunlight because photosensitivity can occur.
- Encourage the patient taking norfloxacin to drink at least 1,500 ml of water per day to ensure proper hydration and adequate urinary output because crystalluria can develop.

METHENAMINE

Physicians prescribe methenamine to suppress chronic bacteriuria. The patient's urinary pH must be maintained at 5 to 5.5 for methenamine to exert its bactericidal effect through ammonia and formaldehyde formation.

History and source

Methenamine was introduced in 1895 to treat UTIs. In 1935, Rosenheim combined methenamine with mandelic acid to increase its bactericidal properties in the urine. The combination of methenamine and mandelic acid is marketed as methenamine mandelate. Methenamine also has been combined with hippuric acid (methenamine hippurate) to enhance its bactericidal properties.

PHARMACOKINETICS

After oral administration, methenamine and its salts are absorbed rapidly from the GI tract and excreted rapidly in the urine. Little methenamine is decomposed in body fluids other than the urine, and methenamine virtually is nontoxic systemically.

Absorption, distribution, metabolism, excretion

The base and salts of methenamine are rapidly absorbed from the GI tract after oral administration. However, 10% to 30% of a dose is hydrolyzed by gastric juices unless the enteric-coated tablet form is used. Methenamine is distributed widely to the body fluids, including cerebrospinal fluid, synovial fluid, and pericardial fluid. Methenamine is hydrolyzed in acid urine to form ammonia and formaldehyde, which is bactericidal. Formaldehyde does not appear in other body fluids because their pH is alkaline and because methenamine does not hydrolyze at a pH greater than 6.8. Methenamine is excreted rapidly in the urine; more than 90% of a dose is excreted within 24 hours.

Onset, peak, duration

The generation of formaldehyde and onset of action depend on the urinary pH, the concentration level of methenamine, and the length of time urine is retained in the bladder. Peak concentration levels of formaldehyde occur at a urinary pH of 5.5 or less about 2 hours after a methenamine hippurate dose and 3 to 8 hours after an enteric-coated methenamine mandelate dose. A urinary formaldehyde concentration of greater than 25 mcg/ml is necessary for antibacterial activity to begin, and steady-state concentration levels will follow in 2 to 3 days.

PHARMACODYNAMICS

Methenamine, which liberates free formaldehyde and ammonia in acid urine with a pH of 5.5 or less, is active against all gram-positive and gram-negative bacteria. It is available in tablet and suspension form.

Mechanism of action

Methenamine's antibacterial effect depends on the drug's release of formaldehyde, a nonspecific bactericidal agent, in acid urine. The acid portions of methenamine salts exhibit some nonspecific bacteriostatic activity and may enhance formaldehyde liberation. Physicians frequently prescribe other substances to acidify the urine, including ascorbic acid, ammonium chloride, and acid-producing food substances such as cranberry juice. During therapy, the nurse monitors the patient's urinary pH to assess the efficacy of methenamine.

PHARMACOTHERAPEUTICS

Methenamine products should not be used alone to treat acute urinary tract infections. They also should not be used in patients with suprapubic or indwelling (Foley) catheters continuously draining urine because methenamine's efficacy requires formaldehyde generation, which takes at least 1 hour to attain sufficient antibacterial concentration levels in the urine.

methenamine (Urised), **methenamine hippurate** (Hiprex, Urex), and **methenamine mandelate** (Mandelamine). Physicians prescribe methenamine prophylactically for recurrent UTIs, especially for long-term therapy. Methenamine is active against all gram-positive and gram-negative bacteria; however, UTIs caused by urea-splitting organisms such as the *Proteus* species may not respond because acidifying the urine is difficult in the presence of these infections that increase urinary pH.
USUAL ADULT DOSAGE: for chronic UTIs, 1 g P.O. every 12 hours (methenamine hippurate or mandelate) or ev-

ery 6 hours (methenamine); for infected residual urine in neuropathic bladder, 1 g P.O. q.i.d. after meals and at bedtime.

Drug interactions

Methenamine combines with sulfonamides in the urine, causing insoluble precipitates and an increasing risk of crystalluria. Methenamine should not be used with urinary alkalinizers (sodium bicarbonate, sodium lactate, potassium citrate), because doing so may decrease the antibacterial effects of methenamine.

ADVERSE DRUG REACTIONS

Methenamine and its salts, which are usually well tolerated, produce few adverse drug reactions.

Predictable reactions

GI reactions, such as gastric distress, nausea, vomiting, and diarrhea, occur most frequently. Patients taking large doses of methenamine may experience bladder irritation, with dysuria, frequency, and hematuria. The methenamine salts should be avoided in patients with gout because the drugs may precipitate urate crystals in the urine.

Unpredictable reactions

Various unpredictable rashes may occur with the administration of methenamine or its salts. Allergic reactions, including bronchial asthma, have occurred with the use of Hiprex, a brand of methenamine hippurate that contains the dye tartrazine. An infrequent reaction, tartrazine sensitivity usually occurs in patients allergic to aspirin.

NURSING IMPLICATIONS

The nurse administering methenamine products should be aware of these implications:
• Do not administer methenamine or its salts to patients with dehydration, severe hepatic impairment, or renal insufficiency because of ammonia production and an inadequate formaldehyde concentration level in the urine.
• Administer methenamine mandelate oral suspension cautiously in elderly or debilitated patients, because the vegetable oil base may induce lipid pneumonia.
• Avoid administering methenamine agents to patients with gout because urate crystals may precipitate in the urine.
• Monitor the patient's urinary pH and encourage the patient to ingest foods that will help maintain an acid pH to facilitate methenamine's effectiveness.

• Advise the patient to avoid excessive intake of alkalinizing foods (vegetables, peanuts, and milk products) or medications (bicarbonate).

NITROFURANTOIN

Nitrofurantoin is used clinically primarily to treat acute and chronic UTIs.

History and source
In 1944, Dodd and Stillman demonstrated the bactericidal property of the furan derivatives. Nitrofurantoin, one of a series of synthetic nitrofuran compounds, has been available for clinical use in a microcrystalline form since 1953. Because nitrofurantoin has limited solubility in water, a macrocrystalline form was prepared for clinical use in 1967.

PHARMACOKINETICS

After oral administration, nitrofurantoin is absorbed rapidly and well from the GI tract and excreted rapidly in the urine. The macrocrystalline form is absorbed and excreted more slowly than the microcrystalline.

Absorption, distribution, metabolism, excretion
Microcrystalline nitrofurantoin is absorbed rapidly and completely from the GI tract. Antibacterial activity in serum is low after oral doses. The macrocrystalline form, with its larger drug particles, was introduced to delay absorption from the GI tract. Delaying the drug's entrance into body fluids lowers the peak concentration levels in serum and decreases the incidence and severity of nausea, without significantly affecting peak concentration levels in the urinary tract.

The concomitant ingestion of food enhances the bioavailability of nitrofurantoin. Antibacterial activity is higher in acid urine. Nitrofurantoin crosses the placenta and appears in breast milk. It is also distributed in bile. Two thirds of a nitrofurantoin dose is metabolized by the liver and one third is excreted unchanged in the urine. The drug's presence in urine decreases as the creatinine clearance decreases.

Onset, peak, duration
Nitrofurantoin does not accumulate in the serum of patients with normal renal function because the serum half-life is 20 minutes. Nitrofurantoin is from 20% to 60% protein-bound. An average dose of nitrofurantoin yields peak concentration levels in the urine of about 200 mcg/ml. Urine concentration levels insufficient to inhibit common urinary tract pathogens occur when creatinine clearance is less than 30 ml/min/1.73 m².

PHARMACODYNAMICS

Usually bacteriostatic, nitrofurantoin may become bactericidal depending on its urinary concentration and the susceptibility of the infecting organisms. Although the exact mechanism of action has not been described, nitrofurantoin appears to inhibit formation of acetyl coenzyme A from pyruvic acid, thereby inhibiting the infecting organism's energy production. Nitrofurantoin may also disrupt bacterial cell wall formation.

PHARMACOTHERAPEUTICS

Physicians use nitrofurantoin to treat UTIs. It is not effective against systemic bacterial infections.

nitrofurantoin (Furadantin, Macrodantin). Used to treat initial or recurrent UTIs, nitrofurantoin is active against a wide spectrum of gram-positive and gram-negative bacteria, especially *E. coli, Klebsiella,* and *Enterobacter* and *Citrobacter* species. The majority of *Proteus* and *Serratia* species are moderately resistant and *P. aeruginosa* almost always is resistant. The drug also is effective against staphylococci and enterococci.
USUAL ADULT DOSAGE: for uncomplicated UTIs, 50 to 100 mg P.O. q.i.d. for 7 to 14 days; for chronic therapy, 50 to 100 mg P.O. daily at bedtime.

Drug interactions
Probenecid and sulfinpyrazone inhibit the renal excretion of nitrofurantoin, reduce the drug's efficacy, and increase its toxic potential. Antacids can decrease the extent and rate of nitrofurantoin absorption. Nitrofurantoin antagonizes the antibacterial effect of nalidixic acid in vitro. Nitrofurantoin may produce false-positive results for urine glucose determinations when Benedict's solution (Clinitest) is used, but does not affect results when glucose oxidase methods (Clinistix, Tes-Tape) are used.

ADVERSE DRUG REACTIONS

Nitrofurantoin use is associated with a number of adverse drug reactions. Some are predictable; others, idiosyncratic.

Predictable reactions
GI irritation is the most frequent adverse effect of nitrofurantoin. Anorexia, nausea, and vomiting occur frequently; diarrhea and abdominal pain, less often. GI

intolerance occurs more frequently in patients receiving nitrofurantoin microcrystalline tablets than in those receiving macrocrystals. Some patients have experienced peripheral neuropathy, which usually begins with paresthesia and dysesthesia of the legs and can progress in severity to a debilitating state.

Unpredictable reactions

Hypersensitivity reactions occur occasionally and involve the skin, lungs, blood, and liver. Chills, fever, arthralgia (a lupus erythematosus syndrome), and anaphylaxis also can occur. Allergic dermatologic reactions include maculopapular, erythematous, or eczematous rashes, urticaria, angioneurotic edema, and pruritus. Pulmonary reactions include asthmatic attacks in patients with a history of asthma, and acute pneumonitis. Acute pneumonitis is manifested by sudden fever, chills, cough, dyspnea, chest pain, eosinophilia, and pulmonary infiltration that may appear as consolidation or pleural effusion on X-rays. Acute pneumonitis occurs most often in elderly patients, with symptoms appearing within the first week of treatment.

Hematologic reactions include leukopenia, granulocytopenia, megaloblastic anemia, and hemolytic anemia. In patients with G6PD deficiency, nitrofurantoin can precipitate an acute episode of hemolytic anemia. Non-dose-related hepatotoxicity can occur, as well as chronic active hepatitis, cholestatic jaundice, and cholestatic hepatitis.

NURSING IMPLICATIONS

Nitrofurantoin is used widely to treat patients in acute and chronic care clinical settings. The nurse administering it must be aware of these nursing implications:
• Administer nitrofurantoin with food or milk.
• Inform the patient that nitrofurantoin may turn urine brown or rust-yellow.
• Do not administer nitrofurantoin to a patient with renal impairment (creatinine clearance less than 40 ml/min/1.73 m²), anemia, diabetes, electrolyte imbalances, vitamin B deficiency, or other debilitating diseases, because the drug may predispose the patient to severe or irreversible peripheral neuropathy.
• Monitor the patient for signs and symptoms of a superinfection caused by bacterial or fungal overgrowth of nonsusceptible organisms, especially *Pseudomonas*.

TRIMETHOPRIM

Physicians prescribe trimethoprim, alone and in combination with sulfamethoxazole, to treat UTIs.

History and source

Researchers synthesized trimethoprim in the early 1940s. The drug was developed as a dihydrofolate reductase inhibitor to enhance sulfonamide activity by sequential inhibition of folic acid synthesis. In the United States, trimethoprim is available as a single agent and in combination with sulfamethoxazole.

PHARMACOKINETICS

As a single agent, trimethoprim is available for oral administration only. It is well absorbed and excreted primarily unchanged in the urine.

Absorption, distribution, metabolism, excretion

After oral administration, trimethoprim is absorbed readily and almost completely from the GI tract. The coadministration of trimethoprim and sulfamethoxazole does not affect trimethoprim's absorption rate or serum concentration levels. Trimethoprim is 44% protein-bound in plasma. Widely distributed to the tissues, it may appear in the kidneys, lungs, and sputum in higher concentration levels than in the plasma. Trimethoprim is also distributed to bile, saliva, breast milk, and seminal fluid.

Trimethoprim distribution to prostatic fluid is 2 to 3 times the serum concentration, but lower levels may occur in patients with chronic prostatitis. The concentration level of trimethoprim in cerebrospinal fluid is about 40% that of serum concentration levels.

About 50% to 60% of a trimethoprim dose is secreted in the urine via tubular secretion within 24 hours; of this amount, about 80% is excreted unchanged. The remainder is excreted by the kidneys as one of four bacteriologically inactive oxide or hydroxyl derivatives. Unlike sulfamethoxazole, trimethoprim's rate of excretion increases with urine acidification. Trimethoprim is also excreted in the bile.

Onset, peak, duration

After oral administration of a 100-mg dose, peak serum concentration levels appear in 2 hours and approach 1 mcg/ml. The serum half-life ranges from 9 to 11 hours in healthy patients. Half-life is prolonged in patients with renal insufficiency. Urine concentration levels in healthy

SELECTED MAJOR DRUGS

Urinary antiseptic agents

Urinary antiseptic agents are used in all types of clinical settings to treat urinary tract infections. The nurse administers these agents and monitors the patient's signs and symptoms to determine a drug's efficacy.

DRUG	MAJOR INDICATIONS	USUAL ADULT DOSAGES	NURSING IMPLICATIONS
nalidixic acid	Acute and chronic UTIs	1 g P.O. q.i.d. for 1 to 2 weeks; 1 g P.O. b.i.d. for long-term treatment	• Do not administer nalidixic acid to patients with a history of convulsive disorders, quinolone allergies, or anuria. • Advise the patient not to operate machinery or drive a car because dizziness may occur. • Instruct the patient to take protective measures against exposure to ultraviolet light or sunlight because photosensitivity can occur. • Advise the patient to take the drug with food if GI upset occurs.
norfloxacin	Uncomplicated UTIs	400 mg P.O. b.i.d. for 7 to 10 days	• Do not administer norfloxacin to patients with quinolone allergies. • Expect to adjust the dosage for a patient with impaired renal function. • Instruct the patient to take protective measures against exposure to ultraviolet light or sunlight because photosensitivity can occur. • Encourage the patient to drink at least 1,500 ml of fluids daily to prevent crystalluria. • Advise the patient not to operate machinery or drive a car because dizziness may occur. • Administer drug 1 hour before or 2 hours after meals. • Do not administer with antacids.
	Complicated UTIs	400 mg P.O. b.i.d. for 10 to 21 days	
methenamine	Chronic UTIs	1 g P.O. every 12 hours (methenamine mandelate or hippurate) or 1 g P.O. every 6 hours (methenamine)	• Administration of methenamine agents is contraindicated in patients with dehydration, severe hepatic impairment, or renal insufficiency. • Administer methenamine mandelate oral suspension cautiously to elderly and debilitated patients because the oil base may induce lipid pneumonia. • Instruct the patient to avoid ingesting excessive amounts of alkalinizing agents such as vegetables, milk, and peanuts. • Monitor the patient's urinary pH; encourage ingestion of cranberry, plum, and prune juices, which will help maintain an acid pH.
	Infected residual urine in neuropathic bladder	1 g P.O. q.i.d. after meals and at bedtime	
nitrofurantoin	Uncomplicated UTIs	50 to 100 mg P.O. q.i.d. for 7 to 14 days	• Administer nitrofurantoin with food or milk to enhance absorption. • Inform the patient that nitrofurantoin may produce brown or rust-yellow colored urine. • Do not administer nitrofurantoin to a patient with renal impairment, anemia, diabetes, electrolyte imbalances, vitamin B deficiency, or other debilitating diseases, because doing so may predispose the patient to severe or irreversible peripheral neuropathy.
	Complicated UTIs	50 to 100 mg P.O. daily at bedtime	
trimethoprim	Acute uncomplicated UTIs	100 mg P.O. every 12 hours, or 200 mg P.O. daily for 10 to 14 days	• Administer trimethoprim cautiously to a patient with renal dysfunction, hepatic dysfunction, or folate deficiency. • Instruct the patient to report to the physician

continued

SELECTED MAJOR DRUGS

Urinary antiseptic agents continued

DRUG	MAJOR INDICATIONS	USUAL ADULT DOSAGES	NURSING IMPLICATIONS
trimethoprim (continued)	UTI prophylaxis	100 mg P.O. daily at bedtime	any fever, sore throat, pallor, or purpura, which may indicate a serious hematologic disorder. • Instruct the patient to take the drug on an empty stomach or, if GI irritation occurs, with meals. • Stress the importance of completing the full course of therapy.

subjects range from 30 to 160 mcg/ml, which exceeds the minimum inhibitory concentration levels for most urinary pathogens.

PHARMACODYNAMICS

Usually, trimethoprim is a slow-acting bactericide. Its effectiveness results from its powerful inhibition of bacterial dihydrofolate reductase. Trimethoprim, which is 50,000 to 100,000 times more active against bacterial dihydrofolate reductase than against the human enzyme, interferes with the conversion of dihydrofolate to tetrahydrofolate. This conversion is necessary for the normal bacterial production of folinic acid, which is necessary for purine and DNA synthesis.

PHARMACOTHERAPEUTICS

Trimethoprim is active against most gram-positive cocci and most gram-negative rods. Using trimethoprim alone for acute uncomplicated UTIs may increase trimethoprim-resistant organisms.

trimethoprim (Proloprim, Trimpex). Physicians use trimethoprim to treat initial episodes of acute uncomplicated UTIs caused by *E. coli, Proteus mirabilis, K. pneumoniae, Enterobacter,* or coagulase-negative staphylococci.
USUAL ADULT DOSAGE: for acute uncomplicated UTIs, 100 mg P.O. every 12 hours, or 200 mg daily for 10 to 14 days; for prophylaxis, 100 mg P.O. daily at bedtime.

Drug interactions
Because trimethoprim possesses antifolate properties, it may increase folate deficiencies induced by other drugs,

such as phenytoin, when used concomitantly. Also, the concurrent administration of trimethoprim and phenytoin may increase serum concentration levels of phenytoin from inhibited hepatic metabolism.

ADVERSE DRUG REACTIONS

The incidence and severity of adverse reactions to trimethoprim therapy are usually dose-related and can be alleviated by decreasing the dosage. The most frequent predictable adverse reactions include epigastric discomfort, nausea, vomiting, glossitis, and an abnormal taste sensation. Also, rash and pruritus occur frequently.

Unpredictable reactions to trimethoprim therapy occur rarely. Hematologic toxicity, resulting from trimethoprim-induced inhibition of dihydrofolate reductase, can lead to thrombocytopenia, neutropenia, megaloblastic anemia, and methemoglobinemia.

NURSING IMPLICATIONS

The nurse administering trimethoprim should be aware of these implications:
• Administer trimethoprim with caution to a patient with renal or hepatic dysfunction or possible folate deficiency.
• Instruct the patient to report fever, sore throat, pallor, or purpura, because these signs may indicate a serious hematologic disorder.
• Instruct the patient to take trimethoprim on an empty stomach. If GI irritation occurs, advise the patient to take the drug with food.
• Stress the importance of completing the full course of therapy.

CHAPTER SUMMARY

Chapter 72 presented the urinary antiseptic agents that can be used against UTIs. Here are the chapter highlights:

• Physicians use the urinary antiseptic agents to treat acute, uncomplicated, symptomatic bacteriuria of the lower urinary tract.

• The quinolones, a major class of urinary antiseptic agents, include nalidixic acid, cinoxacin, and norfloxacin.

• Nalidixic acid may be effective in some patients with recurrent infections, but the patient may develop resistance to the drug.

• Because cinoxacin and norfloxacin provide all the benefits of nalidixic acid without its disadvantages, they may soon replace nalidixic acid in treating UTIs. Cinoxacin and norfloxacin may also be useful as an alternative to penicillins, cephalosporins, and sulfonamides for patients who are allergic to those agents.

• Nitrofurantoin, another urinary antiseptic agent, is effective in upper UTIs and recurrent bacteriuria.

• When used properly, methenamine is effective for treating uncomplicated recurrent bacteriuria involving multiple resistant organisms, and for providing prophylaxis in recurrent infections.

• Used alone, trimethoprim is effective for uncomplicated and recurrent UTIs, especially in patients who are allergic to sulfonamides; however, trimethoprim-resistant organisms may increase with the widespread clinical use of this drug.

BIBLIOGRAPHY

Abramowicz, M. "Adverse Interactions of Drugs," *Medical Letter on Drugs and Therapeutics* 23:17, 1983.

American Hospital Formulary Service. *Drug Information 87.* McEvoy, G.K., et al., eds. Bethesda, Md.: American Society of Hospital Pharmacists, 1987.

Barry, A.L., et al. "Antibacterial Activities of Ciprofloxacin, Norfloxacin, Oxolinic Acid, Cinoxacin, and Nalidixic Acid," *Antimicrobial Agents and Chemotherapy* 25(5):633, May 1984.

Brumfitt, W., and Hamilton-Miller, J.M.T. "A Review of the Problem of Urinary Infection Management and the Evaluation of a Potential New Antibiotic. Symposium on Norfloxacin: A New Quinolone for Urinary Infections," *Journal of Antimicrobial Chemotherapy* 13 (Suppl. B): 121, 1984.

Chantot, J.F., and Bryskier, A. "Antibacterial Activity of Ofloxacin, and Other 4-quinolone Derivatives; In Vitro and In Vivo Comparison," *Journal of Antimicrobial Chemotherapy* 16(4):475, October 1985.

Erickson, S., and Wenzloff, N.J. "An Update on UTIs," *Pharmacy Times* 51(8):106, 1985.

Goldstein, E.J., et al. "Norfloxacin versus Trimethoprim-Sulfamethoxazole in the Therapy of Uncomplicated, Community-Acquired UTIs," *Antimicrobial Agents and Chemotherapy* 27(3):422, 1985.

Holmes, B., et al. "Norfloxacin: A Review of Its Antibacterial Activity, Pharmacokinetic Properties and Therapeutic Use," *Drugs* 30:482, December 1985.

Keys, T., and Edson, R. "Antimicrobial Agents in UTIs," *Mayo Clinic Proceedings* 58:165, 1983.

King, A., et al. "The In Vitro Activity of Ciprofloxacin Compared with That of Norfloxacin and Nalidixic Acid," *Journal of Antimicrobial Chemotherapy* 13(4):325, March 1984.

Krieger, J.N., et al. "Nosocomial UTIs: Secular Trends, Treatment and Economics in a University Hospital," *Journal of Urology* 130:102, July 1983.

Leigh, D.A., and Emmanuel, F.X. "The Treatment of *Pseudomonas aeruginosa* UTIs with Norfloxacin," *Journal of Antimicrobial Chemotherapy* 13 (Suppl. B): 85, May 1984.

Mandel, G., et al., eds. *Principles and Practice of Infectious Diseases*, 2nd ed. New York: John Wiley & Sons, 1985.

Marble, D.A., and Bosso, J.A. "Norfloxacin: A Quinolone Antibiotic," *Drug Intelligence and Clinical Pharmacy* 20(4):261, April 1986.

Norby, R. "Potential Usefulness of Norfloxacin in the Treatment of UTIs, "*European Journal of Clinical Microbiology* 2(3):227, 1983.

Owen, J.A., "Cinoxacin: An Antibacterial Agent for the Treatment of UTI," *Hospital Formulary* 18(3):248, 1983.

Sisca, T.S. et al. "Cinoxacin: A Review of Its Pharmacological Properties and Therapeutic Efficacy in the Treatment of UTIs," *Drugs* 25:544, June 1983.

Wise, R. "Norfloxacin—A Review of Pharmacology and Tissue Penetration," *Journal of Antimicrobial Chemotherapy* 13 (Suppl. B): 59, May 1984.

DRUGS TO TREAT MALIGNANT NEOPLASMS

I n the 1940s, antineoplastic, or chemotherapeutic, drugs were used to treat cancer when all other therapeutic measures failed for disseminated cancers that could not be treated by surgery or radiation therapy. Then, most antineoplastic drugs frequently caused serious adverse reactions. Today, many of their adverse effects can be minimized so that they are not so devastating to the patient. In fact, many childhood cancers now are considered curable because of the advent of chemotherapeutic drugs. Many of these agents are the drugs of choice for different types of cancer and are no longer considered a last resort.

Nurses have actively participated in administering and evaluating more than 50 drugs to treat cancer. In caring for patients receiving these drugs, nurses have helped patients and their families to understand chemotherapy and cope with its adverse effects.

Clinical uses

Antineoplastic agents may be administered to cure, prevent, or relieve cancer symptoms. For patients with systemic cancers, such as leukemia, chemotherapy may be given as a curative treatment. In other patients, it may be given as an adjuvant treatment based on the premise that micrometastases, although undetectable, exist. In patients with advanced neoplastic disorders, chemotherapy may be palliative, reducing tumor size or relieving pain and other symptoms.

Chemotherapy often is combined with other cancer treatments. For example, it may be given preoperatively to reduce tumor size and allow less radical surgery.

The cell cycle

To understand the pharmacodynamics of antineoplastic agents, the nurse needs to know about the cell cycle. All animal cells follow a series of basic steps as they undergo division and replication. This series of steps is called the cell cycle; each step is a phase. During each phase, biochemical events that are necessary for cell division occur. (See *Cell cycle* on page 1149 for a summary of these phases.)

In the first phase, G_1 (G stands for gap), the cell manufactures the enzymes needed for deoxyribonucleic acid (DNA) synthesis. The time a cell spends in G_1 varies greatly but averages about 18 hours.

Next, the cell enters the S phase (S stands for synthesis). In this phase, DNA replication occurs in preparation for mitosis (cell division). This phase lasts from 10 to 20 hours.

Then, the cell enters the G_2 phase, during which specialized DNA proteins and ribonucleic acid (RNA) are synthesized for later mitosis. This phase lasts about 3 hours.

Finally, the cell is ready to divide and enters the M phase (M refers to mitosis). During mitosis, the cell progresses through four subphases: *prophase,* in which the chromosomes aggregate or clump; *metaphase,* in which the chromosomes line up in the middle of the cell; *anaphase,* in which the chromosomes segregate; and *telophase,* in which the cell divides, producing two morphologically identical cells. The entire M phase lasts only 1 hour.

From the M phase, the cell may follow one of three paths. It may differentiate into a functional cell, enter the G_0 (resting) phase, or begin the cycle again by entering the G_1 phase. Resting cells in the G_0 phase may move on to the G_1 phase and progress through the cell cycle.

In different phases of the cycle, cells are susceptible to different drugs, because the drugs interfere with specific biochemical events that occur in these phases.

Mechanisms of action

Although not fully understood, cancer seems to occur when one cell undergoes a malignant transformation and reproduces an abnormal cell. Antineoplastic agents interfere with cell reproduction, leading to tumor destruction. (See *Mechanisms and sites of action of antineoplastic agents* on page 1150 for detailed information.)

During administration of an antineoplastic agent, a fixed percentage of cells die. After treatment, the remaining cells reproduce, and resting cells in the G_0 phase may return to a reproducing phase. (Cells in the G_0 phase are less sensitive to chemotherapy because they are not actively synthesizing DNA.) Total eradication of

Glossary

Adenocarcinoma: malignant tumor that forms in a gland, infiltrates surrounding tissues, and leads to metastases.

Alkylation: linkage between a substance and DNA that causes irreversible inhibition of the DNA molecule by enzyme modification.

Alopecia: loss of hair in areas where it normally appears.

Anemia: blood disorder characterized by a decreased number of erythrocytes, amount of hemoglobin, or volume of packed red cells.

Benign: noncancerous, nonrecurring.

Cancer: general term for the many malignant neoplasms associated with infiltration, metastases, and fatality.

Carcinogenesis: cancer production.

Carcinoma: malignant neoplasm, composed of epithelial cells, that tends to infiltrate surrounding tissues and lead to metastases.

Cell cycle: division pattern of cells characterized by five phases: nonproliferation, G_0; presynthesis, G_1; DNA synthesis, S; RNA production, G_2; and mitosis, M, when the cell divides in two.

Cell-cycle-nonspecific: capable of acting during several or all cell-cycle stages.

Cell-cycle-specific: capable of acting during particular cell-cycle stages only.

Cytostatic: halting cell growth and multiplication.

Cytotoxic: capable of destroying or poisoning cells.

Extravasation: escape of blood or solution from a vessel into surrounding tissues.

Glossitis: tongue inflammation.

Granulocyte: a leukocyte with granules in its cytoplasm; basophils, neutrophils, and eosinophils are types of granulocytes.

Granulocytopoiesis: granulocyte production.

Hepatotoxic: capable of destroying or poisoning liver cells.

Hodgkin's disease: malignant disorder that causes painless, progressive enlargement of the lymph nodes, spleen, and lymphoid tissues, often beginning in the neck; also called malignant granuloma or lymphoma.

Hypercalcemia: excess calcium in the blood.

Intrathecal: within a sheath, as in the cerebrospinal fluid within the subarachnoid space.

Irritant: agent that stimulates cells, producing excitation and undue sensitivity.

Jaundice: yellow appearance of the skin, mucous membranes, and sclera caused by hyperbilirubinemia and bile pigment deposits.

Leukemia: malignant disorder of the blood-forming organs marked by increased leukocytes and leukocyte precursors in the blood and bone marrow.

Leukopenia: decreased leukocytes in the blood, usually under $5,000/mm^3$.

Lymphoblastic: pertaining to lymphoblasts (immature nucleolated lymphocytes).

Lymphocytic: pertaining to lymphocytes.

Lympholysis: lymphocyte destruction.

Lymphoma: any neoplastic disorder of lymphoid tissue.

Malignancy: tendency to grow progressively worse and lead to death.

Melanoma: malignant neoplasm composed of melanin-pigmented cells.

Metastasis: disease transfer from one organ or part to distant parts of the body.

Mitosis: type of cell division that results in two morphologically identical cells.

Mucositis: mucous membrane inflammation.

Mutagenesis: induction of genetic mutation.

Myelocyte: immature white blood cell usually found in the bone marrow that becomes a granular leukocyte in the blood.

Myelogenous: pertaining to cells produced in the bone marrow.

Myeloma: neoplasm composed of cells that normally appear in the bone marrow.

Myeloproliferative: pertaining to or characterized by extramedullary and medullary proliferation of bone marrow constituents.

Nadir: lowest point on a scale or curve, often related to blood counts.

Neoplasm: any new abnormal growth of tissue; may be benign or malignant.

Nephrotoxic: capable of destroying or poisoning kidney cells.

Neuroblastoma: malignant tumor of the nervous system composed primarily of immature nerve cells (neuroblasts).

Neurotoxic: capable of destroying or poisoning nerve cells.

Orchiectomy: surgical removal of one or both testes.

Palliative: providing relief but not cure.

Pancytopenia: deficiency of all cellular elements in the blood; also called aplastic anemia.

Phagocytosis: process of engulfing microorganisms, cells, and foreign particles by reticuloendothelial cells, monocytes, or polymorphonuclear leukocytes.

Pleiotropic: capable of having an affinity for several different types of tissue from different primary germ layers; also a gene's ability to manifest itself in multiple ways.

Polycythemia vera: myeloproliferative disease characterized by increased red blood cells and total

continued

Glossary continued

blood volume, frequently accompanied by spleno-megaly, leukocytosis, thrombocytosis, and bone marrow hyperactivity.

Remission: partial or complete disappearance of the clinical or subjective characteristics of a chronic or malignant disease.

Rhabdomyosarcoma: malignant tumor composed of striated muscle cells.

Sarcoma: malignant tumor composed of a substance similar to embryonic connective tissue.

Stomatitis: mouth inflammation that may affect the buccal mucosa, palate, tongue, floor of the mouth, and gingivae.

Teratogenesis: production of physical defects in the fetus.

Thrombocytopenia: decrease in the number of blood platelets.

Thrombocytosis: excess platelets in the blood.

Tumor: new tissue growth marked by progressive, uncontrolled cell multiplication; neoplasm.

Tumorcidal: destructive to tumors.

Vesicant: agent that produces blisters.

Wilms' tumor: rapidly developing, malignant kidney tumor, composed of embryonic elements, that usually affects children under age 5.

---

cancer cells, therefore, depends on repeated administration of the antineoplastic agent. An interval between treatments permits healthy cells to recover.

Because cancer cells are at various phases in the cell cycle, therapy often combines drugs that act on cells in different phases or that have different sites of action.

Although an antineoplastic agent kills cells as soon as they pass through a specific cell cycle, this action produces no immediate clinical response. Most patients need at least three treatments before a clinical response can be evaluated by a physical examination, an X-ray, a computed tomography (CT) scan, a magnetic resonance imaging (MRI) scan, or biological marker determinations.

Tumor regression depends on several factors, such as the percentage of cells killed, the rate of regrowth, and the development of resistant cells. Evaluation of chemotherapy is difficult, however, because the cancer may be undetected clinically but still may be present. Therefore, treatments may continue for a while after the disease is no longer detectable.

Tumor resistance

Adjuvant chemotherapy for micrometastases and combination drug regimens may be used for patients with tumor resistance. Tumor cell populations are heterogeneous: some cells are sensitive to antineoplastic agents; others are not. When an antineoplastic agent is administered, it kills drug-sensitive cells initially. Repeated administration kills more drug-sensitive cells. Over time, however, tumor cells that are not drug-sensitive remain and replicate, producing a drug-resistant tumor. If these resistant cells are resistant to other drugs also, they will be even more difficult to kill.

Drug resistance may develop by one or more of the following mechanisms: decreased drug entry into the tumor cells, decreased drug-activating enzymes, increased drug-deactivating enzymes, increased levels of target enzymes, decreased target enzyme affinity for the drug, increased DNA repair, or development of alternate pathways that circumvent the drug's action.

Handling antineoplastic agents

Although the safe handling of antineoplastic agents remains controversial, most experts recommend conservative, protective methods. For maximum safety, the nurse should use the following techniques when handling antineoplastic agents:

• Mix chemotherapeutic drugs in a Class II biological safety cabinet only.

• Wear disposable surgical gloves and a protective barrier garment with a closed front and long, cuffed sleeves to protect the body when mixing or administering these agents.

• Reconstitute and administer these agents in syringes or intravenous sets with Luer-Lok connections.

• Use a closed delivery technique when administering these agents.

• Do not prime intravenous lines and syringes into a sink or waste basket; use sterile 2" × 2" gauze pads or alcohol wipes instead.

• Cap needles carefully to prevent accidental skin punctures.

• After mixing and administering these agents, dispose of any waste in a leakproof, punctureproof container labeled "hazardous waste." Such containers may be disposed of by incineration or burial at a hazardous chemical waste site.

• If a spill occurs, follow the institution's policy for cleaning up hazardous materials.

Administering antineoplastic agents

Before administering an antineoplastic agent, the nurse should inform the patient about the benefits and risks of treatment. A patient who consents to investigational chemotherapy should receive additional information. Throughout the patient's therapy, the nurse should continue to teach and reinforce this information to facilitate patient safety and compliance.

To administer an antineoplastic agent safely, the nurse must select an appropriate site and vein, consider drug compatibilities, determine the agent's vesicant potential, consider its sequencing and delivery, and prevent or treat extravasation.

For a patient who must receive several treatments with these potentially damaging agents, site and vein selection is especially important. To select an appropriate intravenous site, the nurse should begin with a distal spot, such as the hand, and proceed to proximal areas, such as up the forearm.

Before administering any antineoplastic agent, the nurse should consider drug compatibilities. As a rule, antineoplastic agents should not be mixed with any other medications. Although little research has been done to determine exact incompatibilities, the agents' nature and toxicity usually prohibit mixing.

To choose the proper drug sequencing and delivery technique, the nurse needs to know the agent's potential to act as a vesicant. (See *Classifications of antineoplastic agents* on page 1151 for a summary of vesicant, irritant,

Cell cycle

Every cell progresses through a series of phases to replicate itself. During each phase, the cell is vulnerable to certain drugs that can interfere with its replication. This concept is the basis of antineoplastic therapy.

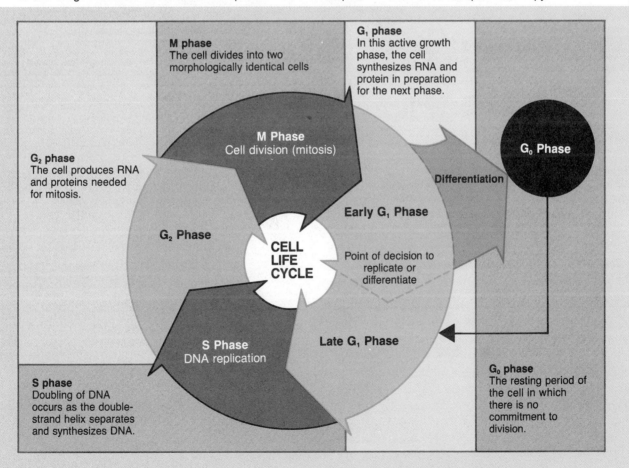

M phase
The cell divides into two morphologically identical cells

G₁ phase
In this active growth phase, the cell synthesizes RNA and protein in preparation for the next phase.

G₂ phase
The cell produces RNA and proteins needed for mitosis.

M Phase
Cell division (mitosis)

G₀ Phase

Differentiation

G₂ Phase

Early G₁ Phase

CELL LIFE CYCLE

Point of decision to replicate or differentiate

S Phase
DNA replication

Late G₁ Phase

S phase
Doubling of DNA occurs as the double-strand helix separates and synthesizes DNA.

G₀ phase
The resting period of the cell in which there is no commitment to division.

Mechanisms and sites of action of antineoplastic agents

Antineoplastic agents act at various phases of a cell to halt its growth or destroy it. Knowing where these agents act will help the nurse understand the basic principles of chemotherapy.

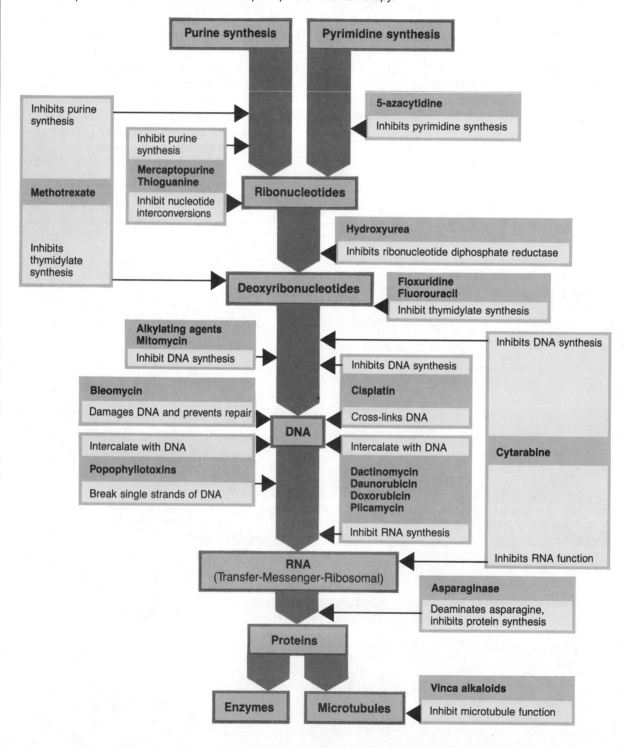

and nonvesicant drugs.) The nurse should administer a vesicant agent by direct push or delivery into the side port of an infusing intravenous line. Nonvesicant agents (including irritants) may be given by direct I.V. push, through the side port of an infusing I.V. line or as a continuous infusion. Some institutions require administration of the vesicant first because vein integrity decreases over time; others require administration of the vesicant last because it may increase vein fragility. Various venous access devices are available and are used when the vesicants are administered. These venous access devices reduce patient discomfort by removing the necessity for multiple I.V. insertions.

During the administration of any intravenous chemotherapeutic agent, the patient's safety depends on the nurse's ability to assess drug delivery into a patent vein. That is why the nurse must elicit a blood return before, during, and after drug administration.

To prevent extravasation, the nurse should use a splint to stabilize the needle and should check frequently for blood returns. Although no definitive measures exist to treat extravasation of an antineoplastic agent, conservative measures include discontinuing the infusion, aspirating any residual drug from the tubing and needle, instilling an intravenous antidote, and removing the needle. After administering an antidote, the nurse may apply heat or cold and may elevate the affected limb.

Adverse reactions

The adverse reactions to antineoplastic agents result from the drugs' systemic effects. Some reactions can be life-threatening, requiring modification of the drug dosage or treatment regimen. Others are less severe but may be stressful to the patient. (See *Frequent adverse reactions and associated nursing implications* on pages 1152 and 1153 for a summary.)

Nausea and vomiting are common adverse reactions. Chemotherapy can cause nausea and vomiting by three basic mechanisms. Orally administered drugs can irritate the gastric mucosa directly, causing nausea and vomiting that is less severe than that caused by the other two mechanisms. Other antineoplastic agents can stimulate the chemoreceptor trigger zone. The incidence of nausea and vomiting from this mechanism depends on the drug's inherent emetic potential. (See *Emetic potential of antineoplastic agents* on page 1154 for more information.) Finally, chemotherapy can cause psychogenic nausea and vomiting, which originates in the cerebral cortex. Known as anticipatory emesis, this reaction can be disabling. A patient who remembers the unpleasantness of previous chemotherapy may feel nauseated or may vomit just by thinking about future treatments. This reaction may become so severe that

---

Classifications of antineoplastic agents

To administer an antineoplastic agent safely, the nurse needs to know whether it is a vesicant (capable of producing blisters), an irritant (capable of producing cell excitation and undue sensitivity), or a nonvesicant drug.

Vesicant agents

- dacarbazine
- dactinomycin
- daunorubicin
- doxorubicin
- mitomycin
- nitrogen mustard
- plicamycin
- vinblastine
- vincristine
- vindesine

Irritant agents

- carmustine
- etoposide
- streptozocin

Nonvesicant agents

- asparaginase
- bleomycin
- cisplatin
- cyclophosphamide
- cytarabine
- floxuridine
- fluorouracil

---

sights, sounds, and smells associated with treatment may induce emesis, no matter how far removed the patient is from the actual treatment setting. Chemotherapy-induced nausea and vomiting is of great concern because it can cause Mallory-Weiss syndrome (tears at the esophageal gastric junction, leading to massive bleeding), wound dehiscence, pathologic fractures, fluid and electrolyte imbalances, and noncompliance with the treatment regimen. It also can cause distress by limiting the patient's ability and motivation to take an active role in life.

To combat the nausea and vomiting caused by chemotherapy, nurses frequently administer drugs, such as dronabinol, droperidol, prochlorperazine, metoclopramide, dexamethasone, and lorazepam. Usually, an antiemetic drug is given in combination with several other antiemetics that act by different mechanisms. A combination regimen is more effective than a single drug, especially for a strong emetic agent, such as cisplatin.

Frequent adverse reactions and associated nursing implications

The antineoplastic agents cause many of the same adverse reactions and require similar nursing implications. To provide quality patient care, the nurse must be aware of these reactions and implications.

ADVERSE REACTIONS	NURSING IMPLICATIONS
Bone marrow suppression	
Bone marrow suppression is the most common and potentially serious adverse reaction to the antineoplastic agents.	• Watch for the blood count nadir because that is when the patient is at greatest risk for complications of leukopenia, thrombocytopenia, and anemia. • Plan a patient-teaching program about bone marrow suppression, including information about blood counts, potential sites of infection, and personal hygiene.
Leukopenia: This reaction increases a patient's risk of infection, especially if the granulocyte count is under 1,000/mm³.	• Because a leukopenic patient is subject to infections, provide information about good hygiene, and assess the patient frequently for signs and symptoms of infection. • Teach the patient to recognize and report the signs and symptoms of infection, such as fever, cough, or a burning sensation on urination. • Teach the patient how to take a temperature. • Caution the patient to avoid crowds and people with colds or the flu during the nadir. • If the patient is receiving corticosteroids, remember that the inflammatory response may be decreased and the complications of leukopenia more difficult to detect.
Thrombocytopenia: This reaction occurs with leukopenia. When the platelet count is under 50,000/mm³, the patient is at risk for bleeding. When it is under 20,000/mm³, the patient is at severe risk and may require a platelet transfusion.	• Assess the patient for bleeding gums, increased bruising or petechiae, hypermenorrhea, tarry stools, hematuria, and coffee-ground emesis. • Advise the patient to avoid cuts and bruises and to use a soft toothbrush and an electric razor. • Instruct the patient to report sudden headaches, which could indicate potentially fatal intracranial bleeding. • Tell the patient to use a stool softener, as prescribed, to prevent colonic irritation and bleeding. • Instruct the patient to avoid using rectal thermometers and I.M. injections, to prevent bleeding.
Anemia: This reaction develops slowly over several courses of treatment.	• Assess the patient for dizziness, fatigue, pallor, and shortness of breath on minimal exertion. • Monitor the patient's hematocrit and hemoglobin, and red blood cell counts. Remember that a patient dehydrated from nausea, vomiting, or anorexia may exhibit a false-normal hematocrit. Once this patient is rehydrated, the hematocrit will decrease. • Be prepared to administer a blood transfusion to a symptomatic patient. • Instruct the patient to rest more frequently and to increase the dietary intake of iron-rich foods. Advise the patient to take a multiple vitamin with iron, as prescribed.
Nausea and vomiting	
These reactions can result from chemical irritation of the central nervous system or from psychogenic factors that may be activated by sensations, suggestions, or anxiety.	• To control the chemical irritation, administer combinations of antiemetics, as ordered. • Monitor the patient for signs and symptoms of aspiration because most antiemetics sedate. • To control psychogenic factors, help the patient perform relaxation techniques before chemotherapy to minimize feelings of isolation and anxiety. • Spend time to encourage the patient to express anxiety. • Encourage the patient to listen to music or to engage in relaxation exercises, meditation, or hypnosis to promote feelings of control and well-being. • Adjust the drug administration time to meet the patient's needs. Some patients prefer treatments in the evening when they find sedation comfortable. Patients who work may prefer their treatments on their days off.

Frequent adverse reactions and associated nursing implications continued

ADVERSE REACTIONS	NURSING IMPLICATIONS
Stomatitis	
Although epithelial tissue damage can affect any mucous membrane, the most common site is the oral mucosa. Stomatitis is temporary and can range from mild and barely noticeable to severe and debilitating. (Debilitation may result from poor nutrition during acute stomatitis.)	• Initiate preventive mouth care before chemotherapy to provide comfort and decrease the severity of the stomatitis. • Provide therapeutic mouth care, including topical antibiotics, if prescribed.
Alopecia	
To the patient, alopecia may be the most distressing adverse reaction.	• Prepare the patient for alopecia. Point out that hair loss usually is gradual and is reversible after treatment ends. • Inform the patient that alopecia may be partial or complete and that it affects men and women. • Advise the patient that alopecia may affect the scalp, eyebrows, eyelashes, and body hair.

Chapter 73
Alkylating Agents

Chapter 73 discusses the cell-cycle-nonspecific alkylating agents used to treat malignant neoplasms: the nitrogen mustards, alkyl sulfonates, nitrosoureas, triazines, and alkylating-like agents. It emphasizes mechanisms of action and pharmacokinetics and describes nursing interventions to help the patient cope with adverse reactions.

Chapter 74
Antimetabolite Agents

Chapter 74 focuses on the cell-cycle-specific antimetabolite antineoplastic agents: the folic acid, pyrimidine, and purine analogues. It explores mechanisms of action and clinical indications of these specific agents. It also discusses adverse reactions, patient education, nursing implications, and leucovorin rescue therapy.

Chapter 75
Antineoplastic Antibiotic Agents

Chapter 75 presents the cell-cycle-nonspecific antibiotic agents that also demonstrate tumorcidal action—such as dactinomycin, mitomycin, and plicamycin—and bleomycine, which is cell-cycle-specific. For these agents, the chapter discusses clinical indications, including their use in treating hypercalcemia. It also details their adverse reactions and associated nursing implications, and provides patient education information.

Chapter 76
Hormonal Antineoplastic Agents

Chapter 76 highlights the hormonal antineoplastic agents, which include estrogens, antiestrogens, androgens, adrenocortical suppressants, progestins, adrenocorticosteroids, and a gonadotropin-releasing hormone analogue. It describes the pharmacokinetics and clinical indications of these cytostatic agents and emphasizes associated nursing interventions and patient education.

Chapter 77
Other Antineoplastic Agents

Chapter 77 investigates several other antineoplastic agents, including the cell-cycle-specific vinca alkaloids, podophyllotoxins, asparaginase, hydroxyurea, and the cell-cycle-nonspecific procarbazine. It discusses their mechanisms of action, the clinical indications for, and adverse reactions to, these agents, along with related nursing interventions, and provides patient education.

Nursing diagnoses

When caring for a patient receiving drugs to treat malignant neoplasms, the following nursing diagnoses may apply:
• Activity intolerance related to neoplastic activity, drug therapy, or nutritional deficits
• Alteration in cardiac output: decreased, related to drug therapy
• Alteration in comfort: pain, related to neoplastic activity or drug therapy

Emetic potential of antineoplastic agents

Some antineoplastic agents are more likely than others to cause nausea and vomiting. Knowing the emetic potential of these agents will help the nurse plan patient care.

Severe (greater than 50% incidence)

- azacytidine
- carmustine
- cisplatin
- cyclophosphamide
- dacarbazine
- dactinomycin
- daunorubicin
- doxorubicin
- mechlorethamine
- mithramycin
- streptozocin

Moderate (25% to 50% incidence)

- 5-azacytidine
- cytarabine
- etoposide
- procarbazine
- thiotepa
- vinblastine

Mild to none (25% incidence)

- asparaginase
- bleomycin
- busulfan
- chlorambucil
- fluorouracil
- hydroxyurea
- mercaptopurine
- methotrexate
- plicamycin
- thioguanine
- vincristine

- Alteration in family process related to neoplastic activity, drug therapy, or life-style changes
- Alteration in fluid volume: excess or deficit, related to neoplastic activity or drug therapy
- Alteration in nutrition: less than body requirement, related to neoplastic activity or drug therapy
- Alteration in oral mucous membrane related to neoplastic activity or drug therapy
- Alteration in thought processes related to neoplastic activity or drug therapy
- Alteration in tissue perfusion related to neoplastic activity or drug therapy
- Alteration in urinary elimination patterns related to neoplastic activity or drug therapy
- Alterations in bowel elimination: constipation or diarrhea, related to neoplastic activity or drug therapy
- Altered growth and development related to neoplastic activity or drug therapy
- Anticipatory grieving related to neoplastic activity, drug therapy, or life-style changes

- Anxiety related to neoplastic activity, drug therapy, or life-style changes
- Disturbance in self-concept related to neoplastic activity, drug therapy, or life-style changes
- Fear related to neoplastic activity, drug therapy, or life-style changes
- Hopelessness related to neoplastic activity, drug therapy, or life-style changes
- Impaired adjustment related to the diagnosis of neoplastic activity, drug therapy, or life-style changes
- Impaired home maintenance management related to neoplastic activity, drug therapy, or life-style changes
- Impaired physical mobility related to neoplastic activity or drug therapy
- Impaired social interaction related to neoplastic activity, drug therapy, or life-style changes
- Impaired swallowing related to neoplastic activity or drug therapy
- Impaired tissue integrity related to neoplastic activity or drug therapy
- Ineffective airway clearance related to neoplastic activity or drug therapy
- Ineffective breathing pattern related to neoplastic activity
- Ineffective family coping: compromised, related to the effects of neoplastic activity or drug therapy on the patient and life-style changes
- Ineffective individual coping related to neoplastic activity, drug therapy, or life-style changes
- Knowledge deficit related to neoplastic activity or drug therapy
- Potential alteration in body temperature related to neoplastic activity or drug therapy
- Potential for infection related to neoplastic activity or drug therapy
- Potential for injury related to neoplastic activity or drug therapy
- Powerlessness related to neoplastic activity or drug therapy
- Self-care deficit related to neoplastic activity or drug therapy
- Sensory-perceptual alteration related to neoplastic activity or drug therapy
- Sexual dysfunction related to neoplastic activity, drug therapy, or life-style changes
- Sleep pattern disturbances related to neoplastic activity or drug therapy
- Social isolation related to neoplastic activity, drug therapy, or life-style changes
- Spiritual distress related to neoplastic activity, drug therapy, or life-style changes.

CHAPTER 73

ALKYLATING AGENTS

OBJECTIVES

After reading and studying this chapter, you should be able to:

1. Explain the alkylation process and its role in the mechanism of action of alkylating agents.

2. Identify the clinical indications for nitrogen mustards, alkyl sulfonates, nitrosoureas, triazines, and alkylating-like agents.

3. Discuss the absorption, distribution, metabolism, and excretion of the nitrogen mustards.

4. Explain how the onset of action, peak concentration levels, and duration of action of the nitrogen mustards, especially mechlorethamine, determine specific nursing implications.

5. Describe the nursing interventions for managing predictable reactions of the alkylating agents, especially nausea and vomiting associated with the therapy.

6. Discuss the pharmacokinetic properties of the nitrosoureas that make these agents especially useful in treating brain tumors and meningeal leukemias.

7. Identify the nursing implications associated with cisplatin, especially those related to drug preparation and administration.

INTRODUCTION

Alkylating agents, which are highly reactive drugs, enter the cell nuclei and disrupt the structure of deoxyribonucleic acid (DNA). These drugs exert cytotoxic activity in a cell-cycle-nonspecific manner but may act more effectively in the late G_1 phase and S phase. Interference with normal cell mitosis in rapidly proliferating tissue explains both the therapeutic action and the adverse effects of alkylating agents.

Alkylating agents, given singly or in combination with other drugs, effectively act against various malignant neoplasms. The sensitive malignant neoplasms include chronic and acute leukemias, non-Hodgkin's lymphomas, multiple melanoma, melanoma, sarcoma, and cancers of the breast, ovaries, uterus, lung, brain, testes, bladder, prostate, and stomach. Protocols for administering these drugs vary from institution to institution.

The major adverse effects produced by alkylating agents include bone marrow suppression, nausea, vomiting, alopecia, and damage to epithelial tissues. The severity of the adverse effects depends on many vari-

Alkylating agents

The following lists the different groups of alkylating agents as well as specific drugs in each group.

Nitrogen mustards

- mechlorethamine (Mustargen)
- cyclophosphamide (Cytoxan)
- melphalan (Alkeran)
- chlorambucil (Leukeran)
- thiotepa (Thiotepa)
- estramustine (Emcyt)
- uracil mustard

Alkyl sulfonate

- busulfan (Myleran)

Nitrosoureas

- carmustine [BCNU] (BiCNU)
- lomustine [CCNU] (CeeNU)
- semustine [methyl-CCNU]
- streptozocin (Zanosar)

Triazine

- dacarbazine (DTIC-Dome)

Alkylating-like agent

- cisplatin [cis-platinum] (Platinol)

ables, including drug dosage, prior chemotherapy treatments, physical condition, and psychological factors. The adverse effects, which are reversible, may occur early or later in the therapeutic regimen.

For a summary of representative drugs, see *Selected major drugs: Alkylating agents* on page 1166.

NITROGEN MUSTARDS

The nitrogen mustards represent the largest group of alkylating agents. Mechlorethamine, which was the first nitrogen mustard introduced, is also the most rapidly acting of all these drugs.

History and source
The history of the alkylating agents originates in 20th-century chemical warfare. Sulfur mustard, first synthesized in 1854, was used as a nerve gas in World War I. In 1919, Krumbhaar and Krumbhaar described the effect of mustard gas on its victims. While surviving soldiers were found to be leukopenic, autopsies of deceased victims revealed aplastic bone marrow. Extensive research occurred between World War I and 1942, when nitrogen mustard was first used to treat patients with advanced lymphomas. Since World War II, researchers have worked toward the synthesis of other nitrogen mustards, also referred to as classic alkylating agents.

PHARMACOKINETICS
The absorption and distribution of nitrogen mustards, as with most alkylating agents, vary widely. The nitrogen mustards are metabolized in the liver and excreted by the kidneys.

Absorption
The nitrogen mustards are administered intravenously, orally, and topically, as well as by instillation. When administered intravenously, the drugs are considered to be 100% bioavailable (absorbed and available in the general circulation). Orally administered nitrogen mustards exhibit variable and incomplete absorption.

Mechlorethamine is sometimes instilled into the pleural, pericardial, and peritoneal cavities to control malignant effusions. Although absorption is variable and incomplete, it may be sufficient to produce systemic toxicity. Systemic absorption from topically applied mechlorethamine for mycosis fungoides is minimal.

When given orally, cyclophosphamide is well absorbed; however, up to 31% of an orally administered dose can be recovered in the stool. Likewise, melphalan is 50% to 70% absorbed after oral administration. Chlorambucil administered orally is adequately but incompletely absorbed.

Thiotepa may be administered into the pleural or peritoneal space to treat malignant effusions. This drug is also administered as a bladder instillation. Significant systemic absorption may occur with these applications, resulting in systemic toxicity.

Estramustine and uracil mustard are administered orally. After administration, 75% of an estramustine dose is absorbed. Uracil mustard is absorbed quickly but incompletely.

Distribution
Mechlorethamine is highly reactive and is hydrolyzed rapidly after I.V. administration. Within a few minutes, less than 10% of the drug remains in the blood.

Cyclophosphamide exhibits limited entry into the central nervous system (CNS), breast milk, sweat, saliva, and synovial fluid. The moderate lipid and water solubility of the drug allows it and its metabolites to be widely distributed to the extracellular fluid spaces of the body.

Melphalan is not well distributed to fat because the volume of distribution approximates total body water at 44 liters. Chlorambucil, however, displays homogenous distribution, being deposited in fatty tissue. The distribution to fatty tissue may explain the prolonged effect of chlorambucil in some patients. By contrast, thiotepa enters the cerebrospinal fluid (CSF), and estramustine exhibits a low volume of distribution because of its extensive plasma protein binding. Plasma concentration levels of uracil mustard decline rapidly after both oral and intravenous administration.

Metabolism
The nitrogen mustards undergo hepatic metabolism. Mechlorethamine is rapidly inactivated as it undergoes chemical transformation in the plasma and other body tissues. Cyclophosphamide is metabolized, then further oxidized to inactive metabolites and phosphoramide mustard, which is cytotoxic.

Excretion
Most nitrogen mustards are excreted in the urine. Within 24 hours of administration, cyclophosphamide is excreted in the urine as 10% cyclophosphamide and 50% metabolites. Only 10% to 15% of a melphalan dose is excreted unchanged in the urine. In 24 hours, 50% of

Administration and excretion routes for alkylating agents

The following chart summarizes the major administration routes and excretion of the alkylating agents, including approximate amounts of the drugs and metabolites excreted.

DRUG	MAJOR ROUTES OF ADMINISTRATION	MAJOR ROUTES OF EXCRETION	AMOUNT EXCRETED
Nitrogen mustards			
mechlorethamine	Intravenous	Urinary	>50% in 24 hours as metabolites
cyclophosphamide	Intravenous, oral	Urinary	60% in 24 hours, mainly as metabolites
melphalan	Oral	Fecal Urinary	20% to 25% in 6 days with oral administration 50% in 24 hours
chlorambucil	Oral	Urinary	60% in 24 hours, mainly as metabolites
thiotepa	Intravesicular	Urinary	Unchanged in urine in 24 to 48 hours
uracil mustard	Oral	Unknown, some urinary	Unknown, less than 19% unchanged in urine
estramustine	Oral	Urinary	23% in 48 hours
Alkyl sulfonate			
busulfan	Oral	Urinary	10% to 50% in 24 hours as metabolites
Nitrosoureas			
carmustine	Intravenous	Urinary	80% in 24 hours as metabolites
lomustine	Oral	Urinary	50% in 24 hours as metabolites
semustine	Oral	Urinary	60% in 48 hours as metabolites
streptozocin	Intravenous	Urinary Pulmonary	10% to 20% Not quantified, probably significant
Triazine			
dacarbazine	Intravenous	Urinary	35% to 40%, half of this as metabolites
Alkylating-like agent			
cisplatin	Intravenous	Urinary	23% in 24 hours 27% to 45% in 5 days

a melphalan dose is excreted in the feces. After undergoing extensive conjugation in the liver and hydrolysis in the liver and prostate, 23% of an estramustine dose appears in the urine. Estramustine is also excreted in the feces and bile as metabolites. (See *Administration and excretion routes for alkylating agents* for more information about the pharmacokinetics of these agents.)

Onset, peak, duration

Mechlorethamine undergoes metabolism in water and body fluids so rapidly that no active drug remains after a few minutes.

Most of the nitrogen mustards possess more intermediate half-lives than mechlorethamine. Cyclophosphamide reaches peak plasma concentration levels approximately 1 hour after an oral dose, with a plasma half-life of approximately 7 hours. However, the alkylating activity of the unbound metabolites lasts for at least 24 hours. The half-life of these alkylating metabolites of cyclophosphamide is significantly prolonged in renal failure.

Melphalan reaches a peak plasma concentration level approximately 1 hour after an oral dose, with a plasma half-life of 90 minutes. Tissue concentration levels of chlorambucil peak in the liver 1 hour after a dose. Chlorambucil has a half-life of 2 hours. Peak concentration levels of thiotepa are not well quantified; however, this drug may have a half-life of up to 1 week or more. After an oral dose, estramustine achieves peak concentration levels in approximately 2 hours or less, and the half-life is 2 hours. Plasma concentration levels of uracil mustard decline rapidly, with no evidence of the drug remaining after 2 hours.

PHARMACODYNAMICS

The nitrogen mustards form covalent bonds with DNA molecules in a chemical reaction known as alkylation. (See *Mechanisms and sites of action of antineoplastic agents* in Unit Fifteen Introduction.) Alkylated DNA cannot replicate properly, resulting in cell death. Unfortunately, tumor cells may develop resistance to the cytotoxic effects of nitrogen mustards.

Mechanism of action

Researchers believe that most nitrogen mustards, like the other alkylating agents, enter cells via active transport systems. Once inside the cell, the drug undergoes strong electrophilic (having an affinity for electrons) chemical reactions with several substances, including phosphate, amino, sulfhydryl, carboxyl, and imidazole groups. These chemical reactions result in covalent bonds. The process is referred to as alkylation, and the alkylation of DNA inhibits its proper functioning. At pharmacologic doses, the nitrogen mustards produce cytotoxic and other effects because of the alkylation of DNA. (See *Alkylation* for a description of this reaction.)

Although the nitrogen mustards are cell-cycle-non-specific, they seem to be most effective against cells in the late G_1 phase or S phase. Alkylation becomes toxic when the cells enter the S phase, during which DNA synthesis occurs, and cell progression through the cycle is blocked by alkylation at the G_2 phase. The alkylation reaction is nontoxic, however, if the cell repairs the DNA damage before cell division. In fact, DNA repair systems may play a key role in the relative resistance of non-proliferating tissue, as well as in the selective action of the drugs against certain cell types and in the tumor's acquired resistance to the drugs. (See *Action of anti-*

Alkylation

Alkylation of DNA can occur as a bifunctional or monofunctional reaction. Bifunctional reactions occur when one molecule of the alkylating agent undergoes two alkylation reactions. That may result in the cross-linking of two DNA molecules, the cross-linking of two strands of a single DNA molecule, or the linking of the DNA molecule to another protein. When bifunctional alkylation occurs, cytotoxic effects predominate.

Monofunctional reactions occur when a single molecule of the alkylating agent undergoes one alkylation reaction. That results in depurination and chain scission, which may later cause permanent damage, such as mutagenesis or carcinogenesis.

---

neoplastic agents on the cell cycle in Unit Fifteen Introduction for more information on how these drugs affect the cell cycle.)

Resistance is an acquired phenomenon whereby previously sensitive tumors are no longer sensitive to the cytotoxic actions of alkylating agents. Resistance usually develops slowly and may result from several biochemical changes. Decreased permeation of the drug into the cell may occur, preventing the drug from reaching its site of action. The tumor cell may also increase production of nucleic substances that compete with the DNA for alkylation. With the increased binding of the drug to these other substances, less drug remains to act on the DNA. The tumor cell may also increase DNA repair systems. If the damage caused by alkylation is repaired before the cell divides, cell death does not occur. Finally, increased metabolism of the active drug may occur, thereby decreasing the contact time between the drug and tumor cell. When resistance of a tumor to one alkylating agent occurs, the tumor cells often become cross-resistant to other alkylating agents.

PHARMACOTHERAPEUTICS

The nitrogen mustards are indicated for various malignant neoplasms. Because they produce leukopenia, the nitrogen mustards are effective in treating malignant neoplasms, such as Hodgkin's disease and leukemias, that have an associated elevated white blood cell count. Also, the nitrogen mustards prove effective against many solid tumors. These drugs can be given singly or in combination with other classes of antineoplastic agents. The activity and effectiveness of each drug depend on many factors, including the type of cancer, the extent of disease, and the patient's condition. Furthermore, the toxicity of the nitrogen mustards depends to a large extent on the dose and administration route. For instance, cyclophosphamide is given in low oral doses and in high intravenous doses, and toxicity is directly related to dose. The nurse administering nitrogen mustards must not only be familiar with the specific pharmacologic data about the drug, but also the protocol being used with the patient.

mechlorethamine (Mustargen). Administered intravenously, mechlorethamine is used primarily to treat advanced Hodgkin's disease (Stages III and IV). The drug is also used to induce brief remissions in the treatment of non-Hodgkin's lymphomas. The I.V. administration can be extremely irritating to the vein. Though mechlorethamine should not be given intramuscularly or subcutaneously, physicians use intracavitary administration to treat malignant pleural effusions.

USUAL ADULT DOSAGE: 0.4 mg/kg I.V. for the course of therapy. Some patients being treated for advanced Hodgkin's disease may receive higher doses. Depending on the protocol, mechlorethamine is administered once every 3 to 6 weeks. With intracavitary administration, the dose is 0.2 to 0.4 mg/kg.

cyclophosphamide (Cytoxan). Alone or in combination therapies, cyclophosphamide is used to treat numerous hematologic and solid tumors. Cyclophosphamide is considered the drug of choice in treating acute lymphoblastic leukemia and neuroblastoma. When used singly, cyclophosphamide has produced a positive response in 30% of patients with multiple myeloma and in 90% of patients with Burkitt's lymphoma. Solid tumors treated with cyclophosphamide include ovarian carcinoma, breast carcinoma, bronchogenic carcinoma, and retinoblastoma. Cyclophosphamide is administered orally or by I.V. injection. It is also given intrapleurally and intraperitoneally.

USUAL ADULT DOSAGE: for patients with no hematologic deficiencies, from 2 to 3 mg/kg to as high as 100 mg/kg. Dosages vary for different types of cancer. Subsequent doses are adjusted according to patient tolerance.

melphalan (Alkeran). Administered orally, melphalan is used primarily to treat multiple myeloma.

USUAL ADULT DOSAGE: initially, 6 mg P.O. daily for 2 to 3 weeks. Subsequent doses may be adjusted depending on the degree of leukopenia induced. Usually, maintenance therapy is 2 to 4 mg P.O. daily to maintain the proper bone marrow suppression.

chlorambucil (Leukeran). Either alone or as a combination agent, chlorambucil is used to treat chronic lymphocytic leukemia, non-Hodgkin's lymphomas, and advanced Hodgkin's disease. Chlorambucil is administered orally.

USUAL ADULT DOSAGE: 4 to 10 mg P.O. daily for 3 to 6 weeks. As clinical improvement occurs and the white blood cell (WBC) count decreases, a maintenance dose of 2 mg/day is prescribed.

thiotepa (Thiotepa). This drug may be given intravesically to treat bladder cancer or parenterally in the palliative treatment of ovarian carcinoma, lymphomas, and breast carcinoma. Thiotepa may also be injected directly into the tumor mass.

USUAL ADULT DOSAGE: for bladder instillation, 60 mg weekly for 4 weeks; for rapid I.V. administration, 0.3 to 0.4 mg/kg should be given at 1- to 4-week intervals; for intratumor administration, initial dose of 0.6 to 0.8 mg/kg; maintenance doses, 0.07 to 0.8 mg/kg at 1- to 4-week intervals.

estramustine (Emcyt). A combination of an estrogen and nitrogen mustard, estramustine was discovered and developed in Sweden and is used to treat advanced prostate cancer.

USUAL ADULT DOSAGE: 10 to 16 mg/kg P.O. in divided daily doses.

uracil mustard. Uracil mustard is used primarily in the palliative treatment of malignant neoplasms of the reticuloendothelial system, such as lymphomas and chronic myelogenous leukemia.

USUAL ADULT DOSAGE: 1 to 2 mg P.O. daily until the desired effect is obtained, usually 3 weeks, followed by a rest period of 1 week; then the protocol is repeated.

Drug interactions

Most drug interactions with antineoplastic agents, including the nitrogen mustards, are theoretical, secondary to animal studies or basic chemical theory. (See Unit Fifteen Introduction for a further discussion.) Mechlorethamine and cyclophosphamide, however, produce known effects when given in combination. (See *Drug interactions: Nitrogen mustards* on page 1160 for details.)

ADVERSE DRUG REACTIONS

Patients receiving nitrogen mustards may experience a wide range of adverse reactions, depending on which drug is given, the dose, the patient's condition and co-morbidity, other drugs being used, and psychological

DRUG INTERACTIONS

Nitrogen mustards

Most of the drug interactions involving nitrogen mustards are based on animal studies and remain theoretical in humans. The following list, however, describes interactions for which human data are available.

DRUG	INTERACTING DRUGS	POSSIBLE EFFECTS	NURSING IMPLICATIONS
cyclophosphamide	allopurinol	Prolongs half-life of cyclophosphamide, resulting in increased bone marrow suppression. Alkylating metabolites unchanged.	• Little clinical significance.
	corticosteroids	May inhibit metabolism of cyclophosphamide	• Decrease of steroids *may* result in increased cyclophosphamide toxicity.
	phenobarbital	Induces enzymes of hepatic oxidase system	• Little clinical significance.

factors. Pharmacologic or nonpharmacologic interventions can manage some reactions, such as nausea and vomiting. Others, such as bone marrow suppression, must resolve on their own. (See *Frequent adverse reactions and associated nursing implications* in Unit Fifteen Introduction.)

Predictable reactions

Bone marrow suppression, evidenced by severe leukopenia and thrombocytopenia, is an anticipated adverse reaction associated with the nitrogen mustards. Depending on the degree of the patient's bone marrow suppression, the physician may modify future drug doses.

Nausea and vomiting from CNS irritation is another common adverse reaction to the nitrogen mustards. Nausea and vomiting may occur 30 minutes after drug administration, as happens with mechlorethamine, or may not begin for hours, as occurs with cyclophosphamide. If used in the right combination and in an effective dosing pattern, antiemetic drugs can control or lessen most nausea and vomiting associated with nitrogen mustards.

Damage to rapidly proliferating cells produces stomatitis and alopecia. The swollen, inflamed mucous membranes that characterize stomatitis can lead to a nutritional problem because of painful swallowing. Alopecia, which results from damage to the hair follicle, results in thinning hair 2 to 3 weeks after the first administration of a nitrogen mustard. However, hair loss is usually not significant for two to three courses of treatment. Once treatment ends, hair growth resumes.

Many patients experience fatigue while receiving nitrogen mustards. Anemia from bone marrow suppression probably produces the fatigue. Some evidence that circulating tumor breakdown products may also contribute to the fatigue exists. Many patients feel most fatigued immediately after treatment and find their energy increases later in the interval between therapeutic courses. However, for patients on protocols that last for months, fatigue is persistent.

Because the nitrogen mustards are powerful local vesicants (blistering agents), direct contact with the drugs or their vapors can cause severe reactions, especially of the skin, eyes, and respiratory tract.

Unpredictable reactions

Hemorrhagic cystitis may develop within 48 hours of an intravenous dose of cyclophosphamide, or it may result after several months of low oral doses of the drug. Cyclophosphamide metabolites in the urine irritate the bladder lining, producing the reaction. Adequate hydration usually prevents this reaction, and the nurse should encourage any patient receiving cyclophosphamide to maintain a fluid intake of at least 2,000 ml daily.

Both men and women may experience alterations in fertility. After several courses of nitrogen mustard treatment, women may experience amenorrhea or irregular menses. Men may have decreased spermatogenesis. Many patients, however, experience no apparent alteration in fertility, and females treated with nitrogen mustards have conceived and given birth to normal children.

Chlorambucil may produce hepatotoxicity, but this reaction rarely occurs. Anaphylaxis is another rare and unpredictable adverse reaction associated with the nitrogen mustards.

NURSING IMPLICATIONS

Because of the potential harmful effects of the nitrogen mustards, the nurse dealing with these drugs must be knowledgeable about administration techniques, precautions, dosages and protocol plans, adverse reactions, and necessary interventions. The nursing implications associated with these agents include the following:

• Use caution when administering nitrogen mustards (vesicants), especially intravenously. In particular, mechlorethamine produces serious tissue damage if extravasated. (See Unit Fifteen Introduction for more information about proper administration principles.)

• Most of these drugs, which are prepared before the administration time, remain quite stable. Mechlorethamine, however, is unstable in solution; therefore, administer mechlorethamine immediately after its reconstitution.

• Altering the infusion rate, further diluting the drug, or warming the injection site to distend the vein increases blood flow and may reduce pain.

• Inform the patient of expected adverse reactions to prepare the patient psychologically for therapy.

• Bone marrow suppression is the most frequent and potentially serious adverse effect of the alkylating agents. Monitor the patient's blood counts carefully, especially the complete blood count (CBC).

• Nitrogen mustards produce alopecia, which may distress the patient even though the condition is physically nonthreatening. Unfortunately, nothing can prevent the alopecia caused by oral alkylating agents. Prepare the patient by discussing when hair loss usually begins and point out that it is reversible when the treatment ends.

• Alopecia affects men and women and may include eyebrows, eyelashes, scalp hair, and body hair.

• Instruct the patient to increase oral fluid intake the day before cyclophosphamide treatment to help prevent hemorrhagic cystitis. Fluid intake should not include coffee or tea, which have diuretic effects.

• Give extra fluid to the patient receiving cyclophosphamide intravenously. After treatment, instruct the patient to maintain increased fluids for 2 to 3 days.

• To prevent cyclophosphamide metabolites from prolonged contact with the bladder, administer the drug earlier in the day rather than at bedtime.

• Encourage patients taking oral cyclophosphamide to take their medications earlier in the day, to maintain good fluid intake, and to void before going to bed.

• Make available to the patient written materials about the drugs for home reference.

See Unit Fifteen Introduction for other important nursing implications concerning bone marrow suppression, leukopenia, thrombocytopenia, anemia, nausea and vomiting, mucositis, and alopecia.

ALKYL SULFONATE

Physicians frequently use the alkyl sulfonate busulfan to treat chronic myelocytic leukemia and less frequently to treat polycythemia vera and other myeloproliferative disorders. Busulfan is not chemically related to the nitrogen mustards.

PHARMACOKINETICS

Busulfan is effective when administered orally.

Absorption, distribution, metabolism, excretion

Busulfan is well absorbed and rapidly distributed throughout the body. The drug disappears from the plasma within minutes. Busulfan is extensively metabolized in the liver before urinary excretion. Within 24 hours, 10% to 50% of busulfan metabolites are excreted in the urine. (See Administration and excretion routes for alkylating agents on page 1157 for more information about the pharmacokinetics of this drug.)

Onset, peak, duration

Precise data concerning the onset of action, peak concentration levels, and duration of action of busulfan are unavailable because analytical methods are insufficient. The only effect of busulfan is myelosuppression, specifically granulocytopoiesis. The effect of the reduced WBC count begins about 10 days after the initiation of therapy and lasts 2 weeks after the discontinuation of the drug.

PHARMACODYNAMICS

The alkyl sulfonate busulfan forms covalent bonds with the DNA molecules in a chemical reaction known as alkylation. (See Mechanisms and sites of action of antineoplastic agents in Unit Fifteen Introduction for more details about the mechanism of action of this drug. Also see Alkylation on page 1158 for a detailed discussion of this process.)

Mechanism of action

Busulfan, in an aqueous medium, undergoes a wide range of nucleophilic substitution reactions, causing alkylation of the DNA and leading to its cytotoxic effects.

PHARMACOTHERAPEUTICS

Busulfan, which is cell-cycle-nonspecific, affects primarily granulocytes and, to a lesser degree, platelets. Because of the drug action on granulocytes, busulfan is the drug of choice for treating chronic myelocytic leukemia. The drug's action also makes busulfan effective for polycythemia vera.

busulfan (Myleran). Administered orally, busulfan is the drug of choice to treat chronic myelocytic leukemia. USUAL ADULT DOSAGE: 4 to 8 mg P.O. daily, until the WBC falls to 10,000/mm³. The drug is then stopped until the WBC rises to 50,000/mm³. Treatment is resumed to maintain the WBC at 10,000 to 20,000/mm³. The maintenance dose is usually 2 mg P.O. daily.

Drug interactions

No significant drug interactions occur with busulfan.

ADVERSE DRUG REACTIONS

Busulfan can cause a wide range of adverse reactions, which may be mild or severe. The nurse can help manage some reactions, such as nausea and vomiting. Within the first 2 weeks after beginning busulfan, the WBC will fall for about 10 days. The decreased WBC may lead to thrombocytopenia, pancytopenia, or anemia. Nausea, vomiting, and diarrhea also usually occur. Hyperuricemia also occurs, and it is treated with hydration and allopurinol. With long-term therapy, an addisonian-like wasting syndrome with hyperpigmentation and weight loss sometimes occurs. Busulfan also may produce irreversible interstitial pulmonary fibrosis (busulfan lung) after long-term use (1 to 3 years).

NURSING IMPLICATIONS

The adverse effects and nursing implications of busulfan resemble those of the other alkylating agents, including the nitrogen mustards. The nurse should be aware of the following during busulfan therapy:
• Be aware that a persistent cough and progressive dyspnea with alveolar exudate may result from drug toxicity, not from pneumonia.
• Recognize that myelosuppression may be uncharacteristically long, from 11 to 30 days, and that recovery may also be prolonged, occurring over 25 to 54 days.

Therefore, monitor all hematologic laboratory values and be prepared to discontinue the drug administration as prescribed if a rapid or significant decrease in those values occurs.
• Monitor uric acid levels and CBC.
• Avoid all I.M. injections when the platelet count is low.
• Use anticoagulants cautiously, and observe for signs of bleeding.

See Unit Fifteen Introduction for additional nursing implications associated with busulfan.

NITROSOUREAS

The nitrosoureas in an aqueous medium are unstable and decompose to alkylating intermediates. The lethal effect of nitrosoureas on cells seems to result from the inhibition of DNA synthesis.

History and source

Scientists at the Southern Research Institute developed the nitrosoureas, which were introduced clinically in the early 1960s.

PHARMACOKINETICS

The nitrosoureas are well absorbed from the gastrointestinal tract. These drugs are lipid-soluble and readily cross the blood-brain barrier. They undergo significant metabolism in the liver. The metabolites of the nitrosoureas are excreted in the urine.

Absorption, distribution, metabolism, excretion

When administered topically for mycosis fungoides, carmustine provides systemic absorption of about 5% to 28%. The nitrosoureas lomustine and semustine are adequately, though incompletely, absorbed after oral administration.

Carmustine, lomustine, semustine, and streptozocin are lipophilic, distributing to fatty tissues and attaining significant CSF levels. Carmustine and lomustine achieve CSF levels of 15% to 30% of plasma levels. Streptozocin and its metabolites enter the CSF to varying degrees. (See *Administration and excretion routes for alkylating agents* on page 1157 for more information about the pharmacokinetics of these agents.)

The nitrosoureas are extensively metabolized before urinary excretion. Within 24 hours, 80% of a carmustine dose appears in the urine as metabolites. Lomustine is rapidly and completely metabolized by the cytochrome P450 enzyme system in the liver. Up to 50% of a lomustine dose is excreted in the urine within 24 hours. Semustine is also metabolized by the cytochrome P450 enzyme system, some to active metabolites. Up to 60% of a semustine dose is excreted in the urine as metabolites within 48 hours. Minor amounts of semustine are excreted in the feces and in the lungs as carbon dioxide. Streptozocin is rapidly metabolized. From 10% to 20% of a dose is excreted in the urine, with minor amounts in the feces. Researchers believe that exhalation may be a significant route of streptozocin excretion.

Onset, peak, duration

The nitrosoureas vary in their peak concentration levels and half-lives. Carmustine peaks instantaneously with I.V. administration and disappears from the plasma, with a half-life of 90 minutes. Peak plasma concentration levels of lomustine metabolites are reached within 3 hours of administration. The half-life of the metabolites ranges from 16 to 48 hours. Semustine peak plasma concentration levels occur in 1 to 6 hours, with the metabolites having a half-life of 36 or more hours. Streptozocin has a plasma half-life of 35 minutes, with some streptozocin metabolites displaying a prolonged terminal half-life of 40 hours.

PHARMACODYNAMICS

The nitrosoureas display bifunctional alkylation of DNA. (See *Alkylation* on page 1158 for a detailed discussion of bifunctional alkylation.)

Mechanism of action

Like the mechanism of action of other alkylating agents, that of the nitrosoureas involves bifunctional alkylation of DNA. (See the section on mechanism of action under nitrogen mustards on page 1158, for a more detailed discussion of this action.)

PHARMACOTHERAPEUTICS

The nitrosoureas display a high degree of lipid solubility, which allows them to cross the blood-brain barrier quite easily. Because of this ability, nitrosoureas are used to treat brain tumors and meningeal leukemias.

carmustine [BCNU] (BiCNU). Since 1963, when carmustine first demonstrated activity against CNS tumors, it has been used for multiple myeloma, refractory Hodgkin's disease, and non-Hodgkin's lymphoma. Administered intravenously, carmustine may irritate the vein and need further dilution. The I.V. dose must be infused

within 2 hours. Two basic dosage schedules have been used for carmustine.
USUAL ADULT DOSAGE: first schedule, 75 to 100 mg/ m² I.V. daily for 2 consecutive days; the alternative schedule, up to 200 mg/m² in a single I.V. infusion, repeated every 6 to 8 weeks.

lomustine [CCNU] (CeeNU). Physicians use lomustine primarily to treat primary brain tumors or brain metastases from other malignant neoplasms.
USUAL ADULT DOSAGE: 100 to 130 mg/m² as a single oral dose, repeated approximately every 6 weeks.

semustine [methyl-CCNU]. Combination treatment of advanced gastrointestinal cancers in clinical research represents the most effective use of semustine.
USUAL ADULT DOSAGE: 125 to 200 mg/m² P.O. no more than every 6 weeks.

streptozocin (Zanosar). The uses of streptozocin include the treatment of pancreatic islet cell tumor, malignant carcinoid lung cancer, and adenocarcimona of the gallbladder.
USUAL ADULT DOSAGE: given singly, from 1 to 1.5 grams/m² I.V. for 6 consecutive weekly doses.

Drug interactions

When combined with cimetidine, carmustine seems to display an increased therapeutic effect via enhanced cellular uptake, leading to increased bone marrow suppression. No significant interactions occur with lomustine and semustine. If given with aminoglycosides, streptozocin exhibits an increased potential for nephrotoxic effects.

ADVERSE DRUG REACTIONS

The nitrosoureas, like all alkylating agents, can produce a range of mild to severe adverse reactions.

Predictable reactions

Carmustine and lomustine produce bone marrow depression, beginning 4 to 6 weeks after treatment and lasting 1 to 2 weeks. Severe nausea lasts 2 to 6 hours after carmustine or lomustine administration. The patient also may experience intense pain at the infusion site during carmustine administration. Renal dysfunction occurs in approximately two thirds of patients receiving streptozocin. Nausea and vomiting also occur with this drug.

Unpredictable reactions

Nephrotoxicity and renal failure have occurred with the nitrosoureas. High-dose carmustine may produce reversible hepatotoxicity. Hematologic toxicity and mild glucose intolerance are possible but rare reactions to streptozocin.

NURSING IMPLICATIONS

Many of the adverse reactions and nursing implications of the nitrosoureas resemble those of the other alkylating agents.
• Alert the patient to watch for signs of infection, such as chills, fever, or sore throat.
• Monitor uric acid level and CBC.
• Inform the patient that carmustine produces pain during injection; dilute and slow the infusion, and use warmth to dilate the veins and increase blood flow to further dilute the drug.
• Renal toxicity with streptozocin therapy is dose-related and cumulative. Monitor urinalysis, blood urea nitrogen (BUN), and creatinine levels. Remember, mild proteinuria is an early sign of renal toxicity.

    See Unit Fifteen Introduction for more nursing implications associated with nitrosoureas.

TRIAZINE

The triazine dacarbazine functions as an alkylating agent after it has been metabolically activated in the liver. Dacarbazine is cell-cycle-nonspecific.

History and source

Dacarbazine was developed under a National Cancer Institute contract by scientists at the Southern Research Institute in the early 1960s.

PHARMACOKINETICS

Physicians administer dacarbazine intravenously because oral administration results in variable, incomplete absorption.

Absorption, distribution, metabolism, excretion

After intravenous injection, the absorption of dacarbazine is rapid. The drug is distributed throughout the body and to the CSF, with the CSF levels being about 14% of the concurrent plasma levels. After metabolism in the liver, cytotoxic metabolites are released. Within 6 hours,

only 35% to 40% of a dose is excreted renally; 50% of the drug is excreted unchanged in the urine. (See *Administration and excretion routes for alkylating agents* on page 1157 to compare dacarbazine with other alkylating drugs.)

Onset, peak, duration

Dacarbazine has a half-life of approximately 5 hours. In patients with renal and hepatic dysfunction, half-life may increase to 7 hours.

PHARMACODYNAMICS

Dacarbazine seems to inhibit both ribonucleic acid (RNA) synthesis and protein synthesis. Like other alkylating agents, dacarbazine is cell-cycle-nonspecific.

Mechanism of action

Dacarbazine must first be metabolized in the liver to become an alkylating agent. The drug then produces a greater effect on RNA synthesis than on DNA synthesis. This characteristic distinguishes dacarbazine from the other alkylating agents.

PHARMACOTHERAPEUTICS

Physicians use dacarbazine primarily in patients with malignant melanoma but also in combination with other drugs to treat Hodgkin's disease.

dacarbazine (DTIC-Dome). Dacarbazine acts most effectively against malignant melanoma and soft-tissue sarcomas. Dacarbazine may cause severe tissue damage if extravasated. Possible pain during administration may necessitate further dilution or a slower rate of administration. Dosage ranges vary greatly according to the protocol.
USUAL ADULT DOSAGE: 150 to 250 mg/m^2 I.V. daily for 5 days; treatment may be repeated in 3 to 4 weeks. Much higher doses are used in some protocols, even as high as 850 mg/m^2 daily.

Drug interactions

No significant drug interactions occur involving dacarbazine.

ADVERSE DRUG REACTIONS

Leukopenia and thrombocytopenia occur as a result of dacarbazine use. Nausea and vomiting begin within 1 to 3 hours of administration in the majority of patients. Infusion of dacarbazine often causes I.V. pain at the site of I.V. infiltration. Phototoxicity also occurs, as do flulike syndrome and alopecia.

NURSING IMPLICATIONS

To administer dacarbazine safely, the nurse must be aware of the following:
- Monitor the patient's temperature daily, and observe for signs of infection.
- Monitor uric acid level and CBC frequently.
- Discard refrigerated solution after 72 hours; discard room-temperature solution after 8 hours.
- Avoid all I.M. injections in patients with low platelet counts.
- Give dacarbazine as an I.V. infusion in 50 to 100 ml of dextrose 5% in water over 30 minutes. To decrease pain at the infusion site, dilute the infusion further, slow the rate of infusion, or apply warmth to the vein.
- Advise the patient to avoid sunlight and sunlamps for the first 2 days after treatment.
- Use anticoagulants cautiously, and observe for signs of bleeding.
- Withhold food 4 to 6 hours prior to dacarbazine therapy, and administer antiemetics to decrease nausea. Nausea and vomiting usually subside after several doses.
- Reassure the patient that the flulike syndrome may be treated with mild antipyretics, such as acetaminophen.

ALKYLATING-LIKE AGENT

Cisplatin is a heavy metal complex that contains platinum. Because the action of cisplatin resembles that of a bifunctional alkylating agent, the drug is referred to as an alkylating-like agent.

History and source

In 1965, cisplatin was discovered by accidental observation by Rosenberg and his co-workers. They noticed that platinum electrodes placed in a bacteria culture produced a bactericidal effect. They later discovered that the bacteria inhibition was caused by the formation of inorganic platinum-containing compounds in the presence of ammonium and chloride ions. Since its introduction, cisplatin has led to major progress in the treatment of testicular cancer, ovarian cancer, and other tumor types as well.

PHARMACOKINETICS

Administered intravenously, cisplatin is highly protein-bound in plasma. It is ineffective when administered orally.

Absorption, distribution, metabolism, excretion

Cisplatin reaches high concentrations in the kidneys, liver, intestines, and testes, but displays poor CNS penetration. When administered intrapleurally and intraperitoneally, cisplatin exhibits significant systemic absorption. Cisplatin undergoes some hepatic metabolism, then renal excretion, with up to 45% of a dose being excreted in 5 days. Initially, cisplatin is excreted mainly as unchanged drug. As time passes, however, more of the excretion products are metabolites. (See *Administration and excretion routes for alkylating agents* on page 1157 for more information about the pharmacokinetics of this drug.)

Onset, peak, duration

The half-life of cisplatin depends on the drug concentration level and the infusion administration rate. After rapid intravenous administration, the initial half-life is 25 to 50 minutes; however, as concentration levels decline, the half-life may extend to 70 hours. When given by slow I.V. infusion, the half-life is shortened and more of the drug is excreted. Platinum is detectable in tissue for at least 4 months after administration.

PHARMACODYNAMICS

Like other alkylating agents, cisplatin is cell-cycle-nonspecific and inhibits DNA synthesis.

Mechanism of action

Cisplatin acts like a bifunctional alkylating agent by cross-linking strands of DNA and inhibiting DNA synthesis. (See the section on mechanism of action under nitrogen mustards on page 1158 for further details.)

PHARMACOTHERAPEUTICS

Physicians prescribe cisplatin to treat metastatic ovarian and testicular cancers; in fact, it is the drug of choice for testicular cancer. Solutions containing mannitol may be administered before and during cisplatin administration to ensure adequate renal output.

cisplatin [cis-platinum] (Platinol). Administered by I.V. infusion, cisplatin is usually used as an adjunctive treatment for metastatic testicular cancer, ovarian tumors, bladder cancer, and lung cancer. This drug has also been

SELECTED MAJOR DRUGS

Alkylating agents

The drugs listed in this chart are the more frequently encountered alkylating agents. Remember that dosages may vary greatly, depending upon the protocol used at the institution.

DRUG	MAJOR INDICATIONS	USUAL ADULT DOSAGES	NURSING IMPLICATIONS
mechlorethamine	Hodgkin's and non-Hodgkin's lymphomas, malignant effusions, mycosis fungoides	0.4 mg/kg I.V.; 0.2 to 0.4 mg/kg intracavitary	• Select a good vein, and check blood return frequently during administration. If extravasation occurs, treat it as quickly as possible. • Administer the drug immediately after reconstituting it. • Give antiemetics and short-acting sedatives as premedication and after administration because nausea and vomiting is severe. • Be aware that, after administration, the patient may experience chills, fever, and diarrhea. • Instruct the patient about the precautions to take associated with leukopenia and thrombocytopenia.
cyclophosphamide	Hodgkin's and non-Hodgkin's lymphomas, breast cancer, oat cell cancer of the lung, multiple myeloma, acute leukemia, sarcoma	2 to 3 mg/kg to 100 mg/kg I.V. or P.O.	• Ensure that the patient is well hydrated to prevent hemorrhagic cystitis. • Instruct the patient in the precautions to take associated with leukopenia and thrombocytopenia. • Give antiemetics routinely during I.V. administration.
carmustine	Primary and metastatic CNS tumors, myeloma, melanoma	75 to 200 mg/m² I.V. (depends on schedule)	• To decrease pain at the injection site, slow the rate or put heat over the site to distend the vein and increase dilution of the drug. • Give antiemetics routinely as prescribed during drug administration.
dacarbazine	Malignant melanoma, Hodgkin's disease, soft-tissue sarcomas	150 to 250 mg/m² I.V. daily for 5 days, repeated in 3 to 4 weeks. (Much higher doses are used in some protocols.)	• Instruct the patient that a flulike syndrome may occur a week after treatment and persist for a week or more and that acetaminophen may be used to treat symptoms. • Be aware that the patient may experience a metallic taste during drug infusion. Select a large vein, and use a slow rate of infusion.
cisplatin	Nonseminomatous testicular cancer; lung, ovarian, and bladder cancers	100 mg/m² I.V. every 3 to 4 weeks	• To minimize renal toxicity, ensure that the patient is well hydrated and that urine output is maintained during treatment. • Give antiemetics routinely as prescribed during drug administration.

administered intraarterially and intraperitoneally. The dosage of cisplatin, which is particularly dependent on renal function, must be reduced if renal dysfunction is indicated by elevations in blood urea nitrogen (BUN), creatinine, and serum uric acid levels and decreased creatinine clearance.

USUAL ADULT DOSAGE: single dose up to 100 mg/m² I.V. once every 3 to 4 weeks. In some protocols, lower doses are given daily for 3 to 5 days.

Drug interactions

Cisplatin and aminoglycosides administered concurrently can result in nephrotoxicity and ototoxicity.

ADVERSE DRUG REACTIONS

Cisplatin produces many of the same adverse reactions as the alkylating agents. Cisplatin therapy usually does not result in leukopenia or thrombocytopenia; however the drug can cause anemia.

Nephrotoxicity occurs in 28% to 36% of patients receiving cisplatin, usually after multiple courses of therapy. Neurotoxicity associated with long-term therapy can also occur, but it is rare. This adverse effect is evidenced by sensory and motor peripheral neuropathies, loss of proprioception, loss of taste, and intestinal ileus. Approximately 30% of patients receiving cisplatin report tinnitus and hearing loss. Renal insufficiency can occur after a single dose but is usually reversible.

NURSING IMPLICATIONS

When administering cisplatin, the nurse should know the following implications:
• Administer cisplatin with caution to patients with renal impairment, myelosuppression, or hearing impairment.
• Hydrate the patient with 1 to 2 liters of fluid before drug administration.
• Administer sufficient fluid to maintain the patient's urine output at 100 ml/hour for 4 consecutive hours before therapy and for 24 hours after therapy.
• Reconstitute the drug with sterile water for injection. Cisplatin remains stable for 24 hours in normal saline solution at room temperature; do not refrigerate solutions.
• Infusions remain most stable in chloride-containing solutions (normal saline, ½ normal saline, ¼ normal saline).
• Do not use aluminum needles for reconstituting or administering cisplatin because cisplatin will interact with the aluminum, forming a black precipitate.
• Mannitol may be prescribed to be given as a 12.5-gram I.V. bolus before cisplatin infusion. The cisplatin infusion also may be followed with an infusion of mannitol, up to 10 grams/hour, as prescribed, to maintain urine output during and for 6 to 24 hours after the cisplatin infusion.
• Monitor CBC, platelet count, and renal function studies before initial and subsequent doses.
• Be aware that repeat doses will not be administered unless the platelets are over 100,000/cu mm, WBC is over 4,000/cu mm, creatinine is under 1.5 mg/dl, and BUN is under 25 mg/dl.
• Instruct the patient to report tinnitus immediately to prevent permanent hearing loss. Schedule audiometry tests before each dose.
• Nausea and vomiting may be severe and protracted (up to 24 hours); therefore, antiemetics should be initiated 24 hours before therapy, as prescribed. Metoclopramide may also be administered, as prescribed, to treat and prevent nausea and vomiting.

• Monitor the patient's fluid intake and output during treatment. Notify the physician if the urine output is less than 100 ml/hour during the first 24 hours.
• Maintain I.V. hydration as prescribed until the patient can tolerate adequate oral intake.
• Avoid all I.M. injections when the platelet count is low.

CHAPTER SUMMARY

The discussion in Chapter 73 centered on the alkylating agents, a class of antineoplastic drugs characterized by an ability to enter the cell nuclei and inhibit DNA synthesis. Here are the highlights of the chapter:
• The alkylating agents include nitrogen mustards, alkyl sulfonates, nitrosoureas, triazines, and alkylating-like agents.
• With the exception of the triazine dacarbazine, the alkylating agents have the same mechanism of action. Most of these drugs enter the cell by active transport systems. The drugs then undergo alkylation, resulting in covalent bonds. The alkylation becomes toxic when the cell enters the S phase, during which DNA synthesis occurs. Dacarbazine acts primarily on RNA synthesis.
• Used singly or in combination with other antineoplastic drugs, alkylating agents are used to treat a wide variety of malignant neoplasms. Nitrogen mustards are indicated for Hodgkin's disease, certain leukemias, and many solid tumors. The alkyl sulfonate busulfan is used to treat chronic myelocytic leukemia and polycythemia vera. Nitrosoureas are effective against brain tumors and meningeal leukemias. The triazine dacarbazine is used for malignant melanoma, and the alkylating-like agent cisplatin is used for metastatic ovarian and testicular cancers.
• The most common and potentially harmful adverse reaction to the alkylating agents is bone marrow suppression, resulting in leukopenia and thrombocytopenia. Other predictable adverse reactions include nausea and vomiting, alopecia, and fatigue. These reactions may be minimized through nursing interventions.
• Unpredictable adverse reactions are specific to certain alkylating agents. For example, cyclophosphamide can produce hemorrhagic cystitis; streptozocin leads to renal dysfunction; and cisplatin can cause nephrotoxicity.
• The nurse can significantly help the patient cope with alkylating agent therapy by: (1) carefully administering the drugs, (2) educating the patient, and (3) using interventions to minimize adverse reactions.

BIBLIOGRAPHY

Carter, S., et al. *Principles of Cancer Treatment.* New York: McGraw-Hill Book Co., 1982.

Cohen, B.E., et al. "Human Plasma Pharmacokinetics and Urinary Excretion of Thiotepa and Its Metabolites," *Cancer Treatment Reports* 70(7):859, July 1986.

Gilman, A.G., et al., eds. *Goodman and Gilman's The Pharmacological Basis of Therapeutics,* 7th ed. New York: Macmillan Publishing Co., 1985.

Gunnarsson, P.O., and Forshell, G.P. "Clinical Pharmacokinetics of Estramustine Phosphate," *Urology* 23(6):22, June (Supplement) 1984.

Hoisaeter, P.A. "Mode of Action of Emcyt," *Urology* 23(6):46, June (Supplement) 1984.

Holland, J., and Frei, E. *Cancer Medicine,* Section XII, 2nd ed. Philadelphia: Lea & Febiger, 1982.

McIntire, S.N., and Cioppa, A.L. *Cancer Nursing: A Developmental Approach.* New York: John Wiley & Sons, 1984.

Mishina, T., et al. "Absorption of Anticancer Drugs Through Bladder Epithelium," *Urology* 27(2):148, February 1986.

CHAPTER 74

ANTIMETABOLITE AGENTS

OBJECTIVES

After reading and studying this chapter, you should be able to:

1. Describe the clinical uses of the antimetabolites.

2. Differentiate among the mechanisms of action of the folic acid, the pyrimidine, and the purine analogues.

3. Identify the frequent drug reactions associated with methotrexate, fluorouracil, 5-azacytidine, floxuridine, cytarabine, mercaptopurine, and thioguanine.

4. Explain the importance of oral care during antimetabolite therapy.

5. Explain the importance of monitoring the patient for leukopenia and thrombocytopenia during folic acid analogue or pyrimidine analogue therapy.

6. Explain the significance of jaundice in a patient receiving a purine analogue.

INTRODUCTION

Because the antimetabolites structurally resemble natural metabolites, they can become involved in processes associated with the natural metabolites; that is, the synthesis of nucleic acids and proteins. However, the antimetabolites differ sufficiently from the natural metabolites to interfere with this synthesis. Because the antimetabolites are cell-cycle specific and primarily affect cells that actively synthesize deoxyribonucleic acid (DNA), they are referred to as S-phase specific. Normal cells that are actively reproducing, as well as the cancer cells, are affected by the antimetabolites. These drugs are further subclassified according to the metabolite affected. (See *Antimetabolites* for the different groups of antimetabolites and the specific drugs in each group.)

Malignancies that respond to the action of antimetabolites include acute leukemia, breast cancer, adenocarcinoma of the gastrointestinal (GI) tract, non-Hodgkin's lymphomas, and squamous cell carcinoma of the head, neck, and cervix. The major adverse reactions occur in the

Antimetabolites

The following list indicates the major groups of antimetabolites and the drugs that comprise each group.

Folic acid analogues
• methotrexate (Folex, Mexate)

Pyrimidine analogues
• fluorouracil [5-fluorouracil or 5-FU] (Adrucil, Efudex) • floxuridine (FUDR) • cytarabine [ARA-C or cytosine arabinoside] (Cytosar-U) • 5-azacytidine

Purine analogues
• mercaptopurine [6-MP] (Purinethol) • thioguanine [6-thioguanine] (Tabloid)

bone marrow, mucosa, skin, and hair follicles. Adverse reactions are usually dose-related and reversible, and many patients may not experience any such reactions.

For a summary of representative drugs, see *Selected major drugs: Antimetabolite agents* on page 1180.

FOLIC ACID ANALOGUES

Although researchers have developed many folic acid analogues, the early compound methotrexate sodium remains the most frequently used.

Administration and excretion routes for antimetabolite agents

This chart provides a quick reference for major routes of administration and excretion of the antimetabolite agents.

DRUG	MAJOR ROUTES OF ADMINISTRATION	MAJOR ROUTES OF EXCRETION	AMOUNT EXCRETED
Folic acid analogues			
methotrexate	Oral, intravenous, intramuscular, intrathecal	Kidneys	40% to 50% in 48 hours Mostly unchanged for low doses Up to 90% for high doses
Pyrimidine analogues			
fluorouracil	Intravenous, topical, intraarterial	Kidneys Lungs	15% in 6 hours unchanged Up to 80% in 24 hours as CO_2
floxuridine	Intraarterial	Kidneys Lungs	10% to 30% in 24 hours Up to 60% as CO_2
cytarabine	Intravenous, subcutaneous, intrathecal	Kidneys	90% in 24 hours as metabolites
5-azacytidine	Intravenous	Kidneys	90% in 24 hours
Purine analogues			
mercaptopurine	Oral	Kidneys	50% in 24 hours
thioguanine	Oral	Kidneys	40% in 24 hours

History and source

The antimetabolites originated in the 1940s during leukemia research. During that time, Heinle and Welch noted that pteroylglutamic acid (folic acid folate) accelerated the course of leukemias. Research groups soon directed their efforts toward creating a folate deficiency by using folate-deficient diets with weak folate antagonists. Aminopterin, a metabolite antagonist, synthesized by Farber and colleagues, produced remissions in patients with acute leukemia. The synthesis and subsequent use of aminopterin demonstrated that metabolite antagonists could serve as effective antineoplastic agents. Methotrexate, which is more therapeutic than aminopterin, is the most frequently used folate antagonist.

PHARMACOKINETICS

Methotrexate is well absorbed and distributed throughout the body. At usual doses, it does not readily enter the central nervous system (CNS). Although methotrexate is partially metabolized, it is excreted primarily unchanged in the urine.

Absorption, distribution, metabolism, excretion

Methotrexate is well absorbed after oral administration and is well distributed throughout the body. When administered intrathecally, methotrexate slowly diffuses into the plasma.

Methotrexate can remain in renal and hepatic tissue for weeks. It does not readily enter the cerebrospinal fluid (CSF) at normal doses, with CSF levels being only 3% to 10% of concurrent plasma levels. To achieve cytotoxic CNS levels requires a high dose of intravenously administered methotrexate. Methotrexate may sequester (deposit) in pleural effusions or ascitic fluid; the sequestered drug may then be slowly released back into the plasma. Methotrexate, which is approximately 50% plasma protein bound, may be displaced from its plasma protein-binding sites by many drugs. The displacement increases free drug levels of methotrexate.

At normal doses, methotrexate is minimally metabolized. At high doses, however, metabolites, including a potentially nephrotoxic one, accumulate.

Methotrexate is excreted primarily unchanged in the urine. At low doses, 40% to 50% is excreted in 48 hours. At high doses, up to 90% may be excreted in 48 hours. Because methotrexate is excreted as a result of glomerular filtration and active tubular secretion, other drugs excreted by tubular secretion may decrease methotrexate secretion. Small amounts of the drug are also excreted in the feces and saliva. (See *Administration and excretion routes for antimetabolite agents* for percentage of drug excretion within specified hours.)

Onset, peak, duration
Methotrexate reaches peak plasma levels 1 hour after an oral dose, with plasma concentration directly dose-related. Following intrathecal administration, peak plasma level is reached in 3 to 12 hours. Methotrexate exhibits a three-part disappearance from plasma; the last part, the terminal half-life, is 7 hours.

PHARMACODYNAMICS

Methotrexate inhibits the action of dihydrofolate reductase, thereby blocking normal biochemical reactions and inhibiting DNA and ribonucleic acid (RNA) synthesis. The result is cell death.

Mechanism of action
Dihydrofolate reductase (DHFR) reduces folic acid to tetrahydrofolic acid (FH_4). The FH_4 then serves as a cofactor in many metabolic reactions requiring the transfer of one-carbon units. Methotrexate enters cells via an active transport system and forms a competitive, high-affinity, noncovalent bond with DHFR. When all of the DHFR becomes bound with methotrexate, the DHFR can no longer reduce folic acid to FH_4. Without FH_4, thymidylate synthesis ceases and purine synthesis becomes inhibited. The blocking of thymidylate and purine synthesis leads to the inhibition of DNA and RNA synthesis and cell death. Methotrexate thus represents a cell-cycle S-phase specific agent.

Tumor cells can develop resistance to the cytotoxic actions of methotrexate. Any one of several biochemical changes can result in resistance. The active transport system that carries methotrexate into the cells may become altered. With the impaired entry of methotrexate into the cells, lower intracellular levels of the drug become available for binding with the DHFR, thereby leading to resistance. Altered forms of DHFR may also be produced. The altered DHFR exhibits a decreased affinity for methotrexate and can function despite normal methotrexate levels. Finally, increased concentrations of

Leucovorin rescue

Methotrexate interferes with cell division in the S phase of the cell cycle by inhibiting dihydrofolate reductase (DHFR), an enzyme involved in DNA synthesis. High-dose methotrexate is most effective against cells that have a high metabolic rate, such as leukemia cells. Used alone, high-dose methotrexate will eventually affect normal cells as well, producing toxicity.

To protect normal cells, physicians often prescribe methotrexate with leucovorin (folinic acid). Leucovorin rescues cells by bypassing methotrexate inhibition of DHFR, as this schematic illustrates, as well as by other mechanisms that are not completely understood. Administer leucovorin exactly on time, as ordered, for the drug to work efficiently. When administered properly, leucovorin rescues cells before they begin active growth and division. Although leucovorin is considered a vitamin, doses must not be skipped, since this drug plays an important role in preventing severe methotrexate toxicity.

Since leucovorin cannot completely prevent methotrexate toxicity, closely watch any patient on high-dose methotrexate therapy for bone marrow depression, stomatitis, pulmonary complications, and renal damage (from precipitation in tubules). Maintain the patient's urine in an alkaline state to avoid precipitation in tubules, and monitor urine output closely.

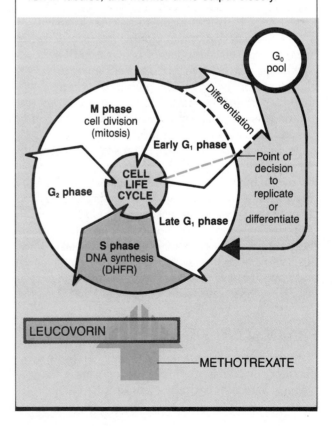

Folic acid analogues

This chart includes drugs that interact with methotrexate, outlining possible effects for each, as well as nursing implications.

DRUG	INTERACTING DRUGS	POSSIBLE EFFECTS	NURSING IMPLICATIONS
methotrexate	oral anticoagulants	May increase anticoagulant effect	• Monitor the patient for increased anticoagulant effect. Educate the patient about bleeding precautions.
	phenytoin	May increase the toxicity of methotrexate by displacing it from protein-binding sites	• Monitor for increased adverse reactions, such as fatigue, bone marrow suppression, and stomatitis.
	probenecid	Inhibits excretion of methotrexate	• Monitor for increased adverse reactions, such as fatigue, bone marrow suppression, and stomatitis.
	salicylates	May increase the toxicity of methotrexate by decreasing tubular secretion	• Monitor for increased adverse reactions, such as fatigue, bone marrow suppression, and stomatitis.
	sulfonamides	May increase the toxicity of methotrexate by displacing the drug from protein-binding sites	• Monitor for increased adverse reactions, such as fatigue, bone marrow suppression, and stomatitis.

DHFR may be produced so that at normal methotrexate levels, free DHFR is available to function normally.

High doses of methotrexate may be given either to overcome resistance produced by increased DHFR concentrations or to achieve cytotoxic CNS levels. With very high doses of methotrexate, physicians prescribe leucovorin, performing what is known as a leucovorin rescue because leucovorin prevents the destruction of normal cells. Leucovorin, a fully reduced folate coenzyme, can function as a carrier of one-carbon units without being reduced by DHFR. By functioning in this way, leucovorin bypasses the biochemical block produced by methotrexate and allows the cell to synthesize DNA and RNA. (See *Leucovorin rescue* on page 1171 for a more detailed discussion.) Leucovorin also enters the cells via the same active transport system as methotrexate. When this active transport system is occupied carrying leucovorin into the cell, less methotrexate enters and intracellular methotrexate levels fall.

PHARMACOTHERAPEUTICS

Methotrexate is especially useful to treat acute lymphoblastic leukemia in children, choriocarcinoma, osteogenic sarcoma, and non-Hodgkin's lymphomas, as well as carcinomas of the head and neck, bladder, testis, and breast. Physicians also prescribe low doses of methotrexate to treat severe psoriasis and rheumatoid arthritis that resist conventional therapy.

methotrexate sodium (Folex, Mexate). This drug is administered orally, intravenously, intramuscularly, and intrathecally.

USUAL ADULT DOSAGE: to maintain remissions in leukemia, 30 mg/m^2 of body-surface area orally or I.M. twice weekly or 175 to 525 mg/m^2 I.M. for 2 days each month; for choriocarcinoma, 15 mg/m^2 P.O. or I.M. daily for 5 days at 1- to 2-week intervals. For meningeal leukemia, methotrexate may also be administered intrathecally 12 mg/m^2 to a maximum of 15 mg/m^2 at 2- to 5-day intervals.

Drug interactions

Methotrexate may increase the effect of oral anticoagulants. Therefore, patients requiring warfarin therapy who are also receiving methotrexate should be monitored for changes in their anticoagulant requirements. Several drugs, including phenytoin, salicylates, and sulfonamides, can displace methotrexate from plasma protein-binding sites. Therefore, the nurse should closely monitor patients on concomitant therapy for methotrexate toxicity. (See *Drug interactions: Folic acid analogues* for the interactions with methotrexate.)

ADVERSE DRUG REACTIONS

A patient receiving methotrexate may experience a wide range of adverse reactions depending on the dosage, the patient's condition, and other drugs the patient may be receiving.

Predictable reactions

Bone marrow suppression can occur with any dosage schedule, with the suppression greatest 10 to 14 days after the administration of methotrexate. Stomatitis may develop 5 to 10 days after therapy begins. Patients receiving high-dose methotrexate are susceptible to severe stomatitis, which may result in a potential nutritional deficit. (See *Care of stomatitis* on page 1179 for information about this adverse effect.) Fatigue, secondary to combined factors such as bone marrow suppression and circulating products of tumor breakdown, may adversely affect a patient's stamina as well as participation in the drug therapy.

Unpredictable reactions

Though unpredictable reactions to methotrexate are relatively rare, they occur in 4% to 10% of patients receiving long-term therapy. Hepatotoxicity, resulting in cirrhosis and the less frequent acute liver atrophy, can occur in patients receiving high-dose methotrexate over a period of time. Hepatotoxicity is related more to the length and frequency of dosing than to the total dose.

Nephrotoxicity, evidenced by rising blood urea nitrogen (BUN) and creatinine values, may be reduced by maintaining alkalinization of the urine and encouraging the ingestion of large quantities of fluid, or by administering sodium bicarbonate intravenously to maintain an alkaline urine and infusing large quantities of fluid.

Photosensitivity may occur in patients despite protection from the sun. A sunburnlike rash is the primary dermatologic reaction. Alopecia occurs in approximately 10% of patients receiving methotrexate. When nausea and vomiting occur with high-dose methotrexate therapy, which is rare, they usually represent the first adverse reactions experienced, often less than 1 hour after administration.

Intrathecal administration of methotrexate warrants special attention because severe adverse reactions, ranging from convulsions and paresis to paralysis and death, have occurred. Because preserved methotrexate preparations have resulted in more adverse reactions, health care professionals should use only unpreserved methotrexate for intrathecal drug administration.

NURSING IMPLICATIONS

High-dose methotrexate with leucovorin rescue is used to treat various tumors. Because this combined therapy intensifies the toxic effects of methotrexate, the nurse should be aware of the following cautions and precautions:

• Because high-dose methotrexate therapy has been associated with reversible nephrotoxicity, monitor the patient's BUN and creatinine levels frequently.
• At high concentrations, methotrexate may precipitate in a renal tubule, causing tubular dilatation and damage.
• Because increasing urine alkalinity and volume may prevent renal toxicity, encourage fluid intake and administer I.V. fluids and sodium bicarbonate as prescribed.
• Maintain strict patient intake and output records, and monitor urinary pH.
• Before each treatment, routinely monitor creatinine and BUN values. If values are abnormal, consult the physician for therapy modification.
• Methotrexate can cause acute reversible allergic pneumonitis with patchy pulmonary infiltrates, fever, cough, and shortness of breath up to 5 months after therapy. Inform patients of the significance of changes in their respiratory function. If they develop fever, a nonproductive cough, or shortness of breath, urge them to notify the physician.
• Patients receiving methotrexate via either a lumbar puncture or reservoir may experience neurotoxicity secondary to increased CSF volume. Symptoms include convulsions, paresis, and a syndrome resembling Guillain-Barré syndrome.
• Because CSF methotrexate levels may help predict appropriate dosing of intrathecal methotrexate, they should be monitored frequently.
• Observe the patient receiving intrathecal methotrexate for potential neurologic adverse reactions, and educate the patient about such reactions.
• Patients receiving methotrexate may experience hepatic cirrhosis and, less commonly, acute liver atrophy. Monitor baseline liver function tests throughout the therapy. (See also *Frequent adverse reactions and associated nursing implications* in Unit XV Introduction.)
• Certain drugs used with methotrexate, such as salicylates and phenytoin, may increase the chance of the patient developing hepatotoxicity and cirrhosis.
• Teach the patient to recognize the symptoms of liver dysfunction, such as yellowing skin or sclera, varnish-colored urine, and clay-colored stools.

PYRIMIDINE ANALOGUES

The pyrimidine analogues include fluorouracil, floxuridine, cytarabine, and 5-azacytidine—a diverse group of drugs that inhibit the biosynthesis of pyrimidine nucleotides by mimicry.

History and source

In the 1950s, researchers observed that tumors absorbed greater quantities of labeled uracil than did normal tissue. Based on these observations, researchers began work on synthesizing an antimetabolite that closely resembled uracil, resulting in the synthesis of fluorouracil (5-fluorouracil or 5-FU). Concurrently, the clinical activity of fluorouracil was noted. Continuing research resulted in modifications of the pyrimidine analogues, producing floxuridine and cytarabine. Ongoing research of fluorinated pyrimidines has resulted in the synthesis of other agents, including 5-azacytidine, which was first reported in 1964 by a group of Czechoslovakian researchers. The analogue 5-azacytidine remains an experimental drug in the United States.

PHARMACOKINETICS

Because the pyrimidine analogues are poorly absorbed when given orally, they are usually administered via other routes. With the exception of 5-azacytidine, the pyrimidine analogues are well distributed throughout the body, achieving therapeutic CSF levels. They are extensively metabolized in the liver and are excreted in the urine. Pyrimidine analogues have short half-lives: the longest, 11 hours.

Absorption, distribution, metabolism, excretion

In most cases, no pyrimidine analogue is administered orally because of the resulting unpredictable and incomplete absorption. For example, fluorouracil is usually administered I.V., but can also be injected into the pleural and peritoneal spaces or applied topically. These routes produce minimal systemic adverse effects. Only 20% of intact cytarabine reaches the circulation after oral administration. However, cytarabine is well absorbed from subcutaneous and intramuscular administration sites, and 5-azacytidine is well absorbed from subcutaneous administration sites.

The pyrimidine analogues are well distributed throughout the body. Fluorouracil is distributed to all areas of body water with a volume of distribution approximately 25% to 33% of body weight. Fluorouracil readily enters the CSF and effusions. Although floxuridine has been less extensively studied, it is believed to enter the CSF also. Cytarabine is also well distributed throughout the body, entering the CSF with levels approximately 50% of concurrent plasma levels. Higher CSF levels occur following continuous infusion than following an intravenous bolus. In contrast, 5-azacytidine is distributed less readily than the other pyrimidine analogues, with little of the drug entering the CSF.

Fluorouracil is metabolized in the liver; its metabolites include carbon dioxide (CO_2), urea, and ammonia. Because floxuridine has a high hepatic extraction ratio, most of the drug administered via the hepatic artery is removed from the systemic circulation on the first pass through the liver. In the liver, floxuridine is metabolized to fluorouracil and its metabolites. Cytarabine is extensively metabolized in the liver, mainly to uracil arabinoside.

Within the first 24 hours, 10% to 30% of a floxuridine dose is excreted in the urine as floxuridine, fluorouracil, urea, and a number of other metabolites. Up to 80% of a dose of fluorouracil is excreted from the lungs as CO_2. Cytarabine is excreted primarily in the urine, with small amounts excreted in the bile. Over 90% of 5-azacytidine is excreted in the urine in 24 hours. (See *Administration and excretion routes for antimetabolite agents* on page 1170 for information related to the administration and excretion of the pyrimidine analogues.)

Onset, peak, duration

After rapid intravenous bolus administration, fluorouracil reaches plasma level concentration of 0.1 to 1 mM. Fluorouracil has a rapid clearance, with a plasma level half-life of only 10 to 20 minutes. The peak concentration time and half-life of floxuridine have not been well quantified. However, floxuridine's high hepatic extraction results in low systemic levels with a short half-life. Peak concentration levels of cytarabine are dose-dependent, and higher concentration levels result from continuous I.V. infusion rather than from bolus injection. Cytarabine has a plasma level half-life of approximately 2½ hours. Following intrathecal administration, cytarabine has a half-life of 2 to 11 hours. After subcutaneous administration, 5-azacytidine reaches peak plasma levels in 1½ hours. It has a half-life of 3½ to 4¼ hours.

PHARMACODYNAMICS

The pyrimidine analogues exhibit their cytotoxic effects by interfering with the natural function of pyrimidine nucleotides. They either interfere with the biosynthesis of the natural pyrimidines or mimic the natural pyrimidines to the point where they interfere with cellular functions. The pyrimidine analogues are cell-cycle S-phase specific.

Mechanism of action

Fluorouracil and floxuridine inhibit the enzyme thymidylate synthetase resulting in a thymidylate deficiency. Thymidylate deficiency inhibits DNA, causing cell death—particularly of those cells which grow rapidly.

Numerous mechanisms may promote resistance to fluorouracil and floxuridine cytotoxicity. These mechanisms include decreased number or activity of enzymes activating fluorouracil, decreased enzymes incorporating the false nucleotide into RNA, and an alteration in thymidylate synthetase preventing its inhibition by the false nucleotide.

Cytarabine must be converted to the nucleotide level to become active. Accumulation of the false nucleotide inhibits DNA synthesis and may also inhibit an enzyme involved in DNA repair. Researchers believe that cell death from cytarabine may result from unbalanced growth, which occurs when the inhibition of DNA synthesis is accompanied by continued RNA and protein synthesis. Resistance to cytarabine may result from decreased intracellular drug levels, decreased activation of cytarabine, or increased levels of molecules that block cytarabine action.

The primary mechanism of action for 5-azacytidine is not well established. The drug may act as a false pyrimidine and become incorporated into both DNA and RNA. It may inhibit the function of RNA, thus interfering with normal protein synthesis. Also, DNA incorporated with 5-azacytidine is more susceptible to breakage than normal DNA.

PHARMACOTHERAPEUTICS

The pyrimidine analogues are used to treat many tumors. The drugs, however, are mostly used to treat acute leukemias, adenocarcinomas of the GI tract, carcinomas of the breast and ovaries, and non-Hodgkin's lymphomas. All of the pyrimidine analogues produce tissue toxicity, mainly myelosuppression and such GI toxicity as stomatitis, glossitis, nausea, vomiting, and diarrhea. Cytarabine and 5-azacytidine may be more toxic than the other drugs in this class.

fluorouracil [5-fluorouracil or 5-FU] (Adrucil, Efudex). Fluorouracil is active against many solid tumors, particularly carcinomas of the breast and GI tract, including oral, gastric, and colorectal tumors. Topically, fluorouracil acts against basal cell carcinomas and other malignant dermatologic entities. Health care professionals use various dosing schedules when administering fluorouracil.

USUAL ADULT DOSAGE: 12 mg/kg of body weight I.V. daily for 4 successive days. Daily dosage should not exceed 800 mg/day if no toxicity, then give 6 mg/kg of body weight on the 6th, 8th, 10th, and 12th day.

floxuridine (FUDR). Administered by continuous infusion, both intravenously and intraarterially, floxuridine acts against adenocarcinomas of the GI tract, including oral, pancreatic, hepatic, and biliary tumors. Unfortunately, only 15% to 20% of the patients treated with fluorouracil or floxuridine for these GI tumors demonstrate objective response.

USUAL ADULT DOSAGE: 0.1 to 0.6 mg/kg/day by continuous arterial infusion for 1 to 6 weeks until toxicity requires discontinuation.

cytarabine [ARA-C or cytosine arabinoside] (Cytosar-U). Cytarabine is primarily used to induce remission of acute leukemias. Over 50% of patients using cytarabine with other drugs have achieved complete remission. Cytarabine also acts effectively against Hodgkin's and other lymphomas.

USUAL ADULT DOSAGE: I.V. bolus injections of 100 to 200 mg/m² of body-surface area daily for 5 to 7 days or continuous I.V. infusions of 100 mg/m²/day or 3 mg/kg daily for 5 to 7 days. For some patients, the physician may prescribe maintenance doses of 1 mg/kg S.C. 1 to 2 times weekly. For meningeal leukemia, intrathecal doses of 30 mg/m² every 4 days are used.

5-azacytidine. 5-azacytidine is beneficial primarily against acute myelogenous leukemia. To a lesser extent, the drug acts against acute lymphocytic leukemia but displays little action against solid tumors. Health care professionals administer 5-azacytidine using various schedules, depending on the protocol used for this experimental agent.

Drug interactions

No significant drug interactions occur involving the pyrimidine analogues.

ADVERSE DRUG REACTIONS

The adverse drug reactions to the pyrimidine analogues resemble those to the other antimetabolites.

Predictable reactions

Bone marrow suppression evidenced by neutropenia and thrombocytopenia is the major dose-limiting adverse reaction to the pyrimidine analogues. This predictable reaction is noticeable 7 to 14 days after the drug's administration, with bone marrow recovery occurring 21 to 28 days after the drug is discontinued.

Stomatitis and esophagopharyngitis may occur 5 to 10 days after the initiation of therapy. This adverse reaction can be particularly distressing to patients since the oral cavity ulcerations and sloughing may be extremely painful and prevent eating. (See *Care of stomatitis* on page 1179 for details on how to manage this adverse reaction.)

The pyrimidine analogues, like most antineoplastic agents, can cause fatigue. Lack of energy can severely limit activities and the roles that cancer patients wish to play in their therapy. With the exception of 5-azacytidine, the pyrimidine analogues do not cause severe nausea and vomiting. Approximately 70% of patients receiving 5-azacytidine, however, experience moderate to severe nausea and vomiting 1½ to 3 hours after I.V. administration. Nausea and anorexia may become problems for patients receiving long-term therapy with fluorouracil or floxuridine. Diarrhea may also occur with fluorouracil administration.

Unpredictable reactions

Although fluorouracil, in most cases, is a relatively well-tolerated drug, it can produce several unpredictable reactions. The patient may experience mild to severe skin reactions, including a pruritic rash on the extremities or trunk, photosensitivity with erythema or increased skin pigmentation, or darkening of the veins with prolonged drug administration. The patient may also experience increased lacrimation, nasal discharge, or epistaxis; these reactions disappear after therapy is discontinued. Within 3 days of fluorouracil administration, diarrhea and cramping may occur and may be severe enough to limit or discontinue therapy.

Both cytarabine and 5-azacytidine administration may precipitate a fever and flulike symptoms within 24 hours of therapy. Cytarabine may also produce a rash in 4% of patients.

NURSING IMPLICATIONS

To safely administer the pyrimidine analogues, the nurse must be familiar with numerous administration precautions as well as possible adverse reactions. The following considerations apply to fluorouracil:

• Administer fluorouracil cautiously after major surgery, when the patient is in a poor nutritional state, or when the patient has a serious infection or bone marrow depression.

• Administer cautiously following high-dose pelvic irradiation or the use of alkylating drugs, as well as in patients with impaired hepatic or renal function or with widespread carcinoma of the bone marrow.

• Give an antiemetic as prescribed before administering fluorouracil to reduce GI adverse reactions.

• Monitor the patient for stomatitis or diarrhea, both signs of toxicity.

• Apply a topical oral anesthetic as prescribed to soothe lesions.

• Monitor white blood cell (WBC) and platelet counts daily, and observe for ecchymoses, petechiae, easy bruising, and anemia.

• Discontinuing the drug reverses the dermatologic adverse effects. Encourage the patient to use protective sun blocks to avoid inflammatory erythematous dermatitis.

• Infuse the drug solution over 2 to 8 hours to lessen toxicity.

• Monitor intake and output, complete blood count (CBC), and renal and hepatic function.

• Store fluorouracil at room temperature, and protect it from light.

• Do not use a cloudy solution. If crystals form, redissolve the solution by warming.

• The solution is more stable in plastic I.V. bags than in glass bottles. Use plastic I.V. containers to administer continuous infusions.

• To prevent bleeding in patients with thrombocytopenia, avoid I.M. injections.

• Warn the patient that reversible alopecia may occur.

The following nursing implications apply to floxuridine:

• Administer cautiously to a patient with a poor nutritional state, bone marrow depression, impaired hepatic or renal function, or serious infection. Administer cautiously after high-dose pelvic irradiation or use of an alkylating drug.

• Explain to the patient that good mouth care can help prevent stomatitis.

• Monitor intake and output, CBC, and renal and hepatic function.

• Administer antacid to ease (not prevent) GI distress.

• Reconstitute floxuridine with sterile water for injection. For the actual infusion, dilute further in 5% dextrose in water (D_5W) or normal saline solution.

- To prevent bleeding in patients with thrombocytopenia, avoid I.M. injections.
- Because refrigerated solution remains stable no more than 2 weeks, discard at that time.
- Inform the patient that the therapeutic effect of floxuridine may be delayed 1 to 6 weeks.

The following nursing implications apply to cytarabine:

- Administer cautiously to patients with inadequate bone marrow reserve or with renal or hepatic disease. Also administer cautiously after other chemotherapy or radiation therapy.
- Observe the patient for signs of infection, such as leukoplakia, fever, and sore throat.
- Nausea and vomiting occur more frequently when large doses are administered rapidly by I.V. push and less frequently with continuous infusion.
- Use preservative-free normal saline solution for intrathecal administration.
- To reduce nausea, administer an antiemetic as prescribed before cytarabine.
- Monitor intake and output carefully. Encourage high fluid intake and give allopurinol, if ordered, to avoid urate nephropathy in leukemia induction therapy.
- Monitor uric acid, CBC, and platelet levels, as well as hepatic function.
- Reconstituted solution remains stable for 48 hours; after that time, discard any cloudy reconstituted solution.
- To prevent bleeding in patients with thrombocytopenia, avoid I.M. injections.
- Explain to the patient that good mouth care can help prevent stomatitis.

The following nursing implications apply to 5-azacytidine:

- 5-azacytidine is contraindicated for patients with hepatic disease.
- Monitor the patient's blood pressure before therapy and at least every 30 minutes after therapy is initiated.
- Monitor the patient's temperature, CBC, and liver function tests.
- Infuse 5-azacytidine using lactated Ringer's solution because the drug is unstable in other types of solutions.
- Infuse slowly to prevent severe hypotension. Continuous infusion decreases nausea and vomiting.
- Discard reconstituted 5-azacytidine.
- Instruct the patient to notify the physician if muscle pain or weakness develop because these signs and symptoms may indicate neurotoxicity.

See also *Frequent adverse reactions and associated nursing implications* in Unit XV Introduction.

PURINE ANALOGUES

The purine analogues, mercaptopurine and thioguanine, are analogues of natural purine bases that must undergo enzymatic conversion to the nucleotide level before they become cytotoxic.

Hitchings and Elion developed the purine analogues in 1952. The drugs are still useful today.

PHARMACOKINETICS

The absorption of the purine analogues is variable and incomplete. They are metabolized in the liver and excreted in the urine.

Absorption, distribution, metabolism, excretion

After oral administration, absorption of both mercaptopurine and thioguanine is incomplete and variable. The distribution of the purine analogues in humans has not been extensively studied. Mercaptopurine is metabolized in the liver by two major pathways: (1) methylation of the sulfhydryl group and (2) oxidation by xanthine oxidase to inactive metabolites. Within 24 hours, up to 50% of a dose of mercaptopurine is excreted in the urine as active drug and metabolites. Thioguanine is metabolized in the liver to several inactive products. Up to 40% of an oral dose of thioguanine is excreted in the urine in 24 hours. (See *Administration and excretion routes for antimetabolite agents* on page 1170 for more information about the purine analogues.)

Onset, peak, duration

Peak blood levels of mercaptopurine have not been quantitatively established. However, a dose of thioguanine reaches peak levels in 6 to 8 hours following an oral dose. Due to cellular uptake, renal excretion, and metabolic degradation, mercaptopurine has a short plasma half-life of 90 minutes. Thioguanine, however, has a plasma half-life of 11 hours.

PHARMACODYNAMICS

Mercaptopurine and thioguanine are analogues of the natural purine bases hypoxanthine and guanine. Because they resemble the natural bases, the purine analogues can enter into biochemical reactions in place of the natural bases. However, because the analogues cannot function exactly like the natural bases, they cause cell death.

Mechanism of action

Like the other antimetabolites, mercaptopurine and thioguanine must first undergo conversion to the nucleotide level to be active. This conversion is facilitated by the enzyme hypoxanthine-guanine phosphoribosyltransferase (HGPRT). The resulting nucleotides are then incorporated into DNA, where they may inhibit DNA and RNA synthesis as well as other metabolic reactions necessary for proper cell growth. The purine analogues are cell-cycle S-phase specific agents.

Cancer cells ultimately resist the cytotoxic effects of the purine analogues. Resistance may be from numerous mechanisms, including: (1) a decreased quantity or complete lack of HGPRT, which converts mercaptopurine and thioguanine to the nucleotide level, (2) decreased affinity of HGPRT for the drugs, (3) decreased drug transport into the cells, and (4) increased degradation of the drugs or their corresponding nucleotides.

PHARMACOTHERAPEUTICS

The purine analogues are used to treat acute and chronic leukemias.

mercaptopurine [6-MP] (Purinethol). Mercaptopurine has been especially useful in achieving remissions in children with acute leukemia. The results have been less impressive in adults with acute leukemia, although remissions are sometimes obtained. Mercaptopurine is also useful for maintaining remissions in acute lymphoblastic leukemia and chronic granulocytic leukemia.

USUAL ADULT DOSAGE: initially, 2.5 mg/kg P.O. daily (range 100 to 200 mg/day); following improvement, may be decreased to a maintenance of 1.2 to 2.5 mg/kg/day. When administered concurrently with allopurinol, the mercaptopurine dose should be reduced to 25% of the usual dose because allopurinol interferes with the oxidation of mercaptopurine, thereby potentiating its antineoplastic effect and increasing toxicity.

thioguanine [6-thioguanine] (Tabloid). Thioguanine is also used to treat acute leukemia, and when combined with cytarabine, is effective in inducing remission in acute granulocytic leukemia.

USUAL ADULT DOSAGE: initially, 2 mg/kg P.O. daily; may be increased to 3 mg/kg/day after 4 weeks if clinical improvement fails to occur or if no toxicity develops. Thioguanine can be administered concurrently with allopurinol without dosage reduction.

Drug interactions

No significant interactions occur with thioguanine. (See *Drug Interactions: Purine analogues* for the significant interactions associated with mercaptopurine.)

ADVERSE DRUG REACTIONS

Both mercaptopurine and thioguanine produce bone marrow suppression, which may not begin for 1 to 6

DRUG INTERACTIONS

Purine analogues

Drug interactions involving mercaptopurine are few although significant. The nurse must be familiar with possible effects and nursing implications before administering mercaptopurine.

DRUG	INTERACTING DRUGS	POSSIBLE EFFECTS	NURSING IMPLICATIONS
mercaptopurine	allopurinol	May increase bone marrow suppression because of decreased mercaptopurine metabolism	• Instruct the patient about the signs and symptoms of infection.
	warfarin	May decrease anticoagulant effect	• Consult the physician regarding warfarin dosage or alternative therapy.

weeks. Leukopenia usually occurs first, followed by thrombocytopenia and anemia.

Thirty-three percent of patients receiving mercaptopurine develop cholestatic jaundice 2 to 5 months after treatment. The patient should report this adverse reaction immediately because the jaundice is usually reversible if the drug is discontinued. Nausea, vomiting, anorexia, mild diarrhea, and stomatitis occur in about 20% of patients.

NURSING IMPLICATIONS

The nurse must be aware of the following implications before administering purine analogues:
• Mercaptopurine hepatotoxicity becomes manifest as cholestatic jaundice, which may progress to hepatic necrosis. Check the patient for pain in the right upper quadrant and elevated liver function enzymes that may indicate hepatic dysfunction.
• Administer cautiously following chemotherapy or radiation therapy, and in patients with depressed neutrophil or platelet counts or those with impaired hepatic or renal function.
• Observe the patient for signs of bleeding and infection.
• Monitor blood counts weekly, watching for a precipitous decrease.
• Avoid administering I.M. injections when the platelet count is low.
• Monitor intake and output, and encourage the patient to drink at least 3 liters of fluids daily.
• Monitor serum uric acid levels. If allopurinol is necessary, administer it cautiously.
• Alert the patient that improvement may take 2 to 4 weeks or longer.

The following nursing implications apply to thioguanine:
• Administer thioguanine cautiously to patients with renal or hepatic dysfunction.
• Observe the patient for jaundice, which may reverse if the drug is stopped promptly.
• Monitor CBC daily during induction, then weekly during maintenance therapy.
• Monitor serum uric acid levels.
• Avoid administering I.M. injections when the platelet count is low.

See also *Frequent adverse reactions and associated nursing implications* in Unit XV Introduction.

Care of stomatitis

Importance of oral care
The oral mucosa is a major first-line defense against significant infections that can compromise nutritional intake and patient comfort.

Symptomatic reaction
Reactions include inflammation of the mucous membrane, local tissue breakdown, bleeding, oral hemorrhage, and infection.

Incidence
Reactions occur in 30% to 60% of patients who receive antimetabolites.

Oral care guidelines

Frequency of oral care	At least twice daily until a special program is required; then after each meal and at bedtime; for severe stomatitis, every 2 hours is routine.
Aids to oral hygiene	Soft toothbrush, foam toothbrush (Toothette), normal saline rinse, lip moisturizer, Water Pik.
Recommendation for rinse	Isotonic solution of normal saline and sodium bicarbonate. Avoid hydrogen peroxide and mouthwash containing alcohol.
Recommendation for pain	Dyclonine hydrochloride (Dyclone), lidocaine (Xylocaine 2% Viscous Solution), or Benadryl and Maalox as a swish. Systemic analgesics for severe pain.

CHAPTER SUMMARY

Here are the highlights of this chapter:
• The antimetabolites are antineoplastic drugs that can interfere with the synthesis of nucleic acids and proteins.
• The antimetabolites, which are cell-cycle specific, are most active in the S phase.
• The major groups of antimetabolites are folic acid analogues, pyrimidine analogues, and purine analogues.

Antimetabolite agents

The following summarizes the important antimetabolites discussed in this chapter.

DRUG	MAJOR INDICATIONS	USUAL ADULT DOSAGES	NURSING IMPLICATIONS
Folic acid analogues			
methotrexate	Leukemia remission	30 mg/m² I.M. twice weekly or 175 to 525 mg/m² I.M. for 2 days monthly	● Explain to the patient the need for strict oral hygiene to alleviate the complications of stomatitis.
	Choriocarcinoma	15 mg/m² P.O. or I.M. daily for 5 days at 1- to 2-week intervals	● Maintain good hydration to prevent nephrotoxicity in high-dose methotrexate therapy. ● Instruct patients on methotrexate about birth control methods.
	Meningeal leukemia	Intrathecally: 12 mg/m² at 2- to 5-day intervals	
Pyrimidine analogues			
cytarabine	Acute nonlymphocytic leukemia, acute lymphocytic leukemia	100 to 200 mg/m²/day for 5 to 7 days by I.V. bolus; 100 mg/m²/day for 5 to 7 days by continuous I.V. infusion	● Instruct the patient about leukopenic and thrombocytopenic care. ● Explain to the patient the need for strict oral hygiene to alleviate the complications of stomatitis.
	Meningeal leukemia	30 mg/m² every 4 days intrathecally	● Injection site may be painful after I.V. dose; apply hot compresses as needed.
fluorouracil	Solid tumors, such as carcinomas of the GI tract and breast; basal cell carcinomas (topical treatment)	12 mg/kg I.V. daily for 4 successive days. Daily dosage should not exceed 800 mg. If no toxicity, give 6 mg/kg/day on the 6th, 8th, 10th, and 12th days.	● Instruct the patient about leukopenic and thrombocytopenic care. ● Explain to the patient the need for strict oral hygiene to prevent the complications of stomatitis. Use antiemetics as necessary for nausea; include high-calorie supplements for anorectic patients. ● Monitor the patient for dehydration secondary to diarrhea. Use antispasmodics for comfort.
Purine analogues			
mercaptopurine	Acute lymphoblastic leukemia, chronic granulocytic leukemia	2.5 mg/kg/day P.O. (100 to 200 mg/day), decreased to 1.2 to 2.5 mg/kg/day for maintenance	● Observe for signs of bleeding and infection. ● Monitor intake and output. Remind the patient to drink 3 liters of fluids a day.
thioguanine	Acute leukemia, acute granulocytic leukemia (used in conjunction with cytarabine)	2 mg/kg/day P.O.; may be increased to 3 mg/kg/day after 4 weeks if no clinical improvement and no signs of toxicity	● Administer cautiously to patients with renal or hepatic dysfunction. ● Monitor for jaundice or hepatic tenderness. ● Monitor CBC and serum uric acid level.

• Antimetabolites, used singly or in combination with other antineoplastic drugs, are used to treat acute leukemia, breast cancer, adenocarcinomas of the GI tract, non-Hodgkin's lymphomas, and squamous cell carcinomas of the head, neck, and cervix.

• The most frequent adverse effects of the antimetabolites include bone marrow suppression and stomatitis.

• During antimetabolite therapy, oral care can minimize injury to the mucosa, which is a first-line defense against infections.

• Unpredictable reactions, specific to each antimetabolite, include mild to severe skin reactions (fluorouracil) and fever and flulike symptoms (cytarabine and 5-azacytidine).

• The nurse can significantly help the patient to cope with chemotherapy through: (1) using caution when administering the antimetabolites, especially in patients with impaired hepatic function or bone marrow depression and following irradiation or chemotherapy, (2) carefully monitoring the patient for any signs of adverse reactions from the antimetabolite being used, and (3) informing the patient about the drug and the patient's role in the therapy.

BIBLIOGRAPHY

Becker, T. *Cancer Chemotherapy: A Manual for Nurses.* Boston: Little, Brown & Co., 1981.

Carter, S., et al. *Principles of Cancer Treatment.* New York: McGraw-Hill Book Co., 1982.

Cline, M., and Haskell, C. *Cancer Chemotherapy.* Philadelphia: W.B. Saunders Co., 1980.

Dorr, R.T., and Fritz, W.L. *Cancer Chemotherapy Handbook.* New York: Elsevier North Holland Inc., 1980.

Gilman, A.G., et al., eds. *Goodman and Gilman's The Pharmacological Basis of Therapeutics,* 7th edition. New York: Macmillan Publishing Co., 1985.

Holland, J., and Frei, E. *Cancer Medicine,* 2nd edition. Philadelphia: Lea & Febiger, 1982.

Lippens, R.J.J. "Methotrexate I. Pharmacology and Pharmacokinetics," *The American Journal of Pediatric Hematology/Oncology.* 6:379, 1984.

Marino, L.B. *Cancer Nursing.* St. Louis: C.V. Mosby Co., 1981.

McIntire, S.N., and Cioppa, A.L. *Cancer Nursing: A Developmental Approach.* New York: John Wiley & Sons, 1984.

Miller, S.A. "Nursing Actions in Cancer Chemotherapy Administration," *Oncology Nursing Forum.* 7:8, Fall 1980.

Sager, D.P., and Bomar, S. *Intravenous Medication: A Guide to Preparation, Administration and Nursing Management.* Philadelphia: J.B. Lippincott Co., 1980.

CHAPTER
75

ANTINEOPLASTIC ANTIBIOTIC AGENTS

OBJECTIVES

After reading and studying this chapter, you should be able to:
1. Describe the primary mechanism of action by which the antineoplastic antibiotics inhibit DNA and RNA synthesis.
2. Identify the major adverse reactions to and nursing implications for the antineoplastic antibiotics.
3. Explain why maximum lifetime doses have been established for bleomycin, daunorubicin, and doxorubicin.
4. Explain the mechanism of action of plicamycin in the treatment of hypercalcemia.
5. Discuss important information about antineoplastic antibiotic therapy that the nurse should include in the patient teaching.

INTRODUCTION

Antineoplastic antibiotics are antimicrobial products that produce tumoricidal effects by binding with deoxyribonucleic acid (DNA). These antineoplastic drugs inhibit the cellular processes of both normal and malignant cells

---

The antineoplastic antibiotics

The following drugs can be used singly or in combination to inhibit the processes of malignant cells.
• bleomycin (Blenoxane)
• dactinomycin [actinomycin D] (Cosmegen)
• daunorubicin [daunomycin] (Cerubidine)
• doxorubicin (Adriamycin)
• mitomycin [mitomycin-C] (Mutamycin)
• plicamycin [mithramycin] (Mithracin)

---

and are cell-cycle–nonspecific, except for bleomycin. Clinically, numerous antineoplastic antibiotics are useful when given singly or with other agents.

For a summary of representative drugs, see *Selected major drugs: Antineoplastic antibiotic agents* on page 1187.

MICROBIAL TUMORCIDAL AGENTS

Physicians prescribe the antineoplastic antibiotics (bleomycin, dactinomycin, daunorubicin, doxorubicin, mitomycin, and plicamycin) to treat many malignant neoplasms. Except for bleomycin, all the antineoplastic antibiotics produce bone marrow suppression resulting in moderate to severe pancytopenia, and all except bleomycin are vesicants that cause tissue damage if extravasated. Nausea, vomiting, and alopecia are common adverse effects caused by the antineoplastic antibiotics.

History and source

Discovered in 1940, dactinomycin acts against various animal tumors. Research in the 1950s produced additional antineoplastic antibiotics, many of them from soil strains of *Streptomyces*. In 1958, Wakaki and co-workers isolated mitomycin from *S. caespitosus*. In 1962, bleomycin was isolated from a soil strain (*S. verticillus)* obtained from a Japanese coal mine. Rao and co-workers isolated plicamycin in 1962 from cultures of *S. tanashiensis*. During independent studies, daunorubicin and doxorubicin were obtained from the fermentation of *S. peucetius* var. *caesius*.

Administration and excretion routes for antineoplastic antibiotic agents

This chart provides a quick reference for major routes of administration and excretion of the antineoplastic antibiotic agents. Because excretion amounts vary widely, the nurse who administers these agents should be familiar with the variations.

DRUG	MAJOR ROUTES OF ADMINISTRATION	MAJOR ROUTES OF EXCRETION	AMOUNT EXCRETED
bleomycin	Intravenous, intramuscular, subcutaneous	Urine	50% in 24 hours, mainly as metabolites
dactinomycin	Intravenous	Urine and feces	30% in 7 days
daunorubicin	Intravenous	Urine Bile	14% to 23% in 7 days Up to 85%
doxorubicin	Intravenous	Urine Bile	5% to 6% unchanged in 5 days 50% in 7 days
mitomycin	Intravenous	Urine	40% in 15 hours
plicamycin	Intravenous	Urine	10% to 30%

PHARMACOKINETICS

The pharmacokinetics of the antineoplastic antibiotics vary widely. Some of these drugs enter the cerebrospinal fluid (CSF); others do not. The extent of metabolism and urinary elimination also varies. The half-lives of the antineoplastic antibiotics range from 35 minutes to 55 hours.

Absorption, distribution, metabolism, excretion

Because the antineoplastic antibiotics are usually administered intravenously, no absorption need occur. They are considered to be 100% bioavailable. Some of the drugs are also administered via intracavitary routes. Bleomycin, doxorubicin, and mitomycin are sometimes given as topical bladder instillations, but significant systemic absorption, as assessed by blood concentration levels or systemic toxicity, does not occur. Bleomycin also has been injected into the pleural space for malignant effusions, with up to 50% of the dose absorbed via this route.

Distribution throughout the body of the antineoplastic antibiotics varies. Bleomycin is rapidly distributed, with a volume of distribution of 20 liters, approximating intracellular and extracellular fluid volume. Bleomycin concentrates in the skin and lungs, which may explain some of the drug's toxicities. Bleomycin's concentration in lung and skin tissue may be from the lack of inacti-

vating enzymes in these tissues. Bleomycin does not enter the CSF.

Dactinomycin is rapidly distributed to tissue-binding sites, with little drug remaining in the plasma 2 minutes after intravenous administration. The drug is distributed to nucleated (bone marrow) cells more than to nonnucleated (plasma) cells. Dactinomycin does not enter the CSF.

Daunorubicin and doxorubicin are rapidly and widely distributed to several organs in the body, including the heart, kidneys, lungs, liver, and spleen. Neither drug enters the CSF. Mitomycin is distributed widely throughout the body, but it does not enter the CSF. Mitomycin concentrates in the nail beds, forming purple bands. Although little is known about the pharmacokinetics of plicamycin, the drug does enter the CSF.

The metabolism of the antineoplastic antibiotics varies widely. Bleomycin undergoes significant tissue inactivation, especially in the liver and kidneys. Dactinomycin undergoes minimal metabolism. Daunorubicin is metabolized in the liver. Doxorubicin is metabolized in the liver, with hepatic clearance approximating 60% of hepatic blood flow. Mitomycin is extensively metabolized in the liver. The metabolism of plicamycin has not been well studied.

The antineoplastic antibiotic agents vary in their excretion. Up to 50% of a bleomycin dose is excreted in the urine in 24 hours, with 20% to 40% excreted as active drug. Dactinomycin is slowly excreted in the feces and urine, with only 30% excreted in 1 week. Daunorubicin is slowly excreted, with 23% of a dose recovered in the urine in 5 days. Daunorubicin is excreted primarily via the biliary route. Doxorubicin is also excreted primarily via the biliary route, with only 5% to 6% of the intact drug being excreted in the urine within 5 days. Small amounts of mitomycin are excreted in bile and feces, while 10% to 30% is excreted in the urine. Up to 40% of a plicamycin dose is excreted in the urine within 15 hours. (See *Administration and excretion routes for antineoplastic antibiotic agents* on page 1183 for a summary of the excretion rates and routes.)

Onset, peak, duration

Bleomycin reaches peak plasma concentration levels of 1 to 10 mU/ml after an intravenous bolus of 15 units/m^2. After an intravenous bolus, bleomycin has a half-life of 3 hours, which extends to 9 hours with a continuous infusion. Dactinomycin concentration levels peak immediately after an intravenous injection, with very little active drug remaining in the circulation after 2 minutes. With slow release from tissue-binding sites, the plasma half-life of dactinomycin is 36 hours.

Daunorubicin has a long half-life of 40 to 55 hours. Doxorubicin has a multiphasic elimination pattern, with a half-life of 24 to 48 hours. Mitomycin reaches a peak plasma concentration level of 1.5 mcg/ml after a dose of 20 mg/m^2. The plasma half-life of mitomycin is 35 minutes. The peak concentration levels and half-life of plicamycin have not been determined.

PHARMACODYNAMICS

With the exception of mitomycin, the antineoplastic antibiotics intercalate, or insert themselves, between adjacent base pairs of a DNA molecule, physically separating them. When the DNA chain replicates, an extra base is inserted opposite the intercalated antibiotic, resulting in a mutant DNA molecule. The overall effect is cell death.

Mechanism of action

Bleomycin's cytotoxic action may be a result of copper-bleomycin and possibly iron-bleomycin complexes that form during intercalation with the DNA molecule. These complexes can generate highly reactive free radicals that cause chain scission (splitting) and fragmentation of DNA molecules. Bleomycin is a cell-cycle–specific drug that causes its major effects in the G$_2$ phase.

Dactinomycin intercalates between adjacent guanine-cytosine pairs in the DNA molecule, where it binds and inhibits the function of DNA-dependent RNA poly-

merase. This inhibiting action blocks transcription of the DNA molecule, which causes cell death. Dactinomycin is a cell-cycle–nonspecific drug.

Daunorubicin and doxorubicin (the anthracycline antibiotics), also intercalate into DNA. This causes many cell changes that ultimately produce the drugs' cytotoxic effects. The drugs inhibit DNA and RNA synthesis. Single- and double-strand breaks in the DNA occur, as does an information exchange between DNA strands known as sister chromatid exchange. These actions account for the mutagenic and carcinogenic actions of the anthracyclines. Finally, daunorubicin and doxorubicin can interfere with cell membrane function, an action that may contribute to cytotoxicity as well as to cardiotoxicity. Daunorubicin and doxorubicin are cell-cycle–nonspecific agents; however, they do appear to be most active in the S phase.

Mitomycin is the one antineoplastic antibiotic that does not intercalate into DNA. Mitomycin is activated intracellulary to a bifunctional or even trifunctional alkylating agent. Mitomycin produces single-strand breakage of DNA; it also cross-links DNA and inhibits DNA synthesis. Mitomycin's ability to cross-link DNA is related to the guanine and cytosine content of the DNA. Mitomycin is cell-cycle nonspecific, although its maximal action occurs in the late G$_1$ and early S phases.

Resembling dactinomycin, plicamycin intercalates between adjacent guanine-cytosine base pairs in the DNA molecule. Plicamycin inhibits RNA, DNA, and protein synthesis, and is cell-cycle–nonspecific. Plicamycin also can lower serum calcium concentration levels, probably because it can inhibit parathyroid hormone action and can act on osteoclasts.

PHARMACOTHERAPEUTICS

The antineoplastic antibiotics are products of microbial fermentation that exhibit antimicrobial activity. Their cytotoxic effects, however, preclude their antimicrobial use. The antineoplastic antibiotics act against many tumors, including Hodgkin's disease and non-Hodgkin's lymphomas; testicular carcinoma; squamous cell carcinoma of the head, neck, and cervix; Wilms' tumor, osteogenic sarcoma, rhabdomyosarcoma; Ewing's tumor and other soft-tissue sarcomas; breast, ovarian, bladder, and bronchogenic carcinomas; acute leukemias; melanoma; carcinomas of the gastrointestinal tract; choriocarcinoma; and hypercalcemia. Mitomycin, doxorubicin, and daunorubicin are the most bone marrow suppressive, whereas bleomycin is the least suppressive. With the exception of bleomycin, all of the antineoplastic antibiotics are vesicants requiring care to avoid extravasation when administered parenterally.

bleomycin (Blenoxane). When combined with vinblastine and cisplatin, bleomycin acts effectively against testicular carcinoma, achieving response rates of over 90%, with complete remissions attained in many patients. Bleomycin also acts effectively against squamous cell carcinomas of the head, neck, esophagus, skin, and genitourinary tract; lung cancer; and Hodgkin's and non-Hodgkin's lymphomas. When combined with other agents, bleomycin may increase the regimen's activity against the cancer without increased bone marrow toxicity.

USUAL ADULT DOSAGE: 10 to 20 units/m^2 I.V. or I.M. once or twice weekly. Bleomycin may also be given subcutaneously or intraarterially. A maximum lifetime dose of 400 units is recommended because of the pulmonary toxicity associated with bleomycin. Dosage reductions should be made in patients with renal failure. Because 1% of lymphoma patients experience an anaphylactic reaction to bleomycin, all lymphoma patients should receive two test doses of 2 to 5 units before the initial dose.

dactinomycin [actinomycin D] (Cosmegen). Effective against rhabdomyosarcoma and Wilms' tumor in children, dactinomycin also acts against Ewing's sarcoma, gestational choriocarcinoma, Kaposi's sarcoma, and testicular carcinoma.

USUAL ADULT DOSAGE: 10 to 15 mcg/kg daily I.V. for 5 days repeated every 3 to 4 weeks. Usually, a total dose of 2.5 to 5 mg is needed to produce antineoplastic effects. Care should be taken to avoid extravasation. Dosage reduction should be considered in patients with hepatic and renal dysfunction.

USUAL PEDIATRIC DOSAGE: 100 to 400 mcg daily I.V. for 10 to 14 days.

daunorubicin [daunomycin] (Cerubidine). When given with cytarabine, daunorubicin is the treatment of choice for acute nonlymphoblastic leukemia in adults. It also acts against numerous tumors in children, including Ewing's sarcoma, rhabdomyosarcoma, Wilms' tumor, and neuroblastoma. Daunorubicin can be given on various treatment schedules.

USUAL ADULT DOSAGE: 30 to 60 mg/m^2 daily I.V. for 2 days, 3 days, or once weekly. Care should be taken to avoid extravasation. A maximum lifetime dose of 500 to 600 mg/m^2 is recommended to prevent cardiotoxicity. Cardiac problems usually preclude daunorubicin use. Dosage reduction is recommended in patients with impaired hepatic or biliary function.

Treating hypercalcemia

The normal serum calcium concentration level is 8.5 to 10.5 mg/dl. Hypercalcemia occurs when the serum concentration level of calcium exceeds 10.5 mg/dl. This abnormal release of calcium occurs in 10% to 20% of all cancer patients and 40% to 50% of patients with multiple myeloma or metastatic breast cancer. The electrolyte imbalance is produced by several bone demineralization mechanisms, including bone destruction by metastases, prolonged immobilization, high concentrations of parathyroid hormone released by some tumors, and high levels of prostaglandin and osteoclast activating factor found in some cancer patients.

The signs and symptoms of hypercalcemia include anorexia, nausea and vomiting, polyuria, deep bone pain, fatigue, depression, loss of memory, stupor, coma, constipation, abdominal pain, dysrhythmias, somnolence, lethargy, weakness, and confusion.

To treat severe hypercalcemia from cancer, physicians first prescribe normal saline solution, diuretics, and oral phosphates; if these fail, then plicamycin. Doses of plicamycin for hypercalcemia range from 12.5 to 25 mcg/kg to inhibit bone resorption of calcium. Adverse effects of this treatment include bone marrow suppression, hypotension, and nephrotoxicity.

---

doxorubicin (Adriamycin). Effective against many hematologic and solid tumors, doxorubicin is also used in combination regimens against acute leukemias as well as non-Hodgkin's and Hodgkin's lymphomas. The solid tumors that are responsive to doxorubicin include breast, lung, ovarian, bladder, and thyroid carcinomas. Doxorubicin is also active against sarcomas, including osteogenic sarcoma, Ewing's tumor, and Wilms' tumor. Like daunorubicin, doxorubicin can be given using various dosing schedules.

USUAL ADULT DOSAGE: 60 to 75 mg/m^2 I.V. every 3 weeks; or 20 to 30 mg/m^2 I.V. daily for 2 to 3 days, repeated every 3 to 4 weeks; or 20 mg/m^2 I.V. weekly. Care should be used to avoid extravasation. A maximum lifetime dose of 550 mg/m^2 is recommended to avoid cardiotoxicity. Cardiac problems usually preclude doxorubicin use. The lifetime dose may be decreased for patients receiving definitive radiation therapy. Dosage reduction is recommended in patients with hepatic or biliary dysfunction.

USUAL PEDIATRIC DOSAGE: 30 mg/m^2 on 3 successive days every 4 weeks.

mitomycin [mitomycin-C] (Mutamycin). Active against various tumors, mitomycin is used particularly in the palliative treatment of gastric adenocarcinoma. It is also active against carcinomas of the cervix, colon, rectum, pancreas, breast, head and neck, and lungs. Mitomycin also exhibits topical activity against bladder carcinoma. USUAL ADULT DOSAGE: as a single I.V. bolus, 10 to 20 mg/m²; or as 2 mg/m² daily for two 5-day periods separated by 2 drug-free days for a total of 20 mg/m² over 12 days. The cycle is repeated in 6 to 8 weeks. Extravasation should be avoided. For topical application for bladder carcinoma, physicians prescribe 20- to 40-mg instillations once weekly, for 8 procedures per course.

plicamycin [mithramycin] (Mithracin). Although plicamycin exhibits its greatest antineoplastic activity against disseminated testicular cancer, its use for this tumor has largely been replaced by other drugs. Plicamycin is primarily used to treat hypercalcemia, especially that from cancer that has metastasized to the bone. (See *Treating hypercalcemia* on page 1185 for further details.) USUAL ADULT DOSAGE: for testicular cancer, 25 to 30 mcg/kg daily I.V. for 8 to 10 days; for hypercalcemia, 25 mcg/kg daily I.V., for 3 to 4 days, repeated weekly as necessary.

Drug interactions
No clinically significant drug interactions occur with the antineoplastic antibiotics.

ADVERSE DRUG REACTIONS

The antineoplastic antibiotics produce many of the same reactions as other drugs used to treat malignant neoplasms.

Predictable reactions
The primary predictable reaction from antineoplastic antibiotics is bone marrow suppression. All of these agents except bleomycin produce moderate to severe pancytopenia. Also, because all except bleomycin are vesicants, extra care is necessary to prevent extravasation.

Bone marrow suppression, stomatitis, and alopecia are produced by the effect of the antineoplastic antibiotics on rapidly proliferating tissues. This is because bone marrow, epithelial tissue, and hair follicles have growth rates faster than many other body tissues; making these cells more vulnerable to antineoplastic agents, causing adverse reactions.

Nausea and vomiting result from the chemical irritation of the thalamic emesis center. Vomiting is also produced by a psychogenic factor that can be triggered by sights, sounds, and smells experienced during chemotherapy. (See *Frequently occurring adverse reactions and associated nursing implications* in Unit Fifteen Introduction.)

Unpredictable reactions
All antineoplastic antibiotics except bleomycin produce severe tissue damage if extravasated. Yet extravasation can occur with even the most careful administration. Bleomycin may produce fever and chills. If these effects become intense, the patient should receive immediate treatment with antihistamines and antipyretics. Patients who develop fever and chills with bleomycin therapy must receive premedication with antihistamines and antipyretics before each bleomycin administration. Bleomycin can result in pulmonary fibrosis, but this effect occurs infrequently and usually in patients over age 70 who have received more than the recommended lifetime dose of 400 units.

The anthracycline antibiotics (daunorubicin and doxorubicin) may cause cardiomyopathy. The potential for cardiomyopathy increases as the patient approaches the lifetime dosage level. Both the pulmonary fibrosis and cardiomyopathy are irreversible effects.

NURSING IMPLICATIONS

The nurse caring for patients receiving antineoplastic antibiotics should aim to alleviate the expected adverse reactions and support the patient through the drug course and recovery period.
- Expect bone marrow suppression with all antineoplastic antibiotics except bleomycin. Expect acute complications when the absolute granulocyte count is below 1,000/mm³. As the count declines, encourage the patient to maintain adequate nutritional and fluid intake. During the nadir, the patient should avoid crowds and anyone with an active contagious infection.
- Teach the patient to watch for, recognize, and report any signs of infection (for example, fever or sore throat) immediately. Hospitalized patients also risk contracting an infection from altered skin integrity, hospital procedures such as I.V. punctures, or urinary drainage devices.
- Evaluate anemia or thrombocytopenia from bone marrow suppression using the hematocrit and the platelet count. Because red blood cells (RBCs) have a longer life than white blood cells and platelets, anemia does not usually occur unless the patient has an occult or overt blood loss. When the platelet count is lower than 50,000 mm³, take additional safety precautions to prevent trauma. Supportive platelet transfusions and packed RBCs may be administered as prescribed.

SELECTED MAJOR DRUGS

Antineoplastic antibiotic agents

This chart summarizes the major antineoplastic antibiotics currently in clinical use, their indications, usual dosages, and nursing implications.

DRUG	MAJOR INDICATIONS	USUAL ADULT DOSAGES	NURSING IMPLICATIONS
bleomycin	Hodgkin's disease; testicular carcinoma; squamous cell carcinoma of the head, neck, and uterine cervix	10 to 20 units/m^2 I.V. or I.M. one to two times weekly	• Monitor the patient for fever and chills; administer an antipyretic as prescribed. • Examine the patient's mouth for signs of stomatitis. • Monitor the cumulative dose, and assess for pulmonary status changes by auscultating lung sounds. • Because the patient may have an anaphylactic reaction, administer a test dose to the patient receiving bleomycin for the first time.
daunorubicin	Acute leukemias	30 to 60 mg/m^2 I.V. for 2 days, 3 days, or once weekly	• Instruct the patient in leukopenic and thrombocytopenic care. • Administer antiemetics as prescribed according to the patient's need. • Monitor the cumulative dose, and assess the patient for symptoms of cardiomyopathy.
doxorubicin	Sarcomas, breast carcinoma, bronchogenic cancer, lymphomas, bladder carcinoma	60 to 75 mg/m^2 I.V. every 3 weeks 20 to 30 mg/m^2 I.V. for 2 to 3 days every 3 to 4 weeks 20 mg/m^2 I.V. weekly	• Inform the patient of potential alopecia, including body hair loss. • Instruct the patient in leukopenic and thrombocytopenic care. • Observe the patient for signs of congestive heart failure. • Administer antiemetics as prescribed according to the patient's need.
plicamycin	Hypercalcemia Testicular tumors	25 mcg/kg/day I.V. for 3 to 4 days 25 to 30 mcg/kg/day I.V. for 8 to 10 days	• Provide routine antiemetic coverage as prescribed during administration of drug. • Monitor the patient's temperature, and administer an antipyretic as prescribed. • Observe the patient for signs of bleeding.

• For nausea and vomiting from chemotherapy, routinely administer prescribed antiemetics in combination with any chemotherapeutic drug with emetic potential.

• Decrease the psychogenic factors of chemotherapy by helping the patient overcome feelings of isolation and anxiety: spend time with the patient, listen supportively, provide music, and use relaxation techniques.

• Assess the patient regularly for stomatitis, or oral mucositis, evidenced by erythema and ulceration of the oral mucosa that may develop 7 to 10 days after therapy. Encourage the patient to use a toothette for mouth care

at least every 4 hours; if the toothette is too painful, provide normal saline solution rinses. Antifungal agents are often prescribed to prevent a candida infection.

• Include patient teaching and support for patients with alopecia, or loss of hair. Inform the patient that the hair loss is temporary, but that hair regrowth may be a different color or texture.

• Before initiating scalp hypothermia to decrease alopecia, consult the physician because the procedure is not appropriate for every patient. Cool the scalp for 15 to 30 minutes before drug administration, and continue to cool it for 15 to 30 minutes after administration. The use of scalp hypothermia is indicated in patients receiving a drug with an immediate onset of action, peak concentration level, and short duration of action.

• Closely monitor patients receiving daunorubicin or doxorubicin for symptoms of congestive heart failure, including dependent edema, tachycardia, dyspnea, decreased urine output, and unexplained weight gain. If the patient exhibits any of the above signs or symptoms, withhold the drug and notify the physician.

• Use pulmonary function tests to monitor the respiratory function of the patient receiving bleomycin before every 100 units of the drug. Inform the patient about potential symptoms of pulmonary fibrosis and interstitial pneumonia, such as dry, unproductive cough and dyspnea.

• Because dactinomycin, daunorubicin, doxorubicin, mitomycin, and plicamycin are powerful vesicants, use extreme caution when administering these agents. Vesicants are most safely given via I.V. push into the side port of a freely infusing I.V., which enables close supervision of the site throughout the administration.

• If infiltration or extravasation is suspected, stop the infusion immediately, apply cold compresses, and elevate the extremity. Instilling hydrocortisone as prescribed into the affected site via an I.V. catheter or subcutaneous injection may decrease tissue damage.

• Inform the patient of the expected adverse reactions to any antineoplastic antibiotic, but caution that the occurrence and severity of such reactions varies among patients. Reassure the patient by describing interventions that may help, should adverse reactions occur.

• When administering an antineoplastic antibiotic, explain to the patient the potential effects of the drug and provide printed handouts to take home.

CHAPTER SUMMARY

Chapter 75 presented the antineoplastic antibiotics, agents that bind to DNA and prevent cellular reproduction. Many of these agents, which are products of microorganisms, have been derived from soil strains of *Streptomyces*. Here are the highlights of the chapter:

• The antineoplastic antibiotics dactinomycin, daunorubicin, doxorubicin, mitomycin, and plicamycin are cell-cycle–nonspecific. Bleomycin is G_2-phase–specific.

• Physicians prescribe antineoplastic antibiotics singly or in combination with other antineoplastic drugs to treat various malignant neoplasms, including Hodgkin's disease, non-Hodgkin's lymphomas, testicular carcinoma, Wilms' tumor, rhabdomyosarcoma, Ewing's sarcoma, breast carcinoma, bladder carcinoma, bronchogenic carcinoma, acute leukemias, and gastrointestinal tract carcinomas.

• The most common adverse reactions to the antineoplastic antibiotics include bone marrow suppression, alopecia, and nausea and vomiting.

• Except for bleomycin, all antineoplastic antibiotics are vesicants and can cause severe tissue damage if extravasated.

• Daunorubicin and doxorubicin may result in cardiomyopathy; bleomycin may produce pulmonary fibrosis. These effects are cumulative, dose-related, and irreversible. Therefore, total lifetime doses of these drugs are limited to prevent the effects. The nurse can assist the patient in coping with chemotherapy through careful drug administration, patient teaching, and interventions to minimize adverse reactions.

BIBLIOGRAPHY

Becker, T. *Cancer Chemotherapy: A Manual for Nurses.* Boston: Little, Brown & Co., 1981.

Carter, S., et al. *Principles of Cancer Treatment.* New York: McGraw-Hill Book Co., 1982.

Cline, M., and Haskell, C. *Cancer Chemotherapy.* Philadelphia: W.B. Saunders Co., 1980.

Cullen, M.L. "Current Interventions for Doxorubicin Extravasations," *Oncology Nursing Forum* 9:52, Winter 1982.

Doroshow, J. "The Usefulness of Noninvasive Cardiac Monitoring in Prevention and Detection of Anthracycline Cardiomyopathy," in *Medical Oncology Controversies in Cancer Treatment.* Edited by Van Scoy-Mosher, M. Boston: G.K. Hall & Co., 1981.

Dorr, R.T., and Fitz, W.L. *Cancer Chemotherapy Handbook.* New York: Elsevier North Holland Inc., 1980.

Frogge, M.H. "Give the Vesicants Last," *Oncology Nursing Forum* 9:53, Winter 1982.

Gilman, A.G., et al., eds. *Goodman and Gilman's The Pharmacological Basis of Therapeutics,* 7th ed. New York: Macmillan Publishing Co., 1985.

Holland, J., and Frei, E. *Cancer Medicine,* 2nd ed. Philadelphia: Lea & Febiger, 1982.

Marino, L.B. *Cancer Nursing.* St. Louis: C.V. Mosby Co., 1981.

McIntire, S.N., and Cioppa, A.L. *Cancer Nursing: A Developmental Approach.* New York: John Wiley & Sons, 1984.

Stuart, M. "Sequence of Administering Vesicant Cytotoxic Drugs," *Oncology Nursing Forum* 9:53, Winter 1982.

Wood, H., and Ellerhorst-Ryan, J. "Delayed Adverse Skin Reactions Associated with Mitomycin-C Administration," *Oncology Nursing Forum* 11:14, July/August 1984.

CHAPTER 76

HORMONAL ANTINEOPLASTIC AGENTS

OBJECTIVES

After reading and studying this chapter, you should be able to:

1. Differentiate among the specific indications for estrogens, antiestrogens, androgens, adrenocortical suppressants, progestins, corticosteroids, and gonadotropin-releasing hormone analogues.

2. Describe how each group of hormonal antineoplastic agents works to inhibit malignant growth.

3. Identify the major adverse reactions to androgens and estrogens and their nursing implications.

4. Describe the pharmacokinetic properties of the progestins and their importance in evaluating patient therapy.

5. Identify adverse reactions to and nursing implications for corticosteroid therapy.

6. Describe the predictable and unpredictable adverse reactions to leuprolide therapy.

INTRODUCTION

Physicians prescribe a wide range of hormonal antineoplastic agents to alter the growth of malignant neoplasms or to manage and treat their physiologic effects. (See *Hormonal antineoplastic agents* for a list of these drugs.) The mechanisms of action are not completely understood and, in fact, the early use of hormonal agents was largely empiric.

The use of hormonal agents as direct or indirect antagonists to inhibit hormonal influence began in 1939 with the use of androgens for breast cancer. However, the earliest therapy for endocrine-related tumors occurred in 1896 when Beatson performed an oophorectomy on a woman with breast cancer. Many advances occurred in the 1940s and 1950s as knowledge of the endocrine system grew rapidly. During that time, procedures that removed glands and eliminated stimulating hormones included orchiectomy in prostatic cancer, 1941; adrenalectomy in breast cancer, 1951; and hypophysectomy in breast cancer, 1952. More recent advances in hormonal therapy include the role of estrogen and progesterone receptors in the treatment of breast cancer. Though not cytotoxic, the hormonal antineoplastic agents can be cytostatic and prevent malignant neoplasm growth. Hormonal therapies prove effective against hormone-dependent tumors, such as cancers of the prostate, breast, and endometrium. Lymphomas and leukemias are usually treated with protocols that include corticosteroids because of their lympholytic potential. (See Chapter 59, Androgenic and Anabolic Steroid Agents, and Chapter 60, Estrogens, Progestins, and Oral Contraceptive Agents, for further information about hormonal agents.)

For a summary of representative drugs, see *Selected major drugs: Hormonal antineoplastic agents* on page 1200.

ESTROGENS

Physicians prescribe estrogens as palliative therapy for metastatic breast cancer in women who are at least 5 years postmenopausal and for whom antiestrogen therapy was ineffective. Estrogens are also prescribed for males with advanced prostate cancers.

History and source

In the late 19th century, physicians recommended castration as a hormone control therapy for breast cancer. In 1919, Loeb castrated mice hoping to find a connection between ovarian secretions and breast cancer. In 1936, Lacassagne used estrogen injections to increase the incidence of breast cancer in mice. Sophisticated research in the 1970s by Jensen, Knight, and others showed that

Hormonal antineoplastic agents

Estrogens

- ethinyl estradiol (Estinyl)
- diethylstilbestrol [DES]
- diethylstilbestrol diphosphate (Stilphostrol)
- conjugated estrogens (Premarin)
- chlorotrianisene (TACE)

Antiestrogens

- tamoxifen citrate (Nolvadex)

Androgens

- fluoxymesterone (Halotestin)
- testolactone (Teslac)
- testosterone propionate (Testex)
- testosterone enanthate (Delatestryl)

Adrenocorticol Suppressants

- aminoglutethimide (Cytadren)

Progestins

- medroxyprogesterone acetate (Depo-Provera, Provera)
- megestrol acetate (Megace)
- hydroxyprogesterone caproate (Delalutin)

Corticosteroids

- hydrocortisone (Cortef)
- prednisone (Deltasone)
- prednisolone (Delta-Cortef)
- methylprednisolone (Medrol, Solu-Medrol)
- dexamethasone (Decadron)

Gonadotropin-Releasing Hormone Analogues

- leuprolide acetate (Lupron)

breast cancer with specific estrogen-binding receptors responds to estrogen therapy.

PHARMACOKINETICS

The estrogens are readily and rapidly absorbed after oral and topical administration. They are well distributed throughout the body. Chlorotrianisene is distributed especially well to fatty tissue, providing a prolonged duration of action. Metabolized in the liver, the estrogens undergo enterohepatic circulation. Chlorotrianisene is metabolized to a more potent compound. After conjugation, the estrogens are excreted in the urine.

Because estrogens have a slow onset of action, they should be administered for 2 to 3 months before their therapeutic efficacy is fully assessed.

PHARMACODYNAMICS

The estrogens act on tumor cells to inhibit hormone-mediated growth; however, the antitumor mechanism of action is not completely understood. The estrogen binds to a receptor on the cell membrane; this complex is then translocated to the nucleus, where it may modulate cell growth. In postmenopausal women with breast cancer, exogenous estrogens may displace endogenous growth-enhancing estrogens from their receptors. Researchers have not yet discovered how high doses of estrogens parodoxically inhibit estrogen production. In men with prostate cancer, the estrogens act on the pituitary to suppress secretion of luteinizing hormone, which in turn decreases testicular androgen secretion.

PHARMACOTHERAPEUTICS

Estrogen therapy is used as a palliative treatment for metastatic breast cancer in women who are at least 5 years postmenopausal and for men with metastatic prostate cancer. Breast cancer tumor cells that are estrogen receptor-positive respond more to hormonal therapy than those that are not. The average duration of remission induced by hormonal therapy is 6 to 12 months.

ethinyl estradiol (Estinyl). Physicians prescribe ethinyl estradiol as a palliative treatment for both breast and prostate cancer.
USUAL ADULT DOSAGE: for breast cancer, 1 mg P.O. t.i.d.; for prostatic cancer, 0.15 to 2 mg P.O. daily.

diethylstilbestrol [DES]. Like ethinyl estradiol, this drug is indicated for the palliative treatment of breast and prostate cancer.
USUAL ADULT DOSAGE: for prostate cancer, 1 to 3 mg P.O. daily; for breast cancer, 5 to 15 mg P.O. daily.

diethylstilbestrol diphosphate (Stilphostrol). Administered orally or intravenously, diethylstilbestrol diphosphate is used to treat prostate cancer.
USUAL ADULT DOSAGE: 50 to 200 mg P.O. t.i.d.; initially 500 mg I.V., then increased to 1,000 mg I.V. daily for 5 days, then 250 to 500 mg I.V. once or twice weekly.

conjugated estrogens (Premarin). Given orally, conjugated estrogens are used to treat breast and prostate cancer.

USUAL ADULT DOSAGE: for breast cancer, 10 mg P.O. t.i.d. for at least 3 months; for prostate cancer, 1.25 to 2.5 mg P.O. t.i.d.

chlorotrianisene (TACE). This drug is used to treat prostate cancer.
USUAL ADULT DOSAGE: 12 to 25 mg P.O. daily.

Drug interactions
Few significant drug interactions occur with the estrogens.

ADVERSE DRUG REACTIONS

Estrogens are relatively well tolerated even in the large doses usually prescribed for cancer treatments. Most of the adverse effects of these agents are extensions of their natural hormonal activities.

Predictable reactions
Estrogen therapy may cause mild nausea, which is more pronounced in women, probably because of the higher dosages used for them. The nausea, which usually disappears after 2 or 3 weeks of therapy, is not severe enough to cause a nutritional deficit. Abdominal cramps, irritability, and frequent urination also occur.

Estrogen therapy causes feminization in male patients, primarily manifested by mammary gland development (gynecomastia) and impotence. Female patients may experience a decreased libido and breast tenderness. Almost all patients display an increased pigmentation of the nipples and areolae.

Unpredictable reactions
Several unpredictable metabolic complications can develop during estrogen therapy. Sodium retention and resulting fluid retention can occur as dose-dependent adverse reactions. Fluid retention can prove extremely serious for patients with congestive heart failure. Patients, especially those with metastatic bone disease, may also develop hypercalcemia. Uterine breakthrough bleeding can occur in postmenopausal women. Patients with metastatic breast cancer may experience a flare of metastatic lesions, manifested by increased skin nodules or worsening bone pain. High doses of estrogens predispose patients to increased risks of thromboembolic complications, including pulmonary embolus, myocardial infarction, and stroke.

NURSING IMPLICATIONS

Estrogen therapy proves effective against neoplastic diseases afflicting organs that depend upon hormones for growth. Prostate and breast cancer are the two primary diseases affected by estrogens. The nurse should be aware of the following implications when treating patients with estrogens:
- Mild nausea is the most common adverse reaction during estrogen therapy. Instruct the patient to report it so that symptomatic treatment may begin: oral antiemetics administered before meals, frequent small meals, and an increased carbohydrate intake. Because estrogens are usually taken daily, a change in therapy may be needed if nausea becomes a continuing problem.
- Inform the patient of the possibility of fluid retention and explain how to observe for edema, especially of the hands, ankles, tibia, and sacrum.
- Inform female patients that breakthrough uterine bleeding is not normal, and instruct them to report any uterine bleeding to the physician. Also, explain that they may notice breast tenderness during therapy.
- Provide emotional support for male patients undergoing estrogen therapy, particularly regarding the effects of estrogens on sexual characteristics. Estrogens may cause temporary gynecomastia and decreased libido, which disappear after therapy ends.
- Because the combined effect of estrogen therapy and bone metastasis may produce hypercalcemia, teach patients and their families to recognize the signs and symptoms of hypercalcemia.
- Instruct the patient to report adverse reactions, such as anorexia, nausea, vomiting, constipation, weakness, loss of muscle tone, lethargy, and polyuria. Emphasize to the patient and family members that these effects may be treatable and are not symptoms of the disease.
- Monitor the patient's serum calcium levels monthly. Mobilize the patient and maintain adequate hydration. Limiting the patient's dietary intake of calcium may have no significant effect on serum calcium levels.
- Thromboemboli have been reported with long-term use of high-dose estrogens. Remind patients to avoid wearing restrictive clothing and sitting for long periods with their legs crossed. Symptoms of thromboemboli may include sudden shortness of breath, partial or complete vision loss, headache, and local pain, tenderness, and swelling in extremities.

ANTIESTROGENS

The antiestrogen, tamoxifen citrate, acts by competing with estradiol for receptor sites. Tamoxifen is the drug of choice for advanced breast cancer involving estrogen receptor-positive tumors.

PHARMACOKINETICS

Tamoxifen is well absorbed after oral administration, undergoing extensive enterohepatic circulation before fecal excretion. Tamoxifen has a half-life of approximately 1 week.

Absorption, distribution, metabolism, excretion

Tamoxifen is well absorbed; however, its distribution has not been thoroughly studied. Tamoxifen is metabolized in the liver to various metabolites displaying cytotoxicity. The monohydroxylated metabolite displays more antiestrogenic activity than does tamoxifen itself or the dihydroxylated derivative. Tamoxifen and its metabolites undergo enterohepatic circulation before being excreted. Most of the drug is excreted in the feces as the conjugated metabolite, with less than 30% excreted as other metabolites or the parent compound. Only minimal amounts are excreted in the urine.

Onset, peak, duration

Peak concentration levels of tamoxifen are achieved in 4 to 7 hours after an oral dose. The half-life of the drug is approximately 7 days. Steady state blood levels are achieved in 4 weeks, with clinical responses usually appearing in 1 to 2 months.

PHARMACODYNAMICS

Estrogen receptors, found in the cancer cells of 50% of premenopausal and 75% of postmenopausal women with breast cancer, respond to estrogenic influence to induce tumor growth. The antiestrogen, tamoxifen, binds to the estrogen receptors and inhibits estrogen-mediated tumor growth. The inhibition may result because the tamoxifen binds to receptors at the nuclear level or because the binding reduces the number of free receptors in the cytoplasm. Ultimately, DNA synthesis and cell growth are inhibited.

PHARMACOTHERAPEUTICS

The antiestrogen, tamoxifen, is the palliative treatment of choice for advanced breast cancer.

tamoxifen citrate (Nolvadex). This drug is indicated for the palliative treatment of metastatic breast cancer that is estrogen receptor-positive. Tumors in postmenopausal women are more responsive to tamoxifen than those in premenopausal women. The drug is used singly or in combination with cytotoxic agents.

USUAL ADULT DOSAGE: 10 to 20 mg P.O. b.i.d.

Drug interactions

No drug interactions have been identified for tamoxifen.

ADVERSE DRUG REACTIONS

Tamoxifen is a relatively nontoxic drug. The most predictable reactions are hot flashes, nausea, and vomiting. Transient mild leukopenia or thrombocytopenia may occur in about 4% of patients.

Tumor flare, an unpredictable reaction, may occur in about 1% of patients treated with tamoxifen. Symptoms may include an increased number and size of lesions, or increased bone pain. Patients receiving high doses of tamoxifen have experienced ocular lesions, retinopathy, and superficial corneal opacity, which reduce visual acuity.

NURSING IMPLICATIONS

The nurse should be aware that tamoxifen, available in tablet form, should be stored at room temperature and protected from light. Other considerations include the following:

• Tamoxifen causes menopausal symptoms such as hot flashes, nausea, and occasional vomiting. Explain to the patient that tolerance to these symptoms develops quite rapidly.

• Tamoxifen can cause slight thrombocytopenia and leukopenia in patients at risk from myelosuppressive therapy. Monitor the patient's blood counts frequently during therapy.

• Instruct female patients to report to the physician any gynecologic adverse reactions, such as vaginal bleeding. The patient may need help quantifying the blood loss.

• Explain to premenopausal women on tamoxifen that they should use some form of mechanical birth control because tamoxifen can induce ovulation. Although tamoxifen's effects on human development are unknown, the drug is teratogenic in animals.

• Tumor flare associated with tamoxifen can be very distressing to patients and families; assure them that this expected adverse effect will subside rapidly. In the meantime, the patient may require increased analgesics.

• Instruct the patient to report immediately to the physician any decreased visual acuity; it may be irreversible. Inform the patient of the need for routine eye examinations by an ophthalmologist, who should be told about the tamoxifen therapy.

ANDROGENS

The therapeutically useful androgens are synthetic derivatives of naturally occurring testosterone. Since 1939, androgens have been used to treat prostate cancer, male breast cancer, and advanced female breast cancer.

PHARMACOKINETICS

The pharmacokinetic properties of therapeutic androgens resemble those of naturally occurring testosterone. The oral androgens, fluoxymesterone and testolactone, are well absorbed. The parenteral dosage forms, testolactone, testosterone propionate, and testosterone enanthate, which are specifically designed for slow absorption, are well distributed throughout the body and extensively metabolized in the liver, conjugated primarily to the glucuronide. Androgens are excreted in the urine.

Because the androgens' onset of action is slow, a 2- to 3-month trial should be completed before a particular agent is considered a therapeutic failure. The oral agents have a short duration of action and require daily dosing. The duration of action of the parenteral forms is longer because the oil suspension is slowly absorbed. Parenteral androgens are administered one to three times weekly.

PHARMACODYNAMICS

Androgens probably act via one or more mechanisms. They may cause a reduced number of prolactin receptors or may competitively bind to those that are available. Also, the androgens may inhibit estrogen synthesis or competitively bind at estrogen receptors. These actions prevent estrogen from affecting estrogen-sensitive tumors.

PHARMACOTHERAPEUTICS

Androgens are indicated for prostate cancer and the palliative treatment of advanced breast cancer, particularly that occurring in postmenopausal women with bone metastases. Because of their easy administration, the oral agents are more commonly used than the parenteral agents.

fluoxymesterone (Halotestin). Of all the androgens, fluoxymesterone is the most commonly prescribed.
USUAL ADULT DOSAGE: 10 to 40 mg P.O. daily in divided doses.

testolactone (Teslac). Physicians prescribe testolactone orally.
USUAL ADULT DOSAGE: 250 mg P.O. q.i.d.

testosterone propionate (Testex). This androgen is administered intramuscularly.
USUAL ADULT DOSAGE: 50 to 100 mg I.M. three times weekly.

testosterone enanthate (Delatestryl). This drug is administered intramuscularly.
USUAL ADULT DOSAGE: 200 to 400 mg I.M. every 2 to 4 weeks.

Drug interactions

No drug interactions have been identified for the androgens.

ADVERSE DRUG REACTIONS

Androgens are generally well tolerated antitumor agents. Dose-related nausea and vomiting are the most common reactions. Fluid retention secondary to sodium retention may also occur; this should be monitored closely in patients with compromised cardiovascular function. Female patients may develop masculine characteristics, including increased facial hair, acne, clitoral hypertrophy, increased libido, and voice deepening.

Prolonged high doses of androgens have produced clinical jaundice, which may limit using these drugs for patients with liver function abnormalities. Also, patients with bony metastases are at greater risk for developing hypercalcemia during prolonged androgen therapy.

NURSING IMPLICATIONS

Occasionally, absorption of orally administered androgens is erratic. Patients who do not benefit from oral administration may receive intramuscular administration. The following nursing implications apply to both routes of administration:
• Use extreme caution with intramuscular injections to avoid inadvertent intravenous or subcutaneous injection. Because intramuscular preparations are oil suspensions, serious oil embolism can occur if intramuscular androgens are administered into a vein.
• When administering androgens intramuscularly, use a 1½-inch (4-cm) needle and inject the drug deep into muscle tissue. If irritation or inflammation develops, apply ice for comfort.
• If maculopapular erythema occurs after parenteral administration, report the reaction to the physician.

• Systemic reactions to oral and intramuscular administration include fluid retention, nausea and vomiting, virilization, and hepatotoxicity. Teach the patient to recognize symptoms and to report them to the physician.

• Symptoms that may indicate fluid retention include edema of the hands, ankles, tibia, or sacrum and sudden unexplained weight gain. Monitor for fluid retention and intravascular overload in patients with a history of congestive heart failure.

• Nausea and vomiting associated with androgen therapy are usually transient and mild. Administer an antiemetic to the severely affected patient before meals.

• Prolonged androgen therapy can cause virilization in female patients. Effects include hirsutism, mild scalp hair loss, deepening of voice, facial acne, clitoral enlargement, increased libido, and breast regression. If therapy is discontinued at the onset of symptoms, the conditions may disappear. If therapy is continued, the conditions may become irreversible. Inform the female patient well in advance about potential virilization and provide necessary emotional support.

• Hepatic dysfunction secondary to androgen therapy is a rare complication. Teach the patient to recognize the signs of jaundice, including yellowing of the skin or sclera, darkened urine, clay-colored stools, and pruritus, and to report any of these symptoms immediately to the nurse or physician.

• The combined effect of an androgen and bone metastasis may result in hypercalcemia. Teach the patient and family members to recognize the signs and symptoms of hypercalcemia, including anorexia, nausea, vomiting, lethargy, and polyuria, and to report any of these symptoms to the nurse or physician. Because the patient and family may attribute these symptoms to the disease, emphasize that such symptoms may be caused by a treatable complication.

• Monitor the patient's serum calcium levels monthly. To help prevent hypercalcemia, mobilize the patient as much as possible and maintain adequate hydration. Limiting dietary calcium intake does not have a significant effect on serum calcium levels.

ADRENOCORTICAL SUPPRESSANTS

The adrenocortical suppressant, aminoglutethimide, has been proven to be as effective as surgical adrenalectomy in treating advanced breast cancer.

PHARMACOKINETICS

Aminoglutethimide is adequately absorbed after oral administration. About 20% to 25% binds to plasma proteins. Approximately 50% of a dose is excreted unchanged in the urine, and 20% to 50% is excreted as metabolites, four of which have been identified.

Data on the onset of action, peak concentration level, and duration of action of aminoglutethimide remain incomplete. The initial plasma half-life is 13 hours, decreasing to 7 hours 1 to 2 weeks after administration.

PHARMACODYNAMICS

Aminoglutethimide acts in the adrenal gland to block the production of cortisol, androgens, and progestins. In extra-adrenal tissues, it also inhibits the conversion of androgens to estrogens. These actions produce a reversible, chemical adrenalectomy.

Because of the compensatory increase in adrenocorticotropic hormone (ACTH) release after aminoglutethimide administration, a pituitary-suppressive glucocorticoid, such as hydrocortisone, must be administered concurrently. Patients treated with aminoglutethimide and hydrocortisone achieve a chemical adrenalectomy; the response is similar to that seen with surgical removal of the adrenal glands.

PHARMACOTHERAPEUTICS

The adrenocortical suppressant, aminoglutethimide, is used for the palliative treatment of hormonally responsive advanced breast and prostate cancers and Cushing's disease.

aminoglutethimide (Cytadren). Skin, soft tissue, and bone lesions respond more frequently to aminoglutethimide therapy than other metastatic sites.
USUAL ADULT DOSAGE: 250 mg P.O. q.i.d.; may be increased in 250 mg daily increments every 1 to 2 weeks to a maximum total dosage of 2 grams/day.

Drug interactions

No drug interactions have been identified for aminoglutethimide.

ADVERSE DRUG REACTIONS

About 50% of patients taking aminoglutethimide experience an adverse reaction that is usually transient.

The most common predictable reaction is a rash that appears in the first weeks of treatment and usually disappears after 5 to 8 days. If the rash persists beyond 8 days, the drug should be discontinued. Fatigue, hypotension, drowsiness, and dizziness also occur.

Unpredictable and rare effects include leukopenia, thrombocytopenia, nausea, vomiting, and anorexia.

NURSING IMPLICATIONS

Because 50% of the patients receiving this drug will have an adverse reaction, nursing implications center on patient teaching.

• Teach the patient to expect a rash the first week of aminoglutethimide treatment and to report it if it does not disappear or begin to clear within 8 days; the drug may need to be reduced or discontinued.

• Lethargy, another adverse reaction to aminoglutethimide, can be severe in elderly patients, who also report visual disturbances and dizziness. Medication-induced lethargy can be especially distressing to patients who may already experience fatigue from cancer. Instruct the patient to rest adequately and to schedule daily activities in order of importance.

• Monitor the patient's blood counts routinely for leukopenia, which is most probable in patients taking cytotoxic antineoplastic agents.

• Administer aminoglutethimide orally in divided doses four times daily, as ordered.

PROGESTINS

In 1949, Hertig and Sommers, who were using progestins, synthetic progesterone derivatives, to treat endometrial cancer, found that some of the cancer cells were affected by normal hormonal controls. In 1961, Kelley and Baker found progestins helpful in treating endometrial cancer patients who had received radiation and surgery.

PHARMACOKINETICS

The pharmacokinetic properties of progestins resemble those of natural progesterone. Oil-based intramuscular injections provide an extended duration of action.

Medroxyprogesterone acetate and megestrol acetate are well absorbed after oral administration. After intramuscular injection in aqueous or oil suspension, medroxyprogesterone and hydroxyprogesterone caproate are slowly absorbed from their deposit sites. These drugs are well distributed throughout the body. The drugs may sequester into fat tissue. Progestins are metabolized in the liver, with a high first-pass extraction. After conjugation in the liver, the progestins are excreted as metabolites in the urine.

Two to three months of progestin therapy may pass before objective responses are observed. These drugs provide varying durations of action, ranging from 1 to 3 days for megestrol, 8 to 14 days for hydroxyprogesterone, 16 days for orally administered medroxyprogesterone, and 4 to 6 weeks for intramuscular medroxyprogesterone.

PHARMACODYNAMICS

The antitumor mechanism of action of the progestins is not completely understood. Researchers believe the drugs bind to a specific receptor to act on hormonally sensitive cells. Because the progestins do not exhibit a cytotoxic activity, they are considered cytostatic.

PHARMACOTHERAPEUTICS

The progestins have been used for the palliative treatment of advanced endometrial, breast, and renal cancers. Of these agents, megestrol is most often used. Up to 30% of patients with advanced endometrial and breast cancers respond to progestin therapy.

medroxyprogesterone acetate (Depo-Provera). This progestin is given intramuscularly.
USUAL ADULT DOSAGE: 400 to 1,000 mg I.M. weekly.

megestrol acetate (Megace). Megestrol is commonly given orally.
USUAL ADULT DOSAGE: 40 mg P.O. daily, up to 40 mg P.O. q.i.d. The maximum recommended daily dose is 320 mg.

hydroxyprogesterone caproate (Delalutin). This drug is given intramuscularly.
USUAL ADULT DOSAGE: 1 gram or more I.M.; repeated one or more times weekly up to 7 grams/week.

Drug interactions
No drug interactions have been identified for the progestins.

ADVERSE DRUG REACTIONS

Progestins are usually well-tolerated antitumor agents. Patients using megestrol have the lowest incidence of adverse effects.

Mild fluid retention with resulting weight gain is probably the most predictable reaction to the progestins. Patients who are allergic to the oil carrier used for injection (usually sesame or castor oil), may have a local or systemic allergic reaction.

Oil in the injectable forms can cause oil embolus if the agent is inadvertently injected intravenously. With high doses of injected progestins, gluteal abscesses can also occur. Because liver function abnormalities have occurred, though rarely, with progestin use, patients with hepatic dysfunction should receive reduced dosages. Thromboemboli can develop with the use of progestins and may cause a cerebrovascular accident, pulmonary dysfunction, blocked blood flow to an extremity, and local, superficial tenderness or swelling.

NURSING IMPLICATIONS

Patients usually begin progestin therapy on high doses to achieve disease control; the doses are then reduced to maintenance levels. Before administering progestins, the nurse should be familiar with the following:
• Progestin therapy is contraindicated in patients with liver failure.
• Do not administer intramuscular injections to patients who are allergic to sesame or castor oil.
• To avoid local adverse reactions to intramuscular injection, inject the progestin deeply and apply pressure and ice after the injection to lessen pain and irritation.
• Monitor the patient for mild fluid retention characterized by edema and weight gain, especially in patients with cardiac insufficiency. Explain the probability of fluid retention to the patient and teach how to recognize it. Explain that fluid retention from progestin therapy is usually mild and not clinically significant.
• Teach the patient to recognize the symptoms of thromboemboli: sudden shortness of breath, loss of vision, severe headache, paresis, or local inflammation and tenderness in an extremity.
• Explain that jaundice may indicate hepatotoxicity. Instruct the patient to report immediately any skin yellowing, varnish-colored urine, clay-colored stools, or pruritus.

CORTICOSTEROIDS

Corticosteroids are naturally occurring hormones secreted by the adrenal cortex or synthetic analogues of these hormones.

The corticosteroids target many different cells. The physiologic effects of these drugs vary widely, depending on the type of cells they act on.

PHARMACOKINETICS

When administered orally, the corticosteroids are absorbed rapidly and distributed throughout the body, including the central nervous system. These drugs are extensively metabolized in the liver and then excreted as conjugated metabolites in the urine. Prednisone must be metabolically activated in the liver.

Hydrocortisone reaches peak concentration levels within 2 hours of administration. The corticosteroids provide varying durations of action: hydrocortisone, 8 to 12 hours; prednisone, 24 hours; prednisolone and methylprednisolone, 36 hours; and dexamethasone, 3 days.

PHARMACODYNAMICS

The antitumor mechanisms of action of the corticosteroids are not well understood. The drugs may inhibit glucose transportation and phosphorylation, two processes that supply cell energy. Without appropriate energy supplies, lymphoid proliferation is inhibited, lymphocytic mitosis is impaired, and cell lysis soon results. Leukemic lymphocyte cells may have specific receptors that selectively bind the corticosteroids, thereby targeting the drugs to the tumor cells.

Physicians prescribe corticosteroids for edema from metastatic cancer because the drugs are anti-inflammatory. (See Chapter 64, Systemic and Topical Corticosteroid and Immunosuppressant Agents, for further explanation of this action.)

PHARMACOTHERAPEUTICS

The corticosteroids differ chiefly in their duration of action and sodium retention activity. Hydrocortisone has the greatest potential for sodium retention; dexamethasone, the least.

The corticosteroids have a lympholytic action that makes them useful in treating lymphatic leukemias, myeloma, and malignant lymphomas. For these indications, these drugs are most often used with cytotoxic agents to induce remissions. Other therapeutic uses include treatment of hypercalcemia, suppression of inflammation from bone or brain metastases, and the treatment of vesicant extravasation.

hydrocortisone (Cortef, Solu-Cortef). Injections of hydrocortisone are used primarily for two indications.
USUAL ADULT DOSAGE: for postadrenalectomy patients or those receiving aminoglutethimide therapy, 20 to 30 mg I.M. or I.V. daily as replacement therapy; as part of a regimen to treat vesicant extravasation, local injections of 50 to 100 mg I.M.

prednisone (Deltasone). Physicians prescribe prednisone for various indications.
USUAL ADULT DOSAGE: to induce leukemia remission, 40 to 50 mg/m²/day P.O.; for Hodgkin's disease, 20 to 30 mg P.O. daily; high doses of 40 to 100 mg/m²/day P.O. may be used in patients with resistant disease; for edema from intracranial metastases and hypercalcemia, 60 to 80 mg P.O. daily.

prednisolone (Delta-Cortef). Prednisolone may be used interchangeably with prednisone.
USUAL ADULT DOSAGE: to induce leukemia remission, 40 to 50 mg/m²/day P.O.; for Hodgkin's disease, 20 to 30 mg P.O. daily; high doses of 40 to 100 mg/m²/day P.O. may be used in patients with resistant disease; for edema from intracranial metastases and hypercalcemia, 60 to 80 mg P.O. daily.

methylprednisolone (Medrol, Solu-Medrol). As an injectable form, methylprednisolone may be used interchangeably with prednisone.
USUAL ADULT DOSAGE: requires dose adjustments using 4 mg I.M. or I.V. of methylprednisolone for 5 mg of prednisone.

dexamethasone (Decadron). Physicians prescribe dexamethasone primarily for its anti-inflammatory properties in patients with intracranial metastases and spinal cord compression.
USUAL ADULT DOSAGE: for intracranial metastases, 3 to 6 mg I.V. or P.O. every 6 hours; for spinal cord compression, 4 to 10 mg I.V. or P.O. immediately, then every 6 hours. (Dosages are highly individualized and may be higher.)

Drug interactions

Many drug interactions of clinical significance are identified with the corticosteroids. (For additional information, see Chapter 64, Systemic and Topical Corticosteroids and Immunosuppressant Agents.)

ADVERSE DRUG REACTIONS

Most adverse reactions to synthetic corticosteroids are similar to those of natural corticosteroids. The large doses required for therapy in cancer patients account for the possible enhanced toxicities.

Predictable reactions

Patients with cardiovascular disease, peptic ulcers, diabetes, and psychological disturbances are more likely to have adverse reactions to the corticosteroids, including fluid and sodium retention and increased potassium and calcium excretion. These may complicate the care of a patient with congestive heart failure. The corticosteroids can also disturb glucose metabolism and promote gluconeogenesis and anti-insulin effects that cause hyperglycemia. Epigastric distress may occur because corticosteroids increase gastric hydrochloric acid secretion and decrease gastric mucus secretion.

Frequent behavioral changes caused by the corticosteroids include mood swings, insomnia, nervousness, euphoria, and psychosis. These reactions may occur with any dose change. Increased appetite is also common.

Unpredictable reactions

Because of their lympholytic effects and their ability to suppress mitosis in lymphocytes, the corticosteroids can cause immunosuppression. They may also mask signs of infection, such as fever and inflammation. During prolonged therapy, patients may develop cataracts, glaucoma, or ocular infections.

Patients risk the complete suppression of the adrenal hormones. Many patients on long-term therapy develop some degree of cushingoid symptomatology: moon face, truncal obesity, purpura, buffalo hump, and acne. Patients withdrawn from long-term corticosteroid therapy may develop depression. The symptoms include fatigue, psychosomatic complaints, crying spells, and insomnia.

NURSING IMPLICATIONS

The nurse needs to be familiar with the following implications when administering corticosteroids:
• Metabolic reactions, such as fluid and sodium retention, combined with electrolyte depletion may cause a significant problem for a patient with cardiac disease. Hypertension may occur secondary to fluid retention.
• Steroid-induced diabetes may occur in patients on long-term therapy, usually only in patients predisposed to diabetes or those with overt diabetes mellitus. Monitor the patient's fasting blood glucose and urine glucose periodically to evaluate for this adverse reaction.

- Most corticosteroid preparations are water-soluble compounds; give by slow intravenous push or intramuscular injection.
- Patients have reported rectal burning from dexamethasone given via intravenous push; minimize this reaction by slow intravenous delivery.
- Administer oral agents with meals to minimize gastric irritation. The patient taking oral corticosteroids should also avoid taking aspirin or other nonsteroidal anti-inflammatory drugs.
- Instruct the patient to report any black or tarry stools or coffee-ground emesis because gastrointestinal bleeding can occur during therapy.
- The behavioral changes associated with corticosteroid therapy may initially benefit some cancer patients. Euphoria and a sense of well-being combined with increased appetite may temporarily improve the patient's life-style. Instruct the patient and family members that such effects may change negatively to mood swings, nervousness, or psychosis. These negative behavioral changes are reversible with the discontinuation of the drug.
- Teach the patient to observe for edema and to notify the physician if it occurs.
- Inform the patient about signs and symptoms of hypocalcemia and hypokalemia. If a potassium supplement has not been prescribed, encourage the patient to eat potassium-rich foods such as bananas, oranges, raisins, prunes, and cranberry juice.
- Instruct the patient to recognize the symptoms of hyperglycemia, such as polyuria and polydipsia.
- Body image changes caused by adrenal hormone suppression are primarily cushingoid symptoms, including moon face, truncal obesity, purpura, buffalo hump, and acne. Inform the patient that such changes are reversible with the discontinuation of therapy.

GONADOTROPIN-RELEASING HORMONE ANALOGUES

Leuprolide acetate, a gonadotropin-releasing hormone analogue, is indicated for advanced prostate cancer.

PHARMACOKINETICS

Not active orally, leuprolide is administered by subcutaneous injection. Leuprolide is well absorbed, but its distribution, metabolism, and excretion have not been determined.

With daily leuprolide injections, the patient's testosterone levels initially rise but fall to castration levels in 2 to 4 weeks. The plasma half-life of leuprolide is about 3 hours.

PHARMACODYNAMICS

Leuprolide acts on a male's pituitary to increase luteinizing hormone secretion, which stimulates testosterone production. Peak testosterone levels are reached approximately 72 hours after daily administration. However, with long-term administration, leuprolide inhibits the release of luteinizing hormone from the pituitary and subsequently inhibits testicular release of testosterone. Because prostate tumor cells are stimulated by testosterone, the reduced testosterone level inhibits tumor growth.

PHARMACOTHERAPEUTICS

Leuprolide is used for the palliative treatment of metastatic prostate cancer. The drug lowers testosterone levels without the adverse psychological effects of castration or the cardiovascular effects of diethylstilbestrol.

leuprolide acetate (Lupron). Used to manage advanced prostate cancer, leuprolide is administered subcutaneously.
USUAL ADULT DOSAGE: 1 mg S.C. daily.

Drug interactions

No drug interactions have been identified with leuprolide.

ADVERSE DRUG REACTIONS

Generally well-tolerated, leuprolide causes fewer adverse reactions than diethylstilbestrol therapy. Hot flashes are the most frequently reported reactions to leuprolide, ranging in severity from mild flushing to frequent sweating for 40% to 70% of patients. Disease symptoms and pain may worsen or flare during the first 2 weeks of leuprolide therapy. The flare can be fatal in patients with bony vertebral metastases because it can increase nerve compression.

Peripheral edema occurs in about 8% of patients. Nausea, vomiting, constipation, or anorexia occur in about 2%. Thromboembolic complications occur infrequently; gynecomastia and breast tenderness occur rarely.

SELECTED MAJOR DRUGS

Hormonal antineoplastic agents

This chart summarizes selected hormonal antineoplastic agents.

DRUG	MAJOR INDICATIONS	USUAL ADULT DOSAGES	NURSING INDICATIONS
diethylstilbestrol [DES]	Breast cancer in females who are at least 5 years postmenopausal Prostate cancer	5 to 15 mg P.O. daily 1 to 3 mg P.O. daily	• Closely monitor patients with cardiac disease for fluid retention. • Quantify and report a patient's breakthrough uterine bleeding. • Closely monitor patients with metastastic bone disease for hypercalcemia. • Inform male patients about potential feminization.
tamoxifen	Advanced breast cancer, best results with estrogen receptor-positive tumors	10 to 20 mg P.O. b.i.d.	• Instruct the patient about potential tumor flare and the need for increased analgesics. • Instruct the patient to report *any* changes in visual acuity. • Administer an antiemetic before meals to the patient who experiences nausea.
fluoxymesterone	Metastatic breast cancer in females and prostate cancer	10 to 40 mg P.O. daily in divided doses	• Monitor the patient with metastatic bone lesions for hypercalcemia. • Inform female patients about potential virilization.
aminoglutethimide	Hormonally responsive breast and prostate cancer	250 mg P.O. q.i.d., may be increased to a maximum of 2 grams/day	• Monitor the patient for a rash or other allergic response. • Instruct the patient to rest more frequently because of increased fatigue.
medroxyprogesterone	Endometrial, breast, and renal cancer	400 to 1000 mg I.M. weekly	• Give intramuscular injections deeply to decrease irritation. • Monitor the patient for signs and symptoms of thromboemboli.

NURSING IMPLICATIONS

The nurse must teach the patient specific techniques for safe administration:

• Teach the patient and a family member to prepare, administer, and rotate the subcutaneous injections of leuprolide. The manufacturer provides the syringes and needles for injection.

• Instruct the patient to keep an accurate record of the doses administered.

• Inform the patient about potential hot flashes and tumor flare.

• Encourage the patient to increase doses of analgesics to control pain, as needed.

• Instruct the patient to report any adverse reaction to the physician.

CHAPTER SUMMARY

Chapter 76 discussed the hormonal agents used to treat malignant tumors. Here are the highlights:

• The hormonal antineoplastic agents are not cytotoxic, but inhibit malignant growth by altering the hormonal environment of the tumor.

• Most hormonal antineoplastic agents have a slow onset of action and require a therapeutic trial of 2 to 3 months.

• Except for corticosteroids, hormonal agents are not used curatively but are given palliatively in combination with other drugs to control malignant growth.

• Estrogen therapy is used as a palliative treatment for metastatic breast cancer in women who are at least 5 years postmenopausal and for metastatic prostate cancer.

- The nurse should inform male patients of the feminization caused by estrogen therapy and female patients of possible decreased libido and breast tenderness.
- The antiestrogen, tamoxifen, is the drug of choice for treating advanced breast cancer of estrogen receptor-positive tumors. The drug can cause tumor flare.
- Usually administered orally, androgens prove effective in treating prostate cancer, male breast cancer, and advanced female breast cancer. Prolonged androgen therapy causes virilization and fluid retention.
- About 50% of patients taking aminoglutethimide experience rash, hypotension, drowsiness, and dizziness.
- The duration of action for progestins varies widely from 1 to 3 days for megestrol to 4 to 6 weeks for intramuscular medroxyprogesterone. The nurse giving intramuscular injections of progestins must be careful to avoid inadvertent intravenous injection.
- The corticosteroids are indicated for lymphatic leukemias, myeloma, and malignant lymphomas.
- Patients taking corticosteroids may experience fluid and sodium retention, behavioral changes, immunosuppression, and cushingoid symptoms.
- Leuprolide treats advanced prostate cancer by decreasing testosterone levels.
- The nurse can significantly help the patient cope with hormonal treatment by teaching about potential adverse reactions and using specific interventions to minimize them.

BIBLIOGRAPHY

Becker, T. *Cancer Chemotherapy: A Manual for Nurses.* Boston: Little, Brown & Co., 1981.

Carbone, P., and Torney, D. "The Clinical Investigation and the Evolution of Treatment of Primary Breast Cancer," *Seminars in Oncology* 13:415, 1986.

Carter, S., et al. *Principles of Cancer Treatment.* New York: McGraw-Hill Book Co., 1982.

Cline, M., and Haskell, C. *Cancer Chemotherapy.* Philadelphia: W.B. Saunders Co., 1980.

Data on file: Medical Department, TAP Pharmaceuticals, North Chicago, Illinois 60064.

Dorr, R.T., and Fitz, W.L. *Cancer Chemotherapy Handbook.* New York: Elsevier North Holland Inc., 1980.

Gilman, A.G., et al., eds. *Goodman and Gilman's The Pharmacological Basis of Therapeutics,* 7th ed. New York: Macmillan Publishing Co., 1985.

Holland, J., and Frei, E. *Cancer Medicine,* 2nd ed. Philadelphia: Lea & Febiger, 1982.

Leuprolide Study Group. "Leuprolide versus Diethylstilbestrol for Metastatic Prostate Cancer," *New England Journal of Medicine* 311:1281, 1984.

Marino, L.B. *Cancer Nursing.* St Louis: C.V. Mosby Co., 1981.

McIntire, S.N., and Cioppa, A.L. *Cancer Nursing: A Developmental Approach.* New York: John Wiley & Sons, 1984.

Smith, J.A., et al. "Clinical Effects of Gonodotropin-Releasing Hormone Analogue in Metastatic Carcinoma of Prostate," *Urology* 25:106, 1985.

Tepperman, G. *Metabolic and Endocrine Physiology.* Chicago: Year Book Medical Pubs., 1980.

CHAPTER
77
OTHER ANTINEOPLASTIC AGENTS

OBJECTIVES

After reading and studying this chapter, you should be able to:

1. Differentiate among the indications for the vinca alkaloids and podophyllotoxins.

2. Describe the mechanisms of action for the vinca alkaloids, the podophyllotoxins, asparaginase, procarbazine, and hydroxyurea.

3. Discuss the major adverse reactions to the vinca alkaloids and the podophyllotoxins and the associated nursing interventions.

4. Discuss the drug and food interactions that occur with procarbazine and their nursing implications.

5. Describe the clinical uses of asparaginase, procarbazine, and hydroxyurea.

INTRODUCTION

This chapter presents a subclass of antineoplastic agents, known as natural products, that includes the vinca alkaloids and the podophyllotoxins. Other antineoplastic agents that cannot be included in the existing classifications also are discussed in this chapter.

For a summary of representative drugs, see *Selected major drugs: Other antineoplastic agents* on page 1212.

VINCA ALKALOIDS

Vinca alkaloids are nitrogenous bases derived from the periwinkle plant. These drugs are cell-cycle-specific for the M phase. (See *Cell cycle* in the Unit Fifteen Introduction for an explanation.) They are used to treat various cancers, including Hodgkin's disease, non-Hodgkin's malignant lymphoma, testicular cancer, lymphosarcoma, breast cancer, acute lymphocytic leukemia, Wilms' tumor, rhabdomyosarcoma, and neuroblastoma.

History and source

Investigation of the periwinkle plant was inspired by the widespread reference to its hypoglycemic effect. Several independent researchers studied periwinkle, and a Canadian group noted that the plant produced bone marrow suppression in rats. Researchers first isolated vinblastine, then vincristine and other experimentally active alkaloids. Vindesine, the synthetic vinca alkaloid derived from vinblastine, is the newest drug in this class.

PHARMACOKINETICS

After I.V. administration, the vinca alkaloids are well distributed throughout the body. The drugs undergo moderate hepatic metabolism before being eliminated, primarily in feces; a small percentage is eliminated in urine.

Absorption, distribution, metabolism, excretion

Because vinblastine, vincristine, and vindesine are unpredictably absorbed after oral administration, they are all administered intravenously. After I.V. administration, the drugs are distributed extensively throughout the body. Vinblastine and vincristine concentrate in platelets and, to a lesser extent, in leukocytes and erythrocytes. Vindesine may be bound extensively in tissue. Neither vinblastine nor vincristine enters the cerebrospinal fluid (CSF) in significant quantities. The extent of CSF penetration by vindesine remains unclear.

The vinca alkaloids are hepatically metabolized. Vinblastine is metabolized to an active metabolite, whereas vincristine is metabolized to inactive metabolites. The drugs then undergo biliary and urinary elimination. Within 72 hours after administration, up to 30% of a vinblastine dose is recovered in the feces, with 21%

appearing in the urine. Up to 70% of a vincristine dose is recovered in the feces within 72 hours, with 12% appearing in the urine. More than 50% of the vincristine dose is excreted unchanged. Vindesine is primarily eliminated via the biliary route, but its elimination has not been well quantified. Because of their biliary elimination, the vinca alkaloids may cause toxicity in the patient with obstructive liver disease. (See *Administration and excretion routes: Other antineoplastic agents* on page 1205 for a summary.)

Onset, peak, duration
The vinca alkaloids have multiphasic clearance rates. The terminal half-life is about 25 hours for vinblastine, 85 hours for vincristine, and 24 hours for vindesine.

PHARMACODYNAMICS
The vinca alkaloids are cell-cycle-specific, inhibiting mitosis and causing cell death. These drugs are structurally similar but vary in their ability to enter specific cells. Generally, a lack of cross-resistance appears among the vinca alkaloids. However, resistance to the vinca alkaloids may result from tubulin protein mutations, which affect drug binding, decrease uptake, and increase the capacity for the drug to flow out of the cell. Drug resistance may include the podophyllotoxins, anthracyclines, and dactinomycin as well as the vinca alkaloids.

Mechanism of action
The vinca alkaloids may disrupt the normal function of the microtubules by binding to the microtubules' protein tubulin. With the microtubules unable to separate chromosomes properly, the chromosomes are either dispersed throughout the cytoplasm or arranged in unusual groupings. As a result, formation of the mitotic spindle is prevented, and the cells are unable to complete mitosis. Cell division is arrested in metaphase, causing cell death. The vinca alkaloids are therefore cell-cycle M-phase–specific. Interruption of the microtubule function also may impair some types of cellular movement, phagocytosis, and central nervous system (CNS) functions.

PHARMACOTHERAPEUTICS
Vinblastine and vincristine have been the most extensively studied vinca alkaloids. Both display various activities and ranges of toxicity. Bone marrow suppression is the major dose-related toxicity produced by vinblastine; neurotoxicity is the major dose-related toxicity produced by vincristine. Vindesine acts effectively against neoplasms that are resistant to vincristine.

vinblastine sulfate (Velban). Vinblastine is most effectively when administered with bleomycin and cisplatin to treat metastatic testicular carcinoma. This combined treatment has produced a significant number of complete remissions. Also, when vinblastine is used to treat lymphomas, up to 90% of the patients show significant improvement. Vinblastine also is effective against Kaposi's sarcoma, neuroblastoma, breast carcinoma, and choriocarcinoma. Vinblastine dosing varies significantly, depending on protocol.
USUAL ADULT DOSAGE: initially, 0.1 mg/kg or 3.7 mg/m^2 I.V. with weekly increases in increments of 0.05 mg/kg or 1.8 mg/m^2 until the leukocyte count falls below 3,000/mm^3, the tumor size decreases, or the maximum dose of 0.5 mg/kg or 18.5 mg/m^2 is reached. For maintenance therapy, give 0.05 mg/kg or 1.8 mg/m^2 I.V. less than the final dosage every 7 to 14 days.

vincristine sulfate (Oncovin). Vincristine's activity resembles that of vinblastine, with important differences. Because the drug does not cause severe bone marrow suppresion, it is commonly used in combination therapy. Vincristine is highly effective in the MOPP (mechlorethamine, vincristine, procarbazine, and prednisone [optional]) regimen used to treat Hodgkin's disease. It is also used to treat non-Hodgkin's lymphoma and acute lymphocytic leukemia in children. It is more effective than vinblastine against lymphocytic leukemia. The dosing schedules vary.
USUAL ADULT DOSAGE: 0.01 to 0.03 mg/kg or 0.4 to 1.4 mg/m^2 I.V. in a single dose, no more often than once weekly. The total single dose for adults should not exceed 2 mg.
USUAL PEDIATRIC DOSAGE: for inducing remission in childhood leukemias, dosage not to exceed 2 mg/m^2 I.V. weekly, given with prednisone.

vindesine (Eldisine). Researchers are still studying the clinical usefulness of vindesine. The drug is effective against lymphomas and chronic granulocytic leukemia in a blastocyte crisis. Vindesine is effective against vincristine-resistant tumors.
USUAL ADULT DOSAGE: 3 to 4 mg/m^2 I.V. weekly.

Drug interactions
Researchers have identified no significant drug interactions with the vinca alkaloids.

ADVERSE DRUG REACTIONS
Minor differences in the chemical structure of the vinca alkaloids cause significant differences in toxicity. Vin-

blastine and vindesine toxicities occur primarily as bone marrow suppression, manifested by predictable leukopenia. Leukopenia increases the patient's risk of infection, especially if the absolute granulocyte count is less than 1,000 mm³. In patients receiving corticosteroids, the inflammatory response may be decreased and complications of leukopenia more difficult to detect.

Alopecia occurs in up to 50% of patients receiving vinca alkaloids, with hair loss more likely with vincristine than vinblastine. Many patients experience partial alopecia; others, total. Men are as affected as women by alopecia of the scalp, eyebrows, eyelashes, and body. Although scalp tourniquets and ice caps have been used to decrease scalp circulation and limit the drug's effect on hair cells, results have been insignificant, and these methods may provide a sanctuary for cancer cells. (See *Frequent adverse reactions and associated nursing implications* in the Unit Fifteen Introduction.)

Neuromuscular abnormalities occur frequently with vincristine and occasionally with vinblastine. Peripheral neuropathies usually are dose-limited with vincristine and vindesine. Other neurotoxicities with vincristine include encephalopathies and cranial nerve dysfunction, such as vocal cord paralysis and ptosis (drooping of the upper eyelid). Prophylactic laxatives can sometimes prevent constipation from vincristine.

The vinca alkaloids may cause severe local necrosis if extravasation occurs. Vindesine may produce pain and phlebitis even without infiltration.

Stomatitis may occur with the vinca alkaloids. Vinblastine may produce tumor pain described as an intense stinging or burning in the tumor bed, with an abrupt onset after 1 to 3 minutes. The pain usually lasts 20 minutes to 3 hours. Nausea and vomiting that may occur can be controlled with antiemetics. Vincristine may induce the syndrome of inappropriate antidiuretic hormone (SIADH) secretion.

NURSING IMPLICATIONS

The vinca alkaloids are complex and potentially harmful drugs. The nurse dealing with these drugs must know specific administration techniques, safety precautions, dosages and protocol plans, potential adverse reactions, and interventions. Specifically, the nurse should:
• Know that neurotoxicity occurs in 5% to 20% of patients, especially those receiving higher dosages. Symptoms include abdominal pain, constipation, paralytic ileus, urinary obstruction, numbness, paresthesia, loss of deep tendon reflexes, footdrop, vocal cord paralysis, headache, and mental depression. Patients receiving narcotics for pain before vinca alkaloid therapy may already be at risk for constipation and require a consistent bowel regimen that includes stool softeners.

• Note the blood count nadir when caring for a patient with bone marrow suppression. At the nadir, which usually occurs 4 to 10 days after administration, the patient is at the greatest risk for problems associated with leukopenia and thrombocytopenia.
• Know that thrombocytopenia occurs in sequence with leukopenia. When the platelet count is under 50,000 mm³, patients are at risk of bleeding. When platelets drop below 20,000 mm³, patients are at severe risk and most likely will require platelet transfusion, as ordered. In patients with thrombocytopenia, monitor for bleeding gums, increased bruising or petechiae, hypermenorrhea, tarry stools, hematuria, and coffee-ground emesis. Rectal temperatures and I.M. injections are contraindicated in thrombocytopenic and leukopenic patients.
• Assess the patient routinely for dizziness, fatigue, pallor, and shortness of breath with minimal exertion, and review laboratory values that would indicate anemia. Remember that patients dehydrated from nausea, vomiting, or anorexia may have a normal hematocrit. Once rehydrated, the hematocrit will fall, revealing anemia. Patients with a history of myocardial infarction may be at an increased risk for further coronary ischemia. If the patient is not experiencing symptoms related to anemia, transfusions may not be ordered; however, the symptomatic patient will be transfused. Instruct the patient to rest more frequently and to be attentive to diet.
• Prepare the patient for alopecia by explaining when hair loss usually begins and that hair loss is gradual and reversible once treatment ends.
• Monitor serum uric acid levels while the patient is on therapy to detect rapid cell lysis. If levels become elevated, allopurinol therapy may be initiated as prescribed. This drug prevents the rapid accumulation of uric acid.
• Explain to the patient that the burning or stinging pain frequently felt at the tumor site after I.V. administration is not caused by a worsening of the tumor but by cellular destruction that causes tissue swelling.
• Know that vinca alkaloids occasionally can cause nausea and vomiting. Antiemetics may be administered in combinations as prescribed, using various delivery routes. Because most antiemetics have a sedative effect, monitor the patient for vomitus aspiration and hypotension.
• Consider the time of drug administration when encouraging patient compliance. Some patients prefer treatments in the evening when they find sedation comfortable; others who work may prefer treatments on their days off.
• Take care in handling intravenous drugs. (See the Unit Fifteen Introduction.) The vinca alkaloids are adminis-

tered intravenously only. Administer them directly into the vein or into the injection port in the tubing of a freely infusing I.V. solution. This method allows for direct observation of the injection site. Because these drugs are vesicants, be aware of the signs and symptoms of extravasation. Also, be familiar with the procedure for treating a suspected extravasation.

• Teach the patient and family about neurotoxicity symptoms.

• Plan an effective teaching program about bone marrow suppression that includes the patient's blood counts, potential sites of infection, and personal habits.

• Ensure that the patient with leukopenia maintains proper hygiene and learns to observe for signs of infection, including fever, cough, and a burning sensation during urination.

• Instruct the patient at risk of developing leukopenia and thrombocytopenia to avoid cuts and bruises and to use a sponge toothbrush and an electric razor.

• Instruct the patient to report sudden headaches, which can indicate potentially lethal intracranial bleeding.

• To prevent colonic irritation and bleeding, recommend a bowel program that includes prophylactic stool softeners.

• Instruct the patient about the potential effects of antineoplastic agents. Provide written materials for home reference.

PODOPHYLLOTOXINS

The podophyllotoxins, etoposide and teniposide, are semisynthetic glycosides of the plant alkaloids derived from the root of *Podophyllum peltatum*, the mayapple plant. This plant was used as a cathartic, an emetic, and an anthelmintic by native Americans and early settlers.

Etoposide and teniposide are cell-cycle-specific. Teniposide, still an investigational agent, has demonstrated some activity in treating Hodgkin's disease, lymphomas, and brain tumors.

PHARMACOKINETICS

With oral administration, the podophyllotoxins are poorly absorbed. Although the drugs are widely distributed throughout the body, they achieve poor CSF levels. The podophyllotoxins are excreted primarily in the urine.

Absorption, distribution, metabolism, excretion

After oral administration, approximately 50% of an etoposide dose is absorbed; that amount for teniposide has not been quantified. After intravesicular administration of teniposide, systemic toxicity does not seem to occur,

---

Administration and excretion routes: Other antineoplastic agents

This chart clarifies the routes of administration and excretion for these drugs.

DRUG	MAJOR ROUTES OF ADMINISTRATION	MAJOR ROUTES OF EXCRETION	AMOUNT EXCRETED
vinblastine	Intravenous	Urine, feces	50% unchanged
vincristine	Intravenous	Urine, feces	50% unchanged
vindesine	Intravenous	Feces	Unknown
etoposide	Intravenous	Urine Feces	67% unchanged; 33% as metabolites 15% unchanged
teniposide	Intravenous	Urine	80% as metabolites
asparaginase	Intravenous, intramuscular	Urine	Unknown
procarbazine	Oral	Urine	20% unchanged; trace amounts as metabolites
hydroxyurea	Oral	Urine, lungs	50% unchanged; 50% as urea and carbon dioxide

which probably indicates minimal systemic absorption. Etoposide and teniposide usually are administered intravenously, making them 100% bioavailable.

Both drugs demonstrate a large volume of distribution because they are extensively bound to plasma albumin, with etoposide 94% bound and teniposide 99% bound. Both drugs are distributed to various tissues, including intestine, liver, kidney, adrenal gland, and lung. Etoposide achieves CSF levels of 1% to 10% of simultaneous plasma levels, whereas teniposide's CSF levels are less than 1% of plasma levels. Teniposide's penetration into intracerebral tumors appears to depend on the type of tumor. Teniposide can penetrate malignant ascites in patients with ovarian carcinoma.

The podophyllotoxins undergo hepatic metabolism. After 72 hours, 40% to 60% of an etoposide dose is eliminated in urine, primarily as unchanged drug. The remainder is eliminated in the feces, predominantly as metabolites. Within 72 hours after administration, approximately 40% of a teniposide dose is excreted in urine, primarily as metabolites; less than 10% is recovered in feces.

Onset, peak, duration

Etoposide achieves peak plasma concentration levels of 30 mcg/ml after intravenous administration. After an intravenous teniposide dose of 30 mg/m², peak plasma concentration levels of 10 mcg/ml are achieved. The terminal half-life of etoposide is 12 hours, whereas teniposide's half-life ranges from 10 to 40 hours.

PHARMACODYNAMICS

Although their mechanism of action is incompletely understood, the podophyllotoxins produce several biochemical changes in tumor cells. At low concentrations, these drugs block cells at the late S or G_2 phase. At higher concentrations, the drugs arrest the cells in the G_2 phase. (See Cell cycle in the Unit Fifteen Introduction.) Etoposide and teniposide can cause single-strand breaks of deoxyribonucleic acid (DNA), and they may stimulate DNA topoisomerase II to cleave DNA. These drugs can also inhibit nucleoside transport and their incorporation into nucleic acids.

PHARMACOTHERAPEUTICS

Physicians have prescribed the podophyllotoxins to treat various tumors, including lymphomas, bladder cancer, leukemias, small-cell lung cancer, and testicular cancer.

etoposide [VP-16] (VePesid). Used primarily to treat testicular cancer that fails to respond completely to vinblastine, bleomycin, and cisplatin, etoposide is also used with cisplatin for treating small-cell lung cancer.
USUAL ADULT DOSAGE: 50 to 100 mg/m² I.V. daily for 5 days, or 100 mg/m² I.V. daily on days 1, 3 and 5. The cycle is repeated every 3 to 4 weeks.

teniposide [VM-26]. Available as an investigational agent, teniposide's activity and toxicity seem similar to etoposide's. Because of its low molecular weight and lipophilicity (affinity for lipids), teniposide may prove useful for CNS tumors. Various dosage regimens have been used for teniposide.
USUAL ADULT DOSAGE: 50 mg/m² I.V. for 5 days, repeated monthly.

Drug interactions

Researchers have identified no significant drug interactions with etoposide or teniposide.

ADVERSE DRUG REACTIONS

The podophyllotoxins and the vinca alkaloids produce similar adverse reactions.

Predictable reactions

The podophyllotoxins suppress bone marrow with nadirs occurring in 10 to 14 days. These drugs can cause leukopenia and, less commonly, thrombocytopenia; leukopenia resolves in about 3 weeks. About 90% of patients receiving podophyllotoxins experience alopecia, which may resolve as the treatment continues.

Approximately one third of patients receiving podophyllotoxins develop nausea and vomiting, which lasts 2 to 6 hours. Anorexia is another common predictable reaction. Stomatitis occurs in 5% of patients. (See Frequent adverse reactions and associated nursing implications in the Unit Fifteen Introduction.)

Acute hypotension may result if the podophyllotoxins are infused too rapidly. Slow administration and close patient monitoring can prevent this adverse reaction.

Unpredictable reactions

Several unpredictable reactions can also occur during podophyllotoxin therapy: acute hypersensitivity, which may be signaled by chills, fever, generalized erythema, pruritus, wheezing, bronchospasm, or tachycardia; transient liver function abnormalities; and elevated alkaline phosphatase that indicates impending hepatotoxicity.

NURSING IMPLICATIONS

Because adverse reactions to the podophyllotoxin agents include bone marrow suppression and leukopenia, the nurse must assess the patient for those complications. The nurse also must:

• Be familiar with the expected nadir of the patient's white blood cell count (7 to 14 days) and platelet count (9 to 16 days). At the nadir, the patient is at the greatest risk for problems associated with leukopenia and thrombocytopenia.

• Advise the patient to maintain nutritional and fluid intake as the absolute granulocyte count declines. Acute complications occur when the absolute granulocyte count is less than $1,000/mm^3$ and when the platelet count is less than $20,000/mm^3$.

• Administer antiemetics as prescribed before administering podophyllotoxins, and every 2 to 4 hours, as needed, to prevent or control nausea and vomiting. Giving the patient light snacks, such as dry crackers or toast and carbonated soda, may alleviate nausea.

• Know that stomatitis, whether mild or severe, is temporary. Prophylactic patient mouth care initiated before chemotherapy may decrease stomatitis severity and provide patient comfort. Therapeutic mouth care, including topical antibiotics and analgesics, may be required, depending on the degree of stomatitis.

• Administer I.V. etoposide and teniposide slowly over 30 to 60 minutes to prevent hypotension. Monitor the patient's blood pressure before the infusion and during treatment if the patient becomes symptomatic.

• Explain to the patient that acute hypersensitivity reactions may occur with podophyllotoxin agents. Instruct the patient to report any symptoms promptly. Have diphenhydramine hydrochloride and epinephrine available when administering these agents.

• Advise the patient to avoid people with active contagious infections, to watch for signs of infection, and to report them immediately to the physician. Hospitalized patients are at risk of contracting an infection from a break in skin integrity, including certain hospital procedures (I.V. punctures, intramuscular or subcutaneous injections, blood draws, or urinary drainage devices).

• Prepare the patient for possible alopecia by explaining when hair loss usually begins and that it is gradual. Alopecia may affect the scalp, eyebrows, eyelashes, or body hair.

• Provide the patient with written materials for home reference about the possible effects of antineoplastic agents.

ASPARAGINASE

Asparaginase, a cell-cycle-specific enzyme, exerts its effect by hydrolyzing exogenous asparagine, which leukemic cells need for survival. Nonleukemic cells can synthesize asparagine and are less affected by asparaginase treatment.

History and source

In 1953, Kidd reported that guinea pig serum inhibited neoplasms in rodents. Subsequently, asparaginase was identified as the active antineoplastic agent. Concurrently, research showed that certain animal neoplasms needed the amino acid asparagine for growth. In 1964, asparaginase from *Escherichia coli* was shown to be as effective as that from guinea pig serum. Today, asparaginase is prepared from *E. coli*. Investigational asparaginase is prepared from *Erwinia caratovora* by the National Cancer Institute for patients allergic to the commercial preparation.

PHARMACOKINETICS

Asparaginase is administered parenterally and is considered 100% bioavailable when administered I.V. and about 50% bioavailable when administered I.M. After administration, it remains in the vascular compartment, with minimal distribution elsewhere. Asparaginase's metabolic route is unknown. Only trace amounts appear in urine.

Peak plasma concentration levels relate to dose and administration route. The half-life of asparaginase varies, from 11 to 23 hours. Cumulative plasma concentration levels may occur with daily dosing, and active enzyme may appear in the blood up to 3 weeks after administration.

PHARMACODYNAMICS

Asparaginase capitalizes on the biochemical differences between normal cells and tumor cells: most normal cells can synthesize asparagine, but some tumor cells depend on exogenous sources. Asparaginase acts as a catalyst in the degrading of asparagine to aspartic acid and ammonia. Deprived of their supply of asparagine, the tumor cells die. Asparaginase is cell-cycle-specific in the G_1 phase.

PHARMACOTHERAPEUTICS

Asparaginase has not proved effective against solid tumors. It is used primarily to induce remission in acute lymphocytic leukemia patients.

asparaginase [L-asparaginase] (Elspar). Administered intravenously or intramuscularly, asparaginase is used primarily in combination therapies to induce remission in acute lymphocytic leukemia.
USUAL ADULT DOSAGE: 200 IU/kg I.V. daily for 28 days; alternately to avoid anaphylaxis, 1,000 IU/kg I.V. daily for up to 10 days.

Drug interactions

Researchers have identified no significant drug interactions with asparaginase.

ADVERSE DRUG REACTIONS

Asparaginase can cause several potentially serious toxicities, which are more severe in adults than in children. Anaphylaxis, the most serious toxicity, is more likely to occur with intermittent I.V. dosing than with daily I.V. dosing or I.M. injections.

Predictable reactions

Approximately 30% of patients receiving asparaginase develop nausea and vomiting shortly after drug administration. Fever, headache, and abdominal pain also may occur. Hepatotoxicity, another predictable adverse reaction, occurs in 68% of patients receiving asparaginase. This hepatotoxicity is manifested by transient and mild liver enzyme elevations, which peak in the 2nd week of therapy.

Unpredictable reactions

Hypersensitivity and anaphylaxis also occur with asparaginase administration. Anaphylaxis occurs in 20% of patients, with the risk for a reaction rising with successive treatment. Pancreatitis, evidenced by epigastric pain and high serum amylase levels, has appeared in 5% of patients taking asparaginase. Consequently, patients with a history of pancreatitis should not receive this drug. Patients may also become hyperglycemic secondary to decreased insulin production. CNS toxicity also may occur in 25% of patients. Personality changes, seizures, and abnormal electroencephalogram tracings have been reported. Coagulation abnormalities, such as hypofibrinogenemia and depression of other coagulation factors, can occur.

NURSING IMPLICATIONS

The nurse administering asparaginase must be alert for the signs of patient hepatotoxicity, hypersensitivity, and anaphylaxis. The nurse also must:
• Know that, because nausea and vomiting are particularly noxious adverse reactions to asparaginase, antiemetics are routinely ordered with therapy. If antiemetic drugs are not ordered, consult with the physician.
• Help alleviate the patient's feelings of isolation and anxiety associated with chemotherapy administration by spending time with the patient, providing supportive listening, providing music, and teaching relaxation techniques.
• Monitor the patient's plasma coagulation factors; as prescribed, withhold asparaginase and administer fresh frozen plasma.
• Handle I.V. preparations of asparaginase with caution. (See Unit Fifteen Introduction.)
• Refrigerate reconstituted asparaginase if the preparation is not used immediately. Use the solution only if it is clear.
• Administer asparaginase in the hospital setting only with a physician present because of the potential for anaphylaxis. Keep available any drugs and equipment necessary to treat cardiac arrest.
• Monitor the patient's baseline vital signs before and during asparaginase administration.
• Educate the patient about the signs and symptoms of CNS toxicity and pancreatitis. CNS toxicity may be evidenced by severe to moderate depression, personality changes, confusion, and tremors. These changes usually disappear when asparaginase is discontinued, but they can appear after therapy has been discontinued. The onset of pancreatitis is marked by abdominal tenderness, midepigastric pain, vomiting, and elevated serum amylase levels. Either CNS toxicity or pancreatitis may cause the physician to discontinue asparaginase treatment.
• Inform the patient of the potential for cardiac arrest, and provide support and reassurance. Instruct the patient to report immediately any symptoms of hypersensitivity, including restlessness, wheezing, facial flushing or edema, hives, itching, tachycardia, hypotension, fever, or dyspnea.
• Instruct the patient to recognize the signs of liver damage and jaundice, such as yellowing skin or eyes, dark varnish-colored urine, clay-colored stools, or itchy skin, and to report these to the physician.
• Provide the patient with written materials for home reference about the possible effects of antineoplastic agents.

PROCARBAZINE

Procarbazine hydrochloride, a methylhydrazine derivative with monoamine oxidase (MAO) inhibitory properties, is used to treat Hodgkin's disease. Because it is lipophilic (having an affinity for fat) and readily enters the cell by diffusion, the drug also is used to treat primary and metastatic brain tumors. Procarbazine causes various changes in the cell and is thought to be cell-cycle-nonspecific.

PHARMACOKINETICS

Procarbazine is well absorbed after oral administration. As a lipophilic molecule, it readily crosses the blood-brain barrier and is well distributed into the CSF. It is rapidly metabolized in the liver and must be metabolically activated by microsomal enzymes. In 24 hours, up to 70% of a procarbazine dose is excreted in urine, primarily as metabolites. Respiratory excretion of the drug occurs as methane and carbon dioxide. Its half-life is 7 minutes.

PHARMACODYNAMICS

An inert drug, procarbazine must be metabolically activated in the liver. After activation, the drug can produce various cell changes. It can cause chromosomal damage,

including chromatid breaks and translocation, produce antimitotic activity, and inhibit DNA, ribonucleic acid (RNA), and protein synthesis. The patient can develop procarbazine resistance quickly, but that mechanism is not well understood.

PHARMACOTHERAPEUTICS

Procarbazine usually is given with other antineoplastic agents. Its lipophilicity makes it useful in treating CNS tumors.

procarbazine (Matulane). Used in combination with other antineoplastic agents, procarbazine is most effective in the MOPP (mechlorethamine, vincristine, procarbazine, and prednisone) regimen for Hodgkin's disease. The drug also is useful against small-cell lung cancer, non-Hodgkin's lymphoma, myeloma, melanoma, and CNS tumors.
USUAL ADULT DOSAGE: initially, 2 to 4 mg/kg P.O. daily for 1 week; may be increased to 4 to 6 mg/kg/day, as tolerated, until maximum response is achieved; maintenance dose, 1 to 2 mg/kg P.O. daily.

Drug interactions

Procarbazine interacts with various drugs. Concurrent use of alcohol and procarbazine may produce a disulfiram-like reaction (headache, nausea, vomiting, and sweating). Procarbazine produces an additive effect when administered with CNS depressants. Hypertensive reactions may occur when procarbazine is administered

DRUG INTERACTIONS

Procarbazine

This chart contains important information that the nurse should include in patient teaching to prevent serious complications during procarbazine therapy.

DRUG	INTERACTING DRUGS	POSSIBLE EFFECTS	NURSING IMPLICATIONS
procarbazine	alcohol	Causes disulfiram-like reaction (nausea, vomiting, flushing, headache, visual disturbances)	• Advise the patient and family to avoid alcohol consumption.
	CNS depressants	Cause increased CNS depression	• Monitor the patient's CNS status for changes such as lethargy and confusion.
	sympathomimetics, antidepressants, tyramine-rich foods	Cause hypertensive crisis, tremors, excitation, tachycardia, angina	• Instruct the patient to avoid pickled herring, chicken or beef liver, ripe or aged cheese, chocolate, cola drinks, and Chianti. • Monitor the patient's vital signs frequently.

concurrently with sympathomimetics, antidepressants, and tyramine-rich foods because of its MAO inhibition. (See *Drug interactions: Procarbazine* on page 1209 for more details and appropriate nursing implications.)

ADVERSE DRUG REACTIONS

Procarbazine is administered orally; however, a crystalline powder for injection is available for investigational use. The following adverse reactions are those associated with oral administration.

Predictable reactions

Late-onset bone marrow suppression is the most common dose-limiting toxicity from procarbazine use. The platelet count nadir occurs after about 4 weeks, followed by the leukocyte count nadir. Complete recovery occurs at about 6 weeks. Nausea and vomiting also occur in 50% of patients. Initial procarbazine therapy may induce a flulike syndrome, including fever, chills, sweating, lethargy, and myalgias. High-dose procarbazine therapy can induce azoospermia or cessation of menses. Because procarbazine may be teratogenic, the patient should avoid pregnancy while on therapy.

Unpredictable reactions

Unpredictable dermatologic reactions have occurred in about 3% of patients. These reactions include pruritus, acneiform rash, and hyperpigmentation.

Various adverse reactions attributed to CNS toxicity may occur. These reactions vary from depression to psychosis. Because procarbazine exhibits MAO-inhibiting properties, patients who eat a tyramine-rich diet while on procarbazine therapy may experience an acute hypertensive episode. Interstitial pneumonitis and pulmonary fibrosis can occur. Postural hypotension has been reported.

NURSING IMPLICATIONS

The nurse administering procarbazine must monitor the patient for bone marrow suppression, nausea and vomiting, flulike symptoms, and CNS toxicity. The nurse also should:

• Help minimize nausea and vomiting occurring with procarbazine use by administering the drug in divided daily doses and at bedtime. If the patient suffers from severe nausea and vomiting, a nonphenothiazine antiemetic may be prescribed.

• Instruct the patient about a tyramine-free diet to help prevent a drug and food interaction. Some foods to avoid include pickled herring, chicken or beef liver, ripe or aged cheeses, beer, Chianti, chocolate, coffee, and cola drinks.

• Know that the bone marrow suppression nadir occurs at 4 weeks; recovery is usual at 6 weeks. Platelets usually reach their nadir first, followed by white and red cells. Acute bone marrow suppression complications can be expected when the absolute granulocyte count is less than 1,000/mm³. Advise the patient to avoid people with active contagious infections. Also, instruct the patient to watch for signs of infection and to report them immediately to the physician.

• Assess the hematocrit and the platelet counts for possible anemia or thrombocytopenia. Because red blood cells have a longer life than white blood cells and platelets, anemia is less of a problem than thrombocytopenia unless the patient has occult or overt blood loss. When the platelet count is below 50,000/mm³, protect the patient from bleeding potential. Expect platelet transfusions and packed red blood cells to be prescribed during times of crisis.

• Help alleviate the patient's feelings of isolation and anxiety associated with chemotherapy administration by spending time with the patient, providing supportive listening, providing music, and teaching relaxation techniques.

• Monitor the patient daily for signs of fingertip paresthesia, footdrop, headache, dizziness, lack of muscle coordination, confusion, and mental depression. Immediately report any of these symptoms to the physician.

• Inform the patient and family about the potential for CNS toxicity.

• Instruct the patient to avoid pregnancy while on procarbazine therapy because the drug may be teratogenic. This is particularly important because procarbazine is used frequently to treat Hodgkin's disease, which affects predominantly young adults.

• Provide the patient with written materials for home reference about the possible effects of antineoplastic agents.

HYDROXYUREA

Hydroxyurea was synthesized in the 1860s and found to be bone marrow suppressive in 1928. However, this miscellaneous antineoplastic agent was not used to treat tumors until the 1960s. Physicians do not widely prescribe hydroxyurea even though it enters the CSF. The drug is used most frequently for patients with chronic myelogenous leukemia (CML).

PHARMACOKINETICS

Hydroxyurea is readily absorbed and well distributed into the CSF after oral administration. Peak CSF concentration levels are reached 3 hours after a dose. Approximately 50% of a dose is metabolized by the liver to either carbon dioxide, which is excreted by the lungs, or urea, which is excreted by the kidneys. The remaining 50% is excreted unchanged in urine. Up to 80% of a dose is recovered in urine in 12 hours.

Hydroxyurea's peak plasma concentration levels are reached 1 to 2 hours after administration. Its plasma half-life is 2 hours. Treatment should be continued for at least 6 weeks before assessing the drug's clinical effectiveness.

PHARMACODYNAMICS

Hydroxyurea exerts its cytotoxic effect by inhibiting the enzyme ribonucleoside diphosphate reductase, which causes ribonucleotides to convert to deoxyribonucleotides. Without deoxyribonucleotides, DNA synthesis cannot occur. In vitro, hydroxyurea kills cells in the S phase of the cell cycle and holds other cells in the G_1 phase, where they are most susceptible to irradiation.

The patient may develop resistance to hydroxyurea, resulting from an increased quantity of ribonucleoside diphosphate reductase or a decreased sensitivity of the enzyme to hydroxyurea. Gene amplification may change the enzyme.

PHARMACOTHERAPEUTICS

Hydroxyurea is used to treat selected myeloproliferative disorders and, with radiation therapy, to treat carcinomas of the cervix, head and neck, and lung. It also has produced temporary remissions in patients with metastatic malignant melanomas.

hydroxyurea (Hydrea). Hydroxyurea primarily is used to manage myeloproliferative disorders, such as acute and chronic granulocytic leukemia, polycythemia vera, and essential thrombocytosis. The drug also has demonstrated slight activity against such solid tumors as malignant melanoma, carcinomas of the head and neck, renal cell carcinoma, and ovarian and advanced prostate carcinomas.
USUAL ADULT DOSAGE: 80 mg/kg P.O. every 3rd day, or 20 to 30 mg/kg P.O. daily. Treatment should be continued for 6 weeks.

Drug interactions

Researchers have identified no significant drug interactions with hydroxyurea.

ADVERSE DRUG REACTIONS

Hydroxyurea causes a dose-related bone marrow suppression characterized primarily by leukopenia. Patients also may experience drowsiness, nausea, headache, vomiting, or anorexia. These adverse reactions are usually dose-related and predictable. Mild dermatologic reactions manifested by pruritus, facial erythema, and a maculopapular rash also may occur.

Rarely, a patient who has received radiation will experience exacerbated radiation erythema when taking hydroxyurea. Stomatitis and alopecia also may occur but are rare. Patients taking hydroxyurea may need to take allopurinol to prevent uric acid nephropathy and its resultant renal damage.

NURSING IMPLICATIONS

The nurse should be familiar with the following implications before administering hydroxyurea:
● Administer oral hydroxyurea either on a daily or every-3rd-day schedule, giving a large single dose rather than divided doses to attain higher blood levels. If the patient has trouble swallowing capsules, dissolve the capsule contents in water.
● Expect bone marrow suppression in patients receiving hydroxyurea. (See *Frequent adverse reactions and associated nursing implications* in the Unit Fifteen Introduction.) Expect acute complications when the absolute granulocyte count is under 1,000/mm³.
● Advise the patient to avoid people with contagious infections.
● Instruct the patient to watch for signs of infection and to report them immediately to the physician.
● Instruct the patient in the use of oral and suppository antiemetic agents as prescribed, should nausea and vomiting develop during hydroxyurea therapy.
● Assess the patient carefully for early identification of stomatitis or oral mucositis — rare but toxic adverse reactions.
● Know that renal insufficiency manifested by rising blood urea nitrogen (BUN) and creatinine levels and uric acid calculi occurs, although rarely, with hydroxyurea therapy. Monitor uric acid, BUN, and creatinine levels throughout therapy.
● Explain to the patient that mild, reversible dermatologic reactions, such as pruritus, maculopapular rash, and facial erythemas, can be treated effectively by over-the-counter lotions or medications. Instruct the patient to keep previously irradiated skin clean, dry, and protected from sunlight. Also instruct the patient to report erythema exacerbation from an irradiated site to the physician.

Other antineoplastic agents

Because most antineoplastic agents can cause bone marrow suppression with anemia, leukopenia, and thrombocytopenia and can result in many adverse reactions, such as nausea, vomiting, alopecia, and CNS toxicity, the nurse must be especially aware of their dosages and nursing implications.

DRUG	MAJOR INDICATIONS	USUAL ADULT DOSAGES	NURSING IMPLICATIONS
vinblastine	Breast carcinoma, neuroblastoma, metastatic testicular cancer, lymphomas, Kaposi's sarcoma, choriocarcinoma	0.1 mg/kg I.V. or 3.7 mg/m^2 I.V. increased by increments of 0.05 mg/kg or 1.8 mg/m^2 to a maximum of 0.5 mg or 18.5 mg/m^2; for maintenance therapy, 0.05 mg/kg I.V. or 1.8 mg/m^2 I.V. less than the final dosage every 7 to 14 days	• Inform the patient about the possibility of alopecia. • Instruct the patient and family about the signs and symptoms of infection.
vincristine	Hodgkin's disease, non-Hodgkin's lymphoma	0.01 to 0.03 mg/kg I.V. or 0.4 to 1.4 mg/m^2 I.V. weekly; dose not to exceed 2 mg/day	• Inform the patient about the possibility of alopecia. • Explain to the patient and family the potential for neurotoxicity. The first symptoms may include fingertip paresthesias, difficulty walking, and constipation.
etoposide	Testicular cancer, small-cell lung cancer	50 to 100 mg/m^2 I.V. daily for 5 days, or 100 mg/m^2 I.V. daily on days 1, 3, and 5, repeated every 3 to 4 weeks	• Inform the patient about the possibility of alopecia. • Administer antiemetics before therapy, as prescribed. • Instruct the patient and family about the signs and symptoms of infection. • Have diphenhydramine hydrochloride, epinephrine, and emergency equipment available in case of a hypersensitivity reaction.
asparaginase	Acute lymphocytic leukemia	200 IU/kg I.V. daily for 28 days, or 1,000 IU/kg I.V. daily for 10 days	• Monitor the patient for signs and symptoms of hepatotoxicity. • Administer antiemetics before therapy, as prescribed. • Have diphenhydramine hydrochloride, epinephrine, and emergency equipment available in case of a hypersensitivity reaction.
procarbazine	Hodgkin's disease, small-cell lung cancer, non-Hodgkin's lymphoma, myeloma, melanoma, and CNS tumors	2 to 4 mg/kg P.O. daily for 1 week, then increased to 4 to 6 mg/kg P.O. daily; maintenance dose, 1 to 2 mg/kg P.O. daily	• Instruct the patient and family about the signs and symptoms of infection. • Instruct the patient to avoid tyramine-rich foods while taking procarbazine.
hydroxyurea	Selected myeloproliferative disorders; malignant melanoma; cervical, head and neck, and lung cancers	80 mg/kg P.O. every 3rd day, or 20 to 30 mg/kg P.O. daily	• Instruct the patient and family about the signs and symptoms of infection. • Instruct the patient in using oral and suppository antiemetic agents for nausea and vomiting, as prescribed. • Explain that dermatologic reactions can be treated with over-the-counter creams and lotions.

CHAPTER SUMMARY

Chapter 77 discussed a variety of antineoplastic agents, including the vinca alkaloids, podophyllotoxins, asparaginase, procarbazine, and hydroxyurea. Here are the chapter highlights:

• The vinca alkaloids and podophyllotoxins are derived from the periwinkle and mayapple plants respectively; both are cell-cycle-specific.

• The vinca alkaloids, vesicants that must be administered carefully to prevent extravasation, are used to treat Hodgkin's disease, lymphomas, testicular cancer, lymphosarcoma, breast cancer, acute lymphocytic leukemia, and Wilms' tumor. The podophyllotoxins are used to treat various tumors, including lymphomas, bladder carcinoma, leukemias, small-cell lung carcinoma, and testicular carcinoma. The vinca alkaloids and podophyllotoxins can produce bone marrow suppression manifested by leukopenia, alopecia, nausea, vomiting, and stomatitis.

• Asparaginase is a cell-cycle-specific agent used primarily to treat acute lymphocytic leukemia. Because asparaginase increases the patient's risk of anaphylaxis, it should be administered with a physician present.

• Procarbazine and hydroxyurea are oral agents that distribute well into the CSF.

• Because procarbazine has MAO-inhibitory properties, patients taking it should avoid eating tyramine-rich foods. The drug is used to treat Hodgkin's disease and primary and metastatic brain tumors.

• Procarbazine interacts with numerous drugs, often causing hypertension.

• Hydroxyurea inhibits DNA synthesis; the drug is used primarily to treat selective myeloproliferative disorders and, with radiation therapy, to treat carcinomas of the cervix, head and neck, and lung. It also has been used to produce temporary remission in patients with metastatic malignant melanomas.

BIBLIOGRAPHY

Becker, T. *Cancer Chemotherapy: A Manual for Nurses.* Boston: Little, Brown & Co., 1981.

Canal, P., et al. "Pharmacokinetics of Teniposide (VM-26) after I.V. Administration in Serum and Malignant Ascites of Patients with Ovarian Carcinoma," *Cancer Chemotherapy and Pharmacology* 15:149, 1985.

Carter, S., et al. *Principles of Cancer Treatment.* New York: McGraw-Hill Book Co., 1982.

Dorr, R.T., and Fritz, W.L. *Cancer Chemotherapy Handbook.* New York: Elsevier North Holland, 1980.

Gilman, A.G., et al. eds. *Goodman and Gilman's The Pharmacological Basis of Therapeutics,* 7th ed. New York: Macmillan Publishing Co., 1985.

Holland, J., and Frei, E. *Cancer Medicine,* 2nd ed. Philadelphia: Lea & Febiger, 1982.

McIntire, S.N., and Cioppa, A.L. *Cancer Nursing: A Developmental Approach.* New York: John Wiley & Sons, 1984.

Marino, L.B. *Cancer Nursing.* St Louis: C.V. Mosby Co., 1981.

Stewart, D.J., et al. "Penetration of Teniposide (VM-26) into Human Intracerebral Tumors," *Journal of Neuro-Oncology* 2:315, 1984.

DRUGS TO TREAT SENSORY SYSTEM DISORDERS

Although oral and parenteral agents may be used to treat certain sensory system disorders, this unit emphasizes the topical agents used to manage disorders of the skin, the eye, and the ear.

Integumentary system agents

The effectiveness of topical therapy depends on drug penetration through the stratum corneum (the outer layer of the skin). This percutaneous drug absorption is greater for lipid-soluble agents than for water-soluble agents, for agents that have a high concentration of drug in a base, and for agents with a base that promotes absorption. Drug absorption is reduced by scaly or crusting skin.

Dermatologic drugs may be wet dressings, powders, lotions, creams, ointments, or aerosols. Wet dressings provide evaporative cooling, which produces vasoconstriction, soothes inflamed skin, dries oozing lesions. softens crusts, aids in debridement, and facilitates drainage. However, wet dressings can lead to skin maceration, necessitating discontinuation of therapy. Powders absorb moisture and dry and cool the skin. Lotions may protect, dry, or cool the skin. Creams, which soften and moisten, are the most common vehicle for dermatologic agents. Ointments relieve dryness. Although aerosols are the most expensive and inefficient topical drug delivery system, they may be useful when touching the skin causes extreme pain.

Ophthalmic agents

In ophthalmology, eye drops and ointments are used to relieve inflammation, reduce intraocular pressure and corneal edema, remove opacified corneal epithelium, and replace tears in dry eyes. They also are used for diagnostic procedures.

Many factors influence a drug's ability to penetrate the eye. When administered topically, ophthalmic preparations are absorbed through the cornea, conjunctiva, and sclera. Because lipid-soluble agents readily penetrate the corneal epithelium and endothelium, and water-soluble agents penetrate the stroma, agents that are lipid- and water-soluble penetrate the cornea best. Wetting agents such as benzalkonium chloride, a preservative in many ophthalmic preparations, can improve corneal drug absorption. Limited absorption into the posterior eye, however, usually restricts the use of topical agents there. For posterior eye disorders, systemic agents usually are required.

Otic agents

Disorders of the external ear include boils, fungal infections, impacted cerumen, acute edematous external otitis (swimmer's ear), and malignant external otitis. These disorders usually require treatment with the same agents that are used to manage dermatitis. Therapy also involves thorough cleansing, restoration of an acidic surface pH, reduction of swelling, elimination of infection, and control of predisposing factors.

Disorders of the middle ear include acute and chronic otitis media. Both disorders usually require a systemic agent to control the infection and possibly a systemic decongestant to restore eustachian tube function and permit fluid drainage from the middle ear.

Chapter 78
Integumentary System Agents

Chapter 78 presents the agents used to treat skin disorders: antibacterials, antifungals, antiseptics, disinfectants, antivirals, scabicides, pediculicides, keratolytics, caustics, antineoplastics, emollients, demulcents, protectants, astringents, and topical tretinoin. It highlights the clinical indications, adverse reactions, and nursing implications for these agents.

Chapter 79
Ophthalmic Agents

Chapter 79 investigates the agents used to diagnose and treat eye disorders. It emphasizes the indications and pharmacodynamics of mydriatics, cycloplegics, miotics, agents that lower intraocular pressure, anesthetics, anti-inflammatory agents, and anti-infectives, as well as the associated nursing implications. It also details administration techniques and patient education.

Glossary

Accommodation: adjustment of the eyes for vision at various distances.

Acne: inflammatory disease of sebaceous glands.

Adnexa oculi: lacrimal apparatus, eyelids, and related structures of the eye.

Amblyopia: reduced vision in an eye that appears to be structurally normal when examined with an ophthalmoscope.

Anisometropia: difference in the refractive power of the eyes.

Cerumen: waxlike secretion in the external opening of the ear; earwax.

Conjunctivitis: inflammation of the conjunctiva.

Cream: semisolid emulsion of oil in water or water in oil; usually used as a base.

Cycloplegia: ciliary muscle paralysis.

Dermatitis: inflammation of the skin.

Dermatosis: skin disorder.

Diplopia: double vision caused by defective function of the intraocular muscles or the nerves that innervate them.

Eczema: inflammatory skin disorder involving primarily the epidermis, characterized by itching oozing lesions, sealing, and crusting.

Esotropia: a kind of strabismus with inward deviation of one eye in relation to the other eye. Also called convergent strabismus.

Exotropia: a kind of strabismus with outward deviation of one eye in relation to the other eye. Also called divergent strabismus.

Folliculitis: inflammation of a follicle; usually hair follicle.

Glaucoma: eye disorder characterized by increased intraocular pressure.

Gonioscopy: examination of the angle of the eye's anterior chamber with a goniscope.

Granuloma: tumor or mass of granulation tissue.

Hyperkeratosis: hypertrophy of the cornea, or a cornified epithelial (horny) layer of the skin characterized by dry, rough, and scaly skin.

Impetigo: inflammatory skin disease caused by bacteria and characterized by pustules.

Iridectomy: surgical excision of part of the iris.

Iridocyclitis: inflammation of the iris and ciliary body.

Iritis: inflammation of the iris.

Keratin: insoluble scleroprotein that is the primary constituent of the epidermis, hair, nails, horny tissues, and tooth enamel.

Keratitis: inflammation of the cornea.

Lotion: suspension of powder and water that requires shaking before application; usually provides a protective, drying, or cooling effect.

Miosis: contraction of the pupil.

Mydriasis: extreme dilatation of the pupil.

Ointment: semisolid oil-based preparation for external application; usually has an occlusive effect.

Otitis: inflammation of the ear.

Otitis externa: inflammation of the external ear.

Otitis media: inflammation of the middle ear.

Ototoxic: having a deleterious effect to the eighth cranial nerve or the organs of hearing and balance.

Paronychia: inflammation of the tissue folds surrounding the fingernail.

Paste: semisolid preparation usually made by incorporating fine powder into an ointment; usually used as a protectant.

Percutaneous: performed through the skin.

Powder: substance made up of an aggregation of small particles; usually produces a drying effect.

Pruritus: itching.

Psoriasis: a chronic, recurrent dermatosis characterized by silver scaling plaques or vivid red macules, papules, or plaques.

Scabies: contagious skin disease caused by *Sarcoptes scabiei*, the itch mite, which bores under the skin, usually producing pruritus and eczema.

Seborrhea: sebaceous gland disorder characterized by excessive secretion of sebum.

Strabismus: each eye's optic axis is misaligned.

Synechia: iris adhesion to the cornea or the lens.

Tonometry: indirect measurement of intraocular pressure by determining the eyeball's resistance to indentation by an applied force.

Trachoma: infectious disease of the conjunctiva and cornea characterized by redness, inflammation, photophobia, and lacrimation.

Uveitis: inflammation of the iris, ciliary body, and choroid.

Chapter 80
Otic Agents

Chapter 80 discusses the anti-infective, anti-inflammatory, local anesthetic, and ceruminolytic agents used to treat ear disorders. Besides the clinical uses and related nursing implications for these agents, the chapter includes information about combination products, administration techniques, and patient education.

Nursing diagnoses

When caring for a patient receiving drugs to treat sensory system disorders, several nursing diagnoses may apply:

● Activity intolerance related to a skin, eye, or ear disorder or drug therapy

● Alteration in comfort: pain, related to a skin, eye, or ear disorder or drug therapy

- Disturbance in self-concept related to a skin, eye, or ear disorder, drug therapy, or life-style changes
- Fear related to a skin, eye, or ear disorder, drug therapy, or life-style changes
- Impaired physical mobility related to an eye or ear disorder or drug therapy
- Impaired social interaction related to a skin, eye, or ear disorder or drug therapy
- Impaired tissue integrity related to a skin, eye, or ear disorder or drug therapy
- Ineffective individual coping related to skin, eye, or ear system disorder, drug therapy, or life-style changes
- Knowledge deficit related to all aspects of a skin, eye, or ear disorder and drug therapy
- Noncompliance related to drug therapy
- Potential alteration in body temperature related to an inflammatory skin, eye, or ear disorder
- Potential for infection related to a skin, eye, or ear disorder or drug therapy
- Potential for injury related to a skin, eye, or ear disorder or drug therapy
- Sensory-perceptual alteration related to a skin, eye, or ear disorder or drug therapy
- Sleep pattern disturbance related to a skin, eye, or ear disorder or drug therapy.

CHAPTER 78

INTEGUMENTARY SYSTEM AGENTS

OBJECTIVES

After reading and studying this chapter, you should be able to:

1. Explain how the skin acts as a barrier and how this action affects the use of topical medications.

2. Describe nursing implications applicable to the administration of all topical medications.

3. Identify clinical indications for antibacterials and antifungals and list nursing implications associated with their use.

4. Differentiate between the functions of antiseptics and disinfectants.

5. Discuss the proper drug treatment for mite infestations and parasite infections.

6. Identify the most common adverse reactions associated with the different classes of topical integumentary system agents.

7. Delineate the uses of keratolytics and caustics in dermatologic therapy.

8. Identify the uses of astringents in dermatologic therapy.

INTRODUCTION

Many drugs are used to treat dermatologic diseases, but topical agents are the mainstay of treatment. This chapter discusses commonly used topical agents, except for topical corticosteroids (see Chapter 64, Corticosteroids and Other Immunosuppressant Agents, for details about topical corticosteroids) and topical anesthetic agents (see Chapter 28, Local and Topical Anesthetic Agents, for details).

The skin has the lowest water permeability index of any biological membrane. This property, combined with the complex protein keratin in the stratum corneum, allows the skin to function as a barrier that slows drug absorption but does not block it. Because the skin is not an absolute barrier, percutaneous absorption may occur.

Application pattern for topical integumentary agents

When applying topical medications, begin at the midline and apply with long, even strokes outward and downward, in the direction of hair growth. This pattern reduces the risk of follicle irritation and skin inflammation.

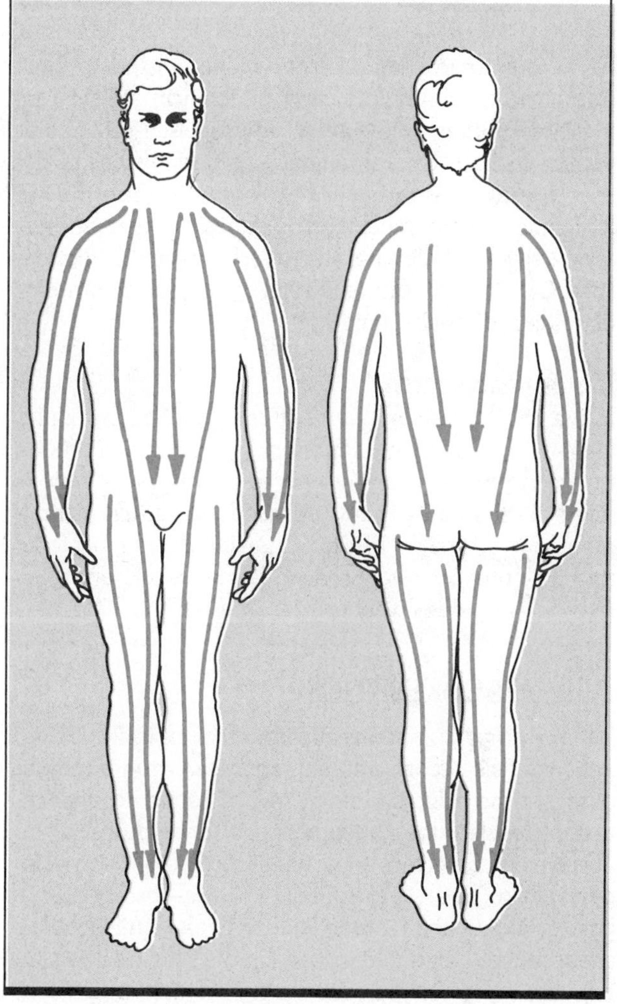

Most drugs that pass through the stratum corneum to the epidermis are metabolized there; this action may decrease a drug's pharmacologic and/or toxicologic activity. Drugs not metabolized in the epidermis pass unchanged into the systemic circulation.

This chapter discusses the following integumentary system agents: antibacterials, antifungals, antivirals, scabicides and pediculicides, keratolytics and caustics, antineoplastics, and other integumentary system agents (antiseptics and disinfectants; astringents; emollients, demulcents, and protectants; and tretinoin). (For information on applying these agents, see *Application pattern for topical integumentary agents* on page 1217.)

For a summary of representative drugs, see *Selected major drugs: Integumentary system agents* on page 1228.

ANTIBACTERIALS

Numerous topical antibacterial agents, including bacitracin, neomycin sulfate, and gentamicin sulfate, are available. Other antibacterial agents discussed in this section include chloramphenicol, chlortetracycline hydrochloride, clindamycin phosphate, erythromycin, mafenide acetate, meclocycline sulfosalicylate, nitrofurazone, silver sulfadiazine, and tetracycline hydrochloride. (See Chapter 66, Antibacterial Agents, for a complete discussion of antibacterials.)

History and source
In the 1870s, contaminants with antagonistic properties were first observed and reported. In 1939, a preparation isolated from a soil bacillus proved active against various gram-positive bacteria and was used successfully in treatment. By the late 1940s, the capacity of fungi, bacteria, and actinomycetes to produce bacteriostatic and bactericidal properties was fully recognized.

PHARMACOKINETICS

Little or no percutaneous absorption of topically applied antibacterials occurs, and any absorbed drug is metabolized in the skin; therefore, few systemic adverse reactions result. If the patient's skin is abraded or broken, absorption of topical antibacterials increases. Neomycin, gentamicin, and silver sulfadiazine are absorbed to a greater extent than other antibacterials. Antibacterials absorbed and then metabolized in the skin are excreted hepatically or renally, depending on the drug. Neo-

mycin, gentamicin and silver sulfadiazine, for example, are excreted through the kidneys.

The onset of action for antibacterials is rapid, usually occurring within a few minutes. However, antibacterials are frequently inactivated by blood, pus, and exudates.

PHARMACODYNAMICS

Antibacterials inhibit or destroy microorganisms by interfering with their metabolic activity. Bacitracin inhibits cell wall synthesis. Other agents disrupt the protein synthesis of bacterial ribosomes.

PHARMACOTHERAPEUTICS

Antibacterials hasten the healing of infected superficial wounds. They may also be used for patients with second- or third-degree burns to hasten healing and retard growth of susceptible bacteria.

neomycin sulfate (Myciguent). A topical aminoglycoside antibacterial, neomycin 0.5% cream or ointment is used to treat aerobic gram-negative and some aerobic gram-postive bacterial skin infections, including infected burns, skin grafts, surgical incisions, otitis externa, and primary pyodermas. Neomycin also is used to treat secondarily infected dermatoses and traumatic lesions that are inflamed or suppurated from bacterial infection.
USUAL ADULT DOSAGE: applied by gently rubbing a small quantity into the cleansed affected area one to three times daily.

bacitracin (Baciguent). This antibacterial is used to treat susceptible gram-positive skin infections, such as impetigo and infected dermatitis, as well as other superficial infections.
USUAL ADULT DOSAGE: applied in a thin film b.i.d. or t.i.d. after cleansing the area.

gentamicin sulfate (Garamycin). Gentamicin 0.1% cream or ointment is used to treat primary bacterial skin infections from aerobic gram-negative and some aerobic gram-postive bacteria, including impetigo, superficial folliculitis, furunculosis, and pyoderma gangrenosum. Gentamicin is also used to treat secondary infections, including infectious eczematoid dermatitis, pustular acne, pustular psoriasis, and infected contact dermatitis.
USUAL ADULT DOSAGE: applied to a cleansed affected area t.i.d. or q.i.d. The area may be covered with a gauze dressing, if desired.

chloramphenicol (Chloromycetin). A broad-spectrum antibacterial with primarily bacteriostatic action, chlor-

amphenicol 1% cream is used to treat superficial skin infections caused by susceptible bacteria.
USUAL ADULT DOSAGE: applied t.i.d. or q.i.d. after cleansing the affected area.

chlortetracycline hydrochloride (Aureomycin). A tetracycline, chlortetracycline is effective against superficial infections with susceptible organisms.
USUAL ADULT AND PEDIATRIC DOSAGE: applied b.i.d. or t.i.d. by rubbing into the affected area.

clindamycin phosphate (Cleocin T). Clindamycin 1% solution is used to treat inflammatory acne vulgaris.
USUAL ADULT DOSAGE: applied to a cleansed affected area b.i.d.

erythromycin (A/T/S, EryDerm, Staticin). This drug, available in 2% ointment, or 1.5% or 2% solution, is used to treat inflammatory conditions, such as acne vulgaris.
USUAL ADULT DOSAGE: applied b.i.d. (a.m. and p.m.) to the affected and surrounding areas after they are cleansed.

mafenide acetate (Sulfamylon). Mafenide 8.5% cream is used as an adjunctive therapy in second- and third-degree burns. The drug promotes spontaneous healing of deep partial-thickness burns and exerts bacteriostatic action against gram-negative and gram-positive bacteria.
USUAL ADULT DOSAGE: 1/16-inch thickness applied by sterile technique one or two times daily to cleansed, debrided wounds.

meclocylcine sulfosalicylate (Meclan). This 1% cream antibacterial is used to treat acne vulgaris.
USUAL ADULT DOSAGE: applied to affected area b.i.d. (a.m. and p.m.).

nitrofurazone (Furacin). This 0.2% cream ointment or solution antibacterial is used to treat surface infections, to provide adjunctive therapy for patients with second- or third-degree burns, and to aid in preventing skin allograft rejection from bacterial contamination.
USUAL ADULT DOSAGE: applied directly to the affected area and reapplied once daily or as indicated.

silver sulfadiazine (Silvadene). A broad-spectrum antibacterial effective against *Candida albicans* at high concentrations, silver sulfadiazine 1% cream is used to control many gram-negative and gram-positive bacteria. It is also used for prophylaxis or adjunctive therapy for patients with second- or third-degree burns who are at risk for wound infection.

USUAL ADULT DOSAGE: applied one or two times daily to a thickness of 1/16 inch, using a sterile-gloved hand. Burned area is covered at all times with the cream.

tetracycline hydrochloride (Topicycline). This drug is used to treat inflammatory acne vulgaris.
USUAL ADULT DOSAGE: applied generously two times daily to the entire affected area.

Drug interactions
The topical antibacterials interact with only a few other drugs. For example, when combined with a topical steroid, neomycin can interact with topical antibiotics, possibly causing an allergic contact dermatitis or a systemic eczematous contact dermatitis.

ADVERSE DRUG REACTIONS

Most adverse reactions to topical antibacterials are limited to local involvement; however, the occurrence of systemic absorption can cause potentially severe reactions.

The antibacterials can cause several predictable reactions. In particular, systemic absorption of neomycin increases when the drug is applied to broken or abraded skin, possibly causing nephrotoxicity or ototoxicity. The topical antibacterials may cause overgrowth of nonsusceptible organisms and dry, scaly skin. Meclocycline may cause temporary follicular staining.

Chloramphenicol can cause several unpredictable reactions, including allergic contact dermatitis, rash, hypersensitivity reactions, photosensitivity, burning sensations, pruritus, urticaria, erythema, and angioneurotic edema.

NURSING IMPLICATIONS

The nurse should be aware of the following considerations when administering topical antibacterials and when teaching the patient:
• Be aware that silver sulfadiazine is inactivated by topical proteolytic enzymes.
• Be aware that ointments may increase percutaneous absorption because they are more occlusive than creams or lotions.
• Be aware that the absorption of bacitracin, silver sulfadiazine, and mafenide acetate increases when these drugs are applied to burned skin. Also, administer these drugs and nitrofurazone cautiously in patients with impaired renal function.
• Administer neomycin sulfate only once daily if applying it to more than 20% of the patient's body area or if the patient has impaired renal function.

• When applying nitrofurazone wet dressings, protect the patient's uninvolved skin with zinc oxide. Store the wet dressings in an airtight, light-resistant container.
• Cleanse suppurated or crusted lesions before applying topical antibacterials.

ANTIFUNGALS

Topical antifungals are used to treat superficial mycotic (fungal) infections. The choice of antifungal agent depends on the causative organism; a distinction must be made between dermatophyte infections (caused by fungi) and candidal infections (caused by *Candida albicans*). Topical agents used to treat dermatophyte infections are clotrimazole, haloprogin, miconazole nitrate, carbol-fuchsin solution, ciclopirox olamine, econazole nitrate, tolnaftate, and zinc undecylenate and undecylenic acid. Agents used to treat candidal, or monilial, infections are amphotericin B and nystatin. Miconazole nitrate, ciclopirox olamine, econazole nitrate, and clotrimazole are used to treat candidal and dermatophyte infections. (See Chapter 69, Antimycotic [Antifungal] Agents, for a complete discussion of the antifungals.)

PHARMACOKINETICS

Topical antifungal agents are usually absorbed only dermally, with little or no systemic absorption unless an agent is applied to broken or abraded skin. Antifungals may have a prolonged onset of action because they must soften and dissolve the cornified epithelium (horny layer of the epidermis) before they can start to exert therapeutic effects. Areas with crusting and oozing require cleansing before application because blood, pus, or exudates may inactivate the drug.

PHARMACODYNAMICS

Most topical antifungal agents are fungistatic at low concentrations and fungicidal at higher concentrations. They inhibit or destroy microorganisms by interfering with their cellular metabolic activity.

PHARMACOTHERAPEUTICS

Antifungals are used topically to treat superficial fungal infections, such as tinea pedis (athlete's foot) tinea cruris, (jock itch), tinea corporis (ringworm of the body), tinea manuum (ringworm of the hands), and tinea versicolor.

clotrimazole (Lotrimin, Lotrisone, Mycelex). Clotrimazole 1% cream, lotion, or solution is used to treat tinea pedis, tinea cruris, tinea corporis, tinea versicolor, and cutaneous candidiasis.
USUAL ADULT DOSAGE: massaged into affected and surrounding skin in the morning and evening.

haloprogin (Halotex). Haloprogin 1% cream or solution is used to treat tinea pedis, tinea cruris, tinea corporis, tinea manuum, and tinea versicolor.
USUAL ADULT DOSAGE: applied liberally to affected area b.i.d. for 2 to 3 weeks; 4 weeks of therapy may be required for intertriginous areas.

miconazole nitrate (Micatin, Monistat-Derm). This synthetic antifungal, available as a 2% cream, lotion, or powder or as an aerosol powder or solution, is used to treat tinea pedis, tinea cruris, tinea corporis, tinea versicolor, and cutaneous candidiasis.
USUAL ADULT DOSAGE: applied sparingly to affected areas b.i.d. (a.m. and p.m.).

carbol-fuchsin solution (Castellani Paint, Castel Plus). This solution is used to treat tinea pedis and tinea cruris.
USUAL ADULT DOSAGE: applied as a thin coat one or two times daily; may be applied more often, depending on the severity of the condition.

ciclopirox olamine (Loprox). This drug is used to treat tinea pedis, tinea corporis, tinea cruris, tinea versicolor, and cutaneous candidiasis (moniliasis).
USUAL ADULT DOSAGE: applied in the morning and evening to affected areas and surrounding skin for up to 4 weeks.

econazole nitrate (Spectazole). Econazole 1% cream is used to treat tinea cruris, tinea corporis, tinea pedis, tinea versicolor, and cutaneous candidiasis.
USUAL ADULT DOSAGE: for tinea cruris, tinea corporis, tinea pedis, and candidiasis, applied b.i.d. (a.m. and p.m.); for tinea versicolor, applied once daily.

tolnaftate (Aftate, Tinactin). Tolnaftate 1% cream, gel, powder, solution, or aerosol is used to treat tinea cruris, tinea corporis, tinea manuum, tinea pedis, and tinea versicolor.

USUAL ADULT DOSAGE: applied to the affected area and massaged into skin b.i.d. for 2 to 3 weeks; treatment for 4 to 6 weeks may be necessary.

zinc undecylenate and **undecylenic acid** (Cruex, Desenex, Quinsana Plus, Ting). Available in cream, ointment, powder, or aerosol form, this drug is used to treat minor skin rashes, such as diaper rash, prickly heat, chafing, tinea pedis, tinea cruris, and tinea corporis.
USUAL ADULT DOSAGE: applied to affected areas b.i.d. or as needed.

amphotericin B (Fungizone). This antifungal, available as a 3% cream, lotion, or ointment, is used topically to treat cutaneous and mucocutaneous candidal infections.
USUAL ADULT DOSAGE: applied liberally to lesions b.i.d. to q.i.d., usually for 1 to 3 weeks; however, treatment may be required for several months.

nystatin (Mycostatin). Available in cream, ointment, or powder form, this drug is used to treat cutaneous candidiasis.
USUAL ADULT DOSAGE: applied by rubbing into or dusting the affected area b.i.d. (a.m. and p.m.).

Drug interactions

No significant interactions occur between topical antifungals and other drugs.

ADVERSE DRUG REACTIONS

The adverse drug reactions associated with topical antifungals are limited to local manifestations. Predictable reactions include an overgrowth of nonsusceptible organisms and occasional mild stinging during application. Unpredictable reactions include hypersensitivity reaction, photosensitivity, edema, erythematous vesicular eruptions, urticaria, pruritus, peeling, blistering, and angioneurotic edema.

NURSING IMPLICATIONS

The nurse administering topical antifungals should be aware of the following considerations:
• Cleanse the affected area before applying antifungal medication.
• Advise the patient who is receiving amphotericin B about the possibility of photosensitivity reactions.
• Advise the patient that topical antifungals can stain clothing. Explain that most stains can be removed by washing the garment with soap and warm water.
• Instruct the patient to report to the physician any skin irritation not present before therapy.

ANTIVIRALS

The topical antiviral acyclovir is used to treat such viral skin conditions as herpes simplex virus types 1 and 2 and varicella zoster virus.

The development of selective antiviral drugs has been difficult and slow. The first virus-coded enzyme was discovered by accident in the 1960s.

PHARMACOKINETICS

Applied directly to viral lesions, acyclovir first penetrates the skin and then begins acting on the virus. Acyclovir penetrates the skin rapidly and must be applied frequently to achieve the maximum therapeutic effect.

Percutaneous absorption of acyclovir is negligible, except when the drug is applied to inflamed, denuded skin.

Acyclovir's onset of action is rapid, but its duration of action is limited; therefore, the drug must be reapplied frequently.

PHARMACODYNAMICS

Acyclovir inhibits viral replication. After conversion to acyclovir triphosphate, acyclovir interferes with herpes simplex virus deoxyribonucleic acid (DNA) polymerase, thereby inhibiting DNA replication.

PHARMACOTHERAPEUTICS

The topical antiviral acyclovir is used to treat herpes simplex skin infections.

acyclovir (Zovirax). Acyclovir 5% ointment is used to manage initial (primary) herpes genitalis and limited non–life-threatening mucocutaneous herpex simplex virus infections in immunocompromised patients. Acyclovir use decreases the healing time and may decrease the duration of viral shedding and pain.
USUAL ADULT DOSAGE: applied in sufficient quantities to cover all lesions every 3 hours, six times daily, for 7 days; therapy should be initiated as soon as possible after onset of signs and symptoms.

Drug Interactions

No drug interactions have been reported with concomitant administration of other drugs with acyclovir.

ADVERSE DRUG REACTIONS

Acyclovir can cause several predictable reactions, including transient burning sensation, stinging, pain, pruritus, and rash.

NURSING IMPLICATIONS

The nurse should administer topical antivirals with the following considerations in mind:
● When applying acyclovir, use a finger cot or glove to apply ointment to prevent spread of infection.
● Keep in mind that acyclovir 5% ointment should not be applied to the eye.
● Report to the physician any burning sensation, stinging, pruritus, or rash that occurs after application.
● Emphasize to the patient the importance of complying with follow-up treatment.
● Explain to the patient that antiviral treatment does not prevent transmission to others.

SCABICIDES AND PEDICULICIDES

Scabicides and pediculicides are used to eradicate scabies and pediculosis (lice infestation). Scabicides and pediculicides include lindane, benzyl benzoate lotion, crotamiton, and pyrethrins with piperonyl butoxide.

PHARMACOKINETICS

Systemic absorption and toxicity rarely occur with the use of scabicides and pediculicides. However, lindane can be absorbed through intact skin; central nervous system (CNS) toxicity may result. Scabicide and pediculicide absorption usually increases when the drugs are applied to the face, scalp, neck; or axillae. Lindane is absorbed readily through intact skin, stored in body fat, metabolized in the liver, and eliminated in the urine and feces. Pyrethrins are poorly absorbed through intact skin; if they are absorbed, they are rapidly metabolized. Distribution is localized. The onset of action for scabicides and pediculicides is usually immediate. The duration of action is limited, and reapplication may be necessary.

PHARMACODYNAMICS

Scabicides and pediculicides usually block or inhibit the CNS functioning of parasites.

Mechanism of action

After absorption through the chitinous exoskeleton of arthropods, lindane stimulates their CNS, resulting in death. Pyrethrins also stimulate the CNS of arthropods by competitively interfering with cationic conductance in the lipid layer of nerve cells. This action blocks nerve impulse transmission, resulting in the parasites' paralysis and death. The mechanisms of action of benzyl benzoate lotion and crotamiton are unknown.

PHARMACOTHERAPEUTICS

Scabicides and pediculicides are used to eradicate parasitic infestations, most commonly scabies and pediculosis. One application is usually sufficient to kill adult arthropods, but reapplication may be necessary to kill nits (eggs).

benzyl benzoate lotion. Benzyl benzoate 28% lotion is used to treat scabies and pediculosis.
USUAL ADULT DOSAGE: bathe the patient using soap and water, leave the skin damp, apply undiluted lotion over the entire body from the neck down (being sure to massage around nails), let dry, reapply to the most involved area, then bathe the patient again after 24 to 48 hours. For scalp treatment, apply lotion to the patient's scalp at night, and shampoo in the morning; repeat one more night if necessary.

crotamiton (Eurax). A scabicidal and antipruritic agent, crotamiton 10% cream or lotion is used to eradicate scabies and to relieve pruritus.
USUAL ADULT DOSAGE: after bathing the patient with soap and water, massage thoroughly into all skin surfaces from the neck down; reapply in 24 hours, and bathe the patient again 48 hours after the last application.

lindane (Kwell, Kwildane, Scabene). An ectoparasiticide and ovicide, lindane 1% cream, lotion, or shampoo is used to treat scabies and pediculosis.
USUAL ADULT DOSAGE: after bathing the patient with soap and water, apply cream or lotion to dry skin in a thin layer and rub it in thoroughly; apply to the entire body from the neck down, leave the lotion on for 8 to 12 hours, then remove it thoroughly by bathing. Alternatively, apply shampoo to the affected area, shampoo for 4 to 5 minutes, rinse and dry hair, then comb the hair with a fine-tooth comb to remove remaining nits.

pyrethrins with piperonyl butoxide (RID). Pyrethrins with piperonyl butoxide are used to treat pediculosis.
USUAL ADULT DOSAGE: apply undiluted gel, shampoo, or solution to the patient's hair, scalp, and any other

infested areas (avoiding eyelashes and eyebrows) until entirely wet; leave on 10 minutes (no longer); wash thoroughly with warm water, soap, or shampoo as appropriate; comb the hair with a fine-tooth comb; reapply in 7 to 10 days.

Drug interactions

No significant interactions occur between scabicides or pediculicides and other drugs.

ADVERSE DRUG REACTIONS

Toxicity from scabicide and pediculicide agents is extremely rare. Adverse reactions are usually limited to skin irritation, pruritus, and stinging and a burning sensation with repeated application. Lindane, however, can cause CNS toxicity manifested by dizziness, muscle spasms, vomiting, restlessness, and seizures. Also, pyrethrins can cause nausea, vomiting, respiratory distress, and muscle paralysis.

NURSING IMPLICATIONS

Although hospital treatment may occur, eradication of lice and scabies infestations is usually performed on the patient at home. Therefore, besides knowing how to apply these medications, the nurse must teach the patient about medication administration as reflected in the following nursing considerations:

• Administer all scabicides and pediculicides with extreme caution to pregnant and lactating women; be aware that lindane is contraindicated for such patients.

• Administer lindane cautiously to infants and small children; do not allow them to suck their fingers after the application.

• Do not apply pyrethrins to children under age 2.

• Be aware that pyrethrins are contraindicated in patients hypersensitive to ragweed.

• Remember that scabicides and pediculicides are contraindicated for raw or inflamed skin.

• Monitor the patient for signs of systemic absorption and CNS toxicity when administering lindane.

• Examine other household members, and treat as prescribed. If the patient has pubic lice, all sexual contacts should also be treated to avoid reinfestation.

• Instruct the patient applying pyrethrins to do so in a well-ventilated area to avoid inhalation.

• Instruct the patient to avoid contact of the medication with the face, eyes, mucous membranes, or uretheal meatus and, if accidental contact occurs, flush the area with water and notify the physician.

• Tell the patient to wash off the drug immediately and to notify the physician if skin irritation or signs of hypersensitivity develop.

• Inform the patient that all linen and clothing that may have been contaminated must be sterilized (boiled, laundered, dry-cleaned, or ironed with a very hot iron) to avoid reinfestation or transmission of the parasites.

• Inform the patient that pruritus may persist for several weeks after treatment.

• Advise the patient that, after the medication is applied to the scalp, nits should be combed out with a fine-tooth comb dipped in vinegar.

KERATOLYTICS AND CAUSTICS

Keratolytics and caustics are used to treat hyperkeratotic diseases such as acne and psoriasis, and benign skin growths, such as warts. They may be used alone or with electrosurgery to treat hyperplastic skin lesions (such as warts, keratoses, or basal cell carcinoma). The most commonly used keratolytics and caustics are anthralin, cantharidin, podophyllum resin, resorcinol, salicylic acid, silver nitrate, and sulfur.

PHARMACOKINETICS

No appreciable percutaneous absorption occurs with most keratolytics and caustics except podophyllum resin, which may be absorbed when applied to mucous membranes. Distribution of keratolytics and caustics is local. No information is available on the metabolism and excretion of these agents because of their minimal percutaneous absorption. Onset of action is immediate upon application. Keratolytics and caustics must be reapplied for continued therapeutic benefit, depending on the disorder and the drug used.

PHARMACODYNAMICS

Keratolytics reduce epidermal mitotic activity, inhibit DNA replication and repair synthesis, and act as irritants. Keratolytics also soften keratin and loosen cornified epithelium (horny layer), causing swelling, softening, and dissolution of viable cells.

All caustics, with the exception of podophyllum resin, precipitate cell proteins, thereby causing scab formation and eventual sloughing. Podophyllum resin

Short-contact anthralin therapy (SCAT)

To apply anthralin to psoriatic or hyperkeratotic lesions, you will need the following equipment: anthralin in the concentration prescribed, cotton-tipped applicators or gloves, petrolatum, mineral oil, and a washcloth.

- Apply petrolatum to the normal skin around the affected areas.
- Apply the prescribed concentration of anthralin directly to the lesions using gloves or a cotton-tipped applicator.
- Be very careful to avoid applying anthralin on normal skin.
- Do not apply anthralin to intertriginous areas; doing so can cause severe burning sensations and blister formation.
- Do not apply anthralin to the patient's face, groin, or axillae.
- Leave the medication on the lesions 20 to 30 minutes.
- Remove the medication with mineral oil and a washcloth.
- After application, apply a lubricant or prescribed medication.

causes cell death by inhibiting cell division and other cellular processes.

PHARMACOTHERAPEUTICS

Keratolytics and caustics are used to treat hyperkeratotic disease and benign skin growths.

anthralin (AnthraDerm, Drithcocreme, Lasan). Anthralin is used to treat psoriasis and other hyperkeratotic conditions.
USUAL ADULT DOSAGE: apply as directed, using a short-contact regimen (see *Short-contact anthralin therapy [SCAT]* for details), beginning with the lowest concentration (0.1%) and gradually increasing the concentration until therapeutic effect is achieved.

cantharidin (Cantharone). This drug is indicated to remove molluscum contagiosum, plantar warts, ordinary and periungual warts, and benign epithelial growths.
USUAL ADULT DOSAGE: for molluscum contagiosum, apply to each lesion, then repeat in 1 week and cover with tape for 4 to 6 hours; for plantar warts, pare down

keratin before applying; for ordinary and periungual warts, apply directly to the lesion (no cutting is required).

podophyllum resin (Podoben). Podophyllum resin is used to treat benign epithelial growths, such as warts, fibroids, and papillomas. It is topically applied, especially to genital and anal warts.
USUAL ADULT DOSAGE: apply podophyllum resin to the lesion for the prescribed period (usually 1 to 6 hours), then wash off; may be repeated once or twice weekly for up to four applications.

resorcinol. Resorcinol is used to treat inflammatory skin diseases, such as eczema, urticaria, acne, seborrhea, psoriasis, and acne scarring.
USUAL ADULT DOSAGE: apply as ordered.

salicylic acid (Occlusal, Keralyt Gel, Salacid). This drug removes excessive keratin in patients with such hyperkeratotic skin disorders as verrucae and various ichthyoses, keratosis palmaris and plantaris, keratosis pilaris, pityriasis rubra pilaris, and psoriasis.
USUAL ADULT DOSAGE: apply thoroughly to the affected area after hydrating the skin for 5 minutes, and occlude at night; wash off the medication in the morning. Apply more frequently to areas where occlusion is impossible.

silver nitrate. A caustic and escharotic agent, this drug is used to treat indolent warts, destroy exuberant granulations, freshen the edges of ulcers and fissures, and touch the basis of vesicular, bullous, or aphthous lesions. It is also used as a cauterizing agent.
USUAL ADULT DOSAGE: apply ointment to the affected area for up to 5 days or as needed; apply solution to the affected area two or three times a week for 2 or 3 weeks, as needed.

sulfur (Fostex, Sebulex, Sulfacet-R). Sulfur is used locally to treat acne and dandruff.
USUAL ADULT DOSAGE: for acne, apply to thoroughly cleansed skin one to three times daily or as directed; for dandruff, apply to wet hair, massage vigorously into the scalp, rinse, then repeat application and rinsing.

Drug interactions
Using podophyllum resin with any other keratolytic may cause extensive skin damage. Salicylic acid may interact with iodine, iron salts, and oxidizing substances. It may also interact with the concomitant use of topical tretinoin.

ADVERSE DRUG REACTIONS

Predictable adverse reactions to keratolytics and caustics include a burning sensation, tingling, irritation, erythema, scaling, and drying. Podophyllum resin may cause thrombocytopenia, leukopenia, and peripheral neuropathy when systemically absorbed.

Unpredictable adverse reactions include extreme skin tenderness, inflammation, and annular warts. When systemically absorbed, salicylic acid may cause salicylism. Silver nitrate causes permanent silver staining of the skin (argyria) with prolonged or frequent use.

NURSING IMPLICATIONS

The use of keratolytics and caustics is considered safe if the following implications are considered:
• Be aware that use of podophyllum resin is contraindicated in pregnant women.
• Administer salicylic acid cautiously to patients with diabetes or impaired circulation; do not use in children under age 12.
• Do not apply keratolytics or caustics to broken or inflamed skin.
• Remember that podophyllum resin may be systemically absorbed when applied to large areas, used for long-term therapy, or used on mucous membranes.
• Protect the patient's surrounding normal skin with petrolatum when using podophyllum resin. After therapy, cleanse the area thoroughly with soap and water to ensure that all of the drug has been removed.
• Avoid applying cantharidin to normal skin. If contact occurs, remove the drug immediately with acetone, alcohol, or tape remover; then scrub the skin with soap and water and rinse well to prevent blistering.
• Do not apply sulfur to a patient using topical acne preparations or preparations containing a peeling agent, such as benzoyl peroxide; combined use of these products may produce severe irritation.
• Apply salicylic acid to well-hydrated skin.
• Do not apply salicylic acid to large areas of the body for prolonged periods; doing so could cause salicylate toxicity.
• Inform the patient receiving podophyllum that the drug may cause soreness 12 to 48 hours after treatment.
• Be aware that prolonged use of sulfur may cause severe dermatitis.
• Explain to the patient receiving cantharidin that if annular warts occur, they will disappear when the effects of the drug wear off.
• Explain to the patient receiving silver nitrate that the drug can stain skin and clothing.

ANTINEOPLASTICS

Two types of antineoplastics, alkylating agents and antimetabolites, are used in dermatologic therapy. The alkylating agent mechlorethamine hydrochloride and the antimetabolite fluorouracil are discussed here. Because they can cause unpleasant adverse reactions, antineoplastics are used primarily in patients with mycosis fungoides, multiple acitinic (solar) keratoses, and superficial basal cell carcinoma. (See Chapter 73, Alkylating Agents, and Chapter 74, Antimetabolite Agents, for a complete discussion of antineoplastic agents.)

History and source

Mechlorethamine, the oldest known anticancer agent, was first synthesized in the 1850s. Nitrogen mustard gases were used during World War I for chemical warfare. Fluorouracil was initially synthesized in 1957.

PHARMCOKINETICS

Mechlorethamine's half-life is reduced with topical administration. The nitrogen mustard molecule is also highly reactive in aqueous solutions and, therefore, relatively safe in topical use. Systemic absorption after topical application of fluorouracil is negligible.

Absorption, distribution, metabolism, excretion

Topical mechlorethamine is not appreciably absorbed; its distribution is local, and any metabolism that occurs is limited to the skin. Fluorouracil, which acts selectively against atypical epidermal cells, is also not appreciably absorbed.

Onset, peak, duration

The topical antineoplastics' onset of action is immediate. However, their duration of action is limited, and reapplication is usually necessary to attain therapeutic benefit.

PHARMACODYNAMICS

Mechlorethamine causes cell death by cross-linking with strands of cellular DNA and ribonucleic acid (RNA). Fluorouracil interferes with DNA synthesis and RNA formation.

Mechanism of action

Mechlorethamine attaches to the nucleic acid inside the cell nucleus, interfering with synthetase activity. Fluorouracil is a pyrimidine analog that inhibits thymidylate synthetase activity, DNA synthesis, and, to a lesser extent, RNA synthesis. All antineoplastic agents are cytotoxic and therefore interfere with the function of normal cells as well as neoplastic cells.

PHARMACOTHERAPEUTICS

Because antineoplastic agents interrupt cell synthesis, they are used to treat disorders characterized by abnormally rapid cell proliferation.

mechlorethamine hydrochloride (Mustargen). This drug is used topically to treat mycosis fungoides.
USUAL ADULT DOSAGE: before use, dissolve 10 mg of mechlorethamine powder in 50 to 100 ml of tap water; apply the total volume as ordered.

fluorouracil (Efudex, Fluoroplex). Fluorouracil is used to treat multiple actinic (solar) keratoses and superficial basal cell carcinoma.
USUAL ADULT DOSAGE: for keratoses, apply 1% to 5% cream or solution to the lesion b.i.d. for 2 to 6 weeks; for superficial basal cell carcinoma, apply 5% cream or solution to the lesion b.i.d. for 3 to 6 weeks.

Drug interactions

Concomitant application of topical preparations containing alcohol, benzoyl peroxide, salicylic acid, or resorcinol may result in increased erythema, desquamation, soreness, or tenderness in patients undergoing therapy with topical mechlorethamine or fluorouracil. No other significant interactions occur between topical mechlorethamine or fluorouracil and other drugs.

ADVERSE DRUG REACTIONS

Topically administered antineoplastics usually cause only local adverse reactions. Mechlorethamine can cause contact dermatitis hypersensitivity reaction with erythema, vesicle formation, and pruritus as well as hyperpigmentation. It can also increase the patient's risk of skin cancer. Fluorouracil can cause pruritus, irritation, burning sensation, photosensitivity, and hyperpigmentation. Fluorouracil can also produce pain, dermatitis, scarring, suppuration, scaling, swelling, and telangiectasia.

NURSING IMPLICATIONS

Topical antineoplastics are used to treat refractory dermatologic diseases, including superficial basal cell carcinoma. Because the antineoplastics are broadly cytotoxic and can cause unpleasant adverse reactions, the nurse should use care in administering them and provide appropriate patient teaching.
• If mechlorethamine is accidentally instilled into the eye, flush the eye with water and notify the physician immediately.
• If the patient develops hypersensitivity to mechlorethamine, discontinue the drug and notify the physician.
• Redilute the mechlorethamine solution before applying it to the patient's face, axillae, or groin.
• Emphasize to the patient the importance of compliance with the topical mechlorethamine regimen.
• Inform family members about the irritating effects of topical mechlorethamine; use gloves when helping the patient administer the drug.
• Advise the patient receiving mechlorethamine that hyperpigmentation may occur but that it is reversible.
• Instruct the patient receiving fluorouracil to avoid applying it to normal skin.
• Advise the patient receiving fluorouracil to avoid exposure to strong sunlight and other sources of ultraviolet rays because such exposure intensifies skin reactions to the drug.
• Explain to the patient that fluorouracil typically causes the following response pattern: erythema followed by vesiculation, erosion of the lesion being treated, ulceration, necrosis, and epithelialization.

OTHER INTEGUMENTARY SYSTEM AGENTS

Other integumentary agents include the antiseptics and disinfectants; astringents; emollients, demulcents, and protectants; and tretinoin.

ANTISEPTICS AND DISINFECTANTS

Antiseptics and disinfectants are used to prevent and control infection. Antiseptics act by killing or inhibiting the growth of microorganisms; disinfectants prevent infection by destroying them. Antiseptics are used mainly on living tissue, whereas disinfectants are generally applied to inanimate objects. Some disinfectants can be used as antiseptics in appropriate concentrations.

Commonly used antiseptics and disinfectants include ethyl alcohol, isopropyl alcohol, chlorhexidine gluconate, iodine, iodine compounds, hexachlorophene, hydrogen peroxide, benzalkonium chloride, and potassium permanganate.

Ethyl alcohol and **isopropyl alcohol** are used as skin antiseptics before procedures that break the skin, such as venipuncture and hypodermic injections. These drugs must remain on the skin for at least 2 minutes to ensure effectiveness.

Chlorhexidine gluconate (Hibiclens, Hibistat) is used as a surgical scrub, hand cleanser, preoperative skin cleanser, and wound cleanser.

Iodine (Iodine Tincture, Iodine Topical Solution) and **iodine compounds,** such as povidone-iodine (Betadine), are used for skin cleansing and for treating minor, superficial skin wounds.

Hexachlorophene (pHisoHex) is used as a sudsing antibacterial skin cleanser and surgical hand scrub but is contraindicated in infants. For preoperative skin cleansing, it should be used at least 3 days before the procedure to ensure its effectiveness.

Hydrogen peroxide is used to cleanse superficial wounds and ulcers. It also may be used as a mouthwash or gargle.

Benzalkonium chloride (Zephiran) is used preoperatively to cleanse unbroken skin, mucous membranes, and denuded skin. It is also used to disinfect surgical equipment and other articles, such as thermometers.

Potassium permanganate is an oxidant antiseptic with broad antimicrobial activity. Besides its use as an antiseptic, it may also be prescribed for athlete's foot or intertriginous candidiasis. Although potassium permanganate can stain clothing and skin, the stains may be removed with dilute acids.

Astringents

Astringents (toners, tonics) are used to provide comfort primarily because of their tightening properties and ability to reduce inflammation and exudation. They also may act as antiseptics. Before applying any of these agents, the affected area should be cleansed. Commonly used astringents include aluminum acetate, aluminum sulfate, and hamamelis water.

Aluminum acetate solution (Burow's solution) is applied as a wet dressing to relieve inflammatory skin conditions, such as insect bites, poison ivy, and athlete's foot.

Aluminum sulfate (Bluboro Powder, Domeboro Powder and Tablets) is used to relieve inflammatory skin conditions. After it is mixed in 1 pint of water, the resulting solution is applied to the affected area for 15 to 30 minutes every 4 to 8 hours.

Hamamelis water [witch hazel] (Tucks) is applied locally t.i.d. or q.i.d. times daily to relieve anal or perineal discomfort.

Emollients, demulcents, and protectants

Emollients, demulcents, and protectants are used to soften, lubricate, provide analgesic effects, and promote healing. They may be used alone or as vehicles for other drugs. Emollients protect and soften the skin; demulcents soothe inflamed or abraded skin and mucous membranes; and protectants occlude and protect skin, ulcers, and wounds. Selected emollients, demulcents, and protectants include vitamins A and D ointment, glycerin, compound benzoin tincture, oatmeal, para-aminobenzoic acid, petrolatum, and zinc oxide gelatin.

Vitamins A and D ointment (Clocream, Desitin) is an emollient and demulcent used for such conditions as superficial burns, abrasions, slow-healing lesions, chapped skin, and diaper rash.

Glycerin (Corn Husker's Lotion), an emollient used for softening dry skin, also serves as a lubricant for inserting tubes and catheters.

Compound benzoin tincture (Benzoin spray) is a demulcent and protectant used for cutaneous ulcers, decubitus ulcers, cracked nipples, and fissures of the lips or anus.

Oatmeal (Aveeno Colloidal, Aveeno Oilated Bath), an emollient and demulcent, softens dry skin by preventing evaporation of perspiration. It also soothes and cools the skin. It may be applied as a lotion or used as a bathtub soak.

Para-aminobenzoic acid (PABA, Pabanol) is a protectant used to prevent sunburn. It also promotes healing by reducing irritation and friction.

Petrolatum (Vaseline) and **liquid petrolatum** (Mineral Oil) are used as protectants and emollients.

SELECTED MAJOR DRUGS

Integumentary system agents

This chart summarizes integumentary system agents commonly used in clinical practice.

DRUG	MAJOR INDICATIONS	USUAL ADULT DOSAGES	NURSING IMPLICATIONS
Antibacterials			
neomycin sulfate	Aerobic gram-negative and some aerobic gram-positive bacterial skin infections	Apply to affected area one to three times daily	• Cleanse the affected area before applying the medication.
Antifungals			
clotrimazole	Tinea pedis, tinea cruris, tinea corporis, tinea versicolor, and cutaneous candidiasis	Massage into affected area and surrounding skin in the morning and evening	• Cleanse the affected area before applying the medication.
Antivirals			
acyclovir	Herpes simplex skin infections	Apply to lesions every 3 hours, six times daily, for 7 days	• Use a finger cot or glove when applying ointment to prevent the spread of infection. • Urge the patient to report to the physician any burning sensation, stinging, pruritus, or rash that occurs after application.
Scabicides and pediculicides			
lindane	Scabies and pediculosis	Apply cream or lotion to the entire body from the neck down, leave on for 8 to 12 hours, then remove; apply shampoo to the affected area, shampoo for 4 to 5 minutes, rinse, then dry hair	• Avoid applying medication to raw or inflamed skin. • Inform the patient that all linens and clothing that may have been contaminated must be sterilized to avoid reinfestation or transmission of the parasite. • Tell the patient to use a fine-tooth comb dipped in vinegar to comb out nits.
Keratolytics and caustics			
podophyllum resin	Benign epithelial growths, such as warts, fibroids, and papillomas	Apply to the lesion for the prescribed period (usually 1 to 6 hours), then wash off; may be repeated once or twice weekly for up to four applications	• Use petrolatum to protect the patient's surrounding normal skin. • After therapy, thoroughly cleanse the area with soap and water to ensure that all of the drug has been removed.
Antineoplastics			
fluorouracil	multiple actinic (solar) keratoses	Apply 1% to 5% cream or solution b.i.d. for 2 to 6 weeks	• Avoid applying the drug to normal skin. • Advise the patient to avoid exposure to strong sunlight and other sources of ultraviolet rays because such exposure intensifies skin reactions to the drug.
	Superficial basal cell carcinoma	Apply 5% cream or solution to the lesion b.i.d. for 3 to 6 weeks	

Zinc oxide gelatin (Dome-Paste, Unna's Boot), a protectant, is used for lesions or injuries of the lower arms or legs. The gelatin is applied as a bandage and worn for about 1 week.

Tretinoin

Tretinoin (Retin-A), a synthetic derivative of vitamin A, is used topically to treat acne vulgaris. It should be applied nightly to the affected area on skin that has been allowed to dry for 15 to 30 minutes after cleansing. The nurse should advise the patient that a transient warm or slight stinging sensation is normal during application and that a mild erythema and peeling of the area is expected after treatment. The nurse should explain that exposure to sunlight or the use of keratolytics or abrasive soaps can aggravate this response.

CHAPTER SUMMARY

Chapter 78 discussed topical integumentary system agents as they are used to treat dermatologic disorders and relieve their signs and symptoms. Here are the highlights of the chapter:

• The major integumentary system agents are the antibacterials, antifungals, antivirals, scabicides and pediculicides, keratolytics and caustics, and antineoplastics. Other integumentary system agents include antiseptics and disinfectants; astringents; emollients, demulcents and protectants; and tretinoin.

• The skin has a low water permeability, which with keratin, makes it an efficient (but not absolute) barrier.

• Absorption of topical agents increases when the agents are applied to abraded or broken skin.

• Antibacterials hasten the healing of infected superficial skin wounds.

• Antifungals are used to treat superficial mycotic skin infections.

• The topical antiviral acyclovir is used to treat herpes simplex skin infections.

• Scabicides and pediculicides are used to eradicate scabies and pediculosis (lice infestation).

• Keratolytics and caustics are used to treat hyperkeratotic skin diseases, such as acne and psoriasis, and benign skin growths, such as warts.

• Two types of antineoplastics are used topically, the alkylating agent mechlorethamine and the antimetabolite fluorouracil.

• Antiseptics kill or inhibit the growth of microorganisms; disinfectants prevent infection by destroying microorganisms.

• Astringents are used as comforting agents primarily because of their tightening properties and their ability to reduce inflammation and exudation.

• Emollients and demulcents may be used alone or as a vehicle for pharmacologically active substances.

• A synthetic vitamin A derivative, tretinoin, is used to treat acne vulgaris.

BIBLIOGRAPHY

Arndt, K. *Manual of Dermatologic Therapeutics.* Boston: Little, Brown & Co., 1983.

Bickers, D.R., *Clinical Pharmacology of Skin Disease.* New York: Churchill Livingstone, 1984.

Block, S. *Disinfection, Sterilization and Preservation.* Philadelphia: Lea & Febiger, 1983.

Bronaugh, R.L., and Malbach, H., eds. *Percutaneous Absorption (Mechanism, Methodology, Drug Delivery).* New York: Marcel Dekker, 1985.

Galasso, G.J., et al., eds. *Antiviral Agents and Viral Diseases of Man.* New York: Raven Press, 1984.

Mandell, G.L., et al. *Anti-Infective Therapy.* New York: John Wiley & Sons, 1985.

Polano, M.K. *Topical Skin Therapeutics.* New York: Churchill Livingstone, 1984.

Rosen, T., et al. *Nurse's Atlas of Dermatology.* Boston: Little, Brown & Co., 1983.

Vonderheid, E.C. "Topical Mechlorethamine: Chemotherapy Considerations on its Use in Mycosis Fungoides," *International Journal of Dermatology* 23(3):180, April 1984.

CHAPTER 79

OPHTHALMIC AGENTS

OBJECTIVES

After reading and studying this chapter, you should be able to:

1. Describe the clinical indications for mydriatic, cycloplegic, and miotic agents.

2. Describe the different types of glaucoma and the therapies used to treat them.

3. Describe the mechanism of action of ophthalmic drugs to lower intraocular pressure.

4. Explain the adverse reactions to ophthalmic anesthetic agents and how to prevent them.

5. Differentiate the ophthalmic conditions that are treated with topical anti-infectives from those that are treated with systemic anti-infectives.

6. Explain how to instill *eye* drops and apply *eye* ointments.

INTRODUCTION

Many ophthalmic agents mimic the action of the autonomic nervous system, which is divided into the sympathetic and parasympathetic nervous systems. (For an additional review of the autonomic nervous system, *see* the introduction to Unit Three). Agents that mimic the actions of the sympathetic nervous system are called *adrenergic*, or *sympathomimetic*, agents; those that mimic the parasympathetic nervous system are called *cholinergic*, or *parasympathomimetic*, agents; those that inhibit the parasympathetic nervous system are called *cholinergic blockers*, or *parasympatholytic* agents.

Adrenergic agents act directly on end-organ (eye) tissues. One example is phenylephrine, used to dilate the pupil. Cholinergic agents act on the eye directly in a manner similar to that of acetylcholine or indirectly by interfering with the action of the enzyme acetylcholinesterase.

The ophthalmic agents discussed in this chapter are primarily instilled as drops or applied as ointments. (See *Ophthalmic agent administration* for explanations and illustrations of those procedures.)

Mydriatics, cycloplegics, and miotics are the three groups of ophthalmic agents that are most commonly used. Besides these three groups, ophthalmic agents that lower intraocular pressure, anesthetic agents, anti-inflammatory agents, and anti-infective preparations also will be reviewed in this chapter.

For a summary of representative drugs, *see Selected major drugs: Ophthalmic agents* on pages 1244 and 1245.

MYDRIATICS AND CYCLOPLEGICS

Mydriatics are used to dilate the pupil for intraocular examinations and to facilitate refraction. Cycloplegics, which have a wide range of uses in ophthalmic diagnosis, are also used to paralyze the accommodative muscle of the ciliary body in patients before refraction. In postoperative patients or patients with intraocular inflammation, mydriatics and cycloplegics are used to dilate the pupils and to paralyze the accommodative muscle of the ciliary body. Mydriatics and cycloplegics include atropine sulfate, clopentolate hydrochloride, dipivefrin, epinephrine bitartrate, epinephrine hydrochloride, epinephryl borate, homatropine hydrobromide, hydroxyamphetamine hydrobromide, phenylephrine hydrochloride, scopolamine hydrobromide, and tropicamide. Of these, epinephrine bitartrate, epinephrine hydrochloride, epinephryl borate, dipivefrin, phenylephrine and hydroxyamphetamine act only as mydriatics, and the rest have combined mydriatic-cycloplegic effects.

Ophthalmic agent administration

Many ophthalmic agents come in two forms: eye drops for instillation and ointments for application. An agent's form determines how it is administered, as shown in the procedures below. With both forms, hand washing is essential before administration to prevent infection and after administration to prevent self-mydriasis.

Applying eye ointment

Place the patient in a supine position or sitting with the neck hyperextended. Clean the eyelashes with saline solution and swabs to remove any secretions. Have the patient look upward; then, with your finger, pull down the lower lid. As the patient continues to look up, apply a thin ribbon of ointment (approximately ¼″) directly into the conjunctival sac, beginning at the inner canthus.

To avoid contamination, do not let the tube touch the eye or conjunctiva. As you approach the outer canthus, rotate the tube to detach the ointment.

Instruct the patient to close the eye gently and to avoid squeezing it shut.

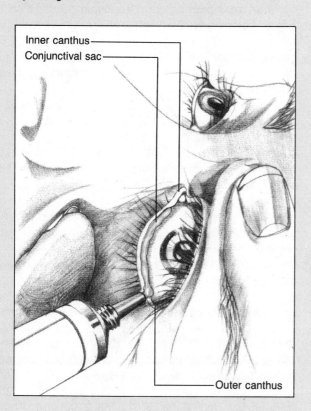

Inner canthus
Conjunctival sac
Outer canthus

Instilling eye drops

Place the patient in a supine position or sitting with the neck hyperextended, looking toward the ceiling.

With your finger, pull down firmly on the lower lid while the patient continues to look upward. This movement exposes the lower conjunctival sac by relaxing the upper tarsal plate as it is retracted into the orbit.

Instill 1 drop of medication into the lower conjunctival sac. Instruct the patient to close the eye gently, but not to squeeze it closed. Wipe away excess tears with a cotton ball or tissue.

The eye can hold only 1 drop (to be exact, ⅙ drop). When instilling more than 1 drop, wait 2 to 3 minutes between drops to avoid losing a drop from tearing or blinking.

Stopping drainage through the nasolacrimal duct when instilling eye drops helps prevent systemic absorption. It also prevents the patient from tasting the drops. After instilling drops, apply digital pressure over the punctum at the inner canthus for 2 to 3 minutes, and have the patient close the eyelids gently for 2 to 3 minutes to prevent drainage through the nasolacrimal duct.

The tip of the container should never touch the lid or eyelashes to avoid contamination.

Discard discolored solutions or solutions with floating particles.

Special attention is needed when instilling mydriatics and cycloplegics to prevent dilation of the unaffected eye.

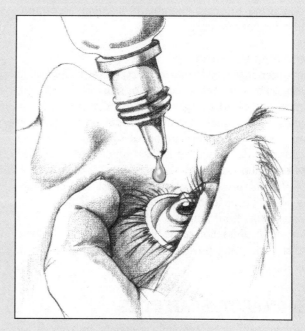

PHARMACOKINETICS

Atropine, cyclopentolate, and scopolamine are absorbed systemically, especially in children and the elderly. Systemic absorption may occur through the conjunctiva or through the gastrointestinal (GI) tract after a drug drains into the nasal sinuses and is swallowed. Other mydriatics and cycloplegics, such as phenylephrine, are less often absorbed systemically. Absorption is enhanced during surgical procedures and treatment of traumatized eyes.

Onset, peak, duration

The onset of action of the adrenergic agents (phenylephrine, hydroxyamphetamine, dipivefrin, and epinephrine) occurs within 10 to 15 minutes. The drugs' peak concentration levels are reached 20 to 40 minutes after instillation, and their duration of action (pupil dilation) is 2 to 3 hours.

The cholinergic-blocking mydriatics and cycloplegics (atropine, cyclopentolate, homatropine, scopolamine, and tropicamide) have an onset of action for mydriatic effects of 10 to 30 minutes and for cycloplegic action from 15 minutes to several hours. Their duration of action is longer than that of the sympathomimetic drugs.

PHARMACODYNAMICS

Mydriatic drops act on the iris to dilate the pupil. Cycloplegic drops act on the ciliary body to paralyze the fine-focusing muscles, thereby preventing accommodation for near vision.

Mechanism of action

The adrenergic mydriatics and cycloplegics stimulate mydriasis by contracting the dilator muscle of the pupil. Topical use of adrenergic drugs also constricts the arterioles and capillaries, thereby producing a whitening (decongesting) of the eye. Intraocular pressure decreases because of decreased aqueous humor and increased flow of aqueous through the meshwork.

The cholinergic-blocking mydriatics and cycloplegics prevent acetylcholine action. With these drugs, mydriasis results from paralysis of the sphincter muscle of the iris and contraction of the dilator muscle. Cycloplegia results from ciliary muscle relaxation, which allows the lens to flatten.

PHARMACOTHERAPEUTICS

Mydriatics are used primarily to dilate the pupils for intraocular examinations. Cycloplegics are essential for performing refraction in children; they also are used before and after ophthalmic surgery and as adjunctive treatment for conditions involving the iris.

Pupil dilation in diabetic patients or in those with darkly pigmented irises requires stronger concentrations of both types of drugs and repeated instillations. Systemic adverse reactions most commonly affect pediatric and geriatric patients.

atropine sulfate (Atropisol, Isopto Atropine). This drug is used to treat acute iris inflammation (iritis) and to facilitate refraction.
USUAL ADULT DOSAGE: for acute iritis, 1 to 2 drops of 0.5% to 2% solution or a small amount of ointment b.i.d. or t.i.d.; for refraction, 1 to 2 drops of 1% solution 1 hour before eye examination.
USUAL PEDIATRIC DOSAGE: for acute iritis, 1 to 2 drops of 0.5% solution b.i.d. or t.i.d.; for refraction in children under age 5, instill 1 to 2 drops of 0.5% solution in each eye for 1 to 3 days before eye examination and again 1 hour before refraction.

cyclopentolate hydrochloride (Cyclogyl). This drug is used for diagnostic procedures that require mydriatic and cycloplegic effects.
USUAL ADULT DOSAGE: 1 drop of 1% solution (2% solution for patients with heavily pigmented irises), then 1 drop 5 minutes later.
USUAL PEDIATRIC DOSAGE: 1 drop of 1% solution; if needed, 1 drop of 1% solution 5 minutes later. For infants under age 1, a 0.5% solution should be used.

dipivefrin (Propine). A topical adrenergic, dipivefrin is used to reduce intraocular pressure in patients with chronic open-angle glaucoma.
USUAL ADULT DOSAGE: 1 drop of 0.1% solution every 12 hours.

epinephrine bitartrate (Epitrate). A topical adrenergic, this drug is used to treat chronic open-angle glaucoma.
USUAL ADULT AND PEDIATRIC DOSAGE: 1 to 2 drops of 1% or 2% solution, frequency usually ranges from one to four times daily every 2 to 4 days.

epinephrine hydrochloride (Epifrin, Glaucon). Physicians administer epinephrine hydrochloride, a topical adrenergic, by intraocular injection during surgery to control bleeding or produce mydriasis. As a topical agent, epinephrine is used to treat chronic open-angle glaucoma and to produce mydriasis before ophthalmologic examination.

USUAL ADULT AND PEDIATRIC DOSAGE: for chronic open-angle glaucoma, 1 drop of 0.25%, 0.5%, 1%, or 2% solution one or two times daily; during surgery, 1 or more drops of 0.1% solution instilled up to three times, or as needed.

epinephryl borate (Epinal, Eppyl/N). A topical adrenergic, epinephryl is used to treat chronic open-angle glaucoma.
USUAL ADULT AND PEDIATRIC DOSAGE: 1 drop of 0.5% or 1% solution b.i.d.

homatropine hydrobromide (Homatrocel Ophthalmic, Isopto Homatropine). Used to facilitate refraction, homatropine is also used to treat uveitis.
USUAL ADULT DOSAGE: for refraction, 1 drop of 2% or 5% solution, repeated in 5 to 10 minutes; for uveitis, 1 drop of 2% or 5% solution b.i.d. or t.i.d.

hydroxyamphetamine hydrobromide (Paredrine). Hydroxyamphetamine is most commonly used to aid diagnosis of Horner's syndrome (unilateral ptosis, miosis, and enophthalmos from destruction of the cervical sympathetic nerves of the affected side).
USUAL ADULT AND PEDIATRIC DOSAGE: 1 drop of 1% solution instilled into the conjunctival sac, repeated in 5 minutes.

phenylephrine hydrochloride (Mydfrin, Neo-Synephrine). This agent is used to achieve mydriasis without cycloplegia.
USUAL ADULT AND PEDIATRIC DOSAGE: for mydriasis, 1 drop of 2.5% solution before examination.

scopolamine hydrobromide (Isopto Hyoscine). Scopolamine is used to achieve postoperative mydriasis, to treat anterior uveitis, and occasionally to facilitate refraction before examination in children.
USUAL ADULT DOSAGE: for postoperative mydriasis, 1 drop of 0.25% solution daily; for anterior uveitis, 1 drop of 0.25% solution once daily or more frequently for severe inflammation.
USUAL PEDIATRIC DOSAGE: for refraction, 1 drop of 0.25% solution or a thin ribbon of 0.25% ointment b.i.d. for 2 days before refraction.

tropicamide (Mydriacyl). This drug is used to facilitate refraction and funduscopic examination.
USUAL ADULT AND PEDIATRIC DOSAGE: for refraction, 1 drop of 1% solution 20 minutes before examination (an additional drop may be instilled in 20 to 30 minutes); for funduscopic examination, 1 drop of 0.5% solution 15 to 20 minutes before examination.

Drug interactions

Among mydriatics and cycloplegics, only phenylephrine interacts significantly with other drugs. For example, use of phenylephrine with guanethidine may increase the mydriatic and pressor effects of phenylephrine, and use of phenylephrine with levodopa may decrease the mydriatic effects. Increased pressor effects also occur when phenylephrine is administered with monoamine oxidase (MAO) inhibitors. The cardiac effects of phenylephrine are potentiated by concomitant administration of tricyclic antidepressants, which should therefore be avoided.

ADVERSE REACTIONS

Many local adverse reactions predictably occur with the mydriatics and cycloplegics, which can include irritation, blurred vision, and transient burning sensations and stinging. With prolonged use, these drugs can increase intraocular pressure and cause ocular congestion, conjunctivitis, contact dermatitis, and eye dryness. Systemic reactions include tachycardia, palpitations, flushing, dry skin, ataxia, and confusion. Dry mouth and tachycardia commonly occur after instillation of atropine, cyclopentolate, or scopolamine. Atropine, cyclopentolate, homatropine, and scopolamine can cause photophobia.

NURSING IMPLICATIONS

The nurse should be aware of the following considerations when administering mydriatics and cycloplegics:
• Mydriatics and cycloplegics are contraindicated in patients with acute closed-angle (narrow-angle) glaucoma.
• Mydriatics and cycloplegics should be used cautiously in infants and the elderly; some agents are contraindicated for pediatric patients.
• These drugs also should be used cautiously in patients with hypertension or cardiac disease.
• To minimize systemic absorption, compress the lacrimal sac of the eye for 1 to 2 minutes after instilling the drops.
• After administration, instruct the patient to wear dark glasses and to avoid operating machinery until blurred vision disappears.
• Teach the patient the proper method of instillation, including hand washing before and after administering the drops, and remind the patient not to touch the dropper to the eye or surrounding tissue.
• Explain to the patient receiving atropine, cyclopentolate, homatropine, or scopolamine that photophobia may occur. Instruct the patient to wear dark glasses for protection.
• Advise the patient to discard any discolored epinephrine solution.

MIOTICS

Miotics constrict the pupils and are used primarily to treat glaucoma and to manage accommodative esotropia. Miotics include direct-acting cholinergics (pilocarpine hydrochloride, pilocarpine nitrate, and carbachol), short-acting anticholinesterases (physostigmine salicylate and physostigmine sulfate), and long-acting anticholinesterases (demecarium bromide, echothiophate iodide, and isoflurophate).

PHARMACOKINETICS

Some systemic absorption is possible with all miotics but seldom occurs.

Onset, peak, duration

Pilocarpine, available in hydrochloride and nitrate forms, has an onset of action of 15 to 30 minutes, reaches peak concentration levels in 2 hours, and has a duration of action of 4 to 8 hours.

Carbachol has a similar duration of action—4 to 8 hours. However, carbachol is poorly absorbed through the cornea and is used only if pilocarpine is ineffective or if the patient is hypersensitive to pilocarpine.

Physostigmine, the short-acting anticholinesterase available in salicylate and sulfate forms, has an onset of action of 10 minutes, reaches peak concentration levels in 3 to 4 hours, and has a duration of action of 12 to 36 hours. The long-acting anticholinesterases, demecarium, echothiophate, and isoflurophate, are potent miotics with a duration of action of days to weeks.

PHARMACODYNAMICS

Miotics stimulate and contract the sphincter muscle of the iris, thereby constricting the pupil. This action is called *miosis*.

Mechanism of action

Miotics are used to treat chronic open-angle glaucoma, because they improve aqueous outflow from the eye's anterior chamber by decreasing both intraocular pressure and resistance to the outflow of aqueous humor. Miotics also are used to treat acute and chronic closed-angle glaucoma. (See *Types of glaucoma* for descriptions; see *Normal flow of aqueous humor* for an illustration.)

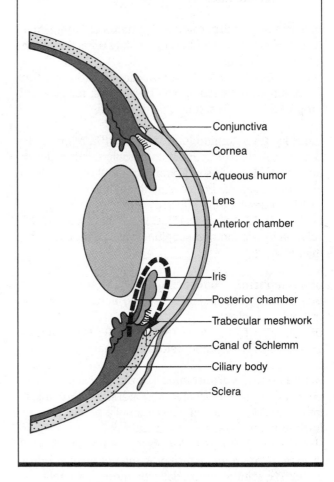

Normal flow of aqueous humor

Aqueous humor, a transparent fluid produced by the ciliary epithelium of the ciliary body, flows from the posterior chamber to the anterior chamber through the pupil. Here it flows peripherally and filters through the trabecular meshwork to the canal of Schlemm. The fluid ultimately enters venous circulation.

- Conjunctiva
- Cornea
- Aqueous humor
- Lens
- Anterior chamber
- Iris
- Posterior chamber
- Trabecular meshwork
- Canal of Schlemm
- Ciliary body
- Sclera

The direct-acting cholinergic miotics constrict the pupil by contracting the sphincter muscles of the iris, contract the ciliary muscle, and widen the trabecular meshwork. These actions open the outflow channels, increasing aqueous outflow. The anticholinesterase miotics inactivate the enzyme cholinesterase, allowing acetylcholine to flow freely and exert its effects, which include pupil constriction and accommodative spasm. Long-acting anticholinesterases combine chemically and irreversibly with cholinesterase for intensified and prolonged action: marked miosis and vasodilation and strong accommodative spasm.

PHARMACOTHERAPEUTICS

The miotics are used to treat chronic open-angle glaucoma, acute and chronic closed-angle glaucoma, and certain cases of secondary glaucoma from disease- or injury-induced increases in intraocular pressure. However, if inflammation such as iritis is present, miotics should not be used because they may increase the inflammation.

Controlling intraocular pressure is the cornerstone of glaucoma therapy, and short-acting miotics such as pilocarpine are usually the drugs of choice. Long-acting miotics such as isoflurophate, which can be toxic, are used only in patients refractory to short-acting agents.

carbachol (Carbacel, Isopto Carbachol). A cholinergic drug, intraocular carbachol is used to achieve miosis for ocular surgery; topical carbachol is used to treat open-angle and closed-angle glaucomas.
USUAL ADULT DOSAGE: for miosis, 0.5 ml of 0.01% solution into the anterior chamber; for open-angle or closed-angle glaucoma, 1 drop of 0.75% to 3% solution instilled into the conjunctival sac every 4 to 8 hours.

demecarium bromide (Humorsol). This long-acting anticholinesterase is used to treat glaucoma and accommodative esotropia in children.
USUAL ADULT DOSAGE: for glaucoma, 1 drop of 0.125% or 0.25% solution every 12 to 48 hours.
USUAL PEDIATRIC DOSAGE: for esotropia, 1 drop of 0.125% solution daily for 2 to 3 weeks, then 1 drop every other day for 3 to 4 weeks, and, if improved, 1 drop twice weekly; therapy should be discontinued after 4 months if condition still requires therapy every other day or if the patient shows no response.

echothiophate iodide (Echodids, Phospholine Iodide). A long-acting anticholinesterase, echothiophate is used to treat open-angle glaucoma, conditions obstructing aqueous outflow, and accommodative esotropia.
USUAL ADULT AND PEDIATRIC DOSAGE: 1 drop of 0.03% to 0.06% solution in the conjunctival sac every 12 to 48 hours. A stronger solution of 0.125% to 0.25% may be required in patients with highly pigmented irises.

isoflurophate (Floropryl). A long-acting anticholinesterase, isoflurophate is used to treat glaucoma and esotropia.
USUAL ADULT AND PEDIATRIC DOSAGE: for open-angle glaucoma, ¼-inch of 0.025% ointment in the conjunctival sac every 8 to 72 hours; for esotropia uncomplicated

Types of glaucoma

Chronic open-angle glaucoma results from overproduction of aqueous humor or obstruction of its outflow through the trabecular meshwork, the canal of Schlemm, or aqueous veins.

Acute closed-angle (narrow-angle) glaucoma results from obstruction of aqueous humor outflow because of anatomically narrow angles between the anterior iris and the posterior corneal surface; shallow anterior chambers; a thickened iris that causes angle closure on pupil dilation; or a bulging iris that presses on the trabeculae, thereby closing the angle.

Chronic closed-angle glaucoma follows an untreated episode of acute closed-angle glaucoma or mild recurring acute episodes that create increased synechiae in the trabecular meshwork.

by amblyopia (loss of vision unrelated to poor refraction) or anisometropia (a difference in refraction between the two eyes), ¼-inch of 0.025% ointment every night for 2 weeks.

physostigmine salicylate (Eserine Salicylate, Isopto Eserine) and **physostigmine sulfate** (Eserine Sulfate). These short-acting anticholinesterases are used to treat open-angle glaucoma.
USUAL ADULT AND PEDIATRIC DOSAGE: ¼-inch of 0.25% ointment in the conjunctival sac or 1 to 2 drops 0.25% or 0.5% solution in the conjunctival sac every 4 to 8 hours.

pilocarpine hydrochloride (Isopto Carpine, Pilocar) and **pilocarpine nitrate** (P.V. Carpine). These cholinergics, considered reliable and highly effective, are the drugs most commonly used to treat chronic open-angle glaucoma and, before surgery, to treat acute closed-angle glaucoma.
USUAL ADULT AND PEDIATRIC DOSAGE: for chronic open-angle glaucoma, 1 to 2 drops of 1% to 2% solution every 4 to 8 hours; for acute closed-angle glaucoma, 1 drop of a 2% solution instilled three to six times over a 30-minute period before surgery.

pilocarpine ocuserts (Ocusert Pilo-20, Ocusert Pilo-40). This form of pilocarpine, an ocular insert, has the same indications as pilocarpine hydrochloride and pilocarpine nitrate and delivers 20 mg/hour or 40 mg/hour for 7 days.
USUAL ADULT DOSAGE: one ocular insert placed in the conjunctival sac every 7 days.

Drug interactions

Carbachol is the only miotic that does not interact significantly with other drugs. See *Drug interactions: Miotics* for information on significant interactions between the miotics and other drugs.

ADVERSE REACTIONS

Miotics commonly cause blurred vision and eye and brow pain. Reversible iris cysts, lid pain, photosensitivity, and cataract formation can also occur. Although uncommon, systemic absorption can lead to abdominal cramps, diarrhea, and increased salivation.

The miotics can also cause unpredictable bronchial constriction and spasm as well as pulmonary edema. In blacks, hypersensitivity reactions to physostigmine can lead to reversible depigmentation of eyelid skin.

NURSING IMPLICATIONS

The nurse administering miotics or instructing the patient in self-administration should be aware of the following considerations, many involving cautions and contraindications:

• Pilocarpine can produce ciliary spasm that some patients, especially younger ones, cannot tolerate. The drug

---

DRUG INTERACTIONS

Miotics

Varied interactions occur between miotics and other drugs (except for carbachol, which interacts with pilocarpine).

DRUG	INTERACTING DRUGS	POSSIBLE EFFECTS	NURSING IMPLICATIONS
demecarium	echothiophate	Decreases duration of miosis	• Administer echothiophate first.
echothiophate	organophosphate insecticides	Cause additive effects	• Advise the patient to avoid exposure to insecticides.
	pilocarpine	Interferes with miosis	• Do not administer concomitantly.
	succinylcholine	Causes respiratory or cardiovascular collapse	• Do not administer concomitantly.
isoflurophate	demecarium, physostigmine	Produce competitive action	• Administer isoflurophate first; decreased miosis occurs if isoflurophate is administered second.
	pilocarpine	Interferes with miosis	• Use caution when administering concomitantly, or avoid such use altogether.
	succinylcholine	Causes respiratory or cardiovascular collapse	• Do not administer concomitantly.
physostigmine	isoflurophate	Produces competitive action	• Administer isoflurophate first; decreased miosis occurs if isoflurophate is administered second.
	organophosphate insecticides	Cause additive effects	• Advise the patient to avoid exposure to insecticides.
	pilocarpine	Interferes with miosis	• Do not administer concomitantly.
	succinylcholine	Causes respiratory or cardiovascular collapse	• Do not administer concomitantly.
pilocarpine	carbachol	Causes additive effect	• Do not administer concomitantly.
	phenylephrine	Decreases mydriasis by phenylephrine	• Do not administer concomitantly.

may also increase myopia. Adding a drop of epinephrine to the regimen, as prescribed, may help these patients adjust to pilocarpine therapy. Epinephrine dilates the pupil, reduces aqueous formation, and increases aqueous outflow.

• Remember that pilocarpine, carbachol, and physostigmine are contraindicated in patients with acute iritis or corneal abrasion. Administer these drugs cautiously to patients with congestive heart failure, bronchial asthma, peptic ulcers, hyperthyroidism, GI spasm, urinary tract obstruction, or parkinsonism.

• Be aware that demecarium, echothiophate, and isoflurophate are contraindicated in patients with uveitis; closed-angle glaucoma; secondary glaucoma resulting from iridocyclitis; ocular hypertension; vasomotor instability; bronchial asthma; or bradycardia.

• Advise the patient to reconstitute echothiophate with the enclosed diluent. Reconstituted echothiophate will remain stable for 1 month at room temperature or 6 months under refrigeration.

• To minimize systemic absorption, press the lacrimal sac for 1 to 2 minutes after instilling drops.

• Explain to the patient that blurred vision will occur after administration; instruct the patient to instill drops at bedtime, if possible, to minimize problems resulting from blurring.

DRUGS THAT LOWER INTRAOCULAR PRESSURE

Topical adrenergic-blocking agents, hyperosmotic agents, and carbonic anhydrase inhibitors are used to lower intraocular pressure. These drugs lower intraocular pressure by either reducing or blocking aqueous humor formation and increasing aqueous humor outflow. Topical adrenergic-blocking agents include timolol maleate, which is a nonselective adrenergic blocker, levobunolol hydrochloride, a nonspecific beta-adrenergic blocker, and betaxolol hydrochloride, a cardioselective receptor blocking agent.

Hyperosmotic agents include anhydrous glycerin, isosorbide, mannitol, and urea. The carbonic anhydrase inhibitors are acetazolamide, acetazolamide sodium, dichlorphenamide, and methazolamide.

PHARMACOKINETICS

The topical adrenergic-blocking agents are less systemically absorbed than other ophthalmic agents.

Absorption, distribution, metabolism, excretion

Timolol and levobunolol are absorbed systemically; betaxolol is not as well absorbed. After oral administration glycerin is not absorbed but isosorbide is readily absorbed. The other hyperosmotic agents, mannitol and urea, are administered I.V. and are distributed immediately. The carbonic anhydrase inhibitors are administered by various routes, so their pharmacokinetics differ accordingly. (See Chapter 38, Diuretic Agents, for additional information about the pharmacokinetic properties of the hyperosmotic agents and the carbonic anhydrase inhibitors.)

Onset, peak, duration

The onset of action of the topical adrenergic-blocking agents occurs 20 minutes after administration, with peak concentration levels usually occurring within 1 to 2 hours. The duration of action of these drugs can range up to 24 hours.

The hyperosmotic agents have an onset of action within 15 minutes and a duration of action of 5 to 8 hours.

The onset of action of the carbonic anhydrase inhibitors varies. The effects of acetazolamide sodium appear within 2 minutes of injection, whereas the onset of oral acetazolamide is 60 to 90 minutes. Oral dichlorphenamide's effects appear within 30 to 60 minutes. The effects of methazolamide do not appear until 2 hours after administration. The duration of action of the carbonic anhydrase inhibitors range from 4 hours to a high of 24 hours for sustained-release acetazolamide.

PHARMACODYNAMICS

Each group of drugs lowers intraocular pressure by a different mechanism of action.

Mechanism of action

The adrenergic-blocking agent timolol decreases intraocular pressure without affecting pupil size or accommodation. Although its action is not well understood, timolol may primarily reduce aqueous humor formation and slightly increase aqueous humor outflow. The action of levobunolol and betaxalol in reducing intraocular pressure has not been established. It is, however, similar to that of timolol.

Hyperosmotic agents, which are reserved for emergencies, increase the absorption of water in the eye into the general circulation, thus lowering intraocular pressure.

The enzyme carbonic anhydrase is involved in the production of aqueous humor in the eye, so drugs that inhibit the action of carbonic anhydrase decrease aqueous production—by 30% to 60%—without affecting aqueous outflow. As less aqueous fluid enters the eye, intraocular pressure decreases. Carbonic anhydrase inhibitors can be used daily for long-term therapy.

PHARMACOTHERAPEUTICS

The topical adrenergic-blocking agents are used to treat chronic open-angle glaucoma, except for timolol, which is used to treat some secondary glaucoma. The hyperosmotic agents are used to treat acute closed-angle glaucoma; they are also used before and after ocular surgery. The carbonic anhydrase inhibitors are used to treat chronic open-angle glaucoma and secondary glaucoma.

betaxolol hydrochloride (Betoptic). This beta$_1$-adrenergic blocking agent is used to treat chronic open-angle glaucoma and increased ocular pressure.
USUAL ADULT DOSAGE: 1 drop of 0.5% solution b.i.d.

timolol maleate (Timoptic). A beta$_1$- and beta$_2$-adrenergic blocking agent, timolol is used to treat chronic open-angle glaucoma, aphakic glaucoma (occurring in an eye with no lens), and increased ocular pressure.
USUAL ADULT DOSAGE: initially, 1 drop of 0.25% solution b.i.d., reduced to once daily for maintenance; if the patient does not respond, 1 drop of 0.5% solution b.i.d.

glycerin, anhydrous (Osmoglyn). This hyperosmotic agent is used to treat corneal edema before ophthalmoscopy or gonioscopy and to treat acute closed-angle glaucoma and keratitis bullosa.
USUAL ADULT DOSAGE: 1 to 1.5 grams/kg P.O. every 5 hours, if necessary.

isosorbide (Ismotic). This oral hyperosmotic agent is used for short-term reduction of increased intraocular pressure from glaucoma and for preoperative reduction of intraocular pressure.
USUAL ADULT DOSAGE: 1.5 grams/kg P.O. up to four times per day.

levobunolol hydrochloride (Betagan). A long-acting, nonselective beta-adrenergic blocking agent, levobunolol is used to treat chronic open-angle glaucoma and increased ocular pressure.
USUAL ADULT DOSAGE: 1 drop of 0.5% solution once or twice daily.

mannitol (Osmitrol). A hyperosmotic agent, mannitol is used to reduce increased intraocular pressure during an episode of acute closed-angle glaucoma.

USUAL ADULT DOSAGE: 0.5 to 2 grams/kg of a 20% solution administered I.V. over 30 to 60 minutes.

urea (Ureaphil). This hyperosmotic agent is used to reduce increased intraocular pressure during an episode of acute closed-angle glaucoma.
USUAL ADULT DOSAGE: 1 to 1.5 grams/kg of 30% solution administered I.V. over 1½ to 2 hours.
USUAL PEDIATRIC DOSAGE: 0.5 to 1.5 grams/kg of 30% solution administered I.V. over 1½ to 2 hours for children over age 2.

acetazolamide (Ak-Zol, Diamox) and **acetazolamide sodium** (Diamox Parenteral, Diamox Sodium). A carbonic anhydrase inhibitor, acetazolamide is used primarily to treat chronic open-angle glaucoma.
USUAL ADULT DOSAGE: 250 mg P.O. daily to q.i.d. For rapid lowering of intraocular pressure, 500 mg I.M. or I.V. initially (may be repeated in 2 to 4 hours).

dichlorphenamide (Daranide, Oratrol). This carbonic anhydrase inhibitor is used as adjunctive therapy for patients with chronic open-angle glaucoma.
USUAL ADULT DOSAGE: initially, 100 to 200 mg P.O., followed by 100 mg every 12 hours until therapeutic response occurs; maintenance dose, 25 to 50 mg P.O. b.i.d. or t.i.d.

methazolamide (Neptazane). This carbonic anhydrase inhibitor is used to treat chronic open-angle glaucoma. Methazolamide is also used preoperatively in patients with acute closed-angle glaucoma.
USUAL ADULT DOSAGE: 50 to 100 mg P.O. b.i.d. or t.i.d.

Drug interactions
No significant interactions occur between hyperosmotic agents and other drugs. Interactions between timolol and such oral beta-adrenergic blocking agents as propranolol increase ocular and systemic effects; caution is required with concomitant use of these drugs. The adrenergic-blocking agents also should be used cautiously with MAO inhibitors. Patients using acetazolamide with a salicylate may need a reduction in salicylate dosage.

ADVERSE REACTIONS

Adverse reactions vary among the topical adrenergic agents, hyperosmotic agents, and carbonic anhydrase inhibitors. The adrenergic-blocking agents can reduce heart rate, causing headaches and fatigue, and the beta blockade effects from systemic timolol absorption may lead to bradycardia and bronchospasm. The hyperosmotic agents can cause stinging when administered. Use of a topical anesthetic is recommended with glycerin administration. (See Chapter 38, Diuretic Agents, for adverse reactions caused by mannitol and urea.) Carbonic anhydrase inhibitors such as acetazolamide can cause drowsiness, hypokalemia, nausea, vomiting, leukopenia, hemolytic anemia, and aplastic anemia.

NURSING IMPLICATIONS

The three groups of drugs that lower intraocular pressure—topical adrenergic agents, hyperosmotic agents, and carbonic anhydrase inhibitors—have distinctive contraindications and precautions, as reflected in the following nursing considerations:
• Be aware that epinephrine is contraindicated in patients with closed-angle glaucoma.
• Be aware that the adrenergic-blocking agents are contraindicated in patients with bronchial asthma or chronic obstructive pulmonary disease; administer them cautiously to patients with sinus bradycardia or heart block.
• Isosorbide, mannitol, and urea are contraindicated in patients with dehydration, pulmonary edema, hemorrhagic glaucoma, or anuria from severe renal disease.
• If appropriate, instruct the patient in self-instillation of eye drops, explaining the importance of not touching the eyedropper to the eye and of hand washing before and after self-instillation.

ANESTHETIC AGENTS

Because the cornea and the conjunctiva contain delicate sensory nerves, surgical (and some diagnostic) procedures involving the eye would be impossible without anesthetics. Topical ophthalmic anesthetics anesthetize the corneal surface so that instruments can be applied to measure intraocular pressure or to remove foreign bodies. Local ophthalmic anesthetics of the globe and eyelid are injected to anesthetize and to paralyze muscles in the eye, eyelid, and face.

Topical ophthalmic anesthetics covered here are proparacaine hydrocholoride, tetracaine, and tetracaine hydrochloride. (For information on uses of other local [regional] anesthetics, such as procaine hydrochloride,

bupivacaine hydrochloride, lidocaine hydrochloride, mepivacaine hydrochloride, prilocaine hydrochloride, and etidocaine hydrochloride, see Chapter 28, Local and Topical Anesthetic Agents.)

Topical cocaine is a natural compound. Because of its corneal toxicity and adverse central nervous system (CNS) reactions, it has been practically replaced by synthetic anesthetics and will not be covered here.

PHARMACOKINETICS

Most of these anesthetics have an onset of action of 1 minute. The duration of action for anesthetics administered by retrobulbar injection is 30 to 60 minutes.

PHARMACODYNAMICS

Proparacaine and tetracaine act by interfering with cell activity. Some ophthalmic anesthetics are effective only when applied topically; others must be injected. More drops may be required to anesthetize an inflamed eye because the blood vessels carry the anesthetic away.

PHARMACOTHERAPEUTICS

Besides anesthetizing the cornea to allow application of instruments for measuring intraocular pressure or removing foreign bodies, topical ophthalmic anesthetics are used for suture removal, for conjunctival or corneal scraping, and for lacrimal canal manipulation. (See Chapter 28, Local and Topical Anesthetic Agents, for dosages used for retrobulbar injection.)

proparacaine hydrochloride (Alcaine, Ophthaine). This topical anesthetic is used for tonometry, gonioscopy, corneal suture removal, and removal of corneal foreign bodies.
USUAL ADULT DOSAGE: 1 to 2 drops of 0.5% solution just before the procedure; for anesthesia for cataract extraction or glaucoma surgery, 1 drop of 0.5% solution every 5 to 10 minutes for five to seven doses; for suture or foreign body removal, 1 drop of 0.5% solution 2 to 3 minutes before the procedure.

tetracaine (Pontocaine) and **tetracaine hydrochloride** (Pontocaine Hydrochloride). These topical anesthetics are used for tonometry, gonioscopy, removal of corneal foreign bodies, corneal suture removal, and other diagnostic and minor surgical procedures. Tetracaine is a 0.5% ointment; tetracaine hydrochloride, a 0.5% solution.
USUAL ADULT AND PEDIATRIC DOSAGE: 1 to 2 drops of 0.5% solution or a ½- to 1-inch ribbon of 0.5% ointment just before the procedure.

Drug interactions

The only significant interaction involving the topical ophthalmic anesthetics occurs with tetracaine, which interferes with the antibacterial action of the sulfonamides. They should be administered ½ hour apart to prevent this interaction. (See Chapter 28, Local and Topical Anesthetic Agents, for drug interactions involving the regional agents.)

ADVERSE REACTIONS

The injectable ophthalmic anesthetics may depress blood pressure and respiration and stimulate the CNS, resulting in nervousness, syncope, nausea, and seizures. Or, respiratory or circulatory collapse may occur from CNS depression. Acute closed-angle glaucoma can also occur.

All four topical ophthalmic anesthetics can cause transient eye pain and redness. Prolonged use can cause keratitis, corneal opacities, scarring, loss of visual acuity, and delayed corneal healing.

NURSING IMPLICATIONS

The nurse should be aware of the following implications when caring for a patient receiving ophthalmic anesthetics:
• Administer proparacaine cautiously to patients with cardiac disease or hyperthyroidism.
• If necessary, provide the patient with a protective eye patch to be worn while the eye is anesthetized.
• After administration, apply digital pressure to the lacrimal sac to prevent systemic absorption and adverse CNS reactions.
• Be prepared to administer emergency care if a patient has an adverse reaction such as edema of the respiratory passages, which may require respiratory resuscitation as well as I.V. administration of hydrocortisone. Have emergency drugs, such as hydrocortisone and epinephrine, available.
• Be prepared to assist if any adverse reaction to the local anesthetic occurs.
• Advise the patient receiving a topical anesthetic not to rub the eye(s); explain that corneal abrasion may occur because the usual pain signal is absent. Also explain that the anesthetic will cause transient blurred vision.

ANTI-INFLAMMATORY AGENTS

Corticosteroids, hormones secreted by the adrenal glands, are produced synthetically for pharmacologic, including ophthalmic, use. Ophthalmic anti-inflammatory agents are corticosteroid solutions or suspensions that decrease leukocyte infiltration at the site of ocular inflammation. Cortisone was the first hormone to be isolated. Investigators used to believe that corticosteroids were contraindicated in patients with infectious diseases. Today, however, corticosteroids may be used cautiously with antimicrobial and antiviral agents when the offending organism has been identified to help prevent serious eye damage caused by inflammation. The topical agents used include dexamethasone, fluorometholone, medrysone, prednisolone acetate, and prednisolone sodium phosphate.

PHARMACOKINETICS

Absorption of topical anti-inflammatory agents through the intact cornea is minimal. Suspensions, such as dexamethasone, are usually more completely absorbed than solutions, such as prednisolone sodium phosphate. Onset and duration of action vary among these anti-inflammatory agents; specific information is unavailable.

PHARMACODYNAMICS

Ophthalmic anti-inflammatory agents' effect of decreasing leukocyte infiltration at inflammation sites reduces the exudative reaction of diseased tissue, leading to reduced edema, redness, and scarring.

PHARMACOTHERAPEUTICS

Corticosteroids are used to treat inflammatory disorders and hypersensitivity-related conditions of the cornea, iris, conjunctiva, sclera, and anterior uvea.

dexamethasone (Maxidex Ophthalmic Suspension). Dexamethasone is used to treat uveitis; iridocyclitis; inflammatory conditions of the eyelid, conjunctiva, cornea, and anterior segment; and corneal injury from chemical or thermal burns, penetration of foreign bodies, and allergic conjunctivitis.
USUAL ADULT AND PEDIATRIC DOSAGE: 1 to 2 drops of 0.1% solution instilled into conjunctival sac; for severe

disease, drops may be used hourly, tapering to discontinuation as condition improves; in mild conditions, drops may be used up to six times daily; treatment may extend from a few days to several weeks.

fluorometholone (Fluor-Op, FML). Fluorometholone is used to treat inflammatory and hypersensitivity-related conditions of the cornea, conjunctiva, sclera, and anterior uvea. It is available as an ointment and as a suspension. Adult and pediatric dosages are the same.
USUAL ADULT DOSAGE: 1 to 2 drops of 0.1% or 0.25% suspension every hour for the first 24 to 48 hours, then 1 to 2 drops of suspension b.i.d. to q.i.d.; or ½" (1.25 cm) of ointment every six hours for 24 to 48 hours, then b.i.d. to daily.

medrysone (HMS Liquifilm Ophthalmic). This anti-inflammatory agent is used to treat allergic conjunctivitis, vernal conjunctivitis, episcleritis, and ophthalmic epinephrine reaction. Adult and pediatric dosages are the same.
USUAL ADULT DOSAGE: 1 drop of 1% solution instilled in the conjunctival sac b.i.d. to q.i.d.; may be used every hour during initial 1 to 2 days, if needed.

prednisolone acetate (Econopred, Pred Mild) and **prednisolone sodium phosphate** (Ak-Pred, Metreton Ophthalmic). Prednisolone is used to treat inflammation of the palpebral and bulbar conjunctiva, the cornea, and the anterior segment. Adult and pediatric dosages are the same.
USUAL ADULT DOSAGE: 1 to 2 drops of 0.12% to 1% suspension; for severe conditions, may be used hourly, tapering to discontinuation; for mild conditions, may be used up to six times daily.

Drug interactions
No significant interactions occur between ophthalmic corticosteroid anti-inflammatory agents and other drugs.

ADVERSE REACTIONS
These drugs can increase intraocular pressure, especially in the elderly. Corneal thinning or ulceration, interference with corneal wound healing, and increased susceptibility to viral or fungal corneal infection can also occur. Long-term or excessive use of these drugs can lead to glaucoma exacerbations, cataracts, reduced visual acuity, and optic nerve damage. Excessive or long-term use of suspensions, which are more readily absorbed, can lead to adrenal suppression.

NURSING IMPLICATIONS
Ophthalmic anti-inflammatory agents are associated with significant contraindications and precautions, including patient-teaching precautions. To administer these drugs safely and effectively, the nurse should be aware of the following considerations:
• Remember that ophthalmic anti-inflammatory agents are contraindicated in patients with vaccinia, varicella, acute superficial herpes simplex, and other fungal and viral diseases that the corticosteroids will worsen; they are also contraindicated in ocular tuberculosis and acute purulent eye infections.
• Administer anti-inflammatory agents cautiously in patients with corneal abrasions, which are commonly contaminated with herpes.
• Be aware that anti-inflammatory agents are not for long-term use.
• Be aware that fluorometholone is less likely than the other anti-inflammatory agents to increase intraocular pressure with long-term use.
• Instruct the patient to notify the physician if any change in visual acuity or visual fields occurs.
• Teach the patient how to instill the drug, including shaking the suspension well before instillation and applying pressure lightly with a finger on the lacrimal sac to minimize systemic absorption.

ANTI-INFECTIVE AGENTS

Ophthalmic anti-infective agents include antibacterial, antiseptic, and antiviral agents. To treat eye diseases, anti-infective agents may be injected beneath the conjunctiva, administered orally, or instilled into the eye. Topical anti-infective therapy will be covered here.

Applied as solution or ointment, topical anti-infective agents including bacitracin, boric acid, chloramphenicol, chlortetracycline hydrochloride, erythromycin, gentamicin sulfate, idoxuridine, natamycin, polymyxin B sulfate, silver nitrate 1%, sulfacetamide, tetracycline hydrochloride, tobramycin, trifluridine, and vidarabine, are often sufficient to treat superficial infections of the conjunctiva, cornea, or eyelids. However, systemic antibacterials may be used along with topical anti-infective agents to treat some patients with conjunctivitis, endophthalmitis, or infections of the ocular adnexa (eyelids and lacrimal apparatus). (For information on systemic antibacterials that achieve therapeutic levels in the eye, see Chapter 66, Antibacterial Agents.)

PHARMACOKINETICS

The pharmacokinetics of the ophthalmic anti-infective agents vary greatly. A physician will prescribe a specific agent based on its spectrum and mechanism of action.

Absorption, distribution, metabolism, excretion
Bacitracin, chloramphenicol, polymyxin B sulfate, and tobramycin penetrate the cornea and conjunctiva; chloramphenicol and tobramycin also penetrate aqueous humor. Silver nitrate does not penetrate intraocularly. Boric acid and idoxuridine are poorly absorbed topically. Erythromycin, gentamicin sulfate, polymyxin B, and the tetracyclines penetrate poorly through an intact cornea but well through corneal abrasions. Natamycin does not reach measurable levels in the deeper corneal layers unless a defect in the epithelium is present. Sulfacetamide's intraocular penetration varies. Trifluridine and vidarabine are found in trace amounts in the aqueous humor after topical application to a cornea with an epithelial defect or inflammation, but neither drug is significantly absorbed systemically.

Bacitracin, chloramphenicol, polymyxin B, and gentamicin are excreted via the nasolacrimal system.

Onset, peak, duration
As a rule, ophthalmic anti-infective agents are administered in frequent doses—as often as every 2 hours. Their onset and duration of action vary according to the patient's disorder and response.

PHARMACODYNAMICS

Antibacterials are chemical substances that inhibit the growth of, or directly kill, bacteria. Antibacterials are selected after the infecting organism is identified; however, withholding therapy until cultures are made is impractical. As a result, most ophthalmologists use broad-spectrum antibacterials until sensitivity has been determined. Broad-spectrum antibacterials provide complete coverage and minimize hypersensitivity reactions. (See Chapter 66, Antibacterial Agents, and Chapter 68, Antiviral Agents, for further information.)

Mechanism of action
Bacitracin, chloramphenicol, erythromycin, gentamicin, polymyxin B, the tetracyclines, and chlortetracycline inhibit protein synthesis in susceptible microorganisms. Tobramycin's mechanism of action is unknown, but it

may inhibit protein synthesis. Boric acid's mechanism of action is unknown. Idoxuridine, trifluridine, and vidarabine interfere with deoxyribonucleic acid (DNA) synthesis in susceptible organisms. Natamycin increases fungal cell membrane permeability. Silver nitrate, instilled in the eyes of neonates, causes protein denaturation that prevents gonorrheal ophthalmia neonatorum. Sulfacetamide prevents uptake of para-aminobenzoic acid, a metabolite of bacterial folic acid synthesis.

PHARMACOTHERAPEUTICS

Bacitracin is effective against infections with gram-positive organisms. Chloramphenicol and gentamicin are used to treat gram-positive and gram-negative bacterial infections. Erythromycin is used to fight infections with gram-positive cocci and gram-positive bacilli. Sulfacetamide provides a wide spectrum of activity and effectiveness against some gram-positive and gram-negative bacterial infections. Natamycin is used to treat fungal infections. Polymyxin B is effective against infections with gram-negative organisms.

The earliest developed antiviral agent, idoxuridine is invaluable in treating herpes simplex of the cornea, because it prevents the herpes virus from feeding off the cells of the corneal epithelium.

The antiviral ophthalmic ointment vidarabine also is used to treat corneal herpes simplex, particularly in early stages.

Trifluridine, an antiviral solution, also is used to treat herpes simplex infections, primary keratoconjunctivitis, and recurrent epithelial keratitis.

bacitracin (Baciguent). This antibacterial agent is used to treat ocular infections.
USUAL ADULT AND PEDIATRIC DOSAGE: apply a ½″ ribbon of ointment into the conjunctival sac several times a day or p.r.n. until a favorable response is achieved.

boric acid (Blinx, Ocu-Boracin). This antiseptic is used for eye irrigation after tonometry, gonioscopy, foreign body removal, or fluorescein use. It is also used to soothe and cleanse the eyes and in connection with contact lens use.
USUAL ADULT DOSAGE: eye irrigation with 2% solution or 5% or 10% ointment, applied two or three times daily.

chloramphenicol (Chloromycetin Ophthalmic, Chloroptic, Chloroptic S.O.P., Econochlor Ophthalmic, Pentamycetin). Chloramphenicol, as a solution or an ointment, is used to treat surface bacterial infections involving the conjunctiva or cornea.

USUAL ADULT AND PEDIATRIC DOSAGE: 2 drops of 0.5% solution instilled every hour until the condition improves or q.i.d., depending on the severity of the infection, or a small amount of 1% ointment applied to the lower conjunctival sac at bedtime as a supplement to drops; ointment may be used alone by applying a small amount to the lower conjunctival sac every 3 to 6 hours or more often, if necessary, until the condition improves.

chlortetracycline hydrochloride (Aureomycin). This antibacterial agent is used to treat superficial ocular infections. Adult and pediatric dosages are the same.

USUAL ADULT DOSAGE: 1% ointment or 1 to 2 drops of 1% solution applied or instilled every 3 to 4 hours or b.i.d. to t.i.d., depending on the severity of the infection.

erythromycin (Ilotycin Ophthalmic). This antibacterial agent is used to treat acute and chronic conjunctivitis, trachoma, and other eye infections.

USUAL ADULT AND PEDIATRIC DOSAGE: 0.5% ointment applied one or more times daily, depending on the severity of the infection.

gentamicin sulfate (Garamycin Ophthalmic, Genoptic). This antibacterial agent is used to treat external ocular infections (conjunctivitis, keratoconjunctivitis, corneal ulcers, blepharitis, blepharoconjunctivitis, meibomianitis, and dacryocystitis) from susceptible organisms, especially *Pseudomonas aeruginosa, Proteus, Klebsiella pneumoniae, Escherichia coli,* and other gram-negative organisms.

USUAL ADULT AND PEDIATRIC DOSAGE: 1 to 2 drops of 0.3% solution instilled every 4 hours; for severe infections, up to 2 drops every hour or 0.3% ointment applied to the lower conjunctival sac b.i.d. or t.i.d.

idoxuridine (Herplex, Stoxil). This antiviral agent is used to treat herpes simplex keratitis.

USUAL ADULT AND PEDIATRIC DOSAGE: 1 drop of 0.1% solution instilled into the conjunctival sac every hour during the day and every 2 hours at night, or 0.5% ointment applied to the conjunctival sac every 4 hours or five times daily, with the last dose at bedtime; response should occur within 7 days, or therapy should be discontinued as ordered and alternate therapy begun; therapy should not be continued longer than 21 days.

natamycin (Natacyn). This antifungal agent is used to treat fungal keratitis, conjunctivitis, and blepharitis.

USUAL ADULT DOSAGE: initially, 1 drop of 5% suspension instilled in the conjunctival sac every 1 to 2 hours; after 3 to 4 days, dosage is reduced to 1 drop six to eight times daily.

polymyxin B sulfate (Neosporin Ophthalmic). This antibacterial agent is used alone or in combination with other agents to treat corneal ulcers from *Pseudomonas* as well as other gram-negative organism infections and for endophthalmitis.

USUAL ADULT AND PEDIATRIC DOSAGE: 1 to 3 drops of 0.1% to 0.25% (10,000 to 25,000 units/ml) solution instilled every hour or 0.5% ointment placed in the conjunctival sac every 3 to 4 hours; interval is increased as ordered, according to patient response. For endophthalmitis, up to 10,000 units injected subconjunctivally daily.

silver nitrate 1%. This antiseptic agent is used to prevent gonorrheal ophthalmia neonatorum.

USUAL PEDIATRIC DOSAGE: for neonates, 1 drop of 1% solution after the eyelids are cleansed.

sulfacetamide sodium 10% (Bleph-10 Liquifilm Ophthalmic, Cetamide Ophthalmic, Sulamyd Sodium 10% Ophthalmic), **sulfacetamide sodium 15%** (Isopto Cetamide Ophthalmic, Sulfair-15 Ophthalmic), and **sulfacetamide sodium 30%** (Sulamyd Sodium 30% Ophthalmic). Sulfacetamide sodium (a sulfonamide antibacterial) is used to treat inclusion conjunctivitis, corneal ulcers, and trachoma. It is also used for prophylaxis against ocular infection after foreign body removal or eye injury.

USUAL ADULT AND PEDIATRIC DOSAGE: 1 to 2 drops of 10% solution instilled into the lower conjunctival sac every 2 to 3 hours during the day, less often at night; or, initially, 1 to 2 drops of 15% solution instilled into the lower conjunctival sac every 1 to 2 hours, then at increasing intervals as the patient responds; or 1 drop of 30% solution instilled into the lower conjunctival sac every 2 hours; ½ inch to 1 inch of 10% ointment applied to the conjunctival sac q.i.d. and at bedtime (ointment may be used at night and drops during the day).

tetracycline hydrochloride (Achromycin Ophthalmic). This anti-infective agent is used to treat superficial ocular infections, inclusion conjunctivitis, and trachoma.

USUAL ADULT AND PEDIATRIC DOSAGE: for superficial ocular infections and inclusion conjunctivitis, a small amount of 1% ointment or 1 to 2 drops of 1% solution instilled b.i.d. to q.i.d. or more often, depending on severity; for trachoma, 2 drops instilled b.i.d., t.i.d., or q.i.d., continued for 3 weeks along with oral therapy.

Ophthalmic agents

The following chart summarizes commonly used ophthalmic agents.

DRUG	MAJOR INDICATIONS	USUAL ADULT DOSAGES	NURSING IMPLICATIONS
Mydriatics and cycloplegics			
atropine	Acute iritis	1 to 2 drops of 0.5 to 2% solution b.i.d. or t.i.d.	● Monitor small children receiving atropine for the following: fever, flushing, increased heart rate, diaphoresis, confusion, and following: fever, flushing, increased heart rate, diaphoresis, confusion and irritability. ● Apply digital pressure on the patient's lacrimal sac to help prevent systemic absorption.
	Refraction	1 to 2 drops of 1% solution 1 hour before eye examination	
cyclopentolate	Mydriasis and cycloplegia	1 drop of 1% solution followed by 1 drop 5 minutes later; use 2% solution in patients with heavily pigmented irises	● This drug is for topical use only; it can produce central nervous system (CNS) disturbances in infants and children. To help prevent systemic absorption, apply digital pressure on the lacrimal sac. ● Apply disposable eye protection to accommodate sensitivity to light. The patient may experience photophobia. ● Advise the patient not to drive or engage in hazardous activities until vision clears.
tropicamide	Refraction	1 drop of 1% solution, 20 minutes before examination, repeated as needed in 20 to 30 minutes	● This drug is contraindicated in patients with glaucoma or a tendency toward glaucoma. ● Monitor infants and children for CNS disturbances. ● Instruct parents to apply digital pressure on the lacrimal sac and to wash hands after administration. ● Provide protection against bright light; the patient may experience photophobia. ● Instruct the patient not to drive or engage in hazardous activities until vision clears.
	Funduscopic examination	1 drop of 0.5% solution 15 to 20 minutes before examination	
Miotics			
carbachol	Miosis	0.5 ml of 0.01% solution into the anterior chamber	● Miosis usually causes difficulty in the dark; instruct the patient to use caution in night driving. ● Carbachol can cause systemic symptoms of a cholinesterase inhibitor. Help prevent absorption by applying digital pressure on the lacrimal sac. ● Use cautiously in patients with cardiac failure, bronchial asthma, active peptic ulcers, GI spasm, or Parkinson's disease.
	Open-angle or closed-angle glaucoma	1 drop of 0.75% to 3% solution instilled into conjunctival sac every 4 to 8 hours	
pilocarpine	Chronic open-angle glaucoma	1 to 2 drops of 1% to 2% solution every 4 to 8 hours	● Pilocarpine can produce skin allergies and conjunctival hypersensitivity reactions. Observe the patient for conjunctival redness and swelling. ● Miosis usually causes difficulty in the dark; instruct the patient to use caution in night driving.
	Before surgery to treat acute closed-angle glaucoma	1 drop of 2% solution instilled three to six times over a 30-minute period before surgery	

SELECTED MAJOR DRUGS

Ophthalmic agents continued

DRUG	MAJOR INDICATIONS	USUAL ADULT DOSAGES	NURSING IMPLICATIONS
Drugs that lower intraocular pressure			
glycerin, anhydrous	Acute closed-angle glaucoma, keratitis bullosa or before intraocular surgery	1 to 1.5 grams/kg P.O. every 5 hours, if necessary	• Administer the drug with orange juice or another juice to make it more palatable. • This drug can cause nausea, vomiting, or headaches. Be prepared to assist the patient if vomiting occurs.
timolol	Chronic open-angle glaucoma, aphakic glaucoma, increased ocular pressure	1 drop of 0.25% solution b.i.d., initially; may be increased to 1 drop of 0.5% solution b.i.d.	• Timolol is contraindicated in patients with bronchial asthma or chronic obstructive pulmonary disease. • Use caution when administering the drug to patients with sinus bradycardia or heart block.

tobramycin (Tobrex). This anti-infective agent is used to treat external ocular infections from susceptible gram-negative bacteria.
USUAL ADULT AND PEDIATRIC DOSAGE: for mild to moderate infections, a 0.4-inch (1-cm) ribbon of 0.3% ointment or 1 to 2 drops of 0.3% solution instilled every 4 hours; for severe infections, 2 drops instilled hourly.

trifluridine (Viroptic Ophthalmic Solution). This antiviral agent is used to treat primary keratoconjunctivitis and recurrent epithelial keratitis resulting from herpes simplex virus, Types I and II.
USUAL ADULT DOSAGE: 1 drop of 1% solution every 2 hours while the patient is awake to a maximum of 9 drops daily until reepithelialization of the corneal ulcer occurs, then 1 drop every 4 hours (minimum 5 drops daily) for an additional 7 days.

vidarabine (Vira-A Ophthalmic). This antiviral agent is used to treat acute keratoconjunctivitis, superficial keratitis, and recurrent epithelial keratitis resulting from herpes simplex virus, Types I and II.
USUAL ADULT AND PEDIATRIC DOSAGE: ½-inch (1.25-cm) ribbon of 3% ointment applied to the lower conjunctival sac five times daily at 3-hour intervals.

Drug interactions
Combined use of bacitracin and silver nitrate inactivates the bacitracin, but no significant interactions occur between most anti-infectives and other drugs. Sulfacetamide action will be decreased if it is used with local anesthetics, such as procaine, tetracaine, and para-aminobenzoic acid derivatives; wait 30 to 60 minutes after anesthetic instillation before instilling sulfacetamide.

ADVERSE DRUG REACTIONS

Hypersensitivity reactions to sulfonamides may ocur; reactions may be severe.

NURSING IMPLICATIONS

The nurse should be aware of the following considerations when caring for patients receiving anti-infectives:
• Advise the patient against indiscriminate or prolonged use of antibacterials; hypersensitivity or bacterial resistance may develop.
• Encourage the patient to see an ophthalmologist if a secondary eye infection occurs and to notify the ophthalmologist if the condition does not improve within 48 hours of initial treatment.
• Teach the patient with herpes simplex infection about the course of this disease. Explain that herpes can and will recur and that, at the first sign of onset, the patient should contact the ophthalmologist and start the prescribed medication.
• Document the patient's history of allergy if sulfacetamide is prescribed; hypersensitivity reactions to sulfonamides can be severe.

CHAPTER SUMMARY

Chapter 79 discussed ophthalmic agents as they are used ·to achieve mydriasis, cycloplegia, miosis, and anesthesia;

to lower intraocular pressure; and to treat ocular inflammation and infection. Here are the highlights of the chapter:

• Ophthalmic agents include (1) mydriatics and cycloplegics, (2) miotics, (3) drugs that lower intraocular pressure, (4) anesthetic agents, (5) anti-inflammatory agents, and (6) anti-infective agents.

• Mydriatics dilate the pupil; cycloplegics paralyze the fine-focusing muscles of the eye. Mydriatics and cycloplegics are used primarily for intraocular examinations and refractions.

• The nurse should not administer mydriatics and cycloplegics to patients with closed-angle glaucoma—pupil dilation can lead to an acute glaucoma episode. Digital pressure on the lacrimal sac helps prevent systemic absorption and decreases the risk of adverse reactions.

• Miotics—including direct-acting cholinergics, short-acting anticholinesterases, and long-acting anticholinesterases—are used primarily to treat glaucoma and to manage accommodative esotropia.

• Pilocarpine is the drug of choice to treat glaucoma. It can be used for prolonged periods of time, and it causes minimal adverse reactions.

• Drugs that lower intraocular pressure include topical adrenergic blocking agents, hyperosmotic agents, and carbonic anhydrase inhibitors.

• The carbonic anhydrase inhibitors decrease aqueous production by inhibiting the action of carbonic anhydrase. When less fluid enters the eye, intraocular pressure decreases.

• Corticosteroid anti-inflammatory agents reduce ocular edema, redness, and scarring.

• Prolonged or indiscriminate use of antibacterial agents can lead to resistant strains of bacteria. Antiviral agents are used to treat ocular herpes simplex.

BIBLIOGRAPHY

Barnhart, E.R., *Physician's Desk Reference for Ophthalmology*. Oradell, N.J.: Medical Economics Books, 1986.

Fraunfelder, F. "Extraocular Fluid Dynamics: How Best to Apply Topical Ocular Medication," *Transactions of the American Ophthalmological Society* vol. LXXIV, 1976.

Nursing88 Drug Handbook. Springhouse, Pa.: Springhouse Corp., 1988.

Smith, J.F., and Nachazel, D.P., Jr. *Ophthalmologic Nursing*. Boston: Little, Brown & Co., 1980.

Stein, H.A., and Slatt, B.J. *The Ophthalmic Assistant*, 4th ed. St. Louis: C.V. Mosby Co., 1983.

CHAPTER
80
OTIC AGENTS

OBJECTIVES

After reading and studying this chapter, you should be able to:
1. Identify the indications for the different classes of otic agents, including anti-infective, anti-inflammatory, local anesthestic, and ceruminolytic agents.
2. Describe the techniques involved in the various administration routes for otic agents.
3. Identify the adverse drug reactions associated with anti-infective otics and describe preventive measures the nurse can take to avoid these reactions.
4. Describe the uses of anti-inflammatory otics.
5. Identify the possible adverse reactions to and contraindications for the anti-inflammatory otics.
6. Explain how benzocaine produces analgesia.
7. Describe the mechanism of action for the ceruminolytic carbamide peroxide.
8. Identify the contraindications for both carbamide peroxide and triethanolamine.

INTRODUCTION

Physicians prescribe otic agents to treat ear infection, inflammation, and pain, and to soften cerumen (earwax). These drugs are categorized as anti-infective agents (single and compound), anti-inflammatory agents, local anesthetics, and ceruminolytic agents. Otic agents are administered via eardrops, ear irrigations, or ear wicks. Several combination products containing both anti-infective and anti-inflammatory agents are available.

For a summary of representative drugs, *See Selected major drugs: Otic agents* on pages 1253 and 1254.

ANTI-INFECTIVE AGENTS

The anti-infective otics represent natural antibiotics or synthetic antibiotic derivatives. Physicians use boric acid and acetic acid, referred to as weak topical anti-infective agents, to treat infections of the external auditory canal (otitis externa) and those of the middle ear (otitis media). These drugs are administered alone or with other anti-infective otics or corticosteroids. Anti-infective otics may also be combined with systemic anti-infective therapy.

The antimicrobial activity of these drugs varies. Most anti-infective otics exhibit a broad spectrum of activity against both gram-positive and gram-negative organisms; a few of the agents have a narrow spectrum.

History and source

Researchers have isolated antibiotics from various microorganisms living in the soil. In 1947, chloramphenicol was isolated in Venezuela from a soil sample containing *Streptomyces venezuelae*, and polymyxin was discovered from *Bacillus polymyxa*, an aerobic spore-forming rod found in the soil. The tetracyclines were introduced in 1948. Neomycin was isolated in 1949 from *Streptomyces fradiae*. Colistin is formed by *Bacillus polymyxa* var. *colistinus*, originally found in Japan.

PHARMACOKINETICS

Long-term use of neomycin may lead to some systemic absorption, but the absorption is not clinically significant. Most anti-infective otics begin to act within 1 hour and have a 4-hour duration of action. The full therapeutic effect of these drugs may not be seen for 2 to 3 days.

PHARMACODYNAMICS

Anti-infective otics are either bactericidal (kill bacteria), or bacteriostatic (inhibit bacterial growth). Both boric acid and acetic acid possess weak bacteriostatic properties and are also fungistatic (inhibit fungal growth).

Mechanism of action

The anti-infective otics kill or inhibit bacterial growth by interfering with the metabolic functions of bacteria. Chloramphenicol primarily inhibits peptide bond formation and protein synthesis in susceptible bacteria. Neomycin inhibits protein synthesis in susceptible bacteria. Polymyxin B and colistin alter the osmotic barrier of the bacterial membrane, enabling essential cellular metabolites to leak out.

Before the administration of an anti-infective otic, the physician identifies the causative organism and conducts drug susceptibility tests to determine the drug's effectiveness and appropriateness. The anti-infective otic should be discontinued if the causative organism becomes resistant to it.

PHARMACOTHERAPEUTICS

Physicians prescribe anti-infective otics for otitis externa caused by various bacteria. Polymyxin B and colistin also prove effective in the treatment of otitis media. Many combination products treat a wide range of microorganisms as well as pain and inflammation.

chloramphenicol (Chloromycetin Otic). A broad-spectrum, bacteriostatic antibiotic, chloramphenicol proves effective against a number of gram-positive and gram-negative bacteria, rickettsiae, and chlamydiae. It is used to treat otitis externa.
USUAL ADULT DOSAGE: 2 to 3 drops into the external auditory canal t.i.d.

neomycin sulfate. An aminoglycoside antibiotic, neomycin is used to treat otitis externa and may be administered as an otic solution or suspension.
USUAL ADULT DOSAGE: 4 drops into the external auditory canal t.i.d. or q.i.d. Therapy should be limited to 10 days.
USUAL PEDIATRIC DOSAGE: 3 drops into the external auditory canal t.i.d. or q.i.d. for no more than 10 days.

polymyxin B sulfate. One of several polymyxin antibiotics active against gram-negative organisms, polymyxin B sulfate appears in several combination products used to treat bacterial infections of the external auditory canal and otitis media. Polymyxin B sulfate may be administered as an otic solution or suspension.

USUAL ADULT DOSAGE: 4 drops into the external auditory canal t.i.d. or q.i.d. The total daily dose for an adult should not exceed 2 million units.
USUAL PEDIATRIC DOSAGE: 3 drops into external auditory canal t.i.d. or q.i.d.

colistin sulfate (Coly-Mycin S Otic). Closely related to polymyxin B sulfate, colistin acts against certain gram-negative organisms. It is combined with neomycin and hydrocortisone to treat otitis externa and otitis media.
USUAL ADULT DOSAGE: 4 drops into the external auditory canal t.i.d. or q.i.d.
USUAL PEDIATRIC DOSAGE: 3 drops into the external auditory canal t.i.d. or q.i.d.

acetic acid (Domeboro Otic, VoSol Otic). Used in superficial infections of the external auditory canal, acetic acid provides antibacterial, antifungal, and hydrophilic actions. Acetic acid with hydrocortisone has anti-inflammatory and antipruritic actions as well.
USUAL ADULT DOSAGE: 5 drops into the ear canal t.i.d. or q.i.d.; an ear wick can be inserted for the first 24 hours.

boric acid (Ear-Dry, Swim-Ear). A weak anti-infective agent with fungistatic and bacteriostatic properties, boric acid is indicated in otitis externa.
USUAL ADULT DOSAGE: 4 to 6 drops in each ear; then plug with cotton t.i.d. or q.i.d.

Drug interactions

Boric acid is incompatible with alkali carbonates, hydroxides, and benzalkonium chloride. Boric acid precipitates in combination with salicylic acid.

ADVERSE DRUG REACTIONS

Superinfections sometimes occur with anti-infective otics, resulting in overgrowth of nonsusceptible organisms. Cumulative nephrotoxicity and neurotoxicity can occur if polymyxin B sulfate is administered topically along with systemic polymyxin B therapy. If topical steroids are combined with anti-infective otics, the clinical signs of bacterial, fungal, or viral infections may be masked.

Patients sensitive to any of the anti-infective otics may experience a hypersensitivity reaction. Neomycin is most likely to produce such a reaction. Hypersensitivity reactions may be suppressed when the anti-infective otic is administered with a topical steroid.

NURSING IMPLICATIONS

Though anti-infective otics can be used safely to treat otitis externa, the nurse should always watch for hypersensitivity reactions. The nurse must teach proper administration techniques because most anti-infective otic agents are used on an outpatient basis. The nurse must be aware of the following considerations:

• Administer neomycin with caution to patients with otitis externa complicated by chronic otitis media.

• Do not instill boric acid or neomycin into the auditory canal if the tympanic membrane is perforated.

• Monitor the patient for a hypersensitivity reaction, which may occur during treatment with anti-infective otics. Symptoms include ear itching or burning, urticaria, and vesicular or maculopapular dermatitis. Notify the physician of any symptoms because another drug may need to be substituted.

• Be alert for symptoms of a superinfection, including continued ear pain, inflammation, and fever. If you suspect a superinfection, contact the physician.

• Before administering an anti-infective otic agent, perform a patch test to determine allergic contact dermatitis in patients who are sensitive to other agents. To perform this test, apply the otic agent onto the flexor surface of the patient's arm or forearm. Cover the area with a small sterile bandage and wait 24 hours before observing for erythema and urticaria.

• Clean and dry the ear canal before administering anti-infective otic solutions or suspensions.

• Before instillation, warm the anti-infective otic to room temperature by rolling the bottle between your hands or allowing it to stand at room temperature for about 30 minutes. A solution that is too hot or cold may stimulate the central nervous system, possibly causing vertigo or nausea.

• Instruct the patient to contact the physician immediately upon experiencing ringing in the ears, decreased hearing acuity, dizziness, or unsteady gait.

• Instruct the patient to discontinue the anti-infective otic and contact the physician if an allergic reaction occurs.

• Teach the patient how to instill eardrops. Tell the patient to fill the dropper with medication and hold it in one hand. Instruct the patient to tilt the head with the affected ear upward, then with the free hand to pull the auricle upward and backward (for a child, the auricle should be pulled downward). The drops can now be instilled into the ear canal. Caution the patient not to touch the ear with the dropper and to remain positioned with the head tilted for 5 to 10 minutes after instilling the drug. Doing so assures that the medication is dispersed to the affected area. (*See Using eardrops* for an illustration of this procedure.)

Using eardrops

Giving drops to an adult

• Shake the bottle if directed, and open it. Fill the dropper and place the bottle within reach.

• Have the patient tilt the head so that the affected ear is up. Then, gently pull the top of the ear up and back to straighten the ear canal.

• Position the dropper above, but not touching the ear, and release the prescribed number of drops.

• Instruct the patient to keep the head tilted for 10 minutes. If desired, plug the ear with cotton moistened with the eardrops. Don't use dry cotton, because it will absorb the drops.

• If ordered, repeat the procedure for the other ear.

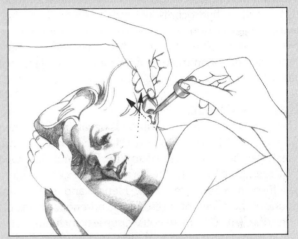

Giving drops to a child

• Lay the child on the side so that the affected ear is turned up.

• Gently pull the ear down and back, then slowly release the prescribed number of drops. (Note the difference in the direction the ear is moved for a child. That is because the child's ear cartilage is immature.)

• If the child experiences any pain after instillation, notify the physician.

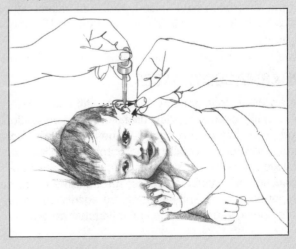

● Instruct the patient not to wash the dropper after use.
● Teach the patient how to insert a cotton pledget moistened with the eardrops, demonstrating how to insert the pledget gently into the ear canal. Inform the patient that the placement of the cotton pledget may impair hearing.

ANTI-INFLAMMATORY AGENTS

The anti-inflammatory agents instilled into the auditory canal include hydrocortisone and its synthetic derivatives. Hydrocortisone is a corticosteroid, a hormone secreted by the adrenal cortex. Anti-inflammatory otics produce anti-inflammatory, antipruritic, and vasoconstrictor effects.

History and source
The development of corticosteroids began in 1855 when Addison and Brown-Séquard established that the adrenal glands were essential to life. Research followed that attempted to isolate the adrenal hormones and identify their functions. In 1949, Hench and others announced the effects of cortisone and adrenocorticotropic hormone (ACTH) in various diseases, including their anti-inflammatory effect in rheumatoid arthritis. Today, physicians widely use synthetic corticosteroids in both systemic and topical forms.

PHARMACOKINETICS
Long-term use of anti-inflammatory otics may cause some systemic absorption, although no clinical effects of the absorption have been noted. Anti-inflammatory otics begin to act within 1 hour, and effects last about 4 hours.

PHARMACODYNAMICS
In an acute inflammatory reaction, anti-inflammatory otics inhibit edema, capillary dilatation, fibrin deposition, and the migration of phagocytes and leukocytes. These drugs also reduce capillary and fibroblast proliferation, collagen deposition, and scar formation. Researchers have not determined the exact mechanisms for these responses. Some anti-inflammatory agents are fluorinated, which enhances the anti-inflammatory action.

PHARMACOTHERAPEUTICS
Anti-inflammatory otics are used for inflammatory conditions of the external ear canal and are administered with a dropper, via an ear wick, or as a cream or ointment.

dexamethasone sodium phosphate (Ak-dex with benzalkonium chloride in otic solution). A fluorinated corticosteroid, dexamethasone sodium phosphate is used to treat inflammatory conditions of the external auditory canal and to relieve symptoms from generalized inflammatory dermatoses.
USUAL ADULT DOSAGE: 3 to 4 drops of solution into the external auditory canal b.i.d. or t.i.d.; when using a gauze wick, first insert the wick into the swollen ear canal, then saturate the wick with the medication. Leave the wick in place for 12 to 24 hours, keeping it moistened with medication while it is in the ear canal.

hydrocortisone and **hydrocortisone acetate** (Cortamed, Otall). For inflammatory conditions of the external auditory canal, hydrocortisone and hydrocortisone acetate are given by dropper or with an ear wick.
USUAL ADULT DOSAGE: 4 to 5 drops into the external auditory canal t.i.d. or q.i.d.; if using a gauze wick, first insert the wick into the ear canal, then saturate the wick with medication, leaving the wick in place for 12 to 24 hours. The wick should be kept moistened with solution while it is in place in the ear canal. The length of treatment will vary from a few days to several weeks.
USUAL PEDIATRIC DOSAGE: for infants and children, 3 drops t.i.d. or q.i.d.

prednisolone sodium phosphate (Metreton). A synthetic glucocorticoid, prednisolone sodium phosphate is used for inflammatory conditions of the external auditory canal.
USUAL ADULT DOSAGE: 3 to 4 drops of solution into the external auditory canal b.i.d. or t.i.d.; if using a gauze wick, first insert the wick, then saturate it with medication, leaving the wick in place for 12 to 24 hours. While in the ear canal, the wick should be kept moistened with solution.

Drug interactions
No significant interactions occur between the anti-inflammatory otics and other drugs.

ADVERSE DRUG REACTIONS
Among predictable adverse reactions, a transient stinging or burning sensation may occur. Anti-inflammatory

agents may also mask or exacerbate an underlying otic infection. A hypersensitivity reaction can occur, though rarely, in patients sensitive to the anti-inflammatory agent.

NURSING IMPLICATIONS

The effectiveness of anti-inflammatory agents may be enhanced with proper cleaning and hygiene of the ear canal. The nurse should also assess for a hypersensitivity reaction and provide patient teaching for proper administration.

• Anti-inflammatory otics are contraindicated in patients with perforated tympanic membranes and in patients with acute, untreated purulent viral, bacterial, or fungal otic conditions.

• Observe the patient for a hypersensitivity reaction. Symptoms include ear itching or burning, urticaria, and vesicular or maculopapular dermatitis.

• Clean and dry the ear canal before administering anti-inflammatory otic agents.

• Administer the anti-inflammatory otic by itself when it is prescribed to treat allergic otitis externa.

• Instill the anti-inflammatory otic sparingly to prevent debris accumulation in the ear canal.

• Anti-inflammatory otics may be administered with anti-infective otics to treat bacterial otitis externa.

• Instruct the patient to discontinue the medication and contact the physician if any signs of an allergic reaction occur.

• Teach the patient how to instill eardrops. (See *Using eardrops* on page 1249 for a description and illustration.)

• Teach the patient how to insert a gauze wick into the ear canal, allowing the loose end of the wick to hang out of the ear canal. The patient then administers the medication, which is absorbed by the wick, taking it to deeper, swollen areas of the canal.

LOCAL ANESTHETIC AGENTS

Local anesthetic agents block nerve conduction at and around the application site to produce an analgesic effect. These drugs affect sensory, motor, and autonomic nerve fibers, and act on small nerve fibers more than on large nerve fibers. The only local anesthetic approved for otic use is benzocaine. It is administered topically as a solution or a gel.

History and source
The first local anesthetic was cocaine. In the 20th century, researchers began to develop substitutes that were safer and less addictive.

PHARMACOKINETICS

Benzocaine is not absorbed systemically. Onset of action is within minutes, and duration of action is only 1 to 2 hours.

PHARMACODYNAMICS

Local anesthetic agents temporarily interrupt the conduction of nerve impulses, reducing the permeability of the nerve cell membrane to sodium and potassium ions. This action interferes with the nerve membrane's ability to depolarize when stimulated.

In an area of mixed nerve fibers, local anesthetics initially affect autonomic nerve fibers, first blocking the small, nonmyelinated C fibers that mediate pain and produce vasoconstrictor responses, then the myelinated A-delta fibers that mediate pain and temperature. The local anesthetics then block the large fibers that carry sensory impulses, thereby blocking impulse conduction in the motor nerves.

PHARMACOTHERAPEUTICS

Benzocaine is used to relieve ear pain temporarily. Benzocaine may be used with anti-infective otics if an ear infection is present.

benzocaine (Americaine Otic, Auralgan Otic, Tympagesic). Ear pain, often caused by infection, can be relieved by instilling benzocaine.
USUAL ADULT DOSAGE: for pain relief, 4 to 5 drops t.i.d. or q.i.d.; benzocaine may be repeated as frequently as 1 to 2 hours. After instilling the drug, insert a cotton pledget moistened with benzocaine into the ear.

Drug interactions
No significant interactions occur between benzocaine and other drugs.

ADVERSE DRUG REACTIONS

Benzocaine may cause ear irritation, itching, and edema. It may also mask the symptoms of a fulminating middle ear infection. It may cause urticaria, a hypersensitivity reaction.

NURSING IMPLICATIONS

Benzocaine can be administered safely, but should be used only temporarily until underlying causes of pain can be treated.
- Caution the patient to seek the physician's attention if pain persists.
- Before administration, irrigate the ear gently to clear it of debris and impacted cerumen.
- Avoid touching the patient's ear with the dropper; do not rinse the dropper.
- Monitor the patient for early signs of an allergic reaction; discontinue the drug immediately and notify the physician if you suspect an allergic reaction.
- Instruct the patient not to use benzocaine for a prolonged time and to contact the physician if the ear problem persists.

CERUMINOLYTIC AGENTS

Ceruminolytic agents emulsify hardened or impacted cerumen, or earwax. They also prevent ceruminosis, or excessive cerumen accumulation.

PHARMACOKINETICS AND PHARMACODYNAMICS

Ceruminolytics are not absorbed systemically. Therapeutic effect occurs in 2 to 4 days.

Ceruminolytics reduce hardened earwax by emulsifying and mechanically loosening it. Carbamide peroxide is combined with anhydrous glycerin to soften cerumen. Exposing the carbamide peroxide to moisture releases oxygen and hydrogen peroxide, which produces an effervescence that mechanically removes cerumen. The ceruminolytic also acts to deodorize odor-causing bacteria.

PHARMACOTHERAPEUTICS

The action of both carbamide peroxide and triethanolamine may mechanically remove some of the cerumen. Nonetheless, the nurse still needs to irrigate the patient's ear after therapy to remove debris.

carbamide peroxide (Benadyne Ear, Debrox, Murine). An equimolar compound of hydrogen peroxide and urea that releases hydrogen peroxide when moistened, carbamide peroxide is used to loosen hardened or impacted earwax and to prevent ceruminosis.
USUAL ADULT DOSAGE: for adults and children age 12 and older, 5 to 10 drops into the external auditory canal b.i.d. for 4 days, then irrigate gently.
USUAL PEDIATRIC DOSAGE: for children under age 12, use with a physician's supervision.

triethanolamine polypeptide oleate-condensate (Cerumenex). Effective with a single 15- to 30-minute treatment, triethanolamine is used to remove excess or impacted earwax. It may also be used before an ear examination, otologic therapy, or audiometry.
USUAL ADULT DOSAGE: fill the patient's ear canal with solution and plug it with cotton for 15 to 30 minutes; then irrigate gently.

Drug interactions

No significant interactions occur between ceruminolytics and other drugs.

ADVERSE DRUG REACTIONS

Adverse reactions to ceruminolytics are usually insignificant. Mild erythema and pruritus may occur with triethanolamine or carbamide peroxide. Some patients using triethanolamine experience hypersensitivity reactions causing severe eczema.

NURSING IMPLICATIONS

The nurse must teach the patient how to administer the ceruminolytics, how to irrigate if necessary, and when to notify the physician. The nurse must also be aware of the following considerations:
- Triethanolamine is contraindicated in patients who have experienced a previous reaction to it, possibly from a positive patch test, or in patients with a perforated tympanic membrane.
- Do not touch the patient's ear with the dropper.
- Keep the container tightly closed and away from moisture.
- Gently irrigate the affected ear with warm water after administering the ceruminolytic agent. Avoid excessive pressure. Irrigation will help remove the cerumen loosened by the ceruminolytic.
- A patch test before the administration of triethanolamine can determine the possibility of an allergic reaction. Perform the patch test by dropping the ceruminolytic agent onto the flexor surface of the arm or forearm. The area is then covered with a small sterile

Otic agents

The drugs discussed in this chapter and presented in this chart are the more frequently used otic agents.

DRUG	MAJOR INDICATIONS	USUAL ADULT DOSAGES	NURSING IMPLICATIONS
Anti-infective agents			
chloramphenicol	Otitis externa	2 to 3 drops t.i.d.	• Assess the patient's past use of and response to the drug. • Observe for signs of superinfection.
neomycin	Otitis externa	4 drops t.i.d. or q.i.d. for no more than 10 days	• Administer cautiously to patients with otitis externa complicated by chronic otitis media. • Neomycin is contraindicated if tympanic membrane is perforated. • Assess the patient's past use of and response to the drug. • Observe for signs of superinfection and allergy.
polymyxin B sulfate	Otitis externa, otitis media	4 drops t.i.d. or q.i.d., not to exceed 2,000,000 units/ day	• Assess the patient's past use of and response to the drug. • Observe for signs of superinfection.
colistin	Otitis externa, otitis media	3 to 4 drops t.i.d. or q.i.d.	• Assess the patient's past use of and response to the drug. • Observe for signs of superinfection.
acetic acid	Superficial infection of the external auditory canal	5 drops t.i.d. or q.i.d.; or use ear wick for first 24 hours, then continue instillations	• Use cautiously in patients with perforated tympanic membrane.
boric acid	Otitis externa	4 to 6 drops in each ear, then plug with cotton t.i.d. or q.i.d.	• Assess the patient's past use of and response to the drug. • Observe for signs of superinfection. • Boric acid is contraindicated if tympanic membrane is perforated.
Anti-inflammatory agents			
dexamethasone sodium phosphate	External auditory canal inflammation, generalized inflammatory dermatoses	3 to 4 drops b.i.d. or t.i.d.	• Drug is contraindicated if tympanic membrane is perforated, or in acute, untreated purulent viral, bacterial, or fungal otic conditions. • Use singly in allergic otitis externa.
hydrocortisone	External auditory canal inflammation	4 to 5 drops t.i.d. or q.i.d.	• Drug is contraindicated in acute, untreated purulent viral, bacterial, or fungal otic conditions. • Use singly in allergic otitis externa.
prednisolone sodium phosphate	External auditory canal inflammation	3 to 4 drops b.i.d. or t.i.d.	• Drug is contraindicated in acute, untreated purulent viral, bacterial, or fungal otic conditions. • Use singly in allergic otitis externa.

continued

SELECTED MAJOR DRUGS

Otic agents continued

DRUG	MAJOR INDICATIONS	USUAL ADULT DOSAGES	NURSING IMPLICATIONS
Local anesthetic agent			
benzocaine	Ear pain from otic infection or other ear conditions	4 to 5 drops t.i.d. or q.i.d., every 1 to 2 hours as needed	• Drug is contraindicated if tympanic membrane is perforated. • Contact physician if ear pain persists for more than 48 hours. • Drug can be used with otic anti-infective agents if ear infection is present.
Ceruminolytic agents			
carbamide peroxide	Hardened or impacted earwax; prevention of ceruminosis	5 to 10 drops b.i.d. for 4 days, then irrigate gently	• Drug is contraindicated after otic surgery or if tympanic membrane is perforated. • Perform a patch test before using.
triethanolamine polypeptide oleate-condensate	Removal of hardened or impacted earwax; before exams, otic therapy, or audiometry	Fill ear canal with solution and allow to remain for 15 to 30 minutes before irrigating	• Drug is contraindicated if previous reaction occurred. • Perform a patch test before using.

bandage and observed, usually after 24 hours, for erythema and swelling.

• Instruct the patient to contact the physician if an allergic reaction develops.

• Instruct the patient not to use carbamide peroxide for more than 4 days unless supervised by a physician, and not to use triethanolamine for more than 15 to 30 minutes unless instructed otherwise by the physician.

• Instruct the patient to allow the ceruminolytic solution to remain in the ear canal for at least 15 minutes.

• Instruct the patient to store the ceruminolytic agent away from high temperature.

• Teach the patient how to administer eardrops. (See *Using eardrops* on page 1249 for proper techniques.)

• Teach the patient how to irrigate the ear. Show the patient how to tilt the head with the affected ear upward. Explain that the tip of the irrigating device is placed inside the meatus and directed toward the roof of the ear canal. Warm water is then allowed to flow into the ear canal. Explain that a basin should be positioned below the ear to collect the irrigating fluid as it flows out of the ear. Instruct the patient to lie on the affected side after irrigation to allow the irrigating solution to flow out.

• Inform the patient that the fizzing sensation heard when the ceruminolytic agent is applied is normal.

• Instruct the patient not to use cotton swabs in an attempt to remove cerumen.

CHAPTER SUMMARY

Chapter 80 presented information on four classes of otic drugs: anti-infective, anti-inflammatory, local anesthetic, and ceruminolytic agents. The discussion covered the drug classes, including the mechanisms of action, therapeutic uses, dosage and administration, interaction between otic agents and drugs, adverse drug reactions, and major nursing implications related to each. Frequently used otic drugs of each class also were listed and described. Here are the highlights of the chapter:

• Otic agents are used to treat external auditory canal infections (otitis externa), middle ear infections (otitis media), inflammation, and pain. They also are used to soften cerumen.

• Otic drugs are instilled topically via drops, irrigations, and ear wicks.

• Anti-infective otics are either bactericidal (kill bacteria) or bacteriostatic (inhibit bacterial growth). Boric acid and acetic acid are also fungistatic (inhibit fungal growth).

• Otic anti-infective agents include chloramphenicol, neomycin, polymyxin B sulfate, colistin, acetic acid, and boric acid.

• Before administering anti-infective otics, the physician identifies the causative organism and conducts susceptibility tests to determine the organism's sensitivity to the agent.

• Adverse reactions to anti-infective otics include a hypersensitivity reaction and a superinfection.

• Anti-inflammatory otics produce anti-inflammatory, antipruritic, and vasoconstrictor effects. Anti-inflammatory otics include dexamethasone sodium phosphate, hydrocortisone, and prednisolone sodium phosphate.

• Anti-inflammatory otics may precipitate a hypersensitivity reaction and may also mask or exacerbate an underlying otic infection.

• Local anesthetics produce analgesia by blocking nerve impulse propagation in a given area. Benzocaine is the local anesthetic approved for otic use.

• Ceruminolytics emulsify hardened or impacted cerumen. They also deodorize odor-causing bacteria.

BIBLIOGRAPHY

American Hospital Formulary Service. *Drug Information '87.* McEvoy, G.K., et al., eds. Bethesda, Md.: American Society of Hospital Pharmacists, 1987.

Malsee, R. *Pharmacology, Drug Therapy, and Nursing Considerations.* Philadelphia: J.B. Lippincott Co., 1985.

Michaels, R., and Brown, G. *Drug Consultant 1985-1986.* New York: John Wiley & Sons, 1985.

Professional Guide to Drugs. Springhouse, Pa.: Springhouse Corporation, 1981.

Scherer, J. *Lippincott's Nurse's Drug Manual.* Philadelphia: J.B. Lippincott Co., 1985.

Sheridan, E., et al. *The Drug, the Nurse, the Patient.* Philadelphia: W.B. Saunders Co., 1985.

DRUGS FOR IMMUNIZATION

The advent of immunizations has eliminated much of the tragedy that occurred before the 19th century when diseases such as diphtheria and pertussis killed thousands of young children. The threat of these diseases, however, persists because many people have become complacent about immunizations.

This unit discusses the agents used to immunize against disease. It presents agents that provide active immunity, including diphtheria and tetanus toxoids, and pertussis, poliovirus, measles, mumps, rubella, rabies (human diploid cell), Haemophilus influenza b, pneu-mococcal, influenza, and hepatitis B vaccines. (Smallpox vaccine is not covered here because it is not routinely administered. It is reserved for those in high-risk categories, such as laboratory workers and scientists, and is administered to some military personnel.) It also describes agents that provide passive immunity, including human plasma and human hepatitis B, rabies, tetanus, and varicella-zoster immune globulins.

To understand how these agents confer immunity, the nurse needs to understand how the immune system functions.

Lymphocyte responses

B lymphocytes, stored in the bone marrow, respond to an antigen by differentiating into plasma cells that secrete antigen-specific antibodies. T lymphocytes, stored in the thymus, become activated when sensitized to an antigen.

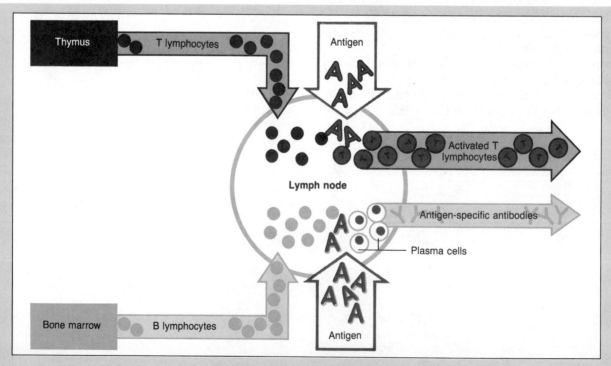

Glossary

Acquired immunity: immunity conferred by the presence of antibodies and by a heightened reactivity of antibody-forming and phagocytic cells; develops after exposure to an antigen or infectious agent or from the passive transfer of antibodies.

Active immunity: form of acquired immunity caused by antibody formation in response to an antigen.

Allergy: hypersensitive reaction caused by exposure to an antigen.

Anaphylaxis: immediate exaggerated hypersensitivity reaction to a foreign protein or other substance.

Antibody: immunoglobulin synthesized by lymphoid tissue in response to a specific antigen.

Antigen: foreign substance, usually a protein or protein-polysaccharide complex, that stimulates formation of a specific antibody to which it reacts.

Antitoxin: antibody to a microorganism's toxin (usually a bacterial exotoxin) that combines with, and neutralizes, the toxin.

Antivenin: suspension of venom-neutralizing antibodies prepared from the serum of immunized horses; confers passive immunity and is given as a part of emergency first-aid treatment for various snake and insect bites.

B lymphocyte: bursal lymphocyte responsible for humoral immunity.

Cell-mediated immunity: acquired immunity in which T lymphocytes play a dominant role.

Complement: enzymatic serum protein that combines with an antigen-antibody complex, causing antigen lysis.

Cytomegalovirus: host-specific virus that infects humans, monkeys, and rodents, producing large cells.

Hepatitis: inflammation of the liver.

Humoral immunity: acquired immunity in which B lymphocytes play a dominant role.

Immune serum: immunizing agent made from the blood of animals inoculated with bacteria or their toxins, producing passive immunity.

Immunity: power to resist or overcome an infection.

Immunoglobulin: gamma globulin in the blood that possesses antibody activity.

Lymphocyte: white blood cell that develops in the bone marrow, characterized by a single nucleus and a nongranular protoplasm.

Macrophage: large mononuclear cell that ingests microorganisms, other cells, or foreign particles.

Monocyte: large white blood cell with a pale, oval nucleus and more protoplasm than a lymphocyte.

Natural immunity: normal human resistance to infection.

Neutrophil: polymorphonuclear white cell easily stained by neutral dyes.

Passive immunity: form of acquired immunity conferred by administration of preformed antibodies.

Phagocytosis: engulfment and disposal of microorganisms, cells, or foreign particles by reticuloendothelial cells, neutrophils, monocytes, or macrophages.

Prophylaxis: prevention of disease.

Tetanus: acute infectious disease produced by a toxin from *Clostridium tetani*, characterized by masseter muscle spasms, trismus (lockjaw), and back muscle spasms that cause opisthotonos.

T lymphocyte: thymic lymphocyte responsible for cell-mediated immunity.

Toxin: poison usually produced by or occurring in a plant or microorganism.

Toxoid: bacterial exotoxin that has lost toxicity but can still combine with antitoxins or stimulate their formation; given to produce immunity.

Vaccine: suspension of attenuated (weakened) or killed microorganisms used to provide immunity against an infectious disease.

Immune system review

The body's immune system is designed to recognize, respond to, and eliminate foreign substances, or antigens. The immune system consists of primary lymphoid organs (thymus, lymph nodes, spleen, and tonsils). Aggregate tissue in nonlymphoid organs, such as Peyer's patches in the gut, and lymphoid cells in the bone marrow, blood, and connective and epithelial tissue make up secondary organs or sites of the immune system.

The responses of the immune system are either nonspecific or specific. Phagocytosis is the primary nonspecific response; the immune system recognizes an antigen, then neutrophils and monocytes, the phagocytic cells, ingest and digest the antigen. The specific responses of the immune system are humoral or cell-mediated immunity. B lymphocytes and T lymphocytes are the antibody-producing cells responsible for specific responses.

Humoral immunity. In humoral immunity, antibodies are produced, primarily by the B lymphocytes. An antigen presence causes the B lymphocytes to divide and differentiate into plasma cells that produce and secrete antigen-specific antibodies. The five types of antibodies, or immunoglobulins, are IgG, IgM, IgA, IgD, and IgE. Each type serves a specific function: IgG, IgM, and IgA antibodies provide bacterial and viral protection; IgD serves as an antigen receptor on B lymphocytes; IgE causes allergic response. The primary antibody response usually occurs when an individual is initially exposed to an antigen. (See *Lymphocyte responses* on page 1256 for an illustration and Unit Thirteen Introduction for more information on antibodies.)

If the individual is exposed to the antigen subsequently, a secondary antibody response occurs and IgG is produced in large quantities within several days. Consecutive immunizations produce memory B lymphocytes that can recognize the same antigen for months or years.

An antigen-antibody complex, which forms after the antibody reacts to the antigen, serves several functions. First, the antigen is processed by a macrophage and presented to antigen-specific B lymphocytes. Then, the antibody activates the nine-factor complement system, causing an enzymatic cascade that destroys the antigen. Activation of the complement system also acts as a bridge between humoral and cell-mediated immunity, resulting in the arrival of neutrophils and macrophages, the phagocytic cells, at the antigen site. This combination of humoral and cell-mediated immune response is the most common.

Cell-mediated immunity. Cell-mediated immunity has various functions involving T lymphocytes. It protects the body against bacterial, viral, and fungal infections, and resists transplanted cells and tumor cells. In the cell-mediated response, a macrophage processes the antigen, which is then presented to T lymphocytes. Some T lymphocytes become sensitized and destroy the antigen; others release lymphokines, which activate macrophages that destroy the antigen.

Immunity acquired from birth. This immunity occurs in the newborn because the fetus receives significant amounts of IgG from the mother during pregnancy. For the first 3 months of life, the newborn is immune to antigens to which the mother was exposed during pregnancy. During this 3-month period, the infant begins to produce IgG, reaching 40% of adult levels by age 1. However, within 6 months of birth, the immunity that was passed on through the mother disappears. Therefore, immunizations must be administered. Although the infant begins to produce IgA, IgD, and IgE, these antibodies will not reach adult levels until early childhood,

Active and passive immunity

Although active and passive immunity provide protection against disease, they differ in many respects. To plan appropriate patient care, the nurse should be aware of the following differences.

	ACTIVE IMMUNITY	PASSIVE IMMUNITY
Source of immunity	Person manufactures antibodies against specific antigens in the body.	Person receives antibodies against specific antigens that have been manufactured in the bodies of other people or animals.
Timing	Immunity takes time to develop and is usually permanent.	Immunity is immediate but temporary.
Cell changes	Body cells undergo change.	Body cells are not changed.
Ways to acquire immunity	A person may acquire immunity naturally as a result of a disease.	A child may receive antibodies from the mother through the placental circulation.
	A person may acquire immunity by inoculation with vaccines or toxoids.	A person may receive antibodies by injection with therapeutic serum.
Immunizing agent	Vaccines may be composed of killed microorganisms (bacteria and viruses) or attenuated living ones; toxoids contain denatured bacterial toxins.	Therapeutic serum is made from the blood of people, horses, or other animals that have been injected with bacteria or bacterial toxins and have developed circulating antibodies.
Adverse reactions to immunizing agent	Vaccines frequently cause local reaction at the injection site, swelling, erythema, and tenderness.	Therapeutic serum may cause serum sickness with such symptoms as fever, malaise, and arthralgia.

which explains why a child may experience a number of colds or minor infections when exposed to new antigens.

The toddler's antibody production is well established. A 2-year-old's production of IgG reaches adult levels. At this point, the toddler is able to neutralize microbial toxins as effectively as the adult.

Immunizations and immunity

Drugs for immunization stimulate the body's immune system to protect against diseases. The goal of immunotherapy is to provide the greatest protection from disease with the fewest adverse reactions. Active immunity aims to protect an individual against a disease for which exposure is likely; passive immunity, against a disease for which exposure has occurred. Either effectively protects an individual from disease.

Active immunity. This immunity can occur naturally, from a clinical or subclinical course of a disease, or artificially, by inoculation with an antigen. Both methods stimulate antibody formation, which can prevent infections and protect individuals from disease.

Passive immunity. Passive immunity results from the administration of exogenous, preformed antibodies to an individual. These antibodies can provide temporary immunity for an unimmunized individual exposed to a disease, or for an immunocompromised individual when the disease's incubation period does not allow enough time for antibody formation or when the disease can be alleviated or modified by passive immunity.

Because passive immunity does not alter body cells, its protection is temporary, from 1 to 6 weeks. (See *Active and passive immunity* for a comparison of these types of immunity.)

Chapter 81
Active Immunity Agents

Chapter 81 investigates agents used to produce active immunity, focusing on the pharmacokinetics, pharmacodynamics, and pharmacotherapeutic properties of specific toxoids and vaccines as well as their associated nursing implications. It also includes the routine immunization schedule for children and information for patient education.

Chapter 82
Passive Immunity Agents

Chapter 82 explores agents used to produce passive immunity. It emphasizes the pharmacokinetic, pharmacodynamic, and pharmacotherapeutic properties of immune globulins and discusses their adverse reactions and related nursing implications. Animal antitoxins, serums, and antivenins are also discussed briefly.

Nursing diagnoses

When caring for a patient receiving drugs for immunization, the nurse can expect to use any of the following nursing diagnoses:

• Alteration in comfort: pain, related to the administration and adverse effects of immunizing agents
• Anxiety related to the administration and effects of immunizing agents.
• Fear related to the administration of and adverse reactions to immunizing agents
• Impaired physical mobility related to the administration and effects of immunizing agents
• Impairment of skin integrity related to the administration of and adverse reactions to immunizing agents
• Ineffective breathing patterns related to adverse reactions to immunizing agents
• Ineffective family coping: compromised, related to the administration of and adverse reactions to immunizing agents
• Ineffective individual coping related to the administration and effects of immunizing agents
• Knowledge deficit related to aspects of immunization therapy
• Noncompliance related to immunization therapy schedules
• Potential activity intolerance related to adverse reactions to immunizing agents
• Potential alteration in body temperature related to effects of immunizing agents
• Potential for infection related to the administration and effects of immunizing agents
• Sleep-pattern disturbance related to the administration and effects of immunizing agents.

CHAPTER 81

ACTIVE IMMUNITY AGENTS

OBJECTIVES

After reading and studying this chapter, you should be able to:

1. Describe how active immunity protects against disease.

2. Discuss the pharmacokinetics of active immunity agents, and explain how these properties determine subsequent treatment.

3. Describe the clinical indications for each active immunity agent.

4. Describe how herd immunity works.

5. Describe the predictable and unpredictable adverse reactions to diphtheria and tetanus toxoids and pertussis vaccine (DTP); measles, mumps, and rubella virus vaccine (MMR); oral poliovirus vaccine (OPV); rabies vaccine, human diploid cell (HDCV); pneumococcal vaccine; influenza virus vaccine; hepatitis B vaccine; and Haemophilus influenza b polysaccharide vaccine (Hib).

INTRODUCTION

A person becomes actively immune when the body develops antibodies against specific antigens. This immunity can be achieved through the administration of the specific antigen, in which case the person is protected before exposure to the disease, or the immunity can be achieved naturally as a result of exposure to the disease. Physicians and nurses provide protection against childhood diseases and certain infectious diseases by administering vaccines and toxoids. For example, tetanus toxoid protects individuals before exposure or after injury; the rabies vaccine protects the person who has possibly been exposed to rabies by an animal bite. Both vaccines and toxoids provide active immunity to either bacteria or viruses. Bacterial vaccines are prepared from whole bacteria (pertussis vaccine) or from purified capsular polysaccharides (pneumococcal vaccine). Viral vaccines are prepared from nonliving viruses (Haemophilus influenza b vaccine) or from living viruses (mumps vaccine). Recombinant hepatitis B vaccine, a recently approved drug, is produced from yeast DNA and is free

of human blood or blood products. Toxoids are prepared from treated bacterial toxins (tetanus toxoid).

The vaccines and toxoids given to provide active immunity are tetanus toxoid, tetanus and diphtheria toxoids (Td), diphtheria and tetanus toxoids and pertussis vaccine (DTP); measles, mumps, and rubella virus vaccines (available separately or in combination as MMR); oral poliovirus vaccine (OPV); rabies vaccine, human diploid cell (HDCV); Haemophilus influenza b polysaccharide vaccine (Hib); pneumococcal vaccine; influenza virus vaccine; and hepatitis B vaccine. Each type of immunization will be discussed in this chapter. (See also *Other vaccines and toxoids* on page 1267 for agents that may be used less frequently.)

For a summary of representative drugs, see *Selected major drugs: Active immunity agents* on pages 1265 and 1266.

PHARMACOKINETICS

The body's antigen-antibody reaction elicits an immunologic response that forms antigen-specific immunoglobulins. Physicians and nurses administer immunizations to provide permanent or long-term immunity against diseases that the individual is likely to encounter.

The onset of action occurs when the immunologic response is elicited, from a few days to a few weeks. Peak action varies among the different immunizations. The durations of action of immunizations also vary. Upon the completion of the OPV series, duration of action is for life. The duration of action of tetanus toxoid is 10 years; that of the pneumococcal vaccine, 3 to 5 years. The duration of action of the influenza vaccine is 1 year.

PHARMACODYNAMICS

Vaccines and toxoids initiate the formation of specific antibodies by stimulating the body's antigen-antibody mechanism. This action provides active, acquired immunity for the individual. Active immunity can also be induced by exposure to an infectious disease or to one of its antigens.

PHARMACOTHERAPEUTICS

Immunizations have been developed that prevent and, in many instances, eradicate commonly occurring communicable diseases. Furthermore, if a high percentage of people are immunized and protected from diseases, those who are not immunized achieve some degree of protection because the people around them are not likely to contract and spread the disease. This type of immunity is referred to as herd immunity.

The timing of immunization for normal healthy children and for those requiring delayed immunization is an important consideration for those caring for infants and children. Every effort should be made to follow the recommended schedule. (See *Recommended schedule for active immunization of normal infants and children* and *Recommended immunization schedules for children not immunized before age 1* on page 1262 for ages and types of immunization.)

diphtheria and tetanus toxoids and pertussis vaccine [DTP] (Tri-Immunol). This vaccine is used to provide immunity to diphtheria, tetanus, and pertussis.
USUAL DOSAGE: 0.5 ml I.M. for children age 2 months to 7 years. Initial dose is followed by two more at 4- to 8-week intervals. One year after the third dose, a fourth is given and a booster is given between ages 4 and 6.

tetanus and diphtheria, adsorbed [Td]. This combination is used to immunize children over age 7 and adults.
USUAL DOSAGE: initially, 0.5 ml I.M., repeated in 4 to 6 weeks. A third 0.5-ml dose is given I.M. in 6 to 12 months and then a booster every 10 years.

tetanus toxoid. This toxoid is inactivated toxin and is given prophylactically for wound management.
USUAL DOSAGE: for children and adults not previously immunized, 0.5 ml I.M. followed in 4 to 6 weeks by 0.5 ml I.M. and a third injection in 1 year. A booster dose is given every 10 years.

measles, mumps, and rubella virus vaccine live [MMR] (M-M-R II). This vaccine is used to provide immunity to measles, mumps, and rubella and contains live viruses.
USUAL DOSAGE: for children age 12 months or older, 0.5 ml S.C. into outer aspect of upper arm.

Recommended schedule for active immunization of normal infants and children

RECOMMENDED AGE	IMMUNIZATION(S)	COMMENTS
2 months	DTP[1], OPV[2]	Can be initiated as early as age 2 weeks in areas of high endemicity or during epidemics
4 months	DTP, OPV	2-month interval desired for OPV to avoid interference from previous dose
6 months	DTP (OPV)	OPV is optional (may be given in areas with increased risk of poliovirus exposure)
15 months	MMR[3]	MMR preferred to individual vaccines; tuberculin testing may be done
18 months	DTP[4,5], OPV[5]	
24 months	Hib	
4 to 6 years	DTP, OPV	At or before school entry
14 to 16 years	Td[8]	Repeat every 10 years throughout life

[1]DTP—Diphtheria and tetanus toxoids with pertussis vaccine.
[2]OPV—Oral poliovirus vaccine contains attenuated poliovirus types 1, 2, and 3.
[3]MMR—Live measles, mumps, and rubella viruses in a combined vaccine.
[4]Should be given 6 to 12 months after the third dose.
[5]May be given simultaneously with MMR at age 15 months.
[6]Haemophilus influenza b polysaccharide vaccine.
[7]Up to the seventh birthday.
[8]Td—Adult tetanus toxoid (full dose) and diphtheria toxoid (reduced dose) in combination.

Recommended immunization schedules for children not immunized before age 1

RECOMMENDED TIME	IMMUNIZATION(S)	COMMENTS
Less than 7 years old		
First visit	DTP, OPV, MMR	MMR if child ≥ age 15 months; tuberculin testing may be done
Interval after first visit		
1 month	Hib*	For children ages 24 to 60 months
2 months	DTP, OPV	
4 months	DTP (OPV)	OPV is optional (may be given in areas with increased risk of poliovirus exposure)
10 to 16 months	DTP, OPV	OPV is not given if third dose was given earlier
Age 4 to 6 years (at or before school entry)	DTP, OPV	DTP is unnecessary if the fourth dose was given after the fourth birthday; OPV is unnecessary if recommended OPV dose at 10 to 16 months after first visit was given after the fourth birthday
Age 14 to 16 years	Td	Repeat every 10 years throughout life
7 years old and older		
First visit	Td, OPV, MMR	
Interval after first visit		
2 months	Td, OPV	
8 to 14 months	Td, OPV	
Age 14 to 16 years	Td	Repeat every 10 years throughout life

*Haemophilus influenza b polysaccharide vaccine can be given, if necessary, simultaneously with DTP (at separate sites). The initial three doses of DTP can be given at 1- to 2-month intervals; so, for the child in whom immunization is initiated at age 24 months or older, one visit could be eliminated by giving DTP, OPV, MMR at the first visit; DTP and Hib at the second visit (1 month later); and DTP and OPV at the third visit (2 months after the first visit). Subsequent DTP and OPV 10 to 16 months after the first visit are still indicated.

Reprinted with permission from the *Report of the Committee on Infectious Diseases,* American Academy of Pediatrics, 20th ed., Elk Grove Village, Ill., 1986.

poliovirus vaccine, live, oral, trivalent [OPV] (Orimune). This vaccine is used to provide immunity to the poliovirus.
USUAL DOSAGE: 0.5 ml P.O.; primary series is administered in three doses. First two doses are given 6 to 8 weeks apart and the third dose is given 12 months later.

rabies vaccine, human diploid cell [HDCV] (Imovax). The rabies vaccine is used to provide active immunity to prevent rabies in high-risk groups such as veterinarians and also after exposure.
USUAL DOSAGE: for preexposure prophylaxis, 1 ml I.M. on days 0, 7, 21, and 28, with booster doses at 6-month to 2-year intervals; for postexposure treatment, 0.5 ml I.M. given as soon as possible after exposure and repeated on days 3, 7, 14, and 28.

influenza virus vaccine [influenza virus vaccine, trivalent types A and B, split virus] (Fluogen) and **[influenza virus vaccine, trivalent types A and B, whole virus]** (Fluzone). This vaccine is given to prevent influenza virus. The split virus vaccines seem to cause less adverse reactions than the whole virus vaccines.
USUAL DOSAGE: for children over age 12 and adults, 0.5 ml of whole or split virus vaccine I.M. in the deltoid. For children 3 to 12 years old, 0.5 ml of split virus vaccine I.M., repeated in 4 weeks; for children age 6 months to 3 years old, 0.25 ml of split virus vaccine I.M., repeated in 4 weeks.

hepatitis B vaccine (Heptavax-B). This vaccine promotes immunity to hepatitis B. Immunization with this vaccine is used against infection caused by all known subtypes of hepatitis B virus. It is recommended for immunization of selected populations who are considered to be at increased risk of contracting hepatitis B infection, such as laboratory technicians and operating room and emergency department nurses.
USUAL DOSAGE: for children over age 10 and adults, initially 1 ml I.M. followed by another 1-ml dose 1 month later and a third 1-ml dose 6 months after the first dose; for children age 3 months to 10 years, initially 0.5 ml I.M. followed by another dose of 0.5 ml I.M. 1 month later and a third 0.5-ml dose 6 months after the first dose; for dialysis and immunocompromised patients, initially 2 ml I.M. followed by another 2-ml dose I.M. 1 month later and a third 2-ml I.M. dose 6 months after the first dose. The 2-ml doses should be divided into two 1-ml doses and administered at two different sites.

Haemophilus influenza b polysaccharide vaccine [Hib] (HibImmune, HibVax). This vaccine is used for pro-

phylactic prevention of *Haemophilus* influenza b and the diseases it causes, such as meningitis, epiglottitis, and pericarditis.
USUAL DOSAGE: for children age 24 months to 6 years, 0.5 ml S.C.

pneumococcal vaccine, polyvalent (Pneumovax-23, Pnu-Immune 23). This polysaccharide vaccine is used to prevent pneumococcal diseases, such as pneumonia and meningitis. It is especially useful for elderly patients and those with chronic cardiac, pulmonary, hepatic, and renal diseases.
USUAL DOSAGE: 0.5 ml I.M. or S.C.

Drug interactions

Some of the active immunity agents interact with other drugs. These interactions can usually be prevented by avoiding concurrent administration or waiting an appropriate length of time after immunization. No significant reactions occur with the pneumococcal, influenza, and hepatitis B vaccines. (See *Drug interactions: Active immunity agents* for further information, including possible effects and nursing implications.)

ADVERSE DRUG REACTIONS

The various immunizations cause many different reactions, from local discomfort at the injection site to mild symptoms of the disease the immunization prevents.

Predictable reactions

DTP produces fever in 50% of children within 48 hours. Local reactions, including erythema, induration, and tenderness at the injection site, may occur within 12 to 24 hours. Mild systemic reactions such as anorexia, fretfulness, and drowsiness can occur.

MMR may produce a transient rash, lymphadenopathy, and fever (up to 103° F. [39.4° C.]) within 6 to 11 days of immunization. Other predictable reactions include arthralgia, arthritis, and painful paresthesias (especially in women). These reactions usually occur 2 to 8 weeks after immunization.

OPV produces no predictable reactions. HDCV can produce local reactions, including pain, swelling, erythema, and itching at the injection site. Systemic reactions to HDCV include headache, nausea, dizziness, muscle aches, and abdominal pain.

DRUG INTERACTIONS

Active immunity agents

The following chart presents the significant drug interactions associated with the active immunity agents. No significant reactions are associated with the pneumococcal, influenza, and hepatitis B vaccines.

DRUG	INTERACTING DRUGS	POSSIBLE EFFECTS	NURSING IMPLICATIONS
diphtheria and tetanus toxoids and pertussis vaccine [DTP]	antimetabolites, alkylating agents, cytotoxic drugs, corticosteroids (large doses)	Decrease immune response; serum antibodies interfere with the immune response	• Avoid concurrent administration.
measles, mumps, and rubella virus vaccine, live [MMR]	other live-virus vaccines	May impair immune response	• Do not administer MMR within 1 month of another live-virus vaccine.
poliovirus vaccine, live, oral, trivalent [OPV]	plasma, whole blood, immune serum globulin, other live-virus vaccines	May impair immune response	• Do not administer OPV within 1 month of another live-virus vaccine.
rabies vaccine, human diploid cell [HDCV]	steroids (in the treatment of anaphylaxis)	Possibly activate the rabies virus	• Be familiar with the manufacturer's recommendations for treating anaphylaxis.
Haemophilus influenza b polysaccharide vaccine [Hib]	chemotherapeutic agents	Impair antibody response	• Avoid concurrent administration.

Pneumococcal vaccine produces soreness at the injection site within 3 days. The vaccine can also produce a fever under 100° F. (37.8° C.) and mild myalgia. The latter reaction can occur within 2 to 14 days of administration and last up to 2 weeks.

The influenza virus vaccine, trivalent types A and B (whole or split virus) can produce fever, malaise, and myalgia within 6 to 24 hours of administration. These reactions may last 1 to 2 days. Hepatitis B vaccine can produce local reactions, including discomfort at the injection site and local inflammation. Systemic reactions to hepatitis B vaccine include slight fever, transient malaise, headache, dizziness, nausea, and vomiting.

Hib can produce local reactions, including erythema, warmth, swelling, and tenderness at the injection site. Systemic reactions occasionally occur and include fever, irritability, and anorexia.

Unpredictable reactions

DTP occasionally produces sterile abcesses. Other reactions, usually associated with the pertussis portion of the immunity agent, include hypotonic-hyporesponsive episodes (shocklike states), onset of new seizures, persistent and abnormally high-pitched cry for over 3 hours in children, and fever up to 105° F. (40.5° C.).

MMR can produce subacute sclerosing panencephalitis and blindness associated with optic neuritis. Rubella may be transmitted by the pregnant patient to the fetus, which presents a risk to normal fetal development. MMR can produce anaphylactic reactions, especially in patients allergic to eggs.

OPV has resulted in poliomyelitis in immunocompromised patients. HDCV may produce unpredictable anaphylactoid reactions, as can the pneumococcal vaccine. Rare anaphylactic reactions sometimes occur with the influenza virus vaccine. This vaccine also but rarely can produce Guillain-Barré syndrome.

Hib can produce unpredictable seizures, rashes, and sleep disturbances. Researchers are not yet sure whether Hib is detrimental to the fetus or whether it appears in breast milk.

NURSING IMPLICATIONS

The nurse should be aware of the following important implications concerning child development and the illnesses that affect immunization:

• Do not expect to immunize the child with a neurologic disorder because immunization may aggravate the disorder. However, children with hydrocephalus or cerebral palsy may receive immunizations on a regular schedule.

• Know that live-virus immunizations may be withheld because of an underlying disease or anticipated immunologic response. In such circumstances, the inactive form of the vaccine may be administered.

• Withhold live-virus immunization for immunocompromised children until they have been off immunosuppressants for 3 months. Administer inactive vaccines as prescribed to avoid a particular naturally occurring disease.

• Withhold DTP and MMR immunization in a child with acute febrile illness until the child is well. Doing so enables the physician to distinguish between a drug reaction and the illness.

• Administer routine immunizations to children with chronic diseases because such children are susceptible to frequent infections.

• Administer immunizations to premature infants based on chronologic age rather than gestational age. For example, a premature infant would receive DTP and OPV at 2 months regardless of gestational age. However, if the infant is still hospitalized, administer only the DTP as prescribed to avoid cross-infection with OPV. The OPV series can be started at discharge.

• Expect to use antipyretics to treat febrile reactions to DTP and MMR immunizations. Do not use heat or cold on local reactions because either is likely to increase the local reaction.

• Change the needle after drawing the medication for DTP out of a vial to prevent local reactions from subcutaneous tissue contamination during I.M. injection.

• Do not administer OPV to immunocompromised patients or to those who are in close contact with immunocompromised individuals; the immunocompromised person will be susceptible to poliovirus infection.

• Obtain a thorough patient history to prevent administration of influenza, pneumococcal, Hib, or rabies vaccine to susceptible patients. Have epinephrine (1:1,000) readily available to treat anaphylaxis should it occur. Any associated fever can be treated with antipyretics as prescribed.

• Provide the immunized patient with information about potential adverse reactions, home treatment of those reactions, and when to call the physician.

• Inform parents of the benefits and risks of the immunization. Explain that severe reactions can occur but are rare.

• Educate the patient and family about the possible adverse effects of the vaccine.

• Discuss with the patient and family the use of antipyretics for fever. Caution about possible erythema and soreness at the injection site.

Active immunity agents

Vaccines and toxoids provide active immunity. The indications for the immunization, recommended dosages, and nursing considerations are presented in the following chart.

DRUG	MAJOR INDICATIONS	USUAL DOSAGES	NURSING IMPLICATIONS
diphtheria and tetanus toxoids and pertussis vaccine [DTP]	Immunity to diphtheria, tetanus, and pertussis	0.5 ml I.M. for children age 2 months to 7 years. Initial dose is followed by two more at 4-to 8-week intervals. One year after the third dose, a fourth is given, and a booster is given at ages 4 and 6.	• Do not administer a live attenuated virus to the immunocompromised patient because the virus can cause the disease. Wait until immunotherapy has been discontinued for 3 months. • Withhold DTP in a patient with an acute febrile illness to avoid the problem of differentiating signs and symptoms of illness from those of reaction; children should return for DTP as soon as they are well. • Document the patient's history of administration of plasma, whole blood, and immune serum globulin; immunization should be administered 3 months after plasma, whole blood, and immune globulin.
measles, mumps, and rubella virus vaccine, live [MMR]	Prevention of measles, mumps, rubella	0.5 ml S.C. for children age 12 months or older	• MMR is contraindicated in patients with severe febrile illness and after the administration of antimetabolites, steroids, or steroid-like medications. • Do not administer MMR if the patient is allergic to eggs or neomycin. • Do not administer to the immunocompromised patient. MMR may be given after chemotherapy has been discontinued for 3 months. • Do not administer to women of childbearing age; if the vaccine is given, the woman must not become pregnant for 3 months. • During a measles outbreak, children age 6 months and older can be immunized but must be reimmunized at age 15 months. • If live-virus vaccines are not administered on the same day, wait at least 1 month before administering another live-virus vaccine. • Have epinephrine (1:1,000) available to treat anaphylactic reactions should they occur. • Do not administer MMR intravenously. • Refrigerate MMR vaccine at 39° F. (4° C.). • Protect the vaccine from heat and light.
poliovirus vaccine, live, oral, trivalent [OPV]	Immunity to poliovirus	0.5 ml P.O.; primary series is administered in three doses. First two doses are given 6 to 8 weeks apart, and a third dose is given 12 months later.	• OPV is contraindicated in the immunocompromised patient; administer the inactivated form. • Avoid administering OPV if the patient has diarrhea, vomiting, or an acute illness, and avoid use in pregnant patients. • Administer by mouth only. • If live-virus vaccines are not administered on the same day, wait at least 1 month before administering another live-virus vaccine. • Store frozen OPV at 7° F. (−13° C.). Once thawed, store it at 36° to 46° F. (2° to 8° C.) and use within 30 days.

continued

Active immunity agents continued

DRUG	MAJOR INDICATIONS	USUAL DOSAGES	NURSING IMPLICATIONS
pneumococcal vaccine, polyvalent	Prevention of pneumococcal diseases such as pneumonia and meningitis	0.5 ml I.M. or S.C.	• Do not administer if the patient has known hypersensitivity to a portion of the vaccine. • Do not administer to patients receiving immunosuppressive therapy. • The influenza and pneumococcal vaccines can be administered to children at the same time in different sites without increased adverse effects.
influenza virus vaccine, trivalent types A and B (whole or split virus)	Prevention of influenza virus	For children over age 12 and adults: 0.5 ml of the whole or split virus vaccine I.M. in the deltoid For children age 3 to 12: 0.5 ml of split virus vaccine I.M. repeated in 4 weeks For children age 6 months to 3 years: 0.25 ml split virus vaccine I.M. repeated in 4 weeks	• Do not administer if the patient is allergic to eggs. • Defer or delay immunization if the patient has an acute respiratory illness. • The influenza and pneumococcal vaccines can be administered to children at the same time in different sites without increased adverse effects.
hepatitis B vaccine	Immunity to hepatitis B and subtypes of hepatitis B	For adults and children over age 10: initially, 1 ml I.M., followed by another 1-ml dose 1 month later, followed by a third 1-ml dose 6 months after the first dose For children age 3 months to 10 years: initially, 0.5 ml I.M., followed by another 0.5-ml dose 1 month later, followed by a third 0.5-ml dose 6 months after the first dose For dialysis and immuno-compromised patients: initially, 2 ml I.M., followed by another 2-ml dose 1 month later, followed by a third 2-ml dose 6 months after the first dose. (The 2-ml doses should be divided into two 1-ml doses and administered at different sites.)	• Administer cautiously to patients with any serious, active infection or compromised cardiac or pulmonary status; use cautiously in those for whom a febrile or systemic reaction could pose a serious risk. • The Centers for Disease Control reports that response to hepatitis B vaccine is significantly better when it is administered in the arm rather than the buttock. • The vaccine may be administered subcutaneously, but only to persons, such as hemophiliacs, who are at risk of hemorrhage. • Thoroughly agitate the vial just before administration to restore suspension. • Store both opened and unopened vials in the refrigerator. Do not freeze the vaccine.

Other vaccines and toxoids

Some other vaccines and toxoids that the nurse may have to administer infrequently are listed here.
- BCG vaccine
- cholera vaccine
- diphtheria toxoid and diphtheria toxoid, adsorbed
- measles virus vaccine, live
- meningococcal polysaccharide vaccines
- mumps virus vaccine, live
- plague vaccine
- rubella and mumps vaccine, live
- rubella virus vaccine, live, attenuated
- typhoid vaccine
- typhus vaccine
- yellow fever vaccine

● Discuss with chronically ill patients and the parents of chronically ill children the advisability of receiving an influenza vaccine regularly. Immunocompromised or immunosuppressed individuals may also benefit from immunization.

CHAPTER SUMMARY

The discussion in Chapter 81 covered agents that provide patients with active immunity. Among their many values, immunizations have helped decrease previously common infectious childhood diseases and other virulent diseases such as smallpox. Patient and family education, indications for the immunization, dosages, adverse reactions, drug interactions, and nursing considerations vary with each drug. Here are the chapter highlights:
● Active immunity is achieved in the body by the formation of antibodies against specific antigens.
● Vaccines and toxoids provide active immunity to bacteria or viruses.
● Some frequently used immunizations include diphtheria and tetanus toxoids and pertussis vaccine (DTP); measles, mumps, and rubella virus vaccines (singly or in combination as MMR); oral poliovirus vaccine (OPV); rabies vaccine, human diploid cell (HDCV); smallpox vaccine; Haemophilus influenza b polysaccharide vac-

cine (Hib); pneumococcal vaccine; influenza virus vaccine; and hepatitis B vaccine.
● Information about possible adverse reactions, how to treat them, and when to call the physician should be presented to the patient or family when the immunizations are given.

BIBLIOGRAPHY

"Adverse Events Following Immunization," *Morbidity and Mortality Weekly Report* 34(3):43-47, January 25, 1985.

Baraff, L.J., et al. "DTP-Associated Reactions: An Analysis by Injection Site, Manufacturer, Prior Reactions, and Dose," *Pediatrics* 73(1):31-36, January 1984.

Behrman, R.E., and Vaughn, V.C., eds. *Nelson's Textbook of Pediatrics,* 12th ed. Philadelphia: W.B. Saunders Co., 1983.

Brunell, P.A., et al. "Hemophilus Type b Polysaccharide Vaccine," *Pediatrics* 76(2):322-24, August 1985.

Brunell, P.A., et al. "Recommendations for Using Pneumococcal Vaccine in Children," *Pediatrics* 75:1153, May 1985.

Church, J.A., and Richards, W. "Recurrent Abscess Formation Following DTP Immunizations: Association with Hypersensitivity to Tetanus Toxoid," *Pediatrics* 75(5):889, May 1985.

Connaught Laboratories Limited. *Poliovirus Vaccine Inactivated* (Drug Insert). Willowdale, Ontario: 1986.

"Diphtheria, Tetanus, and Pertussis: Guidelines for Vaccine Prophylaxis and Other Preventive Measures: Recommendation of the Immunization Practices Advisory Committee," *Annals of Internal Medicine* 103(61):896-905, 1985.

Drugs, 2nd ed. Nurse's Reference Library. Springhouse, Pa.: Springhouse Corp., 1984.

Granoff, D.M., and Cates, K.L. "Haemophilus Influenzae Type b Polysaccharide Vaccines," *Journal of Pediatrics* 107(3):330-36, September 1985.

Karzon, D.T. "A National Compensation Program for Vaccine-Related Injuries," *New England Journal of Medicine* 310:1320, 1984.

Kayhty, H., et al. "Serum Antibodies after Vaccination with Haemophilus Influenzae Type b Capsular Polysaccharide and Responses to Reimmunization: No Evidence of Immunologic Tolerance or Memory," *Pediatrics* 74(5):857-65, November 1984.

Keens, T.G., et al. "Ventilatory Pattern Following Diphtheria-Tetanus-Pertussis Immunization in Infants at Risk for Sudden Infant Death Syndrome," *American Journal of Diseases of Children* 139(10):991-94, October 1985.

Li, K.I., et al. "Haemophilus Influenzae Type b Colonization in Household Contacts of Infected and Colonized Children Enrolled in Day Care," *Pediatrics* 78(1):15-20, July 1986.

McGraw, T.T. "Reimmunization Following Early Immunization with Measles Vaccine: A Prospective Study," *Pediatrics* 77(1):45-48, January 1986.

Mansell, K.A. "New Immunization Against H. Influenzae Type b," *Pediatric Nursing* 11(6):433-35, November/December 1985.

Marshall, G.S., et al. "Diffuse Retinopathy Following Measles, Mumps, and Rubella Vaccination," *Pediatrics* 76(6):989-91, December 1985.

"Measles on a College Campus—Ohio," *Morbidity and Mortality Weekly Report* 34:89, February 1985.

Mitchell, A.A., and Mandell, F. "New Recommended Immunization Schedule for DTP, MMR, and OPV," *Pediatric Alert* 11:77, 1986.

Mott, S.R., et al. *Nursing Care of Children and Families—A Holistic Approach.* Menlo Park, Calif.: Addison-Wesley Publishing Co., 1985.

"Rubella in Colleges—United States, 1983-1984" *Morbidity and Mortality Weekly Report* 34:228, April 1985.

Stetler, H.C., et al. "Impact of Revaccinating Children Who Initially Received Measles Vaccine Before 10 Months of Age," *Pediatrics* 77(4):471-76, April 1986.

Vohr, B.R., and Oh, W. "Age of Diphtheria, Tetanus, and Pertussis Immunization of Special Care Nursery Graduates," *Pediatrics* 77(4):569-71, April 1986.

Waechter, E.H., et al. *Nursing Care of Children.* Philadelphia: J.B. Lippincott Co., 1985.

PASSIVE IMMUNITY AGENTS

OBJECTIVES

After reading and studying this chapter, you should be able to:

1. Describe how passive immunity protects against disease.

2. Discuss the pharmacokinetic properties of passive immunity agents, and explain how these properties determine subsequent treatment.

3. Discuss the effect of passive immunity agents on active immunity agents.

4. Identify the clinical indications for immune globulin (IG), hepatitis B immune globulin (HBIG), rabies immune globulin (RIG), $Rh_o(D)$ immune globulin, tetanus immune globulin (TIG), and varicella-zoster immune globulin (VZIG).

5. Discuss the most common predictable and unpredictable adverse reactions to passive immunity agents and identify related nursing considerations.

INTRODUCTION

Passive immunity can occur naturally, from the mother to the fetus via the placenta, or artificially—via administration of passive immunity agents. These serums, containing preformed antibodies to diseases, are obtained from humans or animals (mainly horses) that have developed antibodies after having the disease or after being injected with live organisms or their toxins. The administration of whole blood, plasma, or specific antibody preparations derived from such humans or animals also confers passive immunity.

The use of serum, whole blood, and plasma can also provide passive immunity. However, these products are more commonly used for their blood product benefits and will not be discussed here. Furthermore, the use of human plasma is severely limited because of the danger of transmitting hepatitis and other infections via contaminated blood. An immunodeficient patient who needs plasma should receive blood from a spouse or a limited number of donors who are free of hepatitis or cytomegalovirus infection.

Passive immunity provides temporary protection against disease to a nonimmunized patient; to a patient exposed to a disease, toxin, or poison for which no other form of immunization exists; or to an immunodeficient patient with a congenital or acquired B-cell defect. Passive immunity agents also may be used to relieve the symptoms caused by some infectious diseases. They also prevent formation of active antibodies in the case of Rh_o-negative mothers who deliver Rh_o-positive infants.

When a patient who has not been immunized against a disease is exposed to it, two options are available. The patient can receive the active form of immunization, which may confer immunity during the incubation period. Or the patient can receive a passive immunity agent for protection during the incubation period, then receive the active agent at the appropriate time. Passive immunity is intended to protect the patient during the incubation period of a disease or until active immunity can be achieved against diseases for which active agents are available, such as rabies.

Physicians use three types of passive immunity agents: (1) immune globulins for general use, (2) immune globulins with known antibodies against certain disease, and (3) animal antitoxins and serums and antivenins. The passive immunity agents discussed in this chapter include IG, HBIG, RIG, $Rh_o(D)$ immune globulin, TIG, and VZIG. (See also *Animal antitoxins, serums, and antivenins* on page 1270 for a list of these agents.)

For a summary of representative drugs, see *Selected major drugs: Passive immunity agents* on pages 1271 and 1272.

PHARMACOKINETICS

Passive immunity agents are administered intravenously (I.V.) or intramuscularly (I.M.): an agent administered I.V. will be distributed immediately.

Although passive immunity is achieved almost immediately, it is temporary, because it does not effect changes in body cells. The duration of passive immunity varies from 1 to 6 weeks.

Animal antitoxins, serums, and antivenins

Antitoxins are used to prevent and treat bacterial toxin infections. Antirabies serum, equine, is used in rabies exposure. Antivenins are used to treat symptoms of insect and spider bites and snakebites. All of these provide passive immunity. Some agents available for use are listed below.

- antirabies serum, equine
- black widow spider antivenin
- botulism antitoxin, bivalent
- crotaline antivenin, polyvalent
- diphtheria antitoxin, equine
- *Micrurus fulvius* antivenin
- tetanus antitoxin (TAT), equine

PHARMACODYNAMICS

Physicians and nurses use passive immunity agents when time does not allow for the production of immunity by active processes and when a disease, such as tetanus, is present and the passive immunity will either alleviate the disease or prevent it from becoming worse. HBIG provides passive immunity to hepatitis B. IG provides passive immunity by increasing antibody titer. RIG provides passive immunity to rabies. $Rh_o(D)$ immune globulin suppresses the active antibody response and formation of anti-$Rh_o(D)$ in Rh_o-negative individuals exposed to Rh_o-positive blood. TIG provides passive immunity to tetanus. VZIG provides passive immunity to varicella-zoster virus.

PHARMACOTHERAPEUTICS

Besides providing temporary immunity against certain diseases, passive immunity agents can be used to relieve disease symptoms after suspected exposure (postexposure prophylaxis). They can also be used to prevent formation of active antibodies, as in Rh_o-negative mothers who deliver Rh_o-positive infants.

immune globulin [IG] (Gamastam, Gammar). This passive immunity agent is used for patients with immunodeficiency syndromes and immunoglobulin deficiency. It may also be administered to patients exposed to hepatitis A.

USUAL ADULT DOSAGE: for exposure to hepatitis A, 0.02 ml/kg I.M. before or soon after exposure, or 0.05 to 0.06 ml/kg at 4- to 5-month intervals for exposure longer than 3 months; for immunoglobulin deficiency, 1.3 ml/kg I.M. initially, then 0.66 ml/kg every 3 to 4 weeks; I.M. dosage administered in divided doses not to exceed 3 ml.

hepatitis B immune globulin [HBIG] (H-BIG, Hyper-Hep). Used for passive immunity and for postexposure prophylaxis against exposure to hepatitis B, HBIG is administered to adults and to newborns whose mothers are hepatitis B surface antigen (HBsAg)-positive.
USUAL ADULT DOSAGE: 0.06 ml/kg I.M., preferably in the deltoid, within 7 days of exposure; a second injection is administered 28 to 30 days later.
USUAL PEDIATRIC DOSAGE: for newborns whose mothers are HBsAg-positive, 0.5 ml I.M. as soon as possible postpartum (no later than 24 hours postpartum); this dose is repeated at ages 3 and 6 months; the injection for infants should be administered in the vastus lateralis.

rabies immune globulin [RIG] (Hyperab, Imogam). This agent provides passive immunity to patients exposed to rabies and is always given with rabies vaccine.
USUAL ADULT DOSAGE: 20 IU/kg; about half the dose should be used to infiltrate the wound, and the remainder should be administered I.M.

$Rh_o(D)$ immune globulin, human (Gamulin Rh, RhoGam). This agent is used to suppress the active antibody response and formation of anti-$Rh_o(D)$ in $Rh_o(D)$–negative individuals exposed to Rh-positive blood.
USUAL ADULT DOSAGE: for women after abortion, miscarriage, or ectopic pregnancy or postpartum, the blood bank determines fetal packed red blood cell (RBC) volume entering the woman's blood; then 1 vial is given I.M. if fetal packed RBC volume is less than 15 ml. More than 1 vial may be required if a large fetomaternal hemorrhage occurs. This agent must be given within 72 hours after delivery or miscarriage.

tetanus immune globulin [TIG] (Hyper-Tet). Used to provide passive immunity against tetanus for nonimmunized patients with susceptible wounds, TIG is also used for post–tetanus exposure prophylaxis and to treat tetanus.
USUAL ADULT AND PEDIATRIC DOSAGE: 250 to 500 units I.M.; for treatment of tetanus, 3,000 to 6,000 units may be used.

varicella-zoster immune globulin [VZIG]. This agent provides passive immunity to immunocompromised children who have been exposed to chicken pox.

Passive immunity agents

The following chart presents key points about each of the drugs used to provide passive immunity discussed in this chapter.

DRUG	MAJOR INDICATIONS	USUAL ADULT DOSAGES	NURSING IMPLICATIONS
hepatitis B immune globulin (HBIG)	Exposure to hepatitis B; post–hepatitis exposure prophylaxis	For postexposure prophylaxis, 0.06 ml/kg I.M. (most adults will receive a dose of 3 to 5 ml), preferably in the deltoid in adults, the vastus lateralis in infants and small children; a second injection is given 28 to 30 days later. For newborns whose mothers are HBsAg-positive: 0.5 ml I.M. as soon as possible postpartum and no later than 24 hours postpartum; this dose is repeated at ages 3 months and 6 months	• Administer HBIG cautiously to patients who have experienced previous systemic allergic reactions to other human immunoglobulins. • Administer HBIG to pregnant women only when clearly indicated and ordered. • Administer HBIG intramuscularly; always aspirate to be sure the injection is not inadvertently administered intravenously. • Store HBIG at 2° to 8° C.; do not freeze. • Instruct an adult patient about the importance of receiving the second dose. Inform parents about the importance of obtaining the second and third doses in children.
rabies immune globulin (RIG)	Exposure to rabies; post–rabies prophylaxis	20 IU/kg; about half the dose should be used to infiltrate the wound and the remainder administered I.M.	• Administer RIG cautiously to patients with a history of systemic hypersensitivity reactions to immunoglobulins and to patients with a known allergy to thimerosal. • Be aware of the risks and benefits of RIG for patients with isolated immunoglobulin A (IgA) deficiency, because hypersensitivity can develop from increased antibodies to IgA. Anaphylaxis can occur with subsequent administration of products that contain IgA. • Teach the patient about the predictable adverse reactions. • Administer the medication I.M. into the deltoid for adults and older children; inject it into the vastus lateralis for infants and young children. • Store RIG at 2° to 8° C. Do not freeze it. • If treatment against rabies is necessary, expect both RIG and human diploid cell rabies vaccine to be administered. Do not administer these medications at the same site or in the same syringe.
tetanus immune globulin (TIG)	Susceptible wounds in nonimmunized patients; post–tetanus prophylaxis, and treatment of tetanus	250 to 500 units I.M. for post–tetanus prophylaxis; for treatment of tetanus, 3,000 to 6,000 units may be used	• TIG is contraindicated in patients with known hypersensitivity to IG or thimerosal. • A skin test should not be performed with TIG, because an area of inflammation may occur after the injection that may be interpreted as a positive skin reaction when actually it is a chemical irritation of the tissues. • Administer TIG intramuscularly to decrease the risk of anaphylaxis. • If TIG is administered intravenously, the patient's blood pressure may decrease sharply, and anaphylaxis may occur. • Store TIG at 2° to 8° C. If the TIG has been frozen, do not use it. • Encourage the patient to schedule follow-up visits if the wound necessitates them.

continued

Passive immunity agents continued

DRUG	MAJOR INDICATIONS	USUAL ADULT DOSAGES	NURSING IMPLICATIONS
varicella-zoster immune globulin (VZIG)	Exposure to chicken pox by immunocompromised children	For children weighing up to 10 kg, 125 units I.M.; 10.1 to 20 kg, 250 units I.M.; 20.1 to 30 kg, 375 units I.M.; 30.1 to 40 kg, 500 units I.M.; over 40 kg, 625 units I.M.	• VZIG is contraindicated in patients with a history of severe hypersensitivity reaction to IG and in patients with severe thrombocytopenia. • VZIG is not recommended for pregnant women. • Administer VZIG intramuscularly to avoid anaphylaxis, which may occur with I.V. injection. • If the child experiences gastrointestinal distress, help the family plan a bland diet.

USUAL PEDIATRIC DOSAGE: for children who weigh up to 10 kg, 125 units; for those from 10.1 to 20 kg, 250 units; for those from 20.1 to 30 kg, 375 units; for those from 30.1 to 40 kg, 500 units; and for those over 40 kg, 625 units. The dose is administered I.M. within 72 hours of exposure.

Drug interactions
No significant drug interactions occur with the use of passive immunity agents.

ADVERSE DRUG REACTIONS
The adverse reactions that occur with use of the passive immunity agents vary from local discomfort at the injection site to anaphylaxis.

Predictable reactions
IG can cause several dose-related predictable reactions. The patient may experience pain at the injection site. A small percentage of patients may experience malaise, fever, chills, headache, nausea and vomiting, chest tightness, dyspnea, faintness, and chest or back pain. If the infusion infiltrates, mild erythema may occur at the site. When IG is administered to patients with idiopathic thrombocytopenic purpura, a few may experience systemic reactions with mild, transient symptoms, including chest tightness, a sense of tachycardia without actual tachycardia, and a burning sensation in the head. Adult patients with idiopathic thrombocytopenic purpura may experience erythema, pain, phlebitis, or eczematous reactions at the infusion site.

HBIG can cause tenderness and pain at the injection site as well as urticaria and angioedema. RIG can cause tenderness at the injection site and mild fever. Patients who are immunoglobulin deficient may develop hypersensitivity after repeated injections.

$Rh_o(D)$ immune globulin and TIG can cause discomfort at the injection site and mild fever.

VZIG can produce both a mild rash and mild fever which will occur, if at all, within 10 to 14 days after passive immunization.

Unpredictable reactions
IG can cause anaphylaxis in patients with a history of severe hypersensitivity reactions to I.M. immunoglobulins. Such reactions have also occurred, though rarely, in patients with no history of previous hypersensitivity reactions. With I.V. administration, anaphylaxis may be related to the infusion rate. HBIG may also cause anaphylaxis, again only rarely.

RIG can produce unpredictable skin rash, angioneurotic edema, nephrotic syndrome, and anaphylaxis: These rare adverse reactions occur after I.M. injection. Some patients receiving VZIG may experience respiratory distress or anaphylaxis.

NURSING IMPLICATIONS
Development of hypersensitivity reactions is a constant concern for nurses administering passive immunity agents, as indicated in the following nursing considerations:

• Do not administer IG to patients with known hypersensitivity to immunoglobulin A or to patients who have had previous anaphylactic reactions. Administer IG to a pregnant woman only if the immunization is clearly indicated and ordered, because safe use during pregnancy has not been determined.

• Regulate the infusion rate of IG to prevent rate-influenced adverse reactions. Begin the infusion at 0.01 to 0.02 ml/minute for the first 30 minutes. If the patient tolerates the rate, gradually increase it to a maximum of 0.08 ml/kg/minute. If adverse reactions occur, interrupt the infusion as ordered, and then resume it as ordered when the adverse reactions resolve.

• Use 5% dextrose in water if dilution is required; do not mix IG with any other fluids or drugs.

• Check the IG product before infusion for particles or any change in color; if either is observed, use another vial. Once a vial has been opened, its contents should be used immediately.

• Store IG at 2° to 8° C. (35° to 46.4° F.). Do not use IG if it has been frozen.

• Inform the patient why the infusion of IG is needed and about the associated symptoms, which include chills and chest pain. Instruct the patient to report occurrence of these symptoms to the physician.

• Administer HBIG cautiously to patients who have experienced previous systemic hypersensitivity reactions to other human immune globulins. Because I.M. injections are contraindicated in patients with thrombocytopenia, the risk of administering the HBIG injection must be carefully considered. Administer HBIG to pregnant women only when the immunization is clearly indicated and ordered.

• Administer HBIG I.M.; always aspirate to ensure that the injection is not inadvertently administered I.V.

• Instruct the adult patient about the importance of receiving the second dose of HBIG. Inform parents about the importance of obtaining the second and third doses for children.

• Administer RIG cautiously to patients with a history of systemic hypersensitivity reactions to immunoglobulins and to patients with known hypersensitivity to thimerosal.

• Know that hypersensitivity can develop with RIG, possibly resulting from the development of increased antibodies to IgA. Anaphylaxis can occur with later administration of products that contain IgA.

• Administer RIG I.M. into the deltoid for adults and older children; use the vastus lateralis for infants and young children.

• If treatment for rabies is necessary, administer RIG and human diploid cell rabies vaccine; do not administer these immunity agents at the same injection site or with the same syringe.

• Explain the possible adverse reactions that may accompany RIG immunization.

• Store RIG at 2° to 8° C. Do not freeze the medication.

• Do not administer $Rh_o(D)$ immune globulin to $Rh_o(D)$-positive patients and those previously immunized against $Rh_o(D)$ blood factor.

• Explain to the mother how $Rh_o(D)$ protects future $Rh_o(D)$-positive infants by preventing the formation of maternal antibodies—that is, by providing active immunity.

• Do not administer TIG to patients with known hypersensitivity to IG or thimerosal.

• Be aware that, if TIG is administered I.V., the patient's blood pressure may decrease sharply; anaphylaxis can also occur.

• Do not use TIG if it is frozen.

• Do not administer VZIG to patients with a history of severe hypersensitivity reactions to IG or to patients with severe thrombocytopenia.

• Know that VZIG should be administered to immunosuppressed children within 72 hours after exposure to chicken pox or herpes zoster. VZIG is not recommended for pregnant women.

• Administer VZIG I.M. to avoid anaphylaxis, which may occur with I.V. injection.

• If a child experiences gastrointestinal distress after VZIG immunization, recommend that the parents provide a bland diet to relieve the effects.

CHAPTER SUMMARY

Chapter 82 discussed the human preparations of passive immunity agents as they are used for temporary prevention or modification of certain diseases after exposure to them. To achieve passive immunity, preformed antibodies from immune human sources are administered. Here are the highlights of the chapter:

• Passive immunity is temporary, intended to last only for the incubation period of the disease or until active immunity agents can be administered safely.

• The three types of passive immunity agents available are general immune globulins, immune globulins with known antibodies for certain diseases, and animal antitoxins and serums and antivenins. The human preparations cause fewer and less severe adverse reactions than the animal preparations.

• The passive immunity agents include human immune globulin (IG), human plasma, hepatitis B immune globulin (HBIG), rabies immune globulin (RIG), tetanus immune globulin (TIG), varicella-zoster immune globulin (VZIG), and $Rh_o(D)$ immune globulin.

• The predictable adverse reactions to passive immunity agents range from fever and tenderness at the injection site to gastrointestinal distress. Anaphylaxis is the unpredictable adverse reaction most commonly associated with these immunizations.

BIBLIOGRAPHY

Azimi, P.H., et al. "Transfusion-Acquired Hepatitis A in a Premature Infant with Secondary Spread in an Intensive Care Nursery," *American Journal of Diseases of Children* 140:23, 1986.

Behrman, R.E., and Vaughn, V.C. "Varicella," in *Nelson Textbook of Pediatrics*, 12th ed. Behrman, R.E., and Vaughn, V.C., eds. Philadelphia: W.B. Saunders Co., 1983.

Brunell, P.A. "Hepatitis," in *Nelson Textbook of Pediatrics,* 12th ed. Behrman, R.E., and Vaughn, V.C., eds. Philadelphia: W.B. Saunders Co., 1983.

Brunell, P.A. "Varicella Vaccine—Where Are We?" *Pediatrics* 78:721, 1986.

Drugs, 2nd ed. Nurse's Reference Library. Springhouse, Pa.: Springhouse Corp., 1984.

Hughes, W.T., et al. "The Immune Compromised Host," *Pediatric Clinics of North America* 30:103, 1983.

Kelin, J.O., et al. "Active and Passive Immunization," in *Report of the Committee on Infectious Disease,* 19th ed. Evanston, Ill.: American Academy of Pediatrics, 1982.

Leff, R.D., and Roberts, R.J. "Host Factors Influencing the Response to Antimicrobial Agents," *Pediatric Clinics of North America* 30:93, 1983.

Lemon, S.M. "Type A Viral Hepatitis," *New England Journal of Medicine* 313:1059, 1985.

Lin, C.Y., et al. "Nephrotic Syndrome Associated with Varicella Infection," *Pediatrics* 75:1127, 1985.

Mott, S.R., et al. *Nursing Care of Children and Families—A Holistic Approach.* Menlo Park, Calif.: Addison-Wesley Publishing Co., 1985.

Plotkin, S.A. "Varicella Vaccine: A Point of Decision," *Pediatrics* 78:705, 1986.

Snydman, D.R. "Current Concept—Hepatitis in Pregnancy," *New England Journal of Medicine* 313: 1398, 1985.

Stiehm, E.R. "Passive Immunization," in *Textbook of Pediatric Infectious Diseases,* vol. 2. Fergin, R.D., and Cherry, J.D., eds. Philadelphia: W.B. Saunders Co., 1981.

"Suboptimal Response to Hepatitis B Vaccine Given by Injection into the Buttock," *Mortality and Morbidity Weekly Report* 34:106, March 1985.

Waechter, F.H., et al. *Nursing Care of Children.* Philadelphia: J.B. Lippincott Co., 1985.

Whaley, L.E., and Wong, D.L. *Nursing Care of Infants and Children,* 2nd ed. St. Louis: C.V. Mosby Co., 1983.

Withers, J., and Bradshaw, E. "Preventing Neonatal Hepatitis-B Infection," *Maternal Child Nursing* 11:270, 1986.

Xu, Z.Y., et al. "Prevention of Perinatal Acquisition of Hepatitis B Virus Carriage Using Vaccine: Preliminary Report of a Randomized Double-Blind, Placebo-Controlled and Comparative Trial," *Pediatrics* 76:714, 1985.

APPENDICES AND INDEX

Diagnostic agents

Pharmaceutical agents, ranging from radioisotopes to synthetic hormones, have diagnostic testing applications. Each classification of such agents carries its specific mechanism and site of action, guidelines for administration, and potential for adverse reactions and interactions with other drugs. To provide optimum care for a patient receiving a diagnostic agent, the nurse must be familiar with these characteristics. This chart lists the most common diagnostic agents and summarizes their uses and related nursing implications.

AGENT	DIAGNOSTIC USES	NURSING IMPLICATIONS
USED FOR STRUCTURAL ASSESSMENT		
barium compounds, including barium sulfate (Baroflave, Barosperse, Esophotrast, Oratrast)	Barium swallow, upper gastrointestinal (GI) and colon series, small-bowel series, hypotonic duodenography, barium enema	● As a radiopaque agent for X-ray visualization, barium is administered P.O. or via enema. ● Barium may be contraindicated in patients with suspected intestinal obstruction or perforation. ● Before testing begins, assess for and report abdominal pain, rigidity, or marked distention. ● Prepare the patient for the thick consistency and chalky taste of oral barium. ● Explain that the testing requires the patient to change positions and hold the breath at certain points. ● As ordered, administer a pre-test laxative or enema. ● Tell the patient to expect gray-colored stools for 24 to 72 hours after the test and to increase fluid intake to prevent constipation.
iodinated compounds, including diatrizoate meglumine, diatrizoate sodium (Gastrografin, Hypaque, Reno-M-60), iocetamic acid (Cholebrine), iodamide meglumine (Renovue), iodipamide meglumine (Cholografin), iohexol (Omnipaque), iopanoic acid (Telepaque), iothalamate meglumine, iothalamate sodium (Angio-Conray, Conray), ipodate sodium, ipodate calcium (Oragrafin), metrizamide (Amipaque), metrizoic acid (Isopaque, Isopaque 280), tyropanoate sodium (Bilopaque), ethiodized oil (Ethiodol), propyliodone (Dionosil Oily)	Angiography, computed tomography scans, urography, pyelography, GI radiology, oral cholecystography, I.V. cholangiography, cystourethrography, myelography, lymphography, hysterosalpingography, visualization of the nasal sinuses, bronchography	● As radiopaque agents for X-ray visualization, these compounds are administered P.O., I.V., intrathecally, intralymphatically, or instilled into the trachea or uterus. ● Before administering iodinated contrast media, document any patient history of asthma or allergies (particularly to iodine or shellfish). ● Tell the patient to expect feelings of warmth and flushing after I.V. injections of iodinated agents. Instruct the patient to report other responses, such as severe nausea or breathing difficulty. ● Closely observe the patient for 30 to 60 minutes after the test, watching for delayed allergic or idiosyncratic reactions. ● Have resuscitation equipment readily available in case of severe reactions. ● Maintain adequate hydration to decrease a possible drug reaction.

Diagnostic agents continued

AGENT	DIAGNOSTIC USES	NURSING IMPLICATIONS
iodinated compounds (continued)		• Metrizamide may react with drugs that decrease the seizure threshold, possibly precipitating seizures. Monitor the patient for increased seizure activity. • Because contrast agents used in urography can alter urinalysis results, obtain any necessary specimens before the test or at least 2 days after the test.
fluorescein sodium	Fluorescein angiography, fluorescein staining of the cornea	• As a nonradiopaque agent for direct visualization, fluorescein is administered I.V. or by instillation into the conjunctiva. • Inform the patient that fluorescein will discolor the skin and urine for 24 to 48 hours. • Explain that I.V. injection may cause flushing, warmth, and nausea. • Inform the patient undergoing fluorescein scanning of the cornea that extravasation of the dye from ophthalmic vessels may be painful.
indigotindisulfonate sodium (indigo carmine)	Cystoscopy	• As a nonradiopaque agent for direct visualization, indigo carmine is administered I.V. • Encourage the patient to increase fluid intake after the test to promote dye excretion.
hysteroscopy fluid (Hyskon)	Hysterosalpingography	• As a nonradiopaque agent for direct visualization, hysteroscopy fluid is administered via uterine instillation. • Assure the patient that uterine cramping is transient.
USED FOR FUNCTIONAL ASSESSMENT		
histamine, including histamine phosphate	Gastric secretion test, diagnosis of pheochromocytoma	• As an agent used in exocrine tests, histamine is administered I.M., S.C., or, rarely, I.V. • Histamine affects many body systems, possibly causing dangerous increases in pulse rate and blood pressure. Monitor the patient's vital signs and observe for signs of anaphylactic reaction. • Have emergency resuscitation equipment available at all times.
pentagastrin (Peptavlon)	Gastric acid stimulation test	• As an agent used in exocrine tests, pentagastrin is administered S.C. • Instruct the patient to avoid eating, drinking, and smoking after midnight on the day of test. • Explain to the patient that the test involves insertion of a nasogastric tube. • Before testing, withhold antacids, anticholinergics, adrenergic blocking agents, and reserpine, as ordered.
pancreatic enzymes and related compounds, including bentiromide (Chymex), cholecystokinin [CCK], secretin (Secretin-Kabi), sincalide (Kinevac), cholecystokinin-pancreozymin [CCK-PZ]	Pancreatic dysfunction tests	• As agents used in exocrine tests, pancreatic enzymes and related compounds are administered P.O., I.M., or I.V. • Before giving bentiromide, withhold acetaminophen, chloramphenicol, sulfonamides,

continued

Diagnostic agents continued

AGENT	DIAGNOSTIC USES	NURSING IMPLICATIONS
pancreatic enzymes and related compounds (continued)		and thiazides, as ordered. These drugs may interfere with test results. • Inform the patient that sincalide may cause abdominal pain and the urge to defecate.
saralasin acetate (Sarenin)	Renin-dependent hypertension	• As an agent used in exocrine tests, saralasin is administered I.V. • A diuretic such as furosemide is usually administered orally the evening before the test. • Monitor the patient's blood pressure during infusion and for 3 hours afterward, because rebound hypertension may occur.
edrophonium chloride (Tensilon)	Myasthenia gravis	• As an agent used in exocrine tests, edrophonium is administered I.V. • Withhold procainamide, muscle relaxants, prednisolone, quinidine, and catecholamines as ordered. These drugs may alter test results. • Have atropine sulfate available for severe adverse reactions, such as bradycardia, hypotension, and wheezing.
arginine hydrochloride (R-Gene 10)	Growth hormone stimulation test	• As an agent used in endocrine tests, arginine is administered I.V. • Advise the patient to restrict activity for 10 to 12 hours before testing. • Withhold steroids, estrogens, progesterones, and other pituitary-based medications, as ordered. These drugs may affect growth hormone levels.
human chorionic gonadotropin [HCG] (Antuitrin, Chorex, Follutein)	HCG-secreting tumors and male primary hypogonadism	• As an agent used in endocrine tests, HCG is administered I.M.
adrenocorticotropic hormone (ACTH), including corticotropin (ACTH, ACTHAR) and cosyntropin (Cortrosyn)	Rapid ACTH test for adrenocortical insufficiency	• As agents used in endocrine tests, corticotropin is administered I.M. or S.C. and cosyntropin (a safer synthetic analog) is administered I.M., I.V., or P.O. • Advise the patient to restrict foods, fluids, and activity for 10 to 12 hours before the test and to maintain a low-cholesterol diet for 2 days before the test. • Before administering ACTH, withhold all other medications as prescribed—particularly estrogens and amphetamines, which interfere with test results.
dexamethasone (Decadron, Hexadrol)	Adrenocortical hyperfunction	• As an agent used in endocrine tests, dexamethasone is administered I.M. or I.V.
glucose	Oral glucose tolerance test (GTT)	• As an agent used in endocrine tests, glucose is administered P.O. • Explain to the patient that GTT requires five urine samples. Teach the patient the proper urine sample collection technique. • Advise the patient to restrict activity for 10 to 12 hours before the test and to avoid eat-

Diagnostic agents continued

AGENT	DIAGNOSTIC USES	NURSING IMPLICATIONS
glucose (continued)		ing, drinking, and smoking after midnight on the day of testing. • Alert the patient that the glucose solution may cause transient nausea.
gonadorelin hydrochloride (Factrel, Synthetic Luteinizing Hormone Releasing Hormone)	Evaluation of hypothalamic-pituitary gonadotropic dysfunction	• As an agent used in endocrine tests, gonadorelin is administered I.V. or S.C. • As ordered, withhold steroid medications (androgens, estrogens, progestins, glucocorticoids) before testing. These drugs may interfere with test results.
metyrapone (Metopirone)	Evaluation of hypothalamic-pituitary dysfunction	• As an agent used in endocrine tests, metyrapone is administered P.O. • Withhold steroid medications before testing, as ordered.
parathyroid hormone (PTH)	Idiopathic hypoparathyroidism	• As an agent used in endocrine tests, PTH is administered I.V., I.M., or S.C. • As ordered, withhold calcium preparations before testing. These agents may interfere with test results.
phentolamine (Regitine)	Pheochromocytoma	• As an agent used in endocrine tests, phentolamine is administered I.V. • This agent may cause hypotension and cardiac dysrhythmias. Monitor the patient's vital signs and keep emergency resuscitation equipment available.
protirelin (Thypinone)	Primary hypothyroidism, pituitary dysfunction, hypothalmic dysfunction	• As an agent used in endocrine tests, protirelin is administered I.V. • Withhold thyroid medication before testing, as ordered. • Radioactive scan performed within 1 week before the test may alter results.
thyrotropin (Thytropar)	Hypothyroidism	• As an agent used in endocrine tests, thyrotropin is administered I.M. or S.C. • Withhold thyroid medications before testing, as ordered.
tolbutamide sodium (Orinase)	Insulinoma test	• As an agent used in endocrine tests, tolbutamide is administered I.V. • Instruct the patient to maintain a high-carbohydrate diet for 3 days before the test, fast overnight, and avoid smoking. • During testing, monitor the patient for signs and symptoms of hypoglycemia.
vasopressin (Pitressin)	Detection of deficient antidiuretic hormone (diabetes insipidus)	• As an agent used in endocrine tests, vasopressin is administered I.M. or S.C. • Alert the patient that vasopressin may cause anginal pain. • Monitor the patient's vital signs and have oxygen available.

continued

Diagnostic agents continued

AGENT	DIAGNOSTIC USES	NURSING IMPLICATIONS
dyes, including indocyanine green (Cardio-Green), bromsulphalein (BSP), phenolsulfon-phthalein (PSP)	Evaluation of cardiac output, hepatic blood flow and function, renal function, lymphatic flow, and ophthalmic circulation	● As agents used to evaluate circulatory-excretory clearance, these dyes are administered I.V. Phenolsulfonphthalein may be administered I.M. ● Alert the patient that skin, sclera, and urine may be discolored after test. Explain that indocyanine green will discolor feces. ● Observe the patient for signs of allergic reaction. Keep epinephrine and emergency resuscitation equipment on hand. ● Morphine, meperidine (Demerol), and methadone yield false-negative results in tests using bromsulphalein; androgens, estrogens, progesterone, and B vitamins yield false-positive results. ● Teach the patient the proper technique for collecting urine samples for renal function tests.
para-aminohippuric acid [PAH]	Measurement of effective renal plasma flow	● As an agent used to evaluate circulatory-excretory clearance, PAH is administered I.V. ● Advise the patient to increase fluid intake during testing. ● Teach the patient to collect urine samples properly. ● Inform the patient of potential adverse reactions, including nausea, vomiting, cramping, and flushing. ● Withhold diuretics, penicillin, probenecid, phenolsulfonphthalein, salicylates, and sulfonamides as prescribed.
dehydrocholic acid (Decholin)	Evaluation of circulation time	● As an agent used to evaluate circulatory-excretory clearance, dehydrocholic acid is administered I.V. ● To determine the circulation time from arm to tongue, tell the patient to report a bitter taste after injection.
inulin	Measurement of glomerular filtration rate	● As an agent used to evaluate circulatory-excretory clearance, inulin is administered I.V. ● Advise the patient to increase fluid intake during testing. ● Teach the patient to collect urine samples properly.
mannitol (Osmitrol)	Measurement of glomerular filtration rate	● As an agent used to evaluate circulatory-excretory clearance, mannitol is administered I.V. ● Teach the patient to collect urine samples properly.
D-xylose (Xylo-Pfan)	Screening for intestinal mal-absorption state	● As an agent used to evaluate circulatory-excretory clearance, D-xylose is administered I.V. or P.O. ● Alert the patient that nausea, vomiting, or diarrhea may occur.

Diagnostic agents continued

AGENT	DIAGNOSTIC USES	NURSING IMPLICATIONS
USED FOR RADIOACTIVE SCANNING		
radioisotopes, including cyanocobalamin [^{57}Co-B$_{12}$] (Rubratope), gallium citrate [^{65}Ga], iodine [^{131}I], iodohippurate sodium [^{131}I] (Hipputope), serum albumin ^{131}I (Albumatope ^{131}I), sodium iodide [^{131}I], iodine [^{125}I], sodium (Iodotope ^{125}I), serum albumin (Albumatope ^{125}I), sodium chromate ^{51}Cr (Chromitope sodium), technetium-99m pyrophosphate kit (Phosphotec), technetium-99m sulfur colloid kit (Tesuloid), technetium-99m medronate kit (MDP-Squibb), technetium-99m pentetate kit (Techneplex), thallous chloride ^{201}TlCl (Thallium 201), phosphorus sodium ^{32}P (Phosphotope), ferrous citrate [^{59}Fe], strontium-87m, xenon [^{133}Xe]	Bone, cardiac, liver, spleen, thyroid, kidney, pancreas, and brain imaging; Schilling test; iron absorption testing; red blood cell volume determination	• As agents used for radioactive scanning, these isotopes are administered I.V. and P.O. • Reassure the patient that these isotopes release only small amounts of radioactivity during diagnostic testing, and that exposure levels are well within safety standards. • Because most radiopharmaceuticals are excreted in the urine, keep the patient well hydrated after administration of a radioisotope to increase its excretion and prevent overexposure of the bladder. Dispose of all patient excretions promptly by flushing them down the sewage system. Keep in mind that this waste is not considered dangerous to the patient or health care personnel. • Technetium, a newer radioisotope with a short half-life, can be given safely in large doses. Its gamma emissions are easily detected.
USED FOR SKIN TESTS		
coccidioidin (Spherulin); histoplasmin; benzyl-penicilloyl-polylysine (Pre-Pen); diphtheria toxin (Schick test toxin); tuberculins, including tuberculin purified protein derivative [Mantoux, PPD] (Aplisol, Tubersol), tuberculin PPD multiple puncture device (Aplitest, Sclavotest-PPD), old tuberculin multiple puncture devices (tine test)	Coccidioidomycosis; histoplasmosis; penicillin sensitivity; diphtheria susceptibility; tuberculin exposure screening	• As agents used for skin tests, these drugs are administered intradermally. • Before administration, document any history of previous testing or any history of reactions to the particular agent. • Instruct the patient to observe for erythema and induration at the administration site, and provide instructions for follow-up examination in 48 to 72 hours.

Serotonin agonists and antagonists

Various endogenous agents produce physiologic responses. One group of these agents—biologically active amines (histamine and serotonin), prostaglandins, and polypeptides—are sometimes referred to as *autacoids,* a term derived from the Greek word meaning "self-remedy." Serotonin (5-hydroxytryptamine or 5-HT), a biologically active amine, represents just one such autacoid.

Serotonin is formed enzymatically from the amino acid tryptophan. Exogenous sources include such foods as pineapples, bananas, plums, avocados, eggplants, and tomatoes. Serotonin is distributed widely in the body and is responsible for numerous physiologic responses. Its biochemical mechanisms have stimulated clinical research in areas ranging from pain management in migraine headache to the treatment of mental disorders, alcoholism, seizure disorders, and Alzheimer's disease.

Although serotonin has no clinical application as a drug, it does exert powerful endogenous effects. Current clinical literature shows an active interest in identifying and developing agents that mimic or reduce the actions of serotonin. Although usually not considered a specific drug class, serotonin agonists and antagonists produce widely varied serotonin-related effects.

Understanding serotonin

Approximately 90% of serotonin is found in the enterochromaffin cells of the gastrointestinal tract. Serotonin located in the brain can be elevated by administering serotonin precursors, but systemic administration will not produce elevated brain levels because serotonin does not cross the blood-brain barrier. When released into the circulation, serotonin binds at once with plasma proteins. The major metabolite, 5-hydroxyindoleacetic acid (5-HIAA), is excreted in the urine.

Serotonin stimulates and inhibits a variety of smooth muscle and nerves. In the central nervous system, increased levels of serotonin will cause a decrease in pain perception. Serotonin has little effect on the myocardium, but slow rate and decreased cardiac output may result from vagal stimulation. Serotonin constricts large arteries and in most vascular beds causes arteriole dilation. Stimulation of carotid and aortic chemoreceptors can cause a short-lived increase in the respiratory rate as well as pulmonary vessel constriction. Serotonin also increases small bowel motility and weakly promotes platelet aggregation.

Serotonin's activity apparently is linked to its relationship with specific endogenous receptors. Reclassification of receptors continues to recognize two types, now referred to as S_1 (5-HT_1) and S_2 (5-HT_2) serotonergic binding sites. S_1 sites are found predominantly in the frontal cortex of the brain, suggesting centrally located receptors.

Serotonin agonists

Several classes of agents have increased serotonergic function. These include serotonin precursors and monoamine oxidase inhibitors, which elevate serotonin stores; uptake inhibitors and serotonin releasers, which increase serotonin concentration in the synaptic cleft; and direct serotonin agonists, which mimic serotonin action on specific receptors.

Direct serotonin agonists, such as the tryptamine structural analogues, and indirect agonists, such as fluoxetine, have been investigated to treat such disorders as depression, obesity, alcoholism, and chronic pain. Some are in use. Fenfluramine, an appetite-suppressant similar to amphetamine but without stimulant properties, can promote rapid serotonin release; it may inhibit serotonin reuptake. Preliminary data indicate that fenfluramine, in doses of 20 to 40 mg three times a day, may be of value in treating chronic alcoholism.

Serotonin may be involved in depressive disorders. Low concentrations of serotonin and 5-HIAA have been found in autopsy studies of brains from suicide victims and in cerebrospinal fluid from depressed patients. Compounds that selectively block neuronal reuptake of serotonin have potential as antidepressant drugs.

Many of the tricyclic antidepressants (TCAs) can inhibit presynaptic uptake of serotonin and of the catecholamines norepinephrine and epinephrine and, in some cases, dopamine. Since development of the classic TCA prototype more than 20 years ago,

Serotonin agonists and antagonists continued

the search has continued for newer agents as effective as these tricyclics but with fewer adverse effects. Fluoxetine, a selective serotonin uptake inhibitor, is currently under review by the Food and Drug Administration (FDA) for use in the United States as an antidepressant.

Clomipramine, a more recent TCA, may possess serotonin uptake inhibition properties. To a lesser extent, clomipramine inhibits norepinephrine reuptake; it appears particularly effective in treating obsessive-compulsive disorders. As of this writing, clinical trials on this agent are being conducted.

Monoamine oxidase (MAO) inhibitors inhibit the enzyme that normally metabolizes the neurotransmitters norepinephrine and serotonin. This action increases the amount of serotonin available and often relieves the symptoms of depression. (See Chapter 31, Antidepressant and Antimanic Agents, for a complete discussion of MAOs and TCAs.)

Serotonin antagonists

Drugs that depress serotonergic function include direct antagonists that block serotonin action on receptors and agents that decrease serotonin release by inhibiting its synthesis or by depleting granular stores.

Serotonin antagonists include methysergide, mianserin, ketanserin, cyproheptadine, metergoline, and ritanserin as well as some indole compounds and histamine H_1 blockers of the ethylenediamine type. The ergot alkaloids (such as methysergide) are antagonists at serotonin receptors, particularly on smooth muscle. (See Chapter 20, Adrenergic Blocking Agents, for a complete discussion of ergot alkaloids.) These compounds have been used for approximately 60 years to treat acute migraine attacks. Besides its serotonin antagonist properties, methysergide produces weak oxytocic effects and possible anticonvulsant activity. Methysergide gained clinical prominence after researchers discovered that migraine attacks were associated with low plasma serotonin levels.

Cyproheptadine is a serotonin and histamine antagonist used effectively to treat various allergic conditions. It also has been used effectively as an appetite stimulant in some patients with anorexia nervosa.

Mianserin, an antidepressant currently under investigation in the United States, is indicated for depression and anxiety. Researchers do not yet understand how serotonin antagonists act as antidepressants. One postulation is that their action shifts the norepinephrine-serotonin balance toward norepinephrine.

Heavy metal antagonists

Poisoning with heavy metals presents unique and difficult diagnostic and treatment problems. Heavy metals commonly have broad systemic impacts and cause irreversible problems. Chronic exposure can lead to the progressive development of symptoms that are quite different from those resulting from acute intoxication.

The treatment of heavy metal poisoning in many cases involves administration of chelating agents—chemicals that form water-soluble, stable complexes by binding with metal ions and allowing renal elimination of heavy metals. Commonly used chelating agents include calcium disodium edetate, deferoxamine mesylate, dimercaprol, and penicillamine. Although in many cases effective in removing heavy metals from the system, chelating agents can produce adverse reactions of their own and should be used cautiously.

Theoretically, *calcium disodium edetate* (CaNa$_2$-EDTA) should bind a variety of metals, but few metals bind strongly enough to alter blood levels. Thus, CaNa$_2$-EDTA is reserved for use in lead poisoning. Adverse reactions include fever, nasal congestion, dermatitis, malaise, and thirst. Severe proximal nephron degeneration may also occur.

Deferoxamine mesylate binds both ferrous and ferric iron. It spares the iron bound tightly to cytochromes and hemoglobin. Histamine release may result from treatment, leading to urticaria, gastrointestinal (GI) irritation, and hypotension. Local irritation at the injection site also occurs. Deferoxamine is contraindicated in patients with severely compromised renal function.

Dimercaprol (British Anti-Lewisite, BAL) effectively binds arsenic, cadmium, lead, gold, thallium, and mercury. Dimercaprol has the potential for extreme toxicity. Serious problems can arise, including hypertension, tachycardia, nausea and vomiting, headache, and fever in children.

Penicillamine binds copper, lead, mercury, and zinc. It is particularly effective in promoting removal of methylmercury and in treating poisoning by mercury vapors. Penicillamine is rarely the first-choice antidote, but it may be used for long-term treatment of chronic poisoning. Allergy to penicillin may predict allergy to this chelator. Other adverse reactions are rare.

Institutional protocols for heavy metal poisoning vary. The following table provides examples of treatments.

HEAVY METAL AND SOURCES OF POISONING	SIGNS AND SYMPTOMS Acute poisoning	Chronic poisoning	TREATMENT
Arsenic			
Accidental or purposeful exposure to weed killers and insecticides used for ant and roach control, as well as some pharmaceuticals; industrial exposure in metallurgy, glass manufacturing, and pigment production	GI effects: severe nausea, projectile vomiting, diarrhea with rice-water stools, abdominal pain; local irritation of eyes, nose, throat; anuria, electrocardiographic abnormalities, hypoxic convulsions	Weight loss, anorexia, GI tract ulcers, garlic breath odor, peripheral neuritis, Mees' lines (white lines on lunulae of nails), hyperpigmentation of skin, chronic liver failure, pancytopenia	● Acute poisoning: symptomatic and supportive treatment with dimercaprol USUAL ADULT AND PEDIATRIC DOSAGE: 3 mg/kg I.M. every 4 hours until abdominal symptoms subside; then penicillamine P.O. in four divided dosages not to exceed 1 gram/day for 4 days. Penicillamine may be repeated if symptoms recur. ● Chronic poisoning: usually penicillamine P.O. is used; length of therapy depends on the patient's condition.
Iron			
Accidental or purposeful ingestion of iron-containing medications	Irritability, restlessness, seizures, abdominal pain, bloody diarrhea, tachypnea, tachy-	Seldom involved in chronic poisoning	● Before absorption: sodium bicarbonate lavage or sodium biphosphate enema

Heavy metal antagonists continued

HEAVY METAL AND SOURCES OF POISONING	SIGNS AND SYMPTOMS Acute poisoning	Chronic poisoning	TREATMENT
Iron (continued)	cardia; after 8 to 16 hours: shock; after 4 days: hepatic necrosis; after 2 to 4 weeks: GI obstruction		• After absorption: chelation with deferoxamine mesylate USUAL ADULT AND PEDIATRIC DOSAGE: 1 gram I.M., followed by 500 mg every 4 hours for two doses, then 500 mg every 4 to 12 hours, depending on clinical response, but not exceeding 6 grams in 24 hours. In an emergency, it can be given as an I.V. infusion at a rate not exceeding 15 mg/kg/hour.
Lead			
Accidental exposure by ingestion of lead-based paint or lead-glazed dishes; industrial exposure in mining, smelting, spray painting, and sheet metal and storage battery production	Acute symptoms rarely seen, but may include: sweet metallic breath, black stools, salivation, vomiting, intestinal colic, muscle weakness, pain, paresthesia	Symptoms in chronic lead poisoning (plumbism): anemia, ataxia, lead palsy, restlessness, irritability, convulsions, coma, anorexia, lead colic, constipation, renal failure, metallic taste	• Administration of CaNa$_2$-EDTA to bind lead from bone and soft tissue USUAL ADULT AND PEDIATRIC DOSAGE: 35 to 50 mg/kg/day in two divided doses deep I.M. or slow I.V. in 250 to 500 ml fluid for up to 5 days. • Administration of dimercaprol to bind lead in serum and cerebrospinal fluid USUAL ADULT AND PEDIATRIC DOSAGE: 4 mg/kg deep I.M. every 4 hours for 48 hours, then every 6 hours for 48 hours, then every 6 to 12 hours for 7 days. Penicillamine: 250 mg P.O. q.i.d. for 5 days; however, chronic therapy should not exceed 40 mg/kg/day.
Mercury			
Industrial exposure in paint and paper manufacturing; agricultural use to retard mold and fungus growth; environmental pollution; rare accidental or purposeful exposure via medications	Elemental mercury (usually inhaled): bronchial irritation, shortness of breath, confusion, chest pain, tremors, nausea and vomiting, metallic taste in mouth	Elemental mercury: variable clinical picture, possibly including central nervous system (CNS) changes, such as irritability or depression; gingivitis; renal dysfunction	• Elemental mercury: Symptomatic treatment; dimercaprol for mercury concentrations in blood and urine as outlined for inorganic mercury poisoning
	Inorganic mercury (usually ingested): GI tract irritation and bleeding	Inorganic mercury: renal dysfunction; hypersensitivity with erythema, tachycardia, photophobia	• Inorganic mercury: Chelation with dimercaprol USUAL ADULT AND PEDIATRIC DOSAGE: 5 mg/kg I.M. initially, then 2.5 mg/kg every 12 hours for 10 days.
	Organic mercurials: usually not involved in acute poisoning	Organic mercurials: CNS changes, such as visual or mental dysfunction, ataxia	• Organic mercurials: no effective treatment, dimercaprol is contraindicated

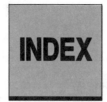

INDEX

Loop diuretics *continued*
 history and source of, 613
 interaction of, with drugs, 614t, 615
 mechanism of action of, 613, 615
 nursing implications for, 616
 patient assessment during therapy with, 616
 patient teaching during therapy with, 616
 pharmacokinetics of, 613
 therapeutic uses of, 615
Lo/Ovral, 944. *See also* Oral contraceptives.
Loperamide, 749-751
 action of, 750
 adverse reactions to, 750-751
 clinical indications for, 750
 contraindications for, 751
 dosage, 750
 interaction of, with drugs, 750
 nursing implications for, 751
 patient assessment during therapy with, 751
 pharmacokinetics of, 750
Lopid, 642. *See also* Gemfibrozil.
Lopressor, 319, 575, 591. *See also* Metoprolol tartrate.
Loprox, 1220. *See also* Antifungal agents.
Lorazepam. *See also* Benzodiazepines *and* Injection anesthetics.
 accumulation of, 481
 adverse reactions to, 516
 for anxiety, 516
 dosage, 440, 481, 516
 for induction of anterograde amnesia, 440
 interaction of, with drugs, 482t
 pharmacokinetics of, 480, 515
 as sedative and hypnotic, 481
Lorelco, 644. *See also* Probucol.
Lotense, 611. *See also* Polythiazide.
Lotrimin, 1220. *See also* Topical glucocorticoids.
Lotrisone, 999, 1220. *See also* Topical glucocorticoids.
Lotusate, 488. *See also* Talbutal.
Lovostatin, 644-645
 action of, 644
 administration considerations for, 645
 adverse reactions to, 645
 dosage, 644
 pharmacokinetics of, 644
Loxapine succinate. *See also* Nonphenothiazines.
 adverse reactions to, 531t
 dosage, 530
Loxitane, 530. *See also* Loxapine succinate.
Lozenge, 93
Lozol, 615. *See also* Indapamide.
L-tryptophan as sleep aid, 493-494
Lubricant laxative, 760, 762-763
Ludiomil, 507. *See also* Maprotiline hydrochloride.
Lufyllin, 707. *See also* Dyphylline.
Lugol's solution, 890
Lumbar block, 449
Luminal, 380, 487. *See also* Phenobarbital.
Lupron, 1199. *See also* Leuprolide acetate.
Luride, 822. *See also* Fluoride.

Luteinizing hormone
 action of, 908i
 as anterior pituitary hormone, 860, 861i
 role of, in menstrual cycle, 930, 931i, 932
 target organ of, 908i
Lymphocyte immune globulin, antithymocyte globulin (equine). *See also* Immunosuppressants.
 action of, 1004
 administration considerations for, 1010
 adverse reactions to, 1005
 dosage, 1004
 history and source of, 1002
 interaction of, with drugs, 1003t
 patient assessment before/during therapy with, 1005
 pharmacokinetics of, 1002-1003
 storage of, 1010
Lymphocyte responses, 1256i
Lymphokines, 998-999
Lypressin. *See also* Posterior pituitary hormones.
 adverse reactions to, 918t
 dosage, 915
 pharmacokinetics of, 913
Lysergic acid diethylamide (LSD) abuse
 general effects of, 89, 89t
 treatment of, 90

Maalox, 785t. *See also* Antacids.
Maalox Plus, 785t. *See also* Antacids.
Maalox TC, 787. *See also* Antacids.
Macrocytic anemia, 657. *See also* Megaloblastic anemia.
Macrodantin, 1141. *See also* Nitrofurantoin.
Mafenide acetate, 1219. *See also* Antibacterial agents.
Magaldrate. *See also* Antacids.
 adverse reactions to, 787
 contraindications for, 787
 in geriatric patient, 787-788
 pharmacokinetics of, 785
Magnesium, 833, 835
 concentration levels of, in fluid compartments, 796t
Magnesium citrate, 754. *See also* Magnesium salts.
Magnesium hydroxide, 754. *See also* Magnesium salts.
 in pregnant patient, 228
Magnesium hydroxide and aluminum hydroxide with simethicone. *See also* Antacids.
 adverse reactions to, 787
 pharmacokinetics of, 785
Magnesium salts. *See also* Hyperosmolar laxatives *and* Saline cathartics.
 action of, 753
 administration considerations for, 755
 adverse reactions to, 755
 chemical name for, 6t
 dosage, 754
 pharmacokinetics of, 753
 in pregnant patient, 228

Magnesium sulfate, 228-229t, 754. *See also* Magnesium salts *and* Tocolytic agents.
 action of, 967
 adverse reactions to, 969
 as anticonvulsant, 391
 contraindications for, 969
 dosage, 967
 effects of magnesium levels on maternal reactions to, 967t
 interaction of, with drugs, 966t
 nursing implications for, 969
 pharmacokinetics of, 966, 967
 for replacement therapy, 833, 835
Magnesium trisilicate, in pregnant patient, 225
Maintenance dose, 35, 36c
Maintenance therapy, 57
Malaria transmission cycle, 1124i
Malignant hypertension, 584
 treatment of, 597
Malignant hyperthermia
 crisis in, 352
 drugs affected by, 73t
 as reaction to inhalant anesthetics, 438
Malignant neoplasms, drugs to treat, 1146-1213. *See also* Antineoplastic agents.
Malnutrition, assessment of, 796-797
Malpractice, medication errors and, 134
Mandelamine, 1140. *See also* Methenamine.
Mandol, 1050. *See also* Cefamandole naftate.
Manganese
 action of, 822
 adverse reactions to, 825
 dosage, 822
 food sources of, 820t
 pharmacokinetics of, 821
Manganese Gluconate, 822. *See also* Manganese.
Mangatrace, 822. *See also* Manganese.
Mania, 499, 500
 treatment of, 507-509
Manic-depressive illness, 499
Mannitol. *See also* Osmotic diuretics.
 administration considerations for, 623
 adverse reactions to, 623
 contraindications for, 1239
 as diagnostic aid, 1280t
 dosage, 623
 pharmacokinetics of, 622
 to reduce intraocular pressure, 1238
 storage of 623
Mantoux, 1281t
MAO inhibitors
 adverse reactions to, 502
 clinical uses of, 500-502
 history and source of, 500
 interaction of
  with drugs, 33c, 501t, 502
  with foods containing tyramine, 66, 74, 502
 mechanism of action of, 500
 nursing implications for, 502-503
 patient teaching during therapy with, 502-503
 pharmacokinetics of, 500
Maolate, 350. *See also* Chlorphenesin carbamate.
Maprotiline hydrochloride. *See also* Second-generation antidepressants.
 action of, 507